Alistair Mackenzie Library
Wishaw General Hospital
50 Netherton Street
Wishaw
ML2 0DP

FEMALE UROLOGY

THIRD EDITION

Shlomo Raz, MD

Professor of Urology, UCLA School of Medicine, Chief Division of Pelvic Medicine and Reconstructive Urology, Los Angeles, California

Larissa V. Rodríguez, MD

Assistant Professor of Urology, Co-Director of the Division of Female Urology, Reconstructive Surgery, and Urodynamics, Director of Female Urology Research, The Geffen School of Medicine at UCLA, Los Angeles, California

SAUNDERS

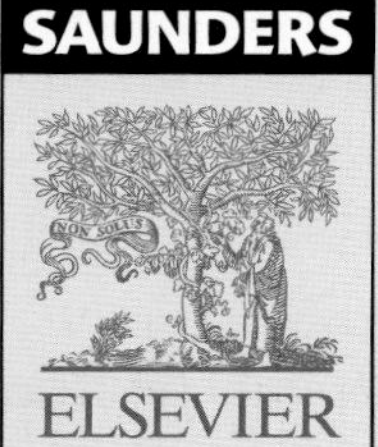

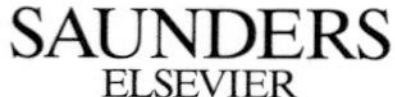

SAUNDERS
ELSEVIER

1600 John F. Kennedy Blvd.
Ste 1800
Philadelphia, PA 19103-2899

FEMALE UROLOGY
ISBN: 978-1-4160-2339-5

Notice

Neither the Publisher nor the Authors assume any responsibility for any loss or injury and/or damage to persons or property arising out of or related to any use of the material contained in this book. It is the responsibility of the treating practitioner, relying on independent expertise and knowledge of the patient, to determine the best treatment and method of application for the patient.

The Publisher

Library of Congress Cataloging-in-Publication Data (in PHL)

Female urology / [edited by] Shlomo Raz, Larissa V. Rodriguez.—3rd ed.
p. ; cm.
Includes bibliographical references and index.
ISBN 978-1-4160-2339-5
1. Urogynecology. I. Raz, Shlomo, 1938- II. Rodríguez, Larissa V.
[DNLM: 1. Genital Diseases, Female. 2. Urologic Diseases. WJ 190 F329 2008]
RG484.F46 2008
616.60082—dc22

2007042440

Acquisitions Editor: Scott Scheidt
Developmental Editor: Elizabeth Hart
Publishing Services Manager: Frank Polizzano
Senior Project Manager: Peter Faber
Design Direction: Steven Stave

Printed in China

Last digit is the print number: 9 8 7 6 5 4 3 2 1

I dedicate this book to my wife Sylvia and our children Alan, Yael, Daniela, and Karyn for their support and sacrifice during this year.

Shlomo Raz

To my sons Marcelo and Andre, because you are the strength of my life, my love, and my inspiration. Thank you for the sacrifices you make to help me fulfill my dreams.

Larissa Rodríguez

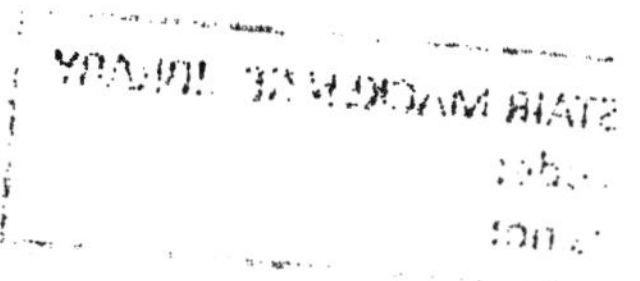

CONTRIBUTORS

Paul Abrams, MD, FRCS
Professor, Bristol Urological Institute, Southmead Hospital, Bristol, United Kingdom
17: *Clinical Diagnosis of Overactive Bladder*

Ilana Beth Addis, MD, MPH
Assistant Professor, University of Arizona College of Medicine, Associate Director, Female Pelvic Medicine and Reconstructive Surgery, University Physicians Healthcare, Tucson, Arizona
6: *Social Impact of Urinary Incontinence and Pelvic Floor Dysfunction*

Danita Harrison Akingba, MD
Fellow, Department of Gynecology, Female Urology, and Pelvic Surgery, Greater Baltimore Medical Center, Baltimore, Maryland
62: *Transabdominal Paravaginal Cystocele Repair*

Michael E. Albo, MD
Associate Clinical Professor of Surgery and Urology, University of California–San Diego, San Diego, California; Co-Director of Women's Pelvic Medical Center, University of California–San Diego Hospital, San Diego, California
29: *Selecting the Best Surgical Option for the Treatment of Stress Urinary Incontinence*

Samih Al-Hayek, MD, MRCS, LMSSA, LRCP, LRCS
Research Registrar, Bristol Urological Institute, Southmead Hospital, Bristol, United Kingdom
17: *Clinical Diagnosis of Overactive Bladder*

Cindy Amundsen, MD
Associate Professor of Obstetrics and Gynecology, Duke University School of Medicine, Durham, North Carolina; Director, Fellowship in Urogynecology and Pelvic Reconstructive Surgery, Department of Obstetrics and Gynecology, Duke University School of Medicine, Durham, North Carolina
77: *Complications of Vaginal Surgery*

Rodney U. Anderson, MD
Professor of Urology, Stanford University, Stanford, California
91: *Focal Neuromuscular Therapies for Chronic Pelvic Pain Syndromes in Women*

Karl-Erik Andersson, MD, PhD
Wake Forest Institute of Regenerative Medicine, Wake Forest University School of Medicine, Winston-Salem, North Carolina
4: *Pharmacologic Basis of Bladder and Urethral Function and Dysfunction*

Rodney A. Appell, MD, FACS
Professor and Chief, Division of Voiding Dysfunction and Female Urology, Baylor College of Medicine, Houston, Texas; Medical Director, Baylor Continence Center, Baylor College of Medicine, Houston, Texas
33: *Vaginal Wall Sling*

Walter Artibani, MD
Full Professor of Urology, University of Padova Medical School, Department of Urology, University of Padova Medical School, Padova, Italy
82: *Abdominal Approach for the Treatment of Vesicovaginal Fistula*

Anthony Atala, MD
Chair, Department of Urology, Wake Forest Institute for Regenerative Medicine, Winston-Salem, North Carolina
98: *Tissue Engineering for Reconstruction of the Urinary Tract and Treatment of Stress Urinary Incontinence*

Richard C. Bennett, MD
Resident, Department of Urology, William Beaumont Hospital, Royal Oak, Michigan
24: *Pudendal Nerve Stimulation*

Alfred Bent, MD
Chairman, Department of Gynecology, Female Urology, and Pelvic Surgery, Greater Baltimore Medical Center, Baltimore, Maryland
62: *Transabdominal Paravaginal Cystocele Repair*

Jerry G. Blaivas, MD
Clinical Professor of Urology, Weill-Cornell Medical College, New York, New York; Attending Surgeon, New York Presbyterian Hospital, New York, New York; Attending Surgeon, Lenox Hill Hospital, New York, New York
7: *Clinical Evaluation of Lower Urinary Tract Dysfunction*;
80: *Reconstruction of the Absent or Damaged Urethra*

David A. Bloom, MD
Jack Lapides Professor of Urology, Department of Pediatric Urology, University of Michigan, Ann Arbor, Michigan
1: *Developmental Anatomy and Urogenital Abnormalities*

Timothy Bolton Boone, MD, PhD
Professor and Chairman, Scott Department of Urology, Baylor College of Medicine, Houston, Texas
11: *Urodynamic Evaluation*

Sylvia M. Botros, MD
Assistant Professor, Evanston Northwestern Healthcare, Northwestern University, Feinberg School of Medicine, Evanston, Illinois
67: *Sacrospinous Ligament Suspension for Vaginal Vault Prolapse*

Alain Bourcier, PT
Tenon Hospital, Department of Urology, University of Paris, Paris, France; Director, Pelvic Floor Rehabilitation Services, Clinique International Monceau, Paris, France
19: *Behavior Modification and Conservative Management of Overactive Bladder*; **28**: *Pathophysiology of Stress Incontinence*

Lousine Boyadzhyan, MD
Resident Physician, Department of Radiology, David Geffen School of Medicine at UCLA, Los Angeles, California
8: *Imaging of the Female Genitourinary Tract*; **55**: *Imaging in the Diagnosis of Pelvic Organ Prolapse*

C. A. Tony Buffington, DVM, PhD, DACVN
Professor, Department of Veterinary Clinical Sciences, Ohio State University College of Veterinary Medicine, Columbus, Ohio
90: *Neuroendocrine Role in Interstitial Cystitis and Chronic Pelvic Pain in Women*

Linda Cardozo, MD
Professor of Urogynaecology, Department of Urogynaecology, King's College Hospital, London, United Kingdom
5: *Hormonal Influences on the Female Genital and Lower Urinary Tract*

Mauro Cervigni, MD
Professor, Catholic University, Rome, Italy; Chief of Urogynecology, San Carlo-IDI Hospital, Rome, Italy
66: *Tension-Free Cystocele Repair Using Prolene Mesh*

R. Duane Cespedes, MD
Associate Professor, Department of Urology, University of Texas Health Sciences Center, San Antonio, Texas; Director of Female Urology and Urodynamics, Wilford Hall Medical Center, Lackland AFB, Texas
97: *Transvaginal Closure of the Bladder Neck in the Treatment of Urinary Incontinence*

Christopher R. Chapple, BSc, MD, FRCS, FEBU
Visiting Professor, Sheffield Hallam University, Sheffield, South Yorkshire, United Kingdom; Consultant Urological Surgeon, Royal Hallamshire Hospital, Sheffield Teaching Hospitals National Health Service Foundation Trust, Sheffield, South Yorkshire, United Kingdom
27: *Pathophysiology of Stress Incontinence*

Chi Chiung Grace Chen, MD
Fellow, Female Pelvic Medicine/Reconstructive Pelvic Surgery and Minimally Invasive Surgery, Department of Obstetrics and Gynecology, Cleveland Clinic, Cleveland, Ohio
54: *Pelvic Organ Prolapse: Clinical Diagnosis and Presentation*;
73: *Open Abdominal Sacral Colpopexy*

Emily E. Cole, MD
Department of Urology, Vanderbilt University Medical Center, Nashville, Tennessee
46: *Radiofrequency for the Management of Genuine Stress Urinary Incontinence*

Craig V. Comiter, MD
Associate Professor, Stanford University, Stanford, California
56: *Dynamic Magnetic Resonance Imaging in the Diagnosis of Pelvic Organ Prolapse*

Matthew Cooperberg, MD
Chief Resident, Department of Urology, University of California–San Francisco, San Francisco, California
23: *Posterior Tibial Nerve Stimulation for Pelvic Floor Dysfunction*

Jaques Corcos, MD
Professor of Urology, Director of the Urology Department, McGill University, Montreal, Quebec, Canada; Director of the Urology Department, Jewish General Hospital, McGill University, Montreal, Quebec, Canada
31: *Urethral Injectables in the Management of Stress Urinary Incontinence*

Firouz Daneshgari, MD
Assistant Professor of Surgery, Department of Urology, Case Western Reserve University, Cleveland, Ohio; Director, Center for Female Pelvic Medicine and Reconstructive Surgery, Cleveland Clinic, Cleveland, Ohio
51: *Epidemiology of Pelvic Organ Prolapse*

William de Groat, PhD
Professor, Department of Pharmacology, University of Pittsburgh. Pittsburgh, Pennsylvania
3: *Neuroanatomy and Neurophysiology: Innervation of the Lower Urinary Tract*

John O. L. DeLancey, MD
Department of Obstetrics and Gynecology, University of Michigan, Women's Hospital, Ann Arbor, Michigan
53: *Functional Anatomy and Pathophysiology of Pelvic Organ Prolapse*

Donna Y. Deng, MD
Assistant Professor of Urology, Division of Pelvic Reconstruction, Incontinence, and Neurourology, Department of Urology, University of California–San Francisco, San Francisco, California
64: *Transvaginal Paravaginal Repair of High-Grade Cystocele*;
68: *Repair of Vaginal Vault Prolapse Using Soft Prolene Mesh;*
83: *Rectovaginal Fistula*

Hans Peter Dietz, MD, PhD
Associate Professor, Department of Obstetrics and Gynaecology, Western Clinical School, University of Sydney, Nepean Hospital, Penrith, NSW, Australia
9: *Pelvic Floor Ultrasound*

Connie DiMarco, MD
Urogynecology Department, Sacred Heart Medical Center, McKenzie Willamette Medical Center, Springfield, Ohio
60: *Managing the Urethra in Vaginal Prolapse*

Ananias Diokno, MD
Department of Urology, William Beaumont Hospital, Royal Oak, Michigan
93: *Epidemiology of Incontinence and Voiding Dysfunction in the Elderly*

Roger Roman Dmochowski, MD
Professor, Department of Urologic Surgery, Vanderbilt University Medical Center, Nashville, Tennessee
46: *Radiofrequency for the Management of Genuine Stress Urinary Incontinence*

Neil T. Dwyer, MD
Fellow, Department of Urology, University of Iowa, Iowa City, Iowa
38: *Fascia Lata Sling*

Daniel Eberli, MD
Wake Forest Institute for Regenerative Medicine, Winston-Salem, North Carolina
98: *Tissue Engineering for Reconstruction of the Urinary Tract and Treatment of Stress Urinary Incontinence*

Karyn Schlunt Eilber, MD
Director, Comprehensive Center for Continence and Pelvic Reconstruction, Los Angeles, California
88: *Benign Cystic Lesions of the Vagina and Vulva*

Ahmad Elbadawi, MD
Departments of Pathology and Urology, State University of New York, Syracuse, New York
2: *Structural Basis of Voiding Dysfunction*

Ahmad Elbadawi, MD
Lecturer in Urology, Alazhar University, Cairo, Egypt; Urology Fellow, Jewish General Hospital, McGill University, Montreal, Quebec, Canada
31: *Urethral Injectables in the Management of Stress Urinary Incontinence*

Raymond T. Foster, Sr., MD, MS, MHSc
Assistant Professor of Obstetrics and Gynecology, University of Missouri–Columbia, School of Medicine, Columbia, Missouri; Director, Missouri Center for Female Continence and Advanced Pelvic Surgery, Department of Obstetrics, Gynecology, and Women's Health, University of Missouri–Columbia, Columbia Missouri
70: *Transvaginal Repair of Apical Prolapse: The Uterosacral Vault Suspension*; 77: *Complications of Vaginal Surgery*

Clare J. Fowler, MBBS, MSc, FRCP
Professor of Neurophysiology, Department of Uro-Neurology, National Hospital of Neurology and Neurosurgery, London, United Kingdom
10: *Electrophysiological Evaluation of the Pelvic Floor*

Joel Funk, MD
Chief Resident, University of Arizona, Tucson, Arizona
56: *Dynamic Magnetic Resonance Imaging in the Diagnosis of Pelvic Organ Prolapse*

Michelle M. Germain, MD
Clinical Instructor, Department of Gynecology, Female Urology, and Pelvic Surgery, Greater Baltimore Medical Center, Baltimore, Maryland
62: *Transabdominal Paravaginal Cystocele Repair*

Jason P. Gilleran, MD
Assistant Professor, Department of Urology, The Ohio State University College of Medicine, Columbus, Ohio
79: *Urethrovaginal Fistula*

David Alan Ginsberg, MD
Assistant Professor of Clinical Urology, Keck School of Medicine of the University of Southern California, Los Angeles, California; Chief of Urology, Rancho Los Amigos National Rehabilitation Center, Downey, California
84: *Ureterovaginal Fistula*

Roger P. Goldberg, MD, MPH
Assistant Professor, Northwestern University, Feinberg School of Medicine, Evanston, Illinois
67: *Sacrospinous Ligament Suspension for Vaginal Vault Prolapse*

Irwin Goldstein, MD
Director, Sexual Medicine, Alvarado Hospital; Clinical Professor of Surgery, University of California, San Diego, California
50: *Female Sexual Function and Dysfunction*

Angelo E. Gousse, MD
Associate Professor of Urology, Chief of Female Urology and Voiding Dysfunction, University of Miami, Miller School of Medicine, Miami, Florida; Attending Urologist, Jackson Memorial Hospital, Miami, Florida
15: *Effect of Pelvic Surgery on Voiding Dysfunction*

Fred E. Govier, MD
Clinical Professor of Urology, University of Washington Medical Center, Seattle, Washington; Chief of Surgery, Virginia Mason Medical Center, Seattle, Washington
59: *Use of Synthetics and Biomaterials in Vaginal Reconstructive Surgery*

Asnat Groutz, MD
Senior Lecturer, The Sackler Faculty of Medicine, Tel Aviv University Tel Aviv, Israel; Urogynecology Unit, Lis Maternity Hospital, Tel Aviv Medical Center, Tel Aviv, Israel
52: *Pregnancy, Childbirth, and Pelvic Floor Injury*

Sender Herschorn, MD, FRCSC
Professor and Chair, Division of Urology, University of Toronto, Martin Barkin Chair in Urological Research, University of Toronto, Toronto, Ontario, Canada; Attending Urologist, Sunnybrook Health Science Center, Toronto, Ontario, Canada
57: *Urodynamics Evaluation of the Prolapse Patient*

Ken Hsiao, BS, MD
Assistant Professor of Urology, Indiana School of Medicine, Indianapolis, Indiana; Staff Urologist, John Muir Medical Center, NorCal Urology, Walnut Creek, California
59: *Use of Synthetics and Biomaterials in Vaginal Reconstructive Surgery*

Yvonne Hsu, MD
Lecturer, University of Michigan, Ann Arbor, Michigan
53: *Functional Anatomy and Pathophysiology of Pelvic Organ Prolapse*

Chad Huckabay, MD
North Shore Long Island Jewish Health System, Smith Institute of Urology, New Hyde Park, New York
49: *Complications of Incontinence Procedures in Women*

Tracy Hull, MD
Staff Colorectal Surgeon, Cleveland Clinic Foundation, Cleveland, Ohio
78: *Pathophysiology, Diagnosis, and Treatment of Defecatory Dysfunction*

Nancy Itano, MD
Assistant Professor and Senior Associate Consultant, Department of Urology, Mayo Clinic, Scottsdale, Arizona
60: *Managing the Urethra in Vaginal Prolapse*

Theodore M. Johnson, II, MD
Associate Professor of Medicine, Emory University, Atlanta, Georgia; Atlanta Site Director, Atlanta VA GRECC, Atlanta VA Medical Center, Decatur, Georgia
94: *Lower Urinary Tract Disorders in the Elderly Female*

Mickey M. Karram, MD
Volunteer Professor of Obstetrics and Gynecology, University of Cincinnati, Cincinnati, Ohio; Director of Urogynecology and Reconstructive Pelvic Surgery, Department of Obstetrics and Gynecology, Good Samaritan Hospital, Cincinnati, Ohio
71: *Vaginal Hysterectomy in the Treatment of Vaginal Prolapse*

Kathleen Kieran, MD
Resident, Department of Urology, University of Michigan Health System, Ann Arbor, Michigan
1: *Developmental Anatomy and Urogenital Abnormalities*

Adam P. Klausner, MD
Assistant Professor, Department of Urology, University of Virginia School of Medicine, Charlottesville, Virginia; Assistant Professor, Department of Surgery, Virginia Commonwealth University, Richmond, Virginia
18: *Pathophysiology of Overactive Bladder*

Carl George Klutke, MD
Division of Urologic Surgery, Washington University School of Medicine, St. Louis, Missouri
39: *Tension-Free Vaginal Tape*; **44**: *Transobturator Approach to Midurethral Sling*

John J. Klutke, MD
Assistant Professor of Clinical Gynecology, Department of Obstetrics and Gynecology, Keck School of Medicine, University of Southern California, Los Angeles, California
39: *Tension-Free Vaginal Tape*; **44**: *Transobturator Approach to Midurethral Sling*

Kathleen C. Kobashi, MD
Clinical Associate Professor, Urology, University of Washington, Seattle, Washington; Co-Director, Clinical Fellowship for Voiding Dysfunction and Pelvic Floor Reconstruction, Continence Center at Virginia Mason, Seattle, Washington
59: *Use of Synthetics and Biomaterials in Vaginal Reconstructive Surgery*

Karl J. Kreder, MD, FACS
Professor of Urology, University of Iowa, Iowa City, Iowa
38: *Fascia Lata Sling*

Henry Lai, MD
Fellow, Female Urology and Neurourology, Scott Department of Urology, Baylor College of Medicine, Houston, Texas
11: *Urodynamic Evaluation*

Jerilyn M. Latini, MD
Assistant Professor of Urology, University of Michigan Health System, Ann Arbor, Michigan
1: *Developmental Anatomy and Urogenital Abnormalities*

Gary E. Leach, MD
Director, Tower Urology Institute for Incontinence, Los Angeles, California
45: *Cadaveric Fascia Using Bone Anchors*; **61**: *Cadaveric Fascial Repair of Cystocele*; **75**: *Posterior Repair Using Cadaveric Fascia*

Monica Lee, MD
David Geffen School of Medicine at the University of California–Los Angeles, Los Angeles, California
87: *Vulvar and Vaginal Pain, Dyspareunia, and Abnormal Vaginal Discharge*

Gary E. Lemack, MD
Associate Professor of Urology and Neurology, University of Texas Southwestern Medical Center, Dallas, Texas
14: *Voiding Dysfunction and Neurological Disorders*

Malcolm A. Lesavoy, MD
Department of Plastic Surgery, University of California–Los Angeles, Encino, California
99: *Reconstruction of Congenital Female Genital Defects*

Amanda M. Macejko, MD
Urology Fellow, Northwestern University School of Medicine, Chicago, Illinois
86: *Urinary Tract Infections in Women*

Mary Grey Maher, MD
Urology Center, Yale Medical Center, New Haven, Connecticut
41: *Distal Urethral Polypropylene Sling*; **47**: *Surgery for Refractory Urinary Incontinence: Spiral Sling*

Francesca Manassero, MD
Doctoral Training, Department of Urology, University of Pisa, Pisa, Italy
27: *Pathophysiology of Stress Incontinence*

Mariangela Mancini, MD
Affiliate Professor, Residency in Urology Program, Department of Urology, University of Padova Medical School, Padova, Italy
82: *Abdominal Approach for the Treatment of Vesicovaginal Fistula*

Edward J. McGuire, MD
Professor, Department of Urology, University of Michigan, Ann Arbor, Michigan
25: *Detrusor Myomectomy*; **26**: *Bladder Augmentation*; **36**: *Autologous Fascial Slings*; **48**: *Mixed Urinary Incontinence*

Sarah E. Moeller, MS
University of Minnesota, Minneapolis, Minnesota
22: *Sacral Neuromodulation Interstim for the Treatment of Overactive Bladder*

Courtenay K. Moore, MD
Assistant Professor, Department of Surgery, Cleveland Clinic Lerner College of Medicine, Case Western Reserve University, Cleveland, Ohio; Staff, Female Pelvic Medicine and Reconstructive Surgery, Glickman Urological and Kidney Institute, Cleveland Ohio
51: *Epidemiology of Pelvic Organ Prolapse*

Arthur Mourtzinos, MD
Assistant Professor of Urology, Tufts University Medical School, Boston, Massachusetts; Senior Staff Physician, Institute of Urology, Continence Center, Lahey Clinic Medical Center, Burlington, Massachusetts
47: *Surgery for Refractory Urinary Incontinence: Spiral Sling*

M. Louis Moy, MD
Assistant Professor, Division of Urology, University of Pennsylvania Health System, Philadelphia, Pennsylvania
13: *Categorization of Voiding Dysfunction*; **20**: *Drug Treatment of Urinary Incontinence in Women*

Tristi W. Muir, MD
Assistant Professor, Uniformed Services University of the Health Sciences; Assistant Chief, Female Pelvic Medicine and Reconstructive Pelvic Medicine, Department of Obstetrics and Gynecology, Brooke Army Hospital, Fort Sam Houston, Texas
63: *Anterior Colporrhaphy for Cystocele Repair*; **74**: *Posterior Repair and Pelvic Floor Repair: Segmental Defect Repair*

Franca Natale, MD
San Carlo–IDI Hospital, Rome, Italy
66: *Tension-Free Cystocele Repair Using Prolene Mesh*

Linda Ng, MD
Assistant Professor of Urology, Boston University School of Medicine, Boston, Massachusetts
25: *Detrusor Myomectomy*; **26**: *Bladder Augmentation*; **36**: *Autologous Fascial Slings*

Victor Nitti, MD
Associate Professor and Vice Chairman, Department of Urology, New York University School of Medicine, New York, New York
49: *Complications of Incontinence Procedures in Women*

Peggy A. Norton, MD
Professor, Department of Obstetrics and Gynecology, and Chief of Urogynecology and Reconstructive Pelvic Surgery, University of Utah School of Medicine, Salt Lake City, Utah
58: *Nonsurgical Treatment of Vaginal Prolapse: Devices for Prolapse and Incontinence*

Pat D. O'Donnell, MD
Professor and Chairman, Department of Urology, University of Arkansas for Medical Sciences, Little Rod, Arkansas
95: *Urodynamics Evaluation in the Elderly*

Joseph G. Ouslander, MD
Director, Division of Geriatrics and Gerontology, Wesley Woods Geriatric Hospital, Atlanta, Georgia
94: *Lower Urinary Tract Disorders in the Elderly Female*

Priya Padmanabhan, MD
Resident, Department of Urology, New York University School of Medicine, New York, New York
16: *Idiopathic Urinary Retention in the Female*

Maria Fidel Paraiso, MD
Staff Physician, Department of Obstetrics and Gynecology and the Glickman Urological Institute, Cleveland Clinic, Cleveland, Ohio; Head, Center of Urogynecology and Reconstructive Pelvic Surgery, Cleveland, Ohio; Co-Director, Program of Female Pelvic Medicine and Reconstructive Surgery, Cleveland Clinic Lerner College of Medicine, Case Western Reserve University, Cleveland, Ohio
72: *Laparoscopic Sacral Colpopexy*; **73**: *Open Abdominal Sacral Colpopexy*

Christopher Kennerly Payne, MD
Associate Professor of Urology, Director, Female Urology and Neurourology, Stanford University Medical Center, Stanford, California
92: *Painful Bladder Syndrome and Interstitial Cystitis*

Virgilio G. Petero, Jr., MD
Urology Research Fellow, William Beaumont Hospital, Royal Oak, Michigan; Clinical Fellow, Division of Immunology and Organ Transplantation, University of Texas, Medical School at Houston, Houston, Texas
93: *Epidemiology of Incontinence and Voiding Dysfunction in the Elderly*

Kenneth M. Peters, MD
Chairman, Department of Urology, Peter and Florine Ministrelli Distinguished Chair in Urology, William Beaumont Hospital, Royal Oak, Michigan
24: *Pudendal Nerve Stimulation*

Peter E. Petros, MBBS, PhD, DS, MD, FRCOG, FRANZCOG CU
Adjunct Professor, Department of Gynaecology, University of Western Australia, Perth, Australia; Consultant Emeritus, Royal Perth Hospital, Perth, Australia
40: *Midurethral to Distal Urethral Slings*; **69**: *Use of IVS Device for Vaginal Vault Prolapse*

Simon Podnar, MD, DSc
Associate Professor of Neurology, University of Ljubljana Medical School, Ljubljana, Slovenia; Staff Neurologist and Clinical Neurophysiologist, Institute of Clinical Neurophysiology, University Medical Center, Ljubljana, Slovenia
10: *Electrophysiologic Evaluation of the Pelvic Floor*

Dimitri U. Pushkar, MD, PhD
Professor and Head, Department of Urology, Moscow State Medical Stomatological University, Moscow, Russia
34: *Free Vaginal Wall Sling*

Raymond Robert Rackley, MD
Co-Head, Section of Voiding Dysfunction and Female Urology; Director, Urothelial Biology Laboratory, Lerner Research Institute, Cleveland Clinic Foundation, Cleveland, Ohio
21: *Pharmacologic Neuromodulation*; **43**: *Percutaneous Vaginal Tape Sling Procedure*

Steven S. Raman, MD
Associate Professor, Division of Abdominal Imaging and Cross Sectional Interventional Radiology, Department of Radiology, David Geffen School of Medicine at UCLA, Los Angeles, California
8: *Imaging of the Female Genitourinary Tract*; **55**: *Imaging in the Diagnosis of Pelvic Organ Prolapse*

Andrea J. Rapkin, MD
Professor, David Geffen School of Medicine, University of California–Los Angeles, Los Angeles, California
87: *Vulvar and Vaginal Disorders: Chronic Pain and Abnormal Discharge*

Shlomo Raz, MD
Professor of Urology, Chief of Female Urology, Urodynamics, and Reconstruction, University of California–Los Angeles, School of Medicine, Los Angeles, California
47: *Surgery for Refractory Urinary Incontinence: Spiral Sling*; **64**: *Transvaginal Paravaginal Repair of High-Grade Cystocele*; **68**: *Repair of Vaginal Vault Prolapse Using Soft Prolene Mesh*; **81**: *Vesicovaginal Fistula: Vaginal Approach*; **83**: *Rectovaginal Fistula*

Dudley Robinson, MRCOG
Consultant Urogynaecologist, Department of Urogynaecology, King's College Hospital, London, United Kingdom
5: *Hormonal Influences on the Female Genital and Lower Urinary Tract*

Larissa V. Rodríguez, MD
Associate Professor of Urology, Division of Female Urology; Co-Director, Division of Pelvic Medicine and Female Urology; Director of Female Urology Research, University of California–Los Angeles, Los Angeles, California
41: *Distal Urethral Polypropylene Sling*; **47**: *Surgery for Refractory Urinary Incontinence: Spiral Sling*; **64**: *Transvaginal Paravaginal Repair of High-Grade Cystocele*; **68**: *Repair of Vaginal Vault Prolapse Using Soft Prolene Mesh*; **81**: *Vesicovaginal Fistula: Vaginal Approach*; **83**: *Rectovaginal Fistula*

Christopher M. Rooney, MD
Instructor, Urogynecology and Pelvic Reconstruction, Department of Obstetrics and Gynecology, Northeastern Ohio Universities College of Medicine, Rootstown, Ohio
71: *Vaginal Hysterectomy in the Treatment of Vaginal Prolapse*

Nirit Rosenblum, MD
Assistant Professor of Urology, New York University School of Medicine, New York, New York
16: *Idiopathic Urinary Retention in the Female*; **76**: *Perineal Hernia and Perineocele*

Eric Scott Rovner, MD
Associate Professor of Urology, Department of Urology, Medical University of South Carolina, Charleston, South Carolina
85: *Urethral Diverticula*

Sarah A. Rueff, MD
Staff Urologist, Director of the Continence Center, Billings Clinic, Billings, Montana
45: *Cadaveric Fascia Using Bone Anchors*; **61**: *Cadaveric Fascial Repair of Cystocele*; **75**: *Posterior Repair Using Cadaveric Fascia*

Matthew P. Rutman, MD
Assistant Professor, Department of Urology, Columbia University Medical Center, New York, New York
64: *Transvaginal Paravaginal Repair of High-Grade Cystocele*; **68**: *Repair of Vaginal Vault Prolapse Using Soft Prolene Mesh*; **81**: *Vesicovaginal Fistula: Vaginal Approach*; **83**: *Rectovaginal Fistula*

Peter K. Sand, MD
Professor, Northwestern University, Feinberg School of Medicine, Evanston, Illinois; Evanston Northwestern Healthcare, Evanston, Illinois
67: *Sacrospinous Ligament Suspension for Vaginal Vault Prolapse*

Jaspreet S. Sandhu, MD
Urology Fellow, Department of Voiding Dysfunction, Neurourology, and Pelvic Reconstructive Surgery, New York Presbyterian Hospital, Weill-Cornell Medical Center, New York, New York
7: *Clinical Evaluation of Lower Urinary Tract Infection*; **80**: *Reconstruction of the Absent or Damaged Urethra*

Anthony J. Schaeffer, MD
Herman L. Kretschmer Professor and Chairman, Department of Urology, Feinberg School of Medicine, Northwestern University; Chairman, Department of Urology, Northeastern Medical Hospital, Chicago, Illinois
86: *Urinary Tract Infections in Women*

Patrick J. Shenot, MD
Assistant Professor, Department of Urology, Thomas Jefferson University, Jefferson Medical College, Philadelphia, Pennsylvania
21: *Pharmacologic Neuromodulation*

Neil D. Sherman, MD
Assistant Professor, Division of Urology, University of Medicine and Dentistry of New Jersey, Newark, New Jersey
37: *Use of Cadaveric Fascia for Pubovaginal Slings*; **65**: *Cystocele Repair Using Biological Material*

Steven W. Siegel, MD
Associate Clinical Professor, Department of Urology, University of Minnesota Medical School, St. Paul, Minnesota; Director, Center for Continence Care, Metropolitan Urologic Specialists, St. Paul, Minnesota
22: *Sacral Neuromodulation Interstim for the Treatment of Overactive Bladder*

Larry Thomas Sirls, MD, FACS
Director, Urodynamic Laboratory, William Beaumont Hospital, Royal Oak, Michigan
12: *The Measurement of Urinary Symptoms, Health related Quality of Life and Outcomes of Treatment for Urinary Incontinence*

Christopher P. Smith, MD
Assistant Professor, Division of Female Urology and Voiding Dysfunction, Scott Department of Urology, Baylor College of Medicine, Houston, Texas
11: *Urodynamic Evaluation*

Karen E. Smith, MD
Kanephe, Hawaii
48: *Mixed Urinary Incontinence*

David Staskin, MD
Associate Professor of Urology, Weill-Cornell Medical College, New York, New York; Director, Female Urology and Voiding Dysfunction, New York Presbyterian Hospital, New York, New York
42: *The SPARC Sling System*

William Donald Steers, MD
Hovey Dabney Professor and Chair, Department of Urology, University of Virginia School of Medicine, Charlottesville, Virginia
18: *Pathophysiology of Overactive Bladder*

Marshall L. Stoller, MD
Professor and Vice-Chair, Department of Urology, University of California–San Francisco, San Francisco, California
23: *Posterior Tibial Nerve Stimulation for Pelvic Floor Dysfunction*

Lynn Stothers, MD, MHSc, FRCSC
Assistant Professor of Surgery and Urology and Associate Member of the Department of Health Care and Epidemiology and Department of Pharmacology, University of British Columbia, Vancouver, British Columbia; Director, Bladder Care Center, University Hospital, British Columbia, Canada
30: *Outcome Measures for Pelvic Organ Prolapse*

Elizabeth B. Takacs, MD
Assistant Professor, University of Iowa, Carver College of Medicine, Iowa City, Iowa
32: *Role of Needle Suspensions*

Emil Tanagho, MD
Professor of Urology, Department of Urology, University of California–San Francisco, San Francisco, California
35: *Colpocystourethropexy*

Joachim W. Thüroff, MD
Chairman, Department of Urology, Johannes Gutenberg University Medical School, Mainz, Germany
96: *Use of Bowel in Lower Urinary Tract Reconstruction in Women*

Hari Siva Gurunadha Rao Tunuguntla, MD
Resident, Department of Urology, University of Miami, Miller School of Medicine, Miami, Florida; Resident Physician in Urology, Jackson Memorial Hospital, Miami, Florida
15: *Effect of Pelvic Surgery on Voiding Dysfunction*

Christian Twiss, MD
Resident, Department of Urology, New York University School of Medicine, New York, New York
76: *Perineocele*

Renuka Tyagi, MD
Assistant Professor of Urology, Assistant Professor of Obstetrics and Gynecology, Weill-Cornell Medical Center, New York Presbyterian Hospitals, New York, New York
42: *The SPARC Sling System*

Sandip P. Vasavada, MD
Associate Professor of Surgery/Urology, Cleveland Clinic Lerner College of Medicine, Cleveland, Ohio; Center for Female Pelvic Medicine and Reconstructive Surgery, Glickman Urological and Kidney Institute, Cleveland, Ohio
43: *Percutaneous Vaginal Tape Sling Procedure*

Mark Walters, MD
Professor of Surgery, Cleveland Clinic Lerner College of Medicine, Case Western Reserve University, Cleveland, Ohio; Professor and Vice-Chair of Gynecology, Center of Urogynecology and Reconstructive Pelvic Surgery, Department of obstetrics and Gynecology, Cleveland Clinic, Cleveland, Ohio
54: *Pelvic Organ Prolapse: Clinical Diagnosis and Presentation*

George D. Webster, MB, FRCS
Professor of Surgery, Duke University Medical Center, Durham, North Carolina; Chief, Section of Urodynamics and Reconstructive Urology, Division of Urology, Department of Surgery, Duke University Medical Center, Durham, North Carolina
37: *Use of Cadaveric Fascia for Pubovaginal Slings*; **65**: *Cystocele Repair Using Biological Material*; **70**: *Transvaginal Repair of Apical Prolapse: The Uterosacral Vault Suspension*; **77**: *Complications of Vaginal Surgery*

Alan J. Wein, MD
Division of Urology, University of Pennsylvania Health System, Philadelphia, Pennsylvania
13: *Categorization of Voiding Dysfunction*; **20**: *Drug Treatment of Urinary Incontinence in Women*

Ursula Wesselmann, MD
Associate Professor of Neurology, Johns Hopkins University School of Medicine, Baltimore, Maryland
89: *Pathophysiology of Pelvic Pain*

Christoph Wiesner, MD
Department of Urology, Johannes Gutenberg University Medical School, Mainz, Germany
96: *Use of Bowel in Lower Urinary Tract Reconstruction in Women*

Nasim Zabihi, MD
Resident, University of California–Los Angeles, Los Angeles, California
41: *Distal Urethral Polypropylene Sling*

Philippe Zimmern, MD
Professor, University of Texas Southwestern Medical Center, Dallas, Texas
32: *Role of Needle Suspensions*; **79**: *Urethrovaginal Fistula*

Massarat Zutshi, MD
Associate Staff Surgeon, Cleveland Clinic Foundation, Cleveland, Ohio
78: *Pathophysiology, Diagnosis, and Treatment of Defecatory Dysfunction*

PREFACE

The mere formulation of a problem is far more essential than its solution, which may be merely a matter of mathematical or experimental skills. To raise new questions, new possibilities, to regard old problems from a new angle requires creative imagination and marks real advances in science. Imagination is more important than knowledge. The important thing is not to stop questioning.

Albert Einstein

During the past 30 years, thanks to the efforts of leading urologists, gynecologists, basic scientists, pharmacologists, neurophysiologists, and geriatricians, we have made unprecedented achievements in female pelvic medicine and reconstruction. These people have worked hard and deserve all the respect and honor they receive. They have done remarkably well in applying new ideas and technologic advances to the field.

Intellectual capital is knowledge, information, and experience that can used to create better medicine. This collective brainpower it is hard to identify and harder still to deploy effectively, but once found and exploited, success is at hand. In this book, we have used this intellectual brainpower of all our collaborators to address simple and complex clinical conditions, with a focus on many medical and surgical specialties.

We have resisted the temptation to offer easy formulas and checklists because the fields of female pelvic medicine and reconstructive surgery are new and continuing to evolve. Although some of the chapters written today may be outdated at the time of publication, we have done our best to provide the most current information available.

The principal contribution of this book is the array of chapters written by leaders in the field that describe the challenges of female pelvic medicine and reconstruction and that offer a framework on which health care professionals can build useful and valuable strategies for treating patients. Although the authors have expressed their own opinions, they also have incorporated the most current scientific and clinical information into accessible formats. They have researched the best evidence for clinical application and have critically appraised that evidence for its validity and usefulness. We thank them all for their great efforts.

We will count this book a success if it inspires many readers to generate ideas far beyond any we have included or we could imagine.

Shlomo Raz and Larissa Rodríguez

CONTENTS

Section 12: RECONSTRUCTION

Section 1

BASIC CONCEPTS

Chapter 1

DEVELOPMENTAL ANATOMY AND UROGENITAL ABNORMALITIES

Kathleen Kieran, Jerilyn M. Latini, and David A. Bloom

Knowledge of the prenatal development of the genitourinary system is essential to understand congenital disorders and normal urinary tract function and anatomy. This chapter summarizes the key milestones in genitourinary tract development at the organ and cellular levels. Many genes appear to play key roles in the molecular signals for development and differentiation of components of the genitourinary system. These genes are temporally and locally expressed during development, and without them, normal development fails.[1] The kidney development database[2] (http://www.ana.ed.ac.uk/anatomy/database/kidbase) provides a list of these genes, and updated or revised designations can be found in the international database (http://www.gene.ucl.ac.uk/nomenclature).

DEVELOPMENT OF THE GENITOURINARY SYSTEM

The genitourinary system begins to take form from intermediate mesoderm in the third week of gestation. At this point, the embryo is a bilaminar disk composed of external ectoderm and internal endoderm. The longitudinal growth of the embryo begins to exceed its transverse growth, such that the resulting tension induces folding of the cranial and caudal ends toward one another around the umbilical stalk. This folding brings the cloacal membrane (a bilaminar membrane in the caudal portion of the embryo, distal to the allantois) ventrally. The endoderm-lined yolk sac dilates, and the cloaca forms.

The cloaca ultimately is divided into the anterior urogenital sinus and the posterior rectum (Fig. 1-1), although the mechanism is debated. It was once believed that urorectal folds on either side of the midline grew caudomedially to fuse with the cloacal membrane and divide the cloacal membrane into the urogenital sinus and the dorsal rectum by week 7. Subsequent regression of the tail then rotated the urogenital sinus and rectum dorsally. Some investigators[3,4] have suggested that the urorectal septum may not exist or may not fuse with the cloacal membrane.

The development of the urinary tracts and portions of the genital system is induced by the mesonephric and paramesonephric (müllerian) ducts. Both ductal systems grow toward the urogenital sinus; the mesonephric ducts grow medially, whereas the müllerian ducts have already fused into a single midline structure. Fusion of the wolffian ducts with the cloaca occurs by the middle of the fourth week (day 24). The junction of the müllerian ducts and the urogenital sinus is a central embryologic location called Müller's tubercle. The mesonephric ducts bend laterally; at this bend, a ureteric bud forms. The portion of the mesonephric duct between the urogenital sinus and the ureteric bud is called the common nephric duct, and by day 33, it is absorbed into the urogenital sinus, providing an island of mesoderm in the otherwise endoderm-based urogenital sinus (Fig. 1-2). This mesodermal island expands laterally to become the trigone of the bladder. The location of the ureteric bud relative to the urogenital sinus determines whether the ureteral

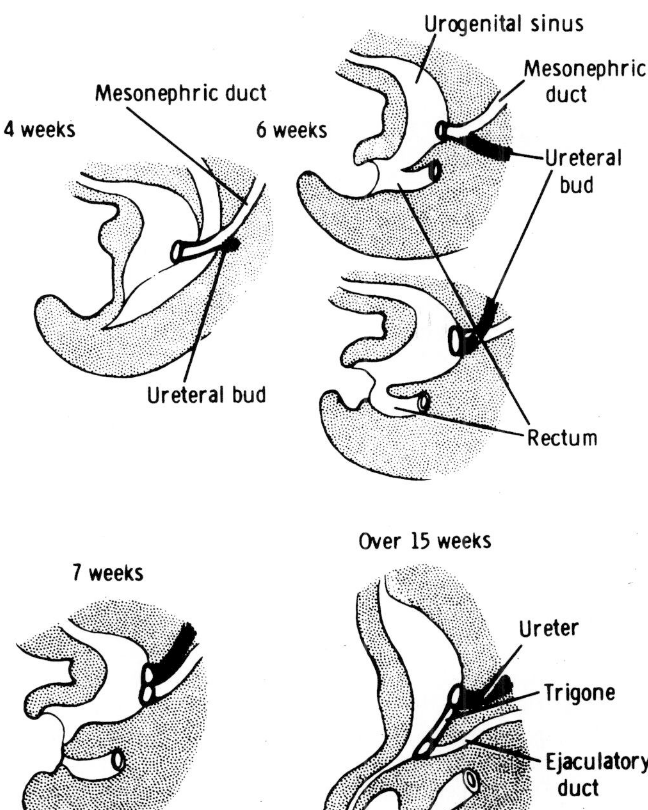

Figure 1-1 Development of the lower urinary tract. At 4 weeks, the cloaca is divided by a septum into an anterior urogenital sinus and posterior rectum. The mesonephric duct already joins the anterior portion of the cloaca, and the ureteral bud has started to develop at the bend of the mesonephric duct as it turns forward and medially to join the urogenital sinus. At 6 weeks, the urorectal septum progressively separates the urogenital sinus anteriorly from the rectum posteriorly. By week 7, the separation is complete, and the ureter and the mesonephric duct acquire separate openings in the urogenital sinus. After the 12th week, the ureter starts its upward and lateral movement as the mesonephric duct moves downward and medially. Tissue absorbed in between forms the trigone.

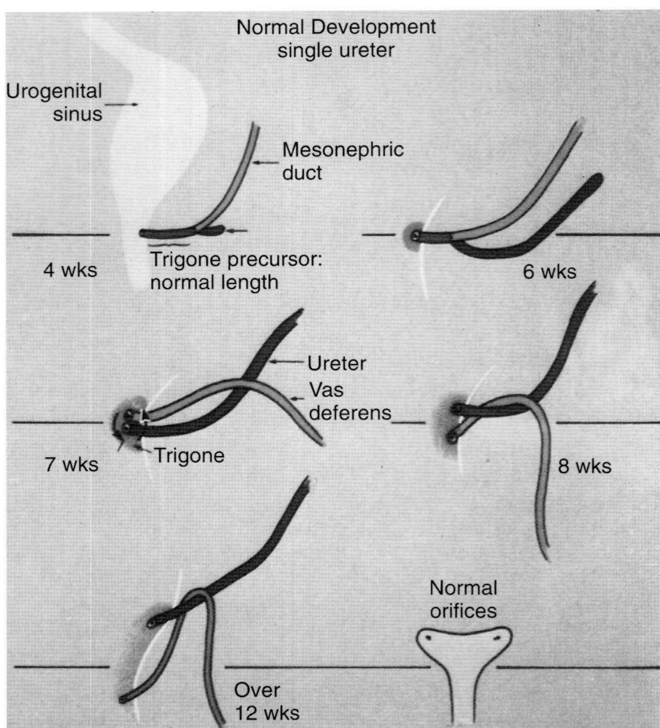

Figure 1-2 The lower end of the mesonephric duct as it joins the anterior division of the cloaca. Notice that the common nephric duct is progressively absorbed into the urogenital sinus. By week 7, the ureter and the mesonephric duct have separate openings, and rotation takes place. The ureter moves upward and laterally, and the mesonephric duct moves downward and medially, expanding the absorbed tissue to form the trigonal structure.

orifices will be orthotopic; a ureteric bud that originates on a short, common nephric duct will be incorporated sooner into the bladder, with resultant lateral displacement of the ureteral orifices. The intramural ureteral tunnel predisposes to vesicoureteral reflux. Conversely, ureteric buds that are located a great distance from the urogenital sinus will be incorporated into the urogenital sinus later and may be associated with ectopic drainage into surrounding structures.

The ureteric bud continues to grow craniolaterally while the mesonephric duct (distal to the bifurcation of the common nephric duct into the mesonephric duct and ureteric bud) grows caudomedially. The ureter undergoes a process of obstruction during the sixth week (37 to 40 days) and then is recanalized from the central portion to the cranial and caudal limits. Incomplete recanalization at either end may account for obstruction at the ureteropelvic junction or at the ureterovesical junction, where a thin transient membrane (i.e., Chwalla's membrane) may fail to dissolve. The cuboidal epithelium of the immature ureter evolves to a lining of transitional cells by 14 weeks.[5]

The urogenital sinus expands caudally to form the bladder and gives rise to the posterior urethra in males or the entire urethra and distal third of the vagina in females. The cranial portion of the urogenital sinus tapers during the third month of gestation so that the allantois forms the urachus and the saccular bladder remains in place. The intramural bladder wall develops throughout the remainder of gestation, with collagen formation beginning in the lamina propria and with subsequent intercalation between intramural muscle fibers. Intramural muscle fibers form as perivesical splanchnic mesoderm matures after induction by epithelial-mesenchymal interactions. Compliance of the fetal bladder increases over time in human fetuses and in animal models.[6,7] Koo and colleagues[7] showed a decreasing ratio of type 3 to type 1 collagen in the fetal bovine bladder; the changing ratios of perivesical collagen and muscle likely account for at least a portion of this evolution.

Renal and Ureteral Development

The renal excretory unit is the result of a complex developmental process influenced by reciprocal induction of mesenchyme and the ureteric bud and by many molecular events. The kidney develops in three stages. The first is the pronephros, which arises late in the third week in the cranial portion of the embryo. Pronephric tubules develop cranially and extend caudally, but they degenerate quickly, and the pronephros is obliterated by the start of the fifth week. By day 24, mesonephric ducts are present at the ninth and tenth somites. These ducts grow caudally to the cloacal membrane by day 28, fuse in the midline, and eventually form the bladder. Caudal canalization and then cranial canalization follows. The mesonephros, unlike its predecessor, is able to accomplish limited excretory function for the growing embryo. Mesonephric tubules along the medial nephrogenic cords form and dissolve, sequentially disappearing by the fourth month of development to leave only remnants. Some tubules develop lumens and vesicles and twist into an S shape, in which the lateral portion becomes the mesonephric duct and the medial portion surrounds capillaries originating in the aorta and forms a primitive renal corpuscle. Cranially, the tubules form efferent ductules. The mesonephric ducts give rise to the epididymis and vas deferens, and in females, remnants persist as the paroöphoron and epoöphoron, which are vestigial mesosalpingeal structures.

The metanephros gives rise to the fetal kidney. It forms in the sacral region as the ureteric buds arise from the mesonephric ducts. As the ureteric buds grow cranially, they encounter metanephric mesenchyme on about day 28. After the ureteric bud contacts the mesenchyme, release of many factors culminates in reciprocal induction of growth factors governing the development of the metanephric system. The ureteric bud divides repeatedly between weeks 6 and 32 of development, ultimately giving rise to the collecting system: the collecting ducts, calyces, renal pelvis, and ureter. The metanephric mesenchyme gives rise to the parenchymal portions of the kidney that perform filtration and clearance: the glomeruli, proximal and distal tubules, and loop of Henle. Because of the lengthy period during which branching of the ureteral bud occurs, the growth of the metanephric mesenchyme that will give rise to renal parenchyma is not uniform; nephrons at the juxtamedullary region are formed earlier and mature sooner than nephrons in more peripheral locations. Nephrons undergo four defined stages of development in the human. Stage I occurs when the metanephric mesenchyme is fully discrete from the ureteral bud. Stage II begins when the S-shaped nephron connects with the ureteral bud. In stage III, an ovoid structure emerges, and in stage IV, a round glomerulus is seen. Most nephrons in humans are stage IV at birth, although maturation is completed fully in the early postnatal period.[5]

As the kidneys grow, their location in the embryo becomes progressively more cranial; this is likely caused by active growth of the kidney parenchyma and by increased differential growth of the caudal portion of the embryo. As a result, the kidneys ascend from their initial pelvic location to the upper retroperitoneum. As renal ascent proceeds, new blood vessels are generated cranially, and the more caudal blood vessels break down. In postnatal patients with renal ectopia, the renal blood supply is typically anomalous because angiogenesis is arrested when renal ascent ceases. The possibility of an aberrant blood supply should be considered in any patient with renal ectopia.

Formation of the Urogenital Sinus and External Genitalia

With dissolution of the tail and further development of the lower abdominal wall, the cloaca returns to a more dorsal position, and mesodermal proliferation in the fifth week forms genital tubercles. These tubercles ultimately fuse in the midline to form the phallus or clitoris. The urogenital sinus remains at the base of the tubercles; the folds of the urogenital sinus ultimately fuse in the male to form the penile urethra and widen in the female to form the vaginal vestibule and the discrete labia minora. The endodermally derived urethral groove develops from the urogenital sinus in the sixth week, and the urethral plate (a deepening of this groove) forms shortly thereafter. Male and female embryos remain morphologically identical until approximately 12 weeks' gestation.

Abnormalities of the Urogenital Sinus

Bladder exstrophy occurs in approximately 1 of 30,000 births and is seven times more likely in children conceived through in vitro fertilization.[8] This disorder is characterized by early rupture of the cloacal membrane, which is sometimes related to an intrinsic defect in the membrane. It is more common in males than in females by a ratio of approximately 2:1 to 6:1,[9] and it is related to epispadias and to cloacal exstrophy. The latter condition is also associated with early rupture of the cloacal membrane, although it occurs much less commonly (1 in 200,000 to 400,000 births[10]). Although no genes associated with either condition have been definitively identified, the risk of bladder exstrophy is substantially greater with an affected relative (1 in 275) or an affected parent (1 in 70).[9] Mesenchymal ingrowth between the ectodermal and endodermal layers of the cloacal membrane ultimately results in formation of the lower anterior abdominal wall and division of the cloaca into the anterior urogenital sinus and posterior rectum. Both disorders are associated with malformations of other organ systems, including the limbs, lower anterior abdominal wall, pelvic girdle, and in the case of cloacal exstrophy, the hindgut. Management of these conditions remains challenging.

Gonadal Development

Development of the testes and ovaries is initiated in the fifth week of gestation, when germ cells from the yolk sac migrate to the posterior body wall, inducing formation of the urogenital ridge medial to the mesonephros (Fig. 1-3). Invasion of the adjacent mesenchyme in the sixth week creates a primitive gonad with epithelium and blastema; the latter is formed from loosened epithelial cells. Persistent growth of the germinal epithelium into the adjacent mesenchyme forms cords that ultimately branch many times and form seminiferous tubules.

Initially, all embryos have the potential to become male or female; the development of internal or external genitalia is an event influenced by genetic, endocrine, and paracrine factors. *SRY*, a gene on the short arm of the Y chromosome, induces formation of the Sertoli and Leydig cells. It also induces secretion of anti-müllerian hormone (AMH), formerly called müllerian-inhibiting substance (MIS), which induces regression of the müllerian system between 8 and 10 weeks' gestation.[5] Remnants of the müllerian system in the male include the prostatic utricle and the appendix testis. AMH has unilateral paracrine activity, and expression is required locally and bilaterally to achieve eradication of müllerian structures. Failure of testicular secretion of AMH or lack of receptive tissue results in persistence of the müllerian structures ipsilaterally as a miniature uterus and fallopian tube, typically associated with an inguinal hernia (i.e., hernia uteri inguinale). In the absence of SRY protein and AMH, ovarian follicles form from the maturing cortex at 3 to 4 months.

Testosterone, which is secreted by the Leydig cells, and dihydrotestosterone, which is a derivative of testosterone arising from the action of 5α-reductase, play key roles in the development of the male ductal anatomy and external genitalia. Testosterone induces formation of the vasa deferentia and efferent ductules. Cranially, the mesonephric ducts degenerate, leaving the epididymis and its appendix. The distal mesonephric ducts give rise to the seminal vesicles. Testosterone stimulation and local conversion to dihydrotestosterone induce development of the prostate. Dihydrotestosterone also is locally responsible for fusion of the labioscrotal folds and the phenotypic development of the male external genitalia. Figure 1-4 illustrates the developmental and phenotypic correlates of male and female external genitalia.

Descent of the fetal gonad is a two-step process. During the third month, the embryonic gonad is retroperitoneal and descends caudally so that by the seventh month, it is at the internal inguinal ring. The gubernaculum forms in the seventh week, and the processus vaginalis develops as a peritoneal outpouching. The second phase of scrotal descent occurs during the eighth and ninth months.

The exact mechanism by which the testicle descends into the scrotum is unknown. Theories include contraction of the cremasteric fibers with resultant shortening of the gubernaculum, swelling of the tissue surrounding the inguinal canal such that the canal is widened sufficiently for passage of the testis, and increased intra-abdominal pressure with subsequent passage of the testis through the inguinal canal.[5] The ovarian gubernaculum attaches to the müllerian ducts in the seventh week when fusion of the paramesonephric structures creates the broad ligament from folds of peritoneum. The gubernaculum then divides into two portions. Superiorly, the ovarian ligament connects the uterus and ovary, and inferiorly, the round ligament connects the ovary and the labioscrotal folds.

Abnormalities in Development of Internal and External Genitalia

Abnormalities in the development of the internal and external genitalia can be divided into those in which only the external genitalia are affected and those in which the internal and external genitalia are affected. Disorders in which the external genitalia are affected are considered ambiguous genitalia ("hermaphroditism") and occur in approximately 1 of 30,000 live births. Male pseudohermaphrodites are genetically 46,XY, with preserved wolffian duct structures and internal testicular tissue but feminized external genitalia.[11,12] Female pseudohermaphrodites (60% to 70% of hermaphrodites) are genetically 46,XX, with preserved müllerian structures and internal ovarian tissue but virilized

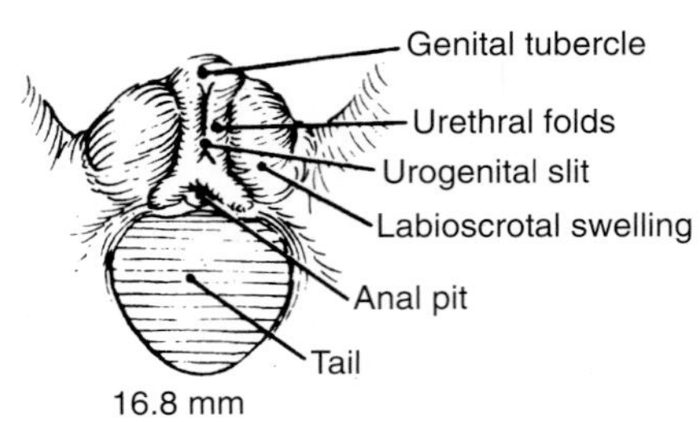

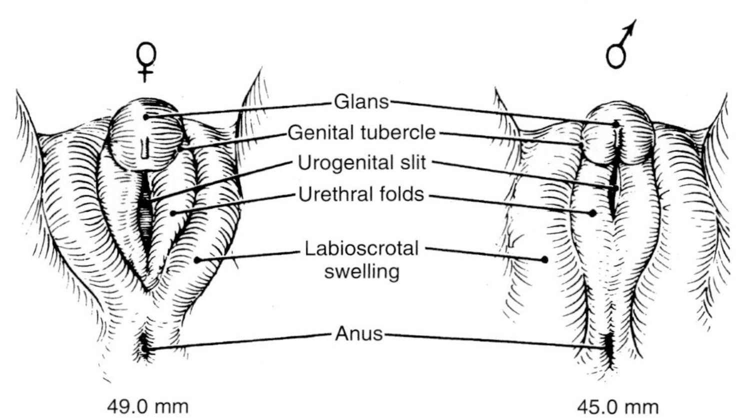

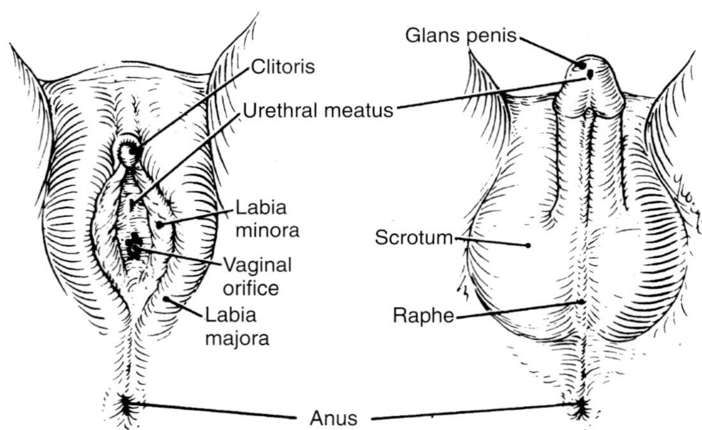

Figure 1-3 The undifferentiated sexual structures early in embryonic life (eighth week) grow and differentiate into female or male forms. The representative segments and their future course (depending on sexual differentiation) are illustrated. (From Tanagho EA: Embryology of the genitourinary system. In Tanagho EA, McAninch JW [eds]: General Urology, 14th ed. Norwalk, CT, Appleton & Lange, 1995.)

external genitalia. True hermaphrodites are rare and have both ovarian and testicular tissue, typically with a 46,XX genotype[11]; there is no consistent appearance of the external genitalia, but about 75% of patients have male external genitalia with hypospadias and variable gonadal descent.[12]

Female pseudohermaphrodites are most commonly the result of 21-hydroxylase deficiency,[11] an autosomal recessive disorder in which insufficiency of this enzyme leads to incomplete synthesis of all products in the steroidogenic pathway in the adrenal gland. The lack of production of the final product yields lack of feedback on the precursors, and intermediate products (many of them androgenic at high doses) accumulate. Less commonly, other enzymes in the steroidogenic pathway are affected; 3β-hydroxylase deficiency is rare, whereas 11-hydroxylase deficiency is associated with salt retention and hypertension rather than the salt wasting observed with 21-hydroxylase deficiency. The end result is virilization of the external genitalia while the normal female internal genitalia are preserved. Less frequently, extrinsic exposure to androgens can be the cause. In either case, management of the affected patient includes correction of the electrolyte abnormalities and reconstruction of functional phenotypic anomalies.

Male pseudohermaphrodites arise through defects in androgen synthesis or recognition in the developing embryo. Androgen resistance is an X-linked abnormality seen in approximately 1 of 60,000 newborns, in which the testes form and function normally

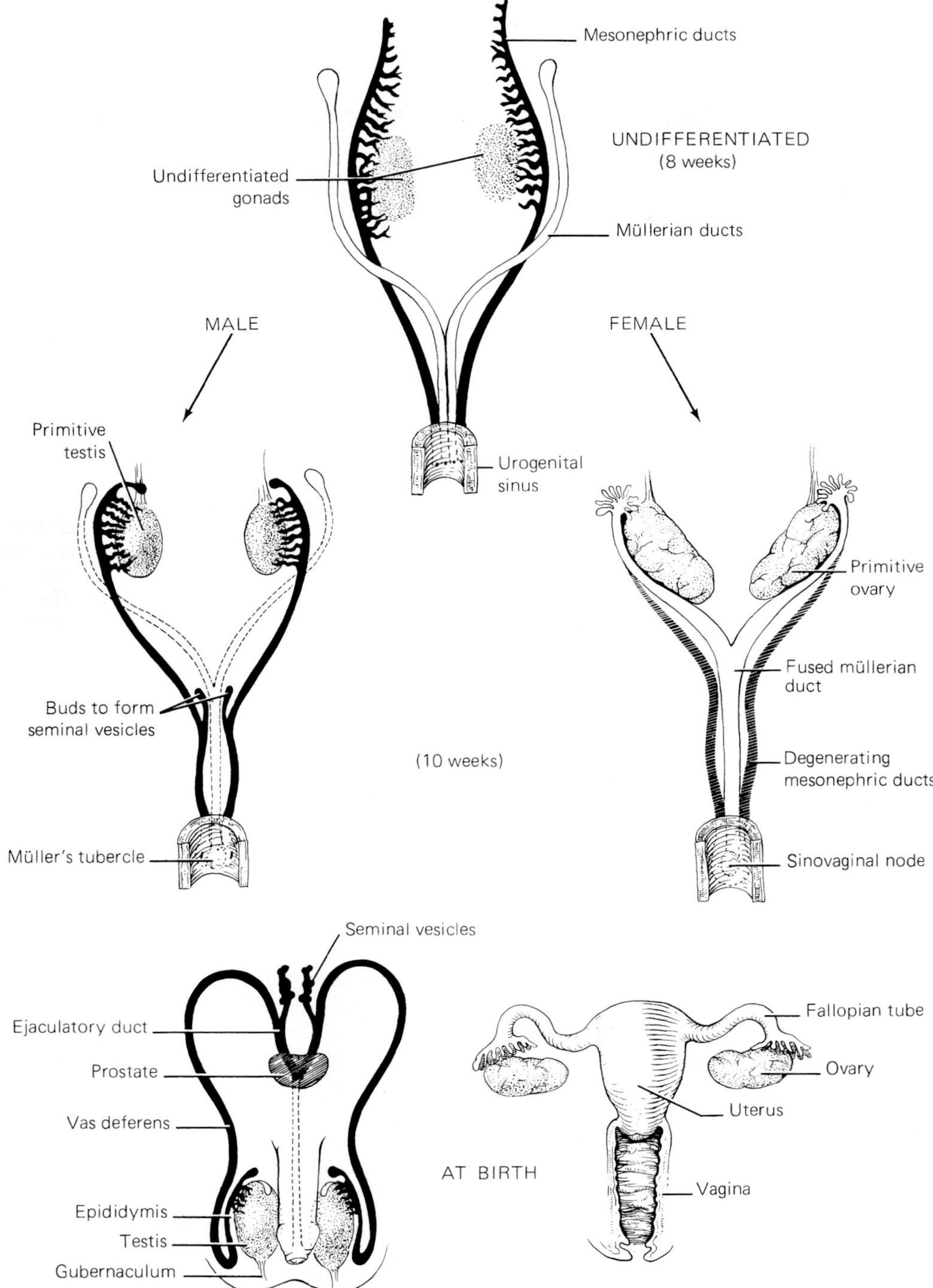

Figure 1-4 Development of the male and female external genitalia. Notice that the genital tubercles that develop on the undersurface of the cloacal membrane progressively enlarge and fuse to form the body of the penis in the male and to form the clitoris in the female. Fusion of the urethral folds completes the urethral formation in the male, whereas the folds remain as the labia in the female. The post-tubercle segment of the urogenital sinus opens to become the vaginal vestibule of the female, whereas in the male, it forms part of the urethra, which is completed by the urethral fold fusion.

but the target tissues have a receptor defect that renders them insensitive to androgens.[11,13] AMH is still secreted by the normal testes, and the müllerian ducts degenerate. Wolffian structures are preserved. Many of these patients present at puberty, but patients who are identified soon after birth can be given testosterone or human chorionic gonadotropin to stimulate phallic growth and determine whether male gender assignment is feasible.[11] Testes should be closely monitored or removed because of the risk of dysgerminoma.

True hermaphroditism is associated with the presence of ovarian and testicular tissue. Lateral hermaphroditism is associated with the presence of an ovary on one side and a testis on the other. Unilateral hermaphroditism is associated with an ovotestis on one side and a normal gonad on the other. Bilateral hermaphroditism is associated with bilateral ovotestes. Like male pseudohermaphroditism, true hermaphroditism is associated with an increased risk of neoplastic conversion in the testis.[11]

Less common abnormalities of gonadal development include mixed gonadal dysgenesis and pure gonadal dysgenesis. In the former, karyotypes are typically 45,X/46,XY, and patients have a single testis accompanied by a streak ovary. These patients are at increased risk for dysgerminoma. In pure gonadal dysgenesis, ambiguous genitalia are not present; these patients are at increased risk for gonadoblastoma.[11,12]

Because formation of the female reproductive system from the müllerian ducts relies on fusion of primitive structures, abnormalities of fusion are not uncommon. Normal development of the müllerian system relies on elongation of the epithelial tubes lateral to the wolffian ducts, fusion of these ducts after reaching Muller's tubercle, independent recanalization of each side, and resorption of the residual septum in a caudad-to-cephalad fashion. Failure at any of these steps may result in disorders such as unicornuate uterus, persistent vaginal septum with resultant septate vagina, or Mayer-Rokitansky-Küster-Hauser syndrome (1 in 5000).[14] In the latter syndrome, failure of müllerian duct fusion gives rise to vaginal agenesis, although the ovaries and fallopian tubes develop normally. Concomitant renal and genitourinary (15% to 40%) or skeletal (12% to 50%) abnormalities occur.[11,15]

MOLECULAR CAUSES OF ABNORMAL DEVELOPMENT

During the past decade, significant advances have been made in the identification of the genes and their proteins involved in the normal and abnormal development of the genitourinary tract. Knowledge of the precise molecular events involved in embryogenesis is evolving rapidly, and key genes and proteins crucial to certain steps in genitourinary development are discussed in the following sections.

FGF10

Fibroblast growth factor 10 (FGF10) is expressed in the mesenchyme of the genital tubercle; FGF8 is expressed by urethral tissues. Interactions between these structures likely induce growth of the male phallus. The lack of FGF10 expression is theorized to account for the hypospadiac morphology with failure of fusion of the distal urethral plate, although the plate itself appears to develop normally because of the presence of FGF-8.[16,17]

GDNF

Glial cell–derived neurotrophic factor (GDNF) is a mesenchyme-derived signaling factor that is a member of the transforming growth factor-β (TGF-β) family. It acts as the ligand for the RET receptor and induces growth of the ureteral bud during its interaction with the metanephric mesenchyme. In *GDNF*-knockout animals, development of the pronephros and mesonephros proceeds normally, but metanephric development is stunted by the lack of reciprocal interactions between the mesenchyme and the ureteral bud.[18] Similar defects are seen in *WT1* mutants[19] and *RET*-deficient mutants, although the latter may have primitive, poorly developed kidneys.[1,19]

WNT4

WNT4 (i.e., wingless-type mouse mammary tumor virus [MMTV] integration site family member 4 protein) is expressed in the mesenchyme adjacent to the mesonephric ducts and in the metanephric mesenchyme. *WNT4* mutants have abnormally small, dysplastic kidneys and arrest of development at the level of formation of the renal tubules and renal epithelium from the mesenchyme.[1] It is theorized that WNT4 signals enable organization of the epithelial cells into tubular structures.[19]

AMH

Behringer and colleagues[20] found that in *AMH* knockouts, testes were bilaterally descended, but the female reproductive organs remained intact, although they were often hypoplastic. Testes had Leydig cell hyperplasia, but spermatogenesis and semen analyses were normal in the affected animals. In contrast, mice that did not produce AMH but who also had a defect in the androgen receptor had absent wolffian structures and bilaterally undescended testes with maturational arrest in spermatogenesis. AMH is thought to exert its effects through paracrine actions, and it must be present before week 8 of gestation to induce müllerian regression.[18]

Bartlett and coworkers[21] evaluated mice heterozygous for the *AMH* gene. These heterozygotes had poor development of the cremaster-gubernacular complex; the gubernaculums did develop but remained fibrotic and had poor cremaster development. Testes descended normally in these mice. The investigators concluded that AMH was not the determinant of gubernacular development or testicular descent but that it did play a key role in cremaster development.

Defects in the type II anti-müllerian hormone receptor gene *(AMHR2)* (formerly referred to as the MIS type II receptor gene) have also been associated with persistent presence of paramesonephric structures. Persistent müllerian duct syndrome (PMDS) is a subtype of male pseudohermaphroditism in which the external genitalia are virilized and are morphologically normal, but paramesonephric structures persist. Hoshiya and associates[22] reported a novel mutation in the *AMHR2* gene caused by abnormal splicing; prior research identified additional abnormalities in the gene caused by base pair mutation in an intron and by deletion of genetic material from an exon.

AMH is a hormone associated with the TGF-β family that is expressed in neonates, with a peak level occurring in male infants and in prepubertal girls. In addition to effects on degeneration of the müllerian system, its exact hormonal effects are unknown. However, it was shown to decrease testosterone production by the Leydig cells by a cytochrome P450–dependent mechanism in one study.[23] Testosterone levels were increased in normal controls compared with hypospadiacs, and AMH protein levels were inversely correlated, suggesting that AMH may influence external genital development and induce the hypospadiac phenotype.

AMH expression has been a useful means of differentiating between patients with extrinsic and those with intrinsic virilization. Because AMH is synthesized by the Sertoli cells, elevated AMH levels in male infants with undescended testes suggest the presence of normal or malignant testicular tissue, whereas the absence of AMH is associated with residual ovarian tissue.[24]

KSP-Cadherin

KSP-cadherin, also designated CHD16 or cadherin 16, is a cell-adhesion molecule expressed solely in the tubular epithelial cells of the kidney and genitourinary tract during prenatal development. Using protein linkage and immunoassays, expression of KSP-cadherin has been localized to the embryonic ureteric bud, wolffian duct, müllerian ducts, and mesonephric and metanephric structures. In adults, expression is limited to the thick ascending loop of Henle, proximal renal tubules, and Bowman's capsules. Shao and colleagues[25] demonstrated that tissue-specific expression of this protein could be established through linkage to a promoter and that a small segment of DNA adjacent to the promoter was adequate for tissue-specific expression. Although the exact function of KSP-cadherin has not been elucidated, its tissue-specific expression during development suggests that it may be involved with organogenesis of the genitourinary system.[25]

PAX2

PAX genes have been linked in previous research to abnormal prenatal development of the renal and visual systems, including Waardenburg's syndrome, aniridia, and alveolar rhabdomyosarcoma. *PAX2* (i.e., paired box gene 2) is localized to chromosome 10. It is expressed in the mesonephric ducts, ureteral bud, and the periureteral mesenchyme, and it is absent in mature nephrons.

Animals heterozygous for the *PAX2* gene had diminished kidney size and disorganized structure, with a thin cortex, decreased number of cortical structures, increased cystic components, and immaturity of mesenchyme-derived tissue.[18] Homozygous *PAX2*-knockout animals manifested renal agenesis associated with failure of wolffian duct formation.[26] These abnormalities are referable to failed branching of the ureteral bud, lack of appropriate differentiation of the metanephric mesenchyme, or failure of reciprocal induction of the mesenchyme and ureteral bud.[26] Sanyanusin and coworkers[27] found similar ultrastructural abnormalities in heterozygotes in a family cohort with a known *PAX2* mutation who were affected by optic nerve colobomas and genitourinary abnormalities, including vesicoureteral reflux and anomalous renal development. Animal models homozygous for *PAX2* mutations failed to develop genitourinary tracts; development of the external genitalia was also abnormal because of limited growth of the mesonephric duct and subsequent failure of the subdivision of the cloaca.[1]

WT1

Wilms' tumor 1 gene *(WT1)* is one of the most well-known genes in renal development. Located on chromosome 11p, its linkage to the appropriate receptor results in blockage of transcription, and abnormal linkage is associated with development of Wilms' tumors. Clarkson and associates[28] demonstrated that mutations in the *WT1* gene were associated with nephric anomalies and genital anomalies, although the latter were not observed independently of the former. Expression of the WT1 protein has been localized to the mesonephric tubules and metanephric mesenchyme, and prenatal lack of expression is associated with failure of metanephric development; *WT1*-knockout mice fail to develop caudal mesonephric tubules, which ultimately give rise to renal structures.[18] The local events surrounding WT1 expression appear to include suppression of insulin-like growth factor 2 (IGF2) expression in the local mesenchyme, because IGF2 is expressed before WT1 activity, and IGF2 expression declines in the presence of WT1.[19]

WT1 has been associated with prenatal expression of PAX2 and AMH. *WT1*-knockout mice fail to express PAX2, and WT1 is thought to exert effects on AMH expression in the developing embryo. Activity of the AMH promoter is known to be under the influence of many substances, including WT1, GATA-binding protein 4 (GATA4), SRY-box 9 (SOX9), and splicing factor 1 (SF1). WT1 expression in the developing embryo parallels that of AMH expression while müllerian regression takes place, and WT1 binds to a specific region of the AMH promoter.[29] Abnormalities in the *WT1* gene are associated with development of Wilms' tumor and with less common syndromes such as the Denys-Drash syndrome (i.e., ambiguous genitalia, rudimentary gonads, nephrotic syndrome, and Wilms' tumor) and Frasier syndrome,[29] which is characterized by dysgenetic gonads and renal anomalies with development of the nephrotic syndrome.[30] Abnormalities in sex differentiation of *WT1* mutants are linked to preservation of a triplet of amino acids (KTS: lysine, threonine, and serine); without KTS preservation, there is decreased synthesis of AMH and SRY. Genetic males with a 46,XY karyotype will be phenotypic females with preservation of müllerian structures.[30]

HOXA

Homeobox genes have been identified in multiple organisms, from mammals to insects and lower organisms, and they appear to affect structural symmetry during organogenesis. Research has identified homeobox genes as important for the normal development of the genitourinary tract. Cohn[31] reviewed the research that found that homeobox genes were needed for the normal growth and differentiation of the urethral plate and distal genital tubercle. Development of the genital tubercle parallels that of development of the limb buds in the embryo; without *HOXA* genes, growth of the distal genital tubercle remains rudimentary.

Mutations in the homeobox genes have also been associated with abnormal development of the external genitalia, often in the setting of a syndrome of developmental abnormalities. One such novel syndrome is X-linked lissencephaly with abnormal genitalia (XLAG), in which patients have frameshift or point mutations in the Aristaless-related homeobox gene *(ARX)*.[32] Affected patients present with neural malformations, including agenesis of the corpus callosum, abnormalities of midline structures in the brain, disorganized and incomplete development of the cerebral cortex, and micropenis with bilateral undescended testicles. Some patients also have associated renal phosphate wasting.[33]

The importance of the homeobox genes in regulating normal organogenesis is underscored by duplication of function. *HOXA* and *HOXD* genes have been found to have compensatory activity for mild mutations such that affected embryos may develop without significant congenital abnormalities. However, more severe or extensive mutations in either gene cannot be compensated by the remaining normal gene.[34] Work by Utsch and colleagues[34] found that novel mutations in the homeobox genes associated with the hand-foot-genital syndrome may reflect the limitations of duplicated function in compensatory genes.

Androgen Receptor

Androgen resistance is associated with decreased growth of the glans and corpora cavernosal structures, but the corpus spongiosum develops normally and may be hypertrophied. This pattern of development suggests that although growth of the corpora cavernosa may be induced by androgens, growth of the corpus spongiosum is androgen independent.[17]

Shapiro and coworkers[35] evaluated an animal model of congenital adrenal hyperplasia by exposing embryos to androgens for different periods. They found that virilization resulting from congenital adrenal hyperplasia could be induced through exogenous androgen exposure between 8 and 13 weeks' gestation. However, even within this time frame, morphologic changes observed after early androgen exposure differed from those induced by later exposure. Exposure to androgens earlier in the critical period was associated with increased virilization, including complete fusion of the labioscrotal folds and clitoromegaly. Clitoromegaly alone was observed with later exposure to androgens. Shapiro's group theorized that somatic growth of the embryo and genital structures later than 13 weeks' gestation was independent of the influence of testosterone and other androgens.

CONCLUSIONS

Development of the genitourinary tract is a complex series of events and interactions over time and space. Common and uncommon errors in these events and interactions result in anomalies and may set the stage for dysfunctions later in life. Understanding the prenatal events involved in the development of the genitourinary tract facilitates comprehension of normal and aberrant postnatal anatomy and informs management of urologic disorders.

References

1. Lipschutz JH: Molecular development of the kidney: A review of the results of gene disruption studies. Am J Kidney Dis 331:383-397, 1998.
2. Davies JA, Brandli A: Kidney development database. Available at http://www.ana.ed.ac.uk/anatomy/database/kidbase
3. Kluth D, Hillen M, Lambrecht W: The principles of normal and abnormal hindgut development. J Pediatr Surg 30:1143-1147, 1995.
4. Nievelstein RA, van der Werff JF, Verbeck FJ, et al: Normal and abnormal development of the anorectum in human embryos. Teratology 57:70-78, 1998.
5. Park JM: Normal and anomalous development of the urogenital system. In Walsh PC, Retik AB, Vaughn ED Jr, Wein WJ (eds): Campbell's Urology, 8th ed. Philadelphia, WB Saunders, 2002, pp 1737-1764.
6. Kim KM, Kogan BA, Massad CA, Huang Y: Collagen and elastin in the normal fetal bladder. J Urol 146:524-527, 1991.
7. Koo HP, Howard PS, Chang SL, et al: Developmental expression of interstitial collagen genes in fetal bladders. J Urol 158:954-961, 1997.
8. Wood HM, Trock BJ, Gearhart JP: In vitro fertilization and the cloacal-bladder exstrophy-epispadias complex: Is there an association? J Urol 69:1512-1515, 2003.
9. Shapiro E, Lepor H, Jeffs RD: The inheritance of the exstrophy-epispadias complex. J Urol 132:308-310, 1984.
10. Casale P, Grady RW, Waldehausen JHT, et al: Cloacal exstrophy variants: Can blighted conjoined twinning play a role? J Urol 172:1103-1107, 2004.
11. Breech LL, Laufer MR: Developmental abnormalities of the female reproductive tract. Curr Opin Obstet Gynecol 11:441-450, 1999.
12. Duckett J, Baskin L: Genitoplasty for intersex anomalies. Eur J Pediatr 152(Suppl 2):S80-S84, 1993.
13. Schweiken HU: The androgen resistance syndromes: Clinical and biochemical aspects. Eur J Pediatr 152(Suppl 2):S50-S57, 1993.
14. Edmonds DK: Vaginal and uterine anomalies in the paediatric and adolescent patient. Curr Opin Obstet Gynecol 13:463-467, 2001.
15. Spevak MR, Cohen HL: Ultrasonography of the Adolescent Female Pelvis. Ultrasound Q 18:275-288, 2002.
16. Haraguchi R, Suzuki K, Murakami R, et al: Molecular analysis of external genitalia formation: The role of fibroblast growth factor (FGF) genes during genital tubercle formation. Development 127:2471-2379, 2000.
17. Yucel S, Liu W, Cordero D, et al: Anatomical studies of the fibroblast growth factor-10 mutant, Sonic Hedge Hog mutant and androgen receptor mutant mouse genital tubercle. Adv Exp Med Biol 545:123-148, 2004.
18. Coplen DE: Molecular aspects of genitourinary development. AUA Update Series 23:13, 2004.
19. Glassberg KI: Normal and abnormal development of the kidney: A clinician's interpretation of current knowledge. J Urol 167:2339-2351, 2002.
20. Behringer RR, Finegold MJ, Cate RL: Mullerian-inhibiting substance function during mammalian sexual development. Cell 79:415-425, 1994.
21. Bartlett JE, Lee SM, Mishina Y, et al: Gubernacular development in mullerian inhibiting substance receptor-deficient mice. BJU Int 89:113-118, 2002.
22. Hoshiya M, Christian BP, Cromie WJ, et al: Persistent Mullerian duct syndrome caused by both a 27-bp deletion and a novel splice mutation in the *MIS* type II receptor gene. Birth Defects Res 67:868-874, 2003.
23. Austin PF, Siow Y, Fallat ME, et al: The relationship between mullerian inhibiting substance and androgens in boys with hypospadias. J Urol 168:1784-1788, 2002.
24. Misra M, MacLaughlin DT, Donahoe PK, Lee MM: The role of müllerian inhibiting substance in the evaluation of phenotypic female patients with mild degrees of virilization. J Clin Endocrinol Metab 88:787-792, 2003.
25. Shao X, Johnson JE, Richardson JA, et al: A minimal KSP-cadherin promoter linked to a green fluorescent protein reporter gene exhibits tissue-specific expression in the developing kidney and genitourinary tract. J Am Soc Nephrol 13:1824-1836, 2002.
26. Piscione TD, Rosenblum ND: The malformed kidney: Disruption of glomerular and tubular development. Clin Genet 56:341-356, 1999.
27. Sanyanusin P, Schimmenti LA, McNue LA, et al: Mutation of the *PAX2* gene in a family with optic nerve colobomas, renal anomalies, and vesicoureteral reflux. Nat Genet 9:358-364, 1995.
28. Clarkson PA, Davies HR, Williams DM, et al: Mutational screening of the Wilms' tumour gene, *WT1*, in males with genital abnormalities. J Med Genet 30:767-772, 1993.
29. Hossain A, Saunders GF: Role of Wilms tumor 1 (WT1) in the transcriptional regulation of the Mullerian-inhibiting substance promoter. Biol Reprod 69:1808-1814, 2003.
30. MacLaughlin DT, Donahoe PK: Sex determination and differentiation. N Engl J Med 350:367-378, 2004.
31. Cohn MJ: Developmental genetics of the external genitalia. Adv Exp Med Biol 545:149-157, 2004.

32. Hartmann H, Uyanik G, Gross C, et al: Agenesis of the corpus callosum, abnormal genitalia and intractable epilepsy due to a novel familial mutation in the Aristaless-related homeobox gene. Neuropediatrics 35:157-160, 2004.
33. Hahn A, Gross C, Uyanik G, et al: X-linked lissencephaly with abnormal genitalia associated with renal phosphate wasting. Neuropediatrics 35:202-205, 2004.
34. Utsch B, Becker K, Brock D, et al: A novel stable polyalanine [poly(A)] expansion in the *HOXA13* gene associated with hand-foot-genital syndrome: Proper function of poly(A)-harbouring transcription factors depends on a critical repeat length? Hum Genet 110:488-494, 2002.
35. Shapiro E, Huang H, Wu, XR: New concepts on the development of the vagina. Adv Exp Med Biol 545:173-185, 2004.

Chapter 2

STRUCTURAL BASIS OF VOIDING DYSFUNCTION

Ahmad Elbadawi

Functional behavior of the urinary bladder has been investigated for more than a century, but several aspects of the mechanism of voiding and the way it is altered in vesical dysfunction remain unresolved. This can largely be attributed to the complexity of structural organization of the bladder and its outlet and the matching complexity of their functions.[1-7]

The storage (i.e., filling) and expulsion (i.e., voiding) phases of micturition involve essentially opposite functions of the bladder and urethra.[8] The bladder acts as a reservoir for urine during filling and as a pump for expelling its stored urine during voiding. The urethra during bladder filling is closed, sealed, and noncompliant, acting as a sphincter to maintain continence, but it opens, dilates, and becomes compliant during voiding, acting as a conduit for the urinary stream. Efficient urine storage requires a compliant and stable detrusor together with a continent bladder outlet.[5,9] Compliance of the detrusor allows distention of the bladder to capacity, and its stability ensures absence of untimely contractions that could involuntarily force some urine past the closed outlet, resulting in incontinence. Complete emptying of the full bladder[9] depends on optimal contractility of the detrusor so that it can mount a strong, speedy, sustained, and unitary voiding contraction; coordinated opening of the bladder outlet; and maintenance of the opened outlet as a free conduit for an uninterrupted and strong urinary stream.

The anatomy and structure of the bladder and urethra must be optimally suited to the complex dynamic events in the micturition cycle.[6] Important elements in this regard are the inherent physical and biomechanical properties of the tissue components of the vesical and urethral walls and their bearing on organ distensibility and contractility.[8,10-12] Two crucial elements are the topographic and microstructural organization of the musculature of the bladder wall and urethra and the elaborate system of vesicourethral innervation, with complex central cephalospinal control and intricate peripheral pathways.[1-6,13,14]

Various disciplines have contributed through experimental and clinical investigation to our knowledge of bladder function and dysfunction. Gross anatomy was the natural start during the previous century, and it prevailed for many decades. It resulted in some fundamental concepts that have been expanded and refined in the current century as the result of improved methods of dissection, neuroanatomic tracing techniques, and microscopic staining procedures. After the initial era of anatomic investigation, the principal approach to studies on voiding has been the characterization of physiologic and muscular responses of the lower urinary tract, mainly the bladder. It is undeniable that definition and measurement of these responses are important for understanding the overall nature of neuromuscular function of the bladder and urethra. Nonetheless, such an approach cannot define the factors that determine function of the effector organ (i.e., smooth muscle of detrusor and urethral wall) in regard to the exact mechanism and balance of their contractility, distensibility, and stability during the filling and expulsion phases of micturition. Attempts to define these factors based purely on physiopharmacologic studies are largely inferential and have generated some misconceptions. One such misconception is the idea that the sympathetic autonomic nervous system has little or no role in vesical or urethral function.[15,16] This dogma prevailed through the mid-1960s, until it was invalidated by microscopic proof of sympathetic innervation of the vesicourethral muscularis, which was subsequently confirmed by innumerable physiopharmacologic observations.[1,4,5,7]

Landmarks in our knowledge of muscular anatomy of the lower urinary tract[3,6,17,18] include continuation of the muscularis of the terminal ureters as the vesical "trigone" and beyond into the dorsal wall of the urethra; the nonlayered, interwoven organization of muscle bundles of the detrusor[13]; identification of a vesical sheath around the terminal ureters,[19] which was eventually refined as the concept of dual ureteral sheath[20,21]; and the concept of the rhabdosphincter as an integral striated muscle component of urethral muscularis.[1,3,6,22] Milestones in our knowledge of the innervation and neural control of the bladder and urethra include[1-5] definition in the spinal cord of a sacral parasympathetic and a lumbar sympathetic nucleus for subcephalic bladder control, as well as a sacral cord nucleus supplying peripheral somatomotor innervation of the volitional urinary sphincter[23-26]; multilevel localization of centers of bladder control in the brain, their interconnections, and their spinal neurotract projections[27-30]; description of the topographic organization of peripheral sympathetic and parasympathetic outflows, respectively, through the hypogastric and pelvic nerve or plexus pathways and their differences in different species[23,31,32]; recognition of dual sympathetic and parasympathetic innervation of the bladder and urethra and introduction of the functional concept of bladder body versus bladder base[33,34]; localization of the origin of intrinsic vesicourethral innervation in peripheral ganglia close to and within the organs, including the concept of sympathetic and parasympathetic effector short neurons[35,36]; concepts of infraspinal interaction of sympathetic and parasympathetic pathways within peripheral ganglia (through collaterals and interneurons)[34-39] and the vesicourethral muscularis (through axoaxonal synapses at the effector cell level)[40-42]; recognition of auxiliary autonomic innervation of the rhabdosphincter in animals and humans[22,43-45]; and recognition of neuropeptides as a class of putative neurotransmitters or modulatory cotransmitters in peripheral vesicourethral innervation.[5-7,46,47]

Full knowledge of the structure of an organ is key to the understanding of how it functions. A corollary of this axiom is that alteration of the structure of an organ is reflected in alteration of its function. The axiom and its corollary should be fundamental premises in studies of the bladder in view of its unique function and intimate anatomic relationship to two other organs of different but closely integrated function—the ureter supplying it with urine and the urethra serving as the conduit for its expulsion. Tacit awareness of these premises stimulated research at the biochemical and molecular levels during the past few decades. This research has yielded important information on the biomechanics, energetics, and neuroreceptor attributes of the bladder and urethra. Not unexpectedly, such information has not fully clarified the basis of normal or abnormal smooth muscle function of either organ.

Microscopic study of the vesicourethral muscularis has yet to attain its full potential for determining the true basis of normal and abnormal voiding. Routine tissue histology and histochemistry have provided only limited information about tissue topography and general organization of this system. The notoriously tedious nature of electron microscopy has in part been responsible for its lagging use in investigation of bladder function and dysfunction until recently. Another major stumbling block has been the lack of clear guidelines and precisely defined criteria for such ultrastructural approaches.

In this chapter, the microstructure of the vesicourethral muscularis and its functional correlates are reviewed. Observations on microstructural defects in various forms of voiding dysfunction are presented, and their bearing on the pathophysiology and management of such disorders is discussed. The information presented is derived largely from overlapping studies on bladder ultrastructure in normal experimental animals, experimental voiding dysfunction, and various clinical disorders of micturition.

ULTRASTRUCTURE OF THE VESICOURETHRAL MUSCULARIS

Until the previous decade, the urinary bladder had received little attention by students of tissue ultrastructure, unlike organs such as the intestine. The rather simplistic ideas about bladder function and its neural control that prevailed until the mid-1960s probably thwarted interest in serious electron microscopic investigation, or perhaps no one suspected that bladder structure and function were sufficiently complex to justify such investigation.

The few reports on vesical ultrastructure available before the 1980s presented general, vague, or imprecise information and therefore were largely noncontributory. A notable exception was a study on the distribution of intrinsic afferent (sensory) nerves in the cat bladder, including the relative contributions of sympathetic and parasympathetic pathways.[48,49] The observations reported in this study confirmed and supplemented earlier accounts of the cholinergic and adrenergic suburothelial nerves demonstrated histochemically in the cat bladder.[33] The existence of nerve terminals within the urothelium is ultrastructurally indisputable in animals and humans.[1] A proposal for distinguishing suburothelial sensory nerves by electron microscopic counting of axonal synaptic vesicles[50] remains unfulfilled.

Studies on the detrusor and "internal sphincter"[51-53] have provided detailed information about their intrinsic innervation and have shown that their muscle cells have the ultrastructural features of smooth muscle in general.[54-56] Definitions of the various terms and structural parameters have been provided in other reports.[51,56-58]

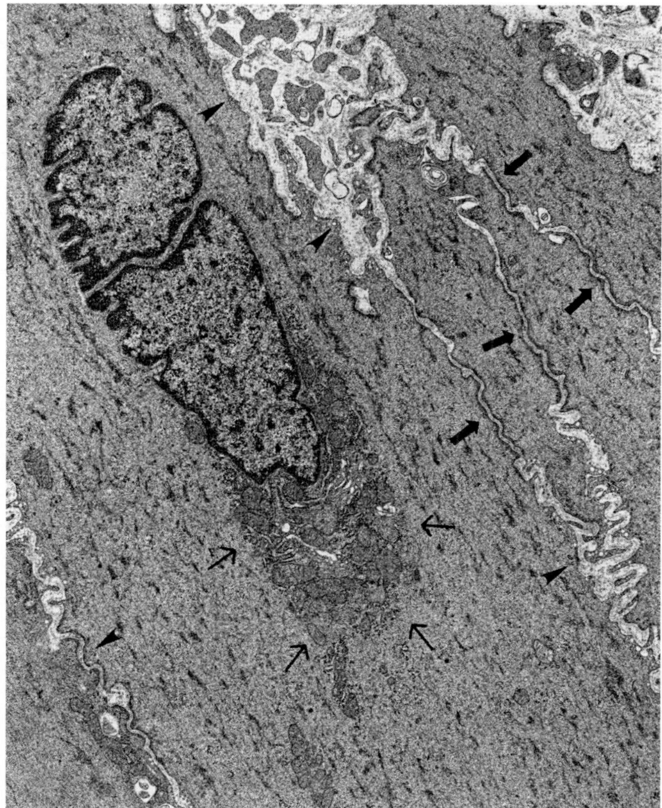

Figure 2-1 Muscle cells of a normal detrusor. The sarcolemma (i.e., cell membrane) has alternating thick, dense bands and interposed thin zones with caveolae, with outlying basal laminae *(arrowheads)*. Cells are adjoined by intermediate junctions *(thick arrows)* and separated by narrow spaces. The nucleus is capped on one side by endoplasmic reticulum and mitochondria *(thin arrows)*. The sarcoplasm is packed with myofilaments and with evenly distributed, cigar-shaped dense bodies and scattered mitochondria (magnification ×13,890). (From Elbadawi A: Functional pathology of urinary bladder muscularis: The new frontier in diagnostic uropathology. Semin Diagn Pathol 10:319, 1993.)

Muscle Cells

Ultrastructurally, each of the grossly recognizable bundles of vesicourethral muscularis in various animals and in humans is composed of incompletely separated and imperfectly outlined compact groups (fascicles) of muscle cells.[51,56,58] The muscle cell profile (Fig. 2-1) has a smooth contour and a polygonal to cylindrical configuration, depending on the plane of sectioning relative to its long axis. Nuclei of typical appearance are centrally located and rarely have nucleoli. Mitoses are ordinarily absent in muscle cells of the adult bladder.[59]

The perimeter of each cell profile is delineated by a continuous cell membrane (i.e., sarcolemma) that displays alternating thick, electron-dense and thinner, less dense zones, with an outlying basal lamina of even thickness and moderate electron density. The thick sarcolemmal zones (i.e., dense bands) are composed of sarcolemma plus subjacent highly dense material in sarcoplasm. The interposed thinner zones consist only of sarcolemma, with strings of caveolae that appear as rows of flask-shaped surface vesicles of uniform size.

The sarcoplasm is packed with evenly distributed myofilaments of uniform orientation and alignment, with evenly dispersed dense bodies of uniform cigar-shaped appearance in cylindrical cell profiles of longitudinally sectioned cells. The myofilaments are slanted at an approximately 10-degree angle from the long cell axis and are anchored to dense bands of sarcolemma. Organelles of typical structure, mainly mitochondria and endoplasmic reticulum, are aggregated in a conical zone capping each nuclear pole (in cylindrical profiles); some mitochondria, cisternae of reticulum, and clusters of ribosomes are also scattered in sarcoplasm, particularly beneath sarcolemmal caveolae.

Individual cells within muscle fascicles are separated by spaces of uniform width (usually <200 nm). The intercellular space contains small amounts of amorphous material similar to basal lamina and a few isolated collagen fibrils that are mainly attached to sarcolemmal dense bands of related muscle cells. Contiguous muscle cells have intermediate-type junctions (e.g., attachment plaques, zonulae adherentes) of typical appearance and length and with 30- to 60-nm separation gaps. Some also have zones (with approximately 15-nm gaps) of simple apposition of sarcolemma.[57,60] Contrary to one report,[61] it is generally accepted that gap junctions (i.e., nexus) are absent or only sparsely encountered in the normal vesicourethral muscularis of animals and humans.[51,53,60,62]

Intrinsic Nerves

Ultrastructural studies have confirmed dual innervation of the normal bladder and urethra by cholinergic and adrenergic axons and provided morphologic details of the relationships between these axons and muscle cells.[1-5] Nerve elements within the vesicourethral muscularis course in its interstitium as Schwann cell–ensheathed axon bundles. Varicosities of some axons become exposed along their course in these bundles to face smooth muscle cells. The main vehicle of muscular innervation is provided by individual preterminal axons that "break away" from the bundles to establish contact with the muscle cells. Many muscle cells have cholinergic or adrenergic neuroeffector junctions, some have both (diautonomic junctions), and some have neither.[2,4,51] Clefts of neuroeffector junctions (i.e., spaces between axon and muscle cell) typically are 15 to 80 nm wide.

It seems certain that no part of the vesicourethral muscularis has a 1 : 1 nerve-to-muscle ratio,[1,5,59] as inferred in the original histochemical study on vesical innervation.[33] The basis for upholding that impression in one study on the human bladder[53] is questionable.[4,6,59] Synaptic contacts between cholinergic and adrenergic or probable copeptidergic axons (i.e., axoaxonal synapses) have been discovered as a unique feature of intrinsic neuroplexuses of vesicourethral muscularis in animals[40,41] and humans (A Elbadawi, unpublished data).

Interstitium

Collagen and elastic fibers are the main components of interstitium in the vesicourethral muscularis. Partitions of interstitium surround and separate muscle bundles.[56,58] These partitions extend into each bundle as microsepta that incompletely delineate its component fascicles. Vascular and neural elements supplying the muscularis are contained in interstitium between and within the muscle bundles.

Microstructural Basis of Vesicourethral Muscular Function

Conceptually, the vesicourethral muscularis comprises three integrated microstructural compartments: one for generating, another for modulating, and a third for coordinating its functional responses.[9,63]

The *generator compartment* consists of smooth muscle cells, which enable the vesicourethral muscularis to respond appropriately to various stimuli, particularly to generate the neurally triggered unitary detrusor contraction of voiding. Several microstructural elements play specific roles in the excitation-contraction coupling mechanism of smooth muscle.[9,52,54-56] Proper composition, organization, and intracellular disposition of myofilaments bearing the contractile proteins actin and myosin ensure generation of an optimal contractile force. A sufficient complement of intact mitochondria provides the enzymes necessary for generating the necessary ATP-dependent energy. Mitochondria and an intact endoplasmic reticulum provide and store intracellular calcium ions (Ca^{2+}), which are necessary for muscle cell contraction. An intact sarcolemma provides anchorage for myofilaments at its dense bands to transmit the contractile force to the cell surface. The function of sarcolemmal caveolae has not yet been established. The close spatial association between caveolae and cisternae of subsarcolemmal endoplasmic reticulum, a site of Ca^{2+} binding and storage,[54,64] suggests that they are involved in the mechanism of muscle contraction. There is evidence that caveolae are sites of active ion (Na^+, K^+, Ca^{2+}) transport, Na^+-Ca^{2+} exchange, or passive Ca^{2+} binding, all of which are involved in the excitation-contraction coupling mechanism.[65]

The *modulator compartment* comprises intrinsic neuroplexuses and their neuroeffector junctions. Neural influence through the latter involves induction, facilitation, inhibition, or disinhibition of chemical neurotransmission to muscle cells under central cephalospinal and peripheral autonomic ganglionic control.[1,5,9] Intact structure of intrinsic axons is necessary for conduction of neural impulses throughout their course within the detrusor. Structural integrity of neuroeffector junctions, including the predominant small (clear or dense-core) vesicle content of their axonal components, is necessary for chemical neurotransmission to the target muscle cells. Axoaxonal synapses modulate prejunctional, reciprocal cholinergic-adrenergic inhibition of effector neural influence in the normal mammalian vesical muscularis, including that of humans.[9,40,41] From the structural standpoint, the efficacy and net effect of neural influence on this muscularis depend mainly on the distribution and relative density of the various functional types of structurally intact axons (i.e., cholinergic versus adrenergic) and the width and content of junctional clefts of preserved neuroeffector junctions. Alteration of the inherent structure or spatial relationship of axons within the bladder may hinder one normal neurally triggered neural response or another, or it may generate incongruous, uncoordinated, or spurious muscle cell responses.[9]

The *coordinator compartment* is in part muscular and in part interstitial. It is responsible for maintaining spatial topographic organization of muscle cells relative to each other within muscle fascicles and bundles of the detrusor and urethral muscularis. Moreover, it provides the basis for tridimensional distensibility of the bladder, which allows it to be filled to capacity with minimal rise in luminal pressure (i.e., compliance).[11,66] Compliance is determined by the relative proportions of muscular and interstitial elements and by the delicate balance of the rigid and elastic components of interstitium—collagen and elastin, respectively.[10,66-68]

The main role of the coordinator compartment is to synergize and unify muscle cell responses in the entire detrusor or urethral wall. The most important functional expression of this role is the neurally triggered, coordinated, unitary detrusor contraction that initiates voiding.[1,4,9] Only a fraction of muscle cells of the detrusor are innervated and are directly excitable by neural stimuli, despite its overall dense innervation.[1,4,6] Voiding contraction of the detrusor, which is in essence a synergized, summated, and sustained contraction of its component fascicles and bundles, requires transmittal of contraction from the innervated to all noninnervated muscle cells (i.e., muscle cell coupling).

Cell coupling in smooth muscle is electrical or mechanical.[54,55,69] Electrical coupling *propagates the electrical signal* (i.e., action potential), heralding contraction of a muscle cell through the gap junctions (and to some extent through simple sarcolemmal appositions) of muscle cells; these junctions (or appositions) provide low-resistance pathways that directly "connect" and allow exchange of ions between sarcoplasms of the adjoined muscle cells. A smooth muscle system endowed with an electrical coupling mechanism behaves functionally as a virtual syncytium through which contraction of the component cells can be elicited in near synchrony. The relatively slower mechanical coupling *transmits the force* generated in a contracting muscle cell through intermediate junctions with adjacent cells. Contrary to one review,[61] cell coupling in normal vesicourethral muscularis is achieved by mechanical cell coupling because its muscle cells have intermediate junctions but no or sparse gap junctions.[51,53,60] Active force generated by the contractile apparatus of a muscle cell is discharged to the entire cell surface through insertions of myofilaments into sarcolemmal dense bands, resulting in cell shortening. The tension developed is transmitted through intermediate junctions to adjoined cells, resulting in their deformation and subsequent contraction. Collagen fibrils juxtaposed to the cell surface in the intercellular space contribute to mechanical transmittal of force from the contracting cell to adjacent cells. Summation of minuscule tensions transmitted from cell to cell and from muscle cells to microsepta of interstitium culminates in contraction of entire muscle bundles—and ultimately in contraction of the entire organ in unison—by subsequent force transmittal through partitions of interstitium between the bundles.[60]

Normal contractility of the vesicourethral muscularis in regard to complete emptying of the bladder depends on three factors in addition to the inherent topographic organization and structural integrity of its cells. These are the ability of a contracting muscle cell to shorten (generating a contraction force), mechanical cell coupling to transmit that force, and a vehicle to summate the transmitted force through the muscularis. All three factors have recognizable ultrastructural correlates. Effective cell shortening requires a normal cylindric configuration of the muscle cell and a normal complement of myofilaments optimally aligned at a narrow angle with sarcolemma. Mechanical cell coupling is largely determined by the geometric spatial disposition of detrusor muscle cells and their structural inter-relationships in regard to their compact arrangement within fascicles, intermediate cell junctions, and narrow interspaces containing few collagen fibrils. Collagen fibers in microsepta and partitions of interstitium, respectively between muscle fascicles and bundles, play a key role in eliciting the summated, unitary voiding contraction.

ULTRASTRUCTURE OF THE RHABDOSPHINCTER

The feline rhabdosphincter is composed of a mixture of fast- and slow-twitch myofibers, which have the same distinguishable ultrastructure as ordinary somatic mammalian striated muscle.[44] Contrary to one report,[70] the human rhabdosphincter appears to be composed of both types of myofibers (Mathews, Light, Wheeler, et al, unpublished data).

The concept of triple (i.e., somatomotor plus dual parasympathetic-sympathetic autonomic) innervation of the feline rhabdosphincter based on histochemical study[22] was validated by electron microscopy in the cat,[44,71] and its adrenergic autonomic component was also confirmed in humans.[45] Two forms of the nerve-myofiber relationship are present in the feline rhabdosphincter with intact innervation. One has the classic sole plate differentiation of the myofiber facing a cholinergic neuroterminal, which is characteristic of somatomotor neuromuscular junctions at large. In the other, a cholinergic or adrenergic axon terminal is closely apposed to the surface of a myofiber and has a functionally plausible, narrow neuromuscular cleft but no sole plate differentiation. These surface contacts are considered autonomic because their morphology is identical to those of autonomic neuroeffector junctions in the vesicourethral muscularis and other mammalian smooth muscle systems and because they persist, despite disappearance of axons innervating sole plates, after bilateral sacral ventral rhizotomy—the known source of somatomotor innervation through the pudendal nerves (discussed later).[71-73]

Functional Pathology of the Detrusor

Changes in the three microstructural compartments of the detrusor have been described in various forms of voiding dysfunction. Those described in histologic preparations are largely nonspecific and have been of limited usefulness in regard to correlation with the functional abnormalities.[56,58] The constellations of changes identified ultrastructurally in different dysfunctions tend to predominate in one compartment or another and are distinctive for each dysfunction.[56,58] For this reason, accurate definition of the microstructural correlates of a voiding dysfunction requires study of the smooth muscle, interstitium, and intrinsic neural compartments of the detrusor with equal attention and scrutiny.[9,56]

NEUROPATHIC VOIDING DYSFUNCTION

Practically all information on the microstructural basis of neuropathic voiding dysfunction has been derived from experimental studies in the cat. These studies have dispelled some traditionally held dogmas and have laid the foundation for a new concept in pathophysiology of the lower motor neuropathic bladder.[74-79] According to this concept, abnormal behavior of such a bladder does not merely reflect its release from cephalospinal neural control but is largely the result of dynamic, profound changes in intrinsic nerves and to some extent muscle cells—the two structural elements that jointly determine that behavior. These neuropathic structural changes can be defined fully and accurately only by electron microscopy,[79] and they readily distinguish a decentralization from a denervation functional type of lower motor neuropathic bladder. The same studies also validate the concept of triple innervation of the feline rhabdosphincter.[71-73,80]

The Decentralized Bladder

For decades, belief that postganglionic nerves within the bladder are unchanged after decentralization by parasympathetic preganglionic neurectomy (e.g., sacral roots, pelvic nerve trunks) remained universal and absolute. The underlying logic was that such neurectomy leaves untouched and structurally intact the ganglion cells that provide the intrinsic vesical nerves. Studies on models of the decentralized bladder, however, revealed dynamic structural changes in intrinsic postganglionic nerves of the detrusor: initial degeneration with eventual regeneration.

Occurring beyond and across preganglionic synapses, short-term degeneration of axons duplicates the well-known phenomenon of primary transsynaptic nerve degeneration in the brain[81] and represents the first example of this phenomenon in the peripheral autonomic nervous system.[74] The axonal degeneration results in loss of cholinergic neuroeffector junctions and is associated with transjunctional degeneration of detrusor muscle cells, a previously unknown phenomenon.[76] The term *transjunctional* underscores the fact that muscle cell degeneration occurs at a site two levels of anatomic discontinuity peripheral to the sacral spinal cord nucleus (i.e., the preganglionic synapse in the peripheral ganglia and the neuroeffector junction at the terminal effector tissue level). The initially degenerating axons eventually regenerate. This regeneration expresses yet another previously unrecognized phenomenon because it is not a simple restitution of the original complement of cholinergic axons but is also associated with[75] sprouting of adrenergic (i.e., postganglionic sympathetic) axons with adrenergic hyperinnervation (also documented histochemically[71,82]) and with emergence of peptide-replete axons and axon terminals. Neuroeffector junctions become reestablished by the latter axonal population in addition to the regenerating cholinergic and sprouting adrenergic axons; muscle cell regeneration occurs concomitantly.[76] Ultrastructural profiles of regenerating muscle cells have expanded rough endoplasmic reticulum replete with clustered ribosomes, prominent subsarcolemmal reticulum, numerous intact paranuclear and subsarcolemmal mitochondria, and frequent nucleoli. It appears that an intact preganglionic sympathetic pathway is necessary for the long-term axonal changes to take place after decentralization because they do not occur when decentralization is combined with hypogastric neurectomy.[78] This fact, together with available pharmacologic evidence,[83] suggests that adrenergic hyperinnervation of the detrusor is an important factor in development of hypertonicity in the lower motor neuropathic bladder.[78]

The Denervated Bladder

Changes in intrinsic axons and muscle cells of the detrusor also occur after postganglionic neurectomy,[77] which severs the pelvic plexus (i.e., parasympathetic plus sympathetic extrinsic nerves) very close to the bladder. Neurectomy mimics the clinical situation of severe neural deficit after major extirpative pelvic surgery.[84] The resultant short-term degenerative changes in axons and muscle cells are similar to those seen in the decentralized bladder but are more profound in scope and degree. Long-term changes, however, are different, including little cholinergic axonal regeneration, sparse adrenergic innervation, and no appreciable population of peptide-rich axons. Similar scarcity of adrenergic nerves has been reported in bladder biopsy specimens from patients who had undergone abdominoperineal resection of the rectum.[85]

The Denervated Rhabdosphincter

Decentralization of the bladder by bilateral sacral ventral rhizotomy deprives the rhabdosphincter of its somatomotor innervation. The somatomotor-denervated rhabdosphincter loses its population of classic neuromuscular junctions, and the ultrastructure of its sole plates becomes markedly simplified, but the autonomic axon contacts with the myofibers lacking sole plates persist.[71] Eventually, the autonomic junctions become prominent and widespread, and many of the residual simplified sole plates become newly innervated by a cholinergic axon or an adrenergic axon, or both.[72] These changes indicate permanent degeneration of somatomotor nerves and persistence plus long-term "propagation" of autonomic innervation in denervated territories of the rhabdosphincter. Along with the axonal changes, the myofibers display a combination of degeneration and regeneration.[80]

The somatomotor-denervated rhabdosphincter appears to be under exclusive autonomic neural control. The nature of this control has not as yet been investigated, nor have responses to autonomic neural stimuli been demonstrated physiologically or pharmacologically in the normal rhabdosphincter, although they are unequivocal in the cat, and their adrenergic component has been proved in humans. The autonomic component may have a subtle, very specific, or precisely timed function in normal micturition that is difficult to duplicate in an investigative setting, or it may be functionally operative or discernible only in abnormal voiding. Available physiopharmacologic methods of study may or may not be sufficiently sensitive to segregate autonomic responses of the rhabdosphincter from those of the intimately associated urethral smooth muscularis in the normal or the neuropathic rhabdosphincter.

The Upper Motor Neuropathic Bladder

As described in the brain, the phenomenon of transsynaptic degeneration may be primary, secondary, tertiary, and so on, depending on the number of synaptic relays between the injured neuron and the neuron providing degenerating terminals in the same pathway.[81] Transsynaptic degeneration in the decentralized bladder is primary because, as far as is known, only one relay station (in a peripheral vesicourethral ganglion) is interposed between the interrupted preganglionic neuron (ventral root) and the corresponding postganglionic neuron providing the degenerating terminals within the bladder. It is conceivable that comparable degeneration may follow interruption of central neuraxial pathways as an expression of secondary or tertiary transsynaptic degeneration (i.e., across one or two central plus the peripheral relay stations). Observations in one study on a spinal cord transection model suggest that such degeneration may occur,[86] but it needs to be confirmed by detailed investigation in experimental models and clinical settings. If such confirmation is obtained, an important concept would emerge: functional derangement in the bladder deprived of cephalic control is in part caused by structural changes in vesicourethral muscularis despite preserved anatomic integrity of the sacral cord and infraspinal neural pathways.

DETRUSOR DYSFUNCTION

Poorly Contractile Detrusor

Impaired contractility may be the only manifestation of a nonneuropathic detrusor dysfunction (e.g., in the elderly[87,88]), or it may occur as an additional abnormality in an obstructed or unstable detrusor.[89,90] The ultrastructural hallmark of a poorly contractile detrusor is the *degeneration pattern* (Fig. 2-2), characterized by widespread degeneration of muscle cells and intrinsic nerves.[52,58] Degeneration of muscle cells can be recognized ultrastructurally by a spectrum of features that reflect its severity. Mild degeneration results in subtle features such as malalignment of myofilaments with patchy stacking, crisscross or swerving patterns, and uneven crowding or clumping of sarcoplasmic dense bodies. Features of moderate degeneration include disorganization or disruption of myofilaments, disruption of sarcoplasmic dense bodies and mitochondria, distention of cisternae of endoplasmic reticulum with loss of ribosomes, appearance in sarcoplasm of highly electron-dense patches or laminate bodies, and occasionally large deposits of glycogen particles. Severe degeneration is manifested by sequestration, extrusion (i.e., blebbing), vacuolation, or floccular appearance of sarcoplasm; loss or electron-dense homogenization of myofilaments; distortion of the nucleus with irregular clumping of chromatin; and thickening or breaching of sarcolemma with replication of the basal lamina. Severely degenerated cells ultimately become shriveled or disintegrated.

Degeneration in intrinsic nerves can be recognized only ultrastructurally by a constellation of features that include[52,58] depletion of synaptic vesicles, axoplasmic dense bodies, breaching of axolemma, and disruption of mitochondria in axon terminals and varicosities of neuroeffector junctions. Severe degeneration of axons results in their retraction from related muscle cells and ultimately in fragmentation or lysis. Axons ensheathed by Schwann cells may undergo vacuolar or floccular change, with disruption of their axoplasmic content of neurofilaments and neurotubules. Loss of ensheathed axons results in the distinctive appearance of collapsed Schwann cells with redundant and replicated basal laminae.

Features of the degeneration pattern can easily explain impaired contractility of the detrusor.[9,52,58] Degeneration of the intrinsic nerves impedes transmission of neural impulses along axons and neuroeffector transmission to muscle cells at their terminals. Degeneration of muscle cells disrupts their contractile elements, energetic machinery, and Ca^{2+} stores, rendering them unable to generate an efficient contraction or any contraction, whether in response to a propagated neural impulse or secondary to mechanical "pull" by a contracting adjacent muscle cell with preserved structure.

Detrusor Overactivity

Several factors have been implicated in the pathogenesis of detrusor instability (i.e., overactivity). Some of these factors are functional, whereas others revolve around a structural change in the unstable detrusor. A change in density of one functional type of intrinsic nerves or another has been reported in histochemical preparations,[91,92] but the methods used to determine nerve density in these studies are questionable.[8,59,89,93] Electron microscopic studies have revealed that the principal structural change in the unstable detrusor, whether obstructed or not, is in the interrelationship of its muscle cells.[58,60,63,89]

Reduction of vasoactive intestinal polypeptide (VIP)–reactive nerves in the detrusor with idiopathic instability (i.e., no outlet obstruction or neural deficit) has been described in one histochemical study.[91] Loss of such nerves was suggested as the cause of instability on the premise that it would deprive the detrusor of an inhibitory role of the neuropeptide as a neurotransmitter or neuromodulator.[94,95] Histochemical observations on VIPergic nerves are not sufficient to determine their structural status; only electron microscopy can determine such status, particularly the content and type of axonal synaptic vesicles.[1,9] No correlation between detrusor function and immunohistochemical reactivity of VIP was found in a study of human bladder biopsies.[96] Loss of inhibitory VIP-reactive nerves as the cause of involuntary detrusor contractions is difficult to reconcile with the clinical observation that they are susceptible to neurally mediated inhibition.[97]

In a later study, "increased appreciation of bladder filling" due to "relative abundance" of "presumptive sensory nerves" in the suburothelium was suggested as an explanation for idiopathic instability.[92] Aside from the questionable counting method used, no adjustment for thickness of suburothelium in the specimens studied was mentioned; such thickness varies in different subjects and can easily be altered even by minor pathologic changes in the bladder wall such as mild cystitis, vascular congestion, or edema.[8] Moreover, there is no basis for the postulated association between the number of nerves and the degree of sensory excitability or perception.[8]

Muscle cells of the overactive (unstable) aging detrusor, whether obstructed or not, have some distinctive ultrastructural features, collectively designated the *dysjunction pattern*.[58,60,89] This pattern is characterized by moderately widened spaces between individual muscle cells, scarce intermediate muscle cell junctions, and abundant distinctive protrusion junctions and ultraclose cell abutments (Figs. 2-3 and 2-4) that are not found in the normal detrusor. The only difference between the obstructed and unobstructed overactive detrusor is a superimposed myohypertrophy pattern (discussed later) in the former (see Fig. 2-4). The dysjunction pattern is not associated with any particular change in intrinsic nerves of the overactive detrusor, whether obstructed or not, except degenerative changes when the detrusor is also poorly contractile.

The protrusion junctions and ultraclose abutments of the dysjunction pattern resemble gap junctions in having a very narrow separation cleft ($\leq$10 nm) and no sarcolemmal thickening at the contact zone of the adjoined muscle cells. These features suggest that both types of junction serve as a vehicle for electrical muscle cell coupling in the overactive detrusor in lieu of the normal mechanism of mechanical cell coupling that is curtailed by reduction of intermediate cell junctions.[58,60] This introduces a new concept of pathogenesis of detrusor overactivity (instability), whether it is associated with outlet obstruction or not. According to this concept, involuntary detrusor contractions in either setting are elicited by a bipartite myogenic mechanism, consisting of irritable loci and a final common pathway. The irritable locus represents muscle cells with heightened inherent spontaneous activity, with or without increased responsiveness to a "trigger for contraction," such as stretch or excitatory neural stimuli. The final common pathway is served by muscle cells linked by protrusion junctions and abutments to acquire the functional properties of a syncytium in and around the irritable loci. Limited, small

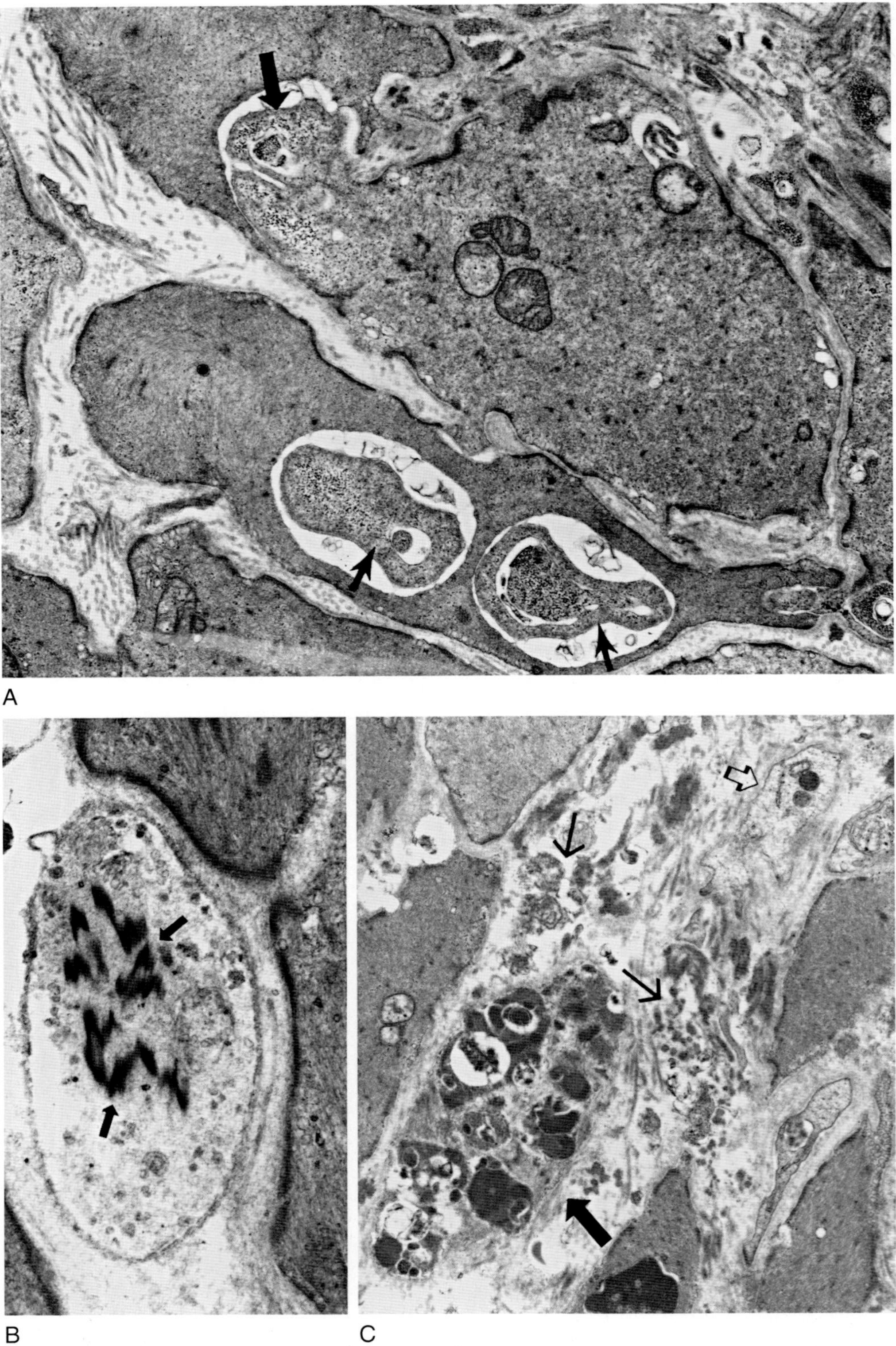

Figure 2-2 Degeneration in poor detrusor contractility. **A,** One degenerating muscle cell has sequestered sarcoplasm *(arrows)*, and another has a sarcoplasmic bleb intruding on an adjacent cell *(thick arrow)* (magnification ×16,500). **B,** In a degenerating muscle cell, the sarcoplasm has a rarefied appearance, with disrupted myofilaments and clustered, thickened, and confluent dense bodies *(arrows)* (magnification ×27,300). **C,** In a severely degenerated muscle cell *(thick arrow)*, the sarcoplasm is completely disrupted and replaced by irregular, large, highly electron-dense patches and multivesiculated bodies; abundant cell debris *(arrows)* is evident in the adjacent interstitium. Notice the profile of a degenerating axon *(open arrow)*, with depleted vesicles, disrupted mitochondria, and a highly electron-dense patch (magnification ×14,000). (From Elbadawi A: Pathology and pathophysiology of detrusor in incontinence. Urol Clin North Am 22:3, 1995.)

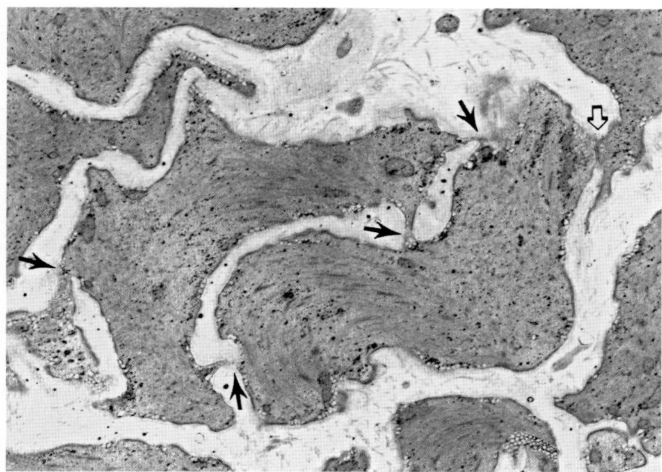

Figure 2-3 Dysjunction pattern in detrusor overactivity. Muscle cells are separated by mildly widened spaces with depleted, normal intermediate junctions, adjoined by protrusion junctions *(arrows)* with indiscernible gaps between the cells and an overall appearance of pseudosyncytium at the junctions. The profile of the residual intermediate junction *(open arrow)* is distinctly different from that of protrusion junction (magnification ×13,500). (From Elbadawi A: Pathology and pathophysiology of detrusor in incontinence. Urol Clin North Am 22:3, 1995.)

contractions originating independently in one or more loci, whether spontaneous or triggered, are propagated electrically through that syncytium to outlying muscle cells, recruiting them to contract in near-synchrony. If the electrical propagation involves a sufficiently large muscle territory, the result would be significant, urodynamically measurable contractions that, by definition, are involuntary. Electrical cell coupling remains partially suppressible by neurally mediated inhibition insofar as its completion, progression, or even initiation is concerned,[60] and it does not hinder the development of neurally triggered, unitary, effective voiding contractions. Preliminary studies indicate the presence of the dysjunction pattern in idiopathic instability in young adults and in the overactive neuropathic (i.e., hyperreflexic) detrusor.

Obstructed Detrusor

Until the previous decade, structure of the obstructed detrusor was investigated almost exclusively by routine histologic methods. The only convincing changes reported were in the interstitium,[98-106] which, not surprisingly, failed to explain why or how the obstructed bladder becomes dysfunctional. Changes in intrinsic nerves of the obstructed detrusor were described in a few histochemical studies, but no meaningful correlation was made with its abnormal functional behavior.[107-111] The validity and significance of these neural changes remain debatable.[8,59,89,93]

Ultrastructural studies revealed characteristic changes in the experimentally or clinically obstructed detrusor,[89,112-116] including the rare entity of outlet obstruction in women.[89] Collectively designated the *myohypertrophy pattern*, these changes predominate in muscle cells and interstitium and can explain practically all functional abnormalities in the obstructed detrusor.[89] Additional changes in the obstructed human detrusor have been correlated with specific superimposed, urodynamically defined

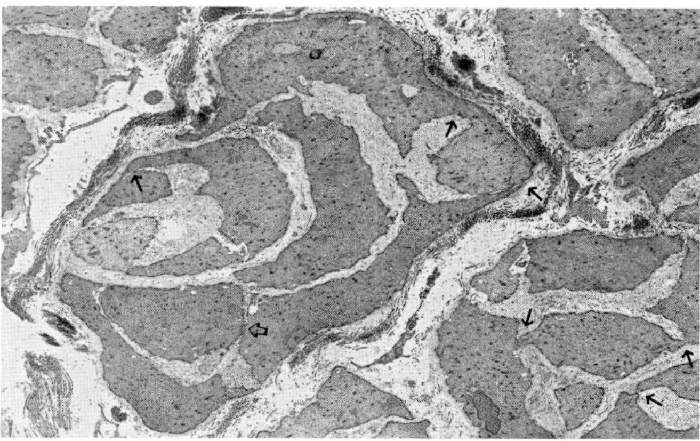

A

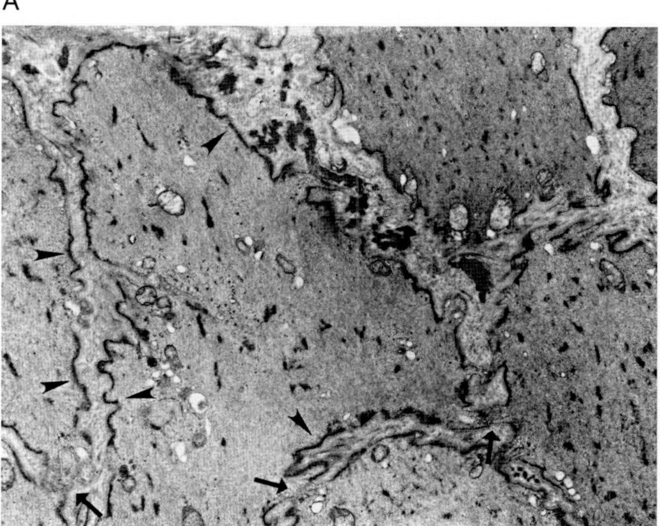

B

Figure 2-4 Myohypertrophy plus dysjunction pattern of an overactive (unstable) obstructed detrusor. **A,** The overview shows the widely variable sizes and shapes of muscle cell profiles, markedly widened intercellular spaces containing abundant collagen, depleted intermediate cell junctions, and numerous protrusion junctions *(arrows);* the open arrow marks a residual intermediate junction (magnification ×4090). **B,** Muscle cell profiles are adjoined as a pseudosyncytium by ultraclose abutments *(arrows);* sarcolemmas (i.e., cell membranes) are dominated by dense bands *(arrowheads)* with depleted caveolae in interposed thinner zones (magnification ×11,800). (**A,** Modified from Elbadawi A: Functional pathology of urinary bladder muscularis: The new frontier in diagnostic uropathology. Semin Diagn Pathol 10:348, 1993; **B,** from Elbadawi A: Pathology and pathophysiology of detrusor in incontinence. Urol Clin North Am 22:3, 1995.)

derangements of its function.[52,60,89] Contrary to some reports,[104,105] there is no correlation between the scope and degree of ultrastructural changes in the detrusor and the degree of bladder trabeculation as observed cystoscopically.[58,89]

Myohypertrophy Pattern

The myohypertrophy pattern has three features (Fig. 2-5): muscle cell hypertrophy, markedly widened spaces between individual muscle cells, and collagenosis.[58,63,89] Characteristically, the extent of cell separation and collagenosis is nonuniform, so that muscle

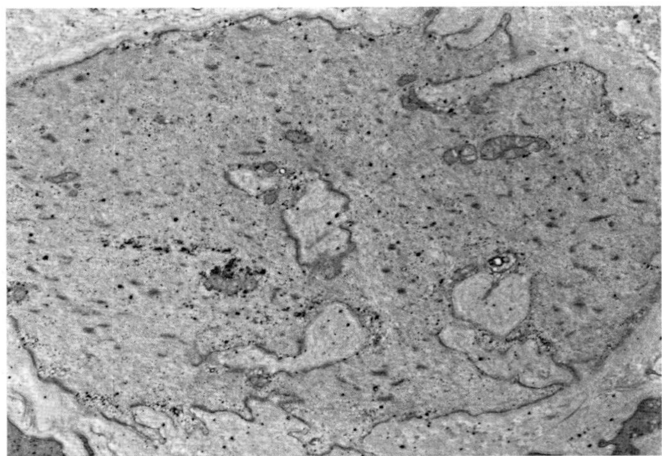

A

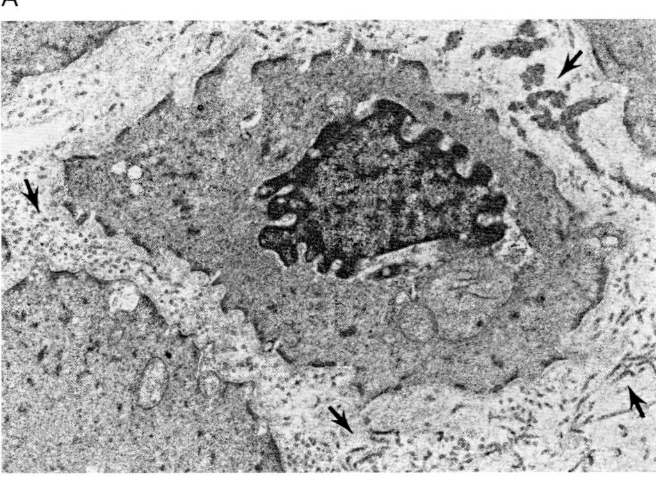

B

Figure 2-5 Myohypertrophy pattern of an obstructed detrusor. **A,** Bizarre, twisted profile of a hypertrophic muscle cell (magnification ×13,000). **B,** Markedly widened spaces between individual muscle cells containing abundant collagen fibrils and some elastic fibers *(arrows)* (magnification ×18,600).

fascicles with different degrees of loosened structure exist side by side in the same section or even microscopic field.

Muscle cell hypertrophy (i.e., increased cell size) is the traditional hallmark of obstruction in hollow viscera.[117,118] Because of its nonlayered meshwork organization,[3,6,13] the detrusor does not lend itself to traditional methods for estimating muscle cell size used in the intestine, such as diameter or length of muscle cell profiles, number of muscle cell nuclei per area, or volume density of muscle cells.[59,93,114] This fact casts doubt on the validity of data indicating the presence of hypertrophy of obstructed detrusor in several studies.[99,103,105,119-121]

A hypertrophied muscle cell cannot be recognized qualitatively on light microscopy, but it has a distinctive, easily discernible ultrastructural profile[58,63,89,113,116] characterized by branching of the tapering ends of the cell, deformed or bizarre cell configuration with irregular infoldings or contortions (see Fig. 2-5A), and occasional reflexive intermediate junctions[122] between contortions or branches of the same cell. Branches of hypertrophic muscle cells appear to interlock as a braid in tridimensional perspective.

Collagenosis designates the presence of abundant collagen fibrils and fibers in markedly widened spaces between individual muscle cells (see Figs. 2-4A and 2-5B).[58,89] These features cannot be recognized by light microscopy. Abundant collagen fibers also expand microsepta and partitions of interstitium, respectively, between muscle fascicles and bundles. This corresponds to the fibrosis mentioned as the main structural change in earlier studies on the obstructed detrusor. Intercellular collagen is generally associated with deposits of basal lamina–like material and a variable number of elastic fibers. Separation of muscle cells results in shearing of their junctions, which consequently become fewer and unevenly distributed. Muscle cell separation results in loosening of the normally compact arrangement of muscle cells in fascicles and bundles of the detrusor. When such separation is excessive, the fascicular arrangement is lost, and the cells lie individually, wide apart, amid a dominant background of collagen.

Structural-Functional Correlations

Traditionally, it has been thought that the obstructed detrusor undergoes compensatory muscular hypertrophy and becomes stronger to overcome the obstruction.[123] This dogma is fallacious. The obstructed detrusor is not stronger; it may actually become weaker, and it has a slower velocity (speed) of contraction than the norm, even in the presence of adequate bladder emptying and absence of retained urine.[63,124-127] Theoretically, a hypertrophic smooth muscle cell can generate a stronger contraction than a normal cell. This, however, does not necessarily mean a stronger contraction of the detrusor as a whole. Several ultrastructural features of the myohypertrophy pattern limit the ability of hypertrophic muscle cells to shorten (i.e., contract). Loss of intermediate cell junctions between widely separated muscle cells greatly restricts the main vehicle for mechanical cell coupling, so that the force of contraction of muscle cells would not be transmitted effectively to outlying cells. Such hindrance of force transmittal is accentuated by excessive collagen in the widened intercellular spaces and the expanded interstitium. The net effect of these impediments is an inability of the obstructed detrusor to mount the speedy, strong, coordinated, or sustained contraction necessary for complete emptying of the full bladder.

Superimposed Structural Changes

Muscle cell degeneration has been described as a constant feature of experimental acute, transient overdistention of the rabbit detrusor,[113,114] the human detrusor after repeated episodes of acute retention with bladder overdistention,[128] and the chronically obstructed human detrusor of both genders when its contractility is overtly impaired with considerable residual urine.[89] Degeneration of intrinsic nerves has also been observed ultrastructurally in the rabbit model and in the chronically obstructed, poorly contractile human detrusor. Widespread degenerative changes superimposed on myohypertrophy and collagenosis further weaken an obstructed detrusor.[89] Reduction in density of intrinsic nerves has been reported in some light microscopic histochemical studies on the obstructed human detrusor[107,109,111] and in a pig model intended to reproduce long-term bladder outlet obstruction.[108] Based primarily on such reduction and on in vitro detrusor responses in the pig model, it was proposed that "cholinergic denervation" with subsequent supersensitivity was the cause of obstruction-associated instability.[129] However, the methods used to assess nerve density in the histochemical studies were questionable.[8,59,93] The conclusion in most of these studies

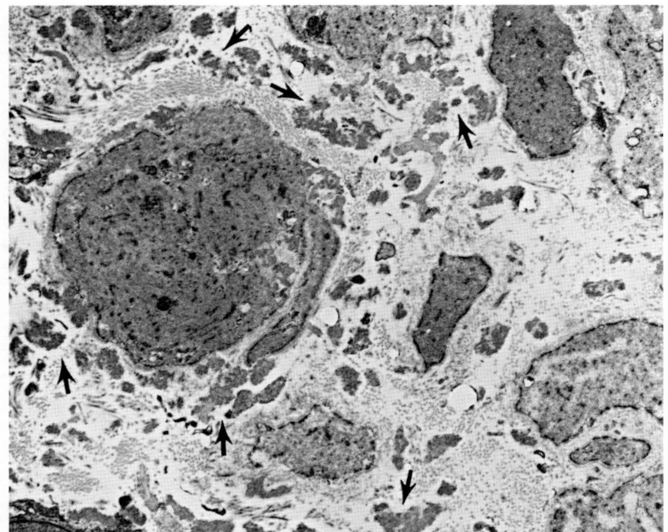

Figure 2-6 Hyperelastosis in an overdistended obstructed detrusor. Muscle cell profiles are far apart (up to 6 μm) in the interstitium with abundant collagen and elastic fibers *(arrows)* (magnification ×10,550). (Modified from Elbadawi A: Functional pathology of urinary bladder muscularis: The new frontier in diagnostic uropathology. Semin Diagn Pathol 10:349, 1993.)

that the observed changes were the result of nerve loss (i.e., denervation) was not substantiated by direct evidence of structural nerve damage or degeneration in any. More reservations about the denervation concept of instability were raised in an ultrastructural study of the obstructed human detrusor,[89] which attributed instability in such detrusors to the presence of the same protrusion junctions and abutments (see Fig. 2-5) that are the cardinal feature of the overactive unobstructed bladder (discussed earlier).

A variable number of elastic fibers accompanies deposits of collagen in intercellular spaces (see Figs. 2-4A and 2-5B) and interstitium of the obstructed detrusor.[89,112] Massive deposits of elastic fibers (i.e., *hyperelastosis*) have been observed in the excessively distended detrusor of patients with chronic urinary retention caused by bladder outlet obstruction (Fig. 2-6).[58,89] Such detrusors also have excessive collagenosis, marked expansion of interstitium, and severe muscle cell degeneration, with scattered residual hypertrophic muscle cells. These changes markedly obscure or eliminate orderly organization of detrusor muscular elements as fascicles.[58,89]

Regeneration of muscle cells and intrinsic axons in the detrusor accompanies degeneration of the corresponding elements after obstruction in the experimental rabbit model of acute transient overdistention and is the most prominent change after relief of that obstruction.[113,114] No regenerative changes were observed in the chronically obstructed human detrusor of either gender, even when degeneration of its muscle cells and axons was evident and widespread in association with overt impaired contractility.[58,63,89] Muscle cell regeneration therefore is not a part of the process leading to myohypertrophy in the obstructed detrusor and probably is not a manifestation of hyperplasia in the rabbit model. In this model, muscle cell regeneration and hypertrophy are probably manifestations of structural adaptation, eventually leading to recovery, that follows the initial damage induced by acute distention of the bladder.[130] Similarly, regeneration of axonal elements in the same model probably represents their eventual structural recovery, as observed earlier in the experimentally decentralized bladder.[75]

The Aging Detrusor

Knowledge about the microstructure of the aging detrusor is crucial for our understanding of the pathology and pathophysiology of voiding dysfunctions and incontinence in the elderly. It has been shown biochemically that collagen content of the detrusor increases with advancing age in women,[131] resulting in reduction of its contractility.[11,68,126] One report stated that neither the amount of smooth muscle nor the size of its individual cells is altered by age, but the density of cholinergic innervation is markedly reduced by age.[132] The validity of these observations has been questioned in an ultrastructural study of truly aging detrusors.[52,56,58] This study defined the microstructural norm of the aging detrusor, which was obtained from asymptomatic subjects who had no urodynamic evidence of obstruction, detrusor hyperactivity, impaired detrusor contractility, or altered bladder compliance.[52,53] In such a detrusor, muscle cells and axons remain virtually intact except for a few subtle ultrastructural changes. These include moderate widening of spaces between individual muscle cells, modest intercellular deposits of basal lamina, considerable depletion of sarcolemmal caveolae with marked elongation of sarcolemmal dense bands, and normal (often elongated) intermediate cell junctions. These changes may be manifestations of a process of dedifferentiation of detrusor muscle cells associated with aging.[52]

CONCLUSIONS

Morphologic evaluation of detrusor microstructure can be truly objective and functionally meaningful only if it includes an analysis of its muscular, interstitial, and neural (MIN) microstructural compartments. Most structural parameters that have direct impact on detrusor function can be defined only by electron microscopy. Studies done so far indicate that the data necessary for correlation of detrusor structure and function can be obtained readily and reproducibly from an endoscopic biopsy, which appears to be truly representative of the whole detrusor insofar as the fine structure of its smooth muscle elements is concerned. The parameters sought are basic and have been defined clearly so that they can be studied and evaluated by any pathologist with a knowledge of diagnostic electron microscopy and smooth muscle ultrastructure.[58]

Different forms of human detrusor dysfunction are associated with changes in one or more of the three MIN compartments but at the same time differ in one or more. This fact emphasizes the great potential of study of detrusor microstructure as the means of better understanding the pathophysiology of various voiding dysfunctions and of developing a valuable tool in the clinical diagnosis and management of such disorders. To gain the full benefit of such study, its goal should be to determine for each dysfunction the presence, spectrum, degree, and extent of distribution of the changes seen in each microstructural compartment. Only through pursuit of this approach can the natural history and the outcome of treatment of various voiding dysfunctions be explained, understood, and perhaps predicted with reasonable accuracy. To this end, the material needed for microstructural study should ideally be obtained at the time of patient presentation, during follow-up of patients managed conservatively, and at various intervals after surgical intervention or other specific therapy aimed at manipulation of bladder behavior. From such information, we can begin to understand the basis for differences in clinical presentation between patients with the same disorder and between different disorders; recognize patterns of the natural course and evolution of different presentations of the same disorder and of different disorders; define structural markers of reversibility or permanence of each disorder; and identify the structural correlates of successful or ineffective treatment in patients with the same disorder and patient groups with different disorders. As information on the various dysfunctional disorders is gathered and correlated, we can begin to identify trends in the natural evolution and prognosis of each dysfunction and to methodically set appropriate indications, contraindications, and predictive indices for available treatment modalities. Eventually, the stage will be set for the use of detrusor structural morphology as a routine modality in the clinical management of vesical dysfunction.

References

1. Elbadawi A: Neuromorphologic basis of vesicourethral function. I. Histochemistry, ultrastructure and function of intrinsic nerves of the bladder and urethra. Neurourol Urodyn 1:3-50, 1982.
2. Elbadawi A: Autonomic innervation of the vesical outlet and its role in micturition. In Hinman F Jr (ed): Benign Prostatic Hypertrophy. New York, Springer-Verlag, 1983, pp 330-348.
3. Elbadawi A: Neuromorphology. Comparative neuromorphology in animals. In Torrens M, Morrison JFB (eds): The Physiology of the Lower Urinary Tract. London, Springer-Verlag, 1987, pp 23-52.
4. Elbadawi A: Le support anatomique de la physiologie des voies urinaires. In Buzelin JM, Richard F, Susset JG (eds): Physiologie et Pathologie de la Dynamique des Voies Urinaires (Haut et Bas Appareil). Paris, FIIS, 1987, pp 43-66.
5. Elbadawi A: Neuromuscular mechanisms of micturition. In Yalla SV, McGuire EJ, Elbadawi A, Blaivas JG (eds): Neurourology and Urodynamics. Principles and Practice. New York, Macmillan, 1988, pp 3-36.
6. Elbadawi A: Anatomy of the neuromuscular apparatus of micturition. In Krane RJ, Siroky MB (eds): Clinical Neurology, 2nd ed. Boston, Little, Brown, 1991, pp 5-24.
7. Van Arsdalen K, Wein AJ: Physiology of micturition and continence. In Krane RJ, Siroky MB (eds): Clinical Neurourology, 2nd ed. Boston, Little, Brown, 1991, pp 25-82.
8. Elbadawi A: Neurophysiology of storage and voiding function. Curr Opin Urol 3:255-261, 1993.
9. Elbadawi A: Structural basis of detrusor contractility. The "MIN" approach to its understanding and study. Neurourol Urodyn 10:77-86, 1989.
10. Coolsaet BLRA: Bladder compliance and detrusor activity during the collection phase. Neurourol Urodyn 4:263-273, 1985.
11. Susset JG, Regnier CH: Viscoelastic properties of the bladder and urethra. In Yalla SV, McGuire EJ, Elbadawi A, Blaivas JG (eds): Neurourology and Urodynamics. Principles and Practice. New York, Macmillan, 1988, pp 106-121.
12. Lose LG: Simultaneous recording of pressure and cross-sectional area in the female urethra: A study of urethral closure function in healthy and stress incontinent women. Neurourol Urodyn 11:55-89, 1992.
13. Hunter deWT: A new concept of the urinary bladder musculature. J Urol 71:695-704, 1954.
14. Uhlenhuth E, Hunter deWT, Loechel WF: Problems in the Anatomy of the Pelvis. Philadelphia, Lippincott, 1953, pp 1-157.
15. Langworthy OR, Kolb LC, Lewis LG: Physiology of Micturition. Baltimore, Williams & Wilkins, 1940.
16. Tanagho EA, Meyers FH: The "internal sphincter." Is it under sympathetic control? Invest Urol 7:79-89, 1969.
17. Gil Vernet S: Morphology and Function of Vesico-Prostato-Urethral Musculature. Treviso, Libreria Editrice Canova, 1968, pp 11-328.
18. Hutch JA: Anatomy and Physiology of the Bladder, Trigone and Urethra. New York, Appleton-Century-Crofts, 1972, pp 71-122.
19. Waldeyer W: Über die sogennante Ureterscheide. Verh Anat Ges 6:259-260, 1892.
20. Elbadawi A: Anatomy and function of the ureteral sheath. J Urol 107:224-229, 1972.
21. Elbadawi A, Amaku EO, Frank IN: Trilaminar musculature of the submucosal ureter. Anatomy and functional implications. Urology 2:409-417, 1973.
22. Elbadawi A, Schenk EA: A new theory of the innervation of bladder musculature. Part IV. Innervation of the vesicourethral junction and external urethral sphincter. J Urol 111:613-615, 1974.
23. Morrison JFB: Neural connections between the lower urinary tract and the spinal cord. In Torrens M, Morrison JFB (eds): The Physiology of the Lower Urinary Tract. London, Springer-Verlag, 1987, pp 53-88.
24. Onufrowicz B: On the arrangement and function of the cell groups in the sacral region of the spinal cord. Arch Neurol Psychopathol 3:387-411, 1900.
24. Shrøder HD: Anatomical and pathoanatomical studies on the spinal efferent systems innervating pelvic structures. J Auton Nerv Syst 14:23-48, 1985.
26. Ueyama T, Mizuno N, Nomura S, et al: Central distribution of afferent and efferent components of the pudendal nerve in the cat. J Comp Neurol 222:38-46, 1984.
27. Kuru M: Nervous control of micturition. Physiol Rev 45:425-494, 1965.
28. Bors E, Comarr AE: Neurological Urology. New York, Karger, 1971, pp 61-128.
29. Morrison JFB: Reflex control of the lower urinary tract. In Torrens M, Morrison JFB (eds): The Physiology of the Lower Urinary Tract. London, Springer-Verlag, 1987, pp 193-235.
30. Morrison JFB: Bladder control: Role of higher levels of the central nervous system. In Torrens M, Morrison JFB (eds): The Physiology of the Lower Urinary Tract. London, Springer-Verlag, 1987, pp 237-274.
31. Kuntz A: The Autonomic Nervous System. Philadelphia, Lea & Febiger, 1945, pp 284-303.
32. Mitchell GAG: Anatomy of the Autonomic Nervous System. Edinburgh, E & S Livingstone, 1853, pp 297-310.
33. Elbadawi A, Schenk EA: Dual innervation of the mammalian urinary bladder. A histochemical study of the distribution of cholinergic and adrenergic nerves. Am J Anat 119:405-428, 1966.
34. Elbadawi A, Schenk EA: A new theory of the innervation of urinary bladder musculature. I. Morphology of the intrinsic vesical innervation apparatus. J Urol 99:585-587, 1968.
35. Elbadawi A, Schenk EA: Intra- and extraganglionic peripheral cholinergic neurons in urogenital organs of the cat. Z Zellforsch Mikrosk Anat 103:26-33, 1970.
36. Elbadawi A, Schenk EA: A new theory of the innervation of urinary bladder musculature. II. The innervation apparatus of the ureterovesical junction. J Urol 105:368-371, 1971.
37. Elbadawi A, Schenk EA: A new theory of the innervation of urinary bladder musculature. III. Postganglionic synapses in ureterovesicourethral autonomic pathways. J Urol 105:372-374, 1971.

38. deGroat WC, Saum WR: Sympathetic inhibition of the urinary bladder and of pelvic ganglionic transmission in the cat. J Physiol 220:297-314, 1972.
39. Elbadawi A, Schenk EA: Parasympathetic and sympathetic postganglionic synapses in ureterovesical autonomic pathways. Z Zellforsch Mikrosk Anat 146:147-156, 1973.
40. Elbadawi A: Ultrastructure of vesicourethral innervation. II. Postganglionic axoaxonal synapses in intrinsic innervation of the vesicourethral lissosphincter: A new structural and functional concept in micturition. J Urol 131:781-790, 1984.
41. Elbadawi A: Ultrastructure of vesicourethral innervation. III. Axoaxonal synapses between postganglionic cholinergic axons and probably SIF-cell derived processes in the feline lissosphincter. J Urol 133:524-528, 1985.
42. Mattiasson A, Andersson KE, Elbadawi A, et al: Interaction between adrenergic and cholinergic nerve terminals in the urinary bladder of rabbit, cat and man. J Urol 137:1017-1019, 1987.
43. Watanabe H, Yamamoto T: Autonomic innervation of the muscles in the wall of the bladder and proximal urethra of male rats. J Anat 128:873-886, 1979.
44. Elbadawi A, Atta MA: Ultrastructure of vesicourethral innervation. IV. Evidence for somatomotor plus autonomic innervation of the male feline rhabdosphincter. Neurourol Urodyn 4:23-26, 1985.
45. Kumagai A, Koyanagi T, Takahashi Y: The innervation of the external urethral sphincter. An ultrastructural study in male human subjects. Eur Res 15:39-43, 1987.
46. Morrison JFB: The functions of efferent nerves to the lower urinary tract. In Torrens M, Morrison JFB (eds): The Physiology of the Lower Urinary Tract. London, Springer-Verlag, 1987, pp 133-159.
47. deGroat WC, Kawatani M, Hisamitsu T, et al: Neural control of micturition: The role of neuropeptides. J Auton Nerv Syst (Suppl):369-387, 1986.
48. Uemura E, Fletcher TF, Dirks VA, et al: Distribution of sacral afferent axons in cat urinary bladder. Am J Anat 136:305-314, 1973.
49. Uemura E, Fletcher TF, Bradley WE: Distribution of lumbar and sacral afferent axons in submucosa of cat urinary bladder. Anat Rec 183:579-588, 1975.
50. Dixon JS, Gilpin CJ: Presumptive sensory axons of the human urinary bladder: A fine structural study. J Anat 151:199-207, 1987.
51. Elbadawi A: Ultrastructure of vesicourethral innervation. I. Neuroeffector and cell junctions in the male internal sphincter. J Urol 128:180-188, 1982.
52. Elbadawi A, Yalla SV, Resnick NM: Structural basis of geriatric voiding dysfunction. II. Aging detrusor: Normal vs impaired contractility. J Urol 150:1657-1667, 1993.
53. Daniel EE, Cowan W, Daniel VP: Structural bases for neural and myogenic control of human detrusor muscle. Can J Physiol Pharmacol 61:1247-1272, 1983.
54. Gabella G: Structure of smooth muscles. In Bülbring E, Brading AF, Jones AW, Tomita T (eds): Smooth Muscle: An Assessment of Current Knowledge. Austin, University of Texas Press, 1981, pp 1-46.
55. Gabella G: General aspects of the fine structure of smooth muscles. In Motta PM (ed): Ultrastructure of Smooth Muscle. Boston, Kluwer Academic Publishers, 1990, pp 1-22.
56. Elbadawi A, Yalla SV, Resnick NM: Structural basis of geriatric voiding dysfunction. I. Methods of a prospective ultrastructural/urodynamic study, and an overview of the findings. J Urol 150:1650-1656, 1993.
57. Henderson RM: Cell-to-cell contacts. In Daniel EE, Paton DM (eds): Methods in Pharmacology, vol 3. New York, Plenum Press, 1975, pp 47-77.
58. Elbadawi A: Functional pathology of urinary bladder muscularis: The new frontier in diagnostic uropathology. Semin Diagn Pathol 10:314-354, 1993.
59. Elbadawi A, Meyer S: Morphometry of the obstructed detrusor: I. Review of the issues. Neurourol Urodyn 8:163-171, 1989.
60. Elbadawi A, Yalla SV, Resnick NM: Structural basis of geriatric voiding dysfunction. III. Detrusor overactivity. J Urol 150:1668-1680, 1993.
61. Brading AF: Physiology of bladder smooth muscle. In Torrens M, Morrison JFB (eds): The Physiology of the Lower Urinary Tract. London, Springer-Verlag, 1987, pp 161-191.
62. Dixon JS, Gosling JA: Ultrastructure of smooth muscle cells in the urinary system. In Motta PM (ed): Ultrastructure of Smooth Muscle. Boston, Kluwer Academic Publishers, 1990, pp 153-169.
63. Elbadawi A: Pathology and pathophysiology of the obstructed detrusor. In Jardin A (ed): Prostate and α-Blockers. Chester, Adis International, 1990, pp 1-25.
64. Inoué T: The three-dimensional ultrastructure of intracellular organization of smooth muscle cells by scanning electron microscopy. In Motta PM (ed): Ultrastructure of Smooth Muscle. Boston, Kluwer Academic Publishers, 1990, pp 63-77.
65. Grover AK: Calcium-handling studies using isolated smooth muscle membranes. In Grover AK, Daniel EE (eds): Calcium and Contractility: Smooth Muscle. Clifton, Humana Press, 1985, pp 245-269.
66. Kondo A, Susset JG, Lefaivre J: Viscoelastic properties of bladder. I. Mechanical model and its mathematical analysis. Invest Urol 10:154-163, 1972.
67. Regnier CH, Kolsky H, Richardson PD, et al: The elastic behavior of the urinary bladder for large deformations. J Biomech 16:915-922, 1983.
68. Susset JG, Regnier CH: Physiologie vésico-sphinctérienne. La phase de remplissage: Properties visco-elastiques de la vessie et de l'urèthre. In Buzelin JM, Richard F, Susset JG (eds): Physiologie et Pathologie de la Dynamique des Voies Urinaires (Haut et Bas Appareil). Paris, FIIS, 1987, pp 66-83.
69. Tomita T: Electrical properties of mammalian smooth muscle. In Bülbring E, Brading AF, Jones AW, Tomita T (eds): Smooth Muscle. Baltimore, Williams & Wilkins, 1970, pp 197-243.
70. Gosling JA, Dixon JS, Critchley HOD, Thompson S-A: A comparative study of the human external sphincter and periurethral levator ani muscles. Br J Urol 53:35-41, 1981.
71. Elbadawi A, Atta MA: Intrinsic neuromuscular defects in the neurogenic bladder. IV. Loss of somatomotor and preservation of autonomic innervation of the male feline rhabdo-sphincter following bilateral sacral ventral rhizotomy. Neurourol Urodyn 4:219-229, 1985.
72. Elbadawi A, Atta MA: Intrinsic neuromuscular defects in the neurogenic bladder. V. Autonomic re-innervation of the male feline rhabdosphincter following somatic denervation by bilateral sacral ventral rhizotomy. Neurourol Urodyn 5:65-85, 1986.
73. Atta MA, Elbadawi A: Intrinsic neuromuscular defects in the neurogenic bladder. VII. Neurohistochemistry of the somatically denervated male feline rhabdosphincter. Neurourol Urodyn 6:47-56, 1987.
74. Elbadawi A, Atta MA, Franck JI: Intrinsic neuromuscular defects in the neurogenic bladder. I. Short-term ultrastructural changes in muscular innervation of the decentralized feline bladder base following unilateral sacral ventral rhizotomy. Neurourol Urodyn 3:93-113, 1984.
75. Atta MA, Franck JI, Elbadawi A: Intrinsic neuromuscular defects in the neurogenic bladder. II. Long-term innervation of the unilaterally decentralized feline bladder base by regenerated cholinergic, increased adrenergic, and emergent probable "peptidergic" nerves. Neurourol Urodyn 3:185-200, 1984.
76. Elbadawi A, Atta MA: Intrinsic neuromuscular defects in the neurogenic bladder. III. Transjunctional, short- and long-term ultrastructural changes in muscle cells of the decentralized bladder base following unilateral sacral ventral rhizotomy. Neurourol Urodyn 3:245-270, 1984.

77. Elbadawi A, Atta MA, Hanno AG-E: Intrinsic neuromuscular defects in the neurogenic bladder. VIII. Effects of unilateral pelvic and pelvic plexus neurectomy on ultrastructure of the feline bladder base. Neurourol Urodyn 7:77-92, 1988.
78. Hanno AGE, Atta MA, Elbadawi A: Intrinsic neuromuscular defects in the neurogenic bladder. IX. Effects of combined parasympathetic decentralization and hypogastric neurectomy on neuromuscular ultrastructure of the feline bladder base. Neurourol Urodyn 7:93-111, 1988.
79. Elbadawi A, Atta MA: Intrinsic neuromuscular defects in the neurogenic bladder. X. Value and limitations of neurohistochemistry. Neurourol Urodyn 8:263-276, 1989.
80. Elbadawi A, Atta MA: Intrinsic neuromuscular defects in the neurogenic bladder. VI. Myofiber ultrastructure in the somatically denervated male feline rhabdosphincter. Neurourol Urodyn 5:453-473, 1986.
81. Cowan WM: Antegrade and retrograde transneuronal degeneration in the central and peripheral nervous system. In Nauta WJH, Ebbesson SOE (eds): Contemporary Research Methods in Neuroanatomy. New York, Springer-Verlag, 1978, pp 217-251.
82. Sundin T, Dahlström A: The sympathetic innervation of the urinary bladder and urethra in the normal state and after parasympathetic denervation at the spinal root level. An experimental study in cats. Scand J Urol Nephrol 7:131-149, 1973.
83. Kawatani M, deGroat WC: The effect of partial denervation on the efferent pathways to the urinary bladder. Proceedings of the Sixth Annual Symposium of the Urodynamics Society. 1984, p 35.
84. McGuire EJ, Yalla SV, Elbadawi A: Abnormalities of vesicourethral dysfunction following radical pelvic extirpative surgery. In Yalla SV, McGuire EJ, Elbadawi A, Blaivas JG (eds): Neurourology and Urodynamics. Principles and Practice. New York, Macmillan, 1988, pp 331-337.
85. Neal DE, Bogue PR, Williams RE: Histological appearances of the nerves of the bladder in patients with denervation of the bladder after excision of the rectum. Br J Urol 54:658-666, 1982.
86. Elbadawi A, Miller LF, Liu JS, et al: Structural detrusor damage in a spinal dog neurostimulation model. Neurourol Urodyn 9:199-200, 1990.
87. Resnick NM: Voiding dysfunction in the elderly. In Yalla SV, McGuire EJ, Elbadawi A, Blaivas JG (eds): Neurourology and Urodynamics: Principles and Practice. New York, Macmillan, 1988, pp 303-330.
88. Resnick NM, Yalla SV, Laurino E: The pathophysiology of urinary incontinence among institutionalized elderly persons. N Engl J Med 320:1-7, 1989.
89. Elbadawi A, Yalla SV, Resnick NM: Structural basis of geriatric voiding dysfunction. IV. Bladder outlet obstruction. J Urol 150:1681-1695, 1993.
90. Resnick NM, Yalla, SV: Detrusor hyperactivity with impaired contractile function. An unrecognized but common cause of incontinence in elderly patients. JAMA 257:3076-3081, 1987.
91. Gu J, Restorick JM, Blank MA, et al: Vasoactive intestinal polypeptide in the normal and unstable bladder. Br J Urol 55:645-647, 1983.
92. Moore KH, Gilpin SA, Dixon JS, et al: Increase in presumptive sensory nerves of the urinary bladder in idiopathic detrusor instability. Br J Urol 70:370-372, 1992.
93. Meyer S, Elbadawi A: Morphometry of the obstructed detrusor. II. Principles of a comprehensive protocol. Neurourol Urodyn 8:173-191, 1989.
94. Kinder RB, Mundy AR: Pathophysiology of idiopathic detrusor instability and detrusor hyper-reflexia. An in vitro study of human detrusor muscle. Br J Urol 60:509-515, 1987.
95. Mundy AR: Detrusor instability. Br J Urol 62:393-397, 1988.
96. Van Poppel H, Stessens R, Baert L, et al: Vasoactive intestinal peptide innervation of human urinary bladder in normal and pathologic conditions. Urol Int 43:205-210, 1988.
97. McGuire EJ: Evaluation of urinary incontinence. In Yalla SV, McGuire EJ, Elbadawi A, Blaivas JG (eds): Neurourology and Urodynamics. Principles and Practice. New York, Macmillan, 1988, pp 211-220.
98. Magasi P, Csontai A, Ruszinkó B: Beiträge zur Blasenwandregeneration. Z Urol Nephrol 62:209-216, 1969.
99. Brent L, Stephens FD: The response of smooth muscle cells in the rabbit urinary bladder to outflow obstruction. Invest Urol 12:494-502, 1975.
100. Ghoniem GM, Regnier CH, Biancani P, et al: The effect of vesical outlet obstruction on detrusor contractility and passive properties in rabbits. J Urol 135:1284-1289, 1986.
101. Clermont A: Etude Ultrastructurale du Muscle Vésical chez l'Homme [thèse, docteur de médecin]. Nice, France, 1978, pp 1-88.
102. Cortivo R, Pagano F, Passerini G, et al: Elastin and collagen in the normal and obstructed bladder. Br J Urol 53:134-137, 1981.
103. Gilpin SA, Gosling JA, Barnard RJ: Morphological and morphometric studies of the human obstructed, trabeculated urinary bladder. Br J Urol 57:525-529, 1985.
104. Gosling JA, Dixon JS: Structure of the trabeculated detrusor smooth muscle in cases of prostatic hypertrophy. Urol Int 35:351-354, 1980.
105. Gosling JA, Dixon JS: Detrusor morphology in relation to bladder outflow obstruction and instability. In Hinman F Jr (ed): Benign prostatic hypertrophy. New York, Springer-Verlag, 1983, pp 666-671.
106. Mayo ME, Lloyd-Davies RW, Shuttleworth KED, Tighe JR: The damaged human detrusor: Functional and electron microscopic changes in disease. Br J Urol 45:116-125, 1973.
107. Gosling JA, Gilpin SA, Dixon JS, Gilpin CJ: Decrease in autonomic innervation of the human detrusor muscle in outflow obstruction. J Urol 136:501-505, 1986.
108. Dixon JS, Gilpin CJ, Gilpin SA, et al: Sequential morphological changes in the pig detrusor in response to chronic partial urethral obstruction. Br J Urol 64:385-390, 1989.
109. Cumming JA, Chisholm GD: Changes in detrusor innervation with relief of outflow tract obstruction. Br J Urol 69:7-11, 1992.
110. Chapple CR, Milner P, Moss HE, Burnstock G: Loss of sensory neuropeptides in the obstructed human bladder. Br J Urol 70:373-381, 1992.
111. Williams JH, Turner WH, Sainsbury GM, Brading AF: Experimental model of bladder outflow tract obstruction in the guinea-pig. Br J Urol 71:543-554, 1993.
112. Mayo ME, Hinman F: Structure and function of the rabbit bladder altered by chronic obstruction or cystitis. Invest Urol 14:6-9, 1976.
113. Elbadawi A, Meyer S, Malkowicz SB, et al: Effects of short-term partial outlet obstruction on the rabbit detrusor: An ultrastructural study. Neurourol Urodyn 8:89-116, 1989.
114. Meyer S, Atta MA, Wein AJ, et al: Morphometric analysis of muscle cell changes in the short-term partially obstructed rabbit detrusor. Neurourol Urodyn 8:117-131, 1989.
115. Meyer S, Levin RM, Ruggieri MR, et al: Quantitative analysis of intercellular changes in the short-term partially obstructed rabbit detrusor. Neurourol Urodyn 8:133-140, 1989.
116. Meyer S, Hassouna M, Mokhless I, et al: Ultrastructural changes in the obstructed pig detrusor: A preliminary report. Neurourol Urodyn 8:141-150, 1989.
117. Gabella G: Hypertrophy of intestinal smooth muscle. Cell Tissue Res 163:199-214, 1975.
118. Gabella G: Hypertrophic smooth muscle. I. Size and shape of cells, occurrence of mitoses. Cell Tissue Res 201:63-78, 1979.
119. Jaske G, Hoffstäder F: Changes in the bladder wall muscle associated with benign prostatic enlargement. Urol Res 5:149-152, 1977.

120. Hoekstra JW, Griffiths DJ, Tauecchio EA, Shroeder TKF: Effects of long-term catheter implantation on the contractile and histological properties of the canine bladder. J Urol 133:709-712, 1985.
121. Uvelius B, Persson L, Mattiasson A: Smooth muscle cell hypertrophy and hyperplasia in the rat detrusor after short-term infravesical outflow obstruction. J Urol 131:173-176, 1984.
122. Gabella G: Hypertrophic smooth muscle. III. Increase in number and size of gap junctions. Cell Tissue Res 201:263-276, 1979.
123. Leriche A: Mécanisme des symptômes fonctionnels de l'hypertrophie bénigne de la prostate. Physiopathologie et symptômes. In Prostate et Alpha-bloquants. Amsterdam, Excerpta Medica, 1989, pp 76-98.
124. Coolsaet B, Elbadawi A: Urodynamics in the management of benign prostatic hypertrophy. World J Urol 6:215-224, 1989.
125. McGuire EJ: Detrusor responses to obstruction. In Rodgers C, Coffey DS, Cuhna G, et al (eds): Benign Prostatic Hypertrophy, II. Bethesda, NIH Publication no. 287-288, 1987, pp 211-220.
126. Susset JG: Effects of aging and prostatic obstruction on detrusor morphology and function. In Hinman F Jr (ed): Benign Prostatic Hypertrophy. New York, Springer-Verlag, 1983, pp 653-665.
127. Susset JG: Effet de l'hypertrophie prostatique bénigne sur la contractilité vésicale. In Prostate et Alpha-bloquants. Amsterdam, Excerpta Medica, 1989, pp 49-72.
128. Lloyd-Davies RW, Hinman F Jr: Structural and functional changes leading to impaired bacterial elimination after overdistension of the rabbit bladder. Invest Urol 9:136-142, 1971.
129. Speakman MJ, Brading AF, Gilpin CJ, et al: Bladder outflow obstruction—a cause of denervation supersensitivity. J Urol 138:1461-1466, 1987.
130. Elbadawi A, Meyer S, Regnier CH: The role of ischemia in structural changes in the rabbit detrusor following partial bladder outlet obstruction. A working hypothesis and a biomechanical/structural model proposal. Neurourol Urodyn 8:151-162, 1989.
131. Susset JG, Servot-Viguier D, Lamy F, et al: Collagen in 155 human bladders. Invest Urol 16:204-206, 1978.
132. Gilpin SA, Gilpin CJ, Dixon JS, et al: The effect of age on the autonomic innervation of the urinary bladder. Br J Urol 58:378-381, 1986.

Chapter 3

NEUROANATOMY AND NEUROPHYSIOLOGY: INNERVATION OF THE LOWER URINARY TRACT

William C. de Groat

The storage and periodic elimination of urine depend on the coordinated activity of two functional units in the lower urinary tract: a reservoir, which is the urinary bladder, and an outlet consisting of the bladder neck, the urethra, and the urethral sphincter. Coordination between these organs is mediated by a complex neural control system located in the brain, spinal cord, and peripheral ganglia. Urine storage and release depend on central nervous system pathways. This distinguishes the lower urinary tract from many other visceral structures (e.g., the gastrointestinal tract, cardiovascular system) that maintain a certain level of function even after extrinsic neural input has been eliminated.

The lower urinary tract is unusual in its pattern of activity and organization of neural control mechanisms. For example, the urinary bladder has only two modes of operation: storage and elimination. Many of the neural circuits have switchlike or phasic patterns of activity, unlike the tonic patterns characteristic of the autonomic pathways to cardiovascular organs. Micturition is under voluntary control and depends on learned behavior that develops during maturation of the nervous system, whereas many other visceral functions are regulated involuntarily. Micturition also requires the integration of autonomic and somatic efferent mechanisms to coordinate the activity of visceral organs (i.e., bladder and urethra) with that of urethral striated muscles.

Because of the complexity of the neural mechanisms regulating the lower urinary tract, micturition is sensitive to a wide variety of injuries, diseases, and chemicals that affect the nervous system. Neurologic mechanisms are an important consideration in the diagnosis and treatment of voiding disorders. This chapter reviews the innervation of the urinary bladder and urethra, the organization of the reflex pathways controlling urine storage and elimination, the neurotransmitters involved in micturition reflex pathways, and neurogenic dysfunctions of the lower urinary tract.

INNERVATION

The innervation of the lower urinary tract is derived from three sets of peripheral nerves: sacral parasympathetic (i.e., pelvic nerves), thoracolumbar sympathetic (i.e., hypogastric nerves and sympathetic chain), and sacral somatic nerves (i.e., primarily pudendal nerves) (Fig. 3-1).[1-5]

Sacral Parasympathetic Pathways

The sacral parasympathetic nerves, which in humans originate from the S2 to S4 segments of the spinal cord, provide most excitatory input to the bladder. Cholinergic preganglionic neurons located in the intermediolateral region of the sacral spinal cord send axons to ganglionic cells in the pelvic plexus and the bladder wall (see Fig. 3-1). Transmission in bladder ganglia is mediated by a nicotinic cholinergic mechanism. In some

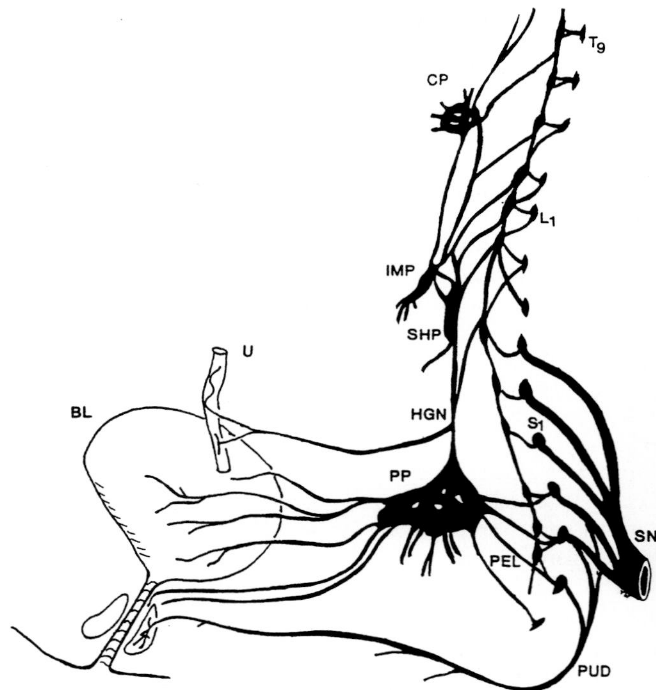

Figure 3-1 Diagram of the innervation of the female lower urinary tract. BL, urinary bladder; CP, celiac plexus; HGN, hypogastric nerve; IMP, inferior mesenteric plexus; L_1, first lumbar root; PEL, pelvic nerves; PP, pelvic plexus; PUD, pudendal nerve; S_1, first sacral root; SN, sciatic nerve; SHP, superior hypogastric plexus; T_9, ninth thoracic root; U, ureter. (Modified from de Groat WC, Booth AM: Autonomic systems to bladder and sex organs. In Dyck PJ, Thomas PK, Griffin JW, et al [eds]: Peripheral Neuropathy, 3rd ed. Philadelphia, WB Saunders, 1993, p 198.)

Table 3-1 Receptors for Putative Transmitters in the Lower Urinary Tract

Tissue	Cholinergic	Adrenergic	Other
Bladder body	+ (M_2)* + (M_3)	− (β_2) − (β_3)	+ Purinergic ($P2X_1$) − VIP + Substance P (NK_2)
Bladder base	+ (M_2) + (M_3)	+ (α_1)	− VIP + Substance P (NK_2) + Purinergic (P2X)
Urothelium	+ (M_2) + (M_3)	+ α + β	+ TRPV1 + TRPM8 + P2X + P2Y + SP +Bradykinin (B_2)
Urethra	+ (M)	+ (α_1) + (α_2) − (β)	+ Purinergic (P2X) − VIP − Nitric oxide
Sphincter striated muscle	+ (N)		
Adrenergic nerve terminals	− (M_2) + (M_1)	− (α_2)	− NPY
Cholinergic nerve terminals	− (M_2) + (M_1)	+ (α_1)	− NPY
Afferent nerve terminals			+ Purinergic ($P2X_{2/3}$) + TRPV1
Ganglia	+ (N) + (M_1)	+ (α_1) − (α_2) + (β)	− Enkephalinergic (δ) − Purinergic (P_1) + Substance P

*Letters in parentheses indicate receptor type, such as muscarinic (M) and nicotinic (N). Plus and minus signs indicate excitatory and inhibitory effects.
NPY, neuropeptide Y; TRP, transient receptor potential; VIP, vasoactive intestinal polypeptide.

species (e.g., cats, rabbits) ganglionic synapses act like gating circuits, exhibiting marked facilitation during repetitive preganglionic activity and modulation by various transmitter systems, including muscarinic, adrenergic, purinergic, and enkephalinergic (Table 3-1).[6,7] The ganglia can have an important role in regulating neural input to the bladder. Whether bladder ganglia in humans have similar properties is not known. Ganglion cells excite the bladder smooth muscle. Histochemical studies of the ganglia and nerves supplying the human lower urinary tract have shown that many ganglion cells contain choline acetyltransferase, acetylcholinesterase, and the vesicular acetylcholine transporter and therefore are cholinergic. Choline acetyltransferase–, acetylcholinesterase-, and acetylcholine transporter–positive nerves are abundant in all parts of the bladder but are less extensive in the urethra.[1,2,5] Neuropeptide Y and nitric oxide synthase also have been identified in 40% to 95% of intramural ganglia of the human bladder. Several populations of axonal varicosities have been detected close to intramural ganglion cells, including substance P–, vasoactive intestinal polypeptide (VIP)–, and calcitonin gene–related peptide (CGRP)–positive axons, which are presumably collaterals of extrinsic sensory nerves; tyrosine hydroxylase and neuropeptide Y axons, which are likely to be sympathetic axons; and galanin- and neuropeptide Y–containing axons.

Parasympathetic neuroeffector transmission in the bladder is mediated by acetylcholine acting on postjunctional muscarinic receptors.[8-11] M_2 and M_3 muscarinic receptors subtypes are expressed in bladder smooth muscle; however, examination of subtype-selective muscarinic receptor antagonists and studies of muscarinic receptor–knockout mice have revealed that the M_3 subtype is the principal receptor involved in excitatory transmission.[8-11] Activation of M_3 receptors triggers intracellular Ca^{2+} release, whereas activation of M_2 receptors inhibits adenylate cyclase.[10] The latter may contribute to bladder contractions by suppressing adrenergic inhibitory mechanisms that are mediated by β_3-adrenergic receptors and stimulation of adenylate cyclase.

In bladders of various animals, stimulation of parasympathetic nerves produces a noncholinergic contraction that is resistant to atropine and other muscarinic receptor–blocking agents. Adenosine triphosphate (ATP) (see Table 3-1) has been identified as the excitatory transmitter mediating the noncholinergic contractions.[10-13] ATP excites the bladder smooth muscle by acting on P2X receptors, which are ligand-gated ion channels. Among the seven types of P2X receptors that have been identified in the bladder, $P2X_1$ is the major subtype expressed in the rat and in human bladder smooth muscle.[12,13] Purinergic agonists also modulate transmission in bladder ganglia.[6,14,15] Although purinergic excitatory transmission is not important in the normal human bladder, it appears to be involved in bladders from patients with pathologic conditions such as detrusor overactivity, chronic urethral outlet obstruction, or interstitial cystitis.[12,16,17]

Parasympathetic pathways to the urethra induce relaxation during voiding.[1,10,11,18-20] In various species, the relaxation is not affected by muscarinic antagonists and therefore is not mediated by acetylcholine. However, inhibitors of nitric oxide synthase block the relaxation in vivo during reflex voiding or block the relaxation of urethral smooth muscle strips induced in vitro by electrical stimulation of intramural nerves, indicating that nitric oxide is the inhibitory transmitter involved in relaxation.[1,2,11,18,19] In some species, neurally evoked contractions of the urethra are reduced by muscarinic receptor antagonists or by desensitization of P2X purinergic receptors, indicating that acetylcholine or ATP are involved in excitatory transmission to urethral smooth muscle.[21]

Thoracolumbar Sympathetic Pathways

Sympathetic preganglionic pathways that arise from the T11 to L2 spinal segments pass to the sympathetic chain ganglia and then to prevertebral ganglia in the superior hypogastric and pelvic plexus and to short adrenergic neurons in the bladder and urethra. Sympathetic postganglionic nerves that release norepinephrine provide excitatory input to smooth muscle of the urethra and bladder base, inhibitory input to smooth muscle in the body of the bladder, and inhibitory and facilitatory input to vesical parasympathetic ganglia.[1,7,11] Radioligand receptor binding studies showed that α-adrenergic receptors are concentrated in the bladder base and proximal urethra, whereas β-adrenergic receptors are most prominent in the bladder body.[1,10] These observations are consistent with pharmacologic studies showing that sympathetic nerve stimulation or exogenous catecholamines produce β-adrenergic receptor–mediated inhibition of the body and α-adrenergic receptor–mediated contraction of the base, dome, and urethra. Molecular and contractility studies have shown that β_3-adrenergic receptors elicit inhibition and α_1-adrenergic receptors elicit contractions in the human bladder.[10] The α_{1A}-adrenergic receptor subtype is most prominent in the normal bladders, but the α_{1D}-adrenergic receptor subtype is upregulated in bladders from patients with outlet obstruction, raising the possibility that α_1-adrenergic receptor excitatory mechanisms in the bladder may contribute to irritative lower urinary tract symptoms in patients with benign prostatic hyperplasia.[10]

Sacral Somatic Pathways

Somatic efferent pathways to the external urethral sphincter are carried in the pudendal nerve from anterior horn cells in the third and fourth sacral segments. Branches of the pudendal nerve and other sacral somatic nerves also carry efferent impulses to muscles of the pelvic floor and proprioceptive afferent signals from these muscles, as well as sensory information from the urethra.[2,22-24] Analysis of urethral closure mechanisms in the female rat during bladder distention or sneeze-induced stress conditions revealed that the major rise in urethral pressure occurred in the middle urethra and was mediated by efferent pathways in the pudendal nerve to the external urethral sphincter and by pathways in nerves to the iliococcygeus and pubococcygeus muscles, although not by pathways in the sympathetic or parasympathetic nerves.[25]

Neural Modulation

Postganglionic nerve terminals are sites of "cross-talk" between sympathetic and parasympathetic nerves and possible sites of gating mechanisms.[26-30] For example, in the rat lower urinary tract, activation of $M_2/_4$ (muscarinic) cholinergic receptors on nerve terminals suppresses acetylcholine and norepinephrine release,[30] whereas activation of M_1 cholinergic receptors or α_1-adrenergic receptors enhances acetylcholine release (see Table 3-1).[26-29] Inhibitory $M_2/_4$ mechanisms are dominant at low frequencies of nerve activity and therefore may contribute to urine storage, whereas M_1 facilitatory mechanisms are dominant at high frequencies of nerve stimulation and may contribute to an enhancement of neurally evoked bladder contractions during micturition to induce complete bladder emptying.

Other putative transmitters that have been identified in efferent pathways to the lower urinary tract of animals and humans may modulate neuroeffector transmission (see Table 3-1).[3,31,32] Neuropeptide Y is present in adrenergic and cholinergic neurons,[32] and when administered exogenously, it acts prejunctionally to suppress the release of norepinephrine and acetylcholine from postganglionic nerve terminals.[21] Although nitric oxide relaxes smooth muscle in the urethra, it is inactive in bladder smooth muscle.[10] However, in the bladder, it may act on afferent nerves to modulate excitability.[10,31] VIP, which is released with acetylcholine, may function as an inhibitory transmitter in the bladder.[10] Efferent control of the bladder and urethra is potentially complex and involves many transmitters and many synaptic gating mechanisms in ganglia and at postganglionic nerve terminals.

Lumbosacral Afferent Pathways

Afferent activity arising in the bladder is transmitted to the central nervous system by both sets of autonomic nerves.[2,33-37] The afferent nerves most important for initiating micturition are those passing in the pelvic nerves to the sacral spinal cord. These afferents consist of small, myelinated (A) and unmyelinated (C) fibers that convey impulses from tension receptors and nociceptors, respectively, in the bladder wall.[2,3,36] Electrophysiologic studies in the cat have shown that A bladder afferents respond in a graded manner to passive distention and to active contraction of the bladder.[35-37] The intravesical pressure threshold for activation of these afferents ranges from 5 to 15 mm Hg, which is consistent with pressures at which humans report the first sensation of bladder filling during cystometry. The A afferents in the cat show a linear increase in firing with increasing intravesical pressures that extend into the noxious range, suggesting that nociceptive stimuli in the bladder may be encoded in part by high rates of firing in polymodal afferents that also transmit nonnoxious information.

High-threshold C-fiber afferents have also been detected in the cat bladder.[34] Under normal conditions, most of these afferents do not respond to bladder distention and therefore have been designated silent C fibers, but many can be activated by chemical irritation of the bladder mucosa[3,34] or cold temperatures (Fig. 3-2).[38] After chemical irritation, C-fiber afferents exhibit spontaneous firing with the bladder empty and increased firing during bladder distention.[34] Activation of C-fiber afferents by chemical irritation facilitates the micturition reflex and decreases bladder capacity.[2,3,39-41] Administration of capsaicin, a neurotoxin that desensitizes C-fiber afferents, blocks this facilitation but does not block micturition reflexes in normal animals, indicating that C-fiber afferent pathways are not essential for normal voiding.[2,42,43]

In the rat, A-fiber and C-fiber bladder afferents are not distinguishable on the basis of stimulus modality; both types of afferents consist of mechanosensitive and chemosensitive popu-

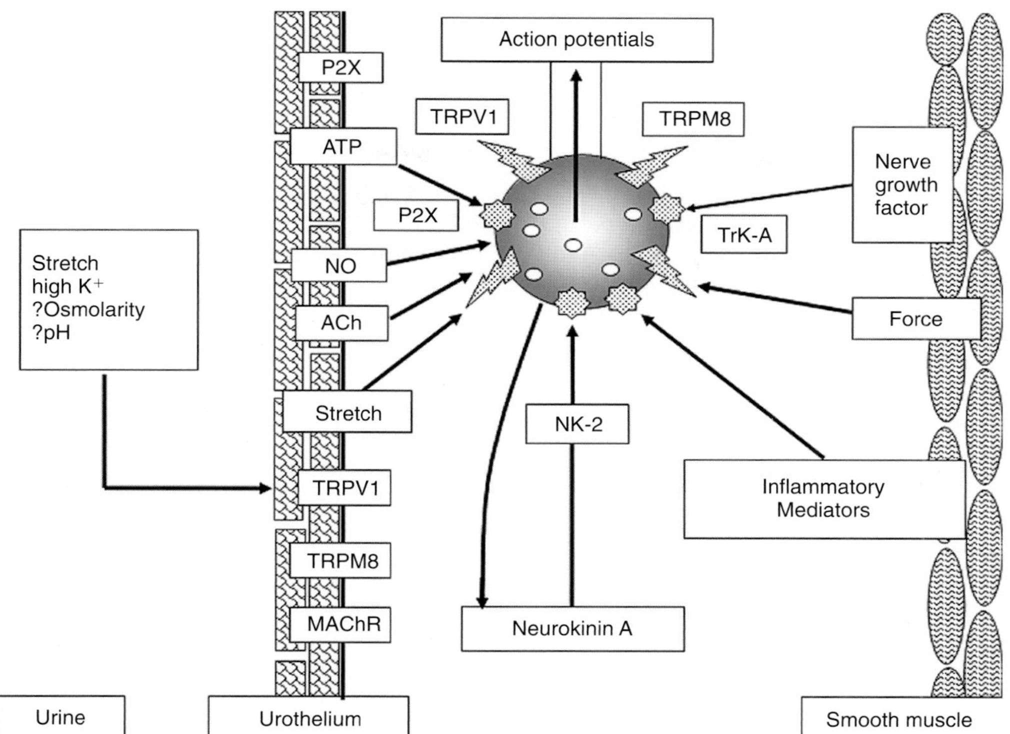

Figure 3-2 The diagram shows the receptors in the urothelium and in sensory nerve endings in the bladder mucosa and the putative chemical mediators that are released by the urothelium, nerves, or smooth muscle that can modulate the excitability of sensory nerves. Urothelial cells and sensory nerves express common receptors (i.e., P2X, TRPV1, and TRPM8). Distention of the bladder activates stretch receptors and triggers the release of urothelial transmitters such as adenosine triphosphate (ATP), acetylcholine (ACh), and nitric oxide (NO) that may interact with adjacent nerves. Receptors in afferent nerves or the urothelium can respond to changes in pH, osmolality, high potassium ion (K^+) concentration, chemicals in the urine, or inflammatory mediators released in the bladder wall. Neuropeptides (e.g., neurokinin A) released from sensory nerves in response to distention or chemical stimulation can act on NK-2 autoreceptors to sensitize the mechanosensitive nerve endings. The smooth muscle can generate a force that may influence some mucosal endings. Nerve growth factor released from muscle or urothelium can exert an acute and chronic influence on the excitability of sensory nerves though an action on tyrosine kinase A (Trk-A) receptors. MAChR, muscarinic acetylcholine receptor; TRPM8, menthol/cold receptor; TRPV1, transient receptor potential vanilloid receptor 1, sensitive to capsaicin.

lations.[44-47] C-fiber afferents that respond only to bladder filling have also been identified in the rat bladder and appear to be volume receptors possibly sensitive to stretch of the mucosa.[2,44] C-fiber afferents are sensitive to the neurotoxins capsaicin and resiniferatoxin and to other substances, such as tachykinins, nitric oxide, ATP, prostaglandins, and neurotrophic factors, released in the bladder by afferent nerves, urothelial cells, and inflammatory cells (see Fig. 3-2).[2,3,41,45,48-54] These substances can sensitize the afferent nerves and change their response to mechanical stimuli.

Mechanosensitive afferents from the bladder and urethra have been identified in sympathetic nerves passing to the lumbar spinal cord.[55] These afferent pathways consist of myelinated and unmyelinated axons that respond to similar stimulus modalities as afferents in the pelvic nerve. The function of sympathetic nerve afferents in the control of micturition is uncertain; however, based on clinical observations, it is clear that in humans they carry nociceptive information from the lower urinary tract.

Afferent pathways from the urethra, which induce the sensations of temperature, pain, and passage of urine, travel in the pudendal nerve to the lumbosacral spinal cord.[2,3] Afferents from the female sex organs, including the clitoris, vagina, and part of the innervation of the uterine cervix, also travel in the pudendal nerve.[56,57] These afferents and pudendal nerve afferents from the striated sphincter muscles have a modulatory influence on micturition.[3,24]

The properties of lumbosacral dorsal root ganglion cells innervating the bladder, urethra, and external urethral sphincter in the rat have been studied with patch-clamp recording techniques in combination with axonal tracing methods to identify the different populations of neurons.[58-65] Based on responsiveness to capsaicin, it is estimated that approximately 70% of bladder afferent neurons in the rat are the C-fiber type. These neurons exhibit high-threshold, tetrodotoxin-resistant sodium channels and action potentials and phasic firing (one to two spikes) in response to prolonged depolarizing current pulses.[58,60,61] Approximately 90% of the bladder C-fiber afferent neurons also are excited by ATP, which induces depolarization and firing of afferent neurons by activating $P2X_3$ or $P2X_{2/3}$ receptors.[65] These neurons express isolectin-B4 binding, which is commonly used as a marker for ATP-responsive sensory neurons.[60] A-fiber afferent neurons are resistant to capsaicin and ATP and exhibit low-threshold, tetrodotoxin-sensitive sodium channels and action potentials and tonic firing (multiple spikes) to depolarizing current pulses. C-fiber bladder afferent neurons also express a slowly decaying A-type K^+ channel that controls spike threshold and firing frequency.[58,62] Suppression of this K^+ channel induces hyperexcitability of bladder afferent nerves.[58] These properties of dorsal root ganglion cells are consistent with the different properties of A-fiber and C-fiber afferent receptors in the bladder.

Immunohistochemical studies have shown that a large percentage of bladder afferent neurons contain peptides: CGRP, VIP, substance P, pituitary adenylate cyclase-activating polypeptide (PACAP), corticotropin-releasing factor (CRF), and enkephalins.[66,67] In the bladder, these peptides are common in nerves in the submucosal and subepithelial layers and around blood vessels. The neurotoxin capsaicin, when applied locally to the bladder in experimental animals, releases peptides from peripheral afferent terminals and produces inflammatory responses, including plasma extravasation and vasodilatation.[41] Afferent peptides can also modulate transmission in bladder ganglia.[6] These findings suggest that the neuropeptides may be important neurotransmitters in afferent pathways in the lower urinary tract.

Urothelial-Afferent Interactions

Studies have revealed that the urothelium, which has been traditionally viewed as a passive barrier at the bladder luminal surface,[2,68,69] has specialized sensory and signaling properties that allows urothelial cells to respond to their chemical and physical environment and to engage in reciprocal chemical communication with neighboring nerves in the bladder wall (see Fig. 3-2).[68-80] These properties include expression of nicotinic, muscarinic, tachykinin, adrenergic, purinergic, and capsaicin (TRPV1) receptors[70-76,80-83]; responsiveness to transmitters released from sensory nerves; close physical association with afferent nerves[74,84,85]; and an ability to release chemical mediators such as ATP, acetylcholine, and nitric oxide that can regulate the activity of adjacent nerves and thereby trigger local vascular changes or reflex bladder contractions.[71,75,77,82,86] The role of ATP in urothelial-afferent communication has attracted considerable attention because bladder or urethral distention releases ATP from the urothelium,[72,77,87,88] and intravesical administration of ATP induces bladder hyperactivity,[86,88] an effect blocked by administration of P2X purinergic receptor antagonists that suppress the excitatory action of ATP on bladder afferent neurons.[65,86,88] Mice in which the $P2X_3$ receptor was knocked out exhibited hypoactive bladder activity and inefficient voiding,[76,88] suggesting that activation of $P2X_3$ receptors on bladder afferent nerves by ATP released from the urothelium was essential for normal bladder function. It has also been reported that urothelial cells obtained from patients or cats with a chronic, painful bladder condition (i.e., interstitial cystitis) released significantly larger amounts of ATP in response to mechanical stretching than urothelial cells from normal patients.[72,89] The release of other substances, including nitric oxide[90] and a nonapeptide glycoprotein called APF,[91-93] is also increased in feline interstitial cystitis and human interstitial cystitis, respectively. This raises the possibility that enhanced signaling between the urothelium and afferent nerves is involved in the triggering of painful bladder sensations (see Fig. 3-2).

Communication between the urothelium and afferent nerves may also involve another cell type, the myofibroblast.[94-96] These cells, which stain intensely for vimentin and gap junction protein connexin 43, have been identified immediately below the urothelium in human and guinea pig bladders. Electron microscopic studies have revealed that the cells make close appositions with unmyelinated suburothelial nerve endings.[95] Exogenous ATP can induce Ca^{+2}-activated chloride currents in myofibroblasts by stimulation of P2Y receptors.[96] It has been suggested that stretch-induced ATP released from urothelial cells may act on myofibroblasts, which modulate the excitability of adjacent afferent nerves.

ANATOMY OF CENTRAL NERVOUS PATHWAYS

Efferent Neurons

Preganglionic neurons in the lumbosacral parasympathetic nucleus have been identified in the intermediolateral region of the spinal cord in several species.[3,97] In the cat, the sacral parasympathetic nucleus is divided into two groups of cells: a dorsal band and a lateral band. Neurons innervating the urinary bladder are located in the lateral band. These neurons have an extensive network of axon collaterals[98] that is involved in a recurrent inhibitory mechanism[99] that regulates reflex bladder activity. The neurons send dendrites to discrete regions of the spinal cord, including the lateral and dorsal lateral funiculus, lamina I on the lateral edge of the dorsal horn, the dorsal gray commissure, and the gray matter and lateral funiculus ventral to the autonomic nucleus (Fig. 3-3).[97] It has been suggested that the dendrites in the lateral funiculus receive inputs from descending pathways from the brain, whereas the other dendrites receive segmental inputs from interneurons or primary afferents. Lumbar sympathetic preganglionic neurons and motor neurons in Onuf's nucleus that innervate the external urethral sphincter have similar dendritic distributions (see Fig. 3-3).[100-102]

Afferent Projections

Afferent pathways from the lower urinary tract project to discrete regions of the dorsal horn that contain the soma or dendrites of efferent neurons innervating the lower urinary tract. Pelvic nerve afferent pathways from the urinary bladder of the cat[103,104] and the rat[105] project into Lissauer's tract at the apex of the dorsal horn and then pass rostrocaudally, giving off collaterals that extend laterally and medially through the superficial layer of the dorsal horn (lamina I) into the deeper layers (laminae V to VII and X) at the base of the dorsal horn (Fig. 3-4A and see Fig. 3-3). The lateral pathway, which is the most prominent projection, terminates in the region of the sacral parasympathetic nucleus and also sends some axons to the dorsal commissure (see Figs. 3-3 and 3-4A).

Pudendal nerve afferent pathways from the external urethral sphincter of the cat have central terminations that overlap in part with those of bladder afferents in lateral laminae, I, V to VII, and X.[100,101] Afferents from the female sexual organs also terminate in these areas.[56,57] The overlap of the central projections of bladder afferents and the afferents in the pudendal nerve to the sex organs and urethra is of interest, because activation of the latter afferents can markedly influence bladder function.[106-109]

Spinal Interneurons

The spinal neurons involved in processing afferent input from the lower urinary tract and the sex organs have been identified by physiologic and anatomic tracing techniques.[110-115] Interneurons that fire in response to bladder distention or mechanical stimulation of the vagina or uterine cervix have been detected in lateral intermediate gray matter near the sacral para-

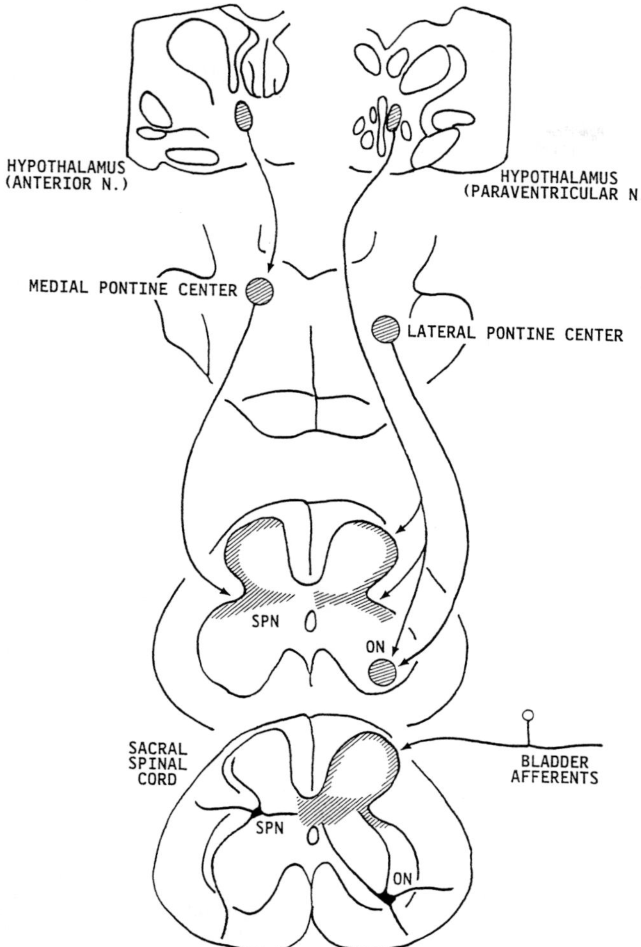

Figure 3-3 Neural connections between the brain and the sacral spinal cord that may be involved in the regulation of the lower urinary tract in the cat. Lower section of the spinal cord shows the location and morphology of a preganglionic neuron in the sacral parasympathetic nucleus (SPN), a sphincter motoneuron in Onuf's nucleus (ON), and the sites of central termination of afferent projections from the urinary bladder. Upper section of the spinal cord shows the sites of termination of descending pathways arising in the pontine micturition center (medial), the pontine sphincter or urine storage center (lateral), and the paraventricular nuclei of the hypothalamus. Section through the pons shows the projection for anterior hypothalamic nuclei to the pontine micturition center. (From de Groat WC: Neural control of urinary bladder and sexual organs. In Bannister R, Mathias, CJ [eds]: Autonomic Failure, 3rd ed. Oxford, Oxford University Press, 1992, p 129.)

sympathetic nucleus and in the region of the dorsal commissure (lamina X).[2,108] Commonly, stimulation of sex organ afferents inhibits neurons activated by bladder distention, which is consistent with the inhibitory effect of these afferents on bladder reflexes.[108,109]

Spinal interneurons have also been identified by the expression of the immediate-early gene *FOS* (see Fig. 3-4B)[110-112] and by transneuronal transport of pseudorabies virus from the bladder (see Fig. 3-4C).[40,113-115] The protein product of the *FOS* gene can be detected immunocytochemically in the nuclei of neurons within 30 to 60 minutes after synaptic activation. In the rat, noxious or non-noxious stimulation of the bladder and urethra and electrical stimulation of the pelvic or pudendal nerves increased the levels of FOS protein, primarily in the dorsal commissure and in the area of the sacral parasympathetic nucleus (see Fig. 3-4B), the major sites of termination of afferents from the lower urinary tract. Neurons in these same regions are labeled by the pseudorabies virus (see Fig. 3-4C), which passes transsynaptically in a sequential manner from postganglionic to preganglionic efferent neurons and then to segmental interneurons and eventually to neurons in the brain (Fig. 3-5) (discussed later).[113-115] Interneurons in the dorsal commissure region also project to the sphincter motor nucleus.[116,117] These results indicate that interneurons in restricted regions of the intermediate gray matter and dorsal commissure play a major role in coordinating the different aspects of lower urinary tract function.

Patch-clamp recordings from parasympathetic preganglionic neurons in the rat spinal slice preparations have revealed that interneurons located immediately dorsal and medial to the parasympathetic nucleus make direct monosynaptic connections with the preganglionic neurons (PGNs).[118-120] Microstimulation of interneurons in both locations elicits glutamatergic, *N*-methyl-D-aspartic acid (NMDA), and non-NMDA excitatory postsynaptic currents in PGNs. Stimulation of a subpopulation of medial interneurons elicits GABAergic and glycinergic inhibitory postsynaptic currents.[118] In this way, local interneurons likely play an important role in excitatory and inhibitory reflex pathways controlling the preganglionic outflow to the lower urinary tract. Glutamatergic excitatory inputs have also been elicited by stimulation of the projections from lamina X and the lateral funiculus.[121,122]

Pathways in the Brain

The neurons in the brain that control the lower urinary tract have been studied with a variety of anatomic tracing techniques in several species. In the rat, transneuronal virus tracing methods[113-115] have identified many populations of central neurons that are involved in the control of the bladder, urethra, and urethral sphincter, including the Barrington nucleus, the pontine micturition center (PMC); the medullary raphe nucleus, which contains serotonergic neurons; the locus ceruleus, which contains noradrenergic neurons; the periaqueductal gray (PAG); and the A5 noradrenergic cell group (see Fig. 3-5). Several regions in the hypothalamus and the cerebral cortex also exhibited virus-infected cells. Neurons in the cortex were located primarily in the medial frontal cortex.

Other anatomic studies in which anterograde tracer substances were injected into brain areas and then identified in terminals in the spinal cord are consistent with the virus-tracing data. Tracer injected into the paraventricular nucleus of the hypothalamus labeled terminals in the sacral parasympathetic nucleus and the sphincter motor nucleus (see Fig. 3-3).[123-125] Neurons in the anterior hypothalamus project to the PMC, and neurons in the PMC project primarily to the sacral parasympathetic nucleus and the lateral edge of the dorsal horn and the dorsal commissure, areas containing dendritic projections from the preganglionic neurons, sphincter motoneurons, and afferent inputs from the bladder. Conversely, projections from neurons in the lateral pons terminate rather selectively in the sphincter motor nucleus (i.e., Onuf's nucleus) (see Fig. 3-3).[125] The sites of termination of descending projections from the PMC are optimally located to regulate reflex mechanisms at the spinal level.

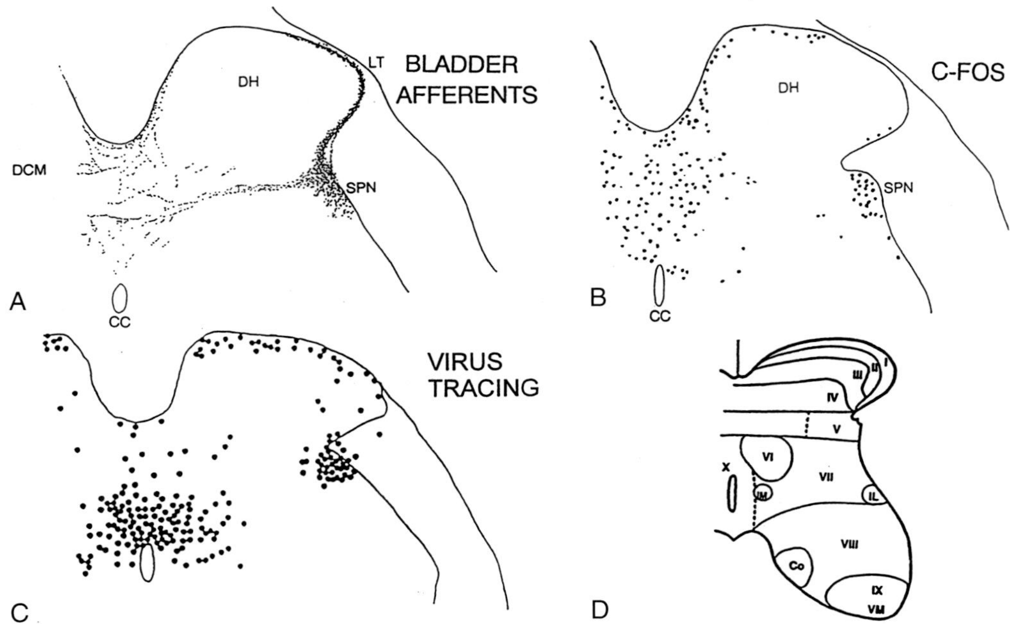

Figure 3-4 The distribution of bladder afferent projections to the L6 spinal cord of the rat **(A)** is shown, with the distribution of Fos-positive cells in the L6 spinal segment after chemical irritation of the lower urinary tract of the rat **(B)** and the distribution of interneurons in the L6 spinal cord labeled by transneuronal transport of pseudorabies virus injected into the urinary bladder **(C).** Afferents labeled by lectin wheat germ agglutinin conjugated to horseradish peroxidase (WGA-HRP) injected into the urinary bladder. Fos immunoreactivity is present in the nuclei of cells. CC central canal; DH, dorsal horn; SPN, sacral parasympathetic nucleus. D, Laminar organization of the cat spinal cord.

Table 3-2 Reflexes to the Lower Urinary Tract

Afferent Pathway	Efferent Pathway	Central Pathway
Urine storage: low-level vesical afferent activity (pelvic nerve)	External sphincter contraction (somatic nerves) Internal sphincter contraction (sympathetic nerves) Detrusor inhibition (sympathetic nerves) Ganglionic inhibition (sympathetic nerves) Sacral parasympathetic outflow, inactive	Spinal reflexes
Micturition: high-level vesical afferent activity (pelvic nerve)	Inhibition of external sphincter activity Inhibition of sympathetic outflow Activation of parasympathetic outflow to the bladder	Spinobulbospinal reflexes

REFLEX MECHANISMS CONTROLLING THE LOWER URINARY TRACT

The central pathways controlling lower urinary tract function are organized as simple on-off switching circuits that maintain a reciprocal relationship between the urinary bladder and the urethral outlet. The principal reflex components of these switching circuits are listed in Table 3-2 and are illustrated in Figure 3-6. Intravesical pressure measurements during bladder filling in humans and animals reveal that bladder pressure is maintained at a low and relatively constant level when bladder volume is below the threshold for inducing voiding (Fig. 3-7A). Accommodation of the bladder to increasing volumes of urine is primarily a passive phenomenon that depends on the intrinsic properties of the vesical smooth muscle and the quiescence of the parasympathetic efferent pathway.[2-4] In some species, urine storage is also facilitated by sympathetic reflexes that mediate inhibition of bladder activity and closure of the urethral outlet (see Table 3-2 and Fig. 3-6).[126,127] During bladder filling, the activity on the sphincter electromyogram also increases (see Fig. 3-7), reflecting an increase in efferent firing in the pudendal nerve and an increase in outlet resistance that contributes to the maintenance of urinary continence.[24]

The storage phase of the urinary bladder can be switched to the voiding phase involuntarily (by reflex) or voluntarily (see Fig. 3-7B). The former is readily demonstrated in the human infant (see Fig. 3-7A) and in the anesthetized animal when the volume of urine exceeds the micturition threshold. At this point, increased afferent firing from tension receptors in the bladder reverses the pattern of efferent outflow, producing firing in the sacral parasympathetic pathways and inhibition of sympathetic and somatic pathways. The expulsion phase consists of an initial relaxation of the urethral sphincter (see Fig. 3-7A) followed in a few seconds by a contraction of the bladder, an increase in bladder pressure,

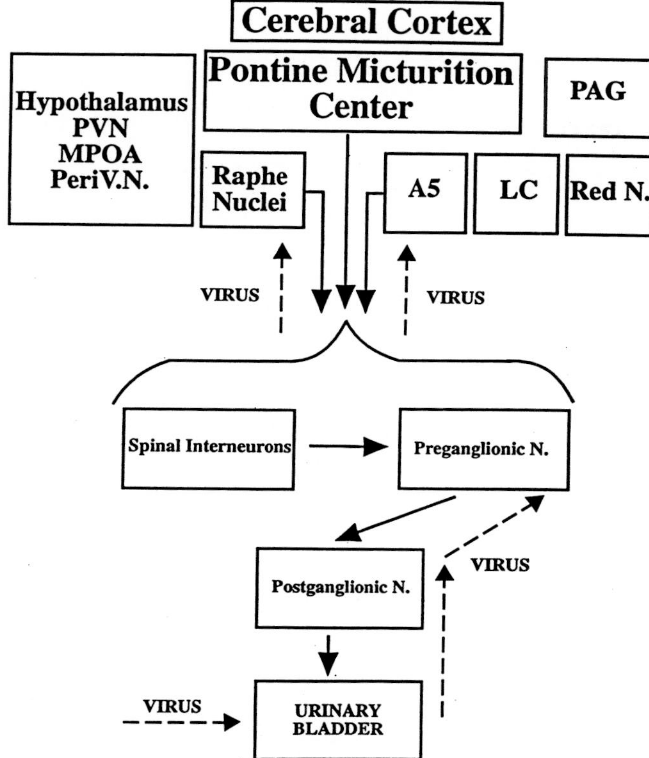

Figure 3-5 Structures in the brain and spinal cord of the adult and neonatal rat were labeled after injection of pseudorabies virus into the urinary bladder or the urethra. Virus is transported transneuronally in a retrograde direction *(dashed arrows)*. Normal synaptic connections are indicated by *solid arrows*. At long survival times, the virus can be detected in neurons at specific sites in the spinal cord and brain, extending to the pontine micturition center in the pons (i.e., Barrington's nucleus) and to the cerebral cortex. Other sites in the brain labeled by the virus are the paraventricular nucleus (PVN), medial preoptic area (MPOA), and periventricular nucleus (Peri.V.N.) of the hypothalamus; periaqueductal gray (PAG); locus ceruleus (LC) and subceruleus; red nucleus (Red N.); medullary raphe nuclei; and the noradrenergic cell group (A5).

and flow of urine. Secondary reflexes elicited by the flow of urine through the urethra facilitate bladder emptying.[4]

These reflexes require the integrated action of neuronal populations at various levels of the neuraxis (Fig. 3-8 and see Fig. 3-6). Certain reflexes, such as those mediating the excitatory input to the sphincters and the sympathetic inhibitory input to the bladder, are organized at the spinal level (see Fig. 3-6A), whereas the parasympathetic input to the detrusor has a more complicated central organization involving spinal and spinobulbospinal pathways (see Fig. 3-6B).

Storage Reflexes

Sympathetic Pathways

Studies in animals indicate that sympathetic input to the lower urinary tract is tonically active during bladder filling.[3] Surgical or pharmacologic blockade of the sympathetic pathways can reduce urethral resistance, bladder capacity, and bladder wall compliance and increase the frequency and amplitude of bladder contractions. Sympathetic firing is initiated at least in part by a sacrolumbar intersegmental spinal reflex pathway triggered by vesical afferent activity in the pelvic nerves (see Table 3-2 and Fig. 3-6A).[126,127] This vesicosympathetic reflex represents a negative-feedback mechanism whereby an increase in bladder pressure triggers an increase in inhibitory input to the bladder, allowing the bladder to accommodate larger volumes of urine. The reflex pathway is inhibited during micturition, and the inhibition is abolished by transection of the spinal cord at the thoracic level, indicating that it originates at a supraspinal site, possibly the PMC (see Fig. 3-6B).[127]

Somatic Efferent Pathways to the Urethral Sphincter

Reflex control of the striated urethral sphincter is similar to control of sympathetic pathways to the lower urinary tract (see Fig. 3-6A). During bladder filling, pudendal motor neurons are activated by vesical afferent input, whereas during micturition, motor neurons are reciprocally inhibited. Inhibition depends in part on supraspinal mechanisms, because in animals with chronic spinal lesions and in paraplegic patients, it is weak or absent. In paraplegics, the uninhibited spinal vesicosphincter excitatory reflex pathway commonly initiates a striated sphincter contraction in concert with a contraction of the bladder (i.e., bladder-sphincter dyssynergia) (see Fig. 3-7C). This reflex interferes with bladder emptying.

Supraspinal control of sphincter motor neurons has been studied with electrophysiologic techniques in animals. Electrical stimulation of the lateral funiculus of the spinal cord or stimulation of various areas of the brain evokes excitatory postsynaptic potentials and firing in sphincter motor neurons and an increase in sphincter electromyographic activity in the cat.[128-132] Stimulation of the lateral pontine reticular formation, an area that has been designated the urine storage center, elicits an increase in sphincter electromyographic activity and inhibits bladder activity.[124,133] Stimulation of dorsal medial pontine sites (e.g., PMC) excites the bladder and inhibits sphincter electromyographic activity at latencies of 40 to 50 ms.[124,132,133] These findings indicate that the spinal reflex pathways that mediate urine storage are strongly modulated by descending input from the brain.

Voiding Reflexes

Spinobulbospinal Micturition Reflex Pathway

Micturition is mediated by activation of the sacral parasympathetic efferent pathway to the bladder and reciprocal inhibition of the somatic pathway to the urethral sphincter (see Table 3-2 and Fig. 3-6B). Studies in animals using brain-lesioning techniques have revealed that neurons in the brainstem at the level of the inferior colliculus play an essential role in the control of the parasympathetic component of micturition (Fig. 3-9 and see Fig. 3-8).[131,134-138] Removal of areas of the brain above the inferior colliculus by intercollicular decerebration usually facilitates micturition by eliminating inhibitory inputs from more rostral areas of the brain (see Fig. 3-8).[3,4,134,135] However, transection at any point below the colliculi abolishes micturition. Bilateral lesions in the rostral pons abolish micturition, whereas electrical stimulation at these sites triggers bladder contractions and micturition.[136,138] These observations led to the concept of a spinobulbospinal micturition reflex pathway that passes through a center in the rostral brainstem, the PMC (see Figs. 3-6B and 3-9). This pathway functions as an on-off switch (see Fig. 3-6)

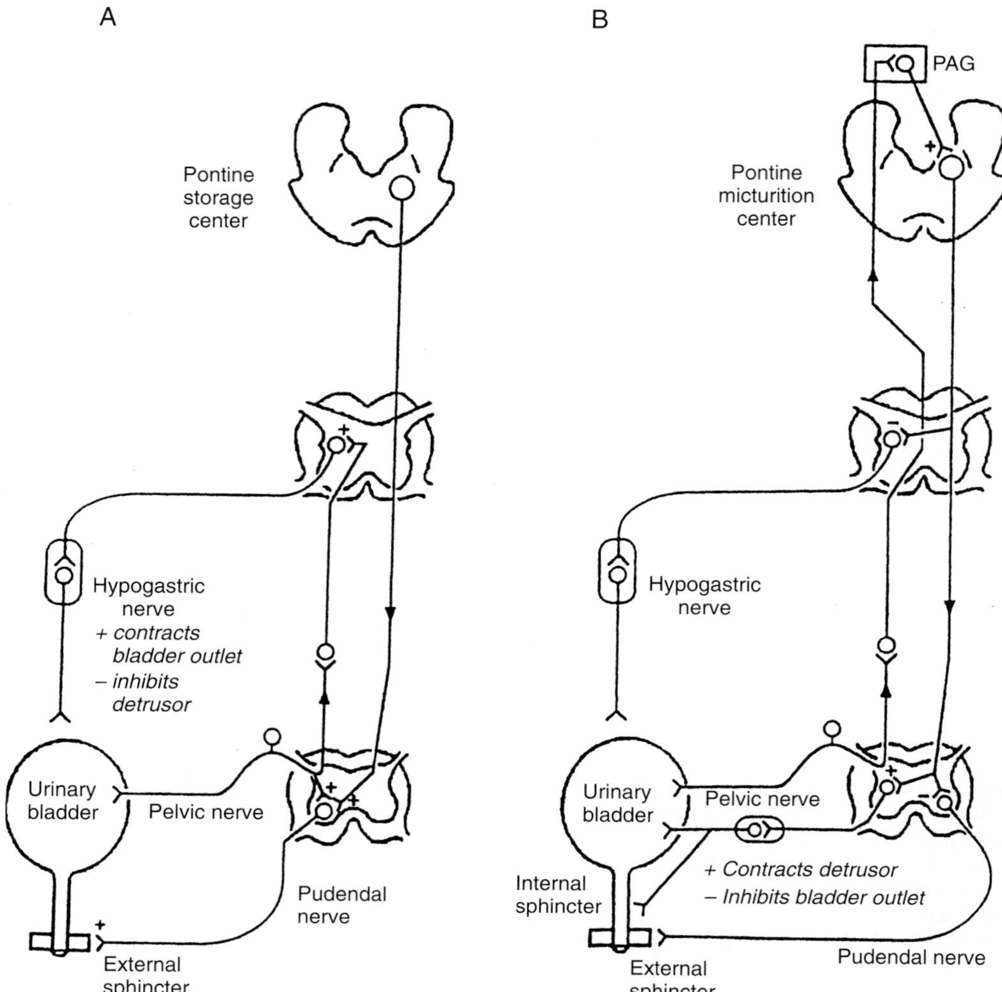

Figure 3-6 Neural circuits controlling continence and micturition. **A,** Urine storage reflexes. During the storage of urine, distention of the bladder produces low-level vesical afferent firing, which stimulates sympathetic outflow to the bladder outlet (i.e., base and urethra) and pudendal outflow to the external urethral sphincter. These responses occur by spinal reflex pathways and represent guarding reflexes, which promote continence. Sympathetic firing also inhibits the detrusor muscle and modulates transmission in the bladder ganglia. A region in the rostral pons (i.e., pontine storage center) increases external urethral sphincter activity. **B,** Voiding reflexes. During elimination of urine, intense bladder afferent firing activates spinobulbospinal reflex pathways passing through the pontine micturition center, which stimulates the parasympathetic outflow to the bladder and internal sphincter smooth muscle and inhibits the sympathetic and pudendal outflow to the urethral outlet. Ascending afferent input from the spinal cord may pass through relay neurons in the periaqueductal gray (PAG) before reaching the pontine micturition center.

that is activated by a critical level of afferent activity arising from tension receptors in the bladder.[136] This switch is modulated by inhibitory and excitatory influences from areas of the brain rostral to the pons (i.e., diencephalon and cerebral cortex) and from other areas of the brainstem (Fig. 3-10 and see Figs. 3-8 and 3-9).[134,135]

Pontine Micturition Center

Physiologic and pharmacologic experiments have provided substantial support for the concept that neuronal circuitry in the PMC functions as a switch in the micturition reflex pathway. The switch seems to regulate bladder capacity and coordinate the activity of the bladder and external urethral sphincter.[2,3,131,138] Electrical or chemical stimulation in the PMC of the rat, cat, or dog induces suppression of urethral sphincter electromyographic activity, firing of sacral preganglionic neurons, bladder contractions, and release of urine.[3,124,131,136,138] Microinjections of putative inhibitory transmitters into the PMC of the cat can increase the volume threshold for inducing micturition and, in high doses, completely block reflex voiding, indicating that synapses in this region are important for regulating the set point for reflex voiding and are an essential link in the reflex pathway.[131] The PMC receives inputs indirectly through relay stations in the PAG or directly from spinal tract neurons (see Fig. 3-10) located in lateral laminae I, V, and VII of the sacral spinal cord.[112,116,139-141] Neurons in the latter areas of the spinal cord receive dense projections from bladder afferent pathways[104,105,110] (see Figs. 3-3 and 3-4) and respond to distention or contraction of the bladder.[108,110] Brain imaging studies in humans using positron emission tomography (PET) or functional magnetic resonance imaging (fMRI) have

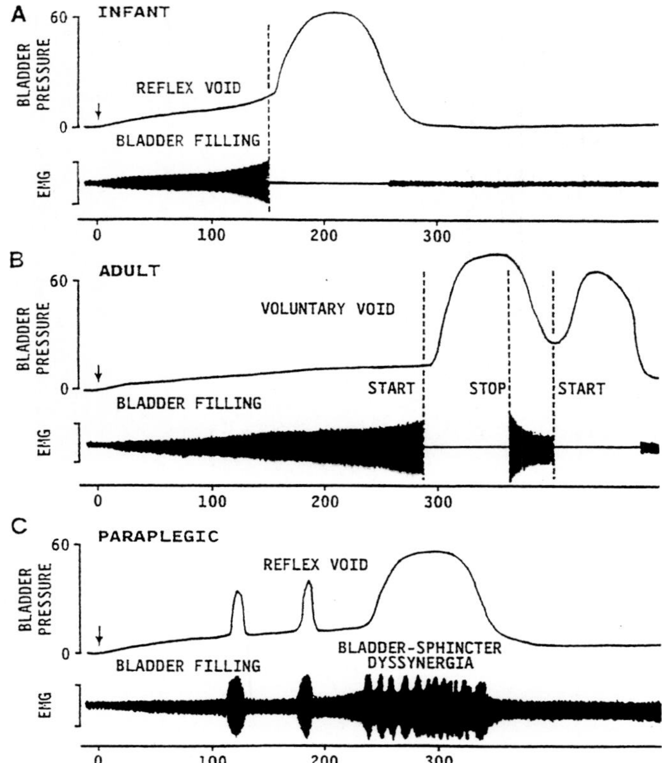

Figure 3-7 Combined cystometrograms and sphincter electromyograms (EMGs) comparing reflex voiding responses in an infant **(A)** and in a paraplegic patient **(C)** with a voluntary voiding response in an adult **(B).** The abscissa in all recordings represents bladder volume (mL), and the ordinates represent bladder pressure (cm H_2O) and electrical activity of the EMG recording. On the left side of each trace, the *arrows* indicate the start of a slow infusion of fluid into the bladder (i.e., bladder filling). Vertical *dashed lines* indicate the start of sphincter relaxation, which precedes by a few seconds the bladder contraction in **A** and **B.** In **B,** notice that a voluntary cessation of voiding (i.e., stop) is associated with an initial increase in the sphincter electromyographic pattern, followed by a reciprocal relaxation of the bladder. A resumption of voiding is associated with sphincter relaxation and a delayed increase in bladder pressure. In the paraplegic patient **(C),** the reciprocal relationship between bladder and sphincter is abolished. During bladder filling, transient uninhibited bladder contractions occur in association with sphincter activity. Further filling leads to more prolonged and simultaneous contractions of the bladder and sphincter (i.e., bladder-sphincter dyssynergia). Loss of the reciprocal relationship between the bladder and sphincter in paraplegic patients interferes with bladder emptying. (From de Groat WC, Steers WD: Autonomic regulation of the urinary bladder and sex organs. In Loewy AD, Spyer KM [eds]: Central Regulation of Autonomic Functions. Oxford, Oxford University Press, 1990, p 310.)

identified increased neuronal activity in the PMC and PAG during voiding (see Fig. 3-9).[142-144]

Spinal Micturition Pathway

Reflex mechanisms in the spinal cord can also mediate bladder contractions and voiding.[2,3,42,43,137] In most species, these mechanisms are weak or absent in adults with an intact nervous system; however, they are prominent in neonates[145] or in mature animals after spinal cord injury above the lumbosacral level.[146,147] In the cat, the spinal micturition reflex is mediated by C-fiber afferents (see Fig. 3-10), whereas the spinobulbospinal reflex in normal animals is triggered by A filer afferent input from tension receptors in the urinary bladder.[43,136,137] Somatic afferent pathways, particularly afferents with receptors in the perineum, can also induce voiding reflexes.[108,145,146] Spinal pathways mediate involuntary or automatic micturition, whereas the spinobulbospinal pathways are involved in voluntary micturition.

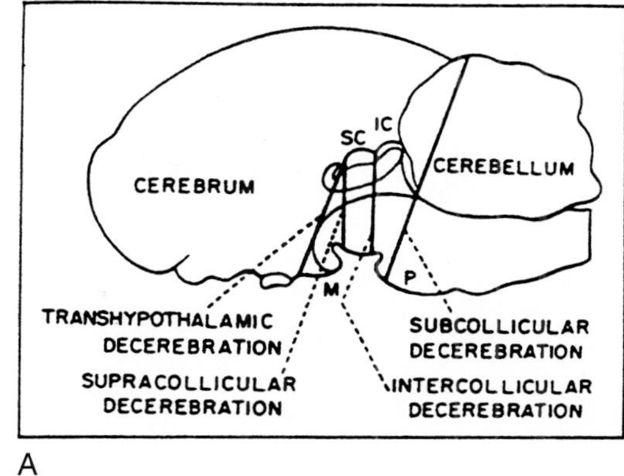

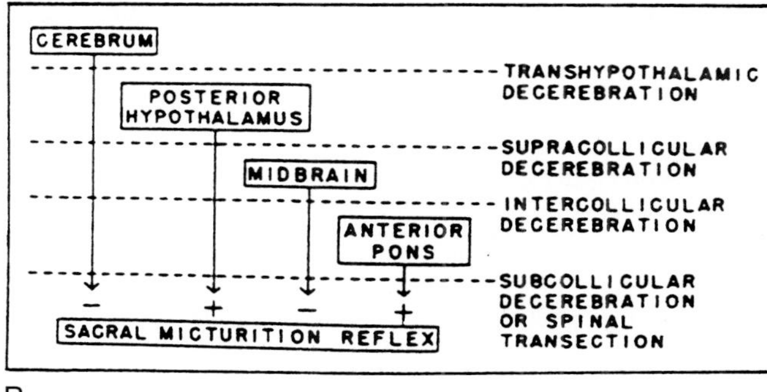

Figure 3-8 A, Sagittal section of the cat brain shows various levels of brain transections made in the study of the supraspinal control of micturition. IC, inferior colliculi; M, midbrain; P, pons; SC superior colliculi. **B,** The net facilitatory and inhibitory actions of various levels of the brain are identified by the transection procedures shown in **A.** (Data from Tang PC: Levels of the brain stem and diencephalon controlling the micturition reflex. J Neurophysiol 18:583, 1955; Tang PC, Ruch TC: Localization of brain stem and diencephalic areas controlling the micturition reflex. J Comp Neurol 106:213, 1956.)

Suprapontine Control of Micturition

Experiments in animals and clinical studies in humans indicate that various sites in the brain in addition to those directly involved in the micturition reflex pathway influence lower urinary tract function. Reviews of the clinical and animal literature concerning the regulation of micturition by the brain have been published.[2-4,125]

Axonal-tracing studies in rats using transsynaptic transport of pseudorabies virus have revealed the presence of direct connections from neurons in many brain areas to the reflex circuitry that regulates bladder function.[113-115] As illustrated in Figure 3-5, after injection of the virus into the bladder wall, preganglionic neurons and interneurons in the spinal cord are labeled at short transport times; at longer transport times, neurons in various areas of the brain, including the PMC, paraventricular and medial

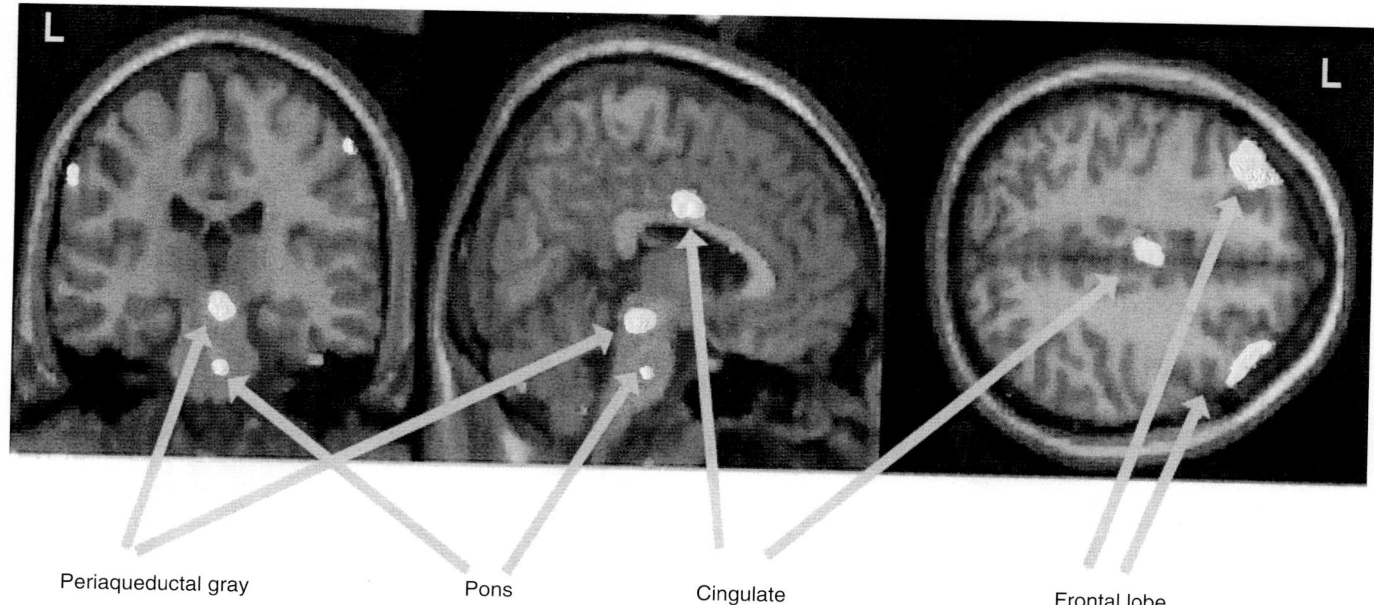

Figure 3-9 Increases in brain activity with increasing volume. Activations are shown superimposed on three orthogonal sections of normalized brain. Increases in brain activity with increases in bladder volume are seen in the periaqueductal gray, pons, cingulate, and frontal lobes (SPM *t*, $P < .05$ uncorrected). (Modified from Athwal BS, Berkley KJ, Hussain I, et al: Brain responses to changes in bladder volume and urge to void in healthy men. Brain 124:369, 2001.)

preoptic nuclei of the hypothalamus, cerebral cortex, red nucleus, and PAG and raphe nuclei in the brainstem, are labeled by the virus. The possible functions of these neurons in the regulation of lower urinary tract function have been revealed by lesion and electrophysiologic studies in animals[134,135] and imaging studies in humans.

Lesion studies in humans[148] and animals[149] indicate that voluntary control of micturition depends on connections between the frontal cortex and forebrain structures, such as the anterior cingulate gyrus, hypothalamus, amygdala, bed nucleus of the stria terminalis, and septal nuclei, in which electrical stimulation elicits excitatory bladder effects.[149,150] Lesions to these areas of cortex resulting from tumors, aneurysms, or cerebrovascular disease appear to remove inhibitory control over the anterior hypothalamic area, which normally provides excitatory input to micturition centers in the brainstem (see Fig. 3-8).[4,148]

The literature on the hypothalamic influences on lower urinary tract function is extensive.[2-4] Electrical stimulation of the anterior or lateral hypothalamus of animals activates the sacral parasympathetic excitatory pathway to the bladder and induces bladder contractions and voiding. In the cat, the effects of hypothalamic stimulation are probably mediated by actions in the brainstem and direct projections to the spinal cord. Axonal tracing studies in cats have shown that hypothalamic areas have diverse projections to areas of the brainstem that have an important role in the control of bladder function. For example, the anterior hypothalamic area projects directly through the medial forebrain bundle to the PMC (see Fig. 3-3). The lateral hypothalamic area projects to the parabrachial nucleus,[151] which reportedly has facilitatory effects on micturition.[4] The anterior, medial, and paraventricular areas of the hypothalamus project to the central gray matter and medullary raphe nuclei. Electrical stimulation of the latter areas and adjacent reticular formation (i.e., nucleus reticularis gigantocellularis) has been shown to exert prominent modulatory effects on bladder and urethral sphincter activity.[3,4] Medial and posterior hypothalamic areas, including the paraventricular nucleus, have direct projections to the sacral parasympathetic nucleus, the sphincter motor nucleus (i.e., Onuf's nucleus), and certain sites in the spinal cord where bladder afferents terminate (i.e., laminae I and X) (see Fig. 3-3).[123] Hypothalamic control may be mediated by direct inputs to pontine and sacral micturition centers or by indirect mechanisms through other brainstem regions.

The influence of the hypothalamus on bladder function may be modulated by afferent input from the bladder. Tracing studies in rats have identified a spinohypothalamic pathway arising from neurons in the region of the sacral parasympathetic nucleus.[112,153] FOS protein studies have shown that a large percentage of these neurons (60%) receive afferent input from the lower urinary tract.[112] This spinohypothalamic pathway may provide one route by which changes in bladder pressure modulate the firing of hypothalamic neurons.[154] This pathway also provides the anatomic substrate for putative spinohypothalamospinal and spinohypothalamopontine loops that may provide important modulatory control over micturition.

In the rat, the prefrontal cortex is considered a visceromotor area, whereas the insular cortex is considered a viscerosensory area. In rats subjected to infarction of the middle cerebral artery on one side, a prominent decrease in bladder capacity was seen, implying that there is tonic cortical inhibition of bladder function.[155-157] However, several types of synaptic changes related to inhibitory and facilitatory mechanisms involving glutamatergic and dopaminergic pathways were observed, attesting to the complexity of cortical influences on bladder control.[155-157]

Medullary centers have been implicated in inhibitory and facilitatory modulation of the micturition reflex pathway. The two most prominent modulatory mechanisms are mediated by descending bulbospinal projections from the nucleus gigantocel-

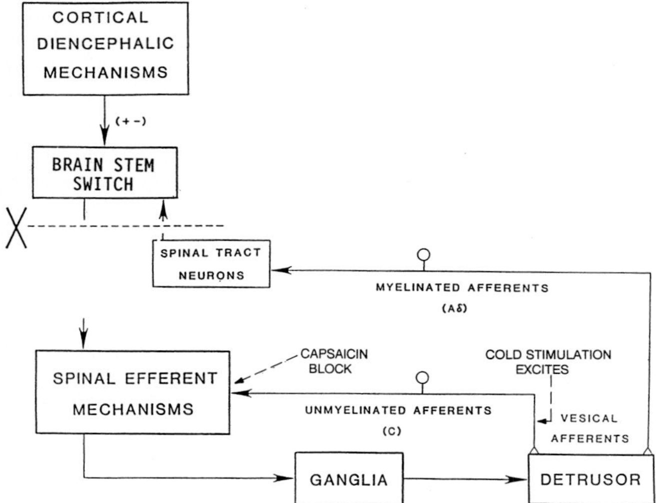

Figure 3-10 Organization of the parasympathetic excitatory reflex pathway to the detrusor muscle. The scheme of micturition reflex pathways is based on electrophysiologic studies in cats. In animals with an intact spinal cord, micturition is initiated by a supraspinal reflex pathway passing through a center in the brainstem. The pathway is triggered by myelinated afferents (A fibers), which are connected to the tension receptors in the bladder wall. Injury to the spinal cord above the sacral segments interrupts the connections between the brain and spinal autonomic centers and initially blocks micturition. However, over a period of several weeks after cord injury, a spinal reflex mechanism emerges, which is triggered by unmyelinated vesical afferents (C fibers); the A-fiber afferent inputs are ineffective. The C-fiber reflex pathway is usually weak or undetectable in animals with an intact nervous system. Stimulation of the C-fiber bladder afferents by instillation of ice water into the bladder (i.e., cold stimulation) activates voiding responses in patients with spinal cord injury. Capsaicin (20 to 30 mg SC) blocks the C-fiber reflex in chronic spinal cats, but it does not block micturition reflexes in intact cats. Intravesical capsaicin also suppresses detrusor hyperreflexia and cold-evoked reflexes in patients with neurogenic bladder dysfunction. (Adapted from de Groat WC, Kawatani M, Hisamitsu T, et al: Mechanisms underlying the recovery of urinary bladder function following spinal cord injury. J Auton Nerv Syst 30[Suppl]:S71, 1990.)

lularis reticularis (NGR) and the caudal raphe nuclei (see Fig. 3-5).[158-160] Electrical stimulation in the NGR inhibits bladder motility, reduces reflex firing in the pelvic nerve efferent pathways,[3,4] and elicits excitatory postsynaptic potentials and inhibitory postsynaptic potentials in sphincter motoneurons.[128] Electrical or chemical stimulation of the nucleus raphe magnus (NRM), which is the origin of descending serotonergic projections to the spinal cord, inhibits reflex bladder contractions and reflex firing in the sacral efferent pathways to the bladder of the cat.[158,159] Stimulation of the NRM also inhibits the firing of spinal dorsal horn neurons activated by afferents in the pelvic nerve.[160] Descending raphe spinal pathways may modulate bladder sensory mechanisms in the spinal cord, and this may account for the inhibitory effect of raphe stimulation on bladder reflexes. In the rat and cat, raphe neurons are activated by bladder distention.[160,161] This raises the possibility that afferent input from the bladder may trigger a reflex loop, resulting in activation of a raphe-spinal inhibitory pathway that may suppress the micturition reflex pathway at the spinal level.

PET studies in humans have revealed that two cortical areas, the right dorsolateral prefrontal cortex and the anterior cingulate gyrus) (see Fig. 3-9), are active (i.e., exhibited increased blood flow) during voiding.[116,143,162-164] The hypothalamus, including the preoptic area, and the pons and the PAG (see Fig. 3-9) also showed activity in concert with bladder filling or voluntary micturition. It is noteworthy that the active areas were predominately on the right side of the brain, which is consistent with reports that urge incontinence is correlated with lesions in the right hemisphere. Other PET studies that examined the changes in brain activity during filling of the bladder revealed that increased activity occurred in the PAG, the midline pons, the mid-cingulate gyrus, and bilaterally in the frontal lobes (see Fig. 3-9).[144,164] The results support the notion that the PAG receives information about bladder fullness and then relays this information to other brain areas involved in the control of bladder storage. A PET study was also conducted in adult female volunteers to identify brain structures involved in voluntary control of pelvic floor muscles.[142] The results revealed that the superomedial precentral gyrus, the most medial portion of the motor cortex, is activated during pelvic floor contraction. The right anterior cingulate gyrus also was activated during sustained pelvic floor straining.

Functional brain imaging has provided the opportunity to study cortical activation in response to different types of sensation arising from the bladder. Recognition of bladder fullness appears to be associated with activation of a network of brain regions that is distinct from that related to the perception of urinary urgency, which is associated with a decrease in activity in the hypothalamus, activation bilaterally in the premotor regions and the cingulate regions, but no activity in the PAG.[164] Activation of the primary somatosensory cortex was not seen with changes in bladder volume or the urge to void, but sensorimotor activity was observed during voiding in the presence of a catheter.[163] A difference was also seen between natural bladder filling to capacity and filling with ice water in that there was no overlap between the areas activated in these two conditions; there was marked somatosensory cortex activity but no PAG activity when filling with ice water.[165]

NEUROTRANSMITTERS IN MICTURITION REFLEX PATHWAYS

Excitatory Transmitters

Glutamic acid plays an essential role as an excitatory transmitter in the central pathways controlling the lower urinary tract of the rat.[2,3] It is involved at the level of the lumbosacral spinal cord in processing afferent input from the bladder,[166,167] at interneuronal synapses on parasympathetic preganglionic neurons,[119,120,122] and in the descending pathway from the PMC to the sacral parasympathetic nucleus (SPN).[168,169] Intrathecal or intravenous administration of NMDA or α-amino-3-hydroxy-5-methylisooxazole-4-propionic acid (AMPA) receptor antagonists in urethane-anesthetized rats depressed reflex bladder contractions and electromyographic activity of the external urethral sphincter in animals with an intact spinal cord and in chronic spinal-injured animals with the cord transected at the midthoracic level.[170-172] These results indicate that spinal reflex pathways controlling bladder and sphincter function use NMDA and AMPA glutamatergic transmitter mechanisms. Glutamate also functions as an excitatory transmitter in the micturition reflex pathways in the brain.[2,3] Administration of glutamatergic agonists into the region of the PMC in cats and rats elicits voiding or increased frequency and amplitude of bladder contractions,[3,131,159,173] whereas injection of agonists at other brainstem nuclei known to have inhibitory functions in micturition elicits inhibitory effects.[159,173] Intracerebroventricular injection of AMPA or NMDA receptor antagonists blocks reflex bladder contractions in anesthetized rats, indicating that glutamatergic transmission in the brain is essential for voiding function.[174]

Substance P is a transmitter in central neurons and in primary afferent neurons innervating the lower urinary tract.[31,41] Studies in various species (e.g., cats, rats, guinea pigs, mice) have shown that substance P or a related tachykinin released from primary afferent terminals and acting on NK_1 receptors in the spinal cord has an excitatory role in the micturition reflex pathways.[175-179] Substance P is thought to act by facilitating the action or enhancing the release of glutamic acid in the spinal cord. Intrathecal or intravenous administration of NK_1 antagonists increased bladder capacity and decreased voiding frequency in animals with normal bladders and in animals with chemically irritated bladders or with neurogenic detrusor overactivity.[175-179] NK_2 receptors also appear to play a role in the generation of chemically induced bladder hyperactivity but not normal bladder activity.[180] NK_1 receptors are upregulated in the spinal cord by chronic irritation of the bladder,[180] and destruction of NK_1 receptor–expressing neurons in the spinal cord of rats by the saporin toxin conjugated with an NK_1 receptor agonist reduces the bladder hyperactivity elicited by intravesical infusion of capsaicin.[181]

Neuronal nitric oxide synthase has been identified in afferent neurons innervating the bladder and in preganglionic neurons in the sacral parasympathetic nucleus.[182-184] Stimulation of bladder afferent nerves with capsaicin releases nitric oxide, and chronic irritation of the bladder, as well as exposure to capsaicin, increases the expression of neuronal nitric oxide synthase in dorsal root ganglion cells.[182,183] Bladder hyperactivity induced by intravesical irritants or capsaicin can be suppressed by intrathecal injection of nitric oxide synthase inhibitors, indicating that nitric oxide release in the spinal cord facilitates the micturition reflex pathway.[185-178]

Injection of ATP or $\alpha\beta$-methylene ATP into the PMC or PAG of the rat increased bladder pressure and elicited a discharge in efferent axons in the pelvic nerve.[173] The effects of the agonists were blocked by pretreatment with the purinergic receptor antagonist suramin, indicating that P2X receptors can mediate excitatory effects in the brainstem pathways underlying micturition.[173]

Inhibitory Transmitters

Several types of transmitters, including inhibitory amino acids (e.g., γ-aminobutyric acid [GABA], glycine) and opioid peptides (e.g., enkephalins) can inhibit the micturition reflex when they are applied to the central nervous system.[2,3,31] In anesthetized animals, GABA and enkephalins exert a tonic inhibitory control in the PMC and regulate bladder capacity. The inhibitory effects are mediated by $GABA_A$ and μ opioid receptors, respectively.[3,31,131,188-191] Administration of $GABA_A$ or opioid receptor antagonists into the PMC reduced the micturition volume threshold, indicating that the set point for reflex voiding is regulated by inhibitory mechanisms in the brain. The amino acids and enkephalins also have inhibitory actions in the spinal cord.[188,189] GABA and glycine are co-released from inhibitory interneurons at synapses on preganglionic neurons.[118] Glycine has also been identified as a transmitter in inhibitory pathways to sphincter motoneurons.[192] Baclofen, a $GABA_B$ agonist that mimics the inhibitory effect of GABA, has been used clinically by intrathecal administration in patients with hyperactive bladders to suppress bladder activity and promote urine storage.[193]

Transmitters with Mixed Excitatory and Inhibitory Actions

Some transmitters have inhibitory and excitatory effects, depending on the type of receptor activated. For example, dopaminergic pathways in the brain exert inhibitory or facilitatory effects on the micturition reflex through D_1-like (D_1 and D_5 receptor subtypes) and D_2-like (D_2, D_3, and D_4 receptor subtypes) dopaminergic receptors, respectively.[194-199] In anesthetized cats, activation of dopaminergic neurons in the substantia nigra inhibits reflex bladder contractions through D_1-like receptors. In awake rats, a D_1-dopamine receptor antagonist (SCH 23390) facilitated the micturition reflex, suggesting that D_1-receptor–mediated suppression of the bladder activity is tonically active in the normal, awake state.[195,198] Activation of central D_2-like dopaminergic receptors with quinpirole or bromocriptine facilitates the micturition reflex pathway in rats, cats, and monkeys.[195,197,198] D_2-like receptor–mediated facilitation of the micturition reflex may involve actions on brainstem and spinal cord because microinjection of dopamine to the PMC reduced bladder capacity and facilitated the micturition reflex in cats,[2] and intrathecal application of quinpirole induced bladder hyperactivity in normal rats and rats with 6-hydroxydopamine–lesioned nigrostriatal pathways.[199]

The monoamines, 5-hydroxytryptamine (5-HT) and norepinephrine, which are present in dense collections of nerve terminals in the lumbosacral spinal autonomic nuclei and in the sphincter motor nucleus,[3,200-202] have a complex role in the regulation of lower urinary tract function. The 5-HT–containing terminals are part of an extensive bulbospinal projection system that arises in the medullary raphe nuclei. Pharmacologic studies in animals indicate that this system may promote urine storage by exciting sympathetic and sphincter efferent pathways and by inhibiting parasympathetic excitatory outflow to the bladder.[200] Many receptors, including $5\text{-}HT_{1a}$, $5\text{-}HT_2$ and $5\text{-}HT_3$ receptors, are involved in these effects.[200-205]

Bulbospinal noradrenergic pathways acting by means of α-adrenergic receptors exert excitatory and inhibitory influences on the lower urinary tract in the rat. Intrathecal administration of an α_1-adrenergic receptor antagonist (doxazosin) decreased the amplitude of bladder contractions,[205,206] an effect that was more prominent in animals with chronic outlet obstruction.[205] Doxazosin also suppressed small amplitude nonvoiding contractions in spontaneously hypertensive rats.[207] However, doxazosin increased the frequency of isovolumetric contractions, indicating the presence of a tonic adrenergic inhibitory mechanism.[205] Intrathecal injection of the α_1-agonist phenylephrine elicited facilitatory and inhibitory effects on micturition.[208,209] Sphincter function is also modulated by the spinal noradrenergic pathways. Striated sphincter reflexes in cats, humans, and rats are inhibited by α_2-adrenergic receptor agonists such as clonidine.[210] Sympathetic and somatic pathways to the lower urinary tract in cats are suppressed by α_1-adrenergic receptor antagonists such as prazosin.[211] These data indicate the existence of α_1-adrenergic receptor–mediated tonic facilitation of sphincter function and a putative α_2-adrenergic receptor inhibitory mechanism in the spinal cord. Duloxetine, a serotonin-norepinephrine reuptake inhibitor that has been developed for the treatment of stress urinary incontinence, appears to act in part by enhancing serotonergic and noradrenergic facilitatory control of motoneurons innervating the external urethral sphincter.[212,213]

Activation of cholinergic mechanisms in the rat central nervous system with nicotinic or muscarinic receptor agonists can modulate bladder activity. Nicotinic agonists administered intracerebroventricularly suppress voiding in awake or anesthetized rats,[214] whereas activation of muscarinic receptors in the brain or spinal cord with oxotremorine stimulates bladder activity during bladder filling but suppresses voluntary voiding.[215-217] Pirenzepine, an M_1-selective blocking agent, antagonized the inhibitory effect of oxotremorine, indicating that inhibition is mediated by M_1 receptors.[218] Atropine blocked the inhibitory and excitatory effects of oxotremorine.[215] Intracerebroventricular administration of atropine alone increased bladder capacity and reduced voiding efficiency, indicating that muscarinic excitatory mechanisms in the brain are tonically active.

Intrathecal administration of various neuropeptides, including VIP, PACAP, and CRF, can influence voiding function. VIP, which is contained in C-fiber bladder afferent neurons,[67] inhibited bladder activity when administered intrathecally to normal cats but excited the bladder when administered to chronically spinal cord–injured cats.[42] These findings raised the possibility that changes in VIP synaptic mechanisms might contribute to the emergence of C-fiber afferent–mediated micturition reflexes in the chronically spinal cord–injured cat (discussed later). PACAP, another member of the secretin/glucagon/VIP peptide family, also facilitates the micturition reflex by actions on the spinal cord.[219] Patch-clamp studies revealed that PACAP has a direct excitatory action on parasympathetic PGNs, in part due to blockade of K^+ channels,[220] and has an indirect action on PGNs mediated by activation of excitatory interneurons.

CRF is contained in neurons in the rat PMC and in axons projecting from the PMC to parasympathetic nucleus in the lumbosacral spinal cord.[221] Initial studies revealed that intrathecal administration of exogenous CRF inhibited micturition and decreased the magnitude of bladder contractions induced by stimulation of the PMC.[222,223] A CRF antagonist blocked the effects of CRF and enhanced the response to PMC stimulation, indicating that endogenous CRF is released by PMC stimulation and exerts an inhibitory effect on the descending limb of the micturition reflex pathway.[223] However, later studies have shown that low doses of CRF have an excitatory effect on micturition, suggesting that CRF also has a facilitatory role in the central control of voiding.[224]

ALTERATIONS IN BLADDER REFLEX PATHWAYS AFTER NEURAL INJURY OR DISEASE

Parkinson's Disease

Degeneration of dopamine-containing neurons in patients with idiopathic Parkinson's disease is often associated with detrusor overactivity.[2,31] Animal models for Parkinson's disease have been developed by administering neurotoxins (MPTP in monkeys[196-197] and 6-hydroxy-dopamine in rats[199]) that destroy dopamine-containing neurons. Animals treated with the neurotoxins show motor symptoms typical of Parkinson's disease, and they have hyperactive bladders. Pharmacologic studies in MPTP-treated monkeys have revealed that bladder hyperactivity was caused by the loss of dopaminergic inhibition mediated by D_1-dopaminergic receptors.[196,197] The bladder hyperactivity was suppressed by stimulation of D_1 receptors with SKF 38393 or pergolide.

Stroke

The transmitter mechanisms involved in bladder dysfunction after stroke have been studied in rats after permanent occlusion of the middle cerebral artery (MCAO) on one side.[155,156,198,225] MCAO produces a dramatic and persistent reduction in bladder capacity in conscious rats. NMDA-glutamatergic mechanisms play a role in this bladder dysfunction because the bladder hyperactivity can be prevented by pretreatment with MK-801, an NMDA receptor antagonist, before MCAO or can be transiently reduced by MK-801 administered after MCAO.[156,198] The bladder hyperactivity appears to occur in two phases that depend on activation of NMDA-glutamatergic receptors. An initiation phase that occurs at the time of infarction seems to function like long-term potentiation to induce a persistent facilitation of micturition, the second phase. The maintained bladder overactivity after infarction is associated with changes in gene expression and RNA synthesis in the PMC induced by glutamatergic synaptic mechanisms.[226,227] D_2 receptors are also involved in the bladder hyperactivity induced by MCAO.[156,198] D_2-receptor antagonists do not alter voiding function in normal rats but suppress the detrusor overactivity after MCAO, indicating that D_2-facilitatory mechanisms are upregulated after cerebral infarction.

Spinal Cord Injury

Electrophysiologic studies in animals have shown that the micturition reflex pathways in neurally intact animals and in those with chronic spinal injuries are markedly different.[42,43,136,137] The most prominent change occurs in the afferent limb of the micturition reflex, which in cats with chronic spinal injuries consists of unmyelinated (C-fiber) axons.[42,43] However, in cats with an intact spinal cord, myelinated (A) afferents activate the micturition reflex (see Fig. 3-10).[136,137] This change in the afferent limb was demonstrated by electrophysiologic recording and by administering capsaicin,[42,43] a neurotoxin known to disrupt the function of C-fiber afferents.[41] In normal cats, capsaicin did not block reflex contractions of the bladder or the A-fiber–evoked bladder reflex. However, in cats with chronic spinal injury, capsaicin completely blocked the rhythmic bladder contractions induced by bladder distention and the C-fiber–evoked reflex firing recorded on bladder postganglionic nerves.[42,43]

The emergence of the C-fiber–evoked reflex in animals with chronic spinal injuries is consistent with the emergence of other types of reflexes in paraplegic humans. For example, introduction of cold water into the bladder of paraplegic patients induces reflex voiding.[228,229] However, cold stimulation has no effect in normal patients. Studies in cats indicate that cold temperatures activate C-fiber afferents (see Fig. 3-10).[38] The positive cold response in paraplegic humans may also reflect emergence of C-fiber–evoked bladder reflexes.

Mechanisms Involved in the Emergence of C-Fiber Afferent–Evoked Bladder Reflexes

The cold water test is positive in infants,[230] patients with multiple sclerosis or Parkinson's disease, and elderly patients with hyperactive bladders.[229] The presence of the cold reflex in neonates, its disappearance with maturation of the nervous system, and its reemergence under conditions in which higher brain functions are disrupted suggests that it may reflect a primitive involuntary voiding reflex organized at the spinal level. Direct evidence of the contribution of C-fiber bladder afferents to bladder hyperactivity and involuntary voiding has been obtained in clinical studies in which capsaicin or resiniferatoxin, C-fiber afferent neurotoxins,[231-233] were administered intravesically to multiple sclerosis patients with hyperreflexic bladders.[233,234] In these patients, capsaicin increased bladder capacity and reduced the frequency of incontinence. These observations suggest that capsaicin-sensitive C-fiber bladder afferents may be involved in several pathologic conditions associated with bladder hyperactivity.

The emergence of C-fiber bladder reflexes is probably mediated by several mechanisms, including changes in central synaptic connections and alterations in the properties of the peripheral afferent receptors that lead to sensitization of the "silent" C fibers and the unmasking of responses to mechanical stimuli.[147,234,235] In rats, bladder afferent neurons undergo morphologic (i.e., neuronal hypertrophy)[236] and physiologic changes (i.e., upregulation of TTX-sensitive Na^+ channels and downregulation of TTR-resistant Na^+ channels) after spinal cord injury.[59] It has been speculated that this neuroplasticity is mediated by the actions of neurotrophic factors released within the spinal cord or the urinary bladder.[234,235] Nerve growth factor (NGF) has been implicated as a chemical mediator of pathology-induced changes in C-fiber afferent nerve excitability and reflex bladder activity (see Fig. 3-2). Chronic administration of NGF into the bladder of rats induced bladder hyperactivity and increased the firing frequency of dissociated bladder afferent neurons,[237] and the production of neurotrophic factors, including NGF, increased in the bladder after spinal cord injury.[238,239] Conversely, intrathecal application of NGF antibodies, which neutralized NGF in the spinal cord, suppressed detrusor hyperreflexia and detrusor-sphincter dyssynergia in spinal cord–injured rats.[240,241] Intrathecal administration of NGF antibodies reportedly blocked autonomic dysreflexia in paraplegic rats.[242] NGF and its receptors represent new targets for the pharmacotherapy of voiding dysfunction after spinal cord injury.

Spinal cord injury alters the urothelium[243,244] and efferent pathways[245] in the bladder. Within 2 hours after spinal cord injury in rats, the apical cell layer of the urothelium is disrupted, and the urea and water permeability of the urothelial layer is increased. These changes were suppressed by a ganglionic blocking agent and therefore thought to be mediated by autonomic nerves.[243] In chronically spinal cord–injured rats, the resting release of ATP from the urothelium measured in the bladder lumen was ninefold higher than in spinal cord–intact rats.[244] Release of ATP evoked by hypo-osmotic stimulation was also increased. Instillation of botulinum toxin A into the bladder lumen reduced the evoked but not the resting release of ATP. Botulinum toxin A also reduced the stretch-induced release of ATP from cultured urothelial cells.[246] These data, coupled with the report that detrusor hyperactivity in the spinal cord–injured rat is reduced by a selective $P2X_{2/3}$ purinergic receptor antagonist,[247] indicate that enhanced purinergic signaling between the urothelium and afferent nerves contributes to neurogenic detrusor overactivity after spinal cord injury. The beneficial effects of intravesical injections of botulinum toxin A in patients with neurogenic bladder dysfunction[248-249] may be mediated by effects on the urothelium and afferent nerves and by effects on the efferent pathways to the bladder smooth muscle.

In chronically spinal cord–injured rats, facilitation of acetylcholine and norepinephrine release by prejunctional muscarinic receptors occurs at lower frequencies, leading to an enhancement of neurally evoked smooth muscle contractions.[245] It was concluded that the hyperreflexic bladder after spinal cord injury in part may reflect modulation of presynaptic mechanisms at bladder postganglionic nerve terminals. The depressant effect of botulinum toxin A on acetylcholine and norepinephrine release in the lower urinary tract[250] is likely to reverse this type of plasticity and promote urine storage in patients with neurogenic bladder dysfunction. More detailed discussions of plasticity in bladder reflex pathways after neural injury can be found in published reviews.[147,239]

CONCLUSIONS

The lower urinary tract has two main functions: storage and periodic elimination of urine. These functions are regulated by a complex neural control system located in the brain and spinal cord. This control system performs like a simple switching circuit to maintain a reciprocal relationship between the reservoir (i.e., bladder) and the outlet components (i.e., urethra and urethral sphincter) of the urinary tract. The switching circuit is modulated by several neurotransmitter systems and is therefore sensitive to a variety of drugs and neurologic diseases. A more complete understanding of the neurohumoral mechanisms involved in bladder and urethral control will no doubt facilitate the development of new diagnostic methods and therapies for lower urinary tract dysfunction.

References

1. Delancey J, Gosling J, Creed K, et al: Gross Anatomy and Cell Biology of the Lower Urinary Tract. In The Second International Consultation on Incontinence. Geneva, World Health Organization, 2002, p 16.
2. Morrison J, Steers WD, Brading A, et al: Neurophysiology and Neuropharmacology. In The Second International Consultation on Incontinence. Geneva, World Health Organization, 2002, p 83.
3. de Groat WC, Booth AM, Yoshimura N: Neurophysiology of micturition and its modification in animal models of human disease. In Maggi CA (ed): The Autonomic Nervous System, vol 3. Nervous Control of the Urogenital System. London, Harwood Academic Publishers, 1993, pp 227.
4. Torrens M, Morrison JFB: The Physiology of the Lower Urinary Tract. Berlin, Springer-Verlag, 1987.
5. Lincoln J, Burnstock G: Autonomic innervation of the urinary bladder and urethra. In Maggi CA (ed): The Autonomic Nervous System, vol 3. Nervous Control of the Urogenital System. London, Harwood Academic Publishers, 1993, p 68.

6. de Groat WC, Booth AM: Synaptic transmission in pelvic ganglia. In Maggi CA (ed): The Autonomic Nervous System, vol 3. Nervous Control of the Urogenital System. London, Harwood Academic Publishers, 1993, p 291.
7. Keast JR, Kawatani M, de Groat WC: Sympathetic modulation of cholinergic transmission in cat vesical ganglia is mediated by alpha-1 and alpha-2 adrenoceptors. Am J Physiol 258:R44, 1990.
8. Matsui M, Motomura D, Fujikawa T, et al: Mice lacking M2 and M3 muscarinic acetylcholine receptors are devoid of cholinergic smooth muscle contractions but still viable. J Neurosci 22:10627, 2002.
9. Matsui M, Motomura D, Karasawa H, et al: Multiple functional defects in peripheral autonomic organs in mice lacking muscarinic acetylcholine receptor gene for the M3 subtype. Proc Nat Acad Sci U S A 97:9579, 2000.
10. Andersson KE, Arner A: Urinary bladder contraction and relaxation: Physiology and pathophysiology. Physiol Rev 84:935, 2004.
11. Andersson KE: Pharmacology of lower urinary tract smooth muscle and penile erection tissues. Pharmacol Rev 45:253, 1993.
12. Burnstock G: Purinergic signaling in the lower urinary tract. In Abbracchio MP, Williams M (eds): Handbook of Experimental Pharmacology. Berlin, Springer-Verlag, 2001, p 423.
13. Ralevic V, Burnstock G: Receptors for purines and pyrimidines. Physiol Rev 50:413, 1998.
14. Theobald RJ, de Groat WC: The effects of purine nucleotides on transmission in vesical parasympathetic ganglia of the cat. J Auton Pharmacol 9:167, 1989.
15. Zhong Y, Dunn PM, Burnstock G: Multiple P2X receptors on guinea-pig pelvic ganglion neurons exhibit novel pharmacological properties. Br J Pharmacol 132:221, 2001.
16. O'Reilly BA, Kosaka AH, Knight GF, et al: P2X receptors and their role in female idiopathic detrusor instability. J Urol 167:157, 2002.
17. Palea S, Artibani W, Ostardo E, et al: Evidence for purinergic neurotransmission in the human urinary bladder affected by interstitial cystitis. J Urol 150:2007, 1993.
18. Ho KM, Ny L, McMurray G, et al: Co-localization of carbon monoxide and nitric oxide synthesizing enzymes in the human urethral sphincter. J Urol 161:1968, 1999.
19. Burnett AL, Calvin DC, Chamness SL, et al: Urinary bladder-urethral sphincter dysfunction in mice with targeted disruption of neuronal nitric oxide synthase models idiopathic voiding disorders in humans. Nature Med 3:571, 1997.
20. Andersson K-E, Garcia-Pascual A, Persson K, et al: Electrically induced, nerve-mediated relaxation of rabbit urethra involves nitric oxide. J Urol 147:253, 1992.
21. Zoubek JA, Somogyi GT, de Groat WC: A comparison of inhibitory effects of neuropeptide Y on rat urinary bladder, urethra and vas deferens. Am J Physiol 265:R537, 1993.
22. Barber MD, Bremer RE, Thor KB, et al: Innervation of the female levator ani muscles. Am J Obstet Gynecol 187:64, 2001.
23. Pierce ML, Reyes M, Thor KB, et al: Innervation of the levator ani muscles in the female squirrel monkey. Am J Obstet Gynecol 188:1141, 2003.
24. de Groat WC, Fraser MO, Yoshiyama M, et al: Neural control of the urethra. Scand J Urol Nephrol 35:35, 2003.
25. Kamo I, Torimoto K, Chancellor MB, et al: Urethral closure mechanisms under sneeze-induced stress condition in rats: A new animal model for evaluation of stress urinary incontinence. Am J Physiol 285:R356, 2003.
26. Somogyi GT, Tanowitz M, de Groat WC: Prejunctional facilitatory α_1-adrenoceptors in the rat urinary bladder. Br J Pharmacol 114:1710, 1995.
27. Somogyi GT, Tanowitz M, Zernova G, et al: M1 muscarinic receptor facilitation of ACh and noradrenaline release in the rat urinary bladder is mediated by protein kinase C. J Physiol (Lond) 496:245, 1996.
28. Somogyi GT, Zernova GV, Tanowitz M, et al: Role of L and N type Ca^{+2} channels in muscarinic receptor mediated facilitation of ACh and noradrenaline release in the rat urinary bladder. J Physiol (Lond) 499:645, 1997.
29. Somogyi GT, Zernova GV, Yoshiyama M, et al: Frequency dependence of muscarinic facilitation of transmitter release in urinary bladder strips from neurally intact or chronic spinal cord transected rats. Br J Pharmacol 125:241, 1998.
30. D'Agostino G, Barbieri A, Chiossa E, et al: M4 muscarinic autoreceptor-mediated inhibition of ^{3}H-acetylcholine release in the rat isolated urinary bladder. J Pharmacol Exp Ther 283:750, 1997.
31. de Groat WC, Yoshimura N: Pharmacology of the lower urinary tract. Annu Rev Pharmacol Toxicol 41:691, 2001.
32. Keast JR, de Groat WC: Immunohistochemical characterization of pelvic neurons which project to the bladder, colon, or penis in rats. J Comp Neurol 288:387, 1989.
33. Jänig W, Koltzenburg M: Pain arising from the urogenital tract. In Maggi CA (ed): The Autonomic Nervous System, vol 3. Nervous Control of the Urogenital System. London, Harwood Academic Publishers, 1993, p 525.
34. Häbler HJ, Jänig W, Koltzenburg M: Activation of unmyelinated afferent fibres by mechanical stimuli and inflammation of the urinary bladder in the cat. J Physiol (Lond) 425:545, 1990.
35. Jänig W, Koltzenburg M: On the function of spinal primary afferent fibres supplying colon and urinary bladder. J Auton Nerv Syst 30(Suppl):S89, 1990.
36. Jänig W, Morrison JFB: Functional properties of spinal visceral afferents supplying abdominal and pelvic organs, with special emphasis on visceral nociception. Prog Brain Res 67:87, 1986.
37. Roppolo JR, Tai C, Booth AM, et al: Bladder δ afferent nerve activity in normal cats and cats with interstitial cystitis. J Urol 173:1011, 2005.
38. Fall M, Lindström S, Mazieres L: A bladder-to-bladder cooling reflex in the cat. J Physiol (Lond) 427:281, 1990.
39. McMahon SB, Abel C: A model for the study of visceral pain states: Chronic inflammation of the chronic decerebrate rat urinary bladder by irritant chemicals. Pain 28:109, 1987.
40. Birder LA, de Groat WC: Increased *c-fos* expression in spinal neurons after chemical irritation of the lower urinary tract of the rat. J Neurosci 12:4878, 1992.
41. Maggi CA: The dual, sensory and efferent function of the capsaicin-sensitive primary sensory nerves in the bladder and urethra. In Maggi CA (ed): The Autonomic Nervous System, vol 3. Nervous Control of the Urogenital System. London, Harwood Academic Publishers, 1993, p 383.
42. de Groat WC, Kawatani M, Hisamitsu T, et al: Mechanisms underlying the recovery of urinary bladder function following spinal cord injury. J Auton Nerv Syst 30(Suppl):S71, 1990.
43. Cheng CL, Liu JC, Chang SY, et al: Effect of capsaicin on the micturition reflex in normal and chronic spinal cats. Am J Physiol 277: R786, 1999.
44. Morrison J, Wen J, Kibble A: Activation of pelvic afferent nerves from the rat bladder during filling. Scand J Urol Nephrol Suppl 201:73, 1999.
45. Rong W, Spyer KM, Burnstock G: Activation and sensitization of low and high threshold afferent fibres mediated by P2X receptors in the mouse urinary bladder. J Physiol (Lond) 541:591, 2002.
46. Sengupta JN, Gebhart GF: Mechanosensitive properties of pelvic afferent nerve fibers innervating the urinary bladder of the rat. J Neurophysiol 72:2420, 1994.
47. Shea VK, Cai R, Crepps B, et al: Sensory fibers of the pelvic nerve innervating the rat's bladder. J Neurophysiol 84:1924, 2000.
48. Namasivayam S, Eardley I, Morrison JFB: Purinergic sensory neurotransmission in the urinary bladder: An in vitro study in the rat. Br J Urol Int 84:854, 1999.
49. Dmitrieva N, Shelton D, Rice AS, et al: The role of nerve growth factor in a model of visceral inflammation. Neuroscience 78:449, 1997.

50. Ozawa H, Chancellor MB, Jung SY, et al: Effect of intravesical nitric oxide therapy on cyclophosphamide-induced cystitis. J Urol 162:2211, 1999.
51. Pandita RK, Mizusawa H, Andersson KE: Intravesical oxyhemoglobin initiates bladder overactivity in conscious normal rats. J Urol 164:545, 2000.
52. Chuang Y, Fraser MO, Yu Y, et al: The role of bladder afferent pathways in the bladder hyperactivity induced by intravesical administration of nerve growth factor. J Urol 165:975, 2001.
53. Jaggar SI, Scott HC, Rice AS: Inflammation of the rat urinary bladder is associated with a referred thermal hyperalgesia which is nerve growth factor dependent. Br J Anesth 83:442, 1999.
54. Ogawa T, Kamo I, Pflug BR, et al: Differential roles of peripheral and spinal endothelin receptors in the micturition reflex in rats. J Urol 172:1533, 2005.
55. Bahns E, Ernsberger U, Janig W, et al: Functional characteristics of lumbar visceral afferent fibers from the urinary bladder and urethra in the cat. Eur J Physiol 407:510, 1998.
56. Kawatani M, Takeshige C, de Groat WC: Central distribution of afferent pathways from the uterus of the cat. J Comp Neurol 302:294, 1990.
57. Kawatani M, Tanowitz M, de Groat WC: Morphological and electrophysiological analysis of the peripheral and central afferent pathways from the clitoris of the cat. Brain Res 646:26, 1994.
58. Yoshimura N, de Groat WC: Increased excitability of afferent neurons innervating rat urinary bladder following chronic bladder inflammation. J Neurosci 19:4644, 1999.
59. Yoshimura N, de Groat WC: Plasticity of Na^+ channels in afferent neurons innervating rat urinary bladder following spinal cord injury. J Physiol (Lond) 503:269, 1997.
60. Yoshimura N, Seki S, Erickson KA, et al: Histological and electrical properties of rat dorsal root ganglion neurons innervating the lower urinary tract. J Neurosci 23:4355, 2003.
61. Yoshimura N, Seki S, Novakovic SD, et al: The role of the tetrodotoxin-resistant sodium channel $Na_v1.8$ (PN3/SNS) in a rat model of visceral pain. J Neurosci 21:8690, 2001.
62. Yoshimura N, White G, Weight FF, et al: Different types of Na^+ and A-type K^+ currents in dorsal root ganglion neurons innervating the rat urinary bladder. J Physiol (Lond) 494:1, 1996.
63. Sculptoreanu A, de Groat WC, Buffington CAT, et al: Protein kinase C contributes to abnormal capsaicin responses in DRG neurons from cats with feline interstitial cystitis. Neurosci Lett 381:42, 2005.
64. Sculptoreanu A, de Groat WC, Buffington CAT, et al: Abnormal excitability in capsaicin-responsive DRG neurons from cats with feline interstitial cystitis. Exp Neurol 193:437, 2005.
65. Zhong Y, Banning AS, Cockayne DA, et al: Bladder and cutaneous sensory neurons of the rat express different functional P2X receptors. Neurosci 120:667, 2003.
66. Keast JR, de Groat WC: Segmental distribution and peptide content of primary afferent neurons innervating the urogenital organs and colon of male rats. J Comp Neurol 319:615, 1992.
67. de Groat WC: Neuropeptides in pelvic afferent pathways. Experientia Suppl 56:334, 1989.
68. Lewis SA: Everything you wanted to know about the bladder epithelium but were afraid to ask. Am J Physiol 278:F867, 2000.
69. Lavelle JP, Meyers S, Ruiz G, et al: Urothelial pathophysiological changes in feline interstitial cystitis: A human model. Am J Physiol 278:F540, 2000.
70. Birder LA, Ruan HZ, Chopra B, et al: Alterations in P2X and P2Y purinergic receptor expression in urinary bladder from normal cats and cats with interstitial cystitis. Am J Physiol 287:F1084, 2004.
71. Birder LA, Apodaca G, de Groat WC, et al: Adrenergic and capsaicin evoked nitric oxide release from urothelium and afferent nerves in urinary bladder. Am J Physiol 275:F226, 1998.
72. Birder LA, Barrick S, Roppolo JR, et al: Feline interstitial cystitis results in mechanical hypersensitivity and altered ATP release from bladder urothelium. Am J Physiol 285:F423, 2003.
73. Birder LA, Kanai AJ, de Groat WC, et al: Vanilloid receptor expression suggest a sensory role for urinary bladder epithelial cells. Proc Natl Acad Sci U S A 98:13396, 2001.
74. Birder LA, Nakamura Y, Kiss S, et al: Altered urinary bladder function in mice lacking the vanilloid receptor TRPV1. Nat Neurosci 5:856, 2002.
75. Birder LA, Nealon M, Kiss S, et al: β-Adrenoceptor agonists stimulate endothelial nitric oxide synthase in rat urinary bladder urothelial cells. J Neurosci 22:8063, 2002.
76. Cockayne DA, Hamilton SG, Zhu QM, et al: Urinary bladder hyporeflexia and reduced pain behaviour in P2X3 deficient mice. Nature 407:1011, 2000.
77. Ferguson DR, Kennedy I, Burton TJ: ATP is released from rabbit urinary bladder cells by hydrostatic pressure changes—A possible sensory mechanism? J Physiol (Lond) 505:503, 1997.
78. Tempest HV, Dixon AK, Turner WH, et al: P2X and P2X receptor expression in human bladder urothelium and changes in interstitial cystitis. BJU Int 93:1344-1348, 2004.
79. Apodaca G: The uroepithelium: Not just a passive barrier. Traffic 5:117, 2004.
80. de Groat WC: The urothelium in overactive bladder: Passive bystander or active participant? Urol 64:7, 2004.
81. Apostolidis A, Brady CM, Yiangou Y, et al: Capsaicin receptor TRPV1 in urothelium of neurogenic human bladders and effect of intravesical resiniferatoxin. Urology 65:400, 2005.
82. Andersson KE, Yoshida M: Antimuscarinics and the overactive detrusor—Which is the main mechanism of action? Eur Urol 43:1, 2003.
83. Stein RJ, Santos S, Nagatomi J, et al: Cool (TRPM8) and hot (TRPV1) receptors in the bladder and male genital tract. J Urol 172:1175, 2004.
84. Brady CM, Apostolidis A, Yiangou Y, et al: P2X3-immunoreactive nerve fibres in neurogenic detrusor overactivity and the effect of intravesical resiniferatoxin. Eur Urol 46:247, 2004.
85. Brady CM, Apostolidis AN, Harper M, et al: Parallel changes in bladder suburothelial vanilloid receptor TRPV1 and pan-neuronal marker PGP9.5 immunoreactivity in patients with neurogenic detrusor overactivity after intravesical resiniferatoxin treatment. BJU Int 93:770, 2004.
86. Pandita RK, Andersson KE: Intravesical adenosine triphosphate stimulates the micturition reflex in awake, freely moving rats. J Urol 168:1230, 2002.
87. Knight GE, Bodin P, de Groat WC, et al: ATP is released from epithelium of the guinea pig ureter upon distension. Am J Physiol 282:F281, 2002.
88. Vlaskovska M, Kasakov L, Rong W, et al: P2X3 knockout mice reveal a major sensory role for urothelially released ATP. J Neurosci 21:5670, 2001.
89. Sun Y, Keay S, De Deyne PG, et al: Augmented stretch activated adenosine triphosphate release from bladder uroepithelial cells in patients with interstitial cystitis. J Urol 166:1951, 2001.
90. Birder LA, Wolf-Johnston A, Buffington CA, et al: Altered inducible nitric oxide synthase expression and nitric oxide production in the bladder of cats with feline interstitial cystitis. J Urol 173:625, 2005.
91. Keay S, Kleinberg M, Zhang CO, et al: Bladder epithelial cells from patients with interstitial cystitis produce an inhibitor of heparin-binding epidermal growth factor-like growth factor production. J Urol 164:2112, 2000.
92. Keay SK, Zhang CO, Shoenfelt J, et al: Sensitivity and specificity of antiproliferative factor, heparin-binding epidermal growth factor-like growth factor, and epidermal growth factor as urine markers for interstitial cystitis. Urology 57:9, 2001.
93. Keay SK, Szekely Z, Conrads TP, et al: An antiproliferative factor from interstitial cystitis patients is a frizzled 8 protein-related sialoglycopeptide. Proc Natl Acad Sci U S A 101:11803, 2004.
94. Sui GP, Rothery S, Dupont E, et al: Gap junctions and connexin expression in human suburothelial interstitial cells. BJU Int 90:118, 2002.

95. Wiseman OJ, Fowler CJ, Landon DN: The role of the human bladder lamina propria myofibroblast. BJU Int 91:89, 2003.
96. Wu C, Sui GP, Fry CH: Purinergic regulation of guinea pig suburothelial myofibroblasts. J Physiol (Lond) 559:231, 2004.
97. Morgan CW, de Groat WC, Felkins LA, et al: Intracellular injection of neurobiotin or horseradish peroxidase reveals separate types of preganglionic neurons in the sacral parasympathetic nucleus of the cat. J Comp Neurol 331:161, 1993.
98. Morgan CW, de Groat WC, Felkins LA, et al: Axon collaterals indicate broad intraspinal role for sacral preganglionic neurons. Proc Nat Acad Sci U S A 88:6888, 1991.
99. de Groat WC: Mechanisms underlying recurrent inhibition in the sacral parasympathetic outflow to the urinary bladder. J Physiol (Lond) 257:503, 1976.
100. Thor KB, Morgan C, Nadelhaft I, et al: Organization of afferent and efferent pathways in the pudendal nerve of the female cat. J Comp Neurol 288:263, 1989.
101. Roppolo JR, Nadelhaft I, de Groat WC: The organization of pudendal motoneurons and primary afferent projections in the spinal cord of the rhesus monkey revealed by horseradish peroxidase. J Comp Neurol 234:475, 1985.
102. Sasaki M: Morphological analysis of external urethral and external anal sphincter motoneurons of cat. J Comp Neurol 349:269, 1994.
103. Morgan C, Nadelhaft I, de Groat WC: The distribution of visceral primary afferents from the pelvic nerve within Lissauer's tract and the spinal gray matter and its relationship to the sacral parasympathetic nucleus. J Comp Neurol 201:415, 1981.
104. de Groat WC: Spinal cord projections of visceral afferent neurones. In Cervero F, Morrison JFB (eds): Visceral Sensation. Amsterdam, Elsevier, 1986, p 165.
105. Steers WD, Ciambotti J, Etzel B, et al: Alterations in afferent pathways from the urinary bladder of the rat in response to partial urethral obstruction. J Comp Neurol 310:401, 1991.
106. Cheng CL, Ma CP, de Groat WC: The effects of capsaicin on micturition and associated reflexes in the rat. Am J Physiol 265:R132, 1993.
107. Gustafson KJ, Creasey GH, Grill WM: A urethral afferent mediated excitatory bladder reflex exists in humans. Neurosci Lett 360:9, 2004.
108. de Groat WC, Nadelhaft I, Milne RJ, et al: Organization of the sacral parasympathetic reflex pathways to the urinary bladder and large intestine. J Auton Nerv Syst 3:135, 1981.
109. de Groat WC: Excitation and inhibition of sacral parasympathetic neurons by visceral and cutaneous stimuli in the cat. Brain Res 33:499, 1971.
110. Birder LA, de Groat WC: Induction of *c-fos* gene expression in spinal neurons in the rat by nociceptive and non-nociceptive stimulation of the lower urinary tract. Am J Physiol 265:R643, 1993.
111. Birder LA, Roppolo JR, Iadarola MJ, et al: Electrical stimulation of visceral afferent pathways in the pelvic nerve increases *c-fos* in the rat lumbosacral spinal cord. Neurosci Lett 129:193, 1991.
112. Birder LA, Roppolo JR, Erickson VL, et al: Increased *c-fos* expression in spinal lumbosacral projection and preganglionic neurons after irritation of the lower urinary tract in the rat. Brain Res 834:55, 1999.
113. Nadelhaft I, Vera PL, Card JP, et al: Central nervous system neurons labeled following the injection of pseudorabies virus into the rat urinary bladder. Neurosci Lett 143:271, 1992.
114. Sugaya K, Roppolo JR, Yoshimura N, et al: The central neural pathways involved in micturition in the neonatal rats as revealed by the injection of pseudorabies virus into the bladder. Neurosci Lett 223:197, 1997.
115. Vizzard MA, Erickson VL, Card JP, et al: Transneuronal labeling of neurons in the adult rat brain and spinal cord after injection of pseudorabies virus into the urethra. J Comp Neurol 355:629, 1995.
116. Blok BFM: Brain control of the lower urinary tract. Scand J Urol Nephrol 36:11, 2002.
117. Sie JA, Blok BF, de Weerd H, et al: Ultrastructural evidence for direct projections from the pontine micturition center to glycine-immunoreactive neurons in the sacral dorsal gray commissure in the cat. J Comp Neurol 429:631, 2001.
118. Araki I: Inhibitory postsynaptic currents and the effects of GABA on visually identified sacral parasympathetic preganglionic neurons in neonatal rats. J Neurophysiol 72:2903, 1994.
119. Araki I, de Groat WC: Unitary excitatory synaptic currents in preganglionic neurons mediated by two distinct groups of interneurons in neonatal rat sacral parasympathetic nucleus. J Neurophysiol 76:215, 1996.
120. Araki I, de Groat WC: Synaptic modulation associated with developmental reorganization of visceral reflex pathways. J Neurosci 17:8402, 1997.
121. Miura A, Kawatani M, de Groat WC: Excitatory synaptic currents in lumbosacral parasympathetic preganglionic neurons elicited from the lateral funiculus. J Neurophysiol 86:1587, 2001.
122. Miura A, Kawatani M, de Groat WC: Excitatory synaptic currents in lumbosacral parasympathetic preganglionic neurons evoked by stimulation of the dorsal commissure. J Neurophysiol 89:382, 2003.
123. Holstege G: Some anatomical observations on the projections from the hypothalamus to brainstem and spinal cord: An HRP and autoradiographic tracing study in the cat. J Comp Neurol 260:98, 1987.
124. Holstege G, Griffiths D, de Wall H, et al: Anatomical and physiological observations on supraspinal control of bladder and urethral sphincter muscles in the cat. J Comp Neurol 250:449, 1986.
125. Holstege G, Mouton LJ: Central nervous system control of micturition. Int Rev Neurobiol 56:123, 2003.
126. de Groat WC, Theobald RJ: Reflex activation of sympathetic pathways to vesical smooth muscle and parasympathetic ganglia by electrical stimulation of vesical afferents. J Physiol (Lond) 259:223, 1976.
127. de Groat WC, Lalley PM: Reflex firing in the lumbar sympathetic outflow to activation of vesical afferent fibres. J Physiol (Lond) 226:289, 1972.
128. Mackel R: Segmental and descending control of the external urethral and anal sphincters in the cat. J Physiol (Lond) 294:105, 1979.
129. Shefchyk SJ: The effects of lumbosacral deafferentation on pontine micturition centre-evoked voiding in the decerebrate cat. Neurosci Lett 99:175, 1989.
130. Kruse MN, Mallory BS, Noto H, et al: Properties of the descending limb of the spinobulbospinal micturition reflex pathway in the cat. Brain Res 556:6, 1991.
131. Mallory BS, Roppolo JR, de Groat WC: Pharmacological modulation of the pontine micturition center. Brain Res 546:310, 1991.
132. Holstege G, Tan J: Supraspinal control of motoneurons innervating the striated muscles of the pelvic floor including urethral and anal sphincters in the cat. Brain 110:1323, 1987.
133. Kruse MN, Noto H, Roppolo JR, et al: Pontine control of the urinary bladder and external urethral sphincter in the rat. Brain Res 532:182, 1990.
134. Tang PC, Ruch TC: Localization of brain stem and diencephalic areas controlling the micturition reflex. J Comp Neurol 106:213, 1956.
135. Tang PC: Levels of the brain stem and diencephalon controlling the micturition reflex. J Neurophysiol 18:583, 1955.
136. de Groat WC: Nervous control of the urinary bladder of the cat. Brain Res 87:201, 1975.
137. de Groat WC, Ryall RW: Reflexes to sacral parasympathetic neurons concerned with micturition in the cat. J Physiol (Lond) 200:87, 1969.

138. Noto H, Roppolo JR, Steers WD, et al: Excitatory and inhibitory influences on bladder activity elicited by electrical stimulation in the pontine micturition center in rat. Brain Res 492:99, 1989.
139. Block BF, de Weerd H, Holstege G: Ultrastructural evidence for a paucity of projections from the lumbosacral cord to the pontine micturition center or M-region in the cat: A new concept for the organization of the micturition reflex with the periaqueductal gray as central relay. J Comp Neurol 359:300, 1995.
140. Blok BF, Holstege G: Direct projections form the periaqueductal gray to the pontine micturition center (M-region). An anterograde and retrograde tracing study in the cat. Neurosci Lett 166:93, 1994.
141. Ding QY, Zheng HX, Gong LW, et al: Direct projections from the lumbosacral spinal cord to Barrington's nucleus in the rat: A special reference to the micturition reflex. J Comp Neurol 389:149-160, 1997.
142. Blok BFM, Sturms LM, Holstege G: A PET study on cortical and subcortical control of the pelvic floor musculature in women. J Comp Neurol 389:535, 1997.
143. Blok BFM, Willemsen ATM, Holstege G: A PET study on the brain control of micturition in humans. Brain 120:111, 1997.
144. Athwal BS, Berkley KJ, Hussain I, et al: Brain responses to changes in bladder volume and urge to void in healthy men. Brain 124:369, 2001.
145. Kruse MN, de Groat WC: Spinal pathways mediate coordinated bladder/urethral sphincter activity during reflex micturition in normal and spinal cord injured neonatal rats. Neurosci Lett 152:141-144, 1993.
146. Kruse MN, de Groat WC: Consequences of spinal cord injury during the neonatal period on micturition reflexes in the rat. Exp Neurol 125:87, 1994.
147. de Groat WC, Yoshimura N: Mechanisms underlying the recovery of lower urinary tract function following spinal cord injury. In Weaver LC, Polosa C (eds): Progress in Brain Research. Autonomic Dysfunction after Spinal Cord Injury 152: 59, 2006.
148. Nathan PW: The central nervous connections of the bladder. In Williams DI, Chisholm GD (eds): Scientific Foundations of Urology, vol II. Chicago, Year Book, 1976, p 51.
149. Gjone R: Excitatory and inhibitory responses to stimulation of 'limbic', diencephalic and mesencephalic structures in the cat. Acta Physiol Scand 66:91, 1966.
150. Langworthy OR, Kolb LC: The encephalic control of tone in the musculature of the urinary bladder. Brain 56:371, 1933.
151. Moga MM, Herbert H, Hurley KM, et al: Organization of cortical, basal forebrain, and hypothalamic afferents to the parabrachial nucleus in the rat. J Comp Neurol 295:624, 1990.
152. McMahon SB, Spillane K: Brain stem influences on the parasympathetic supply to the urinary bladder of the cat. Brain Res 234:237, 1982.
153. Burstein R, Wang JL, Elde RP, et al: Neurons in the sacral parasympathetic nucleus that project to the hypothalamus do not also project through the pelvic nerve—A double labeling study combining Fluoro-gold and cholera toxin B in the rat. Brain Res 506:159, 1990.
154. Stuart DG, Porter RW, Adey WR, et al: Hypothalamic unit activity. I. Visceral and somatic influences. Electroencephalogr Clin Neurophysiol 16:237, 1964.
155. Yokoyama O, Yoshiyama M, Namiki M, et al: Influence of anesthesia on bladder hyperactivity induced by middle cerebral artery occlusion in the rat. Am J Physiol 273:R1900, 1997.
156. Yokoyama O, Yoshiyama M, Namiki M, et al: Changes in dopaminergic and glutamatergic excitatory mechanisms of micturition reflex after middle cerebral artery occlusion in conscious rats. Exp Neurol 173:129, 2002.
157. Yokoyama O, Yoshiyama M, Namiki M, et al: Interaction between D_2 dopaminergic and glutamatergic excitatory influences on lower urinary tract function in normal and cerebral-infarcted rats. Exp Neurol 169:148, 2001.
158. Morrison JFB, Spillane K: Neuropharmacological studies on descending inhibitory controls over the micturition reflex. J Auton Nerv Syst (Suppl):393, 1986.
159. Chen SY, Wang SD, Cheng CL, et al: Glutamate activation of neurons in cardiovascular reactive areas of the cat brain stem affects urinary bladder motility. Am J Physiol 265:F520, 1993.
160. Lumb BM: Brainstem control of visceral afferent pathways in the spinal cord. Prog Brain Res 67:279, 1986.
161. Chandler MJ, Oh UT, Hobbs SF, et al: Response of feline raphe-spinal neurons to urinary bladder distension. J Auton Nerv Sys 47:213, 1994.
162. Blok BF, Sturms LM, Holstege G: Brain activation during micturition in women. Brain 121:2033, 1998
163. Nour S, Svarer C, Kristensen JK, et al: Cerebral activation during micturition in normal men. Brain 123:781, 2000.
164. Athwal BS, Berkley KJ, Brennan A, et al: Brain activity associated with the urge to void and bladder fill volume in normal men: Preliminary data from a PET study. BJU Int 84:148, 1999.
165. Matsuura S, Kakizaki H, Mitsui T, et al: Human brain region response to distention or cold stimulation of the bladder: A positron emission tomography study. J Urol 168:2035, 2002.
166. Birder LA, de Groat WC: The effect of glutamate antagonists on *c-fos* expression induced in spinal neurons by irritation of the lower urinary tract. Brain Res 580:115, 1992.
167. Kakizaki H, Yoshiyama M, de Groat WC: Role of NMDA and AMPA glutamatergic transmission in spinal *c-fos* expression after urinary tract irritation. Am J Physiol 270:R990, 1996.
168. Matsumoto G, Hisamitsu T, de Groat WC: Role of glutamate and NMDA receptors in the descending limb of the spinobulbospinal micturition reflex pathway of the rat. Neurosci Lett 183:58, 1995.
169. Matsumoto G, Hisamitsu T, de Groat WC: Non-NMDA glutamatergic excitatory transmission in the descending limb of the spinobulbospinal micturition reflex pathway in the rat. Brain Res 693:246, 1995.
170. Yoshiyama M, Roppolo JR, de Groat WC: The effects of MK801 on the micturition reflex in the rat: Possible sites of action. J Pharmacol Exp Ther 265:844, 1993.
171. Yoshiyama M, Roppolo JR, de Groat WC: Effects of LY215490, a competitive alpha-amino-3-hydroxy-5-methylisooxazole-4-propionic acid (AMPA) receptor antagonist, on the micturition reflex in the rat. J Pharmacol Exp Ther 280:894, 1997.
172. Yoshiyama M, Roppolo JR, de Groat WC: Alterations by urethane of glutamatergic control of micturition. Eur J Pharmacol 264:417, 1994.
173. Rocha I, Burnstock G, Spyer KM: Effect on urinary bladder function and arterial blood pressure of the activation of putative purine receptors in brainstem areas. Auton Neurosci 88:6, 2001.
174. Yoshiyama M, de Groat WC: Supraspinal and spinal alpha-amino-3-hydroxy-5-methylisooxazole-4-propionic acid and *N*-methyl-D-aspartate glutamatergic control of the micturition reflex in the urethane anesthetized rat. Neuroscience 132:1017, 2005.
175. Lecci A, Giuliani S, Maggi CA: Effect of the NK-1 receptor antagonist GR 82,334 on reflex-induced bladder contractions. Life Sci 51:277, 1992.
176. Kamo I, Doi T: Effect of TAK-637, a tachykinin NK1 receptor antagonist, on lower urinary tract function in cats. Jap J Pharmacol 86:165, 2001.
177. Ishizuka O, Igawa Y, Lecci A, et al: Role of intrathecal tachykinins for micturition in unanaesthetized rats with and without bladder outlet obstruction. Br J Pharmacol 113:111, 1994.
178. Ishizuka O, Mattiasson A, Andersson KE: Effects of neurokinin receptor antagonists on L-dopa induced bladder hyperactivity in normal conscious rats. J Urol 154:1548, 1995.
179. Lecci A, Giuliani S, Tramontana M, et al: MEN 11,420, a peptide tachykinin NK_2 receptor antagonist, reduces motor responses

induced by the intravesical administration of capsaicin in vivo. Naunyn Schmiedebergs Arch Pharmacol 356:182, 1997.

180. Ishigooka M, Zermann DH, Doggweiler R, et al: Spinal NK1 receptor is upregulated after chronic bladder irritation. Pain 93:43, 2001.
181. Seki S, Erickson KE, Seki M, et al: Elimination of lamina I spinal neurons expressing neurokinin 1 receptor using [Sar^9, Met $(O_2)^{11}$] substance-saporin reduces bladder overactivity and spinal *c-fos* expression induced by intravesical instillation of capsaicin. Am J Physiol 288:F466, 2005.
182. Vizzard MA, Erdman SL, de Groat WC: Increased expression of neuronal nitric oxide synthase (NOS) in dorsal rat ganglion neurons after systemic capsaicin administration. Neuroscience 67:1, 1995.
183. Vizzard MA, Erdman SL, de Groat WC: Increased expression of neuronal nitric oxide synthase in bladder afferent pathways following chronic bladder irritation. J Comp Neurol 370:191, 1996.
184. Vizzard MA, Erdman SL, Erickson VL, et al: Localization of NADPH diaphorase in the lumbosacral spinal cord and dorsal root ganglia of the cat. J Comp Neurol 339:62, 1994.
185. Rice AS: Topical spinal administration of a nitric oxide synthase inhibitor prevents the hyper-reflexia associated with a rat model of persistent visceral pain. Neurosci Let 187:111, 1995.
186. Kakizaki H, de Groat WC: Role of spinal nitric oxide in the facilitation of the micturition reflex by bladder irritation. J Urol 155:355, 1996.
187. Pandita RK, Persson K, Andersson KE: Capsaicin-induced bladder overactivity and nociceptive behaviour in conscious rats: Involvement of spinal nitric oxide. J Auton Nerv Syst 67:184, 1997.
188. Hisamitsu T, de Groat WC: The inhibitory effect of opioid peptides and morphine applied intrathecally and intracerebroventricularly on the micturition reflex in the cat. Brain Res 298:51, 1984.
189. Maggi CA, Furio M, Santicioli P, et al: The spinal and supraspinal components of GABAergic inhibition of the micturition reflex in rats. J Pharmacol Exp Ther 240:998, 1987.
190. Kontani H, Kawabata Y, Koshiura R: In vivo effects of gamma-aminobutyric acid on the urinary bladder contraction accompanying micturition. Jpn J Pharmacol 45:45, 1987.
191. Sillën U, Persson B, Rubenson A: Involvement of central GABA receptors in the regulation of the urinary bladder function of anaesthetized rats. Naunyn Schmiedebergs Arch Pharmacol 314:195, 1980.
192. Shefchyk SJ, Espey MJ, Carr P, et al: Evidence for a strychnine-sensitive mechanism and glycine receptors involved in the control of urethral sphincter activity during micturition in the cat. Exp Brain Res 119:297, 1998.
193. Steers WD, Meythaler JM, Haworth C, et al: Effects of acute bolus and chronic continuous intrathecal baclofen on genitourinary dysfunction due to spinal cord pathology. J Urol 148:1849, 1992.
194. Yoshimura N, Sasa M, Yoshida O, et al: Dopamine D-1 receptor-mediated inhibition of micturition reflex by central dopamine from the substantia nigra. Neurourol Urodyn 11:535, 1992.
195. Seki S, Igawa Y, Kaidoh K, et al: Role of dopamine D1 and D2 receptors in the micturition reflex in conscious rats. Neurourol Urodyn 20:105, 2001.
196. Yoshimura N, Mizuta E, Kuno S, et al: The dopamine D1 receptor agonist SKF 38393 suppresses detrusor hyperreflexia in the monkey with parkinsonism induced by 1-methyl-4-phenyl-1,2,3,6-tetrahydropyridine (MPTP). Neuropharmacol 32:315, 1993.
197. Yoshimura N, Mizuta E, Yoshida O, et al: Therapeutic effects of dopamine D_1/D_2 receptor agonists on detrusor hyperreflexia in 1-methyl-4-phenyl-1,2,3,6-tetrahydropyridine-lesioned parkinsonian cynomolgus monkeys. J Pharmacol Exp Ther 286:228, 1998.
198. Yokoyama O, Yoshiyama M, Namiki M, et al: Glutamatergic and dopaminergic contributions to rat bladder hyperactivity following cerebral artery occlusion. Am J Physiol 276:R935, 1999.
199. Yoshimura N, Kuno S, Chancellor MB, et al: Dopaminergic mechanisms underlying bladder hyperactivity in rats with a unilateral 6-hydroxydopamine (6-OHDA) lesion of the nigrostriatal pathway. Br J Pharmacol 139:1425, 2003.
200. de Groat WC: Influence of serotonergic mechanisms in the spinal cord on lower urinary tract function. Urology 59:30, 2002.
201. Thor KB: Targeting serotonin and norepinephrine receptors in stress urinary incontinence. Int J Gynecol Obstet 86(Suppl 1):S38, 2004.
202. Thor KB, Donatucci C: Central nervous system control of the lower urinary tract: New pharmacological approaches to stress urinary incontinence in women. J Urol 172:27, 2004.
203. Guarneri L, Ibba M, Testa R, et al: The effect of mCPP on bladder voiding contractions in rats are mediated by the 5HT2A/5-HT2C receptors. Neurourol Urodyn 15:316, 1996.
204. Espey MJ, Du HJ, Downie JW: Serotonergic modulation of spinal ascending activity and sacral reflex activity evoked by pelvic nerve stimulation in cats. Brain Res 798:101, 1998.
205. Ishizuka O, Persson K, Mattiasson A, et al: Micturition in conscious rats with and without bladder outlet obstruction: Role of spinal alpha 1-adrenoceptors. Br J Pharmacol 117:962, 1996.
206. Ishizuka O, Pandita RK, Mattiasson A, et al: Stimulation of bladder activity by volume, L-dopa and capsaicin in normal conscious rats—Effects of spinal alpha 1-adrenoceptor blockade. Naunyn Schmiedebergs Arch Pharmacol 355:787, 1997.
207. Persson K, Pandita RK, Spitsbergen JM, et al: Spinal and peripheral mechanisms contributing to hyperactive voiding in spontaneously hypertensive rats. Am J Physiol 275:R1366, 1998.
208. de Groat WC, Yoshiyama M, Ramage AG, et al: Modulation of voiding and storage reflexes by activation of alpha1-adrenoceptors. Eur Urol 36:68, 1999.
209. Yoshiyama M, Yamamoto T, de Groat WC: Role of spinal α_1-adrenergic mechanisms in the control of lower urinary tract in the rat. Brain Res 882:36, 2000.
210. Dennys P, Chartier-Kastler E, Azouvi P, et al: Intrathecal clonidine for refractory detrusor hyperreflexia in spinal cord injured patients: A preliminary report. J Urol 160:2137, 1998.
211. Danuser H, Thor KB: Inhibition of central sympathetic and somatic outflow to the urinary tract of the cat by the α_1-adrenergic receptor agonist prazosin. J Urol 153:1308, 1995.
212. Burgard EC, Fraser MO, Thor KB: Serotonergic modulation of bladder afferent pathways. Urology 62:10, 2003.
213. Burgard EC, Fraser MO, Karicheti V, et al: New pharmacological treatments for urinary incontinence and overactive bladder. Curr Opin Investig Drugs 6:81, 2005.
214. Lee SJ, Nakamura Y, de Groat WC: Effect of ±-epibatidine, a nicotinic agonist, on the central pathways controlling voiding function in the rat. Am J Physiol 285:R84, 2003.
215. Ishiura Y, Yoshiyama M, Yokoyama O, et al: Central muscarinic mechanisms regulating voiding in rats. J Pharmacol Exp Ther 297:933, 2001.
216. Nakamura Y, Ishiura Y, Yokoyama O, et al: Role of protein kinase C in central muscarinic inhibitory mechanisms regulating voiding in rats. Neuroscience 116:477, 2003.
217. Ishizuka O, Gu BJ, Yang ZX, et al: Functional role of central muscarinic receptors for micturition in normal conscious rats. J Urol 168:2258, 2002.
218. Yokoyama O, Ootsuka N, Komatsu K, et al: Forebrain muscarinic control of micturition reflex in rats. Neuropharmacology 41:629, 2001.
219. Ishizuka O, Alm P, Larsson B, et al: Facilitatory effect of pituitary adenylate cyclase activating polypeptide on micturition in normal, conscious rats. Neuroscience 66:1009, 1995.
220. Miura A, Kawatani M, de Groat WC: Effect of pituitary adenylate cyclase activating polypeptide on lumbosacral preganglionic neurons in the neonatal rat spinal cord. Brain Res 895:223, 2001.
221. Puder BA, Papka RE: Distribution and origin of corticotropin-releasing factor-immunoreactive axons in the female rat lumbosacral spinal cord. J Neurosci Res 66:1217, 2001.

222. Suzuki T, Kawatani M, Erdman S, et al: Role of CRF and 5HT in central pathways controlling micturition in the rat. Soc Neurosci Abstr 16:1064, 1990.
223. Pavcovich LA, Valentino RJ: Central regulation of micturition in the rat by corticotropin releasing hormone from Barrington's nucleus. Neurosci Lett 196:185, 1995.
224. Klausner AP, Steers WD: Corticotropin releasing factor: A mediator of emotional influences on bladder function. J Urol 172:2570, 2004.
225. Yokoyama O, Yoshiyama M, Namiki M, et al: Role of the forebrain in bladder overactivity following cerebral infarction in the rat. Exp Neurol 163:469, 2000.
226. Yokoyama O, Yotsuyanagi S, Akino H, et al: RNA synthesis in the pons necessary for maintenance of bladder overactivity after cerebral infarction in the rat. J Urol 169:1878, 2003.
227. Yotsuyanagi S, Yokoyama O, Komatsu K, et al: Expression of neural plasticity related gene in the pontine tegmental area of rats with overactive bladder after cerebral infarction. J Urol 166:1148, 2001.
228. Bors E, Comarr AE: Neurological Urology: Physiology of Micturition, and Its Neurological Disorders and Sequelae. Baltimore, University Park Press, 1971.
229. Fall M, Geirsson G, Lindström S: The overactive bladder: Insight into neurophysiology by analysis of cystometric abnormalities. Neurourol Urodyn 10:337, 1991.
230. Geirsson G, Lindstrom S, Fall M, et al: Positive bladder cooling test in neurologically normal young children. J Urol 151:446, 1994.
231. Chancellor MB, de Groat WC: Intravesical capsaicin and resiniferatoxin therapy: Spicing up the ways we treat the overactive bladder. J Urol 162:3,1999.
232. Szallasi A, Fowler CJ: After a decade of intravesical vanilloid therapy: Still more questions than answers. Lancet Neurol 1:167, 2002.
233. Fowler CJ, Jewkes D, McDonald WI, et al: Intravesical capsaicin for neurogenic bladder dysfunction. Lancet 339:1239, 1992.
234. Yoshimura N: Bladder afferent pathway and spinal cord injury: Possible mechanisms inducing hyperreflexia of the urinary bladder. Prog Neurobiol 57:583, 1999.
235. de Groat WC, Kruse MN, Vizzard MA, et al: Modification of urinary bladder function after neural injury. In Seil F (ed): Advances in Neurology, vol 72. Neuronal Regeneration, Reorganization, and Repair. New York, Lippincott-Raven, 1997, p 347.
236. Kruse MN, Bray LA, de Groat WC: Influence of spinal cord injury on the morphology of bladder afferent and efferent neurons. J Auton Nerv Syst 54:215, 1995.
237. Yoshimura N, Bennet NE, Phelan MW, et al: Effects of chronic nerve growth factor treatment on rat urinary bladder and bladder afferent neurons. Soc Neurosci Abstr 25:1946, 1999.
238. Vizzard MA: Changes in urinary bladder neurotrophic factor mRNA and NGF protein following urinary bladder dysfunction. Exp Neurol 161:273, 2000.
239. Vizzard MA: Neurochemical plasticity and the role of neurotrophic factors in bladder reflex pathways after spinal cord injury. In Weaver LC, Polosa C (eds): Autonomic Dysfunction after Spinal Cord Injury: The Problems and Underlying Mechanisms. Amsterdam, Elsevier, 2006.
240. Seki S, Sasaki K, Nishizawa O, et al: Suppression of detrusor-sphincter dyssynergia by immunoneutralization of nerve growth factor in lumbosacral spinal cord in spinal cord injured rats. J Urol 171:478, 2004.
241. Seki S, Sasaki K, Fraser MO, et al: Immunoneutralization of nerve growth factor in lumbosacral spinal cord reduces bladder hyperreflexia in spinal cord injured rats. J Urol 168:2269, 2002.
242. Krenz NR, Meakin SO, Krassioukov AV, et al: Neutralizing intraspinal nerve growth factor blocks autonomic dysreflexia caused by spinal cord injury. J Neurosci 19:7405, 1999.
243. Apodaca G, Kiss S, Ruiz W, et al: Disruption of bladder epithelium barrier function after spinal cord injury. Am J Physiol 284:F966, 2003.
244. Khera M, Somogyi GT, Kiss S, et al: Botulinum toxin A inhibits ATP release from bladder urothelium after chronic spinal cord injury. Neurochem Int 45:987, 2004.
245. Somogyi GT, Zernova GV, Yoshiyama M, et al: Frequency dependence of muscarinic facilitation of transmitter release in urinary bladder strips from neurally intact or chronic spinal cord transected rats. Br J Pharmacol 125:241, 1998.
246. Barrick S, de Groat WC, Birder LA: Regulation of chemical and mechanical-evoked ATP release from urinary bladder urothelium by botulinum toxin A. Soc Neurosci Abstr 541:5, 2004.
247. Lu S, Fraser MO, Chancellor MB, et al: Evaluation of voiding dysfunction and purinergic mechanism in awake long-term spinal cord injured rats: Comparison of metabolism cage and cystometrogram measurements. J Urol 167:276, 2002.
248. Reitz A, Schurch B: Intravesical therapy options for neurogenic detrusor overactivity. Spinal Cord 42:267, 2004.
249. Reitz A, Stohrer M, Kramer G, et al: European experience of 200 cases treated with botulinum-A toxin injections into the detrusor muscle for urinary incontinence due to neurogenic detrusor overactivity. Eur Urol 45:510, 2004.
250. Smith P, Franks ME, McNeil BK, et al: Effect of botulinum toxin A on the autonomic nervous system of the rat lower urinary tract. J Urol 169:1896, 2003.

Chapter 4

PHARMACOLOGIC BASIS OF BLADDER AND URETHRAL FUNCTION AND DYSFUNCTION

Karl-Erik Andersson

The main functions of the bladder and urethra are to collect and store urine at low intravesical pressure and to expel the urine at convenient times. This means that normal voiding is under voluntary control. Urinary continence and voiding depend on the bladder and the urethra working as a functional unit. This is achieved by a complex interplay between the central and peripheral nervous systems and local regulatory factors.[1] Malfunction at various levels may result in micturition disorders, which roughly can be classified as disturbances of storage or emptying. Failure to store urine may lead to various forms of incontinence; the most common forms are urgency and stress incontinence. There are gender differences in these types of bladder dysfunction, which may be related to differences in anatomy and structure of the lower urinary tract.

Because pharmacologic treatment of urinary incontinence (i.e., urgency and stress incontinence) and lower urinary tract symptoms is a main option, several drugs with different modes and sites of action have been tried.[2-5] To optimize treatment, knowledge about the mechanisms of micturition and of the targets for treatment is necessary. This chapter reviews the normal autonomic control of the lower urinary tract and of the pharmacologic basis for some of the principles used for treatment of urinary incontinence and lower urinary tract symptoms.

AUTONOMIC RECEPTOR FUNCTIONS IN THE BLADDER

Contraction and relaxation of detrusor and urethral smooth muscle are mediated mainly through stimulation of autonomic receptors for the main transmitters, acetylcholine and noradrenaline. However, the occurrence of nonadrenergic, noncholinergic (NANC) neurotransmission is well recognized, although, particularly in humans, its physiologic importance remains to be established.[6]

Muscarinic Receptors

Muscarinic receptors comprise five subtypes, encoded by five distinct genes.[7] The five gene products correspond to pharmacologically defined receptors, and M_1 through M_5 are used to describe the molecular and pharmacologic subtypes. In the human bladder, the mRNAs for all muscarinic receptor subtypes have been demonstrated,[8] with a predominance of mRNAs encoding M_2 and M_3 receptors.[8,9] These receptors are functionally coupled to G proteins, but the signal transduction systems vary.[10-12]

Detrusor smooth muscle contains muscarinic receptors of mainly the M_2 and M_3 subtypes, with a predominance (70% to 80%) of M_2 receptors.[10-13] The M_3 receptors are the most important for detrusor contraction. It is generally believed that M_3 receptors are coupled to release of inositol 1,4,5-triphosphate (IP_3) and calcium release from the sarcoplasmic reticulum and that M_2 receptors are linked to inhibition of adenylyl cyclase. This may not be the case in the detrusor.[14] Jezior and colleagues[15] suggested that muscarinic receptor activation of detrusor muscle includes nonselective cation channels and activation of Rho kinase. Supporting a role of Rho kinase in the regulation of rat detrusor contraction and tone, Wibberley and coworkers[16] found that Rho kinase inhibitors (e.g., Y-27632, HA 1077) inhibited contractions evoked by carbachol without affecting the contraction response to KCl. They also demonstrated high levels of Rho kinase isoforms (I and II) in the bladder. Schneider and associates[13] concluded that carbachol-induced contraction of human urinary bladder is mediated by M_3 receptors and largely depends on Ca^{2+} entry through nifedipine-sensitive channels and activation of the Rho kinase pathway. The main pathway for muscarinic receptor activation of the detrusor by means of M_3 receptors may be calcium influx through L-type calcium channels and increased sensitivity to calcium of the contractile machinery produced by inhibition of myosin light chain phosphatase through activation of Rho kinase (Fig. 4-1).[14]

The functional role for the M_2 receptors has not been clarified, but it has been suggested that M_2 receptors may oppose sympathetically mediated smooth muscle relaxation, mediated by β-adrenergic receptors.[17] M_2-receptor stimulation may also activate nonspecific cation channels[18] and inhibit K_{ATP} channels through activation of protein kinase C.[19,20] In certain disease states, M_2 receptors may contribute to contraction of the bladder. In the denervated rat bladder, M_2 receptors or a combination of M_2 and M_3 mediated contractile responses, and the two receptor types seemed to act in a facilitatory manner to mediate contraction.[21-23] In obstructed, hypertrophied rat bladders, there was an increase in total and M_2 receptor density, whereas there was a reduction in M_3 receptor density.[24] The functional significance of this change for voiding function has not been established. Pontari and colleagues[25] analyzed bladder muscle specimens from patients with neurogenic bladder dysfunction to determine whether the muscarinic receptor subtype mediating contraction shifts from M_3 to the M_2 receptor subtype, as found in the denervated, hypertrophied rat bladder. They concluded that whereas normal detrusor contractions are mediated by the M_3 receptor subtype, in patients with neurogenic bladder dysfunction, contractions also can be mediated by the M_2 receptors.

Muscarinic receptors may also be located on the presynaptic nerve terminals and participate in the regulation of transmitter release. The inhibitory prejunctional muscarinic receptors have been classified as M_4 in the human bladder.[26] Prejunctional facili-

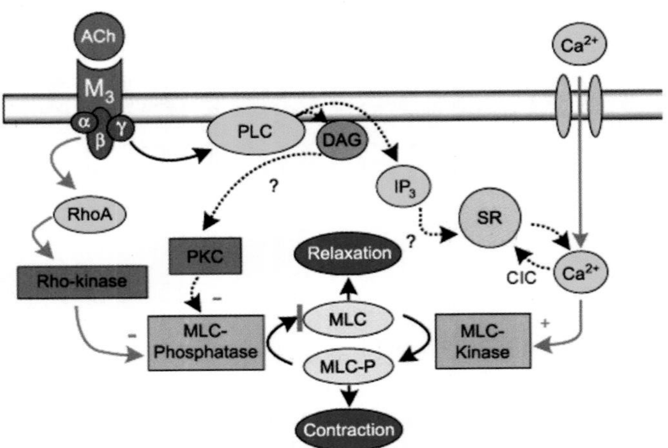

Figure 4-1 Transmitter signal pathways involved in activation of detrusor contraction by means of muscarinic M_3 receptors. ACh, acetylcholine; CIC, calcium-induced calcium release; DAG, diacylglycerol; IP_3, inositol 1,4,5-triphosphate; MLC, myosin light chain; PLC, phospholipase C; PKC, protein kinase C; RhoA, protein encoded by *RAS* homolog gene family member A; SR, sarcoplasmic reticulum. There seem to be differences between species in the contribution of the different pathways in contractile activation. In the human detrusor, Ca^{2+} influx is of major importance.

tatory muscarinic receptors appear to be the M_1 subtype.[27] The muscarinic facilitatory mechanism seems to be upregulated in overactive bladders from chronic spinal cord transected rats. Facilitation in these preparations is primarily mediated by M_3 receptors.[27,28]

Muscarinic receptors have been demonstrated on the urothelium or suburothelium, but their functional importance has not been clarified.[12,29] It has been suggested that they may be involved in the release of an unknown inhibitory factor.[12]

It is well documented[2,3] that antimuscarinic agents are effective for treatment of overactive bladder, which suggests that muscarinic receptors may be involved in its pathogenesis. Contraction of the bladder, whether voluntary or involuntary, involves stimulation of the muscarinic receptors on the detrusor by acetylcholine released from activated cholinergic nerves. However, antimuscarinic agents at clinically recommended doses have little effect on voiding contractions and may act mainly during the bladder storage phase,[30] during which there is normally no parasympathetic outflow from the spinal cord.[31] Supporting this, antimuscarinic agents have been shown to reduce bladder tone during storage and to increase cystometric bladder capacity. A basal release of acetylcholine from non-neuronal (urothelial) and neuronal sources has been demonstrated in isolated human detrusor muscle.[32] It has been suggested that this release, which is increased by stretching the muscle and in the aging bladder, contributes to detrusor overactivity and overactive bladder by eventually increasing bladder afferent activity during storage.[33] This may occur because of a direct effect on suburothelial afferents or stimulation of contraction of detrusor muscle cells, which already have an increased myogenic activity in the overactive detrusor.[34] Enhanced myogenic contractions can generate an enhanced afferent signal, contributing to urge or initiation of the micturition reflex.

Alpha-Adrenoceptors

α-Adrenoceptors may have effects on different locations in the bladder: the detrusor smooth muscle, the detrusor vasculature, the afferent and efferent nerve terminal, and intramural ganglia. The importance of the α_1-adrenoceptors in the human detrusor in the generation of lower urinary tract symptoms has not been established. Most investigators agree on that there is a low-level expression of these receptors.[35,36] In studies of the human detrusor, Malloy and coworkers[36] found that two thirds of the α-adrenoceptor mRNAs expressed were α_{1D}, there was no α_{1B}, and one third was α_{1A}. In the rat detrusor, the α_1-adrenoceptor distribution was different: the α_{1A}-adrenoceptor was the predominant form, one third was the α_{1D}-adrenoceptor, and there was very little of the α_{1B}-adrenoceptor form. This was consistent in the different parts of the detrusor.[37]

A change of subtype distribution may be produced by outflow obstruction. Hampel and associates[37] reported that there was a change in the obstructed bladder from α_{1A}-adrenoceptor to α_{1D}-adrenoceptor mRNA predominance. In humans, there is an α_{1D}-adrenoceptor predominance in the normal detrusor, which means that a change in a similar direction, as in the rat, would be of minor importance provided that the number of receptors did not increase. Studies by Nomiya and colleagues[38] confirmed the low-level expression of α-adrenoceptor mRNA in normal human detrusor, and they further demonstrated that there was no upregulation of any of the adrenergic receptors with obstruction. In functional experiments, they found a small response to phenylephrine at high drug concentrations with no difference between normal and obstructed bladders. In the obstructed human bladder, there seems to be no evidence for α-adrenoceptor upregulation or change in subtype. This finding was challenged by Bouchelouche and coworkers,[39] who found an increased response to α_1-adrenoceptor stimulation in obstructed bladders. Whether this would mean that the α_{1D}-adrenoceptors in the detrusor muscle are responsible for detrusor overactivity or overactive bladder is unclear. Based on available evidence, however, it does not seem likely that in the detrusor muscle these receptors should be an important treatment target, although α_{1D}-adrenoceptors located elsewhere in the bladder may be important.

In the bladder, the function of the detrusor muscle depends on the vasculature and on perfusion. Hypoxia induced by partial outlet obstruction is believed to play a major role in the hypertrophic and degenerative effects of partial outlet obstruction. Das and associates[40] investigated in rats whether doxazosin affected blood flow to the bladder and reduced the level of bladder dysfunction induced by partial outlet obstruction. They found that 4 weeks of treatment with doxazosin increased bladder blood flow in control and obstructed rats. Doxazosin treatment also reduced the severity of the detrusor response to partial outlet obstruction. Doxazosin may reduce the increase in bladder weight in obstructed animals, which may be one of the mechanisms that contributes to a positive effect on detrusor overactivity caused by the obstruction.

Beta-Adrenoceptors

In the human detrusor, the most important β-adrenoceptor for bladder relaxation is the β_3-adrenoceptor.[41] This partly explains why the clinical effects of selective β_2-adrenoceptor agonists in detrusor overactivity have been controversial and largely inconclusive.[2,3] However, the β_2-adrenoceptor agonist clenbuterol inhibited electrically evoked contractions in human "unstable" but not normal bladder,[42] which is in agreement with previous experiences in patients, suggesting that clenbuterol and other β_2-adrenoceptor agonists such as terbutaline may inhibit detrusor overactivity.[43,44]

The β_3-adrenoceptor seems to be an interesting target for drugs aimed for treatment of overactive bladder. Selective β_3-adrenoceptor agonists have relaxant effects on detrusor muscle in vitro and have been effective in animal models of detrusor overactivity.[45-47] However, no proof of concept studies seems to have been performed in humans showing that this is an effective principle to treat overactive bladder.

Purinergic Receptors

In most animal species, bladder contraction induced by stimulation of nerves consists of an atropine-sensitive component and a component mediated by NANC mechanisms.[48] NANC-mediated contractions have been reported to occur in normal human detrusor,[48] even if not representing more than a few percent of the total contraction in response to nerve stimulation. However, a significant degree of NANC-mediated contraction may exist in morphologically or functionally changed human bladders, and it has been reported to occur in several disorders associated with lower urinary tract symptoms, such as bladder hypertrophy,[49-51] idiopathic detrusor overactivity,[51,52] interstitial cystitis,[53] and neurogenic damage[54] and in the aging bladder.[55] In these disorders, the NANC component of the nerve-induced response may be responsible for up to 40% to 50% of the total bladder contraction.

There is good evidence that the transmitter responsible for the NANC component is adenosine triphosphate (ATP)[56] acting on P2X receptors found in the detrusor smooth muscle membranes of rats[57] and humans.[58] The $P2X_1$receptor subtype predominated in both species. Changes in P2X receptor subtypes in bladders from patients with idiopathic detrusor overactivity have been reported.[52,59] O'Reilly and colleagues[52] were unable to detect a purinergic component of nerve-mediated contractions in control (normal) bladder preparations, but they found a significant component in overactive bladder specimens, in which the purinergic component was approximately 50%. They concluded that this abnormal purinergic transmission in the bladder might explain symptoms in these patients. ATP was a more potent contractile agonist in bladder preparations from patients with overactive and obstructive bladders than in specimens from normal bladders,[60] a finding that was suggested to contribute to detrusor overactivity.

O'Reilly and coworkers[61] confirmed that the $P2X_1$ receptor was the predominant purinoceptor subtype in the human male bladder. They also found that the amount of $P2X_1$ receptor per smooth muscle cell was greater in the obstructed than in control bladders. This suggests an increase in purinergic function in the overactive bladder arising from bladder outlet obstruction.

It has not been established whether abnormalities in the purinergic transmission in the bladder can explain overactive bladder symptoms in idiopathic detrusor overactivity in women and in men with bladder outlet obstruction. If this is the case, abnormal purinergic activation of the detrusor may explain why antimuscarinic treatment fails in a number of patients.

Vanilloid Receptors

Appropriate bladder function depends on an intact afferent signaling from the bladder to the central nervous system. This signaling conveys information about bladder filling and the status of the tissue (e.g., presence of infectious agents). The afferent nerves consist of small, slowly conducting, myelinated Aδ fibers and slowly conducting, unmyelinated C fibers. The former are excited by mechanoreceptors and convey information about bladder filling, whereas C fibers mediate painful sensations recognized by chemoreceptors. By means of capsaicin, a subpopulation of primary afferent neurons innervating the bladder and urethra (i.e., capsaicin-sensitive nerves) has been identified. It is believed that capsaicin exerts its effects by acting on specific vanilloid receptors on these nerves.[62] Capsaicin exerts a biphasic effect; initial excitation is followed by a long-lasting blockade, which renders sensitive primary afferents (C fibers) resistant to activation by natural stimuli. In sufficiently high concentrations, capsaicin is believed to cause desensitization, initially by releasing and emptying the stores of neuropeptides and then by blocking further release.[63] Resiniferatoxin, an analogue of capsaicin, is approximately 1000 times more potent for desensitization than capsaicin,[64] but it is only a few hundred times more potent for excitation.[65] Capsaicin and resiniferatoxin also may have effects on Aδ fibers. It is also possible that capsaicin at high concentrations (mM) has additional, nonspecific effects.[66]

Capsaicin and resiniferatoxin have been used successfully to treat bladder function disturbances.[2,3] They are known to bind to the TRPV1 (VR1) receptor, a nonselective cation channel, on the peripheral terminals of nociceptive neurons, but the role of vanilloid receptors in normal bladder function and in the pathogenesis in detrusor overactivity and autonomic dysreflexia has not been established.

Birder and associates[67] investigated bladder function in conscious mice lacking the TRPV1 receptor. TRPV1 receptor–knockout mice seem to have increased voiding frequency compared with wild-type mice. The TRPV1 knockouts also had an increased frequency of nonvoiding bladder contractions. In vitro, stretch-induced ATP release was decreased in bladders from TRPV1-knockout mice, and hypo-osmolality-induced ATP released from cultured urothelial cells was reduced.[67] The investigators suggested that TRPV1 receptors participate in normal bladder function, are essential for normal mechanically evoked purinergic signaling by the urothelium, and are involved in ATP release. Experimental and clinical evidence that capsaicin-sensitive afferents may be involved also in idiopathic detrusor overactivity has been presented.[68,69]

ION CHANNELS

In the detrusor, the two most thoroughly investigated classes of ion channels are calcium channels and potassium channels.[6]

Calcium Channels

Calcium is a key component for cell function in many cells. In smooth muscle, increased intracellular calcium concentrations activate the contractile mechanisms, and in nerve terminals, calcium influx in response to action potentials is an important mechanism for neurotransmitter release. Calcium channels can be divided into at least four different subtypes: L, N, P, and Q channels. The calcium channels present in smooth muscles are L-type (dihydropyridine-sensitive) calcium channels and seem to be involved in contraction of the human bladder irrespective of the mode of activation.[70] A decrease of the membrane potential (i.e., depolarization) increases the open probability for calcium channels, thereby increasing the calcium influx. The channels depend on the membrane potential and are called voltage-operated calcium channels. Elevated intracellular calcium levels are also believed to initiate release of calcium from intracellular stores—calcium-induced calcium release.[71,72] Regulation of the intracellular calcium concentration in smooth muscle cells is a conceivable way to modulate bladder contraction. Dihydropyridines (e.g., nifedipine) have a potent inhibitory effect on isolated detrusor muscle. Inhibitory effects have also been demonstrated on experimentally induced contractions under in vivo conditions in rats and clinically in patients with detrusor overactivity.[48] However, therapeutically, there is no evidence that calcium antagonists have any useful effects in the treatment of overactive bladder or detrusor overactivity.[2,3]

Potassium Channels

Potassium channels represent another mechanism for modulating the excitability of smooth muscle cells. Under normal conditions, the resting membrane potential in smooth muscle cells is determined predominantly by the membrane conductivity for potassium ions. Increased potassium conductivity lowers the membrane potential by increasing the potassium efflux. This increases the threshold for opening of voltage-operated calcium channels and initiation of contraction. There are several different types of K^+ channels, and at least two subtypes have been found in the human detrusor, ATP-sensitive K^+ channels (K_{ATP}) and large-conductance calcium-activated K^+ channels (BK_{Ca}). Studies on isolated human detrusor muscle and on bladder tissue from several animal species have demonstrated that K^+-channel openers reduce spontaneous contractions and contractions induced by carbachol and electrical stimulation.[6] However, the lack of selectivity of the available K^+-channel openers for the bladder versus the vasculature has limited the use of these drugs. No effects of cromakalim or pinacidil on the bladder were found in studies on patients with spinal cord lesions or detrusor overactivity secondary to outflow obstruction.[73,74] Some new K^+-channel openers have been developed and claimed to have selectivity for the bladder.[6] However, there is no evidence that K^+-channels openers are an option for treatment of overactive bladder or detrusor overactivity.[2,3]

AFFERENT SIGNALING FROM THE UROTHELIUM OR SUBUROTHELIUM

Evidence suggests that the urothelium or suburothelium may serve as a mechanosensor that, by producing nitric oxide, ATP, and other mediators, can control the activity in afferent nerves and thereby the initiation of the micturition reflex.[75] Low pH, high K^+ concentration, increased osmolality, and low temperatures can influence afferent nerves, possibly through effects on the vanilloid receptor (i.e., capsaicin-gated ion channel [TRPV1]), which is expressed in afferent nerve terminals and in the epithelial cells that line the bladder lumen.[67,76] A network of interstitial cells, extensively linked by connexin43 (Cx43)–containing gap junctions, was found to be located beneath the urothelium in the human bladder by Sui and colleagues[77,78] This interstitial cellular network was suggested to operate as a functional syncytium, integrating signals and responses in the bladder wall. The firing of suburothelial afferent nerves, conveying sensations and regulating the threshold for bladder activation, may be modified by inhibitory (e.g., nitric oxide) and stimulatory (e.g., ATP, tachykinins, prostanoids) mediators. ATP, generated by the urothelium, has been suggested as an important mediator of urothelial signaling.[56,75] Supporting such a view, intravesical ATP induces detrusor overactivity in conscious rats.[79] Mice lacking the $P2X_3$ receptor were shown to have hypoactive bladders.[80,81]

There seem to be other, unidentified factors in the urothelium that may influence bladder function.[82-89] Fovaeus and coworkers[85] found that a previously unrecognized nonadrenergic, nonnitrergic, nonprostanoid inhibitory mediator is released from the rat urinary bladder by muscarinic receptor stimulation. However, it was not clear whether this factor came from the detrusor muscle or from the detrusor and the urothelium. Hawthorn and associates[86] presented data suggesting the presence of a diffusible, urothelium-derived inhibitory factor, which could not be identified but appeared to be neither nitric oxide, a cyclooxygenase product, a catecholamine, adenosine, γ-aminobutyric acid (GABA), nor any substance sensitive to apamin. The identity and possible physiologic role of the unknown factors remain to be established and should offer an interesting field for further research. These mechanisms can be involved in the pathophysiology of overactive bladder and may be useful targets for pharmacologic intervention.

URETHRAL FUNCTION AND STRESS URINARY INCONTINENCE

Many factors are involved in the pathogenesis of stress urinary incontinence (SUI). Some, such as weak urethral support, vaginal prolapse, and severe vesical neck or urethral dysfunction,[90] cannot be treated pharmacologically. Women with SUI have lower resting urethral pressures than age-matched, continent women,[91,92] and the aim of treatment often is to increase intraurethral pressure.

Factors that may contribute to urethral closure include urethral smooth and striated muscle tone and the passive properties of the urethral lamina propria, in particular the vascular suburothelial layer. The relative contribution to intraurethral pressure of these factors remains a subject of debate. In one study, the contributions to the total intraurethral pressure of the striated muscle component in the urethra and pelvic floor, the urethral vascular bed, and the smooth musculature and connective tissues in urethra and periurethral tissues were found to be one third each.[93]

Many factors have been suggested to contribute to urethral relaxation and to urethral closure, including urethral smooth muscle tone and the properties of the urethral lamina propria. There is ample pharmacologic evidence that a substantial part of urethral tone is mediated through stimulation of α-adrenoceptors in the urethral smooth muscle by released noradrenaline.[48] Nitric oxide has emerged as an important mediator of urethral smooth muscle relaxation, but the roles of other transmitters cannot be excluded.[94-96] However, central nervous control of the smooth and striated urethral muscle is important for the maintenance of continence.[97-99] The nucleus Onuf is the

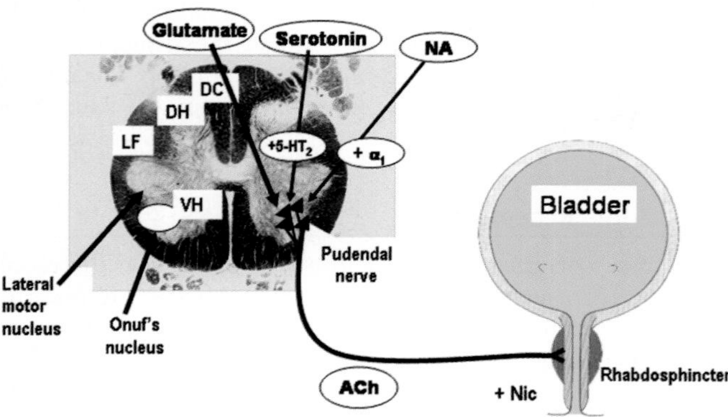

Figure 4-2 The striated urethral sphincter is innervated by the pudendal nerve, which contains the axons of motor neurons whose cell bodies are located in Onuf's nucleus. Glutamate exerts tonic excitatory effects on these motor neurons, and this effect is enhanced by noradrenaline (NA) and serotonin (5-HT), acting on α_1-adrenoceptors and 5-HT_2 receptors, respectively. By inhibition of the reuptake of noradrenaline and serotonin, the contractile activity in the striated sphincter can be increased. ACh, acetylcholine; DC, dorsal commissure; DH, dorsal horn; LF, lateral funiculus; + Nic, nicotinic receptors; VH, ventral horn.

spinal target of reuptake inhibitors of serotonin (5-hydroxytryptamine) and noradrenaline, which may increase the tone of the striated sphincter (Fig. 4-2).

Innervation

The urethra of males and females receives sympathetic (adrenergic), parasympathetic (cholinergic), and sensory innervation. The pelvic nerve conveys parasympathetic fibers to the urethra, and activity in these fibers results in an inhibitory effect on urethral smooth muscle, which relaxes the outflow region. Most of the sympathetic innervation of the bladder and urethra originates from the intermediolateral nuclei in the thoracolumbar region (T10 to L2) of the spinal cord. The axons travel through the inferior mesenteric ganglia and the hypogastric nerve or pass through the paravertebral chain and enter the pelvic nerve. Sympathetic signals are conveyed in the hypogastric and the pelvic nerves.[100]

Adrenergic and cholinergic nerves contain transmitters and transmitter-generating enzymes other than noradrenaline and acetylcholine. These agents, some of which have not been identified, are responsible for the NANC efferent neurotransmission, which can be demonstrated in urethral smooth muscle (discussed later).

Most of the sensory innervation of the urethra reaches the spinal cord through the pelvic nerve and dorsal root ganglia. Some afferents travel in the hypogastric nerve. The sensory nerves of the striated muscle in the rhabdosphincter travel in the pudendal nerve to the sacral region of the spinal cord.[100] These sensory nerves are usually identified by their content of peptides such as calcitonin gene–related peptide and tachykinins.

Adrenergic Nerves

There are well-known anatomic differences between the male and female urethra, which are reflected in the innervation. In the human male, the smooth muscle surrounding the preprostatic part of the urethra is richly innervated by cholinergic and adrenergic nerves.[101] This part is believed to serve as a sexual sphincter, contracting during ejaculation and preventing retrograde transport of sperm. The role of this structure in maintaining continence is unclear, but it probably is not essential.

In the human female, there is no anatomic urethral smooth muscle sphincter, and the muscle bundles run obliquely or longitudinally along the length of the urethra. In the whole human female urethra and in the human male urethra below the preprostatic part, there is a scarce supply of adrenergic nerves.[101,102] Fine varicose terminals can be seen running longitudinally and transversely along the bundles of smooth muscle cells. Adrenergic terminals can also be found around blood vessels. Colocalization studies in animals have revealed that adrenergic nerves, identified by immunohistochemistry (i.e., using tyrosine hydroxylase), also contain neuropeptide Y.[103] Chemical sympathectomy (i.e., using 6-OH-dopamine) in rats resulted in a complete disappearance of tyrosine hydroxylase–immunoreactive nerves, whereas nitric oxide synthase (NOS)–containing nerve fibers did not appear to be affected by the treatment.[104] This result suggests that NOS is not contained within adrenergic nerves.

Cholinergic Nerves

Urethral smooth muscle receives a rich cholinergic innervation. Most probably, the cholinergic nerves cause relaxation of the outflow region at the start of micturition by releasing nitric oxide and other relaxant transmitters, but otherwise, their functional role is largely unknown. The cholinergic nerves of the bladder produce detrusor contraction, and disturbances in the coordination of the contractant effects on the bladder and the relaxation of the outflow region may lead to the detrusor-sphincter dyssynergia, often seen in suprasacral spinal cord injuries.

In the pig urethra, colocalization studies revealed that acetylcholine esterase–positive and some NOS-immunoreactive nerves had profiles that were similar. These nerves also contained neuropeptide Y and vasoactive intestinal polypeptide (VIP) immunoreactivity. NOS-containing nerves were present in a density lower than that of the acetylcholine esterase–positive nerves but higher than the density of any peptidergic nerves.[105] Coexistence of acetylcholine and NOS was also demonstrated in the rat major pelvic ganglion.[106] In the rat urethra, colocalization studies confirmed that NOS and VIP are contained within a population of cholinergic nerves. The distribution of immunoreactivities to neuronal NOS, heme oxygenases, and VIP was assessed by Werkström and colleagues.[107] Heme oxygenase-2 immunoreactivity was found in all nerve cell bodies of intramural ganglia, localized between smooth muscle bundles in the detrusor, bladder base, and proximal urethra. About 70% of the ganglionic cell bodies were also NOS immunoreactive, whereas a minor amount was VIP immunoreactive.

AUTONOMIC RECEPTOR FUNCTIONS

Alpha-Adrenoceptors

In males, up to about 50% of the intraurethral pressure is maintained by stimulation of α-adrenoceptors, as judged from results obtained with α-adrenoceptor antagonists and epidural anesthesia in urodynamic studies.[108,109] In human urethral smooth muscle, functional and receptor binding studies have suggested that the α_1-adrenoceptor subtype is the predominating postjunctional α-adrenoceptor.[48,110] Most in vitro investigations of human urethral α-adrenoceptors have been carried out in the male, and the results support the existence of a sphincter structure in the male proximal urethra, which cannot be found in the female. Other marked differences between sexes in the distribution of α_1- and α_2-adrenoceptors (as can be found in animals such as rabbits) or in the distribution of α_1-adrenoceptor subtypes do not seem to occur.[111] Taki and coworkers[112] separated the entire length of the isolated female human urethra into seven parts, from the external meatus to the bladder neck, and examined regional differences in contractile responses to various agents, including noradrenaline (α_1 and α_2) and clonidine (α_2). Noradrenaline, but not clonidine, produced concentration-dependent contractions in all parts, with a peak response in the middle to proximal urethra. They found a similarity in patterns between noradrenaline-induced contraction and the urethral pressure profile in the human urethra.

Among the three high-affinity α_1-adrenoceptor subtypes identified in molecular cloning and functional studies (α_{1A}, α_{1B}, α_{1D}), α_{1A} seems to predominate in the human lower urinary tract. However, the receptor with low affinity for prazosin (α_{1L}-adrenoceptor), which has not been cloned and may represent a functional phenotype of the α_{1A}-adrenoceptor,[113] was found to be prominent in the human male urethra.[114] In the human female urethra, the expression and distribution of α_1-adrenoceptor subtypes were determined by in situ hybridization and quantitative autoradiography. mRNA for the α_{1A}-adrenoceptor subtype was predominant, and autoradiography confirmed the predominance of the α_{1A}-adrenoceptor.

The studies previously cited suggest that the sympathetic innervation helps to maintain urethral smooth muscle tone through α_1-adrenoceptor receptor stimulation. If urethral α_1-adrenoceptors are contributing to the lower urinary tract symptoms, which can occur also in women,[115-117] an effect of α_1-adrenoceptor antagonists should be expected in women with these symptoms. This was found to be the case in some studies, but it was not confirmed in a randomized, placebo-controlled pilot study,[118] which showed that terazosin was not effective for the treatment of prostatism-like symptoms in aging women.

Urethral α_2-adrenoceptors are able to control the release of noradrenaline from adrenergic nerves, as shown in in vitro studies.[48] In the rabbit urethra incubated with [^{3}H]noradrenaline, electrical stimulation of nerves caused a release of [^{3}H], which was decreased by noradrenaline and clonidine and increased by the α_2-adrenoceptor antagonist rauwolscine. Clonidine was shown to reduce intraurethral pressure in humans,[119] an effect that may be attributed partly to a peripheral effect on adrenergic nerve terminals. More likely, this effect was exerted on the central nervous system, with a resulting decrease in peripheral sympathetic nervous activity. The subtype of prejunctional α_2-adrenoceptor involved in [^{3}H]noradrenaline secretion in the isolated guinea pig urethra was suggested to be of the α_{2A}-adrenoreceptor subtype.[120]

Beta-Adrenoceptors

Both α- and β-adrenoceptors can be demonstrated in isolated urethral smooth muscle from animals and humans.[48] In humans, the β-adrenoceptors in the bladder neck were suggested to be of the β_2-adrenoceptor subtype, as shown by receptor binding studies using subtype-selective antagonists.[121] However, the predominating β-adrenoceptor in the human bladder seems to be the β_3-adrenoceptor subtype,[122-124] and in the striated urethral sphincter, β_3-adrenoceptors can be found.[125] The role of this subtype in urethral function does not seem to have been explored.

Muscarinic Receptors

The number of muscarinic receptor binding sites in the rabbit urethra was lower than in the bladder.[126] Muscarinic receptor agonists contract isolated urethral smooth muscle from several species, including humans, but these responses seem to be mediated mainly by the longitudinal muscle layer.[48] Taki and associates,[112] investigating the whole length of the female human urethra, found that acetylcholine contracted only the proximal part and the bladder neck. If this contractile activation is exerted in the longitudinal direction, it should be expected that the urethra is shortened and that the urethral pressure decreases. Experimentally, in vitro resistance to flow in the urethra was increased only by high concentrations of acetylcholine.[127,128] In humans, tolerable doses of the muscarinic receptor agonist bethanechol[129] and the muscarinic receptor antagonist emeprone[130] had little effect on intraurethral pressure.

Prejunctional muscarinic receptors may influence the release of noradrenaline and acetylcholine in the bladder neck and urethra. In urethral tissue from rabbits and humans, carbachol decreased and scopolamine increased in a concentration-dependent manner the release of [^{3}H]noradrenaline from adrenergic terminals and of [^{3}H]choline from cholinergic nerve terminals.[131] This means that released acetylcholine can inhibit noradrenaline release, thereby decreasing urethral tone and intraurethral pressure. The muscarinic receptor subtypes involved in contractile effects on smooth muscle or controlling transmitter release in the urethra have not been established. This may have clinical ramifications, because subtype-selective antimuscarinic drugs (M_3) have been introduced as a treatment for detrusor overactivity.

NONADRENERGIC, NONCHOLINERGIC RELAXANT MECHANISMS

The normal pattern of voiding in humans is characterized by an initial drop in urethral pressure, followed by an increase in intravesical pressure.[48,132] The mechanism of this relaxant effect has not been established, but several factors may contribute. One possibility is that the fall in intraurethral pressure is caused by stimulation of muscarinic receptors on noradrenergic nerves, diminishing noradrenaline release and thereby tone in the proximal urethra. Another is that contraction of longitudinal urethral smooth muscle in the proximal urethra, produced by released acetylcholine, causes shortening and widening of the urethra, with a concomitant decrease in intraurethral pressure. A third possibility is that a NANC mechanism mediates this response.[48]

Nitric Oxide

Nitric oxide is an important inhibitory neurotransmitter in the lower urinary tract.[133,134] Nitric oxide–mediated responses in smooth muscle preparations are most often linked to an increase in cyclic guanine monophosphate (cGMP) formation. This has

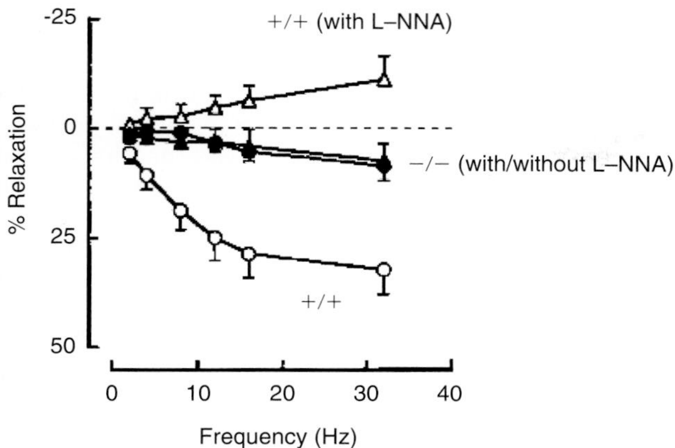

Figure 4-3 Frequency-response curves in response to electrical field stimulation in urethral preparations from mice lacking cyclic cMP-dependent protein kinase (cGKI–/–, *solid symbols*) and wild-type controls (cGKI+/+, *open symbols*) before *(circles)* and after *(triangles)* treatment with the nitric oxide synthase inhibitor, L-NOARG.

been demonstrated in the rabbit urethra.[135-137] The cGMP analogue 8-Br-cGMP was able to induce relaxation of rabbit urethra, further supporting the view of cGMP as a mediator of relaxation in this tissue. cGMP-dependent protein kinase (cGK) phosphorylates K_{Ca} channels and increases their open probability, leading to hyperpolarization.[138] cGMP may affect sequestering of intracellular Ca^{2+}, stimulate Ca^{2+} extrusion pumps, and decrease the sensitivity of the contractile proteins to Ca^{2+}.[139] The latter may occur without changing the membrane potential. In this way, cGMP may be able to induce relaxation in different ways in different tissues. The role of nitric oxide for urethral relaxation was further investigated in mice lacking cGK type I.[140] In urethral preparations of $cGKI^{+/+}$ mice, electrical field stimulation elicited frequency-dependent relaxations. The relaxations were abolished by the NOS inhibitor L-NOARG, and instead, a contractile response to stimulation was generally found (Fig. 4-3). In $cGKI^{-/-}$ urethral strips, the response to electrical field stimulation was practically abolished, but a small relaxation generally appeared at high stimulation frequencies (16 to 32 Hz). This relaxant response was not inhibited by L-NOARG, suggesting the occurrence of additional relaxant transmitters.

The rich occurrence of NOS-immunoreactive nerve fibers supports the current view of nitric oxide as the main inhibitory NANC mediator in rabbit urethra.[133] Waldeck and colleagues[141] demonstrated spindle-shaped cyclic GMP-immunoreactive cells, distinct from the smooth muscle cells, forming a network around and between the smooth muscle bundles. These results confirmed the findings of Smet and coworkers, [142] who found similar cyclic GMP-immunoreactive cells in the guinea pig and human bladder and urethra. The function of these interstitial cells has not been established, but they have been suggested to be pacemaker cells involved in the regulation of urethral tone.[143-145] Based on results obtained in freshly dispersed rabbit urethral interstitial cells, Sergeant and associates[145] suggested that in the urethra, stimulation of α_1-adrenoceptors releases Ca^{2+} from an IP_3-sensitive store. This produces a Ca^{2+}-activated Cl^- current, which elevates the slow-wave frequency in the cells. This may underlie the mechanism responsible for increased urethral tone during nerve stimulation.

Other Nonadrenergic, Noncholinergic Transmitters or Modulators

Additional systems involving ATP, carbon monoxide, and other, unknown mediators have been observed in the urethra. Other agents shown to influence urethral function include neuropeptides, prostanoids, and serotonin.[1] Neuropeptides such as VIP, neuropeptide Y, and endothelins have been suggested to be involved in contraction and relaxation of urethral smooth muscle and, as in the bladder, in afferent signaling, but to a large extent, their functional roles remain to be established.[1]

EFFECTS OF SEX HORMONES ON THE LOWER URINARY TRACT

Estrogen and Progesterone

Lower urinary tract innervation, receptor density and distribution, and contractile function may change significantly during periods of marked changes in female hormone levels, such as puberty, pregnancy, and menopause.[48] The lower urinary tract in animals and humans expresses estrogen receptors.[146,147] However, in human bladders, estrogen receptors were found only in squamous epithelia (i.e., trigone and proximal and distal urethra). No estrogen receptors were found in transitional urothelium or detrusor muscle, and there was no variation with estrogen status.[146] In the urethra, the expression is greater, but it is still inconsistent.[146] In animals, estrogen-α and estrogen-β receptors have been demonstrated in the epithelium, detrusor muscle, and rhabdosphincter, but many of the rapid estrogen-induced changes have been postulated not to be receptor mediated.[147]

The effects of estrogen on lower urinary tract structure and function and on the autonomic nervous control have been examined in many animal studies,[48,148-153] often with conflicting results. In particular, there has been disagreement on how estrogens affect muscarinic receptor functions. Levin and colleagues[154] found that estrogen treatment (i.e., estradiol) of immature female rabbits induced a marked increase in the detrusor response to stimulation of α-adrenoceptors and muscarinic receptors and to ATP, and they found that in the bladder body and midsection, there was a significant increase in the number of α-adrenoceptors and muscarinic receptors. Shapiro[155] reported that treatment of mature female rabbits with estradiol led to a significant decrease in muscarinic receptor density. This observation was confirmed by Batra and Andersson, who found that the decrease in muscarinic receptor number had little effect on the responses to carbachol and electrical stimulation.[156] Elliott and coworkers[157] found a decreased sensitivity to acetylcholine, carbachol, and electrical stimulation, but not to K^+ in isolated detrusor tissue from female rats treated with estradiol. Addition of diethylstilbestrol further reduced these responses, an effect previously investigated by the same group and attributed to a reduction of calcium influx into the detrusor cells.[157] Selective β_3-adrenoceptor agonists relaxed the detrusor muscle of female rats with low estrogen levels,[158] which was suggested to have potential clinical implications.

In nonanesthetized mice lacking estrogen-α, estrogen-β, or both receptor subtypes, in vitro contractility and cystometric values were no different from those in wild-type controls. However, mice lacking estrogen-α receptors did not respond to intravesical capsaicin instillation, suggesting a role of estrogen receptors in afferent signaling in the bladder.[159] In the urethra, estrogens may increase the smooth muscle sensitivity to α-adrenoceptor stimulation and improve the function of the vasculature and connective tissue of the lamina propria.[48]

Taken together, these results suggest that estrogens, at least in animals, can influence lower urinary tract structure and function and modify the responses of the detrusor to autonomic nervous influences. The results are not always consistent, and some of the discrepancies may be attributed to differences in experimental approaches. Even if an estrogen effect on afferent signaling in humans seems possible, available data do not allow conclusions to be drawn that consistently are applicable to treatment (e.g., of urine storage disorders).

Little is known about the effects of progesterone on bladder function, and the functional importance of the progesterone receptors that have been demonstrated in the lower urinary tract has not been established.[160,161] In vitro administration of progesterone reduced the response of bladder strips to electrical field stimulation and KCl.[162] In contrast, long-term in vivo treatment with progesterone increased the maximal response of rabbit bladder preparations to electrical field stimulation and increased the sensitivity to muscarinic receptor stimulation compared with ovariectomized controls.[163] In contrast, Tong and associates[164] found that in vivo treatment with progesterone decreased the maximal response of rat bladder strips to acetylcholine and that there was a decrease in muscarinic receptor density. As for estrogens, available information does not allow conclusions to be drawn that are applicable to treatment of lower urinary tract disorders.

Pregnancy

Urinary incontinence (particularly stress incontinence) is common during pregnancy and has been attributed in part to changes in bladder and urethral function.[165] In rats, pregnancy was reported to increase bladder weight and capacity, decrease the responses to muscarinic and α-adrenoceptor stimulation, and increase the response to ATP.[164] In the presence of bethanechol, bladder strips from pregnant rabbits generated 50% less tension in response to calcium than those from nonpregnant rabbits.[166] The isolated whole bladder from pregnant animals responded to low-frequency stimulation and to ATP with a greater increase in intravesical pressure than did preparations from virgin rabbits, whereas the response to bethanechol was greater in the virgin rabbits.[167] Receptor binding studies in bladder tissue from pregnant animals revealed a significantly reduced muscarinic receptor density (50%), corresponding to the decrease in response to bethanechol of the whole bladder. The results were interpreted to mean that pregnancy induced an increase in the purinergic component and a decrease in the cholinergic component of the urinary bladder response to field stimulation.[167] A reduction of the muscarinic receptor density in the pregnant rabbit bladder was confirmed by other investigators.[168] To what extent the receptor and functional changes demonstrated in the pregnant bladder from different species can explain the voiding disturbances found in pregnant women remains to be established.

References

1. Andersson KE, Wein AJ: Pharmacology of the lower urinary tract: Basis for current and future treatments of urinary incontinence. Pharmacol Rev 56:581, 2004.
2. Andersson KE, Appell R, Awad S, et al: Pharmacological treatment of urinary incontinence. In Abrams P, Khoury S, Wein A (eds): Incontinence. Second International Consultation on Incontinence. Plymouth, UK, Plymbridge Distributors, 2002, pp 479-511.
3. Andersson KE, Appell R, Cardozo L, et al: Pharmacological treatment of urinary incontinence. In Abrams P, Khoury S, Wein A (eds): Incontinence. Second International Consultation on Incontinence. Plymouth, UK, Plymbridge Distributors, 2005.
4. Ouslander JG: Management of overactive bladder. N Engl J Med 350:786, 2004.
5. Zinner NR, Koke SC, Viktrup L: Pharmacotherapy for stress urinary incontinence: Present and future options. Drugs 64:1503, 2004.
6. Andersson KE, Arner A: Urinary bladder contraction and relaxation: Physiology and pathophysiology. Physiol Rev 84:935, 2004.
7. Caulfield MP, Birdsall NJM: International Union of Pharmacology. XVII. Classification of muscarinic acetylcholine receptors. Pharmacol Rev 50:279, 1998.
8. Sigala S, Mirabella G, Peroni A, et al: Differential gene expression of cholinergic muscarinic receptor subtypes in male and female normal human urinary bladder. Urology 60:719, 2002.
9. Yamaguchi O, Shishido K, Tamura K, et al: Evaluation of mRNAs encoding muscarinic receptor subtypes in human detrusor muscle. J Urol 156:1208, 1996.
10. Eglen RM, Hegde SS, Watson N: Muscarinic receptor subtypes and smooth muscle function. Pharmacol Rev 48:531, 1996.
11. Hegde SS, Eglen RM: Muscarinic receptor subtypes modulating smooth muscle contractility in the urinary bladder. Life Sci 64:419, 1999.
12. Chess-Williams R: Muscarinic receptors of the urinary bladder: Detrusor, urothelial and prejunctional. Auton Autacoid Pharmacol 22:133, 2002.
13. Schneider T, Fetscher C, Krege S, Michel MC: Signal transduction underlying carbachol-induced contraction of human urinary bladder. J Pharmacol Exp Ther 309:1148, 2004.
14. Andersson KE: Detrusor contraction—Focus on muscarinic receptors. Scand J Urol Nephrol Suppl 215:54, 2004.
15. Jezior JR, Brady JD, Rosenstein DI, et al: Dependency of detrusor contractions on calcium sensitization and calcium entry through LOE-908-sensitive channels. Br J Pharmacol 134:78, 2001.
16. Wibberley A, Chen Z, Hu E, et al: Expression and functional role of Rho-kinase in rat urinary bladder smooth muscle. Br J Pharmacol 138:757, 2003.
17. Hegde SS, Choppin A, Bonhaus D, et al: Functional role of M-2 and M-3 muscarinic receptors in the urinary bladder of rats in vitro and in vivo. Br J Pharmacol 120:1409, 1997.
18. Kotlikoff MI, Dhulipala P, Wang YX: M2 signaling in smooth muscle cells. Life Sci 64:437, 1999.
19. Bonev AD, Nelson MT: Muscarinic inhibition of ATP-sensitive K^+ channels by protein kinase C in urinary bladder smooth muscle. Am J Physiol 265(Pt 1):C1723, 1993.
20. Nakamura T, Kimura J, Yamaguchi O: Muscarinic M2 receptors inhibit $Ca2^+$-activated K^+ channels in rat bladder smooth muscle. Int J Urol 9:689, 2002.
21. Braverman AS, Luthin GR, Ruggieri MR: M2 muscarinic receptor contributes to contraction of the denervated rat urinary bladder. Am J Physiol 275:R1654, 1998.
22. Braverman A, Legos J, Young W, et al: M2 receptors in genitourinary smooth muscle pathology. Life Sci 64:429, 1999.
23. Braverman AS, Tallarida RJ, Ruggieri MR Sr: Interaction between muscarinic receptor subtype signal transduction pathways mediat-

ing bladder contraction. Am J Physiol Regul Integr Comp Physiol 283:R663, 2002.

24. Braverman AS, Ruggieri MR Sr: Hypertrophy changes the muscarinic receptor subtype mediating bladder contraction from M3 toward M2. Am J Physiol Regul Integr Comp Physiol 285: R701, 2003.
25. Pontari MA, Braverman AS, Ruggieri MR Sr: The M2 muscarinic receptor mediates in vitro bladder contractions from patients with neurogenic bladder dysfunction. Am J Physiol Regul Integr Comp Physiol 286:R874, 2004.
26. D'Agostino G, Bolognesi ML, Lucchelli A, et al: Prejunctional muscarinic inhibitory control of acetylcholine release in the human isolated detrusor: Involvement of the M4 receptor subtype. Br J Pharmacol 129:493, 2000.
27. Somogyi GT, de Groat WC: Function, signal transduction mechanisms and plasticity of presynaptic muscarinic receptors in the urinary bladder. Life Sci 64:411, 1999.
28. Somogyi GT, Zernova GV, Yoshiyama M, et al: Change in muscarinic modulation of transmitter release in the rat urinary bladder after spinal cord injury. Neurochem Int 43:73, 2003.
29. Mansfield KJ, Liu L, Mitchelson FJ, et al: Muscarinic receptor subtypes in human bladder detrusor and mucosa, studied by radioligand binding and quantitative competitive RT-PCR: Changes in ageing. Br J Pharmacol 144:1089, 2005.
30. Andersson KE: Antimuscarinics for treatment of overactive bladder. Lancet Neurol 3:46, 2004.
31. de Groat WC, Booth AM, Yoshimura N: Neurophysiology of micturition and its modification in animal models of human disease. In Maggi CA (ed): Nervous Control of the Urogenital System. London, Harwood Academic Publishers, 1993, pp 227-289.
32. Yoshida M, Inadome A, Murakami S, et al: Effects of age and muscle stretching on acetylcholine release in isolated human bladder smooth muscle [abstract 160]. J Urol 167:40, 2002.
33. Andersson KE, Yoshida M: Antimuscarinics and the overactive detrusor—Which is the main mechanism of action? Eur Urol 43:1, 2003.
34. Brading AF: A myogenic basis for the overactive bladder. Urology 50(Suppl):57, 1997.
35. Goepel M, Wittmann A, Rubben H, Michel MC: Comparison of adrenoceptor subtype expression in porcine and human bladder and prostate. Urol Res 25:199, 1997.
36. Malloy BJ, Price DT, Price RR, et al: Alpha1-adrenergic receptor subtypes in human detrusor. J Urol 160(Pt 1):937, 1998.
37. Hampel C, Dolber PC, Smith MP, et al: Modulation of bladder alpha1-adrenergic receptor subtype expression by bladder outlet obstruction. J Urol 167:1513, 2002.
38. Nomiya M, Shishido K, Uchida H, Yamaguchi O: A quantitative analysis of mRNA expression of α_1- and β-adrenoceptor subtypes and their functional roles in human normal and obstructed bladders. Neurourol Urodyn 21:299, 2002.
39. Bouchelouche K, Andersen L, Alvarez S, et al: Increased contractile response to phenylephrine in detrusor of patients with bladder outlet obstruction: Effect of the alpha1A and alpha1D-adrenergic receptor antagonist tamsulosin. J Urol 173:657, 2005.
40. Das AK, Leggett RE, Whitbeck C, et al: Effect of doxazosin on rat urinary bladder function after partial outlet obstruction. Neurourol Urodyn 21:160, 2002.
41. Yamaguchi O: Beta3-adrenoceptors in human detrusor muscle. Urology 59(Suppl 1):25, 2002.
42. Hudman D, Elliott RA, Norman RI: Inhibition of the contractile response of the rat detrusor muscle by the beta(2)-adrenoceptor agonist clenbuterol. Eur J Pharmacol 392:79, 2000.
43. Grüneberger A: Treatment of motor urge incontinence with clenbuterol and flavoxate hydrochloride. Br J Obstet Gynaecol 91:275, 1984.
44. Lindholm P, Lose G: Terbutaline (Bricanyl) in the treatment of female urge incontinence. Urol Int 41:158, 1986.
45. Woods M, Carson N, Norton NW, et al: Efficacy of the beta3-adrenergic receptor agonist CL-316243 on experimental bladder hyperreflexia and detrusor instability in the rat. J Urol 166:1142, 2001.
46. Kaidoh K, Igawa Y, Takeda H, et al. Effects of selective beta2 and beta3-adrenoceptor agonists on detrusor hyperreflexia in conscious cerebral infarcted rats. J Urol 168:1247, 2002.
47. Takeda H, Yamazaki Y, Igawa Y, et al: Effects of beta(3)-adrenoceptor stimulation on prostaglandin E(2)-induced bladder hyperactivity and on the cardiovascular system in conscious rats. Neurourol Urodyn 21:558, 2002.
48. Andersson KE: Pharmacology of lower urinary tract smooth muscles and penile erectile tissues. Pharmacol Rev 45:253, 1993.
49. Sjögren C, Andersson KE, Husted S, et al: Atropine resistance of transmurally stimulated isolated human bladder muscle. J Urol 128:1368, 1982.
50. Husted S, Sjøgren C, Andersson KE: Direct effects of adenosine and adenine nucleotides on isolated human urinary bladder and their influence on electrically induced contractions. J Urol 130:392, 1983.
51. Bayliss M, Wu C, Newgreen D, et al: A quantitative study of atropine-resistant contractile responses in human detrusor smooth muscle, from stable, unstable and obstructed bladders. J Urol 162:1833, 1999.
52. O'Reilly BA, Kosaka AH, Knight GF, et al: P2X receptors and their role in female idiopathic detrusor instability. J Urol 167:157, 2002.
53. Palea S, Artibani W, Ostardo E, et al: Evidence for purinergic neurotransmission in human urinary bladder affected by interstitial cystitis. J Urol 150:2007, 1993.
54. Wammack R, Weihe E, Dienes H-P, Hohenfellner R: Die Neurogene Blase in vitro. Akt Urol 26:16, 1995.
55. Yoshida M, Homma Y, Inadome A, et al: Age-related changes in cholinergic and purinergic neurotransmission in human isolated bladder smooth muscles. Exp Gerontol 36:99, 2001.
56. Burnstock G: Purinergic signalling in lower urinary tract. In Abbracchio MP, Berlin WM (eds): Purinergic and Pyrimidinergic Signalling. I. Molecular, Nervous and Urogenitary System Function. New York, Springer-Verlag, 2001, pp 423-515.
57. Lee HY, Bardini M, Burnstock G: Distribution of P2X receptors in the urinary bladder and the ureter of the rat. J Urol 163:2002, 2000.
58. O'Reilly BA, Kosaka AH, Chang TK, et al: A quantitative analysis of purinoceptor expression in human fetal and adult bladders. J Urol 165:1730, 2001.
59. Moore KH, Ray FR, Barden JA: Loss of purinergic P2X(3) and P2X(5) receptor innervation in human detrusor from adults with urge incontinence. J Neurosci 21:RC166, 2001.
60. Harvey RA, Skennerton DE, Newgreen D, Fry CH: The contractile potency of adenosine triphosphate and ecto-adenosine triphosphatase activity in guinea pig detrusor and detrusor from patients with a stable, unstable or obstructed bladder. J Urol 168:1235, 2002.
61. O'Reilly BA, Kosaka AH, Chang TK, et al: A quantitative analysis of purinoceptor expression in the bladders of patients with symptomatic outlet obstruction. BJU Int 87:617, 2001.
62. Szallasi A: The vanilloid (capsaicin) receptor: Receptor types and species differences. Gen Pharmacol 25:223, 1994.
63. Maggi CA: The dual sensory and 'efferent' function of the capsaicin-sensitive primary sensory neurons in the urinary bladder and urethra. In Maggi CA (ed): Nervous Control of the Urogenital System. London, Harwood Academic, 1993, pp 383-422.
64. Ishizuka O, Mattiasson A, Andersson KE: Urodynamic effects of intravesical resiniferatoxin and capsaicin in conscious rats with and without outflow obstruction. J Urol 154:611, 1995.
65. Szallazi A, Blumberg PM: Vanilloid receptors: New insights enhance potential as a therapeutic target. Pain 68:195, 1996.
66. Kuo HC: Inhibitory effect of capsaicin on detrusor contractility: Further study in the presence of ganglionic blocker and neurokinin

receptor antagonist in the rat urinary bladder. Urol Int 59:95, 1997.
67. Birder LA, Nakamura Y, Kiss S, et al: Altered urinary bladder function in mice lacking the vanilloid receptor TRPV1. Nat Neurosci 5:856, 2002.
68. Cruz F: Vanilloid receptor and detrusor instability. Urology 59(Suppl 1):51, 2002.
69. Silva C, Ribeiro MJ, Cruz F: The effect of intravesical resiniferatoxin in patients with idiopathic detrusor instability suggests that involuntary detrusor contractions are triggered by C-fiber input. J Urol 168:575, 2002.
70. Forman A, Andersson KE, Henriksson L, et al: Effects of nifedipine on the smooth muscle of the human urinary tract in vitro and in vivo. Acta Pharmacol Toxicol 43:111, 1978.
71. Ganitkevich VY, Isenberg G: Contribution of Ca(2+)-induced Ca2+ release to the [Ca2+]i transients in myocytes from guinea-pig urinary bladder. J Physiol (Lond) 458:119, 1992.
72. Isenberg G, Wendt-Gallitelli MF, Ganitkevich V: Contribution of Ca(2+)-induced Ca2+ release to depolarization-induced Ca2+ transients of myocytes from guinea-pig urinary bladder myocytes. Jpn J Pharmacol 58:81P, 1992.
73. Hedlund H, Mattiasson A, Andersson KE: Effects of pinacidil on detrusor instability in men with bladder outlet obstruction. J Urol 146:1345, 1991.
74. Komersova K, Rogerson JW, Conway EL, et al: The effect of levcromakalim (BRL 38227) on bladder function in patients with high spinal cord lesions. Br J Clin Pharmacol 39:207, 1995.
75. Andersson KE: Bladder activation: Afferent mechanisms. Urology 59(Suppl 1):43, 2002.
76. Birder LA, Kanai AJ, de Groat WC, et al: Vanilloid receptor expression suggests a sensory role for urinary bladder epithelial cells. Proc Natl Acad Sci U S A 98:13396, 2001.
77. Sui GP, Rothery S, Dupont E, et al: Gap junctions and connexin expression in human suburothelial interstitial cells. BJU Int 90:118, 2002.
78. Sui GP, Wu C, Fry CH: Electrical characteristics of suburothelial cells isolated from the human bladder. J Urol 171(Pt 1):938, 2004.
79. Pandita RK, Andersson KE: Intravesical adenosine triphosphate stimulates the micturition reflex in awake, freely moving rats. J Urol 168:1230, 2002.
80. Cockayne DA, Hamilton SG, Zhu QM, et al: Urinary bladder hyporeflexia and reduced pain-related behaviour in P2X3-deficient mice. Nature 407:1011, 2000.
81. Vlaskovska M, Kasakov L, Rong W, et al: P2X3 knock-out mice reveal a major sensory role for urothelially released ATP. J Neurosci 21:5670, 2001.
82. Pinna C, Caratozzolo O, Puglisi L: A possible role for urinary bladder epithelium in bradykinin-induced contraction in diabetic rats. Eur J Pharmacol 214:143, 1992.
83. Pinna C, Ventura S, Puglisi L, Burnstock G: A pharmacological and histochemical study of hamster urethra and the role of urothelium. Br J Pharmacol 119:655, 1996.
84. Hypolite JA, Longhurst PA, Gong C, et al: Metabolic studies on rabbit bladder smooth muscle and mucosa. Mol Cell Biochem 125:35, 1993.
85. Fovaeus M, Fujiwara M, Hogestatt ED, et al: A non-nitrergic smooth muscle relaxant factor released from rat urinary bladder by muscarinic receptor stimulation. J Urol 161:649, 1999.
86. Hawthorn MH, Chapple CR, Cock M, Chess-Williams R: Urothelium-derived inhibitory factor(s) influences on detrusor muscle contractility in vitro. Br J Pharmacol 129:416, 2000.
87. Templeman L, Chapple CR, Chess-Williams R: Urothelium derived inhibitory factor and cross-talk among receptors in the trigone of the bladder of the pig. J Urol 167(Pt 1):742, 2002.
88. Warner FJ, Shang F, Millard RJ, Burcher E: Enhancement of neurokinin A-induced smooth muscle contraction in human urinary bladder by mucosal removal and phosphoramidon: Relationship to peptidase inhibition. Eur J Pharmacol 438:171, 2002.
89. Chaiyaprasithi B, Mang CF, Kilbinger H, Hohenfellner M: Inhibition of human detrusor contraction by a urothelium derived factor. J Urol 170:1897, 2003.
90. DeLancey JO, Fowler CJ, Keane D, et al: Pathophysiology. In Abrams P, Khoury S, Wein AJ (eds): Incontinence. First International Consultation of Incontinence. Plymouth, UK, Plymbridge Distributors, 1999, pp 227-294.
91. Henriksson L, Andersson K-E, Ulmsten U: The urethral pressure profiles in continent and stress-incontinent women. Scand J Urol Nephrol 13:5, 1979.
92. Hilton P, Stanton SL: Urethral pressure measurement by microtransducer: The results in symptom-free women and in those with genuine stress incontinence. Br J Obstet Gynaecol 90:919, 1983.
93. Rud T, Andersson KE, Asmussen M, et al: Factors maintaining the intraurethral pressure in women. Invest Urol 17:343, 1980.
94. Bridgewater M, Brading AF: Evidence for a non-nitrergic inhibitory innervation in the pig urethra. Neurourol Urodyn 12:357, 1993.
95. Hashimoto S, Kigoshi S, Muramatsu I: Nitric oxide-dependent and -independent neurogenic relaxation of isolated dog urethra. Eur J Pharmacol 231:209, 1993.
96. Werkstrom V, Persson K, Ny L, et al: Factors involved in the relaxation of female pig urethra evoked by electrical field stimulation. Br J Pharmacol 116:1599, 1995.
97. Fraser MO, Chancellor MB: Neural control of the urethra and development of pharmacotherapy for stress urinary incontinence. BJU Int 91:743, 2003.
98. Michel MC, Peters SL: Role of serotonin and noradrenaline in stress urinary incontinence. BJU Int 94(Suppl 1):23, 2004.
99. Thor KB, Donatucci CF: Central nervous system control of the lower urinary tract: New pharmacological approaches to stress urinary incontinence in women. J Urol 172:27, 2004.
100. Lincoln J, Burnstock G: Autonomic innervation of the urinary bladder and urethra. In Maggi CA (ed): Nervous Control of the Urogenital System. London, Harwood Academic Publisher, 1993, pp 33-68.
101. Gosling JA, Dixon JS, Lendon RG: The autonomic innervation of the human male and female bladder neck and proximal urethra. J Urol 118:302, 1977.
102. Ek A, Alm P, Andersson KE, Persson CG: Adrenergic and cholinergic nerves of the human urethra and urinary bladder. A histochemical study. Acta Physiol Scand 99:345, 1977.
103. Alm P, Zygmunt PK, Iselin C, et al: Nitric oxide synthase-immunoreactive, adrenergic, cholinergic, and peptidergic nerves of the female rat urinary tract: A comparative study. J Auton Nerv Syst 56:105, 1995.
104. Persson K, Johansson K, Alm P, et al: Morphological and functional evidence against a sensory and sympathetic origin of nitric oxide synthase-containing nerves in the rat lower urinary tract. Neuroscience 77:271, 1997.
105. Persson K, Alm, P, Johansson K, et al: Co-existence of nitrergic, peptidergic and acetylcholine esterase-positive nerves in the pig lower urinary tract. J Auton Nerv Syst 52:225, 1995.
106. Persson K, Alm P, Uvelius B, Andersson KE: Nitrergic and cholinergic innervation of the rat lower urinary tract after pelvic ganglionectomy. Am J Physiol 274:R389, 1998.
107. Werkstrom V, Alm P, Persson K, Andersson KE: Inhibitory innervation of the guinea-pig urethra; roles of CO, NO and VIP. J Auton Nerv Syst 74:33, 1998.
108. Appell RA, England HR, Hussell AR, McGuire EJ: The effects of epidural anesthesia on the urethral closure pressure profile in patients with prostatic enlargement. J Urol 124:410, 1980.
109. Furuya S, Kumamoto Y, Yokoyama E, et al: Alpha-adrenergic activity and urethral pressure in prostatic zone in benign prostatic hypertrophy. J Urol 128:836, 1982.

110. Brading AF, McCoy R, Dass N: Alpha1-adrenoceptors in urethral function. Eur Urol 36 Suppl 1:74, 1999.
111. Nasu K, Moriyama N, Fukasawa R, et al: Quantification and distribution of alpha1-adrenoceptor subtype mRNAs in human proximal urethra. Br J Pharmacol 123:1289, 1998.
112. Taki N, Taniguchi T, Okada K, et al: Evidence for predominant mediation of alpha1-adrenoceptor in the tonus of entire urethra of women. J Urol 162:1829, 1999.
113. Daniels DV, Gever JR, Jasper JR, et al: Human cloned alpha1A-adrenoceptor isoforms display alpha1L-adrenoceptor pharmacology in functional studies. Eur J Pharmacol 370:337, 1999.
114. Fukasawa R, Taniguchi N, Moriyama N, et al: The alpha1L-adrenoceptor subtype in the lower urinary tract: A comparison of human urethra and prostate. Br J Urol 82:733, 1998.
115. Chai TC, Belville WD, McGuire EJ, Nyquist L: Specificity of the American Urological Association voiding symptom index: Comparison of unselected and selected samples of both. J Urol 150:1710, 1993.
116. Jollys JV, Jollys JC, Wilson J, et al: Does sexual equality extend to urinary symptoms? Neurourol Urodyn 12:391, 1993.
117. Lepor H, Machi G: Comparison of AUA symptom index in unselected males and females between fifty-five and seventy-nine years of age. Urology 42:36, 1993.
118. Lepor H, Theune C: Randomized double-blind study comparing the efficacy of terazosin versus placebo in women with prostatism-like symptoms. J Urol 154:116, 1995.
119. Nordling J: Effects of clonidine (Catapresan) on urethral pressure. Invest Urol 16:289, 1979.
120. Alberts P: Subtype classification of the presynaptic alpha-adrenoceptors which regulate [^{3}H]-noradrenaline secretion in guinea-pig isolated urethra. Br J Pharmacol 105:142, 1992.
121. Levin RM, Ruggieri MR, Wein AJ: Identification of receptor subtypes in the rabbit and human urinary bladder by selective radioligand binding. J Urol 139:844, 1988.
122. Fujimura T, Tamura K, Tsutsumi T, et al: Expression and possible functional role of the beta3-adrenoceptor in human and rat detrusor muscle. J Urol 161:680, 1999.
123. Igawa Y, Yamazaki Y, Takeda H, et al: Functional and molecular biological evidence for a possible beta3-adrenoceptor in the human detrusor muscle. Br J Pharmacol 126:819, 1999.
124. Takeda M, Obara K, Mizusawa T, et al: Evidence for beta3-adrenoceptor subtypes in relaxation of the human urinary bladder detrusor: Analysis by molecular biological and pharmacological methods. J Pharmacol Exp Ther 288:1367, 1999.
125. Morita T, Iizuka H, Iwata T, Kondo S: Function and distribution of beta3-adrenoceptors in rat, rabbit and human urinary bladder and external urethral sphincter. J Smooth Muscle Res 36:21, 2000.
126. Johns A: Alpha- and beta-adrenergic and muscarinic cholinergic binding sites in the bladder and urethra of the rabbit. Can J Physiol Pharmacol 61:61, 1983.
127. Persson CG, Andersson KE: Adrenoceptor and cholinoceptor mediated effects in the isolated urethra of cat and guinea-pig. Clin Exp Pharmacol Physiol 3:415, 1976.
128. Andersson KE, Persson CG, Alm P, et al: Effects of acetylcholine, noradrenaline, and prostaglandins on the isolated, perfused human fetal urethra. Acta Physiol Scand 104:394, 1978.
129. Ek A, Andersson KE, Ulmsten U: The effects of norephedrine and bethanechol on the human urethral closure pressure profile. Scand J Urol Nephrol 12:97, 1978.
130. Ulmsten U, Andersson KE: The effects of emeprone on intravesical and intra-urethral pressure in women with urgency incontinence. Scand J Urol Nephrol 11:103, 1977.
131. Mattiasson A, Andersson KE, Sjögren C: Adrenoceptors and cholinoceptors controlling noradrenaline release from adrenergic nerves in the urethra of rabbit and man. J Urol 131:1190, 1984.
132. Tanagho EA, Miller ER: Initiation of voiding. Br J Urol 42:175, 1970.
133. Andersson KE, Persson K: The L-arginine/nitric oxide pathway and non-adrenergic, non-cholinergic relaxation of the lower urinary tract. Gen Pharmacol 24:833, 1993.
134. Burnett AL: Nitric oxide control of lower genitourinary tract functions: A review. Urology 45:1071, 1995.
135. Dokita S, Smith SD, Nishimoto T, et al: Involvement of nitric oxide and cyclic GMP in rabbit urethral relaxation. Eur J Pharmacol 269:269, 1994.
136. Morita T, Tsujii T, Dokita S: Regional difference in functional roles of cAMP and cGMP in lower urinary tract smooth muscle contractility. Urol Int 49:191, 192.
137. Persson K, Andersson KE: Non-adrenergic, non-cholinergic relaxation and levels of cyclic nucleotides in rabbit lower urinary tract. Eur J Pharmacol 268:159, 1994.
138. Robertson BE, Schubert R, Hescheler J, Nelson MT: cGMP-dependent protein kinase activates Ca-activated K-channels in cerebral artery smooth muscle cells. Am J Physiol 265:C299, 1993.
139. Warner T, Mitchell JA, Sheng H, Murad F: Effects of cyclic GMP on smooth muscle relaxation. Adv Pharmacol 26:171, 1994.
140. Persson K, Kumar Pandita R, et al: Functional characteristics of lower urinary tract smooth muscles in mice lacking cyclic GMP protein kinase type I. Am J Physiol Regul Integr Comp Physiol 279: R1112, 2000.
141. Waldeck K, Ny L, Persson K, Andersson KE: Mediators and mechanisms of relaxation in rabbit urethral smooth muscle. Br J Pharmacol 123:617, 1998.
142. Smet PJ, Jonavicius J, Marshall VR, De Vente J: Distribution of nitric oxide synthase-immunoreactive nerves and identification of the cellular targets of nitric oxide in guinea-pig and human urinary bladder by cGMP immunohistochemistry. Neuroscience 71:337, 1996.
143. Sergeant GP, Hollywood MA, McCloskey KD, et al: Specialised pacemaking cells in the rabbit urethra. J Physiol 526(Pt 2):359, 2000.
144. Sergeant GP, Hollywood MA, McCloskey KD, et al: Role of IP(3) in modulation of spontaneous activity in pacemaker cells of rabbit urethra. Am J Physiol Cell Physiol 280:C1349, 2001.
145. Sergeant GP, Thornbury KD, McHale NG, Hollywood MA: Characterization of norepinephrine-evoked inward currents in interstitial cells isolated from the rabbit urethra. Am J Physiol Cell Physiol 283:C885, 2002.
146. Blakeman PJ, Hilton P, Bulmer JN: Oestrogen and progesterone receptor expression in the female lower urinary tract, with reference to oestrogen status. BJU Int 86:32, 2000.
147. Nilsson S, Mäkelä S, Treuter E, et al: Mechanisms of estrogen action. Physiol Rev 81:1535, 2001.
148. Liang W, Afshar K, Stothers L, Laher I: The influence of ovariectomy and estrogen replacement on voiding patterns and detrusor muscarinic receptor affinity in the rat. Life Sci 71:351, 2002.
149. Longhurst PA, Levendusky M: Influence of gender and the oestrus cycle on in vitro contractile response of rat urinary bladder to cholinergic stimulation. Br J Pharmacol 131:177, 2000.
150. Yono M, Yoshida M, Takahashi W, et al: Effects of ovarian hormones on beta-adrenergic receptor-mediated relaxation in the female rabbit bladder. Urol Res 28:38, 2000.
151. Fleischmann N, Christ G, Sclafani T, Melman A: The effect of ovariectomy and long-term estrogen replacement on bladder structure and function in the rat. J Urol 168:1265, 2002.
152. Longhurst PA: In vitro rat bladder function after neonatal estrogenization. J Urol 168:2695, 2002.
153. Aikawa K, Sugino T, Matsumoto S, et al: The effect of ovariectomy and estradiol on rabbit bladder smooth muscle contraction and morphology. J Urol 170:634, 2003.

154. Levin RM, Shofer FS, Wein AJ: Estrogen-induced alterations in the autonomic responses of the rabbit urinary bladder. J Pharmacol Exp Ther 215:614, 1980.
155. Shapiro E: Effect of estrogens on the weight and muscarinic cholinergic receptor density of the rabbit bladder and urethra. J Urol 135:1084, 1986.
156. Batra S, Andersson KE: Oestrogen-induced changes in muscarinic receptor density and contractile responses in the female rabbit urinary bladder. Acta Physiol Scand 137:135, 1989.
157. Elliott RA, Castleden CM, Miodrag A: The effect of in vivo oestrogen treatment on the contractile response of rat isolated detrusor muscle. Br J Pharmacol 107:766, 1992.
158. Matsubara S, Okada H, Shirakawa T, et al: Estrogen levels influence beta-3-adrenoceptor-mediated relaxation of the female rat detrusor muscle. Urology 59:621, 2002.
159. Schröder A, Pandita RK, Hedlund P, et al: Estrogen receptor subtypes and afferent signaling in the bladder. J Urol 170:1013, 2003.
160. Batra S, Iosif CS: Progesterone receptors in the female lower urinary tract. J Urol 138:1301, 1987.
161. Wolf H, Wandt H, Jonat W: Immunohistochemical evidence of estrogen and progesterone receptors in the female lower urinary tract and comparison with the vagina. Gynecol Obstet Invest 32:227, 1991.
162. Elliott RA, Castleden CM: Effect of progestogens and oestrogens on the contractile response of rat detrusor muscle to electrical field stimulation. Clin Sci 87:337, 1994.
163. Ekström J, Iosif CS, Malmberg L: Effects of long-term treatment with estrogen and progesterone on in vitro muscle responses of the female rabbit urinary bladder and urethra to autonomic drugs and nerve stimulation. J Urol 150:1284, 1993.
164. Tong YC, Hung YC, Lin JSN, et al: Effects of pregnancy and progesterone on autonomic functioning the rat urinary bladder. Pharmacology 50:192, 1995.
165. Toozs-Hobson P, Cutner A: Pregnancy and childbirth. In Cardozo L, Staskin D (eds): Textbook of Female Urology and Urogynaecology. London, Isis Medical Media, 2002, pp 978-992, 2002.
166. Zderic SA, Plazak JE, Duckett JW, et al: Effect of pregnancy on rabbit urinary bladder physiology. I. Effects of extracellular calcium. Pharmacology 41:124, 1990.
167. Levin RM, Zderic SA, Ewalt DH, et al: Effects of pregnancy on muscarinic receptor density and function in the rabbit urinary bladder. Pharmacology 43:69, 1991.
168. Baselli EC, Brandes SB, Luthin GR, Ruggieri MR: The effect of pregnancy and contractile activity on bladder muscarinic receptor subtypes. Neurourol Urodyn 18:511, 1999.

Chapter 5

HORMONAL INFLUENCES ON THE FEMALE GENITAL AND LOWER URINARY TRACTS

Dudley Robinson and Linda Cardozo

The female genital tract and lower urinary tract share a common embryologic origin, arising from the urogenital sinus. Both are sensitive to the effects of female sex steroid hormones. Estrogen has an important role in the function of the lower urinary tract throughout adult life, and estrogen and progesterone receptors have been demonstrated in the vagina, urethra, bladder, and pelvic floor musculature.[1-4] This role is supported by the fact that estrogen deficiency occurring after menopause is known to cause atrophic changes within the urogenital tract[5] and is associated with urinary symptoms such as frequency, urgency, nocturia, incontinence, and recurrent infection. These effects may also coexist with symptoms of vaginal atrophy such as dyspareunia, itching, burning, and dryness. This chapter reviews the roles of estrogen and progesterone in lower urinary tract function and assesses the role of estrogens in the management of lower urinary tract dysfunction.

ESTROGEN RECEPTORS AND HORMONAL FACTORS

The effects of the steroid hormone 17β-estradiol are mediated by ligand-activated transcription factors known as estrogen receptors. They are glycoproteins that share common features with androgen and progesterone receptors, and they can be divided into several functional domains.[6] The classic estrogen receptor (ERα) was first discovered by Elwood Jensen in 1958 and cloned from uterine tissue in 1986,[7] although it was not until 1996 that the second estrogen receptor (ERβ) was identified.[8] The precise role of the two different receptors remains to be elucidated, although estrogen receptor-α appears to play a major role in the regulation of reproduction, whereas estrogen receptor-β has a more minor role.[9]

Estrogen receptors have been demonstrated throughout the lower urinary tract and are expressed in the squamous epithelium of the proximal and distal urethra, vagina, and trigone of the bladder[3,10] although not in the dome of the bladder, reflecting its different embryologic origin. The pubococcygeus and the musculature of the pelvic floor also are estrogen sensitive,[11] although estrogen receptors have not yet been identified in the levator ani muscles.[12]

The distribution of estrogen receptors throughout the urogenital tract has been studied, and ERα and ERβ receptors have been found in the vaginal walls and uterosacral ligaments of premenopausal women, although the latter were absent in the vaginal walls of postmenopausal women.[13] The ERα receptors are localized in the urethral sphincter, and when sensitized by estrogens, they are thought to help maintain muscular tone.[14]

In addition to estrogen receptors, androgen and progesterone receptors are expressed in the lower urinary tract, although their role is less clear. Progesterone receptors are expressed inconsistently, and they have been reported in the bladder, trigone, and vagina. Their presence may depend on estrogen status.[5] Androgen receptors are present in the bladder and urethra, although their role has not yet been defined.[15] Estrogen receptors have also been identified in mast cells in women with interstitial cystitis[16,17] and in the male lower urinary tract.[18]

The incidence of both estrogen and progesterone expression has been examined throughout the lower urinary tract in 90 women undergoing gynecologic surgery; 33 were premenopausal, 26 were postmenopausal without hormone replacement therapy (HRT), and 31 were postmenopausal and taking HRT.[19] Biopsies were taken from the bladder dome, trigone, proximal urethra, distal urethra, vagina, and vesicovaginal fascia adjacent to the bladder neck. Estrogen receptors were consistently expressed in the squamous epithelia, but they were absent in the urothelial tissues of the lower urinary tract of all women, irrespective of estrogen status. Progesterone receptor expression, however, showed more variability because it was mostly subepithelial and was significantly lower in postmenopausal women not taking estrogen replacement therapy.

HORMONAL INFLUENCES ON LOWER URINARY TRACT SYMPTOMS

To maintain continence, the urethral pressure must remain higher than the intravesical pressure at all times, except during micturition.[20] Estrogens play an important role in the continence mechanism, with bladder and urethral function becoming less efficient with age.[21] Elderly women have been found to have a reduced flow rate, increased urinary residuals, higher filling pressures, reduced bladder capacity, and lower maximum voiding pressures.[22] Estrogens may affect continence by increasing urethral resistance, raising the sensory threshold of the bladder or by increasing α-adrenoreceptor sensitivity in the urethral smooth muscle.[23,24] Exogenous estrogens have been shown to increase the number of intermediate and superficial cells in the vagina of postmenopausal women.[25] These changes have also been demonstrated in the bladder and urethra.[26]

A prospective, observational study was performed to assess cell proliferation rates throughout the tissues of the lower urinary tract.[27] Fifty-nine women were studied; 23 were premenopausal, 20 were postmenopausal and not taking HRT and 20 were postmenopausal and taking HRT. Biopsies were taken from the bladder dome, trigone, proximal urethra, distal urethra, vagina, and vesicovaginal fascia adjacent to the bladder neck. The squamous epithelium of estrogen-replete women was shown to exhibit greater levels of cellular proliferation than in those women who were estrogen deficient.

Cyclic variations in the levels of estrogen and progesterone during the menstrual cycle lead to changes in urodynamic variables and lower urinary tract symptoms, with 37% of women noticing a deterioration in symptoms before menstruation.[28] Measurement of the urethral pressure profile in nulliparous premenopausal women shows there is an increase in functional urethral length midcycle and early in the luteal phase, corresponding to an increase in plasma estradiol.[29] Progestogens have been associated with an increase in irritating bladder symptoms[30,31] and urinary incontinence in women taking combined HRT.[32] The incidence of detrusor overactivity in the luteal phase of the menstrual cycle may be associated with raised plasma progesterone levels after ovulation, and progesterone has been shown to antagonize the inhibitory effect of estradiol on rat detrusor contractions.[33] This may help to explain the increased prevalence of detrusor overactivity found in pregnancy.[34]

The role of estrogen therapy in the management of women with fecal incontinence has been investigated in a prospective, observational study using symptom questionnaires and anorectal physiologic testing before and after 6 months of estrogen replacement therapy. At follow-up, 25% of women were asymptomatic, and another 65% were improved in terms of flatus control, urgency, and fecal staining. Anal resting pressures and voluntary squeeze increments were significantly increased after estrogen therapy, although there were no changes in pudendal nerve terminal latency. The investigators concluded that estrogen replacement therapy may have a beneficial effect, although larger studies are needed to confirm these findings.[35]

HORMONAL INFLUENCES ON URINARY TRACT INFECTION

Urinary tract infection is a common cause of urinary symptoms in women of all ages. This is a particular problem in the elderly, with a reported incidence of 20% in the community and more than 50% among institutionalized patients.[36,37] Pathophysiologic changes such as impairment of bladder emptying, poor perineal hygiene, and fecal and urinary incontinence may partly account for the high prevalence observed. Changes in the vaginal flora due to estrogen depletion lead to colonization with gram-negative bacilli, which cause locally irritating symptoms and act as uropathogens. These microbiologic changes may be reversed with estrogen replacement after menopause, offering a rationale for treatment and prophylaxis.

HORMONAL INFLUENCES ON LOWER URINARY TRACT FUNCTION

Neurologic Control

Sex hormones are known to influence the central neurologic control of micturition, although their exact role in the micturition pathway has yet to be elucidated. Estrogen receptors have been demonstrated in the cerebral cortex, limbic system, hippocampus, and cerebellum,[38,39] and androgen receptors have been demonstrated in the pontine micturition center and the preoptic area of the hypothalamus.[40]

Bladder Function

Estrogen receptors, although absent in the transitional epithelium at the dome of the bladder, are present in the areas of the trigone that have undergone squamous metaplasia.[10] Estrogen is known to have a direct effect on detrusor function through modifications in muscarinic receptors[41,42] and by inhibition of movement of extracellular calcium ions into muscle cells.[43] Consequently, estradiol has been shown to reduce the amplitude and frequency of spontaneous rhythmic detrusor contractions,[44] and there is evidence that it may increase the sensory threshold of the bladder in some women.[45]

Urethral Function

Estrogen receptors have been demonstrated in the squamous epithelium of the proximal and distal urethra,[10] and estrogen has been shown to improve the maturation index of urethral squamous epithelium.[46] It has been suggested that estrogen increases urethral closure pressure and improves pressure transmission to the proximal urethra, both promoting continence.[47-50] Estrogens have been shown to cause vasodilatation in the systemic and cerebral circulation, and these changes are also seen in the urethra.[51-53]

The vascular pulsations seen on urethral pressure profilometry resulting from blood flow in the urethral submucosa and urethral sphincter have been shown to increase in size after estrogen administration,[54] and the effect is lost after estrogen withdrawal at menopause. The urethral vascular bed is thought to account for about one third of the urethral closure pressure, and estrogen replacement therapy in postmenopausal women with stress incontinence has been shown to increase the number of periurethral vessels.[55]

Collagen Metabolism

Estrogens affect collagen synthesis, and they have a direct effect on collagen metabolism in the lower genital tract.[56] Changes found in women with urogenital atrophy may represent an alteration in systemic collagenase activity,[57] and urodynamic stress incontinence and urogenital prolapse have been associated with a reduction in vaginal and periurethral collagen levels.[58-60] There is a reduction in skin collagen content after menopause,[61] and the rectus muscle fascia becomes less elastic with increasing age, resulting in a lower energy requirement to cause irreversible damage.[62] Changes in collagen content have also been identified, the hydroxyproline content in connective tissue from women with stress incontinence being 40% lower than in continent controls.[63]

LOWER URINARY TRACT SYMPTOMS

Urinary Incontinence

The prevalence of urinary incontinence increases with age, affecting 15% to 35% of community-dwelling women older than 60 years,[64] and other studies have reported a prevalence of 49% among women older than 65 years.[65] Rates of 50% have been reported in elderly nursing home residents.[66] A cross-sectional population prevalence survey of 146 women between the ages of 15 and 97 years found that 46% experienced symptoms of pelvic floor dysfunction, defined as stress or urge incontinence, flatus or fecal incontinence, symptomatic prolapse, or previous pelvic floor surgery.[67]

Little work has been done to examine the incidence of urinary incontinence. However, a study in New Zealand of women older than 65 years found 10% of the originally continent developed urinary incontinence in the 3-year study period.[68]

Epidemiologic studies have implicated estrogen deficiency in the cause of lower urinary tract symptoms, with 70% of women relating the onset of urinary incontinence to their final menstrual period.[5] Lower urinary tract symptoms are common in postmenopausal women attending a menopause clinic, with 20% complaining of severe urgency and almost 50% complaining of stress incontinence.[69] Urge incontinence in particular is more prevalent after menopause, and the prevalence appears to rise with increasing years of estrogen deficiency.[70] There is, however, conflicting evidence regarding the role of estrogen withdrawal at the time of menopause. Some studies have shown a peak incidence in perimenopausal women,[71,72] and other evidence suggests that many women develop incontinence at least 10 years before the cessation of menstruation, with significantly more premenopausal women than postmenopausal women being affected.[73]

Urogenital Atrophy

Urogenital atrophy is a manifestation of estrogen withdrawal after menopause, and symptoms may appear for the first time more than 10 years after the last menstrual period.[74] Increasing life expectancy has led to an increasingly elderly population, and with the average age of the menopause being 50 years,[76] it is now common for women to spend one third of their lives in the estrogen-deficient postmenopausal state.[75]

Postmenopausal women comprise 15% of the population in industrialized countries, with a predicted growth rate of 1.5% over the next 20 years. Overall, in the developed world, 8% of the total population is estimated to have urogenital symptoms.[77] This represents 200 million women in the United States alone.

It has been estimated that 10% to 40% of all postmenopausal women are symptomatic,[78] although only 25% are thought to seek medical help. Two out of three women report vaginal symptoms associated with urogenital atrophy by the age of 75 years.[79] However, the prevalence of symptomatic urogenital atrophy is difficult to estimate, because many women accept the changes as being an inevitable consequence of the aging process and do not seek help, leading to considerable underreporting.

In a study assessing the prevalence of urogenital symptoms in 2157 Dutch women,[80] 27% complained of vaginal dryness, soreness, and dyspareunia, and the prevalence of urinary symptoms such as leakage and recurrent infections was 36%. When considering severity, almost 50% reported moderate to severe discomfort, although only a third had received medical intervention. Women who had had a hysterectomy reported moderate to severe complaints more often than those who had not.

The prevalence of urogenital atrophy and urogenital prolapse was examined in a population of 285 women attending a menopause clinic.[81] Overall, 51% of women had anterior vaginal wall prolapse, 27% had posterior vaginal prolapse, and 20% had apical prolapse. In this same group, 34% of women had urogenital atrophy, and 40% complained of dyspareunia. Although urogenital atrophy and symptoms of dyspareunia were related to menopausal age, the prevalence of prolapse showed no association.

Although urogenital atrophy is an inevitable consequence of menopause, women may not always be symptomatic. In one study, 69 women attending a gynecology clinic were asked to fill out a symptom questionnaire before examination and undergoing vaginal cytology.[82] Urogenital symptoms were found to be relatively low and were poorly correlated with age and physical examination findings, although not with vaginal cytologic maturation index. Women who were taking estrogen replacement therapy had higher symptom scores and physical examination scores.

From this evidence, it appears that urogenital atrophy is a universal consequence of menopause, although elderly women often may be minimally symptomatic. Treatment therefore should not be the only indication for replacement therapy.

MANAGEMENT OF LOWER URINARY DYSFUNCTION

Estrogens in the Management of Incontinence

Estrogen preparations have been used for many years in the treatment of urinary incontinence,[83,84] although their precise role remains controversial. Many of the studies performed have been uncontrolled, observational series examining the use of a wide range of different preparations, doses, and routes of administration. The inconsistent use of progestogens to provide endometrial protection is another confounding factor, making interpretation of the results difficult.

To clarify the situation, a meta-analysis was conducted by the Hormones and Urogenital Therapy (HUT) Committee.[85] Of 166 articles identified that were published in English between 1969 and 1992, only 6 were controlled trials, and 17 were uncontrolled series. Meta-analysis found an overall significant effect of estrogen therapy on subjective improvement in all patients and for patients with urodynamic stress incontinence alone. Subjective improvement rates with estrogen therapy in randomized, controlled trials ranged from 64% to 75%, although placebo groups also reported an improvement of 10% to 56%. In uncontrolled series, subjective improvement rates were 8% to 89%, with patients with urodynamic stress incontinence showing improvement rates of 34% to 73%. However, when assessing objective fluid loss, there was no significant effect. Maximum urethral closure pressure was found to increase significantly with estrogen therapy, although this outcome was influenced by a single study showing a large effect.[86]

Another meta-analysis performed in Italy analyzed the results of randomized, controlled clinical trials on the efficacy of estrogen treatment in postmenopausal women with urinary incontinence.[87] A search of the literature (1965-1996) revealed 72 articles, of which only four were considered to meet the meta-analysis criteria. There was a statistically significant difference in subjective outcome between estrogen and placebo, although there was no such difference in objective or urodynamic outcome. The investigators concluded that this difference could be relevant, although the studies may have lacked objective sensitivity to detect this effect.

The role of estrogen replacement therapy in the prevention of ischemic heart disease was assessed in a 4-year, randomized trial, the Heart and Estrogen/Progestin Replacement Study (HERS),[88] involving 2763 postmenopausal women younger than 80 years with intact uteri and ischemic heart disease. In the study, 55% of women reported at least one episode of urinary incontinence

Table 5-1 Randomized, Controlled Trials Assessing the Use of Estrogens in the Management of Urinary Incontinence

Study	Year	Type of Incontinence	Estrogen	Route
Henalla et al[88]	1989	Stress	Conjugated estrogen	Vaginal
Hilton et al[100]	1990	Stress	Conjugated estrogen	Vaginal
Beisland et al[99]	1984	Stress	Estriol	Vaginal
Judge[126]	1969	Mixed	Quinestradol	Oral
Kinn and Lindskog[127]	1988	Stress	Estriol	Oral
Samsioe et al[103]	1985	Mixed	Estriol	Oral
Walter et al[95]	1978	Urge	Estradiol and estriol	Oral
Walter et al[128]	1990	Stress	Estriol	Oral
Wilson et al[94]	1987	Stress	Piperazine estrone sulfate	Oral

each week, and they were randomly assigned to oral conjugated estrogen plus medroxyprogesterone acetate or to placebo daily. Incontinence improved in 26% of women assigned to placebo and in 21% receiving HRT, and 27% of the placebo group complained of worsening symptoms, compared with 39% in the HRT group ($P = .001$). The incidence of incontinent episodes per week increased an average of 0.7 in the HRT group and decreased by 0.1 in the placebo group ($P < .001$). Overall, combined HRT was associated with worsening stress and urge urinary incontinence, although there was no significant difference in daytime frequency, nocturia, or number of urinary tract infections.

These findings were confirmed in the Nurse's Health Study, which followed 39,436 postmenopausal women between 50 and 75 years old over a 4-year period. The risk of incontinence was found to be elevated for those women taking HRT compared with those who had never taken HRT. There was an increase in risk for women taking oral estrogen (RR = 1.54; 95% CI: 1.44 to 1.65), transdermal estrogen (RR = 1.68; 95% CI: 1.41 to 2.00), oral estrogen and progesterone (RR = 1.34; 95% CI: 1.24 to 1.34), and transdermal estrogen and progesterone (RR = 1.46; 95% CI: 1.16 to 1.84). Although there remained a small risk after the cessation of HRT (RR = 1.14; 95% CI: 1.06 to 1.23), by 10 years, the risk was identical to that for women who had never taken HRT (RR = 1.02; 95% CI: 0.91 to 1.41).[89]

The effects of oral estrogens and progestogens on the lower urinary tract were assessed in 32 female nursing home residents[90] with an average age of 88 years. Subjects were randomized to oral estrogen and progesterone or to placebo for 6 months. At follow-up, there was no difference in severity of incontinence, prevalence of bacteriuria, or the results of vaginal cultures, although there was an improvement in atrophic vaginitis in the placebo group.

A meta-analysis of the effect of estrogen therapy on the lower urinary tract was performed by the Cochrane group.[91] Overall, 28 trials were identified that included 2926 women. In the 15 trials comparing estrogen with placebo, there was a higher subjective impression of improvement rate in women taking estrogen, and this was the case for all types of incontinence (RR for cure = 1.61; 95% CI: 1.04 to 2.49). When subjective cure and improvement were taken together, there was a statistically higher cure and improvement rate for urge (57% versus 28%) and stress (43% versus 27%) incontinence. In women with urge incontinence, the chance of improvement was 25% higher than in women with stress incontinence, and overall, about 50% of women treated with estrogen were cured or improved, compared with 25% on placebo. The investigators conclude that estrogens can improve or cure incontinence and that the effect may be most useful in women complaining of urge incontinence.

Estrogens in the Management of Stress Incontinence

In addition to the studies included in the HUT meta-analysis, several investigators have also assessed the role of estrogen therapy in the management of urodynamic stress incontinence only (Table 5-1). Oral estrogens have been reported to increase the maximum urethral pressures and to lead to symptomatic improvement in 65% to 70% of women,[92,93] although other work has not confirmed this finding.[94,95] Two placebo-controlled studies examined the use of oral estrogens in the treatment of urodynamic stress incontinence in postmenopausal women. Neither conjugated equine estrogens plus medroxyprogesterone[96] nor unopposed estradiol valerate[97] showed a significant difference in subjective or objective outcomes. A review of 8 controlled and 14 uncontrolled, prospective trials concluded that estrogen therapy was not an efficacious treatment for stress incontinence but that it could be useful for symptoms of urgency and frequency.[98]

From the available evidence, estrogen does not appear to be an effective treatment for stress incontinence, although it may have a synergistic role in combination therapy. Two placebo-controlled studies examined the use of oral and vaginal estrogens with the α-adrenergic agonist phenylpropanolamine, used separately and in combination. Both studies found that combination therapy was superior to either drug given alone; although there was subjective improvement in all groups,[99] there was objective improvement only in the combination therapy group.[100] This may offer an alternative conservative treatment for women who have mild urodynamic stress incontinence; however, because of its pressor effects, phenylpropanolamine has been withdrawn in the United States.[101]

One meta-analysis has helped determine the role of estrogen replacement in women with stress incontinence.[102] Of the papers reviewed, 14 were nonrandomized studies, 6 were randomized trials (of which 4 were placebo controlled), and 2 were meta-analyses. There was symptomatic or clinical improvement identified only in the nonrandomized studies, whereas there was no such effect found in the randomized trials. The study authors concluded that the evidence does not support the use of estrogen replacement alone in the management of stress incontinence.

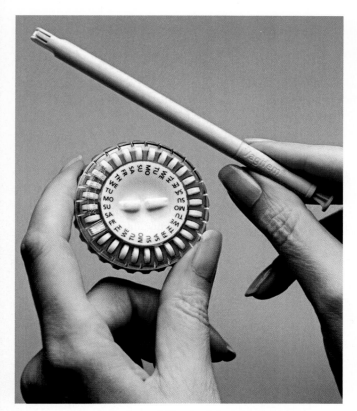

Figure 5-1 Sustained release 17β-estradiol vaginal tablets. (Courtesy of Novo Nordisk, Denmark.)

Estrogens in the Management of Urge Incontinence

Estrogens have been used in the treatment of urinary urgency and urge incontinence for many years, although there have been few controlled trials to confirm their efficacy (see Table 5-1). A double-blind, placebo-controlled, crossover study using oral estriol in 34 postmenopausal women produced subjective improvement in 8 women with mixed incontinence and in 12 with urge incontinence.[103] However, a double-blind, multicenter study of the use of estriol (3 mg/day) in postmenopausal women complaining of urgency has failed to confirm these findings,[104] showing subjective and objective improvement but not significantly better than placebo. Estriol is a naturally occurring, weak estrogen that has little effect on the endometrium and does not prevent osteoporosis, although it has been used in the treatment of urogenital atrophy. Consequently, it is possible that the dosage or route of administration in this study was not appropriate in the treatment of urinary symptoms, and higher systemic levels may be required.

The use of sustained release 17β-estradiol vaginal tablets (Vagifem, Novo Nordisk) (Fig. 5-1) has been examined in postmenopausal women with urgency and urge incontinence or a urodynamic diagnosis of sensory urgency or detrusor overactivity. These vaginal tablets were well absorbed from the vagina and induced maturation of the vaginal epithelium within 14 days.[105] However, after a 6-month course of treatment, the only significant difference between active and placebo groups was an improvement in the symptom of urgency in women with a urodynamic diagnosis of sensory urgency.[106] Another double-blind, randomized, placebo-controlled trial of 17β-estradiol vaginal tablets showed lower urinary tract symptoms of frequency, urgency, and urge and stress incontinence to be significantly improved, although no objective urodynamic assessment was performed.[107] In both of these studies, the subjective improvement in symptoms may represent local estrogenic effects reversing urogenital atrophy rather than a direct effect on bladder function.

A randomized, parallel-group, controlled trial compared the estradiol-releasing vaginal ring (Estring, Pharmacia, Uppsala, Sweden) with estriol vaginal pessaries in the treatment of postmenopausal women with bothersome lower urinary tract symptoms.[108] Low-dose, vaginally administered estradiol and estriol were found to be equally efficacious in alleviating lower urinary tract symptoms of urge incontinence (58% versus 58%), stress incontinence (53% versus 59%), and nocturia (51% versus 54%), although the vaginal ring was found to have greater patient acceptability.

To clarify the role of estrogen therapy in the management of women with urge incontinence, a meta-analysis of the use of estrogen in women with symptoms of overactive bladder was conducted by the HUT Committee.[109] In a review of 10 randomized, placebo-controlled trials, estrogen was found to be superior to placebo when considering symptoms of urge incontinence, frequency, and nocturia, and vaginal estrogen administration was found to be superior for symptoms of urgency. In those taking estrogens, there was also a significant increase in first sensation and bladder capacity compared with those taking placebo.

Estrogens in the Management of Recurrent Urinary Tract Infection

Estrogen therapy has been shown to increase vaginal pH and reverse the microbiologic changes that occur in the vagina after menopause.[110] Initial small, uncontrolled studies using oral or vaginal estrogens in the treatment of recurrent urinary tract infection appeared to give promising results,[111,112] although unfortunately this has not been supported by larger, randomized trials. Several studies have examined the use of oral and vaginal estrogens, and they have had mixed results (Table 5-2).

Kjaergaard and colleagues[113] compared vaginal estriol tablets with placebo in 21 postmenopausal women over a 5-month period and found no significant difference between the two groups. However, a subsequent randomized, double-blind, placebo-controlled study assessing the use of estriol vaginal cream in 93 postmenopausal women during an 8-month period did reveal a significant effect.[114]

Kirkengen randomized 40 postmenopausal women to receive placebo or oral estriol and found that although both groups initially had a significantly decreased incidence of recurrent infections, estriol was shown after 12 weeks to be significantly more effective.[115] These findings were not confirmed subsequently in a trial of 72 postmenopausal women with recurrent urinary tract infections randomized to oral estriol or placebo. After a 6-month treatment period and another 6-month follow-up, estriol was found to be no more effective than placebo.[116]

A randomized, open, parallel-group study assessing the use of an estradiol-releasing silicone vaginal ring (Estring) in postmenopausal women with recurrent infections showed the cumulative likelihood of remaining infection free was 45% in the active group and 20% in the placebo group.[117] Estring was also shown to decrease the number of recurrences per year and to prolong the interval between infection episodes.

Table 5-2 Randomized, Controlled Trials Assessing the Use of Estrogens in the Management of Recurrent Lower Urinary Tract Infections

Study	Study Group	Type of Estrogen	Route of Delivery	Duration of Therapy	Results
Kjaergaard et al, 1990[113]	21 Postmenopausal women with recurrent cystitis *10 active group* *11 placebo*	Estradiol	Vaginal tablets	5 months	Number of positive cultures not statistically different between the two groups
Kirkengen et al, 1992[115]	40 Postmenopausal women with recurrent UTIs *20 active group* *20 placebo*	Estriol	Oral	12 weeks	Both estriol and placebo significantly reduced the incidence of UTIs ($P < .05$). After 12 weeks, estriol was significantly more effective than placebo ($P < .05$).
Raz and Stamm, 1993[114]	93 Postmenopausal women with recurrent UTIs *50 active group* *43 placebo*	Estriol	Vaginal cream	8 months	Significant reduction in the incidence of UTIs in the group given estriol compared with placebo ($P < .001$)
Cardozo et al, 1998[116]	72 Postmenopausal women with recurrent UTIs *36 active group* *36 placebo*	Estriol	Oral	6-month treatment period with another 6 months of follow-up	Reduction in urinary symptoms and incidence of UTIs in both groups; estriol no better than placebo
Eriksen, 1999[117]	108 Women with recurrent UTIs *53 active group* *55 no treatment*	Estradiol	Estring	36 weeks for the active group; 36 weeks or until first recurrence for the controls	Cumulative likelihood of remaining free of infection was 45% in active group and 20% in control group ($P = .008$)

UTI, urinary tract infection.

Estrogens in the Management of Urogenital Atrophy

Symptoms of urogenital atrophy do not occur until the levels of endogenous estrogen are lower than those required to promote endometrial proliferation.[118] Consequently, it is possible to use a low dose of estrogen replacement therapy to alleviate urogenital symptoms while avoiding the risk of endometrial proliferation and removing the necessity of providing endometrial protection with progestogens.[119] The dose of estradiol commonly used in systemic estrogen replacement is usually 25 μg to 100 μg, although studies investigating the use of estrogens in the management of urogenital symptoms have shown that 8 μg to 10 μg of vaginal estradiol are effective.[120] Only 10% to 30% of the dose used to treat vasomotor symptoms may be effective in the management of urogenital symptoms. Because 10% to 25% of women receiving systemic HRT still experience the symptoms of urogenital atrophy,[121] low-dose local preparations may have an additional beneficial effect.

The HUT Committee[122] reviewed estrogen therapy in the management of urogenital atrophy. Ten randomized trials and 54 uncontrolled series conducted between 1969 and 1995 assessed 24 treatment regimens. Meta-analysis of 10 placebo-controlled trials confirmed the significant effect of estrogens in the management of urogenital atrophy (Table 5-3).

The route of administration was assessed, and oral, vaginal, and parenteral (i.e., transcutaneous patches and subcutaneous implants) were compared. Overall, the vaginal route of administration correlated with better symptom relief, greater improvement in cytologic findings, and higher serum estradiol levels.

Estradiol was found to be the most effective type of estrogen preparation in reducing patient symptoms. Conjugated estrogens produced the most cytologic change and the greatest increase in serum levels of estradiol and estrone.

The effect of different dosages was examined. Low-dose vaginal estradiol was found to be the most efficacious according to symptom relief, although oral estriol was also effective. Estriol had no effect on the serum levels of estradiol or estrone, and vaginal estriol had a minimal effect. Vaginal estradiol was found to have a small effect on serum estrogen levels, although not as great as systemic preparations. These findings indicate that estrogen is efficacious in the treatment of urogenital atrophy and that low-dose vaginal preparations are as effective as systemic therapy.

The use of a low-dose, estradiol-releasing silicone vaginal ring (Estring) continuously releasing estradiol (5 to 10 μg/24 hr) was investigated in postmenopausal women with symptomatic urogenital atrophy.[111] There was a significant effect on symptoms of vaginal dryness, pruritus vulvae, dyspareunia, and urinary urgency, with improvement reported for more than 90% of women in an uncontrolled study. Patient acceptability was high, and although the maturation of vaginal epithelium was significantly improved, there was no effect on endometrial proliferation.

Table 5-3 Randomized, Controlled Trials Assessing the Use of Estrogens in the Management of Urogenital Atrophy

Study	Year	Estrogen	Route
Bellatoni et al[129]	1991	Estradiol	Transdermal
Campbell et al[130]	1977	Conjugated estrogen	Oral
Campbell et al[130]	1977	Conjugated estrogen	Oral
Eriksen and Rasmussen[107]	1992	Estradiol	Pessary
Felding et al[131]	1992	Estradiol	Pessary
Foidart et al[132]	1991	Estriol	Vaginal cream
Laufer et al[133]	1983	Estradiol	Transdermal
Mettler and Olsen[119]	1991	Estradiol	Pessary
Molander et al[134]	1990	Estriol	Oral
Raz and Stamm[114]	1993	Estriol	Vaginal cream
Van der Linden et al[135]	1993	Estriol	Oral

These findings were supported by a 1-year multicenter study of Estring in postmenopausal women with urogenital atrophy, which found subjective and objective improvement in 90% of patients up to 1 year. However, there was a 20% withdrawal rate, with 7% of women reporting vaginal irritation, two having vaginal ulceration, and three complaining of vaginal bleeding, although there were no cases of endometrial proliferation.[123] Long-term safety was confirmed by a 10-year review of the use of the estradiol ring delivery system, which found its safety, efficacy, and acceptability to be comparable to other forms of vaginal administration.[124] A comparative study of safety and efficacy of Estring with conjugated equine estrogen vaginal cream in 194 postmenopausal women complaining of urogenital atrophy found no significant difference in vaginal dryness, dyspareunia, and resolution of atrophic signs between the two treatment groups. There was similar improvement in the vaginal mucosal maturation index and a reduction in pH in both groups, with the vaginal ring found to be preferable to the cream.[125]

CONCLUSIONS

Estrogens have important physiologic effects on the female lower genital tract throughout adult life, leading to symptomatic, histologic, and functional changes. Urogenital atrophy occurs with estrogen withdrawal after menopause, manifesting with vaginal and urinary symptoms. The use of estrogen replacement therapy has been examined in the management of lower urinary tract symptoms and in the treatment of urogenital atrophy, although only recently has it been subjected to randomized, placebo-controlled trials and meta-analyses.

Estrogen therapy alone has been shown to have little effect in the management of urodynamic stress incontinence, but when used in combination with α-adrenergic agonists, it may lead to an improvement in urinary leakage. For the overactive bladder symptoms of urinary urgency, frequency, and urge incontinence, estrogen therapy may be of benefit, although it may cause reversal of urogenital atrophy rather than having a direct effect on the lower urinary tract. The role of estrogen replacement therapy in the management of women with recurrent lower urinary tract infections remains to be determined, but there is some evidence that vaginal administration may be efficacious. Low-dose vaginal estrogens have been shown to have a role in the treatment of urogenital atrophy in postmenopausal women and appear to be as effective as systemic preparations.

References

1. Cardozo LD: Role of oestrogens in the treatment of female urinary incontinence. J Am Geriatr Soc 38:326-328, 1990.
2. Iosif CS, Batra S, Ek A, Astedt B: Estrogen receptors in the human female lower urinary tract. Am J Obstet Gynecol 141:817-820, 1981.
3. Batra SC, Fossil CS: Female urethra, a target for oestrogen action. J Urol 129:418-420, 1983.
4. Batra SC, Iosif LS: Progesterone receptors in the female urinary tract. J Urol 138:130-134, 1987.
5. Iosif C, Bekassy Z: Prevalence of genitourinary symptoms in the late menopause. Acta Obstet Gynaecol Scand 63:257-260, 1984.
6. Beato M, Herrich P, Schutz G: Steroid hormone receptors: Many actors in search of a plot. Cell 83:851-857, 1995.
7. Green S, Walter P, Kumar V, et al: Human oestrogen receptor cDNA: Sequence, expression and homology to v-erbA. Nature 320:134-139, 1986.
8. Kuiper G, Enmark E, Pelto-Huikko M, et al: Cloning of a novel receptor expressed in rat prostate and ovary. Proc Natl Acad Sci U S A 93:5925-5930, 1996.
9. Warner M, Nilsson S, Gustafsson JA: The oestrogen receptor family. Curr Opin Obstet Gynecol 11:249-254, 1999.
10. Blakeman PJ, Hilton P, Bulmer JN: Mapping oestrogen and progesterone receptors throughout the female lower urinary tract. Neurourol Urodyn 15:324-325, 1996.
11. Ingelman-Sundberg A, Rosen J, Gustafsson SA: Cytosol oestrogen receptors in urogenital tissues in stress incontinent women. Acta Obstet Gynecol Scand 60:585-586, 1981.
12. Bernstein IT: The pelvic floor muscles: Muscle thickness in healthy and urinary-incontinent women measured by perineal ultrasonography with reference to the effect of pelvic floor training. Oestrogen receptor studies. Neurourol Urodyn 16:237-275, 1997.
13. Chen GD, Oliver RH, Leung BS, et al: Oestrogen receptor α and β expression in the vaginal walls and uterosacral ligaments of premenopausal and postmenopausal women. Fertil Steril 71:1099-1102, 1999.
14. Screiter F, Fuchs P, Stockamp K: Oestrogenic sensitivity of α receptors in the urethral musculature. Urol Int 31:13-19, 1976.

15. Blakeman PJ, Hilton P, Bulmer JN: Androgen receptors in the female lower urinary tract. Int Urogynaecol J 8:S54, 1997.
16. Pang X, Cotreau-Bibbo MM, Sant GR, Theoharides TC: Bladder mast cell expression of high affinity oestrogen receptors in receptors in patients with interstitial cystitis. Br J Urol 75:154-161, 1995.
17. Letourneau R, Pang X, Sant GR, Theoharides TC: Intragranular activation of bladder mast cells and their association with nerve processes in interstitial cystitis. Br J Urol 77:41-54, 1996.
18. Bodker A, Balsev E, Juul BR, et al: Oestrogen receptors in the human male bladder, prostatic urethra and prostate. Scand J Urol Nephrol 29:161-165, 1995.
19. Blakeman PJ, Hilton P, Bulmer JN: Oestrogen and progesterone receptor expression in the female lower urinary tract, with reference to oestrogen status. BJU Int 86:32-38, 2000.
20. Abrams P, Blaivas JG, Stanton SL, et al: The standardisation of terminology of lower urinary tract dysfunction. Br J Obstet Gynaecol 97:1-16, 1990.
21. Rud T, Anderson KE, Asmussen M, et al: Factors maintaining the urethral pressure in women. Invest Urol 17:343-347, 1980.
22. Malone-Lee J: Urodynamic measurement and urinary incontinence in the elderly. In Brocklehurst JC (ed): Managing and Measuring Incontinence. Proceedings of the Geriatric Workshop on Incontinence, July 1988.
23. Versi E, Cardozo LD: Oestrogens and lower urinary tract function. In Studd JWW, Whitehead MI (eds): The Menopause. Oxford, Blackwell Scientific Publications, 1988, pp 76-84.
24. Kinn AC, Lindskog M: Oestrogens and phenylpropanolamine in combination for stress incontinence. Urology 32:273-280, 1988.
25. Smith PJB: The effect of oestrogens on bladder function in the female. In Campbell S (ed): The Management of the Menopause and Postmenopausal Years. Carnforth, MTP, 1976, pp 291-298.
26. Samsioe G, Jansson I, Mellström D, Svandborg A: Occurrence, nature and treatment of urinary incontinence in a 70 year old female population. Maturitas 7:335-342, 1985.
27. Blakeman PJ, Hilton P, Bulmer JN: Cellular proliferation in the female lower urinary tract with reference to oestrogen status. Br J Obstet Gynaecol 8:813-816, 2001.
28. Hextall A, Bidmead J, Cardozo L, Hooper R: Hormonal influences on the human female lower urinary tract: A prospective evaluation of the effects of the menstrual cycle on symptomatology and the results of urodynamic investigation. Neurourol Urodyn 18:282-283, 1999.
29. Van Geelen JM, Doesburg WH, Thomas CMG: Urodynamic studies in the normal menstrual cycle: The relationship between hormonal changes during the menstrual cycle and the urethral pressure profile. Am J Obstet Gynecol 141:384-392, 1981.
30. Burton G, Cardozo LD, Abdalla H, et al: The hormonal effects on the lower urinary tract in 282 women with premature ovarian failure. Neurourol Urodyn 10:318-319, 1992.
31. Cutner A, Burton G, Cardozo LD, et al: Does progesterone cause an irritable bladder? Int Urogynaecol J 4:259-261, 1993.
32. Benness C, Gangar K, Cardozo LD, Cutner A: Do progestogens exacerbate urinary incontinence in women on HRT? Neurourol Urodyn 10:316-318, 1991.
33. Elliot RA, Castleden CM: Effect of progestagens and oestrogens on the contractile response of rat detrusor muscle to electrical field stimulation. Clin Sci 87:342, 1994.
34. Cutner A: The urinary tract in pregnancy [MD thesis]. London, University of London, 1993.
35. Donnelly V, O'Connell PR, O'Herlihy C: The influence of hormonal replacement on faecal incontinence in post menopausal women. Br J Obstet Gynaecol 104:311-315, 1997.
36. Sandford JP: Urinary tract symptoms and infection. Annu Rev Med 26:485-505, 1975.
37. Boscia JA, Kaye D: Asymptomatic bacteria in the elderly. Infect Dis Clin North Am 1:893-903, 1987.
38. Maggi A, Perez J: Role of female gonadal hormones in the CNS. Life Sci 37:893-906, 1985.
39. Smith SS, Berg G, Hammar M (eds): The Modern Management of the Menopause. Hormones, Mood and Neurobiology—A Summary. Carnforth, UK, Parthenon Publishing, 1993, p 204.
40. Blok EFM, Holstege G: Androgen receptor immunoreactive neurones in the hypothalamic preoptic area project to the pontine micturition centre in the male cat. Neurourol Urodyn 17:404-405, 1998.
41. Shapiro E: Effect of oestrogens on the weight and muscarinic receptor density of the rabbit bladder and urethra. J Urol 135:1084-1087, 1986.
42. Batra S, Anderson KE: Oestrogen induced changes in muscarinic receptor density and contractile responses in the female rat urinary bladder. Acta Physiol Scand 137:135-141, 1989.
43. Elliott RA, Castleden CM, Miodrag A, Kirwan P: The direct effects of diethylstilboestrol and nifedipine on the contractile responses of isolated human and rat detrusor muscles. Eur J Clin Pharmacol 43:149-155, 1992.
44. Shenfield OZ, Blackmore PF, Morgan CW, et al: Rapid effects of oestriol and progesterone on tone and spontaneous rhythmic contractions of the rabbit bladder. Neurourol Urodyn 17:408-409, 1998.
45. Fantl JA, Wyman JF, Anderson RL, et al: Postmenopausal urinary incontinence: Comparison between non-oestrogen and oestrogen supplemented women. Obstet Gynecol 71:823-828, 1988.
46. Bergman A, Karram MM, Bhatia NN: Changes in urethral cytology following oestrogen administration. Gynecol Obstet Invest 29:211-213, 1990.
47. Rud T: The effects of oestrogens and gestagens on the urethral pressure profile in urinary continent and stress incontinent women. Acta Obstet Gynaecol Scand 59:265-270, 1980.
48. Hilton P, Stanton SL: The use of intravaginal oestrogen cream in genuine stress incontinence. Br J Obstet Gynaecol 90:940-944, 1983.
49. Bhatia NN, Bergman A, Karram MM, et al: Effects of estrogen on urethral function in women with urinary incontinence. Am J Obstet Gynecol 160:176-180, 1989.
50. Karram MM, Yeko TR, Sauer MV, et al: Urodynamic changes following hormone replacement therapy in women with premature ovarian failure. Obstet Gynecol 74:208-211, 1989.
51. Ganger KF, Vyas S, Whitehead RW, et al: Pulsitility index in the internal carotid artery in relation to transdermal oestradiol and time since the menopause. Lancet 338:839-842, 1991.
52. Jackson S, Vyas S: A double blind, placebo controlled study of postmenopausal oestrogen replacement therapy and carotid artery pulsatility index. Br J Obstet Gynaecol 105:408-412, 1998.
53. Penotti M, Farina M, Sironi L, et al: Long term effects of postmenopausal hormone replacement therapy on pulsatility index of the internal carotid and middle cerebral arteries. Menopause 4:101-104, 1997.
54. Versi E, Cardozo LD: Urethral instability: Diagnosis based on variations in the maximum urethral pressure in normal climacteric women. Neurourol Urodyn 5:535-541, 1986.
55. Girao MJ, Jarmy-Di Bella ZI, Sartori MG, et al: Doppler velocimetry parameters of periurethral vessels in postmenopausal incontinent women receiving oestrogen replacement. Int Urogynaecol 12:241-246, 2001.
56. Falconer C, Ekman-Ordeberg G, Ulmsten U, et al: Changes in paraurethral connective tissue at menopause are counteracted by oestrogen. Maturitas 24:197-204, 1996.
57. Kushner L, Chen Y, Desautel M, et al: Collagenase activity is elevated in conditioned media from fibroblasts of women with pelvic floor weakening. Int Urogynaecol 10(Suppl 1):34, 1999.
58. Jackson S, Avery N, Shepherd A, et al: The effect of oestradiol on vaginal collagen in postmenopausal women with stress urinary incontinence. Nurourol Urodyn 15:327-328, 1996.

59. James M, Avery N, Jackson S, et al: The pathophysiological changes of vaginal skin tissue in women with stress urinary incontinence: A controlled trial. Int Urogynaecol J 10(Suppl 1):35, 1999.
60. James M, Avery N, Jackson S, et al: The biochemical profile of vaginal tissue in women with genitourinary prolapse: A controlled trial. Neurourol Urodyn 18:284-285, 1999.
61. Brincat M, Moniz CF, Studd JWW: Long term effects of the menopause and sex hormones on skin thickness. Br J Obstet Gynaecol 92:256-259, 1985.
62. Landon CR, Smith ARB, Crofts CE, Trowbridge EA: Biochemical properties of connective tissue in women with stress incontinence of urine. Neurourol Urodyn 8:369-370, 1989.
63. Ulmsten U, Ekman G, Giertz G, Malmström A: Different biochemical composition of connective tissue in continent and stress incontinent women. Acta Obstet Gynaecol Scand 66:455-457, 1987.
64. Diokno AC, Brook BM, Brown MB: Prevalence of urinary incontinence and other urological symptoms in the non-institutionalised elderly. J Urol 136:1022, 1986.
65. Yarnell J, Voyle G, Richards C, Stephenson T: The prevalence and severity of urinary incontinence in women. J Epidemiol Community Health 35:71-74, 1981.
66. Ouslander JG: Urinary incontinence in nursing homes. J Am Geriatr Soc 38:289-291, 1990.
67. MacLennan AH, Taylor AW, Wilson AW, Wilson D: The prevalence of pelvic floor disorders and their relationship to gender, age, parity, and mode of delivery. Br J Obstet Gynaecol 107:1460-1470, 2000.
68. Kok AL, Voorhorst FJ, Burger CW, et al: Urinary and faecal incontinence in community residing elderly women. Age Ageing 21:211, 1992.
69. Cardozo LD, Tapp A, Versi E, et al (eds): The lower urinary tract in peri- and postmenopausal women. In The Urogenital Deficiency Syndrome. Bagsverd, Denmark, Novo Industries, 1987, pp 10-17.
70. Kondo A, Kato K, Saito M, et al: Prevalence of hand washing incontinence in females in comparison with stress and urge incontinence. Neurourol Urodyn 9:330-331, 1990.
71. Thomas TM, Plymat KR, Blannin J, et al: Prevalence of urinary incontinence. Br Med J 281:1243-1245, 1980.
72. Jolleys JV: Reported prevalence of urinary incontinence in a general practice. Br Med J 296:1300-1302, 1988.
73. Burgio KL, Matthews KA, Engel B: Prevalence, incidence and correlates of urinary incontinence in healthy, middle aged women. J Urol 146:1255-1259, 1991.
74. Iosif CS: Effects of protracted administration of oestriol on the lower genitourinary tract in postmenopausal women. Acta Obstet Gynaecol Scand 251:115-120, 1992.
75. U.S. Treasury Department: American National Institute of Health Population Figures. Bethesda, National Institutes of Health, 1991.
76. Research on the menopause in the 1990s. Report of a WHO Scientific Group. In WHO Technical Report, series 866. Geneva, Switzerland, World Health Organization, 1994.
77. Barlow D, Samsioe G, van Geelan H: Prevalence of urinary problems in European countries. Maturitas 27:239-248, 1997.
78. Greendale GA, Judd JL: The menopause: Health implications and clinical management. J Am Geriatr Soc 41:426-436, 1993.
79. Samsioe G, Jansson I, Mellstrom D, Svanborg A: The occurrence, nature and treatment of urinary incontinence in a 70 year old population. Maturitas 7:335-343, 1985.
80. Van Geelen JM, Van de Weijer PH, Arnolds HT: Urogenital symptoms and resulting discomfort in non-institutionalised Dutch women aged 50-75 years. Int Urogynecol J Pelvic Floor Dysfunct 11:9-14, 2000.
81. Versi E, Harvey MA, Cardozo L, et al: Urogenital prolapse and atrophy at menopause: A prevalence study. Int Urogynaecol J Pelvic Dysfunct 12:107-110, 2001.
82. Davila GW, Karapanagiotou I, Woodhouse S, et al: Are women with urogenital atrophy symptomatic? Obstet Gynecol 97(Suppl 1): S48, 2001.
83. Salmon UL, Walter RI, Gast SH: The use of oestrogen in the treatment of dysuria and incontinence in postmenopausal women. Am J Obstet Gynecol 14:23-31, 1941.
84. Youngblood VH, Tomlin EM, Davis JB: Senile urethritis in women. J Urol 78:150-152, 1957.
85. Fantl JA, Cardozo LD, McClish DK, for the Hormones and Urogenital Therapy Committee: Oestrogen therapy in the management of incontinence in postmenopausal women: A meta-analysis. First report of the Hormones and Urogenital Therapy Committee. Obstet Gynecol 83:12-18, 1994.
86. Henalla SM, Hutchins CJ, Robinson P, Macivar J: Non-operative methods in the treatment of female genuine stress incontinence of urine. Br J Obstet Gynaecol 9:222-225, 1989.
87. Zullo MA, Oliva C, Falconi G, et al: Efficacy of oestrogen therapy in urinary incontinence: A meta-analytic study. Minerva Ginecol 50:199-205, 1998.
88. Grady D, Brown JS, Vittinghoff E, et al: Postmenopausal hormones and incontinence: The Heart and Estrogen/Progestin Replacement Study. Obstet Gynecol 97:116-120, 2001.
89. Grodstein F, Lifford K, Resnick NM, Curhan GC: Postmenopausal hormone therapy and risk of developing urinary incontinence. Obstet Gynecol 103:254-260, 2004.
90. Ouslander JG, Greendale GA, Uman G, et al: Effects of oral estrogen and progestin on the lower urinary tract among female nursing home residents. Am Geriatr Soc 49:803-807, 2001.
91. Moehrer B, Hextall A, Jackson S: Oestrogens for urinary incontinence in women. Cochrane Database Syst Rev (2):CD001405, 2003.
92. Caine M, Raz S: The role of female hormones in stress incontinence. Proceedings of the 16th Congress of the International Society of Urology, Amsterdam, Netherlands.
93. Rud T: The effects of oestrogens and gestagens on the urethral pressure profile in urinary continent and stress incontinent women. Acta Obstet Gynaecol Scand 59:265-270, 1980.
94. Wilson PD, Faragher B, Butler B, et al: Treatment with oral piperazine oestrone sulphate for genuine stress incontinence in postmenopausal women. Br J Obstet Gynaecol 94:568-574, 1987.
95. Walter S, Wolf H, Barlebo H, Jansen H. Urinary incontinence in postmenopausal women treated with oestrogens: A double-blind clinical trial. J Urol 33:135-143, 1978.
96. Fantl JA, Bump RC, Robinson D, et al: Efficacy of oestrogen supplementation in the treatment of urinary incontinence. Obstet Gynecol 88:745-749, 1996.
97. Jackson S, Shepherd A, Brookes S, Abrams P: The effect of oestrogen supplementation on post-menopausal urinary stress incontinence: A double-blind, placebo controlled trial. Br J Obstet Gynaecol 106:711-718, 1999.
98. Sultana CJ, Walters MD: Oestrogen and urinary incontinence in women. Maturitas 20:129-138, 1995.
99. Beisland HO, Fossberg E, Moer A, et al: Urethral insufficiency in post-menopausal females: Treatment with phenylpropanolamine and oestriol separately and in combination. Urol Int 39:211-216, 1984.
100. Hilton P, Tweddel AL, Mayne C: Oral and intravaginal oestrogens alone and in combination with alpha adrenergic stimulation in genuine stress incontinence. Int Urogynecol J 12:80-86, 1990.
101. Horwitz RI, Brass LM, Kernan WN, Viscoli CM: Phenylpropanolamine and risk of hemorrhagic stroke: Final report of The Hemorrhagic Stroke Project, May 10, 2000. N Eng J Med 343:1826-1832, 2000.
102. Ahmed Al-Badr, Ross S, Soroka D, Drutz HP: What is the available evidence for hormone replacement therapy in women with stress urinary incontinence? J Obstet Gynaecol Can 25:567-574, 2003.
103. Samsicoe G, Jansson I, Mellström D, Svanberg A: Urinary incontinence in 75 year old women. Effects of oestriol. Acta Obstet Gynaecol Scand 93:57, 1985.

104. Cardozo LD, Rekers H, Tapp A, et al: Oestriol in the treatment of postmenopausal urgency: A multicentre study. Maturitas 18:47-53, 1993.
105. Nilsson K, Heimer G: Low dose oestradiol in the treatment of urogenital oestrogen deficiency—A pharmacokinetic and pharmacodynamic study. Maturitas 15:121-127, 1992.
106. Benness C, Wise BG, Cutner A, Cardozo LD: Does low dose vaginal oestradiol improve frequency and urgency in postmenopausal women. Int Urogynaecol J 3:281, 1992.
107. Eriksen PS, Rasmussen H: Low dose 17 beta-estradiol vaginal tablets in the treatment of atrophic vaginitis: A double-blind placebo controlled study. Eur J Obstet Gynecol Reprod Biol 44: 137-144, 1992.
108. Lose G, Englev E: Oestradiol-releasing vaginal ring versus oestriol vaginal pessaries in the treatment of bothersome lower urinary tract symptoms. Br J Obstet Gynaecol 107:1029-1034, 2000.
109. Cardozo L, Lose G, McClish D, Versi E: Estrogen treatment for symptoms of an overactive bladder, results of a meta analysis. Int J Urogynaecol 12:3 V, 2001.
110. Brandberg A, Mellstrom D, Samsioe G: Low dose oral oestriol treatment in elderly women with urogenital infections. Acta Obstet Gynaecol Scand 140:33-38, 1987.
111. Parsons CL, Schmidt JD: Control of recurrent urinary tract infections in postmenopausal women. J Urol 128:1224-1226, 1982.
112. Privette M, Cade R, Peterson J, et al: Prevention of recurrent urinary tract infections in postmenopausal women. Nephron 50:24-27, 1988.
113. Kjaergaard B, Walter S, Knudsen A, et al: Treatment with low dose vaginal oestradiol in postmenopausal women. A double blind controlled trial. Ugeskr Laeger 152:658-659, 1990.
114. Raz R, Stamm WE: A controlled trial of intravaginal oestriol in postmenopausal women with recurrent urinary tract infections. N Engl J Med 329:753-756, 1993.
115. Kirkengen AL, Anderson P, Gjersoe E, et al: Oestriol in the prophylactic treatment of recurrent urinary tract infections in postmenopausal women. Scand J Prim Health Care 10:142, 1992.
116. Cardozo LD, Benness C, Abbott D: Low dose oestrogen prophylaxis for recurrent urinary tract infections in elderly women. Br J Obstet Gynaecol 105:403-407, 1998.
117. Eriksen B: A randomised, open, parallel-group study on the preventative effect of an estradiol-releasing vaginal ring (Estring) on recurrent urinary tract infections in postmenopausal women. Am J Obstet Gynecol 180:1072-1079, 1999.
118. Samisoe G: Urogenital aging—A hidden problem. Am J Obstet Gynecol 178:S245-S249, 1998.
119. Mettler L, Olsen PG: Long term treatment of atrophic vaginitis with low dose oestradiol vaginal tablets. Maturitas 14:23-31, 1991.
120. Smith P, Heimer G, Lindskog, Ulmsten U: Oestradiol releasing vaginal ring for treatment of postmenopausal urogenital atrophy. Maturitas 16:145-154, 1993.
121. Smith RJN, Studd JWW: Recent advances in hormone replacement therapy. Br J Hosp Med 49:799-809, 1993.
122. Cardozo LD, Bachmann G, McClish D, et al: Meta-analysis of oestrogen therapy in the management of urogenital atrophy in postmenopausal women: Second report of the Hormones and Urogenital Therapy Committee. Obstet Gynecol 92:722-727, 1998.
123. Henriksson L, Stjernquist M, Boquist L, et al: A one-year multicentre study of efficacy and safety of a continuous, low dose, estradiol-releasing vaginal ring (Estring) in postmenopausal women with symptoms and signs of urogenital aging. Am J Obstet Gynecol 174:85-92, 1996.
124. Bachmann G: Oestradiol-releasing vaginal ring delivery system for urogenital atrophy. Experience over the last decade. J Reprod Med 43:991-998, 1998.
125. Ayton RA, Darling GM, Murkies AL, et al: A comparative study of safety and efficacy of low dose oestradiol released from a vaginal ring compared with conjugated equine oestrogen vaginal cream in the treatment of postmenopausal vaginal atrophy. Br J Obstet Gynaecol 103:351-358, 1996.
126. Judge TG: The use of quinestradol in elderly incontinent women: A preliminary report. Gerontol Clin 11:159-164, 1969.
127. Kinn AC, Lindskog M: Oestrogens and phenylpropanolamine in combination for stress incontinence in postmenopausal women. Urology 32:273-280, 1988.
128. Walter S, Kjaergaard B, Lose G, et al: Stress urinary incontinence in postmenopausal women treated with oral oestrogen (oestriol) and an α-adrenoceptor stimulating agent (phenylpropanolamine): A randomised double-blind placebo-controlled study. Int Urogynaecol J 1:74-79, 1990.
129. Bellatoni MF, Harman SM, Cullins VE, et al: Transdermal oestradiol with oral progestin: Biological and clinical effects in younger and older postmenopausal women. J Gerontol 46:M216-M222, 1991.
130. Campbell S, Whitehead M: Oestrogen therapy and the menopausal syndrome. Clin Obstet Gynaecol 4:31-47, 1977.
131. Felding C, Mikkelse AL, Chausen HV, et al: Preoperative treatment with oestradiol in women scheduled for vaginal operations for genital prolapse. A randomised double blind trial. Maturitas 15:241-249, 1992.
132. Foidart JM, Vervliet J, Buytaert P: Efficacy of sustained release vaginal formulation of oestriol in alleviating urogenital and systemic climacteric complaints. Maturitas 13:99-107, 1991.
133. Laufer LR, Defazio JL, Lu JK, et al: Estrogen replacement therapy by transdermal oestradiol administration. Am J Obstet Gynecol 146:533-540, 1983.
134. Molander U, Milson I, Ekelund P, Mellstrom D: An epidemiological study of urinary incontinence and related urogenital symptoms in elderly women. Maturitas 12:51-60, 1990.
135. Van der Linden MC, Gerretsen G, Brandhorst MS, et al: The effect of estriol on the cytology of urethra and vagina in postmenopausal women with genitourinary symptoms. Eur J Obstet Gynecol Reprod Biol 51:29-33, 1993.

Chapter 6

SOCIAL IMPACT OF URINARY INCONTINENCE AND PELVIC FLOOR DYSFUNCTION

Ilana Beth Addis

Urinary incontinence is a common condition in women that in the past was considered an inevitable result of aging. As a result, little attention was paid to women who complained of the condition. They were expected to suffer silently, and because they were concerned about leakage, they often became housebound. Urinary incontinence is defined by the International Continence Society as an "involuntary loss of urine which is objectively demonstrable and a social or hygienic problem."[1] With more focus placed on the problems of aging, specifically of aging women, we now know that urinary incontinence has many, wide-ranging effects on a woman's daily activities, social interactions, and personal perceptions of wellness. Women with urinary incontinence, especially urgency, have a lower sense of general well-being compared with similar-aged women without this problem. Urinary incontinence does not have to be endured by every aging woman. It is often curable, and it is certainly manageable by a multitude of therapies.

Normal support of the vagina and pelvic organs is provided by an interaction between the levator ani muscle and the connective tissue supports constituting the pelvic diaphragm. When muscular function in the pelvis is normal, the pelvic organs are held over the levator plate and away from the genital hiatus, with increased intra-abdominal pressure pushing the pelvic organs into the hollow of the sacrum. The purpose of the connective tissue is to provide stabilization of the pelvic organs in relation to the pelvic muscles and to provide temporary support when the pelvic muscles are relaxed. *Pelvic floor dysfunction* is a term that is applied to a wide variety of clinical conditions, including urinary incontinence, pelvic organ prolapse, sensory abnormalities of the lower urinary tract, defecatory dysfunction, sexual dysfunction, and chronic pain syndromes. The most common conditions are urinary and fecal incontinence and pelvic organ prolapse. The pathophysiology of pelvic floor disorders includes a combination of genetic predisposition and acquired dysfunction of the muscular and connective tissue support systems.

This chapter provides a review of the epidemiology of urinary incontinence and pelvic floor dysfunction. In it, I discuss the prevalence, incidence, and risk factors of urinary incontinence and pelvic organ prolapse. The social, psychologic, sexual, and economic effects of female urinary incontinence and pelvic floor dysfunction also are addressed.

URINARY INCONTINENCE

Defining Urinary Incontinence

It is difficult to discuss urinary incontinence without discussing the definition of urinary incontinence. Various definitions have been used, depending on the goals of the definer, and according to the International Continence Society, the definition of urinary incontinence has changed in the past 25 years. In 1979, urinary incontinence was "the involuntary loss of urine that is a social or hygienic problem and is objectively demonstrable."[2] By 2002, urinary incontinence became "the complaint of any involuntary leakage of urine" with further description of frequency, severity, risk factors, social and hygienic impact, and effect on quality of life.[1] These changes were made to promote treatments based on symptoms, to facilitate comparison of results in research, and to help with effective communication between researchers. The most recent definition does not require incontinence to be demonstrable; rather, a complaint of urinary incontinence is enough to support a diagnosis of urinary incontinence, allowing for the fact that each woman's perception of her incontinence is different.

Incidence and Prevalence

Despite approved definitions of urinary incontinence, every study uses a slightly different definition. For example, in four studies published in 2000, the prevalence of incontinence ranged from 11% to 72%.[3-6] This wide range probably reflects the different populations studied and the differences in definitions of urinary incontinence that were used in each study. One review found that a study with a broad definition of urinary incontinence, such as any loss of urine in a 12-month period, had a higher prevalence rate than one defining urinary incontinence over a shorter period, such as the number of episodes in the past month.[7] When the definition of urinary incontinence in a study becomes even more specific, the result is that the prevalence numbers decrease. For example, in one study, incontinence was assessed by asking a series of detailed questions modified from epidemiologic studies, as opposed to asking just one or two questions. The result of this more detailed ascertainment was a slightly lower number of women with incontinence in the population than identified in previous studies, with only 21% of women over the age of 70 complaining of at least weekly urinary incontinence.[8] These differences speak loudly to the need for standardized definitions of urinary incontinence to achieve a more precise assessment of the scope of the problem.

Three types of incontinence are usually assessed in survey questionnaires. *Urge urinary incontinence* is urine loss associated with an overwhelming urge to void associated with rushing to the bathroom and not making it there in time. These women wear a pad to go out and often limit their social schedule. *Stress urinary incontinence* is loss of urine caused by increased physical activity, coughing, sneezing, or laughing. These women have limited their physical activity because of their incontinence. *Mixed urinary incontinence* incorporates aspects of stress and urge incontinence in a woman's complaints. Mixed incontinence is often difficult to assess until certain therapies have been attempted. For example, a woman with stress and urge symptoms may be so significantly improved with behavioral modification, pelvic floor exercises, and medication for urgency that she does not notice her stress incontinence. Most studies report a higher rate of stress and mixed incontinence compared with urge incontinence.[9,10] An analysis of the world literature reports that stress incontinence is predominant at 49%, followed by mixed incontinence at 29% and urge incontinence at 22%.[11]

The various prevalence numbers for different varieties of incontinence also result from the inconsistent ages of populations studied and from the diverse populations evaluated. Each study has a new group of women with differences in age, ethnicity, and history such that it is difficult to generalize the results of the study to any other population. Incorrect estimates can also result from bias in data collection and underreporting due to embarrassment. In simple population surveys, most adult women report that they occasionally leak drops of urine with physical exercise, and up to 46% of community-dwelling women complain about some degree of urinary incontinence.[12,13] These numbers underscore the magnitude of this issue and the importance of reporting valid data.

Risk Factors

Women who exercise report more urinary incontinence. Studies by Nygaard and associates[14,15] found that as many as 30% of women complain of urinary leakage during physical activity. The highest rate (38%) was reported in runners. The same researchers demonstrated that even among young, nulliparous women, up to 28% report incontinence with exercise.[14,15] Another study found that up to 80% of elite trampolinists reported involuntary urine leakage.[16] Although this is an extreme example, it does make the point that high-impact sports lead to more urinary incontinence in women.

As our population ages, the prevalence of urinary incontinence will increase. According to the United States Bureau of Census, the number of postmenopausal women in the population will increase from 23% of the total population in 1995 to 33% in 2050, and the proportion of women older than 85 years will triple in the same period.[17] In women with incontinence, the rate of stress incontinence peaks between 45 and 49 years of age and then begins to slowly decrease with further aging.[3] This decrease in stress urinary incontinence may reflect the decrease in activity that usually occurs with aging, leading to a concomitant decrease in urinary incontinence. Although there is a decrease in stress urinary incontinence, the prevalence of any incontinence increases with age in a linear fashion from 3% to 34.7% in young women to 25% to 59.5% in women older than 60 years. This statistic highlights the increase in urge urinary incontinence and the prevalence of that problem later in life.

More than 70% of women living in nursing homes report urinary incontinence.[18-20] Urinary incontinence reported by nursing home residents often has causes other than detrusor overactivity or hypermobility of the urethra. These women can have problems with chronic disease, decreased mobility, and medications that cause urinary incontinence.

Urinary incontinence is two to three times more common in women than in men. There is a very low prevalence of urinary incontinence in men younger than 60 years, whereas incontinence in women steadily increases starting at a much younger age. Men are very unlikely to report stress incontinence, severe incontinence, or irritative bladder symptoms. The anatomic differences between men and women and the risk factors that women face, such as childbirth and hysterectomy, cause them to have more problems with stress urinary incontinence. Men are, however, much more likely to report voiding difficulties due to prostate problems as they age and their prostates enlarge.[21]

Several studies have shown an association between childbirth and urinary incontinence.[22-24] Stress incontinence shows the strongest correlation with parity, whereas there is little correlation between parity and urgency incontinence; rather, aging is more strongly associated with this problem. Vaginal birth may directly damage the pelvic muscles and connective tissues that are necessary for pelvic floor support and for functioning of the urethra. Vaginal birth also leads to a loss of pelvic muscle strength in the immediate postpartum period that gradually returns, something not seen after cesarean section. Studies have also shown that there is an increased risk of urinary incontinence after surgical vaginal delivery compared with cesarean section that lasts for at least 3 years.[25] The debate over whether cesarean section prevents urinary incontinence is ongoing, with arguments from both sides and many physicians caught in the middle.

It had been thought that menopause was a risk factor for lower urinary tract symptoms and urinary incontinence. Atrophic vaginitis of menopause is associated with a multitude of symptoms, including vaginal dryness, burning, and irritation; urinary urgency and frequency; stress urinary incontinence; and recurrent urinary tract infections. The atrophy caused by estrogen deficiency is in part responsible for sensory urogenital symptoms and for the decreased resistance to infection seen in menopausal women. The value of estrogen replacement in this situation, however, is debatable. In two randomized, controlled trials of estrogen and progestin or estrogen alone versus placebo in menopausal women, there was no difference in urinary tract infection rates in the patients who received hormone therapy.[26,27] In another trial, low-dose estriol reduced the frequency of urinary tract infections in menopausal women.[28] Another study showed that intravaginal estriol reduced the risk of recurrent urinary tract infections.[29] Hormone therapy for urinary incontinence has been evaluated in many randomized, controlled trials. In the Heart and Estrogen/Progestin Replacement Study (HERS), no difference was found in incontinence improvement between the hormone therapy group and the placebo group, and hormone therapy seemed to exacerbate incontinence more than the placebo group.[30] Another randomized trial also demonstrated no difference between the estrogen group and the placebo group for improvement of stress urinary incontinence.[31] In a trial of estrogen for urgency incontinence, there was no difference between the hormone group and the placebo group.[32] The conclusion can be made that frequent urinary tract infection in menopausal women can be treated with intravaginal estrogen if there is an element of atrophy involved with the bladder infection.

Obesity and hysterectomy have been thought to be risk factors for urinary incontinence, although much of the evidence is conflicting. Obesity is more common in women with urinary incontinence than in continent women. It is possible that obese women have higher intra-abdominal pressures that overwhelm the continence mechanism. Weight loss has been shown to improve incontinence that is primarily stress related.[33-38] Hysterectomy has been associated with incontinence in some observational studies, but in others, there was no difference between women who had had a hysterectomy and those who had not had surgery.[24,39,40]

Psychosocial Impact

Approximately 31% to 38% of community-dwelling, middle-aged and older women have urinary incontinence, making it a very common chronic health condition among women of many ages.[41,42] The International Continence Society defines urinary incontinence as "a condition in which involuntary loss of urine is a social or hygienic problem." By this definition, every woman with urinary incontinence has some social distress.[12,43,44] Because many women believe that urinary incontinence is a normal consequence of childbirth and aging, they avoid seeking therapy.[45] The burden of urinary incontinence reflects experiences from many aspects of life. Urinary incontinence can affect physical, psychosocial, and economic well-being. Women with urinary incontinence can experience psychologic distress, social isolation and loneliness, increased falls, and increased health care use.[46-50] The monetary costs of urinary incontinence have been estimated at $3565 per incontinent person.[51]

Many studies suggest an association between urinary incontinence and depression and anxiety,[52-54] whereas some suggest only a weak association between urinary incontinence and psychological well-being.[48] There seem to be ethnic differences in distress about urinary incontinence. African American women with urinary incontinence have higher rates of psychological distress than those without urinary incontinence, whereas there is a much weaker association between urinary incontinence and psychological distress among white women.[46] This difference in reactions may reflect the fact that urinary incontinence is less common in African American women and therefore is seen as more of a problem. Despite the apparent bother of urinary incontinence, many women do not discuss this problem with their physicians. The reasons include embarrassment, feelings that incontinence is a natural part of aging, and a belief that there is nothing to help the problem.

Almost 75% of women with stress urinary incontinence are at least slightly bothered by their symptoms, and about 29% moderately to extremely bothered by their incontinence. The frequency and duration of symptoms and the existence of comorbid conditions are associated with increased annoyance by stress urinary incontinence. Fifty-four percent of women who are bothered by their symptoms feel that their symptoms have at least a moderate impact on certain aspects of their lives, including physical activity, self-confidence, daily activities, and social activities.[10] Urinary incontinence does not just affect older women in the psychosocial realm. One study demonstrated that urinary stress incontinence negatively affected the quality of life, work performance, and sexual activity of young and middle-aged women. Urinary incontinence in this group of women caused distress for them emotionally, physically, and socially.[55]

Some forms of urinary incontinence have a more detrimental social impact than others.[56] Urge urinary incontinence has a greater effect on quality of life than stress incontinence.[57-60] In a study of primarily urge urinary incontinence, the women reported generalized anxiety and concern about location of the bathroom. They also reported concern about dating and sexual activity. Women younger than 70 years reported feeling unattractive and having more feelings of low self-esteem.[61]

Loss of urinary control affects the social, psychological, domestic, occupational, physical, and sexual lives of 15% to 30% of women of all ages.[62] Women who perceive urinary incontinence as a disease and those with a higher degree of quality-of-life impact are more likely to seek medical help.[63] Quality-of-life issues seem to be more important than objective outcome measures for most patients.[64] One study demonstrated that the perceived degree of urinary incontinence significantly affected quality of life. Women who perceive their symptoms as being moderate or severe have a significantly lower quality of life.[65] This response was entirely independent of the severity of symptoms determined by objective measures such as a diary or urodynamic testing.

In assessing the economic impacts of urinary incontinence, many studies focus on the cost of caring for elderly incontinent people in nursing homes. This type of data is easier to obtain than that from patients in a community setting.[66] When estimating costs of urinary incontinence, direct and indirect expenses should be included. Direct costs are the resources used to diagnose, treat, care for, and rehabilitate incontinent patients. Indirect costs include lost productivity, missed days of work, time spent by caregivers, and the consequences of incontinence from problems such as skin breakdown or falls and its impact on death rates.[67] A study conducted in 2005 found that although admissions and inpatient stays for urinary incontinence decreased from 1994 to 2000, outpatient visits more than doubled for the same period. While inpatient surgery rates decreased during this time, rates of outpatient surgery were more than doubled. Medical expenditures for urinary incontinence also greatly increased during the 1990s, doubling from 1992 to 1998 for Medicare beneficiaries.[68] Urinary incontinence increases the risk of hospitalization by more than 30% and is believed to be a significant factor for institutionalization among the elderly.[69] One study shows that urinary incontinence doubles the risk of admissions to nursing homes, independent of age and the presence of other diseases.[50]

PELVIC ORGAN PROLAPSE

Definition and Prevalence

Pelvic organ prolapse can be defined as any descent of the uterus or anterior or posterior vagina into the potential space of the vagina. With this definition, 30% to 40% of older women have had some degree of prolapse.[70,71] A newer definition uses the stages of prolapse proposed by the International Continence Society using the pelvic organ prolapse quantification system. This definition is translated into a 0 to 4 staging system. Stage 1is minor vaginal descensus, and stages 2 and above are believed to be more clinically relevant degrees of prolapse. Prevalence estimates for pelvic organ prolapse range from 2% to 50%, depending on the severity of the prolapse and the definition that is used.[72] In a group of women from the Women's Health Initiative Study, 65.5% had prolapse of stage 2 or above. Risk factors for significant pelvic organ prolapse include a history of hysterectomy, lower education level, and a greater number of vaginal deliveries.[73]

Women with prolapse can be asymptomatic with regard to bladder, bowel, and sexual dysfunction, or they can have various complaints. Some of the symptoms associated with advanced prolapse are urgency, frequency, and voiding difficulties. It is difficult to tell whether other symptoms, such as sexual dysfunction, have any relation to severity of prolapse or are multifactorial, with one aspect of the sexual dysfunction being related to prolapse.[74-77] Pelvic organ prolapse is the most common indication for hysterectomy in women older than 55 years.[78] In the United States, rates of surgery for pelvic organ prolapse vary by age, race, and region of the country. Approximately 200,000 women underwent surgery for pelvic organ prolapse between 1979 and 1997, making prolapse one of the most common surgical indications in women.[73,79] The lifetime risk for undergoing surgery for prolapse or incontinence is 11%.[80] Surgery for prolapse, because it is so common, likely has its own impact on quality of life when immediate and long-term postoperative recovery is taken into account.

As with urinary incontinence, pelvic organ prolapse reduces the quality of life.[81] One study found that surgery for pelvic organ prolapse or urinary incontinence improved the quality of life for women who received this treatment.[82] Research shows that conservative therapy also greatly improves the quality of life of these women.[83,84] The use of nonsurgical therapy, such as biofeedback and pelvic floor rehabilitation, for urinary incontinence and pelvic organ prolapse can greatly help with very little risk to the patient.

PSYCHOSOCIAL IMPACT OF URINARY INCONTINENCE AND PELVIC FLOOR DYSFUNCTION IN CLINICAL PRACTICE

It is difficult to interpret the research on the social implications of urinary incontinence and pelvic floor dysfunction and apply this information to current clinical practice. The experience of each woman is different, and the actuality of incontinence should be separated from the woman's experience of the problem. The lived experience of incontinence is very dissimilar for different groups of women and for women of different ages.[41,85]

Incontinent women do share some burdens. Many do not report their incontinence to their health care provider and may live for years without medical treatment. Only one of four eventually seeks help from her physician. Reasons for not discussing this problem with a physician include social embarrassment, fear of surgery, belief that urinary incontinence is a natural part of aging, and lack of knowledge or information about the condition and its management.[7] In the past, urinary incontinence has been marginalized by physicians, and patients have been dissatisfied with their interactions with health care professionals, making them wary of presenting for treatment or returning for worsening of symptoms.[86] Only recently has innovative therapy been introduced for urinary incontinence and pelvic floor dysfunction, so that women now have a choice of treatment options.

A sensitive approach to the subject of urine leakage is required while taking a woman's history and performing the physical examination. It is sometimes helpful to have a woman complete her pelvic floor history form and voiding diary before her initial visit to help her feel more at ease with the subject. Women often are able to describe the problem in more detail when given adequate time to think about it. Continuing public information and patient education allow women to recognize incontinence as a treatable symptom and encourage them to seek solutions for this problem. The complaint of urinary incontinence should be addressed at every annual visit and should then be taken as seriously as any other health problem.

References

1. Abrams P, Cardozo L, Fall M, et al: The standardization of terminology of lower urinary tract function: Report from the Standardisation Sub-committee of the International Continence Society. Am J Obstet Gynecol 187:116-126, 2002.
2. Bates P, Bradley WE, Glen E, et al: The standardization of terminology of lower urinary tract function. J Urol 121:551-554, 1979.
3. Hannestad YS, Rortveit G, Sandvik H, et al: A community-based epidemiological survey of female urinary incontinence: The Norwegian EPINCONT study. Epidemiology of Incontinence in the County of Nord-Trondelag. J Clin Epidemiol 53:1150-1157, 2000.
4. Temml C, Haidinger G, Schmidbauer J, et al: Urinary incontinence in both sexes: Prevalence rates and impact on quality of life and sexual life. Neurourol Urodyn 19:259-271, 2000.
5. Bortolotti A, Bernardini B, Colli E, et al: Prevalence and risk factors for urinary incontinence in Italy. Eur Urol 37:30-35, 2000.
6. Moller LA, Lose G, Jorgensen T: The prevalence and bothersomeness of lower urinary tract symptoms in women 40-60 years of age. Acta Obstet Gynecol Scand 79:298-305, 2000.
7. Minassian VA, Drutz HP, Al-Badr A: Urinary incontinence as a worldwide problem. Int J Gynaecol Obstet 82:327-338, 2003.
8. Jackson RA, Vittinghoff E, Kanaya AM, et al: Urinary incontinence in elderly women: Findings from the Health, Aging, and Body Composition Study. Obstet Gynecol 104:301-307, 2004.
9. Hunskaar S, Lose G, Sykes D, Voss S: The prevalence of urinary incontinence in women in four European countries. BJU Int 93:324-330, 2004.
10. Fultz NH, Burgio K, Diokno AC, et al: Burden of stress urinary incontinence for community-dwelling women. Am J Obstet Gynecol 189:1275-1282, 2003.
11. Hampel C, Wienhold D, Benken N: Prevalence and natural history of female incontinence. Eur Urol 32(Suppl 2):3-12, 1997.
12. Vandoninck V, Bemelmans BL, Mazzetta C, et al: The prevalence of urinary incontinence in community-dwelling married women: A matter of definition. BJU Int 94:1291-1295, 2004.
13. Adelmann PK: Prevalence and detection of urinary incontinence among older Medicaid recipients. J Health Care Poor Underserved 15:99-112, 2004.
14. Nygaard I, DeLancey JO, Arnsdorf L, Murphy E: Exercise and incontinence. Obstet Gynecol 75:848-851, 1990.
15. Nygaard IE, Thompson FL, Svengalis SL, Albright JP: Urinary incontinence in elite nulliparous athletes. Obstet Gynecol 84:183-187, 1994.
16. Eliasson K, Larsson T, Mattsson E: Prevalence of stress incontinence in nulliparous elite trampolinists. Scand J Med Sci Sports 12:106-110, 2002.
17. Projected Population of the United States, by Age and Sex: 2000 to 2050. Washington, DC, United States Census Bureau, 2004.
18. Harrison GL, Memel DS: Urinary incontinence in women: Its prevalence and its management in a health promotion clinic. Br J Gen Pract 44:149-152, 1994.
19. Hellstrom L, Ekelund P, Milsom I, Mellstrom D: The prevalence of urinary incontinence and use of incontinence aids in 85-year-old men and women. Age Ageing 19:383-389, 1990.
20. Lagace EA, Hansen W, Hickner JM: Prevalence and severity of urinary incontinence in ambulatory adults: An UPRNet study. J Fam Pract 36:610-614, 1993.
21. Teunissen TA, van den Bosch WJ, van den Hoogen HJ, Lagro-Janssen AL: Prevalence of urinary, fecal and double incontinence in the elderly living at home. Int Urogynecol J Pelvic Floor Dysfunct 15:10-3; discussion 13, 2004.

22. Elving LB, Foldspang A, Lam GW, Mommsen S: Descriptive epidemiology of urinary incontinence in 3,100 women age 30-59. Scand J Urol Nephrol Suppl 125:37-43, 1989.
23. Burgio KL, Locher JL, Zyczynski H, et al: Urinary incontinence during pregnancy in a racially mixed sample: Characteristics and predisposing factors. Int Urogynecol J Pelvic Floor Dysfunct 7:69-73, 1996.
24. Melville JL, Katon W, Delaney K, Newton K: Urinary incontinence in US women: A population-based study. Arch Intern Med 165:537-542, 2005.
25. Bahl R, Strachan B, Murphy DJ: Pelvic floor morbidity at 3 years after instrumental delivery and cesarean delivery in the second stage of labor and the impact of a subsequent delivery. Am J Obstet Gynecol 192:789-794, 2005.
26. Brown JS, Vittinghoff E, Kanaya AM, et al: Urinary tract infections in postmenopausal women: Effect of hormone therapy and risk factors. Obstet Gynecol 98:1045-1052, 2001.
27. Cardozo L, Benness C, Abbott D: Low dose oestrogen prophylaxis for recurrent urinary tract infections in elderly women. Br J Obstet Gynaecol 105:403-407, 1998.
28. Kirkengen AL, Andersen P, Gjersøe E, et al: Oestriol in the prophylactic treatment of recurrent urinary tract infections in postmenopausal women. Scand J Prim Health Care 10:139-142, 1992.
29. Raz R, Stamm WE: A controlled trial of intravaginal estriol in postmenopausal women with recurrent urinary tract infections. N Engl J Med 329:753-756, 1993.
30. Grady D, Brown JS, Vittinghoff E, et al: Postmenopausal hormones and incontinence: The Heart and Estrogen/Progestin Replacement Study. Obstet Gynecol 97:116-120, 2001.
31. Jackson S, Shepherd A, Brookes S, Abrams P: The effect of oestrogen supplementation on post-menopausal urinary stress incontinence: A double-blind placebo-controlled trial. Br J Obstet Gynaecol 106:711-718, 1999.
32. Cardozo L, Rekers H, Tapp A, et al: Oestriol in the treatment of postmenopausal urgency: A multicentre study. Maturitas 18:47-53, 1993.
33. Thom DH, Brown JS: Reproductive and hormonal risk factors for urinary incontinence in later life: A review of the clinical and epidemiologic literature. J Am Geriatr Soc 46:1411-1417, 1998.
34. Thom DH, van den Eeden SK, Brown JS: Evaluation of parturition and other reproductive variables as risk factors for urinary incontinence in later life. Obstet Gynecol 90:983-989, 1997.
35. Hording U, Pedersen KH, Sidenius K, Hedegaard L: Urinary incontinence in 45-year-old women. An epidemiological survey. Scand J Urol Nephrol 20:183-186, 1986.
36. Weber AM, Walters MD, Shover LR, et al: Functional outcomes and satisfaction after abdominal hysterectomy. Am J Obstet Gynecol 181:530-535, 1999.
37. Bump RC, Sugerman HJ, Fantl JA, McClish DK: Obesity and lower urinary tract function in women: Effect of surgically induced weight loss. Am J Obstet Gynecol 167:392-397; discussion 397-399, 1992.
38. Oskay UY, Beji NK, Yalcin O: A study on urogenital complaints of postmenopausal women aged 50 and over. Acta Obstet Gynecol Scand 84:72-78, 2005.
39. Gimbel H, Zobbe V, Andersen BM, et al: Total versus subtotal hysterectomy: An observational study with one-year follow-up. Aust N Z J Obstet Gynaecol 45:64-67, 2005.
40. de Tayrac R, Chevalier N, Chauveaud-Limbling A, et al: Risk of urge and stress urinary incontinence at long-term follow-up after vaginal hysterectomy. Am J Obstet Gynecol 191:90-94, 2004.
41. Burgio KL, Matthews KA, Engel BT: Prevalence, incidence and correlates of urinary incontinence in healthy, middle-aged women. J Urol 146:1255-1259, 1991.
42. Diokno AC, Brock BM, Brown MB, Herzog AR: Prevalence of urinary incontinence and other urological symptoms in the noninstitutionalized elderly. J Urol 136:1022-1025, 1986.
43. Abrams P, Blaivas JG, Stanton SL, Andersen JT: The standardisation of terminology of lower urinary tract function. The International Continence Society Committee on Standardisation of Terminology. Scand J Urol Nephrol Suppl 114:5-19, 1988.
44. Valerius AJ: The psychosocial impact of urinary incontinence on women aged 25 to 45 years. Urol Nurs 17:96-103, 1997.
45. Bush TA, Castellucci DT, Phillips C: Exploring women's beliefs regarding urinary incontinence. Urol Nurs 21:211-218, 2001.
46. Bogner HR: Urinary incontinence and psychological distress in community-dwelling older African Americans and whites. J Am Geriatr Soc 52:1870-1874, 2004.
47. Lam GW, Foldspang, Elving LB, Mommsen S: Social context, social abstention, and problem recognition correlated with adult female urinary incontinence. Dan Med Bull 39:565-570, 1992.
48. Fultz NH, Herzog AR: Self-reported social and emotional impact of urinary incontinence. J Am Geriatr Soc 49:892-899, 2001.
49. Brown JS, Vuittinghoff E, Wyman JF, et al: Urinary incontinence: Does it increase risk for falls and fractures? Study of Osteoporotic Fractures Research Group. J Am Geriatr Soc 48:721-725, 2000.
50. Thom DH, Haan MN, Van Den Eeden SK: Medically recognized urinary incontinence and risks of hospitalization, nursing home admission and mortality. Age Ageing 26:367-374, 1997.
51. Wagner TH, Hu TW: Economic costs of urinary incontinence in 1995. Urology 51:355-361, 1998.
52. Walters MD, Taylor S, Schoenfeld LS: Psychosexual study of women with detrusor instability. Obstet Gynecol 75:22-26, 1990.
53. Norton KR, Bhat AV, Stanton SL: Psychiatric aspects of urinary incontinence in women attending an outpatient urodynamic clinic. BMJ 301:271-272, 1990.
54. Dugan E, Cohen SJ, Bland DR, et al: The association of depressive symptoms and urinary incontinence among older adults. J Am Geriatr Soc 48:413-416, 2000.
55. Margalith I, Gillon G, Gordon D: Urinary incontinence in women under 65: Quality of life, stress related to incontinence and patterns of seeking health care. Qual Life Res 13:1381-1390, 2004.
56. Kulseng-Hanssen S, Berild GH: Subjective and objective incontinence 5 to 10 years after Burch colposuspension. Neurourol Urodyn 21:100-105, 2002.
57. Wyman JF, Harkins SW, Choi SC, et al: Psychosocial impact of urinary incontinence in women. Obstet Gynecol 70(Pt 1):378-381, 1987.
58. Hunskaar S, Vinsnes A: The quality of life in women with urinary incontinence as measured by the sickness impact profile. J Am Geriatr Soc 39:378-382, 1991.
59. Robinson D, Pearce KF, Priesser JS, et al: Relationship between patient reports of urinary incontinence symptoms and quality of life measures. Obstet Gynecol 91:224-228, 1998.
60. Coyne KS, Payne C, Bhattacharyya SK, et al: The impact of urinary urgency and frequency on health-related quality of life in overactive bladder: Results from a national community survey. Value Health 7:455-463, 2004.
61. Brown JS, Subak LL, Gras J, et al: Urge incontinence: The patient's perspective. J Womens Health 7:1263-1269, 1998.
62. Thomas TM, Plymat KR, Blannin J, Meade TW: Prevalence of urinary incontinence. Br Med J 281:1243-1245, 1980.
63. Yu HJ, Wong WY, Chen J, Chie WC: Quality of life impact and treatment seeking of Chinese women with urinary incontinence. Qual Life Res 12:327-333, 2003.
64. Fialkow MF, Melville JL, Lentz GM, et al: The functional and psychosocial impact of fecal incontinence on women with urinary incontinence. Am J Obstet Gynecol 189:127-129, 2003.
65. Oh SJ, Ku JH, Hong SK, et al: Factors influencing self-perceived disease severity in women with stress urinary incontinence combined with or without urge incontinence. Neurourol Urodyn 24:341-347, 2005.
66. Borrie MJ, Davidson HA: Incontinence in institutions: Costs and contributing factors. CMAJ 147:322-328, 1992.

67. Hu TW: Impact of urinary incontinence on health-care costs. J Am Geriatr Soc 38:292-295, 1990.
68. Thom DH, Nygaard IE, Calhoun EA: Urologic diseases in America project: Urinary incontinence in women—national trends in hospitalizations, office visits, treatment and economic impact. J Urol 173:1295-1301, 2005.
69. Newman DK: What's new: The AHCPR guideline update on urinary incontinence. Ostomy Wound Manage 42:46-50; 52-54; 56; 1996.
70. Coates KW, Harris RL, Cundiff GW, Bum RC: Uroflometry in women with urinary incontinence and pelvic organ prolapse. Br J Urol 80:217-221, 1997.
71. Mouritsen L, Larsen JP: Symptoms, bother and POPQ in women referred with pelvic organ prolapse. Int Urogynecol J Pelvic Floor Dysfunct 14:122-127, 2003.
72. Samuelsson EC, Victor FT, Tibblin G, Svärdsudd KF: Signs of genital prolapse in a Swedish population of women 20 to 59 years of age and possible related factors. Am J Obstet Gynecol 180(Pt 1):299-305, 1999.
73. Nygaard I, Bradley C, Brandt D: Pelvic organ prolapse in older women: Prevalence and risk factors. Obstet Gynecol 104:489-497, 2004.
74. Romanzi LJ, Chaikin DC, Blaivas JG: The effect of genital prolapse on voiding. J Urol 161:581-586, 1999.
75. Barber MD, Visco AG, Wyman JF, et al: Sexual function in women with urinary incontinence and pelvic organ prolapse. Obstet Gynecol 99:281-289, 2002.
76. Rogers GR, Villarreal A, Kammerer-Doak D, Qualls C: Sexual function in women with and without urinary incontinence and/or pelvic organ prolapse. Int Urogynecol J Pelvic Floor Dysfunct 12:361-365, 2001.
77. Weber AM, Walters MD, Piedmonte MR: Sexual function and vaginal anatomy in women before and after surgery for pelvic organ prolapse and urinary incontinence. Am J Obstet Gynecol 182:1610-1615, 2000.
78. Wilcox LS, Koonin LM, Pokras R, et al: Hysterectomy in the United States, 1988-1990. Obstet Gynecol 83:549-555, 1994.
79. Brown JS, Waetjen LE, Subak LL, et al: Pelvic organ prolapse surgery in the United States, 1997. Am J Obstet Gynecol 186:712-716, 2002.
80. Olsen AL, Smith VJ, Bergstrom JO, et al: Epidemiology of surgically managed pelvic organ prolapse and urinary incontinence. Obstet Gynecol 89:501-506, 1997.
81. Wagner TH, Patrick DL, Bavendam TG, et al: Quality of life of persons with urinary incontinence: Development of a new measure. Urology 47:67-71; discussion 71-72, 1996.
82. Helstrom L, Nilsson B: Impact of vaginal surgery on sexuality and quality of life in women with urinary incontinence or genital descensus. Acta Obstet Gynecol Scand 84:79-84, 2005.
83. Bo K, Talseth T, Vinsnes A: Randomized controlled trial on the effect of pelvic floor muscle training on quality of life and sexual problems in genuine stress incontinent women. Acta Obstet Gynecol Scand 79:598-603, 2000.
84. Beji NK, Yalcin O, Erkan HA: The effect of pelvic floor training on sexual function of treated patients. Int Urogynecol J Pelvic Floor Dysfunct 14:234-238; discussion 238, 2003.
85. Klemm LW, Creason NS: Self-care practices of women with urinary incontinence—A preliminary study. Health Care Women Int 12:199-209, 1991.
86. Rosenzweig BA, Hischke D, Thomas S, et al: Stress incontinence in women. Psychological status before and after treatment. J Reprod Med 36:835-838, 1991.

Section 2

EVALUATION AND DIAGNOSIS

Chapter 7

CLINICAL EVALUATION OF LOWER URINARY TRACT SYMPTOMS

Jerry G. Blaivas and Jaspreet Sandha

Diagnostic evaluation of voiding dysfunction in women commences with a focused but detailed history and physical examination. Various diagnostic tests and instruments are used to determine the nature and severity of the symptoms. These may be divided into subjective, semi-objective, and objective instruments. Subjective information is obtained from the patient's history. Semi-objective data are obtained from self-reported diaries, pad tests, and validated questionnaires. Objective data are obtained by physical examination, laboratory tests, radiologic studies, ultrasound imaging, urodynamic studies, and cystoscopy. The collection of subjective, semi-objective, and objective data should continue during and after treatment to determine outcomes.

The spectrum of voiding dysfunction ranges from mild stress urinary incontinence to severe neurologic disease resulting in upper tract deterioration. Because the patient's symptoms are not necessarily proportional to the degree of bladder or renal involvement, a systematic approach should be taken in assessing all aspects of voiding dysfunction.

LOWER URINARY TRACT SYMPTOMS

Standardization

What follows is based on the International Continence Society (ICS) Standardization Report, except where specifically stated to be otherwise.[1] The ICS divides lower urinary tract symptoms into three groups: storage, voiding, and postmicturition. However, the ICS also recognizes a number of pain syndromes that are poorly defined and cannot be easily classified. Storage symptoms include daytime frequency, urgency, incontinence, nocturia, and pain. Voiding symptoms are experienced during the voiding phase and include slow stream, splitting or spraying of the stream, intermittent stream, hesitancy, straining to void, and terminal dribble. Postmicturition symptoms are experienced immediately after micturition and include a feeling of incomplete emptying, postmicturition dribble, or pain.

Storage Symptoms

Urinary frequency (i.e., pollakisuria) is defined as eight or more voids per 24 hours. *Urinary urgency* is defined by the ICS as "the complaint of a sudden, compelling desire to pass urine, which is difficult to defer." We think this definition is too restrictive. Many patients feel a "compelling desire to void" that is not sudden, and others feel uncomfortable, annoying feelings in their bladder that make them think they should void frequently, but the desire is really not compelling. There are currently no single other words or phrases to capture these symptoms.

Urinary incontinence is the involuntary loss of urine. It denotes a symptom, a sign, and a condition. It indicates the patient's (or caregiver's) statement of involuntary urine loss. The sign is the objective demonstration of urine loss. The condition is the pathophysiology underlying incontinence as demonstrated by clinical, cystoscopic, or urodynamic techniques. The symptoms of incontinence include stress, urge, mixed, unaware, continuous, and nocturnal enuresis.[1,2]

Stress urinary incontinence is the complaint of involuntary leakage on effort or exertion or on sneezing or coughing, and *urge incontinence* is the complaint of involuntary leakage accompanied by or immediately preceded by urgency. *Mixed urinary incontinence* is the complaint of involuntary leakage associated with urgency and with exertion, effort, sneezing, or coughing. *Enuresis* means any involuntary loss of urine, and *nocturnal enuresis* is the complaint of loss of urine occurring during sleep. *Continuous urinary incontinence* is the complaint of continuous leakage. *Other types of urinary incontinence* may be situational, such as the report of incontinence during sexual intercourse or giggle incontinence.

CAUSES OF URINARY INCONTINENCE

Urinary incontinence can be further divided into urethral and extraurethral incontinence. Extraurethral causes of incontinence include an ectopic ureter opening into the vagina and urinary fistula. Urethral incontinence is caused by bladder abnormalities, sphincter abnormalities, or combinations of both. Cognitive abnormalities and physical immobility, although not the proximate causes of incontinence, are important cofactors that should be taken into account for the diagnosis and treatment. For example, a woman with mild urgency and severe Parkinson's disease may develop disabling incontinence because it takes her too long to get to the bathroom.

The conditions causing urinary incontinence may be presumed or definite.[2] Definite conditions are documented by urodynamic or other objective techniques. Presumed conditions are documented clinically. For example, a neurologically normal woman who complains of urge incontinence despite a normal cystometrogram is considered to have presumed detrusor overactivity provided that sphincter abnormalities and overflow incontinence have been excluded. If the cystometrogram documents involuntary detrusor contractions, the diagnosis is definite detrusor overactivity.

Urethral Incontinence

Bladder abnormalities causing urinary incontinence include detrusor overactivity and low bladder compliance. *Detrusor*

Table 7-1 Detrusor Overactivity: Causes and Associated Conditions

Idiopathic detrusor overactivity
Non-neurogenic detrusor overactivity
- Bladder outlet obstruction
- Sphincteric incontinence
- Postoperative (anti-incontinence, prolapse)
- Bladder infection
- Bladder tumor
- Bladder stones
- Foreign body

Neurogenic detrusor overactivity
- Supraspinal neurologic lesions
  - Stroke
  - Parkinson's disease
  - Hydrocephalus
  - Brain tumor
  - Traumatic brain injury
  - Multiple sclerosis
- Suprasacral spinal lesions
  - Spinal cord injury
  - Spinal cord tumor
  - Multiple sclerosis
  - Myelodysplasia
  - Transverse myelitis

overactivity is a generic term for involuntary detrusor contractions, defined by the ICS as a "urodynamic observation characterized by involuntary detrusor contractions during the filling phase which may be spontaneous or provoked." The ICS subdivides detrusor overactivity into idiopathic (i.e., non-neurogenic) and neurogenic detrusor overactivity. We have modified this classification as follows:

Idiopathic detrusor overactivity denotes involuntary detrusor contractions that are not associated with neurologic disorders or other conditions known to be associated with involuntary detrusor contractions.

Neurogenic detrusor overactivity denotes involuntary detrusor contractions that are caused by neurologic conditions.

Non-neurogenic detrusor overactivity denotes involuntary detrusor contractions that are associated with conditions thought to be related to detrusor overactivity, such as urethral obstruction and stress incontinence.[3,28,29] The causes of detrusor overactivity are depicted in Table 7-1.

Low bladder compliance denotes an abnormal (decreased) volume-pressure relationship during bladder filling. Low bladder compliance is recognized by a steep rise in detrusor pressure during bladder filling. Causes of low bladder compliance are provided in Table 7-2.

Sphincter Abnormalities Causing Urinary Incontinence

It has long been thought that sphincter abnormalities that cause urinary incontinence were of two generic types—urethral hypermobility and intrinsic sphincter deficiency—and many clinicians still adhere to this concept.[4-6] According to this classification, urethral hypermobility is characterized by rotational descent of the vesical neck and proximal urethra during increases in abdominal pressure.[4-11] If the urethra opens concomitantly, stress urinary

Table 7-2 Causes of Low Bladder Compliance

Neurogenic causes
- Myelodysplasia
- Shy-Drager syndrome
- Suprasacral spinal cord injury or lesion
- Radical hysterectomy
- Abdominoperineal resection

Non-neurogenic causes (i.e., increased collagen)
- Chronic indwelling catheter
- Bladder outlet obstruction
- Chronic cystitis (e.g., radiation, tuberculous, bilharzial)

incontinence ensues. The basic abnormality causing urethral hypermobility is a weakness of the pelvic floor. Intrinsic sphincteric deficiency denotes an intrinsic malfunction of the urethral sphincter itself.[4,12] Clinically, intrinsic sphincter deficiency manifests by a low leak point pressure and is most commonly seen in three circumstances: after surgery on the urethra, vagina, or bladder neck; as a consequence of a neurologic lesion that involves the nerves to the vesical neck and proximal urethra; and in the elderly.[4,12,13] It had also been accepted that urethral hypermobility and intrinsic sphincter deficiency often coexist in the same patient.[14]

The validity of the concept of urethral hypermobility as a sole cause of urinary incontinence has been challenged, and several investigators have shown that there is no relationship between vesical leak point pressure and urethral mobility.[15,16] For that reason, we no longer use the term *intrinsic sphincter deficiency*, but instead characterize sphincteric incontinence by two parameters, vesical leak point pressure and urethral mobility, as measured by the Q-tip test.[7,17]

Overflow Incontinence

Overflow incontinence is the leakage of urine associated with incomplete bladder emptying caused by impaired detrusor contractility or bladder outlet obstruction. The pathophysiology of overflow incontinence has not been studied very well. Conceptually, the leakage must be caused by an overactive detrusor or a relative sphincter deficiency.

SYMPTOMS, SIGNS, AND CONDITIONS CAUSING INCONTINENCE

The symptoms of incontinence are elicited by the patient's history, questionnaires, voiding diaries, and pad test. Symptoms can and should be reproduced during urodynamic studies. The signs are assessed by examination and urodynamic studies. The conditions are the underlying pathophysiologies. Table 7-3 lists symptoms and conditions that cause urinary incontinence.

Urge incontinence has the following characteristics:

Symptom: The symptom of urge incontinence is the complaint of the involuntary loss of urine immediately preceded by urgency.

Sign: The sign of urge incontinence is the observation of involuntary urine loss from the urethra synchronous with an uncontrollable urge to void. Urodynamically, the sign is the presence of detrusor overactivity incon-

Table 7-3 Storage Symptoms and the Conditions That Cause Urinary Incontinence

Symptom	Conditions
Urinary frequency	Polyuria Sensory urgency Detrusor overactivity Low bladder compliance Acquired behavior (e.g., defensive voiding)
Urgency or urge incontinence	Sensory urgency Detrusor overactivity Low bladder compliance
Stress incontinence	Urethral hypermobility Intrinsic sphincter deficiency Stress hyperreflexia
Unaware incontinence*	Detrusor overactivity Sphincter weakness Extra-urethral incontinence
Continuous leakage	Sphincter weakness Extra-urethral incontinence
Nocturnal enuresis	Detrusor overactivity Sphincter weakness Extra-urethral incontinence
Postvoid dribble	Urethral diverticulum Urethral obstruction Vaginal voiding
Extra-urethral incontinence	Urinary fistula Ectopic ureter

*Not part of International Continence Society (ICS) definitions.

tinence (i.e., incontinence due to an involuntary detrusor contraction).

Condition: The condition of urge incontinence is caused by detrusor overactivity.

Stress incontinence has the following characteristics:

Symptom: The symptom of stress incontinence is the complaint of involuntary loss of urine during coughing, sneezing, or physical exertion, such as sport activities or sudden changes of position.

Sign: The sign of stress incontinence is the observation of loss of urine from the urethra synchronous with coughing, sneezing, or physical exertion.

Condition: The condition of stress incontinence may be caused by an underactive sphincter or detrusor overactivity, presumably caused by an increase in abdominal pressure. This is called *stress hyperreflexia*, but it is not part of the ICS lexicon.

Unconscious incontinence has the following characteristics:

Symptom: The symptom of unconscious incontinence is the involuntary loss of urine that is unaccompanied by urge or stress. The patient may be aware of the incontinent episode by feeling wetness or by other associated symptoms such as the onset of autonomic dysreflexia with spinal cord injury.

Sign: The sign of unconscious incontinence is the observation of loss of urine without patient awareness of urge or stress.

Condition: The condition of unconscious incontinence may be caused by detrusor overactivity, sphincter abnormalities, overflow, or extraurethral incontinence.

Continuous leakage has the following characteristics:

Symptom: The symptom of continuous leakage is the complaint of a continuous, involuntary loss of urine.

Sign: The sign of continuous leakage is the observation of a continuous urinary loss.

Condition: The condition of continuous leakage may be caused by sphincter abnormalities or extraurethral incontinence.

Nocturnal enuresis has the following characteristics:

Symptom: The symptom of nocturnal enuresis is the complaint of urinary loss that occurs only during sleep.

Sign: The sign of nocturnal enuresis is the observation of urinary loss during sleep.

Condition: The condition of nocturnal enuresis may be caused by a sphincter abnormality, detrusor overactivity, or extraurethral incontinence.

A precise diagnosis of urinary incontinence is best attained when it is witnessed by the examiner. In most instances, it makes little difference whether the urinary loss is visualized during physical examination with a full bladder (i.e., Marshall or Bonney test), at cystoscopy, cystometry, or by x-ray imaging. Regardless of the method of observation, when urinary loss is visualized from the urethral meatus, the observations and measurements of the astute clinician usually can pinpoint the underlying abnormality and direct appropriate treatment.

Voiding Symptoms

Voiding symptoms are experienced during the voiding phase and include slow stream, splitting or spraying of the urine stream, intermittent stream (i.e., stopping and starting during micturition), hesitancy (i.e., difficulty in initiating micturition, resulting in a delay in the onset of voiding after the individual is ready to pass urine), straining to void, and terminal dribble (i.e., prolonged final part of micturition when the flow has slowed to a trickle or dribble). The conditions underlying these symptoms include urethral obstruction, impaired or absent detrusor contractility, detrusor–external sphincter dyssynergia, and voiding at low bladder volumes. Pain during voiding may be caused by urinary tract infection, urethral stricture, urethral diverticulum, foreign body, or stone.

Pain

During storage, suprapubic or retropubic pain that increases with bladder filling and subsides immediately after voiding is most likely caused by the bladder; if the pain persists after voiding, the source is more difficult to assess. The relationship between other sites of pain is confounding, and a cause-and-effect relationship usually can only be inferred for the urethra, vulva (in and around the external genitalia), vaginal (internally, above the introitus), and perineum (between the posterior fourchette and the anus). The term *pelvic pain* is used when patients describe a pain "down there" but cannot pinpoint its location.

Painful bladder syndrome is the complaint of suprapubic pain related to bladder filling, accompanied by other symptoms such as increased daytime and nighttime frequency, in the absence of proven urinary infection or other obvious pathology. We think interstitial cystitis should be considered in this category because, in contradistinction to the National Institutes of Health consensus recommendations,[18] there are no diagnostic cystoscopic or histologic features that can be used to distinguish these two terms. Interstitial cystitis has connotations of incurability and chronicity—allusions that are not necessarily warranted in many of the patients burdened by such a diagnosis. The differential diagnosis includes pelvic floor myalgia, endometriosis, chronic cystitis (e.g., radiation, tuberculous, bilharzial), low bladder compliance, urethral diverticulum, bladder cancer, bladder stones, and a foreign body.

Urethral pain syndrome is recurrent episodic urethral pain that usually occurs on voiding, often with daytime frequency and nocturia. The differential diagnosis includes urethritis (unspecified), vaginitis, pelvic floor myalgia, urethral diverticulum, urethral stricture, and tumor.

Vulvar pain syndrome (i.e., vulvodynia) is the occurrence of persistent or recurrent episodic vulval pain. The differential diagnosis includes pelvic organ prolapse, vaginitis, and tumor.

Vaginal pain syndrome is the occurrence of persistent or recurrent episodic vaginal pain that is associated with symptoms suggesting urinary tract or sexual dysfunction. The differential diagnosis includes vaginitis, prolapse, urethral diverticulum, endometriosis, pelvic floor myalgia, and tumor.

Perineal pain syndrome is the occurrence of persistent or recurrent episodic perineal pain, which is related to the micturition cycle or associated with symptoms suggesting urinary tract or sexual dysfunction. The differential diagnosis includes pelvic organ prolapse, endometriosis, pelvic floor myalgia, urethral diverticulum, and tumor.

In addition to the specific symptoms listed previously, several clinical symptoms and syndromes warrant special mention. For most of the pain symptoms, the cause remains speculative. The ICS suggests that these terms be used when "there is no proven infection or other obvious pathology."[1] We disagree. We find these terms useful to describe symptoms just as one would use the word *headache* to describe pain in the head from any source, even migraine, brain tumor, or stroke. Moreover, some experts believe that all of these pain syndromes can be the result of a kind of pelvic floor myalgia that results from muscular spasm associated with emotional stress or an acquired behavior resulting from prior painful experiences that could be as simple as bacterial cystitis.

Detrusor Sphincter Dyssynergia

Detrusor–external sphincter dyssynergia is a condition characterized by involuntary sphincter contractions during involuntary detrusor contractions. It is seen exclusively in patients with neurologic disorders that interrupt the normal spinal neuronal circuits of micturition (between the pontine and sacral micturition centers).[20,21] It is essentially a urodynamic diagnosis characterized by increased sphincter electromyographic activity during an involuntary detrusor contraction and narrowing of the distal third of the urethra on voiding cystourethrography.[21] Detrusor–external sphincter dyssynergia is a serious condition that, untreated, leads to urinary retention, ureteral obstruction, vesicoureteral reflux, stones, infection, upper tract deterioration, and renal failure. It should not be confused with acquired voiding dysfunction.

Acquired Voiding Dysfunction

Acquired voiding dysfunction (i.e., learned voiding dysfunction, dysfunctional voiding, or Hinman's syndrome) is often confused with detrusor–external sphincter dyssynergia because the urodynamic findings are similar.[22,25-28] In detrusor–external sphincter dyssynergia, the increased electromyographic activity (when detected by needle electrodes placed directly in the urethral or periurethral striated muscles) precedes the onset of the involuntary detrusor contraction.[21] In acquired voiding dysfunction, there is a period of electromyographic silence that precedes the involuntary detrusor contraction, followed by increased electromyographic activity during the contraction (i.e., the acquired dysfunction). In childhood, acquired voiding dysfunction (i.e., Hinman's syndrome) is postulated to be caused by improper toilet training, resulting in prolonged times between voiding, or "holding urine" to prevent urinary loss, resulting in increased sphincter tone while voiding. It can also be associated with constipation, recurrent urinary tract infection, low bladder compliance, hydronephrosis, and vesicourethral reflux. In children and adults, it can be caused by recurrent painful experiences associated with voiding, such as cystitis and local trauma.

Overactive Bladder

Overactive bladder is defined by the ICS as "urgency, with or without urge incontinence, usually with frequency and nocturia . . . if there is no proven infection or other etiology."[1] From a practical standpoint, we believe that this definition is much too restrictive, and in contradistinction to the ICS definition consider overactive bladder to be a symptom complex caused by one or more of the following conditions: detrusor overactivity, sensory urgency, and low bladder compliance. *Sensory urgency* is a term (abandoned by the ICS) that refers to an uncomfortable need to void that is unassociated with detrusor overactivity. Common conditions causing or associated with overactive bladder are diverse and include urinary tract infection, urethral obstruction, pelvic organ prolapse, sphincteric incontinence, urethral diverticulum, bladder stones or a foreign body, and bladder cancer. In women with overactive bladder, diagnostic evaluation should be directed at early detection of these conditions, because in many instances, the symptoms are reversible if the underlying cause is successfully treated.

Pelvic Prolapse

Prolapse refers to a protrusion of the bladder (i.e., cystocele), urethra (i.e., urethrocele), rectum (i.e., rectocele), intestine (i.e., enterocele), or uterus (i.e., uterine prolapse) past the ordinary anatomic confines of the affected organ. Women with pelvic prolapse may be asymptomatic, or they may complain of concomitant voiding, bowel, or other pelvic symptoms. The severity of symptoms may not correlate at all with the degree of prolapse. A large prolapse can cause extrinsic urethral or ureteral obstruction with resultant hydronephrosis and recurrent urinary tract infection due to incomplete emptying. Prolapse may mask sphincteric incontinence, which becomes evident only after the prolapse is reduced manually or by a pessary or surgery.[29] Failure to take this into account can result in a high rate of incontinence after prolapse surgery. The ICS has described an objective, validated system for quantifying pelvic organ prolapse (POPQ).[30] The POPQ describes the topographic position of six vaginal sites and gives information regarding perineal descent and the change in axis of the levator plate based on increases in the genital hiatus and perineal body measurements. Table 7-4 and Figure 7-1 depict the ICS POP quantification and staging system.

Table 7-4 International Continence Society Pelvic Organ Prolapse Quantification and Staging System

Stage	Description
0	No prolapse is demonstrated.
1	The most distal portion of the prolapse is greater than 1 cm above the level of the hymen.
2	The most distal portion of the prolapse is less than 1 cm above or below the level of the hymen.
3	The most distal portion of the prolapse is greater than 1 cm below the level of the hymen but protrudes no more than 2 cm less than the total vaginal length.
4	There is complete eversion of the total length of the lower genital tract. The distal portion of the prolapse protrudes by at least 2 cm less than the total vaginal length.

From Bump et al.[30]

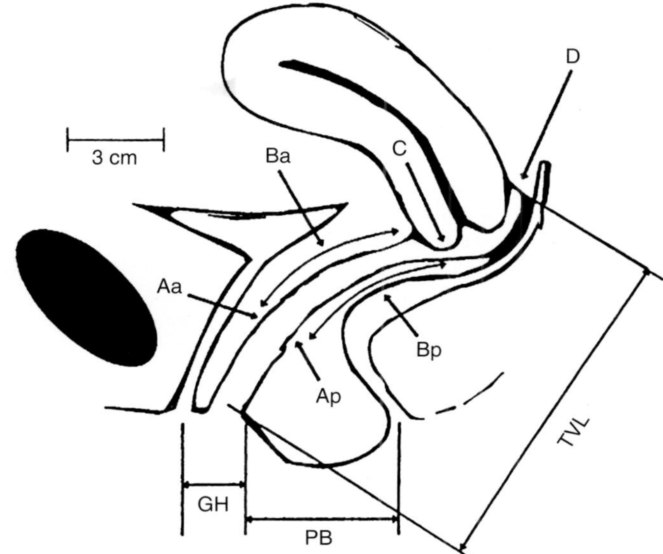

Figure 7-1 Pelvic organ prolapse grading system. The Aa point is located in the midline of the anterior vaginal wall 3 cm proximal to the external urethral meatus. The Ba point represents the most distal (i.e., most dependent) position of any part of the upper anterior vaginal wall from the vaginal cuff or anterior vaginal fornix to point Aa. By definition, point Ba is at –8 cm in the absence of prolapse. The C point represents the most distal (i.e., most dependent) edge of the cervix or the leading edge of the vaginal cuff (i.e., hysterectomy scar) after total hysterectomy. Point D represents the location of the posterior fornix (or pouch of Douglas) in a woman who still has a cervix. It represents the level of uterosacral ligament attachment to the proximal posterior cervix. It is included as a point of measurement to differentiate suspensory failure of the uterosacral-cardinal ligament complex from cervical elongation. When the location of point C is significantly more positive than the location of point D, it indicates cervical elongation that may be symmetric or eccentric. Point D is omitted in the absence of the cervix. Point Bp represents the most distal (i.e., most dependent) position of any part of the upper posterior vaginal wall from the vaginal cuff or posterior vaginal fornix to point Ap. By definition, point Bp is at –3 cm in the absence of prolapse. Point Ap is located in the midline of the posterior vaginal wall 3 cm proximal to the hymen. By definition, the range of position of point Ap relative to the hymen is –3 to +3 cm. The genital hiatus (GH) is measured from the middle of the external urethral meatus to the posterior midline hymen. The perineal body (PB) is measured from the posterior margin of the genital hiatus to the mid-anal opening. The total vaginal length (TVL) is the greatest depth of the vagina (in centimeters) when point C or D is reduced to its full normal position. (Modified from Bump RC, Mattiasson A, Bo K, et al: The standardization of terminology of female pelvic organ prolapse and pelvic floor dysfunction. Am J Obstet Gynecol 175:10, 1996.)

Prolapse is caused by loss of vaginal wall support and weakness in suspensory ligaments. Enterocele may be further classified as congenital, acquired, pulsion, and traction. Congenital enteroceles result from an incomplete closure of the rectovaginal septum. Acquired enteroceles occur after bladder suspension procedures that cause widening of the pouch of Douglas or cul-de-sac, and traction enteroceles are associated with uterine prolapse. Pulsion enteroceles occur after hysterectomy, and they are associated with weakness of the vaginal vault. Another term for pulsion enterocele is a *true enterocele*, because it is filled with bowel, whereas a traction enterocele may contain only the cul-de-sac.[30-33]

EVALUATION OF LOWER URINARY TRACT DYSFUNCTION

Subjective Data

History

The history begins with a detailed account of the precise nature of the patient's symptoms. Each symptom should be characterized and quantified as accurately as possible by anamnesis, questionnaire, bladder diary, and for incontinence, a pad test. When more than one symptom is present, the patient's assessment of the relative severity of each should be considered. The examiner should not rely on any one of these tools, but rather use each as a test of the other.

The patient should be asked how often she urinates during the day and night, how long she can comfortably go between urinations, and how long micturition can be postponed after she gets the urge. It should be determined why she voids as often as she does. Is it because of a severe urge, or is it merely out of convenience or an attempt to prevent incontinence? The severity of incontinence should be graded. Does stress incontinence occur during coughing, sneezing, or rising from a sitting to standing position or only during heavy physical exercise? If the incontinence is associated with stress, is urine lost only for an instant during the stress, or is there uncontrollable voiding? Is the incontinence positional? Does it ever occur in the lying or sitting positions? Is there a sense of urgency first? Does urge incontinence occur? Is the patient aware of the act of incontinence, or does she just find herself wet (i.e., unconscious incontinence)? Is there continuous, involuntary loss of urine? Does the patient lose a few drops or saturate her outer clothing? Does she have postvoid dribbling or enuresis? Are protective pads worn? Do they become saturated? How often are they changed? Is there difficulty initiating the stream requiring pushing or straining to start? Is the stream weak or interrupted? Is there postvoid dribbling? Has the patient ever been in urinary retention?

The symptoms of prolapse do not necessarily correlate with the degree of prolapse. The patient may notice or feel the protrusion or feel like she is "sitting on a ball." There may be a pressure sensation in the vagina, rectum, or groin. She may feel perineal wetness or bleeding from vaginal ulceration, or she may perceive a sensation of pelvic insecurity.[31] There may be a sacral backache that resolves when the patient is lying down.

Prolapse may manifest with a spectrum of lower urinary tract symptoms ranging from urinary retention to overt stress incontinence. Between the two ends of this spectrum fall symptoms of urgency, frequency, straining to void, and a dribbling stream. Most women with prolapse are less symptomatic when supine during the night, with the prolapse reduced. Some patients enhance voiding by applying pressure on the anterior wall of the vagina. When a pessary is inserted, a previously continent woman may develop stress incontinence, a condition called *occult stress incontinence*. A history of stress incontinence that spontaneously subsides suggests occult stress urinary incontinence. Rarely, in severe prolapse, the intestines can become irreducible or even strangulated, which is a surgical emergency. Unmonitored pessaries can erode into the bladder, urethra, bowel, or uterus.

Symptoms caused by a rectocele include the sensation of an inability to evacuate stool from the rectum or the need to apply digital pressure on the posterior vaginal wall to evacuate. Constipation usually is not caused by a rectocele, although the patient may misinterpret her symptoms as constipation. Blood in the stool or changes in the caliber of the stools should prompt colon and rectal examination to rule out neoplasm.[29-33]

Medical History

The patient should be specifically queried about neurologic conditions that are known to affect bladder and sphincteric function, such as multiple sclerosis, spinal cord injury, lumbar disk disease, myelodysplasia, diabetes, stroke, Parkinson's disease, or multisystem atrophy. If she does not have a previously diagnosed neurologic disease, it is important to ask about double vision, muscular weakness, paralysis or poor coordination, tremor, numbness, and tingling. A history of vaginal surgery or previous surgical repair of incontinence should suggest the possibility of sphincteric injury. Abdominoperineal resection of the rectum or radical hysterectomy may be associated with neurologic injury to the bladder and sphincter, resulting in sphincteric incontinence, urinary retention (due to detrusor areflexia), or hydronephrosis (due to low bladder compliance). Radiation therapy may cause a small-capacity, low-compliance bladder or radiation cystitis.

Medications are a rare cause of urinary incontinence. α-Adrenergic antagonists may cause stress incontinence. α-Adrenergic agonists such as histamine and tricyclic antidepressants may cause bladder outlet obstruction, urinary retention, and overflow incontinence. Parasympathomimetics such as bethanechol may cause involuntary detrusor contractions and bladder pain.

Bladder Questionnaire

Questionnaires can expedite the retrieval of all information. In the past decade, there has been a plethora of questionnaires, but no single one has met with widespread approval.[34,35] However, even well-constructed questionnaires with highly significant validation cannot supplant the medical history. Each should supplement the other, and final judgment about the nature of symptoms should be attained by resolving conflicts in the questionnaire, bladder diary, pad tests, and anamnestic responses. We have fashioned two questionnaires for our practice; one is directed toward bladder symptoms, and the other addresses the medical history, medications, and allergies. These questionnaires are sent to the patient before the office visit. The patient has the opportunity to ponder the questions and to acquire information, such as the names of medications and dates of previous operations, before the office visit.

Semi-objective Data

Bladder Diary

To document the nature and severity of urinary symptoms, we find a bladder diary indispensable. The reproducibility of the diary has been confirmed.[23,36-42] The particular information recorded in the diary depends on the patient's symptoms, but all diaries should include at least the time and amount of each micturition. From such a diary, the following information can be calculated: the total 24-hour urinary output, number of voids, longest intervoiding interval, largest single voided volume, diurnal distribution, and diuresis. Depending on the patient's complaints, notations about the characterization, time, and severity of incontinence; the need to push or strain to void; and associated pain or urgency can be compiled. The ICS has advised that the inclusion of a frequency-volume chart is an essential component of the patient's clinical assessment.[8]

Pad Tests

A number of pad tests have been described, but none has met with widespread approval. The reliability of 24-hour pad tests has been reasonably well established, but most 1- and 2-hour tests have considerable test-retest variability.[23-24,43-47] Despite these shortcomings, the pad test is exceedingly useful, but it must be put in perspective with the patient's symptoms. The most direct way of doing this is to ask the patient whether the pad test was representative of her usual symptoms; if not, it should be repeated. The relationship between pad loss and degree of incontinence has been described by a number of studies. A rate of less than 8 g/24 hours is considered normal (e.g., sweat, secretions), and more than 20 g/24 hours is considered to be moderate to severe incontinence.[24,45]

Objective Data

Physical Examination

The physical examination begins by observing the patient's gait and demeanor as she first enters the office. A slight limp or lack of coordination, an abnormal speech pattern, facial asymmetry, or other abnormalities may be subtle signs of a neurologic condition.

The abdomen and flanks should be examined for masses, hernias, and a distended bladder. A pelvic examination is performed with the bladder comfortably full and the patient in the lithotomy position; in patients with prolapse and incontinence it usually should be repeated with the patient standing or sitting. The patient is asked to cough or strain to reproduce symptoms of incontinence. The degree of hypermobility may be assessed by examination with a full bladder and by the Q-tip test. However, examination alone is insufficient for accurate assessment. The Q-tip test is performed by inserting a well-lubricated, sterile, cotton-tipped applicator gently into the urethra while the patient is in lithotomy position. During a Valsalva maneuver or while coughing, the arc of the end of the Q-tip may be estimated or measured from the resting position with a goniometer or approximated by the examiner in terms of degrees from the 0 axis (i.e., position of the applicator at rest). Some examiners use a shortened, red-rubber catheter to obtain a residual volume and then check for mobility during stress. Mobility of the end of the instrument from the resting position to more than 30 degrees with straining indicates urethral hypermobility.[7,17]

Pelvic organ prolapse is best evaluated according to the POPQ protocol as depicted in Table 7-4 and Figure 7-1.[30] The anterior vaginal wall is inspected by applying gentle pressure on the posterior vaginal wall with the posterior blade from a split speculum or with examining fingers. The blade, if metal, should be warmed with water and inserted into the vagina toward the posterior wall. While the patient is straining, the presence of anterior vaginal wall and cervical or uterine mobility are assessed. The design of some examination and urodynamics tables allows the perineum to be visualized and examined while the patient is sitting. In many instances, prolapse and incontinence are appreciated only in one or the other position. Moreover, in some patients, incontinence can be reproduced only with the cystocele reduced. The cervix is normally mobile, but descent to within 1 cm of the hymenal ring is considered grade 1 prolapse.

After examination of the anterior vaginal wall and cervix or uterus, the speculum blade is rotated, and the anterior vagina is gently retracted. The posterior vaginal wall and vault are examined for the presence of an enterocele and rectocele. As the speculum is slowly withdrawn, a transverse groove separating an enterocele from a rectocele below may be visible, and a finger inserted into the rectum can "tent up" a rectocele but not an enterocele.[38]

The sacral dermatomes are evaluated by assessing anal sphincter tone and control, perianal sensation, and the bulbocavernosus reflex. With a finger in the rectum, the patient is asked to squeeze as if she were in the middle of urinating and trying to stop. A lax or weakened anal sphincter and the inability to voluntarily contract and relax may be signs of neurologic damage. The bulbocavernosus reflex is checked by suddenly squeezing the clitoris and feeling (or seeing) the anal sphincter and perineal muscles contract. Alternatively, the reflex may be initiated by suddenly pulling the balloon of the Foley catheter against the vesical neck. The absence of this reflex in men is almost always associated with a neurologic lesion, but the reflex is not detectable in up to 30% of otherwise normal women.[19]

If the patient complains of prolapse or incontinence that is not demonstrated in the lithotomy or sitting position, she is asked to cough and strain while standing. She should be positioned standing in front of the examiner with one foot elevated on a short standing stool. An enterocele is palpable between the forefinger (in the rectum) and the thumb (in the vagina). The perineal body and vaginal rectal septum are examined by palpating the septum through the vagina and rectum.

If a patient has been fitted with a pessary, the pessary should ideally be removed on the day before the office visit; if not, it should be removed and the patient examined. If she states that the prolapse is not at its maximum descent, she should be asked to return later in the day (after she feels the prolapse has fallen down again). The vagina should be examined for any erosions or pudendal nerve injury from an ill-fitted pessary.

The diagnosis of urinary fistula depends on a high index of suspicion, and it should be suspected if there is new onset of incontinence after pelvic surgery or childbirth or after pelvic irradiation for gynecologic malignancy. In most instances, vesicovaginal and urethrovaginal fistulas are apparent on examination of the patient with a full bladder or at the time of cystoscopy, but ectopic ureter and ureterovaginal or vesicouterine fistula are usually not apparent on examination. If a vesicovaginal fistula is suspected but not seen on examination, it almost always is apparent at cystoscopy. If detection defies these simple steps, the bladder can be filled with saline or water to which a dye such as indigo carmine has been added. The vagina should then be inspected for signs of urinary leakage with the urethra occluded with a Foley balloon catheter or with the surgeon's examining finger to prevent urethral leakage. Cystoscopy and pelvic examination are essential to evaluate the extent of the anatomic defect, the possibility of unrecognized secondary fistulas, the pliability of local tissue, the need for securing bulk-ensuring tissue pedicle flaps, the need for concomitant pelvic reconstructive surgery, and the timing of surgery. At the time of cystoscopy, retrograde pyelography may be performed when indicated, and the integrity of the urethral sphincter should be tested while the bladder is full.

To confirm the presence of an ectopic ureter or of a ureterovaginal or vesicouterine fistula, intravenous pyelography, retrograde pyelography, cystography, and hysterosalpingography may be necessary. In doubtful cases, Pyridium may be given orally and the patient instructed to wear a tampon and pads. If the Pyridium stains the tampon but not the pad, a vaginal fistula should be excluded. Urinary incontinence is not always caused by what appears to be the most overt lesion. For example, neither a urethrovaginal fistula nor a destroyed distal urethra should cause urinary incontinence unless the proximal urethra and vesical neck are also damaged. A careful, stepwise evaluation should be carried out in all patients to delineate the pathophysiology underlying incontinence. Other causes of urinary incontinence commonly seen in these patients include a previously undiagnosed vesicovaginal or ureterovaginal fistula, detrusor overactivity, low bladder compliance, and sphincteric abnormalities.

Routine Urologic Assessment

Routine laboratory studies include urinalysis, urine culture, and, in selected patients, renal function tests. Positive urine cultures should be treated with culture-specific antibiotics, but patients with persistent bacteriuria or recurrent infections may require invasive testing while on antibiotics. Hematuria should be evaluated by upper tract imaging (i.e., computed tomography with intravenous contrast or intravenous pyelography) and cystourethroscopy.

Urodynamic Study

The main purpose of urodynamic investigation is to determine the precise cause of the patient's voiding dysfunction, and to this end, it is important that the symptoms be reproduced during the ex-amination. Urodynamic technique varies from "eyeball urodynamics" to sophisticated multichannel, synchronous video, pressure-flow, and electromyographic studies. Using synchronous, multichannel video urodynamics offers the most comprehensive, artifact-free means of arriving at a precise diagnosis, and we perform these techniques routinely when urodynamics are indicated. When multichannel studies are not routinely performed, they should be considered under the following circumstances:

1. When simpler diagnostic tests have been inconclusive
2. When the patient complains of incontinence, but it cannot be demonstrated clinically
3. In patients who have previously undergone corrective surgery for incontinence
4. In patients who have previously undergone radical pelvic surgery, such as abdominoperineal resection of the rectum or radical hysterectomy
5. In patients with known or suspected neurologic disorders that may interfere with bladder or sphincter function (e.g., myelodysplasia, spinal cord injury, multiple sclerosis, herniated disk, cerebrovascular accident, Parkinson's disease, multisystem atrophy).

Laboratory urodynamics are discussed in Chapter 11. The use of eyeball urodynamics is discussed here.

Eyeball Urodynamics

Eyeball urodynamics are performed with the patient in the lithotomy position. The patient should already have completed a bladder diary and, if incontinent, a pad test. The examiner should know the patient's history and symptoms. She should be asked to void (and uroflow measured, if available). After voiding, she should be asked whether that void was typical and if she felt that she emptied her bladder; if not, the data should not be considered with that perspective. A regional neurologic examination, including the assessment of perineal sensation, anal tone and control, and bulbocavernosus reflex,[47] is performed. A Foley catheter or (preferably) a cystoscope is inserted, and postvoid residual urine is measured. A fluid reservoir (i.e., 60-mL catheter tip syringe with its barrel removed or irrigation bag or bottle) is connected, and water or saline is then infused into the bladder by gravity. The syringe, bag, or bottle is lowered, and the meniscus is observed at the height that fluid inflow stops. The height (in centimeters) of the meniscus above the symphysis pubis is the resting intravesical pressure. The bladder is filled, and in contradistinction to the recommendations of the ICS, the patient is told to neither void nor try to inhibit micturition; rather, she is instructed to report her sensations to the examiner. When she perceives the urge to void, she is asked if that is the usual feeling that she experiences when she needs to urinate. Changes in intravesical pressure are apparent as a slowing down in the rate of fall or a rise in the level of the fluid meniscus. A change in pressure may be caused by a detrusor contraction, an increase in abdominal pressure, or low bladder wall compliance. As soon as a change in pressure occurs, the examiner should attempt to determine the cause. Visual inspection usually belies abdominal straining, but in doubtful cases, the abdomen should be palpated. In most instances, the cause of the rise in intravesical pressure is obvious, but when in doubt, formal cystometry with rectal pressure monitoring is necessary.

Any sudden rise in pressure that is accompanied by an urge to void or by incontinence is an involuntary detrusor contraction. In some instances, the cause of the patient's incontinence is easily discernable because she voids uncontrollably around the catheter during an involuntary detrusor contraction. If involuntary detrusor contractions do not occur, the bladder is filled until a normal urge to void is experienced. The bladder is left full, and the catheter is removed. The presence or absence of gravitational urinary loss is noted. The patient is asked to cough and bear down with gradually increasing force to determine the ease with which incontinence is produced, and the vagina is inspected for signs of prolapse.

Incontinence that occurs during stress is not always caused by sphincter abnormalities. In some patients, the stress initiates a reflex detrusor contraction. This condition has been called *stress hyperreflexia*. It is important to determine whether the leakage is accompanied by descent of the bladder base and urethra. It should be further noticed whether the leakage stops as soon as the stress is over or the patient continues to void uncontrollably. In the former case, the patient has stress incontinence; in the latter, it is stress hyperreflexia.

If the patient complains of urinary incontinence, but it has not been demonstrated, the examination should be repeated in the standing position as described previously. Under ordinary circumstances, no patient should undergo invasive or irreversible treatment until the cause of the incontinence has been clearly demonstrated.

References

1. Abrams P, Cardozo L, Fall M, et al: The standardization of terminology of lower urinary tract function: Report from the Standardisation Sub-committee of the International Continence Society. Neurourol Urodyn 21:167, 2002.
2. Blaivas JG, Appell RA, Fantl JA, et al: Definition and classification of urinary incontinence: Recommendations of the urodynamic society. Neurourol Urodyn 16:149, 1997.
3. Chou EC, Flisser AJ, Panagopoulos G, Blaivas JG: Effective Treatment for mixed urinary Incontinence with Pubovaginal sling, J Urol, 170:494-497, 2003.
4. Blaivas JG, Olsson CA: Stress incontinence: Classification and surgical approach. J Urol 139:727, 1988.
5. Green TH: The problem of stress urinary incontinence in the female: An appraisal of its current status. Obstet Gynecol Surg 23:603, 1968.
6. McGuire EJ, Lytton B, Pepe V, Kohorn EI: Stress urinary incontinence. Obstet Gynecol 47:255, 1976.
7. Bergman A, McCarthy TA, Ballard CA, Yanai J: Role of the Q-tip test in evaluating stress urinary incontinence. J Reprod Med 32:273, 1987.
8. Brandt FT, Albuquerque CDC, Lorenzato FR, Amaral FJ: Perineal assessment of urethrovesical junction mobility in young continent females. Int Urogynecol J 11:97, 2000.
9. Montella JM, Ewing S, Carter J: Visual assessment of urethrovesical junction mobility. Int Urogynecol J 8:13, 1997.
10. Mostwin JL, Yang A, Sanders R, Genadry R: Radiography, sonography and magnetic resonance imaging for stress incontinence. Urol Clin North Am 22:539, 1995.
11. Yang A, Mostwin JL, Rosenshein N: Dynamic evaluation of pelvic floor descent using fast MRI and cinematic display. Radiology 179:25, 1991.
12. McGuire EJ, Fitzpatrick CC, Wan J, et al: Clinical assessment of urethral sphincter function. J Urol 150:1452, 1993.
13. Barbalias GA, Blaivas JG: Neurologic implications of the pathologically open bladder neck. J Urol 129:780, 1983.
14. Kaygil O, Ahmed SI, Metin A: The co-existence of intrinsic sphincter deficiency with type II stress incontinence. J Urol 162:1365, 1999.
15. Fleischmann N, Flisser AJ, Blaivas JG, Panagopoulos G: Sphincteric urinary incontinence: Relationship of vesical leak point pressure,

urethral mobility and severity of incontinence. J Urol 169:999, 2003.

16. Nitti VW, Combs AJ: Correlation of Valsalva leak point pressure with subjective degree of stress urinary incontinence in women. J Urol 155:281, 1996.
17. Crystle C, Charme L, Copeland W: Q-tip test in stress urinary incontinence. Obstet Gynecol 38:313, 1971.
18. Kusek JW, Nyberg LM: The epidemiology of interstitial cystitis: Is it time to expand our definition? Urology 57(Suppl 1):95, 2001.
19. Blaivas JG: The bulbocavernosus reflex in urology: A prospective study of 299 patients. J Urol 126:197, 1981.
20. Blaivas JG: The neurophysiology of micturition: A clinical study of 550 patients. J Urol 127:958, 1982.
21. Blaivas JG, Sinha HPM, Zayed AAH, Labib KB: Detrusor external sphincter dyssynergia. J Urol 125:542, 1981.
22. Allen TA: The non-neurogenic neurogenic bladder. J Urol 117:232, 1977.
23. Groutz A, Blaivas JG, Chaikin DC, et al: Noninvasive outcome measures of urinary incontinence and lower urinary tract symptoms: A multicenter study of micturition diaries and pad tests. J Urol 164:698, 2000.
24. Groutz A, Blaivas JG, Rosenthal JD: A simplified urinary incontinence score for the evaluation of treatment outcomes. Neurourol Urodyn 19:127, 2000.
25. Groutz A, Blaivas JG: Non-neurogenic female voiding dysfunction [review]. Curr Opin Urol 12:311, 2002.
26. Groutz A, Blaivas JG, Chaikin DC: Bladder outlet obstruction in women: Definition and characteristics. Neurourol Urodyn 19:213, 2000.
27. Hinman F Jr, Baumann FW: Vesical and urethral damage from voiding dysfunction in boys without neurologic or obstructive disease. J Urol 109:727, 1973.
28. Patel R, Nitti V: Bladder outlet obstruction in women: Prevalence, recognition, and management [review]. Curr Urol Rep 2:379, 2001.
29. Chaikin DC, Romanzi LJ, Rosenthal J, et al: The effects of genital prolapse on micturition. Neurourol Urodyn 17:426, 1998.
30. Bump RC, Mattiasson A, Bo K, et al: The standardization of terminology of female pelvic organ prolapse and pelvic floor dysfunction. Am J Obstet Gynecol 175:10, 1996.
31. Wall LL, Norton PA, DeLancey JOL: Prolapse and the lower urinary tract. In Wall LL, Norton PA, DeLancey JOL (eds): Practical Urogynecology. Baltimore, Williams & Wilkins, 1993, pp 293-315.
32. Zacharin RF: The clinical features of enterocoele. In Zacharin RF (ed): Pelvic Floor Anatomy and the Surgery of Pulsion Enterocoele. Vienna, Springer-Verlag, 1985, pp 77-101.
33. Zimmern PE, Leach GE, Ganabathi K: The urological aspects of vaginal wall prolapse. Part I. Diagnosis and Surgical Indications, Lesson 25. Houston, TX, American Urological Association, Office of Education, 1993, pp 194-199.
34. Graham CW, Dmochowski RR: Questionnaires for women with urinary symptoms. Neurourol Urodyn 21:473, 2002.
35. Jackson S, Donovan J, Kent L, et al: The reliability and validity of a new female urinary symptoms questionnaire. Neurourol Urodyn 5:536, 1995.
36. Abrams P, Klevmark B: Frequency volume charts: An indispensable part of lower urinary tract assessment. Scand J Urol Nephrol Suppl 179:47, 1996.
37. DeWachter S, Wyndaele JJ: Frequency-volume charts: A tool to evaluate bladder sensation. Neurourol Urodyn 22:638, 2003.
38. Diokno AC, Wells TJ, Brink CA: Comparison of self-reported voided volume with cystometric bladder capacity. J Urol 137:698, 1987.
39. Fink D, Perucchini D, Schaer GN, Haller U: The role of the frequency-volume chart in the differential diagnosis of female urinary incontinence. Acta Obstet Gynecol Scand 78:254, 1999.
40. Fitzgerald MP, Brubaker L: Variability of 24-hour voiding diary variables among asymptomatic women. J Urol 169:207, 2003.
41. Kassis A, Schick E: Frequency-volume chart pattern in a healthy female population. Br J Urol 72:708, 1993.
42. Larsson G, Victor A: Micturition patterns in a healthy female population, studied with a frequency/volume chart. Scand J Urol Nephrol Suppl 114:53, 1988.
43. Christensen SJ, Colstrup H, Hertz JB, et al: Inter- and intradepartmental variations of the perineal pad-weighing test. Neurourol Urodyn 5:23, 1986.
44. Lose G, Gammelgaard J, Jorgensen TJ: The one-hour pad-weighing test: Reproducibility and the correlation between the test result, start volume in the bladder and the diuresis. Neurourol Urodyn 5:17, 1986.
45. O'Sullivan R, Karantanis E, Stevermuer TL, et al: Definition of mild, moderate, and severe incontinence of the 24-hour pad test. BJOG 111:859, 2004.
46. Siltberg H, Victor A, Larsson G: Pad weighing tests: The best way to quantify urine loss in patients with incontinence. Acta Obstet Gynecol Scand Suppl 166:28, 1997.
47. Diokno AC, Hollander JB, Bennett CJ: Bladder neck obstruction in women: A real entity. J Urol 132:294, 1984.

Chapter 8

IMAGING OF THE FEMALE GENITOURINARY TRACT

Steven S. Raman and Lousine Boyadzhyan

REVIEW OF IMAGING MODALITIES

Projectional Radiography

In uroradiology, the role of projectional radiography, once an integral part of diagnosis, has been steadily diminishing as cross-sectional techniques have become more advanced (Fig. 8-1). X-ray–based images are now routinely captured on digital media instead of film, enabling rapid storage on a central server with multiple display options, including a picture archiving and retrieval system (PACS), or for distribution on the Internet. However, the principles of x-ray–based diagnosis have not changed. An image is formed when diagnostic-range x-ray energy interacts with the electron cloud of different human tissues (i.e., bone, soft tissue [water], fat, and air). The different electron densities of these tissues allow various degrees of x-ray beam penetration, resulting in differences in exposure (i.e., shades of gray) on the receptor film or digital media. Most naturally occurring electron-dense structures, such as calcified bone or dental enamel, attenuate x-ray energy strongly and by convention appear white on the conventional or digital receptor. Conversely, the least electron-dense substances, such as gas, allow almost 99% of x-ray energy to penetrate the tissue and reach the receptor, and by convention, these images are black. Between these two extremes are the shades of gray, which represent the summation of various three-dimensional (3D) electron densities on a two-dimensional (2D) receptor. Perception and interpretation of projectional images is highly operator dependent and requires a large degree of experience for proper interpretation.

Because it is easy to visualize structures at extremes of the spectrum of beam penetrance, calcified structures such as most urologic stones (i.e., white) or gas (i.e., black) can be seen well. However, most solid and fluid-filled organs are essentially of water density and are distinguished on radiographs by the relative contrast provided by relatively radiolucent fat.

A patterned approach to the abdominal radiograph is useful for instruction. On most radiographs, the lower poles of the kidneys are apparent with a laterally divergent axis that usually parallels the psoas muscles when visualized. Renal calculi are usually seen as ovoid or toothlike opacities overlying the kidneys or proximal ureters. They are more difficult to detect over the distal ureter because contrast is reduced by overlying bony pelvis. Gas projecting over the bladder is usually seen after recent Foley catheterization, but it may be caused by infections and fistulas. Bony abnormalities should not be overlooked because they can represent metastatic disease or suggest a neurogenic bladder, especially in patients with spinal abnormalities.[1]

To address the problem of poor soft tissue attenuation differences and to image gross pathologic conditions, various radiographic contrast agents (usually iodinated agents with high electron density especially suited for x-ray interaction) were introduced into the field of uroradiology. The first introduction of retrograde urothelial injection agents in the 1920s was followed by the development of intravascular contrast agents, giving rise to intravenous urography, a mainstay of uroradiology for renal and ureteral evaluation for almost 50 years (Figs. 8-2 and 8-3).[2] A large variety of catheter-injected uroradiologic studies were developed for niche applications, including urethrograms, cystograms, pyelograms, loopograms, nephrostograms, and suprapubic cystograms.

Fluoroscopy

Fluoroscopy is the dynamic counterpart of static projectional radiography because it displays real-time images of a particular process under investigation. During fluoroscopic studies, a low dose of continuous x-ray beams passes through the patient to an image intensifier to generate images on a high-resolution television monitor.[3] The examiner can obtain a series of individual snapshots (i.e., frames per second) of the process, so-called spot films, or a real-time movie such as evaluation of dynamic processes for storage and review. However, fluoroscopic imaging is best performed with iodinated contrast material for genitourinary applications. Fluoroscopy is most useful for vascular applications, but it may be used for real-time evaluation of ureteral peristalsis; bladder filling and emptying, especially during voiding (i.e., voiding cystourethrography [VCUG]); and guiding a variety of genitourinary interventions, such as nephrostomy tube placement.

Cystography and Voiding Cystoureterography

Cystography can be done in a static fashion or as VCUG. During static cystography, contrast material is instilled into the bladder through a Foley catheter, and various views of the full bladder are taken along with postdrainage views. This examination is usually indicated in cases of suspected bladder rupture, low-pressure vesicoureteral reflux, or a vesical fistula. It can also be useful in the assessment of intravesical filling defects, bladder diverticula, or lower urinary tract congenital anomalies. In an update to conventional cystography, the study may be modified and performed as a computed tomography (CT)–based examination for almost all indications, especially in the setting of trauma.

VCUG is performed as an adjunct to a cystogram to determine the morphology of the bladder and urethra, especially if high-pressure vesicoureteral reflux and related complications are suspected. The bladder is filled, as in static cystography, followed by fluoroscopy and/or a video recording of the voiding process once the catheter is removed.[1]

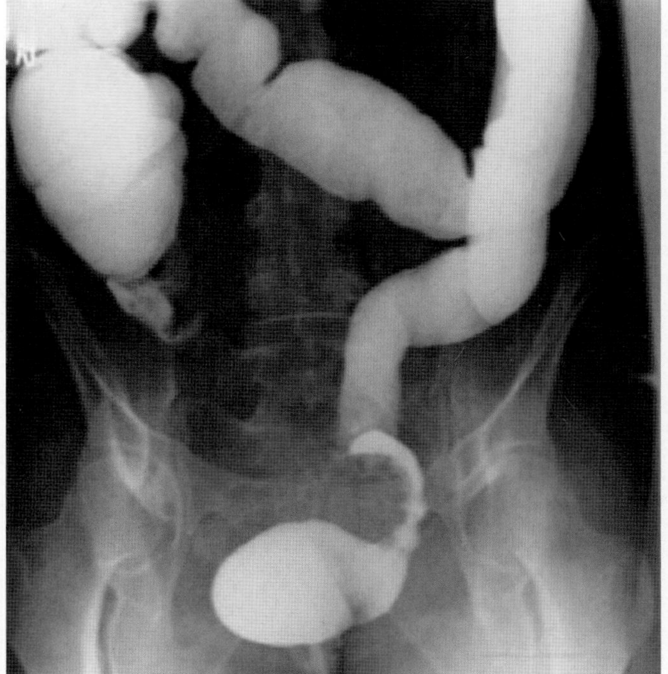
A

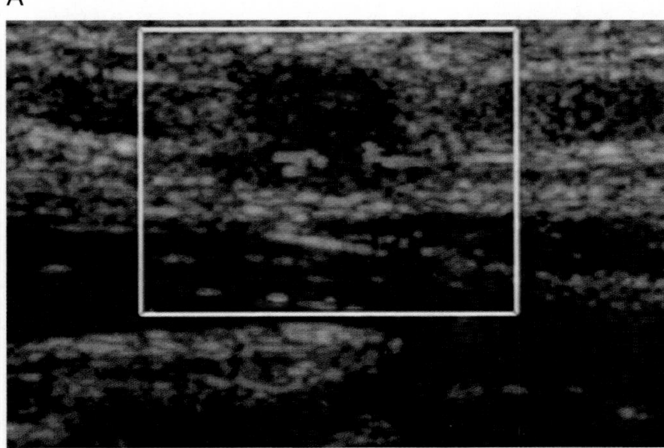
B

Figure 8-1 Endometriosis implants in the colon are seen on a plain film **(A)** as filling defects, which were later confirmed with transabdominal ultrasound **(B).**

Video Urodynamics

In video urodynamics (VUDs), multichannel urodynamic measurements are combined with concomitant fluoroscopic VCUG to determine whether morphologic findings with regard to bladder function and its outlet correlate with physiologic measurements. It is therefore possible to go beyond the level of a simple VCUG or cystometry by obtaining simultaneous measurements of abdominal and vesical pressures under fluoroscopic guidance. In addition to revealing a great deal about dynamics of the bladder and its outlet, VUDs has led to greater diagnostic and therapeutic efficacy. With modern advent of digital recording, the examiner can manipulate the data with various software packages with incorporation of other clinical information and statistical calculations to maximize the yield even further. Some of the most common indications for VUDs in women are various

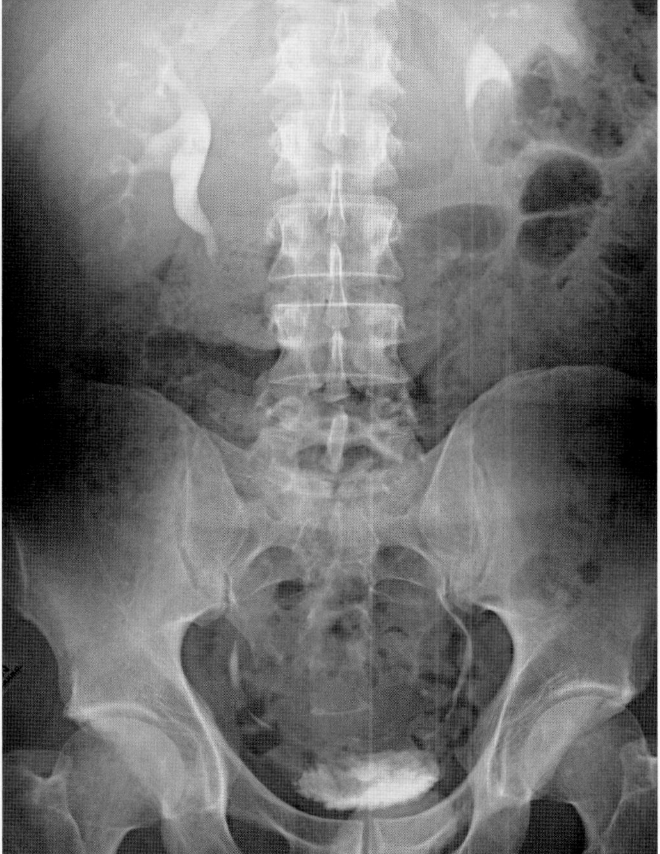
A

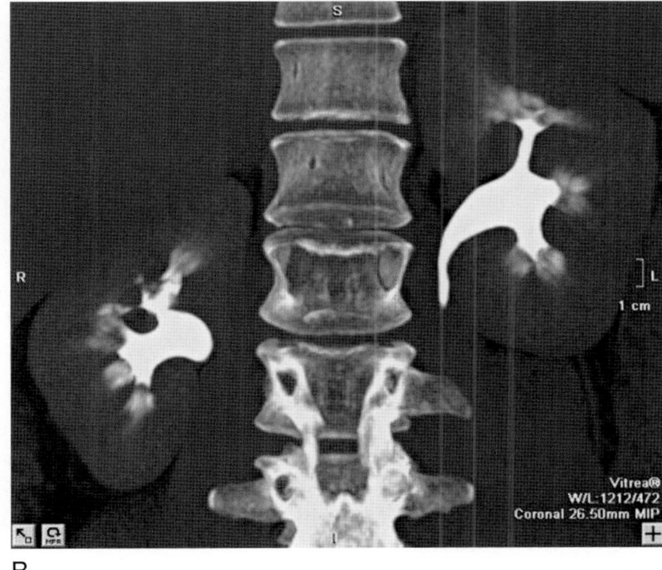

B

Figure 8-2 Tubular ectasia in the kidney is shown by traditional intravenous pyelogram **(A)** and computed tomography **(B).**

kinds of incontinence; bladder outlet obstruction, as can be seen in urethral obstruction; neuropathic bladder due to a variety of neurologic disorders; geriatric incontinence; urinary diversion; and unidiversion.[4]

The main problem with VUDs is that it often may not reproduce the presenting symptoms of the patient because it is

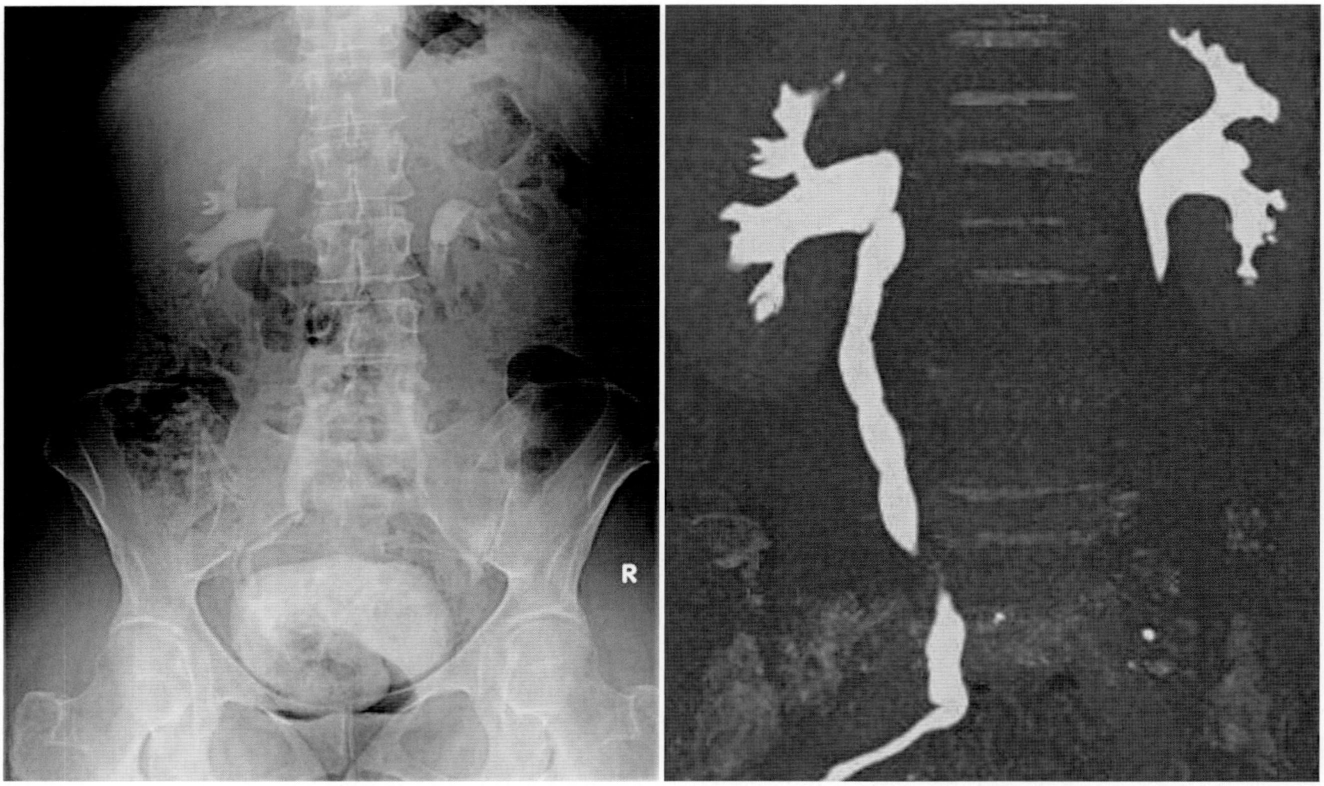

Figure 8-3 Papillary necrosis is shown by traditional intravenous pyelogram **(A)** and maximum intensity projection (MIP), from CTP urogram computed tomography **(B).** Note that they defect in the renal papilla in the liver poles are more easily seen on the MIP CT image.

nonphysiologic in nature and is performed in surroundings unfamiliar to the patient. The presence of severe grades of cystoceles, rectoceles, enteroceles, and uterine prolapse can lead to a rather unreliable interpretation of the examination results. In such clinical scenarios, it is especially important to repeat the study in a variety of positions to assess the severity of the pelvic floor pathology present in a given patient. Despite these limitations, VUDs is still highly recommended in patients with postoperative incontinence and in neuropathic and refractory cases.[4]

Intravenous Urography and Pyelography

The traditional intravenous urogram (IVU), which is used to evaluate the kidneys, kidney function, and ureteral excretion and function, has undergone a radical transformation over the past 10 years, with increasing resolution and performance of CT, magnetic resonance imaging (MRI), and ultrasound (see Figs. 8-2 and 8-3). Evaluation of the kidneys is best performed with contrast-enhanced CT or MRI (Figs. 8-4 and 8-5). Evaluation of the ureters also may be performed with CT or MRI, although a fluoroscopic or radiographic examination, if performed properly, may be adequate, especially when detecting urothelial malignancies. Advances in competing technologies have limited or severely restricted the clinical application of the IVU. The intravenous urogram is no longer indicated for many upper tract indications, such as renal mass evaluation and evaluation of acute renal colic, and is best reserved for evaluation of hollow parts of the urinary system, such as follow-up of patients with transitional cell carcinoma.[1]

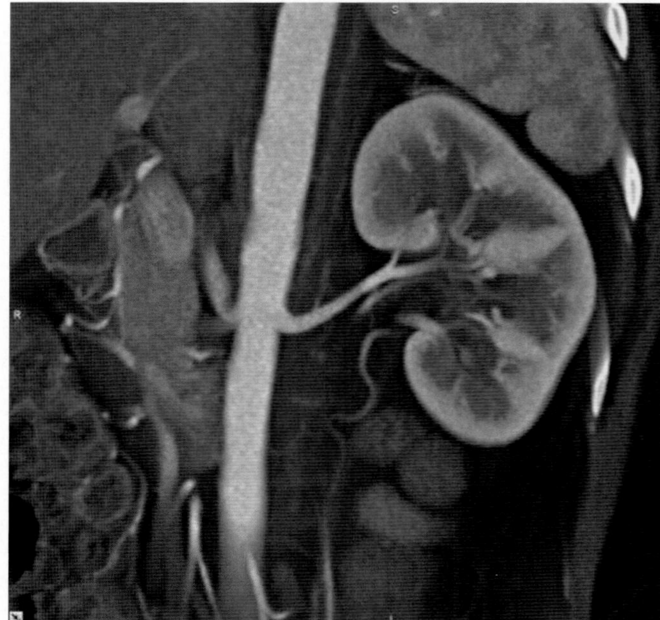

Figure 8-4 Oblique coronal virtually rendered image shows detailed renal and vascular anatomy. Notice the small renal vein draining into the gonadal vein in the lower abdomen.

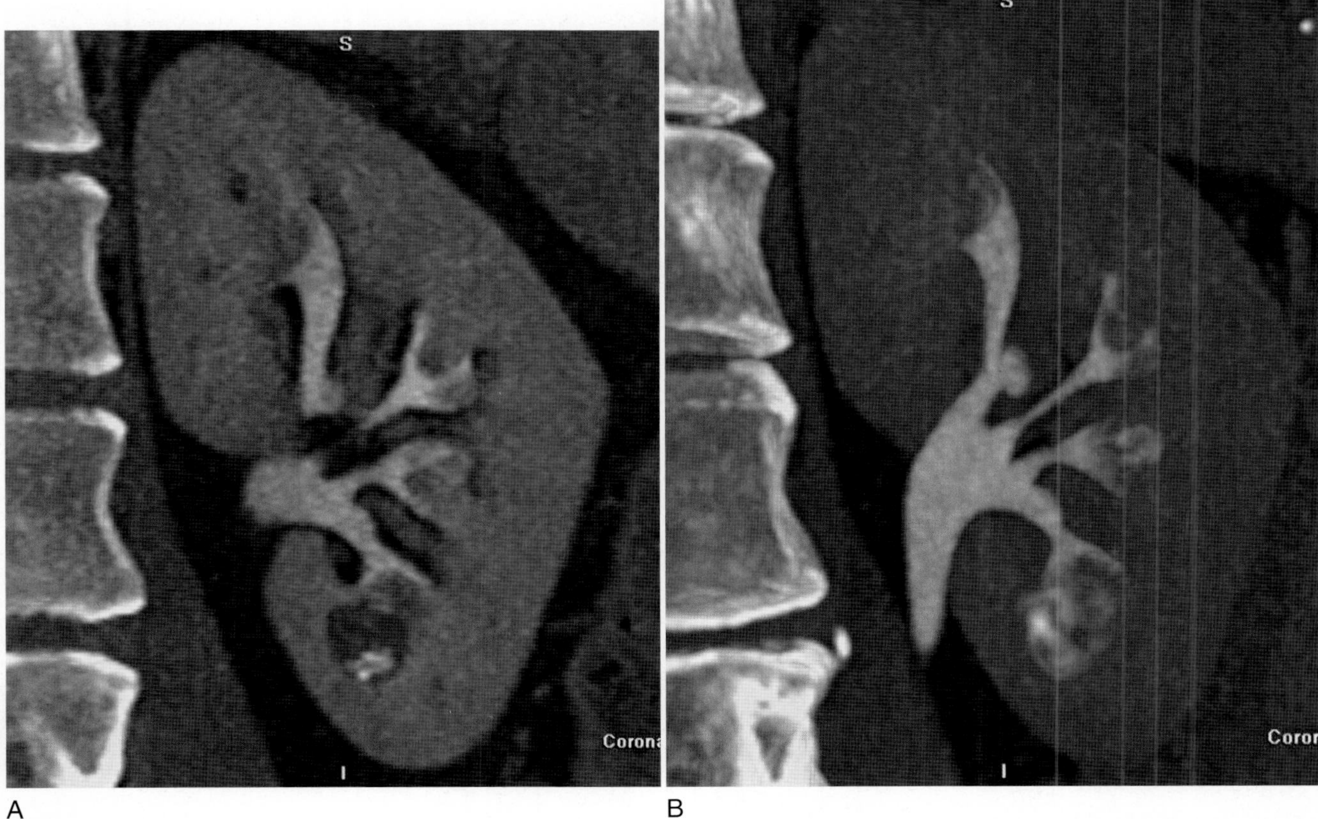

A B

Figure 8-5 Coronal maximum intensity projection (MIP) image generated with a 64-detector CT scanner in nephrographic **(A)** and excretory **(B)** phase demonstrates a cystic structure. It contains a stone adjacent to the fornix of the lower pole calyx on the left kidney, which displays delayed-contrast filling, suggesting a calyceal diverticulum.

Retrograde Pyelography

Retrograde pyelography allows morphologic evaluation of the collecting system and ureters. It involves retrograde injection of contrast material directly into the ureters after their cystoscopic cannulation to visualize the collecting system and the ureter without reliance on renal contrast excretion. It also is possible to biopsy suspected urothelial lesions in the course of the examination. Some of the most common indications for retrograde pyelography are further evaluation of congenital anomalies, urinary obstruction, and possible filling defects detected during other studies. However, because this is a rather invasive diagnostic study associated with several potential complications, it usually is not used as an initial diagnostic procedure.[1]

Urethrography

Although most commonly used in male patients, urethrography occasionally is used in female patients by injecting contrast material into the urethra directly. This examination can be especially useful in cases of urethral fistulas and suspected urethral diverticula that failed to opacify during voiding studies, as described in the preceding section.

Ultrasonography

In sonography, also referred to as ultrasound or ultrasonography, sound waves with frequencies in the range of 2 to 20 MHz are generated by an array of piezoelectric crystals in a hand-held transducer. These tightly focused, high-frequency sound waves are propagated through human tissues and reflected back at tissue interfaces to the transducer's crystals, subsequently producing a diagnostic medical image.[3] The choice of imaging frequencies is determined by the size and composition of the tissue involved. Higher frequencies (>7 MHz) usually lead to improved spatial resolution at the expense of depth of imaging, whereas lower frequencies (2 to 5 MHz) enable imaging of deeper tissues with lower spatial resolution. The chief advantages of sonography are its lack of ionizing radiation, its real-time imaging capability, its 2D and 3D imaging capability, and its ability to depict flow direction and velocity in blood vessels and tissues.[4] Disadvantages of sonography are its operator dependence and its inability to image through hollow viscera or bone. In urology, ultrasound is the initial test of choice for adult and pediatric renal and bladder imaging. A wide variety of pathologies, such as congenital anomalies, hydronephrosis, and vascular disorders, may be diagnosed. In bladder applications, it may be used to determine residual postvoid urine volume and to delineate the urethrovesical anatomy (Figs. 8-6 and 8-7).[5]

Sonography is integral to diagnosis in obstetrics and gynecology (Figs. 8-8 and 8-9; see Fig. 8-1). The reproductive organs may be evaluated by means of transabdominal, transvaginal, or transrectal approaches, as appropriate. Transvaginal and transrectal sonography enable high-resolution imaging of the uterus, adnexa, bladder, and pelvic side wall. For endometrial abnormalities,

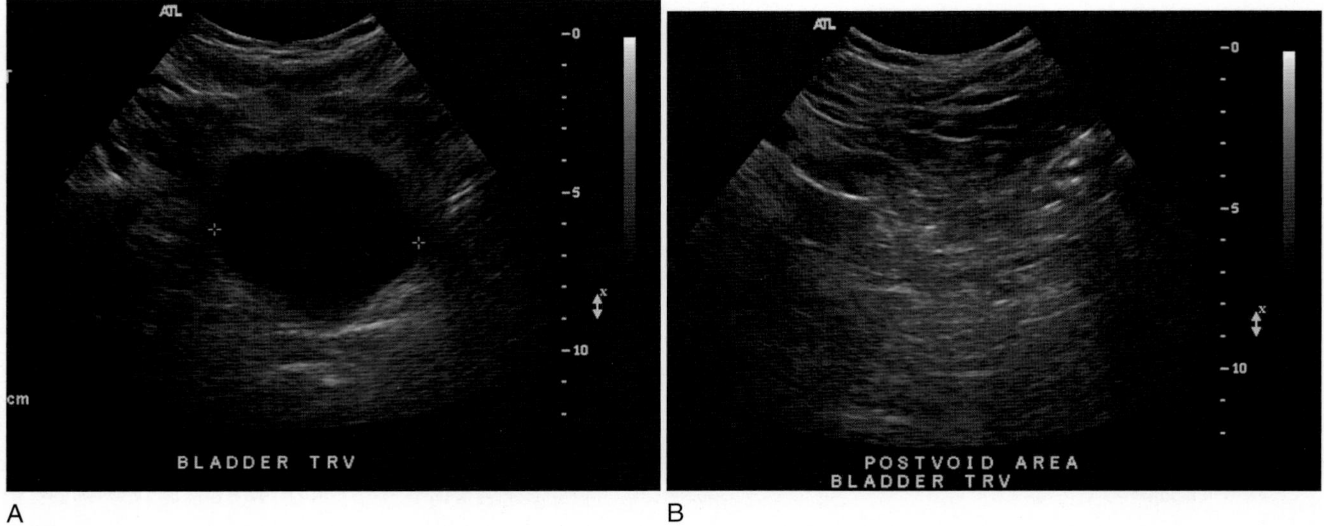

Figure 8-6 Transverse views of the bladder on ultrasound show prevoid **(A)** and postvoid **(B)** bladder volume of urine.

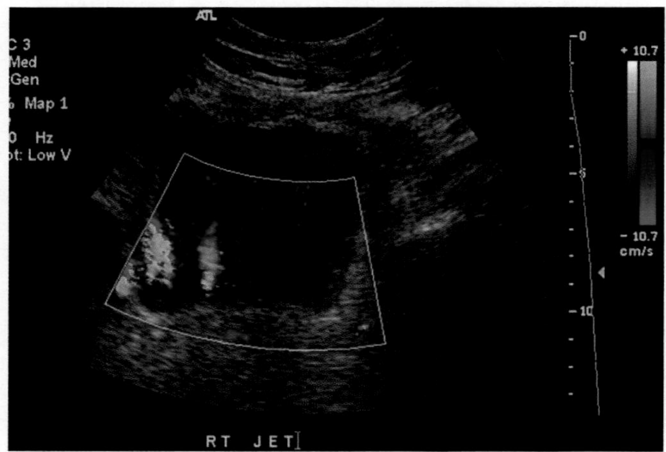

Figure 8-7 Color doppler ultrasound of the bladder shows the urinary jet, which indicating urine flow from the right ureter in the blatter.

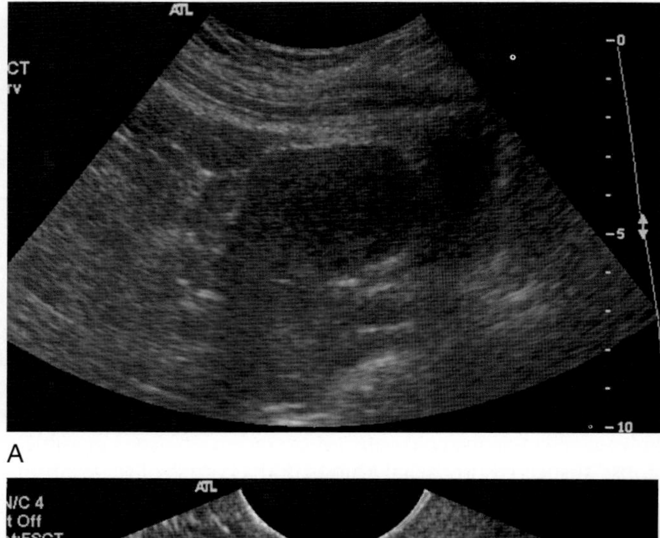

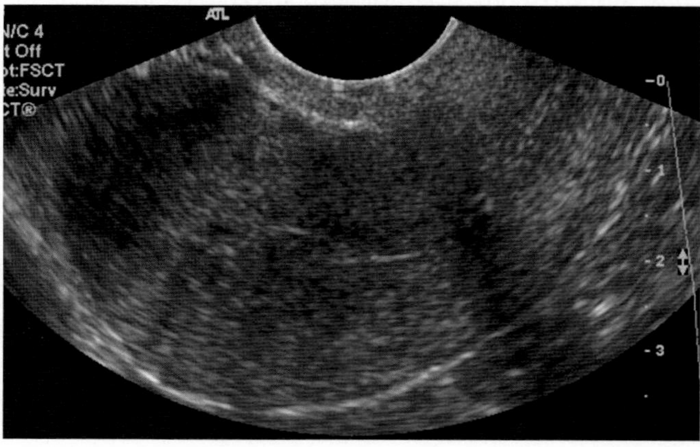

Figure 8-8 Sagittal views of the uterus in a female patient with menometrorrhagia were obtained from transabdominal **(A)** and transvaginal **(B)** approaches. In *B*, notice some endometrial displacement, which led to additional studies in this patient (see Fig. 8-9).

especially in the setting of vaginal bleeding, saline infusion hysterosonography, which involves catheterizing the endometrium and infusing saline during imaging, has become the initial test of choice in the evaluation of endometrial and subendometrial disorders such as polyps, fibroids, and cancer (see Fig. 8-9).[6,7] Endoanal ultrasonography enables high-resolution visualization of the anal sphincter muscles in patients with incontinence, as well as delineation of fistulas, abscesses, and anal malignancies.[5]

Computed Tomography

Introduction of CT revolutionalized evaluation of the retroperitoneum and disorders of the upper urinary tract, essentially replacing most indications for the intravenous urogram (see Figs. 8-2 to 8-5). Although many systems have been devised, on most CT scanners, a thin narrowly collimated beam of x-rays from a

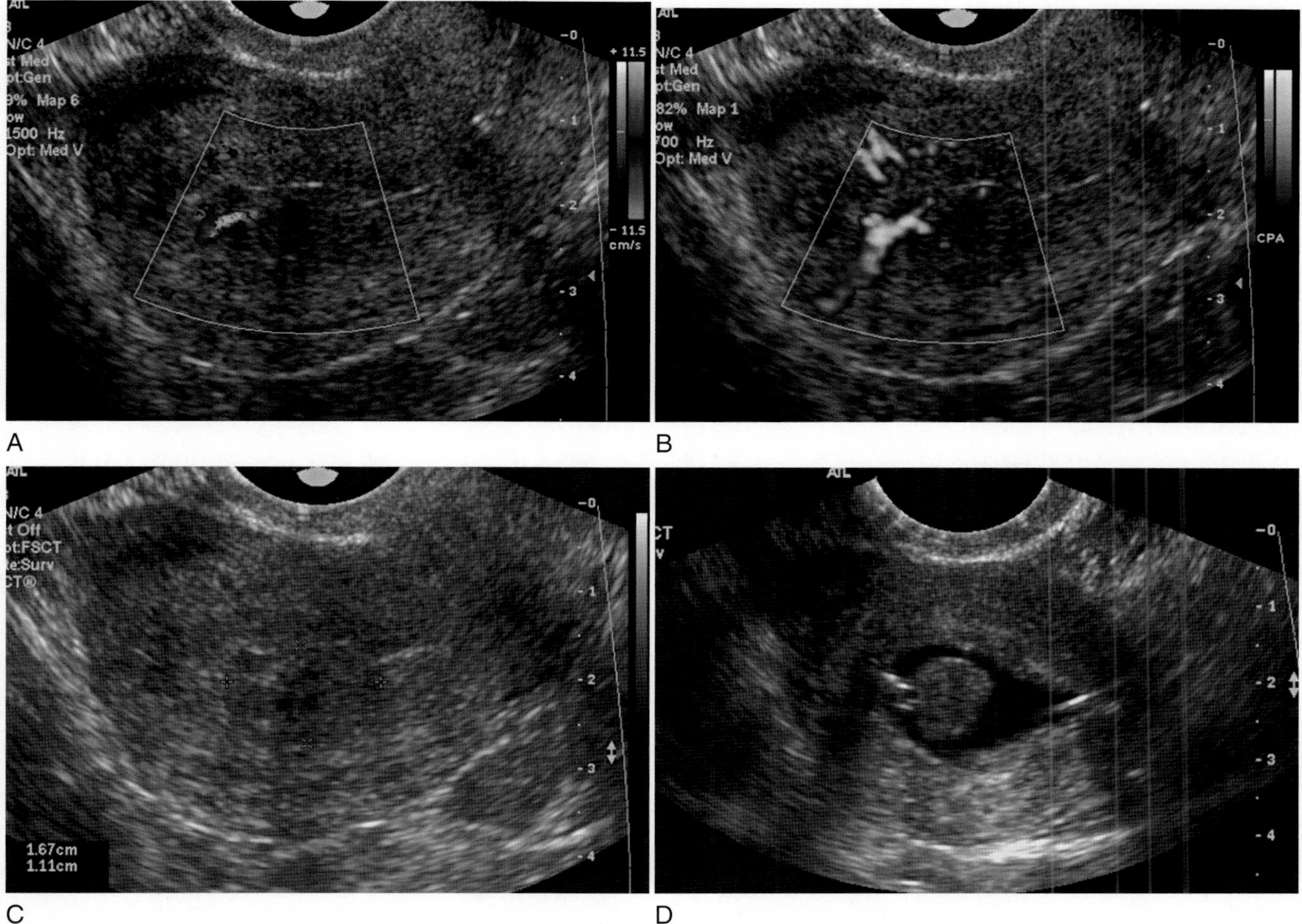

Figure 8-9 Series of transvaginal studies in a female patient presenting for a gynecologic evaluation of menometrorrhagia. Color **(A)** and power Doppler **(B)** images show a displaced endometrium with a heterogeneous structure demarcated **(C)**, which has Doppler flow to it. After infusion of saline **(D)**, an intracavitary solid mass can be seen protruding into the endometrial cavity. The mass was shown to be a submucosal myoma during surgery.

generator rotates around a patient's body on a ring in a continuous circular arc. A panel of electronic x-ray detectors lies directly opposite the x-ray tube on the ring and converts the x-ray beams exiting the patient's body into electronic signals, which are converted by a computer to display the density of each point (i.e., voxel) of the region being scanned, eventually generating a cross-sectional image. Helical multidetector CT (MDCT) scanners are configured to scan a volume of the body continuously. With MDCT, the principal advantages compared with conventional "step and shoot" CT are rapid, near-isotropic voxel ($x = y = z$) data acquisition with greater radiation dose efficiency. With isotropic voxels and sophisticated software, multiplanar and 3D imaging has become routine. Many postprocessing techniques exist, and two of the most useful are known as multiplanar reformation (MPR) and volume rendering (VR). These display techniques that are especially important for determining renal vascular anatomy, determining the relation of tumors to collecting system and vessels, and detecting fine filling defects on excretory CT urography. In the realm of female uroradiology, CT has become a well-established imaging modality for conditions such as congenital anomalies, tumors, acute and chronic inflammatory diseases, and abscesses.

Magnetic Resonance Imaging

MRI provides unparalleled tissue contrast and multiplanar, high-resolution imaging of urologic and pelvic floor structures without ionizing radiation. With MRI, a variety of tissues, such as muscle, fat, fluid, blood, blood vessels, and bone marrow, may be delineated with exceptional clarity (Figs. 8-10 to 8-12).[8] In MRI, the water protons in the human body are magnetized by a main magnetic field ranging between 1 and 3 Tesla. Using a variety of supplemental magnetic fields, a region of interest may be selected, and based on subtle magnetic field perturbations of water protons and their various relaxation times, diagnostic images are obtained. Tissues such as fat and fluid are differentiated based on their different relaxation properties by a variety of excitation algorithms known as MR sequences. One of the most useful in urology and pelvic floor imaging is the half-Fourier acquisition turbo spin-echo (HASTE) or single-shot fast spin-echo (SSFSE) T2-weighted sequence. This is a rapid, cost-effective, and noninvasive sequence that allows a multiplanar survey of the entire abdomen and pelvis within less than 1 minute. It may also be used to provide a dynamic study of the pelvic floor during relaxation and straining, providing superb anatomic detail survey of

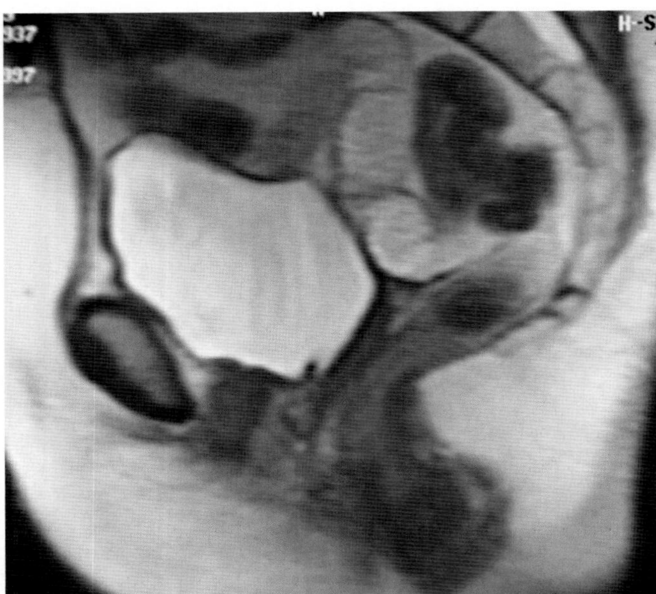

Figure 8-10 Sagittal magnetic resonance image shows the detailed anatomy of a post-hysterectomy patient.

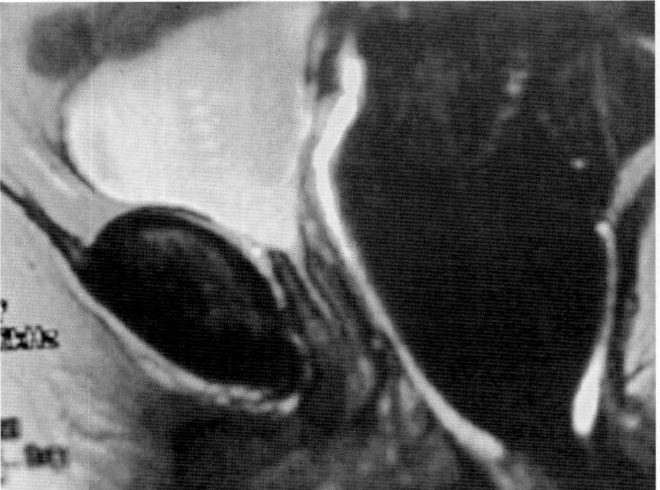

Figure 8-11 Vaginal coil magnetic resonance imaging provides a detailed view of the urethral mucosa.

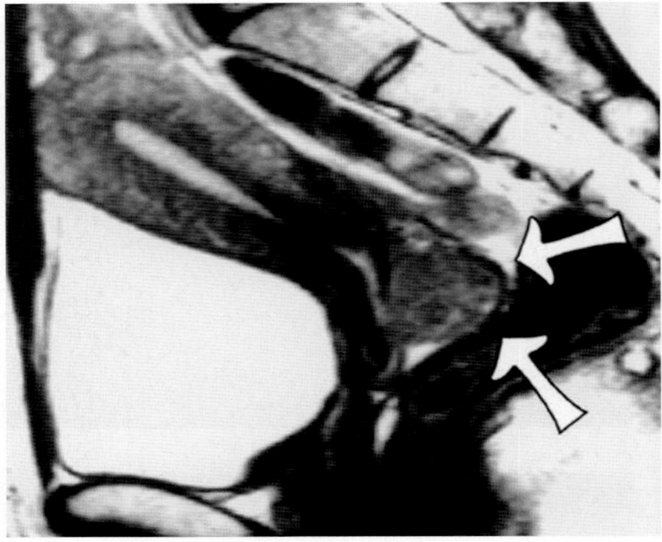

A

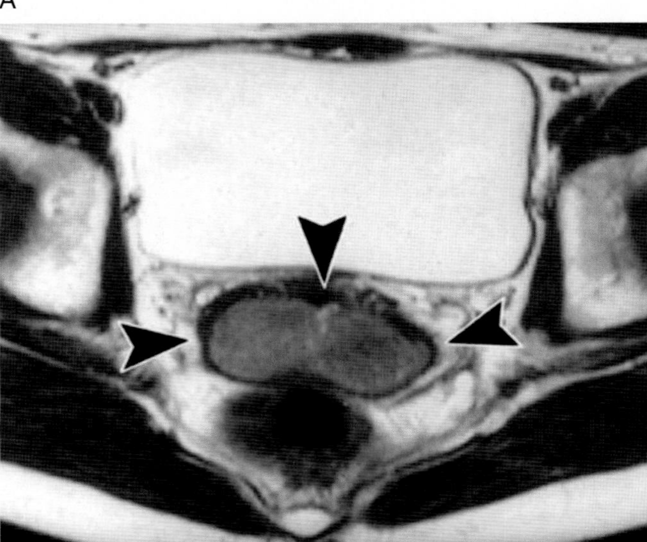

B

Figure 8-12 Magnetic resonance imaging used in staging cervical cancer. The tumor is shown to protrude into the vaginal fornix (**A,** *arrows*) with its walls clearly intact (**B,** *arrowheads*).

the extent of suspected pelvic floor relaxation and pelvic organ prolapse. It is very likely that it will replace ultrasound for evaluating women, even those with pelvic pain.[9]

Like CT, MRI may be performed with the use of contrast agents; gadolinium-diethylenetriamine penta-acetic acid (Gd-DTPA), which is a water-soluble, inert agent excreted primarily through the kidneys. Advantages compared with iodinated agents include a much lower incidence of dose-related and idiosyncratic reactions. T1-weighted, gradient-echo MR sequences in combination with a small dose of gadolinium contrast enables a comprehensive evaluation of the kidneys and ureters, similar to CT and CT urography, without ionizing radiation or iodinated contrast risk. T2-weighted sequences enable differentiation of cysts, tumors, and normal tissue parenchyma.

In patients with hydronephrosis, use of the HASTE T2-weighted sequence enables acquisition of the collecting system, including the calyces, pelvis, and ureters. MRI with T1- and T2-weighted sequences can be used for urinary tract disorders in pregnant patients without any radiation exposure risk to the fetus.[10] Endoanal MRI is an invaluable method for assessing the integrity of the anal sphincter components in patients with incontinence.

CLINICAL APPLICATIONS

Bladder Imaging

MDCT and MRI have enabled more sophisticated, noninvasive bladder imaging primarily because of their unparalleled resolution and multiplanar display (Figs. 8-13 to 8-15). Both methods

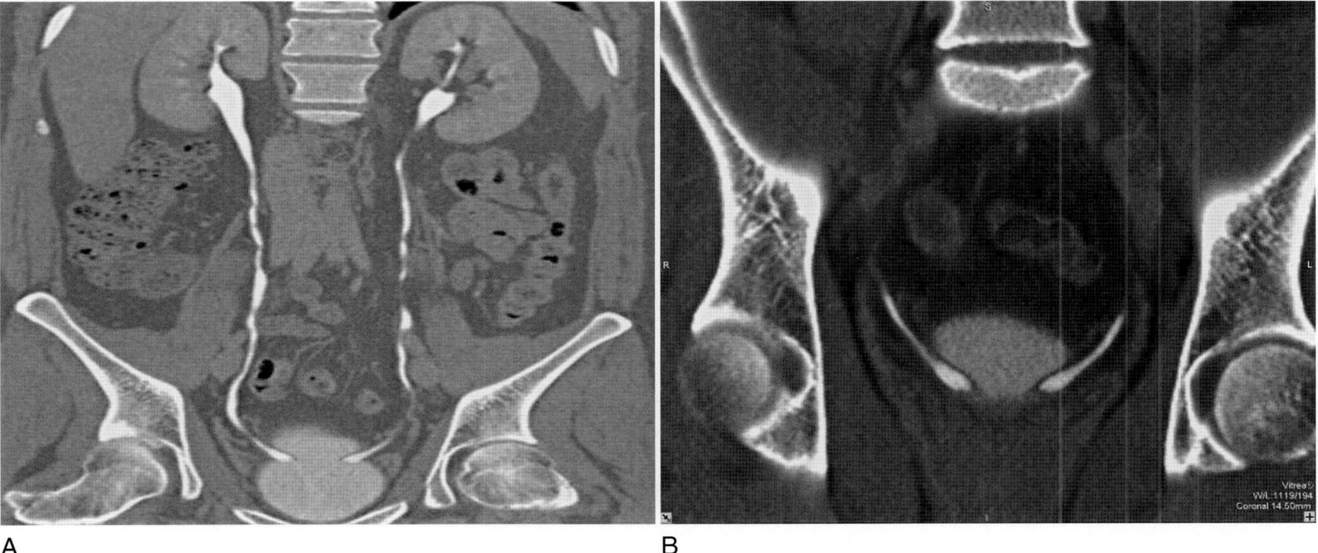

Figure 8-13 Coronal virtually rendered images of bilateral, simple ureteroceles obtained with multidetector computed tomography show bilateral, mild intramural dilation at the opening into the urinary bladder filled with contrast medium **(A).** Radiolucent layers of adjacent mucosa and contrast-filled surrounding bladder resemble a cobra head **(B).**

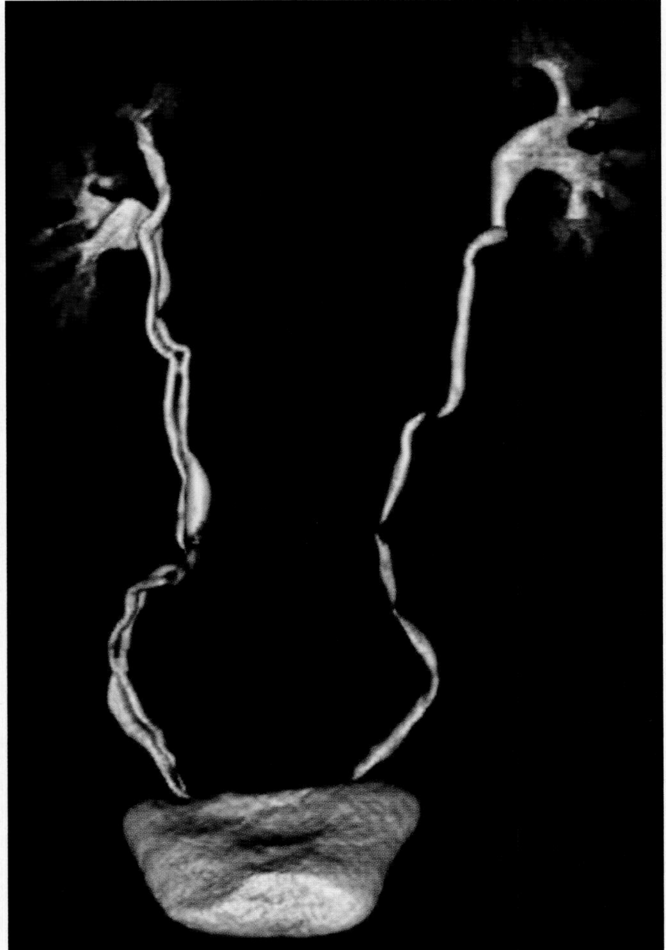

Figure 8-14 A coronal virtually rendered image obtained with multidetector computed tomography shows a double collecting system on the right.

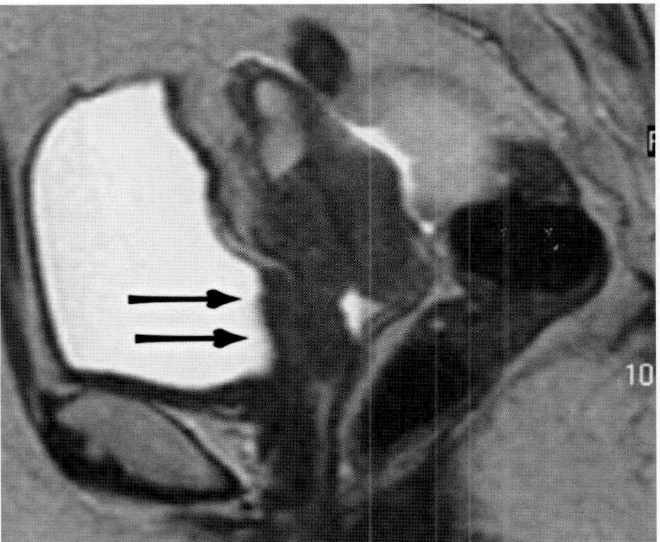

Figure 8-15 A sagittal magnetic resonance image shows cervical carcinoma in the lower third of the vagina invading the bladder *(arrows).*

can easily detect bladder filling defects, demonstrate bladder-related fistulas, and determine the extent of extravesicular tumor invasion. Based on the isotropic MR or CT 3D data sets, a virtual cystogram, similar to more clinically accepted virtual colonoscopy techniques, can be performed. Using 2D and 3D methods, CT and MRI have shown very high correlation with conventional cystoscopy in the detection of bladder lesions that are 0.5 cm or larger. Although CT and MRI are limited in detecting small and intramuscular lesions of the muscle layer of the bladder, contrast-enhanced techniques may help improve this approach. However, in cases of invasive neoplasms, MRI has been shown to be superior to transvesical ultrasound, clinical staging, and CT.[11,12]

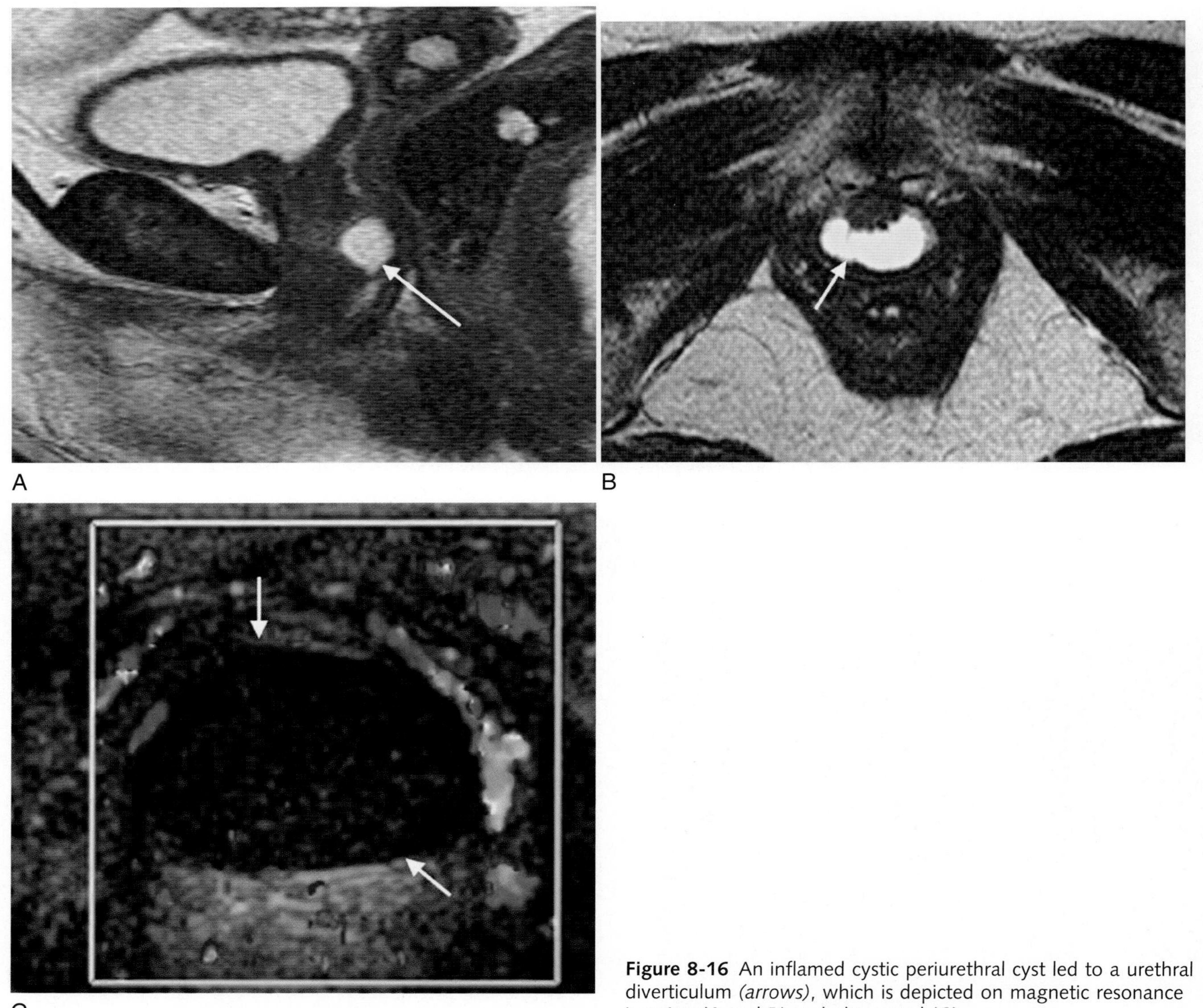

Figure 8-16 An inflamed cystic periurethral cyst led to a urethral diverticulum *(arrows)*, which is depicted on magnetic resonance imaging **(A** and **B)** and ultrasound **(C)**.

Although intraluminal ultrasound has been reported as an imaging technique for staging of bladder neoplasms, this application is limited to a handful of medical centers in the country and has not gained widespread acceptance.[4]

MRI can be used for dynamic imaging studies of the pelvic floor, enabling assessment of pelvic floor musculature and organs during relaxation phases and Valsalva maneuvers. MRI produces superb soft tissue detail without radiation or contrast exposure to help triage patients with a range of difficult-to-manage problems such as pelvic floor disorders and urinary and rectal incontinence. In the daily practice of uroradiology, ultrasonography has remained a rather useful modality in the determination of the postvoid residual urine volume and for characterizing the size and location of bladder diverticula, neoplasms, and radiolucent calculi.[4]

Urethral Imaging: Urethral Diverticula

Traditionally, VCUG has been the imaging study of choice for urethral diverticula. However, some investigators have shown that high-resolution, fast spin-echo MRI has a higher sensitivity for detecting such diverticula and a higher negative predictive rate than double-balloon urethrography. Other experts in the field believe that a combination of VCUG and MRI leads to a more accurate diagnosis and localization of the lesion (Fig. 8-16).[13]

Vaginal Imaging: Benign Cystic Lesions

Benign cystic lesions of the vagina are a relatively common finding in female urologic practice and represent a spectrum of abnormalities ranging from an asymptomatic small finding to a cyst large enough to cause incontinence or urinary obstruction. They can originate in the vagina or the urethra and the surrounding tissues. Some of the more common examples of vaginal lesions are müllerian cysts, epidermal inclusion cysts, Gartner's duct cysts, Bartholin's gland cysts, and endometriotic-type cysts (Figs. 8-17 and 8-18).[14]

In addition to a careful physical examination, an imaging study is warranted to characterize lesions. Overall, the most

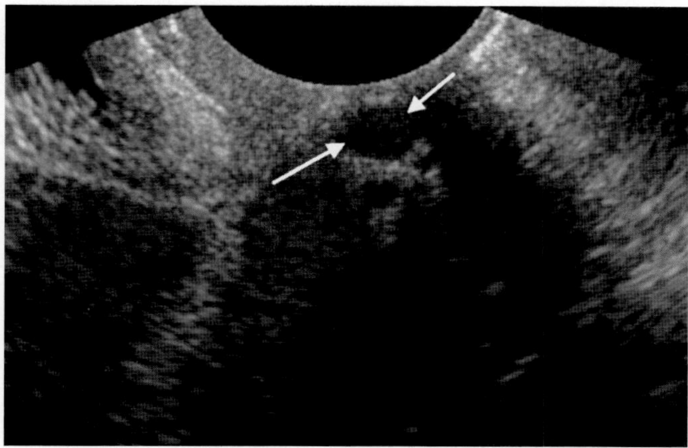

A

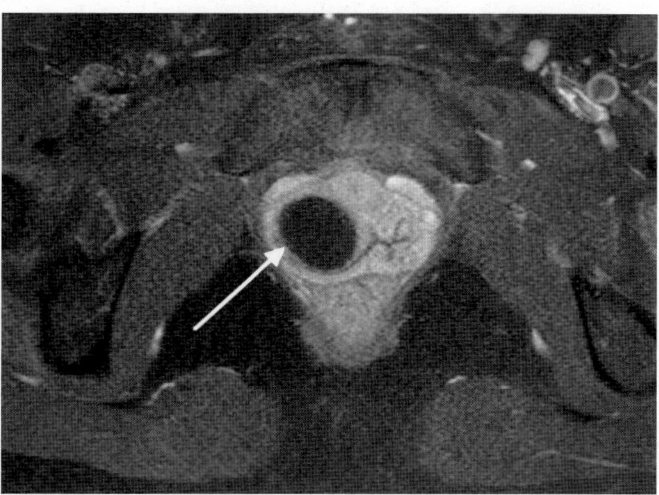

B

Figure 8-17 A Gartner's duct is depicted on ultrasound (**A,** *arrows*) and magnetic resonance (MR) imaging (**B,** *arrow*). Notice the usual anterolateral paravaginal location, with the cyst typically bright on T1-weighted and dark on T2-weighted MR sequences.

useful imaging modalities are sonography and MRI, although CT and VCUG may be useful on occasion.[15] For instance, when evaluating a Skene duct cyst, it must be differentiated from a urethral diverticulum to assist in proper surgical planning, potentially preventing complications such as urethrovaginal fistulas. Pelvic MRI is useful for this purpose, because it enables the clinician to determine whether there is a communication between the lesion and the urethra, leading to the correct diagnosis.[15] Ultrasound, CT, or MRI can be used to detect a Bartholin duct cyst.

Uterine Imaging

Transvaginal and transabdominal sonography are the most widely used imaging modalities for the detection and characterization of a wide variety of uterine anomalies and pathologies. Common indications include evaluation of congenital uterine anomalies; assessment of uterine leiomyomas in women with related symptoms such as pelvic pain, pressure, or heavy bleeding; and assessment of the endometrium. Hysterosonography, which involves instilling saline during continuous endovaginal sonographic uterine imaging, is particularly useful for detecting endometrial polyps, tumors, and leiomyomas.[16,17] However, over the past few years, MRI has emerged as the definitive imaging modality for evaluation of uterine disorders. MRI enables evaluation of the uterine zonal anatomy with clear T2-weighted signal differences between endometrium (i.e., bright), junctional zone (i.e., dark), and myometrium (i.e., intermediate). If the appropriate views are acquired, a variety of congenital fusion anomalies, such as septate uterus and bicornuate uterus with obstructed horns, can be demonstrated.[18] Associated anomalies of the kidneys are also easily demonstrated. MRI is considered to be the best noninvasive method of assessment for women with symptoms related to uterine leiomyomas and adenomyosis (Fig. 8-19 and Fig. 8-20). MRI is the best modality to determine the vascular supply of pelvic vascular malformations and has been shown to be highly accurate in local staging of endometrial and cervical cancer.

MR angiography is performed with MRI to assess the arterial supply and venous drainage to the uterus. It is especially useful in delineating the collateral supply through the gonadal arterial branches.

Endometriosis Imaging

Laparoscopy has traditionally been the gold standard for diagnosis of endometriosis, which most commonly manifests as small implants with or without related adhesions on the parametrial surfaces, uterosacral ligament, ovaries, serosal surface of the uterus, and the cul-de-sac. Because laparoscopy is an invasive technique and visual inspection of the pelvis has limitations, especially in the diagnosis of retroperitoneal implants, major efforts are being made in the field of female urogynecology to improve the diagnostic utility of current noninvasive imaging modalities. Transvaginal ultrasonography and contrast-enhanced MRI have been used for noninvasive diagnosis and clinical follow-up of patients with endometriosis (Fig. 8-21; see Fig. 8-1). They allow imaging of the retroperitoneal space for determining the presence and characterization of deep pelvic endometriosis and bowel involvement.[19,20]

Although patients with endometriosis more commonly present to their gynecologists, these ectopic endometrial implants can create urinary symptoms due to direct bladder involvement or deep pelvic involvement causing ureteral obstruction. These patients therefore often present to urologists for clinical and radiographic evaluation. Bladder endometriosis, which is not easily palpable on vaginal examination, may mimic interstitial cystitis and interfere with bladder function.[21,22] In experienced hands, transvaginal ultrasonography performed on a slightly filled bladder can detect solid nodules (>0.5 cm) within the posterior bladder wall that cause urinary symptoms in these patients with dysmenorrhea. The presence of low to moderate vascularity demonstrated by color Doppler signal within these nodules and focal pain precipitated by mild pressure applied with the vaginal probe in the involved area helps confirm the diagnosis when suspected.[19,20] Nodules in the cul-de-sac may be biopsied transvaginally or percutaneously for confirmation. A high-resolution, contrast-enhanced MR scan of the pelvis at a field strength of 1.5 or 3 Tesla may help diagnose large, focal implants or confluent, small implants on the peritoneal surfaces by the findings of a concomitant thickened peritoneum and enhancement.

Adnexal Imaging

A comprehensive examination of the female pelvis mandates evaluation of the adnexa for determining the ovarian volume,

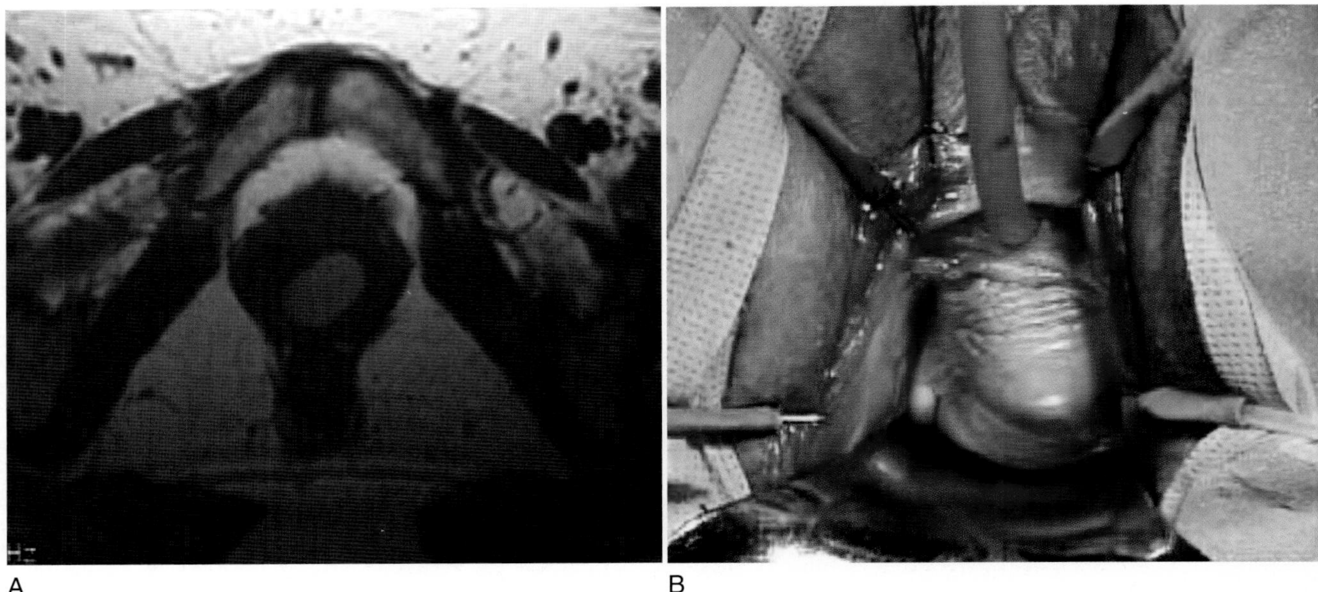

Figure 8-18 An inclusion cyst is shown first on a magnetic resonance image **(A)** and then in the operating room **(B)**.

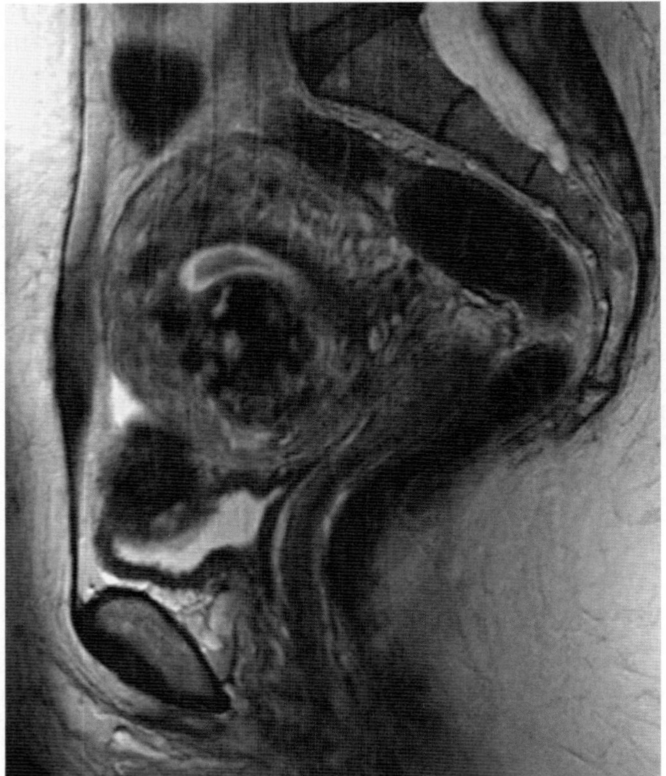

Figure 8-19 Leiomyomas are appreciated on a sagittal magnetic resonance image.

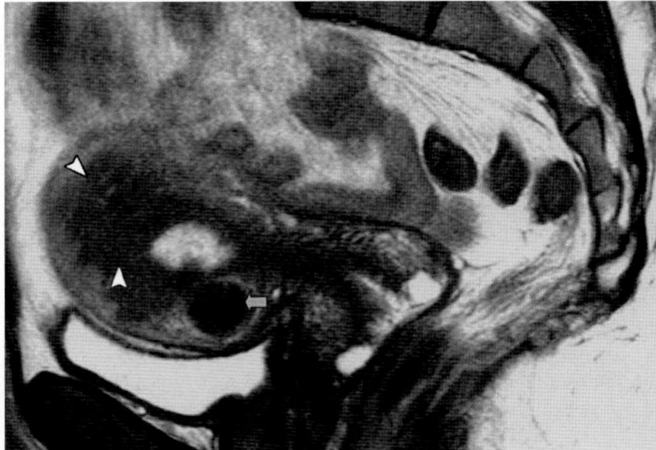

Figure 8-20 Focal adenomyoma *(arrowheads)* and leiomyoma *(arrow)* are present on the same sagittal T2 Haste magnetic resonance image.

assessing blood flow, and detecting and characterizing masses, especially in any evaluation of pelvic pain and other genitourinary symptoms. Functional ovarian disorders such as polycystic ovary syndrome also may be detected with limited sensitivity. In premenopausal women, ovarian ultrasonography has been the primary imaging modality for benign and pathologic adnexal entities. However, MRI has become an invaluable addition in this field because of its superb soft tissue characterization, contrast resolution, and multiplanar capabilities. MRI enables the imager to determine with certainty whether a given mass is ovarian or extraovarian, which is an important distinction in evaluating the malignant potential of a tumor. It also plays an essential role in characterizing benign adnexal diseases such as mature teratomas, endometriomas, and ovarian fibromas because of their specific MR features (Fig. 8-22). For instance, MRI can delineate the internal architecture of cystic masses, such as thick internal septations and enhancing mural nodularity, especially after administration of Gd-DTPA-based contrast.[8]

Pelvic Inflammatory Disease Imaging

Most ovarian infections in the Western world result from pelvic inflammatory disease of bacterial origin. They classically manifest

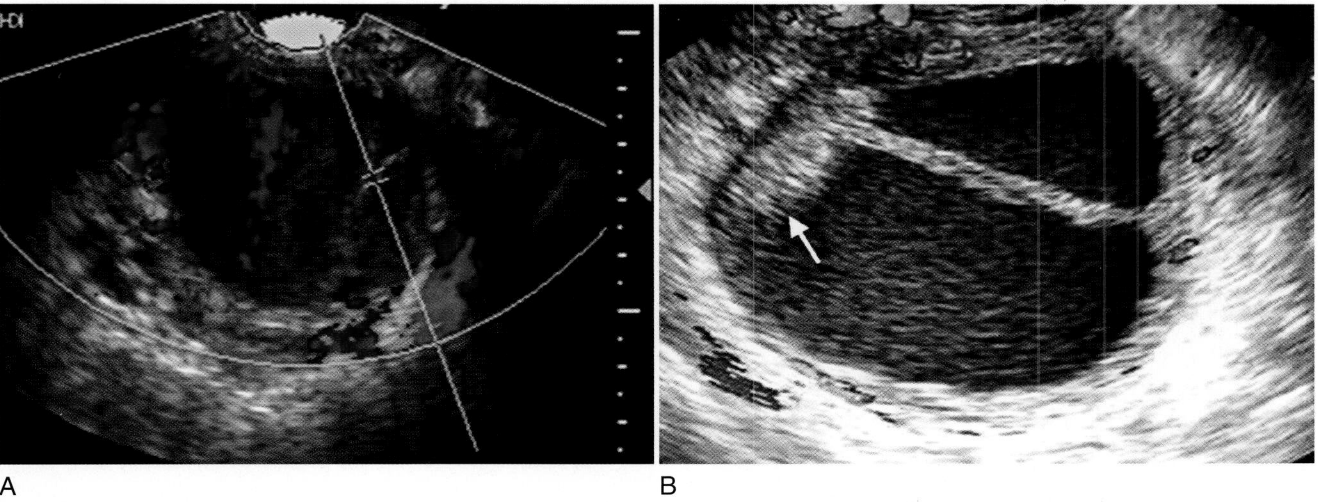

Figure 8-21 Endometriosis is appreciated on ultrasound (**A** and **B**, *arrow*), which classically manifests as a cystic mass with diffuse, low-level echoes. Notice the septations, fluid-fluid levels, unilocularity or multilocularity, and an echogenic retracting clot.

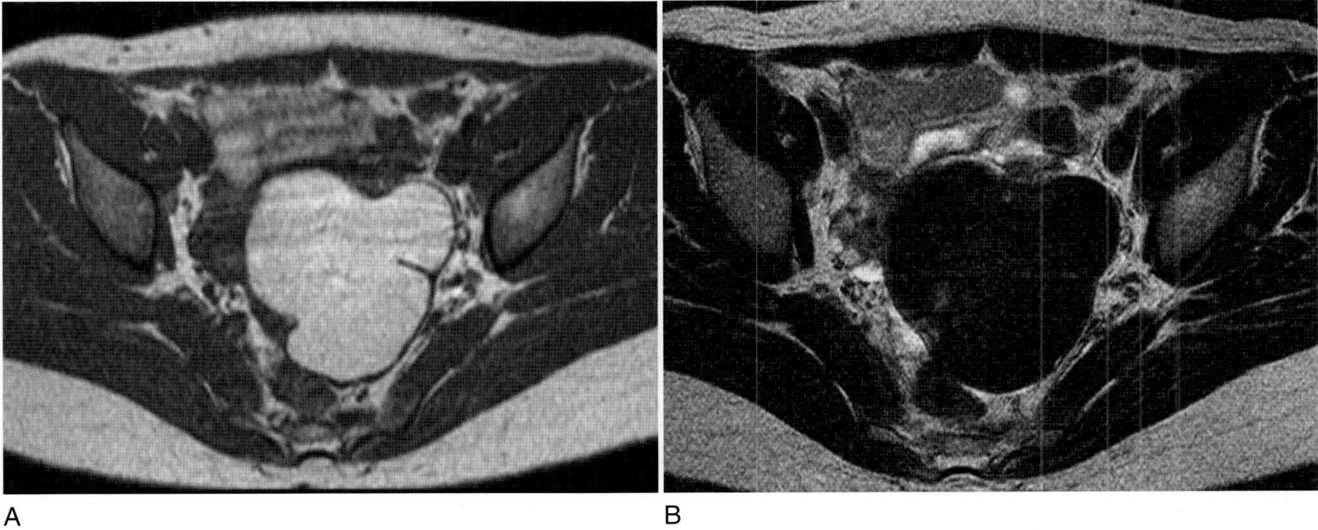

Figure 8-22 Endometrioma is appreciated on magnetic resonance imaging with T1-weighted **(A)** and T2-weighted **(B)** sequences. Notice characteristic high T1 and low T2 appearances, caused by high protein and iron content from recurrent bleeding and grading within the lesion.

with abdominal pain, fever, and an elevated white blood cell count. Some patients may present with vaginal discharge and urinary complaints. Involvement of the ovaries in this process usually results from salpingitis. In cases of delayed diagnosis and inadequate treatment, disease can progress to cause a tubo-ovarian abscess (TOA) (Fig. 8-23). In up to 20% of cases of infection that result in TOAs, the patients are afebrile and have normal white blood cell counts.[23]

The gold standard for the diagnosis of pelvic inflammatory disease is laparoscopy and tubal culture; the sensitivity and specificity of transvaginal ultrasound has not been reported in the literature.[23] Sonography is relied on heavily in the initial evaluation of a patient, because it can show pelvic and endometrial fluid in addition to other characteristic findings. Pyosalpinx and hydrosalpinx appear as cystic structures, with internal echoes resulting in adnexal distortion.[24] A TOA usually appears as a well-defined, thick-walled, tubular structure, containing fluid-debris levels within the abscess. Most clinicians advocate a follow-up CT scan of the abdomen and pelvis to fully characterize any other intra-abdominal collections to prepare for a subsequent drainage procedure, especially when the abscesses do not respond to an antimicrobial treatment.[25]

When the clinical and ultrasonographic findings are questionable, MRI can play an important role (see Fig. 8-23). Pyosalpinx typically appears as a fluid-filled, tortuous, and dilated structure, and the signal intensity of the fluid depends on its viscosity and protein concentration. It is usually appreciated as a hypointense area on T2-weighted sequences in the peripheral area of a hyperintense, pus-filled cavity. The adjacent inflamed structures usually have low signal intensity

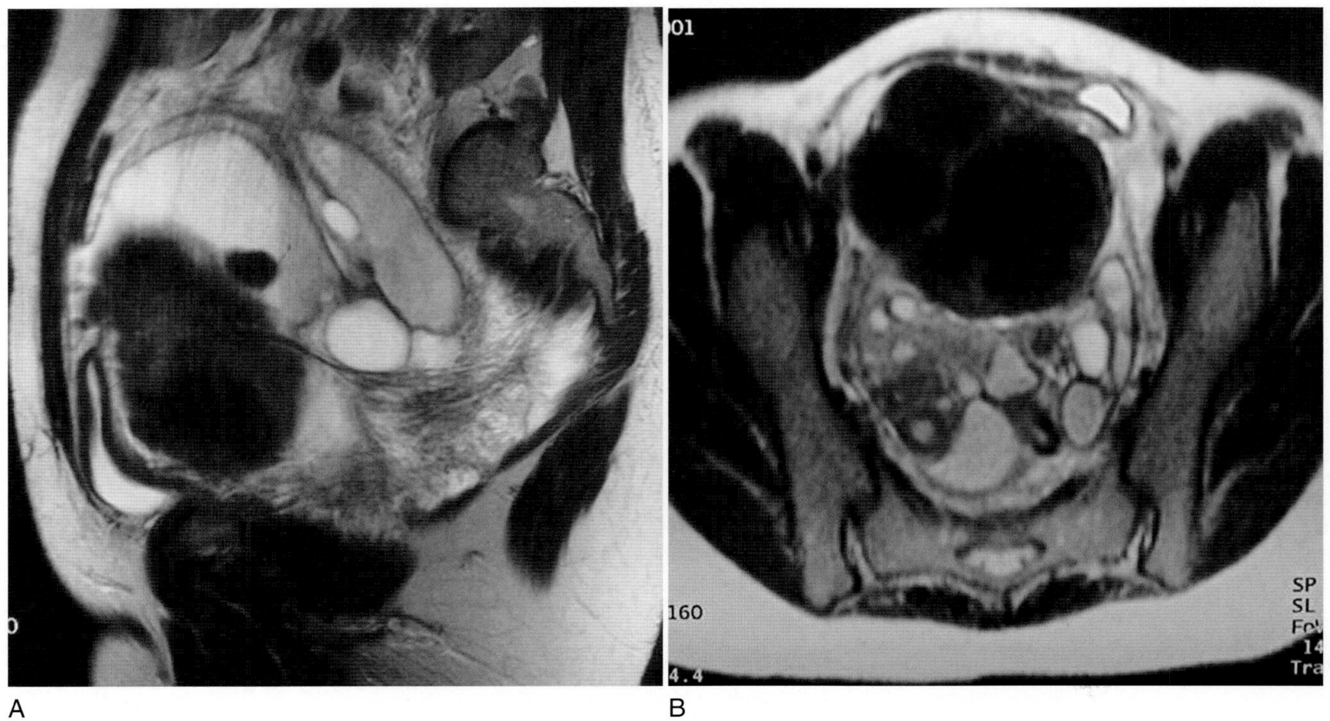

Figure 8-23 A tubo-ovarian abscess is appreciated on sagittal **(A)** and axial **(B)** magnetic resonance images in a patient who presented with fever and chills after a uterine artery embolization procedure.

on T1-weighted sequences and intermediate to high signal intensity on T2-weighted MR images. Wall enhancement and thickening usually have greater signal intensity than those observed with hydrosalpinx. The TOA is usually a thick-walled, fluid-filled mass in an adnexal location with significant wall enhancement and adjacent soft tissue inflammation characterized by similarly intense enhancement.[8] The most specific sign of an abscess is the presence of internal gas bubbles, best appreciated on T2-weighted sequences due to differences in magnetic susceptibility.[26]

References

1. Dunnick MR, Sandler CM, Newhouse JH, Amis ES: Textbook of Uroradiology, 3rd ed. Philadelphia, Lippincott Williams & Wilkins, 2001.
2. Goldman SM, Sandler CM: Genitourinary imaging: The past 40 years. Radiology 215:313-324, 2000.
3. Novelline RA: Squire's Fundamentals of Radiology, 6th ed. Cambridge, MA, Harvard University Press, 2004.
4. Marinkovic SP, Badlani GH: Imaging of the lower urinary tract in adults. J Endourol 15:75-86, 2001.
5. Weidner AC, Low VHS: Imaging studies of the pelvic floor. Obstet Gynecol Clin North Am 25:825-848, 1998.
6. Berridge DL, Winter TC: Saline infusion sonohysterography. J Ultrasound Med 23:97-112, 2004.
7. Laifer-Narin S, Ragavendra N, Parmenter EK, Grant EG: False-normal appearance of the endometrium on conventional transvaginal sonography: Comparison with saline hysterosonography. AJR Am J Roentgenol 178:129-133, 2002.
8. Sala EJS, Atri M: Magnetic resonance imaging of benign adnexal disease. Top Magn Reson Imaging 14:305-328, 2003.
9. Gousse AE, Barbaric ZL, Safir MH, et al: Dynamic half-Fourier acquisition single shot turbo spin-echo magnetic resonance imaging for evaluating the female pelvis. J Urol 164:1606-1613, 2000.
10. Nolte-Ernsting CCA, Staatz G, Tacke J, Gunther RW: MR urography today. Abdom Imaging 28:191-209, 2003.
11. Bernhardt TM, Rapp-Bernhardt U: Virtual cystoscopy of the bladder based on CT and MRI data. Abdom Imaging 26:325-332, 2001.
12. Lawler LP, Fishman EK: Bladder imaging using multidetector row computed tomography, volume rendering, and magnetic resonance imaging. J Comput Assist Tomogr 27:553-563, 2003.
13. Neitlich JD, Foster HE Jr, Glickman MG, Smith RC: Detection of urethral diverticula in women: Comparison of a high resolution fast spin echo technique with double balloon urethrography. J Urol 159:408-410, 1998.
14. Pradhan S, Tobon H: Vaginal cysts: A clinicopathological study of 41 cases. Int J Gynecol Pathol 5:35-46, 1986.
15. Eilber KS, Raz S: Benign cystic lesions of the vagina: A literature review. J Urol 170:717-722, 2003.
16. Farquhar C, Ekeroma A, Furness S, Arroll B: A systematic review of transvaginal ultrasonography, sonohysterography and hysteroscopy for the investigation of abnormal uterine bleeding in premenopausal women. Acta Obstet Gynecol Scand 82:493-504, 2003.
17. Fleischer AC: Color Doppler sonography of uterine disorders. Ultrasound Q 19:179-189, 2003.
18. Togashi K, Nakai A, Sugimura K: Anatomy and physiology of the female pelvis: MR imaging revisited. J Magn Reson Imaging 13:842-849, 2001.
19. Brosens I, Puttemans P, Campo R, et al: Non-invasive methods of diagnosis of endometriosis. Curr Opin Obstet Gynecol 15:519-522, 2003.
20. Brosens J, Timmerman D, Starzinski-Powitz A, Brosens I: Non-invasive diagnosis of endometriosis: The role of imaging and markers. Obstet Gynecol Clin North Am 30:95-114, 2003.

21. Siegelman ES, Outwater E, Wang T, Mitchell DG: Solid pelvic masses caused by endometriosis: MR imaging features. AJR Am J Roentgenol 163:357-361, 1994.
22. Sircus SI, Sant GR, Ucci AA Jr: Bladder detrusor endometriosis mimicking interstitial cystitis. Urology 32:339-342, 1988.
23. Cartwright PS: Pelvic inflammatory disease. In Beck JS (ed): Novak's Textbook of Gynecology, 11th ed. Baltimore, Williams & Wilkins, 1988.
24. Bulas DI, Ahlstrom PA, Sivit CJ, et al: Pelvic inflammatory disease in the adolescent: Comparison of transabdominal and transvaginal sonographic evaluation. Radiology 183:435-439, 1992.
25. Varghese JC, O'Neill MJ, Gervais DA, et al: Transvaginal catheter drainage of tubo-ovarian abscess using the trocar method: Technique and literature review. AJR Am J Roentgenol 177:139-144, 2001.
26. Dohke M, Watanabe Y, Okumura A, et al: Comprehensive MR imaging of acute gynecologic diseases. Radiographics 20:1551-1566, 2000.

Chapter 9

PELVIC FLOOR ULTRASOUND

Hans Peter Dietz

The increasing availability of ultrasound and magnetic resonance imaging (MRI) equipment has triggered a renewed interest in diagnostic imaging in female urology and urogynecology, after radiologic methods, developed since the 1920s,[1-6] had largely fallen into disuse. Because of cost and access problems, MRI has had limited clinical use in the evaluation of pelvic floor disorders, and until recently, slow acquisition speeds have precluded dynamic imaging. In contrast, ultrasound is almost universally available and provides real-time observation of diagnostic maneuvers. Beginning in the 1980s, transabdominal,[7,8] perineal,[9,10] transrectal,[11] and transvaginal ultrasound[12] have been investigated for use in women with urinary incontinence and pelvic organ prolapse. Because of its noninvasive nature, ready availability, and the absence of distortion, perineal or translabial ultrasound has become the most widely used method.

The development of three-dimensional (3D) ultrasound[13,14] has opened up new diagnostic possibilities. The first attempts at producing 3D-capable systems were made in the 1970s, when processing a single volume of data required 24 hours of computer time on a system that filled a small room.[15] Such data processing is now possible on a laptop computer and is achieved in real time. Transvaginal, transrectal, and translabial 3D ultrasound techniques have been reported, and significant development in this field is likely to occur in the next few years.

TWO-DIMENSIONAL PELVIC FLOOR ULTRASOUND

Basic Methodology

Because translabial ultrasound is the most commonly used modality for pelvic floor evaluation, it is the focus of this chapter. A modification of the translabial or transperineal technique is introital imaging, which typically uses high-frequency endocavitary transducers placed in the introitus. This results in higher resolution of urethra and paraurethral tissues or of the anal sphincter complex, but it does not allow simultaneous imaging of all three compartments and may complicate quantification of findings because the symphysis pubis may not be included in the field of vision. Distortion of tissues is also more likely. However, most of the following discussion also applies to this technique.

A midsagittal view is obtained by placing a transducer (usually a curved array with frequencies between 3.5 and 9 MHz) on the perineum (Fig. 9-1) after covering the transducer with a glove or thin plastic wrap for hygienic reasons. Powdered gloves can markedly impair imaging quality because of reverberations and should be avoided. Imaging can be performed with the patient in the dorsal lithotomy position, with the hips flexed and slightly abducted, or in the standing position. Bladder filling should be specified; for some applications, prior voiding is preferable, and a full bladder can prevent complete development of a prolapse. The presence of a full rectum may also impair diagnostic accuracy and sometimes necessitates a repeat assessment after bowel emptying. Parting of the labia can improve image quality, which is optimal in pregnancy and poorest in menopausal women with marked atrophy, most likely due to various levels of tissue hydration. The transducer usually can be placed quite firmly against the symphysis pubis without causing significant discomfort, unless there is marked atrophy. The resulting image includes the symphysis pubis (specifically, the interpubic disk) anteriorly, the urethra and bladder neck, the vagina, cervix, rectum, and anal canal (see Fig. 9-1) with the internal and external anal sphincter. Posterior to the anorectal junction, a hyperechogenic area indicates the central portion of the levator plate, the puborectalis-pubococcygeus (or pubovisceral) muscle. The cul-de-sac may also be seen as filled with a small amount of fluid, echogenic fat, or peristalsing small bowel. Parasagittal or transverse views may yield additional information, such as enabling assessment of the puborectalis muscle and its insertion on the on the pelvic sidewall and imaging of transobturator implants.

There has been disagreement regarding image orientation in the midsagittal plane. Some clinicians prefer orientation as in the standing patient facing right,[16] which requires image inversion on the ultrasound system, a facility that is not universally available. Others (including me) prefer an orientation as on conventional transvaginal ultrasound (i.e., cranioventral aspects to the left, dorsocaudal to the right). The latter orientation seems more convenient when using 3D or 4D systems because it automatically results in rendered volumes that are oriented as on conventional MRI of the pelvic floor (discussed later). Because

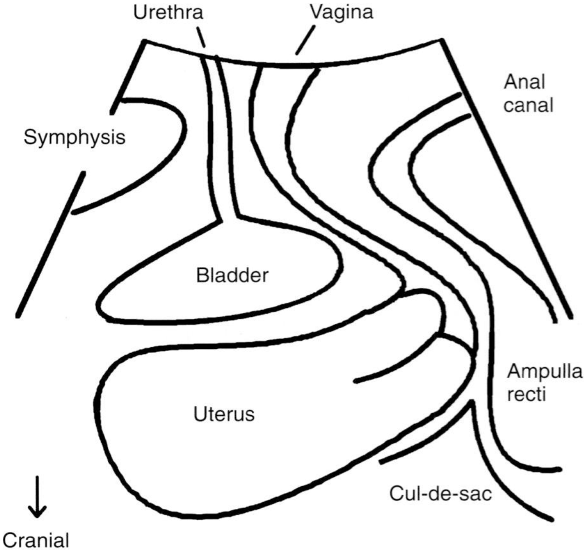

Figure 9-1 Drawing of the field of vision for translabial or perineal ultrasound in the midsagittal plane. Image adapted from Ultrasound Obstet Gynecol 2004; 23:80-92, with permission.

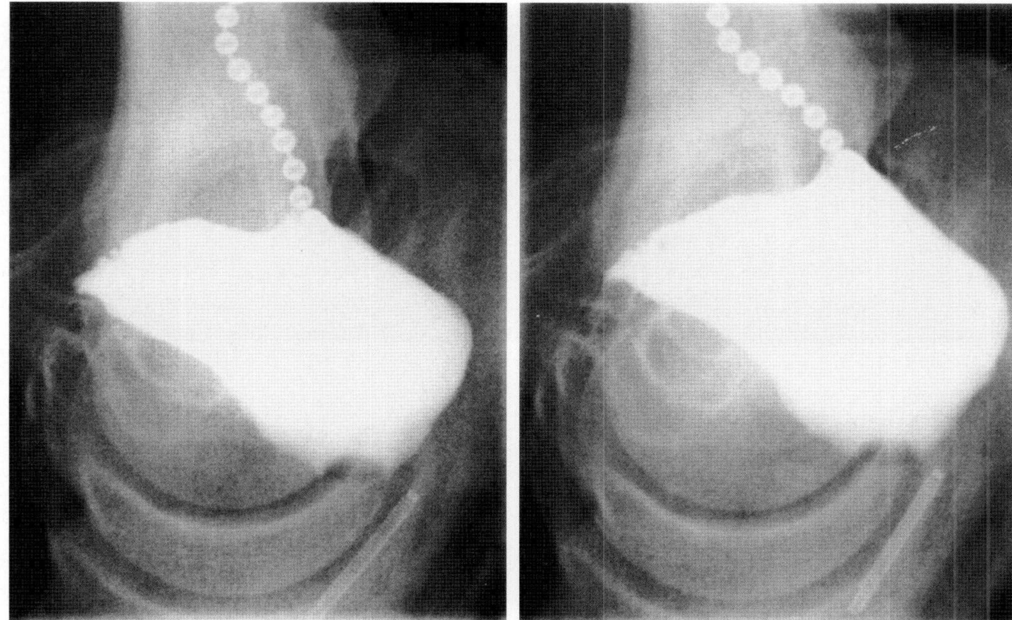

Figure 9-2 Lateral urethrocystogram with a bead chain outlining the urethra. The images are rotated by 180 degrees to allow comparison with standard translabial ultrasound views. The image on the *left* was obtained with the patient at rest; the image on the *right* was obtained during a Valsalva maneuver. Reproduced from Ultrasound Obstet Gynecol 2004; 23:80-92, with permission.

any image reproduced in one of these orientations can be converted to the other by rotation through 180 degrees, formal standardization may be unnecessary. Orientations that require mirroring for conversion should be avoided.

Translabial ultrasound of the lower urinary tract, even if limited to B-mode imaging in the midsagittal plane, yields information equivalent or superior to the lateral urethrocystogram (Fig. 9-2, shown rotated by 180 degrees for comparison) or fluoroscopic imaging. Comparative studies have mostly shown good correlation between radiologic and ultrasound data.[11,17-22] The one remaining advantage of x-ray fluoroscopy may be the ease with which the voiding phase can be observed, although some investigators have used specially constructed equipment to document voiding with ultrasound.[23]

Bladder Neck Position and Mobility

Bladder neck position and mobility can be assessed with a high degree of reliability. Points of reference are the central axis of the symphysis pubis[24] or its inferoposterior margin.[17] The former may be more accurate because measurements are independent of transducer position or movement; however, because of calcification of the interpubic disk, the central axis is often difficult to obtain in older women, reducing reliability. Imaging can be undertaken with the patient supine or erect and with a full or empty bladder. The full bladder is less mobile[25] and may prevent complete development of pelvic organ prolapse. In the standing position, the bladder is situated lower at rest but descends about as far as in the supine patient during a Valsalva maneuver.[26] Either way, it is essential to not exert undue pressure on the perineum to allow full development of pelvic organ descent, although this may be difficult in women with severe prolapse, such as vaginal eversion or procidentia.

Measurements of bladder neck position are generally performed at rest and during maximal Valsalva maneuver. The difference yields a numeric value for bladder neck descent. During a Valsalva maneuver, the proximal urethra may rotate in a posteroinferior direction. The extent of rotation can be measured by comparing the angle of inclination between the proximal urethra and any other fixed axis (Fig. 9-3). Some investigators measure the retrovesical (or posterior urethrovesical) angle between proximal urethra and trigone (see Fig. 9-3).[27] Others determine the angle γ between the central axis of the symphysis pubis and a line from the inferior symphyseal margin to the bladder neck.[28,29] Of all the ultrasound parameters of hypermobility, bladder neck descent may have the strongest association with urodynamic stress incontinence.[30] The reproducibility of this dynamic measurement has been assessed,[31] with a percent variation or coefficient of variation of 0.16 between multiple effective Valsalva maneuvers, 0.21 for interobserver variability, and 0.219 for a test-retest series at an average interval of 46 days. Intraclass correlations were between 0.75 and 0.98, indicating excellent agreement.[31]

There is no definition of *normal* for bladder neck descent, although cutoffs of 20 and 25 mm have been proposed to define hypermobility. Average measurements in stress-incontinent women are consistently around 30 mm (HP Dietz, unpublished data). Figure 9-4 shows a relatively immobile bladder neck before a first delivery and a marked increase in bladder neck mobility after childbirth. Figure 9-5 demonstrates typical ultrasound findings in a stress-incontinent patient with a first-degree cystourethrocele, 25.5 mm of bladder neck descent, and funneling. Bladder filling, patient position, and catheterization influence measurements,[25,26,32,33] and it sometimes is difficult to obtain an effective Valsalva maneuver, especially in nulliparous women. Perhaps not surprisingly, publications have presented widely different reference measurements in nulliparous women. Although two series documented mean or median bladder neck descent of only 5.1 mm[34] and 5.3 mm[35] in continent, nulliparous women, another study of 39 continent, nulliparous volunteers measured

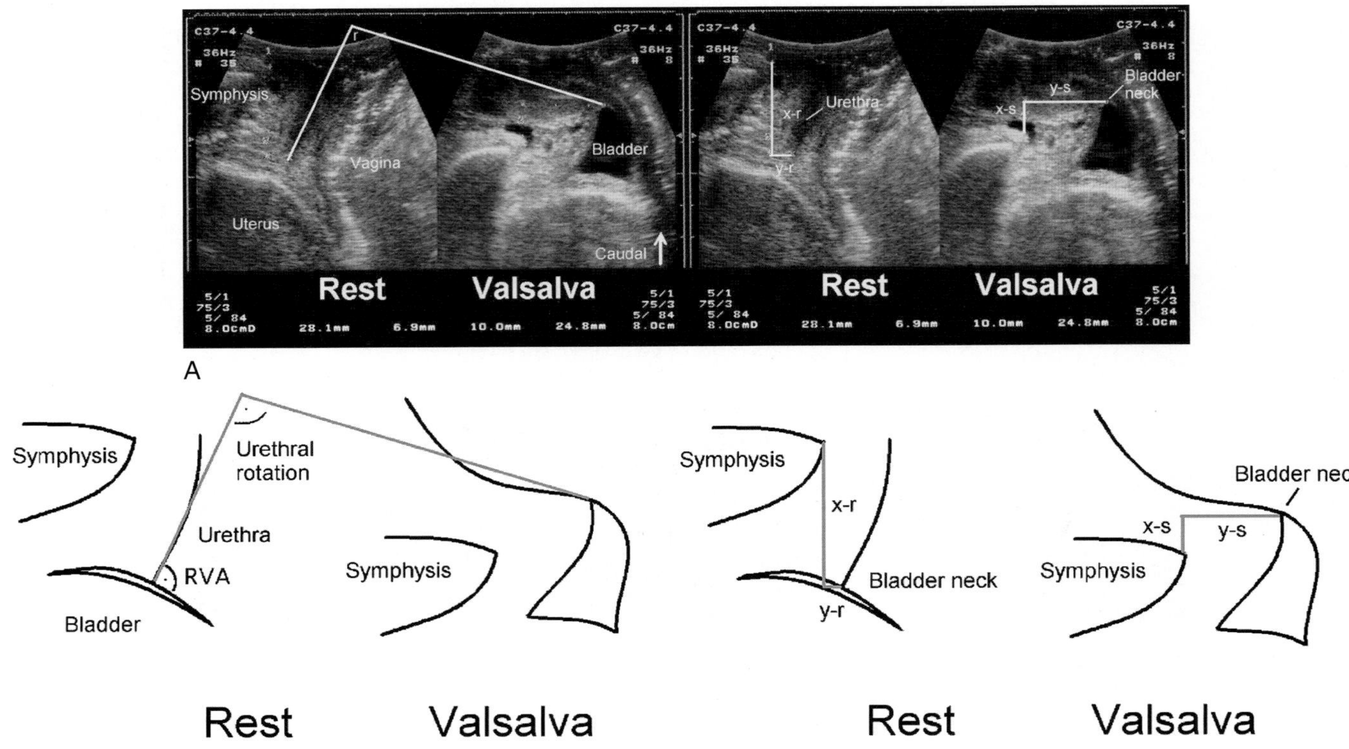

Figure 9-3 The ultrasound image **(A)** and line drawing **(B)** illustrate some of the parameters measured to quantify bladder and urethral mobility: the location of the bladder neck relative to the symphysis pubis (coordinates x-r, y-r, x-s, y-s), urethral rotation and retrovesical angle (RVA). This figure is reproduced from Br J Obstet Gynecol 2005; 112:334-339, with permission.

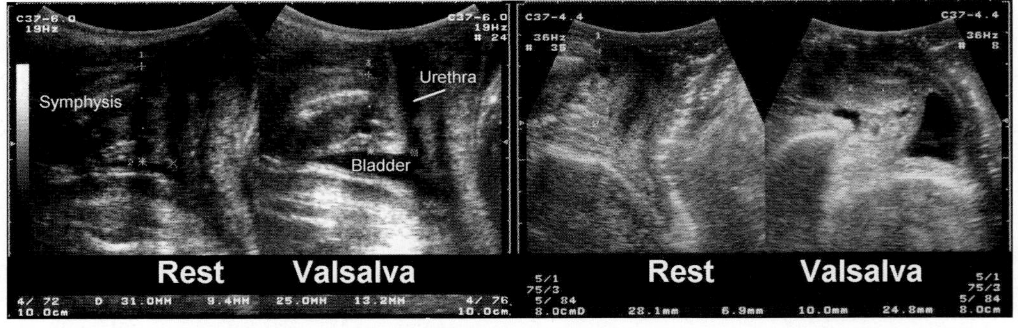

Figure 9-4 Immobile bladder neck (bladder neck distance [BND] = 6 mm) before childbirth *(left pair of images)* and a marked increase in bladder neck mobility (BND = 38.1 mm) after vaginal delivery *(right pair of images)*. The figure is reproduced from Obstet Gynecol 2003; 102:223-228, with permission.

an average bladder neck descent of 15 mm.[36] The author has obtained bladder neck descent measurements of 1.2 to 40.2 mm (mean, 17.3 mm) in a group of 106 stress-continent, nulligravid women between the ages of 18 and 23 years.[37] It is likely that methodologic differences, such as patient position, bladder filling, and quality of the Valsalva maneuver (i.e., controlling for confounders such as concomitant levator activation), account for the measurement discrepancies, with all known confounders tending to reduce descent. Attempts at standardizing Valsalva maneuvers[38,39] have not found widespread application because this requires intra-abdominal pressure measurement (i.e., use of a rectal balloon catheter). Other methods, such as the use of a spirometer, are likely to lead to suboptimal Valsalva maneuvers; the pressures used in the one study describing the use of such a device[38] were clearly insufficient to achieve maximal or even near-maximal descent.[39]

The cause of increased bladder neck descent is likely to be multifactorial. The wide range of values obtained in young, nulliparous women suggests a congenital component, and a twin study has confirmed a high degree of heritability for anterior vaginal wall mobility.[44] Vaginal childbirth[45-47] is probably the most significant environmental factor (see Fig. 9-4), with a long second stage of labor and vaginal operative delivery associated with increased postpartum descent of the bladder neck.[47] This association between increased bladder descent and vaginal parity is also evident in older women with symptoms of pelvic floor dysfunction.[48] While the pelvic floor is undoubtedly affected by labor and delivery, it has been speculated that progress in labor

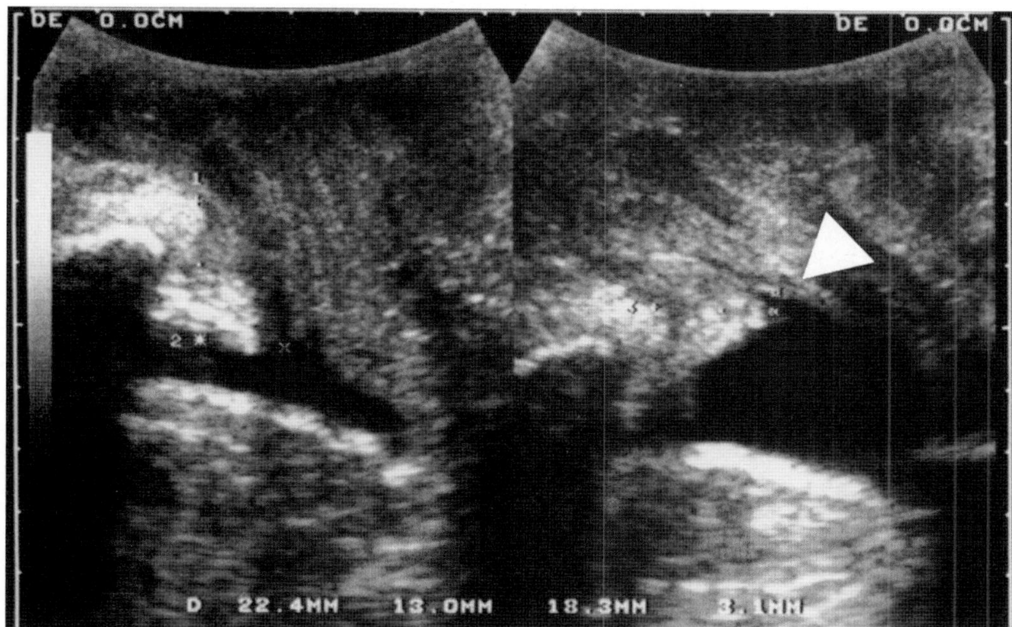

Figure 9-5 Typical findings in a patient with stress incontinence and mild anterior vaginal wall descent (i.e., cystourethrocele grade 1): posteroinferior rotation of the urethra, opening of the retrovesical angle, and funneling of the proximal urethra *(arrow)*. Figure reproduced from Ultrasound Obstet Gynecol 2004; 23:80-92, with permission.

may not be independent of pelvic floor biomechanics.[49] Anterior vaginal wall mobility during a Valsalva maneuver was found to be a potential predictor of progress in labor in two independent studies.[50,51]

Funneling

In patients with stress incontinence and in asymptomatic women,[40] funneling of the internal urethral meatus may be observed during a Valsalva maneuver (see Fig. 9-5) and sometimes even at rest. Funneling is often associated with leakage. Other indirect signs of urine leakage on B-mode real-time imaging are weak gray-scale echoes (i.e., streaming) and the appearance of two linear echoes defining the lumen of a fluid-filled urethra. However, funneling may also be observed in patients with urge incontinence, and it cannot be used to prove urodynamic stress incontinence. Its anatomic basis is unclear, but marked funneling is associated with poor urethral closure pressures.[41,42]

Classifications developed for the evaluation of radiologic imaging[43] can be modified for ultrasound; however, this approach is not generally accepted. The most common finding in cases of bladder neck hypermobility is a so-called rotational descent of the internal meatus (i.e., proximal urethra and trigone rotate around the symphysis pubis in a posteroinferior direction). In these cases, the retrovesical angle opens to up to 160 to 180 degrees from a normal value of 90 to 120 degrees, and the change in the retrovesical angle usually is associated with funneling. Often, there seems to be increased mobility of the entire urethra. A cystocele with intact retrovesical angle (90 to 120 degrees) is frequently seen in continent patients with prolapse (Fig. 9-6), and distal and central urethral fixation to the pubic rami usually seems to be relatively normal, resulting in urethral kinking. It has been surmised that this configuration distinguishes a central from a lateral defect of the endopelvic fascia,[16] although proof for this hypothesis is lacking. Marked urethral kinking in these patients may protect against stress incontinence but can lead to voiding dysfunction and urinary retention. Occult stress incontinence may be unmasked once a successful prolapse repair prevents urethral kinking.

Color Doppler

Color Doppler ultrasound has been used to demonstrate urine leakage through the urethra during a Valsalva maneuver or coughing.[58] Agreement between color Doppler and fluoroscopy results was high in a controlled group with indwelling catheters and identical bladder volumes.[59] Color Doppler ultrasound velocity (Fig. 9-7) and energy mapping (Color Doppler or power Doppler) (Fig. 9-8) were able to document leakage. Color Doppler ultrasound velocity was slightly more likely to show a positive result, probably because of its better motion discrimination. This results in less flash artifact and better orientation, particularly on coughing, although imaging quality depends on the systems used and selected color Doppler settings. As a result, routine sonographic documentation of stress incontinence during urodynamic testing has become feasible. Color Doppler imaging may also facilitate documentation of leak point pressures.[60] Whether this is desired depends on the clinician's preferences, because it may be argued that urine leakage and leak point pressures can be determined more easily with other methods.

Bladder Wall Thickness

There has been considerable interest in the quantification of bladder wall thickness by transvaginal or translabial ultrasound.[61,62] Measurements are obtained after bladder emptying, and they are acquired perpendicular to the mucosa (Fig. 9-9). In the original description, three sites were assessed—anterior wall, trigone, and dome of the bladder—and the mean of all three was

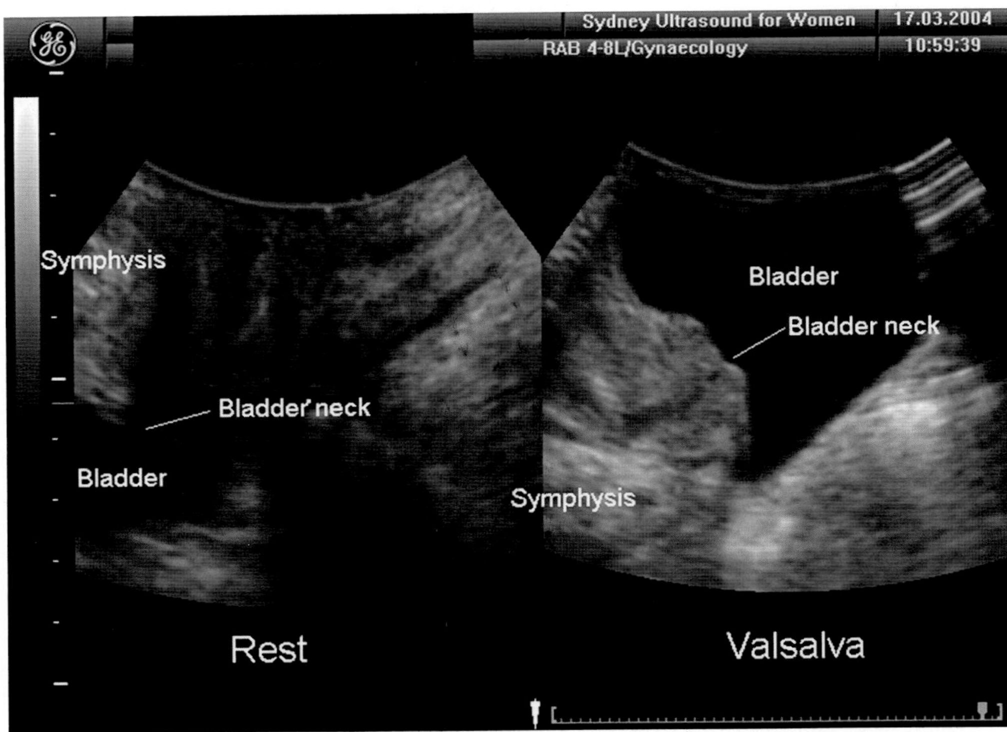

Figure 9-6 A cystocele with an intact retrovesical angle. Notice the absence of funneling. The bladder neck and proximal urethra are virtually inverted compared with their position at rest. Reproduced from Textbook of Female Urology and Urogynecology, Abingdon UK, 2006.

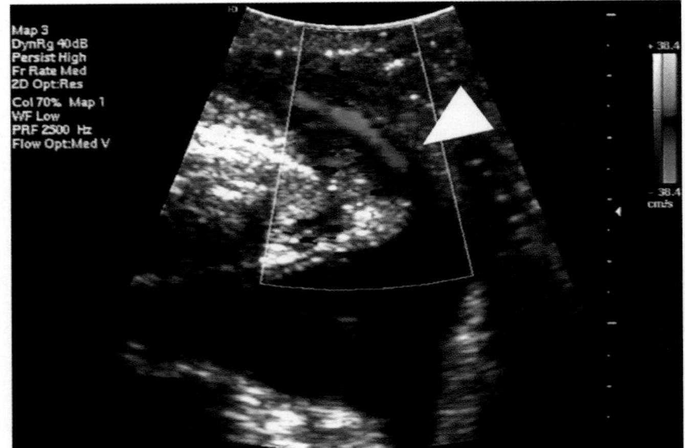

Figure 9-7 Color Doppler velocity (CDV) demonstrates urine leakage *(arrowhead)* through the urethra during a Valsalva maneuver. Reproduced from Ultrasound Obstet Gynecol 2004; 23:80-92, with permission.

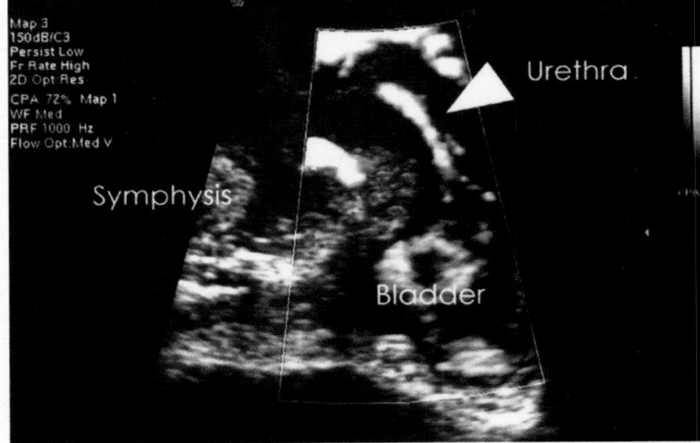

Figure 9-8 Color Doppler energy mapping (CDE) of stress urinary incontinence. The Doppler signal outlines most of the proximal urethra *(arrowhead)*. Reproduced from Ultrasound Obstet Gynecol 2004; 23:80-92, with permission.

calculated. A bladder wall thickness of more than 5 mm seems to be associated with detrusor instability,[61,63] although this has been disputed.[64] Increased bladder wall thickness is likely caused by hypertrophy of the detrusor muscle,[64] which is most evident at the dome; this may be the cause of symptoms or the effect of an underlying abnormality. Although bladder wall thickness on its own seems only moderately predictive of detrusor instability and is not in itself a useful diagnostic test, the method may be of value when combined with symptoms of the overactive bladder.[65] It remains to be seen whether determination of this parameter can contribute to the workup of a patient with pelvic floor and bladder dysfunction, such as serving as a predictor of postoperative voiding function or de novo or worsened detrusor overactivity.

Levator Activity

Perineal ultrasound has been used for the quantification of pelvic floor muscle function in women with stress incontinence and in continent controls[66] before and after childbirth.[67,68] A cranioventral shift of pelvic organs imaged in a sagittal midline orientation is taken as evidence of a levator contraction. The resulting dis-

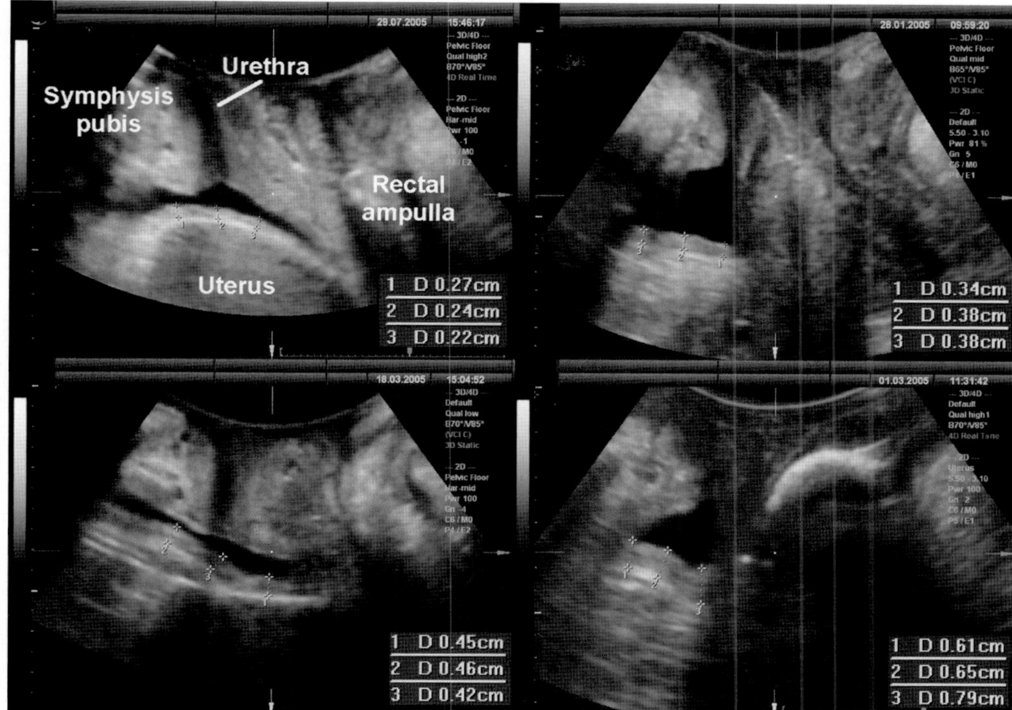

Figure 9-9 Measurement of bladder wall thickness at the dome in four women with non-neuropathic bladder dysfunction. In all cases, the residual urine volume is well below 50 mL.

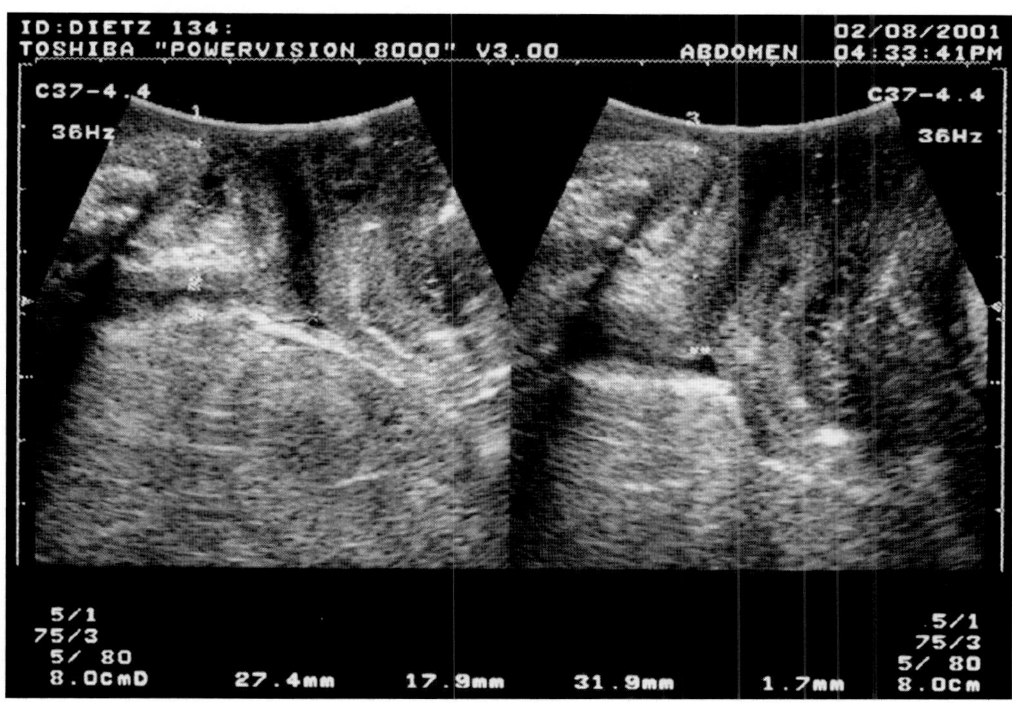

Figure 9-10 Quantification of levator contraction. Cranioventral displacement of the bladder neck is measured relative to the inferoposterior symphyseal margin. The measurements indicate 4.5 (range, 31.9 minus 27.4) mm of cranial displacement and 16.2 (range, 17.9 minus 1.7) mm of ventral displacement of the bladder neck. Figure reproduced from Ultrasound Obstet Gynecol 2004; 23:80-92, with permission.

placement of the internal urethral meatus is measured relative to the inferoposterior symphyseal margin (Fig. 9-10). In this way, pelvic floor activity is assessed at the bladder neck, where its effect as part of the continence mechanism is most likely to be relevant.[69] Another means of quantifying levator activity is to measure reduction of the levator hiatus in the midsagittal plane or to determine the changing angle of the hiatal plane relative to the symphyseal axis. The method can also be used for pelvic floor muscle exercise teaching by providing visual biofeedback.[70] The technique has helped validate the concept of *the knack*, a reflex levator contraction immediately before increases in intra-abdominal pressure, such as those resulting

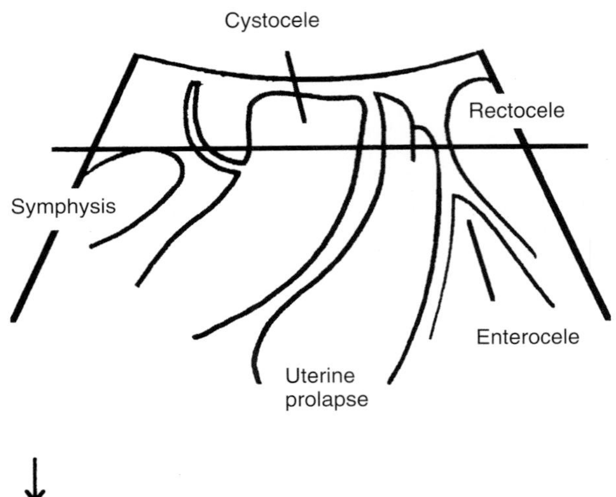

Figure 9-11 Line drawing demonstrating the ultrasound quantification of uterovaginal prolapse. The inferior margin of the symphysis pubis serves as a line of reference against which the maximal descent of the bladder, uterus, cul-de-sac, and rectal ampulla on Valsalva maneuver can be measured. Figure reproduced from Ultrasound Obstet Gynecol 2004; 23:80-92, with permission.

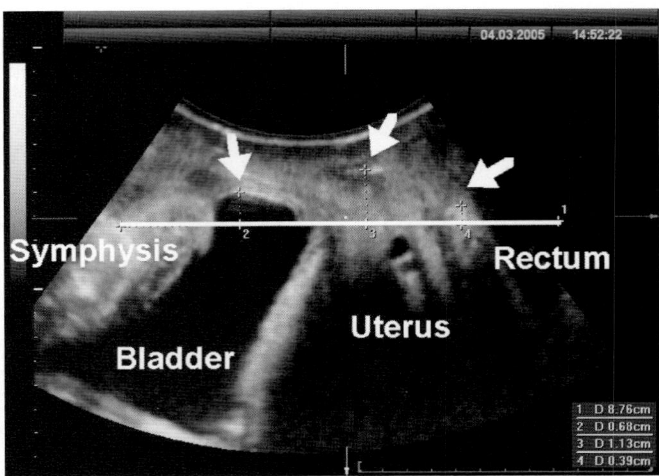

Figure 9-12 Three-compartment prolapse on translabial ultrasound. The line of reference is placed through the inferior margin of the symphysis pubis. Measurements indicate descent of the bladder to 6.8 mm below the symphysis pubis, of the uterus to 11.3 mm, and of the rectal ampulla to 3.9 mm below. *Arrows* indicate the leading edges of those organs. The clinical examination showed a second-degree uterine prolapse and first-degree anterior and posterior compartment descent.

from coughing.[71] Good correlations have been found between cranioventral shift of the bladder neck and palpation or perineometry.[72]

Prolapse Quantification

Translabial ultrasound can demonstrate uterovaginal prolapse.[73,74] The inferior margin of the symphysis pubis serves as a convenient (if arbitrary) line of reference against which the maximal descent of the bladder, uterus, cul-de-sac, and rectal ampulla during a Valsalva maneuver can be measured (Fig. 9-11). On Valsalva the transducer is withdrawn to allow full development of the prolapse, while retaining contact with the insonated tissues. Angling of the transducer should be avoided in order to prevent changes in the relative position of transducer and symphysea axes. Figure 9-12 shows a three-compartment prolapse, with the uterus leading. Findings have been compared with clinical staging and the results of a standardized assessment according to criteria developed by the International Continence Society,[75] with good correlations shown for the anterior and central compartments.[76] Although there may be poorer correlation between posterior compartment clinical assessment and ultrasound, not the least due to variable rectal filling, it is possible to distinguish between true rectocele (i.e., defect of the rectovaginal septum) (Fig. 9-13A) and perineal hypermobility without fascial defects (see Fig. 9-13B). True rectoceles may be present in young, nulliparous women but are more common in parous women. In some instances, they arise in childbirth.[77] From imaging experience, fascial defects seem to almost always be found in the same area (i.e., very close to the anorectal junction), and they most commonly are transverse. Many are asymptomatic. Routine posterior repair often results in reduction or distortion of such defects without effecting closure.

The ability to differentiate different forms of posterior compartment descent should allow better surgical management in the future, especially because enterocele (Fig. 9-14) can easily be distinguished from rectocele. It appears that colorectal surgeons are starting to use the technique to complement or replace defecography,[78] and perineal ultrasound can also be used for exoanal imaging of the anal sphincter.[79,80]

Disadvantages of the method include incomplete imaging of bladder neck, cervix, and vault with large rectoceles and possible underestimation of severe prolapse due to transducer pressure. Occasionally, apparent anterior vaginal wall prolapse turns out to be caused by a urethral diverticulum[81,82] (Fig. 9-15) or a paravaginal cyst.

The main use of this technique may prove to be in outcome assessment after prolapse and incontinence surgery for clinical and research applications. Elevation and distortion of the bladder neck arising from a colposuspension is easily documented.[83,84] Fascial and synthetic slings are visible posterior to the trigone or the urethra (Figs. 9-16 and 9-17). Bulking agents such as Macroplastique (Fig. 9-18) show up anterior, lateral, and posterior to the proximal urethra. It has been demonstrated that overelevation of the bladder neck on colposuspension is unnecessary for cure of urodynamic stress incontinence, and elevation may also have a bearing on postoperative symptoms of voiding dysfunction and de novo detrusor instability.[83,84]

Implants

Ultrasound has contributed significantly to the investigation of new surgical procedures, such as wide-weave suburethral Prolene slings, showing that they act by urethral kinking or *dynamic compression* against the posterior surface of the symphysis pubis.[85] Available synthetic slings are easily visualized posterior to the urethra[86-93] (see Fig. 9-16). Wide-weave monofilament mesh such as tension-free vaginal tape (e.g., Gynecare TVT), SPARC sling, and Monarc Subfascial Hammock or transobturator (TOT) sling are more echogenic than more tightly woven multifilament implants, such as the IVS (i.e., polypropylene mesh) (see Fig.

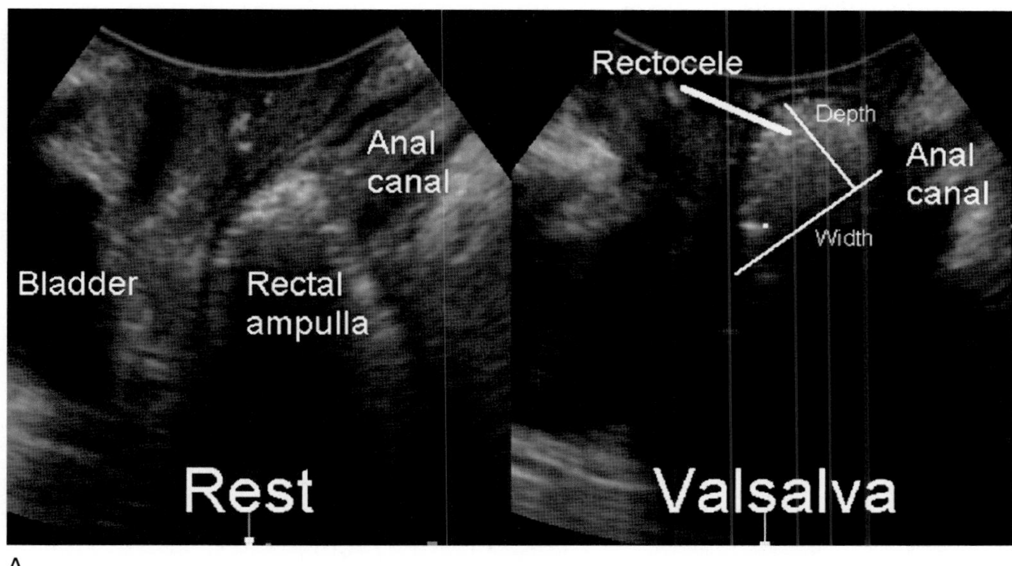

A

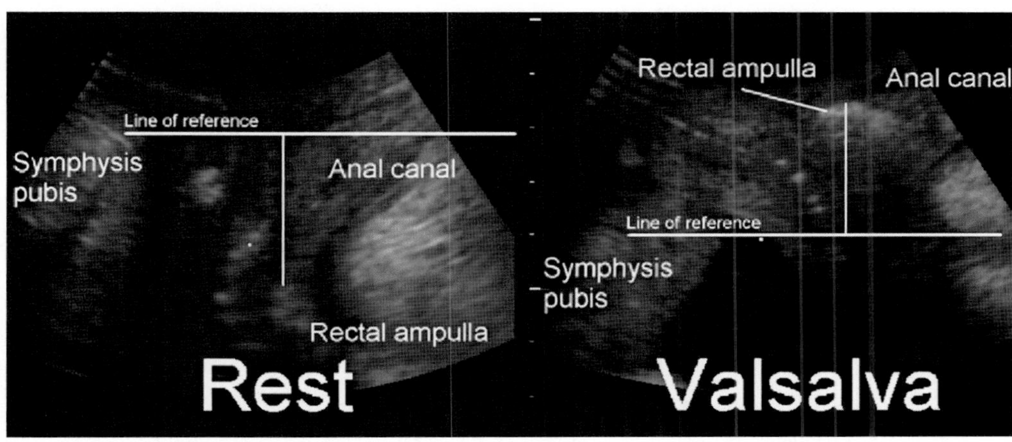

B

Figure 9-13 **A,** The top pair of images shows a first-degree rectocele. The anal canal is seen to the right of both images, with a small rectocele (deep 2 cm) clearly visible during a Valsalva maneuver *(right)*. **B,** The lower pair of images demonstrates descent of the rectal ampulla without herniation of rectal contents into the vagina, a condition that may mimic rectocele and that has been called *perineal hypermobility* or *pseudorectocele*. Figure reproduced from Textbook of Female Urology and Urogynecology, Abingdon UK, 2006.

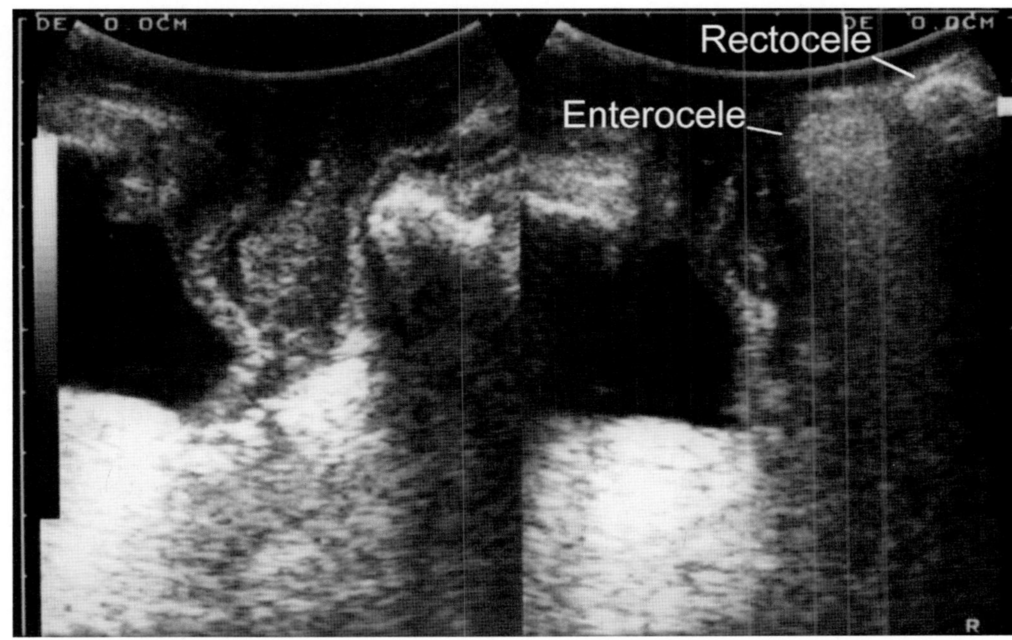

Figure 9-14 Rectocele after Burch colposuspension with the patient at rest *(left)* and during a Valsalva maneuver *(right)*. Usually, enteroceles (filled by peristalsing small bowel, epiploic fat, or omentum) appear more homogeneous and nearly isoechoic, whereas the rectocele is filled by a stool bolus and/or air, resulting in hyperechogenicity with distal shadowing. Figure reproduced from Ultrasound Obstet Gynecol 2005; 26:73-77, with permission.

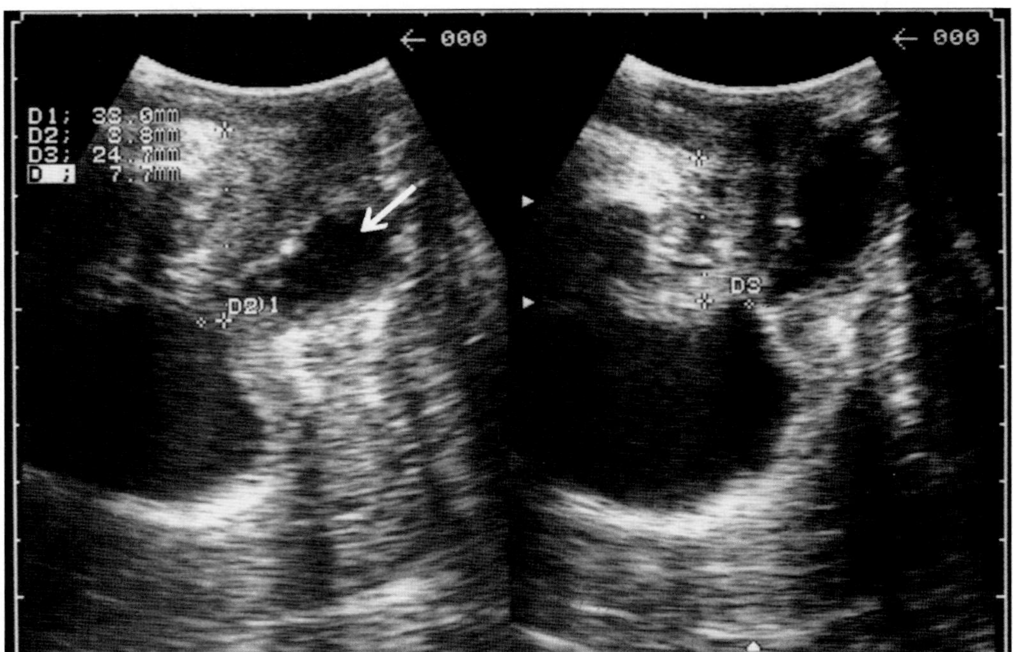

Figure 9-15 Urethral diverticulum *(arrow)*, herniating downward and clinically simulating a cystourethrocele during a Valsalva maneuver. The neck of the diverticulum is close to the bladder neck. Reproduced from Ultrasound Obstet Gynecol 2004; 23:80-92, with permission.

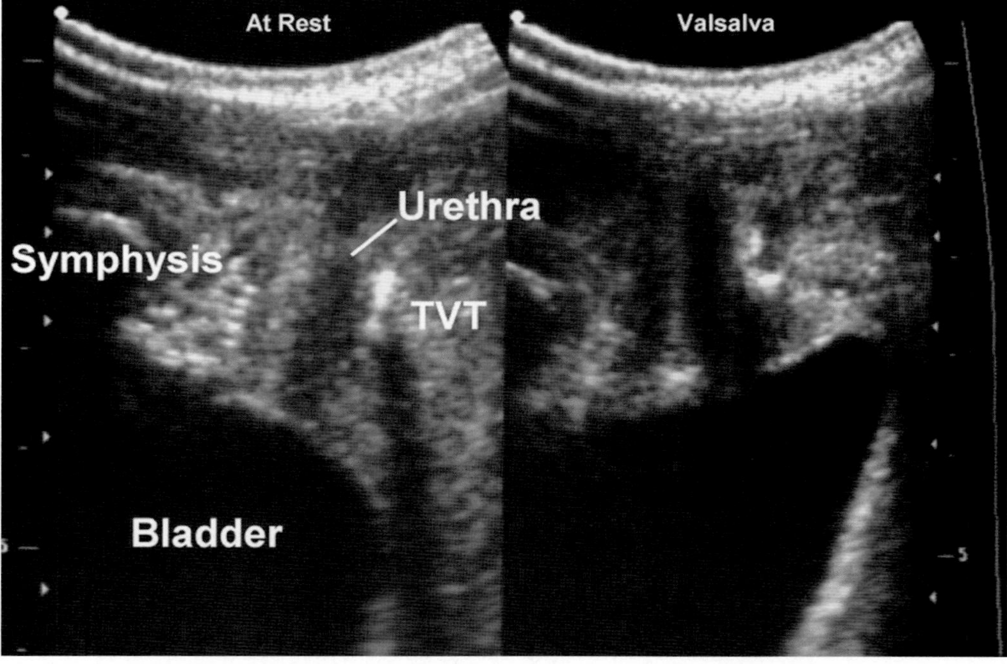

Figure 9-16 Synthetic implants such as the tension-free vaginal tape or SPARC are easily visualized as highly echogenic structures posterior to the urethra. The images illustrate tape position relative to the symphysis pubis and urethra with the patient at rest *(left)* and during a Valsalva maneuver *(right)*. Reproduced from Ultrasound Obstet Gynecol 2004; 23:80-92, with permission.

9-17), but virtually all can be identified and followed in their course from the pubic rami laterally to the urethra centrally. The difference between transobturator tapes (e.g., Monarc, TOT) and tapes placed through the space of Retzius (e.g., TVT, SPARC, IVS) is evident when following the tapes in the parasagittal or axial planes. In the parasagittal plane, transobturator tapes often can be seen to perforate the obturator fascia and muscle close to the insertion of the pubovisceral muscle; sometimes, they traverse the most inferomedial component of the levator before exiting the pelvis.[93] Wide-weave mesh implants used in procedures, such as the Perigee, Apogee or Prolift implants, are very echogenic and easily identified,[94] and their transobturator or

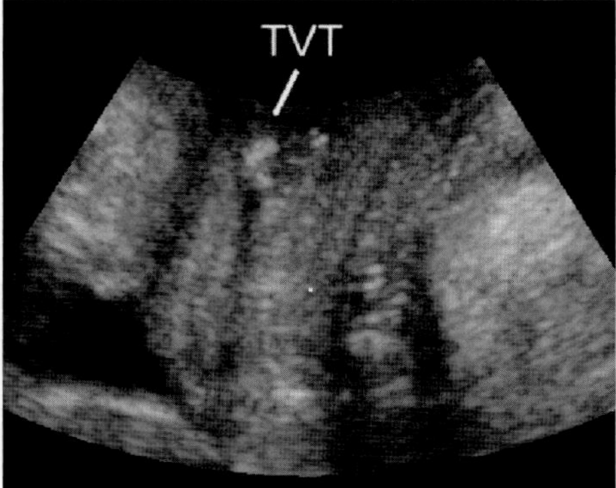

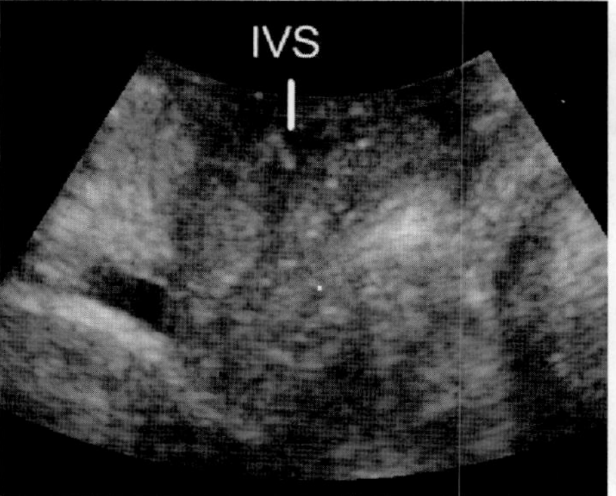

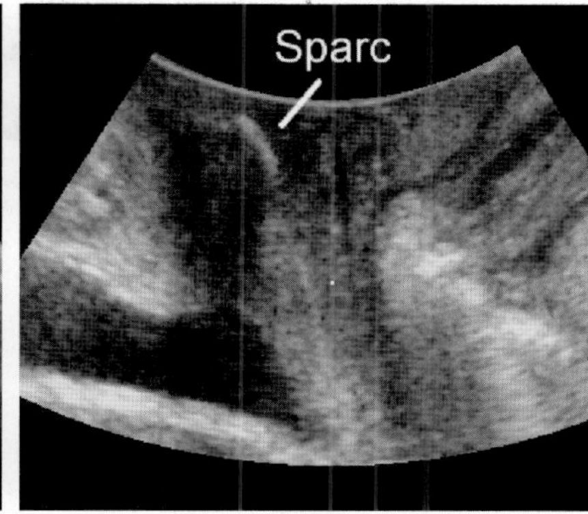

Figure 9-17 A comparison of tension-free vaginal tape (TVT), SPARC mesh, and IVS mesh *(left to right)* on midsagittal imaging. The TVT often appears slightly curled, signifying a greater degree of tension compared with the SPARC material, which often is under less tension because of a central suture that avoids pretensioning of the tape on removal of plastic sheaths during surgery. Reproduced from Ultrasound Obstet Gynecol 2005; 26:175-179, with permission.

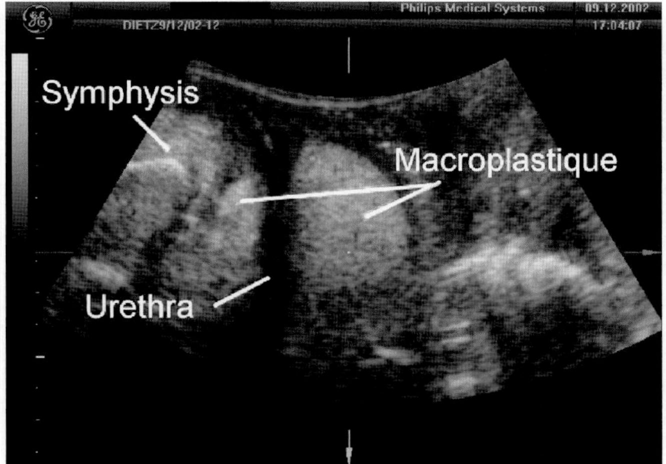

Figure 9-18 Macroplastique (silicone macroparticles), an injectable used in USI surgery, is very echogenic and can be located ventral, dorsal and lateral to the proximal and mid-urethra. Figure reproduced from Ultrasound Obstet Gynecol 2004; 23:80-92, with permission.

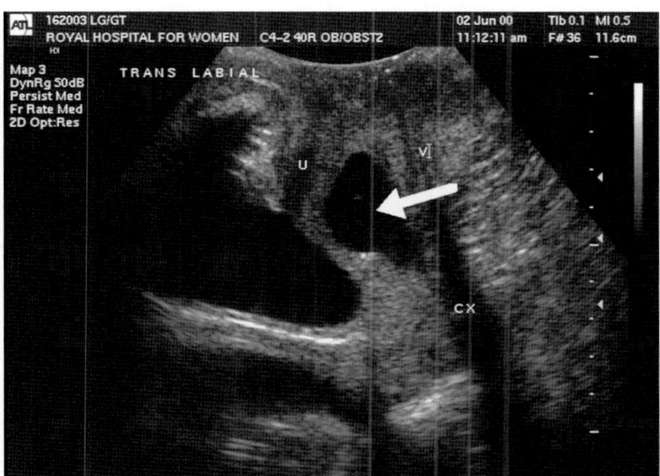

Figure 9-19 A Gartner duct cyst is shown close to the bladder neck *(arrow)*. Reproduced from Ultrasound Obstet Gynecol 2004; 23:80-92, with permission.

pararectal extensions can be followed for some distance, although 3D or 4D imaging allows much more comprehensive evaluation.

Ultrasound has demonstrated the wide margin of safety and efficacy of suburethral tapes in regard to placement (which helps explain their extraordinary success) and allayed concerns regarding tape shrinkage and tightening due to scar formation.[90,91] The assessment of bladder neck mobility before implantation of a suburethral sling may predict success or failure,[95] an observation that makes perfect sense considering that dynamic compression relies on relative movement of implant and native tissues.

Paravaginal Defect Imaging

Transabdominal ultrasound has been used to demonstrate lateral defects of the endopelvic fascia, also called *paravaginal defects*. However, this method has not been fully validated, and a prospective study showed poor correlation with clinically observed defects.[96] Several factors may limit the predictive value of transabdominal ultrasound in the identification of paravaginal defects: the poor definition of an optimal scanning plane, the influence of uterine prolapse or a full rectum, and the inability to observe the effect of a Valsalva maneuver (which would dislodge the transducer) by transabdominal imaging. It is likely that levator trauma (see below) is frequently misinterpreted as a "paravaginal defect." Fascial trauma is highly likely in patients with a full avulsion, but it is conceivable that fascial defects may occur in women with intact muscle. Much work remains to be done in this field.

Other Findings

A range of other abnormalities, incidental or expected, may sometimes be detected on translabial ultrasound, although a full pelvic ultrasound assessment does require a transvaginal approach. Urethral diverticula (see Fig. 9-15),[78,97] labial cysts, Gartner's duct cysts (Fig. 9-19), or bladder tumors (Fig. 9-20) may be identified, and intravesical stents and bladder diverticula also can be visualized.[16] Postoperative hematomas may be visible after vaginal surgery or TVT placement and sometimes explain clinical symptoms such as voiding dysfunction or persistent pain (Fig. 9-21).

Most recently, it has become clear that rectal intussusception and rectal prolapse can be diagnosed on pelvic floor ultrasound in the midsagittal plane. The pathognomonic feature of intussusception is splaying of the anal canal and inversion of the anterior rectal wall into the anal canal (see Figure 9-21). The intussuscipiens is propelled by small bowel or sigmoid colon, resulting in inversion of the rectal wall: an enterocele that does not develop into the vagina, but down the anal canal. Mucosal prolapse, on the other hand, is much more discrete as it does not involve the full thickness of the rectal wall, and seems limited to the area immediately proximal to the anal canal. The usefulness of translabial ultrasound in patients with symptoms of obstructed defecation, in particular as compared to defecation proctography, is not yet clear however. Several comparative studies are in progress in urogynaecological and colorectal units at the time of writing.

THREE-DIMENSIONAL PELVIC FLOOR IMAGING

Technical Overview

Two main engineering solutions have been developed to allow integration of two-dimensional (2D) sectional images into 3D volume data: motorized acquisition and external electromagnetic position sensors. A simplified technique is the freehand acquisition of volumes without any reference to transducer position. In essence, this means that a cine loop of images is collated to form a volume data set; because the system has no information on transducer position relative to the insonated tissues, measurements on volume data are impossible. Nevertheless, qualitative information may be obtained, and such systems have been used for clinical research in urogynecology.[98]

Quantitative evaluation of volumes requires information on transducer position at the time of acquisition. If probe movement is achieved with the help of a motor, its characteristics will determine imaging data coordinates. Motorized acquisition may take the shape of automatic withdrawal of an endocavitary probe, motorized rotation of such a probe, or motor action within the transducer itself. The first such motorized probe was developed in 1974, and by 1987, transducers for clinical use were developed that allowed motorized acquisition of imaging data.[99] The first commercially available platform, the Kretz Voluson system, was developed around such a "fan scan" probe. Endocavitary probes make a freehand acquisition technique impractical, which is why the company did not develop this alternative approach further[99] and instead concentrated on a technology reminiscent of (otherwise obsolete) mechanical sector transducers. The results have been the abdominal and endovaginal probes used in systems such as the GE Kretz Voluson 530, 730, 730 expert, E8 and Volusoni System. The widespread acceptance of 3D ultrasound in obstetrics and gynecology was helped considerably by this development because these transducers do not require any movement relative to the investigated tissue during acquisition. Most of the major suppliers of ultrasound equipment have developed their own transducers along such lines, although it is widely recognized that this technology will probably be replaced by matrix array transducers within the next 5 to 10 years. Such transducers are already available for echocardiography.[100]

With current mechanical 3D transducers, automatic image acquisition is achieved by rapid oscillation of a group of elements within the transducer. This allows the registration of multiple sectional planes that can be integrated into a volume as the location of a given voxel (i.e., a pixel that has a defined location in space) is determined by transducer and insonation characteristics. Fortuitously, transducer characteristics on available systems for transabdominal use have been highly suitable for pelvic floor imaging. A single volume obtained at rest with an acquisition angle of 70 degrees or higher includes the entire levator hiatus

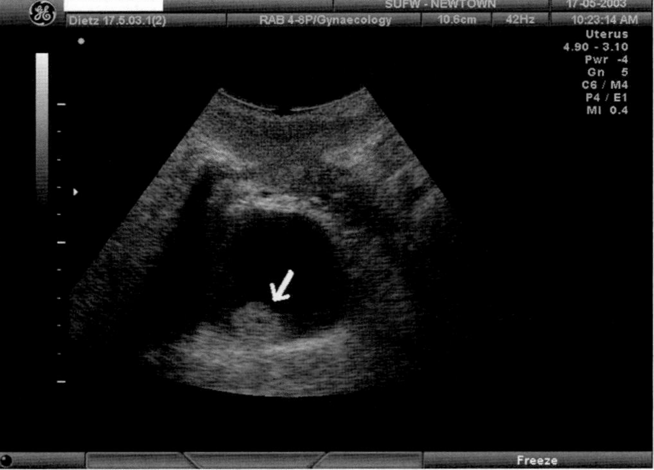

Figure 9-20 A transitional cell carcinoma *(arrow)* of the bladder is seen on parasagittal translabial ultrasound. Reproduced from Ultrasound Ostet Gynecol 2004; 23:80-92, with permission.

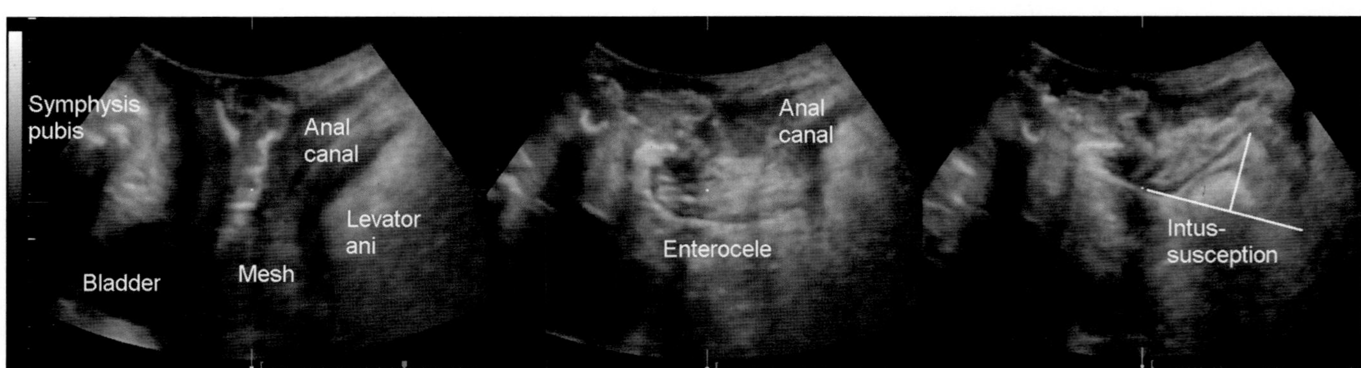

Figure 9-21 Retroperitoneal hematoma and subcutaneous vaginal hematoma after mesh sacrocolpopexy and posterior repair. Reproduced from ASUM Bulletin 2007; 10:17-23, with permission.

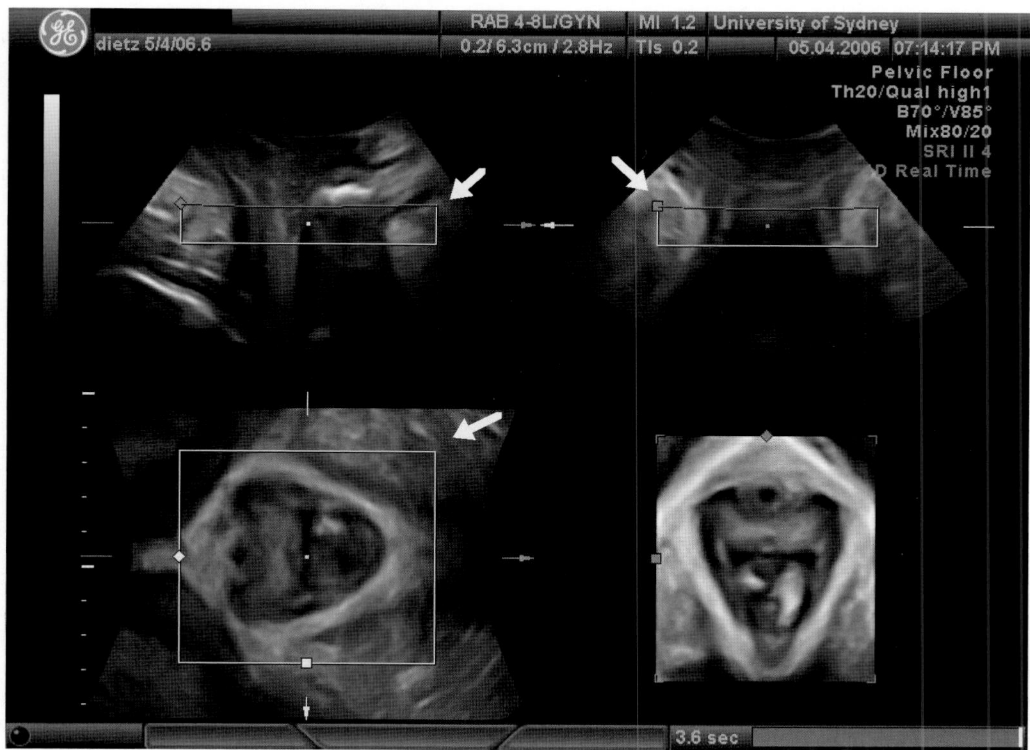

Figure 9-22 The usual acquisition or evaluation screen on Voluson-type systems shows the three orthogonal planes: sagittal *(top left)*, coronal *(top right)*, and axial *(bottom left)*. It also shows a rendered volume *(bottom right)*, which is a semitransparent representation of all gray-scale data in the region of interest *(arrows)*.

with the symphysis pubis, urethra, paravaginal tissues, the vagina, anorectum, and pubovisceral (i.e., puborectalis or pubococcygeus part of the levator ani) muscle from the pelvic side wall in the area of the arcus tendineus of the levator ani (ATLA) to the posterior aspect of the anorectal junction (Fig. 9-22). Depending on the anteroposterior dimensions of the pubovisceral muscle, it may also include the anal canal and the external anal sphincter. This also holds true for volumes acquired on levator contraction. A Valsalva maneuver may result in lateral or posterior parts of the puborectalis being pushed outside the field of vision, especially in women with significant prolapse (discussed later). The abdominal 8-4-MHz volume transducer for Voluson systems allows acquisition angles of up to 85 degrees, ensuring that the levator hiatus can be imaged in its entirety, even in women with significant enlargement (i.e., ballooning) of the hiatus during a Valsalva maneuver.

Display Modes

Figure 9-22 demonstrates the two basic display modes used on 3D ultrasound systems. The multiplanar or orthogonal display mode shows cross-sectional planes through the volume in question. For pelvic floor imaging, this most conveniently means the midsagittal, the coronal, and the axial or transverse plane.

One of the main advantages of volume ultrasound for pelvic floor imaging is that the method gives access to the axial plane. Until recently, pelvic floor ultrasound was limited to the midsagittal plane.[9,101,102] Parasagittal and coronal plane imaging have not been reported, perhaps because there are no obvious points of reference, unlike the convenient reference point of the symphysis pubis on midsagittal views. The axial plane was accessible only on MRI; Figure 9-23 provides an axial view of the levator hiatus on MRI and 3D ultrasound.[103] Pelvic floor MRI is an established investigational method, at least for research applications, with a multitude of papers published over the past 10 years.[104-113]

Imaging planes on 3D ultrasound can be varied in a completely arbitrary fashion to enhance the visibility of a given anatomical structure at the time of acquisition or offline at a later time. The levator ani, for example, usually requires an axial plane that is slightly tilted in a cranioventral to dorsocaudal direction. The three orthogonal images are complemented by a rendered image, which is a semitransparent representation of all voxels in an arbitrarily definable box, termed the Region of Interest (ROI). Figure 9-22 (bottom right image) shows a standard rendered volume of the levator hiatus, with the rendering direction set caudally to cranially, which seems to be most convenient for pelvic floor imaging. The possibilities for postprocessing are restricted only by the software used for this purpose; programs such as GE Kretz 4D View (GE Medical Systems Kretztechnik, Zipf, Austria) allow extensive manipulation of image characteristics and output of stills, cine loops, and rotational volumes in bitmap and AVI formats.

FOUR-DIMENSIONAL IMAGING

The use of 4D imaging implies the real-time acquisition of volume ultrasound data, which can then be represented in orthogonal planes or rendered volumes. It has become possible

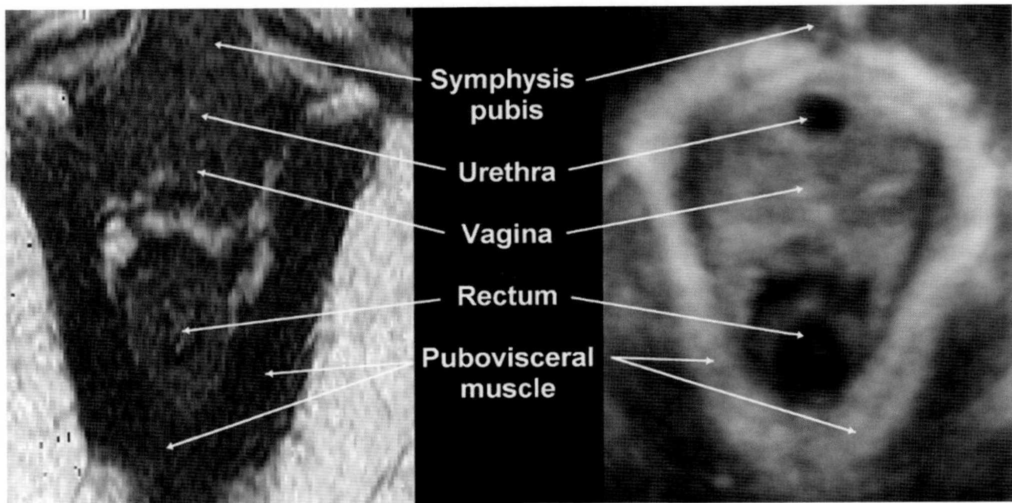

Figure 9-23 The axial plane on magnetic resonance imaging (MRI) and ultrasound (rendered volume) in a young nulliparous volunteer. (MRI courtesy of J Kruger, Auckland.) Reproduced from Obstet Gynecol 2005; 106:707-712, with permission.

to save cine loops of volumes, which is important in pelvic floor imaging because it allows enhanced documentation of functional anatomy. Even on 2D, single-plane imaging, a static assessment at rest gives little information compared with the evaluation of maneuvers such as a levator contraction and Valsalva. Observation enables better assessment of levator function and improved delineation of levator or fascial trauma. Avulsion of the pubovisceral muscle from the arcus tendineus of the levator ani is often more evident on levator contraction, and most significant pelvic organ prolapse is not visible with the patient at rest in the supine position. Fascial defects such as those defining a true rectocele often only become visible during a Valsalva maneuver.

The ability to perform a real-time 3D (or 4D) assessment of pelvic floor structures makes the technology clearly superior to MRI. Prolapse assessment by MRI requires ultrafast acquisition,[107,109] which is of limited availability and does not allow optimal resolutions. Alternatively, some systems allow imaging of the sitting or erect patient,[108] but accessibility will remain limited for the foreseeable future. The sheer physical characteristics of MRI systems make it much harder for the operator to ensure efficient maneuvers because more than 50% of women do not perform a proper pelvic floor contraction when asked[114] and a Valsalva maneuver is often confounded by concomitant levator activation.[115] Without real-time imaging, it is impossible to control for these confounders. Ultrasound therefore has major potential advantages when it comes to describing prolapse, especially when it is associated with fascial or muscular defects, and for defining functional anatomy. Offline analysis packages such as the GE Kretz 4D View or Philips QL AB software allow distance, area, and volume measurements in any user-defined plane (e.g., oblique, orthogonal), which is superior to what is possible with Digital Imaging and Communications in Medicine (DICOM) viewer software on a standard set of single-plane MRI images. DICOM is a standard for distributing and viewing any kind of medical image, regardless of the origin.

Speckle Reduction Techniques

Technical developments such as volume-contrast imaging (VCI) and speckle-reduction imaging (SRI) employ rendering algorithms as a means of improving resolutions in the coronal plane. As a result, speckle artifact is markedly reduced.[116] Measuring in the axial or C plane has been limited to raw data without significant postprocessing. Consequently, resolutions were much poorer than in the sagittal plane, reducing the accuracy of measurements and our ability to identify structural changes. By using VCI on slices 1 to 3 mm thick, resolutions of about 1 mm can be reached on axial or oblique axial slices that allow distance and area measurements on the ultrasound system and offline on a computer. Figure 9-24 shows normal C-plane imaging and VCI in the axial plane in a patient with major bilateral levator trauma after rotational forceps delivery. Another technique using rendering algorithms to enhance single plane resolutions, Speckle Reduction Imaging or "SRI," results in improved tissue discrimination, which should help to improve detection of morphologic abnormalities. Figure 9-22 provides an example of image quality using SRI for orthogonal planes and rendered volumes.

Tomographic Ultrasound Imaging

During or after acquisition of volumes, it is possible to process imaging information into slices of predetermined number and spacing, reminiscent of computed tomography (CT) or nuclear MRI. This technique has been called *multislice imaging* or *tomographic ultrasound imaging* (TUI) by manufacturers. Unlike CT or MRI, the location, number, depth, and tilt of slices can be adjusted at will after volume acquisition. The combination of true 4D (volume cine loop) capability and TUI or multislice imaging allows simultaneous observation of the effect of maneuvers at many different levels.

The pelvic floor easily lends itself to such techniques, and I suggest using the plane of minimal dimensions as plane of reference: an oblique axial plane that is defined in the midsagittal plane by the shortest line between the posterior symphyseal margin and the levator ani immediately posterior to the anorectal angle (Fig. 9-25). For the sake of convenience, I use 8 × 2.5-mm steps recorded from 5 mm below this plane to 12.5 mm above, which should encompass the entire puborectalis muscle.

Figure 9-26 shows the standard TUI format most appropriate to pelvic floor imaging, with the coronal plane for reference

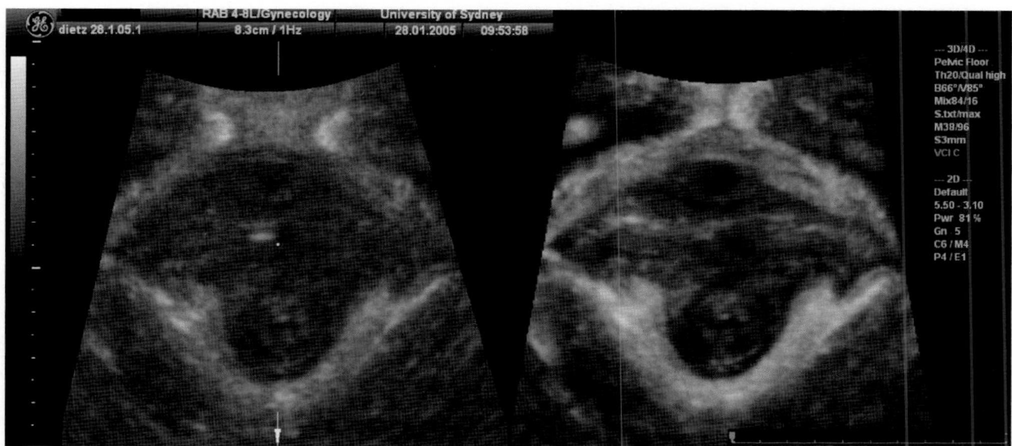

Figure 9-24 Axial plane translabial imaging with the patient at rest, illustrating a severe case of delivery-related pelvic floor trauma. A bilateral avulsion and complete loss of tenting bilaterally is shown on conventional axial-plane, 3D ultrasound *(left)*. The same plane in the same volume data set *(right)* is shown using volume-contrast imaging (VCI). This patient has severe stress incontinence and prolapse 3 years after a rotational forceps delivery.

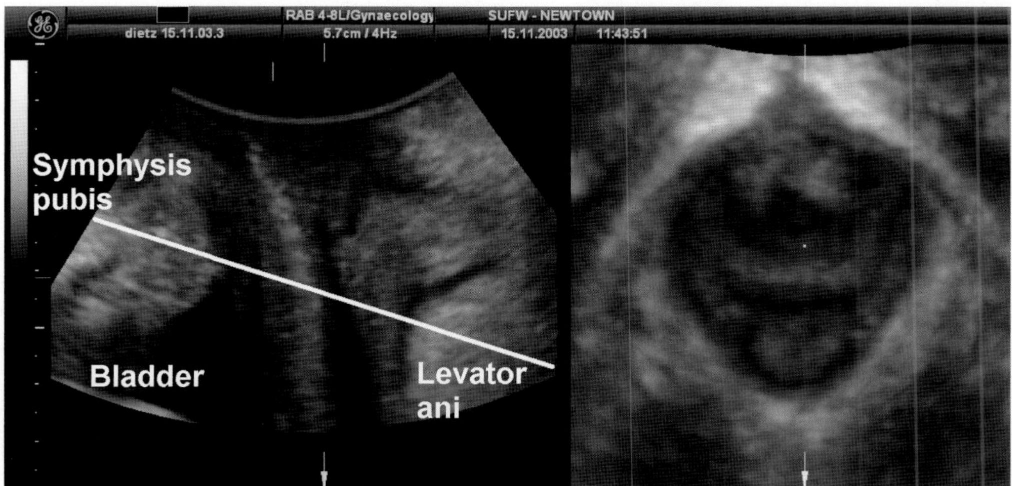

Figure 9-25 Determination of the plane of minimal hiatal dimensions. The minimal distance between the posterior symphyseal margin and the levator ani immediately posterior to the anorectal angle (*left,* midsagittal plane) identifies the correct axial plane *(right)*, which in this case was obtained by volume-contrast C-plane imaging.

in the top left corner and eight axial-plane slices at a distance of 2.5 mm each, in a nulliparous patient with normal pelvic floor function and anatomy. The presence and extent of injuries is evident at a glance from one printout or film, without requiring any further manipulation of data, as is familiar from radiologic cross-sectional techniques. It is likely that such techniques will help with the standardization of assessment methods and allow more accurate classification and quantification of morphologic abnormalities.[117]

PRACTICAL CONSIDERATIONS

Pelvic floor ultrasound is highly operator dependent, as is true for all real-time ultrasound procedures. The 3D systems have the potential to reduce this operator dependence because volume acquisition is easily taught and should be within the capabilities of every sonographer or sonologist after a day's training. Although the method does require postprocessing (and the skills involved in this are more significant), static volume data typically of 1 to 6 MB can be de-identified and transmitted electronically so that evaluation may be obtained by e-mail, and this opens up new possibilities for local and international cooperation. Unfortunately, the de facto software standard of 3D image files provided by licensing of original technology has been lost, with many companies developing their own standards, which are incompatible with the others. A DICOM standard for 3D imaging data would be the solution, but standardization does not appear to be imminent. Consequently, increasing numbers of clinicians and researchers are frustrated by the inability to exchange volume data. Users need to exert significant pressure on manufacturers, who may not be inclined to cooperate with competitors on this issue.

Most publications on 3D ultrasound in obstetrics and gynecology deal with obstetric applications.[15] The visualization of fetal structures such as extremities, skeleton, and face has to a large

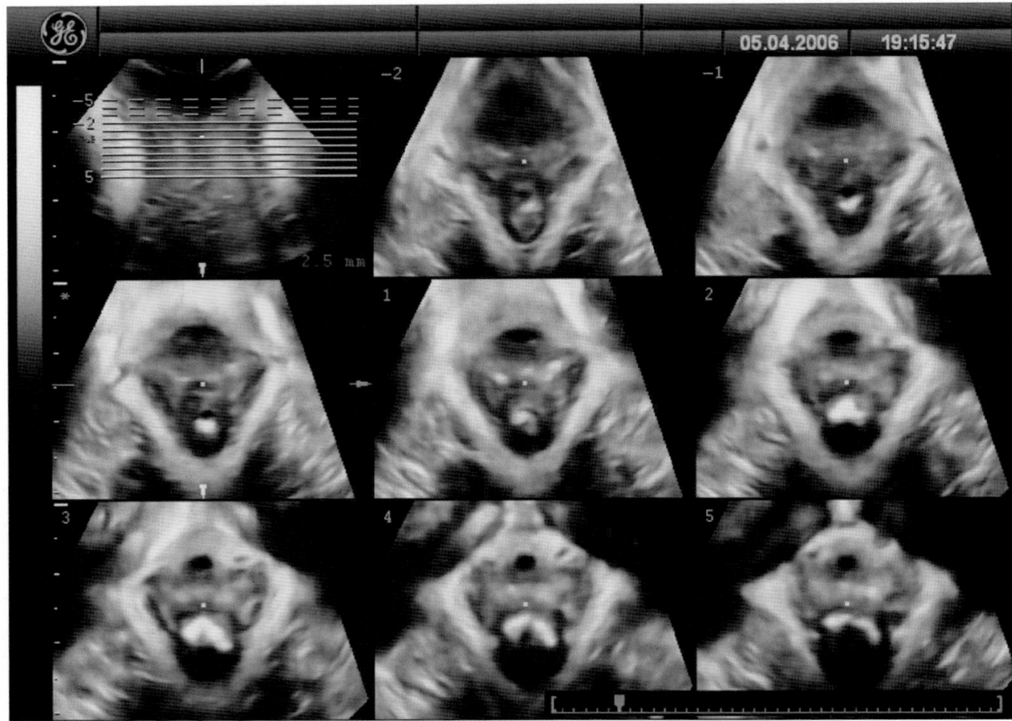

Figure 9-26 Normal pelvic floor. Tomographic ultrasound imaging provides cross-sectional imaging at user-definable depths and intervals and at arbitrarily definable angles or tilts within the acquired volume. A cine loop of volumes allows observation of the effect of maneuvers in multiple cross sections at any time.

extent driven the research, development, and marketing of these systems. Although well-selected 3D data may enhance the understanding of certain conditions or abnormalities for patients and caregivers,[15] some critics contend that 3D ultrasound has been a technology searching for an application.

Pelvic floor imaging is a minor niche within the field of ultrasound diagnostics, but it may provide one of the first true indications for 3D and 4D volume ultrasound imaging. Pelvic floor 3D ultrasound has been used for the evaluation of the urethra and its structures, for imaging of the more inferior aspects of the levator ani complex (i.e., pubococcygeus and puborectalis), for the visualization of paravaginal supports, and for prolapse and implant imaging.

Three-Dimensional Imaging of the Urethra

Technically, 3D pelvic floor ultrasound imaging became feasible in 1989 with the advent of the Kretz Voluson 530 system. However, there are no records of the early use of such systems; the first publication on 3D ultrasound in urogynecology was in 1994,[118] when Khullar et al demonstrated that this technique could be employed to assess the urethra.[118] They used transvaginal probes with motorized withdrawal to allow the use of calipers in all three planes. Subsequently, it was shown that urethral volumetric data correlated with urethral pressure profilometry[118] and that urethral volume decreased with parity. This technique has been used to assess delivery-related changes,[119] and 3D ultrasound with intracavitary transducers may also aid in identifying paraurethral support structures such as the pubourethral ligaments. Probes designed for prostatic imaging have also been employed for the assessment of the urethra and paraurethral structures by the transrectal route.[120]

Three-Dimensional Imaging of the Levator Ani Complex

The inferior aspects of the levator ani were identified on early studies using transvaginal techniques[14] and translabial freehand volume acquisition,[98] as well as on translabial ultrasound using a Voluson system,[13] but the focus of these reports was on the urethra and paraurethral tissues. With translabial acquisition, the whole levator hiatus and surrounding muscle (i.e., pubococcygeus and puborectalis) can be visualized, provided acquisition angles are at or above 70 degrees. Similar to MRI, it is impossible to distinguish the different components of the pubovisceral or puborectalis-pubococcygeus complex. In a series of 52 young, nulligravid women, no significant asymmetry of the levator was observed, supporting the hypothesis that morphologic abnormalities of the levator are likely to be evidence of delivery- related trauma.[121] Contrary to MRI data,[112] there was no significant side difference in thickness or area.

A number of biometric parameters of the puborectalis-pubococcygeus complex itself and of the levator hiatus have been defined.[121] Results agreed with MRI data obtained in small numbers of nulliparous women for the dimensions of the levator hiatus[112] and levator thickness.[110] Hiatal depth, width, and area measurements seem highly reproducible (intraclass correlation coefficients of 0.70 to 0.82) and correlate strongly with pelvic organ descent at rest and during a Valsalva maneuver.[121] This study was replicated in a Chinese population, with very similar results for repeatability measures and intriguing differences in

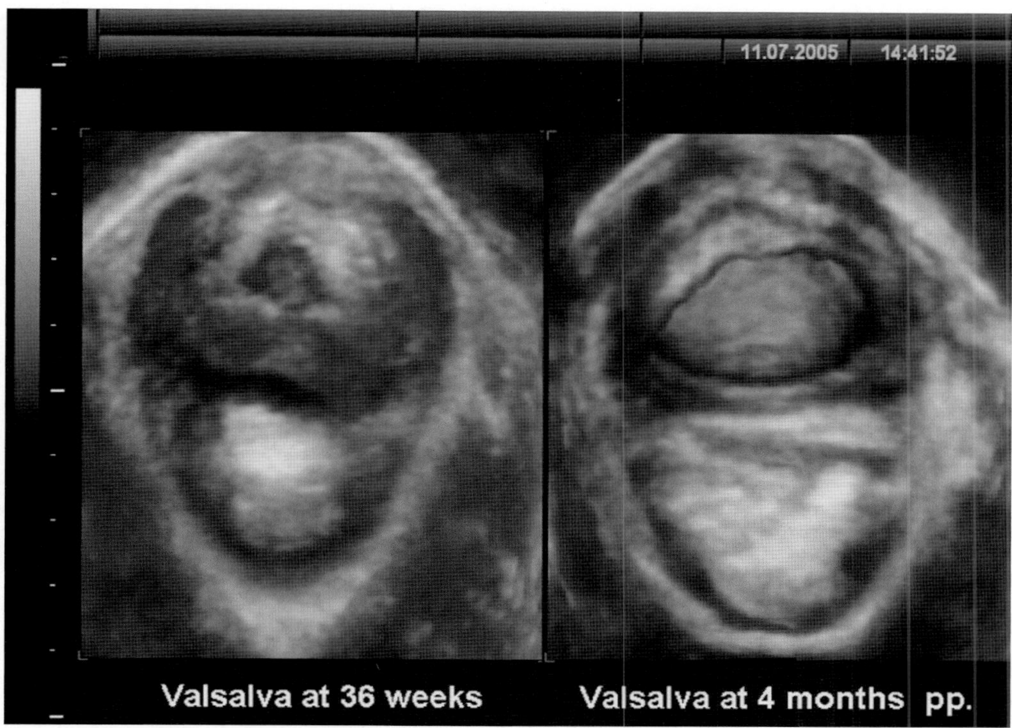

Figure 9-27 Hiatal appearance in a patient during a Valsalva maneuver. At 36 weeks, the hiatus measured 25 cm², and this had increased to 32 cm² 4 months after a normal vaginal delivery.

the shape of the hiatus.[122] Other investigators have confirmed good repeatability of this technique[123-125], and a comparison with measures obtained on magnetic resonance imaging showed high levels of agreement.[126]

Although it is not surprising that the hiatal area during a Valsalva maneuver correlates with descent (because downward displacement of organs may displace the levator laterally), it is much more interesting that hiatal area at rest seems associated with pelvic organ descent during a Valsalva maneuver. These data constitute the first real evidence for the hypothesis that the state of the levator ani is important for pelvic organ support,[127] even in the absence of levator trauma. Relative enlargement of the hiatus during Valsalva maneuvers, or rather distention or elongation of its muscular component, may be a measure of compliance or elasticity and seems to correlate with resting tone as determined by palpation.[128] The population distribution for hiatal area enlargement during Valsalva maneuvers in nulligravid white women seems to be remarkably wide, with measurements from 6 to 36 cm² in one study.[121] The 95th percentile of the distribution seems to lie at about 25 cm², and based on this and receiver operator characteristics,[129] the author considers hiatal enlargement in excess of this cutoff to be ballooning of the hiatus, indicating abnormal biomechanical properties. Figure 9-27 shows a case of de novo ballooning of the hiatus after vaginal childbirth. It is not clear whether such changes are due to myopathy, neuropathy or microtrauma to connective tissue structures. Pelvic floor compliance or distensibility deserves further study because it may be important for the progress of labor and in the diagnosis and treatment of pelvic organ prolapse. In fact, it is likely that surgical reduction of the levator hiatus, now feasible as a minimally invasive technique, will become an entirely new concept in pelvic reconstructive surgery.

The most common form of levator trauma, a unilateral avulsion of the pubococcygeus muscle off the pelvic side wall, is related to childbirth (Figs. 9-28 to 9-30; see Fig. 9-24) and is generally palpable as an asymmetric loss of substance in the inferomedial portion of the muscle at the site of its insertion on the pelvic side wall. It is usually occult but may occasionally be observed directly in women after major vaginal tears (see Fig. 9-28). Bilateral defects (see Figs. 9-24 and 9-30) are more difficult to palpate because of the lack of asymmetry and are much less common, probably in the order of 1% to 4% of the vaginally parous population. In one study,[129] the investigators found that more than one third of women delivering vaginally suffered avulsion injuries, an incidence that is unexpectedly high compared with observations in older, symptomatic women.[130]

The clinical significance of such defects is being studied. Our data[130,131] and evidence from MR studies[132,133] suggest that levator avulsion is common (affecting about 15% to 20% of vaginally parous women) and that it is associated with maternal age at first delivery, which is a concern in view of the continuing trend toward delayed childbearing in Western societies. It seems that the likelihood of major levator trauma at vaginal delivery triples during the reproductive years, from 15% at about 18 years of age to 45% at 40 years. Forceps seem to double the risk.[131] Taken together with the increasing likelihood of cesarean section, it seems that the likelihood of a successful vaginal delivery without levator trauma decreases from more than 80% at age 20 to less than 30% at age 40 (our unpublished data).

Levator avulsion is associated with anterior and central compartment prolapses,[117,129,130] and it likely represents the missing link between childbirth and prolapse, but the relationship with bladder dysfunction is not as obvious.[130] The larger a defect

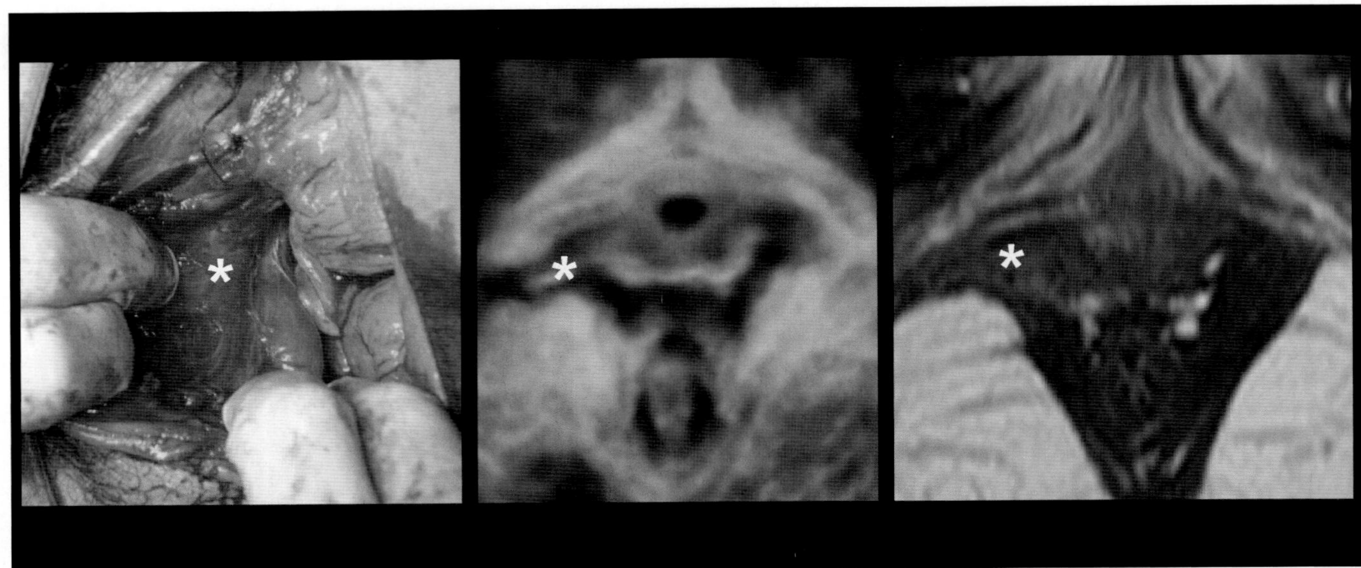

Figure 9-28 A comparison of intrapartum appearances *(left)*, 4D pelvic floor ultrasound findings *(middle)* and magnetic resonance *(right)* imaging in the axial plane after a normal vaginal delivery that resulted in a right-sided levator avulsion *. (MRI courtesy of Dr. Lennox Hoyte, Boston, MA.)

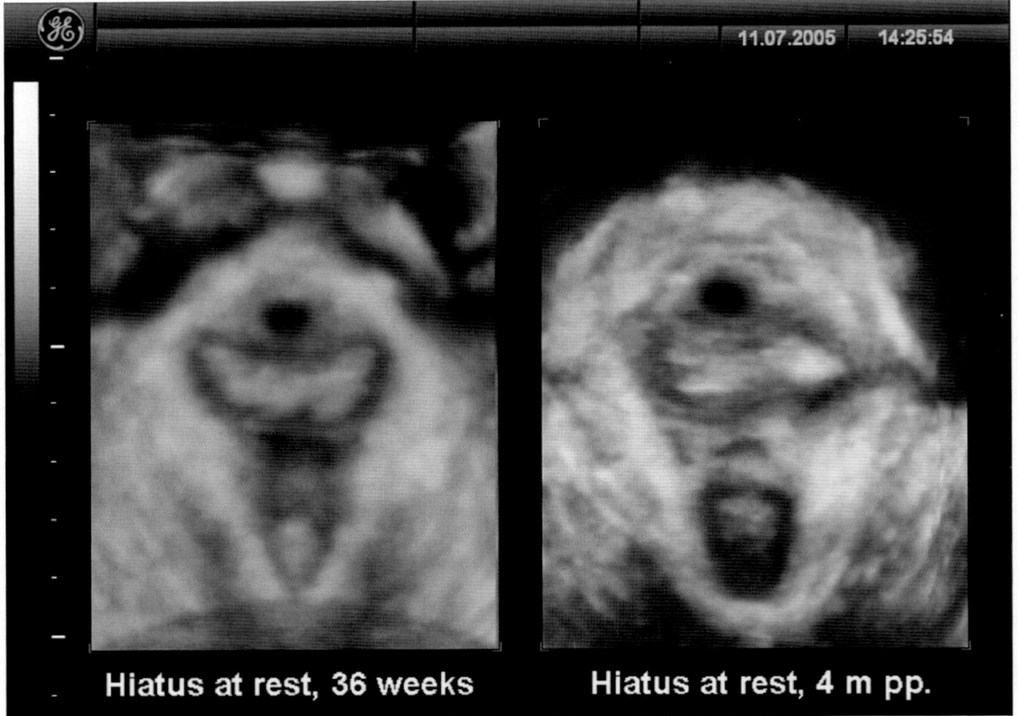

Figure 9-29 Small, left-sided, unilateral levator avulsion. Normal antepartum findings are shown on the *left*, and the postpartum state is demonstrated on the *right*.

(width and depth), the more likely are symptoms and signs of prolapse.[117] However, cross-sectional studies of levator anatomy in asymptomatic and symptomatic older women are needed to determine whether such abnormalities are associated with clinical symptoms or conditions in the general population. Another interesting question is whether major morphologic abnormalities of the levator ani affect surgical outcomes. A study using MRI demonstrated that recurrence after anterior colporrhaphy was much more likely in women with levator trauma.[135] From our experience, it appears that major levator trauma (i.e., avulsion of the puborectalis or pubococcygeus from the pelvic side wall) is associated with early presentation and recurrent prolapse after surgical repair. If this is the case, we should create in vitro models for such trauma and start thinking about surgical intervention.

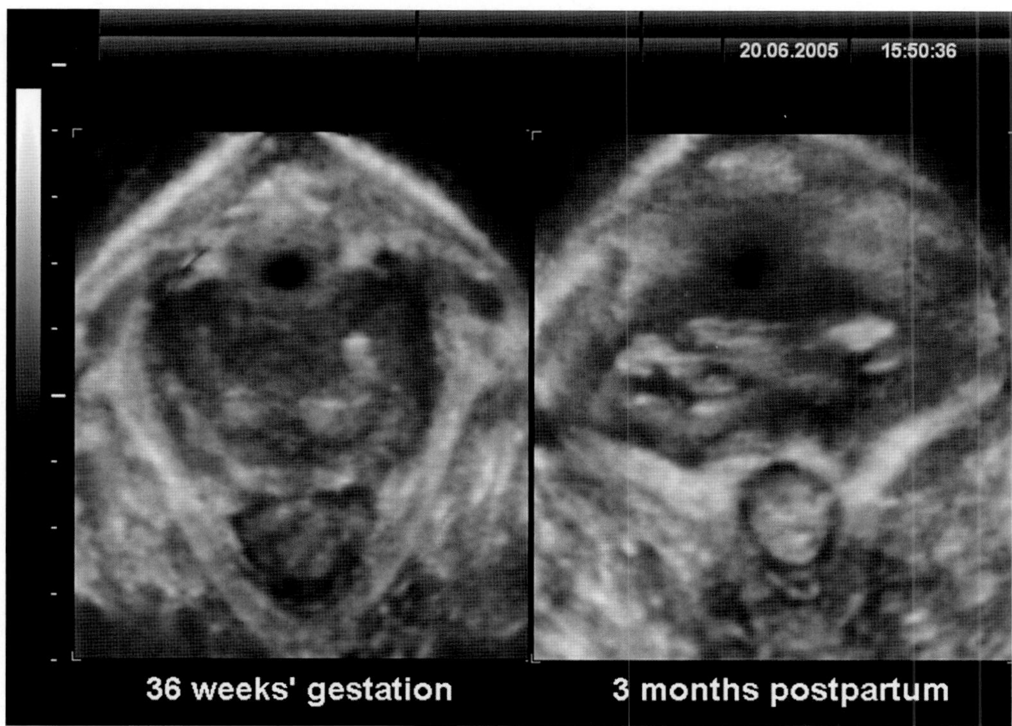

Figure 9-30 Major bilateral levator avulsion. Normal antepartum findings are shown on the *left*, and the postpartum state is demonstrated on the *right*.

The presence of levator avulsion may indicate the need for something other than conventional surgical management.

Three-Dimensional Imaging of Paravaginal Supports

It has been assumed that anterior vaginal wall prolapse and stress urinary incontinence are at least partly caused by disruption of paravaginal and paraurethral support structures (i.e., endopelvic fascia and pubourethral ligaments) at the time of vaginal delivery. In a pilot study using the now-obsolete technology of freehand acquisition of 3D volumes, alterations in paravaginal supports were observed in 5 of 21 women seen before and after delivery, and the interobserver variability of the qualitative assessment of paravaginal supports was shown to be good.[98] In light of current knowledge, the loss of tenting documented in this study was probably at least partly caused by levator avulsion. Paravaginal tissues also can be assessed by transrectal or transvaginal 3D ultrasound using probes designed for pelvic or prostatic imaging.[14] One study using transrectal, high-frequency, 3D ultrasound suggested that defects of the subvesical or paravaginal fascia might be similar in appearance to striae gravidarum, making direct surgical repair impractical.[136]

Three-Dimensional Imaging of Prolapse

The downward displacement of pelvic organs during a Valsalva maneuver in itself does not require MRI or ultrasound 3D imaging technology. Descent of the urethra, bladder, cervix, cul-de-sac, and rectum is easily documented in the midsagittal plane.[76] However, rendered volumes may allow a complete 3D visualization of a cystocele or rectocele (Figs. 9-31 to 9-33) and help with operative planning. When processed into rotational volumes, hyperechoic structures such as a rectocele become particularly evident (see Fig. 9-33). The ease with which preoperative and postoperative data can be compared with the help of stored imaging volumes can be especially useful in audit activities.

Three-Dimensional Imaging of Synthetic Implant Materials

The imaging of synthetic implants may prove to be a major factor in the uptake of this new investigational technique into clinical practice. Suburethral slings such as the TVT, SPARC, IVS, Monarc, and TOT have become very popular during the past 10 years[137-139] and have become the primary anti-incontinence procedure in many developed countries. These slings are not without their problems, even if biocompatibility is markedly better than for previously used synthetic slings, and they differ in some important aspects. Imaging may be indicated in research to determine the location and function of such slings and possibly for assessing in vivo biomechanical characteristics. Clinically, complications such as sling failure, voiding dysfunction, erosion, and postoperative symptoms of the irritable bladder may benefit from imaging assessment. Often, patients do not remember the exact nature of an incontinence or prolapse procedure, and implants may be identified in women who are not aware of their presence or type.

Most modern synthetic implant materials are highly echogenic; TVT Sparc, TVT-O, Monarc and TOT are usually more visible than the IVS sling. Implants can be located with 3D ultrasound, usually over most of thier intrapelvic course.[140] (Fig 9-34). Variations in placement, such as asymmetry, varying width, the effect of tape division, and tape twisting, can be visualized. The difference between transobturator tapes and the TVT-type

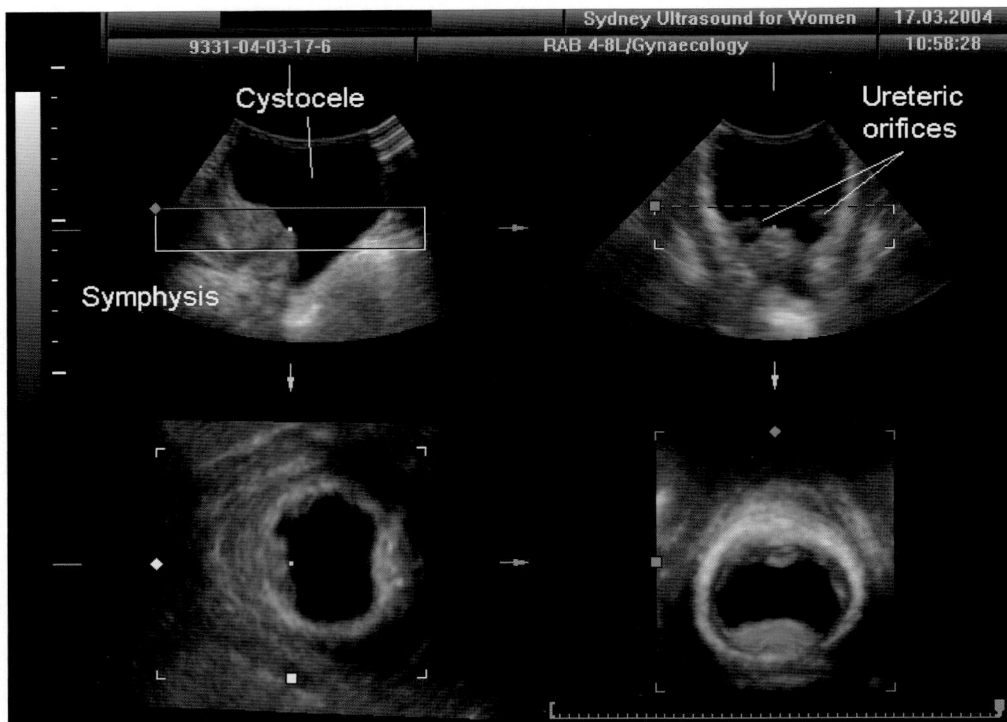

Figure 9-31 A large cystocele *(arrow)* is seen in the three standard planes (sagittal, *top left;* coronal, *top right*; axial, *bottom left*) and in a rendered image (axial, caudocranial rendering), showing a view through the cystocele onto the bladder roof. Reproduced from Textbook of Female Urology and Urogynecology, Chapter 26; Informa Healthcare, Abingdon UK, 2006.

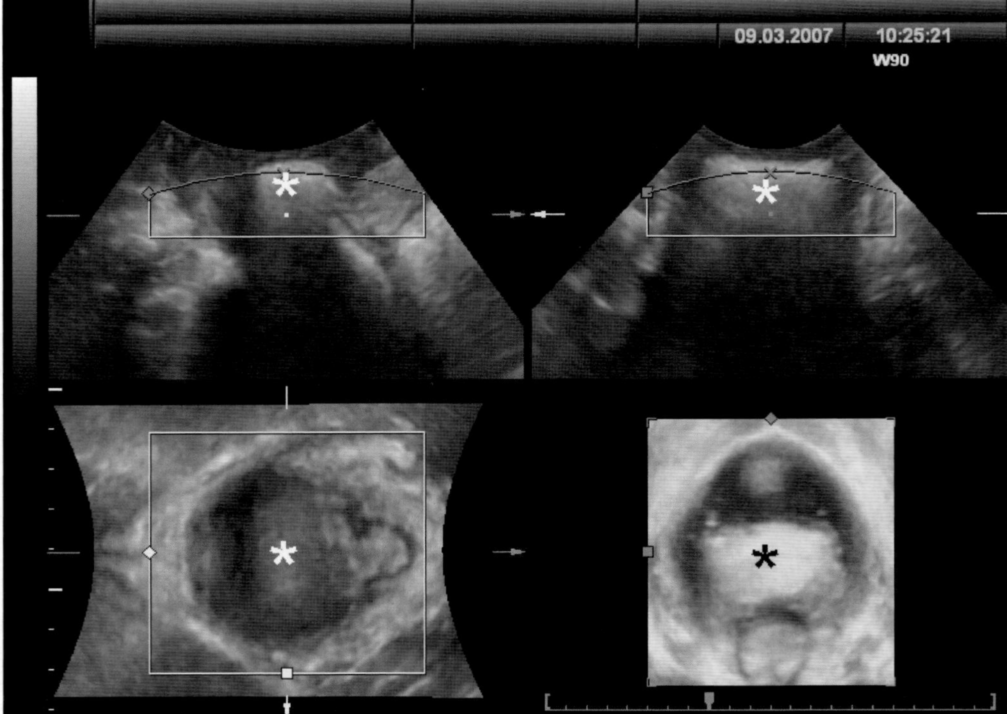

Figure 9-32 Second-degree true rectocele imaged in the three orthogonal planes and a rendered volume *(bottom right)*. Stars indicate the rectocele, showing it to be symmetrical, arising from the anorectal junction, and filling most of the hiatus.

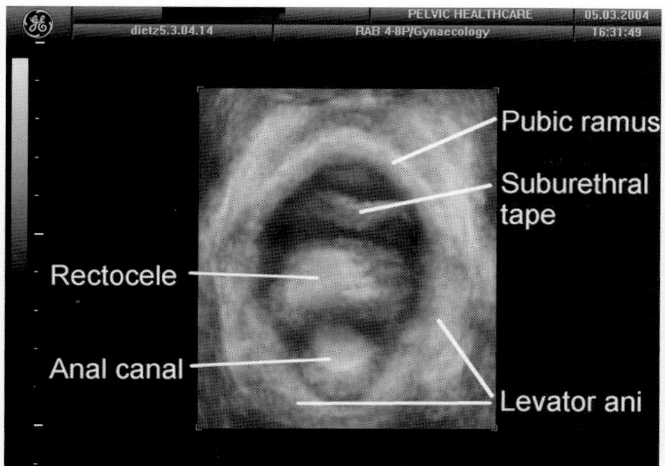

Figure 9-33 A rectocele is shown in a rendered volume of the levator hiatus during a Valsalva maneuver. Reproduced from Textbook of Female Urology and Urogynecology, Chapter 26, Informa Healthcare, Abingdon UK, 2006.

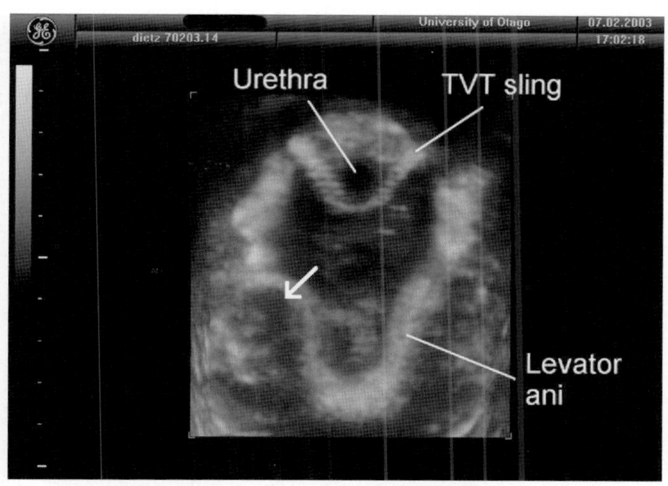

Figure 9-34 The tension-free vaginal tape (TVT) sling is imaged on an oblique rendered volume of the levator hiatus. The mesh structure of the tape is clearly visible. There is also a very unusual local abnormality of the levator on the patient's right side (i.e., left side of the image, *arrow*). Reproduced from Obstet Gynecol 2004; 23:615-625, with permission.

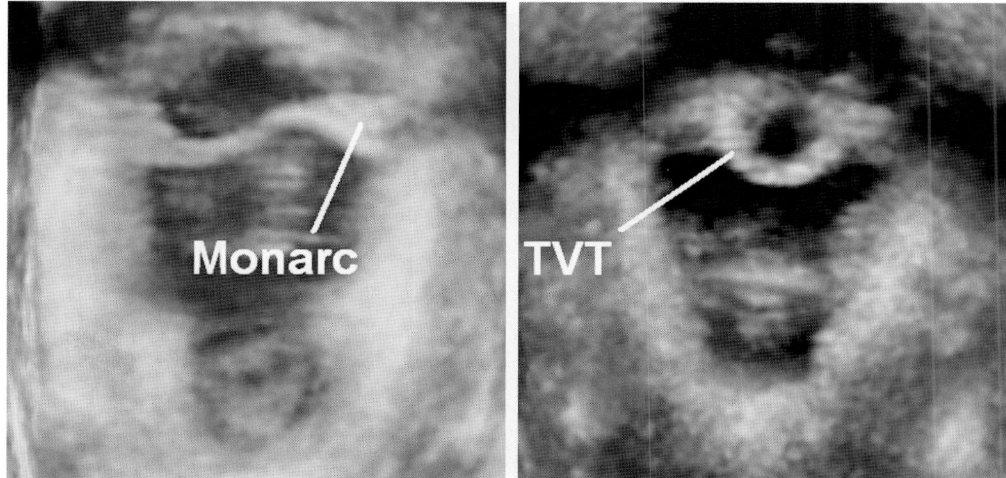

Figure 9-35 Monarc sling (left) compared with tension-free vaginal tape (TVT) sling in rendered volumes of the levator hiatus. Notice the difference in placement. The Monarc sling is inserted through the obturator foramen, and the TVT sling is inserted through the space of Retzius. As a result, the TVT sling arms are situated much more medially. Reproduced from Obstet Gynecol 2004; 23:615-625, with permission.

implants, which is difficult to distinguish on 2D imaging, is readily apparent in the axial plane (Fig. 9-35). It is therefore likely that 3D imaging will turn out to be very helpful in the assessment of patients with suburethral slings.

The same holds true for mesh implants used in prolapse surgery. There is a worldwide trend toward mesh implantation, especially for recurrent prolapse, and complications such as failure and mesh erosion are not uncommon.[141,142] Polypropylene meshes such as the Perigee, Prolift, and Apogee are highly echogenic, and their visibility is limited only by persistent prolapse and transducer distance. Translabial 3D ultrasound has demonstrated that the implanted mesh often does not remain as flat as it was on implantation (Fig. 9-36).[143] Surgical technique seems to play some role, because fixation of mesh to underlying tissues results in a flatter, more even appearance (Fig. 9-37). The position, extent, and mobility of anterior vaginal wall mesh can be determined and may sometimes uncover complications such as dislodgment of anchoring arms.[94]

Translabial 4D ultrasound can be useful in determining functional outcome and the location of implants, and it can help in optimizing implant design and surgical technique. Although it is not much more than an afterthought in this age of minimally invasive slings, most of the injectables used in anti-incontinence surgery are highly echogenic and can be visualized as a hyperechoic donut shape surrounding the urethra (Fig. 9-38).

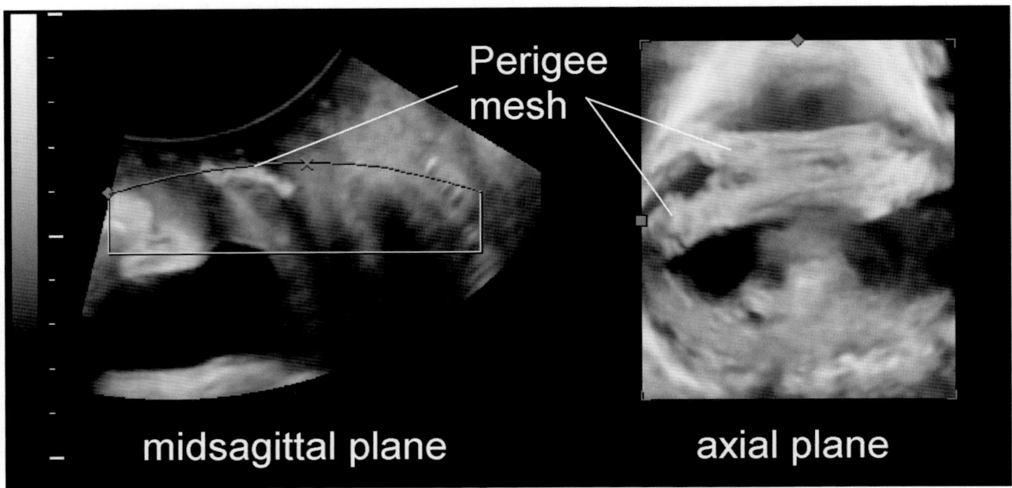

Figure 9-36 A Perigee transobturator mesh implant is imaged in the midsagittal plane *(left)* and as an oblique axial rendered volume *(right)*. Reproduced from ASUM Bulletin 2007; 10:17-23, with permission.

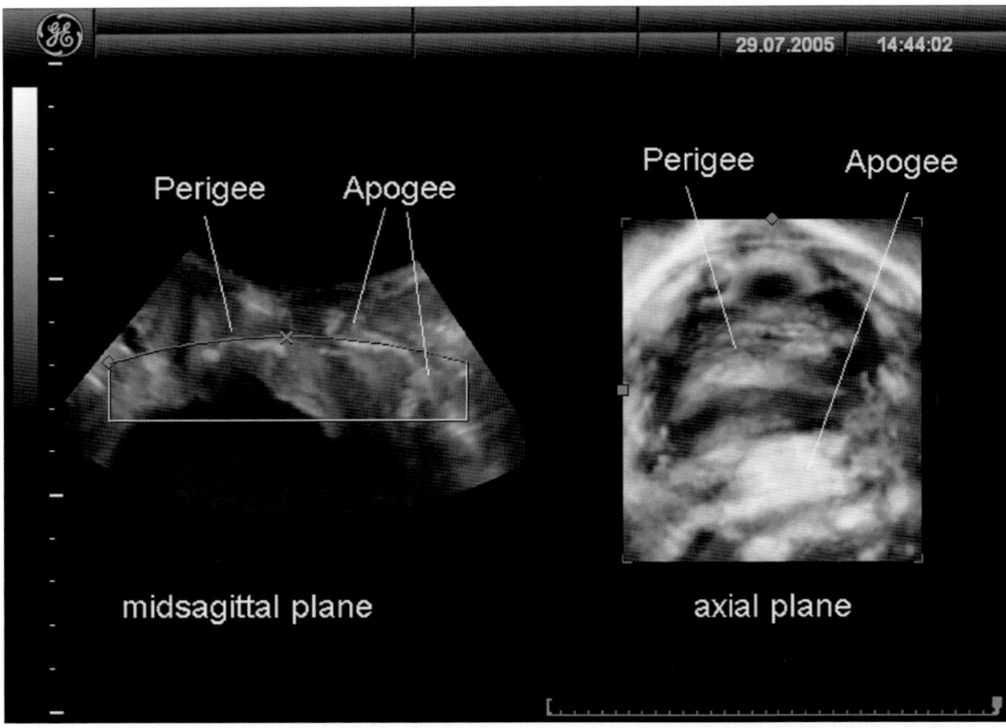

Figure 9-37 Perigee and Apogee mesh implants are seen in a patient with massive levator ballooning, and despite this, prolapse repair was successful. Both implants appear flat and smooth, and both are functional, blocking a large part of the hiatus during a Valsalva maneuver.

CONCLUSIONS

Ultrasound imaging, particularly translabial or transperineal ultrasound, is becoming the new diagnostic standard in urogynecology. Several factors have contributed to its acceptance, but the most important is the availability of suitable equipment. Developments such as the assessment of levator activity and prolapse and the use of color Doppler to document urine leakage enhance the clinical usefulness of the method. Increasing standardization of parameters should make it easier for clinicians and researchers to compare data.

The convenience with which pretreatment and post-treatment imaging data is obtained can simplify outcome studies after prolapse and incontinence surgery. Ultrasound imaging may be able to significantly enhance our understanding of the different mechanisms by which conservative and surgical methods achieve—or fail to achieve—continence. It may even be possible to identify distinct fascial defects, such as defects of the rectovaginal septum in true rectoceles, which should generate new surgical possibilities.

Regardless of which methodology is used to determine descent of pelvic organs, it is evident that there is a wide variation in

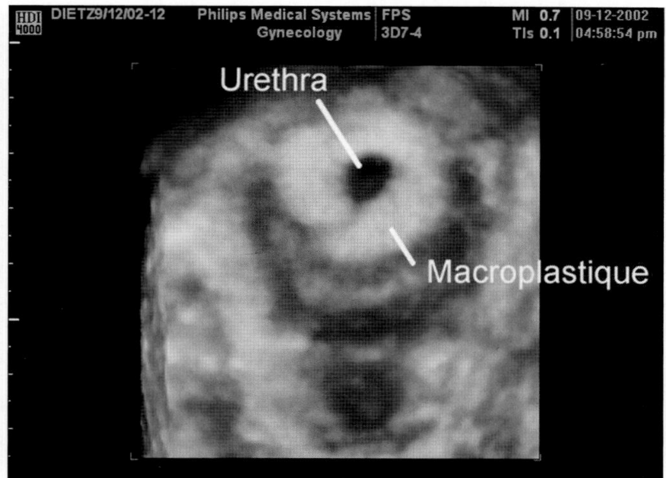

Figure 9-38 Macroplastique as demonstrated in a rendered axial volume, axial plane, surrounding the uretha in a donut shape. Figure reproduced from Obstet Gynecol 2004; 23:615-625, with permission.

pelvic organ mobility, even in young, nulliparous women. This variation is likely to be at least partly genetic in origin. Ultrasound imaging allows quantification of the phenotype of pelvic organ prolapse, which will facilitate molecular and population genetic approaches to evaluate the cause of pelvic floor and bladder dysfunction.

Childbirth causes significant alterations of pelvic organ support and levator structure and function, and there is some relationship between the prior state of pelvic organ supports and labor outcome. Pelvic floor ultrasound can help us in identify women at high risk of emergency operative delivery,[144] and in the future we will be able to predict significant pelvic floor trauma. It remains to be seen, however, whether such information can have a positive effect on clinical outcomes in what is no doubt a highly politicized environment.

The use of 3D volume ultrasound adds several dimensions to pelvic floor imaging, particularly in its most recent incarnations using automatic volume acquisition, 4D cine volume ultrasound, SRI techniques, and TUI. Spatial resolutions now equal or exceed those obtained on static MRI, and temporal resolutions are far superior, although most clinicians working in this field are largely unaware of recent developments because of a traditional lack of access to imaging techniques. The technology opens up new possibilities for observing functional anatomy and examining muscular and fascial structures of the pelvic floor. Data acquisition can be simplified and research capabilities enhanced, and surgical audits in this field are likely to undergo a significant change. Modern imaging will allow us to optimize current surgical techniques and to develop new ones.

There is no evidence to prove that modern imaging techniques can improve outcomes in pelvic floor medicine for patients. However, this limitation is true for many diagnostic modalities in clinical medicine. Because of methodologic problems, the situation is unlikely to improve soon. In the meantime, it must be recognized that any diagnostic method is only as good as the operator behind the machine, and diagnostic ultrasound is well known for its operator-dependent nature. Training is essential to ensure that imaging techniques are used appropriately and effectively.

Acknowledgments

This chapter is based on three review articles published in *Ultrasound in Obstetrics and Gynecology*, John Wiley & Sons, 2004.

References

1. Schubert E: Topographie des Uterus und der Harnblase im Roentgenprofilbild. Zentralbl Gynakol 53:1182-1193, 1929.
2. Mikulicz-Radecki J: Roentgenologische Studien zur Aetiologie der urethralen Inkontinenz. Zentralbl Gynakol 55:795-810, 1931.
3. Jeffcoate TNA, Roberts H: Observations on stress incontinence of urine. Am J Obstet Gynecol 64:721-738, 1952.
4. Hodgkinson CP: "Recurrent" stress urinary incontinence. Am J Obstet Gynecol 132:844-860, 1978.
5. Noll LE, Hutch JA: The SCIPP line—An aid in interpreting the voiding lateral cystourethrogram. Obstet Gynecol 33:680-689, 1969.
6. Richter K: Die Bedeutung der radiologischen Beckenviszerographie für eine rationelle Therapie der weiblichen Stressinkontinenz. Geburtshilfe Frauenheilkd 47:509-517, 1987.
7. White RD, McQuown D, McCarthy TA, Ostergard DR: Real-time ultrasonography in the evaluation of urinary stress incontinence. Am J Obstet Gynecol 138:235-237, 1980.
8. Bernaschek G, Spernol R, Wolf G, Kratochwil A: Comparative determination of the vesico-urethral angle in incontinence via ultrasound and lateral urethro-cystogram [in German]. Geburtshilfe Frauenheilkd 41:339-342, 1981.
9. Kohorn EI, Scioscia AL, Jeanty P, Hobbins JC: Ultrasound cystourethrography by perineal scanning for the assessment of female stress urinary incontinence. Obstet Gynecol 68:269-272, 1986.
10. Grischke EM, Dietz HP, Jeanty P, Schmidt W. A new study method: The perineal scan in obstetrics and gynecology [in German]. Ultraschall Med 7:154-161, 1986.
11. Bergman A, McKenzie CJ, Richmond J, et al: Transrectal ultrasound versus cystography in the evaluation of anatomical stress urinary incontinence. Br J Urol 62:228-234, 1988.
12. Quinn MJ, Beynon J, Mortensen NJ, Smith PJ: Transvaginal endosonography: A new method to study the anatomy of the lower urinary tract in urinary stress incontinence. Br J Urol 62:414-418, 1988.
13. Khullar V, Cardozo L: Three-dimensional ultrasound in urogynecology. In Merz E (ed): 3-D Ultrasound in Obstetrics and Gynecology. Philadelphia, Lippincott Williams & Wilkins Healthcare, 1998, pp 65-71.
14. Wisser J, Schaer G, Kurmanavicius J, et al: Use of 3D ultrasound as a new approach to assess obstetrical trauma to the pelvic floor. Ultraschall Med 20:15-18, 1999.
15. Timor-Tritsch IE, Platt LD: Three-dimensional ultrasound experience in obstetrics [review]. Curr Opin Obstet Gynecol 14:569-575, 2002.
16. Tunn R, Petri E: Introital and transvaginal ultrasound as the main tool in the assessment of urogenital and pelvic floor dysfunction: An imaging panel and practical approach. Ultrasound Obstet Gynecol 22:205-213, 2003.
17. Dietz HP, Wilson PD: Anatomical assessment of the bladder outlet and proximal urethra using ultrasound and videocystourethrography. Neurourol Urodyn 15:363-364, 1996.
18. Gordon D, Pearce M, Norton P, Stanton SL: Comparison of ultrasound and lateral chain urethrocystography in the determination of bladder neck descent. Am J Obstet Gynecol 160:182-185, 1989.

19. Koelbl H, Bernaschek G, Wolf G: A comparative study of perineal ultrasound scanning and urethrocystography in patients with genuine stress incontinence. Arch Gynecol Obstet 244:39-45, 1988.
20. Voigt R, Halaska M, Michels W, et al: Examination of the urethrovesical junction using perineal sonography compared to urethrocystography using a bead chain. Int Urogynecol J 5:212-214. 1994.
21. Grischke EM, Anton HW, Dietz P, Schmidt W: Perinealsonographie und roentgenologische Verfahren im Rahmen der weiblichen Harninkontinenzdiagnostik. Geburtshilfe Frauenheilkd 49:733-736, 1989.
22. Ammann ME, Winkelbauer F, Fitzal P: The urethrocystogram and perineal sonography compared [in German]. Rofo Fortschr Geb Rontgenstr Neuen Bildgeb Verfahr 156:309-312, 1992.
23. Schaer GN, Siegwart R, Perucchini D, DeLancey JO: Examination of voiding in seated women using a remote-controlled ultrasound probe. Obstet Gynecol 91:297-301, 1998.
24. Schaer GN, Koechli OR, Schuessler B, Haller U: Perineal ultrasound for evaluating the bladder neck in urinary stress incontinence. Obstet Gynecol 85:220-224, 1995.
25. Dietz HP, Wilson PD: The influence of bladder volume on the position and mobility of the urethrovesical junction. Int Urogynecol J 10:3-6, 1999.
26. Dietz HP, Clarke B: The influence of posture on perineal ultrasound imaging parameters. Int Urogynecol J 12:104-106, 2001.
27. Alper T, Cetinkaya M, Okutgen S, et al: Evaluation of urethrovesical angle by ultrasound in women with and without urinary stress incontinence. Int Urogynecol J 12:308-311, 2001.
28. Martan A, Halaska M, Voigt R, Drbohlav B: Ultrasound of the bladder neck-urethra transition before and after pelvic floor training with Kolpexin [in German]. Zentralbl Gynakol 116:416-418, 1994.
29. Martan A, Masata J, Halaska M, Voigt R: Ultrasound imaging of the lower urinary system in women after Burch colposuspension. Ultrasound Obstet Gynecol 17:58-64, 2001.
30. Dietz HP, Clarke B, Herbison P: Bladder neck mobility and urethral closure pressure as predictors of genuine stress incontinence. Int Urogynecol J 13:289-293, 2002.
31. Dietz HP, Eldridge A, Grace M, Clarke B: Test-retest reliability of the ultrasound assessment of bladder neck mobility. Int Urogynecol J 14(Suppl 1):S57-S58, 2003.
32. Mouritsen L, Bach P: Ultrasonic evaluation of bladder neck position and mobility: The influence of urethral catheter, bladder volume, and body position. Neurourol Urodyn 13:637-646, 1994.
33. Schaer GN, Koechli OR, Schuessler B, Haller U: Perineal ultrasound: Determination of reliable examination procedures. Ultrasound Obstet Gynecol 7:347-352, 1996.
34. Reed H, Waterfield A, Freeman RM, Adekanmi OA: Bladder neck mobility in continent nulliparous women: Normal references. Int Urogynecol J 13:S4, 2002.
35. Brandt FT, Albuquerque CD, Lorenzato FR, Amaral FJ: Perineal assessment of urethrovesical junction mobility in young continent females. Int Urogynecol J 11:18-22, 2000.
36. Peschers UM, Fanger G, Schaer GN, et al: Bladder neck mobility in continent nulliparous women. Br J Obstet Gynaecol 108:320-324, 2001.
37. Dietz HP, Eldridge A, Grace M, Clarke B: Normal values for pelvic organ descent in healthy nulligravid young Caucasian women. Neurourol Urodyn 22:420-421, 2003.
38. King JK, Freeman RM: Is antenatal bladder neck mobility a risk factor for postpartum stress incontinence? Br J Obstet Gynaecol 105:1300-1307, 1998.
39. Martan A, Masata J, Halaska M, et al: The effect of increasing of intraabdominal pressure on the position of the bladder neck in ultrasound imaging. In: Proceedings of the 30th Annual Meeting, International Continence Society; 2001, Seoul, South Korea.
40. Schaer GN, Perucchini D, Munz E, et al: Sonographic evaluation of the bladder neck in continent and stress-incontinent women. Obstet Gynecol 93:412-416, 1999.
41. Dietz HP, Clarke B: The urethral pressure profile and ultrasound imaging of the lower urinary tract. Int Urogynecol J 12:38-41, 2001.
42. Huang WC, Yang JM: Bladder neck funneling on ultrasound cystourethrography in primary stress urinary incontinence: A sign associated with urethral hypermobility and intrinsic sphincter deficiency. Urology 61:936-941, 2003.
43. Green TH: Urinary stress incontinence: Differential diagnosis, pathophysiology, and management. Am J Obstet Gynecol 122:378-400, 1975.
44. Dietz HP, Hansell N, Grace M, et al: Bladder neck mobility is a heritable trait. Br J Obstet Gynaecol 112:334-339, 2005.
45. Peschers U, Schaer G, Anthuber C, et al: Changes in vesical neck mobility following vaginal delivery. Obstet Gynecol 88:1001-1006, 1996.
46. Meyer S, Schreyer A, De Grandi P, Hohlfeld P: The effects of birth on urinary continence mechanisms and other pelvic-floor characteristics. Obstet Gynecol 92:613-618, 1998.
47. Dietz HP, Bennett MJ: The effect of childbirth on pelvic organ mobility [comment]. Obstet Gynecol 102:223-228, 2003.
48. Dietz HP, Clarke B, Vancaillie TG: Vaginal childbirth and bladder neck mobility. Aust N Z J Obstet Gynaecol 42:522-525, 2002.
49. Digesu GA, Toosz-Hobson P, Bidmead J, et al: Pregnancy, childbirth and urinary incontinence: Caesarean for all? Neurourol Urodyn 19:508-509, 2000.
50. Dietz HP, Moore KH, Steensma AB: Antenatal pelvic organ mobility is associated with delivery mode. Aust N Z J Obstet Gynaecol 43:70-74, 2003.
51. Balmforth J, Toosz-Hobson P, Cardozo L: Ask not what childbirth can do to your pelvic floor but what your pelvic floor can do in childbirth. Neurourol Urodyn 22:540-542, 2003.
52. Reilly ET, Freeman RM, Waterfield MR, et al: Prevention of postpartum stress incontinence in primigravidae with increased bladder neck mobility: A randomised controlled trial of antenatal pelvic floor exercises. BJOG 109:68-76, 2002.
53. Dietz HP, Steensma AB: Which women are most affected by delivery-related changes in pelvic organ mobility? Eur J Obstet Gynecol Reprod Biol 111:15-18, 2003.
54. Kim SJ, Choi JH, Kim DK, Lee KS: The significance of an open bladder neck in the evaluation of the female stress urinary incontinence. Int Urogynecol J 10(Suppl 1):S59, 1999.
55. Schaer GN, Koechli OR, Schuessler B, Haller U: Improvement of perineal sonographic bladder neck imaging with ultrasound contrast medium. Obstet Gynecol 86:950-954, 1995.
56. Schaer GN, Koechli OR, Schuessler B, Haller U: Usefulness of ultrasound contrast medium in perineal sonography for visualization of bladder neck funneling—First observations. Urology 47:452-453, 1996.
57. Masata J, Martan A, Halaska M, et al: Ultrasound imaging of urethral funneling. Int Urogynecol J 10(Suppl 1):S62, 1999.
58. Dietz HP, McKnoulty L, Clarke B: Translabial color Doppler for imaging in urogynecology: A preliminary report. Ultrasound Obstet Gynecol 14:144-147, 1999.
59. Dietz HP, Clarke B: Translabial color Doppler urodynamics. Int Urogynecol J 12:304-307, 2001.
60. Masata J, Martan A, Halaska M, et al: Detection of Valsalva leak point pressure with colour Doppler—New method for routine use. Neurourol Urodyn 20:494-496, 2001.
61. Khullar V, Cardozo LD, Salvatore S, Hill S: Ultrasound: A non-invasive screening test for detrusor instability. Br J Obstet Gynaecol 103:904-908, 1996.
62. Khullar V. Ultrasonography. In Cardozo L, Staskin D (eds): Textbook of Female Urology and Urogynaecology. London, Isis Medical Media, 2001, pp 300-312.

63. Robinson D, Anders K, Cardozo L, et al: Can ultrasound replace ambulatory urodynamics when investigating women with irritative urinary symptoms? Br J Obstet Gynaecol 109:145-148, 2002.
64. Yang JM, Huang WC: Bladder wall thickness on ultrasound cystourethrography. J Ultrasound Med 22:777-782, 2003.
65. Soligo M, Khullar V, Salvatore S, Luppino G, et al: Overactive bladder definition and ultrasound measurement of bladder wall thickness: The right way without urodynamics. Neurourol Urodyn 21:284-285, 2002.
66. Wijma J, Tinga DJ, Visser GH: Perineal ultrasonography in women with stress incontinence and controls: The role of the pelvic floor muscles. Gynecol Obstet Invest 32:176-179, 1991.
67. Peschers UM, Schaer GN, DeLancey JO, Schuessler B: Levator ani function before and after childbirth. Br J Obstet Gynaecol 104:1004-1008, 1997.
68. Dietz HP: Levator function before and after childbirth. Aust N Z J Obstet Gynaecol 44:19-23, 2004.
69. DeLancey JO: Stress urinary incontinence: Where are we now, where should we go? Am J Obstet Gynecol 175:311-319, 1996.
70. Dietz HP, Wilson PD, Clarke B: The use of perineal ultrasound to quantify levator activity and teach pelvic floor muscle exercises. Int Urogynecol J 12:166-168; discussion 168-169, 2001.
71. Miller JM, Perucchini D, Carchidi LT, et al: Pelvic floor muscle contraction during a cough and decreased vesical neck mobility. Obstet Gynecol 97:255-260, 2001.
72. Dietz HP, Jarvis SK, Vancaillie TG: The assessment of levator muscle strength: A validation of three ultrasound techniques. Int Urogynecol J 13:156-159, 2002.
73. Creighton SM, Pearce JM, Stanton SL: Perineal videoultrasonography in the assessment of vaginal prolapse: Early observations. Br J Obstet Gynaecol 99:310-313, 1992.
74. Petri E, Koelbl H, Schaer G: What is the place of ultrasound in urogynecology? A written panel. Int Urogynecol J 10:262-273, 1999.
75. Bump RC, Mattiasson A, Bø K, et al: The standardization of terminology of female pelvic organ prolapse and pelvic floor dysfunction. Am J Obstet Gynecol 175:10-17, 1996.
76. Dietz HP, Haylen BT, Broome J: Ultrasound in the quantification of female pelvic organ prolapse. Ultrasound Obstet Gynecol 18:511-514, 2001.
77. Dietz HP, Steensma A: The role of childbirth in the aetiology of rectocele. Br J Obstet Gynaecol 2006; 113:264-267, 2006.
78. Beer-Gabel M, Teshler M, Barzilai N, et al: Dynamic transperineal ultrasound in the diagnosis of pelvic floor disorders: Pilot study. Dis Colon Rectum 45:239-245, 2002.
79. Peschers UM, DeLancey JO, Schaer GN, Schuessler B: Exoanal ultrasound of the anal sphincter: Normal anatomy and sphincter defects. Br J Obstet Gynaecol 104:999-1003, 1997.
80. Starck M, Bohe M, Valentin L: The extent of endosonographic anal sphincter defects after primary repair of obstetric sphincter tears increases over time and is related to anal incontinence. Ultrasound Obstet Gynaecol 27:188-197, 2006.
81. Mouritsen L, Bernstein I. Vaginal ultrasonography: A diagnostic tool for urethral diverticulum. Acta Obstet Gynecol Scand 75:188-190, 1996.
82. Siegel CL, Middleton WD, Teefey SA, et al: Sonography of the female urethra. AJR Am J Roentgenol 170:1269-1274, 1998.
83. Bombieri L, Freeman RM: Do bladder neck position and amount of elevation influence the surgical outcome of colposuspension? Neurourol Urodyn 18:316-317, 1999.
84. Viereck V, Pauer HU, Bader W, et al: Introital ultrasound of the lower genital tract before and after colposuspension: A 4-year objective follow-up. Ultrasound Obstet Gynecol 23:277-283, 2004.
85. Dietz HP, Wilson PD, Gillies K, Vancaillie TG: How does the TVT achieve continence? Neurourol Urodyn 19:393-394, 2000.
86. Lo TS, Wang AC, Horng SG, et al: Ultrasonographic and urodynamic evaluation after tension free vagina tape procedure (TVT). Acta Obstet Gynecol Scand 80:65-70, 2001.
87. Martan A, Masata J, Svabik K, Halaska M, Voigt P: The ultrasound imaging of the tape after TVT procedure. Neurourol Urodyn 21:322-324, 2002.
88. Masata J, Martan A, Kasikova E, et al: Ultrasound study of the effect of TVT operation on the mobility of the whole urethra. Neurourol Urodyn 21:286-288, 2002.
89. Geiss IM, Dungl A, Riss PA: Position of the prolene tape after TVT—A sonographic and urodynamic study. Int Urogynecol J 11: S30, 2000.
90. Dietz HP, Mouritsen L, Ellis G, Wilson P: How important is TVT location? Acta Obstet Gynecol Scand 83:904-908, 2004.
91. Dietz HP, Mouritsen L, Ellis G, Wilson PD: Does the tension-free vaginal tape stay where you put it? Am J Obstet Gynecol 188:950-953, 2003.
92. Lo TS, Horng SG, Liang CC, et al: Ultrasound assessment of mid-urethra tape at three-year follow-up after tension-free vaginal tape procedure. Urology 63:671-675, 2004.
93. Greenland H, Dietz HP, Barry C, Rane A: An independent assessment of the location of the Transobturator (Monarc®) tape in relation to the levator ani muscle using 3 dimensional ultrasound scanning techniques. Int Urogynecol J 16(Suppl 2):S59, 2005.
94. Shek KL, Dietz HP, Rane A: Transobturator mesh anchoring for the repair of large or recurrent cystocele. Neurourol Urodyn 25:554-555, 2006.
95. Fritel X, Zabak K, Pigne A, Benifla J: Predictive value of the urethra mobility before sub-urethra tape procedure for urinary stress incontinence in women. J of Urology 168(6):2472-2475, 2002.
96. Dietz HP, Pang S, Korda A, Benness C: Paravaginal defects: A comparison of clinical examination and 2D/3D ultrasound imaging. Aust N Z J Obstet Gynaecol 45:187-190, 2005.
97. Fortunato P, Schettini M, Gallucci M: Diagnosis and therapy of the female urethral diverticula. Int Urogynecol J 12:51-57, 2001.
98. Dietz HP, Steensma AB: Three-dimensional ultrasound imaging of the pelvic floor: The effect of parturition on paravaginal support structures. Ultrasound Obstet Gynecol 21:589-595, 2003.
99. Gritzky A, Brandl H: The Voluson (Kretz) technique. In Merz E (ed): 3-D Ultrasound in Obstetrics and Gynecology. Philadelphia, Lippincott Williams & Wilkins Healthcare, 1998, pp 9-15.
100. Stetten G, Tamburo R: Real-time three-dimensional ultrasound methods for shape analysis and visualization [review]. Methods 25:221-230, 2001.
101. Koelbl H, Hanzal E: Imaging of the lower urinary tract. Curr Opin Obstet Gynecol 7:382-385, 1995.
102. Schaer GN: Ultrasonography of the lower urinary tract. Curr Opin Obstet Gynecol 9:313-316, 1997.
103. Klutke C, Golomb J, Barbaric Z, Raz S: The anatomy of stress incontinence: Magnetic resonance imaging of the female bladder neck and urethra. J Urol 143:563-566, 1990.
104. Yang A, Mostwin JL, Rosenshein NB, Zerhouni EA: Pelvic floor descent in women: Dynamic evaluation with fast MR imaging and cinematic display. Radiology 179:25-33, 1991.
105. Debus-Thiede G: Magnetic resonance imaging (MRI) of the pelvic floor. In Schuessler B, Laycock J, Norton P, Stanton SL (eds): Pelvic Floor Reeducation—Principles and Practice. London, Springer Verlag, 1994, pp 78-82.
106. Aronson MP, Bates SM, Jacoby AF, et al: Periurethral and paravaginal anatomy: An endovaginal magnetic resonance imaging study. Am J Obstet Gynecol 173:1702-1708, 1995.
107. Dohke M, Mitchell DG, Vasavada SP: Fast magnetic resonance imaging of pelvic organ prolapse [review]. Tech Urol 7:133-138, 2001.
108. Law PA, Danin JC, Lamb GM, et al: Dynamic imaging of the pelvic floor using an open-configuration magnetic resonance scanner. J Magn Reson Imaging 13:923-929, 2001.
109. Lienemann A, Sprenger D, Anthuber C, et al: Functional cine magnetic resonance imaging in women after abdominal sacrocolpopexy. Obstet Gynecol 97:81-85, 2001.

110. Tunn R, DeLancey JO, Howard D, et al: MR imaging of levator ani muscle recovery following vaginal delivery. Int Urogynecol J 10:300-307, 1999.
111. Hoyte L, Schierlitz L, Zou K, et al: Two- and 3-dimensional MRI comparison of levator ani structure, volume, and integrity in women with stress incontinence and prolapse. Am J Obstet Gynecol 185:11-19, 2001.
112. Fielding JR, Dumanli H, Schreyer AG, et al: MR-based three-dimensional modeling of the normal pelvic floor in women: Quantification of muscle mass. AJR Am J Roentgenol 174:657-660, 2000.
113. Tunn R, Paris S, Fischer W, et al: Static magnetic resonance imaging of the pelvic floor muscle morphology in women with stress urinary incontinence and pelvic prolapse. Neurourol Urodyn 17:579-589, 1998.
114. Bo K, Larson S, Oseid S, et al: Knowledge about and ability to do correct pelvic floor muscle exercises in women with urinary stress incontinence. Neurourol Urodyn 7:261-262, 1988.
115. Oerno A, Dietz HP: Levator co-activation is an important confounder of pelvic organ descent on Valsalva maneuver. Ultrasound Obstet Gynecol 30:346-350, 2007.
116. Ruano R, Benachi A, Aubry MC, et al: Volume contrast imaging: A new approach to identify fetal thoracic structures. J Ultrasound Med 23:403-408, 2004.
117. Dietz HP: Quantification of major morphological abnormalities of the levator ani. Ultrasound Obstet Gynecol 29:329-334, 2007.
118. Khullar V, Salvatore S, Cardozo LD: Three dimensional ultrasound of the urethra and urethral pressure profiles. Int Urogynecol J 5:319, 1994.
119. Toozs-Hobson P, Khullar V, Cardozo L: Three-dimensional ultrasound: A novel technique for investigating the urethral sphincter in the third trimester of pregnancy. Ultrasound Obstet Gynecol 17:421-424, 2001.
120. Umek W, Kratochwil A, Obermair A, et al: Three-dimensional ultrasound of the female urethra comparing transvaginal and transrectal scanning. Int Urogynecol J 10(Suppl 1):S109, 1999.
121. Dietz HP, Shek C, Clarke B: Biometry of the pubovisceral muscle and levator hiatus by 3D pelvic floor ultrasound. Ultrasound Obstet Gynaecol 25:580-585, 2005.
122. Yang JM, Yang SH, Huang WC: Biometry of the pubovisceral muscle and levator hiatus in nulliparous Chinese women. Ultrasound Obstet Gynaecol 28:710-716, 2006.
123. Guaderrama N, Liu J, Nager C, et al: Evidence for the innervation of pelvic floor muscles by the pudendal nerve. Obstet Gynecol 106(4):774-781, 2006.
124. Hoff Braekken I, Majida M, Ellstrom Engh M, et al: Test-retest and intra-observer reliability of two-, three-, and four-dimensional perineal ultrasound of pelvic floor muscle anatomy and function. In print, Int Urogynecol J.
125. Kruger J, Dietz HP, Murphy BA: Pelvic floor function in elite nulliparous athletes and controls. Ultrasound Obstet Gynaecol 30(1):81-85, 2007.
126. Kruger J, Dietz HP, Heap S, Murphy B: Comparative study of pelvic floor function in nulliparous women using 3D ultrasound and magnetic resonance imaging. Int Urogynecol J 18(S1):S7, 2007.
127. DeLancey JO: Anatomy. In Cardozo L, Staskin D (eds): Textbook of Female Urology and Urogynaecology. London, Isis Medical Media, 2001, pp 112-124.
128. Thyer I, Dietz HP, Shek KL: Clinical validation of a new imaging method for assessing pelvic floor biomechanics [abstract]. Paper presented at the ISUOG International Meeting, Hong Kong, 2007.
129. De Leon J, Shek KL, Dietz HP: Ballooning: can we define pathological distensibility of the levator hiatus? Int Urogynecol J 18(S1): S102, 2007.
130. Dietz HP, Steensma A: The prevalence and clinical significance of major morphological abnormalities of the levator ani. BJOG 113:225-230, 2006.
131. Dietz HP: Does delayed childbearing increase the risk of levator injury in labour? Neurourol Urodyn (in press).
132. DeLancey JO, Kearney R, Chou Q, et al: The appearance of levator ani muscle abnormalities in magnetic resonance images after vaginal delivery. Obstet Gynecol 101:46-53, 2003.
133. Kearney R, Miller JM, Ashton-Miller JA, Delancey JO: Obstetric factors associated with levator ani muscle injury after vaginal birth. Obstet Gynecol 107:144-149, 2006.
134. Adekanmi B, Freeman R, Puckett M, Jackson S: Cystocele: Does anterior repair fail because we fail to correct the fascial defects? A clinical and radiological study. Int Urogynecol J 16(Suppl 2):S73, 2005.
135. Reisinger E, Stummvoll W. Visualization of the endopelvic fascia by transrectal three-dimensional ultrasound. Int Urogynecol J 17:165-169, 2006.
136. Ulmsten U, Falconer C, Johnson P, et al: A multicenter study of tension-free vaginal tape (TVT) for surgical treatment of stress urinary incontinence. Int Urogynecol J 9:210-213, 1998.
137. Nilsson CG: The tension-free vaginal tape procedure (TVT) for treatment of female urinary incontinence. A minimal invasive surgical procedure. Acta Obstet Gynecol Scand Suppl 168:34-37, 1998.
138. Ward KL, Hilton P, for United Kingdom and Ireland Tension-free Vaginal Tape Trial Group: Prospective multicentre randomised trial of tension-free vaginal tape and colposuspension as primary treatment for stress incontinence. Br Med J 325:67, 2002.
139. Dietz HP, Wilson PD: The Iris effect: How 2D and 3D volume ultrasound can help us understand anti-incontinence procedures. Ultrasound Obstet Gynecol 22:999, 2004.
140. Iglesia CB, Fenner DE, Brubaker L: The use of mesh in gynecologic surgery. Int Urogynecol J 8:105-115, 1997.
141. Fenner DE: New surgical mesh. Clin Obstet Gynecol 43:650-658, 2000.
142. Tunn R, Picot A, Marschke J, Gauruder-Burmester A: Sonomorphological evaluation of polypropylene mesh implants after vaginal mesh repair in women with recurrent prolapse. Ultrasound Obstet Gynecol 29:449-452, 2007.
143. Shek KL, Dietz HP, Rane A: Transobturator mesh anchoring for the repair of large or recurrent cystocele. Neurourol Urodyn (in press).
144. Dietz HP, Lanzarone V, Simpson JM: Predicting Operative Delivery. Ultrasound Obstet Gynecol 27:419-415, 2006.

Chapter 10

ELECTROPHYSIOLOGIC EVALUATION OF THE PELVIC FLOOR

Simon Podnar and Clare J. Fowler

Clinical neurophysiologic tests have been proposed for research applications in patients with sacral dysfunction, but the emphasis in this chapter is on describing investigations with established diagnostic value. The roles of electrodiagnostic tests in various clinical conditions are described first, and brief descriptions of these investigative procedures are given at the end of the chapter.

CLINICAL APPLICATION OF SACRAL ELECTRODIAGNOSTIC TESTS

Electrodiagnostic tests are an extension of the clinical neurologic examination, and they are helpful in evaluating patients in whom a neurologic lesion is suspected. An international consensus statement proposes that sacral electrodiagnostic studies are most useful in patients with focal peripheral sacral lesions (i.e., conus medullaris, cauda equina, sacral plexus, and pudendal nerve lesions), in patients with multiple system atrophy, and in women with urinary retention.[1] They can document the severity of a clinically diagnosed lesion and provide data on the integrity of various neurologic structures. However, these tests have limitations. They require trained personnel to be properly performed, they are not useful for screening, and they are uncomfortable for the patient. The results do not correlate well with clinical bladder, anorectal, or sexual dysfunction.

Neurogenic sacral organ dysfunction can be caused by a variety of neurologic disorders, but the value of sacral electrodiagnostic studies in such patients may be minor. In patients with brain and spinal cord disease, who may have pronounced pelvic organ complaints, imaging studies—magnetic resonance imaging (MRI) in particular—are more useful for establishing the underlying neurologic diagnosis. In this context, neurophysiologic testing outside the pelvic region may provide information about relevant abnormal spinal conduction, and somatosensory evoked potentials (SEPs) elicited by stimulation of the tibial nerve are more useful in these circumstances than pudendal SEPs.[2,3] Similarly, in patients with sacral dysfunction due to a generalized peripheral neuropathy such as diabetes, nerve conduction studies in the lower limbs are a more sensitive adjunct to clinical examination than are sacral electrodiagnostic studies.[4]

ASSESSMENT OF PATIENTS BEFORE ELECTRODIAGNOSTIC TESTING

Clinical and laboratory evaluation of a woman with pelvic organ dysfunction is necessary before electrodiagnostic investigations can be considered. This order is followed so that there can be proper formulation of the questions for those in the clinical neurophysiology laboratory carrying out the tests. Examples of such questions are listed in Box 10-1.

Necessary preliminary investigations may include urodynamics, anorectal manometry, cine defecography, or colonic transit studies. Imaging studies such as ultrasound, computed tomography (CT), and MRI of the anorectum and the lower urinary and genital tracts may aid the diagnosis because they can exclude structural abnormalities (e.g., anal sphincter tears, abnormal position of the bladder neck, vaginal wall prolapse) that can cause or contribute to sacral organ dysfunction.

ELECTRODIAGNOSTIC TESTING IN WOMEN WITH SACRAL COMPLAINTS

Incontinence after Childbirth

Research studies have used needle electromyography to examine the extent of nerve damage contributing to urinary stress incontinence after childbirth. The first studies using single-fiber electromyography (SFEMG) to look at fiber density showed partial reinnervation changes in the external anal sphincter (EAS)[5] and pubococcygeus muscles in women with stress incontinence and genital prolapse.[6] Needle electromyographic examination of the pubococcygeus muscle revealed a significant increase in motor unit potential (MUP) duration (i.e., an indication of reinnervation) after vaginal delivery, which was most marked in women with urinary incontinence 8 weeks after delivery, a prolonged second stage, and heavier babies.[7] However, an electromyographic study, using less biased methods of automated MUPs and interference pattern analysis, questioned the widely held notion that significant damage to the innervation of the EAS occurs even during uncomplicated deliveries. Although vaginal delivery was related to minor electromyographic abnormalities, there was no indication that this correlated with loss of sphincter function.[8] A

Box 10-1 Questions to Consider before Requesting Electrodiagnostic Testing

Is there a neurogenic component to this patient's complaint?
How severe is the neurologic damage?
Are there signs of acute denervation or chronic reinnervation?
Is there abnormal sphincter electromyographic activity suggesting a cause for obstructed voiding or urinary retention?

histomorphologic study supported these data by failing to demonstrate significant neuropathic changes in pelvic floor muscles.[9] In the urethral sphincter, in contrast, electromyography and muscle biopsy showed more neuropathic changes in women with stress incontinence than in controls.[10] Even uncomplicated delivery may cause some distal pudendal nerve damage. Significant neurogenic damage proximal to the EAS muscle innervation probably occurs only rarely,[11] and it is mainly caused by compression of the sacral plexus by fetal head.[12] The prevalence and relevance of minor proximal injuries is unknown.

Kinesiologic electromyography performed using hook electrodes so that a prolonged recording could be made without causing discomfort showed some loss of coordination between the two sides of the pubococcygeus muscle in women with stress incontinence, implying an abnormal primary role of the central nervous system or a neurologic response to muscle or tendon damage.[13] In addition to age-related neurogenic changes, the interference pattern changes consistent with motor unit loss, and failure of central activation has been found in the levator ani and EAS muscles of women with stress incontinence.[14]

Sufficient research data exist for us to know that the changes of denervation in pelvic floor in stress incontinence do occur, but they are quite subtle. Sphincter electromyography does not have an important role in the routine investigation in stress incontinence.

Although extensively used in the past,[15,16] the pudendal nerve terminal motor latency test is probably of no clinical use in women with urinary stress incontinence.[11] Nerve latencies evaluate only the fastest nerve fibers and are therefore not sensitive to axonal loss, which is the major type of damage causing muscle denervation.

Detrusor Overactivity

Detrusor overactivity may result from neurologic disease or occur in an otherwise healthy individual, in which case the condition is called *idiopathic detrusor overactivity*. Clinical neurologic examination is the most useful means of differentiating these two entities. In addition to the clinical examination, imaging studies and electrodiagnostic tests of central nervous system conduction (i.e., motor evoked potentials [MEPs] and SEPs) may reveal underlying spinal cord disease, such as multiple sclerosis. In this respect, tibial SEPs are the most useful investigation.[2,3]

Extensive neurophysiologic investigations (e.g., electromyography of the EAS, bulbocavernosus reflex after dorsal clitoral nerve stimulation, tibial and pudendal SEPs, MEPs on cortical magnetic stimulation, recording from the EAS and abductor hallucis brevis muscles) in women with idiopathic detrusor overactivity failed to reveal any abnormality.[17] No significant differences were reported in comparing this group with a group of 13 age-matched, healthy control women, thereby excluding even an occult neurologic abnormality. This result supports the view that idiopathic detrusor overactivity is caused by intrinsic bladder defects (i.e., neurogenic or myogenic). The role of electrodiagnostic investigations in detrusor overactivity is limited to establishing or excluding an underlying neurologic disease.

Urinary Retention

Isolated urinary retention in young women was formerly considered to be psychogenic or the first symptom of multiple sclerosis. However, needle electromyography of the urethral sphincter muscle has demonstrated that many such patients have profuse, complex, repetitive discharges and decelerating burst activity (Fig. 10-1).[18] The cause of this activity is unknown, but an association with polycystic ovaries was described in a syndrome by Fowler and colleagues.[19] The explanation probably lies with some unidentified hormonal susceptibility of the female striated urethral sphincter muscle that causes a loss of stability of the muscle membrane and permits direct muscle fiber to muscle fiber (ephaptic) transmission to develop, which manifests as complex, repetitive discharges. The current hypothesis is that the sustained contraction of the urethral sphincter has an inhibitory effect on the detrusor, resulting in urinary retention.

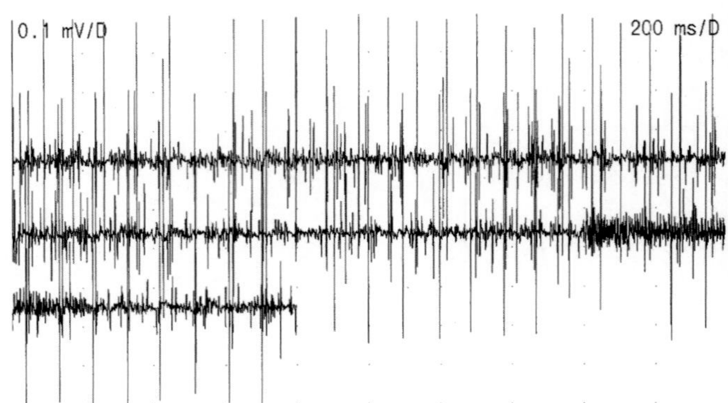

Figure 10-1 Profuse pathologic spontaneous activity (i.e., complex repetitive discharges) in the urethral sphincter muscle of a 26-year-old, otherwise healthy woman with an 8-year history of difficult emptying of the bladder. Her sister has similar problems and electromyographic abnormalities of the urethral sphincter muscle. Activity was provoked by movement of the concentric needle electrode or by voluntary muscle contraction.

When recording from the striated urethral sphincter in this condition, only complex repetitive discharges (which sound like helicopters) may be heard, and the distinction between these and reinnervated motor units can be problematic, but if decelerating bursts (which sound like underwater recordings of whales) are also present, it is easier to be certain that the characteristic electromyographic activity has been recorded. Although electromyography may indicate the presence of an abnormality, it is inevitably only a very limited sample of the muscle activity in the immediate vicinity, and it is difficult to know whether the abnormality is sufficient to account for the clinical finding of complete or partial urinary retention. The investigations that have proved to be useful adjuncts are measurement of the urethral pressure profile and volume of the urethral sphincter muscle estimated with ultrasound.[20] Young women with urinary retention due to the urethral sphincter abnormality often have urethral pressure profiles in excess of 100 cm H_2O.

The typical clinical presentation of Fowler's syndrome is of a young woman with spontaneous onset of urinary retention or retention after some sort of operative intervention. The mean age of a series of women with this problem was 27 years, and a spontaneous onset appears to be more common in women younger than 30 years.[21] The woman may present with a bladder capacity in excess of 1 L, and although this may cause painful distention, she lacks any of the expected sensations of urinary urgency. There may or may not be a history of infrequent voiding before the onset of urinary retention. These women are taught to do clean, intermittent self-catheterization and commonly experience difficulties with the technique, particularly pain and difficulty in removing the catheter. A retrospective study of 248 women presenting with urinary retention over a 5-year period showed that this was by far the most common cause for urinary retention in young women.[22]

Patients with Fowler's syndrome seem to respond particularly well to sacral neuromodulation.[23] Although the mechanism of its action is still the subject of research using functional brain imaging methods,[24] stimulation does not appear to lower the urethral pressure profile or cause a cessation of the abnormal electromyographic activity.[25]

The same type of abnormal spontaneous electromyographic activity may also occur in women with obstructed voiding. The electromyographic abnormality may persist during attempts at micturition,[26] leading to interrupted flow, high detrusor pressure, low flow, and incomplete bladder emptying. It is thought that in this condition, the overactive urethral sphincter, although it produces obstruction, does not have the same inhibitory effect on the detrusor muscle as it does in women who become unable to void and develop urinary retention. Because needle electromyography of the urethral sphincter detects changes related to denervation and reinnervation, as well as this peculiar abnormal, spontaneous activity, it has been proposed that needle electromyography of the urethral sphincter muscle should always be undertaken in women with unexplained urinary retention.[1,18]

Anal Incontinence

Needle electromyography of the EAS was thought to be useful in patients with anal incontinence.[27] However, there is no consensus regarding the utility of electrophysiologic testing in neurologically normal patients with isolated anal incontinence. In a series evaluated by Podnar and coworkers,[28] patients with isolated anal incontinence rarely had neuropathic electromyographic changes in sacral segments. In a subgroup of patients in whom no cause of anal incontinence could be established (i.e., idiopathic anal incontinence), the only electrophysiologic abnormality found was a diminished number (absence) of continuously firing, low-threshold motor units during relaxation.[28] In patients with fecal incontinence and an increased fiber density on SFEMG, lower anal squeeze pressures and diminished rectal sensation have been demonstrated. If marked changes of denervation and reinnervation are found in the EAS in the appropriate clinical setting, a more generalized disorder, such as multiple system atrophy or a cauda equina or conus medullaris lesion, should be considered. If performed, it is probably better that needle electromyography follows an anal ultrasound examination that excludes structural lesions of the sphincter mechanism.[29]

Chronic Constipation

Constipation occurs for a variety of reasons. Its prevalence depends on the diagnostic criteria applied. Radiographic methods can demonstrate prolonged colonic transit (using radiopaque markers) and abnormal pelvic floor movement during defecation (using cine defecography), which are the main mechanisms.[30] Electromyography can be used to demonstrate continuous puborectalis muscle contraction characteristic of a subtype of obstructed defecation (i.e., nonrelaxing puborectalis syndrome),[31] but this would be considered only if other investigations suggested that particular pathophysiology.

Chronic constipation with repetitive straining was thought to be the main cause of advancing pudendal neuropathy and increased fiber density identified on SFEMG in patients with urinary and anal incontinence.[32] Semiquantitative or quantitative MUP changes on conventional electromyography of the EAS muscles of severely constipated subjects have been reported by some investigators. In a study using advanced MUP and interference pattern analysis, no abnormalities were demonstrated in the EAS muscles of patients with mild chronic constipation. This finding is important for the interpretation of electromyographic findings in patients with other conditions, a significant proportion of whom also suffer from chronic constipation.[33]

Sexual Dysfunction

Neurophysiologic techniques have been applied extensively in the research of male erectile dysfunction, but much less research has gone into female sexual dysfunction. Pudendal SEP recordings have been employed in women with sexual dysfunction due to spinal cord lesions, multiple sclerosis, and diabetes,[34] but in a placebo-controlled trial of the effect of sildenafil citrate in women with sexual dysfunction and multiple sclerosis, the pudendal SEP was not found to be contributory.[35] Pudendal SEPs usually have been found to be of no greater value than clinical examination in detecting relevant spinal cord disease.[3]

ELECTRODIAGNOSTIC TESTING IN WOMEN WITH ESTABLISHED NEUROLOGIC DISEASE

Cauda Equina and Conus Medullaris Lesions

Lesions of the cauda equina or conus medullaris may cause severe bladder, bowel, and sexual dysfunction. The sacral roots that innervate pelvic organs may be compressed within the spinal canal by intervertebral disk herniation, spinal fractures, hematomas, and tumors or may be a result of lumbar disk surgery.

After detailed clinical examination of the lumbosacral segments (with particular emphasis on perianal sensation), neurophysiologic testing can assess the severity of the lesion and clarify the diagnosis. In our series, approximately 10% of patients with cauda equina lesions reported normal perianal sensation. Bilateral needle electromyography of the EAS muscle (Fig. 10-2) and sometimes of the bulbocavernosus muscle and electrophysiologic evaluation of the bulbocavernosus reflex (Fig. 10-3) are the electrodiagnostic tests that should be considered. Most of these lesions cause partial denervation. Three weeks to several months after injury, spontaneous denervation activity and later reinnervation MUP changes can be demonstrated by needle electromyography (Fig. 10-4). The bulbocavernosus reflex complements electromyography and increases sensitivity of electrodiagnostic studies in patients with cauda equina or conus medullaris lesions.

Sacral Plexus and Pudendal Nerve Lesions

After uncomplicated deliveries, electromyographic changes in the EAS are minor,[8] but they may be more pronounced in the urethral sphincter muscle.[10] It is commonly assumed that these lesions may be contributory to some degree in the pathogenesis of urinary stress incontinence and pelvic organ prolapse in women.[11] However, electrodiagnostic testing in these women is recommended only when a proximal peripheral sacral neurogenic lesion is a possibility.[1]

Other lesions of the sacral plexus and pudendal nerves are less common than are cauda equina or conus medullaris lesions. They can be caused by pelvic fractures, hip surgery, complicated deliveries,[12] malignant infiltration, local radiotherapy, and use of orthopedic traction tables. They are usually unilateral. There are no validated techniques for differentiating cauda equina lesions from more distal lesions.

Parkinsonism and Multiple System Atrophy

Multiple system atrophy is a progressive neurodegenerative disease of unknown origin that is often mistaken for Parkinson's disease in its early stages. It is characterized at onset by an akinetic, rigid parkinsonian syndrome; cerebellar ataxia; or autonomic failure, usually accompanied by severe incontinence. In the advanced stages of the disease (formerly called Shy-Drager syndrome), all these features may be present. The severe and early incontinence probably results from neuronal atrophy in the brainstem, which causes detrusor overactivity, and in the sacral spinal cord, where degeneration of the parasympathetic intermediolateral cell columns causes incomplete emptying and degeneration of the somatic anterior horn cells forming Onuf's nucleus causes incontinence.

Using needle electromyography of the sphincter muscles prolonged duration of MUPs has been described as the main electrodiagnostic marker for degeneration of Onuf's nucleus.[36-38] Changes consistent with chronic reinnervation can also be demonstrated as an increase in fiber density on SFEMG. Sphincter electromyography may not be sensitive in the early phase of the disease, and it is not specific after 5 years of parkinsonism. The changes of chronic reinnervation may also be found in another parkinsonian syndrome, progressive supranuclear palsy,[39] a disease in which neuronal loss in Onuf's nucleus has been demonstrated histologically.[40]

Unilateral needle electromyography, including observation of denervation activity and quantitative MUP analysis, is indicated in patients with suspected multisystem atrophy, particularly in its early stages if the diagnosis is unclear.[38,41] If the test result is normal, but suspicion of the diagnosis persists, it may be of value to repeat the test later. Kinesiologic electromyography performed during urodynamics can also help to document detrusor-sphincter dyssynergia in patients with Parkinson's disease or multiple system atrophy.[42]

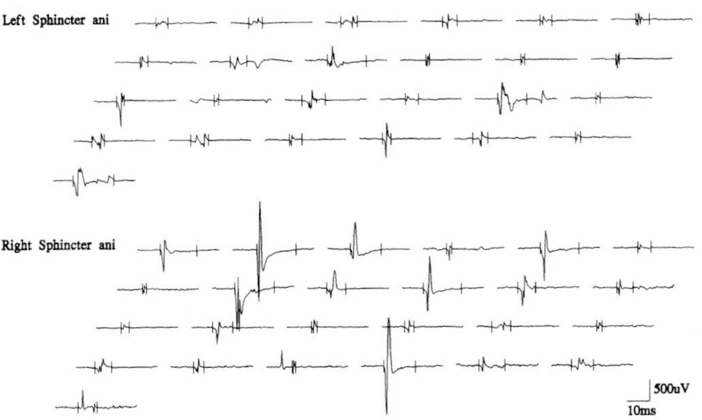

Figure 10-2 Motor unit potential (MUP) analysis of the external anal sphincter (EAS) muscles of a 53-year-old woman 8 years after a traumatic fracture of the L4 vertebra. She continues to have back pain radiating to the right leg, right leg weakness with paresthesia, and moderate bladder, bowel, and sexual dysfunction. MUPs were within normal limits in the left EAS muscle and definitely abnormal in the right EAS muscle. Quantitative sphincter electromyography findings were compatible with a lesion of the right half of the cauda equina.

Primary Muscle Diseases

There are no reports of a myopathy manifesting or remaining confined to the pelvic floor or sphincter muscles. Even in patients with a generalized myopathy, normal and abnormal muscle biopsy and needle electromyographic findings and abnormal histology with normal electromyographic findings have been reported.

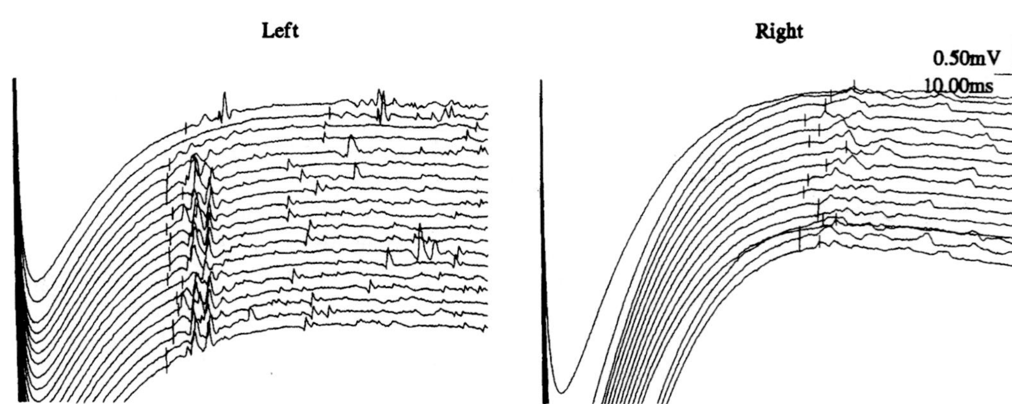

Figure 10-3 Bulbocavernosus reflex (BCR) on electrical stimulation in a 42-year-old woman with a sudden onset of urinary frequency, urgency, and incontinence 4 years earlier. On clinical examination, she reported normal sensation of touch and abnormal sensation of temperature and pinprick (i.e., dissociated sensory loss) in sacral segments on the right. Notice a very prolonged latency of the BCR on the *right* (56 ms) and a normal latency response on the *left* (34 ms). On concentric needle electromyography, definite motor unit potential abnormalities were found in the right and normal results in the left external anal sphincter muscle. She had an episode of right-sided retrobulbar neuritis 6 years before the onset of transient urinary dysfunction. Brain magnetic resonance imaging revealed several lesions in the white substance of the brain consistent with demyelinization. Based on these data, the diagnosis of multiple sclerosis was made.

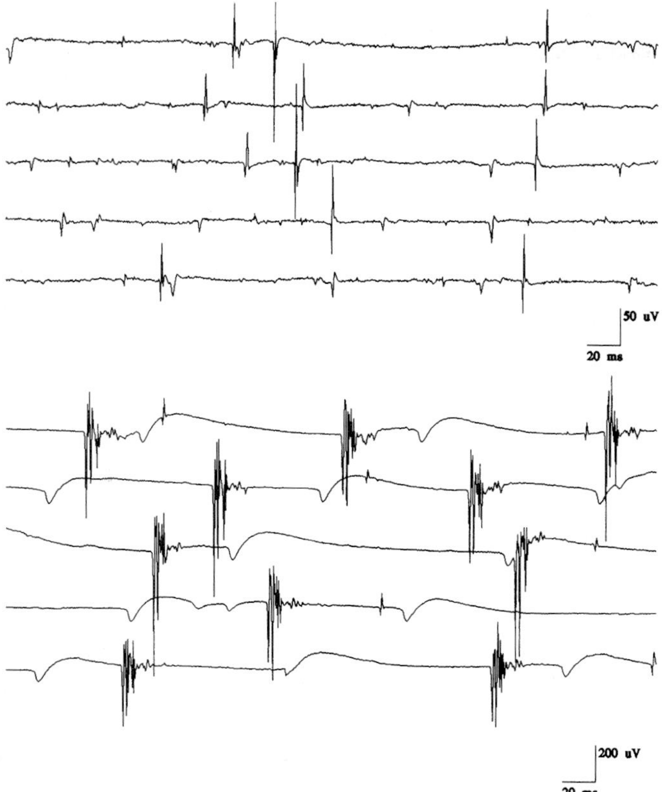

Figure 10-4 Spontaneous denervation electromyographic (EMG) activity is seen during relaxation *(top)*, and a single, extremely polyphasic motor unit potential (MUP) is recruited on maximal voluntary contraction *(bottom)*. The former is a sign of muscle fiber denervation, and the latter is a sign of collateral reinnervation. Both signals were recorded by a concentric EMG needle in the left subcutaneous external anal sphincter muscle of a 50-year-old woman 3 months after surgery for a large, centrally herniated intervertebral disk (between L5 and S1).

Exclusion of a Neurologic Lesion

Occasionally, it may be necessary to exclude a neurologic basis for bladder dysfunction. A normal EAS muscle electromyographic pattern indicates integrity of the sacral lower motor neuron, a normal bulbocavernosus reflex indicates preservation of the sacral reflex arc (including conus medullaris with parasympathetic sacral center), a normal sympathetic skin response indicates preservation of the sympathetic lumbosacral center, and a normal pudendal SEP correlates with preserved spinal somatosensory pathways.[43]

ELECTRODIAGNOSTIC TESTS

Electromyography

Electromyography relies on the extracellular recording of spontaneous and reflexively or voluntarily provoked bioelectrical activity generated by muscle fibers. Bioelectrical activity consisting of action potentials is generated by depolarization of muscle fibers. Motor neurons that innervate striated pelvic floor and sphincter muscle lie in the anterior horn of the sacral spinal cord (i.e., conus medullaris). Within the muscle, the motor axon tapers and then branches to innervate muscle fibers constituting an individual motor unit. In health, muscle fibers that belong to the same motor unit do not lie adjacent to one another (i.e., checkerboard pattern of muscle innervation).

Concentric Needle Electromyography

The needle electrode most commonly used in electromyography is the single-use, disposable, concentric needle electrode. It can provide information on insertion activity, spontaneous activity, MUPs, and interference patterns.[41]

In healthy skeletal muscle, initial placement of the needle elicits a short burst of insertion activity due to mechanical stimulation of excitable membranes. Absence of insertion activity with an appropriately placed needle electrode (if all technical causes have been excluded) may mean complete denervation of the muscle being examined. In contrast to most other skeletal muscles, the sphincter muscles exhibit continuous firing of low-threshold motor units. This activity can be quantified most easily and reproducibly by template-operated MUP sampling techniques (e.g., multi-MUP analysis), which provides information on excitability and loss of motor units.[28] An abnormal, spontaneously active type of activity may be recorded from the urethral sphincter muscle in some young women with retention or obstructed voiding, so-called decelerating bursts and complex repetitive discharges (see Fig. 10-1).[18,21]

Between 10 and 20 days after an acute denervating injury, the abnormal, spontaneous activity appears: fibrillation potentials and positive sharp waves (Fig. 10-4). This type of activity originates from denervated, single muscle fibers. In partially denervated sphincter muscle, this activity is mingled with continuously firing MUPs, and examination of the bulbocavernosus muscle, which in contrast to sphincter muscles lacks on-going MUP firing during relaxation, is particularly useful.[41]

Examination of MUPs recorded by a needle electrode has proved to be the most valuable process in the neurophysiologic assessment of the pelvic floor. A MUP is generated by summation of action potentials of all muscle fibers constituting individual motor unit, and MUP morphology is determined by the bioelectrical characteristics of muscle fibers constituting the motor unit and by their spatial distribution. In partially denervated muscle, collateral reinnervation tends to take place, and surviving motor nerves sprout and grow out to reinnervate muscle fibers that have lost their nerve supply. This results in a change in the arrangement of muscle fibers within the motor unit and in a consequent change in MUP shape (see Figs. 10-2 and 10-4), which can be quantitatively described by several MUP parameters (Fig. 10-5). For diagnosis of neuropathic changes in the EAS muscle, an optimal set of MUP parameters (i.e., area, duration, and number of turns) was identified.[44] In addition to duration, MUP amplitude and number of phases traditionally were used.

MUPs are identified by their repetitive appearance in a prolonged recording of electromyographic activity (i.e., manual-MUP analysis), using a trigger and delay line (i.e., single-MUP analysis) or using the template-based multi-MUP analysis. The multi-MUP analysis is an automated computer operated analysis, and is fast (5 to 10 minutes per muscle), easy to apply, and minimizes examiner's bias.[45] A representative sample of 20 MUPs (i.e., standard number in limb muscles) must be analyzed for the test to be valid (see Fig. 10-2).

The EAS muscle is regarded as the best indicator muscle for proximal neuropathic sacral lesion, and bilateral examination of only the subcutaneous EAS muscle usually suffices.[46] Normative

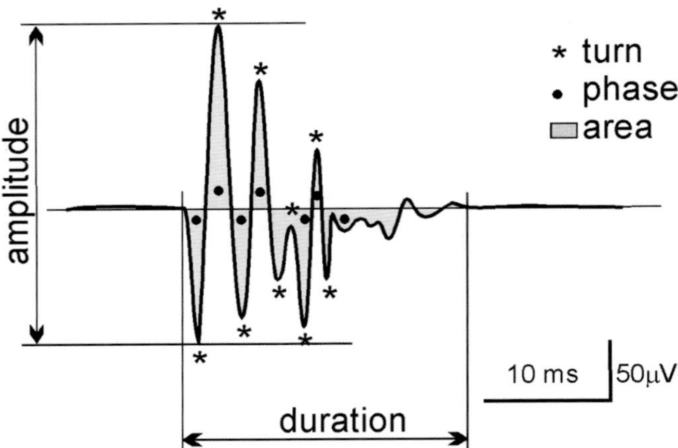

Figure 10-5 Motor unit potential (MUP) parameters. Amplitude is the voltage difference (µV) between the most positive and most negative point of the MUP trace. The MUP duration is the time (ms) between the first deflection and the point when MUP waveform finally returns to the baseline. The number of MUP phases *(circles)* is defined by the number of MUP areas alternately below and above the baseline and can be counted as the number of baseline crossings plus one. Turns *(asterisks)* are defined as changes in direction of the MUP trace that are larger than the specified amplitude (50 µV). MUP area measures the integrated surface of the MUP waveform *(shaded area)*.

data for the EAS muscle have been published and show no significant changes with age, gender, number of uncomplicated vaginal deliveries,[8] and mild, chronic constipation.[33] Similar in-depth analysis of normative data from standardized technique for other pelvic floor and perineal muscles is not available.

At increased levels of voluntary and reflex activation, a more dense interference pattern can be seen. This can be quantitatively assessed, but its sensitivity for detecting neuropathic EAS muscles is only about one half of that for MUP analysis techniques.[45] Qualitative assessment of the interference pattern has been recommended for sphincter and pelvic floor muscles to assess motor unit loss.[41]

Kinesiologic Electromyography

The aim of kinesiologic electromyography is to assess patterns of individual muscle activity during physiologic maneuvers (e.g., electromyographic activity patterns of pelvic floor muscle during bladder filling and voiding). Various types of surface or intramuscular (needle or hook wire) electrodes can be used for recording kinesiologic electromyography, but there are often technical problems to overcome, such as electrical artifacts and contamination with electromyographic signals from other muscles. Large pelvic floor muscles are not adequately represented by the signal measured with intramuscular electrodes.

Little is known about the normal activity patterns of different pelvic floor and sphincter muscles. It is assumed that they all act in a coordinated fashion, which is frequently lost in abnormal conditions.[26] On voiding, disappearance of all electromyographic activity in the urethral sphincter precedes detrusor contraction. In central nervous system disorders, however, detrusor contractions may be associated with an increase of sphincter electromyographic activity (i.e., detrusor-sphincter dyssynergia),[47] which can be most easily demonstrated by kinesiologic electromyography performed during cystometry.

Conduction Studies

Conduction studies examine the capacity of a nerve (or a nervous pathway) to transmit a test volley of depolarization along its length. If the tested nerve contains motor fibers, its responsiveness can be recorded from the muscle as a compound muscle action potential (CMAP).[48] The time taken from stimulation to muscle response (i.e., latency) and the amplitude of the muscle response can be measured. The latency reflects the conduction speed of only the fastest motor fibers and is therefore a poor guide to the overall function of the nerve. The amplitude of the CMAP reflects the number of intact motor units and gives a somewhat better guide to the severity of a neuropathic lesion. However, in anatomically complex muscles of the pelvis, recording of a well-formed CMAP is difficult.[49]

Pudendal Nerve Terminal Motor Latency

Terminal motor latency of the pudendal nerve can be measured by recording with a concentric needle electrode from the bulbocavernosus, EAS, or urethral sphincter muscles in response to bipolar stimulation placed on the perianal or perineal surface. The latencies of MEPs obtained by this means are between 4.7 and 5.1 ms.[50]

The more widely employed technique of obtaining the pudendal terminal motor latency relies on a bipolar stimulating electrode fixed to the tip of the gloved index finger, with the recording electrode pair placed 8 cm proximally on the base of the finger (i.e., St. Mark's stimulator).[51] The finger is inserted into the rectum or vagina, and stimulation is performed close to the ischial spine. Using this stimulator, the terminal motor latency for the EAS CMAP is typically about 2 ms.[51] If a catheter-mounted electrode is used, responses from the urethral sphincter can also be obtained. The difference in latencies obtained by the perineal and transrectal methods has not yet been explained. Unfortunately, amplitudes of the pudendal CMAP have not proved contributory because of their large variability.[1]

Electrical and Magnetic Stimulation of Sacral Roots

With development of special electrical and magnetic stimulators, transcutaneous stimulation of deeply situated nervous tissue became possible. When applied over the spine, the roots at the exit from the vertebral canal mainly are stimulated.[49] Recording of MEPs with magnetic stimulation has been less successful, at least with standard coils, than with electrical stimulation, and there is often a large stimulus artifact. Positioning of the ground electrode between the recording electrodes and the stimulating coil should decrease the artifact.[49,52]

Sacral Reflexes

Sacral reflexes refer to electrophysiologically recordable responses of perineal or pelvic floor muscles to electrical stimulation in the urinary-genital-anal region. Two reflexes, the anal and the bulbocavernosus reflex, are commonly clinically elicited in the lower sacral segments. Both have the afferent and efferent limb of their reflex arc in the pudendal nerve, and both are centrally integrated at the S2 to S4 cord levels.[49,53] In women, the bulbocavernosus reflex is clinically elicited by squeezing or taping of the clitoris and observing movement of the perineum or anal sphincter. It is, however, much less reliable than in men,[53,54] and in our opinion, is not useful. The anal reflex is elicited by a pinprick of the perianal skin, producing an anal wink.

Electrophysiologic correlates of these reflexes have been described using electrical, mechanical, and magnetic stimulation. Whereas the latter two modalities have been applied only to the clitoris, electrical stimulation can be applied to other sites, such as the dorsal clitoral nerve and perianal area. Responses are usually detected by needle electrode inserted into the EAS or bulbocavernosus muscle. The bulbocavernosus detection site is preferred because traces do not contain continuously firing, low-threshold MUPs.

The bladder neck or proximal urethra can be stimulated using a catheter-mounted ring electrode, and reflex responses can be obtained from perineal muscles. With visceral denervation, such as after radical hysterectomy, these reflexes may be lost while the sacral reflex mediated by pudendal nerve is preserved. Loss of vesicourethral reflex with preservation of vesicoanal reflex has been described for patients with urethral afferent injury after recurrent urethral operations.

Reports of sacral reflexes obtained after electrical stimulation of the clitoral nerve give consistent mean latencies of between 31 and 39 ms (see Fig. 10-3). Sacral reflex responses obtained on perianal, bladder neck, or proximal urethra stimulation have latencies between 50 and 65 ms.[49] This more prolonged response is thought to be caused by the afferent limb of the reflex being conveyed by thinner myelinated pelvic nerves with slower conduction velocities than the thicker myelinated pudendal afferents. The longer-latency anal reflex, the contraction of the EAS on stimulation of the perianal region, may also have thinner myelinated fibers in its afferent limb because it is produced by a nociceptive stimulus.[49]

Sympathetic Skin Response

The sympathetic skin response is a reflex served by myelinated sensory fibers (i.e., afferent limb), a complex central integrative mechanism, and sympathetic postganglionic nonmyelinated C fibers (i.e., efferent limb).[55] The responses can be recorded from the perineum with some difficulty. The stimulus used in clinical practice typically is an electrical pulse delivered to a peripheral nerve in the limbs, but the genital organs also can be stimulated. Only an absent sympathetic skin response can be considered abnormal. The response is reportedly useful in the assessment of patients with neuropathies involving unmyelinated nerve fibers[56] and patients with spinal cord injury. In the latter group, it may serve as an indicator of the preserved sympathetic lumbosacral center, which is particularly important for bladder neck competence.[57]

Cerebral Somatosensory Evoked Potentials

The pudendal evoked response is easily recorded after electrical stimulation of the dorsal clitoral nerves. The first positive peak at 41 ± 2.3 ms (called P1 or P40) is usually clearly defined in healthy subjects. This SEP is of the highest amplitude (0.5 to 12 μV) at a site central over the sensory cortex and is highly reproducible. Later negative (at about 55 ms) and then additional positive waves are quite variable in amplitude and expression and have little known clinical relevance.[49]

Cerebral SEPs can be obtained on stimulation of the bladder urothelium. These cerebral SEPs have low amplitudes (≤1 μV), have variable configurations, and may be difficult to identify in some control subjects. The typical latency of the most prominent negative potential (N1) is about 100 ms. The responses are of more relevance to neurogenic bladder dysfunction than the pudendal SEP, because the Aδ sensory afferents from bladder and proximal urethra accompany the autonomic fibers in the pelvic nerves. Another stimulation site is the anal canal; after stimulation, cerebral SEPs with a slightly longer latency than those obtained after stimulation of the clitoris have been reported. However, because it is not possible to record this response from all control subjects, these tests have not proved clinically useful. The rectum and sigmoid colon have also been stimulated, and cerebral SEPs of two types have been recorded. One was similar in shape and latency to the pudendal SEP, and the other was similar to the SEP recorded on stimulation of bladder and posterior urethra.

CONCLUSIONS

Several electrodiagnostic tests have been proposed for evaluation of the sacral nervous system in women with bladder, bowel, and sexual dysfunction. Although all of the tests discussed here are of research interest, concentric needle electromyography is of greatest value in the diagnostic evaluation of selected groups of patients with pelvic floor dysfunction: those with traumatic lesions and those with atypical parkinsonism. Bulbocavernosus reflex and pudendal SEP studies are useful in the evaluation of selected patients with suspected peripheral or central neurogenic sacral lesions. Probably the only patients in whom sacral dysfunction in itself should be considered an indication for electromyography of the urethral sphincter are young women with unexplained urinary retention.

References

1. Fowler CJ, Benson JT, Craggs MD, et al: Clinical neurophysiology. In Abrams P, Cardozo L, Khoury S (eds): Incontinence. The Second International Consultation on Incontinence, 2001 July 1-3, Paris. Plymouth, UK, Health Publication, 2002, p 389.
2. Rodi Z, Vodusek DB, Denislic M: Clinical uro-neurophysiological investigation in multiple sclerosis. Eur J Neurol 3:574, 1996.
3. Delodovici ML, Fowler CJ: Clinical value of the pudendal somatosensory evoked potential. Electroencephalogr Clin Neurophysiol 96:509, 1995.
4. Hecht MJ, Neundorfer B, Kiesewetter F, et al: Neuropathy is a major contributing factor to diabetic erectile dysfunction. Neurol Res 23:651, 2001.
5. Anderson RS: A neurogenic element to urinary genuine stress incontinence. Br J Obstet Gynaecol 91:41, 1984.
6. Smith AR, Hosker GL, Warrell DW: The role of partial denervation of the pelvic floor in the aetiology of genitourinary prolapse and stress incontinence of urine. A neurophysiological study. Br J Obstet Gynaecol 96:24, 1989.
7. Allen RE, Hosker GL, Smith AR, et al: Pelvic floor damage and childbirth: A neurophysiological study. Br J Obstet Gynaecol 97:770, 1990.
8. Podnar S, Lukanovic A, Vodusek DB: Anal sphincter electromyography after vaginal delivery: Neuropathic insufficiency or normal wear and tear? Neurourol Urodyn 19:249, 2000.
9. Jundt K, Kiening M, Fischer P, et al: Is the histomorphological concept of the female pelvic floor and its changes due to age and vaginal delivery correct? Neurourol Urodyn 24:44, 2005.
10. Hale DS, Benson JT, Brubaker L, et al: Histologic analysis of needle biopsy of urethral sphincter from women with normal and stress

incontinence with comparison of electromyographic findings. Am J Obstet Gynecol 180:342, 1999.
11. Vodusek DB: The role of electrophysiology in the evaluation of incontinence and prolapse. Curr Opin Obstet Gynecol 14:509, 2002.
12. Feasby TE, Burton SR, Hahn AF: Obstetrical lumbosacral plexus injury. Muscle Nerve 15:937, 1992.
13. Deindl FM, Vodusek DB, Hesse U, et al: Pelvic floor activity patterns: Comparison of nulliparous continent and parous urinary stress incontinent women. A kinesiological EMG study. Br J Urol 73:413, 1994.
14. Weidner AC, Barber MD, Visco AG, et al: Pelvic muscle electromyography of levator ani and external anal sphincter in nulliparous women and women with pelvic floor dysfunction. Am J Obstet Gynecol 183:1390, 2000.
15. Snooks SJ, Setchell M, Swash M, et al: Injury to innervation of pelvic floor sphincter musculature in childbirth. Lancet 2:546, 1984.
16. Smith AR, Hosker GL, Warrell DW: The role of pudendal nerve damage in the aetiology of genuine stress incontinence in women. Br J Obstet Gynaecol 96:29, 1989.
17. Del Carro U, Riva D, Comi GC, et al: Neurophysiological evaluation in detrusor instability. Neurourol Urodyn 12:455, 1993.
18. Fowler CJ, Kirby RS: Electromyography of urethral sphincter in women with urinary retention. Lancet 1:1455, 1986.
19. Fowler CJ, Christmas TJ, Chapple CR, et al: Abnormal electromyographic activity of the urethral sphincter, voiding dysfunction, and polycystic ovaries: A new syndrome? Br Med J 297:1436, 1988.
20. Wiseman OJ, Swinn MJ, Brady CM, et al: Maximum urethral closure pressure and sphincter volume in women with urinary retention. J Urol 167:1348, 2002.
21. Swinn MJ, Wiseman OJ, Lowe E, et al: The cause and natural history of isolated urinary retention in young women. J Urol 167:151, 2002.
22. Kavia R, Datta S, DasGupta R, et al: Urinary retention in women: Its causes and its management. BJU Int 97:281, 2006.
23. Swinn MJ, Kitchen ND, Goodwin RJ, et al: Sacral neuromodulation for women with Fowler's syndrome. Eur Urol 38:439, 2000.
24. DasGupta R, Critchley HD, Dolan RJ, Fowler CJ: Changes in brain activity following sacral neuromodulation for urinary retention. J Urol 174:2268, 2005.
25. DasGupta R, Fowler CJ: Urodynamic study of women in urinary retention treated with sacral neuromodulation. J Urol 171:1161, 2004.
26. Deindl FM, Vodusek DB, Bischoff C, et al: Dysfunctional voiding in women: Which muscles are responsible? Br J Urol 82:814, 1998.
27. Aanestad O, Flink R: Interference pattern in perineal muscles. A quantitative electromyographic study in patients with faecal incontinence. Eur J Surg 160:111, 1994.
28. Podnar S, Mrkaic M, Vodusek DB: Standardization of anal sphincter electromyography: quantification of continuous activity during relaxation. Neurourol Urodyn 21:540, 2002.
29. Sultan AH, Kamm MA, Hudson CN, et al: Anal-sphincter disruption during vaginal delivery. N Engl J Med 329:1905, 1993.
30. Snape WJ Jr: Role of colonic motility in guiding therapy in patients with constipation. Dig Dis 15(Suppl 1):104, 1997.
31. Jorge JM, Wexner SD, Ger GC, et al: Cinedefecography and electromyography in the diagnosis of nonrelaxing puborectalis syndrome. Dis Colon Rectum 36:668, 1993.
32. Snooks SJ, Barnes PR, Swash M, et al: Damage to the innervation of the pelvic floor musculature in chronic constipation. Gastroenterology 89:977, 1985.
33. Podnar S, Vodusek DB: Standardization of anal sphincter electromyography: Effect of chronic constipation. Muscle Nerve 23:1748, 2000.
34. Yang CC, Bowen JR, Kraft GH: Cortical evoked potentials of the dorsal nerve of the clitoris and female sexual dysfunction in multiple sclerosis. J Urol 164:2010, 2000.
35. DasGupta R, Wiseman OJ, Kanabar G, et al: Efficacy of sildenafil in the treatment of female sexual dysfunction due to multiple sclerosis. J Urol 171:1189, 2004.
36. Palace J, Chandiramani VA, Fowler CJ: Value of sphincter electromyography in the diagnosis of multiple system atrophy. Muscle Nerve 20:1396, 1997.
37. Libelius R, Johansson F: Quantitative electromyography of the external anal sphincter in Parkinson's disease and multiple system atrophy. Muscle Nerve 23:1250, 2000.
38. Vodusek DB: Sphincter EMG and differential diagnosis of multiple system atrophy. Mov Disord 16:600, 2001.
39. Valldeoriola F, Valls-Sole J, Tolosa ES, et al: Striated anal sphincter denervation in patients with progressive supranuclear palsy. Mov Disord 10:550, 1995.
40. Scaravilli T, Pramstaller PP, Salerno A, et al: Neuronal loss in Onuf's nucleus in three patients with progressive supranuclear palsy. Ann Neurol 48:97, 2000.
41. Podnar S, Vodusek DB: Protocol for clinical neurophysiologic examination of the pelvic floor. Neurourol Urodyn 20:669, 2001.
42. Sakakibara R, Hattori T, Uchiyama T, et al: Urinary dysfunction and orthostatic hypotension in multiple system atrophy: Which is the more common and earlier manifestation? J Neurol Neurosurg Psychiatry 68:25, 2000.
43. Schmid DM, Curt A, Hauri D, et al: Clinical value of combined electrophysiological and urodynamic recordings to assess sexual disorders in spinal cord injured men. Neurourol Urodyn 22:314, 2003.
44. Podnar S, Mrkaic M: Predictive power of motor unit potential parameters in anal sphincter electromyography. Muscle Nerve 26:389, 2002.
45. Podnar S, Vodusek DB, Stalberg E: Comparison of quantitative techniques in anal sphincter electromyography. Muscle Nerve 25:83, 2002.
46. Podnar S: Electromyography of the anal sphincter: Which muscle to examine? Muscle Nerve 28:377, 2003.
47. Chancellor MB, Kaplan SA, Blaivas JG: Detrusor-external sphincter dyssynergia. Ciba Found Symp 151:195, 1990.
48. AAEE glossary of terms in clinical electromyography. Muscle Nerve 10:G1, 1987.
49. Vodusek DB: Evoked potential testing. Urol Clin North Am 23:427, 1996.
50. Vodusek DB, Janko M, Lokar J: Direct and reflex responses in perineal muscles on electrical stimulation. J Neurol Neurosurg Psychiatry 46:67, 1983.
51. Kiff ES, Swash M: Normal proximal and delayed distal conduction in the pudendal nerves of patients with idiopathic (neurogenic) faecal incontinence. J Neurol Neurosurg Psychiatry 47:820, 1984.
52. Lefaucheur JP: Intrarectal ground electrode improves the reliability of motor evoked potentials recorded in the anal sphincter. Muscle Nerve 32:110, 2005.
53. Blaivas JG, Zayed AA, Labib KB: The bulbocavernosus reflex in urology: A prospective study of 299 patients. J Urol 126:197, 1981.
54. Wester C, FitzGerald MP, Brubaker L, et al: Validation of the clinical bulbocavernosus reflex. Neurourol Urodyn 22:589, 2003.
55. Arunodaya GR, Taly AB: Sympathetic skin response: A decade later. J Neurol Sci 129:81, 1995.
56. Ertekin C, Ertekin N, Mutlu S, et al: Skin potentials (SP) recorded from the extremities and genital regions in normal and impotent subjects. Acta Neurol Scand 76:28, 1987.
57. Rodic B, Curt A, Dietz V, et al: Bladder neck incompetence in patients with spinal cord injury: Significance of sympathetic skin response. J Urol 163:1223, 2000.

Chapter 11

URODYNAMICS

H. Henry Lai, Christopher P. Smith, and Timothy B. Boone

The term *urodynamics* was first coined by Davis[1] in 1953 to define the study of the storage and emptying phases of the lower urinary tract. Patients with voiding and storage symptoms cannot be reliably diagnosed by history and physical examination alone.[2,3] Urodynamic studies offer objective measurements of bladder and urethral functions and dysfunctions while reproducing the patient's presenting symptoms.

REPRODUCTION OF SYMPTOMS FOR URODYNAMIC EVALUATION

The urodynamic armamentarium is extensive, including bedside eyeball urodynamics, noninvasive uroflowmetry, and multichannel fluoroscopic studies (Table 11-1). A "reflex hammer" approach to urodynamic testing is condemned. Before any urodynamic evaluation, the clinician must formulate specific questions about the case, and a working diagnosis must be in place. The most accurate and least invasive study tailored to answer specific questions and to confirm the diagnosis is performed. It is crucial that urodynamic tests reproduce the patient's presenting symptoms. A study that does not duplicate the patient's symptoms is not diagnostic.[4] For instance, if a patient states that she loses urine only in an upright position, little is gained by a supine cystometrogram.[5] Failure to record an abnormality on urodynamic assessment does not rule out its clinical existence.[4] Conversely, not all abnormalities detected on urodynamic tests are clinically significant.[4] If urodynamic testing reveals information that is totally unexpected, the history and working diagnosis should be re-evaluated.

Urodynamic testing should be done in a quiet, private, and orderly suite with as little distraction and as few observers as possible so that patients can relax to replicate their usual voiding habits. Patients must be told what to expect, how the tests are done, and what information the clinician is seeking. For example, in evaluating incontinence, patients need to understand that the goal of the study is to demonstrate leakage characteristic of their experience, so that they do not voluntarily and mistakenly contract the external sphincter to avoid the embarrassment of incontinence and falsely elevate the abdominal leak point pressure (ALPP). In evaluating outlet obstruction, patients are encouraged to void as close to their normal pattern as possible so that they does not strain excessively nor involuntarily tighten the pelvic floor out of anxiety. Accurate interpretation of urodynamic studies is an art. It relies on patient cooperation and open communication between the patient and the clinician during the procedure, allowing urodynamic events to be correlated with the patient's symptoms in real time.

INDICATIONS, CONTRAINDICATIONS, AND PATIENT PREPARATION

Urodynamic assessment is indicated if the diagnosis is uncertain, empirical treatment has failed, or an invasive procedure or surgery is contemplated. Urodynamic testing is deferred during an active urinary tract infection or after recent instrumentation. When possible, patients with a chronically indwelling catheter should be started on intermittent catheterization before the study because bladder sensation, capacity, and compliance may be altered by a chronic Foley catheter. Routine antibiotic prophylaxis is unnecessary unless the patient is at high risk for urinary infection, endocarditis, or prosthetic infection.[6] Patients with a history of or at risk for autonomic dysreflexia (i.e., T6 or above spinal cord injury) should be pretreated with oral nifedipine or α-blockers and have their blood pressures monitored during urodynamic studies.[7,8] If sweating, headache, flushing, severe hypertension, and reflex bradycardia do not respond to bladder drainage, oral nifedipine or intravenous hydralazine, or both, should be administrated immediately. Pharmacologic agents may alter bladder and sphincter functions. Whether these medications should be stopped before the study depends on the goal of the study. If the goal is to evaluate the response to medications (e.g., response of bladder compliance to anticholinergics), the medications should be taken. If the goal is to uncover the cause of urge symptoms, the medications should be stopped before the study.

Table 11-1 The Urodynamic Armamentarium

Phase	Study of Bladder Functions	Study of Urethral Functions
Storage	Eyeball urodynamics Cystometrogram Video urodynamics	Detrusor leak point pressure Abdominal leak point pressure Resting urethral pressure profilometry Stress urethral pressure profilometry Video urodynamics
Voiding	Uroflowmetry Pressure-flow study Video urodynamics	Uroflowmetry Pressure-flow study Micturitional urethral pressure profilometry Video urodynamics Electromyography

Urodynamic Evaluation for Stress Urinary Incontinence

The indications for urodynamic evaluation of stress urinary incontinence (SUI) are controversial and deserve special consideration. Many investigators argued that patients with classic SUI symptoms and obvious urethral hypermobility without associated irritative symptoms (e.g., urge, urge continence, nocturia), voiding dysfunction (e.g., weak stream, high postvoid residual volume), pelvic organ prolapse, neurologic disease, or history of incontinence surgery or radical pelvic surgery require no invasive urodynamic testing if they choose nonoperative treatments. Urodynamic tests are indicated when empirical therapy is ineffective and surgery is planned; patients complain of a confusing mix of urge and stress incontinence symptoms or significant emptying symptoms; or patients have equivocal urethral hypermobility, large prolapse, neurologic disease, or a history of failed incontinence surgery or pelvic surgery.

Classically, preoperative urodynamic assessments help to define the exact cause of incontinence and therefore guide the SUI surgical approach; evaluate detrusor function (e.g., capacity, instability, poor contractility) and identify patients at risk for voiding dysfunction (i.e., instability, retention) after SUI surgery; predict the impact of prolapse and its correction on storage and voiding functions; and identify urodynamic factors (e.g., high detrusor leak point pressure) that place the upper tract at risk postoperatively.[9] In the modern era of minimally invasive pubovaginal and mid-urethral slings, the roles of preoperative urodynamics become more controversial. Although few would argue that additional information could be gleaned from preoperative testing (albeit with a finite risk of urinary infection), it remains unclear whether urodynamics can improve SUI surgical success or alter the surgical approach.[10,11] Pubovaginal and mid-urethral slings appear to have reasonable success for any type and severity of SUI.[12-15] Patients without preoperative urodynamic evaluation before mid-urethral synthetic slings appear to do as well as those who underwent preoperative urodynamics routinely.[16] Nevertheless, urodynamics may identify subpopulation of patients at risk for postoperative failure or voiding complications (e.g., urge, retention).[17-19]

EVALUATION OF STORAGE FUNCTION

Eyeball Urodynamics

The so-called bedside eyeball urodynamics is the simplest of all tests. It enables detection of bladder sensation, overactivity, and capacity without sophisticated instruments. It requires only a catheter, filling syringe, normal saline, and careful observation. After voiding, a red rubber catheter is inserted, and the postvoid residual (PVR) volume is measured. A 60-mL syringe (with its barrel removed) is then used to fill the bladder under gravity. Intravesical pressure is estimated by the height of the saline column above the pubic symphysis. Changes in intravesical pressure are detected as slowing of the rate of fall or a rise in the fluid meniscus. Rising intravesical pressure may result from involuntary detrusor contraction (i.e., associated with a sudden urge to void and possibly leakage around the catheter), abdominal straining (i.e., the abdomen can be palpated or inspected to confirm a Valsalva response), or poor bladder compliance. The bladder is filled until the patient is comfortably full. The catheter is removed, and the patient is asked to cough and perform a Valsalva maneuver with increasing abdominal force. Stress incontinence, urethral hypermobility, and pelvic organ prolapse are assessed in the lithotomy and upright positions. Pure SUI and stress-induced detrusor instability may be distinguished by the characteristics of the incontinence; the former is associated with a few drops of leakage, and the latter is associated with urge and continuous, uncontrollable voiding after the stress maneuver.

Cystometrography

A cystometrogram measures the intravesical pressure (P_{ves}) during bladder filling. The bladder is filled physiologically (i.e., diuresis) or through a catheter using room-temperature saline, water, or contrast (for video urodynamic studies [VUDS]). Fluid infusion is preferred over gas (CO_2) infusion because the fluid is less irritative to the bladder than CO_2, fluid is noncompressible and can detect smaller detrusor contractions than CO_2, fluid leakage (i.e., incontinence) can be easily demonstrated, and leak point pressures, pressure-flow studies (PFSs), and anatomic studies can be performed using fluid but not a gaseous medium. Pressure is transmitted through an intravenous line to an external strain gauge transducer, or it is measured directly on a catheter-mounted, solid-state microtip transducer or fiberoptic transducer.[20]

In the single-channel cystometrogram, only P_{ves} is monitored, whereas in the multichannel cystometrogram, the P_{ves} and intra-abdominal pressure (P_{abd}) are measured. A rectal balloon catheter is advanced well past the anal sphincter to measure P_{abd} to avoid interference with rectal contractions.[21] In patients with no anus (e.g., after abdominoperineal resection), P_{abd} can be monitored inside a colostomy, ileostomy, or vagina. Detrusor pressure (P_{det}) is calculated by subtracting intra-abdominal pressure from intravesical pressure ($P_{det} = P_{ves} - P_{abd}$) (Fig. 11-1). P_{det} is a computer-generated number and is subject to error if negative abdominal pressures are recorded. Having both P_{ves} and P_{abd} monitored simultaneously allows the examiner to differentiate bladder

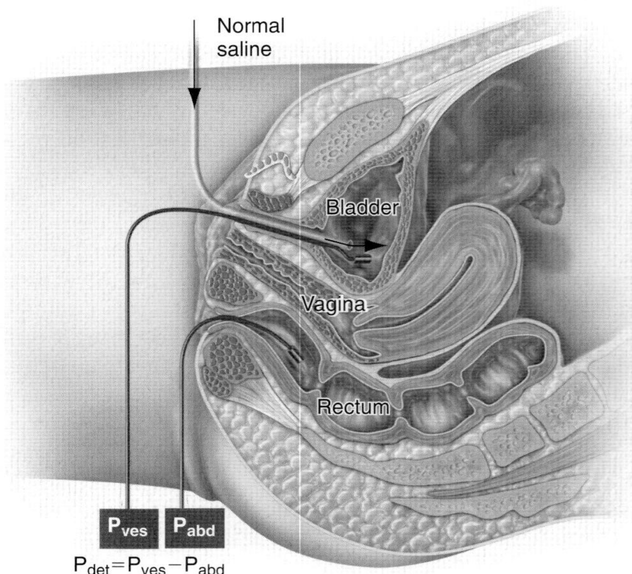

Figure 11-1 Intravesical pressure (P_{ves}) and intra-abdominal pressure (P_{abd}) are measured independently during multichannel cystometrography. Detrusor pressure (P_{det}) is calculated by subtracting P_{abd} from P_{ves}.

contractions from abdominal straining. This is particularly useful in the evaluation of SUI to differentiate stress-induced detrusor overactivity from genuine SUI during cystometrography; in the evaluation of obstruction to distinguish bladder hypocontraction or straining from high-pressure detrusor contraction during PFSs; and to monitor bladder behavior during leak point pressure determinations and VUDS.

The rate of bladder filling (slow: <10 mL/min; medium: 10 to 100 mL/min; fast: >100 mL/min; physiologic: ≤body weight [kg]/4 [mL/min]; nonphysiologic) and the size of urethral catheter must be specified. Most patients are filled at medium rate initially. Filling is slowed if poor compliance, neurogenic bladder, decreased capacity, or excessive detrusor overactivity is encountered. Filling is increased during provocative maneuvers. Because large catheters may cause obstruction, smaller catheters (<10 Fr) are used.[22] A two-catheter technique, in which the larger, infusing catheter (8 to 12 Fr) is removed before voiding (i.e., voids along the smaller, pressure-monitoring catheter [3 to 4 Fr), has been described.[23]

To avoid artifacts, all lines are flushed to remove any air, and all transducers are zeroed at the superior edge of the pubic symphysis.[25] The patient is then asked to perform a Valsalva maneuver to ensure equal pressure transmission to the P_{ves} and P_{abd} catheters. Changes in P_{abd} must be accompanied by corresponding changes in P_{ves}; otherwise, the calculated ΔP_{det} represents artifacts rather than true detrusor contractions. Potential source of errors include pressure measurement artifacts (e.g., air bubbles and kinks in tubing, incorrect placement or migration of catheters, rectal contractions, incorrect zeroing), infusion artifacts (e.g., too rapid infusion in neurogenic and overactive bladders), unanticipated "pop-off" mechanisms (e.g., incompetent urethra that leaks, large bladder diverticulum or vesicoureteral reflux that falsely improves bladder compliance), and patient-related issues (e.g., lack of cooperation, ineffective communication, anxiety, psychological inhibition).[21,24]

Parameters that are measured by cystometrography include the following:

1. *Sensation.* Volumes at first sensation of bladder filling, first desire to void, strong desire to void, urgency, and pain are recorded.[25] These values are subjective, and the absolute volumes at which these symptoms occur are clinically less relevant. The more important issues are whether bladder sensation is increased, decreased, or absent and whether a particular sensation (e.g., urgency) is correlated or not with urodynamic findings (e.g., inhibited bladder contraction) during cystometrography.
2. *Capacity.* Functional bladder capacity measured on the voiding diary dictates the volume that the bladder should be filled during cystometrography. Maximal cystometric capacity measured on cystometrography tends to be larger than the functional bladder capacity. Urodynamic findings and symptoms experienced at filling volume beyond the functional bladder capacity should be interpreted with caution. Before surgical correction for SUI, it is prudent to ensure that bladder capacity and compliance are adequate.
3. *Compliance.* Bladder compliance ($\Delta V/\Delta P_{det}$) describes the relationship between changes in bladder volume (ΔV) and changes in detrusor pressure (ΔP_{det}).[25] It is a measure of bladder vesicoelasticity and reflects the sum of two factors: the passive mechanoelastic property of the bladder wall

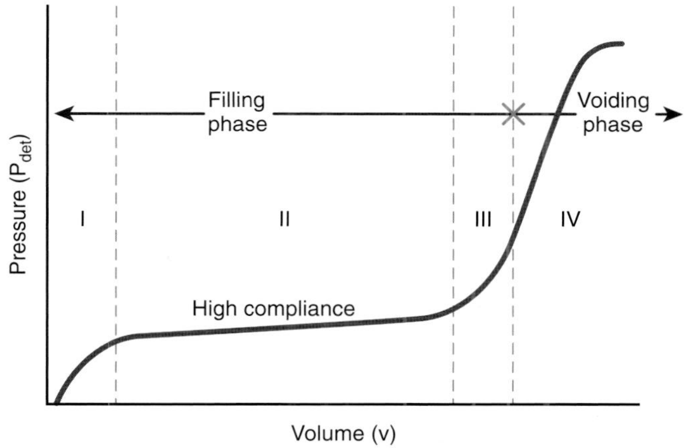

Figure 11-2 Detrusor compliance ($\Delta V/\Delta P_{det}$) remains high during the flat filling phase (phase II) of the cystometrogram in a normal subject. (Adapted from Steers WD, Barrett DM, Wein AJ: Voiding dysfunction: Diagnosis, classification and management. In Gillenwater JY, Grayhack JT, Howards SS, Duckett JW (eds): Adult and Pediatric Urology, 3rd ed. St. Louis, Mosby–Year Book, 1996.)

(correlated with collagen content) and the active neuromuscular force called *tonus* under neural modulation. The normal bladder has high compliance and is able to expand to capacity (large ΔV) with minimal changes in intravesical pressure ($\Delta P_{det} < 15$ to 20 cm H_2O) (Fig. 11-2, flat slope). Decreased compliance is defined as $\Delta V/\Delta P_{det}$ less than 20 mL/cm H_2O, measured from the moment of bladder filling to the point of cystometric capacity or immediately before the start of detrusor contraction that causes significant leakage.[25] Poor compliance may be caused by infection (e.g., cystitis, tuberculosis, schistosomiasis), inflammation (e.g., calculus, interstitial cystitis, carcinoma, radiation), obstruction, chronic indwelling catheter, neurologic disease (e.g., spinal cord injury, Shy-Drager disease), or surgical denervation (e.g., after hysterectomy, abdominoperineal resection), or it may be an artifact of too-rapid bladder filling. The rate of filling should be slowed if poor compliance is encountered. Compliance may be falsely overestimated if a pop-off mechanism prevents adequate bladder filling (e.g., intrinsic sphincter deficiency or vesicoureteral reflux). Low bladder compliance is a harbinger of upper tract disease in neurogenic patients. Patients with poor compliance who are slated for potentially obstructive outlet surgery (e.g., sling, artificial sphincter) need their compliance corrected before or concurrent with the outlet surgery to protect the upper tracts.
4. *Detrusor overactivity.* Involuntary bladder contraction due to neurogenic disorders is called *neurogenic detrusor overactivity* (formerly designated detrusor hyperreflexia), and that not attributed to neurogenic causes is called *idiopathic detrusor overactivity* (formerly designated detrusor instability).[25] Historically a ΔP_{det} of more than15 cm H_2O was necessary to diagnose detrusor overactivity, but any involuntary pressure increase that is associated with urgency now qualifies as overactivity.[21] In patients in whom detrusor overactivity is suspected but not detected on the cystometrogram, provocative maneuvers such as rapid filling (>100 mL/min), filling with cold saline, coughing, heel bouncing, squatting, and hand washing may unmask the

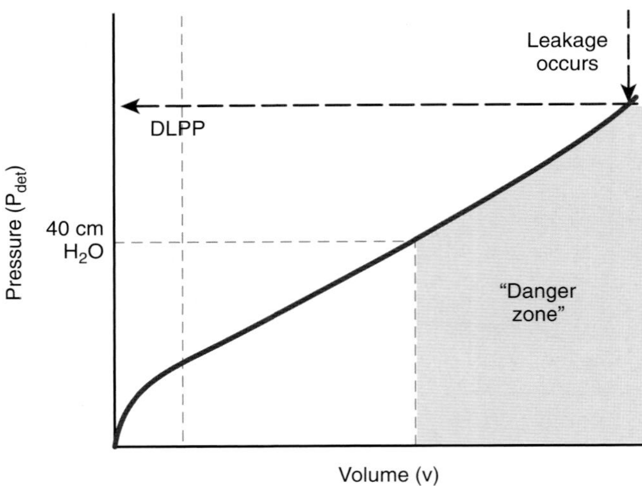

Figure 11-3 Detrusor leak point pressure (DLPP) measurement in the absence of straining or detrusor contraction. The *shaded area* represents the "danger zone," with the DLPP and filling pressure higher than 40 cm H_2O.

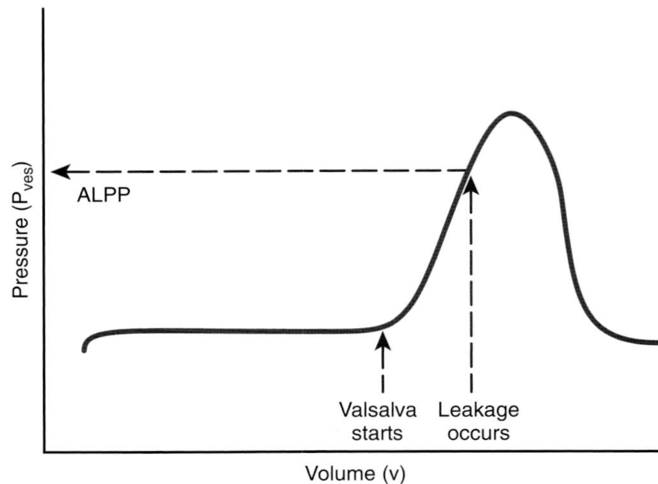

Figure 11-4 Abdominal leak point pressure (ALPP) measurement in the presence of straining but without detrusor contraction.

abnormalities. Up to 40% of patients with urge incontinence fail to demonstrate detrusor overactivity on conventional cystometrography.[26] The absence of documented detrusor overactivity on cystometrography does not rule out its existence. Conversely, patients with detrusor overactivity may not have any symptoms, and its documentation on cystometrography may have no clinical significance.[27] Even though patients with irritative symptoms and stress-induced detrusor overactivity often improve after bladder neck suspension surgery,[28] presumably as a result of eliminating the entrance of urine into the proximal urethra,[29] patients with mixed incontinence as a group appear to fare worse than those with pure SUI after tension-free tape surgery (69% versus 97% cure).[16] There is no consensus about whether the finding of detrusor overactivity in addition to SUI on preoperative cystometrography alters the outcome after surgery.[30]

Detrusor Leak Point Pressure

A concept first introduced by McGuire and associates[31] in 1981 in the evaluation of myelodysplasia patients, detrusor leak point pressure (DLPP) is defined as the lowest detrusor pressure (P_{det}) at which leakage occurs in the absence of detrusor contraction or increased abdominal pressure (Fig. 11-3).[25] The bladder is filled until overflow incontinence occurs, and the instantaneous P_{det} at which leakage occurs (i.e., DLPP) reflects the resistance of the urethra against the expulsive force of bladder storage pressure. When outlet resistance is high, high bladder pressure is needed to overcome this resistance and cause leakage. Bladder pressure higher than 40 cm H_2O impedes ureteral peristalsis, causes hydroureters, and damages the upper tracts. In the classic study of McGuire and colleagues,[31] 81% and 68% of myelodysplasia patients with DLPP greater than 40 cm H_2O developed hydronephrosis and vesicoureteral reflux, respectively. In long-term follow-up, 100% of patients with DLPP greater than 40 cm H_2O exhibited upper tract deterioration or reflux, or both.[32] A DLPP higher than 40 cm H_2O is a prognostic marker for upper tract damage.

Patients with low bladder compliance and a low DLPP may be floridly incontinent, but their upper tracts are safe because the low-resistance urethra functions as a pop-off mechanism to relieve the high detrusor pressure. Patients with low bladder compliance and a DLPP higher than 40 cm H_2O risk upper tract damage unless the outlet resistance is reduced or compliance is improved with medication or surgery. Correction of outlet resistance in patients with detrusor–external sphincter dyssynergia (DESD) by sphincter dilation results in an immediate decrease in DLPP and a gradual but significant improvement of bladder compliance over time.[33] Failure to reduce DLPP to below 40 cm H_2O after sphincterotomy predicts surgical failure, persistent DESD, and upper tract deterioration.[34] The use of intermittent catheterization, anticholinergics, and vesicostomy are effective in protecting the upper tracts of neonates with myelodysplasia.[35] Plotting the danger zone on a filling cystometrogram is an effective method to establish a storage baseline for patients with neurogenic dysfunction and subsequently track effective management by reducing the danger zone.

Abdominal Leak Point Pressure

The idea of ALPP emerged from McGuire's group a decade after the description of DLPP.[36] Originally designed to categorize women with SUI into two groups—urethral hypermobility and intrinsic sphincter deficiency (ISD)—ALPP measurement and Q-tip examination became indispensable tools in the diagnosis of SUI. The International Continence Society defined ALPP as the intravesical pressure (P_{ves}) at which urine leakage occurs due to increased abdominal pressure in the absence of a detrusor contraction.[25] The bladder is half-filled to an arbitrary volume of 200 to 250 mL. The patient is then asked to perform a Valsalva maneuver or cough until leakage occurs. If no leakage is observed, the bladder is filled in 50-mL increments. The smallest recorded P_{ves} associated with urodynamic demonstration of SUI is the ALPP (Fig. 11-4). ALPP (leakage) usually occurs on the upward slope of the curve and not at the peak pressure generated unless the peak pressure represents the exact ALPP (i.e., exact moment of incontinence).

Abdominal Leak Point Pressure versus Detrusor Leak Point Pressure

Unlike DLPP, which is a static reflection of urethral resistance to bladder intrinsic storage pressure, ALPP measures the dynamic urethral resistance to brief increases in abdominal pressure. Abdominal pressure (ALPP) and detrusor pressure (DLPP) are different expulsive forces with respect to the urethra. Whereas detrusor pressure tends to open the bladder neck, abdominal pressure tends to close the internal sphincter shut. Normally, the internal sphincter does not leak or open, regardless of how much abdominal pressure is exerted. For instance, during blunt trauma to a full bladder, the bladder will rupture before the bladder neck is forced open. If SUI occurs as a result of an increase in abdominal pressure, the proximal urethra and bladder neck are rotated and descended away from its resting intra-abdominal position during a Valsalva maneuver (i.e., urethral hypermobility), or there is an intrinsic malfunction of the internal urethral sphincter (i.e., ISD).[37] All women with urethral hypermobility and SUI are considered to have some degree of ISD, because the normal internal sphincter should remain closed no matter how much stress and rotational descent it experiences.[23] ISD is a spectrum of urethral dysfunction.

Abdominal Leak Point Pressure, Urethral Hypermobility, and Internal Urethral Sphincter

SUI patients with urethral hypermobility leak at considerably higher abdominal pressures than those with pure ISD. Leakage at an ALPP less than 60 cm H_2O is characteristic of ISD. Eighty-one percent of patients with an ALPP less than 60 cm H_2O reported a history of severe incontinence, and 76% of patients with an ALPP less than 60 cm H_2O demonstrated type III SUI on fluoroscopic studies (i.e., no urethral hypermobility). Leakage at an ALPP greater than 90 cm H_2O is indicative of urethral hypermobility. These patients reported lesser degrees of incontinence and exhibited type I or type II SUI on VUDS (i.e., minimal to gross hypermobility).[36] Patients with an ALPP between 60 and 90 cm H_2O have type II or type III SUI. Patients with an ALPP less than 60 cm H_2O classically failed to respond to suspension operations designed for the hypermobile urethra. They should be treated with pubovaginal slings, periurethral bulking agents (if there is no associated hypermobility), or artificial sphincters. Subdividing patients into hypermobility or ISD groups based on ALPP measurement and Q-tip test results on physical examination may become less important because pubovaginal slings and mid-urethral slings have been shown to be effective for anatomic incontinence.[12-15]

Abdominal Leak Point Pressure and Pelvic Organ Prolapse

ALPP measurements are more difficult to interpret in the presence of pelvic organ prolapse. Anterior vaginal wall prolapse may falsely elevate the ALPP because the prolapse functions as a sink to dissipate and absorb the effect of abdominal pressure on the proximal urethra.[38] The urethra may be kinked or compressed by the prolapsed organ, causing partial obstruction and elevating the ALPP. This is why patients with high-grade cystoceles rarely complain of clinical SUI. When the prolapse is reduced, up to 60% of patients with grade 1 to 2 cystocele and 91% of patients with grade 3 to 4 cystocele who do not complain of incontinence demonstrate SUI on urodynamic evaluations.[39] If the cystocele is repaired without addressing the urethra, occult stress incontinence may be unmasked postoperatively. It is unclear what percentage of patients with no symptoms of SUI will be symptomatic after a prolapse repair. It is also unclear whether performing ALPP with a pessary helps to predict that population. Whether prophylactic sling should be placed at the time of concomitant prolapse surgery and what roles preoperative ALPP plays in that decision remain controversial. Nevertheless, all patients undergoing ALPP measurements should have a pelvic examination in supine and upright positions to determine whether prolapse exists. If significant prolapse is found, upright ALPP measurements should be repeated with the prolapse reduced.[40]

Abdominal Leak Point Pressure Measurement

The technique for ALPP determination has not been standardized. ALPP decreases significantly as the bladder volume increases.[41] There is no consensus about whether ALPP should be measured at an absolute volume (e.g., 150 mL),[36] one-half the functional bladder capacity,[42] or near capacity.[43] Most expects agree that testing should be done at a "moderate filling volume" that is sufficient to provide a urine bolus for abdominal pressure to act on but not full enough to induce a detrusor contraction, which opens the bladder neck and gives a false impression of ISD.[38] Cough leak point pressure is significantly higher and more variable than Valsalva leak point pressure,[44] possibly due to reflex contraction of the pelvic floor during cough.[45] The size and necessity of bladder catheters have not been standardized. Larger catheters correlate with higher ALPP values, presumably due to partial obstruction.[45] Patients with a history of SUI who do not leak with a urethral catheter in place should have ALPP measurements repeated with the catheter removed.[46] Some investigators recommended measuring ALPP using a rectal catheter alone to measure P_{abd}.[46,47] Others argued that P_{det} should be monitored to ensure that that the detrusor is stable during a Valsalva maneuver.

It is unclear whether the *absolute pressure value*[48] or the *subtracted pressure value from baseline pressure*[49] should be used. It is recommended that the location of pressure sensors, type of catheters, position of patient, status of prolapse (reduced or not), methods in which the bladder is filled (e.g., diuresis, catheter fill), types of ALPP (e.g., cough, Valsalva maneuver), and volume at which measurements are made should be specified. ALPP measurement is inaccurate if the patient cannot generate adequate abdominal pressure.

Resting Urethral Pressure Profilometry

Urethral pressure profilometry (UPP) is a topographic curve that plots the urethral closure pressure (UCP) along the length of the urethra. Intravesical pressure (P_{ves}) and intraluminal urethral pressure (P_{ure}) are measured simultaneously while a mechanical puller withdraws the pressure transducer from the urethra at a set rate (1 to 2 mm/sec). The difference between these two pressures is defined as UCP ($UCP = P_{ure} - P_{ves}$), and it is plotted on the *y*-axis. The urethral length is plotted on the *x*-axis. UPP attempts to quantify the contributions of urinary sphincters and periurethral structures to urethral closure at rest (i.e., resting UPP), during periods of straining (i.e., stress UPP), and during voiding (i.e., micturitional UPP).

Resting UPP measures the static urethral pressure along its length in a resting patient with a full bladder (i.e., no Valsalva maneuver and no voiding). It is measured using the technique of Brown and Wickham.[50] A urethral catheter with radially drilled side holes is slowly withdrawn from the urethra while being

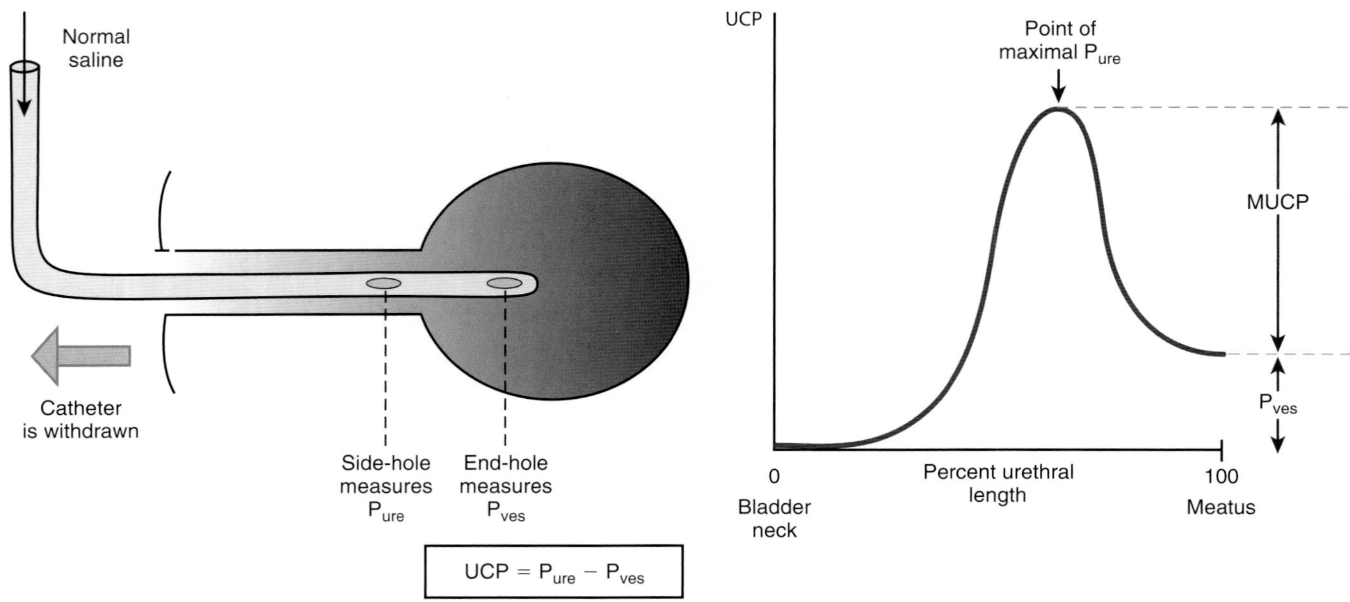

Figure 11-5 Schematic diagram of the resting urethral pressure profile (UPP) shows the calculated urethral closure pressure (UCP), which is equal to the urethral pressure minus the intravesical pressure ($P_{ure} - P_{ves}$) along the length of the urethra.

infused. The intraluminal urethral pressure that is recorded corresponds to the pressure needed to lift the urethral wall off the catheter side holes, and it is presumed that this reflects the radial stress at the urethral surface.[51] The intravesical pressure is simultaneously measured with the end holes of the same catheter. The maximal urethral closure pressure (MUCP), the highest point along the UCP curve, corresponds anatomically to the area of mid-urethra where the striated and smooth muscle sphincters overlap (Fig. 11-5).

Resting UPP has no role in the evaluation of the patient with SUI.[52,53] MUCP lacks the sensitivity and specificity to diagnose and classify incontinence.[54] MUCP cannot be used to distinguish continent from incontinent patients. A low MUCP (<20 cm H_2O) does not predict stress incontinence; many continent women have a low MUCP, and the MUCP cannot characterize the severity of incontinence.[55] An MUCP less than 20 cm H_2O, however, does predict failure of classic retropubic suspension surgery.[56-59] This "low-pressure urethra" was considered to be associated with ISD. No change in UPP has been recorded in patients achieving continence after successful collagen injections[60] or urethropexy.[61] Studies have repeatedly demonstrated that there is no relationship between ALPP and MUCP.[54] This is not surprising because many believe that continence is maintained at the bladder neck, not at the mid-urethral high-pressure zone where MUCP is recorded. (The success of mid-urethral sling surgery challenges this view). Incontinence or continence is not determined by urethral pressure at rest (i.e., MUCP) but by urethral resistance to abdominal pressure during straining (i.e., ALPP). Resting UPP is a rudimentary measurement of urethral closure at rest, and it cannot capture the complex interactions among the detrusor, the sphincters, and the pelvic floor during the dynamic moment of straining. The reproducibility of resting UPP is poor because techniques of its measurement have not been standardized.[55]

Stress Urethral Pressure Profilometry

Stress UPP measures the dynamic urethral resistance along its length as the patient strains. It reflects the patient's ability to maintain continence in the face of abdominal pressure. Pressure spikes are generated intravesically (ΔP_{ves}) and intraurethrally (ΔP_{ure}) during a Valsalva maneuver or coughing. The pressure-transmission ratio (PTR) is calculated as the ratio ($\Delta P_{ure}/\Delta P_{ves}$) along the urethral length during the pressure spikes (Fig. 11-6). A PTR greater than 100% implies positive-pressure transmission (i.e., the urethral pressure spikes exceed the bladder pressure spikes), whereas a PTR less than 100% suggests that more pressure is transmitted to the bladder than to the urethra.

Normally, the proximal urethra remains intra-abdominal during straining, with equal pressure transmission to the bladder and the urethra ($\Delta P_{ure} \geq \Delta P_{ves}$, or PTR $\geq$ 100%). In patients with SUI and urethral hypermobility, posterior rotation and descent of the proximal urethra during straining results in unequal pressure transmission[62] and therefore a PTR less than 100% ($\Delta P_{ure} < \Delta P_{ves}$). Although it is true that patients with anatomic SUI tend to have lower PTR values (usually < 90%) than continent subjects,[63,64] there are significant overlaps between the PTR values of continent and incontinent patients,[65,66] rendering the test insensitive in diagnosing anatomic SUI.[67] The reason for the large overlap may be explained by the observation that not all patients with urethral hypermobility and low PTR are incontinent; a certain degree of ISD must exist for leakage to occur. Unlike MUCP, PTR increases after successful bladder suspension[68-71] and mid-urethral sling procedures.[72]

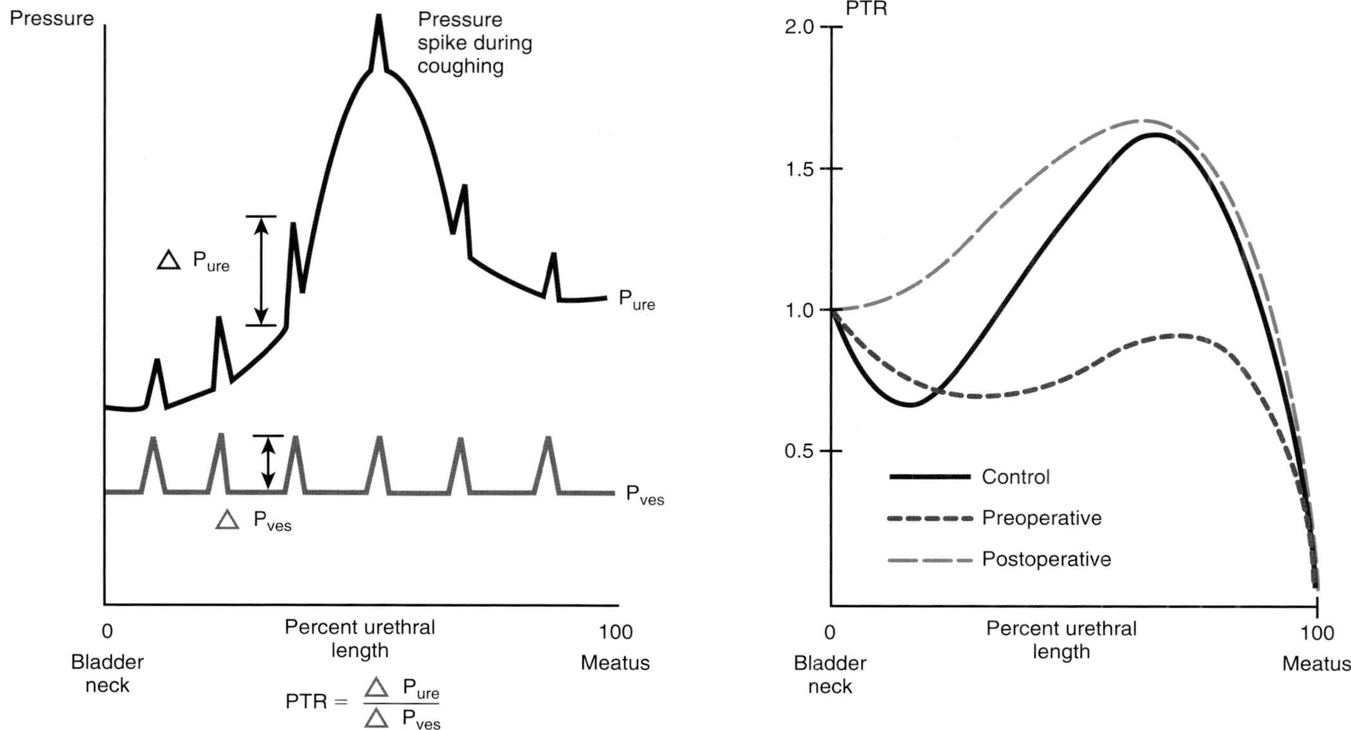

Figure 11-6 The pressure-transmission ratio (PTR) is plotted along the urethral length as the ratio between urethral pressure spikes (ΔP_{ure}) and bladder pressure spikes (ΔP_{ves}): PTR = $\Delta P_{ure}/\Delta P_{ves}$. *Controls* are defined as normal, healthy volunteers with no symptoms of urinary incontinence. *Preoperative* indicates patients with stress incontinence. *Postoperative* indicates the same patients after bladder neck suspension. (Adapted from Constantinou CE: Urethrometry: Consideration of static dynamic and stability characteristics of the female urethra. Neuroradiol Urodyn 7:521, 1998.)

EVALUATION OF VOIDING FUNCTION

Uroflowmetry

Uroflowmetry Measurement

First described by von Garrelts in the 1950s,[73] uroflowmetry is the measurement of the rate of urine flow (Q) over time. Urine flow rate can be measured by weight transducers, rotating disks, or electronic capacitance dipsticks.[74] The seated position is recommended for female patients. Patients should be well hydrated and have a reasonably full bladder before the study. An overly distended bladder may decompensate and result in reduced urine flow. However, a small voided volume (<150 mL) may affect flow rate interpretation. Voiding should be done in privacy, with as little distraction and as few observers as possible so that the patient can relax to replicate her usual urine flow. An anxious and tense patient may be psychologically inhibited and involuntarily contract her pelvic floor. Her flow rate may be altered, or she may not be able to empty at all. The patients should always be asked if the void is typical with respect to its volume, force, and pattern.[74] If in doubt, several measurements may be obtained to exclude variations. Studies have shown that between 20% and 40% of patients have a difference of $Q_{max} \pm 2$ mL/sec between successive voids.[75,76] Maximal flow rate (Q_{max}) is the most commonly reported parameter (Fig. 11-7). It is important to visually confirm the Q_{max} value on the flow curve because machine-read values are on average 1.5 mL/sec higher than manually read (true) values due to wag artifacts.[77] It is also crucial to interpret the quantitative measurements in the context of the shape of the flow curve (i.e., normal versus intermittent versus obstructive patterns).

Normal Uroflowmetry in Females

Normal uroflow patterns in female patients have been described in the literature.[78,79] Unlike men, in whom Q_{max} decreases with age, the Q_{max} is not influenced by age in women.[80] As in men, Q_{max} in women is influenced by bladder volume. The Liverpool nomogram plots the Q_{max} and Q_{ave} values against bladder volumes based on measurements from 249 normal female volunteers.[81] The 10th percentile curve was picked arbitrarily as the lower limit of normality. Other uroflow nomograms (e.g., Siroky, Bristol) do not apply to females because they were based on male patients.[82] A small voided volume (<150 mL) may affect flow rate interpretation. In women with frequency or urgency syndromes, the flow rate curves may be nondiagnostic because of small voided volumes. In general, normal women have a higher Q_{max} value for a given voided volume than age-matched men, usually on the order of 5 mL/sec,[83,84] because of lower outlet resistance.

Clinical Applications of Uroflowmetry

Uroflow reflects the final summation of detrusor contraction, abdominal straining, urethral resistance, and sphincteric or pelvic floor relaxation. A Q_{max} greater than 15 mL/sec with a voided volume greater than 100 mL and minimal PVR essentially rules out obstruction in female patients.[86] However, it is not possible

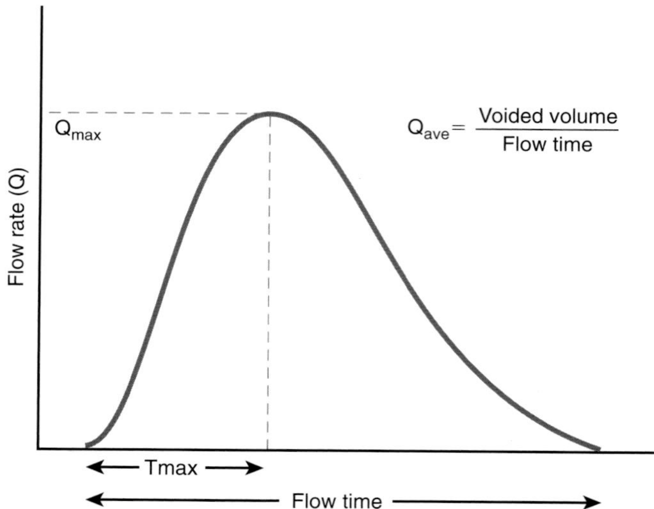

Figure 11-7 Uroflowmetry. The voided volume is the total volume of urine expelled through the urethra. The maximal flow rate (Q_{max}) is the maximal measured rate of flow, and the time to maximal flow (T_{max}) is the time elapsed from onset of flow to maximal flow. The flow time is the time during which flow occurs, and the average flow rate (Q_{ave}) is determined by dividing the voided volume by the flow time. In patients with intermittent flow patterns, the flow time is measured by disregarding the time intervals between flow episodes. Q_{ave} cannot be accurately calculated if the flow is intermittent or dribbling.

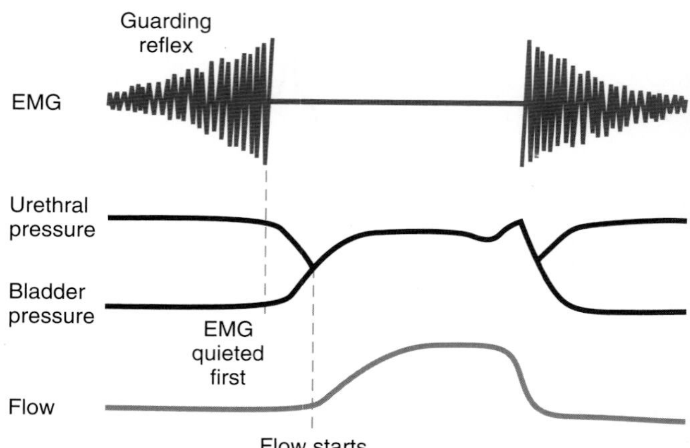

Figure 11-8 Normal electromyographic pattern. The electromyographic signals become more intense and frequent as the bladder fills because of recruitment of the pelvic floor and urinary sphincter during filling (i.e., guarding reflex). The signal is quieted before actual detrusor contraction and flow. (Adapted from Blaivas JG: Pathophysiology of lower urinary tract dysfunction. Clin Obstet Gynaecol 12:295, 1985.)

to tell from a low Q_{max} whether there is bladder outlet obstruction or impaired detrusor contractility.[87] PFSs, micturitional UPP, and video-urodynamic or sphincteric electromyography are needed to differentiate obstruction from detrusor underactivity. Flow rate does not tell whether or why a female patient is incontinent. Patients with SUI and low outlet resistance may present with a superflow pattern. Patients with SUI who are slated for surgery should be screened with uroflowmetry and PVR. Those with an abnormally low Q_{max} and high PVR deserve further urodynamic evaluations to rule out detrusor underactivity or outlet obstruction before SUI surgery. This is particularly important for patients who had prior posterior pelvic exenteration, radical hysterectomy, abdominoperineal resection, or pelvic reconstructive surgery. These procedures are associated with a high incidence of voiding dysfunction due to vascular, neural, and anatomic disruption to the lower urinary tract.[88] In summary, uroflow is a fast, cheap, and noninvasive urodynamic screening test for voiding dysfunction.

Pressure-Flow Studies

A PFS is usually performed after cystometrography. The patient is instructed to void while bladder pressure and flow rate are simultaneously measured throughout the micturition cycle. The flow pattern should be representative of that observed during uroflowmetry. The flow rate measured by PFS (with a catheter) may be slightly lower than the free flow rate measured during uroflowmetry (without a catheter).[89] The patient should be specifically asked if the void is typical with respect to its volume, force, and pattern.[74] PFS allows bladder outlet obstruction to be differentiated from detrusor underactivity when a low Q_{max} is detected. High-pressure low flow is diagnostic of functional or anatomic outlet obstruction. However, low-pressure low flow does not rule out obstruction in female patients (Fig. 11-8). PFS alone cannot identify the site or mechanism of obstruction; VUDS or sphincteric electromyography is needed instead.

Female Outlet Obstruction

Female outlet obstruction is most commonly encountered after anti-incontinence surgery, particularly if an associated anterior wall defect (e.g., cystocele) was not repaired at the time of anti-incontinence surgery. Large prolapse can also cause outlet obstruction by kinking the urethra, distorting the bladder neck anatomy, or direct compression. There is no consensus regarding a critical value of pressure and flow that is diagnostic for obstruction in females. Commonly used pressure-flow plots (i.e., Abrams-Griffith, Schafer, urethral resistance factor, and International Continence Society provisional nomograms) are not applicable to female patients because they were developed for use in men with bladder outlet obstruction.[90-93] Nomograms for obstruction in females have been published but are not widely used.[94] Massey and Abrams[95] proposed a definition of obstruction if two of the following conditions exist: Q_{max} less than 12 mL/sec; P_{det} greater than 50 cm H_2O; resistive index greater than 0.2, which is defined as $P_{det}/(Q_{max})^2$; or a high PVR volume. Axelrod[96] defined primary bladder neck obstruction as P_{det} greater than 20 cm H_2O and Q_{max} less than 12 mL/sec. In light of the low specificity and lack of standardization of PFS results, Nitti[97] proposed the use of VUDS to diagnose obstruction, which was defined as radiographic evidence of obstruction between the bladder neck and the external sphincter in the presence of sustained bladder contraction.

The voiding dynamics of women are different from those of men. In men, a significant P_{det} is recorded during voiding because the detrusor has to exert a force strong enough to move the urine bolus through a relatively high-resistance conduit (i.e., prostatic urethra). In normal women, however, there is very little increase in P_{det} during voiding, even when bladder contractility is normal, because the flow of urine encounters minimal resistance against the female urethra. Inability to record a strong detrusor contrac-

Table 11-2 Stress Urinary Incontinence Types Based on Video Urodynamics Appearance

		Bladder Neck at Rest		*Bladder Neck During Valsalva*		
Type of SUI	**SUI Seen on VUDS?**	**Status**	**Position**	**Status**	**Position**	**Cystocele Present?**
0	No	Closed	At/above PS	Open	Descends < 2 cm	No
I	Yes	Closed	At/above PS	Open	Descends < 2 cm	No
IIA	Yes	Closed	At/above PS	Open	Rotational descent	No or small
IIB	Yes	Closed	Below PS	Open	Rotational descent	Large
III	Yes	Open	—	Open	—	—

PS, pubic symphysis; SUI, stress urinary incontinence, VUDS, video urodynamics.
From Blaivas JG, Olsson CA: Stress incontinence: Classification and surgical approach. J Urol 139:727, 1988.

tion in females is common during PFS and should not be a cause for alarm if the patient's history, physical examination, and voiding diary are otherwise normal.[98] Even in the setting of bladder outlet obstruction, many patients fail to generate a high P_{det} on PFS, probably because women void by pelvic floor relaxation rather than high-pressure detrusor contraction. Habitual Valsalva-induced voiding across a relaxed pelvic floor is a common pattern seen in women. For instance, in patients who underwent bladder suspension complicated by obstruction and irritative voiding who improved after successful urethrolysis, only one third to one half have obstructive PFS patterns before urethrolysis.[99-101] Although a high-pressure, low-flow PFS result is diagnostic of obstruction, a low-pressure, low-flow PFS result does not necessarily rule out obstruction (depending on the definition of obstruction). This observation calls into question the need to perform urodynamic evaluation of patients who are presumably obstructed after anti-incontinence surgery and who are slated for urethrolysis. Patients unable to generate adequate P_{det} on preoperative a PFS may be at higher risk for prolonged postoperative retention after cadaveric pubovaginal slings.[102] Patients most likely to report de novo urgency, presumably due to partial obstruction, after tension-free tape procedures are those in whom Valsalva-induced voiding or low P_{det} was present on preoperative PFSs.[18] Patients with preoperative dysfunctional voiding on the PFS ($P_{det} > 20$ cm H_2O and $Q_{max} < 12$ mL/sec) are less likely to be cured (based on pad tests) and more likely to have a diminished quality of life after tension-free tape surgery.[103] The role of the preoperative PFS in the evaluation of SUI is evolving.

Micturitional Urethral Pressure Profilometry

Described originally by Yalla and associates,[104] micturitional urethral pressure profilometry (MUPP) is used to diagnose and localize the site of urethral obstruction. During steady midstream voiding, P_{ves} and P_{det} are the same (i.e., isobaric). If an obstruction exists in the urethra, the intraurethral pressure distal to the obstruction is lower, and the pressures in the urethra proximal to the obstruction and in the bladder are higher. When a significant pressure drop is encountered on catheter withdrawal, it corresponds to the site of the obstruction. In a patient with a normal urethra, the bladder and almost the entire length of urethra are isobaric, except the terminal 1 cm of the distal urethra.[105] This normal pressure drop occurs distal to the point of MUCP and proximal to the external meatus. In an obstructed urethra, the site of obstruction can be identified by *an additional* drop in urethral pressure that occurs *proximal* to the normal pressure drop point. Even though the concept is elegant, MUPP lacks anatomic resolution to define the exact location and mechanism of obstruction (VUDS is far superior). The exact location of the pressure being transduced is difficult to ascertain without fluoroscopy. MUPP is difficult to perform correctly because it is prone to micturitional artifacts.[106]

VIDEO URODYNAMICS

First described in the late 1960s,[107] the use of VUDS adds real-time, high-resolution anatomic details to a cystometrogram and PFS. Regarded as the gold standard of urodynamic evaluation, VUDS allow structural-functional correlations to be investigated because transducer pressures, patients' symptoms, and live fluoroscopic images are studied simultaneously. Historically, SUI was classified as type 0, I, II, or III based on the fluoroscopic appearance of the bladder neck on VUDS (Table 11-2).[108] ALPP measurements and Q-tip tests are commonly used to classify patients with urethral hypermobility or ISD, or both. VUDS are not indicated in many situations.[109] For instance, VUDS are rarely needed to diagnose detrusor overactivity. If obstruction is suspected, PFS can be obtained. VUDS are not indicated in SUI patients with obvious hypermobility and no overactive bladder symptoms. If ISD is suspected, ALPP can be performed. Because of the expense and radiographic exposure, VUDS are reserved for patients with complex pathophysiology, as in the following circumstances:

1. *Neurogenic bladder*. VUDS can detect vesicoureteral reflux and the pressure and volume at which it occurs. With cystometrography alone (without fluoroscopy), the reflux pop-off mechanism can artificially overestimate the bladder compliance and capacity and falsely decrease the DLPP, making the compliance, capacity, and DLPP appear better than they really are. Other "bladder hostile factors," such as bladder diverticulum, trabeculation, and detrusor–external sphincter dyssynergia (DESD) or detrusor–internal sphincter dyssynergia (DISD), can also be easily identified on VUDS.
2. *Failed prior anti-incontinence surgery*. VUDS allow simultaneous determination of the presence and degree of vesical neck hypermobility, the degree and presence of ISD, the degree and type of cystocele, the presence and location of obstruction, and ALPP simultaneously. Although these characteristics can be identified with a simple cystogram, the presence of an open bladder neck on radiography has little significance without knowing whether the detrusor is

contracting. In the presence of a detrusor contraction, an open bladder neck is a normal response, whereas an open bladder neck in the absence of a detrusor contraction in a woman with SUI may be a sign of ISD. Only by simultaneously recording the detrusor behavior by VUDS can such a distinction be made.[23] Fluoroscopy may also improve the accuracy of ALPP measurement because it is easier to observe leakage of contrast agent than it is to observe leakage from an upright patient directly using a flashlight.

3. *Obstructive voiding.* It is easier to define the exact anatomic location and mechanism of obstruction (e.g., stricture, DESD, DISD, pseudo-dyssynergia, urethral kinking) by VUDS. Filling is done in a standing position, and voiding is done seated.
4. *Significant pelvic organ prolapse.* VUDS demonstrates the real-time anatomic effects of prolapse on bladder and urethral function. Dynamic magnetic resonance imaging may also offer additional insights on the effect of posterior or apical vaginal wall defects on voiding.
5. *Urinary diversion and augmentation.* VUDS can be used to investigate the cause of incontinence and hydronephrosis after continent urinary diversion, orthotopic bladder substitution, or bladder augmentation. Incontinence may be caused by an incompetent outlet in the native sphincter or the reconstructed continence mechanism, high-pressure intestinal or bladder contraction, or poor neobladder or augmented bladder compliance (often caused by ischemia). These possibilities can be distinguished on VUDS. The sphincteric mechanism in orthotopic bladder may be evaluated in the same manner as ISD in the native bladder. Vesicoureteral reflux causing hydronephrosis can be easily detected. DLPP measurement (at catheterization volume) should be measured regularly after bladder augmentation in neurogenic patients to ensure that the goal of low-pressure filling is accomplished.[110,111]

SPHINCTER ELECTROMYOGRAPHY

Electromyographic Measurement

Electromyography measures the electrical activities of the striated urinary sphincter through an electrode. It provides kinesiologic information about the urethral sphincter and the pelvic floor muscles. Needle electrodes or surface electrodes can be used. The needle electrode is inserted directly into the striated urinary sphincter and records activities directly from that muscle group. Needle insertion causes discomfort, and it is easily dislodged during posture change, but it provides high-quality signals directly from the muscle of interest. Surface electrodes are placed on the skin or mucosa overlying the muscle of interest, and they pick up the potentials produced by various muscles in the vicinity. Commonly, the surface electrode is applied around the anus and records activities from the striated anal sphincter. Usually, anal sphincter activity and urinary sphincter activity are congruent. In patients with neurologic disease, this relationship cannot be assumed, and when possible, needle electrodes should be used instead. Before bladder filling, the examiner should ensure that sphincteric activity is recorded appropriately by eliciting a burst of electromyographic activity by asking the patient to contract her sphincter voluntarily, asking the patient to perform a Valsalva maneuver or cough, or stimulating the bulbocavernosus reflex.

Clinical Applications of Electromyography

Electromyography is indicated in the evaluation of spinal cord injury; neurologic disease, such as multiple sclerosis or Parkinson's disease; voiding dysfunction after radical pelvic surgery or back surgery; and in young women with idiopathic urinary retention. Clinically, the most important information is whether bladder contraction and sphincter relaxation are coordinated during volitional voiding. During normal voiding, electromyographic activity is quieted (i.e., relaxation of striated sphincter and pelvic floor) before initiation of detrusor contraction (see Fig. 11-8). Increased electromyographic activity and sphincter closure at the time of volitional voiding is detrimental to the bladder (e.g., poor compliance, diverticulum formation, trabeculation) and the upper tract (e.g., renal insufficiency, hydronephrosis, vesicoureteral reflux, recurrent sepsis, stone formation) due to high voiding pressure.

In DESD, there is true discoordination between the detrusor and the external sphincter due to suprasacral spinal cord injury. The sphincter involuntarily closes shut when the bladder contracts. DESD should not be confused with the pseudo-dyssynergia commonly seen after a stroke. In pseudo-dyssynergia, there is a voluntary increase in sphincter activity with the sudden onset of a bladder contraction and sense of urgency. Pseudo-dyssynergia is a volitional response to urgency to prevent urge incontinence rather than a true discoordination between the bladder and the sphincter. DESD can be differentiated from pseudo-dyssynergia by asking the patient if she is voluntarily contracting the sphincter or pelvic floor in response to urgency during periods of increased electromyographic activities. Hinman's syndrome is a subconscious contraction of the sphincter with a bladder contraction. Unlike true DESD, no spinal cord injury or neurologic disease exists in Hinman's syndrome. For this reason, Hinman's syndrome is also called *non-neurogenic neurogenic bladder,* and it is thought to be a learned voiding dysfunction.[112] DESD can be treated with sphincterotomy,[34] external sphincter dilation,[34] urinary diversion, or a combination of clean intermittent catheterization and anticholinergic drugs.[35] Hinman's syndrome can be treated by behavioral modification combined with medications. Sphincteric bradykinesia in patients with Parkinson's disease can be diagnosed with electromyography in conjunction with fluoroscopic imaging.

AMBULATORY URODYNAMICS

Conventional cystometrography may fail to reproduce the patient's symptoms and may provoke symptoms or findings not usually experienced by the patient. Ambulatory urodynamic tests offer the theoretical advantage of being able to monitor the patient's storage and voiding function in a more physiologic manner. The bladder is filled naturally (i.e., diuresis), and the patient has the freedom to move freely and to perform daily activities that normally trigger the presenting symptoms (e.g., incontinence, urgency). Nonphysiologic bladder filling through a catheter is avoided. The psychological inhibition and intimidation associated with voiding in front of strangers in an unfamiliar laboratory is minimized.

Different methods of recording have been described.[113,114] Cystometry is monitored through intravesical and rectal catheters, and the signal is transmitted to a portable, battery-powered recorder. Flow measurements can be made using home uroflowmetry. Incontinence is measured using regular pads or electronic moisture-sensitive pads. The premise of ambulatory urodynamics is that it may offer additional insights when conventional urodynamics is unable to reproduce the patient's presenting symptoms.

Because the investigator is not present during the telemetry, significant problems may arise in the proper interpretation of the tracing. For events (e.g., urgency, incontinence, voiding) to be properly recorded, the patient must take an active role and conscientiously press an event marker or write in a diary every time the event happens. This reliance on patient compliance may be a source of significant error. Detrusor after-contractions, aberrant rectal pressures, movement artifacts, and catheter movements are common.[115] It may be difficult to distinguish these artifacts from physiologic events. It remains difficult to resolve the different findings with conventional and ambulatory cystometrography and explain what these differences mean clinically.

A higher incidence of unstable detrusor contractions was recorded during ambulatory urodynamics compared with conventional cystometrography in symptomatic and asymptomatic patients. Van Waalwijk van Doorn and associates[116] found unstable detrusor contractions in 69% of asymptomatic women using ambulatory urodynamics, whereas conventional cystometrography detected detrusor instability in only 18% of asymptomatic women. Robertson's group[115] similarly found significantly more detrusor instability on ambulatory studies compared with cystometrography (38% versus 17%) in asymptomatic men and women. Ambulatory urodynamics can also detect detrusor instability in patients for whom a cystometrogram is nondiagnostic. The significance of this increased detection of detrusor instability is unclear, given the high incidence found in asymptomatic patients. It is unclear whether ambulatory cystometrography is more sensitive or it has a higher false-positive rate of diagnosing detrusor overactivity than conventional cystometrography. Whether this increased phasic detrusor activity is a physiologic finding or caused by movement artifacts of the catheter or interpretation ambiguity is debated. Although the terminology, methodology, analysis, and reporting of ambulatory urodynamics have been standardized by the International Continence Society,[116] widespread adoption of the technique has been limited by its technical complexity, time consumption, potential artifacts, difficult result interpretation, and uncertain clinical applicability.

In patients with chronic retention and neurogenic bladder, bladder compliance measured by ambulatory urodynamics is much higher than that measured by conventional cystometrography.[117,118] Patients with hydronephrosis and high filling pressures on conventional cystometrography were found to have normal filling pressures and better bladder compliance on ambulatory urodynamics. It is possible that the low compliance seen on conventional cystometrography in some patients may be an artifact related to too-rapid bladder filling.

References

1. Davis DM: The Mechanisms of Urology Disease. Philadelphia, WB Saunders, 1953.
2. Amundsen C, Lau M, English SF, McGuire EJ: Do urinary symptoms correlate with urodynamic findings? J Urol 161:1871, 1999.
3. Madersbacher S, Pycha A, Klimgler CH, et al: The International Prostate Symptom Score in both sexes: A urodynamics-based comparison. Neurourol Urodyn 18:173, 1999.
4. Nitti VW, Combs AJ: Urodynamics: When, why, and how. In Nitti VW (ed): Practical Urodynamics. Philadelphia, WB Saunders, 1998, pp 15-26.
5. Winters JC, Appell RA: Urinary incontinence and frequency and urgency syndromes in women. In Nitti VW (ed): Practical Urodynamics. Philadelphia, WB Saunders, 1998, pp 184-196.
6. Cheng TO: Prevention of bacterial endocarditis: American Heart Association recommendations. JAMA 278:1233, 1997.
7. Krum H, Louis WJ, Brown DJ, Howes LG: A study of the alpha-1 adrenoreceptor blocker prazosin in the prophylactic management of autonomic dysreflexia in high spinal cord injury patients. Clin Auton Res 2:83, 1992.
8. Thyberg M, Ertgaard P, Gylling M, Granerus G: Effect of nifedipine on cystometry-induced elevation of blood pressure in patients with reflex urinary bladder after high spinal cord injury. Paraplegia 32:308, 1994.
9. Blaivas JG, Groutz A: Urinary incontinence: Pathophysiology, evaluation, and management overview In Walsh PC, Retik AB, Vaughan ED, Wein AW (eds): Campbell's Urology, 8th ed. Philadelphia, WB Saunders, 2002, pp 1027-1052.
10. Glazener CM, Lapitan MC: Urodynamic investigation for management of urinary incontinence in adults. Cochrane Database Sys Rev (3):CD003195, 2002.
11. Lemack GE: Urodynamic assessment of patients with stress incontinence: How effective are urethral pressure profilometry and abdominal leak point pressures at case selection and predict outcome. Curr Opin Urol 14:307, 2004.
12. Zaragoza MR: Expanded indications for the pubovaginal sling: Treatment of type 2 or 3 stress incontinence. J Urol 156:1620, 1996.
13. Chaikin DC, Rosenthal J, Blaivas JG: Pubovaginal fascial sling for all types of stress urinary incontinence. J Urol 160:1312, 1998.
14. Morgan TO, Westney OL, McGuire EJ: Pubovaginal sling: 4-year outcome analysis and quality of life assessment. J Urol 163:1845, 2000.
15. Rodriguez LV, de Almeida F, Dorey F, Raz S: Does Valsalva leak point pressure predict outcome after the distal urethral polypropylene sling? Role of urodynamics in the sling era. J Urol 172:210, 2004.
16. Laurikainen E, Kiilholma P: The tension free vaginal tape procedure for female urinary incontinence without preoperative urodynamic evaluation. J Am Coll Surg 196:579, 2003
17. Miller EA, Amundsen CL, Toh KL, et al: Preoperative urodynamic evaluation may predict voiding dysfunction in women undergoing pubovaginal sling. J Urol 169:2234, 2003.
18. Gateau T, Faramarzi-Roques R, Le Normand L, et al: Clinical and urodynamic repercussions after TVT procedure and how to diminish patients complaints. Eur Urol 44:372, 2003.
19. Wang AC, Chen M-C: The correlation between preoperative voiding mechanism and surgical outcome of the tension-free vaginal tape procedure, with reference to quality of life. BJU Int 91:502, 2003.
20. Kaula N: Practical engineering aspects of urodynamics. In Nitti VW (ed): Practical Urodynamics. Philadelphia, WB Saunders, 1998, pp 5-14.
21. Nitti VW: Cystometry and abdominal pressure monitoring. In Nitti VW (ed): Practical Urodynamics. Philadelphia, WB Saunders, 1998, pp 38-51.
22. Tessier J, Schick E: Does urethral instrumentation affect uroflowmetry measurements. Br J Urol 65:261, 1990.

23. Webster GD, Guralnick ML: The neurourologic evaluation. In Walsh PC, Retik AB, Vaughan ED, Wein AW (eds): Campbell's Urology, 8th ed. Philadelphia, WB Saunders, 2002, pp 900-930.
24. Smith CP, Boone TB, Nitti VW: Pitfalls and artifacts in urodynamic studies: In Nitti VW (ed): Practical Urodynamics. Philadelphia, WB Saunders, 1998, pp 131-139.
25. Abrams P, Cardozo L, Fall M, et al: The standardization of terminology of lower urinary tract function: Report from the Standardization Sub-committee of the International Continence Society. Neurourol Urodyn 21:167, 2002.
26. McGuire EJ: Urodynamic evaluation of stress incontinence. Urol Clin North Am 22:551, 1995.
27. van Waalwijk van Doorn ESC, Meier AH, Ambergen AW, Janknegt RA: Ambulatory urodynamics: Extramural testing of the lower and upper urinary tract by Holter monitoring of cystometrogram, uroflowmetry, and renal pelvic pressures. Urol Clin North Am 23:345, 1996.
28. McGuire EJ, Lytton B, Kohorn E, et al: The value of urodynamic testing in stress urinary incontinence. J Urol 124:256, 1980.
29. Mahoney D, Laferte R, Blais D: Incontinence of urine due to instability of micturition reflexes. Urology 15:229, 1980.
30. Griffith D: Clinical aspects of detrusor instability and the value of urodynamics: A review of the evidence. Eur Urol 34(Supp 1):13, 1998.
31. McGuire EJ, Woodside JR, Borden TA, Weiss RM: Prognostic value of urodynamic testing in myelodysplastic patients. J Urol 126:205, 1981.
32. McGuire EJ, Woodside JR, Borden TA: Upper urinary tract deterioration in patients with myelodysplasia and detrusor hypotonia: A follow-up study. J Urol 129:823, 1983.
33. Park JM, McGuire EJ, Koo HP, et al: External urethral sphincter dilation for the management of high risk myelomeningocele: 15-year experience. J Urol 165:2383, 2001.
34. Kim YH, Kattan MW, Boone TB: Bladder leak point pressure: The measure for sphincterotomy success in spinal cord injured patients with external detrusor-sphincter dyssynergia. J Urol 159:493, 1998.
35. Sidi AA, Dykstra DD, Gonzalez R: The value of urodynamic testing and the management of neonates with myelodysplasia: A prospective study. J Urol 135:90, 1986.
36. McGuire EJ, Fitzpatrick CC, Wan J, et al: Clinical assessment of urethral sphincter function. J Urol 150:1452, 1993.
37. McGuire EJ, Gormley EA: Clinical assessment of urethral sphincter and conduit function by measurement of abdominal and detrusor pressures required to induce leakage. In Raz S (ed): Female Urology. Philadelphia, WB Saunders, 1996, pp 106-114.
38. McGuire EJ, Cespedes RD, O'Connell HE: Leak-point pressures. Urol Clin North Am 23:253, 1996.
39. Gardy M, Kozminski M, DeLancey J, et al: Stress incontinence and cystoceles. J Urol 145:1211, 1991.
40. Ghoniem GM, Walters F, Lewis V: The value of the vaginal pack test in large cystoceles. J Urol 152:931, 1994.
41. Theofrastous JP, Cundiff GW, Harris RL, Bump RC: The effect of vesical volume on Valsalva leak-point pressures in women with genuine stress urinary incontinence. Obstet Gynecol 87:711, 1996.
42. Nitti VW, Combs AJ: Correlation of Valsalva leak point pressure with subjective degree of stress urinary incontinence in women. J Urol 155:281, 1996.
43. Bump RC, Elser DM, Theofrastus JP, McClish DK: Valsalva leak point pressures in women with genuine stress incontinence: Reproducibility, effect of catheter caliber, and correlations with other measures of urethral resistance. Am J Obstet Gynecol 173:551, 1995.
44. Peschers UM, Jundt K, Dimpfl T: Differences between cough and Valsalva leak-point pressure in stress incontinent women. Neurourol Urodyn 19:677, 2000.
45. Bump RC, Copeland WE, Hurt WG, Fantl JA: Dynamic urethral pressure/profilometry pressure transmission ratio determination in stress-incontinent and stress-continent subjects. Am J Obstet Gynecol 159:749, 1988.
46. Chaikin DC, Blaivas JG, Rosenthal JE, Weiss JP: Results of pubovaginal sling for stress incontinence: A prospective comparison of instruments for outcome analysis. J Urol 162:1670, 1999.
47. Stohrer M, Goepel M, Kondo A, et al: The standardization of terminology in neurogenic lower urinary tract dysfunction with suggestions for diagnostic procedures. Neurourol Urodyn 18:139, 1999.
48. Appell RA: Sphincter insufficiency: Testing and treatment. Curr Opin Urol 7:197, 1997.
49. Bump RC, Coates KW, Cundiff GW, et al: Diagnosing intrinsic sphincter deficiency: Comparing urethral closure pressure, urethral axis, and Valsalva leak point pressures. Am J Obstet Gynecol 177:303, 1997.
50. Brown M, Wickham JEA: The urethral pressure profile. Br J Urol 41:211, 1969.
51. Steele GS, Sullivan MP, Yalla SV: Urethral pressure profilometry: Vesicourethral pressure measurements under resting and voiding conditions. In Nitti VW (ed): Practical Urodynamics. Philadelphia, WB Saunders, 1998, pp 108-130.
52. Blaivas JG, Awad SA, Bissada N: Urodynamic procedure: Recommendations of the Urodynamics Society. I. Procedures that should be available for routine urologic practice. Neurourol Urodyn 1:51, 1982.
53. McGuire EJ, Gormley EA: Abdominal fascial slings. In Raz S (ed): Female Urology, 2nd ed. Philadelphia, WB Saunders, 1986, pp 369-375.
54. McGuire EJ: Urodynamic evaluation of stress incontinence. Urol Clin North Am 22:551, 1995.
55. Weber AM: Is urethral pressure profilometry a useful diagnostic test for stress urinary incontinence? Obstet Gynecol Surv 56:720, 2001.
56. McGuire EJ: Urodynamic findings in patients after failure of stress incontinence operations. Prog Clin Biol Res 78:351, 1981.
57. Sand PK, Bowen LW, Panganiban R, Ostergard DR: The low pressure urethra as a factor in failed retropubic urethropexy. Obstet Gynecol 69:399, 1987.
58. Bowen LW, Sand PK, Ostergard DR: Unsuccessful Burch retropubic urethropexy: A case controlled urodynamic study. Am J Obstet Gynecol 160:451, 1989.
59. Koonings PP, Bergman A, Ballard CA: Low urethral pressure and stress urinary incontinence in women: Risk factor for failed retropubic surgical procedure. Urology 16:245, 1990.
60. McGuire EJ, Appell RA: Transurethral collagen injection for urinary incontinence. Urology 43:413, 1994.
61. Rydhstrom H, Iosif S: Urodynamic studies before and after retropubic colpo-urethral cystopexy in fertile women with stress urinary incontinence. Arch Gynecol Obstet 241:201, 1988.
62. Einhorning G: Simultaneous recording of intravesical and intraurethral pressure. Acta Chir Scand 276:1, 1961.
63. Hilton P, Stanton SL: Urethral pressure measurements by microtransducer: The results in symptom-free women and those with genuine stress incontinence. Br J Obstet Gynaecol 90:919, 1983.
64. Bump RC, Copeland WE, Hurt WG, Fantl JA: Dynamic urethral pressure profilometry pressure transmission ratio determinations in stress-incontinent and stress-continent subjects. Am J Obstet Gynecol 159:749, 1988.
65. Rosenzweig BA, Bhatia NN, Nelson AL: Dynamic urethral pressure profilometry pressure transmission ratios: What do the numbers really mean? Obstet Gynecol 77:586, 1991.
66. Lose G, Thind P, Colstrup H: The value of pressure transmission ratio in the diagnosis of stress incontinence. Neurourol Urodyn 9:323, 1990.

67. Hanzal E, Berger E, Koelbl H: Reliability of the urethral closure pressure profile during stress in the diagnosis of genuine stress incontinence. Br J Urol 68:369, 1991.
68. Constantinou CE: Urethrometry: Consideration of static dynamic and stability characteristics of the female urethra. Neuroradiol Urodyn 7:521, 1998.
69. Leach GE, Yip CM, Donovan BJ: Mechanism of continence after modified Pereyra bladder-neck suspension. Urology 24:328, 1987.
70. Constantinou CE, Faysal MH, Rother L: The impact of bladder neck suspension on the mode of distribution of abdominal pressure along the female urethra. In Zinner NR, Sterling AM (eds): Female Incontinence. New York, Alan Liss, 1981, pp 121-132.
71. Penttinen J, Kaark K, Kauppila A: Effect of suprapubic operation on urethral closure-evaluation by single cough: Urethrocystometry. Br J Urol 63:384, 1989.
72. Mutone N, Mastropietro M, Brizendine E, Hale D: Effect of tension-free vaginal tape procedure on urodynamic continence indices. Obstet Gynecol 98:638, 2001.
73. Von Garrelts B: Analysis of micturition: A new method of recording the voiding of the bladder. Acta Chir Scand 112:326, 1956.
74. Boone TB, Kim YH: Uroflowmetry. In Nitti VW (ed): Practical Urodynamics. Philadelphia, WB Saunders, 1998, pp 28-37.
75. Barry MJ, Girman CJ, O'Leary MP, et al: Using repeated measures of symptom score, uroflowmetry and prostatic specific antigen in the clinical management of prostate disease. J Urol 153:99, 1995.
76. Feneley MR, Dunsmuir WD, Pearce J, Kirby RS: Reproducibility of uroflow measurement: Experience during a double-blind placebo-controlled study of doxazosin in benign prostatic hyperplasia. Urology 47:658, 1996.
77. Grino PB, Bruskewitz R, Blaivas JG, et al: Maximum urinary flow rate by uroflowmetry: Automatic or visual interpretation. J Urol 149:339, 1993.
78. Bottaccini MR, Gleason DM: Urodynamic norms in women. I. Normal versus stress incontinence. J Urol 124:659, 1980.
79. Gleason DM, Bottaccini MR: Urodynamic norms in female voiding. II. The flow modulating zone and voiding dysfunction. J Urol 127:495, 1982.
80. Jorgensen JB, Jensen KM-E: Uroflowmetry. Urol Clin North Am 26:237, 1996.
81. Haylen BT, Ashby D, Suthers JR: Maximum and average urine flow rates in normal male and female populations—The Liverpool nomograms. Br J Urol 64:30, 1989.
82. Siroky MB, Olsson CA, Krane RJ: The flow rate nomogram. I. Development. J Urol 122:665, 1979.
83. Drach GW, Ignatoff J, Layton TN: Peak urinary flow rate: Observations in female subjects and comparison to male subjects. J Urol 1979 122:215, 1979.
84. Beckman KA: Urinary flow during micturition in normal women. Acta Chir Scand 130:357, 965.
85. Abrams PH, Torrens M: Urine flow studies. Urol Clin North Am 6:71, 1979.
86. Bass JS, Leach GE: Bladder outlet obstruction in women. Probl Urol 5:141, 1991.
87. Chancellor MB, Blaivas JG, Kaplan SA, Axelrod S: Bladder outlet obstruction versus impaired detrusor contractility: Role of uroflow. J Urol 145:810, 1991.
88. Golomb J: Uroflowmetry. In Raz S (ed): Female Urology, 2nd ed. Philadelphia, WB Saunders, 1996, pp 97-105.
89. Griffiths DJ: Pressure-flow studies of micturition. Urol Clin North Am 23:279, 1996.
90. Abrams PH, Griffiths DJ: The assessment of prostatic obstruction from urodynamic measurements and from residual urine. Br J Urol 51:129, 1979.
91. Schafer W: Analysis of bladder-outlet function with the linearized passive urethral resistance relation, linPURR, and a disease-specific approach for grading obstruction: From complex to simple. World J Urol 13:47, 1995.
92. Griffiths D, van Mastrigt R, Bosch R: Quantification of urethral resistance and bladder function during voiding, with special reference to the effects of prostate size reduction on urethral obstruction due to benign prostatic hyperplasia. Neurourol Urodyn 8:12, 1989.
93. Griffiths D, Hofner K, van Mastrigt R, et al: Standardization of terminology of lower urinary tract function: Pressure-flow studies of voiding, urethral resistance, and urethral obstruction. Neurourol Urodyn 16:1, 1997.
94. Blaivas JG, Groutz A: Bladder outlet obstruction nomogram for women with lower urinary tract symptomatology. Neurourol Urodyn 19:533, 2000.
95. Massey JA, Abrams PA: Obstructed voiding in the female. Br J Urol 61:36, 1988.
96. Axelrod SI, Alaivas JG: Bladder neck obstruction in women. J Urol 137:497, 1987.
97. Nitti VW: Bladder outlet obstruction in women. In Nitti VW (ed): Practical Urodynamics. Philadelphia, WB Saunders, 1998, pp 197-210.
98. Kerr LA, Statkin DR: The use of artificial material for sling surgery n the treatment of female stress urinary incontinence. In Raz S (ed): Female Urology, 2nd ed. Philadelphia, WB Saunders, 1986, pp 382-391.
99. Webster GD, Kreder KJ: Voiding dysfunction following cystourethropexy: Its evaluation and management. J Urol 144:670, 1990.
100. Nitti VW, Raz S: Obstruction following anti-incontinence procedures: Diagnosis and treatment with transvaginal urethrolysis. J Urol 152:93, 1994.
101. Amundsen CL, Guralnick ML, Webster GD: Variations in strategy for the treatment of urethral obstruction after a pubovaginal sling procedure. J Urol 164:434, 2000.
102. Miller EA, Amundsen CL, Toh KL, et al: Preoperative urodynamic evaluation may predict voiding dysfunction in women undergoing pubovaginal sling. J Urol 169:2234, 2003.
103. Wang AC, Chen M-C: The correlation between preoperative voiding mechanism and surgical outcome of the tension free vaginal tape procedure, with reference to quality of life. BJU Int 91:502, 2003.
104. Yalla SV, Sharma GVRK, Barsamian EM: Micturitional urethral pressure profile during voiding and the implications. J Urol 124:649, 1980.
105. Yalla SV, Resnick N, Dyro FM: The response of bladder neck and external sphincter regions during initiation of voiding. J Urol 131:167, 1984.
106. Sullivan MP, Comiter CV, Yalla SV: Micturitional urethral pressure profilometry. Urol Clin North Am 23:263, 1996.
107. Bates CP, Whiteside CG, Turner-Warwick R: Synchronous cine-pressure-slow cystourethrography with special reference to stress and urge incontinence. Br J Urol 42:714, 1970.
108. Blaivas JG, Olsson CA: Stress incontinence: Classification and surgical approach. J Urol 139:727, 1988.
109. Blaivas JG: Videourodynamic studies. In Nitti VW (ed): Practical Urodynamics. Philadelphia, WB Saunders, 1998, pp 78-93.
110. Knapp PM Jr: Urodynamic evaluation of ileal loop function. J Urol 137:929, 1987.
111. Ordorica RC: Evaluation and management of mechanical dysfunction in continence colonic urinary reservoirs. J Urol 163:1679, 2000.
112. Hinman F Jr: Nonneurogenic neurogenic bladder (the Hinman syndrome)—15 years later. J Urol 136:796, 1986.
113. Robertson A, Neal DE: Ambulatory urodynamics. In Nitti VW (ed): Practical Urodynamics. Philadelphia, WB Saunders, 1998, pp 273-286.
114. James ED, Flack FC, Caldwell KPS, Martin MR: Continuous measurement of urine loss and frequency in incontinent patients. Br J Urol 43:233, 1971.
115. Robertson AS, Griffiths CJ, Ramsden PD, Neal DE: Bladder function in healthy volunteers: Ambulatory monitoring and conventional urodynamic studies. Br J Urol 73:242, 1994.

116. van Waalwijk van Doorn E, Anders K, Khullar V, Kulseng-Hanssen S, et al: Standardisation of ambulatory urodynamic monitoring: Report of the Standardisation Sub-committee of the International Continence Society for Ambulatory Urodynamic Studies. Neurourol Urodyn 19:113, 2000.
117. Webb RJ, Styles RA, Griffiths CJ, et al: Ambulatory monitoring of bladder pressures in patients with low compliance as a result of neurogenic bladder dysfunction. Br J Urol 64:150, 1989.
118. Webb RJ, Griffiths CJ, Ramsden PD, Neal DE: Ambulatory monitoring of bladder pressure in low compliance neurogenic bladder dysfunction. J Urol 148:1477, 1992.
119. Steers WD, Barrett DM, Wein AJ: Voiding dysfunction: Diagnosis, classification and management. In Gillenwater JY, Grayhack JT, Howards SS, Duckett JW (eds): Adult and Pediatric Urology, 3rd ed. St. Louis, Mosby–Year Book, 1996.
120. Constantinou CE: Urethrometry: Consideration of static dynamic and stability characteristics of the female urethra. Neuroradiol Urodyn 7:521, 1988.
121. Blaivas JG: Pathophysiology of lower urinary tract dysfunction. Clin Obstet Gynaecol 12:295, 1985.

Chapter 12

MEASUREMENT OF URINARY SYMPTOMS, HEALTH-RELATED QUALITY OF LIFE, AND OUTCOMES OF TREATMENT FOR URINARY INCONTINENCE

Larry T. Sirls

The evaluation of lower urinary tract symptoms (LUTS) in women involves several objective and subjective parameters. The difficulty in evaluating treatment outcomes for urinary incontinence is that the objective measures of improvement and cure do not necessarily correlate with the subjective outcomes patients report. This becomes complicated when we consider that the outcomes after surgery for stress urinary incontinence (SUI) include assessment of the surgery (e.g., success, persistent or recurrent SUI); the resolution, persistence, or development of urgency and urge incontinence (UUI); and evaluation of voiding dysfunction. This is an almost overwhelming task, and it remains controversial. Most agree that measuring treatment outcomes requires the collection of objective data to help evaluate the success of treatment and the incidence of complications, as well as subjective patient reports of their outcomes and the influence of post-treatment changes on their health-related quality of life (HRQOL).

To improve the initial evaluation and post-treatment assessment of urinary incontinence, noninvasive outcome measures, including pad tests,[1] voiding diaries,[2] and questionnaires, have been developed.[3,4] A critical addition to the measurement of subjective outcome is the symptom questionnaire.[5,6] Although limitations remain in what can be accomplished through the use of a symptom questionnaire, they are clearly more objective than retrospective reviews and can be validated in a systematic fashion. Retrospective chart reviews and the opinions of the surgeons or their surrogates have several limitations, including patient reluctance to complain to surgeons about minor symptoms,[7,8] different definitions of success by patients and physicians,[9] and potential loss to follow-up of symptomatic patients who seek medical attention elsewhere.[7]

Although various outcome measures have been proposed, no single tool has met with widespread acceptance. There are no standard definitions of cure or failure, and there are no standardized widely accepted clinical tools to assess outcomes after anti-incontinence surgery. Although attempts to standardize the evaluation of treatment outcomes in urinary incontinence have been made, these recommendations are often not followed. There are no specific recommendations on how to assess patient HRQOL or gather this information.[10]

In this chapter, we discuss the development and composition of many questionnaires used to evaluate LUTS and the impact of those symptoms on patients' HRQOL. We discuss the difficulty in evaluating patients after treatment for urinary incontinence and the apparent dissociation of objective measures of SUI such as cure and complicating symptoms such as UUI. We then address the role of combined objective and subjective data to evaluate treatment outcomes.

HEALTH-RELATED QUALITY OF LIFE

The most common outcome measures for urinary incontinence assess the quantity and frequency of urine loss through voiding diaries, pad tests, or urodynamic testing such as leak point pressure and pressure-flow studies. These observations may confirm the degree of leakage, but they do not reflect the impact of the symptoms on the patients' quality of life. Norton[11] first reported that there was no direct relationship of objective measures of urinary incontinence with the degree of improvement experienced by the patient. Several others have found only weak relationships of the perceived impact of incontinence with measures of frequency and quantity of urine loss.[12-15] Consequently, quality-of-life instruments have become an important outcome measure for surgical interventions.[16] It is mainly in the past decade that researchers have developed and used several different self-administered questionnaires for urinary incontinence that measure of bother, symptom impact, and HRQOL.

HRQOL is a multidimensional paradigm defined as the impact of health status, including disease and treatment on physical, psychologic, and social functioning. HRQOL can be assessed with generic or condition-specific measures. Generic measures are developed for use with patients regardless of their medical condition and can be used for patients with different disease processes to compare the HRQOL impacts of various diseases. In contrast, condition-specific measures assess aspects of disease and treatment that are unique to the specific disease. Compared with generic measures, condition-specific instruments tend to be more sensitive to clinically relevant changes and treatment effects.

DEVELOPMENT AND VALIDATION OF QUESTIONNAIRES

Questionnaires to evaluate LUTS may provide information about the nature of the patient's problem, the frequency of symptoms, the extent of symptoms, and the impact of symptoms on HRQOL.

The ideal questionnaire would help the clinician establish the cause of the problem (i.e., differentiate SUI from UUI) and limit the need for invasive and expensive testing. Questionnaires may include a wide range of items depending on the purpose and target subjects of the study population.

Measurement of Symptoms on Questionnaires

Applying scientific methods to evaluate symptoms that are generated by a great variety of underlying conditions can be complicated. How can the physician be sure that the score from a symptom questionnaire accurately reflects the symptoms the subject reports? Psychometrics is the science of measurement of responses to phenomena that are not easily quantifiable, and the principles of psychometrics govern the development of symptom questionnaires. Symptom scores are only as good as the instrument measuring the symptoms, and psychometric testing provides assurance that symptoms questionnaires measure symptoms.[17]

Validity

Validity refers to the degree that an instrument measures what it is intended to measure. *Content validity* is usually evaluated early in development of the questionnaire and assesses how representative the contents are. This is often done with literature review and through consultation with experts and patients. The questions chosen should cover all of the important aspects of the condition, and all items should be relevant to the condition. *Criterion validity* determines how accurately the new instrument predicts findings of the gold standard, and it can be determined by using several methods. Correlation coefficients are frequently used, the choice of which depends on the nature of the data under analysis. *Sensitivity* is the proportion of people identified by the questionnaire as having the condition who do suffer from the condition. *Specificity* refers to the ability of the questionnaire to correctly identify subjects who do not have the condition. Related measurements include predictive values, accuracy, and receiver operation characteristic (ROC) curves. These measures are only accurate if the gold standard is highly accurate.

Although urodynamic evaluation is generally accepted as the best available diagnostic test for LUTS, many other standards—history, voiding diary, demonstration of incontinence on examination, and pad testing—have been used for criterion validation of LUTS questionnaires. No one method accurately assesses the scope of LUTS, the severity of the problem, and the cause of LUTS well enough to be the undisputed gold standard.[18-21] Nevertheless, results from questionnaires should be compared with several of these objective measures, particularly urodynamic findings, as part of the validation process.

When no gold standard is available for comparison, *construct validity* is used to assess questionnaires. One approach to establishing construct validity is to examine hypothetical associations of the measure with other domains, such as pain, anxiety, and life satisfaction. For example, anxiety may correlate moderately with quality of life. The Spearman or Pearson correlation coefficients typically are used. *Convergent validity* (similar to sensitivity) may be determined by demonstrating good correlation with a measure known to be related to the subject of the questionnaire, and it should have high correlation coefficients. *Discriminant validity* (similar to specificity) may be confirmed by showing poor correlation to characteristics unrelated to the subject of the questionnaire.

Reliability

Questionnaires that measure the same characteristics should produce similar responses from a subject. The same questionnaire also should produce similar results for a subject over short intervals of time. Reliability is the quantifiable assessment of these sources of error in a questionnaire. Reliability implies the instrument is dependable.[17] *Internal reliability* estimates how the individual items of a questionnaire relate to each other and to the total score. Questionnaires may be divided into two similar tools, each of which may give results similar to each other and to the parent questionnaire. Selected items may be used to construct a short form that is consistent with the original long form of the questionnaire. Cronbach's α (0-1) indicates the level of internal consistency; values greater that 0.7 are considered acceptable, greater than 0.8 are good, and greater than 0.9 are excellent. Although high internal consistency is desirable, removing redundant items from questionnaires improves clinical speed but diminishes internal consistency. Longer or multiple questionnaires are probably needed for research purposes, but in most clinical situations, we are looking for brevity. *Test-retest reliability* is evaluated by repeat administration of the questionnaire to subjects over time. Enough time should have elapsed for the subjects to forget their responses to the items, but no change in their symptoms should be evident. A Pearson and Spearman correlation coefficient value of greater that 0.8 indicates high reliability.

Responsiveness is evaluated to confirm that a questionnaire reflects a clinically important change in the patient's condition. The questionnaire is used before and after treatment of known efficacy, and the patient's perception of change is correlated with the quality of life scores. The Student *t* test is often used to report responsiveness.

The psychometric evaluation of a questionnaire must be evaluated in the context of the study subjects used. Questionnaires may perform very differently after translation to another language or when used in different countries with different races or socioeconomic groups.[22] The accuracy of questionnaire data depends on choosing the appropriate tool for the population under study.

The method of data collection can dramatically influence the cure rates reported after anti-incontinence surgery.[6,23] Physicians' biases with the use of retrospective chart review have been repeatedly documented. To eliminate this bias, prospective studies that contain HRQOL assessments have nearly replaced the retrospective chart review. Rodriguez and colleagues[24] addressed the question of whether medical personnel (physicians in particular) could reliably fill out HRQOL questionnaires with information obtained from medical interviews? Seventy-nine patients completed the Urogenital Distress Inventory (UDI-6) and a quality-of-life survey. An interviewing physician then completed these same instruments based on the interview of the patient. Overall, the physicians underestimated the patient's degree of bother by 25% to 37%. Self-administered questionnaires minimize bias and are preferred over medical personnel–administered instruments because of labor, time, and cost.

TYPES OF QUESTIONNAIRES

Questionnaires for Lower Urinary Tract Symptoms

Self-administered symptom questionnaires are designed to accomplish at least one of three objectives: discriminate between SUI and UUI, quantify the amount of symptoms, or assess the impact of symptoms on daily activity and HRQOL. Brief descriptive information and references for each questionnaire are presented in Table 12-1.

Questionnaires for Differentiating Stress Urinary Incontinence from Urgency Urinary Incontinence

The Detrusor Instability Score (DIS) quantifies the extent of detrusor instability symptoms to discriminate stress from urge as the cause for incontinence. The tool is translated from Finnish but has been validated for use in English. DIS scores have been compared with urodynamic findings, demonstrating a low DIS score (0-5) had reasonable predictive value for the absence of detrusor instability. Although sensitivity and specificity are

Table 12-1 Symptom Questionnaires for Lower Urinary Tract Symptoms

Instrument	Purpose	Items	Subscales	References
Bristol Female Lower Urinary Tract Symptoms (BFLUTS) Questionnaire	Impact, amount of UI, women	33	Severity, associated symptoms, impact symptoms, sexual function; many items have bother component	Jackson et al[33]
CONTILIFE: a quality-of-life questionnaire for urinary incontinence	Impact, response to SUI, women	28	Daily activities, effort activities, self-image, emotional consequences, sexuality, well-being, global score	Amarenco et al[53]
International Consultation on Incontinence Questionnaire (ICIQ)	Impact, amount of UI, women, men	4	Not applicable	Avery et al[34] Karantanis et al[35]
Incontinence Impact Questionnaire (IIQ)	Impact, response to UI, women	30	Physical activity, travel, social, emotional	Shumaker et al[3] van der Vaart et al[39] Uebersax et al[41]
Incontinence Impact Questionnaire-Revised (IIQ-R)		30	Physical activity, travel, social, emotional, embarrassment	
Incontinence Impact Questionnaire-Short Form (IIQ-7)		7	Not applicable	
Incontinence Quality-of-Life Questionnaire (I-QOL)	Impact, response to UI, women, men	22	Avoidance and limiting behaviors, psychosocial, social embarrassment	Wagner et al[44]
Incontinence Stress Questionnaire for Patients (IQS-P)	Impact, response to UUI, elderly women	20	Depressive, aesthetic or somatic, social	Yu et al[56]
King's Health Questionnaire (KHQ)	Impact, response to UI, women, men	21	Role limitations, physical limitations, social limitations, personal limitations, emotional problems, sleep and energy disturbance, severity (coping) measures, symptom severity, incontinence impact (single item), general health perception (single item)	Kelleher et al[51]
Leicester Impact Scale	Impact, response to LUTS, women, men	21	Travel, activities, social, hobbies, family life, feelings	Shaw et al[59]
Overactive Bladder Questionnaire (OAB-Q)	Continent and incontinent OAB	33	Symptom bother, coping, concern, social interaction, sleep	Coyne et al[54]
Quality-of-life Questionnaire for Urinary Urge Incontinence	Impact, response to UUI, women	24	Activities, emotional impact, self-image, sleep, well-being	Marquis et al[57]

Continued

Table 12-1 Symptom Questionnaires for Lower Urinary Tract Symptoms—cont'd

Instrument	Purpose	Items	Subscales	References
Symptom Impact Index for Stress Incontinence in Women	Impact, response to SUI, women	3	Not applicable	Black et al[32]
Severity Index	Amount of SUI, women	2	Not applicable	Sandvik et al[30] Sandvik et al[31]
Severity Index & Symptom Impact Index (SII-SI)	Amount, impact of SUI, women	5 (severity) 3 (impact)	Not applicable	Black et al[32]
Stress Incontinence Questionnaire (SIQ)	Amount of SUI, women	18	Maneuvers for SUI, active, passive planned, unplanned	Nochajski et al[29]
Urogenital Distress Inventory (UDI)	Impact, response to UUI, women	19	Irritative, obstructive, or discomfort stress	Shumaker et al[3] Brown et al[22]
Urge Urogenital Distress Inventory (U-UDI)		9	Not applicable	
Urogenital Distress Inventory–Short Form (UDI-6)		6	Not applicable	
Urge Impact Scale (URIS-24)	Elderly, UI	24	Psychologic burden, perception of personal control, self-concept	DuBeau et al[47]
Urge Incontinence Impact Questionnaire (U-IIQ)	Impact, response to UUI, women, men	32	Travel, activities, physical activities, feelings, relationships, sexual function, nighttime bladder control	Lubeck et al[40]
Urinary Incontinence Handicap Inventory (UIHI)	Elderly women, UI	17	Not applicable	Rai et al[56]
Urinary Incontinence Severity Score (UISS)	Women, UI	10	Not applicable	Stach-Lempinen et al[37]
York Incontinence Perceptions Scale (YIPS)	Women, UI	8	Not applicable	Lee et al[48]

LUTS, lower urinary tract symptoms; OAB, overactive bladder; SUI, stress urinary incontinence; UI, urinary incontinence; UUI, urge urinary incontinence.

marginal, the DIS has a positive predictive value of 0.82 for determining which patients would not demonstrate detrusor instability on urodynamic evaluation.[25,26]

The Gaudenz Incontinence Questionnaire has been used widely in Europe as a diagnostic tool to discriminate between SUI and UUI. Initial studies demonstrated high validity. A validation study evaluated the ability of the two subscales to predict urodynamic findings in 1938 women with incontinence. The strict urodynamic criteria used demonstrated detrusor instability in only 2% of women, with 5% having mixed incontinence, making interpretation of this questionnaires performance difficult.[27] A shorter, English-language variation of the Gaudenz Incontinence Questionnaire used in Japan was compared with physical examination, pad test, and urodynamic data before and after intervention. Post-treatment scores for both parameters were significantly reduced.[28]

Questionnaires that Quantify the Amount of Urinary Symptoms

The Stress Incontinence Questionnaire (SIQ) was created to evaluate whether specific activities women routinely perform that result in SUI have diagnostic value. Subjects use a 4-point scale to respond about urinary leakage when performing 18 specific maneuvers. Statistical analysis identified four subscales or factors designated active maneuvers, passive maneuvers, planned maneuvers, and unplanned maneuvers. Psychometric testing using clinical and urodynamic data demonstrated good reliability. The correlation of the four factors with different clinical characteristics suggests that the factors identify different aspects of incontinence.[29]

The Severity Index attempts to determine the extent that women are bothered by incontinence.[30] There are two questions;

one asks about the frequency of urinary incontinence, and the second assesses the amount of leakage per urinary incontinence event. The numeric values 1 to 4 for the frequency and 1 to 3 for the amount are multiplied to give the score ranging from 1 to 12. The scores are then divided into four levels of severity. The severity level correlated reasonably well with leakage by 48-hour pad tests, but there was overlap between the severity groups. An updated version includes a *very severe* category, which identified a subgroup of older women when used in an epidemiologic study. The investigators recommend adding a *no leakage* response if the questions are being used to monitor outcome.[31]

Questionnaires that Assess the Amount of Symptoms and the Impact of Symptoms

The Severity Index and the Symptom Impact Index for stress incontinence are paired indices specific for SUI that divide *severity* and *impact* into separate scores. The three items of the Symptom Impact Index assess the degree to which women avoid activities because of stress incontinence. After a comprehensive development process, the instrument was found to have good reliability, but convergent validity was demonstrated only through a significant correlation with body mass index. The instrument was not significantly related to the more relevant characteristic of whether a woman had undergone previous surgery for stress incontinence. Conversely, discriminant validity was shown by the lack of correlation between index scores, demographic variables, and unrelated medical history.[32]

The Bristol Female Lower Urinary Tract Symptoms Questionnaire (BFLUTS) was developed from the International Continence Society male questionnaire, retaining the same format and many of the items. Thirty-three questions evaluate four domains: incontinence severity, associated symptoms, quality of life, and sexual function. Many of the questions have an additional component assessing the level of associated bother.[33] Initial psychometric testing compared BFLUTS scores with voiding diaries and pad tests in 85 incontinent women and control subjects. The frequency of reported symptoms and the degree of bother were significantly higher for all symptoms in the clinical cohort. Criterion validity was confirmed by comparing items assessing urinary frequency and incontinent episodes to the voiding diaries. All voiding diary parameters except daytime frequency correlated well with BFLUTS scores. Subjective assessment of the degree of incontinence correlated with pad test results. Internal consistency and test-retest reliability were confirmed. The BFLUTS questionnaire is a comprehensive tool for evaluating urinary incontinence in women. Its large size may limit general use by clinicians.

The International Consultation on Incontinence Questionnaire (ICIQ) is a four-item questionnaire composed of three scored items and an unscored self-diagnostic item that assesses the prevalence, frequency, and perceived cause of urinary incontinence and its impact on everyday life. It was developed for a wide range of patients for clinical practice and research settings. The ICIQ is easily completed, with low levels of missing data (mean, 1.6%), and it is able to discriminate among different groups of individuals, indicating good construct validity. Convergent validity was acceptable, and reliability was good, with "moderate" to "very good" stability in test-retest analysis and a Cronbach's α value of 0.95. Statistically significant reductions in symptoms from baseline after surgical and conservative treatment were observed, demonstrating that the ICIQ is responsive.[34]

The ICIQ, a 24-hour pad test, Stamey grade, and 3-day frequency volume diary used to assess severity were further evaluated in 95 women with primary or recurrent SUI. In the primary SUI group, there was a strong correlation between the ICIQ and the 24-hour pad test results. The ICIQ and 24-hour pad test results also correlated with the mean frequency of urinary loss on the diary but not with the Stamey grade. Although good correlation between the 24-hour pad test and ICIQ in women with primary SUI was demonstrated, no subjective or objective tests correlated for women with recurrent SUI.[35] Intraobserver and interobserver reliabilities of the ICIQ have been established by observing that the results obtained from administering the ICIQ at the office or at home were not different from those obtained by the physician during an interview, a potentially unique advantage of this tool.

The ICIQ has been shown to be an effective tool for the assessment of the frequency, severity, and impact on quality of life of urinary incontinence in a wide range of patients. Because it is brief and simple, is responsive to treatment, and includes a measure of quality-of-life impact, the ICIQ may prove to be extremely useful as an outcome measure in patients in clinical and research settings.[36]

Four of 10 items on the Urinary Incontinence Severity Score assess the amount of leakage, and the other six items refer to the impact of urinary incontinence on a woman's daily life.[37] Although this measure was found to have adequate psychometric properties, the instrument yields only a total score that combines the four symptom items and six symptom impact items. This instrument therefore does not provide a pure indication of symptom impact or quality of life.

Questionnaires that Assess the Impact of Urinary Symptoms

The Incontinence Impact Questionnaire (IIQ) and the Urogenital Distress Inventory (UDI) are paired symptom questionnaires that measure the HRQOL effect and the level of distress in women with stress incontinence.[3] Variations of these two products include short forms and urge-specific forms. The 30-question IIQ has four domains: physical activity, travel, social or relationships, and emotional health. The UDI is more of a measure of "bothersomeness" and contains three domains of irritative, obstructive or discomfort, and stress symptoms. Validation was established with convergent and discriminant correlation with several clinical parameters, including final diagnosis, pad test results, and voiding diaries. However, a subsequent study found it to have poor construct validity as indicated by weak correlations with a clinical measure.[38] The instrument recently was re-examined using factor analysis, and a new subscale assessing embarrassment was identified. This revised version (IIQ-R) was found to have good psychometric properties.[38] A version of the IIQ with two additional items has been shown to perform well in assessing men with urinary incontinence.[39]

In 1995, the original psychometric test data was re-analyzed to produce the short forms of both the IIQ and the UDI. The seven-item IIQ (IIQ-7) retains the four subscales. The UDI-6 was constructed by taking two items from each of the three original subscales. Regression analysis confirmed adequate validity and consistency. Correlation between the long and short forms of both indices (total scores and subscale scores) was high.[40]

The original IIQ and UDI were validated primarily among patients with stress incontinence and subsequently have been adapted to be more specific for the urge component of incontinence. The Urge IIQ (U-IIQ) domains are travel, activities, feelings, physical activity, relationships, and sexual function. The Urge-UDI (U-UDI) has 9 items, some of which have an associated bother question. Eighty-three women with racial and socioeconomic diversity were used for initial psychometric testing. All women had pure or predominantly urge UUI. A large percentage of women did not answer some questions on physical and sexual activity. Only minimal correlation was seen between these questionnaires and the general quality-of-life index Short Form-36 Item Health Survey (SF-36). All subscales demonstrated high internal consistency. Test-retest correlation was adequate for the U-IIQ subscales and low for the U-UDI.[22,40]

The Incontinence Quality of Life Measure (I-QOL) is a 22-item questionnaire designed to assess the quality of life of men and women with urinary incontinence. There are three subscales of avoidance and limiting behaviors, psychosocial impact, and social embarrassment. A number of items address worry about certain things that may happen, such as worry about not getting to the toilet or worry about being embarrassed. Reliability and validity have been demonstrated, but the reported psychometric results have focused primarily on the total score rather than the subscales.[41,42] Construct and discriminant validity were demonstrated further in later studies.[43,44] Although the I-QOL was designed for use in men and women, it has been used primarily in women. The instrument has been translated into more than 20 languages. The I-QOL has been used as an outcome measure in clinical trials of treatment for SUI, and it has been used as a fundamental tool to validate patient global impression questionnaires.[45]

The Urge Impact Scale (URIS-24) is a 24-item quality-of-life measure specifically for older persons (65 years or older) with UUI. The original 32-item questionnaire was developed from comprehensive interviews with 21 older men and women with UUI. Questions were formulated by using language recorded during the interviews.[46] Analysis revealed three factors or subscales: psychological burden, perception of personal control, and self-concept. URIS-24 scores demonstrated moderate correlation with mean incontinent episodes per day. Reliability was acceptable. Although there was some test-retest variability for individual items, the composite score was reproducible. As is common with HRQOL questionnaires, criterion validity is lacking. This seems to be a well-constructed tool with a defined target population of older adults.[47]

The York Incontinence Perception Scale (YIPS) is a one-dimensional index of eight items that measures the psychosocial impact of incontinence in women. Psychometric techniques were used to select the items. Voiding diaries, response to treatment, and comparison with the IIQ were used for validation. Responsiveness was tested in a randomized trial of behavioral therapy for incontinence. YIPS scores substantially increased in the treatment group relative to the control group.[48] The YIPS is a brief incontinence impact questionnaire with good psychometric characteristics.

The King's Health Questionnaire (KHQ) is a 21-item quality-of-life index specific for women and for urinary incontinence.[49] The KHQ was developed to assess HRQOL in women with general symptoms of incontinence, but it has since been shown to be valid and reliable for use in men and women with overactive bladder symptoms.[50] Eight domains were identified: general health, incontinence impact, role limitations, physical limitations, social limitations, personal limitations, emotional problems, and sleep or energy disturbances and severity measures. The reliability and validity were assessed in 285 women before urodynamic evaluation. Internal consistency and test-retest reliability were excellent. Common domains between the KHQ and the SF-36 correlated highly. Scores were analyzed relative to urodynamic diagnosis. Although women with genuine SUI tended to report more severe leakage, those suffering from detrusor instability reported poorer general health and greater impact of incontinence on their lives. The KHQ is reliable and valid in women with incontinence and in men and women with overactive bladder.

The CONTILIFE is an HRQOL questionnaire that has been validated in five languages among women with SUI.[51] Psychometric properties were good with some exceptions, including internal consistency of the effort activities, responsiveness of sexuality, and well-being dimensions.

The Overactive Bladder Questionnaire (OAB-q) consists of an eight-item symptom bother scale and 25 items assessing HRQOL in four domains: coping, concern, sleep, and social interaction. This instrument is unique in that it was directly based on perceptions of continent and incontinent patients with overactive bladder.[52] In community and clinical samples, it has been shown to have strong psychometric properties, including responsiveness to change in the continent overactive bladder symptoms of urgency and frequency and nocturia.[52] The OAB-q has been shown to discriminate between patients with different levels of nocturia and among patients with stress, urge, or mixed incontinence in a community sample.[53]

The Incontinence Stress Questionnaire for Patients (ISQ-P) was developed to evaluate patients psychologic distress associated with urinary incontinence in long-term care.[54] The final 20-item version of the questionnaire was derived from a broad item pool of 109 items based on interviews with patients and factor analyses. The published validation study reports good internal consistency and construct validity, although test-retest reliability was assessed over a longer period (11 weeks) than is preferred. The instrument was validated among a sample of 96 elderly women with cognitive impairment and therefore may not be applicable to a more general sample of patients with urinary incontinence.

The 24-item Quality-of-life Questionnaire for Urinary Urge Incontinence questionnaire is grouped into five dimensions: activities, emotional repercussions, self-image, sleep, and well-being.[57] Although the instrument appears to have sound psychometric properties, subsequent instruments have been developed and validated specifically for patients with urge incontinence.

The Urinary Incontinence Handicap Inventory (UIHI) was based on the perceptions of 10 individuals in the target population (i.e., elderly women with urinary incontinence) on emotions, activities, social interaction, and physical functioning.[56] The instrument demonstrated good internal consistency reliability, test-retest reliability, and construct validity.

The Leicester Impact Scale is a 21-item, condition-specific quality-of-life measure for men and women with LUTS, with or without incontinence. The questionnaire was interviewer administered to a community sample of men and women older than 40 years. The distribution of scores was skewed with low levels of impact, which may reflect a community sample rather than a treatment sample, but it was responsive to conservative treatment. Limitations include the length, the fact that it is interviewer administered (e.g., costly, time intensive, bias,) and the poor interrater reliability for some items, specifically the "depressed" and "angry" items.[57]

THE ROLE OF INCONTINENCE QUESTIONNAIRES

The perfect LUTS symptom questionnaire would be short, easily administered and scored, discriminate between SUI and UUI, measure severity, and measure the effect of the symptoms on HRQOL. It would minimize the need for invasive and expensive testing. All clinicians treating incontinence would regularly use this tool, helping create a standardized means for evaluating LUTS and measuring the outcomes of treatment. Unfortunately, this questionnaire does not exist, and using more than one questionnaire may be necessary. Because stress and urge incontinence probably represent different disease processes, scales that discriminate between them or score them separately may more accurately reflect a patient's condition than a more general scale.

To reduce bias and inadvertent outside influence when using HRQOL questionnaires, several guidelines should be followed. The questionnaire should be self-administered by the patient, and the patient should be given a specific timeframe for their answers. Usually, patients are asked to think about their symptoms over the past 4 weeks. Longer timeframes may predispose patients to report how they act or feel, decreasing responsiveness.[58] The psychologic effect of surgical intervention must be considered because it has been shown there may be a false sense of well-being immediately after surgery (from anxiety and stress relief), regardless of the effect of the surgery.[59] Surgeons reporting on this subject would agree that the outcomes of incontinence therapy should not be evaluated too soon after surgery. Patients must complete the questionnaire in the same setting, which may be most practical in the office while waiting for the physician. Patients must not have assistance, unless by trained personnel, to eliminate inadvertent bias through personal interpretation or explanation of the questions.

When selecting which HRQOL instrument to use in a specific situation, several factors should be considered. The functional domains assessed by items and subscales among different tools vary, and one instrument may be preferable over another. For example, because the IIQ has a travel subscale, it can be used to evaluate the impact of treatment on patients' ability to travel.

It is critical to match the questionnaire with the intended study sample. There are inherent differences between urinary symptoms in terms of causes and HROQL impacts. For example, SUI has less HROQL impact than urge or mixed urinary incontinence, and mixed urinary incontinence has a greater impact than urge alone.[60] Because different urinary symptoms affect patients in different ways, it is necessary to choose a questionnaire that has been developed and validated for use among the study population. Instruments validated among samples with SUI include the CONTILIFE and the Symptom Impact Index for Stress Incontinence in Women, whereas the URIS and U-IIQ were designed specifically for patients with urge urinary incontinence. The ISQ-P would be useful to study a population of cognitively impaired older women in long a term care facility.

Of the urinary incontinence-specific HRQOL instruments, the KHQ has been validated in a large and diverse population, and many translations are available. Other sound urinary incontinence-specific instruments for women include the IIQ, UDI, I-QOL, and ICIQ. When a brief questionnaire is desired, the IIQ-7 and UDI-6 or the ICIQ would be appropriate. The OAB-q is an HRQOL instrument that was specifically developed and validated for use in continent and incontinent patients with overactive bladder, and it may be appropriate for diverse populations of patients with symptoms of urgency, frequency, or nocturia, but not incontinence.

The ICIQ has been shown to be an effective tool for the assessment of the frequency, severity, and impact on quality of life of urinary incontinence in a wide range of patients. Because it is brief and simple, is responsive to treatment, and includes a measure of quality-of-life impact, the ICIQ may prove to be extremely useful as an outcome measure.

Many have reported that urinary incontinence HRQOL questionnaires do not always correlate with *preoperative* objective measures of urinary incontinence There is poor correlation between the severity of scores in the IIQ and UDI and the 1-hour pad test in a community population.[15] The poor predictive value of the IIQ and the UDI for patients with the urodynamic diagnosis of stress or urge incontinence has been reported,[61] but these tools have been shown to be responsive to treatment of SUI after reconstructive pelvic surgery.[62] Others have shown poor correlation between the severity of incontinence determined by Valsalva leak point pressure and scores on the UDI-6, but specific items from the UDI-6 were able to provide predictive information regarding urodynamic findings in women.[63] For example, 85% of patients with detrusor overactivity reported a moderate or great response to urge-related leakage (item 2) of the UDI-6. Preoperative use of the UDI-6 could therefore have avoided 52 of 128 urodynamic studies, and only six patients with detrusor overactivity would have been missed. This type of information may help eliminate the discomfort and potential complications of invasive urodynamic testing and reduce the associated costs.

The *postoperative* evaluation of incontinence treatment is complicated. Our objective tools that evaluate incontinence are extremely insensitive and miss the incontinence in many of patients, or our symptom questionnaires reveal some unknown characteristics that do not relate to objective urinary incontinence. We know that women may report satisfaction with surgery even if they have not achieved continence. Satisfaction rates decrease with pad use, with the increasing frequency of stress symptoms, and with urge incontinence.[64] Can this be measured accurately, and does it predict or correlate with patients' subjective outcomes?

A comprehensive discussion of the role of urodynamic testing is beyond the scope of this chapter, but several observations can be offered. In a prospective, randomized study comparing the use of tension-free vaginal tape with colposuspension, the objective cure rate (defined as negative pad test and negative cystometric results) was 66% in the tension-free vaginal tape group and 57% in the colposuspension group.[65] When patients completed validated questionnaires, only 59% and 53%, respectively, reported cure of their SUI. Only 36% and 28%, respectively, reported no urine leakage under any circumstance. However, 84% in the tension-free vaginal tape group and 82% in the colposuspension group reported being satisfied or very satisfied with their surgery and were willing to recommend it to a friend. Fulford and colleagues[66] identified six patients with demonstrable stress incontinence on postoperative video urodynamics who had no subjective complaints of stress incontinence. In the same study, despite 83 of 85 patients reporting symptomatic resolution of stress incontinence, only 66 were satisfied with the surgical result, mainly because of persistent urge symptoms. These data are similar to those of Litwiller and coworkers,[67] who reported just over one half of patients subjectively satisfied in the presence of persistent urgency or urge incontinence, compared with a 100% satisfaction rate for those without an urge component.

Although postoperative stress incontinence may not correlate with patient satisfaction, detrusor overactivity and urgency symptoms are important factors in poor subjective outcomes after surgery. Rodriguez and coworkers[68] evaluated postoperative patients who had preoperative detrusor overactivity on urodynamic study. Although these patients reported similar improvement in SUI symptoms, their postoperative symptoms of frequency, urgency, urge incontinence, and use of pads for protection were significantly more severe than those without preoperative detrusor overactivity. In this study, perception of overall quality of life was not different for patients with or without detrusor overactivity on urodynamic studies, regardless of their worse outcome. This finding may reflect realistic patient expectations that UUI symptoms may not improve after surgery (perhaps because of good preoperative counseling) or the fact that overall improvement (85% versus 88%) and decrease in daily pad use (69% versus 71%) was similar between groups.

Many investigators have evaluated patients' expectations for surgery[9,69-74] and have shown that the patients' goals can range from improvement of a specific symptom to restoration of a general lifestyle. Patients' expectations for surgery to improve quality of life are critical, and preoperative counseling is essential to clarify and negotiate reasonable surgical outcomes. Failure to meet these expectations is an important reason why patients report dissatisfaction after surgery. Lifestyle factors may include the goal of return to missed activities ("I want to be able to play with my grandchildren" or "I want to go back to an exercise routine"), whereas other patients may desire resolution of a particular problem ("I want the bulge gone" or "I don't want to leak when I cough").

Although we cannot predict individual goals, achievement of specific goals appears to be a primary reason for undergoing surgery. Elkadry and associates[74] observed that women's expectations of goal achievement are so strong that even extensive preoperative counseling did not eliminate unrealistic hopes such as relief of urinary frequency and urgency from the personal goals list. Further study is needed to establish whether the inclusion of patient goals into preoperative evaluation improves patient outcomes.

Box 12-1 Groutz-Blaivas Anti-Incontinence Surgery Response Score

The Groutz-Blaivas anti-incontinence surgery response score combines the patient's objective clinical data with their subjective report of outcome. The three measures of incontinence—the patient questionnaire, 24-hour pad test, and 24-hour voiding diary—are scored from 0 to 2, and the cumulative score determines the outcome category of cure, good, fair, poor, or failure.

Postoperative 24-Hour Voiding Diary

0 = No urinary incontinence (urge or stress) episodes.
1 = 1 or 2 incontinence episodes
2 = ≥3 incontinence episodes

Postoperative 24-Hour Pad Test

0 = Total weight gain of the pads: ≤8 g
1 = Total weight gain of the pads: 9 to 20 g
2 = Total weight gain of the pads: >20 g

Patient Questionnaire

0 = The patient considers herself cured.
1 = The patient considers herself improved.
2 = The patient considers the operation to have failed.

Cumulative Score

Outcome	Total score
Cure	0
Good response	1-2
Fair response	3-4
Poor response	5
Failure	6

From Groutz A, Blaivas JG, Rosenthal JE: A simplified urinary incontinence score for the evaluation of treatment outcomes. Neurourol Urodyn 19:127-135, 2000.

COMBINED MEASURES OF TREATMENT OUTCOMES

Most clinicians would agree that the ultimate definition of success is the patient's subjective outcome. However, objective data obtained through testing are critical to assess a procedure's efficacy and its complications, allow accurate comparison of different procedures, and ultimately allow the clinician to provide realistic outcomes expectations and counseling to patients. Although the perfect questionnaire could help us sort out these symptoms without invasive testing, it does not exist. We are left with a dilemma about how to evaluate and report patient outcomes after incontinence therapy. The Urodynamics Society recommended that the post-treatment evaluation of incontinence should include at least the patient's opinion of treatment outcome, a micturition questionnaire, a voiding diary, a pad test, a physical examination, uroflowmetry, and postvoid residual volume.[10]

An innovative system to combine subjective and objective evaluation of incontinence, the SEAPI QMM, was published by Raz and Erickson in 1992.[4] This system is conceptually similar to the TNM system, with each letter of SEAPI QMM representing an aspect of incontinence (*s*tress-related leakage, bladder *e*mptying ability, *a*natomy, *p*rotection, *i*nhibition of bladder activity, *q*uality of life, *m*obility, and *m*ental status) and each factor assigned a number grade.[4]

The quality-of-life measure consists of a 15-item questionnaire that looks at several domains, including social interactions, personal strain, global health and quality of life, satisfaction and financial impact. This quality-of-life measure was further assessed for reliability and secondarily evaluated the gender differences in the impact of incontinence before and after treatment. The self-directed SEAPI QMM quality-of-life index was evaluated in 315 patients (102 men and 213 women) with incontinence and 35 without incontinence.[75] A voiding diary reported the frequency of incontinence episodes and the number of pads or type of protection used daily for incontinence. Mean scores before and after treatment with medical or surgical management were significantly different for both genders. Women reported that urinary incontinence had the greatest impact in the social domain, and men reported the greatest impact was on sexual relations. This instrument demonstrated a high degree of reliability relating to stability and internal consistency across a wide age range in men and women. The length of this instrument may limit its general acceptance by clinicians.

Groutz and Blaivas[76] developed and presented a compilation of noninvasive outcome measures to better assess and report the combination of the patients' objective clinical data with their subjective reports of outcome. They use three measures of incontinence: patient questionnaire, 24-hour pad test (which the patient completes before the postoperative visit), and 24-hour voiding diary. Ninety-four patients who underwent pubovaginal sling procedures had their outcomes evaluated twice, first by each of these three measures separately and by assigned outcome categories of cure, improvement, and failure and, second, by combining the three outcome tools into a new response score. The new response score summed these three incontinence measures from 0 to 2, with the total score added from the three categories (therefore combining the objective and subjective outcome data) to determine the new outcome categories of cure, good, fair, poor, and failure (Box 12-1). The strict criterion for cure in the new response score category was no incontinence episode, a negative pad test result, and subjective cure. Using the new response score, 44.7% of patients were classified as cured, whereas the old system had classified 64% as cured by pad test and questionnaire results and 69% according to voiding diary information. Seven patients who were reclassified as having a poor response reported subjective improvement by means of the questionnaire. The 44.7 % cure from this combined score correlates well with previous reports of subjective outcome after pubovaginal sling of 46% by Haaband colleagues[77] and of 47% after modified Pereyra procedures by Sirls and associates.[7] The incorporation of these noninvasive objective data with patient questionnaires to generate a global outcome score seems to be an effective tool in evaluating treatment outcomes for SUI. More sophisticated urodynamic testing and the addition of a validated HRQOL tool would strengthen the outcome data but may discourage patient follow-up.

CONCLUSIONS

Evaluating treatment outcome for urinary incontinence is complicated by studies that have different surgical technique, patient selection, length of follow-up, study methodology, and investigator definition of cure. Standardizing outcomes measures would be a great stride in achieving comparable data for treatment evaluation. Until the evaluation of urinary incontinence is standardized, it is most reasonable to suggest that investigators present complete data sets, including any urodynamic data (e.g., Valsalva leak point pressure, pressure-flow data), postvoid residual volume, pad test weights, voiding diary data, and HRQOL questionnaire data for review. This would allow more accurate interpretation and evaluation of the effect and complications of different treatments. Choosing a single questionnaire may not be sufficient for most purposes, and combining two or more questionnaires may prove comprehensive and practical for most clinical environments. Longer symptom questionnaires may be necessary to provide the data set for clinical research to help understand urinary incontinence and the impact of treatment on symptoms. The incorporation of noninvasive objective data with patient questionnaires, such as that presented in the response score of Groutz and Blaivas,[76] seems to be the most effective means of evaluating treatment outcomes for SUI.

References

1. Nygaard I, Zmolek G: Exercise pad testing in continent exercisers: Reproducibility and correlation with voided volume, Pyridium staining and type of exercise. Neurourol Urodyn 14:125-129, 1995.
2. Ouslander JG, Urman HN, Uman GC: Development and testing of an incontinence monitoring record. J Am Geriatr Soc 34:83-90, 1986.
3. Shumaker SA, Wyman JF, Uebersax JS, et al: Health-related quality of life measures for women with urinary incontinence: The Incontinence Impact Questionnaire and the Urogenital Distress Inventory. Continence Program in Women (CPW) Research Group. Qual Life Res 3:291-306, 1994.
4. Raz S, Erickson DR: SEAPI QMM incontinence classification system. Neurourol Urodyn 11:187-199, 1992.
5. Korman HK, Sirls LT, Kirkemo AK: Success rate of modified Pereyra bladder neck suspension determined by outcomes analysis. J Urol 152:1453-1457, 1994.
6. Sirls LT, Keoleian CM, Korman HK, et al: The effect of study methodology on reported success rates of the modified Pereyra bladder neck suspension. J Urol 154:1732-1735, 1995.
7. Conrad S, Pieper A, de la Maza SF, et al: Long-term results of the Stamey bladder neck suspension procedure: A patient questionnaire based outcome analysis. J Urol 157:1672-1677, 1997.
8. Bidmead J, Cardozo L, McLellan A, et al: A comparison of the objective and subjective outcomes of colposuspension for stress incontinence in women. BJOG 108:408-413, 2001.
9. Hullfish KL, Bovbjerg VE, Gibson J, Steers WD: Patient-centered goals for pelvic floor dysfunction surgery: Is success, and is it achieved? Am J Obstet Gynecol 187:88-92, 2002.
10. Blaivas JG, Appell RA, Fantyl JA, et al: Standards of efficacy for the evaluation of treatment outcomes in urinary incontinence: Recommendations of the Urodynamics Society. Neurourol Urodyn 16:145-147, 1997.
11. Norton C: The effects of urinary incontinence in women. Int Rehabil Med 4:9-14, 1982.
12. Hunskaar S, Vinsnes A: The quality of life in women with urinary incontinence as measured by the sickness impact profile. J Am Geriatr Soc 39:378-382, 1991.
13. Uebersax JS, Wyman JF, Shumaker SA, et al: Short forms to assess life quality and symptom distress for urinary incontinence in women: The Incontinence Impact Questionnaire and the Urogenital Distress Inventory. Neurourol Urodyn 14:131-139, 1995.
14. Wyman JF, Harkins SW, Choi SC, et al: Psychosocial impact of urinary incontinence in women. Obstet Gynecol 70:378-381, 1987.
15. Harvey MA, Kristjansson B, Griffith D, Versi E: The Incontinence Impact Questionnaire and the Urogenital Distress Inventory: A revisit of their validity in women without a urodynamic diagnosis. Am J Obstet Gynecol 185:25-31, 2001.
16. Wood-Dauphinee S, Troidl H: Endpoints for clinical studies: Conventional and innovative variables. In Troidl H, Spitzer WO, McPeek B, et al (eds): Principles and Practice of Research. New York, Springer-Verlag, 1991.
17. McDowell I, Newell C: Measuring health: A guide to rating scales and questionnaires. New York, Oxford University Press, 1996, pp 10-36.
18. Sand PK, Hill RC, Ostergard DR: Incontinence history as a predictor of detrusor stability. Obstet Gynecol 71:257-260, 1988.

19. Wyman JF, Choi SC, Harkins SW, et al: The urinary diary in evaluation of incontinent women: A test-retest analysis. Obstet Gynecol 71:812-8817, 1988.
20. Mouritsen L, Berild G, Hertz J: Comparison of different methods for quantification of urinary leakage in incontinent women. Neurourol Urodyn 8:579-587, 1989.
21. Jackson S: Female urinary incontinence—Symptom evaluation and diagnosis. Eur Urol 32(Suppl 2):20-24, 1997.
22. Brown, JS, Posner SF, Stewart AL: Urge incontinence: new health related quality of life measures. J Am Geriatr Soc 7:980-989, 1999.
23. Chaikin DC, Blaivas JG, Rosenthal JE, Weiss JP: Results of pubovaginal sling for stress incontinence: a prospective comparison of 4 instruments for outcome analysis. J Urol 162:1670-1673, 1999.
24. Rodriguez LV, Blander DS, Dorey F, et al: Discrepancy in patient and physician perception of patient's quality of life related to urinary symptoms. Urology 62:49-53, 2003.
25. Kujansuu E, Kauppila A: Scored urological history and urethrocystometry in the differential diagnosis of female urinary incontinence. Ann Chri Gynaecol 71:197-202, 1982.
26. Klovning A, Hunskaar S, Eriksen BC: Validity of a scored urological history in detecting detrusor instability in female incontinence. Acta Obstet Gynecol Scand 75:941, 1996.
27. Haeusler G, Hanzal E, Joura E, et al: Differential diagnosis of detrusor instability and stress incontinence by patient history: The Gaudenz Incontinence Questionnaire revisited. Acta Obset Gynecol Scand 74:636-637, 1995.
28. Ishiko O, Hirai K, Sumi T, et al: The urinary incontinence score in the diagnosis of female urinary incontinence. Int J Gynaecol Obstet 68:131-137, 2000.
29. Nochajski TH, Burns PA, Pranikoff K, Dittmar SS: Dimensions of urine loss among older women with genuine stress incontinence. Neurourol Urodyn 12:223-233, 1993.
30. Sandvik H, Hunskaar S, Seim A, et al: Validation of a severity index in female urinary incontinence and its implementation in an epidemiological surgery. Epidemiol Community Health 47:497-499, 1993.
31. Sandvik H, Seim A, Vanvik A, Hunskaar S: A severity index for epidemiological surveys of female urinary incontinence: Comparison with 48-hour pad-weighing tests. Neurourol Urodyn 19:137-146, 2000.
32. Black N, Griffiths J, Pope C: Development of a symptom severity index and a symptom impact index for stress incontinence in women. Neurourol Urodyn 15:630-640, 1996.
33. Jackson S, Donovan J, Kent L, Abrams P: The reliability and validity of a new female urinary symptoms questionnaire. Neurourol Urodyn 5:536-537, 1995.
34. Avery K, Donovan J, Peters J, et al: ICIQ: A brief and robust measure for evaluating the symptoms and impact of urinary incontinence, Neurourol Urodyn 23:322-330, 2004.
35. Karantanis E, Fynes M, Moore KH, Stanton SL: Comparison of the ICIQ-SF and 24-hour pad test with other measures for evaluating the severity of urodynamic stress incontinence. Int Urogynecol J Pelvic Floor Dysfunct 15:111-116, 2004.
36. Hajebrahimi S, Corcos J, Lemieux MC: International consultation on incontinence questionnaire short form: Comparison of physician versus patient completion and immediate and delayed self-administration. Urology 63:1076-1078, 2004.
37. Stach-Lempinen B, Kujansuu E, Laippala P, Metsanoja R: Visual analogue scale, urinary incontinence severity score and 15 D—Psychometric testing of three different health-related quality of life instruments for urinary incontinent women. Scand U Urol Nephrol 35:476-483, 2001.
38. van der Vaart CH, de Leeuw JR, Roovers JP, Heintz AP: The effect of urinary incontinence and overactive bladder symptoms on quality of life in young women. BJU Int 90:544-549, 2002.
39. Robinson JP, Shea JA: Development and testing of a measure of health-related quality of life for men with urinary incontinence. J Am Geriatr Soc 50:935-945, 2002.
40. Lubeck DP, Prebil LA, Peeples P, Brown JS: A health related quality of life measure for use in patients with urge urinary incontinence: A validation study. Qual Life Res 8:337-344, 1999.
41. Patrick DL, Martin ML, Bushnell DM, et al: Quality of life of women with urinary incontinence: Further development of the incontinence quality of life instrument (I-QOL). Urology 53:71-76, 1999.
42. Wagner TH, Patrick DL, Bavendam DM, et al: Quality of life of persons with urinary incontinence: development of a new measure. Urology 47:67-71, 1996.
43. Bump RC, Norton PA, Sinner NR, Yalcin I: Mixed urinary incontinience symptoms: urodynamic findings, incontinence severity, and treatment response. Obstet Gynecol 102:76-83, 2003.
44. Melville JL, Miller EA, Fialkow MF, et al: Relationship between patient report and physician assessment of urinary incontinence severity. Am J Obstet Gynecol 189:76-80, 2003.
45. Yalcin I, Bump RC: Validaton of two global impression questionnaires for incontinence. Am J Obstet Gynecol 189:98-101, 2003.
46. DuBeau CE, Levy B Mangione CM, Resnick NM: The impact of urge urinary incontinence on quality of life: Importance of patients' perspective and explanatory style. J Am Geriatr Soc 46:683-692, 1998.
47. DuBeau CE, Keily DK, Resnick NM: Quality of life impact of urge incontinence in older persons: A new measure and conceptual structure. J Am Geriatr Soc 47:989-994, 1999.
48. Lee PS, Reid DW, Saltmarche A, Linton LJ: Measuring the psychosocial impact of urinary incontinence: The York Incontinence Perception Scale (YIPS). Am Geriatr Soc 43:1275-1278, 1995.
49. Kelleher CJ, Cardozo LD, Khullar V, Salvatore S: A new questionnaire to assess the quality of life of urinary incontinent women. Br J Obstet Gynaecol 104:1374-1379, 1997.
50. Reese P, Pleil A, Okano G, Kelleher C: Multinational study of Reliability and validity of the King's Health Questionnaire in patients with overactive bladder. Qual Life Res 12:427-442, 2004.
51. Amarenco G, Arnould B, Carita P, et al: European psychometrics validation of CONTILIFE: A quality of life questionnaire for urinary incontinence. Eur Urol 43:391-404, 2003.
52. Coyne K, Revicki D, Hunt T, et al: Psychometric validation of an overactive bladder symptom and health-related quality of life questionnaire: The OAB-q. Qual Life Res 11:563-574, 2002.
53. Coyne KS, Zhou Z, Bhattacharyya SK, et al: The prevalence of nocturia and its effect on health-related quality of life and sleep in a community sample in the USA. BJU Int 92:948-954, 2003.
54. Yu LC, Kaltreider DL, Hu T, et al: The ISQ-P tool: Measuring stress associated with incontinence. J Gerontol Nurs 15:9-15, 1989.
55. Marquis P, Amarenco G, Sapede C, et al: development and validation of a disease specific quality of life questionnaire for urinary urge incontinency. Qual Life Res 4:458-459, 1995.
56. Rai GS, Kiniors M, Wientjes H: Urinary incontinence handicap inventory. Arch Gerontol Geriatr 19:7-10, 1994.
57. Shaw C, Matthews RJ, Perry SI, et al: Validity and reliability of a questionnaire to measure impact of lower urinary tract symptoms on quality of life: The Leicester Impact Scale. Neurol Urodyn 23:229-236, 2004.
58. Huisman SJ, van Dam FSAM, Aaronson NK, Hanewald GJFP: On measuring complaints of cancer patients: Some remarks on the time span of the question. In Aaronson NK, Beckmann J (eds): The Quality of Life of Cancer Patients. New York, Raven Press, 1987.
59. Cohen C: On the quality of life: Some philosophical reflections. Circulation 66 (Suppl III):29-33, 1982.
60. Coyne KS, Zhou Z, Thompson C, Versi E: The impact on health-related quality of life of stress, urge, and mixed urinary incontinence. BJU Int 92:731-735, 2003.
61. Fitzgerald MP, Brubaker L. Urinary incontinence symptom scores and urodynamic diagnoses. Neurourol Urodyn 21:30-35, 2002.
62. Fitzgerald MP, Kenton K, Shott S, Brubaker L: Responsiveness of quality of life measurements to change after reconstructive pelvic surgery. Am J Obstet Gynecol 185:20-24, 2001.

63. Lemack GE, Zimmern PE: Predictability of urodynamic findings based on the Urogenital Distress Inventory-6 questionnaire. Urology 54:461-466, 1999.
64. Diokno AD, Burgio K, Fultz NH, et al: Prevalence and outcomes of continence surgery in community dwelling women. J Urol 170:507-511, 2003.
65. Ward K, Hilton P, for the United Kingdom and Ireland Tension-free Vaginal Tape Trial Group: Prospective multicentre randomised trial of tension-free vaginal tape and colposuspension as primary treatment for stress incontinence. BMJ 325:67-72, 2002.
66. Fulford SCV, Flynn R, Barrington J, et al: An assessment of the surgical outcome and urodynamic effects of the pubovaginal sling for stress incontinence and the associated urge syndrome. J Urol 162:135-137, 1999.
67. Litwiller SE, Nelson RS, Fone PD, et al: Vaginal wall sling: Long-term outcome analysis of factors contributing to patients satisfaction and surgical success. J Urol 157:1287-1282, 1997.
68. Rodriguex LV, de Almeida F, Dorey F, Raz S: Does Valsalva leak point pressure predict outcome after the distal urethral polypropylene sling? Role of urodynamics in the sling era. J Urol 172:210-214, 2004.
69. Jones KR, Burney RE, Christy B: Patient expectations for surgery: Are they being met? Jt Comm J Qual Improv 26:349-360, 2000.
70. Jeffry L, Deval B, Birsan A, et al: Objective and subjective cure rates after tension-free vaginal tape for treatment of urinary incontinence. Urology 58:702-706, 2001.
71. Khullar V, Cardozo L, Boos K, et al: Impact of surgery for stress incontinence on morbidity: Effects of confounding variables on outcomes of incontinence surgery must be considered. BMJ 317:143, 1998.
72. McKinley RK, Stevenson K, Adams S, Manku-Scott TK: Meeting patient expectations of care: The major determinant of satisfaction with out-of-hours primary medical care? Fam Pract 19:333-338, 2002.
73. Mondloch MV, Cole DC, Frank JW: Does how you do depend on how you think you'll do? A systematic review of the evidence for a relation between patients' recovery expectations and health outcomes. CMAJ 165:174-179, 2001.
74. Elkadry EA, Kenton KS, FitzGerald MP, et al: Patient-selected goals: A new perspective on surgical outcome. Am J Obstet Gynecol 189:1551-1558. 2003.
75. Stothers L: Reliability, validity, and gender differences in the quality of life index of the SEAPI-QMM incontinence classification system. Neurourol Urodyn 23:223-228, 2004.
76. Groutz A, Blaivas JG, Rosenthal JE: A simplified urinary incontinence score for the evaluation of treatment outcomes. Neurourol Urodyn 19:127-135, 2000.
77. Haab F, Trockman BA, Zimmern PE, Leach G: Results of pubovaginal sling for the treatment of intrinsic sphincter deficiency determined by questionnaire analysis. J Urol 158:1738-1742, 1997.

Section 3

PATHOPHYSIOLOGY OF VOIDING DYSFUNCTION

Chapter 13

CATEGORIZATION OF VOIDING DYSFUNCTION

Alan J. Wein and M. Louis Moy

The lower urinary tract functions as a group of interrelated structures in the adult to bring about efficient and low-pressure bladder filling, low-pressure urine storage with perfect continence, and periodic, complete, voluntary urine expulsion at low pressure. Because in the adult the lower urinary tract is normally under voluntary neural control, it is different from other visceral organs, whose regulation is solely by involuntary mechanisms.

For the purposes of description and teaching, the micturition cycle is best divided into two relatively discrete phases: bladder filling with urine storage and bladder emptying or voiding. The micturition cycle normally displays these two modes of operation in a simple on-off fashion. The cycle involves switching from inhibition of the voiding reflex and activation of storage reflexes to inhibition of the storage reflexes and activation of the voiding reflex—and back again.

This chapter begins with a functional, physiologic, and pharmacologic overview of normal and abnormal lower urinary tract function. A simple way of looking at the pathophysiology of all types of voiding dysfunction is presented, followed by a discussion of various systems of classification and categorization.

NORMAL LOWER URINARY TRACT FUNCTION

Two-Phase Concept of Function: Filling or Storage and Emptying or Voiding

Whatever disagreements exist regarding the anatomic, morphologic, physiologic, pharmacologic, and mechanical details involved in the storage and expulsion of urine by the lower urinary tract, most experts agree on certain points.[1] The first is that the micturition cycle involves two relatively discrete processes: bladder filling with urine storage and bladder emptying. The second is that, whatever the details involved, these processes can be summarized from a conceptual point of view as follows.

Bladder filling and urine storage require the following:

1. Accommodation of increasing volumes of urine at a low intravesical pressure and with appropriate sensation
2. A bladder outlet that is closed at rest and remains so during increases in intra-abdominal pressure
3. Absence of involuntary bladder contractions

Bladder emptying requires the following:

1. Coordinated contraction of the bladder smooth musculature of adequate magnitude and duration
2. Concomitant lowering of resistance at the level of the smooth and striated sphincter
3. Absence of anatomic (as opposed to functional) obstruction

The smooth sphincter refers to the smooth musculature of the bladder neck and proximal urethra. This is a physiologic but not an anatomic sphincter and one that is not under voluntary control. The striated sphincter refers to the striated musculature, which is a part of the outer wall of the proximal urethra in males and females (this portion is often referred to as the *intrinsic* or *intramural striated sphincter*), and the bulky skeletal muscle group that surrounds the urethra at the level of the membranous portion in the male and the middle segment in the female (often referred to as the *extrinsic* or *extramural striated sphincter*). The extramural portion is the classically described *external urethral sphincter* and is under voluntary control.[2]

Any type of voiding dysfunction must result from an abnormality of one or more of the factors just listed. This two-phase concept of micturition, with the three components of each, related to the bladder or to the outlet provides a logical framework for a functional categorization of all types of voiding dysfunction and disorders of filling and storage or to voiding (Boxes 13-1 and 13-2). Some types of voiding dysfunction represent combinations of filling with storage and voiding abnormalities. Within this scheme, however, these become readily understandable, and their detection and treatment can be logically described. Various aspects of physiology and pathophysiology are always related more to one phase of micturition than another. All aspects of urodynamic and video-urodynamic evaluation can be conceptualized in this functional manner according to what they evaluate in terms of bladder or outlet activity during filling with storage or voiding (Table 13-1). All known treatments for voiding dysfunction can be classified in the broad categories of whether they facilitate filling with storage or voiding and whether they do so by an action primarily on the bladder or on one or more of the components of the bladder outlet (see Box 13-2 and Table 13-1).

Mechanisms Underlying the Two Phases of Function

This section summarizes pertinent points regarding the physiology of the various mechanisms underlying normal bladder filling with storage and voiding, abnormalities of which constitute the

Box 13-1 Functional Classification

Failure to store
- Because of the bladder
- Because of the outlet

Failure to empty
- Because of the bladder
- Because of the outlet

Box 13-2 Expanded Functional Classification

Failure to Store

- Because of the bladder
  - Overactivity
    - Involuntary contractions
    - Neurologic disease or injury
    - Bladder outlet obstruction (myogenic)
    - Inflammation
    - Idiopathic cause
  - Decreased compliance
    - Neurologic disease or injury
    - Fibrosis
    - Idiopathic cause
  - Combination of overactivity and decreased compliance
  - Hypersensitivity
    - Inflammation or infection
    - Neurologic disease or injury
    - Psychological origin
    - Idiopathic cause
- Because of the outlet
  - Genuine stress urinary incontinence
  - Lack of suburethral support
  - Pelvic floor laxity or hypermobility
  - Intrinsic sphincter deficiency
    - Neurologic disease or injury
    - Fibrosis
  - Combination of causes

Failure to Empty

- Because of the bladder
  - Neurologic cause
  - Myogenic cause
  - Psychogenic cause
  - Idiopathic cause
- Because of the outlet
  - Anatomic causes
    - Prostatic obstruction
    - Bladder neck contracture
    - Urethral stricture
    - Urethral compression
  - Functional causes
    - Smooth sphincter dyssynergia
    - Striated sphincter dyssynergia
  - Combination of causes

pathophysiologic mechanisms of the various types of dysfunction of the lower urinary tract. The information is consistent with that detailed by de Groat and associates,[3,4] Zderic and colleagues,[2] and Steers,[5] and references are provided only when particularly applicable.

Bladder Response during Filling

The normal adult bladder response to filling at a physiologic rate is an almost imperceptible change in intravesical pressure. During at least the initial stages of bladder filling, after unfolding of the bladder wall from its collapsed state, this very high compliance (Δ volume/Δ pressure) of the bladder primarily results from its elastic and viscoelastic properties. *Elasticity* allows the constituents of the bladder wall to stretch to a certain degree without any increase in tension. *Viscoelasticity* allows stretch to induce a rise in tension, followed by a decay (i.e., stress relaxation) when the filling (i.e., stretch stimulus) slows or stops. Brading and colleagues[6] think there is continuous contractile activity in the smooth muscle cells to adjust their length during filling but without (normally) synchronous activity that would increase intravesical pressure, would impede filling, and could cause urinary leakage. Clinically and urodynamically, the bladder seems relaxed. The urothelium also expands but must preserve its barrier function while doing so. There may be an active component to the storage properties of the bladder. The mucosa and lamina propria are normally the most compliant layers of the bladder. Coplen and associates[7] have hypothesized that the smooth muscle layer may have a chronic effect on compliance in the midportion of the cystometric filling curve through a complex interaction between muscle and extracellular matrix. This layer may acutely affect compliance in response to neurologic input as well.

In the usual clinical setting, filling cystometry seems to show a slight increase in intravesical pressure, but Klevmark[8,9] elegantly showed that this pressure rise is a function of the fact that cystometric filling is carried out at a greater than physiologic rate and, at physiologic filling rates, there is essentially no rise in bladder pressure until bladder capacity is reached.

The viscoelastic properties of the stroma (i.e., bladder wall less smooth muscle and epithelium) and the urodynamically relaxed detrusor muscle account for the passive mechanical properties and normal bladder compliance seen during filling. The main components of the stroma are collagen and elastin. When the collagen component increases, compliance decreases. This can occur with various types of injury, chronic inflammation, bladder outlet obstruction, and neurologic decentralization. After decreased compliance has occurred because of a replacement by collagen of other components of the stroma, it is generally unresponsive to pharmacologic manipulation, hydraulic distention, or nerve section. Most often, under those circumstances, augmentation cystoplasty is required to achieve satisfactory reservoir function.

Does the nervous system affect the normal bladder response to filling? At a certain level of bladder filling, spinal sympathetic reflexes facilitatory to bladder filling and storage are evoked in animals, a concept developed over the years by de Groat and associates,[3] who have also cited indirect evidence to support such a role in humans. This inhibitory effect is likely mediated primarily by sympathetic modulation of cholinergic ganglionic transmission. Through this reflex mechanism, two other possibilities exist for promoting filling and storage. One is neurally mediated stimulation of the predominantly α-adrenergic receptors in the area of the smooth sphincter, the net result of which would be to cause an increase in resistance in that area. The second is neurally mediated stimulation of the predominantly β-adrenergic receptors (inhibitory) in the bladder body smooth musculature, which would cause a decrease in bladder wall tension. McGuire and colleagues[10] also cited evidence for direct inhibition of detrusor motor neurons in the sacral spinal cord during bladder filling that results from increased afferent pudendal nerve activity generated by receptors in the striated sphincter. Good evidence exists to support a tonic inhibitory effect of other neurotransmitters on the micturition reflex at various levels of the neural axis. Bladder filling and consequent wall distention may also release autocrine-like factors (e.g., nitric oxide, prostaglandins, peptides) that influence contractility.

Table 13-1 Urodynamics Simplified

Phase Assessed*	Bladder Assessment	Outlet Assessment
Filling and storage phase	Total P_{ves} and P_{det} during a filling cystometrogram	Urethral pressure profilometry
	Detrusor leak point pressure	Valsalva leak point pressure
		Fluoroscopy
Emptying phase	Total P_{ves} and P_{det} during a voiding cystometrogram	Micturitional urethral pressure profilometry
		Fluoroscopy
		Electromyography of periurethral striated musculature
	Flowmetry†	Flowmetry†
	Residual urine†	Residual urine†

P_{det}, detrusor pressure; P_{ves}, bladder pressure.

*This functional conceptualization of urodynamics categorizes each study according to whether it examines bladder or outlet activity during the filling and storage phase or emptying phase of micturition.

†In this scheme, uroflow and residual urine integrate the activity of the bladder and the outlet during the emptying phase.

Outlet Response during Filling

There is a gradual increase in urethral pressure during bladder filling, contributed to by at least the striated sphincteric element and perhaps by the smooth sphincteric element as well. The rise in urethral pressure seen during the filling and storage phase of micturition can be correlated with an increase in efferent pudendal nerve impulse frequency and in electromyographic activity of the periurethral striated musculature. This constitutes the efferent limb of a spinal somatic reflex, the so-called guarding reflex, which results in a gradual increase in striated sphincter activity.

Although it seems logical and compatible with neuropharmacologic, neurophysiologic, and neuromorphologic data to assume that the muscular component of the smooth sphincter also contributes to the change in urethral response during bladder filling, it is extremely difficult to prove this experimentally or clinically. The direct and circumstantial evidence in favor of such a hypothesis has been summarized by Wein and Barrett,[1] Elbadawi,[11] and Brading.[12] The passive properties of the urethral wall deserve mention because they undoubtedly play a large role in the maintenance of continence.[6,13] Urethral wall tension develops within the outer layers of the urethra; however, urethral pressure is a product of the active characteristics of smooth and striated muscle and of the passive characteristics of the elastic, collagenous, and vascular components of the urethral wall, because this tension must be exerted on a soft or plastic inner layer capable of being compressed to a closed configuration—the "filler material" representing the submucosal portion of the urethra. The softer and more plastic this area is, the less pressure required by the tension-producing area to produce continence. Whatever the compressive forces, the lumen of the urethra must be capable of being obliterated by a watertight seal. This mucosal seal mechanism explains why a thin-walled rubber tube requires less pressure to close an open end when the inner layer is coated with a fine layer of grease than when it is not, and the latter case is much like scarred or atrophic urethral mucosa.

Voiding with a Normal Bladder Contraction

Although many factors are involved in the initiation of micturition, intravesical pressure producing the sensation of distention is primarily responsible for the initiation of voluntarily induced emptying of the lower urinary tract in adults. Although the origin of the parasympathetic neural outflow to the bladder, the pelvic nerve, is in the sacral spinal cord, the organizational center for the micturition reflex in an intact neural axis is in the brainstem, and the complete neural circuit for normal micturition includes the ascending and descending spinal cord pathways to and from this area and the facilitatory and inhibitory influences from other parts of the brain.

The final step in voluntarily induced micturition involves inhibition of the somatic neural efferent activity to the striated sphincter and an inhibition of all aspects of any spinal sympathetic reflex evoked during filling. Efferent parasympathetic pelvic nerve activity is ultimately responsible for a highly coordinated contraction of the bulk of the bladder smooth musculature. A decrease in outlet resistance occurs, with adaptive shaping or funneling of the relaxed bladder outlet. Besides the inhibition of any continence-promoting reflexes that have occurred during bladder filling, the change in outlet resistance may also involve active relaxation of the smooth sphincter area through a nonadrenergic, noncholinergic mechanism, probably mediated by nitric oxide. The adaptive changes that occur in the outlet in part result from the anatomic interrelationships of the smooth muscle of the bladder base and proximal urethra (i.e., longitudinal smooth muscle continuity). Other reflexes that are elicited by bladder contraction and by the passage of urine through the urethra may reinforce and facilitate complete bladder emptying. Superimposed on these autonomic and somatic reflexes are complex, modifying supraspinal inputs from other central neuronal networks. These facilitatory and inhibitory impulses, which originate from several areas of the nervous system, allow for the full conscious control of micturition in the adult.

Urinary Continence during Abdominal Pressure Increases

During voluntarily initiated micturition, the bladder pressure becomes higher than the outlet pressure, and certain adaptive changes occur in the shape of the bladder outlet, with consequent passage of urine into and through the proximal urethra. Why do such changes not occur with increases in intravesical pressure that are similar in magnitude but that are produced only by changes in intra-abdominal pressure, such as straining or coughing? A coordinated bladder contraction does not occur in response to such stimuli, emphasizing the fact that increases in total intravesical pressure are by no means equivalent to emptying ability. Normally, for urine to flow into the proximal urethra, there be an increase in intravesical pressure; the increase must be a product of a coordinated bladder contraction, occurring through a neurally mediated reflex mechanism; and it must be associated with characteristic conformational and tension changes in the bladder neck and proximal urethral area.

Assuming that the bladder outlet is competent at rest, a major factor in the prevention of urinary leakage during increases in intra-abdominal pressure is the fact that there is at least equal pressure transmission to the proximal urethra during such activity. This phenomenon was first described by Enhorning[14] and has been confirmed in virtually every urodynamic laboratory since then. Failure of this mechanism, generally associated with hypermobility of the bladder neck and proximal urethra (another way of describing pathologic descent with abdominal straining), is an almost invariable correlate of genuine stress urinary incontinence in the female. No such hypermobility occurs in the male. The increase in urethral closure pressure that is seen with increments in intra-abdominal pressure normally exceeds the intra-abdominal pressure increase, indicating that active muscular function due to a reflex increase in striated sphincter activity or other factors that increase urethral resistance, in addition to simple transmission of pressure, is also involved in preventing such leakage. Tanagho[15] was the first to provide direct evidence of this.

OVERVIEW OF THE MICTURITION CYCLE

Bladder accommodation during filling is a primarily passive phenomenon that depends on the elastic and viscoelastic properties of the bladder wall and the lack of parasympathetic excitatory input. An increase in outlet resistance occurs by means of the striated sphincter somatic guarding reflex. In some species, a sympathetic reflex also contributes to storage by increasing outlet resistance by increasing tension on the smooth sphincter, inhibiting bladder contractility through an inhibitory effect on parasympathetic ganglia, and causing a decrease in tension of bladder smooth muscle. Continence is maintained during increases in intra-abdominal pressure by the intrinsic competence of the bladder outlet and the pressure transmission ratio to this area with respect to the intravesical contents. A further increase in striated sphincter activity, on a reflex basis, is also contributory.

Voiding can be voluntary or involuntary and involves inhibition of the spinal somatic and sympathetic reflexes and activation of the vesical parasympathetic pathways, the organizational center for which is in the brainstem. Initially, there is a relaxation of the outlet musculature, mediated by the cessation of the somatic and sympathetic spinal reflexes and probably by a relaxing factor, possibly nitric oxide, released by parasympathetic stimulation or by some effect of bladder smooth muscle contraction itself. A highly coordinated, parasympathetically induced contraction of the bulk of the bladder smooth musculature occurs, with shaping or funneling of the relaxed outlet, caused in part by a smooth muscle continuity between the bladder base and the proximal urethra. With amplification and facilitation of the bladder contraction from other peripheral reflexes and from spinal cord supraspinal sources and the absence of anatomic obstruction between the bladder and the urethral meatus, complete emptying occurs.

OVERVIEW OF PATHOPHYSIOLOGY: ABNORMALITIES OF FILLING OR STORAGE AND EMPTYING OR VOIDING

The failure of the lower urinary tract to fill with or store urine adequately is caused by pathologic conditions of the bladder or the outlet, or both.[1,16] Overactivity of the bladder during filling can be expressed as phasic involuntary contractions, as low compliance, or as a combination. Involuntary contractions are most commonly associated with suprasacral neurologic disease or occur after suprasacral neurologic injury; however, they also may be associated with aging, inflammation, or irritation of the bladder wall, bladder outlet obstruction, or stress urinary incontinence, or they may be idiopathic. Decreased compliance during filling may result from neurologic injury or disease, usually at a sacral or infrasacral level, but it may also result from any process that destroys the viscoelastic or elastic properties of the bladder wall. Storage failure may also occur in the absence of hyperactivity resulting from hypersensitivity or pain during filling. Inflammation and irritation can be responsible, as can neurologic, psychological, or idiopathic causes. The classic clinical example is interstitial cystitis.

Decreased outlet resistance may result from any process that damages the innervation, structural elements, or support of the smooth or striated sphincter. This may occur with neurologic disease or injury, surgical or other mechanical trauma, or aging. Classically, sphincteric incontinence in the female patient has been categorized as genuine stress incontinence and as what was originally described as type III stress incontinence, which is now referred to as intrinsic sphincter dysfunction. Genuine stress incontinence in the female is associated with hypermobility of the vesicourethral junction, with poor pelvic support, and with an outlet that is competent at rest but loses its competence only during increases in intra-abdominal pressure. Intrinsic sphincter dysfunction describes a nonfunctional or very poorly functional bladder neck and proximal urethra at rest. The division between these two situations is not absolute, and virtually every case of sphincteric incontinence involves various proportions of genuine stress incontinence and intrinsic sphincter dysfunction. The implication of classic intrinsic sphincter dysfunction is that a surgical procedure designed to correct only urethral hypermobility will have a relatively high failure rate compared with one designed to improve urethral coaptation and compression; however, this approach has become less dogmatic with newer surgical therapies for urinary incontinence.

Stress urinary incontinence is a symptom that arises from damage to muscles, nerves, and connective tissue within the pelvic floor.[17] Urethral support is important; the urethra normally is supported by the action of the levator ani muscles through their connection to the endopelvic fascia of the anterior vaginal wall. Damage to the connection between this fascia and this muscle, damage to the nerve supply, or direct muscle damage can influence continence. Bladder neck function is likewise important, and loss of normal bladder neck closure can result in incontinence despite normal urethral support. In older reports, the urethra was sometimes ignored as a factor contributing to continence in women, and the site of continence was thought to be exclusively the bladder neck. However, in approximately 50% of continent women, urine enters the urethra during increases in abdominal pressure. The continence point in these women is at the middle of the urethra, where urine is stopped before it can escape from the urethral meatus.

With urethral hypermobility, there is weakness of the pelvic floor. During increases in intra-abdominal pressure, there is descent of the bladder neck and proximal urethra. If the outlet opens concomitantly, stress urinary incontinence ensues. In the classic form of urethral hypermobility, there is rotational descent of the bladder neck and urethra. However, the urethra may also descend without rotation (i.e., it shortens and widens), or the posterior wall of the urethra may be pulled open while the anterior wall remains fixed. However, urethral hypermobility is often present in women who are not incontinent, and the mere presence of urethral hypermobility is not sufficient to make a diagnosis of a sphincter abnormality unless urinary incontinence is also demonstrated. The *hammock hypothesis* of John DeLancey[18] proposes that for stress incontinence to occur with hypermobility, there must be a lack of stability of the suburethral supportive layer. This theory proposes that the effect of abdominal pressure increases on the normal bladder outlet, if the suburethral supportive layer is firm, is to compress the urethra rapidly and effectively. If the supportive suburethral layer is lax or movable, compression is not as effective. Intrinsic sphincter dysfunction denotes an intrinsic malfunction of the urethral a misnomer, because many believe that the drop in urethral pressure represents simply the urethral component of a normal voiding reflex in an individual whose bladder does not measurably contract because of myogenic or neurogenic reasons.

In theory, categories of outlet-related incontinence in the male are similar to those in the female. In reality, there is little information regarding the topic of urethral instability in the male. Sphincteric incontinence in the male is not associated with hypermobility of the bladder neck and proximal urethra but is rather more similar to what is called intrinsic sphincter dysfunction in the female.

The treatment of filling and storage abnormalities is directed toward inhibiting bladder contractility, decreasing sensory input, or mechanically increasing bladder capacity and toward increasing outlet resistance, continuously or only during increases in intra-abdominal pressure.

Absolute or relative failure to empty the bladder results from decreased bladder contractility (i.e., decrease in magnitude or duration) or increased outlet resistance, or both. Absolute or relative failure of bladder contractility may result from temporary or permanent alteration in one of the neuromuscular mechanisms necessary for initiating and maintaining a normal detrusor contraction. Inhibition of the voiding reflex in a neurologically normal individual may also occur; it may be inhibited by a reflex mechanism resulting from painful stimuli, especially from the pelvic and perineal areas, or it may be psychogenic. Non-neurogenic causes include impairment of bladder smooth muscle function, which may result from overdistention, various drugs, severe infection, or fibrosis.

Pathologically, decrease outlet resistance is the result of change to the sphincter mechanism itself. In its most overt form, it is characterized by a bladder neck that is open at rest and at a low Valsalva leak point pressure and urethral closure pressure, and it is usually the result of prior surgery, trauma with scarring, or a neurologic lesion.

Urethral instability refers to the rare phenomenon of episodic decreases in outlet pressure unrelated to increases in bladder or abdominal pressure. The term *urethral instability* is probably more common in men than in women. Although it is most often caused by anatomic obstruction, it may result from a failure of relaxation or active contraction of the striated or smooth sphincter during bladder contraction. Striated sphincter dyssynergia is a common cause of functional or nonanatomic (as opposed to fixed anatomic) obstruction in patients with neurologic disease or injury.

The treatment of emptying failure consists of attempts to increase intravesical pressure or facilitate the micturition reflex or to decrease outlet resistance, or both. If other means fail or are impractical, intermittent catheterization is an effective way to circumvent emptying failure.

CATEGORIZATION OF VOIDING DYSFUNCTIONS

Based on the data obtained from the neurourologic evaluation, a given voiding dysfunction can be categorized by an ever-increasing number of descriptive systems. The purpose of any classification system should be to facilitate understanding and management and to avoid confusion among those who are concerned with the problem for which the system was designed. A good classification should serve as intellectual shorthand and should convey in a few key words or phrases the essence of a clinical situation. An ideal system for all types of voiding dysfunction would include or imply several factors: the conclusions reached from urodynamic testing, expected clinical symptoms, and approximate site and type of a neurologic lesion or a lack of one. If the various categories accurately portray pathophysiology, the treatment options should be evident. Most systems of classification for voiding dysfunction were formulated primarily to describe dysfunction caused by neurologic disease or injury. The ideal system should be applicable to all types of voiding dysfunction. No one system is perfect. Most major systems or types of systems in use are reviewed, along with their advantages, disadvantages, and applicability. Understanding the rationale and shortcomings of each system significantly improves the urologist's knowledge of voiding function and dysfunction.

Bors-Comarr Classification

Bors and Comarr[19] made a remarkable contribution by logically deducing a classification system from clinical observation of their patients with traumatic spinal cord injury (Box 13-3). This system applies only to patients with neurologic dysfunction and considers three factors: anatomic localization of the lesion, neurologic completeness or incompleteness of the lesion, and whether lower urinary tract function is *balanced* or *unbalanced*. The latter terms are based solely on the percentage of residual urine relative to bladder capacity. *Unbalanced* signifies the presence of more than 20% residual urine in a patient with an upper motor neuron (UMN) lesion or 10% in a patient with a lower motor neuron (LMN) lesion. This relative residual urine volume was ideally meant to imply coordination (i.e., synergy) or dyssynergia between the smooth and the striated sphincters of the outlet and the bladder during bladder contraction or during attempted micturition by abdominal straining or the Credé maneuver. Determination of the completeness of the lesion is made on the basis of a thorough neurologic examination.

The system erroneously assumes that the sacral spinal cord is the primary reflex center for micturition. *LMN* implies collectively the preganglionic and postganglionic parasympathetic autonomic fibers that innervate the bladder and outlet and originate as preganglionic fibers in the sacral spinal cord. The term is used in an analogy to efferent somatic nerve fibers, such as those of the pudendal nerve, which originate in the same sacral cord

Box 13-3 Bors-Comarr Classification

Sensory Neuron Lesion
Incomplete, balanced
Complete, balanced

Motor Neuron Lesion
Balanced
Imbalanced

Sensory-Motor Neuron Lesion
Upper motor neuron lesion
- Complete, balanced
- Complete, imbalanced
- Incomplete, balanced
- Incomplete, imbalanced

Lower motor neuron lesion
- Complete, balanced
- Complete, imbalanced
- Incomplete, balanced
- Incomplete, imbalanced

Mixed lesion
- Upper somatomotor neuron, lower visceromotor neuron
- Lower somatomotor neuron, upper visceromotor neuron
- Normal somatomotor neuron, lower visceromotor neuron

From Bors E, Comarr AE: Neurological Urology. Baltimore, University Park Press, 1971.

segment but terminate directly on pelvic floor striated musculature without the interposition of ganglia. *UMN* is used in a similar analogy to the somatic nervous system to describe the descending autonomic pathways above the sacral spinal cord, the origin of the motor efferent supply to the bladder.

In this system, *UMN bladder* refers to the pattern of micturition that results from an injury to the suprasacral spinal cord after the period of spinal shock has passed, assuming that the sacral spinal cord and the sacral nerve roots are intact and that the pelvic and pudendal nerve reflexes are intact. *LMN bladder* refers to the pattern resulting if the sacral spinal cord or sacral roots are damaged and the reflex pattern through the autonomic and somatic nerves that emanate from these segments is absent. This system implies that if skeletal muscle spasticity exists below the level of the lesion, the lesion is above the sacral spinal cord and is by definition a UMN lesion. This type of lesion is characterized by involuntary bladder contraction during filling. If flaccidity of the skeletal musculature below the level of a lesion exists, an LMN lesion is assumed to be present, implying detrusor areflexia. Exceptions occur and are classified in a *mixed lesion* group characterized by involuntary bladder contraction with a flaccid paralysis below the level of the lesion or by detrusor areflexia with spasticity or normal skeletal muscle tone neurologically below the lesion level.

The use of this system is illustrated as follows. A *UMN lesion, complete, imbalanced*, implies a neurologically complete lesion above the level of the sacral spinal cord that results in skeletal muscle spasticity below the level of the injury. Involuntary bladder contraction occurs during filling, but a residual urine volume of more than 20% of the bladder capacity is left after bladder contraction, implying obstruction in the area of the bladder outlet during the involuntary detrusor contraction. This obstruction usually is caused by striated sphincter dyssynergia, typically occurring in patients who are paraplegic and quadriplegic with lesions between the cervical and the sacral spinal cord. Smooth sphincter dyssynergia also may be seen in patients with lesions above the level of T6, usually in association with autonomic hyperreflexia. An *LMN lesion, complete, imbalanced*, implies a neurologically complete lesion at the level of the sacral spinal cord or of the sacral roots, resulting in skeletal muscle flaccidity below that level. Detrusor areflexia results, and whatever measures the patient may use to increase intravesical pressure during attempted voiding are not sufficient to decrease residual urine to less than 10% of bladder capacity.

This classification system is best applied to spinal cord injury patients with complete neurologic lesions after spinal shock has passed. It is difficult to apply to patients with multicentric neurologic disease and cannot be used for patients with non-neurologic disease. The system fails to reconcile the clinical and urodynamic variability exhibited by patients who, by neurologic examination alone, seem to have similar lesions. The period of spinal shock that immediately follows severe cord injury usually is associated with bladder areflexia, whatever the status of the sacral somatic reflexes. Temporary or permanent changes in bladder or outlet activity during filling and storage or voiding may because by several factors, such as chronic overdistention, infection, and reinnervation or reorganization of neural pathways after injury or disease; such changes make it impossible to always accurately predict lower urinary tract activity solely on the basis of the level of the neurologic lesion. Although the terms *balanced* and *imbalanced* are helpful because they describe the presence or absence of a certain relative percentage of residual urine, they do not necessarily imply the true functional significance of a lesion, which depends on the potential for damage to the lower or upper urinary tracts and on the social and vocational disability that results.

Box 13-4 Hald-Bradley Classification

Suprasacral lesion
Suprasacral spinal lesion
Infrasacral lesion
Peripheral autonomic neuropathy
Muscular lesion

From Hald T, Bradley WE: The Urinary Bladder: Neurology and Dynamics. Baltimore, Williams & Wilkins, 1982.

Hald-Bradley Classification

Hald and Bradley[20] described what they called a simple neurotopographic classification (Box 13-4). A supraspinal lesion is characterized by synergy between detrusor contraction and the smooth and striated sphincters, but defective inhibition of the voiding reflex exists. Involuntary bladder contraction typically occurs, and sensation is usually preserved. However, depending on the site of the lesion, detrusor areflexia and defective sensation may occur. A suprasacral spinal lesion is roughly equivalent to what is described as a UMN lesion in the Bors-Comarr classification. An infrasacral lesion is roughly equivalent to an LMN lesion. Peripheral autonomic neuropathy is most frequently encountered in the diabetic patient and is characterized by deficient bladder sensation, gradually increasing residual urine volumes, and ultimate decompensation, with loss of detrusor contractility. A muscular lesion can involve the detrusor itself, the smooth sphincter, or any portion or all of the striated sphincter. The resultant dysfunction depends on which structure is affected. Detrusor dysfunction is the most common, and it usually results from decompensation after long-standing bladder outlet obstruction.

Bradley Classification

Bradley's "loop system" of classification is a primarily neurologic system based on his conceptualization of central nervous system control of the lower urinary tract that identifies four neurologic loops.[20] Dysfunctions are classified according to the loop affected.

Loop 1 consists of neuronal connections between the cerebral cortex and the pontine-mesencephalic micturition center, which coordinate voluntary control of the detrusor reflex. Loop 1 lesions are seen in conditions such as brain tumor, cerebrovascular accident or disease, and cerebral atrophy with dementia. The final result is characteristically involuntary bladder contraction.

Loop 2 includes the intraspinal pathway of detrusor muscle afferents to the brainstem micturition center and the motor impulses from this center to the sacral spinal cord. Loop 2 is thought to coordinate and provide a detrusor reflex of adequate temporal duration to allow complete voiding. Partial interruption by spinal cord injury results in a detrusor reflex of low threshold and in poor emptying with residual urine. Spinal cord transection of loop 2 acutely produces detrusor areflexia and urinary retention (i.e., spinal shock). After this has passed, involuntary bladder contraction results.

Loop 3 consists of the peripheral detrusor afferent axons and their pathways in the spinal cord; these terminate by synapsing on pudendal motor neurons that ultimately innervate periurethral striated muscle. Loop 3 was thought to provide a neurologic substrate for coordinated reciprocal action of the bladder and striated sphincter. Loop 3 dysfunction could be responsible for detrusor–striated sphincter dyssynergia or involuntary sphincter relaxation.

Loop 4 consists of two components. Loop 4A is the suprasacral afferent and efferent innervation of the pudendal motor neurons to the periurethral striated musculature. Loop 4B consists of afferent fibers from the periurethral striated musculature that synapse on pudendal motor neurons in Onuf's nucleus—the segmental innervation of the periurethral striated muscle. In contrast to the stimulation of detrusor afferent fibers, which produce inhibitory postsynaptic potentials in pudendal motor neurons through loop 3, pudendal nerve afferents produce excitatory postsynaptic potentials in the motor neurons through loop 4B. They enable contraction of the periurethral striated muscle during bladder filling and urine storage. The related sensory impulses arise from muscle spindles and tendon organs in the pelvic floor musculature. Loop 4 provides volitional control of the striated sphincter. Abnormalities of the suprasacral portion result in abnormal responses of the pudendal motor neurons to bladder filling and emptying, manifested as detrusor-striated sphincter dyssynergia or loss of the ability to voluntarily contract the striated sphincter.

The Bradley system is sophisticated and reflects the ingenuity and neurophysiologic expertise of its originator, himself a neurologist. For neurologists, this method may be an excellent way to conceptualize the neurophysiology involved, assuming that there is agreement on the existence and significance of all four loops. Most urologists find this system difficult to use for many types of neurogenic voiding dysfunction and not at all applicable to non-neurogenic voiding dysfunction. Urodynamically, it may be extremely difficult to test the intactness of each loop system, and multicentric and partial lesions are difficult to describe.

Box 13-5 Lapides Classification

Sensory neurogenic bladder
Motor paralytic bladder (i.e., motor neurogenic bladder)
Uninhibited neurogenic bladder
Reflex neurogenic bladder
Autonomous neurogenic bladder

From McLellan FC: The Neurogenic Bladder. Springfield, IL, Charles C Thomas, 1939, pp 116-185.

Lapides Classification

Lapides[21] contributed significantly to the classification and care of the patient with neuropathic voiding dysfunction by slightly modifying and popularizing a system originally proposed by McLellan in 1939 (Box 13-5).[22]

Lapides' classification differs from that of McLellan in only one respect: the division of the group of "atonic neurogenic bladder" into sensory neurogenic and motor neurogenic bladder. This remains one of the most familiar systems to urologists and nonurologists because it describes in recognizable shorthand the clinical and cystometric conditions of many types of neurogenic voiding dysfunction.

A sensory neurogenic bladder results from disease that selectively interrupts the sensory fibers between the bladder and the spinal cord or the afferent tracts to the brain. Diabetes mellitus, tabes dorsalis, and pernicious anemia are most commonly responsible. The first clinical changes are described as those of impaired sensation of bladder distention. Unless voiding is initiated on a timed basis, various degrees of bladder overdistention can result, producing hypotonicity. If bladder decompensation occurs, significant amounts of residual urine are found, and at this point, the cystometric curve usually demonstrates a large-capacity bladder with a flat, high-compliance, low-pressure filling curve.

A motor paralytic bladder results from disease processes that destroy the parasympathetic motor innervation of the bladder. Extensive pelvic surgery or trauma may produce this. Herpes zoster has been listed as a cause, but evidence suggests that the voiding dysfunction seen with herpes infection is more related to a problem with afferent pathways. The early symptoms of a motor paralytic bladder vary from painful urinary retention to only a relative inability to initiate and maintain normal micturition. Early cystometric filling is normal but without a voluntary bladder contraction at capacity. Chronic overdistention and decompensation may occur, resulting in a large-capacity bladder with a flat, low-pressure filling curve; a large residual urine volume may result.

An uninhibited neurogenic bladder was described originally as resulting from injury to or disease of the "corticoregulatory tract." The sacral spinal cord was presumed to be the micturition reflex center, and this corticoregulatory tract was believed to normally exert an inhibitory influence on the sacral micturition reflex center. A destructive lesion in this tract would then result in overfacilitation of the micturition reflex. Cerebrovascular accident, brain or spinal cord tumor, Parkinson's disease, and demyelinating disease were listed as the most common causes in this category. The voiding dysfunction is most often characterized symptomatically by frequency, urgency, and urge incontinence, and it is urodynamically characterized by normal sensation with involuntary contraction at low filling volumes. The residual urine volume typically is low unless anatomic outlet obstruction or true smooth or striated sphincter dyssynergia occurs. The patient usually can initiate a bladder contraction voluntarily but is often unable to do so during cystometry because sufficient urine storage cannot occur before involuntary contraction is stimulated.

Reflex neurogenic bladder describes the post-spinal shock condition that exists after complete interruption of the sensory and motor pathways between the sacral spinal cord and the brain stem. Most commonly, this occurs in traumatic spinal cord injury and transverse myelitis, but it may occur with extensive demyelinating disease or any process that produces significant spinal cord destruction. Typically, there is no bladder sensation, and there is an inability to initiate voluntary micturition. Incontinence without sensation generally results because of low-volume involuntary contraction. Striated sphincter dyssynergia is the rule. This type of lesion is essentially equivalent to a complete UMN lesion in the Bors-Comarr system.

An autonomous neurogenic bladder results from complete motor and sensory separation of the bladder from the sacral spinal cord. This may be caused by any disease that destroys the sacral cord or causes extensive damage to the sacral roots or pelvic nerves. There is an inability to voluntarily initiate micturition, no bladder reflex activity, and no specific bladder sensation. This type of bladder is equivalent to a complete LMN lesion in the Bors-Comarr system and is the type of dysfunction seen in patients with spinal shock. The characteristic cystometric pattern is initially similar to the late stages of the motor or sensory paralytic bladder, with a marked shift to the right of the cystometric filling curve and a large bladder capacity at low intravesical pressure. However, decreased compliance may develop from chronic inflammatory changes or the effects of denervation and centralization with secondary neuromorphologic and neuropharmacologic reorganizational changes. Emptying capacity may vary widely, depending on the ability of the patient to increase intravesical pressure and on the resistance offered during this increase by the smooth and striated sphincters.

These classic categories in their usual settings are generally easily understood and remembered, which is why this system provides an excellent framework for teaching some fundamentals of neurogenic voiding dysfunction to students and nonurologists. Unfortunately, many patients do not exactly fit into a Lapides category. Gradations of sensory, motor, and mixed lesions occur, and the patterns produced after different types of peripheral denervation or defunctionalization may vary widely from those that are classically described. The system is applicable only to neuropathic dysfunction.

Urodynamic Classification

As urodynamic techniques have become more accepted and sophisticated, systems of classification have evolved based solely on objective urodynamic data (Box 13-6). Among the first to popularize this concept were Krane and Siroky.[23] When exact urodynamic classification is possible, this system provides a precise description of the voiding dysfunction that occurs. If a normal or hyperreflexic detrusor exists with coordinated smooth and striated sphincter function and without anatomic obstruction, normal bladder emptying should occur.

Box 13-6 Urodynamic Classification

Detrusor hyperreflexia (or normoreflexia)
- Coordinated sphincters
- Striated sphincter dyssynergia
- Smooth sphincter dyssynergia
- Nonrelaxing smooth sphincter

Detrusor areflexia
- Coordinated sphincters
- Nonrelaxing striated sphincter
- Denervated striated sphincter
- Nonrelaxing smooth sphincter

From Krane RJ, Siroky MB: Classification of voiding dysfunction: Value of classification systems. In Barrett DM, Wein AJ (eds): Controversies in Neuro-Urology. New York, Churchill Livingstone, 1984, pp 223-23.

Detrusor hyperreflexia is most commonly associated with neurologic lesions above the sacral spinal cord. Striated sphincter dyssynergia is most commonly seen after complete suprasacral spinal cord injury following the period of spinal shock. Smooth sphincter dyssynergia is seen most classically in autonomic dysreflexia, when it is characteristically associated with detrusor hyperreflexia and striated sphincter dyssynergia.

Detrusor areflexia may result from bladder muscle decompensation or other conditions that produce inhibition at the level of the brainstem micturition center, the sacral spinal cord, bladder ganglia, or bladder smooth muscle. Patients with a voiding dysfunction caused by detrusor areflexia usually attempt bladder emptying by abdominal straining, and their continence status and the efficiency of their emptying efforts are determined by the status of their smooth and striated sphincter mechanisms.

This classification system is easiest to use when detrusor hyperreflexia or normoreflexia exists. A typical T10-level paraplegic patient after spinal shock exhibits detrusor hyperreflexia, smooth sphincter synergia, and striated sphincter dyssynergia. When a voluntary or a hyperreflexic contraction cannot be elicited, the system is more difficult to use, because it is not appropriate to speak of true sphincter dyssynergia in the absence of an opposing bladder contraction. There are many variations and extensions of such a system. These systems work well when total urodynamic agreement exists among classifiers. Unfortunately, many voiding dysfunctions do not fit neatly into a urodynamic classification system that is agreed on by all experts. As sophisticated urodynamic technology and understanding improve, this type of classification system may supplant some others in general use.

International Continence Society Classification

The classification system proposed by the International Continence Society (ICS) is in essence an extension of a urodynamic classification system. The storage and voiding phases of micturition are described separately, and within each, various designations are applied to describe bladder and urethral function.[24]

Normal detrusor function during filling and storage implies no significant increases in detrusor pressure with filling . *Detrusor overactivity* is the urodynamic observation of involuntary detrusor contractions during the filling phase that may be spontaneous or provoked. If caused by a neurologic disease, the term *neurogenic detrusor overactivity* (which replaces detrusor hyperreflexia) is used; if there is no defined cause, the term *idiopathic detrusor overactivity* (which replaces detrusor instability) is applied. Bladder sensation can be categorized only in qualitative terms as indicated. Bladder capacity and compliance (Δ volume/Δ pressure) are cystometric measurements. Normal urethral function during filling and storage indicates a positive urethral closure pressure (i.e., urethral pressure minus bladder pressure) even with increases in intra-abdominal pressure. Incompetent urethral function during filling or storage implies urine leakage in the absence of a detrusor contraction. This may be caused by genuine stress incontinence, intrinsic sphincter dysfunction, or an involuntary decrease in urethral pressure in the absence of a detrusor contraction.

During the voiding phase of micturition, normal detrusor activity implies voiding by a voluntarily initiated sustained contraction that also can be suppressed voluntarily. Detrusor underactivity defines a contraction of inadequate magnitude or duration to empty the bladder within a normal time span. An acontractile detrusor is one that cannot be demonstrated to contract during urodynamic testing. Normal urethral function during voiding indicates a urethra that opens and is continually relaxed to allow bladder emptying at normal pressures. An obstructed urethra is one that contracts against a detrusor contraction or fails to open (nonrelaxation) with attempted micturition. Contraction may result from smooth or striated sphincter dyssynergia. *Detrusor-sphincter dyssynergia*, the occurrence of an involuntary contraction of the urethral or periurethral striated muscle with a detrusor contraction, is a term that should be applied only when neurologic disease is present. A similar syndrome but without neurologic disease is called *dysfunctional voiding. Nonrelaxing urethral sphincter* occurs in individuals with a neurologic lesion who have reduced urine flow because of a nonrelaxing, obstructing urethra. *Bladder outlet obstruction* is defined as an increased detrusor pressure and low urine flow rate due to obstruction during voiding. This is a generic term that has been poorly defined in women and children.

Voiding dysfunction in a classic T10-level paraplegic patient after spinal shock has passed is classified as follows:

1. Storage phase: neurogenic detrusor overactivity, absent sensation, low capacity, normal compliance, and normal urethral closure function
2. Voiding phase: overactive obstructive urethral function and normal (?) detrusor activity (i.e., hyperreflexic)

The voiding dysfunction of a stroke patient with urgency incontinence would most likely be classified during storage as neurogenic detrusor overactivity, normal sensation, low capacity, normal compliance, and normal urethral closure function. During voiding, the dysfunction would be classified as normal detrusor activity and normal urethral function, assuming that no anatomic obstruction existed.

Functional System of Classification

Classification of voiding dysfunction can be formulated on a simple functional basis, describing the dysfunction in terms of whether the deficit produced is primarily one of the filing and storage phase or the voiding phase of micturition (see Box 13-1).[1,16] The system was proposed initially by Quesada and associates.[25] This type of system is an excellent alternative when a particular dysfunction does not readily lend itself to a generally agreed on classification elsewhere. This simple scheme assumes only that, whatever their differences, all experts would agree on the two-phase concept of micturition (i.e., filling with storage and voiding) and on simple overall mechanisms underlying the normality of each phase (discussed earlier).

Storage failure results because of bladder or outlet abnormalities or a combination. The bladder abnormalities include involuntary bladder contractions, low compliance, and hypersensitivity. The outlet abnormalities can include an intermittent or continuous decrease in outlet resistance.

Emptying failure can occur because of bladder or outlet abnormalities or a combination. The bladder abnormalities include inadequate or unsustained bladder contractility, and the outlet problems include anatomic obstruction and sphincter dyssynergia.

Failure in either category usually is not absolute, but more often relative. This functional system can easily be expanded to include etiologic or specific urodynamic connotations (see Box 13-2). However, the simplified system is workable and avoids argument about complex situations in which the exact cause or urodynamic mechanism for a voiding dysfunction cannot be agreed on.

Proper use of the functional system for a given voiding dysfunction requires a reasonably accurate notion of what the urodynamic data show. However, an exact diagnosis is not required for treatment. Some patients do not have only a discrete storage or emptying failure, and the existence of combination deficits must be recognized to properly use this system of classification. For instance, the classic T10-level paraplegic patient after spinal shock typically exhibits a relative failure to store urine because of involuntary bladder contractions and a relative failure to empty the bladder because of striated sphincter dyssynergia. With such a combination deficit, to use this classification system as a guide to treatment, the physician must assume that one of the deficits is primary and that significant improvement will result from its treatment alone or that the voiding dysfunction can be converted primarily to a disorder of storage or emptying by means of nonsurgical or surgical therapy. The resultant deficit can then be treated or circumvented.

Using the same example, the combined deficit in a T10-level paraplegic patient can be converted primarily to a storage failure by procedures directed at the dyssynergic striated sphincter; the resultant incontinence (caused by involuntary contraction) can be circumvented (in a male) with an external collecting device. Alternatively, the deficit can be converted primarily to an emptying failure by pharmacologic or surgical measures designed to abolish or reduce the involuntary contraction, and the resultant emptying failure can then be circumvented with clean intermittent catheterization. Other examples of combination deficits include impaired bladder contractility with sphincter dysfunction, bladder outlet obstruction with detrusor overactivity, bladder outlet obstruction with sphincter malfunction, and detrusor overactivity with impaired contractility.

One of the advantages of this functional classification is that it allows the clinician the liberty of using the system to suit his or her preferences without an alteration in the basic concept of keeping it simple but accurate and informative. For instance, the physician can substitute the terms *overactive or oversensitive bladder* and *outlet insufficiency* for *because of the bladder* and *because of the outlet* under "Failure to Store" in Box 13-1. A urologist can further categorize the bladder reasons for overactivity (see Box 13-2) in terms of neurogenic, myogenic, or anatomic causes and further subcategorize *neurogenic* in terms of decreased inhibitory control, increased afferent activity, increased sensitivity to efferent activity, and so on. The system is flexible.

THE OVERACTIVE BLADDER: DEFINITIONS

There is some confusion about and misuse of the terms *overactive detrusor* and *overactive bladder*. The term *overactive detrusor function*, commonly shortened to *overactive detrusor*, is a term that was originated and defined by the ICS to describe a urodynamic finding of involuntary detrusor contractions during filling. The term *overactive bladder* is frequently substituted for *overactive detrusor*, even though this is not a part of the ICS lexicon. *Overactive bladder* can be defined in terms of urodynamic findings or symptoms. The urodynamic definition of overactive bladder approximates that of the ICS term *overactive detrusor* or *overactive detrusor function*.

Using a strict urodynamic definition has limitations.[26,27] On a worldwide basis, it is impossible, impractical, and unnecessary for all patients with symptoms compatible with overactive detrusor function (e.g., urgency, frequency, incontinence due to involuntary bladder contraction) to be initially evaluated and treated by the type of specialist capable of performing and interpreting urodynamic studies. However, with the current urodynamic-based definition, these specialists are the only ones capable of making this exact diagnosis. Critics of a solely urodynamic-based definition also point out that the demonstration of involuntary contraction during urodynamic studies varies with the type of study done. Most individuals who have symptoms of overactive detrusor function but who fail to demonstrate intraventricular contraction on conventional urodynamic studies will do so on repeated or more complex urodynamic studies.[28] A substantial portion of individuals who, by symptoms and bother index, do not have characteristics of overactive detrusor function do exhibit involuntary bladder contractions on urodynamic studies (38% to 69% of normal asymptomatic patients).[29,30] Many believe that overactive bladder also should be defined by symptoms.[31,32]

We have suggested that the overactive bladder is a medical condition referring to the symptoms of frequency and urgency, with or without urge or reflex incontinence, when appearing in the absence of local pathologic or metabolic factors that would account for these symptoms. Incontinence is not a necessary condition for diagnosis, because roughly two thirds of the people with overactive bladder do not have incontinence. Nevertheless, there is a profound impairment in their quality of life because of urge and frequency symptoms. These local or metabolic factors may include urinary tract infection, malignant or premalignant conditions of the bladder, calculi, interstitial cystitis, diabetes, polydipsia, diuretics, and pregnancy. The urodynamic definition of overactive bladder would then describe the demonstration of involuntary bladder contraction causing symptoms or signs of frequency and urgency.

References

1. Wein AJ, Barrett DM: Voiding Function and Dysfunction: A Logical and Practical Approach. Chicago, Year Book Medical, 1988.
2. Zderic SA, Levin RM, Wein AJ: Voiding function: Relevant anatomy, physiology, pharmacology and molecular aspects. In Gillenwater JY, Grayhack JT, Howards SS, Ducket JW Jr (eds): Adult and Pediatric Urology. Chicago, Year Book Medical, 1996, pp 1159-1219.
3. de Groat WC, Booth AM, Yoshimura N: Neurophysiology of micturition and its modifications in animal models of human disease. In Maggi CA (ed): The Autonomic Nervous System, vol 3. London, Harwood Academic, 1993, pp 227-2990.
4. de Groat WC, Downie JW, Levin RM, et al: Basic neurophysiology and neuropharmacology. In Abrams P, Khoury S, Wein A (eds): Incontinence. First International Consultation on Incontinence, June 28-July 1, 1998, Monaco. Co-sponsored by the World Health Organization and International Union Against Cancer. Plymouth, UK, Health Publications, 1999, pp 105-154.
5. Steers WD: Physiology and pharmacology of the bladder and urethra. In Walsh PC, Retik AB, Vaughan ED Jr, Wein AJ (eds): Campbell's Urology, 7th ed. Philadelphia, WB Saunders, 1998, pp 870-916.
6. Brading AF: The physiology of the mammalian outflow tract. Exp Physiol 84:215-221, 1999.
7. Coplen D, Macarek E, Levin RM: Developmental changes in normal fetal bovine whole bladder physiology. J Urol 151:1391-1395, 1994.
8. Klevmark B: Motility of the urinary bladder in cats during filling at physiological rates. I. Intravesical pressure patterns studied by new methods of cystometry. Acta Physiol Scand 90:565-569, 1974.
9. Klevmark B: Natural pressure-volume curves and conventional cystometry. Scand J Urol Nephrol Suppl 201:1-4, 1999.
10. McGuire EJ, Shi-Chun Z, Horwinski ER: Treatment for motor and sensory detrusor instability by electrical stimulation. J Urol 129:78-79, 1983.
11. Elbadawi A: Neuromuscular mechanisms of micturition. In Yalla SV, McGuire EJ, Elbadawi A, Blaivas JG (eds): Neurourology and Urodynamics: Principles and Practice. New York, Macmillan, 1988, pp 3-35.
12. Brading AF, Fry CHI, Maggi CA, et al: Cellular biology. In Abrams P, Khoury S, Wein A (eds): Incontinence. First International Consultation on Incontinence, June 28-July 1, 1998, Monaco. Co-sponsored by the World Health Organization and International Union Against Cancer. Plymouth, UK, Health Publications, 1999, pp 57-104.
13. Zinner NR, Sterling AM, Ritter R: Structure and forces of continence. In Raz S (ed): Female Urology. Philadelphia, WB Saunders, 1983, pp 33-41.
14. Enhorning G: Simultaneous recording of intravesical and intraurethral pressure. Acta Chir Scand 276(Suppl):1-68, 1961.
15. Tanagho EA: The anatomy and physiology of micturition. Clin Obstet Gynecol 5:3-9, 1978.
16. Wein AJ: Classification of neurogenic voiding dysfunction. J Urol 125:605-609, 1981.
17. DeLancey JOL, Fowler CJ, Keane D, et al: Pathophysiology. In Abrams P, Khoury S, Wein A (eds): Incontinence. First International Consultation on Incontinence, June 28-July 1, 1998, Monaco. Co-sponsored by the World Health Organization and International Union Against Cancer. Plymouth, UK, Health Publications, 1999, pp 227-294.
18. DeLancey JOL: Structural support of the urethra as it relates to stress urinary incontinence: The hammock hypothesis. Am J Obstet Gynecol 170:1713-1717, 1994.
19. Bors E, Comarr AE: Neurological Urology. Baltimore, University Park Press, 1971.
20. Hald T, Bradley WE: The Urinary Bladder: Neurology and Dynamics. Baltimore, Williams & Wilkins, 1982.
21. Lapides J: Neuromuscular, vesical and ureteral dysfunction. In Campbell MF, Harrison JHG (eds): Urology. Philadelphia, WB Saunders, 1970, pp 1343-1279.

22. McLellan FC: The Neurogenic Bladder. Springfield, IL, Charles C Thomas, 1939, pp 116-185.
23. Krane RJ, Siroky MB: Classification of voiding dysfunction: Value of classification systems. In Barrett DM, Wein AJ (eds): Controversies in Neuro-Urology. New York, Churchill Livingstone, 1984, pp 223-238.
24. Abrams P, Cardoza L, Fall M, et al: The standardization of terminology of lower urinary tract function: Report from the Standardization Sub-committee of the International Continence Society. Neurourol Urodyn 21:167-178, 2002.
25. Quesada EM, Scott FB, Cardus D: Functional classification of neurogenic bladder dysfunction. Arch Phys Med Rehabil 49:692-697, 1968.
26. Hampel C, Wienhold D, Benkan N, et al: Definition of overactive bladder and epidemiology of urinary incontinence. Urology 50(Suppl 6A):4-14, 1997.
27. Payne CK: Advances in non-surgical treatment of urinary incontinence and overactive bladder. In Walsh PC, Retik A, Vaughan ED Jr, Wein AJ (eds): Campbell's Urology Updates. Philadelphia, WB Saunders, 1999, pp 1-20.
28. Artibani W: Diagnosis and significance of idiopathic overactive bladder. Urology 50(Suppl 6A):25-32, 1997.
30. Heslington K, Hilton P: A comparison of ambulatory monitoring and conventional cystometry in asymptomatic female volunteers. Neurourol Urodyn 14:533-534, 1995.
31. Abrams P, Wein AJ: The overactive bladder and incontinence: Definitions and a plea for discussion. Neurourol Urodyn 18:413-416, 1999.
32. Abrams P, Wein AJ (eds): Overactive Bladder and Its Treatments Consensus Conference, London, July 4, 1999. Urology 55(Suppl 5A): 1-84, 2000.

Chapter 14

VOIDING DYSFUNCTION AND NEUROLOGIC DISORDERS

Gary E. Lemack

Perhaps more than any other situation facing physicians who care for patients with bladder dysfunction, care of the neurologic patient requires a thorough initial investigation, frequently with upper and lower urinary tract evaluations in addition to periodic assessments to minimize the urologic morbidity often associated with these conditions. Development and refinement of urodynamic techniques to assess bladder function in patients with neurogenic voiding dysfunction have enhanced our understanding of their condition and improved our ability to identify when these patients require more intense monitoring and intervention. As new treatment strategies for these conditions have surfaced and as patients at risk for morbidity associated with neurogenic voiding dysfunction are recognized more promptly, the likelihood of finding advanced urologic dysfunction at the time of initial presentation is gradually decreasing. This chapter focuses on evaluation of patients with neurogenic voiding dysfunction and discusses specific aspects of some of the more common subgroups.

EVALUATION OF THE NEUROLOGIC PATIENT

Neurologic History

Establishing the onset of bladder and systemic symptoms in patients with progressive neurologic conditions (which often predate the diagnosis) and documenting recent changes in symptom severity are essential, because this information usually influences treatment recommendations. Disease duration has been correlated with the development of urinary symptoms, particularly in patients with multiple sclerosis or Parkinson's disease.[1] Even those with presumably fixed neurologic conditions (e.g., spinal cord injury, myelomeningocele) may have insidious but progressive symptomatic deterioration (e.g., from development of a syrinx or tethered cord), and therefore any recent changes in sensory or motor function should be directly assessed.

Patients with movement disorders should be carefully questioned about the onset of their neurologic symptoms compared with their urinary symptoms, because those with more progressive syndromes, such as multiple systems atrophy, often develop autonomic disturbances such as bladder and erectile dysfunction early during the course of their illness. Every attempt should be made to identify these patients because their overall response to surgical urologic interventions is poor.[2] The Hoehn and Yahr stage should be documented in patients with Parkinson's disease. This staging information can be useful in predicting the severity of bladder dysfunction and prospects for further deterioration.[3]

Patients with multiple sclerosis should be queried about the timing of the onset of symptoms and about recent exacerbations, because such exacerbations frequently are initiated by urologic events.[4] Patients should be specifically questioned about the development of lower extremity motor dysfunction, because there is a strong correlation between pyramidal symptoms, such as weakness and spasticity, and bladder dysfunction in patients with multiple sclerosis.[5] Symptoms of urge incontinence, urgency, and nocturia are strongly correlated with severe pyramidal dysfunction as measured by Kurtzke scores.[6] Inquiring about the classification of their condition (e.g., relapsing remitting, primary progressive, secondary progressive) and the timing and findings of their most recent magnetic resonance imaging (MRI) studies may be important in planning therapy, particularly when considering surgical options, which may require considerable dexterity.

In patients with recent acute events, such as cerebrovascular accidents (CVAs), information about the stroke location and the recovery since the event is useful because stroke location impacts theprognosis.[7] Specific questions regarding the presence of voiding disturbance and urinary leakage episodes before the stroke are required, because the persistence of new-onset urinary incontinence after stroke can indicate a poor overall prognosis and is a strong indicator of eventual functional dependence in patients after stroke.[8]

Patients with history of back surgery and intervertebral disk protrusion should be questioned about the vertebral level of the surgery or affected disk and about the presence of ongoing sensory deficit because patients with multiple operations or advanced disk prolapse may be at higher risk for voiding disturbances.[9] Patients should also be evaluated for a diagnosis of cervical myelopathy, because these patients frequently have symptomatic bladder dysfunction that may be independent of the severity of other symptoms associated with this condition, such as spacticity.[10]

Current treatments should be documented, with particular attention to medications. Medications with properties that can affect the bladder outlet (typically those with α-agonist or α-antagonist properties) or detrusor contractility (typically those with anticholinergic properties) should be recorded, along with the use of narcotics and skeletal muscle relaxants. Diuretic use should also be documented. Altering the timing of diuretic intake may affect the severity of nocturia. Patients on diuretics and those with a history of congestive heart failure probably are not suitable candidates for treatment with vasopressin for nocturia and nocturnal enuresis.

Physical Examination

General Observations

Although most patients with neurologic impairment are followed elsewhere for the primary condition, certain aspects of the physical examination are essential to document when evaluating them urologically, particularly if surgical intervention is being considered. Patients should be assessed for ambulatory disturbances at the initial visit. The degree of physical dependence of the patient, particularly as it relates to the ability to void independently, may affect the frequency of leakage episodes. Self-catheterization of the urethra may be impossible in patients who are not ambulatory, particularly those with severe lower extremity spasticity or contractures.

Hand function in patients with cervical spinal cord injury, particularly the ability to grasp firmly between the thumb and index or middle finger, must be carefully judged in patients who may require intermittent catheterization after treatment. With the advent of single-system catheterization techniques, it is not mandatory that patients have bilateral hand function, although a careful assessment of the patient's ability to work with such products is essential, particularly before considering surgery that will require clean intermittent catheterization postoperatively.

An evaluation of the skin, particularly in the gluteal region, should be carried out, because localized skin and subcutaneous infections and even more severe skin breakdown can occur in patients with restricted mobility. These issues need to be addressed before major reconstructive procedures are considered. Some patients may have intrathecal pumps in place, and their location and that of the tubing should be assessed before surgical endeavors.

Neurologic Examination

A brief neurologic examination is essential when first evaluating patients with presumed neurovesical dysfunction. Mental status should be assessed because significant cognitive dysfunction and memory disturbances have been independently associated with abnormal voiding function. An appreciation of past and current intellectual capacity may provide insight into the progression of lower urinary tract disorders and thereby guide the degree of complexity of treatment strategies. Motor strength and sensory level should be determined because distribution of motor and sensory disturbances can often predict lower urinary tract dysfunction, particularly in patients with multiple sclerosis.[5]

Cutaneous and motor reflexes require a thorough evaluation at the time of the initial encounter. The bulbocavernosus reflex, which is elicited by gently squeezing the glans penis in men or gentle compression of the clitoris against the pubis in women and simultaneously feeling for an anal sphincter contraction (by placing a finger in the rectum), assesses the integrity of the S2-S4 reflex arc. The anal reflex, which assesses integrity of S2 to S5, can be checked by applying a pinprick to the mucocutaneous junction of the anus and evaluating for anal sphincter contraction. The cremasteric reflex may be somewhat less reliable, but it assesses sensory dermatomes supplied by L1 to L2.

Muscle motor reflexes should be routinely evaluated. The most common of these are the biceps reflex (assesses C5 to C6), patellar reflex (L2 to L4), and Achilles (ankle) reflex (L5 to S2). Evidence of an upper motor neurologic injury includes spasticity of the involved skeletal muscle, heightened response to reflex testing, and an upgoing toe on gentle stroking of the plantar surface of the foot (i.e., positive Babinski's sign).

Other Testing

A thorough investigation for upper tract abnormalities (imaging) and lower urinary tract dysfunction (video urodynamic testing) is mandatory when first evaluating patients with neurogenic voiding dysfunction and at periodic intervals thereafter. The frequency of testing is not readily agreed on, although many experts recommend annual upper tract evaluation (nuclear renal scan or renal ultrasound) and at least biannual urodynamic testing in high-risk patients (e.g., traumatic spinal cord injury).[11] Others have advocated less frequent evaluations in stable patients.[12] Regardless of the frequency of evaluations, the most important aspect of testing is to identify patients at risk for upper tract deterioration and to monitor them closely. Although a description of the technique of urodynamic testing is beyond the scope of this chapter, it is clear that in no other situation in urology is the importance of properly performed urodynamic testing as important as it is when evaluating the patient with neurogenic voiding dysfunction.

BLADDER DYSFUNCTION IN SPECIFIC NEUROLOGIC CONDITIONS

Traumatic Spinal Cord Injury

Suprasacral Injuries

The classification scheme most commonly used for patients with spinal cord injury is that developed by the American Spinal Injury Association (ASIA). Using this scheme, the level and completeness of the injury are assessed by careful examination of the affected dermatomes and muscle groups (Table 14-1). Normally, at least 3 months must pass from the time of injury to assess the patient's neurologic status, because the spinal shock phase can last this long or longer. During this time, spinal reflex activity below the level of the lesion is rendered inactive, resulting in transient skeletal muscle paralysis. Smooth muscle activity (i.e., detrusor) is similarly depressed, whereas in most situations, the bladder neck and external sphincter remain closed, and as a result, most patients are in retention or dribbling small amounts of urine. Immediate management therefore focuses on bladder drainage (i.e., indwelling or clean intermittent catheterization) until reflex bladder activity returns.

After suprasacral injuries, several pathologic bladder reflexes occur. In most situations, neurogenic detrusor overactivity

Table 14-1 American Spinal Injury Association Classification of Spinal Cord Injury

Class	Description
A	*Complete*: No motor or sensory function is preserved in the sacral segments from S4 to S5.
B	*Incomplete*: Sensory but not motor function is preserved below the neurologic level and includes the sacral segments from S4 to S5.
C	*Incomplete*: Motor function is preserved below the neurological level, and more than one half of key muscles below the neurologic level have a muscle grade less than 3.
D	*Incomplete*: Motor function is preserved below the neurologic level, and at least one half of key muscles below the neurologic level have a muscle grade of 3 or more.
E	*Normal*: Motor and sensory function are normal.

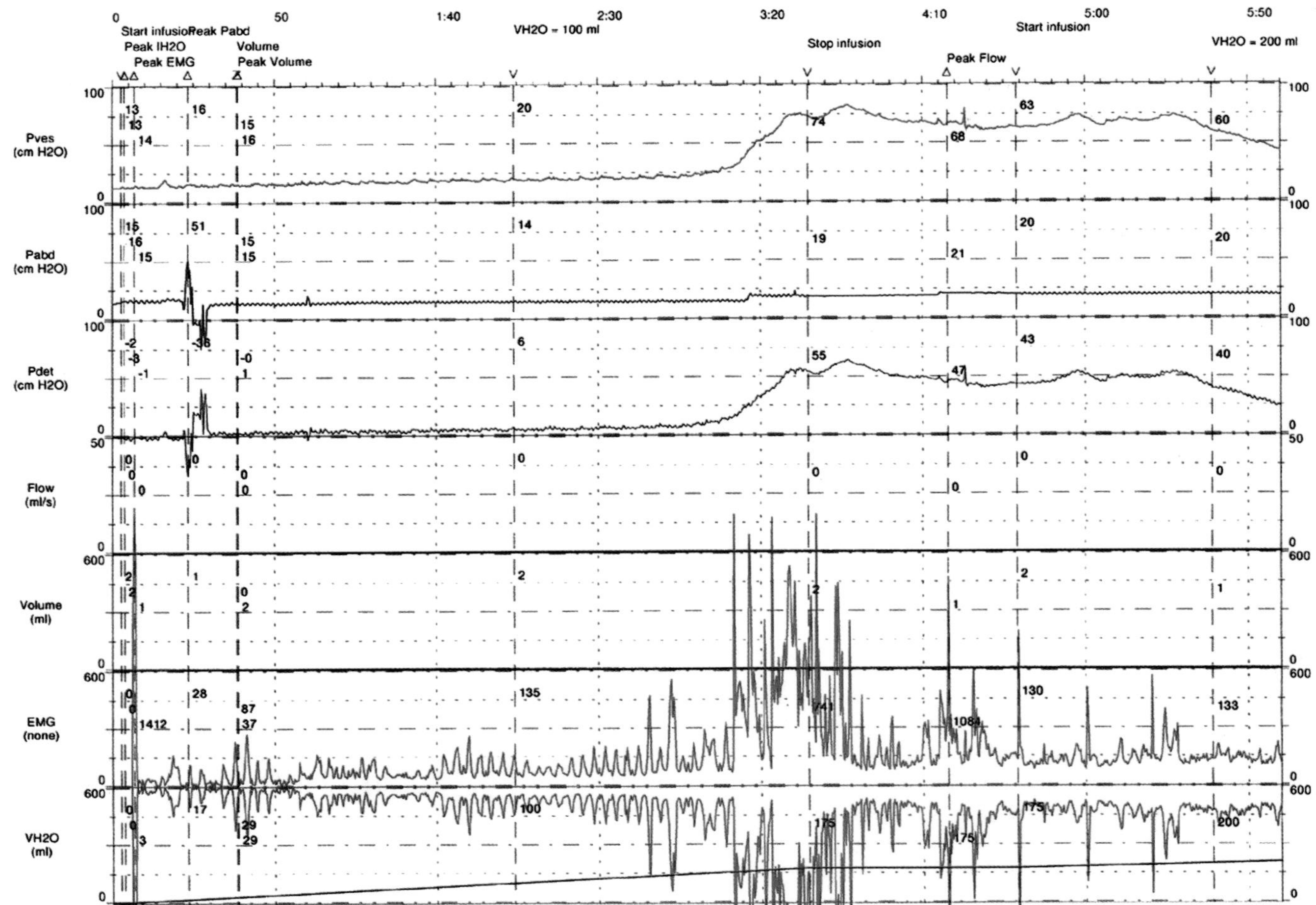

Figure 14-1 Detrusor external sphincter dyssynergia in patient with T5 level spinal cord injury.

replaces the flaccid detrusor of the spinal shock phase, resulting in a small-capacity, overactive bladder, which cannot be inhibited by the patient. With an interruption of the spinobulbospinal reflex, there is loss of coordination between the normal detrusor contraction and simultaneous inhibition of the pudendal-mediated external sphincter contraction. Detrusor–external sphincter dyssynergia (DESD) emerges, resulting in a staccato-type voiding pattern, impaired bladder emptying, and sustained increases in intravesical pressure (Fig. 14-1). These sustained elevations in pressure are thought to be responsible for upper tract damage in patients with spinal cord lesions.[13] In patients with lesions above spinal cord level T6-T8, smooth muscle dyssynergia of the bladder neck generally occurs in conjunction with DESD because of a loss of the normal inhibition provided by supraspinal sympathetic activity at the level of the bladder neck.

Afferent fibers are altered after traumatic spinal cord injury. Whereas in the normal micturition reflex, Aδ afferent fibers are active in bladder sensation, unmyelinated C fibers appear to become active in inflammatory conditions of the bladder and after spinal cord injury. Although the emergence of C fibers may not be essential to the micturition reflex after a spinal cord injury, their presence does contribute to the emergence of overactivity and dyssynergia,[14] and treatment with agonists of the vanilloid receptor (found mainly on unmyelinated C fibers), such as capsaicin and resiniferatoxin, can desensitize (after initially exciting, in the case of capsaicin) the receptor and attenuate the clinical effects of spinal cord injury on bladder function.[15]

Any discussion of bladder dysfunction in spinal cord injury would not be complete without reference to autonomic dysreflexia, the syndrome of unopposed sympathetic outflow normally initiated by a visceral disturbance in patients with spinal cord injury. Typically, it is seen in patients with spinal cord injury above the level of T6 to T8, and it may result in profound hypertension, headache, flushing, and sweating. Bradycardia is the most likely arrhythmia to be seen, although tachyarrhythmias have also been described. The most common stimulus for this syndrome is distention of the bladder or rectum, or both, during cystoscopy or urodynamic assessment. All patients at risk should be hemodynamically monitored during bladder studies, and some authorities have advocated the administration of oral nifedipine approximately 30 minutes before urologic procedures.[16] Alternatively, sublingual nifedipine can halt an acute episode if removing the offending stimulus does result in immediate improvement.[17]

Sacral Injuries

Injuries affecting the sacral spinal cord (usually below the vertebral level of T12 to L1) cause a loss of parasympathetic innerva-

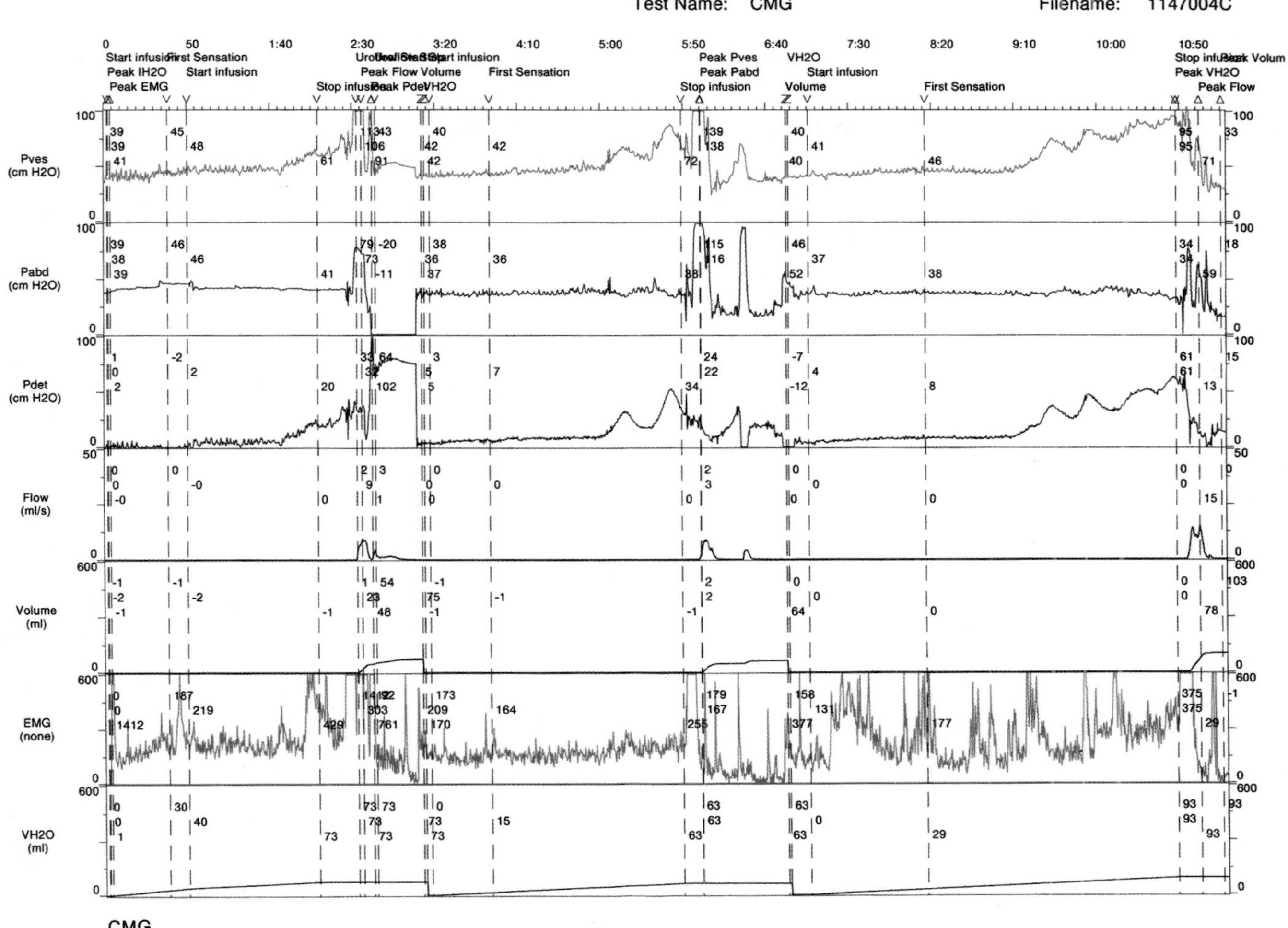

Figure 14-2 Phasic neurogenic detrusor overactivity in patient with multiple sclerosis. Notice the pseudo-dyssynergic electromyographic pattern in the patient attempting to prevent leakage.

tion of the detrusor smooth muscle and resultant areflexia and urinary retention. In most cases, the bladder neck appears to be competent, and the external sphincter maintains fixed tone, although volitional control is lacking. There exists some variability because certain patients have leaks due to sphincteric deficiency, and reduced urethral closure pressures have been documented in patients with lower spinal cord lesions.[18]

Multiple Sclerosis

Although only 2% to 10% of patients with multiple sclerosis present with lower urinary tract symptoms (LUTS) as their initial complaint, up to 97% eventually develop symptoms during the course of their disease. The most common subjective complaints include urinary frequency, urgency, and urge-related incontinence. Urinary hesitancy, recurrent urinary tract infections, and voiding dysfunction (e.g., straining, incomplete emptying) may also typify the symptoms of up to 40% of patients.

Although it is difficult to predict who will develop LUTS, it is rare to develop the symptoms in the absence of pyramidal dysfunction involving the lower extremities. In a study of 186 patients with multiple sclerosis, Betts and colleagues[5] found only two patients had LUTS in the absence of pyramidal dysfunction affecting the legs. There is a strong correlation between the presence of LUTS and Kurtzke scores for pyramidal dysfunction and total disability scores.[6]

The most common urodynamic finding in patients with multiple sclerosis is neurogenic detrusor overactivity. In general, 60% to 90% of patients undergoing urodynamics will be found to have neurogenic detrusor overactivity (Fig. 14-2). Symptoms of urgency and frequency commonly are associated with the finding of detrusor overactivity, accompanied by urge incontinence if high-grade, unstable contractions or insufficient outlet resistance (typically, pelvic floor voluntary contractions are impaired) are present. Detrusor-sphincter dyssynergia, which may lead to poor emptying and elevated intravesical pressures, is seen in approximately 25% to 40% of patients. Both bladder neck (smooth muscle) and external sphincter dyssynergia seem to contribute to the voiding dysfunction in many of these patients. Recurrent bladder infections, prolonged voiding, extreme hesitancy, and incontinence typify the symptoms of multiple sclerosis patients with DESD, although symptoms are not always a reliable indicator of the type of bladder dysfunction responsible in these patients.. Detrusor hyporeflexia, which is the lack of a sufficient contraction during voiding to facilitate bladder emptying, occurs in approximately 20% of patients with multiple sclerosis.

Renal insufficiency due to bladder dysfunction is fairly uncommon among multiple sclerosis patients. However, certain multiple sclerosis populations, including those with untreated DESD, those with elevated intravesical filling pressures, and those with indwelling catheters, may be at risk for renal deterioration over time.[19] Nonetheless, in a series of 120 patients undergoing initial urologic evaluation, we found abnormal ultrasonographic results of any clinical significance to be extremely uncommon, regardless of the urodynamic diagnosis, age, sex, and duration of multiple sclerosis.[20] This apparent improvement may be a result of earlier recognition of patients at risk for urologic dysfunction and prompt treatment.

Movement Disorders: Parkinson's Disease and Multiple Systems Atrophy

It has been estimated that 70% of patients with movement disorders develop LUTS. Although it is believed that patients with Parkinson's disease tend to develop symptoms later in the course of the disease, it has been shown that patients with mild to moderate Hoehn and Yahr symptom scores still are more symptomatic than age-matched counterparts.[3] In contrast, patients with multiple systems atrophy typically do show signs of autonomic dysfunction early in the course of their disease, and men may report erectile dysfunction before other neurologic disturbances are noticed.

Overall, most patients with Parkinson's disease, when studied urodynamically, are found to have detrusor overactivity. Cell loss in the substantia nigra, which is thought to inhibit detrusor activity at baseline, is believed to be responsible for the emergence of detrusor overactivity in patients with Parkinson's disease. Reflecting the diffuse neuronal cell loss seen in multiple systems atrophy, patients with this condition can have a variety of conditions affecting the bladder and sphincter. In particular, neuronal cell loss in Onuf's nucleus leads to sphincteric denervation and insufficiency, whereas neuronal cell loss in the intermediolateral cell columns may lead to detrusor hyporeflexia. Although the risk of postprostatectomy incontinence in men with Parkinson's disease is high (approximately 20%), the risks may be prohibitively high (80%) in patients with multiple systems atrophy due to specific sphincteric disturbances.[21] It is thought that a relative bradykinesia, which is a failure to relax the external sphincter, is present in some patients with Parkinson's disease, manifesting as an obstructive picture that is unrelated to prostate encroachment. These patients, although perhaps presenting with elevated residual volumes and voiding disturbances, are unlikely to be helped by surgical therapy to relieve outlet obstruction.

Several trials have investigated the impact of Parkinson's disease therapies on LUTS. The dopamine receptor agonist apomorphine has no reliable effect on detrusor overactivity, although it has been shown to improve urodynamic indices of bladder outlet obstruction.[22] The effects of levodopa on bladder function appear to be somewhat mixed. One hour after administering levodopa in patients with more advanced disease, urodynamics revealed diminish bladder capacity and a reduced threshold volume for overactivity, thereby worsening urgency, although an improvement in voiding efficiency occurred because of enhanced detrusor contractility.[23] Patients undergoing subthalamic nucleus stimulation were found to have improved bladder capacity and threshold volume for detrusor overactivity during active treatment.[24]

Cerebrovascular Accident

The development or progression of LUTS after a CVA may be found in up to 70% of patients. Because most patients affected by CVA are elderly and may have preexisting disturbances of micturition or incontinence, it is often difficult to decipher what is acute and what chronic in the weeks to months after a stroke. This is particularly troublesome when patients have difficulty communicating after a CVA because of aphasia, and preexisting symptoms are unknown. Because many strokes can affect the suprapontine centers, which provide input (largely inhibitory) to the pontine micturition center, such as the thalamus, basal ganglia, cerebellum, and cerebral cortex, the development of new urinary symptoms after a stroke is common.

From a clinical standpoint, the development of urinary retention shortly after a CVA is quite common. Generally, unless preexisting detrusor dysfunction or coexisting outlet obstruction is present, retention is later replaced by frequency, urgency, and often, urge incontinence. Urodynamically, neurogenic detrusor overactivity is the most common finding, with the external sphincter being synergic in most cases, although patients with internal capsule or cerebral cortex CVA may be more vulnerable to incontinence due to uninhibited sphincteric relaxation.[7] True detrusor-sphincter dyssynergia is quite uncommon after CVA. Detrusor areflexia may also be seen in a significant number of patients after CVA, regardless of CVA location, and overall, it is not clear that stroke location can accurately predict the nature of bladder dysfunction.[25]

Data have emerged regarding the pathogenesis of detrusor dysfunction after CVA, opening the door for new treatments. In animal models, occlusion of the middle cerebral artery has been associated with increases in nitric oxide production at the level of the bladder and spinal cord (by neuronal nitric oxide synthase), and intracerebral injections of nitric oxide inhibitors have rapidly increased bladder capacity that had been diminished after middle cerebral artery occlusion.[26,27] Treatment with an ATP-dependent potassium channel opener has improved bladder capacity after cerebral infarction in rats, whereas others have found that specific alterations in the glutamatergic and dopaminergic pathways may be responsible for detrusor overactivity after a CVA.[28,29] These findings and others have provided hope that alternative treatment strategies may be available to help reduce the impact of CVA on bladder function when used in the acute setting.

Cervical Spondylosis

Cervical spondylosis is most commonly associated with intermittent but severe neck pain, and it can lead to gait disturbance and progressive LUTS. A form of degenerative disk disease, cervical spondylosis can result in a significant myelopathy, causing loss of manual dexterity, arm and hand weakness, sensory abnormalities (C3 to C5 levels), lower extremity spasticity, loss of proprioception, and ultimately, gait imbalance (C5 to C8). Shooting electric shock sensations may occur in the extremities (i.e., Lhermitte's sign) on neck flexion and extension in some patients with cervical spondylosis. The development of radiculopathy symptoms (typically neck or arm pain with paresthesias) may also occur.

Urinary symptoms seem to be present in most patients with cervical spondylosis; however, as with CVA, the presence of preexisting non-neurogenic LUTS must also be considered. Frequency, urgency, and nocturia are most commonly reported (60%), and neurogenic detrusor overactivity is the most common urodynamic finding (40% to 73%).[30] Outlet obstruction resulting from DESD occurs in 0% to 36% of patient series.[10] It is believed that patients with more advanced forms of cervical spondylosis tend to have more debilitating urologic symptoms and are more likely to experience DESD.[31]

CONCLUSIONS

Patients with neurogenic voiding dysfunction are challenging to treat because of the progressive nature of the disease process. Common treatment approaches often do not render the same quality results seen in other patients. The treating urologist must use all tools available to pinpoint the nature of the bladder dysfunction, including complex video urodynamic testing. The physician must have a good understanding of the underlying neurologic disorder to be able to offer appropriate and reasonable solutions to what are often very complex voiding disorders.

References

1. Koldewijn EL, Hommes OR, Lemmens WAJG, et al: Relationship between lower urinary tract abnormalities and disease related parameters in multiple sclerosis. J Urol 154:169-173, 1995.
2. Sakakibara R. Hattori T. Uchiyama T. Yamanishi T: Videourodynamic and sphincter motor unit potential analyses in Parkinson's disease and multiple system atrophy. J Neurol Neurosurg Psychiatry 71:600-606, 2001.
3. Lemack GE, Dewey RB, Roehrborn CG, et al: Questionnaire-based assessment of bladder dysfunction in patients with mild to moderate Parkinson's disease. Urology 56:250-254, 2000.
4. Rapp NS, Gilroy J, Lerner AM: Role of bacterial infection in exacerbation of multiple sclerosis. Am J Phys Med Rehab 74:415-418, 1995.
5. Betts CD, D'Mellow MT, Fowler CJ: Urinary symptoms and the neurological features of bladder dysfunction in multiple sclerosis. J Neurol Neurosurg Psychiatry 56:245-250, 1993.
6. Awad SA, Gajewski JB, Sogbein SK, et al: Relationship between neurological and urological status in multiple sclerosis. J Urol 132:499-502, 1984.
7. Khan Z, Starer P, Yang YC, Bhola A: Analysis of voiding disorders in patients with cerebrovascular accidents. Urology 32:265-270, 1990.
8. Wade D, Langton-Hewer R: Outlook after an acute stroke: Urinary incontinence and loss of consciousness compared in 532 patients. Q J Med 56:601-608, 1985.
9. Bartolin Z, Savic I, Persec Z: Relationship between clinical data and urodynamics findings in patients with lumbar intervertebral disk protrusion. Urol Res 30:219-222, 2002.
10. Tammela TL, Heiskari MJ, Lukkarinen OA: Voiding dysfunction and urodynamic findings in patients with cervical spondylotic spinal stenosis compared with severity of disease. Br J Urol 70:144-148, 1992.
11. Razdan S, Leboeuf L, Mienbach DS, et al: Current practice patterns in the urologic surveillance and management of patients with spinal cord injury. Urology 61:893-896, 2003.
12. Schick E, Corcos J: Practical guide to diagnosis and follow-up of patients with neurogenic bladder dysfunction. In Corcos J, Schick E (eds): The Neurogenic Bladder. London, Martin Dunitz, 2004.
13. McGuire EJ, Savastano JA: Long term follow-up of spinal cord injury patients managed by intermittent catheterization. J Urol 129:775-776, 1983.
14. Cheng CL, deGroat WC: The role of capsaicin-sensitive afferent fibers in the lower urinary tract dysfunction induced by chronic spinal cord injury in rats. Exp Neurol 187:445-454, 2004.
15. de Seze M, Wiart L, de Seze MP, et al: Intravesical capsaicin versus resiniferatoxin for the treatment of detrusor hyperreflexia in spinal cord injured patients: A double-blind, randomized, controlled study. J Urol 171:251-255, 2004.
16. Steinberger RE, Ohl DA, Bennett CJ, et al: Nifedipine pretreatment for autonomic dysreflexia during electroejaculation. Urology 36:228-231, 1990.
17. Consortium for Spinal Cord Medicine: Acute management of autonomic dysreflexia: Individuals with spinal cord injury presenting to health-care facilities. J Spinal Cord Med 25(Suppl 1):S67-S88, 2002.
18. Gajewski JB, Awad SA, Jeffernan LPH, et al: Neurogenic bladder in lower motor neuron lesion: Long term assessment. Neurourol Urodyn 11:509-518, 1999.
19. Chancellor MB, Blaivas JG: Multiple sclerosis. Problems in Urology 1993;7:15-33.
20. Lemack GE, Hawker K, Frohman E: Incidence of upper tract abnormalities in patients with neurovesical dysfunction secondary to multiple sclerosis: Analysis of risk factors at initial urologic presentation. Urology 65:854-857, 2005.
21. Chandiramani VA, Palace J, Fowler CJ. How to recognize patients with parkinsonism who should not have urological surgery. J Urol 80:100-104, 1997.
22. Christmas TJ, Chapple CR, Lees AJ, et al: Role of subcutaneous apomorphine in parkinsonian voiding dysfunction. Lancet 2:1451-1453, 1988.
23. Uchiyama T, Sakakibara R, Hattori T, Yamanishi T: Short-term effect of a single levodopa dose on micturition disturbance in Parkinson's disease patients with wearing off phenomenon. Mov Disord 18:573-578, 2003.
24. Finazzi-Agro E, Peppe A, D'Amico A, et al: Effects of subthalamic nucleus stimulation on urodynamic findings in patients with Parkinson's disease. J Urol 169:1388-1391, 2003.
25. Burney TL, Senepati M, Desai S, et al: Acute cerebrovascular accident and lower urinary tract dysfunction: A prospective correlation of the site of brain injury with urodynamic findings. J Urol 156:1748-1750, 1996.
26. Fu D, Ng YK, Gan P, Ling EA: Permanent occlusion of the middle cerebral artery upregulates expression of cytokines and neuronal nitric oxide synthase in the spinal cord and urinary bladder in the adult rat. Neuroscience 125:819-831, 2004.
27. Kodama K, Yokoyama O, Komatsu K, et al: Contribution of cerebral nitric oxide to bladder overactivity after cerebral infarction in rats. J Urol 167:391-396, 2002.
28. Nakamrua Y, Kontani H, Tanaka T, et al: Effects of adenosine triphosphate dependent potassium channel opener on bladder overactivity in rats with cerebral infarction. J Urol 168:2275-2279, 2002.
29. Yokoyama O, Yoshiyama M, Namiki M, de Groat WC: Changes in dopaminergic and glutamateric excitatory mechanisms of micturition reflex after middle cerebral artery occlusion in conscious rate. Exp Neurol 173:129-135, 2002.
30. Hattori T, Sakakibara R, Yasuda K, et al: Micturitional disturbance in cervical spondylotic myelopathy. J Spinal Disord 3:16-18, 1990.
31. Katz PG, Alberico AM, Zampieri TA, Foz L: Voiding dysfunction associated with cervical spondylotic myelopathy. Neurourol Urodyn 6:419-424, 1988.

Chapter 15

VOIDING DYSFUNCTION AFTER PELVIC SURGERY

Hari Siva Gurunadha Rao Tunuguntla, and Angelo E. Gousse

Pelvic surgery can result in urinary retention or other voiding dysfunction by causing inadvertent damage to the pelvic plexus. It occurs most often after abdominoperineal resection and radical hysterectomy, although it may be seen after transvaginal or abdominal surgery for urinary incontinence (e.g., colposuspension, use of tension-free vaginal tape [TVT]) and pelvic organ prolapse, hysterectomy for benign disease, and laparoscopic hysterectomy.

SURGICAL ANATOMY OF THE PELVIC NERVOUS SYSTEM

The bladder receives innervation from the pelvic plexus (i.e., input from the S2 to S4 spinal cord segments by way of the presacral nerve), which is situated on the lateral aspect of the rectum. The portion of the pelvic plexus that specifically supplies the bladder is also called the vesical plexus.

The primary supply to the detrusor is by parasympathetic nerves that are uniformly and diffusely distributed throughout the detrusor. In contrast, the sympathetic nerve supply to the detrusor is rather sparse.[1] In women, numerous parasympathetic nerves, identical to those innervating the detrusor, supply the bladder neck and urethral muscle. The female bladder muscle and urethra receive a poor supply of sympathetic innervation.[2] The sympathetic preganglionic nuclei are located in the L1 and L2 spinal segments and possibly in the T12 segment. Afferent sensory fibers from the bladder exit along the sympathetic or parasympathetic pathways.

The superior hypogastric plexus is a fenestrated network of fibers anterior to the lower abdominal aorta. The hypogastric nerves exit bilaterally at the inferior poles of the superior hypogastric plexus that lie at the level of the sacral promontory. The network of nerve structures is located between the endopelvic fascia and the peritoneum. The hypogastric nerves unite the superior hypogastric plexus and the inferior hypogastric plexus or pelvic plexus bilaterally. The inferior hypogastric plexus has connections with the sacral roots from S3 and some contributions from S4 and S2.[3] The superior hypogastric plexus and hypogastric nerves are mainly sympathetic, the pelvic splanchnic nerves are mainly parasympathetic, and the inferior hypogastric plexus contains both types of fibers.

Bladder afferent fibers convey mechanoreceptive input essential for voiding. These visceral afferent fibers also transmit sensations of bladder fullness, urgency, and pain.

Ablative pelvic surgery may result in injury to the pelvic plexus and pudendal nerve, leading to abnormal function of parasympathetic, sympathetic, and somatic function. The resultant urodynamic abnormalities include any combination of reduced compliance, hypocontractile detrusor, bladder neck incompetence identified on fluoroscopic screening, reduced urethral closure pressure, and electromyographic changes in the perineal musculature.[4-6]

PATHOPHYSIOLOGY OF VOIDING DYSFUNCTION

Voiding dysfunction after pelvic surgery may be caused by anatomic or functional disturbances of the lower urinary tract. The causes may be divided into two broad categories: failure to store (i.e., altered bladder or bladder outlet function) and failure to empty (i.e., altered bladder or bladder outlet function).

Failure to store may be caused by detrusor overactivity, which may result from denervation supersensitivity after pelvic dissection or from surgery-related bladder outlet obstruction (e.g., after tight suburethral slingplasty). Bladder outlet obstruction may be the most common factor in the development of postoperative voiding dysfunction.[7] Bladder outlet obstruction is intimately involved with the onset of postoperative voiding dysfunction. Harrison and associates[8] and Speakman and colleagues[9] proposed that parasympathetic denervation supersensitivity develops as a result of bladder outlet obstruction, and others[10] have postulated that denervation hypersensitivity may develop from the surgical dissection alone in the absence of bladder outlet obstruction. Other studies suggested that bladder outlet obstruction might result in changes in cholinergic and purinergic signaling. Likewise, inadequate tension during sling placement, although uncommon, may result in failure of the bladder to store.

Postvoid residual (PVR) volume (achieved by a Valsalva maneuver or effective detrusor contraction) is an indicator of voiding efficiency. Preoperatively, increased PVR volumes due to loss of contractility or obstruction, or both, can be a demonstration of efficiency loss, and consequently, it is a risk factor for postoperative voiding dysfunction.

Bladder outlet obstruction after sling surgery is related to increased tension resulting in urethral compression.[7] It may result from different causes after different procedures for incontinence. Retropubic and transvaginal needle suspensions stabilize lateral juxtaurethral tissues; obstruction is often related to hyperelevation of the bladder neck and kinking of the proximal urethra. Pubovaginal slings provide suburethral support to augment urethral coaptation during periods of increased intra-abdominal pressure. Midurethral slings using TVT (Gynecare, Ethicon,

Somerville, NJ) or SPARC mesh material (American Medical Systems, Minnetonka, MN) are the new class of anti-incontinence procedures and are placed without tension at the mid-urethral level to simulate the supportive function of the pubourethral ligaments. Obstruction after these procedures has been attributed to compression from excessive tension or sling misplacement or migration.[7]

Voiding with a weak detrusor contraction (identified by cystometrogram) or during a Valsalva maneuver has been associated with a higher risk of urinary retention and surgical failure.[11-13] Miller and colleagues[11] observed that of 21 women who voided without contraction on the preoperative test, 4 (19%) presented with postoperative urinary retention, compared with none of 48 other women with normal contraction. In the same study, no patient with a contraction pressure greater than 12 cm H_2O presented with retention. Among the parameters tested for voiding dysfunction, only PVR volume was a significant factor. However, the investigators emphasized that the small sample limited the conclusions of the study.[11]

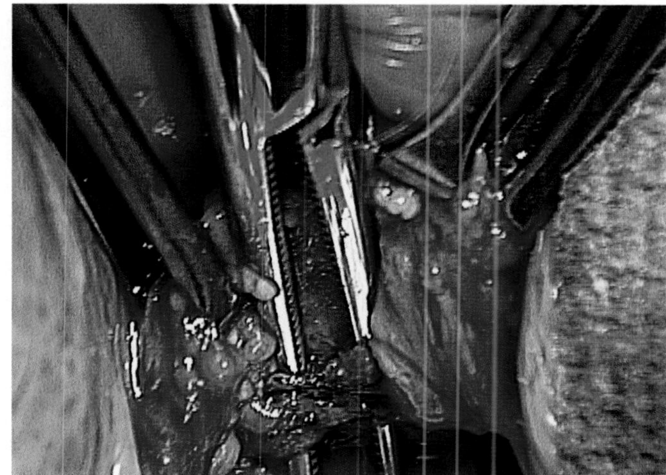

Figure 15-1 Urethral erosion by a tension-free vaginal tape suburethral sling.

EVALUATION OF VOIDING DYSFUNCTION

The presence and extent of preoperative storage and voiding symptoms are useful for comparison with de novo or persistent symptoms after incontinence surgery. Important factors include preoperative emptying status and PVR volume. These assessments are important for those with elevated PVR volumes after slingplasty. If preoperative voiding parameters and emptying are normal, incomplete emptying or retention after surgery increases the suspicion of obstruction.

Studies have found that patients with poor detrusor contractility and those who void with abdominal straining may require a longer period of postoperative catheterization (e.g., after retropubic suspensions and pubovaginal sling) and take longer to resume normal voiding.[14,15] However, McLennan and coworkers[16] found no association between returning to normal voiding and length of postoperative catheterization in those undergoing autologous fascia lata sling surgery. Urethral erosion (Fig. 15-1) and bladder perforation (Fig. 15-2) during placement of a synthetic sling should be excluded by a thorough cystourethroscopy (if necessary, by a retroflexed flexible cystoscope) during the evaluation of a patient with urgency, urge incontinence, UTI, and or hematuria after slingplasty.

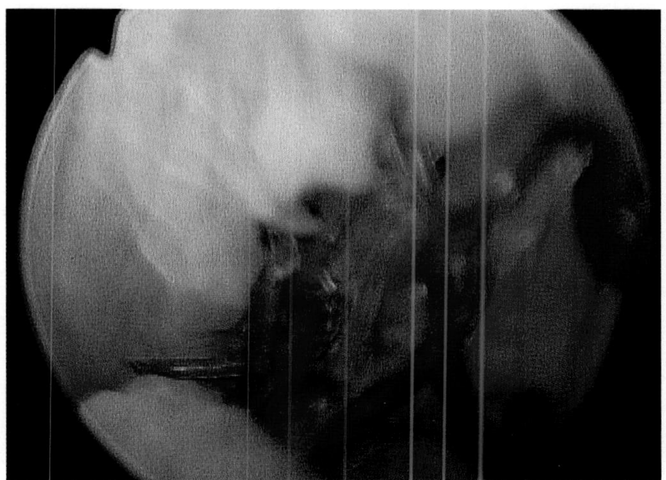

Figure 15-2 Bladder perforation by a tension-free vaginal tape suburethral sling.

History and Physical Examination

Postoperative evaluation demands a thorough history that includes assessment of storage symptoms such as frequency, dysuria, urgency, and urge incontinence and voiding symptoms such as hesitancy, incomplete emptying, straining, positional voiding, and complete urinary retention. The physical examination evaluates symptoms or signs of hyperelevated bladder neck, frank stress urinary incontinence (SUI), worsening or new-onset pelvic organ prolapse, and erosion of the mesh in the vaginal canal. UTI should be ruled out with urinalysis and culture. The PVR volume should be documented, although an elevated PVR volume cannot accurately separate bladder outlet obstruction from impaired detrusor contractility.

The findings on physical examination may vary from normal to a frankly hypersuspended urethra. Midurethral slings (e.g., SPARC suburethral sling, TVT) typically do not result in overcorrection of the urethrovesical angle.[17] Bladder neck slings, however, can pull or scar the urethra against the pubic bone and result in a negative urethrovesical angle. The surgeon may also encounter an iatrogenic obstruction without hypersuspension or elevation of the bladder neck or urethra. Any additional outlet resistance may be enough to cause retention or de novo obstruction in patients with a hypocontractile detrusor.

Cystocele may create a fulcrum or point of obstruction and should be excluded in the evaluation of voiding dysfunction after sling surgery. Urethral or vaginal erosion of the sling, SUI, and persistent urethral hypermobility also should be considered.

Video Urodynamic Study

Although commonly performed by most clinicians, the evidence-based value of urodynamic study in the evaluation of voiding dysfunction after incontinence surgery remains controversial. Most studies have shown a poor correlation between findings on urodynamics and outcomes after urethrolysis.[17]

Urodynamic studies may provide information on detrusor overactivity or impaired compliance in patients in urinary retention or increased PVR capacity.[18] They may also confirm the diagnosis of obstruction as demonstrated by high pressure or low flow. McGuire and colleagues,[19] Nitti and coworkers,[20] and Cross and associates[21] have shown that presence of an adequate detrusor contraction has no association with successful voiding after transvaginal urethrolysis and sling takedown. Urodynamic study may provide a specific diagnosis of voiding dysfunction (e.g., impaired pelvic floor relaxation during voiding) and therefore can be helpful in directing therapy. It may also ascertain the cause of concomitant incontinence, guiding concurrent surgery during urethrolysis.

Absolute urodynamic criteria for obstruction in women have not been defined despite several proposed cutoff values. Chassagne and associates[22] noticed that at a cutoff value of 15 mL/sec or less, flow with a combined detrusor pressure of at least 20 cm H_2O was able to define bladder outlet obstruction in women with a sensitivity of 74% and specificity of 91%. Blaivas and Groutz[23] used a "free uroflow" parameter in 600 women to provide useful information for those unable to void during the study. They classified obstruction on the basis of a detrusor pressure of more than 20 cm H_2O despite no flow or an inability to void with a catheter in place. Nitti and coworkers[24] used a combination of multichannel urodynamic study and videofluoroscopy to aid in the diagnosis of bladder outlet obstruction as a sustained detrusor contraction with reduced flow and radiographic evidence of obstruction between the bladder neck and urethra. However, if a patient does not demonstrate a contraction during the voiding phase with concomitant uroflow, it is not as useful. Notwithstanding these limitations, a urodynamic study confirming obstruction can make the surgeon feel more confident in his or her decision to perform urethrolysis. Urodynamic study provides information regarding bladder capacity, SUI, compliance, detrusor overactivity, or learned voiding dysfunction.

Cystoscopy

All patients with persistent storage symptoms after pelvic surgery should undergo cystoscopy to rule out urethral erosion (see Fig. 15-1) and bladder perforation (see Fig. 15-2) from sutures, the suture passer, or sling material. Cystoscopy may also show a hypersuspended mid-urethra or bladder neck (indicating excessive sling tension), scarring, deviation of the urethra, misplacement or migration, or even a fistula. Vaginoscopy also can be performed to exclude vaginal erosion of a sling.

Postoperative Recovery

Some delay in initiating volitional voiding may occur up to 4 weeks after any anti-incontinence surgery. Management depends on the nature of symptoms. Those with high PVR volumes or complete retention should be initially treated with intermittent or continuous catheterization for up to 3 or 4 weeks. The clinician can use his or her judgment to intervene sooner. Significant incomplete emptying or total retention persisting beyond this period rarely resolves without intervention. Evaluation and treatment can therefore be considered at this point. Experience with midurethral polypropylene slings suggests that incomplete emptying or urinary retention can be addressed as early as 1 week postoperatively.[25] However, the outcomes after earlier intervention have not been established. In patients with voiding symptoms alone, a temporal relationship of severe symptoms after surgery, and normal preoperative voiding and emptying, urethrolysis may be undertaken without urodynamic assessment. This principle also applies to obstruction after any incontinence procedure when a temporal or causal relationship between surgery and voiding dysfunction exists.

Evaluation in those with de novo or worsening storage symptoms and normal emptying is based on the severity of bother compared with that from preoperative symptoms. Such patients should initially undergo conservative treatment with fluid restriction and antimuscarinic agents. If symptoms persist, urodynamic study and cystoscopy should be performed. If symptoms fail to resolve over an arbitrary 3 months' waiting period and obstruction is the cause of the storage symptoms, urethrolysis should be considered. Although 3 months is the minimal period before surgical intervention in most urethrolysis series,[26] we feel that treatment should be individualized for each patient with storage symptoms after pelvic organ prolapse or sling surgery.

PELVIC SURGERY

Radical Hysterectomy

Short-term and long-term bladder dysfunction remains a common side effect after radical hysterectomy, with bladder atony (requiring indwelling catheter drainage for more than 2 weeks) reported in as many as 42% of patients.[27] Mundy and colleagues[28] reported voiding dysfunction in 52% to 85% of patients after radical total hysterectomy.

Mundy and colleagues[28] reported urinary retention in only 0.5% of patients after radical hysterectomy, whereas straining was required by 85%. Buchsbaum and associates[29] reported urinary retention in 10% to 60% of patients after radical hysterectomy. Compared with surgery, adjuvant pelvic irradiation is more often associated with contracted and overactive bladders. Retention is usually treated with clean intermittent self-catheterization. Bandy and assocaites[30] have shown that prolonged indwelling catheterization (>30 days) after radical hysterectomy is associated with worse long-term PVR and total bladder capacity. Fortunately, this voiding dysfunction becomes permanent in less than 5% of patients. [30]

In a prospective study of 18 patients who underwent modified radical hysterectomy (involving restricted dissection of the anterior parts of the cardinal ligament and preservation of the posterior cardinal ligament), Chuang and coworkers[31] demonstrated only temporary (<6 months) vesicourethral dysfunction attributable to transient somatic and autonomic demyelination with or without denervation. These investigators studied the patients by pudendal motor nerve conduction and urodynamic studies, including urethral pressure profiling, cystometry, and uroflowmetry.

Central Compartment Surgery and Voiding Dysfunction

Hysterectomy for Benign Disease

Urologic complications occur after 0.1% of the abdominal and 0.05% of the vaginal procedures.[32] Most controlled, prospective studies have found minimal effect of hysterectomy for benign disease on bladder function, and urinary retention therefore appears to be related to other factors.[33] Voiding dysfunction is more common after total than after subtotal hysterectomy performed for benign causes (see Fig. 15-1).[34]

Loss of bladder-filling sensation is the suggested pathophysiologic mechanism of urinary retention after hysterectomy.[35] Everaert and colleagues[35] showed that urinary retention after hysterectomy for benign disease was associated with deafferentiation of the bladder wall in four patients and of the bladder neck in one. Decreased visceral sensation of the bladder or bladder neck is associated with neurogenic disease.[36] Functionally, these patients have absent filling sensation on cystometry, together with partial or complete sensory denervation of the bladder, resulting in increased bladder capacity and secondary urinary retention. Compared with subtotal hysterectomy, total hysterectomy has been associated with a more prominent decrease in voiding frequency and increased bladder capacity.[34] Mild symptoms of deafferentiation are more frequent after hysterectomy but are temporary.[33] Partial or complete deafferentiation, together with a concomitant factor (e.g., preexisting pelvic floor dysfunction, histrionic personality, medications) may result in urinary retention.

Although retention is rare after hysterectomy for benign disease, it is bothersome for the patient. Selected patients may be candidates for sacral nerve neuromodulation.[35] Everaert and associates[35] reported good response in 50% and partial long-term success in 33% of 15 patients.

Laparoscopic Hysterectomy and Voiding Function

Most women undergoing hysterectomy are in the perimenopausal age group, and urinary symptoms are common in all women in this age group. Long and colleagues[37] have shown improvement in urinary symptoms after laparoscopic hysterectomy. These investigators showed a significant decrease in the number of women with one or more urinary symptoms, from 81 (53.6%) of 151 preoperatively to 58 (38.4%) of 151 postoperatively. Urinary frequency, SUI, and nocturia were the most common preoperative symptoms that improved after surgery. This improvement may result from the postoperative changes in the urodynamics and mobility of the bladder neck.[38] The investigators suggest that these effects may be attributed to the anchoring of the vaginal cuff to the cardinal-uterosacral ligament complex during hysterectomy. Similarly, Virtanen and coworkers[39] noticed a decrease in the incidence of urinary frequency and SUI after total hysterectomy.

Anterior Compartment Surgery and Voiding Dysfunction

Anti-incontinence Surgery and Voiding Dysfunction

Anti-incontinence procedures are designed to correct SUI by restoring support to the urethrovesical junction and, in cases of intrinsic sphincter dysfunction, by improving coaptation of the urethra. Persistent voiding dysfunction from postoperative urethral hypersuspension is a known but not well-characterized complication after female anti-incontinence surgery. It has been reported to occur in 2.5% to 24% of patients.[40] In a large series of 503 patients comparing the Burch colposuspension with Stamey endoscopic needle suspension, voiding dysfunction was found to be the most common complication (12.1%).[41]

In most patients, postoperative voiding dysfunction is caused by obstruction from the incontinence procedure itself.[42] Urodynamic obstruction has been reported in 2.5% to 24% of patients after incontinence operations.[43,44] Some of these patients have "clinical obstruction." Others may have obvious voiding symptoms or retention de novo after surgery. However, storage symptoms without incomplete emptying also may be a manifestation of obstruction. Carr and Webster[45] reported irritative symptoms as the most common presenting symptoms, occurring in 75% of women, most of whom emptied their bladder satisfactorily.

Bladder outlet obstruction occurs in 5% to 20% of patients after a Marshall-Marchetti-Krantz procedure,[46] in 4% to 7% after a Burch colposuspension,[47,48] in 5% to 7% after a needle suspension,[49] and in 4% to 10% after pubovaginal sling operations.[50] Although the vaginal TVT is placed without tension at the midurethra, studies have shown that it may still be associated with voiding dysfunction in 4.9% to 10% of patients.[51,52]

Postoperative voiding and storage symptoms are common in the immediate postoperative period, although most resolve within the first 4 weeks. Workup and intervention is warranted in patients with persistent symptoms. Contemporary sling series[53-55] revealed a less than 5% rate of postoperative retention or urodynamically proven obstruction requiring surgical intervention.

Incidence of voiding dysfunction after anti-incontinence surgery is likely greater than reported. Although this is not a common outcome, it is possible to underestimate its actual incidence because there exists a spectrum of bladder outlet obstruction from frank retention to obstructive (i.e., weak stream, intermittency, or straining to void) or irritative voiding symptoms (i.e., frequency, urgency, or urge incontinence) alone.[17] Some patients may develop de novo instability or detrusor overactivity after surgery. Patients with preoperative irritative voiding symptoms may be at risk for continued symptoms after surgery. Which patients need correction of potential bladder outlet obstruction or alternative therapy rests on the clinician's judgment.

Carr and Webster[45] found that among 51 patients presenting for urethrolysis, 75% had irritative complaints, 61% had obstructive symptoms, and 55% experienced de no urge. Urinary retention as the sole symptom (with or without the need for intermittent self catheterization) was uncommon, occurring only in 24%. Urethral erosion (see Fig. 15-1) may occasionally manifest with obstructive or irritative voiding symptoms.[56]

Patients with long-term retention may choose to continue intermittent or continuous catheterization rather than risk recurrent incontinence from urethrolysis. Surgery has been reserved for patients with frank voiding symptoms, whereas patients with de novo or worsening storage symptoms are more often managed nonoperatively. Initial therapy includes fluid management, timed voiding, and antimuscarinic medications. Surgical procedures such as sacral neuromodulation and augmentation cystoplasty are reserved for the more refractory cases. Botulinum toxin type A intradetrusor injection may have a role in these cases in the future.

Surgical Intervention for Retention after Slingplasty

Urethrolysis (Fig. 15-3) performed in patients with persistent voiding dysfunction has consistently been shown to ameliorate voiding complaints and urinary retention after sling surgery for SUI. Factors important for decision-making include the type of sling or anti-incontinence procedure used, the nature of voiding dysfunction (i.e., frank retention versus irritative voiding), and the patient's desired outcome. If a patient is content with the current status of retention compared with her severe preoperative incontinence and is not willing to take the risk of recurrent

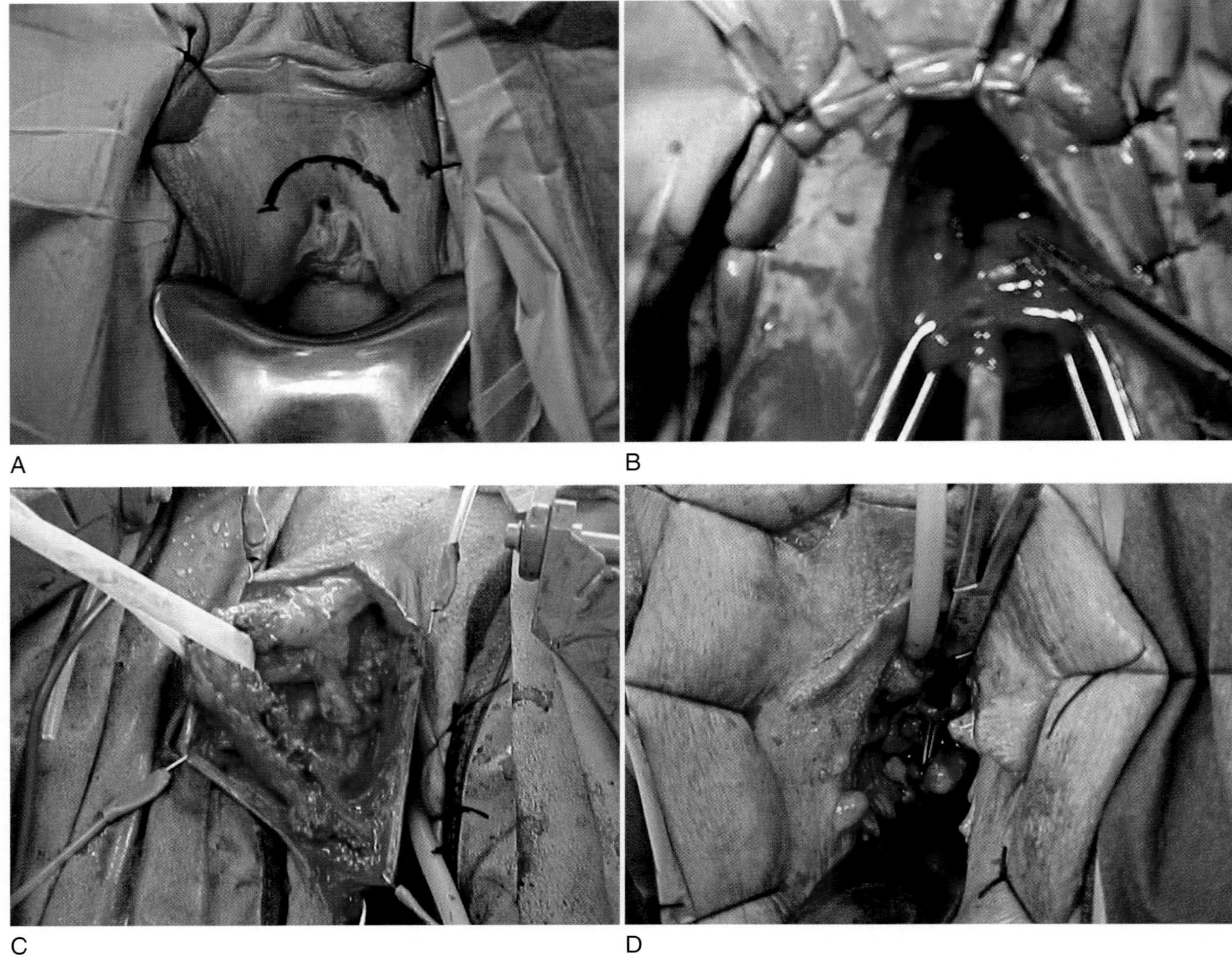

Figure 15-3 Transvaginal suprameatal urethrolysis. **A,** Inverted U incision is made between 9 and 3 o'clock positions 1 cm from urethral meatus. **B,** plane is dissected above urethra to base of symphysis pubis. **C,** Lateral dissection identifies wings of fibrous tissue overlying obstructing suburethral sling. **D,** Residual obstructing tissue ventral to midurethra.

SUI after urethrolysis, she may decide to manage the problem with clean intermittent self-catheterization.

The 3-month waiting period for surgical intervention arose from data on autologous fascia slings that might have loosened with time, allowing the patient to void to completion. Many question whether the patient who "'opens up"' at 3 months is actually achieving balanced voiding with a low detrusor pressure (i.e., unobstructed). The trend has been to perform urethrolysis as soon as 4 weeks into the postoperative period. The available literature suggests short-term symptomatic success.[7,17]

Surgical technique depends on type of material or approach used for initial surgery, duration of symptoms after surgery, and any associated surgery (e.g., cystocele repair). Operative approaches include sling incision, transvaginal urethrolysis, retropubic urethrolysis, suprameatal (see Fig. 15-3) transvaginal urethrolysis, and interposition grafts.[17] The overall success rate of urethrolysis is acceptable (Table 15-1).

In surgery for retention after slingplasty, a midline incision over the sling (see Fig. 15-1) should be attempted initially. If the sling cannot be identified or bladder neck mobility is not restored, formal transvaginal urethrolysis (see Fig. 15-3) should be performed.[7] Suprameatal dissection (see Fig. 15-3) may be helpful in lysing scarred fibrous attachments between the urethra and pubis. Retropubic urethrolysis is reserved for patients with voiding dysfunction after retropubic suspension and for initial transvaginal urethrolysis failures. Resuspension of the urethra may be considered if the patient has concomitant SUI. Patients with persistent obstruction or voiding dysfunction after initial urethrolysis should undergo a workup similar to that for primary voiding dysfunction after anti-incontinence surgery and may be considered for aggressive repeat urethrolysis if obstruction is diagnosed. This approach may prevent chronic bladder dysfunction.[57]

Leng and coworkers[57] observed an association between prolonged time to urethrolysis for obstructive voiding symptoms after slingplasty and greater likelihood of persistent bladder dysfunction after urethrolysis. Time to urethrolysis for the whole cohort ranged from 2 to 66 months, with a mean follow-up after urethrolysis of 17.3 ± 22.9 months. If their observation can be corroborated by other studies, it would be prudent to lower the threshold of clinical suspicion to detect bladder outlet obstruction after slingplasty. Video urodynamics testing can help differ-

Table 15-1 Results of Urethrolysis

Study	No. of Patients	Type of Urethrolysis	Success Rate (%)	Stress Urinary Incontinence (%)
Foster and McGuire[76]	48	Transvaginal	65	0
Nitti and Raz[20]	42	Transvaginal	71	0
Cross et al[21]	39	Transvaginal	72	3
Goldman et al[77]	32	Transvaginal	84	19
Petrou et al[75]	32	Suprameatal	67	3
Carr and Webster[45]	15	Retropubic	93	13
Carr and Webster[45]	54	Mixed	78	14

Adapted from Vasavada SP: Evaluation and management of postoperative bladder outlet obstruction in women. Issues Incontinence Fall:5-7, 2002.

entiate between outlet obstruction and de novo urge incontinence. Rather than curtailing evaluation before urethrolysis, routine urodynamic testing can help us obtain the data for the pathologic condition of female bladder outlet obstruction. We do not know the role of sacral neuromodulation in nonobstructive retention after sling surgery.

Colposuspension and Voiding Function

Wang[58] attributed the postoperative voiding dysfunction (i.e., frequency, urgency, and obstructive voiding symptoms) to outflow obstruction. He reported higher postoperative voiding dysfunction after a Stamey bladder neck suspension procedure.

Bombieri and associates[59] demonstrated that bladder neck elevation and compression (anterior and lateral) during colposuspension were responsible for voiding symptoms using magnetic resonance imaging. Postoperative voiding was assessed clinically and by voiding cystometry. At 3 months, 21.4% of patients developed de novo symptoms of overactive bladder. Bump and colleagues[60] demonstrated higher pressure transmission ratios in women with postoperative detrusor overactivity compared with women without detrusor overactivity after colposuspension and controls with overactive bladder symptoms who did not undergo surgery.

Pelvic Organ Prolapse Surgery and Voiding Function

Uterine prolapse may negatively affect pelvic floor function, resulting in voiding symptoms, defecation symptoms, and sexual dysfunction.[61] In a multicenter, randomized, controlled trial comparing abdominal and vaginal prolapse surgery in their effects on urogenital function, Roovers and coworkers[62] found higher (indicating more discomfort) Urogenital Distress Inventory scores (i.e., discomfort/pain domains and obstructive micturition domains) in the abdominal group than in the vaginal group. The investigators concluded that vaginal hysterectomy with anterior or posterior colporrhaphy, or both, was preferable to abdominal sacrocolpopexy with preservation of the uterus as surgical correction in patients with uterine prolapse stages II to IV. Urinary frequency, urgency, nocturia, and obstructive voiding symptoms requiring doctor's visits occurred in 7% of patients after vaginal repair and in 20% of patients after abdominal repair.

Rosenzweig and colleagues[63] reported improvement in urgency and urinary incontinence after simple anterior repair. However, in a study of the functional and anatomic outcome of anterior and posterior vaginal prolapse repair with Prolene mesh, Milani and associates[64] reported persistent urge incontinence (16% before and after surgery) and clinical SUI (25% before surgery and 22% after surgery) but improved urgency (50% before surgery and 40% after surgery) and urodynamically confirmed SUI (54% before surgery and 44% after surgery), whereas urodynamic detrusor overactivity worsened after surgery (56% versus 22%). The investigators attributed these outcomes to a "reduced capacity of the bladder to expand because of the anelasticity of the Prolene mesh." Larger, prospective studies may settle the issue.

Theofrastous and coworkers[65] reported improvement in the length of postoperative bladder catheterization in postmenopausal women undergoing pelvic organ prolapse repair with preoperative estrogen replacement.

Cystocele Repair and Voiding Dysfunction

Most patients with advanced pelvic organ prolapse and elevated RVR volumes demonstrate normalization of the PVR volumes after surgical correction of the pelvic organ prolapse.[66] Patients who had stress or urge urinary incontinence 8 weeks after grade 4 cystocele repair are evaluated with cystoscopy and video urodynamic evaluation when indicated.[67]

Voiding function (in terms of SUI) improves after cystocele repair. None of the patients in the series by Safir and colleagues[67] had de novo SUI. For 112 patients in this study, urinary incontinence resolved in 39 (87%) of 45, whereas 5 (7%) of the remaining 67 patients with no detrusor overactivity preoperatively had de novo urinary incontinence.

One study[68] enrolled 45 women (mean age, 65 years) who underwent grade 4 cystocele repair and had preoperative parameters of grade 4 cystocele in 43 (100.0%), SUI in 24 (55.8%), urge urinary incontinence in 26 (60.4%), and obstructive voiding symptoms in 26 (60.4%).[68] Patients were evaluated using the stress, emptying, anatomic, protection, and instability (SEAPI) test, with a follow-up of 15 months. Leboeuf and associates[68] demonstrated statistically significant improvement in all the SEAPI domains. Two patients (4.7%) had postoperative urinary retention, and de novo urge incontinence occurred in two patients (11.7%).

In a study by Frederick and Leach,[69] 8.5% of patients experienced de novo urge incontinence after acadaveric prolapse repair with sling procedure for combined SUI and cystocele. Three of 251 patients experienced prolonged urinary retention (>1 month); one required urethrolysis.

Enterocele Repair and Voiding Dysfunction

Enterocele was consistently found to be associated with reduced maximum and average uroflow rate centiles.[70]. Winters and colleagues[71] reported the outcomes for 20 women between 45 and 82 years old (mean age, 67.9 years) with complex pelvic floor prolapse (all patients had cystocele, enterocele, and vaginal vault prolapse) managed by abdominal sacral colpopexy and abdominal enterocele repair. Three patients developed SUI postoperatively, two despite having a Burch suspension and one after a pubovaginal sling. Two patients were successfully managed by collagen injection. No complications involving the mesh have been encountered.

Sacrospinous Ligament Fixation and Voiding Dysfunction

Cespedes[72] reported outcomes of treating total vault prolapse using bilateral sacrospinous ligament fixation through an anterior vaginal approach in 28 patients. All patients had grade 3 or 4 vault prolapse, and all patients had associated enteroceles, cystoceles, and rectoceles. At a mean follow-up of 17 months (range, 5 to 35 months), SUI had been cured in all patients; however, two patients continued to have mild urge incontinence requiring less than 1 pad per day. One patient had elevated PVR volumes requiring intermittent catheterization for 2 months.

Orthotopic Neobladders and Voiding Function

In a multicenter study of orthotopic neobladders, Carrion and coworkers[73] did not show any difference in outcomes after ileal neobladder versus colonic neobladder. Even a moderate degree of nocturnal incontinence is a significant problem for these patients. The incidences of diurnal incontinence, nocturnal incontinence, and intermittent catheterization were 7%, 31%, and 14% of patients undergoing ileal neobladder, respectively. The corresponding figures for those that underwent colonic neobladder are 12%, 30%, and 11%, respectively.

Fujisawa and colleagues[74] have shown that the location of the neobladder and avoidance of angulation (>90 degrees) of the outlet are important for obtaining normal voiding after neobladder reconstruction in women. These investigators showed that intrareservoir pressure is less critical for normal voiding function. Although an increased intrareservoir pressure (contributed mostly by abdominal straining) was associated with increased frequency, it did not correlate with the peak urinary flow rate (Table 15-2).

CONCLUSIONS

Female bladder outlet obstruction after pelvic surgery is a multifaceted topic because of the lack of defined criteria for the evaluation. The long-term outcome is often not as good as expected. Short-term and long-term bladder dysfunction remains a common side effect after radical hysterectomy, with bladder atony reported in as many as 42% of patients. Bladder outlet obstruction can occur after a Marshall-Marchetti-Krantz procedure, Burch colposuspension, and pubovaginal sling procedure. Although the vaginal TVT is placed without tension at the midurethra, studies have shown that it may still be associated with voiding dysfunction in 4.9% to 10% of patients. Urethral erosion may occasionally manifest with obstructive or irritative voiding symptoms. Most patients with advanced pelvic organ prolapse and elevated PVR volumes had normalization of PVR volumes after surgical correction of the pelvic organ prolapse. De novo urge incontinence occurs in 11% of patients after high-grade cystocele repair. Postoperative urinary retention after sacrospinous ligament fixation is less affected by the vault suspension than by the preoperative and postoperative management and

Table 15-2 Incidence of Voiding Dysfunction after Pelvic Surgery

Type of Surgery	Incidence of Voiding Dysfunction (%)	Study
Radical hysterectomy	42	Artman et al[27]
Hysterectomy for benign causes	0.1 (abdominal) 0.05 (vaginal)	Diels et al[32]
Slings for urinary incontinence	2.5-24	Dorflinger et al[40] Morgan et al[53] Chaiken et al[55] Klutke et al[55]
Marshall-Marchetti-Krantz colposuspension	5-20	Zimmern et al[46]
Burch colposuspension	4-7 21.4	Akpinalr et al[47] Ward et al[48] Bombieri et al[59]
Tension-free vaginal tape (TVT)	4.9-10	Dorflinger et al[51] Karram et al[52]
Anterior plus posterior compartment pelvic organ prolapse repair	16*	Milani et al[64]
Cystocele repair	4.7† 11.7‡	Leboeuf et al[68]
Ileal neobladder	7 (diurnal incontinence) 31 (nocturnal incontinence) 14 (clean catheterization)	Carrion et al[73]
Colonic neobladder	12 (diurnal incontinence) 30 (nocturnal incontinence) 11 (clean catheterization)	Carrion et al[73]

*Incidence of persistent urge incontinence.
†Incidence of urinary retention.
‡Incidence of de novo urge incontinence.

concurrent pelvic surgical procedures (e.g., cystocele repair). Postoperative stress incontinence may occur in 10% of patients when the bladder neck and urethra are not adequately supported.

Guidelines on postoperative outcome measures offer a more effective way to manage this problem. Quality-of-life scores, including the 7-item Incontinence Impact Questionnaire (IIQ-7), 6-item Urogenital Distress Inventory (UDI-6), and American Urological Association (AUA) symptom scores may be used to gain more information on the quality-of-life changes that may be induced with management of bladder outlet obstruction in these patients.

References

1. Gosling J: The structure of the bladder and urethra in relation to function. Urol Clin North Am 6:31-38, 1979.
2. American College of Obstetricians and Gynecologists: Chronic pelvic pain. ACOG technical bulletin no. 223. Int J Gynecol Obstet 54:59-68, 1996.
3. Havenga K, DeRuiter MC, Enker WE, Welvaart K: Anatomical basis of autonomic nerve-preserving total mesorectal excision for rectal cancer. Br J Surg 83:384-388, 1996.
4. Woodside JR, Crawford ED: Urodynamic features of pelvic plexus injury. J Urol 124:657-658, 1980.
5. Blaivas JG, Barbalias GA: Characteristics of neural injury after abdomino-perineal resection. J Urol 129:84-87, 1983.
6. Pavlkis AJ: Cauda equine and pelvic plexus injury. In Krane RJ, Siroky ME (eds): Clinical Neuro-Urology, 2nd ed. Boston, Little, Brown, 1991, pp 333-344.
7. Gomelsky A, Nitti VW, Dmochowski RR: Management of obstructive voiding dysfunction after incontinence surgery: Lessons learned. Urology 62:391-399, 2003.
8. Harrison SC, Hunnam GR, Farman P, et al: Bladder instability and denervation in patients with bladder outflow obstruction. Br J Urol 60:519-522, 1987.
9. Speakman MJ, Brading AF, Guilpin CJ, et al: Bladder outflow obstruction: A cause of denervation supersensitivity. J Urol 138:1461-1466, 1987.
10. Cardozo LD, Stanton SL, Williams JE: Detrusor instability following surgery for genuine stress incontinence. Br J Urol 51:204-207, 1979.
11. Miller EA, Amundsen CL, Toh KL, et al: Preoperative urodynamic evaluation may predict voiding dysfunction in women undergoing pubovaginal sling. J Urol 169:2234-2237, 2003.
12. Mutone N, Brizendine E, Hale D: Factors that influence voiding function after the tension-free vaginal tape procedure for stress urinary incontinence. Am J Obstet Gynecol 188:1477-1481, 2003.
13. Wang AC, Chen MC: Comparison of tension-free vaginal taping versus modified Burch colposuspension on urethral obstruction: A randomized controlled trial. Neurourol Urodyn 22:185-190, 2003.
14. Iglesia CB, Shott S, Fenner DE, et al: Effect of preoperative voiding mechanism on success rate of autologous rectus fascia suburethral sling procedure. Obstet Gynecol 91:577-581, 1998.
15. Sze EH, Miklos JR, Karram MM: Voiding after Burch colposuspension and effects of concomitant pelvic surgery: Correlation with preoperative voiding mechanism. Obstet Gynecol 88:564-567, 1996.
16. McLennan MT, Melick CF, Bent AE: Clinical and urodynamic predictors of delayed voiding after fascia lata suburethral sling. Obstet Gynecol 92:608-612, 1998.
17. Vasavada SP: Evaluation and management of postoperative bladder outlet obstruction in women. Issues Incontinence Fall:1, 5-7, 2002.
18. Petrou SP, Nitti VW: Urethrolysis. Lession 22. AUA Update Series 20:169-176, 2001.
19. McGuire EJ, Letson W, Wang S: Transvaginal urethrolysis after obstructive urethral suspension procedures. J Urol 142:1037-1039, 1989.
20. Nitti VW, Raz S: Obstruction following anti-incontinence procedures: Diagnosis and treatment with transvaginal urethrolysis. J Urol 152:93-98, 1994.
21. Cross CA, Cespedes RD, English SF, et al: Transvaginal urethrolysis for urethral obstruction after anti-incontinence surgery. J Urol 159:1199-1201, 1998.
22. Chassagne S, Bernier PA, Haab F, et al: Proposed cutoff values to determine bladder outlet obstruction in females. Urology 51:408-411, 1998.
23. Blaivas JG, Groutz A: Bladder outlet obstruction nomogram for women with lower urinary tract symptomatology. Neurourol Urodyn 19:553-564, 2000.
24. Nitti VW, Tu LM, Gitlin J: Diagnosing bladder outlet obstruction in women. J Urol 161:1535-1540, 1999.
25. Klutke C, Siegel S, Carlin B, et al: Urinary retention after tension-free vaginal tape procedure: Incidence and treatment. Urology 58:697-701, 2001.
26. Abouassally R, Steinberg JR, Corcos J: Complications of tension-free vaginal tape surgery: A multi-institutional review of 242 cases [abstract 416]. J Urol 167(Suppl):104, 2002.
27. Artman LE, Hoskins WJ, Bibro MC, et al: Radical hysterectomy and pelvic lymphadenectomy for stage 1B carcinoma of the cervix: 21 year experience. Gynecol Oncol 28:8-13, 1987.
28. Mundy AR: An anatomical explanation for bladder dysfunction following rectal and uterine surgery. Br J Urol 54:501-504, 1982.
29. Buchsbaum HJ, Plaxe SC: The urinary tract and radical hysterectomy. In Buchsbaum HJ, Schmidt JD (eds): Gynecologic and Obstetric Urology. Philadelphia, WB Saunders, 1993.
30. Bandy LC, Clarke-Pearson DL, Soper JT, et al: Long-term effects on bladder function following radical hysterectomy with and without postoperative radiation. Gynecol Oncol 26:160-168, 1987.
31. Chuang TY, Yu KJ, Penn IW, et al: Neurourological changes before and after radical hysterectomy in patients with cervical cancer. Acta Obstet Gynecol Scand 82:954-959, 2003.
32. Diels J, Cluyse L, Gaussin C, Mertens R: Hysterectomy in Belgium. Thematic files. Leuven, Christelijk Ziekenfonds, 1999.
33. Weber AM, Walters MD, Schover LR, et al: Functional outcomes and satisfaction after abdominal hysterectomy. Am J Obstet Gynecol 181:530-535, 1999.
34. Roovers JP, van der Brom JG, Huub van der Vaart C, et al: Does mode of hysterectomy influence micturition and defecation? Acta Obstet Gynecol Scand 80:945-951, 2001.
35. Everaert K, De Muynck M, Rimbaut S, Weyers S: Urinary retention after hysterectomy benign disease: Extended diagnostic evaluation and treatment with sacral nerve stimulation. BJU Int 91:497-501, 2003.
36. Wyndaele JJ: Is abnormal electrosensitivity in the lower urinary tract a sign of neuropathy? Br J Urol 72:575-579, 1993.
37. Long C, Hsu SC, Wu TP, et al: Effect of laparoscopic hysterectomy on bladder neck and urinary symptoms. Aust N Z J Obstet Gynaecol 43:65-69, 2004.
38. Long CY, Jang MY, Chen SC, et al: Changes in vesicourethral function following laparoscopic hysterectomy versus abdominal hysterectomy. Aust N Z J Obstet Gynaecol 42:259-263, 2002.
39. Virtanen H, Makinen J, Tenho T, et al: Effects of abdominal hysterectomy on urinary and sexual symptoms. Br J Urol 72:868-872, 1993.
40. Dorflinger A, Monga A: Voiding dysfunction. Curr Opin Obstet Gynecol 13:507-512, 2001.
41. Wang AC: Burch colposuspension vs. Stamey bladder neck suspension: A comparison of complications with special emphasis on

detrusor instability and voiding dysfunction. J Reprod Med 41:529-533, 1996.

42. Gomelsky A, Nitti VW, Dmochowski RR: Management of obstructive voiding dysfunction after incontinence surgery: Lessons learned. Urology 62:391-399, 2003.
43. Mundy AR: A trial comparing the Stamey bladder neck suspension with colposuspension for the treatment of stress incontinence. Br J Urol 55:687-690, 1983.
44. Juma S, Sdrales L: Etiology of urinary retention after bladder neck suspension [abstract]. J Urol 149:400A, 1993.
45. Carr LK, Webster GD: Voiding dysfunction following incontinence surgery: Diagnosis and treatment with retropubic or vaginal urethrolysis. J Urol 157:821-823, 1997.
46. Zimmern PE, Hadley HR, Leach GE, Raz S: Female urethral obstruction after Marshall-Marchetti-Krantz operation. J Urol 138:517-520, 1987.
47. Akpinalr H, Cetinel B, Demirkesen O: Long-term results in Burch colposuspension. Int J Urol 7:119-125, 2000.
48. Ward KL, Hilton P, Browning J: A randomized trial of colposuspension and tension free vaginal tape for primary stress incontinence. Neurourol Urodyn 19:386-388, 2000.
49. Holschneider CH, Solh S, Lebhertz TB, Montz FJ: The modified Pereyra procedure in recurrent stress urinary incontinence: A 15 year review. Obstet Gynecol 83:573-578, 1994.
50. Horbach NS: Suburethral sling procedures. In Ostergard D, Bent AE (eds): Urogynecology and Urodynamics Theory and Practice, 3rd ed. Baltimore, Williams & Wilkins, 1991, pp 413-421.
51. Dorflinger A, Monga A: Voiding dysfunction. Curr Opinion Obstet Gynecol 13:507-512, 2001.
52. Karram MM, Segal JL, Vassallo BJ, Kleeman SD: Complications and untoward effects of the tension-free vaginal tape procedure. Obstet Gynecol 101:929-932, 2003.
53. Morgan TO, Westney OL, McGuire EJ: Pubovaginal sling: 4-year outcome analysis and quality of life assessment. J Urol 163:1645-1648, 2000.
54. Chaiken DC, Rosenthal J, Blaivas JG: Pubovaginal fascial sling for all types of stress urinary incontinence: Long-term analysis. J Urol 160:1312-1316, 1998.
55. Klutke C, Siegel S, Carlin B, et al: Urinary retention after tension-free vaginal tape procedure: Incidence and treatment. Urology 58:697-701, 2001.
56. Kobashi KC, Dmochowski R, Mee SL, et al: Erosion of woven polyester pubovaginal sling. J Urol 162:2070-2072, 1999.
57. Leng WW, Davies BJ, Tarin T, et al: Delayed treatment of bladder outlet obstruction after sling surgery: Association with irreversible bladder dysfunction. J Urol 172(Pt 1):1379-1381, 2004.
58. Wang AC: Burch colposuspension vs. Stamey bladder neck suspension. A comparison of complications with special emphasis on detrusor overactivity and voiding dysfunction. J Reprod Med 41:529-533, 1996.
59. Bombieri L, Freeman RM, Perkins EP, et al: Why do women have voiding dysfunction and de novo detrusor instability after colposuspension? Br J Obstet Gynaecol 109:402-412, 2002.
60. Bump RC, Fantl JA, Hurt WG: Dynamic urethral pressure profilometry. Pressure transmission ratio determinations after continence surgery: Understanding the mechanism of success, failure and complications. Obstet Gynecol 72:870-874, 1988.
61. Hudson CN: Female genital prolapse and pelvic floor deficiency. Int J Colorectal Dis 3:181-185, 1988.
62. Roovers JPWR, van der Vaart CH, van der Bom JG, et al: A randomised controlled trial comparing abdominal and vaginal prolapse surgery: effects on urogenital function. BJOG 111:50-56, 2004.
63. Rosenzweig BA, Pushkin S, Blumenfeld D, Bhatia NN: Prevalence of abnormal urodynamic test results in continent women with severe genitourinary prolapse. Obstet Gynecol 79:539-542, 1992.
64. Milani R, Salvatore S, Soligo M, et al: Functional and anatomical outcome of anterior and posterior vaginal prolapse repair with prolene mesh. BJOG 111:1-5, 2004.
65. Theofrastous JP, Addison WA, Timmons MC: Voiding function following prolapse surgery. Impact of estrogen replacement. J Reprod Med 41:881-884, 1996.
66. FitzGerald MP, Kulkarni N, Fenner D: Postoperative resolution of urinary retention in patients with advanced pelvic organ prolapse. Am J Obstet Gynecol 183:1361-1364, 2000.
67. Safir MH, Gousse AE, Rovner ES, et al: 4-Defect repair of grade 4 cystocele. J Urol 161:587-594, 1999.
68. Leboeuf L, Miles RA, Kim SS, Gousse AE: Grade 4 cystocele repair using four-defect repair and porcine xenograft acellular matrix (Pelvicol): Outcome measures using SEAPI. Urology 64:282-286, 2004.
69. Frederick RW, Leach GE: Cadaveric prolapse repair with sling: Intermediate outcomes with 6 months to 5 years of follow-up. J Urol 173:1229-1233, 2005.
70. Dietz HP, Haylen BT, Vancaillie TG: Female pelvic organ prolapse and voiding function. Int Urogynecol J 13:284-288, 2002.
71. Winters JC, Cespedes RD, Vanlangendonck R: Abdominal sacral colpopexy and abdominal enterocele repair in the management of vaginal vault prolapse. Urology 56:55-63, 2000.
72. Cespedes RD: Anterior approach bilateral sacrospinous ligament fixation for vaginal vault prolapse. Urology 56:70-75, 2000.
73. Carrion R, Arap S, Corcione G, et al, for the Confederation of American Urology: A multi-institutional study of orthotopic neobladders: Functional results in men and women. BJU Int 93:803-806, 2004.
74. Fujisawa M, Isotani S, Gotoh A, et al: Voiding dysfunction of sigmoid neobladder in women: a comparative study with men. Eur Urol 40:191-195, 2001.
75. Petrou SP, Broderick GA: Valsalva leak point pressure changes after successful suburethral sling. Int Urogynecol J Pelvic Floor Dysfuct 13:299-302, 2002.
76. Foster HE, McGuire EJ: Management of urethral obstruction with transvaginal urethrolysis. J Urol 150(5 pt 1):1448-1451, 1993.
77. Goldman HB, Rackley PR, Appell RA: The efficacy of urethrolysis without resuspension for iatrogenic urethral obstruction. J Urol 161(1):196-198; discussion 198-199, 1999.

Chapter 16

IDIOPATHIC URINARY RETENTION IN THE FEMALE

Priya Padmanabhan and Nirit Rosenblum

Urinary retention describes the inability to void voluntarily with a bladder volume exceeding the expected bladder capacity. More attention has been placed on male urinary retention caused by benign prostatic hypertrophy than urinary retention in women. Causes of incomplete bladder emptying in women are as variable and numerous as in men, but the presumed infrequency and difficulty in diagnosis accounts for less focus on them.[1] The largest body of medical literature on causes of female urinary retention, even in the past decade, assumes a psychogenic or hysterical basis to the problem.[2] The exact incidence of female urinary retention is unknown, but proper workup ensures that psychogenic retention is a diagnosis of exclusion and not an assumption. Excellent reviews of causes, workup, and management of urinary retention in females were published by Nitti and Raz[1] and Smith and coworkers.[3] Classically cited causes of urinary retention include neurologic, pharmacologic, anatomic, myopathic, functional, and psychogenic origins.

There are no quantitative definitions for bladder volumes associated with urinary retention. Instead, it is the effects of the urinary retention on the female patient that is of clinical concern. Diagnosis and management are not directed at addressing a specific volume or postvoid residual (PVR) volume; instead, the focus is on treating the effects of urinary retention. The symptomatic female patient may present with abdominal discomfort, irritative voiding symptoms, recurrent urinary tract infections, and incontinence and may eventually suffer from the sequelae of long-term retention, upper tract deterioration.

Instead of describing all of the causes of urinary retention in women, we focus on the area of idiopathic urinary retention, a group of causes that was previously gathered under the term *psychogenic retention*. The following sections provide an overview of common causes of urinary retention, discuss the history and basis of idiopathic retention, and describe the diagnostic tools and treatment options for the management of *pseudomyotonia*, a term coined by Fowler in 1986.

ETIOLOGY AND PATHOPHYSIOLOGY OF URINARY RETENTION

Reviews have classified urinary retention as transient or established (i.e., requiring a more comprehensive workup). Transient causes include immobility (especially postoperative), constipation or fecal impaction, medications, urinary tract infections, delirium, endocrine abnormalities, and psychological problems. After the underlying cause is treated or the offending agent is removed, there is usually a return to normal voiding.[1,3] Common causes of established urinary retention are listed in Box 16-1.

Neurogenic Causes

Disruption in neural pathways and non-neurogenic causes can cause bladder outlet obstruction and decreased bladder contractility, leading to urinary retention. Normal voiding requires the coordinated contraction by the detrusor of adequate magnitude and concomitant lowering of resistance at the smooth and striated sphincters, with an absence of obstruction.[4] The pontine micturition center controls voiding by stimulating parasympathetic fibers at S2 to S4, causing a detrusor contraction and inhibiting sympathetic fibers (T11 to L2) and somatic fibers of the pudendal nerve (S2 to S4). This causes relaxation of the bladder neck and proximal urethra and the external urethral sphincter, respectively.[3]

Detrusor–external sphincter dyssynergia (DESD) is a neurogenic cause of bladder outlet obstruction resulting from a suprasacral spinal cord lesion. DESD is associated with myelitis, spinal cord injury (i.e., upper motor neuron), and multiple sclerosis. Video urodynamics studies (VUDS) demonstrate detrusor hyperreflexia, high detrusor pressures, an increase in external sphincter activity, and small voided volumes. The ideal treatment for DESD is anticholinergics with clean intermittent catheterization (CIC).[1,5]

Multiple sclerosis is a focal demyelinating disease with a predilection for women between the ages of 20 and 50 years. Multiple sclerosis is associated with upper motor neuron and lower motor neuron lesions and therefore causes bladder outlet obstruction and decreased bladder contractility. Between 50% and 90% of patients with multiple sclerosis complain of voiding symptoms, usually urinary retention.[6] Detrusor hyperreflexia is the most common findings on VUDS, with areflexia identified in up to 40% and DESD in up to 66%.[7] The most important factors predisposing a multiple sclerosis patient to complications are high detrusor filling pressure (>40 cm H_2O) and an indwelling Foley catheter.[8] Management includes anticholinergics with or without CIC and behavioral therapy.[9]

Cauda equina syndrome is caused by distal spinal cord injury, intervertebral disk protrusion, myelodysplasia, neoplasms, and vascular malformations, leading to decreased bladder contractility. It is associated with a complex of lower back pain, sciatica, saddle anesthesia, lower extremity weakness, sexual dysfunction, and bowel or bladder dysfunction. Urinary retention and straining are the most common urologic presentation. Diagnosis is made by computed tomography, magnetic resonance imaging (MRI), or myelography.[1,3] VUDS indicate an areflexic bladder, variable detrusor pressures, and sphincter denervation on electromyography.[10] The extent of sensory deficit in the perineal or saddle area is the most significant negative predictor of bladder function recovery.[11] Recovery of bladder function occurs

Box 16-1 Causes of Urinary Retention in Females

I. Neurogenic causes
  A. Obstruction
    1. Detrusor-sphincter dyssynergia
      a. Suprasacral spinal cord injury
      b. Myelitis
      c. Multiple sclerosis
    2. Parkinson's disease
  B. Decreased bladder contractility
    1. Lower motor neuron lesion
      a. Cauda equina injury (e.g., distal spinal cord, intervertebral disk protrusion, myelodysplasia, primary and metastatic neoplasms, vascular malformations)
      b. Pelvic plexus injury
      c. Peripheral neuropathy (e.g., diabetes mellitus, pernicious anemia, alcoholic neuropathy, tabes dorsalis, herpes zoster, Guilland-Barré syndrome, Shy-Drager syndrome)
    2. Multiple sclerosis
II. Non-neurogenic causes
  A. Obstruction
    1. Anatomic causes
      a. Primary bladder neck obstruction
      b. Inflammatory processes (e.g., bladder neck fibrosis, urethral stricture, meatal stenosis, urethral caruncle, Skene's gland cyst or abscess, urethral diverticulum)
      c. Pelvic prolapse
      d. Neoplasm (e.g., urethral carcinoma)
      e. Gynecologic, extrinsic compression (e.g., retroverted uterus, vaginal carcinoma, cervical carcinoma, ovarian mass)
      f. Iatrogenic obstruction (e.g., anti-incontinence procedures, multiple urethral dilations, urethral excision or reconstruction)
      g. Miscellaneous causes (e.g., urethral valves, ectopic ureterocele, bladder calculi, atrophic vaginitis, reconstruction)
    2. Functional causes
      a. Dysfunctional voiding
      b. External sphincter spasticity
  B. Decreased bladder contractility
    1. Hypotonia or atony
      a. Chronic obstruction
      b. Radiation cystitis
      c. Tuberculosis
    2. Detrusor hyperactivity with impaired contractility
    3. Psychogenic retention
    4. Infrequent voider's syndrome
III. Idiopathic causes (e.g., Fowler's syndrome)

over 3 to 4 years in 25% of patients with prompt surgical intervention.[3]

Pelvic plexus injury is most common during abdominoperineal resection, radical hysterectomy, proctocolectomy, and low anterior resection after injury or malignant extension to pelvic, hypogastric, and pudendal nerves. Findings of VUDS are similar to those for cauda equina syndrome. Urinary retention usually resolves within months, with one third of patients having permanent voiding dysfunction. Urodynamically, permanent voiding dysfunction is characterized by fixed, residual, striated sphincter tone and an open, nonfunctional smooth sphincter. CIC is the management of choice until normal voiding returns.[1,12]

Multiple infectious, endocrine, and nutritional abnormalities cause peripheral neuropathy and decreased bladder contractility, leading to urinary retention. The classic example is diabetic cystopathy, but others include pernicious anemia, alcoholic neuropathy, tabes dorsalis, herpes zoster infection, Guillain-Barré syndrome, and Shy-Drager syndrome. Diabetic cystopathy often has insidious loss or impairment of bladder sensation, with progressive increase in bladder volumes and hypocontractility.[13-16] Management combines behavioral modification (e.g., timed voiding, Credé voiding) and CIC to facilitate emptying.[1]

Non-neurogenic Causes

There are many non-neurogenic causes of bladder outlet obstruction and decreased bladder contractility that lead to urinary retention in the female patient (see Box 16-1). Most obstruction is classified as anatomic and functional. Anatomic obstruction includes primary bladder neck obstruction, inflammatory processes, prolapse, neoplasm, gynecologic, iatrogenic, and other causes. Functional obstruction is usually described in terms of dysfunctional voiding and external sphincter spasticity.

Primary bladder neck obstruction was introduced in 1933 by Marion[17] as a diagnosis of exclusion. Typically, these women present with irritative voiding symptoms and are given a trial of anticholinergics or antispasmodics; the course is eventual progression to periodic urinary retention or high PVR urine volumes. The exact cause is unknown, but the advent of video urodynamic testing has made diagnosis more accurate. The hallmark of primary bladder neck obstruction is incomplete opening or funneling of the bladder neck in the setting of sustained detrusor contraction of normal or high amplitude. There is resultant poor or nonexistent flow but a synergic external urethral sphincter. Management is medical and surgical. Terazosin has been used with improvement in flow rate and reduction of PVR volumes. Surgical options include transurethral incision of the bladder neck and Y-V-plasty of the bladder neck. Care is taken to avoid injury to the external sphincter, which can lead to stress urinary incontinence.[1,3,18-20]

Inflammatory processes, such as bladder neck fibrosis, urethral stricture, meatal stenosis, urethral caruncle, Skene's gland cyst or abscess, and urethral diverticulum, are associated with anatomic obstruction. Management usually involves treatment of the offending infection and surgical excision of obstructing lesions.

Patients with pelvic prolapse (e.g., uterine, cystocele, enterocele, rectocele) usually present with incomplete emptying, lower urinary tract symptoms, and recurrent urinary tract infections with or without stress urinary incontinence. They may describe positional changes or the need to reduce the prolapse to void. Bladder outlet obstruction is caused by kinking or compression of the urethra during voiding. VUDS are useful in making the diagnosis. After the initial diagnosis, a pessary or packing should be used to reduce the prolapse and confirm the diagnosis. This helps predict the outcome of prolapse repair. Treatment of symptomatic prolapse is usually surgical.[1,21] In cases of significant morbidity or age, a pessary alone may be used.

There are multiple neoplastic, obstetric, and gynecologic causes of bladder outlet obstruction in women. Urethral carcinoma is the only urologic malignancy more frequent in women (0.2%), although it remains rare. Patients present with bleeding and develop irritative and obstructive symptoms. Treatment ranges from local excision to anterior exenteration with complementary radiation therapy.[22] Gynecologic neoplasms and masses usually cause urinary retention by external compression or direct invasion. A retroverted, impacted uterus that occurs in the first trimester of pregnancy is associated with urinary retention. Gravid females are usually managed with manual dislodging of the uterus or a pessary until voiding resumes.[1]

The most common iatrogenic cause of urinary retention is surgical correction of stress urinary incontinence. The published incidence ranges from 2.5% to 24%, which may be underestimated. The irritative or obstructive voiding symptoms and recurrent urinary tract infections that result may be overlooked if the patient demonstrates normal emptying. The placement of sutures is the key factor determining a procedure's likelihood of causing obstruction. For example, sutures placed too medially cause urethral deviation or periurethral scarring; those placed too distally can cause kinking, leading to stress urinary incontinence; and tying sutures too tightly leads to hypersuspension, closing the bladder neck.[1] Newer mid-urethral slings can cause bladder outlet obstruction if the urethra is injured or the tape is placed under tension. The diagnosis is made by a patient's history before the procedure, physical examination, VUDS, endoscopy, and imaging. Urethrolysis is the treatment of choice. However, several studies have not correlated urodynamics and successful voiding after urethrolysis.[23-25]

Other iatrogenic causes of bladder outlet obstruction include a history of recurrent urethral dilation and postoperative urethral strictures. Urethral dilation leads to postdilatation bleeding or urine extravasation into periurethral tissue, causing scarring of the urethral wall and periurethral fibrosis.[26] This is diagnosed with VUDS and managed with transurethral resection or incision. Urethral strictures are rare in women, but they are seen endoscopically after urethral surgery and prior instrumentation. They are usually managed with periodic self-catheterization, permanent CIC, transurethral incision, or urethral reconstruction.[1]

Dysfunctional voiding and external sphincter spasticity are non-neurogenic functional causes of bladder outlet obstruction. Both conditions have been associated with inappropriate electromyographic activity during micturition with decreased urinary flow[27] and with high pressure increases in the urethral pressure profile. Dysfunctional voiding is referred to as *pseudodyssynergia* (which mimics DESD), because it is a learned behavior that can be treated and cured. Treatment combines timed voiding, biofeedback, and anticholinergics.[1] External sphincter spasticity, characterized by "spasticity of the external sphincter and pelvic floor"[28] results from introital or vaginal infections, Skene's gland abscesses, adnexal disease, or cystitis. Pudendal nerve block improves voiding. VUDS reveal a bladder with intact sensation without the ability to contract due to cortical inhibition from the spastic pelvic floor.[21] After managing painful or inflammatory lesions, treatment involves pharmacologic agents, including muscle relaxants and α-blockers. α-Blockers relax the bladder neck and urethra and enhance pelvic ganglionic transmission, which improves detrusor contraction. α-Blockers also treat the urinary retention that develops from transient spasticity.[1,26,28]

Non-neurogenic bladder hypocontractility is associated with radiation cystitis, chronic obstruction, and tuberculosis. Irradiation causes fibrosis of the lamina propria and muscular layers, leading to muscle cell death. The enlarged intercellular gaps in circular and longitudinal muscle fibers cause spasms and poorly coordinated detrusor contractions, with eventual hypocontractility or areflexia.[29-31] In chronic obstruction, the detrusor develops smooth muscle hypertrophy, a reduction in myofilaments, and damaged mitochondria within detrusor smooth muscle cells. This leads to a progressive decrease in detrusor contractility.[32] In all of these cases, complete VUDS are required for diagnosis and treatment of the urinary retention.

Decreased bladder contractility occurs in the detrusor hyperactivity with impaired contractility syndrome. This was discovered in a nursing home population; the women had opposite bladder reflex and contractile functions. Uninhibited contractions emptied less than one half of the bladder. Impaired neuromuscular transmission at the detrusor or myopathic processes (e.g., cellular degeneration) are proposed causes of the decreased contractility.[33,34] VUDS are essential for diagnosis, with the addition of fluoroscopically monitored synchronous cystosphincterometry to rule out other conditions. CIC is the mainstay of therapy.[33]

When urinary retention occurs with no organic disease but with centrally mediated, subconscious inhibition of detrusor contraction or sphincter relaxation, it is referred to as *psychogenic retention*. Psychological trauma (e.g., sexual) is one cause. Findings of VUDS are normal except for delayed sensation and a large-capacity bladder. It is usually temporary and responds well to supportive management. Treatment includes psychiatric support and CIC until normal voiding returns. With severe detrusor degeneration, some patients become dependent on CIC.[35]

IDIOPATHIC URINARY RETENTION: FOWLER'S SYNDROME

Pathogenesis

Historically, women with chronic, painless bladder distention were labeled as having a psychological problem. In 1986, Fowler and Kirby[36] identified a group of 19 young women with longstanding urinary retention who had distinctive electromyographic activity and impaired urethral relaxation. Electromyography with a concentric-needle electrode was used to study the striated muscle of the urethral sphincters in these patients. Concentric needle electromyography is useful in testing the integrity of the motor innervation arising from the S2 to S4 spinal levels and the activity associated with urethral sphincter striated muscle impairment. The impairment identified by Fowler and Kirby[36] was referred to as decelerating bursts and complex repetitive discharges (CRDs). CRDs are caused by direct spread of electrical activity form one muscle fiber to another, producing a low "jitter" sound on the audio output of the electromyographic machine. The decelerating bursts produce a sound similar to whales singing in the ocean, and laboratory research describes patients in retention with these findings as "whale noise, positive or negative."[37-39] The bursts of depolarizing activity in the semicircular urethral sphincter muscle impair normal relaxation of the muscle. This impedes normal bladder emptying, causing an insidious increase in residual volumes and bladder distention. The investigators noticed the similarity of this electromyographic activity and the bizarre, high-frequency discharges associated with reinnervation.[36] However, reinnervation was thought unlikely, because abnormal burst discharges are infrequent in patients with cauda equina lesions or Shy-Drager syndrome.[40,41]

Fowler and colleagues[42] further associated these electromyographic abnormalities with endocrine dysfunction and polycystic ovarian disease (PCOD). Thirty-three of 57 women with urinary retention or voiding dysfunction had abnormal electromyographic activity. Sixty-four percent of this group had polycystic ovaries, seen on pelvic ultrasound. The other women in the group also demonstrated ovarian disturbances (e.g., single or bilateral oophorectomy, premature ovarian failure). High concentrations of circulating androgens and estrogens and low levels of progesterone are seen in women with PCOD. Progesterone stabilizes membranes. Progesterone deficiency in PCOD was hypothesized to reduce urethral sphincter muscle membrane stability, enabling the establishment of a circuitous excitatory pathway between muscle fibers.[42]

Concentric needle electromyographic measurements of the external urethral sphincter during micturition in women with voiding dysfunction and proximal urethral dilation (on VUDS) by Deindl and coworkers[43] confirmed the correlation between abnormal bursts of CRD and poor urinary stream. This provided support for the association between sphincter electromyographic overactivity and impaired relaxation.[44] A significant number of women with voiding dysfunction also have symptoms of fecal incontinence. Webb and colleagues[45] described the dysfunction of the urethral sphincter in idiopathic urinary retention as part of a more widespread disorder of the entire pelvic floor. All of the women studied had undergone urethral dilation in the past and were performing CIC. Similar abnormalities in the urethral and anal sphincters were seen, including polyphasic and abnormally long duration of potentials and CRD.[45] Anatomically, the striated sphincter muscle of the urethra and the anal sphincter receive their nerve supply through the pudendal nerve from the sacral plexus, explaining the correlation in electromyographic abnormalities.[46]

Clinical Presentation

Using a survey questionnaire, Swinn and associates[2] described the typical profile of a woman with idiopathic urinary retention. Of 91 women who completed the survey, the mean age at retention onset was 27.7 years (range, 10 to 50 years), with a mean maximal bladder capacity of 1208 mL at the initial episode of retention. Thirty-five percent of these women developed retention spontaneously, 43% developed retention after a surgical procedure (usually gynecologic), and in 15%, childbirth was the preceding event. Eighty-six (94%) of the 91 women performed CIC, with 69% complaining of difficulty passing the catheter because of “something gripping” it. Fifty percent of the study group had PCOD. Voiding spontaneously returned in 38 patients. Sacral neuromodulation was the only therapy that restored function in the other 53 patients.[2]

Diagnosis

There are no universally accepted criteria for diagnosing bladder outlet obstruction in women. Many investigators[47-51] have proposed urodynamic criteria for classification of bladder outlet obstruction, attempting to identify cutoffs for maximal flow rate, maximal detrusor pressure, and PVR volumes. Consistently, the absolute values were not as dramatic as seen in men, and diagnosis relied on imaging of the bladder outlet during micturition.[47-51] Based on the criteria used to evaluate bladder outlet obstruction, women with idiopathic retention are within the mildly obstructed range. VUDS in these patients typically show a prolonged filling phase and large bladder capacity, with reduced sensations of filling and limited detrusor pressure rise during the voiding phase. However, there are no definite urodynamic criteria to diagnose idiopathic retention in women. The basis for diagnosis remains a typical history and the abnormalities of the sphincter electromyographic activity as described earlier.[52,53]

Other ancillary indicators used in the diagnosis of idiopathic retention include urethral pressures and urethral sphincter volumes. Urethral pressure measurements have been used for almost a century to assess urethral closure function,[54] representing the urethra’s ability to leak. Urethral pressures are criticized for not being a “real physical pressure” in a fluid, based on Griffiths’ definition of urethral pressure as the fluid pressure needed to open a closed (collapsed) tube.[55,56] Measurement of urethral pressure (UPM) requires introduction of a Foley catheter, which introduces a nonzero cross-sectional area (zero cross-sectional area when urethra collapses) and changes the shape of the urethral lumen.[57] Historically, these measurements have not been standardized and fluctuate based on catheter type, cross section of the probe, patient position, and bladder filling pressures. The standard parameters do not discriminate between voiding dysfunctions, identify underlying pathophysiology, return to normal after surgery (as seen after incontinence procedures), or provide a reliable indicator of surgical success. UPM is useful in identifying strictures or diverticula and targeting interventions (e.g., low-pressure urethra).[55] In 2002, The Standardisation Sub-committee of the International Continence Society attempted to define UPM and recommend standards for measurement.[57]

The abnormal, myotonia-like electromyographic activity seen in women with idiopathic retention is theoretically expected to increase the bulk of urethral sphincter muscle by work-induced hypertrophy. Transvaginal or transrectal ultrasound (TRUS) has been used to image bladder outlet obstruction and identify pelvic pathology.[58,59] Later, MRI was used for the diagnosis of female urethral pathology.[60] Noble and associates[61]. used TRUS to compare urethral sphincter volumes in women with obstructed voiding with age-matched controls. The volume of the urethral sphincter in obstructed women was more than 2 cm^3 greater ($P < .001$) than in the control group. TRUS was unable to visualize the three layers of the urethral sphincter, which is elucidated better with MRI.[61] Wiseman and colleagues.[62] evaluated urethral closure pressure and sphincter volume transvaginally in women with electromyographic abnormalities and idiopathic urinary retention. The maximum urethral closure pressure and ultrasound volume were significantly higher in the group with electromyographic abnormalities.[62] These studies support the concept of sphincter electromyographic overactivity producing sphincteric hypertrophy. These assessments may be improved with the use of MRI instead of ultrasound for volume measurement.[53]

Treatment

All management strategies are directed at successful bladder emptying. Successful treatment abolishes the myotonia-like electromyographic activity and improves urethral relaxation. CIC, rather than indwelling or suprapubic cystotomy, is traditionally the option given to many women with idiopathic retention. Other medical and surgical options, such as oral agents, urethral botulinum toxin, sacral neuromodulation, and biofeedback, have been used. The only treatment that has conclusively restored voiding is sacral neuromodulation.[53]

Oral Agents

There are limited data on the use of oral agents, such as α-blockers or β-agonists, in the treatment of functional bladder neck obstruction. In a study of 24 women with retention treated with α-blockers and initial CIC, only 50% had a significantly sustained improvement in PVR and peak flow. The group that failed α-blocker treatment returned to CIC or had a bladder neck incision.[63]

The effects of tamsulosin on urethral pressures in healthy women were studied at rest and after sacral magnetic stimulation. Tamsulosin did significantly reduce the mean and maximal urethral pressures acquired in all three segments (i.e., proximal, middle and distal) of the urethra. The amplitude of urethral contractions after sacral magnetic stimulation was unchanged after tamsulosin. These results may support tamsulosin's use in female retention from an overactive or nonrelaxing urethra.[64]

Bethanechol has been used as treatment for retention caused by detrusor acontractility, but it has not been used in women with sphincteric overactivity.[65] Its treatment value is therefore unknown.

Botulinum A Toxin

There has been mixed success with the use of botulinum toxin in treating chronic urinary retention in women. Botulinum A toxin is an inhibitor of acetylcholine release at the presynaptic neuromuscular junction, which decreases regional muscle contractility and causes muscle atrophy at the site of injection.[66,67] Fowler and coworkers[68] evaluated six women with a characteristic pattern of electromyographic activity by injecting botulinum toxin into each of their striated urethral sphincters. Three of the six women experienced stress incontinence for 10 days, and three had no change. Although the botulinum toxin did not have a beneficial effect, the result of stress incontinence did ensure that sufficient botulinum was given to weaken the striated sphincter muscle. This supported the hypothesis that abnormal sphincteric activity results from an "ephaptic transmission of impulses between muscle fibers" and not repetitive firing of reinnervated motor units.[68]

Phelan and colleagues[66] were the first to report successful outcomes with botulinum A injections in women and in nonneurogenic voiding dysfunction. They studied 21 patients (13 women) with impaired bladder emptying who were dependent on catheterization. All except one were able to void spontaneously after an injection of 80 to 100 units of botulinum toxin.[66] This denervation by botulinum is reversible because new axons sprout in 3 to 6 months.[69] Patients had repeat injections at intervals consistent with this regrowth. In some cases, the injection had clinical efficacy beyond 6 months, suggesting neural plasticity or altered neuromuscular junction dynamics.[66] Kuo and associates[70] repeated this study in 20 patients with urinary retention or dysuria due to detrusor hypocontractility and nonrelaxing urethral sphincter who were refractory to conservative therapy. This study clearly showed that botulinum toxin is effective in decreasing urethral sphincter resistance and improving voiding efficiency in patients with various type of lower urinary tract dysfunction.[70] Botulinum A toxin injections do have therapeutic value in urethral spasticity, but larger, controlled trials are necessary to establish their role.[71]

Tanagho and Schmidt[72] are responsible for the first implantable sacral nerve stimulators (SNSs). The effects of SNSs depend on the electrical stimulation of somatic afferent axons in spinal roots, which modulate voiding and continence reflex pathways in the central nervous system. In urinary retention, SNSs are responsible for turning off excitatory outflow to the urethral outlet, which promotes bladder emptying.[73] Traditionally, a test percutaneous nerve evaluation is performed under local anesthesia by inserting a stimulating electrode through the S3 foramen. This lead is left in place for 4 to 7 days, during which a voiding diary is kept. If the patient has a more than 50% improvement in voiding function, the implant is considered effective, and a permanent implantable pulse generator (IPG) is placed.

Recognized complications of neuromodulation include lead migration, pain at the IPG box site or ipsilateral leg, infection, and lack of efficacy.[53] To improve the efficacy of chronic sacral neuromodulation, the placement of bilateral SNSs has been proposed. Scheepens and colleagues[74] compared unilateral with bilateral SNSs in a series of women with urinary retention and found no significant differences, except for two patients with complete obstruction, who voided only with bilateral stimulation.

Sacral Neuromodulation

Sacral neuromodulation has been shown in many studies to restore voiding function in women with urinary retention. The results of peripheral nerve evaluation testing in 34 patients with Fowler's syndrome revealed an overall success rate of 68%. This compares favorably with a reported success rate of 30% to 50% for the period of trial stimulation of all lower urinary tract dysfunctions.[75] Shaker and Hassouna[76] treated 20 patients (19 women) with idiopathic, nonobstructing, chronic urinary retention dependent on CIC who had at least a 50% improvement on percutaneous nerve evaluation screening. These patients were followed for a mean of 15.2 months and had significant improvement in voiding function, pelvic pain, and sensation of emptiness after voiding. The study authors emphasize that the lack of change in cystometrography after SNS implantation indicates that the cause of the problem is not the bladder but the pelvic floor musculature.[76]

Investigators have reported good results after SNS when there are pelvic floor electromyographic activity abnormalities. Their explanation is that patients with chronic urinary retention fail to identify their pelvic floor muscles and are incapable of relaxing the pelvic floor to initiate the voiding reflex. The permanent contraction of the pelvic floor is thought responsible for detrusor inhibition. Neuromodulation provides increased awareness of the pelvic floor and allows relaxation of the hypertonic pelvic floor musculature. The mechanism involves sacral stimulation of presynaptic inhibition of afferents to the spastic muscle motor neurons at the level of the dorsal column.[77-80]

A prospective, randomized, multicenter trial enrolled 177 patients with urinary retention (74% were female), with a follow-up of 18 months. Sixty-eight of these women qualified for an IPG and were divided into treatment and control groups. At 6 months, 83% of the implant groups had successful results, compared with 9% of the controls. Temporary inactivation of the SNS resulted in a significant increase in the PVR volume. This supports the idea that the SNS does not cure the underlying mechanism of urinary retention, but instead controls aberrant dysfunctional reflexes causing voiding dysfunction.[77,81]

Dasgupta and colleagues[82] provided long-term results of SNSs in women with Fowler's syndrome. This retrospective study included 26 women who were followed for more than 6 years. Seventy-seven percent were voiding successfully more than 5 years postoperatively; 54% required revision surgery. The longevity of an IPG battery is 7 to 10 years. This study supported the effectiveness of SNSs for at least 5 years after implantation.[82]

Behavioral Treatment and Biofeedback

Behavioral and biofeedback treatments are safe, noninvasive, and effective interventions that are useful in the management of idiopathic urinary retention. Behavioral changes enlighten patients about their fluid intake and voiding behavior. Biofeedback involves surface or internal (vaginal or rectal) electrodes that transduce muscle potentials into auditory or visual signals. This helps the patient learn to increase or decrease voluntary muscle activity.[83]

CONCLUSIONS

There are many neurogenic and non-neurogenic causes of urinary retention in the female patient. Idiopathic urinary retention and Fowler's syndrome should be considered in any young female with insidious, painless retention and urethral sphincter overactivity identified on electromyography. The diagnosis combines a thorough history with abnormal electromyographic and urodynamic findings. Sacral neuromodulation offers the best option in restoring voiding function. Although the exact mechanism of action of sacral stimulation is not established, evidence supports action through the afferent pathways. Other accessory treatment options, such as botulinum and tamsulosin, have some therapeutic merits, but they require larger, long-term, case-controlled studies in women with urethral overactivity. Behavioral modification and biofeedback are safe and effective and should be considered as first-line treatment for voiding dysfunction.

References

1. Nitti VW, Raz S: Urinary Retention in Female Urology, 2nd ed. Philadelphia, WB Saunders, 1996, pp 197-213.
2. Swinn MJ, Wiseman OJ, Lowe E, Folwer CJ: The causes of and natural history of isolated urinary retention in young women. J Urol 167:151-156, 2002.
3. Smith CP, Kraus SR, Boone TB: Urinary retention in the young female. AUA Update Series 18:145-152, 1999.
4. Wein AJ, Levin RM, Barrett DM: Voiding function and dysfunction. Voiding function relevant to anatomy, physiology and pharmacology. In Gillenwater JY, Grayhack JT, Howards SS, Duckett JW (eds): Adult and Pediatric Urology, 2nd ed, vol I. St. Louis, Mosby–Year Book, 1991, p 933.
5. O'Donnell PD: Electromyography. In Nitti VW (ed): Practical Urodynamics. Philadelphia, WB Saunders, 1998, p 70.
6. Litwiller SE, Frohman EM, Zimmern PE: Multiple sclerosis and the urologist. J Urol 61:743-757, 1999.
7. Hinson JL, Boone TB: Urodynamics and multiple sclerosis. Urol Clin North Am 12:475-481, 1996.
8. Chancellor MB, Blaivas JG: Multiple sclerosis. Probl Urol 7:15-33, 1993.
9. Sirls LT, Zimmern PE, Leach GE: Role of limited evaluation and aggressive medical management in multiple sclerosis: A review of 113 patients. J Urol 151:946-950, 1994.
10. Watanabe T, Chancellor MB, Rivas DA: Neurogenic voiding dysfunction. In Nitti VW (ed): Practical Urodynamics. Philadelphia, WB Saunders, 1998, p 148.
11. Kostuik JP, Harrington I, Alexander D, et al: Cauda equina syndrome and lumbar disc herniation. J Bone Joint Surg Am 68:386-391, 1986.
12. Wein AJ: Neuromuscular dysfunction of the lower urinary tract and its management. In Walsh PC, Retik AB, Vaughan ED, Wein AJ (eds): Campbell's Urology, 8th ed, vol II. Philadelphia, Saunders, 2002, p 955.
13. Frimodt-Moller C, Mortensen S: Diabetic cystopathy: Epidemiology and related disorders. Ann Intern Med 92:327-328, 1980.
14. Ellenberg M: Development of urinary bladder dysfunction in diabetes mellitus. Ann Intern Med 92(Pt 2):321-323, 1980.
15. Bradley WE: Diagnosis of urinary bladder dysfunction in diabetes mellitus. Ann Intern Med 92(Pt 2):323-326, 1980.
16. Frimodt-Moller C, Mortensen S: Treatment of diabetic cystopathy. Ann Intern Med 92(Pt 2):327-328, 1980.
17. Marion G: Surgery of the neck of the bladder. Br J Urol 5:351, 1933.
18. Axelrod SL, Blaivas JG: Bladder neck obstruction in women. J Urol 137:497-499, 1987.
19. Gronbaek K, Struckmann JR, Frimodt-Moller C: The treatment of female bladder neck dysfunction. Scand J Urol Nephrol 26:113-118, 1992.
20. Diokno AC, Hollander JB, Bennett CJ: Bladder neck obstruction in women: A real entity. J Urol 132:294-298, 1984.
21. Nitti VW: Bladder outlet obstruction in women. In Nitti VW (ed): Practical Urodynamics. Philadelphia, WB Saunders, 1998, pp 207-209.
22. Sardosky MF: Urethral carcinoma. AUA Update Series 6:13, 1987.
23. Nitti VW, Raz S: Obstruction following anti-incontinence procedures: Diagnosis and treatment with transvaginal urethrolysis. J Urol 152:93-98, 1994.
24. Foster HE, McGuire EJ: Management of urethral obstruction with transvaginal urethrolysis. J Urol 150:1448-1451, 1993.
25. Webster GD, Kreder KJ: Voiding dysfunction following cystourethropexy: Its evaluation and management. J Urol 144:670-673, 1990.
26. Bass JS, Leach GE: Bladder outlet obstruction in women. Probl Urol 5:141, 1991.
27. Kaplan W, Firlit CF, Schoenber HW: The female urethral syndrome: External sphincter spasm as etiology. J Urol 124:48-49, 1980.
28. Raz S, Smith RB: External sphincter spasticity syndrome in female patients. J Urol 115:443-446, 1976.
29. Antonakopoulous GN, Hicks RM, Berry RJ: The subcellular basis of damage to the human urinary bladder induced by radiation. J Pathol 143:103-116, 1984.
30. Mikhailov MCH, Elsaber E, Welscher UE: Immediate mechanical reactions of isolated human detrusor muscle on x-irradiation. Strahlentherapie 155:284-286, 1979.
31. Zoubek J, McGuire EJ, Noll F, et al: The late occurrence of urinary tract damage in patients successfully treated by radiotherapy for cervical carcinoma. J Urol 141:1347-1349, 1989.
32. Gosling JA, Kung LS, Dixon JS, et al: Correlation between the structure and function of the rabbit urinary bladder following partial outlet obstruction. J Urol 163:1349-1356, 2000.
33. Resnick NM, Yalla SV: Detrusor hyperactivity with impaired contractile function—An unrecognized but common cause of incontinence in elderly patients. JAMA 257:3076-3081, 1987.
34. Elbadawi A, Yalla SV, Resnick NM: Structural basis of geriatric voiding dysfunction. III. Detrusor overactivity. J Urol 150:1668-1680, 1993.
35. Barrett DM: Evaluation of psychogenic urinary retention. J Urol 120:191-192, 1978.
36. Fowler CJ, Kirby RS: Electromyography of urethral sphincter in women with urinary retention. Lancet 1:1455-1456, 1986.

37. Butler WJ: Pseudomyotonia of the periurethral sphincter in women with urinary incontinence. J Urol 122:838-840, 1979.
38. Fowler CJ, Kirby RS, Harrison MJG: Decelerating bursts and complex repetitive discharges in the striated muscle of the urethral sphincter associated with urinary retention in women. J Neurol Neurosurg Psychiatry 48:1004-1009, 1985.
39. Trontelj J, Stolberg E: Bizarre repetitive discharges recorded with single fibre EMG. J Neurol Neurosurg Psychiatry 46:310-316, 1983.
40. Fowler CJ, Kirby RS, Harrison MJG et al: Individual motor unit analysis in the diagnosis of disorders of urethral sphincter innervation. J Neurol Neurosurg Psychiatry 47:637-641, 1984.
41. Kirby R, Fowler C, Gosling J, Bannister R: Urethro-vesical dysfunction in progressive autonomic failure with multiple system atrophy. J Neurol Neurosurg Psychiatry 49:554-562, 1986.
42. Fowler CJ, Christmas TJ, Chapple CR, et al: Abnormal electromyographic activity of the urethral sphincter, voiding dysfunction, and polycystic ovaries: A new syndrome? BMJ 297:1436-1438, 1988.
43. Deindl FM, Vodusek DB, Bischoff C, et al: Dysfunctional voiding in women: Which muscles are responsible? Br J Urol 82:814-819, 1998.
44. DasGupta R, Fowler CJ: The management of female voiding dysfunction: Fowler's syndrome—A contemporary update. Curr Opin Urol 13:293-299, 2003.
45. Webb RJ, Fawcett PRW, Neal DE: Electromyographic abnormalities in the urethral and anal sphincters of women with idiopathic retention of urine. 70:22-25, 1992.
46. Brooks JD: Anatomy of the lower urinary tract and male genitalia. In Walsh PC, Retik AB, Vaughan ED, Wein AJ (eds): Campbell's Urology, 8th ed, vol 1. Philadelphia, WB Saunders, 2002, pp 54-55.
47. Farrar DJ, Osborne JL, Stephenson TP, et al: A urodynamic view of bladder outflow obstruction in the female: Factors influencing the results of treatment. Br J Urol 47:815-822, 1976.
48. Axelrod SL, Blaivas JG: Bladder neck obstruction in women. J Urol 137:497-499, 1987.
49. Massey JA, Abrams PH: Obstructed voiding in the female. Br J Urol 61:36-39, 1988.
50. Nitti VN, TU LM, Gitlin J: Diagnosing bladder outlet obstruction in women. J Urol 161:1535-1540, 1999.
51. Blaivas JG, Groutz A: Bladder outlet obstruction nomogram for women with lower urinary tract symptomatology. Neurourol Urodyn 19:553-564, 2000.
52. DasGupta R, Fowler CJ: Urodynamic study of women in urinary retention treated with sacral neuromodulation. 171:1161-1164, 2004.
53. DasGupta R, Fowler CJ: The management of female voiding dysfunction: Fowler's syndrome—A contemporary update. Curr Opin Urol 13:293-299, 2003.
54. Bonney V: On diurnal incontinence of urine in women. J Obstet Gynaecol Br Emp 30:358-365, 1923.
55. Lose G: Urethral pressure measurement—Problems and clinical value. Scand J Urol Nephrol 207(Suppl):61-66, 2001.
56. Griffiths D: The pressure within a collapsible tube with special reference to urethral pressure. Phys Med Biol 9;951-961, 1985.
57. Lose G, Griffiths D, Hosker G, et al: Standardisation of urethral pressure measurement: Report from the Standardisation Sub-Committee of the International Continence Society. 21:258-260, 2002.
58. Hennigan HW, DuBose TJ: Sonography of the normal female urethra. AJR Am J Roentgenol 145:839-841, 1985.
59. Leonor de Gonzalez E, Cosgrove DO, Joseph AE, et al: The appearances on ultrasound of the female urethral sphincter. Br J Radiol 61:687-690, 1988.
60. Klutke C, Golomb J, Barbaric Z, Raz S: The anatomy of stress incontinence: Magnetic resonance imaging of the female bladder neck and urethra. J Urol 143:563-566, 1990.
61. Noble JG, Dixon PJ, Rickards D, et al: Urethral sphincter volumes in women with obstructed voiding and abnormal sphincter electromyographic activity. Br J Urol 76:741-746, 1995.
62. Wiseman OJ, Swinn MJ, Brady C, et al: Maximum urethral closure pressure and sphincter volume in women with urinary retention. J Urol 167:1348-1352, 2002.
63. Kumar A, Mandhani A, Gogoi S, et al: Management of functional bladder neck obstruction in women: Use of α-blockers and pediatric resectoscope for bladder neck incision. J Urol 162:2061-2065, 1999.
64. Reitz A, Haferkamp A, Kyburz T, et al: The effect of tamsulosin on the resting tone and the contractile behaviour of the female urethra: A functional urodynamic study in healthy women. Eur Urol 46:235-240, 2004.
65. Riedl CR, Stephen RL, Daha LK, et al: Electromotive administration of intravesical bethanechol and the clinical impact on acontractile detrusor management: Introduction of a new test. J Urol 164:2108-2111, 2000.
66. Phelan MW, Franks M, Somogyi GT, et al: Botulinum toxin urethral sphincter injection to restore bladder emptying in men and women with voiding dysfunction. J Urol 165:1107-1110, 2001.
67. Duchen LW: Changes in motor innervation and cholinesterase localization induced by botulinum toxin in skeletal muscle of mouse: Differences between fast and slow muscles. J Neurol Neurosurg Psychiatry 33:40-54, 1970.
68. Fowler CJ, Betts CD, Swash CM, et al: Botulinum toxin in the treatment of chronic urinary retention in women. Br J Urol 70:387-389, 1992.
69. Borodic GE, Joseph M, Fay L, et al: Botulinum A toxin for the treatment of spasmodic torticollis—Dysphagia and regional toxin spread. Head Neck 12:392-399, 1990.
70. Kuo H-C: Botulinum A toxin urethral injection for the treatment of lower urinary tract dysfunction. J Urol 170:1908-1912, 2003.
71. Leippold T, Reitz A, Schurch B: Botulinum toxin as a new therapy option for voiding disorders: Current state of the art. Eur Urol 44:165-174, 2003.
72. Tanagho E, Schmidt R: Electrical stimulation in the clinical management of the neurogenic bladder. J Urol 140:1331-1339, 1988.
73. Leng WW, Chancellor MB: How sacral nerve stimulation neuromodulation works. Urol Clin North Am 32:11-18, 2005.
74. Scheepens WA, de Bie RA, Weil EH, et al: Unilateral versus bilateral sacral neuromodulation in patients with chronic voiding dysfunction. J Urol 168:2046-2050, 2002.
75. Swinn MJ, Kitchen ND, Goodwin RJ, et al: Sacral neuromodulation for women with Fowler's syndrome. Eur Urol 38:439-443, 2000.
76. Shaker H, Hassouna M: Sacral root neuromodulation in idiopathic nonobstructive chronic urinary retention. J Urol 159:1476-1478, 1998.
77. Schultz-Lampel D, Jiang C, Lindstrom S, et al: Experimental results on mechanism of action of electrical neuromodulation in chronic urinary retention. World J Urol 16:301-304, 1998.
78. De Ridder D, Van Poppel H, Baert L: Sacral nerve stimulation is a successful treatment for Fowler syndrome. Neurourol Urodyn 15:120, 1996.
79. Everaert K, Plancke H, Oosterlinck W: Urodynamic evaluation of neuromodulation (subchronic) in patients with voiding dysfunctions. Neurourol Urodyn 14:114, 1996.
80. Schmidt RA, Vapnek J, Tanagho EA: Restoration of voiding in chronic retention states. Neurourol Urodyn 15:365, 1996.
81. Jonas U, Fowler CJ, Chancellor MB, et al: Efficacy of sacral nerve stimulation for urinary retention: Results 18 months after implantation. J Urol 165:15-19, 2001.
82. Dasgupta R, Wiseman OJ, Kitchen N, et al: Long-term result of sacral neuromodulation for women with urinary retention. BJU Int 94:335-337, 2004.
83. Doggweiler-Wiygul R, Sellhorn E: Role of behavioral changes and biofeedback in urology. World J Urol 20:302-305, 2002.

Section 4

OVERACTIVE BLADDER

Chapter 17

CLINICAL DIAGNOSIS OF OVERACTIVE BLADDER

Samih Al-Hayek and Paul Abrams

TERMINOLOGY

Overactive bladder (OAB) is a newly described condition. It was probably first alluded to by Dudley in 1905 when he distinguished between active and passive incontinence due to sphincter weakness.[1] In 1917, Taylor and Watt reported the importance of urgency, as a symptom, during history taking, to distinguish incontinence with and without urgency.[2] Bates and colleagues introduced the term *unstable bladder* in 1970 when they used cinecysturethrography to investigate urge incontinence.[3]

The International Continence Society (ICS) established a committee for the standardization of terminology of lower urinary tract function to facilitate comparison of results and enable effective communication by investigators. Since 1976, a large number of standardization reports have been published, the latest in 2002.[4-19]

In 2002, the ICS subcommittee restated the principle of describing any lower urinary tract dysfunction from four aspects: as a symptom (taken by detailed history), a sign (physical examination and bedside tests), a condition, and a urodynamic observation in addition to the terminology related to therapies.[1]

The lower urinary tract is composed of the bladder and the urethra. When reference is made to the whole anatomic organ, "vesica urinaria," the correct term is *bladder*. When the smooth muscle structure known as the "m. detrusor urinae" is being discussed, the correct term is *detrusor*.

OAB was defined by the ICS in 2002 as urgency, with or without urge incontinence, usually with frequency and nocturia, in the absence of local pathologic or endocrine factors.

The OAB term was introduced for use in a consensus conference in 1996, as an alternative to "unstable bladder." It was believed that the term "overactive bladder" would facilitate communication between patients and health care staff.

OAB symptoms are part of the storage symptoms that are experienced during the storage phase of the bladder and include the following:

- *Urgency* is the complaint of a sudden compelling desire to pass urine that is difficult to defer.
- *Increased daytime frequency* is the complaint by the patient who considers that she voids too often by day. This term is equivalent to "pollakisuria," a term used in many countries.
- *Nocturia* is the complaint that the patient has to wake at night one or more times to void. The term *nighttime frequency* differs from nocturia, because it includes voids that occur after the patient has gone to bed but before he or she has gone to sleep, as well as voids that occur in the early morning and prevent the patient from getting back to sleep as he or she wishes. These voids before and after sleep may need to be considered in research studies (e.g., nocturnal polyuria). If this definition were used, then an adapted definition of daytime frequency would need to be used with it.
- *Urinary incontinence* (UI) is the complaint of any involuntary leakage of urine. In each specific circumstance, UI should be further described by specifying relevant factors such as type, frequency, severity, precipitating factors, social impact, effect on hygiene and quality of life, measures used to contain the leakage, and whether the patient seeks or desires help because of UI. Urinary leakage may need to be distinguished from sweating or vaginal discharge.
- *Urgency urinary incontinence* (UUI) is the complaint of involuntary leakage accompanied by or immediately preceded by urgency. UUI can manifest in various symptomatic forms; for example, as frequent small losses between micturitions or as a catastrophic leak with complete bladder emptying.

These symptom combinations of OAB are suggestive of *detrusor overactivity* (DO), a urodynamic diagnosis, which is characterized by involuntary detrusor contractions during bladder filling; it may be spontaneous or provoked. Figure 17-1 represents the relationships among OAB, UUI, and DO.

EPIDEMIOLOGY

Until recently, most studies have looked at the prevalence of UI; as a result, prevalence data on OAB are lacking. The other difficulty in estimating the scale of the problem is the variation among studies in definitions used, methods of collecting data, and populations studied.

Almost all surveys on UI concluded that stress urinary incontinence (SUI) is the most common type of UI in women. In the large Epidemiology of Incontinence in the County of Nord-Trondelag (EPINCONT) study, 50% of the incontinent women had SUI, 36% had mixed urinary incontinence (MUI), and 11% had UUI.[20] The recent literature review by Minassian and colleagues reported similar prevalence rates for the various types of UI.[21] The survey carried out by Diokno and associates[22] showed that symptoms of MUI were most frequently reported; however, this study differed from the others in that only elderly people were assessed.

The results of these studies were based on symptoms only; if urodynamics had been used to confirm the diagnosis, the results might have been different. In one study with 863 women, most of the subjects with symptoms of MUI were diagnosed to have pure SUI (42%) during urodynamic testing.[23] Weidner and

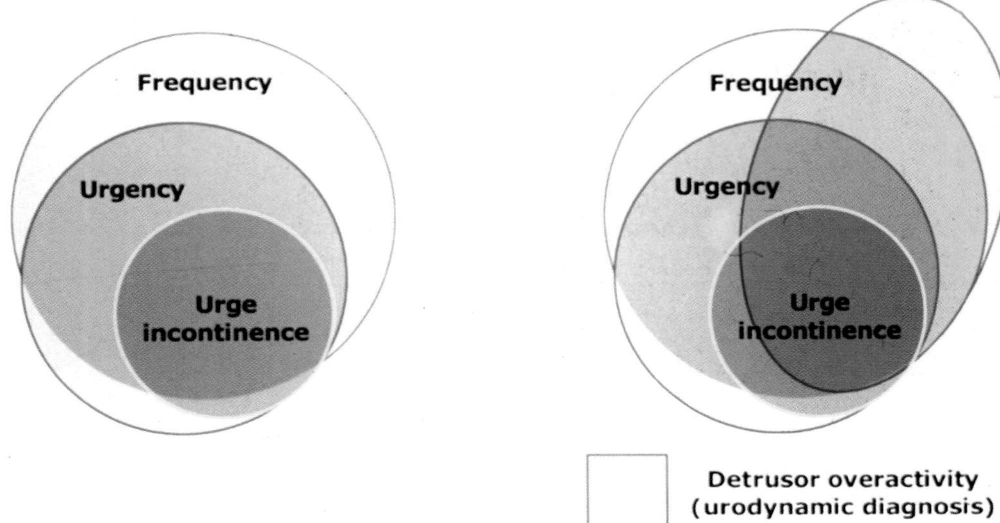

Figure 17-1 The relationships among symptoms of overactive bladder (OAB), urgency urinary incontinence (UUI), and detrusor overactivity (DO).

Sanvik and their colleagues showed similar results.[24,25] This reinforces the fact that SUI is the major type of UI in women.

A large population-based survey that was conducted in France, Germany, Italy, Spain, Sweden, and the United Kingdom defined OAB as the presence of chronic frequency, urgency, and urge incontinence (either alone or in any combination). This definition is somewhat different from the new ICS definition, which uses urgency as the cornerstone of the diagnosis. The authors reported that the overall prevalence of OAB symptoms in subjects aged 40 years or older was 16.6%. Frequency (85%) was the most commonly reported symptom, followed by urgency (54%) and urge incontinence (36%). The prevalence of OAB symptoms increased with advancing age. Overall, 60% of respondents with symptoms had consulted a doctor, but only 27% were currently receiving treatment.[26]

The National Overactive Bladder Evaluation (NOBLE) Program that was undertaken in the United States used the new ICS definition from 2002 in a clinically validated interview and a follow-up nested study. A sample of 5204 adults aged 18 years or older was studied. The overall prevalence of OAB was similar between men (16.0%) and women (16.9%), but sex-specific prevalence differed substantially by severity of symptoms: 55% of the women with OAB symptoms had OAB associated with urge incontinence ("wet OAB"), and the rest had OAB without incontinence ("dry OAB"). In women, prevalence of urge incontinence increased with age, from 2.0% among those 18 to 24 years of age to 19% among those 65 to 74 years of age, with a marked increase after 44 years of age. However, the dry OAB tended to have gradual increase before 44 years of age and reached a plateau at that point. The prevalence of urge incontinence increased in relation to increased body mass index across all age groups. Dry OAB was more common in men than in women.

The NOBLE study does not support the commonly held notion that women are considerably more likely than men to have urgency-related symptoms. However, sex-specific anatomic differences may increase the probability that OAB is expressed as urge incontinence among women compared with men.[27] The prevalence of OAB among women in this study was higher than what was reported by Milsom[26] but similar to the prevalence of UI reported by Simeonova[28] and by Samuelsson (20- to 59-year-olds).[29]

Not all studies distinguish wet from dry OAB. On average, urgency without UI appears to be as common as urgency with UI (Table 17-1).

EVALUATION

History

Because OAB is a symptomatic diagnosis, history plays an important part in assessing the patient. The purpose of the clinical history is to have an empiric diagnosis, to exclude other causes for the patient's symptoms, and to assess the effects of the problem on the patient's daily activities that would help in deciding the treatment strategy. Excluding secondary causes is important; these include diabetes, congestive heart failure, bladder cancer, urinary tract infection (UTI), medications, and pregnancy or recent birth.

Questions should include details of the following:

- Nature and duration of symptoms
- Which symptoms are most bothersome
- Current management, including pad usage
- Previous medical or surgical treatment for the condition
- History of radiation exposure
- Environmental issues
- Patient mobility
- Mental status
- Other disease status, especially neurologic conditions (stoke, trauma)
- Patient medication
- Sexual function
- Bowel function, bearing in mind that irritable bowel syndrome may be associated with OAB[35]

Table 17-1 Prevalence of Urgency and Urgency Urinary Incontinence (UUI) in Community-Dwelling Women*

First Author and Ref. No.	Year	Age (yr)	Sample size	Definition of urgency or UUI	Prevalence of urgency (%)	Prevalence of UUI (%)	Ratio†
Swithinbank[30]	1999	19+	2,075	Any	61	46	1.3
Lapitan[31]	2001	18+	5,502	Any	35	11	3.2
Milsom[26]	2001	40+	16,776	Current	54	36	1.5
Van Der Vaart[32]	2002	20-45	1,393	Any	45	15	3.0
Chen[33]	2003	20+	1,253	Any	13	9	1.4

*There are few data on the incidence of new cases of overactive bladder (OAB), the incidence of new cases of detrusor overactivity (DO), or the natural history of established cases of OAB or DO (or the combination of both).
†Overall median: 2.1.
From Hunskaar H, Burgio K, Diakno AC, et al: Epidemiology and natural history of urinary incontinence. In Abrams P, Cardozo L, Khoury S, Wein A (eds): Incontinence. Plymouth, UK, Health Publication Ltd., 2002, pp 515-551.

- Gynecologic and obstetric history, especially pelvic organ prolapse
- The effect of the condition on daily activity (social restriction, reduced physical activities)
- Patient's goals or expectations of treatment
- Patient's fitness for possible surgical procedures
- For a complicated history, other symptoms, such as the presence of pain or hematuria

Quantification of Symptoms

Questionnaires

Taking a detailed history from the patient depends to a great deal on the physician's skills. The questions, and the aspects tackled, are different for each clinician. Another issue is the embarrassment of the patient, which can lead her to avoid talking about some or all of her symptoms. In addition, clinicians tend to rate the patient's quality of life lower than the patients themselves do.[36] For all of these reasons, patient-completed questionnaires were developed. They provide details regarding the presence of symptoms, their frequency, their severity, and the bother caused to the patient. Questionnaires also assess quality of life in general and in relation to the symptoms. In theory, validated questionnaires can be used for making the diagnosis, as a tool in prevalence studies, and to measure the outcome of treatment.

Several questionnaires have been developed to assess UI. The modular International Consultation on Incontinence Questionnaire (ICIQ) has been validated and includes modules for lower urinary tract symptoms (LUTS) as well as OAB.[37] ICIQ-OAB is a short form based on the Bristol Female Lower Urinary Tract Symptoms Questionnaire (BFLUTS) and should be a helpful tool in assessing these patients (Box 17-1).[38,39] The full list of ICI questionnaires may be found by visiting the web site, www.iciq.net.

Box 17-1 Questions Included in the International Consultation on Incontinence Modular Questionnaire on Overactive Bladder

Do you have to rush to the toilet to urinate?
Does urine leak before you can get to the toilet?
How often do you pass urine during the day?
During the night, on average, how many times do you have to get up to urinate?
Do you have a sudden need to rush to the toilet to urinate?
Does urine leak after you feel a sudden need to go to the toilet?

Fluid Input/Output Charts

Asking the patient to record each micturition for a period of days provides valuable information. For some women, it may be therapeutic, because it provides them with insight into their bladder behavior. Micturition events can be recorded in three main forms:

- *Micturition time chart:* records only the times of micturitions, day and night, for at least 24 hours.
- *Frequency-volume chart (FVC):* records the volumes voided as well as the time of each micturition, day and night, for at least 24 hours.
- *Bladder diary:* records the times of micturitions and voided volumes, incontinence episodes, pad usage, and other information such as fluid intake, degree of urgency, and degree of incontinence.

It is useful to ask the patient to make an estimate of liquid intake in a 24-hour period. Consumption of significant quantities of water-containing foods (vegetables, fruit, and salads) should be taken into account. The time at which any diuretic therapy is taken should be marked on the chart or diary.

The following measurements can be abstracted from FVCs and bladder diaries using the 2002 ICS definitions[40]:

- *Daytime frequency* is the number of voids recorded during waking hours and includes the last void before sleep and the first void after waking and rising in the morning.
- *Nocturia* is the number of voids recorded during a night's sleep: each void is preceded and followed by sleep.
- *24-Hour frequency* is the total number of daytime voids and episodes of nocturia during a specified 24-hour period.
- *24-Hour production* is measured by collecting all urine for 24 hours. This is usually commenced after the first void produced after rising in the morning and is completed by including the first void produced after rising the following morning. *Polyuria* is defined as the measured production of more than 2.8 L of urine in 24 hours in adults. It may be useful to look at output over shorter time frames.[41]

- *Nocturnal urine volume* is defined as the total volume of urine passed between the time the patient goes to bed with the intention of sleeping and the time of waking with the intention of rising. Therefore, it excludes the last void before going to bed but includes the first void after rising in the morning. *Nocturnal polyuria* is present when an increased proportion of the 24-hour output occurs at night (normally during the 8 hours while the patient is in bed). The nighttime urine output excludes the last void before sleep but includes the first void of the morning. The normal range of nocturnal urine production differs with age, and the normal ranges remain to be defined. Therefore, nocturnal polyuria is present when greater than 20% (young adults) to 33% (>65 years) is produced at night. Hence, the precise definition is dependent on age.
- *Maximum voided volume* is the largest volume of urine voided during a single micturition and is determined from the FVC or bladder diary. The term "functional bladder capacity" is no longer recommended by the ICS, because "voided volume" is a clearer and less confusing term, particularly if qualified (e.g., "maximum voided volume"). If the term "bladder capacity" is used, in any situation, it implies that this has been measured in some way, if only by abdominal ultrasonography. In adults, voided volumes vary considerably.

In OAB /DO, the patient has reduced variable volumes of urine during the day. The nighttime volumes and the first void on waking in the morning are often larger and of normal quantity.[42]

In a recent study, the authors correlated the patients' symptoms of frequency, urgency, nocturia, and urge incontinence with the parameters on the bladder diary. They found that frequency and urgency symptoms were associated with a higher 24-hour frequency, lower maximum volume voided, and lower mean voided volume.[43,44]

There has been wide variation in the number of days over which the patient is complete a bladder diary, ranging from 1 day to 2 weeks, with 7 days probably being the previous "gold standard." A recent study by Schick and coworkers indicated that a 4-day chart in women is as reliable as a 7-day chart. They suggested that a 4 day chart optimizes patients' compliance without compromising the diagnostic value of the FVC.[43]

It is advised that a simple FVC with the additional recording of incontinent episodes, pad usage, and overall assessment of fluid intake be used for routine clinical use. In a research setting, urinary diaries may add significant additional information, allowing a more complete evaluation of novel therapies.[45]

Quality of Life Assessment

Severe OAB is a disabling condition that may render the patient housebound to avoid the embarrassment of leakage episodes. Assessing the severity and the impact of the symptoms on the patient's daily activity is an essential part of evaluating these patients. OAB symptoms can have an effect on the psychological, occupational, and sexual function of the patient.[46] In the study by Milsolm and colleagues, 67% of women with OAB reported that their symptoms had a deleterious effect on daily living.[26] The OABqol is a quality-of-life questionnaire that is specifically designed to assess the effect of OAB on the patients' life.[47]

Physical Examination

In addition to the general examination, there are a number of other essential components in the examination of patients with OAB:

Abdominal examination after voiding in an effort to detect a palpable bladder or abnormal masses.

Focused neurologic examination, in particular of the lower limbs, looking for any focal signs that might suggest a neurologic cause for OAB. Patients with a history suggestive of possible neurogenic OAB require a more extensive neurologic examination.

Rectal examination to assess anal tone, pelvic floor function, and the consistency of stool as a sign of constipation.

External genitalia and perineal examination allows inspection of the skin (e.g., atrophy, excoriation) or any abnormal anatomic features. In addition, the area should be tested for normal sensation

Vaginal examination to assess pelvic organ prolapse, with the patient bearing down, and pelvic floor function as described in the ICS report on Pelvic Organ Prolapse.[48] Pelvic floor muscle function can be qualitatively defined by the tone at rest and the strength of a voluntary or reflex contraction (strong, weak, or absent) or by a validated grading system (e.g., modified Oxford scale).[49] A pelvic muscle contraction may be assessed by visual inspection, palpation, electromyography, or perineometry. Factors to be assessed include strength, duration, displacement, and repeatability. Changes due to lack of estrogen should also be noted

Simple Investigations

Urinalysis

Because UTI is a readily detected and easily treatable cause of LUTS, urine testing is highly recommended. Patients with UTI often suffer from frequency and have urgency to pass urine, with nocturia and sometimes urge incontinence that mimics OAB. Therefore, all patients with OAB should have their urine tested to exclude UTI. Testing may range from examination of urine in a clear glass container, to dipstick testing, to urine microscopy.

Estimation of Postvoid Residual Urine

In patients with suspected voiding dysfunction, the postvoid residual urine (PVR) estimation is part of the initial assessment. The result is likely to influence management; for example, in patients with neurologic disorders. PVR can be estimated by noninvasive methods such as the standard ultrasound scan or hand-held bladder scan, or invasively with the use of a urethral catheter; the latter method has the advantage of taking a clean specimen of urine for microbiologic testing.

Urinary Tract Imaging

Routine imaging of the urinary tract in patients with OAB symptoms is not recommended. However, if the history or the initial assessment indicate a complex problem or is suspicious for an associated pathology, then imaging could be used to exclude it. To start with, an ultrasound scan or plain radiographic study should be used.

Imaging of the lower urinary tract is recommended in those women with suspected lower tract or pelvic pathology (e.g., bladder stone, pelvic mass).

Imaging of the upper urinary tract is recommended only in specific situations, including

- Neurogenic UI (e.g., myelodysplasia, spinal cord trauma)
- Incontinence associated with significant PVR
- Coexistent loin or kidney pain
- Severe pelvic organ prolapse, not being treated
- Suspected extraurethral UI
- Hematuria

Invasive Investigations

Invasive investigations are used only after the initial workup has failed to make the diagnosis.

Endoscopy

Flexible or rigid cystoscopy has a limited role in patients with pure symptoms of OAB unless other pathology is suspected. Hence, endoscopy is recommended in the following situations:

- When initial testing suggests other pathologies, such as microscopic hematuria (possibility of bladder tumor)
- When pain or discomfort occurs in a patient with OAB (suggesting a possible intravesical lesion)

Urodynamics

There is some controversy in regard to the use of urodynamic testing in patients with LUTS, particularly those with OAB, based on several issues:

- Urodynamics is an invasive test with possible side effects, mainly UTI.
- The test is uncomfortable and could be embarrassing for the patient.
- The test has a considerable false-negative rate.

Urodynamic evaluation is recommended in the following situations:

- Before invasive treatments
- After treatment failure
- As part of a long-term surveillance program in neurogenic OAB
- In "complicated incontinence"

The aims of routine urodynamic evaluation are

- The detection of detrusor overactivity
- The assessment of urethral competence during filling
- The determination of detrusor function during voiding
- The assessment of outlet function during voiding
- The measurement of residual urine

It is recommended that routine urodynamic evaluation should consist of

- Filling cystometry (with provocation, and tailored to the individual patient's requirements)
- Voiding cystometry

The symptom combinations of OAB are suggestive of urodynamically demonstrable DO, which is characterized by involuntary detrusor contractions during bladder filling that may be spontaneous or provoked. Provocative maneuvers are defined as techniques used during urodynamics in an effort to provoke detrusor overactivity, such as rapid filling, use of cooled or acid medium, postural changes, and hand washing.

DO incontinence is incontinence caused by an involuntary detrusor contraction. In a patient with normal sensation, urgency is likely to be experienced just before the leakage episode. ICS recommends that the terms "motor urge incontinence" and "reflex incontinence" should no longer be used, because they have no intuitive meaning and are often misused.

In everyday life, the patient attempts to inhibit detrusor activity until he or she is in a position to void. Normally, after the aims of the filling study have been achieved and the patient has a desire to void, the "permission to void" is given. That moment is indicated on the urodynamic trace, and all detrusor activity before this point of "permission" is defined as "involuntary detrusor activity."[40]

Normal detrusor function allows bladder filling with little or no change in pressure. No involuntary phasic contractions occur despite provocation. There is no lower limit for the amplitude of an involuntary detrusor contraction, but confident interpretation of low-pressure waves (amplitude <5 cm H_2O) depends on "high-quality" urodynamic technique. The phrase "which the patient cannot completely suppress" has been deleted from the old definition.

Classification of Detrusor Overactivity

DO can be phasic or terminal, idiopathic or neurogenic, symptomatic or asymptomatic. There are certain patterns of DO:

- *Phasic DO* is defined by a characteristic wave form and may or may not lead to UI. Phasic detrusor contractions are not always accompanied by any sensation, or they may be interpreted as a first sensation of bladder filling or as a normal desire to void.
- *Terminal DO* is defined as a single, involuntary detrusor contraction, occurring at cystometric capacity, that cannot be suppressed and results in incontinence, usually leading to bladder emptying (voiding). This is a new ICS term; it is typically associated with reduced bladder sensation; for example, in the elderly stroke patient, when urgency may be felt as the voiding contraction occurs. However, in patients with complete spinal cord injury, there may be no sensation whatsoever.

DO may also be qualified, when possible, according to cause:

- *Neurogenic DO* is the term used when there is a relevant neurologic condition; it replaces the term "detrusor hyperreflexia."
- *Idiopathic DO* is the term used when there is no defined cause; it replaces the term "detrusor instability."

The terms "detrusor instability" and "detrusor hyperreflexia" were both used as generic terms, in the English speaking world and in Scandinavia, before the first ICS report in 1976. As a compromise, they were allocated to idiopathic and neurogenic overactivity, respectively. Because there is no real logic or intuitive meaning to the terms, the ICS believes they should be abandoned.

Other patterns of DO are seen, such as the combination of phasic and terminal DO and the sustained high-pressure detrusor contractions seen in patients with spinal cord injury when attempted voiding occurs against a dyssynergic sphincter.

CONCLUSIONS

Patients with OAB symptoms should be assessed systematically, should be investigated according to treatment intentions, and should have high-quality urodynamic studies performed if the diagnosis is obscure or if invasive treatment is contemplated, but only after a full basic assessment.

References

1. Dudley EC: The expansion of gynecology and a suggestion for the surgical treatment of incontinence in women. Trans Am Gynecol Soc 30:3, 1905.
2. Taylor HC, Watt CH: Incontinence of urine in women. Surg Gynecol Obstet 24:296, 1917.
3. Bates CP, Whiteside CG, Turner-Warwick R: Synchronous cine-pressure-flow-cysto-urethrography with special reference to stress and urge incontinence. Br J Urol 42:714-723, 1970.
4. (Standardisation of the terminology of function of the lower urinary tract: Incontinence, cystometry, ureteral profile, units of measurement [author's translation]). J Urol Nephrol (Paris) 82:429-436, 1976.
5. First report on the standardisation of terminology of lower urinary tract function. Br J Urol 48:39-42, 1976.
6. Second report on the standardisation of terminology of lower urinary tract function. Br J Urol 49:207-210, 1977.
7. Second report on the standardisation of terminology of lower urinary tract function. International Continence Society Committee on Standardisation of Terminology, Copenhagen, August 1976. Eur Urol 3:168-170, 1977.
8. Second report on the standardisation of terminology of lower urinary tract function. Procedures related to the evaluation of micturition: Flow rate, pressure measurement. Symbols. Scand J Urol Nephrol 11:197-199, 1977.
9. First report on the standardisation of terminology of lower urinary tract function: Incontinence, cystometry, urethral closure pressure profile, and units of measurement. Scand J Urol Nephrol 11:193-196, 1977.
10. Third report on the standardisation of terminology of lower urinary tract function procedures related to the evaluation of micturition: Pressure-flow relationships, residual urine. Produced by the International Continence Society, February 1977. Br J Urol 52:348-350, 1980.
11. Third report on the standardisation of terminology of lower urinary tract function: Procedures related to the evaluation of micturition, pressure-flow relationships, residual urine. Produced by the International Continence Society Committee on Standardisation of Terminology, Nottingham, February 1977. Eur Urol 6:170-171, 1980.
12. Fourth report on the standardisation of terminology of lower urinary tract function: Terminology related to neuromuscular dysfunction of the lower urinary tract. Produced by the International Continence Society. Br J Urol 53:333-335, 1981.
13. Fourth report on the standardisation of terminology of lower urinary tract function: Terminology related to neuromuscular dysfunction of the lower urinary tract. The International Continence Society Committee on Standardisation of Terminology. Scand J Urol Nephrol 15:169-171, 1981.
14. Sixth report on the standardisation of terminology of lower urinary tract function. Procedures related to neurophysiological investigations: Electromyography, nerve conduction studies, reflex latencies, evoked potentials and sensory testing. The International Continence Society Committee on Standardisation of Terminology, New York, May 1985. Int Urol Nephrol 18:349-356, 1986.
15. Seventh report on the standardisation of terminology of lower urinary tract function: Lower urinary tract rehabilitation techniques. International Continence Society Committee on Standardisation of Terminology. Scand J Urol Nephrol 26:99-106, 1992.
16. Abrams P, Blaivas JG, Stanton SL, et al: Sixth report on the standardisation of terminology of lower urinary tract function. Procedures related to neurophysiological investigations: Electromyography, nerve conduction studies, reflex latencies, evoked potentials and sensory testing. The International Continence Society Committee on Standardisation of Terminology, New York, May 1985. Scand J Urol Nephrol 20:161-164, 1986.
17. Abrams P, Blaivas JG, Stanton SL, et al: Sixth report on the standardisation of terminology of lower urinary tract function. Procedures related to neurophysiological investigations: Electromyography, nerve conduction studies, reflex latencies, evoked potentials and sensory testing. The International Continence Society. Br J Urol 59:300-304, 1987.
18. Abrams P, Blaivas JG, Stanton SL, Andersen JT: The standardisation of terminology of lower urinary tract function. The International Continence Society Committee on Standardisation of Terminology. Scand J Urol Nephrol Suppl 114:5-19, 1988.
19. Abrams P, Cardozo L, Fall M, et al: The standardisation of terminology of lower urinary tract function: Report from the Standardisation Sub-committee of the International Continence Society. Neurourol Urodyn 21:167-178, 2002.
20. Hannestad YS, Rortveit G, Sandvik H, Hunskaar S: A community-based epidemiological survey of female urinary incontinence: The Norwegian EPINCONT study. Epidemiology of Incontinence in the County of Nord-Trondelag. J Clin Epidemiol 53:1150-1157, 2000.
21. Minassian VA, Drutz HP, Al-Badr A: Urinary incontinence as a worldwide problem. Int J Gynaecol Obstet 82:327-338, 2003.
22. Diokno AC, Brock BM, Brown MB, Herzog AR: Prevalence of urinary incontinence and other urological symptoms in the noninstitutionalized elderly. J Urol 136:1022-1025, 1986.
23. Carey MP, Dwyer PL, Glenning PP: The sign of stress incontinence—Should we believe what we see? Aust N Z J Obstet Gynaecol 37:436-439, 1997.
24. Sandvik H, Hunskaar S, Vanvik A, et al: Diagnostic classification of female urinary incontinence: An epidemiological survey corrected for validity. J Clin Epidemiol 48:339-343, 1995.
25. Weidner AC, Myers ER, Visco AG, et al: Which women with stress incontinence require urodynamic evaluation? Am J Obstet Gynecol 184:20-27, 2001.
26. Milsom I, Abrams P, Cardozo L, et al: How widespread are the symptoms of an overactive bladder and how are they managed? A population-based prevalence study. BJU Int 87:760-766, 2001.
27. Stewart WF, Van Rooyen JB, Cundiff GW, et al: Prevalence and burden of overactive bladder in the United States. World J Urol 20:327-336, 2003.
28. Simeonova Z, Milsom I, Kullendorff AM, et al: The prevalence of urinary incontinence and its influence on the quality of life in women from an urban Swedish population. Acta Obstet Gynecol Scand 78:546-551, 1999.
29. Samuelsson E, Victor A, Tibblin G: A population study of urinary incontinence and nocturia among women aged 20-59 years: Prevalence, well-being and wish for treatment. Acta Obstet Gynecol Scand 76:74-80, 1997.
30. Swithinbank LV, Donovan JL, du Heaume JC, et al: Urinary symptoms and incontinence in women: Relationships between occurrence, age, and perceived impact. Br J Gen Pract 49:897-900, 1999.
31. Lapitan MC, Chye PL: The epidemiology of overactive bladder among females in Asia: A questionnaire survey. Int Urogynecol J Pelvic Floor Dysfunct 12:226-231, 2001.

32. Van der Vaart CH, de Leeuw JR, Roovers JP, Heintz AP: The effect of urinary incontinence and overactive bladder symptoms on quality of life in young women. BJU Int 90:544-549, 2002.
33. Chen GD, Hu SW, Chen YC, et al: Prevalence and correlations of anal incontinence and constipation in Taiwanese women. Neurourol Urodyn 22:664-669, 2003.
34. Hunskaar H, Burgio K, Diakno AC, et al: Epidemiology and natural history of urinary incontinence. In Abrams P, Cardozo L, Khoury S, Wein A (eds): Incontinence. Plymouth, UK, Health Publication Ltd., 2002, pp 515-551.
35. Cukier JM, Cortina-Borja M, Brading AF: A case-control study to examine any association between idiopathic detrusor instability and gastrointestinal tract disorder, and between irritable bowel syndrome and urinary tract disorder. Br J Urol 79:865-878, 1997.
36. Pearlman RA, Uhlmann RF: Quality of life in chronic diseases: Perceptions of elderly patients. J Gerontol 43:M25-M30, 1988.
37. Avery K, Donovan J, Peters TJ, et al: ICIQ: A brief and robust measure for evaluating the symptoms and impact of urinary incontinence. Neurourol Urodyn 23:322-330, 2004.
38. Brookes ST, Donovan JL, Wright M, et al: A scored form of the Bristol Female Lower Urinary Tract Symptoms questionnaire: Data from a randomized controlled trial of surgery for women with stress incontinence. Am J Obstet Gynecol 191:73-82, 2004.
39. Coyne K, Revicki D, Hunt T, et al: Psychometric validation of an overactive bladder symptom and health-related quality of life questionnaire: The OAB-q. Qual Life Res 11:563-574, 2002.
40. Abrams P, Cardozo L, Fall M, et al: The standardisation of terminology of lower urinary tract function: Report from the Standardisation Sub-committee of the International Continence Society. Neurourol Urodyn 21:167-178, 2002.
41. Van KP, Abrams P, Chaikin D, et al: The standardization of terminology in nocturia: Report from the standardization subcommittee of the International Continence Society. BJU Int 90(Suppl 3):11-15, 2002.
42. Abrams P: Urodynamics, 2nd ed. London, Springer, 2002.
43. Schick E, Jolivet-Tremblay M, Dupont C, et al: Frequency-volume chart: The minimum number of days required to obtain reliable results. Neurourol Urodyn 22:92-96, 2003.
44. van Brummen HJ, Heintz AP, van der Vaart CH: The association between overactive bladder symptoms and objective parameters from bladder diary and filling cystometry. Neurourol Urodyn 23:38-42, 2004.
45. Abrams P, Klevmark B: Frequency volume charts: An indispensable part of lower urinary tract assessment. Scand J Urol Nephrol Suppl 179:47-53, 1996.
46. Diokno AC: Epidemiology and psychosocial aspects of incontinence. Urol Clin North Am 22:481-485, 1995.
47. Coyne K, Revicki D, Hunt T, et al: Psychometric validation of an overactive bladder symptom and health-related quality of life questionnaire: The OAB-q. Qual Life Res 11:563-574, 2002.
48. Bump RC, Mattiasson A, Bo K, et al: The standardization of terminology of female pelvic organ prolapse and pelvic floor dysfunction. Am J Obstet Gynecol 175:10-17, 1996.
49. Brink CA, Sampselle CM, Wells TJ, et al: A digital test for pelvic muscle strength in older women with urinary incontinence. Nurs Res 38:196-199, 1989.

Chapter 18

PATHOPHYSIOLOGY OF OVERACTIVE BLADDER

William D. Steers and Adam P. Klausner

The term *overactive bladder* (OAB) refers to the symptom complex of urgency, usually with frequency, and nocturia, with or without urge urinary incontinence. However, this definition, supported by the International Continence Society subcommittee on terminology,[1] is based on expert opinion and fails to account for causation or pathophysiology. Initially limited to the idiopathic condition, the term OAB has been used to describe the described constellation of symptoms regardless of their etiology. The term has gained widespread acceptance by the nonmedical community as well as health care professionals. Furthermore, there has been a dramatic increase in awareness of OAB because of marketing strategies focused on patient-directed advertising of pharmaceutical products. This chapter reviews the causes of OAB and describes possible linkages with other conditions that may provide insight into its pathogenesis. By shedding light on the pathophysiology of OAB, we hope to highlight new targets for therapeutic intervention and directions for further investigation.

The bladder functions as a cohesive unit for the purpose of urine storage and elimination. Several disparate elements contribute in concert to yield normal bladder function. These elements include the detrusor muscle, the urothelium, the vascular supply, interstitial cells, and innervation. A balance between these elements is requisite for normal bladder function. General factors such as mechanical obstruction, inflammation, injury, and the psychological state of the host can alter this balance and lead to OAB (Fig. 18-1). Specific etiologic entities of known importance in the pathophysiology of OAB, such as urinary tract infections, interstitial cystitis, benign prostatic obstruction, spinal cord injury, transitional cell carcinoma, and anxiety disorders, can be viewed as distinct "perturbations" that affect one or more of these elements. The end result is often the symptom complex known as OAB.

Experimental data continue to reveal that, with time, an alteration in one cell type often leads to changes in other cell types. Therefore, a single explanation for the pathophysiology of OAB is unlikely.

EPIDEMIOLOGY

A detailed review of the epidemiology of OAB is beyond the scope of this review. However, a few key points are worth mentioning. The first is that the prevalence of OAB has generally been underestimated, because many studies have been limited to patients with incontinence, which is only one subset of OAB. The second is that, contrary to popular belief, the prevalence of OAB is similar in men and women. The third is that OAB is a chronic condition that adversely affects the quality of life.

Several well-done, large-scale studies have attempted to provide solid epidemiologic data for OAB. In a European study spanning six nations, telephone interviews of subjects older than 40 years of age were used to determine OAB prevalence. In this study, OAB was defined as urinary frequency greater than eight times per day and urgency, with or without urge incontinence. Using this definition, the prevalence of OAB was found to be 16.6%.[2] Symptoms increased with advancing age and, surprisingly, were of similar prevalence in men (15.6%) and women (17.4%). In addition, 40% of those who met criteria for OAB had never sought medical care for this condition. Of the 60% who had spoken to a physician, only 27% were currently taking medication to control their symptoms.

In an OAB prevalence study conducted in the United States, strikingly similar results were found. The overall prevalence of OAB was 16.0% in men and 16.9% in women.[3] Based on the combined results of these works, a reasonable estimate for the prevalence of OAB is approximately 17% of the adult female population. These studies highlight the relatively high prevalence of OAB, the substantial degree of underreporting, and the possibility of poor treatment efficacy. Although the epidemiology of OAB is complex, these numbers emphasize the dramatic social and economic impact of this condition.

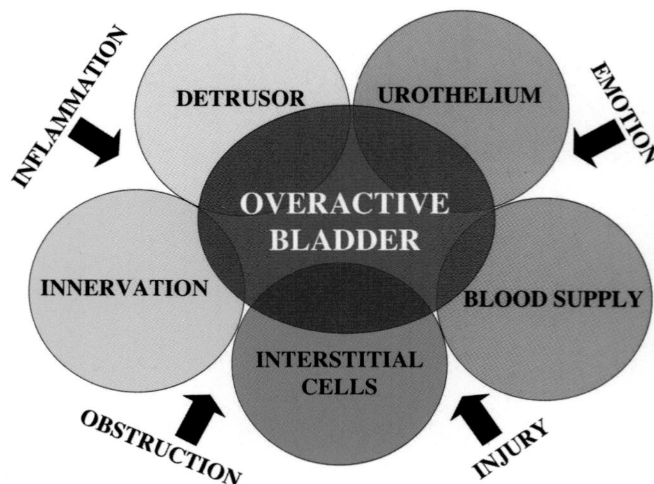

Figure 18-1 Diagram showing intrinsic and extrinsic factors that may contribute to the pathophysiology of overactive bladder (OAB). Substantial overlap between factors suggests that a single etiology for OAB is unlikely.

CONTRIBUTORS TO OVERACTIVE BLADDER

Role of the Detrusor Muscle

Most experimental research pertaining to OAB, urge incontinence, and detrusor overactivity (DO) has relied on increased detrusor contractions on cystometry as a surrogate for this disorder. Insight into urgency is lacking. In addition, the clinical findings that almost a quarter of patients with OAB and urge incontinence do not demonstrate DO on urodynamic testing[4] and, conversely, that almost a quarter of asymptomatic men and women demonstrate DO suggest that this symptom complex may not universally affect the detrusor per se.[5-7] This observation may explain in some patients the lack of efficacy of drugs such as antimuscarinics that target receptors on the detrusor.

Autonomous Activity

New research in detrusor physiology has added to our understanding of how this muscle contracts in a coordinated fashion. In a study by Gillespie and colleagues,[8] two distinct types of detrusor muscle activity were identified—phasic activity and global contractions (Fig. 18-2). During phasic activity, small regions of the detrusor muscle undergo localized "stretches" that are associated with phasic increases in bladder pressure. The investigators found that these phasic responses were triggered by low-dose muscarinics, low-dose nicotinics, and low-frequency nerve stimulation. In contrast, during global contractions, most of the bladder smooth muscle is involved. These global contractions were triggered by high-dose muscarinics and high-frequency nerve stimulation and were unresponsive to nicotinics. Immunohistochemistry confirmed the presence of two distinct smooth muscle cell populations. A thin layer of cells was found to reside just beneath the bladder mucosa. A larger layer was found to comprise the bulk of the detrusor. The authors postulated that the thin, submucosal layer may be responsible for autonomous pacemaker activity in the bladder, and the remaining detrusor may be responsible for the classically understood parasympathetic nerve–stimulated bladder contraction.

Interstitial Cells

Interstitial cells with spontaneous pacemaker activity have been found in gut smooth muscle. In the gut, these pacemaker cells, known as interstitial cells of Cajal (ICCs), have been identified by their immunohistochemical (Kit-positive) and morphologic (presence of dendritic processes) properties. The search for these cells in the bladder dome has been prompted by research showing bladder electrical waves that start at the dome and propagate in a caudad fashion.[9,10] Shafik and coworkers[9] identified cells with these characteristics in bladder strips harvested from cystectomy specimens obtained from patients with bladder cancer. ICC cells were found to exist in isolation or in interconnected networks in the bladder dome of all specimens. The authors suggested that changes in the number or functionality of this cell population may be important in motility disorders involving the bladder.

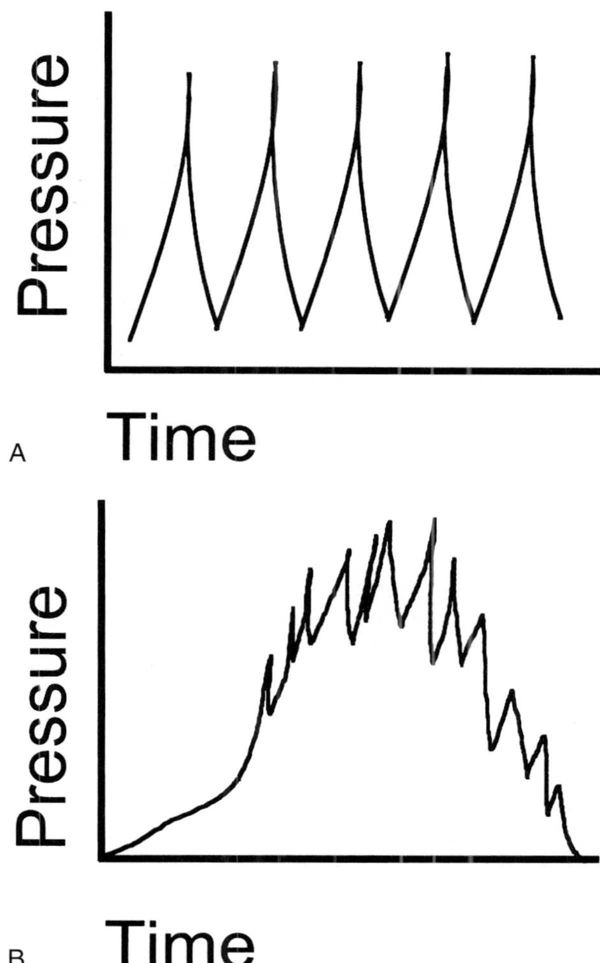

Figure 18-2 Comparison of phasic and global bladder contractions. **A,** During phasic contractions, localized stretches lead to short, nonsustained bursts of increased bladder pressure. **B,** During global contractions, the majority of detrusor muscle is involved, and a sustained rise in bladder pressure is observed.

Table 18-1 Electrical Properties of the Detrusor Muscle in Overactive Bladder (OAB)

Property	Idiopathic OAB	OAB of Obstruction
Spontaneous activity	↑	↑
KCl^- sensitivity	↑	↑
Response to electrical stimulation	↓	↓
Response to muscarinics	Normal	↑

Electrical Properties of the Detrusor

Tissue from unstable bladder shows enhanced spontaneous contractile activity. This has been documented in human bladder strips from obstructed unstable bladders[11,12] and from those with neuropathy.[13] However, depending on the etiology of OAB, important differences exist. In both idiopathic DO and obstruction, bladder strips demonstrate increased sensitivity to potassium chloride and reduced response to electrical stimulation.[11,12,14,15] However, strips from obstructed bladders appear to be supersensitive to muscarinic agonists, whereas strips from bladders with idiopathic DO do not demonstrate this response (Table 18-1).[11,12]

Increased electrical coupling has been identified in bladders with OAB. Gap junctions are believed to be important in the

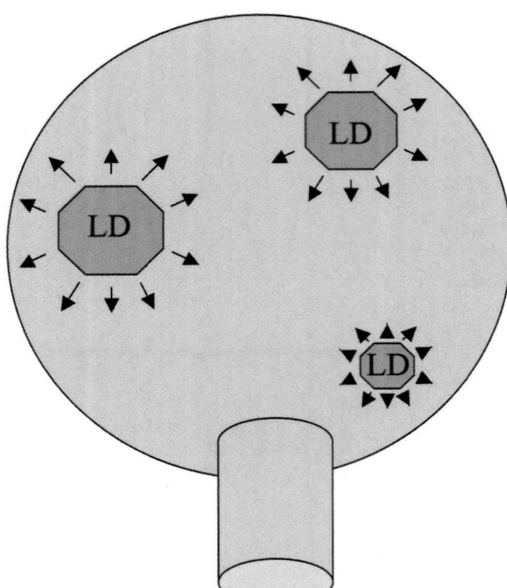

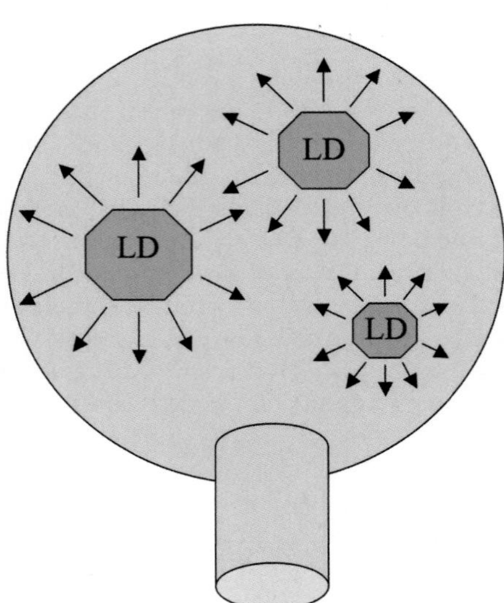

Figure 18-3 Mechanism of overactive bladder (OAB) initiated by local distortions (LD) in the bladder wall. In the normal bladder *(left)*, lack of coupling limits the spread of activity initiated by LD. In OAB *(right)*, increased coupling allows LD to propagate. Accordingly, in the setting of increased coupling, LD could lead to involuntary contractions.

electrical coupling of detrusor smooth muscle cells. In a study by Haferkamp and associates,[16] increased gap junction expression was identified by testing for the gap junction marker, connexin-43. Biopsy specimens from patients with neurogenic DO were compared to control specimens obtained from women with pure stress urinary incontinence. Connexin-43 RNA expression was determined by using a polymerase chain reaction method. A statistically significant increase in connexin-43 RNA was found in specimens from patients with neurogenic DO. These results suggest that increased electrical coupling via heightened expression of gap junctions may be important in the pathophysiology of certain forms of OAB.

One theory of OAB is based on the observation[17] that localized distortions of the bladder wall occur during filling. These distortions are probably activated by sporadic populations of low-threshold postganglionic parasympathetic neurons. In the normal detrusor, poor coupling between smooth muscle bundles would limit the spread of this activity, and only a localized distortion of the bladder wall would occur. However, in the setting of increased coupling, as seen in OAB, localized distortions would spread throughout the bladder (Fig. 18-3). In this scenario, intravesical pressure would rise, and involuntary contractions might occur.

Morphologic Changes

Morphologic changes in the structure of the detrusor muscle have also been identified in the setting of OAB. Patchy denervation of muscle bundles can be identified. Furthermore, areas of reduced innervation become infiltrated with connective tissue, and, after compete denervation, smooth muscle cell hypertrophy occurs.[18] At the ultrastructural level, detrusor muscle that demonstrates OAB contains protrusion junctions and ultra-close abutments between myocytes. This ultrastructural pattern is not typically present in normal detrusor muscle and may represent an additional mechanism through which increased electrical coupling in OAB might occur (Table 18-2).[19]

Table 18-2 EMorphologic Changes in the Detrusor Muscle in Overactive Bladder (OAB)

Cellular Level	Ultrastructural Level
Connective tissue infiltration	Increased protrusion junctions
Smooth muscle cell hypertrophy	Increased ultra-close myocyte abutments
Patchy denervation	Increased gap junctions (connexin-43)

Role of the Urothelium

The previous notion of the urothelium as an inert, impermeable barrier has been challenged in recent years. New research focuses on the urothelium as a biologically active layer that functions as a luminal sensor. In the bladder, the presence of afferent nerve terminals just beneath the urothelium highlights the importance of this sensory communication. One theory to explain the presence of OAB symptoms is that urothelial signals may lead to heightened sensitivity of submucosal afferents. Accordingly, isolated sensitization of submucosal afferents would trigger symptoms of urgency. Further sensitization of submucosal afferents would then lead to enhanced smooth muscle coupling, and urgency with associated unstable detrusor contractions might ensue. Signaling most likely occurs through mediators such as nitric oxide,[20-22] neurokinin A,[23,24] and adenosine triphosphate (ATP).[25,26] These mediators are released by the urothelium in response to low urinary pH, high urinary potassium, and increased urinary osmolality. Furthermore, urothelial signaling is probably a dynamic process. In studies by Sun and colleagues, the presence of increased urinary ATP, as seen in conditions of OAB such as interstitial cystitis, was associated with increased ATP production from stretched urothelial cells (Fig. 18-4).[25-27] Identification of feed-forward processes such as these may

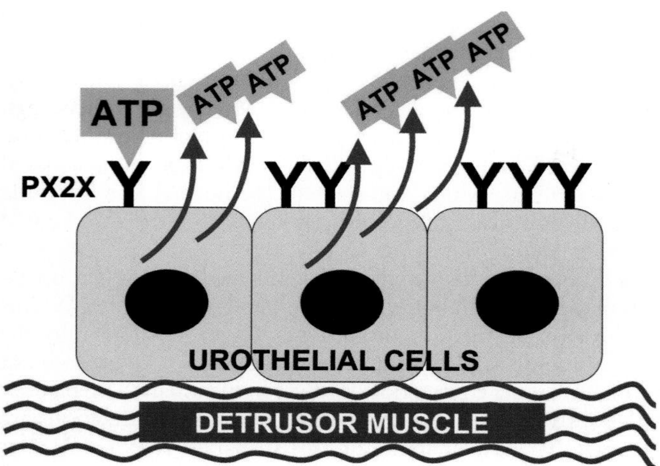

Figure 18-4 Mechanism of overactive bladder (OAB) initiated by feed-forward stimulation of afferent nerve terminals through adenosine triphosphate (ATP) signaling, based on work from Sun and colleagues.[25-27] In this model, urinary ATP leads to increased ATP release from stretched urothelial cells. ATP then stimulates additional afferent nerve terminals by binding to the purinergic receptor, P_X2_X. As a result, new afferent fibers are "turned on," a condition that could lead to the occurrence of OAB.

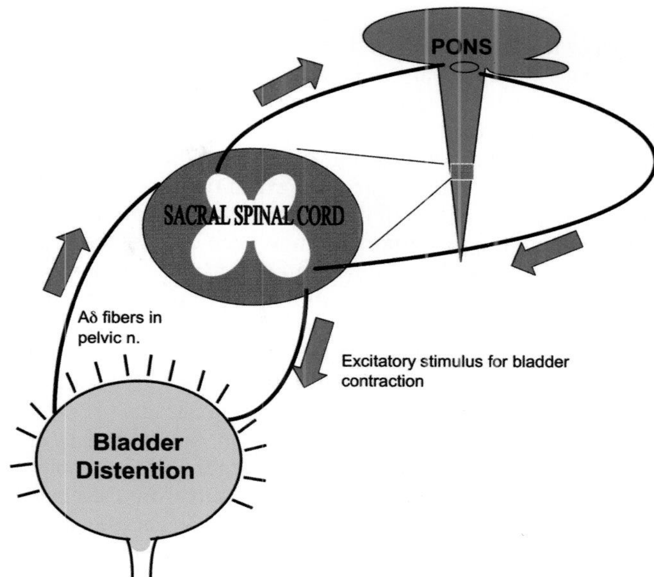

Figure 18-5 Neural circuitry involved in micturition. In response to bladder distention, mechanosensitive afferent nerve terminals in the bladder wall are stimulated. Signals ascend in the spinal cord via a spinobulbospinal pathway. In the brainstem, the pontine micturition center coordinates processing of ascending and descending signals. The excitatory motor stimulus exits the sacral cord via the pelvic nerve and leads to detrusor contraction.

help to explain the self-sustaining nature of many forms of OAB.

Role of Blood Flow

Research demonstrates that reduction in blood flow is related to the level of bladder decompensation.[28] OAB in the elderly is associated with various changes in the bladder, including reduced compliance, ultrastructural changes of detrusor myocytes, and ischemia.[29,30] Reduced blood flow to the bladder triggers a cascade of events that include apoptosis of smooth muscle cells and damage to intrinsic bladder nerves. Importantly, nerve tissue is far more sensitive to ischemic damage than detrusor muscle itself, and damage that occurs to nerve tissue is generally irreversible. In the setting of OAB associated with obstruction, damage and degeneration of the intrinsic bladder nerves is a common finding. Hypertrophy of detrusor myocytes is also prevalent, and this creates increased metabolic demand on the cells and the surrounding nerve tissue. Therefore, the effects of reduced blood flow, coupled with increased metabolic demand, can produce an anoxic environment and lead to increased neuronal death.[31]

In an animal model of bladder outflow obstruction, high-pressure urination was associated with prolonged periods of detrusor ischemia. This ischemic state may play a role in the metabolic and structural changes in smooth muscle and nerve tissues found in the setting of OAB.[32] The effects of acute ischemia have also been studied. Bratslavsky and colleagues[33] produced complete ischemia to the bladder for up to 18 hours. Strips of bladder were then harvested and tested in organ bath experiments. The bladder strips showed altered contractile responses to a variety of stimulants, and the most pronounced alteration was seen with electrical field stimulation. In another model, bilateral iliac artery injury was created to produce a state of chronic bladder ischemia. When tested urodynamically, animals with severe ischemia were found to have reduced bladder contractility and evidence of bladder decompensation. Animals with moderate ischemia were found to have DO only.[34] Again, this highlights the point that ischemia may contribute to the pathophysiology of OAB.

Role of Innervation

Voiding occurs as the result of a spinobulbospinal micturition reflex that is initiated by afferents from the bladder and culminates in efferent outflow via the pelvic nerve (Fig. 18-5). Micturition may be initiated by three events: bladder distention triggering mechanoreceptive afferents, autonomous myogenic activity activating afferents in the detrusor, and urothelial/interstitial cell interaction with chemosensitive or mechanoreceptive suburothelial afferents. In many instances, DO has been attributed to activation of a micturition reflex. It is not difficult to envision that the key symptom of urgency may be caused by activation of afferents that is consciously perceived but insufficient for micturition. A threshold for afferent firing is determined by the balance between myogenic, urothelial, and interstitial cell factors that are designed to limit the spread of inadvertent neural impulses and neural mechanisms that are designed to ensure the efficient transmission of impulses across synapses. In response to injury or disease, it has been postulated that either the trigger for firing is changed, the type of fiber is altered, or the threshold for firing is lowered. Any of these hypothetical scenarios could manifest as a sensation of fullness or precipitate detrusor contractions at lower bladder volumes. The abnormal sensation of urgency may derive from a change in the stimulus or in the type of afferents that are activated. Plasticity in afferents may be a protective mechanism whereby a noxious stimulus or injury facilitates the elimination of toxins and potentially shortens the duration of disease processes.

Neuroplasticity

Neuroplasticity is the term that describes the mechanisms whereby the nervous system changes in response to injury or disease. Unfortunately, these mechanisms may continue long after the elimination of the inciting events. As an example, neuroplasticity may occur in women with chronic bladder infections to promote the rapid elimination of urinary bacteria in times of active infection. However, in a subset of these women, symptoms of urinary frequency and urgency may continue even in the absence of active bacterial infection. These women are said to have idiopathic DO or simply OAB. A comprehensive understanding of why this occurs (e.g., ATP release) and to whom (e.g., genomic predisposition) simply does not exist. Ongoing research in this area is critical and will undoubtedly result in the identification of novel therapeutic strategies in the upcoming decade.

Currently, researchers have focused on the role of neurotrophic factors in bladder neuroplasticity. In this regard, molecular triggers for changes in sensory nerve inputs from the bladder or neural transmission directly in the central nervous system could involve nerve growth factor (NGF) or other neurotrophins such as brain-derived neurotrophin factor (BDNF), glia-derived neurotrophin factor (GDNF), neurotrophin 3 and 4, and various cytokines. NGF has been shown to promote neuronal regrowth after injury and is important for the growth and sustenance of both sensory and sympathetic nerves.[35,36] In fact, elevations in NGF have been identified in patients with OAB, benign prostatic hyperplasia,[37,38] and interstitial cystitis.[39]

Neuroplasticity resulting in symptoms of OAB occurs in experimental animals after spinal cord injury or urethral obstruction. In these situations, a size increase in both sensory and motor neurons to the bladder has been found.[40,41] The transmission time of the micturition reflex becomes shorter after spinal cord injury.[42,43] At the neuronal level, significant reorganization occurs. The micturition pathway changes from a spinobulbospinal loop to a network that is mainly spinal. In addition, unmyelinated sensory C fibers, which are silent in the normal state, become active and contribute to the reduced micturition threshold noted after spinal cord injury (Fig. 18-6).

In humans, the ice water test provides evidence for neuroplasticity associated with both obstruction and neurogenic DO. This test involves instillation of ice-cold water or saline into the bladder. In normal subjects, the instillation of cold fluid does not stimulate bladder contractions. However, in patients with bladder outlet obstruction and neurogenic DO, bladder contractions are triggered. The explanation for this disparate response is that cold-sensitive C fibers are silent in the normal state and become active in various conditions associated with OAB.[44,45] Additional evidence for C-fiber neuroplasticity is demonstrated by the occasional clinical efficacy of capsaicin[46] and resiniferatoxin[47] in the amelioration of OAB. These neurotoxins selectively block C fibers.[46] Therefore, they likely act to suppress the heightened C-fiber activity that occurs in many forms of OAB.

Capsaicin, an ingredient found in chile peppers that is responsible for their hot or pungent taste, acts as a neurotoxin to selectively desensitize C-fiber afferents.[48] As described earlier, C-fiber neurons are typically silent in the normal bladder but become active in many conditions that result in neurogenic DO. Capsaicin and the more potent resiniferatoxin have been used for

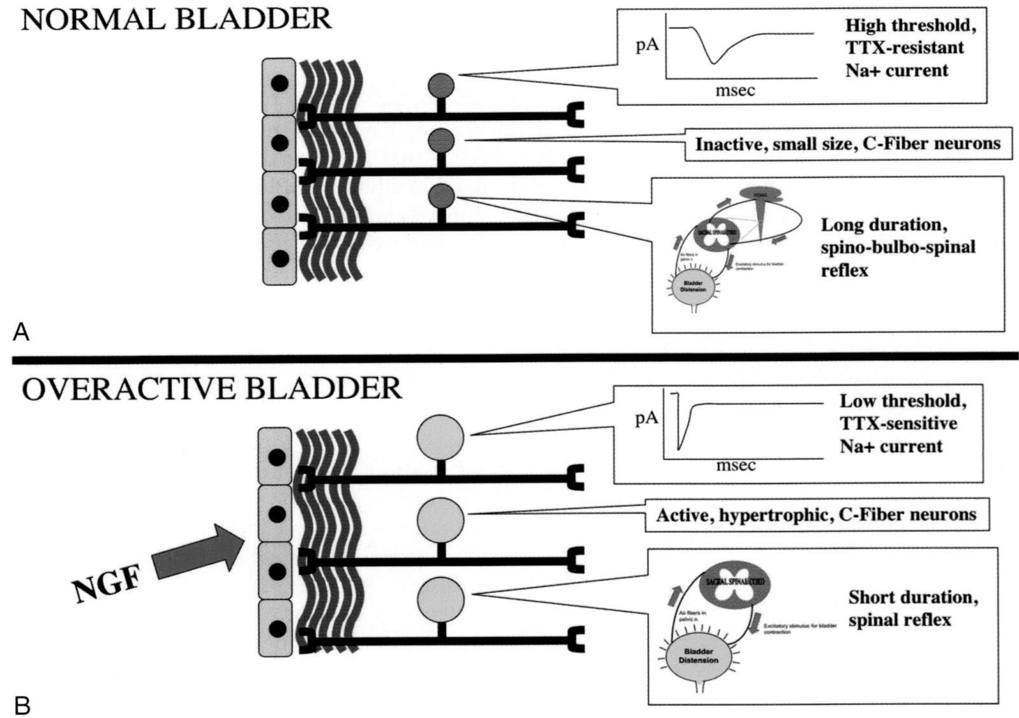

Figure 18-6 Neuroplasticity. Simplified view of several nerve growth factor (NGF)-mediated processes that are probably involved in neuroplasticity associated with overactive bladder (**B**) compared with the normal bladder (**A**). These mechanisms include changing from high-threshold, tetrodotoxin (TTX)-resistant Na^+ currents to low-threshold, TTX-sensitive Na^+ currents in bladder afferent neurons *(top insets)*; changing from inactive, small size C-fiber neurons to active, hypertrophic C-fiber neurons *(middle insets)*; and changing from a long duration, spino-bulbo-spinal reflex to a short duration spinal reflex *(bottom insets)*.

several years in clinical trials in patients with DO. The success of this C fiber–directed therapy highlights the importance of activated C-fiber afferent neurons as a key element in the pathophysiology of neurogenic DO.

Spinal Cord Injury

After spinal cord injury, neurogenic DO often occurs. The exact sequence of molecular events leading to this clinical picture remains unknown. However, it is clear that, after spinal cord injury, C-fiber afferents in the bladder develop increased mechanosensitivity. Cell bodies of these afferents located in dorsal root ganglia become hypertrophied.[49] Furthermore, patch clamp experiments demonstrate that expression of sodium (Na^+) channels shifts from the high-threshold, tetrodotoxin-resistant type channel to the low-threshold, tetrodotoxin-sensitive type channel.[50,51] Because conductances via Na^+ and potassium (K^+) channels are crucial to neuronal excitability, the ability of disorders to alter these channels, possibly through cytokines and neurotrophins, may underlie the mechanism of OAB in conditions ranging from spinal cord injury and bladder outlet obstruction to inflammation. In fact, such plasticity in channel function or expression could mediate the reduction in firing threshold for chemo/thermo/mechano-sensitive afferents demonstrated in OAB. Therefore, Na^+ and K^+ channels are attractive targets for OAB therapy.

The presence of these changes in neuron morphology and electrophysiology suggests that transport of signals from the injured spinal cord to nerve terminals in the bladder or vice versa must be occurring in the setting of spinal cord injury. NGF and GDNF have been investigated in this regard. Indeed, NGF is associated with hypertrophy of cell bodies of bladder afferents seen in various forms of OAB.[40,41] In addition, experimental blockage of NGF in the setting of spinal cord injury prevents the occurrence of DO. GDNF may also be important in the setting of spinal cord injury, because a small population of bladder C-fiber neurons responds only to GDNF and are unresponsive to NGF.[52]

Role of Obstruction and Inflammation

In the setting of mechanical obstruction of the bladder outlet, symptoms of OAB are frequently present. This is most commonly seen in men with bladder outlet obstruction due to prostatic enlargement. However, women with functional obstruction of the bladder neck or mechanical obstruction due to trauma or surgery can display similar symptomatology. Insight into the pathophysiology of OAB can be gleaned from urodynamic studies in patients who present with persistent lower urinary tract symptoms after surgical resection of the prostate. These studies demonstrate that persistent symptoms are related more to DO than to recurrent or residual bladder outlet obstruction.[53,54]

The explanation for this persistent symptomatology is that the effects of bladder outlet obstruction are not purely mechanical. Rather, obstruction causes enhancement of a facilitory spinal reflex mediated by C-fiber afferent bladder nerves. Evidence for this reflex is seen in the positive response of patients with bladder outlet obstruction to the ice water test. Again, the presence of involuntary contractions after instillation of ice-cold water into the bladder demonstrates an activated C-fiber reflex. In addition, bladder outlet obstruction triggers heightened expression of growth-associated protein-43, a phosphoprotein whose expression is induced in the setting of axonal sprouting and neuronal remodeling.[55] New spinal circuits may arise after bladder outlet obstruction, and failure to revert to a normal voiding pattern after obstruction is relieved suggests that these new circuits can sometimes persist.

NGF probably plays an important role in the activation of these de novo circuits after bladder outlet obstruction. Levels of NGF are elevated in obstructed bladders of humans and experimental animals.[56] In animal models of bladder outlet obstruction, blockade of NGF prevents the activation of C-fiber reflexes, and DO does not occur. Importantly, the rise in NGF precedes the development of neuronal hypertrophy and the clinical development of OAB. This suggests that NGF is involved in the initiation of the obstruction-induced neuroplastic process.

Likewise, NGF is also increased in the setting of bladder inflammation. This increase is seen in both the urine and the bladder tissue itself. It has been identified in animal models of experimental bladder inflammation and also in patients with interstitial cystitis.[39,57,58] Inflammation of the bladder results in enlargement of cell bodies of bladder afferent nerves, a finding that is seen in other forms of OAB and that is associated with increased expression of NGF. Changes in the neurons within the spinal cord have also been identified in the setting of bladder inflammation. After experimental inflammation of the bladder induced by mechanical irritation or chemically by systemic treatment with cyclophosphamide, neurons in the lumbosacral spinal cord displayed increased expression of FOS, a nonspecific marker for neuronal activation.[59,60]

These findings suggest that inflammatory stimuli within the bladder trigger changes in afferent nerve endings. These changes are then communicated to cell bodies that reside in dorsal root ganglia and ultimately are relayed to spinal cord neurons and to higher-order neurons in the brain. NGF is probably an important mediator in this signaling process. However, the exact cascade of molecular events remains unknown, and elaboration of this cascade will certainly lead to the identification of novel targets for pharmacologic intervention in OAB.

Role of Psychological Factors

Depression

In 1978, Stone and colleagues[61] first documented the association of psychiatric symptoms and voiding dysfunction. Subsequent researchers noted this association specifically for disorders of idiopathic DO and urge incontinence[62,63] and suggested that these voiding symptoms might be psychosomatic in nature. Chiverton and Judd[64] found a higher incidence of depression among women with urinary incontinence compared with women in the general population. Zorn and coworkers[65] performed a case-control study in which 115 consecutive patients presenting to an incontinence clinic were compared with 80 continent controls. Patients with incontinence had significantly higher scores on the Beck Depression Inventory and reported a history of depression more frequently. Interestingly, when stratified by type of incontinence, patients with stress incontinence and those with urge incontinence due to obstruction or neurogenic causes did not demonstrate these differences. However, 60% of patients with idiopathic urge incontinence reported a history of depression, compared with only 17% of continent control patients. In addition, a history of depression often preceded the development of urine loss, suggesting that incontinence or OAB symptoms per se did not cause depression. Recently, several large cross-sectional studies examined the association of depression and incontinence. Dugan and colleagues[66] found a strong association in elderly patients. Nygaard and colleagues[67] performed a cross-sectional survey study of almost 6000 women comparing incontinence with depressive symptoms. After adjusting for medical morbidity, functional status, and demographic variables, women with severe incontinence or mild to moderate incontinence were 80% and 40% more likely, respectively, to have depression than continent women.

One possible explanation for an association between depression and OAB or urge incontinence may be altered central transmitter function, especially monoamines, in certain areas of the brain that influence micturition. Recently, our group and others[68] identified a significant increased relative risk for OAB and urge incontinence in postpartum women with severe depression ("baby blues"), compared with nondepressed cohorts. Postpartum depression may herald future depressive episodes that are associated with altered serotonin function. This association is intriguing and is consistent with animal studies demonstrating that lowered serotonin induces urinary frequency and intermicturition contractions on cystometry.[69]

Anxiety and Panic Disorders

Melville and coworkers[70] examined the association of incontinence and panic disorder in a prospective study of 218 consecutive women presenting to a urogynecology clinic with a diagnosis of urinary incontinence. All patients underwent a history, physical examination, multichannel urodynamics to assess the type of incontinence and completed validated instruments to diagnose psychiatric disorders and disease-specific quality-of-life effects. Overall, 11% of patients with urge incontinence or mixed incontinence suffered from panic disorder, compared with 0% of patients with stress incontinence. After adjusting for potential confounding variables such as medical comorbidities, marital status, and age, patients with urge incontinence were found to be 9.2 times more likely than those with stress incontinence to have a panic disorder. Patients with mixed incontinence were found to be 13.5 times more likely to have a panic disorder than patients with stress incontinence. Furthermore, Weissman and associates[71] identified a potential genetic syndrome in which families manifest both panic disorder and urinary frequency. Using genetic linkage analysis, they identified a clinical syndrome in certain families with panic disorder that included voiding dysfunction, migraine headaches, mitral valve prolapse, and hypothyroid conditions. The association of this mental condition with seemingly unrelated medical conditions prompted the authors to advocate for more extensive clinical evaluation of patients with psychiatric conditions, in order to identify this type of phenotypic clustering.

Some investigators have found that patients with anxiety and panic disorders may simply experience greater "bother" from their symptoms. For this reason, they might present more frequently for medical evaluation. Watson and coworkers[72] performed a prospective study on women with symptoms of incontinence presenting for urodynamics testing. The 48-hour pad test and the Hospital Anxiety and Depression (HAD) scale were administered. Patients with high anxiety scores had statistically significant lower mean urine loss on the 48-hour pad test (44 versus 97 mL) compared with patients without high anxiety scores. The investigators concluded that anxious patients present with a lesser degree of incontinence than nonanxious patients. However, most data appear to support the notion that anxiety and panic disorders are significant risk factors for OAB and urge incontinence.

These clinical associations are consistent with laboratory investigations showing that anxiety models such as the spontaneously hypertensive rat exhibit urinary frequency and intermicturition contractions on cystometry.[38] Central neurotransmitters that activate the stress response (e.g., corticotropin-releasing factor) also increase bladder activity. Conversely, corticotropin-releasing factor antagonists reduce bladder activity in certain animal models of OAB.[73]

CONCLUSIONS

The pathophysiology of OAB is diverse and involves an interplay between urothelial, myogenic, and neurogenic mechanisms. Ultimately, the ability to effectively combat the symptoms of OAB depends on success in identifying the underlying mechanisms in each affected patient. Unique therapeutic strategies targeting individual pathologies can then be crafted. In the future, the use of bioimaging modalities such as positron emission tomographic (PET) scanning or functional, local blood oxygen level–dependent (fBOLD) magnetic resonance imaging (MRI); risk factor or hazard scoring; genetic profiling; and molecular techniques will allow clinicians to better categorize patients and individualize therapy. As advances are made in molecular medicine, clinical applications in the treatment of OAB will evolve. However, more effective treatments for this pervasive, costly, and debilitating condition can be achieved only by the pursuit of translational research aimed at a comprehensive understanding of the pathophysiology of OAB.

References

1. Abrams P, Cardozo L, Fall M, et al: The standardisation of terminology of lower urinary tract function: Report from the Standardisation Sub-committee of the International Continence Society. Neurourol Urodyn 21:167-178, 2002.
2. Milsom I, Abrams P, Cardozo L, et al: How widespread are the symptoms of an overactive bladder and how are they managed? A population-based prevalence study. BJU Int 87:760-766, 2001.
3. Stewart WF, Van Rooyen JB, Cundiff GW, et al: Prevalence and burden of overactive bladder in the United States. World J Urol 20:327-336, 2003.
4. McGuire EJ: Urodynamic evaluation of stress incontinence. Urol Clin North Am 22:551-555, 1995.
5. Zinner NR: Clinical aspects of detrusor instability and the value of urodynamics. Eur Urol 34(Suppl 1):16-19, 1998.
6. Heslington K, Hilton P: Ambulatory monitoring and conventional cystometry in asymptomatic female volunteers. Br J Obstet Gynaecol 103:434-441, 1996.
7. Robertson AS, Griffiths CJ, Ramsden PD, Neal DE: Bladder function in healthy volunteers: Ambulatory monitoring and conventional urodynamic studies. Br J Urol 73:242-249, 1994.
8. Gillespie JI, Harvey IJ, Drake MJ: Agonist- and nerve-induced phasic activity in the isolated whole bladder of the guinea pig: Evidence for two types of bladder activity. Exp Physiol 88:343-357, 2003.

9. Shafik A, El-Sibai O, Shafik AA, Shafik I: Identification of interstitial cells of Cajal in human urinary bladder: Concept of vesical pacemaker. Urology 64:809-813, 2004.
10. McCloskey KD, Gurney AM: Kit positive cells in the guinea pig bladder. J Urol 168:832-836, 2002.
11. Sibley GN: Developments in our understanding of detrusor instability. Br J Urol 80(Suppl 1):54-61, 1997.
12. Sibley GN: The physiological response of the detrusor muscle to experimental bladder outflow obstruction in the pig. Br J Urol 60:332-336, 1987.
13. German K, Bedwani J, Davies J, et al: Physiological and morphometric studies into the pathophysiology of detrusor hyperreflexia in neuropathic patients. J Urol 153:1678-1683, 1995.
14. Brading AF, Turner WH: The unstable bladder: Towards a common mechanism. Br J Urol 73:3-8, 1994.
15. Mills IW, Greenland JE, McMurray G, et al: Studies of the pathophysiology of idiopathic detrusor instability: The physiological properties of the detrusor smooth muscle and its pattern of innervation. J Urol 163:646-651, 2000.
16. Haferkamp A, Mundhenk J, Bastian PJ, et al: Increased expression of connexin 43 in the overactive neurogenic detrusor. Eur Urol 46:799-805, 2000.
17. Coolsaet BL, Van Duyl WA, Van Os-Bossagh P, De Bakker HV: New concepts in relation to urge and detrusor activity. Neurourol Urodyn 12:463-471, 1993.
18. Charlton RG, Morley AR, Chambers P, Gillespie JI: Focal changes in nerve, muscle and connective tissue in normal and unstable human bladder. BJU Int 84:953-960, 1999.
19. Elbadawi A, Yalla SV, Resnick NM: Structural basis of geriatric voiding dysfunction: III. Detrusor overactivity. J Urol 150(5 Pt 2):1668-1680, 1993.
20. Pandita RK, Mizusawa H, Andersson KE: Intravesical oxyhemoglobin initiates bladder overactivity in conscious, normal rats. J Urol 164:545-550, 2000.
21. Persson K, Poljakovic M, Johansson K, Larsson B: Morphological and biochemical investigation of nitric oxide synthase and related enzymes in the rat and pig urothelium. J Histochem Cytochem 47:739-750, 1999.
22. Birder LA, Apodaca G, De Groat WC, Kanai AJ: Adrenergic- and capsaicin-evoked nitric oxide release from urothelium and afferent nerves in urinary bladder. Am J Physiol 275(2 Pt 2):F226-F229, 1998.
23. Ishizuka O, Mattiasson A, Andersson KE: Tachykinin effects on bladder activity in conscious normal rats. J Urol 154:257-261, 1995.
24. Maggi CA, Giuliani S, Santicioli P, et al: Facilitation of reflex micturition by intravesical administration of [beta Ala8]-neurokinin A (4-10), a selective NK-2 tachykinin receptor agonist. J Urol 145:184-187, 1991.
25. Sun Y, Keay S, De Deyne PG, Chai TC : Augmented stretch activated adenosine triphosphate release from bladder uroepithelial cells in patients with interstitial cystitis. J Urol 166:1951-1956, 2001.
26. Sun Y, Chai TC: Effects of dimethyl sulphoxide and heparin on stretch-activated ATP release by bladder urothelial cells from patients with interstitial cystitis. BJU Int 90:381-385, 2002.
27. Sun Y, Chai TC: Up-regulation of P2X3 receptor during stretch of bladder urothelial cells from patients with interstitial cystitis. J Urol 171:448-452, 2004.
28. Schroder A, Chichester P, Kogan BA, et al: Effect of chronic bladder outlet obstruction on blood flow of the rabbit bladder. J Urol 165:640-646, 2001.
29. Elbadawi A, Yalla SV, Resnick NM: Structural basis of geriatric voiding dysfunction: II. Aging detrusor: Normal versus impaired contractility. J Urol 150(5 Pt 2):1657-1667, 1993.
30. Elbadawi A, Hailemariam S, Yalla SV, Resnick NM: Structural basis of geriatric voiding dysfunction: VII. Prospective ultrastructural/urodynamic evaluation of its natural evolution. J Urol 157:1814-1822, 1997.
31. Levin RM, Haugaard N, Hypolite JA, et al: Metabolic factors influencing lower urinary tract function. Exp Physiol 84:171-194, 1999.
32. Greenland JE, Brading AF: The effect of bladder outflow obstruction on detrusor blood flow changes during the voiding cycle in conscious pigs. J Urol 165:245-248, 2001.
33. Bratslavsky G, Whitbeck C, Horan P, Levin RM: Effects of in vivo ischemia on contractile responses of rabbit bladder to field stimulation, carbachol, ATP and KCl. Pharmacology 59:221-226, 1999.
34. Azadzoi KM, Tarcan T, Kozlowski R, et al: Overactivity and structural changes in the chronically ischemic bladder. J Urol 162:1768-1778, 1999.
35. Yuen EC, Howe CL, Li Y, et al: Nerve growth factor and the neurotrophic factor hypothesis. Brain Dev 18:362-368, 1996.
36. Bennet MR, Gibson WG, Lemon G: Neuronal cell death, nerve growth factor and neurotrophic models: 50 Years on. Auton Neurosci 95:1-23, 2002.
37. Graham CW, Lynch JH, Djakiew D: Distribution of nerve growth factor-like protein and nerve growth factor receptor in human benign prostatic hyperplasia and prostatic adenocarcinoma. J Urol 147:1444-1447, 1992.
38. Steers WD, Clemow DB, Persson K, et al: The spontaneously hypertensive rat: Insight into the pathogenesis of irritative symptoms in benign prostatic hyperplasia and young anxious males. Exp Physiol 84:137-147, 1999.
39. Lowe EM, Anand P, Terenghi G, et al: Increased nerve growth factor levels in the urinary bladder of women with idiopathic sensory urgency and interstitial cystitis. Br J Urol 79:572-577, 1997.
40. Steers WD, Ciambotti J, Erdman S, de Groat WC: Morphological plasticity in efferent pathways to the urinary bladder of the rat following urethral obstruction. J Neurosci 10:1943-1951, 1990.
41. Gabella G, Berggren T, Uvelius B: Hypertrophy and reversal of hypertrophy in rat pelvic ganglion neurons. J Neurocytol 21:649-662, 1992.
42. Kruse MN, Belton AL, de Groat WC: Changes in bladder and external urethral sphincter function after spinal cord injury in the rat. Am J Physiol 264(6 Pt 2):R1157-R1163, 1993.
43. de Groat WC: A neurologic basis for the overactive bladder. Urology 50(6A Suppl):36-52; discussion 53-36, 1997.
44. Geirsson G, Lindstrom S, Fall M: The bladder cooling reflex in man—Characteristics and sensitivity to temperature. Br J Urol 71:675-680, 1993.
45. Geirsson G, Fall M, Lindstrom S: The ice-water test—A simple and valuable supplement to routine cystometry. Br J Urol 71:681-685, 1993.
46. Dasgupta P, Chandiramani VA, Beckett A, et al: The effect of intravesical capsaicin on the suburothelial innervation in patients with detrusor hyper-reflexia. BJU Int 85:238-245, 2000.
47. Kim JH, Rivas DA, Shenot PJ, et al: Intravesical resiniferatoxin for refractory detrusor hyperreflexia: A multicenter, blinded, randomized, placebo-controlled trial. J Spinal Cord Med 26:358-363, 2003.
48. Chancellor MB, de Groat WC: Intravesical capsaicin and resiniferatoxin therapy: Spicing up the ways to treat the overactive bladder. J Urol 162:3-11, 1999.
49. Aguayo LG, White G: Effects of nerve growth factor on TTX- and capsaicin-sensitivity in adult rat sensory neurons. Brain Res 570: 61-67, 1992.
50. Yoshimura N: Bladder afferent pathway and spinal cord injury: Possible mechanisms inducing hyperreflexia of the urinary bladder. Prog Neurobiol 57:583-606, 1999.
51. Black JA, Cummins TR, Yoshimura N, et al:. Tetrodotoxin-resistant sodium channels Na(v)1.8/SNS and Na(v)1.9/NaN in afferent neurons innervating urinary bladder in control and spinal cord injured rats. Brain Res 963:132-138, 2003.
52. Vizzard MA: Changes in urinary bladder neurotrophic factor mRNA and NGF protein following urinary bladder dysfunction. Exp Neurol 161:273-284, 2000.

53. Nitti VW, Kim Y, Combs AJ: Voiding dysfunction following transurethral resection of the prostate: Symptoms and urodynamic findings. J Urol 157:600-603, 1997.
54. Kuo HC: Analysis of the pathophysiology of lower urinary tract symptoms in patients after prostatectomy. Urol Int 68:99-104, 2002.
55. De Moliner KL, Wolfson ML, Perrone Bizzozero N, Adamo AM: Growth-associated protein-43 is degraded via the ubiquitin-proteasome system. J Neurosci Res 79:652-660, 2005.
56. Tanner R, Chambers P, Khadra MH, Gillespie JI: The production of nerve growth factor by human bladder smooth muscle cells in vivo and in vitro. BJU Int 85:1115-1119, 2000.
57. Dupont MC, Spitsbergen JM, Kim KB, et al: Histological and neurotrophic changes triggered by varying models of bladder inflammation. J Urol 166:1111-1118, 2001.
58. Bjorling DE, Jacobsen HE, Blum JR, et al: Intravesical Escherichia coli lipopolysaccharide stimulates an increase in bladder nerve growth factor. BJU Int 87:697-702, 2001.
59. Vizzard MA: Increased expression of spinal cord Fos protein induced by bladder stimulation after spinal cord injury. Am J Physiol Regul Integr Comp Physiol 279:R295-R305, 2000.
60. Lagos P, Ballejo G: Role of spinal nitric oxide synthase-dependent processes in the initiation of the micturition hyperreflexia associated with cyclophosphamide-induced cystitis. Neuroscience 125:663-670, 2004.
61. Stone CB, Judd GE: Psychogenic aspects of urinary incontinence in women. Clin Obstet Gynecol 21:807-815, 1978.
62. Freeman RM, McPherson FM, Baxby K: Psychological features of women with idiopathic detrusor instability. Urol Int 40:257-259, 1985.
63. Walters MD, Taylor S, Schoenfeld LS: Psychosexual study of women with detrusor instability. Obstet Gynecol 75:22-26, 1990.
64. Chiverton PA, Wells TJ, Brink CA, Mayer R: Psychological factors associated with urinary incontinence [comment]. Clin Nurse Specialist 10:229-233, 1996.
65. Zorn BH, Montgomery H, Pieper K, et al: Urinary incontinence and depression. J Urol 162:82-84, 1999.
66. Dugan E, Cohen SJ, Bland DR, et al: The association of depressive symptoms and urinary incontinence among older adults. J Am Geriatr Soc 48:413-416, 2000.
67. Nygaard I, Turvey C, Burns TL, et al: Urinary incontinence and depression in middle-aged United States women. Obstet Gynecol 101:149-156, 2003.
68. Brown S, Lumley J: Physical health problems after childbirth and maternal depression at six to seven months postpartum. BJOG 107:1194-1201, 2000.
69. Lee KS, Na YG, Dean-McKinney T, et al: Alterations in voiding frequency and cystometry in the clomipramine induced model of endogenous depression and reversal with fluoxetine. J Urol 170:2067-2071, 2003.
70. Melville JL, Walker E, Katon W, et al: Prevalence of comorbid psychiatric illness and its impact on symptom perception, quality of life, and functional status in women with urinary incontinence. Am J Obstet Gynecol 187:80-87, 2002.
71. Weissman MM, Fyer AJ, Haghighi F, et al: Potential panic disorder syndrome: Clinical and genetic linkage evidence. Am J Med Genet 96:24-35, 2000.
72. Watson AJ, Currie I, Curran S, Jarvis GJ: A prospective study examining the association between the symptoms of anxiety and depression and severity of urinary incontinence. Eur J Obstet Gynecol Reprod Biol 88:7-9, 2000.
73. Klausner AP, Steers WD: Corticotropin releasing factor: A mediator of emotional influences on bladder function. J Urol 172(Pt 2):2570-2573, 2004.

Chapter 19

BEHAVIORAL MODIFICATION AND CONSERVATIVE MANAGEMENT OF OVERACTIVE BLADDER

Alain P. Bourcier

Millions of people throughout the world are affected by overactive bladder (OAB) syndrome, a serious condition that can have dramatic personal and social costs. Symptoms of OAB increase with age and are slightly more common in women. The median prevalence of incontinence in women has been reported as varying from 14% to 40.5%; using the definition of the International Continence Society (ICS), it is 23.5%. In women, urge and mixed incontinence accounted for a median relative share of 51% of cases.

These estimates have varied based on the differing methodologies of the studies and the previously uncertain definition of OAB. OAB is characterized by the ICS as a syndrome encompassing urgency (with or without urge incontinence), usually with frequency and nocturia.[1] OAB syndrome is a well-recognized complex of symptoms that is usually suggestive of detrusor overactivity but can also be caused by urethrovesical dysfunction of another type.

According to the ICS,[1] urgency, with or without urge incontinence, usually with frequency and nocturia, can be described as OAB syndrome, urge syndrome, or urgency-frequency syndrome. Lower urinary tract symptoms are the subjective indicator of a disease or change in condition as perceived by the patient, caregiver, or partner. In this context, urgency is the complaint of a sudden compelling desire to pass urine that is difficult to defer, increased daytime frequency is the complaint of voiding more than to seven times a day, and nocturia is the complaint of awakening one or more times at night to void. Urge incontinence is characterized by a strong desire to void coupled with an involuntary loss of urine.[2] OAB patients are likely to require long-term or even lifelong therapy to control their symptoms. Patients with OAB symptoms are at elevated risk for other conditions that increase their use of health care resources. Common patient reactions to OAB symptoms and incontinence are embarrassment, frustration, anxiety, depression, and fear of odor from urine leakage.[2]

Nonpharmacologic approaches include education and explanation of normal lower urinary tract structure and function, lifestyle changes, toileting programs, bladder retraining, and pelvic muscle training or rehabilitation. Behavior modification, which involves learning new skills and strategies for preventing urine loss and other symptoms, has a growing body of clinical research.

LIFESTYLE INTERVENTIONS

Behavior modification is a treatment option for persons with urinary incontinence (UI) and OAB. Changing a patient's behavior, environment, or lifestyle can mitigate or reduce symptoms (urine leakage or incontinence, urgency, frequency, and nocturia).

The interventions include lifestyle changes: cessation of smoking, weight reduction, elimination of dietary bladder irritants, adequate fluid intake, bowel regulation, moderation of physical activities, and exercises. Lifestyle changes and behavior modification are integral to clinical management of UI and OAB. In the United States, therapies have been combined to include interventions called behavioral treatments.

Behavioral interventions are a group of therapies used to modify stress, urge, or mixed UI by changing the patient's bladder habits or by teaching new skills. The interventions include lifestyle changes, toileting programs (e.g., habit training, prompted voiding), bladder retraining, and pelvic muscle training or rehabilitation (using methods such as biofeedback, vaginal weights, and electrical stimulation). Although research showing the effectiveness of changes in certain lifestyle behaviors on UI, urgency, and frequency may not be conclusive, many health care providers frequently recommend alterations in lifestyle and behavior.

Smoking

Increased intra-abdominal pressure may promote the development of UI and urinary urgency, particularly in women. This increased pressure exists with conditions that include pulmonary diseases such as asthma, emphysema, and chronic coughing such as seen in smokers.[3] Smoking, in particular, increases the risk of developing all forms of UI, and especially stress urinary incontinence (SUI); the level of risk depends on the number of cigarettes smoked. There may be several causes of the increased risk of SUI in smokers. Compared with nonsmokers, smokers have stronger, more frequent, and more violent coughing, which may lead to earlier development of damage to the urethral sphincteric mechanism and vaginal supports.[4] Violent and frequent prolonged coughing can increase downward pressure on the pelvic floor, causing repeated stretch injury to the pudendal and pelvic nerves. In addition, elements of tobacco products may have antiestrogenic hormonal effects, which may influence collagen synthesis. Nicotine contributes to large phasic bladder contractions, as shown in animal studies through the activation of purinergic receptors; nicotine seems to affect the human bladder similarly.[5] There may also be an association between nicotine and increased detrusor contractions. Bump and McClish[6] showed that women who previously smoked had a 2.2-fold increased incidence, and those who currently smoked had a 2.5-fold increased incidence of SUI. The risk of UI in women caused by cigarette smoking was estimated to be 28%. This study indicated that the risk of genuine SUI is positively correlated with both the current intensity of cigarette consumption and the degree of lifetime exposure to cigarette smoking. The increased prevalence of SUI in smokers is independent of other risk factors such as older age, parity, obesity, and hypoestrogenism. Smoking habits indicate that smoking can cause symptoms of urge incontinence and urgency and frequency.[3] Nuotio and colleagues[7] showed a correlation between smoking and urinary urgency in a population-based survey of 1059 women and men aged 60 to 89 years. Smokers were more likely to report incontinence than nonsmokers. In a survey of 2128 middle-aged and elderly men who smoked or formerly smoked, Koskimaki and colleagues showed an increased risk of lower urinary tract symptoms.[8]

Obesity

Obesity is an independent risk factor for the development of SUI and mixed UI in women.[9,10] Excessive body weight, specifically measured by sagittal abdominal diameter, affects bladder pressure. The SUI that occurs with obesity may be secondary to increases in intra-abdominal pressure on the bladder and greater urethral mobility. Also, obesity may impair blood flow or nerve innervation to the bladder. A woman with a body mass index (BMI) of 29 or less is considered to be of normal or low weight; a woman with a BMI of 30 or greater is obese.[3] Elia and associates[9] reported on 540 women who responded to a questionnaire and whose BMI status was obtained. The association between BMI and UI was statistically significant. Poor personal hygiene in obese women may lead to an infectious process. Mommsen and Foldspang found a relationship between SUI and an increased BMI.[11] Roe and Doll[12] reported on 6139 (53% response rate) respondents to a postal survey on incontinence status. Significantly more respondents with UI had a higher mean BMI when compared with continent respondents. This association was more prevalent in women than men. Brown and colleagues[13] studied 2763 women who completed questionnaires about prevalence and type of incontinence as part of a randomized trial of hormone therapy. A higher BMI and higher waist-to-hip ratio were found to be predictors of SUI and also of mixed UI when the major component was stress. This study found that the prevalence of at least weekly SUI increased by 10% for every 5 units of increased BMI. At this time, there is little information on whether weight loss resolves incontinence in women who are moderately obese. Obese women should lose weight before surgery to improve the technical ease, increase the durability, and decrease the failure rate of the surgery.[14] Maintaining normal weight through adulthood may be an important factor in the prevention of UI. Given the high prevalence of both incontinence and obesity in women, weight reduction should be recommended as part of the conservative management and behavior modification for obese women with UI.[3]

Dietary Habits

Fluid Management

Patients with UI and OAB symptoms may subscribe to either restrictive or excessive fluid intake behaviors. It is important to teach the patient that adequate fluid intake is necessary to eliminate irritants from the bladder and prevent UI.[3] Surveys of community-residing elders report self-care practices that include the self-imposed restrictions of fluid intake because of fears of UI, urinary urgency, and urinary frequency.[15] Adequate fluid intake is very important for older adults, who already have a decrease in their total body weight and are at increased risk for dehydration. Institutionalized patients are chronically dehydrated, because most require assistance to eat and drink. Although drinking less liquid does result in less urine in the bladder, the smaller amount of urine may be more highly concentrated and irritating to the bladder mucosa. In addition, inadequate fluid intake is a risk factor for constipation, another problem common in older adults. Nygaard and Linder[16] surveyed teachers and questioned their voiding habits at work, allotted breaks, and bladder complaints including urinary tract infections and incontinence. Teachers who drank less while working to decrease their voiding frequency had a twofold higher risk of urinary tract infection than those who did not report self-imposed fluid restriction. There was no association between urinary tract infection and either voiding infrequently at work or mean number of voids at work. Fitzgerald and colleagues[17] surveyed women who worked for a large academic center. Of the 1113 women surveyed, 232 (21%) reported UI at least monthly.

Incontinent women were significantly older and had a higher BMI than continent women. The strategies used by women in this study to avoid urinary symptoms included limiting fluids and avoiding caffeinated beverages. The recommended daily fluid intake is 1500 mL, but many believe that a more appropriate intake is 1800 mL to 2400 mL per day.[3] To be adequately hydrated, older patients must consume at least 1500 to 2000 mL per day of liquids.[18] It is suggesting by the renal physicians, that a total fluid intake of 24 mL/kg/day in a temperature climate is appropriate to normal requirements, and of course there are variations depending on factors such as amount of exercise or presence of air-conditioning at home.[19]

Influence of Bladder Irritants

The type of fluid or food is important. Caffeine is a xanthine derivative, a natural diuretic and bladder irritant. It acts similarly to thiazide diuretics. Caffeine is a central nervous system stimulant that reaches peak blood concentrations within 30 to 60 minutes after ingestion and has an average half-life of 4 to 6 hours.[3] Caffeine can cause a significant rise in detrusor pressure, leading to urinary urgency and frequency after caffeine ingestion.[20] Caffeine has an excitatory effect on the detrusor muscles.[21] Caffeine is found in liquids such as sodas (e.g., Pepsi, Coca-cola) and foods and candy that contain milk chocolate (e.g., 7 mg in 10 ounces of milk chocolate). Carbonated drinks that are identified as "caffeinated colas" have been associated with an increased risk of SUI.[22]

Alcohol also has a diuretic effect. Alcohol causes a release of antidiuretic hormone from the posterior pituitary.[20] Anecdotal evidence suggests that elimination of dietary factors such as artificial sweeteners (aspartame) and certain foods (e.g., highly spiced foods, citrus juices, tomato-based products) may promote continence.[3,23,24] Arya and colleagues[25] found that women ($n = 20$) with higher caffeine intake (361 to 607 mg per day) had a 2.4-fold increased risk for detrusor instability than women ($n = 10$) with a low caffeine intake (110 to 278 mg per day). There was also a correlation between current smoking and caffeine intake.

Bryant and coworkers[26] conducted a prospective randomized trial of persons with symptoms of urgency, frequency, and urge

UI who routinely ingested 100 mg or more of caffeine per day. Both groups were taught bladder training, but the intervention group was also instructed to reduce caffeine intake to less than 100 mg/day. Significant improvement in urgency (61% decrease), in voiding frequency (35% decrease), and in urine leakage (55% decrease) was seen in the treatment group compared to baseline. Even though current research is not conclusive, patients with UI and OAB should be assessed for amount of caffeine intake. They should be advised about the possible adverse effects caffeine may have on the detrusor muscle and the possible benefits of reduction of caffeine intake.[3,27] They also should be instructed to switch to caffeine-free beverages and foods or to eliminate them and see if urinary urgency and frequency decrease. If they continue to consume caffeine, clients with incontinence and OAB should take no more than 100 mg/day to decrease urgency and frequency.

Nutrient Composition of the Diet

Storage symptoms can affect quality of life and activities of daily living and have large resource implications for both the individual and the health service. Clinically, a number of foods and drinks are thought to have adverse or beneficial effects on certain urinary symptoms. However, little scientific evidence exists, and no studies have investigated the association between nutrient intake and urinary storage symptoms. The origin of detrusor overactivity may be neurogenic, with a variety of neurologic causes[28]; some of these may be related to diet, such as neuropathies resulting from vitamin B_{12} deficiency.[29,30] Another proposed pathologic mechanism is myogenic bladder overactivity,[31] possibly due to ischemia. Associations with diseases such as stroke and diabetes[32] suggest that OAB may be linked to a number of systemic conditions related to nutrition. In an earlier publication, Dallosso and colleagues[33] reported possible dietary associations with OAB in terms of food groups and individual food items and showed that lower intakes of three food groups (vegetables, $P < .02$; chicken, $P < .005$; breads, $P < .001$) were independently associated with increased risks of OAB onset. A higher intake of vitamin D was significantly associated with reduced risk of OAB onset ($P = .008$). There was some evidence of a trend toward decreased risk of onset with increasing vitamin D intake: those in the 4th quintile were 0.51 times less likely to experience OAB onset, compared with the lowest intake quintile (95% confidence interval: 0.34 to 0.78).

Evidence for an association between diet and the OAB symptom syndrome would be valuable in understanding its etiology. In a very recent study, Dallosso and associates[34] investigated prospectively the association between the nutrient composition of the diet and the onset of OAB. A random sample of community-dwelling women aged 40 years or older was studied. Baseline data on urinary symptoms and diet were collected from 6371 women using a postal questionnaire and food frequency questionnaire. Follow-up data on urinary symptoms were collected from 5816 of the women in a postal survey 1 year later. Logistic regression was used to investigate the association of diet (daily intakes of energy, macronutrients, and micronutrients) with 1-year incidence of OAB. There was evidence that three nutrients may be associated with OAB onset. Higher intakes of vitamin D ($P = .008$), protein ($P = .03$), and potassium ($P = .05$) were significantly associated with decreased risks of onset. Although overall the associations with vitamin B_6 and niacin were not significant ($P = .08$ and $P = .13$, respectively), there was some evidence of a decreased risk of onset with higher intakes. This study was the first to consider an association between the nutrient composition of the diet and OAB onset, and it provided some evidence that lower intakes of a number of nutrients may be associated with an increased risk of OAB onset. The association was strongest for vitamin D. Further studies are needed using additional validated indicators of OAB status and diet to confirm the associations found.

The observed associations of a number of nutrients with OAB onset present an overall pattern of low intake levels associated with increased risk of onset, possibly suggesting that general inadequacy of the diet may be an important factor. Although clinical deficiencies of protein and vitamins are very uncommon in Western countries, suboptimal levels of intake may be important.[35] Comparisons with the literature are difficult, because the only published work on diet and urinary symptoms comes from studies looking at prostatic enlargement in men, defined either clinically[36,37] or by reporting of symptoms.[38]

The Dallosso study[34] results suggested that low intake levels of certain micronutrients may be associated with increased risk of OAB onset, the most significant association being with vitamin D. Vitamin D and its metabolites are steroid hormones and have many important functions. Low vitamin D status is involved in the pathogenesis of several chronic diseases. Muscle wasting is a symptom of osteomalacia, the clinical condition resulting from vitamin D deficiency in adults, and muscle atrophy has been described histopathologically in type II fibers. The potential role of vitamin D in the function of the detrusor muscle needs to be considered. Because it is produced phytochemically in the skin by exposure to ultraviolet light, the level of dietary intake is not usually very important. Apart from the elderly and other at-risk groups, there is no recommended level of vitamin D intake in the United Kingdom.

This study[34] also provided some evidence that lower intake levels of the B vitamins niacin and B_6 may be associated with OAB onset. Bread and chicken are sizeable sources of niacin in the diet,[39] and lower intake levels of both of these food groups showed an association with greater onset of OAB in our earlier analysis.[33] Niacin is involved in energy metabolism and is essential for normal functioning of various systems of the body, including the central nervous system. However, the literature also reports strong associations with folate and vitamin B_{12}; this suggests that the B_6 association with homocysteine may be due to the fact that the three vitamins share the same food sources.[40] Potassium is very widespread in the diet, and a low intake is rare, sometimes occurring in people with bizarre or extremely low energy intakes. Potassium depletion in the body never results solely from an inadequate intake and is always associated with abnormal losses from the body. The largest sources in the diet are fruit and vegetables (30%) and refined grains (21%)[41]; in our earlier analysis, high intakes of vegetables and breads were associated with a reduced risk of OAB onset. A high potassium intake is generally considered an indicator of a "good quality diet," mainly because of its association with high fruit and vegetable content. The associated reduced risk of OAB onset could therefore be related to some aspect of a "healthy diet."

Dietary Changes with Improvement of Defecation

Lubowski and colleagues[42] reported that denervation of the external anal sphincter and pelvic floor muscles (PFMs) may occur in association with a history of excessive straining on defecation. Many believe that, if these are lifetime habits, they may have a cumulative effect on pelvic floor and bladder function. There is very little research that assesses the effect of regulating bowel function on incontinence and OAB. Spence-Jones and colleagues[43] found that straining excessively at stool was significantly more common in women with SUI and in women with prolapse than in women who experienced neither condition. Moller and coworkers[44] reported an almost uniform positive association between straining at stool and constipation and lower urinary tract symptoms in women ($N = 487$) 40 to 60 years of age. Moller believed that chronic constipation and repeated straining efforts induce progressive neuropathy in the pelvic floor. Because research suggests that chronic constipation and straining may be risk factors for the development of incontinence and OAB, self-care practices that promote bowel regularity should be an integral part of any treatment program.[3]

Treatment of elderly patients can significantly improve lower urinary tract symptoms, which include urgency and frequency.[45] Suggestions to reduce constipation include the addition of fiber to the diet, increased fluid intake, regular exercise, external stimulation, and establishment of a routine defecation schedule. Improved bowel function can also be achieved by determining a schedule for bowel evacuation so that the client can take advantage of the "call to stool," or the urge to defecate. The schedule should be determined by the client's bowel elimination pattern and previous time pattern for defecation. Dougherty and colleagues[46] conducted a randomized, controlled trial that incorporated reduction of caffeine consumption, adjustments in the amount and timing of intake of fluids, and dietary changes to promote bowel regularity, which were termed "self-monitoring activities." Women in the intervention group also received bladder training and biofeedback-assisted pelvic muscle exercises. A total of 218 women with stress, urge, or mixed UI were randomized, and 178 completed one or more follow-ups. At 2 years, the intervention group's UI severity had decreased by 61%. Self-monitoring and bladder training accounted for most of the improvement.

Epidemiologic research has revealed several factors associated with UI in women, the most commonly reported being age, pregnancy, and childbirth. Risk factors that may be modifiable have not been investigated to the same extent. Inadequate control for confounding factors is a weakness of several studies, and many investigations have been performed in selected populations. The aim of one large population-based study[47] was to evaluate the role of smoking and other modifiable lifestyle factors potentially associated with UI in women. A total of 27,936 women completed the incontinence part of the questionnaire. For the 6876 incontinent women (24.6 %), a severity index was calculated based on the answers regarding frequency and amount of leakage, and the incontinence was categorized as slight, moderate, or severe. The incontinence was also classified into three different subtypes: stress, urge, and mixed UI. The participating women answered additional questions about many other topics, including smoking habits; intake of alcohol, tea, and coffee; and amount of physical activity. BMI was derived from the measurements of height and weight (kg/m^2) at the screening station. Proportions were used to describe the univariate relationship between UI and the ordered variables. Where relevant, possible interaction or confounding was evaluated by stratified table analyses and logistic regression. Logistic regression analyses were used to adjust for confounding and to establish the factors independently associated with the outcome, and odds ratios (ORs) were the effect measure.

Effects were denoted as strong if the ORs were 1.8 or greater and weak if they were between 1.2 and 1.7. In all logistic regression analyses, women without incontinence served as the reference group. All analyses were performed separately for each of the different outcomes under investigation: any incontinence (all incontinent women), severe incontinence, and the different subtypes. The crude analyses showed that the prevalence of any UI increased with increasing age and increasing BMI. Former smokers reported incontinence more frequently than did current or never smokers. An increasing intake of tea and coffee seemed to be associated with a higher prevalence of incontinence, whereas the inverse relationship was true for intake of alcoholic beverages. The crude prevalences also suggested an association between physical activity and any incontinence.

The prevalence of severe incontinence and of the different subtypes of incontinence varied in a pattern parallel to that for any incontinence, according to the factor in question. When smoking status was explored, there was no association between any incontinence and former or current smoking of less than 20 cigarettes a day, but there was an increased and significant OR for both former and current smoking of 20 cigarettes or more daily. The effect was stronger for severe incontinence. For the different subtypes of incontinence, smoking status showed an weak and significant association only with mixed incontinence. Increasing BMI was strongly associated with any UI, with severe symptoms and with all subtypes An increasing amount of low-intensity physical activity was related to slightly lowered odds for any incontinence, severe incontinence, and both SUI and mixed types of incontinence. High-intensity physical activity showed only weak and insignificant associations to either of the outcomes. Daily tea drinkers had an increased risk for incontinence. The intake of tea was weakly associated with all three types, although not significantly for the urge type. Coffee had no effect on any incontinence and a weak but significant negative effect on severe incontinence and severe mixed type. The intake of alcohol showed no association with any of the outcomes under analysis.

Hannestad and colleagues[47] found that former and current smoking was associated with incontinence only for those who smoked more than 20 cigarettes per day. Severe incontinence was weakly associated with smoking regardless of number of cigarettes. The association between increasing BMI and incontinence was strong and was present for all subtypes. Increasing amounts of low-intensity physical activity had a weak and negative association with incontinence. Tea drinkers had raised risk for all types of incontinence. No important effects of high-intensity activity or of intake of alcohol or coffee were found. This study was designed to describe associations, and accordingly no conclusions could be drawn regarding causality. It remains for future research to establish whether modification of associated lifestyle factors alters the prevalence of incontinence. Nevertheless, strategies to discourage women from smoking should be implemented. At the very least, women should be educated on the relationship between smoking, UI, and OAB.[3]

Physical and Occupational Stressors: Sports and Fitness Activities

Another lifestyle behavior associated with triggering of SUI in young, healthy women is physical exertion. This is more common than health care professionals estimated, and it is one of the chief complaints in the younger female population. Physically active women are more likely than sedentary women to experience incontinence, and the problem is most common in high-impact sports, such as running and basketball, because repetitive bouncing can increase abdominal pressure and transmit the impact to the bladder. Because SUI occurs during physical exertion, we could say that this condition represents a major problem for females participating in fitness programs or sports activities.

Regarding the problem of PFMs, there are two contradicting theories about female athletes and the strength of their PFM.[48] The first theory is to consider that general physical activities strengthen all the body muscles, including the pelvic floor, and female athletes could have a strong pelvic musculature. The second theory is that heavy activities with repetitive pressure on the pelvic floor support may overload the pelvic floor and weaken these muscles over time. The PFMs play a major role in the continence control system. The speed and strength of PFM contractions may be one of the main causes.[49] During stressful situations (physical exertion, strain), the levator ani muscles pull the vesical neck upward, and the urethra is compressed against a supportive layer composed of the endopelvic fascia and the anterior vaginal wall. The theory of Petros and Ulstem, with their prediction that defects of the vagina or its supporting ligaments adversely affect the dynamics of the pelvic floor and the ability of interacting forces to coordinate closing of the urethra, is another explanation of the SUI associated with physical activities.[50] The high intra-abdominal pressure and/or weakness or nonfunctioning of the levator ani leads to loss of support of the bladder neck and urethra. These two parameters represent the mechanical hypothesis in the pathophysiology of SUI related to sports. Because of the rigidity of the abdominal wall, the pelvic diaphragm cannot play its role of "shock absorber." Prevalence of SUI in young female athletes and women who exercise ranges from 8% to 47%.

Nygard and associates[51] studied the relationship between exercise and incontinence. A self-administered questionnaire assessed the prevalence of both exercise and incontinence in 326 regularly exercising women (mean age, 38.5 years) attending private gynecologic offices. Eighty-nine percent exercised at least once a week, with an average practice of three times per week for 30 to 60 minutes per session. Researchers found that 47% of regularly exercising women reported some degree of incontinence. In another study[52] involved a group of 156 nulliparous, elite college varsity female athletes (mean age, 19.9 years), who were asked to fill out a questionnaire about the occurrence of UI during participation in their sport and during activities of daily life. Overall, 40 athletes (28 %) reported urine loss while participating in their sport. Activities most likely to provoke incontinence included jumping (basketball), running, and making impact on the floor as gymnasts do with dismounting or after flips.

Bourcier and Juras[53] studied SUI in sports and fitness activities in 59 women, whom they divided into two groups: group I (n = 28) represented female athletes, and group II (n = 31) represented women who practiced sports on a regular basis. In group I, the mean age was 25.5 years (range, 21 to 29) and mean parity was 0.5 (range, 0 to 1); in group II, mean age was 28 years (range, 23 to 32), and mean parity was 1 (range, 0 to 2). The degree of SUI was defined as severe (dripping incontinence on exercising), moderate (incontinence with heavy lifting, running), or mild (incontinence in jumping). In the athlete group, the prevalence of SUI symptoms was 7% for severe, 24% for moderate, and 33% for mild incontinence. Bourcier and coworkers[48] studied the relationship between physical activity and incontinence. A self-administered questionnaire assessed the prevalence of both exercise and incontinence in two groups of patients; 480 women (group I; mean age, 48.5 years) with no regular practice of sports and 120 women (group II; mean age, 28 years) who practiced sports on regular basis (>5 hr/wk) were investigated. The investigators reported that urine loss in group I was related to sneezing or coughing in 87% of the women; in group II, urine loss was related to running or tennis in 38% and aerobics in 35%.

The purpose of the study by Larsen and Yavorek[54] was to determine the prevalence of UI and to assess the stages of pelvic support in a population of nulliparous, physically active college students at the United States Military Academy. This was an observational study of 143 female cadets. Cadets in the freshman and sophomore classes were asked to participate in an ongoing study comparing UI and pelvic organ support before and after attending military jump school. The results were as follows. Overall, the group of women were found to be very physically active, with 69.2% (99/143) exercising four or more times per week and 91.6% (131/143) working out three or more times. Additionally, 49.7% (60/131) of those exercising spent 60 minutes or more per session. Running was the most common form of exercise, with 77.6% (111/143) running for at least part of their workout. Of the women examined, 50.3% (72/143) were found to be at pelvic prolapse stage 0 and 49.7% (71/143) at stage I. A total of 18.8% (27/143) women who reported recurrent incontinence, with the largest percentage (44%) being SUI by history. The conclusion of the authors was that 50% of nulliparous cadets had stage I prolapse on standardized pelvic support examination, primarily in the anterior compartment. A small percentage admitted to incontinence at the time of examination. This study indicates that trauma from physical activity might cause pelvic support defects that could predispose women to incontinence problems later in life.

Because the percentage of women who exercise and participate in sports is increasing, it is important to determine what effect this increase has on pelvic support. Jorgensen and coworkers[55] reported that Danish nursing assistants, who are exposed to frequent heavy lifting, were 1.6-fold more likely to undergo surgery for pelvic organ prolapse or UI than women in the general population. Fitzgerald and colleagues[17] surveyed women who worked for a large academic center. Of the 1113 women surveyed, 21% (n = 232) reported UI at least monthly. Incontinent women were significantly older and had a higher BMI than continent women. Women in this study used self-care practices such as using absorbent products or limiting fluids.

Several studies have reported on the relationship between UI and military training and activities. Women in the military have physically demanding roles, and the presence of UI can interfere with lifestyle as well as ability to perform assigned duties. Sherman and associates[56] found that 27% (N = 450) of U.S. female army soldiers (average age, 28.5 years) experienced problematic UI, with 19.9% saying they leaked significantly during training tests. However, only 5.3% felt that urine leakage had a significant impact on their regular duties. This may due to the fact that 30.7% women stated that they took precautions such as voiding before training, wearing "extra-thick" pads, and limiting fluid intake. A very disturbing finding in this study was that 13.3% of women restricted fluid intake while participating in strenuous field training. A third study[57] looked at women flying in high-performance combat aircraft. Aircrews who fly in high-gravity aircraft perform an M-1 maneuver, which is a modified Valsalva with an isometric contraction of the lower extremities. This movement may place women pilots at risk for urine loss due to increased intra-abdominal pressure and increased gravity load. Results of a questionnaire of aircrew ($N = 274$) indicated that 26.3% had experienced urine loss at some time. However, pilots did not have higher UI rates than women in other positions (e.g., navigators, weapon systems operators). In this study, as in others, crew position, history of vaginal delivery, and age were found to be significant risk factors.[3]

The data from these studies demonstrate that UI is not rare among young women. We think that young incontinent women need an appropriate treatment to prevent the possible worsening of symptoms, and it seems logical to develop strategies for screening those with high risk factors.[58] We assume that UI is a female disease with much higher prevalence than medical literature has demonstrated and with a surprisingly high prevalence in groups of physically active women.[48,53] Based on our current knowledge of the effect of pelvic floor muscle training (PFMT), we recommend that specific training pelvic programs be proposed as the first choice of treatment. The perineal blockage technique and the Knack technique appear to be effective adjunctive modalities for pelvic floor rehabilitation and can be proposed for active women.[48,53] The impact of carefully instructed pelvic floor exercises on sports incontinence has not been as beneficial as that in a normal female population.

BLADDER RETRAINING AND PELVIC FLOOR MUSCLE EXERCISES

Bladder Retraining

No single treatment modality should be considered the first choice of treatment in the management of either the unstable bladder or the urge syndrome. Bladder retraining, sometimes termed bladder drill, is a noninvasive treatment modality that has been used not only for these two conditions but also for mixed incontinence and even SUI.[59] It has been widely studied over the last 20 to 25 years, although little scientific work has been published recently. An excellent review of the subject is available in the Cochrane Library.[60] Bladder retraining is a form of behavioral therapy in which a patient with an intact nervous system "relearns" to inhibit a detrusor contraction or a sensation of urgency. Such behavioral therapies include biofeedback, hypnotherapy, and acupuncture. There are good reasons why behavioral methods or therapies may be of value in idiopathic urge syndromes. Although these have been a subject of review,[59,61] they can be summarized as follows:

- A strong emotive event in a patient' life may be the initial trigger for urinary symptoms.
- Patients with detrusor instability have a higher neuroticism score on formal testing than do patients with genuine SUI.
- There is relationship between detrusor instability and hysterical personality trait.
- Patients with detrusor instability are more likely to have psychosexual problems than patients with genuine SUI.
- Other behavioral forms of therapy, such as hypnosis, are effective methods of treatment.
- Treatment is itself associated with a strong placebo effect, which has been estimated at between 4% and 47% in clinical trials.

A frequently used treatment regimen[59] can be broken into the following components:

- Exclude pathology.
- Explain the condition to the patient.
- Explain the treatment and its rationale to the patient.
- Instruct the patient to void at set times during the day, for instance, every hour. The patient must not void between these times; she must wait or be incontinent.
- The voiding interval is increased by increments (of perhaps 30 minutes) after the initial goal is achieved, and the process is then repeated.
- The patient should have a normal fluid intake.
- The patient should keep her own input and output chart. The increasing volumes of urinary output at increasing intervals act as a reinforcement reward.
- The patient should receive praise and encouragement on reaching her daily targets.

Typical results note that up to 90% of patients become continent, although there is a relapse rate up to 40% within 3 years of treatment. Such relapses could be treated by reinstitution of a retraining program.

Most patients with a urodynamically demonstrable unstable bladder who were rendered symptom free also became stable on urodynamic assessment.[59] Several studies have compared bladder retraining regimens with pharmacologic treatment. Further studies have addressed the issue of supplementing bladder retraining with drug treatment. Although the data from such studies are currently limited, there is no evidence so far that supplemental drug therapy is superior to bladder retraining alone.[59,61] Therefore, bladder retraining appears to be equal or superior to drug treatment and may have greater long-term benefits.

There are numerous areas for future study. There is a lack of consistency in bladder retraining programs. There is a need not only to evaluate an optimal program but also, most importantly, to identify the optimal increment in both the voiding interval and the rate at which the voiding interval is iterated after attainment of each stage of the regimen. A shorter initial voiding interval, for instance, may be necessary for women with more intense frequency or with less confidence. There is clearly a popular benefit from widespread treatment in a community as opposed to treatment of a small number of patients in hospital, but there is a need to determine the optimal supervision in the community. There is a need for comparison between bladder retraining and other physical interventions. There are limited data, for instance, comparing bladder retraining with PFMT, estrogen replacement, and electrical stimulation. Bladder retraining is an effective treatment for women with urge, stress, or mixed UI. It is not yet clear whether the urodynamic diagnosis specifically affects the likelihood of success. There is a lack of consistency in bladder retraining programs, and an optimal regimen needs to be identified. However, it is possible that regimens will need to be tailored to the individual patient.[59] Bladder retraining appears to have benefits similar to those of drug treatment; it does not appear to be benefited by supplementary drug treatment; and it may have greater long-term benefits than drug therapy. Bladder retraining appears to be largely free of adverse effects and is acceptable to patients.[59]

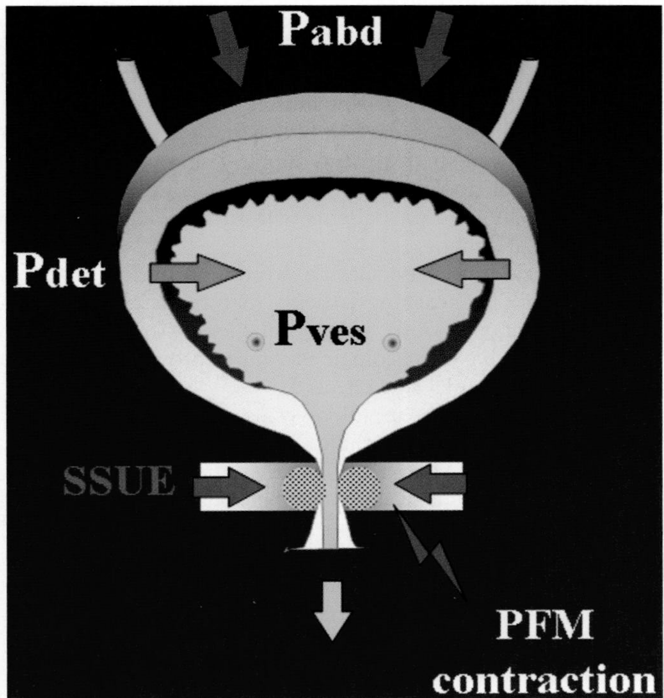

Figure 19-1 Pelvic floor muscle strength is important to the control of urge incontinence. Patients are taught "urge strategies" to prevent loss of urine. The goal is to challenge the urgency by using pelvic floor muscles to inhibit the involuntary detrusor contraction; this is accomplished by rapidly contracting the pelvic floor muscles and taking a deep breath. Pabd: Intra-abdominal pressure; Pdet: Detrusor pressure; Pves: Intra vesical pessure; SSUE: Externam Striated Urethral Sphincter; PFM: Pelvic Floor Muscles.

Pelvic Floor Muscle Exercises

The role of the PFMs in urge incontinence is less clear. Therapy is usually based on improving PFM function—in particular, the ability to sustain a contraction—and then using the improved muscle function in a bladder retraining program. Reflex inhibition of a detrusor contraction may be possible by producing a voluntary contraction of the striated muscles of the pelvic floor and activating the perineodetrusor inhibitory reflex, as described by Mahony and colleagues.[62] PFM exercises are also used for the treatment of OAB. The rationale behind the use of PFMT to treat urge incontinence is the observation that electrical stimulation of the pelvic floor inhibits detrusor contractions. The aims of this approach are to inhibit detrusor muscle contraction by voluntary contraction of the PFMs when the patient has the urge to void and to counteract the fall in urethral pressure or urethral relaxation that occurs with an involuntary detrusor contraction.[63] It has been suggested that reflex inhibition of detrusor contractions may accompany repeated voluntary PFM contraction or maximum contractions (Fig. 19-1).

Clinical Results: Bladder Retraining and Pelvic Floor Muscle Exercises

Berghmans and associates[64] recently reviewed the literature concerning the effectiveness of pelvic floor exercises for the treatment of OAB and concluded that, although bladder retraining seems to yield some benefit, the available data are insufficient to fully evaluate the efficacy of this strategy. Conservative treatment of women with UI, specifically PFMT and bladder retraining, is recognized as effective therapy.[65] Only three published reports of a single-session group education were identified, but none assessed improvement of pelvic floor contraction strength, an expected outcome of PFMT, or lengthening of intervoid interval, an expected outcome of bladder retraining.[66-68]

Frequency-volume charts (FVCs) are an important tool in the investigation of patients with lower urinary tract dysfunction, because they provide the ability to study lower urinary tract function during normal daily activities. The information obtained by FVCs is currently limited to the number of voidings, the voided volumes, the distribution of voidings between daytime and nighttime, the registration of episodes of urgency and leakage, and the number of incontinence pads used. Little research has been done to incorporate a sensory evaluation into these charts. However adequate sensation of bladder filling is important for proper bladder function. Currently, sensory information related to bladder filling is mainly deducted from cystometric studies in which the patient is catheterized and, in case of conventional cystometry, the bladder is artificially filled. To what extent these factors confound the sensory evaluation remains unknown. De Wachter and Wyndaele[69] studied whether FVCs can be used as a noninvasive tool for sensory evaluation. Furthermore, they studied the agreement between sensory data derived from these charts and data obtained during conventional cystometry. Fifteen healthy female, nulliparous students, without urologic history, between 18 and 24 years old, were asked to fill out a 3-day FVC during normal daily activities. They noted the time and volume of each micturition and scored the grade of perception of bladder fullness according to predefined grades before each micturition. All volunteers also underwent a conventional cystometric bladder filling at 30 mL/min and were asked to describe all sensations related to bladder filling. They also correlated these sensations to the same predefined grades of perception of bladder fullness that were used on the FVCs. Data from this pilot study showed that the information obtained from FVCs can be extended beyond just recording "classic" parameters such as voided volumes: these charts can be used as a noninvasive, inexpensive tool to evaluate sensations of bladder filling during normal daily activities. Moreover, sensory data deducted from FVCs show good agreement with sensory data from cystometric bladder filling. Because the largest proportion of the micturitions was made without a desire to void in the healthy female population we studied, the distribution of sensation-related micturitions may provide a new parameter to study bladder behavior. Including a sensory evaluation into FVCs and evaluating the distribution between sensation-related and non–sensation-related micturitions may improve the power of these charts to discriminate among different pathologies. The use of these "sensation-related FVCs" is currently being investigated in groups of incontinent patients.[64]

In a randomized controlled trial, Sampselle and colleagues[70] examined changes in pelvic floor contraction strength and intervoid interval at 12 months after intervention in women who attended a single group teaching session followed up with a single brief individual visit. They further examined the treatment group's knowledge of PFMT and bladder training as well as technique and adherence. Volunteers who qualified from telephone screening were randomly assigned to a control (no treatment) group or to a treatment group that received the behavioral modification program. Both groups underwent clinical baseline screening and evaluation of pelvic floor contraction strength (measured by palpation of pressure and displacement), as well as documentation of intervoid interval (measured by a 3-day voiding diary). The treatment group received a 2-hour classroom presentation of the anatomy and physiology of continence, with an explanation of the rationale and verbal instruction in PFMT and bladder training. This was followed in 2 to 4 weeks with an individualized evaluation to test knowledge (measured by response to eight multiple-choice items), technique (measured by palpation), and adherence (measured by report of practice). Brief additional instruction in PFMT and bladder training was provided as needed. Follow-up was by phone and mail every 3 months except at the 12th month, when all participants underwent a final clinical examination.

A total of 195 control and 164 treated participants completed the study.[70] In the treatment group, mean knowledge at 2 to 4 weeks after instruction was 87% for PFMT and 89% for bladder training. Palpation of PFMT technique revealed that 65% of participants needed no further instruction, and 32% required brief individual instruction (approximately 5 minutes); 3% were unable to demonstrate effective PFM contraction techniques after individual instruction and were excluded from the study. With respect to adherence, participants in the behavioral modification program were encouraged to practice PFMT every day throughout the 12-month postinstruction period. At the 3-month data point, 82% of participants reported practicing PFMT two to three or more times per week. At 12 months, the treatment group demonstrated significant increases in pelvic floor contraction pressure ($P = .0008$) and displacement ($P < .0001$), compared with controls. Intervoid interval also was significantly lengthened for those in the treatment group compared with the control group ($P < .0001$). A regression model that adjusted for UI level at baseline and other covariants, including race, age, and education, revealed a treatment group effect that was significant at $P < .0001$ for each of the three outcomes (i.e., pelvic floor contraction pressure, displacement, and intervoid interval). The authors concluded[70] that this randomized controlled trial of the effectiveness of group teaching of behavioral therapies followed by brief individual instruction as needed demonstrated positive effects on knowledge, technique, and adherence. The significant 12-month outcome differences between treatment and control groups provided evidence that this was an effective method to teach these behavioral therapies.

Clearly, the necessary knowledge and skills were imparted to enable women to perform PFMT and bladder training at levels that resulted in significant differences in pelvic floor contraction strength and lengthened intervoid interval. The greater efficiency of instruction when provided to groups rather than individually warrants further study to document cost-effectiveness outcomes.

BIOFEEDBACK THERAPY

Biofeedback can be defined as the use of monitoring equipment to measure internal physiologic events, or various body conditions of which the person is usually unaware, to develop conscious control of body processes. Biofeedback uses instruments to detect, measure, and amplify internal physiologic responses to provide the patient with feedback concerning those responses.[71,72]

The most common modalities of biofeedback involve electromyography (EMG), manometry, thermal measurement, electroencephalography (EEG), electrodermal feedback, and respiration rate. The instruments include sensors (EMG, pressure sensors) for detecting and measuring the activity of anal or urinary sphincters and PFMs, and techniques also have been developed to measure activity of the detrusor muscle for treatment of UI. A major reason for high interest in biofeedback is that the patient is actively involved in treatment. Biofeedback has now gained several potential applications for urologic conditions, having been successfully used for patients with urologic disorders such as detrusor instability.

Biofeedback is a very specific treatment that can restore bladder control by teaching patients to modulate the mechanisms of continence. Also, behavioral therapy can be used in combination with pharmacologic therapy to provide an excellent response with minimal side effects.[73]

For biofeedback to be useful, several conditions must be met. There must be a readily detectable and measurable response (e.g., bladder pressure, PFM activity), and there must be a perceptible cue (e.g., the sensation of urgency) that indicates to the patient when control should be performed. Of particular importance is the patient's ability to modify bladder function through operant conditioning. In the application of biofeedback to the treatment of UI, the concepts of neurophysiology of voiding and learning and conditioning are combined to accomplish the clinical objective of voluntary control of bladder function.[74,75]

Cystometric Biofeedback

During cystometry, bladder pressure readings are available to the patients and may provide a mechanism for feedback that allows them to acquire better control. An overactive detrusor contraction with imperative urge should be inhibited before it escalates. Cystometric biofeedback is used to teach the patient how to recognize and inhibit detrusor contractions. Other authors have described similar methods.[76]

The original technique for biofeedback in the management of idiopathic detrusor instability was described by Cardozo and colleagues.[77] After an initial explanation, the patient's detrusor pressure was measured cystometrically and recorded on a chart recorder. A voltage-to-frequency converter was connected to the detrusor pressure strain-gauge amplifier. This emitted an auditory signal rather like a siren. Alternatively, for patients who exhibited confusing rectal contractions during the treatment sessions, the auditory feedback could be transferred to the intravesical-pressure strain gauge. The gain and frequency range were adjusted to suit the individual patient, but once a baseline tone was decided upon, the note emitted through the loudspeaker increased in pitch as the detrusor pressure rose and decreased as it fell. A mirror was positioned in such a way that the patient could observe the detrusor (or intravesical) pressure tracing. Female patients attended four to eight 1-hour sessions, during which the bladder was filled two or three times with 0.9% saline prewarmed to body temperature. When detrusor contractions occurred, they could be heard and seen, and these signals were associated with the symptoms of urgency and urge incontinence.

The women were instructed to attempt to control the pitch of the auditory signal by deep breathing, general relaxation, tightening certain muscle groups, or any other means they found helpful. As patients learned to control their detrusor pressure during supine cystometry, provocative maneuvers such as erect cystometry, laughing, coughing, and running the water taps were employed.[78] Burgio and colleagues[79] used a similar technique of bladder biofeedback in a behavioral training program for older

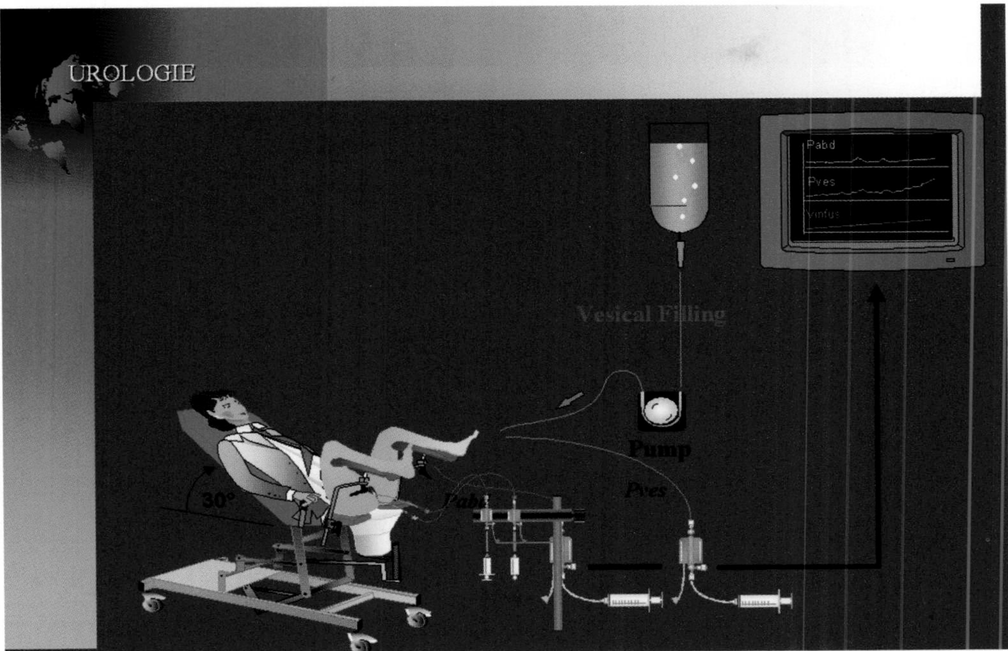

Figure 19-2 During cystometric biofeedback, bladder pressure readings are available to the patient and may provide feedback that allows the patient to acquire better control. The rectal catheter measures and subtracts the intra-abdominal pressure. When detrusor contraction occurs, it can be seen on the screen. The patient is requested to produce a voluntary pelvic floor contraction when she feels the strong urge to void. Pabd *(top)*: Intra-abdominal pressure; Pves *(middle)*: Intra-vesical pressure.

men and women with urge incontinence. During training sessions, patients observed bladder pressure during retrograde filling and practiced keeping bladder pressure low. Cystometric biofeedback requires the use of a transurethral bladder catheter and a rectal pressure monitor for suppression of the uninhibited contractions (Fig. 19-2). The bladder catheter measures increases in intravesical pressure indicative of uninhibited contractions. The rectal catheter measures and subtracts the intra-abdominal pressure. Artificial filling of the bladder is necessary for this technique of biofeedback and represents more accurately the conditions under which continence must be achieved during regular daily activities. Although this concept appears to be clinically relevant, filling of the bladder requires catheterization, with its associated discomfort and a small degree of risk. Such therapy could be proposed using urodynamics equipment with the biofeedback included.

Pelvic Floor Muscle Biofeedback

The three common signal sources (bladder pressure, anal sphincter pressure, and vaginal EMG) are significantly altered by increases in intra-abdominal pressure. Simultaneous measurement of abdominal activity should be done with all biofeedback therapy techniques. Intra-abdominal pressure can be measured easily using an internal rectal balloon. Electromyographic activity of the rectus abdominis muscles can be determined by surface electrodes. The abdominal muscle activity is displayed via two active electrodes placed 3 cm apart just below the umbilicus. A ground electrode is placed on a convenient bony prominence, such as the iliac crest.[73,80,81] Myographic biofeedback training has a twofold purpose: to increase the activity of weak muscle groups and to promote relaxation of spastic or tense muscles. Biofeedback equipment has become sophisticated, and there are two basic types designed to suit the setting in which biofeedback is implemented: the outpatient clinic, where the patient is trained using a comprehensive clinic system, and the individual's home, where a smaller unit is used, generally on a more frequent basis. Abdominal muscle activity should be monitored simultaneously with PFMs so that patients can learn to contract the PFMs selectively. These measurements can be accomplished through a two-channel system.

Another approach to biofeedback for UI[79,82] combines bladder pressure and pelvic floor musculature biofeedback in a procedure that provides simultaneous visual feedback of bladder, external anal sphincter, and intra-abdominal pressures. Using two-channel biofeedback (one with surface electrodes and one using an internal rectal balloon), patients are taught to contract and relax the PFMs selectively without increasing bladder pressure or intra-abdominal pressure.

The initial step in treatment is to help the patient identify the PFMs. It is important to test contractility and to know how the patient contracts the PFMs when instructed to squeeze around the examining fingers. Very often, the contraction is performed incorrectly (Fig. 19-3). Instead of lifting up with the muscles, the patient is observed to be bearing down, which is counterproductive because it increases intra-abdominal pressure and therefore bladder pressure.[82-84] This response has been referred to as a "reversed perineal command"[82,85] or a "paradoxical perineal command." The frequency of such incorrect contraction is about 22% in women after childbirth, and it decreases to about 10% in women in the perimenopausal period. Bump and colleagues[86] reported that 50% of women were unable to perform a voluntary PFM contraction after brief verbal instruction, and as many as 25% mistakenly performed a Valsalva maneuver. This type of

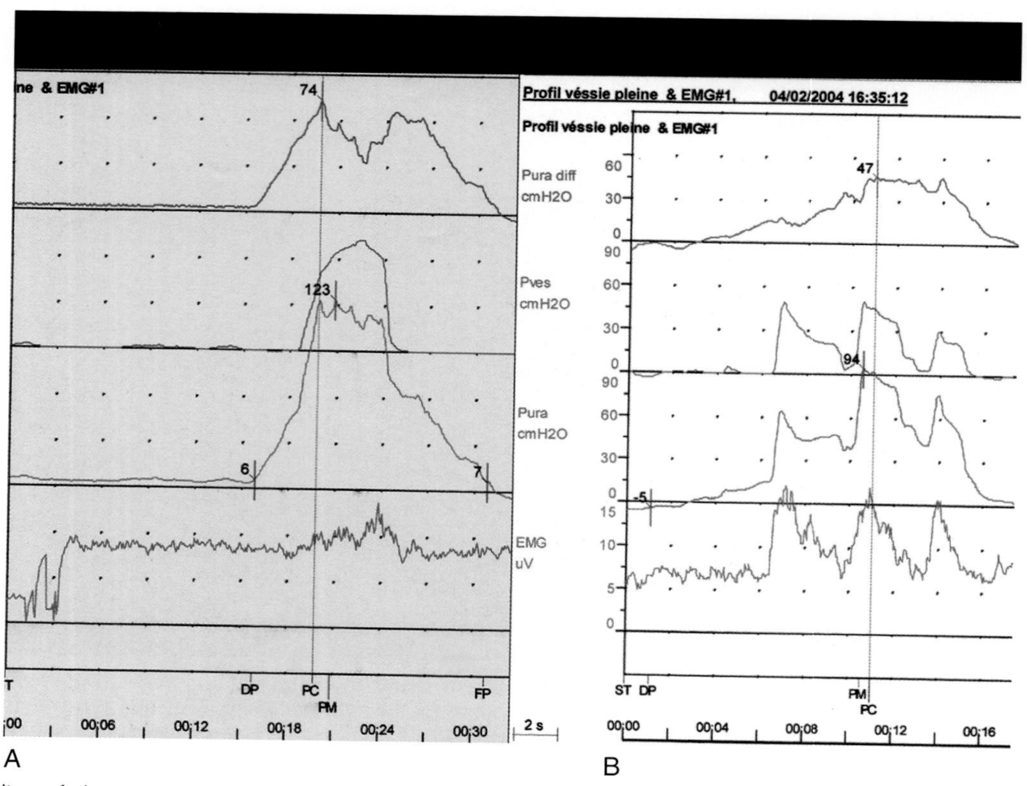

Figure 19-3 Recording of electromyographic (EMG) surface activity of pelvic floor muscles *(bottom)*, urethral pressure *(middle)*, and vesical pressure *(top)* during a hold maneuver. The graphs demonstrate abnormal voluntary perineal contractions. **A,** Paradoxical Perineal Command: Instead of lifting up the anus and vagina in drawing up, the patient is observed to be bearing down or pushing, which is counterproductive because it increases intra-abdominal pressure and therefore bladder pressure. From bottom to top, four tracings: Surface EMG of Pelvic floor muscles activity *(bottom)*; Urethral pressure Profile *(second)*; Vesical Pressure *(third)*; Differential pressure: Urethral Pressure minus Vesical Pressure *(top)*. **B,** Co-contraction of abdominal muscles. Some patients use antagonist muscles when contracting the pelvic floor From bottom to top, four tracings: Surface EMG of Pelvic floor muscles activity *(bottom)*; Urethral Pressure Profile *(second)*; Vesical pressure *(third)*; Differential pressure: Urethral Pressure minus Vesical Pressure *(top)*.

improper PFM activity needs to be identified and eliminated as soon as possible.

It seems clear that patients who bear down in this way must be identified before being asked to practice Kegel exercises at home, or the efforts will be futile. In addition, such maneuvers might increase vaginal wall descent or worsen UI by increasing intra-abdominal pressure. Except for the group of patients who are unable to perform a proper voluntary pelvic floor contraction, it seems very rare to perform a voluntary pelvic floor contraction without a co-contraction of the abdominal muscles. Research suggests that it is not possible to maximally contract the PFM without co-contraction of transverse abdominal muscle (transversus abdominis). Contraction of this muscle can be observed as a pulling in of the abdominal wall with no movement of the pelvis. During the initial biofeedback session, it is also common to observe patients perform pelvic muscle contractions accompanied by contraction of synergistic muscles such as adductors (pressing the knees), or gluteal muscles (squeezing the buttocks). This natural substitution of the stronger muscles for the weakened or minimally perceived motor response can also have negative consequences.

An instrumentation system allows multiple measurements and modalities to be displayed on a monitor and stored in a computer database. Feedback must be relevant in order to enhance learning and to focus on agonist (levator ani) and antagonist (abdominal) muscles. Patients should be able to recognize that the proper muscles are being used appropriately. Therapy is first concentrated on inhibition of the antagonist muscles and decreasing the activity of surrounding muscles while increasing the response of the agonists. Because the aim of performing the contraction is to contract the PFMs correctly, the proprioceptive signals generated by the substituting muscles can easily be misinterpreted as originating from the pelvic floor rather than from the strong antagonist muscles. When the substituting muscles contract, their afferents can mask low-intensity sensory signals that may be generated by the weakened PFMs. This faulty maneuver perpetuates the substitution pattern and delays the development of increased awareness of the isolated PFMs. During the initial session (Fig. 19-4), this pattern occurs quite often as the patient attempts to contract her PFMs by moving the upper part of the abdomen, even rising off the table.

When the patient is instructed to relax the abdominal muscles or the surrounding muscles (adductors/gluteal), substitution of the interfering muscles may be detected by the biofeedback equipment. An abdominal substitution pattern used when attempting to "hold back" leads to a false maneuver of pushing down, which causes a rise in intra-abdominal pressure. With such recruitment, the contraction would only maximize a rise of intra-abdominal pressure, resulting in an increase in EMG abdominal signals.

To minimize inappropriate tensing, it is helpful to train patients to keep these muscles relaxed when trying to prevent urine loss. For this purpose, patients are instructed to breathe evenly and to relax abdominal muscles. During the training

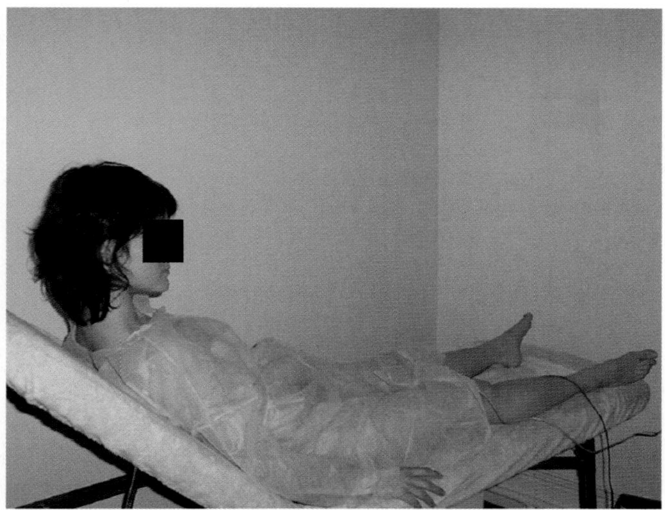

Figure 19-4 The initial step in treatment is to help the patient identify the pelvic floor muscles. During the session, the patient needs to be comfortably installed with legs slightly apart and abducted. Patient is instructed to breathe evenly and to relax abdominal muscles.

sessions, the patient is also asked to place one hand on her lower abdomen to palpate the faulty abdominal contraction.

Biofeedback therapy provides the patient with better volitional control over skeletal muscles such as levator ani and urinary sphincter, heightened sensory awareness of the pelvic floor area, and decreased muscle antagonist contractions. PFM strength and control are also important to the control of urge incontinence.[79,82] Patients with urge incontinence are taught "urge strategies" to prevent loss of urine during detrusor contractions. Patients with urge incontinence typically report that they rush to the toilet when they experience a sensation of urgency to void. Voluntary PFM contraction to control urge has been shown to be effective in the management of urge incontinence.[79,82,87,88] Godec and colleagues[89] inhibited reflex contraction of the detrusor muscle with an electrically stimulated contraction of the PFM. Reflex inhibition of detrusor contractions may accompany repeated voluntary pelvic floor contractions.[90] Patients are taught a more effective pattern of responding to urgency. They are told not to rush to the toilet, because this movement increases abdominal pressure on the bladder, increasing the likelihood of incontinence. Instead, they are encouraged to pause, sit down if possible, practice relaxing, and contract the PFMs maximally several times in an effort to diminish urgency, inhibit detrusor contraction, and prevent urine loss. When urgency subsides, they then proceed at a normal pace to the toilet.[79,82,87] Multichannel systems (Figs. 19-5 and 19-6) allow pressure and EMG measurements as well as abdominal measurements, thereby providing the clinician with multiple methods of biofeedback.

Clinical Results

Many studies have demonstrated that treatment with biofeedback reduces incontinence. The data show clearly that the treatments are safe and effective, and they yield high levels of patient satisfaction. Cardozo and colleagues[91] reported a study of 34 women between the ages of 16 and 65 years treated by bladder biofeedback. They were given an average of 5.4 sessions of cystometric biofeedback. Female patients were treated in 4- to 8-hour sessions at weekly intervals, during which the bladder was filled two to three times using 0.9% saline prewarmed to body temperature. A total of 87% were cured or improved subjectively and 60% objectively. No patient's condition was worsened by biofeedback. The six patients who failed to improve had severe detrusor instability, with detrusor contractions greater than 60 cm H_2O and a cystometric capacity of less than 200 mL. They found it impossible to inhibit detrusor activity. One of them was later found to have multiple sclerosis. Patient follow-up proved difficult, but of 11 women who were initially cured or improved, 4 remained completely cured and 2 had undergone surgery. These long-term results seem disappointing, but all the patients in the group had previously failed drug therapy.[92]

Millard and Oldenburg[93] used bladder training, bladder biofeedback, or a combination of both to treat 59 women with frequency, nocturia, urgency, and urge incontinence. The women underwent urodynamic testing, which revealed detrusor instability alone in 38 women, detrusor instability and sphincter incompetence in 6, sensory urgency in 12, and sensory urgency and sphincter incompetence in 3. All patients were initially hospitalized for 5 to 14 days and then assigned to either a Frewen-type bladder training program or a weekly outpatient biofeedback program. Millard and Oldenburg stated that "biofeedback was undoubtedly the most useful of the techniques."[55] They claimed a 74% rate of cure or major improvement for patients with detrusor instability. None of the patients with detrusor instability and urethral incompetence was cured, although three of them improved, with conversion to stable cystometry. Of the women with sensory urgency, 92% benefited. It is difficult to see how biofeedback could have helped them, because their symptoms could not have been associated with cystometric changes. We think that patients were using their inhibition skills to abort detrusor contractions and give themselves enough time to reach the bathroom; it is difficult to separate components of treatment (bladder retraining, biofeedback).

Kjolseth and colleagues[94] assessed the outcome of biofeedback therapy (bladder filling with visual stimuli) in 15 children (6 to 12 years of age) and 7 adults (aged 20 to 50 years) with cystometrically proven detrusor instability. Detrusor pressure was visually conveyed to the patient during repeated bladder fillings.

Patients were instructed to inhibit detrusor pressure incrementally by tensing the pelvic floor musculature. None of the children was completely cured, but nine showed a marked decrease in the number or extent of symptoms. Two children showed moderate improvement, and for four children the treatment failed. One adult was completely cured, two showed moderate improvement, and four remained the same. None of these patients was converted to stable bladder.

In an uncontrolled study, Burgio and colleagues[79,82] demonstrated an 88% reduction in incontinence episodes in elderly men with urge incontinence who participated in an average of four 30-minute biofeedback training sessions. O'Donnell and Doyle[95] treated 20 male patients (>65 years old) with urge incontinence using 1-hour sessions twice weekly for 5 weeks. The mean number of incontinence episodes was decreased from 5.1 to 2.0 per day after treatment. Burns and colleagues[96,97] conducted a randomized clinical trial of vaginal EMG biofeedback in the treatment of SUI or mixed UI.[9] As part of this trial, older women (>55 years old) were assigned to 8 weeks of biofeedback-assisted PFMT. A no-treatment control group contained 38 subjects. Biofeedback combined with daily practice resulted in a mean 61% reduction in frequency of urine losses; this was not significantly better than

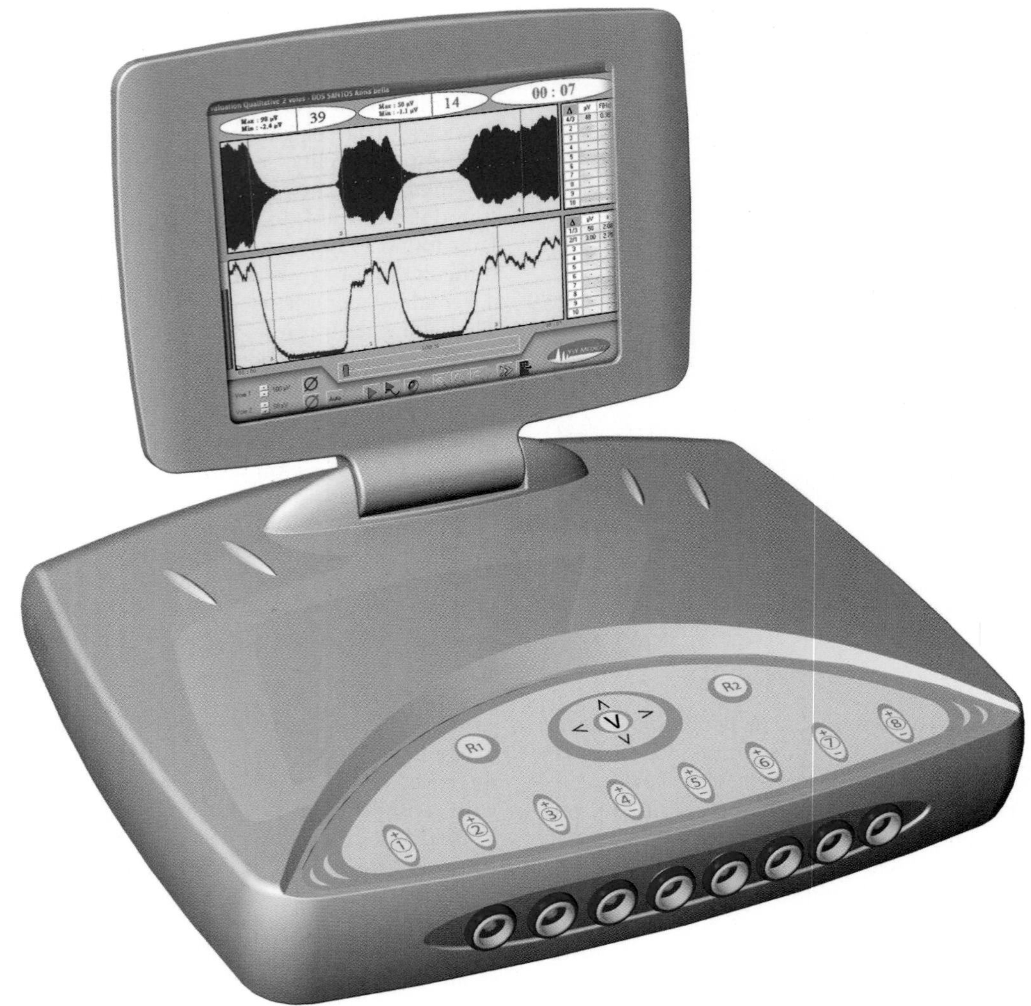

Figure 19-5 The unit used by the patient at home could be connected the stationary device. (Courtesy of HMT Inc.)

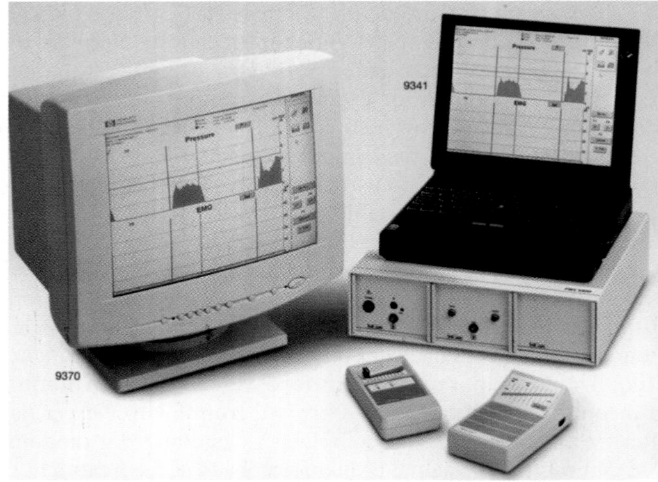

Figure 19-6 Multichannel system allows pressure and electromyographic measurements as well as abdominal measurements. (Courtesy of Incare Medical Products Inc.).

training without biofeedback, which resulted in a mean 59% reduction of incontinence. Both results were significantly better than the mean 9% increase in incontinence demonstrated by the control group.

Because the mechanisms of urge incontinence are in some ways different from the mechanisms for SUI, the role that biofeedback plays in treating these conditions may be different as well. The contribution of biofeedback in the treatment of urge incontinence was examined in a randomized study of 20 older men and women with persistent urge incontinence.[98] Patients who were trained without biofeedback responded as well to treatment as those trained with bladder-sphincter biofeedback. Later, a larger randomized controlled trial corroborated this finding. Burgio and colleagues[82,88] studied 222 older women with predominantly urge incontinence. Patients were randomly assigned to behavioral training with biofeedback, behavioral training without biofeedback, or behavioral training with a self-help booklet. Instead of biofeedback, training was done with verbal feedback based on vaginal palpation. Patients in the biofeedback group showed a 63% reduction of incontinence, which was not significantly different from the 69% reduction in the verbal feedback group. These findings indicate that careful training with verbal feedback is as effective as biofeedback in the first-line treatment of urge incontinence, and that biofeedback can be reserved for those cases in which women cannot successfully identify their muscles. Stein and colleagues evaluated the long-term effectiveness of transvaginal or transrectal EMG biofeedback in 28 patients with stress and urge incontinence.[99] Sixty percent of the patients had detrusor instability, as demonstrated by urodynamics. Biofeedback successfully treated 5 (36%) of 14 patients with SUI and 9 (43%) of 21 with urge incontinence. The treatment response was durable throughout follow-up, from 3 to 36 months, in all of the responding patients. The authors concluded that biofeedback is a moderately effective treatment for stress and urge incontinence and should be offered to patients as a treatment option.

PFMT with biofeedback is also effective for treatment of predominantly urge incontinence. Burgio and colleagues[82,87] conducted a randomized clinical trial to compare biofeedback-assisted behavioral training with drug therapy (oxybutynin chloride) for treatment of urge incontinence in ambulatory, community-dwelling older women. A volunteer sample of 197 older women (55 to 92 years of age) was evaluated. Subjects were randomized to four sessions (8 weeks) of biofeedback-assisted behavioral treatment, drug treatment, or a placebo control condition. Daily bladder diaries were completed by patients before, during, and after treatment. Behavioral training, which resulted in a mean 80.7% improvement, was significantly more effective than drug treatment (mean, 68.5% improvement; P = .009). Similarly, a larger proportion of subjects in the behavioral group achieved at least 50% and 75% reductions of incontinence (P = .002 and P = .001, respectively). Although the values for full recovery of continence (100%) followed a similar pattern, the differences were not statistically significant (P = .07). Several secondary outcome measures were used to assess the patients' perceptions of treatment. On every parameter, the behavioral group reported the highest perceived improvement and satisfaction with treatment progress ($P < .001$).

Wyman and colleagues compared the efficacy of bladder training, PFM exercise with biofeedback-assisted instruction, and combination therapy in women with genuine SUI and in those with detrusor instability.[100] This was a large randomized clinical trial with three treatment groups. Women with incontinence (N = 204: 145 with SUI and 59 with urge incontinence due to instability) received a 12-week intervention program, including six weekly office visits and six weekly mail or telephone contacts. They were followed up immediately and after 3 months. The combination therapy group had significantly fewer incontinent episodes, better quality of life, and greater treatment satisfaction immediately after the therapy. No differences between groups were observed at the 3-month follow-up. The authors concluded that combination therapy consisting of bladder training and PFMT with biofeedback had the greatest immediate efficacy in the management of female UI.

ELECTRICAL STIMULATION

Basic Principles and Mechanism of Action

Electrical currents are applied therapeutically to stimulate muscle contraction, usually through activation of nerves that supply muscles. Electrical stimulation was first used in the management of UI in 1952, when Bors[101] described the influence of electrical stimulation on the pudendal nerves, and in 1963, when Caldwell[102] developed electrodes that were permanently implanted into the pelvic floor and controlled by radiofrequency.

Godec and associates[103] first described the use of nonimplanted stimulators specifically for bladder inhibition. Initial work in animals indicated the potential of this therapy, and early clinical experience in Europe supported its likely efficacy. Much confusion surrounds electrical stimulation, and some is the result of inconsistent nomenclature. Commonly used terms include "functional electrical stimulation" and "neuromuscular electrical stimulation." Further confusion has arisen because of the wide range of stimulators, probes, and applications used.

Electrical stimulation is an effective treatment for urge incontinence. This technique uses natural pathways and the micturition reflexes , and its efficacy relies on a preserved reflex arc, with complete or partial integrity of the PFM innervation.[104] Based on animal experiments, direct stimulation of afferent or efferent fibers appears to be the most important mechanism to enhance the reflex response.

The mechanism of electrical stimulation for urge incontinence is a reflex inhibition of detrusor contraction. Bladder inhibition is accomplished through three mechanisms[105,106]:

1. Activation of afferent fibers within the pudendal nerve by activation of the hypogastric nerve at low intravesical pressure, corresponding to the filling phase
2. Direct inhibition of the pelvic nerve within the sacral cord at high intravesical pressure
3. Supraspinal inhibition of the detrusor reflex

In principle, defective control of the urinary bladder, resulting in urge incontinence, is caused by a central nervous dysfunction that affects central inhibitory control of the micturition reflex. Appropriate electrical stimulation may restore the inhibition effect.[107] Threshold intensity varies inversely with fiber diameter.

Any pulse configuration can provide nerve activation, and many stimulation waveforms have been used to cause neural excitation.[105,107] These include biphasic capacitively coupled pulses, monophasic square pulses, biphasic square pulses, and monophasic capacitively coupled spike pulses. Pulse durations ranged from 0.08 milliseconds up to 100 milliseconds but the most common used pulse duration is 0.2 milliseconds. To minimize electrochemical reactions at the electrode-mucosa interface, biphasic or alternating pulses are recommended.[108] The effects of electrical stimulation on detrusor inhibition are optimal with different stimulation parameters: 10 to 20 Hz. The sacral afferent nerves, particularly the autonomic nerves of the pelvic organs, are poorly myelinated (Aδ) or unmyelinated (C) fibers, which conduct current at a slow rate of 5 to 20 Hz. Thus, in the treatment of bladder instability and hyperreflexia, low-frequency stimulation is applied to the pudendal nerve afferents through probes. In both forms of electrical stimulation, the frequencies are chosen based on the clinical diagnosis. In mixed incontinence, two strategies are used. One strategy involves the use of a compromise setting of approximately 20 Hz; the other involves delivering both low-frequency and high-frequency stimuli.[109] Low frequencies (1 to 5 Hz) generate twitch contractions, allowing little sustained tension to develop in the muscle. Slow-twitch muscle fibers have a natural firing rate of 10 to 20 Hz, whereas fast-twitch fibers fire at 30 to 60 Hz.

Treatment of chronic lower urinary tract dysfunction can be challenging and difficult. Behavioral and medical therapies in

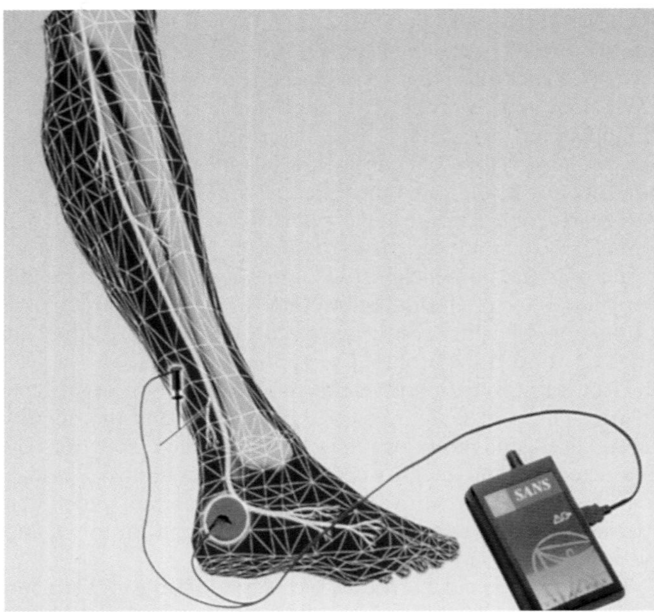

Figure 19-7 Transcutaneous electrical stimulation of the peripheral nerves may facilitate inhibition of detrusor activity, with specific parameters: intensity of 5 to 8 V, frequency of 10 Hz, and pulse width of 5 to 20 msec. Transcutaneous posterior nerve stimulation is performed with a needle inserted 5 cm cephalad to the medial malleolus.

patients with urge incontinence often result in unsatisfactory outcomes, leaving the patient with refractory incontinence no other option but surgery (e.g., bladder transsection phenolization, clam-ileocystoplasty).[110] To sidestep surgery, electrostimulation offers an alternative for therapy-resistant urge incontinence. During the past decades, electrical stimulation of the bladder, sacral roots, and pudendal nerves has been explored with varying success. However, these treatments involve technical problems, high cost, or low patient compliance because of the discomfort associated with treatment procedures.[111-113]

Transcutaneous electrical nerve stimulation (TENS) of the S3 segment is a useful alternative in patients with detrusor instability.[114] Okada and coworkers stimulated thigh muscles and observed clinical improvement for several weeks to months.[115] However, TENS therapy can induce skin irritation and allergy at the stimulation site due to chemical and mechanical irritation. Consequently, other stimulation approaches have been explored. Research has focused on the effect of stimulation of afferent nerves in the lower limb. In cat experiments, Lindstrom and Sudsuang demonstrated detrusor inhibition through stimulation of the myelinated afferents of the hip adductor muscles.[116] Inspired by acupuncture points over the tibial and peroneal nerves, McGuire and Zhang applied TENS to these nerves to treat bladder overactivity. They reported restoration of bladder control in a small group of patients.[117] Stoller proposed percutaneous posterior tibial nerve stimulation (PTNS) for treatment of bladder and pelvic floor dysfunction.[118] In this multicenter study, PTNS was used for the treatment of symptoms related to bladder overactivity. The posterior tibial nerve is a mixed nerve, containing motor and sensory nerve fibers. Correct placement of the needle electrode induces a motor and sensory response (Fig. 19-7). Centrally, the posterior tibial nerve projects to the sacral spinal cord in the same area where bladder projections are found (i.e., the sacral micturition center and the nucleus of Onuf). These are most probably the areas where the therapeutic effect of neuromodulation of the bladder through PTNS takes place.

PTNS has a clear carry-over effect: 30 minutes of stimulation induces a lasting beneficial effect. In cat experiments, a 5-minute stimulation of afferent nerves resulted in more than 1 hour of bladder inhibition.[119] Perhaps some kind of learned behavior is activated by intermittent stimulation such as PTNS. This supposition suggests that higher regions within the cortical central nervous system are also involved. Furthermore, in rats, PTNS exerted its influence on FOS expression, suggesting neuromodulating action.[120] In addition, activation of endorphin pathways at sites within the spinal cord could affect detrusor behavior.[121] Parallel to the gate control theory for pain, it can be suggested that stimulation of large somatic fibers modulates or inhibits the thinner afferent Aδ or C fibers, thus decreasing the perception of urgency.[122]

Clinical Practice and Selection of Patients

Different types of electrical stimulation (see Figs. 19-4 and 19-5) include office therapy and the home treatment program.[123,124] Office therapy is also called the outpatient program or in-clinic treatment. With this approach, a stationary device with a wide range of electrical parameters is used in the office or clinic under the control of the therapist. The system can be modified to suit the needs of each patient. Devices with microcomputers allow the caregiver to change the stimulation parameters (e.g., waveform, pulse width, frequency) based on patient history and urodynamic data.

Many probes are available (Fig. 19-8), including a standard two-ring vaginal probe; an intra-anal probe; and a two-channel vaginal and anal insertion probe. Special conditions that affect the choice of probe include the following:

- Vaginal size (depth of 4 to 12 cm) and shape (e.g., atresia or gaping vagina)
- Vaginal angle (10 to 45 degrees) and quality of the levator ani (thin or thick fibers)
- Type and degree of vaginal wall descent

Accurate assessment of individual anatomic differences allows the therapist to select the appropriate electrodes to obtain the most effective results. Low frequencies (10 to 20 Hz) are used for urge incontinence. Some stimulators have controls that are used to adjust frequency, duty cycle, and timing. The stimulus and intensity of the current are also adjustable, and all of these systems allow easy graduation in the intensity of contraction.

Therapeutic stimulation is recommended for women with UI who have undergone unsuccessful PFMT as a first-line treatment.[125,126] Pelvic floor electrical stimulation is one of the nonsurgical approaches when treating UI. The stimulation decreases detrusor contractions in cases of OAB. Electrical stimulation must be performed in conjunction with a bladder drill and biofeedback.

The main contraindications to electrical stimulation are as follows:

1. Demand heart pacemakers
2. Pregnancy, if the risk of pregnancy exists
3. Postvolume residual (PVR) greater than 100 mL
4. Obstruction of the urethra, a fixed and radiated urethra, or a heavily scarred urethra

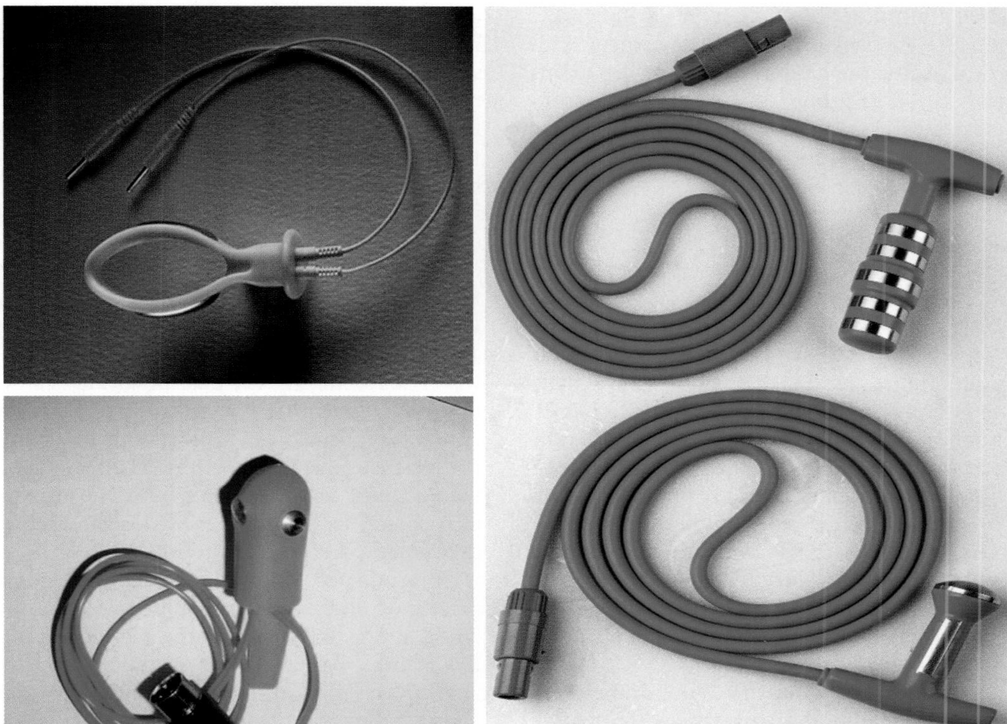

Figure 19-8 Many probes are available with special conditions that affect the choice of probe. **A,** A probe designed specifically for patients with a wide vaginal hiatus *(top left)*. **B,** The reference electrode is inserted in the middle of the vaginal probe *(top right)*. **C,** During a severe relaxation of the pelvic floor or an important defect of levator ani muscles, the "finger" probe is used *(bottom left)*. The patient is in lithotomy position with a one leg well supported while the therapist stimulates one side of the pubococcygeal portion of the levator ani with the "finger probe," which is a two channel probe. **D,** An anal probe with the reference electrode inserted in the middle *(bottom right)*.

5. Bleeding
6. Urinary tract infection or vaginal discharge
7. Complete peripheral denervation of the pelvic floor
8. Severe genital prolapse with complete eversion of the vagina

There are a few strict contraindications,[1,2,6,7] and there is general agreement that a patient with pelvic floor disorder associated with other conditions[4,5,8] will not respond to treatment. Although patients with severe genital prolapse are poor candidates, mild prolapse is not a significant problem. Many patients will not accept treatment with vaginal or anal probes because of ethical and religious beliefs. These concerns must be taken into account before this therapy is advocated. This issue is especially relevant when home treatment is being considered, because some patients will not agree to insert the device themselves, and some will refuse this type of treatment altogether. Functional, anatomic, and attitudinal barriers are more common in frail elderly people. Cognitively or functionally impaired subjects require a participating caregiver. In the elderly, home care treatment could be performed by a nurse or a physical therapist.

Patients with mild to moderate incontinence are the best candidates for this treatment, regardless of age. Because of the slight discomfort and embarrassment that may occur during stimulation, motivated patients of any age are the best candidates for this therapy. For unmotivated patients, another technique may be recommended, such as PTNS or electromagnetic stimulation.

In PTNS, the posterior tibial nerve is stimulated. This nerve closely relates to pelvic nerves for bladder and perineal floor; therefore, a retrograde stimulation of S3 roots and of sacral spinal cord can be obtained. Several studies on the effects of this treatment on OAB syndrome have been published.[127,128] TENS of acupuncture points (see Fig. 19-7) may be used to inhibit detrusor activity. Surface electrodes are placed bilaterally over both tibial nerves or both common peroneal nerves.[129] Percutaneous stimulation of peripheral S2 and S3 afferents by way of the posterior tibial nerve modulates unstable detrusor activity. PTNS[130] is performed with a 34-gauge needle inserted 5 cm cephalad to the medial malleolus TENS of the peripheral nerves may facilitate inhibition of detrusor activity with specific parameters, such as intensity of 5 to 8 V, frequency of 2 to 10 Hz, and pulse width of 5 to 20 msec.

Clinical Results

One major problem in reviewing the literature on incontinence is the lack of data on the pretreatment status of patients, particularly when noninvasive forms of therapy are studied.[131] The interpretation of data may be limited because patients often are not classified urodynamically. Nonimplanted stimulators are effective in treating UI: overall, an improvement or cure rate of approximately 50% is common. No serious morbidity is reported with this type of therapy. Side effects that are common with drug therapy (e.g., anticholinergics, α-adrenergics) do not occur with electrical stimulation.

Eriksen and Eik-Nes[132] performed a study of chronic stimulation with a dual vaginal-anal electrode in 55 patients. They found an initial response rate of 68%, with 47% of the overall group becoming dry. The objective response was an improved stress profile. Kralj[133] studied the influence of the type of idiopathic urge incontinence on the efficient outcome of treatment with acute maximal electrical stimulation. Eighty-eight female patients were divided into a motor urge group (n = 40) and a sensory group (n= 48). Both groups underwent vaginal stimulation for 20 minutes. Of the 40 patients in the motor urge group, 55% were cured and 20% showed improvement, whereas 25% showed no change. Of the 48 patients in the sensory group, 87.5% were cured and 12.5% showed improvement.

Bent and associates[134] conducted a study of 45 patients with genuine SUI (n = 14), detrusor instability (n = 10), or mixed incontinence (n = 21) and assessed the applicability of electrical stimulation and patient response to short-term electrical home therapy. Treatment was administered for 15 minutes twice daily for 6 weeks. Treatment consisted of biphasic stimulation at 20 Hz for urge incontinence and at 50 Hz for genuine SUI. The ratio of the duty cycle was 2 seconds "on" and 4 seconds "off." Subjective results showed improvement in 71% of patients with genuine SUI, 70% of patients with urge incontinence, and 52% of patients with mixed incontinence. The pressure-transmission ratio improved in four patients, and urethral pressure profiles improved in five patients with genuine SUI. Bladder capacity during cystometry improved in only one patient with detrusor instability.

Bourcier and Juras[135] conducted a study to establish the effectiveness of two different modalities: home treatment, consisting of treatment for 20 minutes twice daily for a 6-week period, and office therapy, consisting of twice-weekly treatment administered in the clinic for an average of 12 sessions. Of the 95 patients included in the study, 50 received home treatment and 45 received office therapy. Twelve patients had undergone a hysterectomy, and six had previously undergone colposuspension. All were evaluated with urodynamic tests. Patients with urge incontinence received biphasic capacity-coupled pulses with a continuous current of 20 Hz at a pulse width of 0.75 msec. Patients with genuine SUI received biphasic square pulses of 50 Hz at a pulse width of 1 msec. Current intensity was 0 to 90 mA or 0 to 24 V. During the first follow-up period (3 months), 71% of patients in the office therapy group reported subjective improvement, as did 51% of patients in the home treatment group. During the late follow-up period (6 months), 85 patients were studied (7 patients in the home treatment group and 3 in the office therapy group withdrew). Of the patients who participated in late follow-up, 47 were in the office therapy group (28 patients with genuine SUI and 19 with urge incontinence) and 38 were in the home treatment group (23 patients with genuine SUI and 15 with urge incontinence). The cure rate was approximately 50%. This study showed that both office therapy and home treatment are effective forms of treatment for patients with genuine SUI or urge incontinence. In addition, this treatment has no side effects. The results showed a higher degree of improvement with office therapy than with home treatment. The number of patients who did not continue physiotherapy was much higher in the group with urge incontinence (43%) than in the group with genuine SUI (15%). Patients with urge incontinence had less motivation to continue with therapy and also had a higher degree of psychological factors (e.g., chronic depression, psychosomatic disturbances, hysterical personality), which included reluctance to cooperate actively with treatment.

Many factors (e.g., age, severity of incontinence) are less crucial than previously thought, but the single factor that is consistently associated with positive outcome is greater motivation and/or compliance with the intervention.[136] Brubaker and colleagues[137] compared electrical stimulation with sham electrical stimulation in women with urodynamically proven detrusor instability and found a significant reduction in detrusor overactivity in the electrical stimulation group only. This prospective double-blind, randomized control trial included 121 women who had genuine SUI (n = 60), urge incontinence (n = 28), or mixed incontinence (n = 33). The study had two groups: a treated group (n = 61) and a placebo-controlled group (n = 60) with sham electrical stimulation. Patients underwent 8 weeks of treatment. Electrical stimulation was administered twice daily for 20 minutes with a vaginal probe at 20 Hz, a pulse duration of 0.1 msec, and a duty cycle of 2 seconds "on" and 4 seconds "off." The output was 0 to 100 mA; in the placebo group, sham electrical stimulation was characterized by no current in patient circuit. Objective cure was reported in 49% of patients in the treatment group who had detrusor instability, but no change was observed in patients with genuine SUI in either group. The authors found no significant change in the number of women who had genuine SUI on urodynamic testing at 2 months.

In a prospective multicenter study,[138] 35 patients with complaints of urge incontinence underwent 12 weekly sessions of PTNS at one of five sites in the Netherlands and one site in Italy. FVCs and I-QoL and SF-36 questionnaires were completed at 0 and 12 weeks. Success was analyzed by using subjective and objective criteria. Overall subjective success was defined as the willingness to continue treatment, whereas objective success was defined as a significant decrease (to <50%) in total number of leakage episodes. Twenty-two patients (63%) reported a subjective success. Twenty-four patients (70%) showed a 50% or greater reduction in total number of leakage episodes. Sixteen (46%) of these patients were completely cured (i.e., no leakage episodes) after 12 sessions. Quality-of-life parameters improved significantly. The authors concluded that PTNS is an effective, minimally invasive option for treatment of patients with complaints of urge incontinence, because improvement was seen in subjective as well as objective parameters.

One of the latest studies compared the three different approaches of conservative treatment: PFMT, biofeedback-assisted PFMT, and electrical stimulation (ES) in the management of OAB in women.[139] Exclusion criteria included pregnancy, deafness, neurologic disorders, diabetes mellitus, use of a pacemaker or intrauterine device, genital prolapse greater than stage two of the ICS grading system, residual urine volume 100 mL or greater, and urinary tract infection. Inclusion criteria included age between 16 and 75 years, symptoms and/or signs of OAB for more than 6 months, frequency of voiding eight or more times per day, and urgency of voiding one or more times per day. After the calculation of sample size, which disclosed that the total sample size should be at least 102 women, randomization of the eligible participants into the three treatment groups was performed. Initial assessment included a detailed medical history, a pelvic examination in the dorsal lithotomy position, a 1-hour pad test, and a filling and voiding cystometry, as well as a 4-day 24-hour FVC. Other assessments were evaluation of PFM strength using internal digital assessment according to the Oxford grading system and measurement of vaginal pressure with a balloon probe connected to a pressure transducer, as well as the Kings Health Questionnaire. The interventions included a PFMT program, an EMG-based biofeedback-assisted PFMT program with an intravaginal probe accompanied by a home program, and an electrical stimulation program using a biphasic symmetric probe current with a frequency of 10 Hz, a pulse width of 400 milliseconds, and a duty cycle of 5 sec "on" and 10 sec "off."

The treatment period consisted of 12 weeks. Patients also returned twice a week to the physiotherapy unit for mentoring of their progress. The treatment protocol for the biofeedback-assisted PFMT and electrical stimulation groups was conducted twice a week at the physiotherapy unit. The main outcome measures were post-treatment PFM strength, the record of the FVC, and the Kings Health Questionnaire. A total of 137 women with clinically proven OAB were recruited for the study; 120 subjects were randomly allocated to the three different treatment groups after 17 women were excluded for various reasons. Another 17 women dropped out during the treatment, leaving 34 women in the PFMT group, 34 in the biofeedback-assisted PFMT group, and 35 in the electrical stimulation to complete the study. Significant differences were noted between the biofeedback-assisted PFMT and electrical stimulation groups and also between the electrical stimulation and PFMT groups in specific gravity ($P = 0.22$ and $P = .003$, respectively) and the number of subjects in menopause ($P = .025$ and $P = .001$, respectively). A significant difference in parity ($P = .01$) was also noted between the electrical stimulation and PFMT groups. With regard to PFM strength, compared to the electrical stimulation group, the biofeedback-assisted PFMT group and the PFMT group both showed significant post-treatment versus pretreatment improvements in scale of power ($P = .001$ and $P = .001$, respectively), time of fast contraction ($P = .007$ and $P = .012$, respectively), and degree of vaginal pressure ($P = .001$ and $P = .001$, respectively). However, between the biofeedback-assisted PFMT and PFMT groups there were no significant pretreatment or post-treatment differences in these three variables. Based on comparison of the main outcome measures, either biofeedback-assisted PFMT or PFMT resulted in significantly better PFM strength and better quality of life than electrical stimulation and therefore was more effective than electrical stimulation in the management of OAB in women.

CONCLUSION

Although adjunctive therapies are useful because they may actively involve the patient in treatment, a combination of behavioral and pharmacologic approaches to the OAB syndrome offers the greatest chance of success.[140] Bladder training is a modification of bladder drill that is conducted more gradually on an outpatient basis and has resulted in significant reduction of incontinence in older, community-dwelling women. Multicomponent behavioral training is another form of behavioral treatment that includes PFM exercises. Patients may learn strategies to inhibit bladder contraction using PFM contraction and other suppression strategies.[19] Biofeedback is a treatment methodology that has considerable potential application for urogynecologic conditions and represents an important consideration in the initial treatment of UI for women of all ages. Further, it may be used to help relieve symptoms such as urge incontinence, detrusor instability, and irritative symptoms. Biofeedback-assisted training may be used as a conservative first-line therapy for urge or mixed incontinence, either alone or in combination with other behavioral or pharmacologic therapy.

Correction of continence with electrical stimulation has been achieved with various techniques, with results showing bladder inhibition. Electrical stimulation is indicated for patients who are not strongly motivated to perform pelvic floor exercises and for those with weak PFM activity. As the use of electrotherapy grows due to advances in technology, it is necessary that health care professionals carefully analyze innovative applications and demand a demonstration of the efficacy of this therapy.

Behavioral treatments are effective in only half of patients with OAB syndrome. It is not yet clear whether these approaches should be the first-line treatment for all patients with OAB syndrome or whether they should be used in conjunction with anticholinergic agents. In addition, it is not yet known which behavioral therapies are most appropriate for various subgroups of patients with OAB.[141]

References

1. Abrams P, Cardozo L, Fall M, et al: The standardisation of terminology in lower urinary tract function: OAB dramatically disrupts and diminishes the quality of life. Neurourol Urodyn 21:167-178, 2002.
2. McGham WF: Cost effectiveness and quality of life considerations in the treatment of patients with overactive bladder. Am J Manag Care 7(Suppl 2):562-575, 2001.
3. Newman DK: Lifestyle interventions. In Bourcier AP, Mc Guire EJ, Abrams P: Pelvic Floor Disorders. Philadelphia, Elsevier Saunders, 2004, pp 269-276.
4. Bump RC, McClish DM: Cigarette smoking and pure genuine stress incontinence of urine: A comparison of risk factors and determinants between smokers and nonsmokers. Am J Obstet Gynecol 170:579-582, 1994.
5. Ruggieri MR, Whitmore KE, Levine RM: Bladder purinergic receptors. J Urol 144:176-181, 1990.
6. Bump RC, McClish DM: Cigarette smoking and urinary incontinence. Am J Obstet Gynecol 167:1214-1218, 1992.
7. Nuotio M, Jylha M, Koivisto AM, Tammela TLJ: Association of smoking with urgency in older people. Eur Urol 40:206-212, 2001.
8. Koskimaki J, Hakama M, Huhtala H, Tammela TLJ: Association of smoking with lower urinary tract symptoms. J Urol 159:1580-1582, 1998.
9. Elia G, Dye TD, Scariati PD: Body mass index and urinary symptoms in women. Int Urogynecol J 12:366-369, 2001.
10. Burgio KL, Matthews KA, Engel BT: Prevalence, incidence and correlates of urinary incontinence in healthy, middle-aged women. J Urol 146:1255-1259, 1991.
11. Mommsen S, Foldspang A: Body mass index and adult female urinary incontinence. World J Urol 19:319-322, 1994.
12. Roe B, Doll H: Lifestyle factors and continence status: Comparison of self-report data from a postal survey in England. J Wound Ostomy Continence Nurs 26:312-319, 1999.
13. Brown JS, Grady D, Ouslander JG, et al: Prevalence of urinary incontinence and associated risk factors in postmenopausal women. Obstet Gynecol 94:66-70, 1999.
14. Dwyer PL, Lee ETC, Hay DM: Obesity and urinary incontinence in women. Br J Obstet Gynecol 95:91-96, 1988.
15. Johnson TM, Kincade JE, Bernard SL, et al: Self-care practices used by older men and women to manage urinary incontinence: Results from the national follow-up survey on self-care and aging. J Am Geriatr Soc 48:894-902, 2000.
16. Nygaard IE, Linder M: Thirst at work: An occupational hazard? Int Urogynecol J Pelvic Floor Dysfunct 8:340-343, 1997.
17. Fitzgerald S, Palmer MH, Berry SJ, Hart K: Urinary incontinence: Impact on working women. AAOHN J 48:112-118, 2000.
18. Kayser-Jones J, Schell ES, Porter C, et al: Factors contributing to dehydration in nursing homes: Inadequate staffing and lack of professional supervision. J Am Geriatr Soc 47:1187-1194, 1999.

19. Wells TJ: Nursing management. In O'Donnel PD (ed): Urinary Incontinence. St Louis, Mosby, 1997, pp 439-433.
20. Creighton SM, Stanton SL: Caffeine: Does it affect your bladder? Br J Urol 66:613-614, 1990.
21. Lee JG, Wein AJ, Levin RM: The effect of caffeine on the contractile response of the rabbit urinary bladder to field stimulation. Gen Pharmacol 24:1007-1011, 1993.
22. Dallosso HM, McGrother CW, Matthews RJ, Donaldson MK: The association of diet and other lifestyle factors with overactive bladder and stress incontinence: A longitudinal study in women. BJU Int 92:69-77, 2003.
23. Newman DK: The Urinary Incontinence Sourcebook, 2nd ed. Chicago, Lowell House, 1999.
24. Newman DK: Managing and Treating Urinary Incontinence. Baltimore, Health Professions Press, 2002.
25. Arya LA, Myers DL, Jackson ND: Dietary caffeine intake and the risk for detrusor instability: A case-control study. Obstet Gynecol 96:85-89, 2000.
26. Bryant CM, Dowell CJ, Fairbrother G: Caffeine reduction education to improve urinary symptoms. Br J Nurs 11:560-565, 2002.
27. Gray M: Caffeine and urinary continence. J WOCN 28:66-69, 2001.
28. De Groat WC. A neurologic basis for the overactive bladder. Urology 50:36-52, 1997.
29. Campellone JV, Bosley TM, Malloy TR. Neuropathic bladder in setting of severe vitamin B12 deficiency : A case report. J Urol 154:199-200, 1995.
30. Rana S, D'amico F, Merenstein JH. Relationship of vitamin B-12 deficiency with incontinence in older people. J Am Geriatr Soc 46:931-932, 1998.
31. Artibani W. Diagnosis and significance of idiopathic overactive bladder. Urology 50:25-35, 1997.
32. McGrother CW, Donaldson MMK, Wagg A: Continence. In Stevens A, Raftery J, Mant J (eds): Health Care Needs Assessment: The Epidemiologically Based Needs Assessment Reviews. Abingdon, Radcliffe Medical Press, 2003.
33. Dallosso HM, McGrother CW, Matthews RJ, et al: The association of diet and other lifestyle factors with overactive bladder and stress incontinence: A longitudinal study in women. BJU Int 92:69-77, 2003.
34. Dallosso HM, McGrother CW, Matthews RJ, Donaldson MK: Nutrient composition of the diet and the development of overactive bladder: A longitudinal study in women. Neurourol Urodyn 23:204-210, 2004.
35. Elia G: Guidelines for Detection and Management of Malnutrition: A Report by the Malnutrition Advisory Group. Maidenhead, BAPEN, 2000.
36. Chyou P, Nomura A: A prospective study of alcohol, diet, and other lifestyle factors in relation to obstructive uropathy. Prostate 22:253-264, 1993.
37. Lagiou P, Wuu J, Trichopoulou A, et al: Diet and benign prostatic hyperplasia: A study in Greece. Urology 54:284-290, 1999.
38. Suzuki S, Platz EA, Kawachi I, et al: Intakes of energy and macronutrients and the risk of benign prostatic hyperplasia. Am J Clin Nutr 75:689-697, 2002.
39. Gregory J, Foster K, Tyler H: The Dietary and Nutritional Survey of British Adults. London: HMSO, 1990.
40. De Bree A, Verschuren WMM, Blom HJ, et al: Association between B vitamin intake and plasma homocysteine concentration in the general Dutch population aged 20 65 y. Am J Clin Nutr 73:1027-1033, 2001.
41. Lin P, Aickin M, Champagne C: Food group sources of nutrients in the dietary patterns of the DASH-Sodium trial. J Am Diet Assoc 103:488-496, 2003.
42. Lubowski DZ, Swash M, Nicholls RJ, Henry MM: Increase in pudendal nerve terminal motor latency with defaecation straining. Br J Surg 75:1095-1097, 1988.
43. Spence-Jones C, Kamm MA, Henry MM, Hudson CN: Bowel dysfunction: A pathogenic factor in uterovaginal prolapse and urinary stress incontinence. Br J Obstet Gynecol 101:147-152, 1994.
44. Moller LA, Lose G, Jorgensen T: Risk factors for lower urinary tract symptoms in women 40 to 60 years of age. Obstet Gynecol 96:446-451, 2000.
45. Charach G, Greenstein A, Rabinovich P, et al: Alleviating constipation in the elderly improves lower urinary tract symptoms. Gerontology 47:72-76, 2001.
46. Dougherty MC, Dwyer JW, Pendergast JF, et al: A randomized trial of behavioral management for continence with older rural women. Res Nurs Health 25:3-13, 2002.
47. Hannestad Y, Rortveit G, Daltveit AK, Hunskar S: Are Smoking and Other Lifestyle Factors Associated with Urinary Incontinence? Proceedings of the International Continence Society, 32nd Annual Meeting, Heidelberg, Germany, August 28-30, 2002, Vol 21, No. 4.
48. Bourcier AP, Juras JC, Jacquetin B: Urinary incontinence in physically active and sportswomen. In Appell RA, Bourcier AP, La Torre F (eds): Pelvic Floor Dysfunction: Investigations and Conservative Treatment. Rome, C.E.S.I., 1999, pp 9-17.
49. Lose G: Simultaneous recording of pressure and cross-sectional area in the female urethra: A study of urethral closure function in healthy and stress incontinent women. Neurourol Urodyn 11:54-89, 1992.
50. Petros PE, Ulstem U: An integral theory of female urinary incontinence. Acta Obstet Gynecol Scan 69(Suppl 153):1-79, 1990.
51. Nygard IE, DeLancey JOL, Arnsdorf L, Murphy E: Exercise and incontinence. Obstet Gynecol 75:848-851, 1990.
52. Nygard IE: Prevention of exercise incontinence with mechanical devices. J Reprod Med 40:89, 1995.
53. Miller J, Ashton–Miller JA, De Lancey JOL: The knack: Use of precisely timed pelvic floor muscle contraction can reduce leakage in USI. Neurourol 15, 4, 1Bs 90, Proceedings of I.C.S. Athens, 1996.
54. Larsen W, Yavorek T: Pelvic organ prolapse and urinary incontinence in nulliparous women at the United States Military Academy. London: Springer, 2004.
55. Jorgensen S, Heiin HO, Gyntelberg F: Heavy lifting at work and risk of genital prolapse and herniated lumbar disc in assistant nurses. Occup Med 44:47-49, 1997.
56. Sherman RA, Davis GD, Wong MF: Behavioral treatment of exercise-induced urinary incontinence among female soldiers. Mil Med 162:690-694, 1997.
57. Fischer JR, Berg PH: Urinary incontinence in United States Air Force female aircrew. Obstet Gynecol 94:532-536, 1999.
58. Bourcier AP: Nulliparous. In Cardozo I, Staskin D (eds): Textbook of Female Urology and Urogynecology. London, Isis Medical Media, 2001, pp 969-977.
59. Jarvis GJ: Bladder retraining. In Bourcier AP, McGuire EJ, Abrams P: Pelvic Floor Disorders. Philadelphia, Elsevier Saunders, 2004, pp 311-313.
60. Roe B: Bladder training for urinary incontinence in adults. In Cochrane Library, issue 3, 2000.
61. Jarvis G: Investigations and management of the unstable bladder. In Bonnar J (ed): Recent Advances in Obstetrics and Gynecology, Vol 19. Churchill Livingstone, 1995.
62. Mahony DT, Laferte RO, Blais DJ: Incontinence of urine due to instability of micturition reflexes: Part I. Detrusor reflex instability. Urology 15:229-239, 1980.
63. Bo K, Berghmans LCM: Nonpharmacologic treatments for overactive bladder: Pelvic floor exercises. Urology 55(Suppl 5A):7-11, 2000.
64. Berghmans LCM, Hendriks HJ, De Bie RA, van Waalwijk, et al: Conservative treatment or urge urinary incontinence in women: A systematic review of randomized clinical trials. BJU Int 85:254-263, 2000.

65. Wilson PD, Bo K, Hay-Smith J, et al: Conservative management in women. In Abrams P, Cardozo L, Khoury S, Wein A (eds): International Consultation Incontinence, 2nd ed. Plymouth, Plymbridge Distributors, 2002.
66. Girard L: Group learning behavior modification and exercise for women with urinary incontinence. Urol Nurs 17:17-22, 1997.
67. McFall SC, Yerkes AM, Cowan LD: Outcomes of a small group educational intervention for urinary incontinence, episodes of incontinence and other urinary symptoms. J Aging Health 12:250-267, 2000.
68. Janson CC, Lagro-Janssen AL, Felling AJ: The effects of physiotherapy for female urinary incontinence: Individual compared with group therapy. Br J Urol Intern 87:201-206, 2001.
69. De Wachter S, Wyndaele JJ: Exploring the use of frequency/volume charts. Proceedings of the ICS 33rd Annual Meeting, Florence, 5-9, 2004. Neurourol Urodyn 22(5), 2004.
70. Sampelle CM, Messer KL, Herzog R, et al: Group teaching of pelvic floor and bladder training: Function and knowledge outcomes. Proceedings of the ICS 33rd Annual Meeting, Florence, 5-9, 2004. Neurourol Urodyn 22(5), 2004.
71. Basmajian JV: Biofeedback: Principles and Practice for Clinicians, 2nd ed. Baltimore, Williams & Wilkins, 1978.
72. Olson RP: Definitions of biofeedback. In Schwartz MS (ed): Biofeedback: A Practitioner's Guide. New York, Guilford Press, 1987, pp 33-37.
73. Burgio KL: Urinary incontinence: Biofeedback therapy. In Benson JT (ed): Female Pelvic Floor Disorders. New York, Norton Medical Books, 1992, pp 210-218.
74. O'Donnell PD: Biofeedback therapy. In Raz S (ed): Female Urology. Philadelphia, WB Saunders, 1996, pp 253-262.
75. Norgard JP, Djurhuus JC: Treatment of detrusor sphincter dyssynergia by biofeedback. Urol Int 37:236-239, 1982.
76. Willington FL: Urinary incontinence: A practical approach. Geriatrics 35:41-48, 1980.
77. Cardozo LD, Stanton SL, Hafner J: Biofeedback in the treatment of detrusor instability. Br J Urol 50(Suppl 5A):250-254, 1978.
78. Cardozo LD: Biofeedback in overactive bladder. Br J Urol 85(Suppl 3):24-28, 2000.
79. Burgio KL, Whitehead WE, Engel BT: Urinary incontinence in the elderly: Bladder/sphincter biofeedback and toileting skills training. Ann Intern Med 103:507-515, 1985.
80. O'Donnell PD, Doyle R: Biofeedback therapy technique for treatment of urinary incontinence. Urology 37:432-436, 1991.
81. Burns PA: Biofeedback therapy. In O'Donnell PD (ed): Urinary Incontinence. St Louis, Mosby-Year Book, 1997, pp 273-277.
82. Bourcier AP, Burgio KL: Bourcier AP, Burgio KL: Biofeedback therapy. In: Bourcier AP, McGuire EJ, Abrams P (eds): Pelvic Floor Disorders. Philadelphia, Elsevier-Saunders, 2004, pp 297-311.
83. Bourcier AP: Pelvic floor rehabilitation. In Raz S (ed): Female Urology. Philadelphia, WB Saunders, 1996, pp 263-281.
84. Bourcier AP: Applied biofeedback in pelvic floor re-education. In Appell RA, Bourcier AP, La Torre F (eds): Pelvic Floor Dysfunction: Investigations and Conservative Treatment. Rome, Casa Editrice Scientifica Internazionale, 1999, pp 241-248.
85. Bourcier AP, Bonde B, Haab F: Functional assessment of pelvic floor muscles. In Appell RA, Bourcier AP, La Torre F (eds): Pelvic Floor Dysfunction: Investigations and Conservative Treatment. Rome, Casa Editrice Scientifica Internazionale, 1999, pp 97-106.
86. Bump RC, Hurt G, Fantl A, Wyman J: Assessment of Kegel muscle exercise performance after brief verbal instruction. Am J Obstet Gynecol 165:332-329, 1991.
87. Burgio KL, Locher JL, Goode PS, et al: Behavioral versus drug treatment for urge incontinence in older women: A randomized clinical trial. JAMA 23:1995-2000, 1998.
88. Burgio KL, Goode PS, Locher JL, et al: Behavioral training with and without biofeedback in the treatment of urge incontinence in older women: A randomized controlled trial. JAMA 288:2293-2299, 2002.
89. Godec C, Cass AS, Ayala GF: Bladder inhibition with functional electrical stimulation. Urology 6:663-666, 1975.
90. Berghmans LCM, Van Doorn ESC, Nieman F, et al: Efficacy of extramural physical therapy modalities in women with proven bladder overactivity: A randomized clinical trial. Neurourol Urodyn 19:496-497, 2000.
91. Cardozo LD, Abrams PD, Stanton SL: Idiopathic detrusor instability treated by biofeedback. Br J Urol 50:521-523, 1978.
92. Cardozo LD, Stanton SL: Biofeedback: A 5 year review. Br J Urol 56:220, 1984.
93. Millard RJ, Oldenburg BF: The symptomatic, urodynamic and psychodynamic results of bladder re-education programmes. J Urol 130:715-719, 1983.
94. Kjolseth D, Madsen B, Knudsen LM: Biofeedback treatment of children and adults with idiopathic detrusor instability. Scand J Urol Nephrol 28:243-247, 1994.
95. O'Donnell PD, Doyle R: Biofeedback therapy technique for treatment of urinary incontinence. Urology 37:432-436, 1991.
96. Burns PA, Pranikoff K, Nochajksi TH, et al: A comparison of effectiveness of biofeedback and pelvic muscle exercise treatment of stress incontinence in older community-dwelling women. J Gerontol 48:167-174, 1993.
97. Burns PA, Pranikoff K, Nochakski T, et al: Treatment of stress incontinence with pelvic floor exercises and biofeedback. J Am Geriatr Soc 38:341-344, 1990.
98. Burton JR, Pearce KL, Burgio KL, et al: Behavioral training for urinary incontinence in elderly ambulatory patients. J Am Geriatr Soc 36:693-698, 1988.
99. Stein M, Discippio W, Davia M: Biofeedback for the treatment of stress and urge incontinence. J Urol 153:641-643, 1995.
100. Wyman JF, Fantl JA, McClish DK: Comparative efficacy of behavioural interventions in the management of female urinary incontinence. Continence Program for Women Research Group. Am J Obstet Gynecol 179:999-1007, 1998.
101. Bors E: Effect of electrical stimulation of the pudendal nerves on the vesical neck: Its significance for the function of cord bladders. J Urol 167:925, 1952.
102. Caldwell KPS, Cook PJ, Flack FC, James ED: Stress incontinence in females: Report on 31 cases of treated electrical implants. J Obstet Gynaecol Br Commonwealth 75:777, 1968.
103. Godec C, Cass AS, Ayala G: Bladder inhibition with functional, electrical stimulation. Urology 6:663-666, 1975.
104. Fall M, Lindstrom S: Electrical stimulation: A physiologic approach to the treatment of urinary incontinence. Urol Clin North Am 18:393-407, 1991.
105. Fall M, Lindstrom SHG: Inhibition of overactive bladder by functional electrical stimulation. In Appell RA, Bourcier AP, La Torre F (eds): Pelvic Floor Dysfunction: Investigations and Conservative Treatment. Rome, Casa Editrice Scientifica Internazionale, 1999, pp 267-272.
106. Vodusek DB, Light JK, Libby JM: Detrusor inhibition induced by stimulation of pudendal nerve afferents. Neurourol Urodyn 5:381-389, 1986.
107. Sundin T, Carlsson CA: Reconstruction of severed dorsal roots innervating the urinary bladder: An experimental study in cats. Studies on the normal afferent pathways in the pelvic and pudendal nerves. Scand J Urol Nephrol 6:176-184, 1972.
108. Plevnik S, Janez J, Vrtacnick P, et al: Short-term electrical stimulation: Home treatment for urinary incontinence. World J Urol 4:24-26, 1986.
109. Bazed MA, Thüroff JW, Schmidt RA: Effect of chronic electrostimulation of the sacral roots on the striated urethral sphincter. J Urol 128:1357, 1982.
110. Stephenson TP, Mundy AR: The urge syndrome. In Mundy AR (ed): Urodynamics: Principles, Practice and Application, 2nd ed. Edinburgh, Churchill Livingstone, 2001, pp 263-275.

111. Janez J, Plevnik S, Suhel P: Urethral and bladder responses to anal electrical stimulation Urol 122:192-194, 1979.
112. Schmidt RA: Application of neurostimulation in urology. Neurourol Urodyn 7:585-592, 1988.
113. Bemelmans BL, Mundy AR, Craggs MD: Neuromodulation by implant for treating lower urinary tract symptoms and dysfunction. Eur Urol 36:81-91, 1999.
114. Walsh IK, Thompson T, Loughridge WG, et al: Non-invasive antidromic neurostimulation: A simple effective method for improving bladder storage. Neurourol Urodyn 20:73-84, 2001.
115. Okada N, Igawa Y, Ogawa A, Nishizawa O: Transcutaneous electrical stimulation of thigh muscles in the treatment of detrusor overactivity. Br J Urol 81:560-564, 1998.
116. Lindstrom S, Sudsuang R: Functionally specific bladder reflexes from pelvic and pudendal nerve branches: An experimental study in cat. Neurourol Urodyn 8:392-393, 1989.
117. McGuire EJ, Zhang SC, Horwinski ER, Lytton B: Treatment of motor and sensory detrusor instability by electrical stimulation. J Urol 129:78-79, 1983.
118. Stoller ML: Afferent nerve stimulation for pelvic floor dysfunction [abstract]. Eur Urol 35:132, 1999.
119. Jiang CH, Lindstrom S: Prolonged enhancement of the micturition reflex in the cat by repetitive stimulation of bladder afferents. J Physiol (Lond) 517(Pt 2):599-605, 1999.
120. Chang CJ, Huang ST, Hsu K, et al: Electroacupuncture decreases c-fos expression in the spinal cord induced by noxious stimulation of the rat bladder. J Urol 160(Pt 1):2274-2279, 1998.
121. Oosterwijk R, Meyler W, Henley E, et al: Pain control with TENS and TEAM nerve stimulators: A review. Physiol Rehabil Med 6:219-258, 1994.
122. Melzack R, Wall PD: Pain mechanisms: A new theory. Science 150:971-979, 1965.
123. Bourcier AP: Office therapy and home care perineal stimulation. Urodynam Neurourodynam Continence 2:83-85, 1992.
124. Bourcier AP, Juras JC: Electrical stimulation: Home treatment versus office therapy. Eighty-ninth Annual Meeting of American Urological Association, San Francisco, May 14-19, 1994. J Urol 151:1171, 1994.
125. Bourcier AP, Mamberti-Dias A, Susset J: Functional electrical stimulation in uro-gynecology. In Appell RA, Bourcier AP, La Torre F (eds): Pelvic Floor Dysfunction: Investigations and Conservative Treatment. Rome, Casa Editrice Scientifica Internazionale, 1999, pp 259-266.
126. Bourcier AP, Park TAE: Electrical stimulation. In Bourcier AP, McGuire EJ, Abrams P (eds): Pelvic Floor Disorders. Philadelphia, Elsevier-Saunders, 2004, pp 281-291.
127. Van Balken MR, Vandoninck V, Gisolf KW, et al: Posterior tibial nerve stimulation as neuromodulative treatment of lower urinary tract dysfunction. J Urol 166:914-918, 2001.
128. Govier FE, Litwiller S, Nitti V, et al: Percutaneous afferent neuromodulation for the refractory overactive bladder: Results of a multicenter study. J Urol 165:1193-1198, 2001.
129. McGuire EJ: Treatment of motor and sensory detrusor instability by electrical stimulation. J Urol 129:78, 1983.
130. Fynes M, Cleaver S, Murray C, et al: Evaluation of the effect of posterior tibial nerve stimulation in women with intractable urge urinary incontinence. In Proceedings of the 31st Annual Meeting of the International Continence Society. Neurourol Urodyn 20:116, 2001.
131. Mantle J: Physiotherapy for incontinence. In Cardozo L, Staskin D (eds): Textbook of Female Urology and Urogynecology. London, Isis Medical Media, 2001, pp 351-358.
132. Eriksen BC, Eik-Nes SH: Long-term electrostimulation of the pelvic floor: Primary therapy in female stress incontinence. Urol Int 44:90-95, 1989.
133. Kralj B: Treatment of idiopathic urge incontinence with functional electrical stimulation. Proceedings of the International Uro Gynecological Association 18th Annual Meeting, Nîmes, France, 1993, p 323.
134. Bent AE, Sand PK, Ostergard DR, Brubaker LT: Transvaginal electrical stimulation in the treatment of genuine stress incontinence and detrusor instability. Int Gynecol J 4:9-13, 1993.
135. Bourcier AP, Juras JC: Electrical stimulation: Home treatment versus office therapy. Eighty-ninth Annual Meeting of the American Urological Association, San Francisco, May 14-19, 1994. J Urol 151:1171, 1994.
136. Lagro-Jansen ALM, Debryune FMJ, Smith AJA, Van Weel C: The effects of treatment of urinary incontinence in general practice. Fam Pract 9:284-289, 1992.
137. Brubaker L, Benson T, Bent A, et al: Transvaginal electrical stimulation for female urinary incontinence. Am J Obstet Gynecol 177:536-540, 1997.
138. Vandoninck V, van Balken MR, Agro EF, et al: Posterior tibial nerve stimulation in the treatment of urge incontinence. Neurourol Urodyn 22:17-23, 2003.
139. Wang A, Wang Y: Single blind, randomized trial of pelvic floor muscle training (PFMT), biofeedback assisted pelvic floor muscle training (BAPFMT) and electrical stimulation (ES) in the management of overactive bladder (OAB). Proceedings of the ICS 33rd Annual Meeting, Florence, 5-9, 2004. Neurourol Urodyn 22(5), 2004.
140. Burgio KE, Locher JL, Goode PS: Combined behavioral and drug therapy for urge incontinence in women. J Am Geriatr Soc 48:370-374, 2000.
141. Payne CK: Behavioral therapy of overactive bladder. Urology 55(Suppl 5A):3-6, 2000.

Chapter 20

DRUG TREATMENT OF URINARY INCONTINENCE IN WOMEN

Alan J. Wein and M. Louis Moy

The lower urinary tract has two basic functions: the storage and emptying of urine. The physiology and pharmacology of micturition have been described by many qualified authors, each of whom has reported his or her own particular concept of the neuroanatomy, neurophysiology, and neuropharmacology of the smooth and striated muscle structures involved; of the peripheral, autonomic, and somatic neural factors; and of the spinal and supraspinal influences that are necessary for normal function.[1-5] Although there are significant disagreements about the finer details, it is important to realize that exact agreement about neuromorphology, neurophysiology, and neuropharmacology is not necessary for an understanding of the pharmacologic principles and applications involved in drug-induced alterations of voiding function and dysfunction. Despite such disagreements, "experts" would agree that, for the purposes of description and teaching, urinary continence requires, first, accommodation of increasing volumes of urine at a low intravesical pressure and with appropriate sensation; second, a bladder outlet that is closed at rest and remains so during increases in intra-abdominal pressure; and third, absence of involuntary bladder contractions (IVCs), including non-neurogenic and neurogenic detrusor overactivity (DO).

As a result of advances in understanding of the neuropharmacology and neurophysiology of the lower urinary tract, effective pharmacologic therapy now exists for the management of urinary incontinence. Because of the number of drug therapies available along with the varying quality and quantity of studies performed using them, the International Consultation on Incontinence has assessed many of the available agents for voiding dysfunction and made recommendations regarding their use (Table 20-1).

This chapter summarizes the pharmacologic treatments available for female urinary incontinence within this functional classification. As an apology to others in the field whose works have not been specifically cited in this chapter, it should be noted that citations have generally been chosen primarily because of their review or informational content, or sometimes for their controversial nature, and not because of originality or initial publication on a particular subject.

CLINICAL UROPHARMACOLOGY OF THE LOWER URINARY TRACT

Some Useful Concepts

Clinical uropharmacology of the lower urinary tract is based primarily on an appreciation of the innervation and receptor content of the bladder and its related anatomic structures. The targets of pharmacologic intervention in the bladder body, base, or outlet include nerve terminals that alter the release of specific neurotransmitters, receptor subtypes, cellular second-messenger systems, and ion channels identified in the bladder and urethra. Peripheral nerves and ganglia, spinal cord, and supraspinal areas are also sites of action of some agents discussed. Because autonomic innervation and receptor content are ubiquitous throughout the human body's organ systems, there are no agents in clinical use that are purely selective for action on the lower urinary tract. The majority of side effects attributed to drugs facilitating bladder storage or emptying are collateral effects on organ systems that share some of the same neurophysiologic or neuropharmacologic characteristics as the bladder.

Table 20-1 International Consultation on Incontinence Assessments of Pharmacotherapy for Voiding Dysfunction, 2004

Drug	Level*	Grade†
Antimuscarinics		
Tolterodine	1	A
Trospium	1	A
Darifenacin	1	A
Solifenacin	1	A
Propantheline	2	B
Atropine, hyoscyamine	3	C
Drugs with mixed actions		
Oxybutynin	1	A
Propiverine	1	A
Dicyclomine	3	C
Flavoxate	2	D
Antidepressants		
Imipramine	3	C
Vasopressin analogues		
Desmopressin	1	A
β-Adrenergic receptor agonists‡	3	C
Baclofen	3	C
Capsaicin	2	C
Resiniferatoxin	2	C
Botulinum toxin	2	B

*Levels: 1—systematic reviews, meta-analyses, good-quality randomized controlled clinical trials; 2—randomized controlled trials, good-quality prospective cohort studies; 3—case-controlled studies, case series; 4—expert opinion.
†Grades: A—based on level 1 evidence (highly recommended); B—consistent level 2 or 3 evidence (recommended); C—level 4 studies or "majority evidence" (optional); D—evidence inconsistent or inconclusive (no recommendation possible).
‡Class includes terbutaline, salbutamol, and clenbuterol.

Generally speaking, the simplest and least hazardous form of treatment should be tried first. A combination of therapeutic maneuvers or pharmacologic agents can sometimes be used to achieve a particular effect, especially if their mechanisms of action are different and their side effects are not synergistic. At the outset it should be noted that, in our experience, although great improvement often occurs with rational pharmacologic therapy, a perfect result (restoration to "normal" status) is seldom, if ever, achieved.

Facilitation of Urine Storage

The pathophysiology of failure of the lower urinary tract to fill with or to store urine adequately may be secondary to problems related to the bladder, the outlet, or both.[6] DO can be expressed as discrete IVCs or as reduced compliance with or without phasic contractions. It may manifest symptomatically as overactive bladder (OAB) syndrome, a syndrome of urgency that may be associated with frequency and nocturia. IVCs are most commonly associated with inflammatory or irritating processes in the bladder wall or with bladder outlet obstruction, or they may be idiopathic. Decreased compliance during filling may be secondary to the sequelae of neurologic injury or disease but may also result from any process that destroys the elastic or viscoelastic properties of the bladder wall. Purely sensory urgency may result from inflammatory, infectious, neurologic, or psychological factors, or it may be idiopathic. A fixed decrease in outlet resistance may result from degeneration of or damage to innervation of the structural elements of the smooth or striated sphincter or from neurologic disease or injury, surgical or other mechanical trauma, or aging. Classic stress urinary incontinence (SUI) or genuine SUI in women implies a failure of the normal transmission of increases in intra-abdominal pressure to the area of the bladder neck and proximal urethra due to changes in the anatomic position of the vesicourethral junction and proximal urethra during increases in intra-abdominal pressure (hypermobility). The pathophysiology of SUI may also involve a decrease in the reflex striated sphincter contraction, which occurs with a number of maneuvers that increase intra-abdominal pressure. Treatment of abnormalities related to the filling or storage phase of micturition are directed toward inhibiting bladder contractility, increasing bladder capacity, decreasing sensory input during filling, or increasing outlet resistance, either continuously or only during abdominal straining.

DECREASING BLADDER CONTRACTILITY

Anticholinergic Agents

Physiologic bladder contractions are thought to be primarily triggered by acetylcholine-induced stimulation of postganglionic parasympathetic muscarinic cholinergic receptor sites on bladder smooth muscle.[1,5] Atropine and atropine-like agents should depress normal bladder contractions and IVCs of any cause.[6-8] In patients taking such agents, the volume accumulated before the first IVC is generally increased, the amplitude of the IVC is decreased, and the maximum bladder capacity is increased. However, although the volume and pressure thresholds at which an IVC is elicited may increase, the "warning time" (the time between perception of an IVC about to occur and its occurrence) and the ability to suppress an IVC are not increased. Therefore, urgency and incontinence still occur unless such therapy is combined with a regimen of timed voiding or toileting. McGuire and Savastano[9] reported that atropine increased both the compliance and the capacity of the neurologically decentralized primate bladder.[10] However, the effect of pure antimuscarinics in those who exhibit only decreased compliance has not been well studied. Outlet resistance, at least as reflected by urethral pressure measurements, does not seem to be clinically affected by anticholinergic therapy.

Although antimuscarinic agents can produce significant clinical improvement in patients with IVCs and associated symptoms, only partial inhibition results. In many animal models, atropine only partially antagonizes the response of the whole bladder to pelvic nerve stimulation and of bladder strips to field stimulation, although it does completely inhibit the response of bladder smooth muscle to exogenous cholinergic stimulation. Of the theories proposed to explain this phenomenon, termed *atropine resistance*, the most attractive and most commonly cited is the idea that a portion of the neurotransmission involved in the final common pathway of bladder contraction is nonadrenergic noncholinergic (NANC)—that is, it occurs secondary to a release of a transmitter other than acetylcholine or noradrenaline.[1,2,5] Although the existence of atropine resistance in human bladder muscle is by no means agreed on, this concept is the most common hypothesis invoked to explain clinical difficulty in abolishing IVCs with anticholinergic agents alone, and it is also used to support the rationale of treatment of such types of bladder activity with agents that have different mechanisms of action. Brading[11,12] and Andersson[5] both discussed the difficulty of evaluating apparently conflicting data in the literature with respect to atropine resistance. Brading[12] stated that the size of the atropine-resistant component varies markedly among species and, in a given preparation, also depends on the frequency of nerve stimulation. Andersson[5] stated that "most probably normal human detrusor muscle exhibits little atropine resistance," but that this does not exclude its existence in morphologically or functionally abnormal bladders.

At least five different genetically established muscarinic subtypes (M_1 through M_5) exist, as determined by cloning experiments[13]; the cholinergic muscarinic receptor genes are designated *CHRM1* through *CHRM5*. The protein products of the M_1 through M_4 subtypes have been defined pharmacologically with the use of receptor subtype agonists and antagonists.[5,14,15] A physiologic role for the product of the M_5 coding region remains undefined.[15] Pirenzepine (a selective muscarinic blocker) was originally used to subdivide muscarinic receptors into M_1 and M_2 categories; using this subclassification, detrusor muscarinic receptors were classified as the M_2 type.[5,16,17] On further analysis of the M_2 receptor population, a small proportion of glandular M_2 receptors were found which could represent the pharmacologic type responsible for muscarinic agonist-induced contractions. This subtype is now called the M_3 receptor.[5,14] Although it appears that the majority of the muscarinic receptors in human smooth muscle, including bladder, are of the M_2 subtype,[18] in vitro data indicate that most smooth muscle contraction, including that of the urinary bladder, is mediated by the M_3 receptor subtype.[18,19] Muscarinic receptor subtyping becomes important when considering the possibility of pharmacologically selecting (and blocking) those receptors responsible for urinary bladder smooth muscle contraction while minimally affecting other muscarinic receptor sites throughout the body. Ideally, this approach would effectively treat the underlying problem (DO) while eliminating the unpleasant systemic side effects of most nonspecific antimuscarinic agents (e.g., dry mouth, constipation, blurred vision), which, in many cases, are worse than the problem they are treating and result in patient noncompliance.

Specific Drugs

Propantheline bromide is the classically described oral agent used for producing an antimuscarinic effect in the lower urinary tract. The usual adult oral dose is 15 to 30 mg every 4 to 6 hours, although higher doses are often necessary. Propantheline is a quaternary ammonium compound that is poorly absorbed after oral administration. No available oral drug has a direct in vitro antimuscarinic binding potential that is closer to that of atropine than propantheline bromide.[20,21] There is a surprising lack of valuable data on the effectiveness of propantheline for the treatment of bladder overactivity. As Andersson pointed out,[8] anticholinergic drugs in general have been reported to have both great and poor efficacy for this indication. Zorzitto and colleagues[22] concluded that propantheline bromide administered orally in doses of 30 mg four times a day to a group of institutionalized incontinent geriatric patients had marginal benefits that were outweighed by the side effects. Blaivas and colleagues,[7] on the other hand, increased the dose of propantheline (up to 60 mg four times a day) until incontinence was eliminated or side effects precluded further use and obtained a complete response in 25 of 26 patients with IVCs. Differences in bioavailability, selective drug delivery, receptor selectivity, receptor density, atropine resistance, pathophysiology, susceptibility to dose-limiting side effects, and mental status are all potential factors that could explain such disparate results. The Agency for Health Care Policy and Research (AHCPR) Clinical Practice Guidelines[23] listed five randomized controlled trials for propantheline, in which 82% of the patients were women. The percentage of cure was listed as ranging from zero to 5%, reduction in urge incontinence from zero to 53%, side effects from zero to 50%, and dropouts from zero to 9% (all figures refer to overall percentage minus percentage on placebo).

Atropine is reported to be available in a 0.5-mg tablet, although we have yet to find it. Atropine and all related belladonna alkaloids are well absorbed from the gastrointestinal tract. Atropine is said to have almost no detectable central nervous system (CNS) effects at clinically used doses.[24] It has a half-life of about 4 hours.

Scopolamine is another belladonna alkaloid marketed as a soluble salt. It has prominent central depressive effects at low doses, probably because of its greater penetration (compared with atropine) through the blood-brain barrier. Transdermal scopolamine has been used for treatment of IVCs.[25] The "patch" provides continuous delivery of 0.5 mg daily to the circulation for 3 days. Cornella and associates,[26] however, reported poor results with this dosage in 10 patients with DO: only 2 patients showed a positive response; 1 showed a slight improvement, and the drug was discontinued in 8 patients because of side effects. Side effects were related to the CNS (ataxia, dizziness) and included blurred vision and dry mouth. A double-blind placebo-controlled study using transdermal scopolamine was performed on 20 patients with DO: after a 14-day treatment period, the 10 patients randomized to transdermal scopolamine treatment showed statistically significant improvements in frequency, nocturia, urgency, and urge incontinence compared with the placebo group; no adverse effects of the therapy were reported.[27] A double-blind placebo study on the effects of transdermal scopolamine in patients who had undergone suprapubic prostatectomy was performed to investigate its use in the treatment or prevention of pain, IVCs, urgency, and bladder pressure rises of 15 cm H_2O. No statistical differences were found.[28] In our experience of treating IVCs with this method, results were very erratic, and skin irritation with the patch was a problem for some patients. Because of the fixed dose, caution should be exercised in the use of the patch in elderly and young patients.

Hyoscyamine and hyoscyamine sulphate are reported to have anticholinergic actions and side effects similar to those of other belladonna alkaloids. Hyoscyamine sulphate is available as a sublingual formulation, a theoretical advantage, but controlled studies of its effects on bladder overactivity are lacking. Glycopyrrolate is a synthetic quaternary ammonium compound that is a potent inhibitor of both M_1 and M_2 receptors but has a preference for the M_2 subtype.[29] It is available in both oral and parenteral preparations; the latter is commonly used as an antisialagogue during anesthesia. An anticholinergic agent with a significant ganglionic-blocking action as well as such action at the peripheral receptor level might be more effective in suppressing bladder contractility. Although methantheline has a higher ratio of ganglionic blocking to antimuscarinic activity than does propantheline, the latter drug seems to be at least as potent in each respect, clinical dose for dose. Methantheline does have similar effects on the lower urinary tract, and some clinicians still prefer it over other anticholinergic agents. Few solid data are available regarding its efficacy.

The potential side effects of all antimuscarinic agents include inhibition of salivary secretion (dry mouth), blockade of the ciliary muscle of the lens to cholinergic stimulation (blurred vision for near objects), tachycardia, drowsiness, and inhibition of gut motility. Those agents that possess some ganglionic-blocking activity may also cause orthostatic hypotension and erectile dysfunction at high doses (at which nicotinic activity becomes manifest). Antimuscarinic agents are contraindicated in patients with narrow-angle glaucoma and should be used with caution in patients with significant bladder outlet obstruction, because complete urinary retention may be precipitated.

A lack of selectivity is a major problem with all antimuscarinic compounds, because they tend to affect parasympathetically innervated organs in the same order; in general, larger doses are required to inhibit bladder activity than to affect salivary, bronchial, nasopharyngeal, and sweat secretions. Several new receptor antagonists with varying degrees of specificity for the lower urinary tract show some promise in decreasing the side effect profiles of this class of medications without compromising efficacy.

Tolterodine and its primary metabolite, PNU-200577,[30] have shown some selectivity for bladder tissue over salivary tissue in in vitro and in vivo studies in the anesthetized cat.[31,32] These tissue-selective effects do not appear to be related to muscarinic receptor subtype selectivity[30,31] but may be the result of differential affinities of the receptors in the salivary gland and detrusor muscle for tolterodine compared with oxybutynin. Although it appears that the binding affinity of tolterodine and oxybutynin to muscarinic receptors in the urinary bladder (in the guinea pig) are very similar, the affinity of tolterodine for muscarinic receptors in the parotid gland is eight times lower than that of oxybutynin.[33] Tolterodine is available in two formulations: an immediate-release (IR) form (2 mg twice daily) and an extended-release (ER) form (2 mg or 4 mg once daily).

In a pilot study in 12 healthy men, tolterodine was shown to have a greater objective and subjective effect on bladder function than on salivation.[34] Jonas and colleagues[35] looked at the urodynamic effects of tolterodine in a multicenter, randomized, double-blind, placebo-controlled study: 242 patients were enrolled and treated over a 4-week period with 1 or 2 mg tolterodine or placebo twice daily. Compared with placebo, 2 mg tolterodine (but not 1 mg) produced statistically significant improvements in mean volume to first IVC (from 141 to 230 mL in the 2-mg group, 142 to 210 mL in the 1-mg group, and 140 to 181 mL in the placebo group), mean maximal strength of IVC (52 to 37 cm H_2O, 41 to 35 cm H_2O, and 47 to 40 cm H_2O in the three groups, respectively), and maximal cystometric capacity (272 to 316 mL, 276 to 294 mL, and 264 to 268 mL, respectively). The proportion of adverse effects in the treated groups, compared with placebo, was not statistically significant; however, dry mouth, the most common event, was reported in 9% of treated patients, significantly less than the 50% incidence reported in the literature for other commonly used anticholinergic preparations.[36] Furthermore, the dry mouth was classified as "severe" by only 1% of patients. At higher doses, the incidence of side effects of tolterodine may be more significant and may approach that of other commonly used anticholinergic drugs.

Rentzhog and colleagues[37] noted that, at a dose of 2 mg or less, the incidence of adverse effects (including dry mouth) due to tolterodine was comparable to that of placebo (2/13 patients in the placebo group versus 9/51 patients in the tolterodine group reported dry mouth); however, when the dose of tolterodine was increased to 4 mg, a substantial increase in the incidence of dry mouth occurred (9/16 patients). Overall, it appears that tolterodine is safe and efficacious for the treatment of DO. A favorable side-effect profile exists at lower doses (less effect on salivary glands), which may diminish in a dose-dependent fashion.

There have been have been several randomized controlled studies documenting the effectiveness of tolterodine in reducing micturition frequency and incontinence episodes.[38,39] There have also been comparative trials comparing it to other agents.

The Overactive Bladder: Judging Effective Control and Treatment (OBJECT) trial performed by Appell and colleagues[40] compared tolterodine IR 2 mg twice daily to oxybutynin ER 10 mg daily. This was a randomized, double blind, parallel-group study that included 378 patients with OAB. Patients were treated for 12 weeks. The outcome measures included number of episodes of urge incontinence, total incontinence, and micturition frequency. The study showed oxybutynin ER to be significantly more effective than tolterodine in each of the outcome measures when adjusted for baseline. The most common adverse event was dry mouth, which was reported by 28% and 33% of those taking oxybutynin ER and tolterodine IR, respectively. Rates of other adverse events including CNS side effects were generally low and comparable between the two groups.

In the Overactive Bladder: Performance of Extended Release Agents (OPERA) study, Diokno and colleagues[41] compared tolterodine ER 4 mg daily to oxybutynin ER 10 mg daily in 790 women with OAB symptoms. This too was a randomized, double-blind study with a duration of 12 weeks. Patients kept 24-hour voiding diaries to document the number of incontinence episodes (primary outcome), total incontinence, and micturition frequency at weeks 2, 4, 8, and 12. Improvements in weekly urge incontinence episodes were similar between the two treatment groups. Oxybutynin ER was more effective in reducing micturition frequency, and 23.0% of women taking it reported no episodes of urinary incontinence, compared with to 16.8% of women taking tolterodine ER. Dry mouth was more common in the oxybutynin ER group, with both groups having similar discontinuation rates. The conclusions were that the two drugs had similar reductions in weekly urge incontinence and total incontinence episodes. Those taking oxybutynin ER had more dry mouth, but the tolerability between the two drugs was comparable.

In the Antimuscarinic Clinical Effectiveness Trial (ACET), Sussman and Garely[42] performed an open-label trial in patients with OAB comparing tolterodine ER 2 mg or 4 mg to oxybutynin ER 5 mg or 10 mg. A total of 1289 subjects participated in the study. After 8 weeks, 70% of patients taking tolterodine ER 4 mg perceived an improved bladder condition, compared with about 60% in the other groups. There were fewer withdrawals from the study in the tolterodine ER 4 mg group (12%) than in either the oxybutynin ER 5 mg group (19%) or the oxybutynin 10 mg group (21%). Patients taking tolterodine ER 4 mg reported significantly less dry mouth than those taking oxybutynin ER 10 mg. Although the findings suggest that tolterodine ER 4 mg may have improved clinical efficacy and tolerability compared with oxybutynin ER 10 mg, the open-label design of this study makes for a less convincing conclusion.

Zinner and colleagues[43] performed a 12-week randomized, double-blind, placebo-controlled study to evaluate the efficacy, safety, and tolerability of tolterodine ER in treating OAB symptoms in older (≥65 years) and younger (<65 years) patients. Objective measures by micturition diaries as well as subjective measures were evaluated. There were significant improvements among patients taking tolterodine ER in micturition chart variables, compared with placebo. There were no age-related differences. Dry mouth was the most common adverse event in both arms. No CNS or cardiac events were seen. Tolterodine ER appeared to be well tolerated by both age groups.

Freeman et al[44] presented a secondary analysis of a double-blind, placebo-controlled study looking at the effects of tolterodine ER 4 mg on the symptoms of urinary urgency in patients with OAB. A total of 772 patients with eight or more micturitions per 24 hours and urge incontinence (≥5/week) were randomized to drug or placebo therapy and treated for 12 weeks. Efficacy was assessed by using patient perception evaluations. Patients taking tolterodine ER 4 mg had a greater improvement in urgency (44% versus 32%) and bladder symptoms (62% versus 48%) than those taking placebo. Patients taking tolterodine ER 4 mg were also significantly more likely to hold their urine after experiencing urgency.

Recently, several pharmacologic agents have been approved by the Food and Drug Administration (FDA) for use in the United States. Darifenacin, a tertiary amine, is a selective muscarinic M_3 receptor antagonist. Its theoretical advantage is its ability to selectively block the M_3 receptor, which is the most important subtype in bladder contraction, and thereby decrease the adverse events related to blockade of other muscarinic subtypes.

Darifenacin has been studied in several randomized controlled studies. Haab and colleagues performed a multicenter, randomized, double-blind, placebo-controlled study comparing darifenacin 3.75 mg, 7.5 mg, 15 mg, and placebo once daily.[45] The treatment period was 12 weeks. Using an electronic voiding diary, patients recorded daily incontinence episodes, micturition frequency, volume voided, frequency and severity of urgency, incontinence episodes necessitating a change of clothing or pads, and nocturnal awakenings due to bladder symptoms. The

7.5- and 15-mg doses of darifenacin had a quick onset of action, with significant improvements over placebo being seen at week 2. The clinical parameters in which the treatment arm were significantly better than placebo included improvements in micturition frequency, bladder capacity, frequency of urgency, severity of urgency, and number of incontinence episodes. No significant change occurred in nocturnal awakening due to bladder symptoms. The most common side effects seen were mild-to-moderate dry mouth and constipation. No patients withdrew from the study due to dry mouth, and the discontinuation rate due to constipation was rare (0.9% for darifenacin versus 0.6% for placebo). The CNS and safety profile were similar for darifenacin and placebo.

An analysis of the pooled data from phase 3 trials was performed by Chapple and associates.[46] A total of 1059 patients (85% female) with symptoms of urgency, urge incontinence, and frequency were randomized to into three arms: darifenacin 7.5 mg, darifenacin 15 mg, or placebo daily for 12 weeks. Once again, patient voiding diaries were maintained electronically. The parameters monitored included incontinence episodes, frequency and severity of urgency, micturition frequency, and volume voided. Compared to baseline, there was a significant dose-related decrease in the number of incontinence episodes per week, with darifenacin 7.5 mg reducing episodes by 8.8, and darifenacin 15 mg reducing episodes by 10.6 per week. Significant decreases in the frequency and severity of urgency, micturition frequency, and number of incontinent episodes requiring a change of clothing or pads were seen, as well as an increase in bladder capacity. Although the most common side effect was dry mouth, this led to few discontinuations (darifenacin 7.5 mg, 0.5%; darifenacin, 15 mg, 2.1%; placebo, 0.3%), and the incidence of CNS and cardiovascular adverse events was similar to placebo.

Cardozo and colleagues[47] performed a study to determine the effects of darifenacin on "warning time," or the ability of the medication to allow patients to postpone micturition once urge was sensed. This was a multicenter, randomized, double-blind, placebo-controlled study with a 2-week treatment phase of darifenacin 30 mg daily or placebo. Darifenacin treatment resulted in a significant increase in the mean warning time (median increase, 4.3 minutes) compared with placebo. Overall, 47% of darifenacin-treated subjects and 20% of those receiving placebo achieved a greater than 30% increase in mean warning time. Although this study used a higher than usual dose of therapeutic agent and the treatment period was short, it was the first to evaluate changes in warning time. This effect may be particularly germane to patients with severe symptoms of urgency and urge incontinence.

Solifenacin (YM-905) is a tertiary amine, once-daily antimuscarinic. It is well absorbed from the gastrointestinal tract and undergoes significant hepatic metabolism by the cytochrome P450 enzyme system. There have been several large trials examining the effects of solifenacin.

Chapple and colleagues performed a multinational study comparing various does of solifenacin (2.5, 5, 10, and 20 mg) to tolterodine IR 2 mg twice daily and placebo[48] in patients with OAB. A total of 225 patients were treated for 4 weeks and monitored for an additional 2 weeks. To be included in the study, all patients had to have at least eight micturitions in 24 hours and one episode of incontinence or one episode of urgency daily, as recorded by a 3-day voiding diary. Micturition frequency was the primary outcome. In patients treated with solifenacin, there was a statistically significant reduction in micturition frequency for those taking 5, 10, or 20 mg. This was not seen in the other two arms of the study. Additionally, these doses of solifenacin, when compared with placebo, resulted in a significant increase in volume voided and a reduction in episodes of frequency and incontinence. The onset of action was rapid, occurring at 2 weeks, the earliest follow-up point in the study. Discontinuation rates were similar among the various treatments except for solifenacin 20 mg, which was higher. The 5- and 10-mg doses of solifenacin had a lower rate of dry mouth than tolterodine did.

Another dose-ranging, placebo-controlled study of solifenacin 2.5 to 20 mg, was performed by Smith and colleagues in the United States.[49] The treatment duration was 4 weeks, with 2 weeks of follow-up. There was a significant reduction in micturition frequency in the solifenacin 10-mg and 20-mg groups, compared with placebo. The onset of efficacy was seen at 7 days, with continued improvement at 28 days. Significant increases in volume voided were seen in those taking 5, 10, or 20 mg of solifenacin. The 10 mg solifenacin dose also had a significant decrease in incontinent episodes.

There were four phase 3 trials to evaluate efficacy, safety, and tolerability of solifenacin in adult patients with OAB. The primary outcome in all the studies was 24-hour micturition frequency. Secondary outcomes included change in number of urgency and incontinence episodes and mean volume voided.

Chapple and colleagues[50] performed a multicenter, randomized, placebo-controlled and tolterodine-controlled study. Subjects were treated for 12 weeks with solifenacin 5 mg daily, solifenacin 10 mg daily, tolterodine IR 2 mg twice daily, or placebo. Both doses of solifenacin resulted in a significant decrease in urgency episodes at 24 hours, compared with placebo, but tolterodine did not. In the solifenacin group, there was a significant decrease in incontinence episodes; and the mean number of voids in 24 hours was significantly lower in all three active treatment arms. As with most antimuscarinics, the most common side effect was dry mouth, occurring in 14% in the solifenacin 5 mg group and in 21.3% of the solifenacin 10 mg group.

Cardozo and colleagues[51] performed a multicenter randomized, placebo-controlled study comparing solifenacin 5 mg and 10 mg once daily with placebo. They found that both of the doses significantly improved frequency compared with placebo. Solifenacin was also better than placebo in improving urgency, increasing volume voided, and decreasing incontinence episodes over 24 hours. The reduction in urgency was slightly greater than 50% for both doses of solifenacin, whereas placebo resulted in a reduction of 33%. The percentage increases in voided volume per micturition were 25.4%, 29.7%, and 11% for solifenacin 5 mg, 10 mg, and placebo, respectively. The percentage decreases in overall incontinence episodes were 60.7%, 51.9%, and 27.9%, respectively. Only a small percentage of patients (2% to 4%) did not complete the study due to adverse events, which were comparable in all groups. The incidence of dry mouth was 2.3%, 7.7%, and 23.1% in placebo, solifenacin 10 mg, and solifenacin 20 mg groups, respectively. There were no changes in electrocardiographic parameters.

Two double-blind trials of solifenacin were performed[52] in the United States, in which a total of 1208 patients participated. Findings included a reduction in the number of micturitions per 24 hours, a decrease in the number of incontinence and urgency episodes per 24 hours, and an increase in the volume voided per micturition. Among patients who were incontinent at baseline, a significant percentage of those taking solifenacin became continent, compared to those taking placebo (53% versus 31%, respectively).

Musculotropic Relaxants

Musculotropic relaxants affect smooth muscle directly at a site that is metabolically distal to the cholinergic or other contractile receptor mechanism. Although the agents discussed in this section do relax smooth muscle in vitro by papaverine-like (direct) action, all have also been found to possess variable anticholinergic and local-anesthetic properties. There is still some uncertainty about how much of their clinical efficacy is due only to their atropine-like effect. If, in fact, any of these agents do exert a clinically significant inhibitory effect that is independent of antimuscarinic action, a therapeutic rationale exists for combining them with a relatively pure anticholinergic agent.

Oxybutynin chloride is a moderately potent anticholinergic agent that has strong independent musculotropic relaxant activity as well as local-anesthetic activity. The recommended oral adult dose is 5 mg three or four times a day; side effects are antimuscarinic and dose-related. Initial reports documented success in depressing neurogenic DO,[53] and subsequent reports documented success in inhibiting other types of bladder overactivity as well.[8] A randomized double-blind, placebo-controlled study comparing 5 mg oxybutynin three times a day with placebo in 30 patients with DO was carried out by Moisey and colleagues: 17 of 23 patients who completed the study with oxybutynin had symptomatic improvement, and 9 showed evidence of urodynamic improvement, mainly an increase in maximum bladder capacity.[54] Hehir and Fitzpatrick[55] reported that 16 of 24 patients with neuropathic voiding dysfunction secondary to myelomeningocele were cured or improved (17% dry, 50% improved) with oxybutynin treatment; average bladder capacity increased from 197 to 299 mL with oxybutynin compared to 218 mL with placebo, and maximum bladder filling pressure decreased from 47 to 37 cm H_2O with oxybutynin versus 45 cm H_2O with placebo. In a prospective randomized study of 34 patients with voiding dysfunction secondary to multiple sclerosis, Gajewski and Awad[56] found that 5 mg oral oxybutynin three times a day produced a good response more frequently than 15 mg propantheline three times a day; they concluded that oxybutynin was more effective in the treatment of neurogenic DO secondary to multiple sclerosis. Holmes and associates[57] compared the results of oxybutynin and propantheline in a small group of women with DO. The experimental design was a randomized crossover trial with a patient-regulated variable-dose regimen. This kind of dose-titration study allows the patient to increase the drug dose to whatever she perceives to be the optimum ratio between clinical improvement and side effects—an interesting way of comparing two drugs while minimizing differences in oral absorption. Of the 23 women in the trial, 14 reported subjective improvement with oxybutynin as opposed to 11 with propantheline. Both drugs significantly increased the maximum cystometric capacity and reduced the maximum detrusor pressure on filling. The only significant objective difference was a greater increase in the maximum cystometric capacity with oxybutynin. The mean total daily dose of oxybutynin tolerated was 15 mg (range, 7.5 to 30 mg), and that of propantheline was 90 mg (range, 45 to 145 mg).

Thuroff and colleagues[58] compared oxybutynin with propantheline and placebo in a group of patients with symptoms of instability and either neurogenic and non-neurogenic DO. Oxybutynin (5 mg three times a day) performed best, but propantheline was used at a relatively low dose (15 mg three times a day). The incidence of side effects was higher for oxybutynin at approximately the level of clinical and urodynamic improvement. The mean grade of improvement on a visual analogue scale was higher for oxybutynin (58.2%) than for propantheline (44.7%) or placebo (43.4%). Urodynamic volume at the first IVC increased more with oxybutynin (51 mL, versus 11.2 mL for propantheline and 9.7 mL for placebo), as did the change in maximum cystometric capacity (80.1, 48.9, and 22.5 mL, respectively). Residual urine volume also increased more (27.0, 2.2, and 1.9 mL, respectively). The authors further subdivided their overall results into the categories of excellent (>75% improvement), good (50% to 74%), fair (25% to 49%), and poor (<25%). Results for treatment with oxybutynin were 42% excellent, 25% good, 15% fair, and 18% poor. The authors concluded that their 67% rate of good or excellent results compared favorably with those reported in seven other oxybutynin series in the literature (some admittedly poorer studies included), which ranged from 61% to 86%. The results of propantheline treatment generally ranked between those of oxybutynin and placebo but did not reach significant levels over placebo in any variable. Subdivision of propantheline results into excellent, good, fair, and poor categories yielded percentages of 20%, 30%, 14%, and 36%, respectively. The 50% ratio of good or excellent results were consistent with those achieved in six other propantheline studies reported in the literature (30% to 57%). Although this study was better than most in the literature, it did have drawbacks, and anyone using it in a meta-analysis would be well advised to read it and the other cited studies very carefully.

Zeegers and colleagues[59] reported on a double-blind, prospective, crossover study comparing oxybutynin, flavoxate, emepronium, and placebo. Although there was a high dropout rate (19 of 60 patients) and the entry criteria were vague (frequency, urgency, urge incontinence), the results, scored as 5 (excellent overall effect) to 1 (no improvement) by both patient and physician, were combined into a single number. The percentages of results in categories 3 to 5 for the agents used were oxybutynin, 61%; placebo, 41%; emepronium, 34%; and flavoxate, 31%. The results of the first treatment gave corresponding percentages of only 63%, 29%, 18% (probably reflecting eight dropouts due to side effects), and 44%, respectively.

Ambulatory urodynamic monitoring and pad weighing were used to assess the effects of oxybutynin on DO by Von Doorn and Zwiers.[60] The 24-hour average frequency of IVCs decreased from 8.7 to 3.4; the maximum contraction amplitude decreased from 32 to 22 cm H_2O, and the duration of the average IVC decreased from 90 to 60 seconds. However, the daily micturition frequency did not change (11 to 10), nor did the amount of urine lost—findings the authors tried to minimize by pointing out that some patients also had sphincteric incontinence and that, during treatment, there may have been a higher fluid intake.

The AHCPR guidelines[23] list six randomized controlled trials for oxybutynin; 90% of patients were women. The percentage of cure was listed as ranging from 28% to 44%, reduction in urge incontinence from 9% to 56%, side effects from 2% and 66%, and dropouts from 3% to 45% (all figures refer to overall percentage minus percentage on placebo). There were some negative reports on the efficacy of oxybutynin. Zorzitto and colleagues[61] came to conclusions similar to those resulting from their study of propantheline in a double-blind placebo-controlled trial conducted in 24 incontinent geriatric institutionalized patients:

oxybutynin 5 mg twice a day was no more effective than placebo with scheduled toileting in treating incontinence in this type of population with DO. An incontinence profile was used to assess results, and the only significant difference noted was an increase in residual urine volume (from 159 to 92 mL). Ouslander and colleagues[62] reported similar conclusions in a smaller study of geriatric patients, and in an accompanying article they concluded simply that the drug is safe for use in the elderly at doses of 2.5 to 5 mg three times a day.[62,63]

An ER form of oxybutynin is available that releases the active compound over a period of 24 hours. Aside from the ease of once-daily administration, the potential benefit of the ER formulation is that stabilization of serum levels throughout the day should lower the incidence of side effects.[64] Another theoretical advantage may be that less absorption occurs in the proximal portion of the gastrointestinal tract which drains into the portal system, so there is less first-pass metabolism.

IR and ER oxybutynin were compared in a multicenter randomized, double-blind trial of 106 patients, all of whom had previously responded to IR oxybutynin.[65] For patients currently taking anticholinergic therapy, after a 1-week washout period, a dose-titration schedule was used to reach the maximum allowable dose (20 mg IR or 30 mg ER daily), or to the dose at which no urge urinary incontinence (UUI) episodes occurred over the course of 2 days (as measured from a diary) or until a dose was reached with intolerable side effects (at which point, the final dose was decreased by 5 mg). Thirteen patients discontinued therapy during the trial, four because of anticholinergic events. Overall, similar efficacy was noted for both formulations of oxybutynin in overall number of episodes (27.4 to 4.8 for ER and 23.4 to 3.1 for IR), in the percentage decrease in weekly UUI episodes (84% for ER and 88% for IR), and in overall incontinence episodes (urge, stress, and mixed). The number and proportion of patients achieving continence was also similar between the groups (41% for ER, and 40% for IR). Curiously, voiding frequency increased in both groups, with a statistically significant percentage increase of voiding frequency in patients receiving the ER compared with those receiving the IR formulation (54% versus 17%; $P < .001$). Anticholinergic side effects were noted in both groups. Dry mouth was the most frequent symptom, occurring in a majority of patients. Dry mouth was reported as moderate or severe by 25% and 46% of patients receiving the ER and IR formulations, respectively ($P = .03$). Other anticholinergic side effects were reported with similar frequency in the ER and IR groups: somnolence (38% versus 40%), blurred vision (28% versus 17%), constipation (30% versus 31%), dizziness (28% versus 38%), impaired urination (25% versus 29%), nervousness (25% versus 23 %), and nausea (19% versus 17%).

In an open-label trial[66] with 256 patients (23.4 % of whom were taking an anti-incontinence medication at baseline and switched over to oxybutynin ER for the study), oxybutynin ER reduced the number of incontinence episodes per week from 18.8 at baseline to 2.8 at the end of the study (83.1% reduction); 31% of patients remained free of UUI throughout the study. A 14.7% reduction in voiding frequency was noted on therapy compared with baseline, as measured from the voiding diary. Dry mouth was reported by 58.6% of patients; 23.0% reported moderate or severe dry mouth. Only 1.6% of patients discontinued therapy because of dry mouth. Overall, 7.8% of patients discontinued therapy because of adverse events, of which nausea, dry mouth, and somnolence were most frequent.

Topical application of oxybutynin and other agents to normal or unstable bladders has been suggested and implemented.[67] This conceptually attractive form of alternative drug administration, delivered by periodic intravesical instillation of either liquid or timed-released pellets, awaits further clinical trials and the development of preparations specifically formulated for this purpose. Several nonrandomized, unblinded and non–placebo-controlled studies have demonstrated the efficacy of this therapy in a variety of patients with neurogenic bladders, showing statistically significant improvements in cystometric capacity, volume at first IVC, bladder compliance, and overall continence.[68-70]

Madersbacher and Jilg reviewed the intravesical usage of 5 mg of oxybutynin dissolved in 30 mL distilled water in 13 patients with complete suprasacral cord lesions who were on clean intermittent catheterization.[71] Of the 10 patients who were incontinent, 9 remained dry for 6 hours. For the group, the changes in bladder capacity and maximum detrusor pressure were statistically significant. Some of the more interesting data were given in a figure showing plasma oxybutynin levels for a group of patients in whom administration was intravesical or oral. The level achieved after an oral dose rose to 7.3 mg/mL within 2 hours and then precipitously dropped to slightly less than 2 mg/mL at 4 hours. After intravesical administration, the level rose gradually to a peak of about 6.2 mg/mL at 3.5 hours, but at 6 hours it was still greater than 4 mg/mL and at 9 hours it was still between 3 and 4 mg/mL. From these data, it is unclear whether the intravesically applied drug acted locally or systemically.

In a later study, Madersbacher and Knoll[72] administered oxybutynin intravesically and then, 1 week later, gave oxybutynin orally to six patients with neurogenic bladders in order to study the pharmacokinetics of the drug and investigate the pharmacologic properties responsible for its clinical effects. Serum drug levels were correlated with urodynamic effects 20 minutes and 2 hours after administration of the drug. The authors concluded that the main effect of intravesical oxybutynin was a result of systemic absorption; however, a secondary direct local effect (smooth muscle relaxation or topical anesthetic effect) could not be excluded.

Weese and colleagues[73] reported use of a similar dose of oxybutynin (5 mg in 30 mL sterile water) to treat 42 patients with IVCs for whom oral anticholinergic therapy had failed (11 patients) or who had intolerable side effects (31 patients): 20 had neurogenic DO, 19 had non-neurogenic DO, and 3 had bowel or DO after augmentation. The drug was instilled two or three times each day for 10 minutes by catheter. Nine patients (21%) withdrew from the study because they were unable to tolerate clean intermittent catheterization or to retain the solution properly, but there were no reported side effects. Of the patients (33) who were able to follow the protocol, 18 (55%) reported at least a moderate subjective improvement in incontinence and urgency. Nine patients became totally continent and experienced complete resolution of their symptoms; 18 patients improved and experienced a decrease of 2.5 pads per day. There were no urodynamic data. Follow-up ranged from 5 to 35 months (mean, 18.4 months).

The lack of side effects prompted some speculation about the mechanism of drug action: one possibility was simply a more prolonged rate of absorption; another was a decreased pass through the liver and therefore a decrease in metabolites, the hypothesis being that perhaps the metabolites and not the primary compound are responsible for the side effects.

Enzelsberger and associates[74] reported on the use of intravesical oxybutynin in the treatment of DO in 52 women. In the only published randomized, double-blind, placebo-controlled study of this intravesical administration, patients received once-daily intravesical oxybutynin (20 mg in 40 mL sterile water) or placebo for 12 days. The results revealed statistically significant differences in first desire to void (from 95 mL before treatment to 150 mL after treatment), cystometric capacity (205 to 310 mL), maximal pressure during filling (16 to 9 cm H_2O), daytime frequency (7.5 to 4), and nocturia (5.1 to 1.8). Side effects were similar in the treated and placebo groups (17% versus 10%, respectively). For unexplained reasons, 19 of 23 patients in the treated group continued to have symptomatic relief after termination of the study.

In an increasing effort to maintain or improve the efficacy of oxybutynin while minimizing its side effects, the use of transdermal oxybutynin has been investigated. In one study,[75] the daily-dose patch significantly reduced the number of weekly incontinence episodes while reducing average daily urinary frequency by increasing the average voided volume. Dry mouth rates were similar to those reported with placebo (7% versus 8.3%). A recent study[76] comparing transdermal oxybutynin and oxybutynin IR demonstrated equivalent reduction in incontinent episodes but significantly less dry mouth with the patch (38% versus 94%). In a third study,[77] transdermal oxybutynin was compared to placebo and tolterodine ER. The two drugs had similarly significant reduced daily incontinence episodes and increased voided volume, but tolterodine ER was associated with a higher rate of antimuscarinic adverse events. The major side effect for transdermal oxybutynin was pruritus at the application site in 14% and erythema in 8.3% of patients.

Dicyclomine hydrochloride is also reported to exert a direct relaxant effect on smooth muscle in addition to an antimuscarinic action.[78] An oral dose of 20 mg three times a day in adults has been reported to increase bladder capacity in patients with neurogenic DO.[79] Beck and coworkers[80] compared the use of 10 mg dicyclomine, 15 mg propantheline, and placebo three times a day in patients with DO[81]: the rates of cure or improvement were 62%, 73%, and 20%, respectively. Awad and associates[82] reported that 20 mg dicyclomine three times a day caused resolution or significant improvement in 24 of 27 patients with IVCs.

Flavoxate hydrochloride has a direct inhibitory action on smooth muscle but very weak anticholinergic properties.[8,83] In cats, at least, there is some evidence that flavoxate may also have central effects on the inhibition of the micturition reflex in addition to its effects on the relaxation of smooth muscle.[84] Clinical studies addressing the efficacy of flavoxate in the treatment of DO have been mixed. Milani and colleagues[85] performed a double-blind, crossover study comparing flavoxate 1200 mg/day with oxybutynin 15 mg daily in 41 women with idiopathic motor or sensory urgency, using clinical and urodynamic criteria. The two drugs had similar efficacy, with flavoxate having fewer side effects. However, Briggs and colleagues[86] reported that this drug had essentially no effect on non-neurogenic DO in an elderly population, an experience that coincides with the laboratory effects obtained by Benson and associates.[87] There were few reported side effects. Although the efficacy of flavoxate compared with other agents in this group has not been proven, a short clinical trial may be worthwhile.

Trospium and propiverine are classified as predominantly antispasmodic agents (smooth muscle relaxants) with some anticholinergic effects as well. Although both drugs have been used in Europe for years, trospium chloride has been recently approved by the FDA and is now available for use in the United States. It is a quaternary amine and has limited ability to cross the blood-brain barrier, therefore in theory leading to minimal cognitive dysfunction.[88-90] Trospium has no selectivity for a muscarinic subtype.

Several randomized controlled trials have shown the beneficial effects of trospium[91,92] in both neurogenic and non-neurogenic DO.[93-97] Stohrer and colleagues performed a multicenter, placebo controlled, double-blind study to determine the effects of trospium on urodynamic parameters in patients with neurogenic DO secondary to spinal cord injury.[91] Patients were randomized to either trospium 20 mg twice daily or placebo for 3 weeks. The treatment group showed an increase in maximum cystometric capacity, decreased maximal detrusor pressure, and increased compliance. No such effects were seen in the placebo group. A similar study by Madersbacher and coworkers[92] compared the use of trospium and oxybutynin in the treatment of neurogenic DO. The two medications appeared to have equal effects, but those patients taking trospium had fewer side effects.

The effectiveness of trospium in the treatment of non-neurogenic DO has also been well documented. Allouis and colleagues[93] performed a randomized, double-blind, placebo-controlled study in 309 patients with non-neurogenic DO. The treatment group received trospium 20 mg twice daily, and the study length was 3 weeks. They found a significant increase over placebo in volume at first involuntary detrusor contraction and in maximum bladder capacity. Cardozo and colleagues[94] also performed a randomized, placebo-controlled, double-blind study in patients with non-neurogenic DO. A total of 208 patients participated in the study and were given placebo or trospium 20 mg twice daily for 2 weeks. They similarly found an increase in volume at which the first involuntary detrusor contraction took place as well as an increase in maximum cystometric capacity.

In a study comparing the efficacy of trospium 20 mg twice daily with tolterodine 2 mg twice daily and placebo in patients with urodynamically proven DO, Junemann and colleagues found trospium to be significantly more effective in decreasing the frequency of micturition than either tolterodine or placebo.[95] Trospium was also found to cause a greater reduction in the number of incontinence episodes and produced similar rates of dry mouth as tolterodine.

Halaska and associates[96] performed a long-term tolerability and efficacy study comparing trospium 20 mg twice daily and oxybutynin 5 mg twice daily in patients with DO. Patients were treated for 52 weeks. Urodynamic studies were performed at baseline, 26 weeks, and 52 weeks, and patient voiding diaries were also kept at baseline, 2, 26, and 52 weeks. A significant increase in mean maximum cystometric capacity was found, with 92 mL at 26 weeks and 115 mL at 52 weeks in the trospium group. No other significant difference in urodynamic parameters was noted between the two treatment groups. Voiding diaries revealed a decrease in frequency, frequency of incontinence, and urgency episodes in both groups. At least one adverse event occurred in patients (64.8% and 76.6% in the trospium and oxybutynin groups, respectively). The most common side effect in both groups was dry mouth. Overall, the two drugs were comparable in efficacy in improving urinary symptoms, but trospium had a better benefit-risk ratio than oxybutynin due to better tolerability.

In a large multicenter, placebo controlled, randomized, parallel study, Zinner and colleagues, from the Trospium Study Group,[97] compared the effects of trospium 20 mg twice daily and placebo in patients with OAB and urge incontinence. The study length was 12 weeks, with the primary end points being a change in the mean number of voids and a change in urge incontinent episodes in a 24-hour period. Other variables, such as mean volume per void, urge severity, diurnal and nocturnal micturition episodes, and onset of action, were also examined. Compared with placebo, trospium produced a significant reduction in the mean frequency of toilet voids and in urge incontinent episodes. A significant increase in volume voided and decrease in urge severity and diurnal frequency were also seen. The effects were seen after 1 week of treatment and were maintained throughout the remainder of the study. Once again, the most common side effect was dry mouth, occurring in 21.8% of patients, followed by constipation in 9.5% and headache in 6.5%. Similar results were confirmed by Rudy and colleagues[98] in a large multicenter study in the United States that included 658 patients.

Propiverine is a musculotropic smooth muscle relaxant with anticholinergic activity. It is rapidly absorbed and has a high first-pass metabolism.[99] Thuroff and associates[100] reviewed nine randomized studies on a total of 230 patients and found reductions in frequency and micturitions per 24 hours of 30% and 17%, respectively. There was a 77% subjective improvement, and side effects were found in 14% of the patients. In a study by Stohrer and colleagues,[101] superiority of propiverine over placebo was documented in patients with neurogenic DO. In controlled trials comparing propiverine, flavoxate, and placebo or propiverine, oxybutynin, and placebo,[102] they confirmed the efficacy of propiverine and suggested that the drug may have equal efficacy and fewer side effects than oxybutynin.

Madersbacher and colleagues[103] compared the tolerability and efficacy of propiverine (15 mg three times daily), oxybutynin (5 mg twice daily) and placebo in 366 patients with urgency and urge incontinence in a randomized, double-blind, placebo-controlled clinical trial. The urodynamic efficacy of propiverine was similar to that of oxybutynin, but the incidence and severity of dry mouth was less. Dorschner and colleagues[104] performed a double-blind, multicenter, placebo-controlled randomized study to test the efficacy and cardiac safety of propiverine in elderly patients with urgency, urge, or mixed incontinence. There were 98 patients with a mean age of 68 years who received propiverine 15 mg or placebo three times daily for 4 weeks. Propiverine resulted in a significant reduction in micturition frequency and a decrease in incontinence episodes. The adverse events were very low. Therefore, propiverine appears to have an acceptable side effect profile and reasonable efficacy.

Calcium Antagonists

The role of calcium as a messenger in linking extracellular stimuli to the intracellular environment is well established, including its involvement in excitation-contraction coupling in striated, cardiac, and smooth muscle.[1,5] Interference with calcium inflow or intracellular release is a very potent potential mechanism for bladder smooth muscle relaxation.

Nifedipine has been shown to be an effective inhibitor of contraction induced by several mechanisms in human and guinea pig bladder muscle.[8,105] It has also been shown to block completely the noncholinergic portion of the contraction produced by electrical field stimulation in rabbit bladder.[106] Nifedipine more effectively inhibited contractions induced by potassium than those induced by carbachol in rabbit bladder strips, whereas terodiline, an agent with both calcium-antagonistic and anticholinergic properties, had the opposite effect. However, terodiline did cause complete inhibition of the response of rabbit bladder to electrical field stimulation. At low concentrations, terodiline has mainly an antimuscarinic action, whereas at higher concentration a calcium-antagonistic effect becomes evident. Experiments in vitro appeared to show that these two effects were at least additive with regard to bladder contractility. Other experimental studies confirmed the inhibitory effect of the calcium antagonists nifedipine, verapamil, and diltiazem on a variety of experimental models of the activity of spontaneous and induced bladder muscle strips and whole bladder preparations.[101,108] Andersson and colleagues[109] showed that nifedipine effectively (and with some selectivity) inhibited the nonmuscarinic portion of the contraction of rabbit detrusor strips, whereas verapamil, diltiazem, flunarizine, and lidoflazine caused a marked depression of both the total and the nonmuscarinic part of contraction, suggesting that differences exist between various calcium-channel blockers with respect to their effects, at least on electrically induced bladder muscle contraction. These results were used as support for the view that, even if "atropine-resistant" contractions in rabbit and human bladder had different causes, combined muscarinic-receptor and calcium-channel blockade might offer a more effective way of treating bladder overactivity than the single-mechanism therapies currently available.

A number of clinical studies on the inhibitory action of terodiline on bladder overactivity have shown clinical effectiveness.[110] In a double-blind crossover study of 12 women with motor urge incontinence, Ekman and colleagues[111] reported increases in bladder capacity and the volume at which sensation of urgency was experienced in all but one of the patients treated with terodiline, whereas placebo treatment had no objective or subjective effect. Peters[112] reported the results of a multicenter study that ultimately included data from 89 patients (from an original 128) and compared terodiline and placebo in women with motor urge incontinence. The daily dose in this study was 12.5 mg in the morning and 25 mg at night. The authors concluded that terodiline was more effective than placebo but noted that this improvement was much more apparent on subjective than on objective assessment of cystometric and micturition data; 63% of patients preferred terodiline, regardless of treatment sequence. Although statistically significant objective differences between terodiline and placebo were recorded, they were not very impressive. Tapp and colleagues[113] reported on a double-blind placebo-controlled study that used a dose-titration technique and included 70 women with urodynamically proven DO and bladder capacities of less than 400 mL. Of the 34 women in the terodiline group, 62% considered themselves improved, and 38% were unchanged; of the 36 women in the placebo group, 42% considered themselves improved, 47% unchanged, and 11% worse—a statistically significant response in favor of terodiline with regard to the improvement percentage. Micturition variables of daytime frequency, daytime incontinence episodes, number of pads used, and average voided volumes were statistically changed in favor of terodiline, but the absolute changes were relatively small (e.g., a change in daytime incontinence episodes among patients taking placebo from 2.5 to 1.9 per day, as opposed to a reduction from 3.7 to 1.6 for those taking terodiline). Urodynamic data, although showing a trend in favor of terodiline in each parameter, showed no statistically significant differences in any category. Side effects were noted in a large number of patients and with equal frequency in both groups after the dose-titration phase. However, the incidence of anticholinergic side effects was higher in the drug group: 29% of the terodiline group and 11% of the placebo group spontaneously complained of a dry mouth, and 20% of the terodiline group but none of the placebo group complained of blurred vision. The AHCPR guidelines[23] list seven randomized controlled trials for terodiline; 94% of patients were women. The percentage of cure was listed as ranging from 18% to 33%, reduction in urge incontinence from 14% to 83%, side effects from 14% to 40%, and dropouts from 2% to 8% (all figures refer to overall percentage minus percentage on placebo).

Terodiline also exhibited an inhibitory effect on experimental neurogenic DO in the rabbit whole-bladder model, suggesting a possible role for local administration as well.[114] Terodiline is almost completely absorbed from the gastrointestinal tract and has a low serum clearance. The recommended dosage in adults is 25 mg twice a day, reduced to an initial dose of 12 mg twice a day in geriatric patients. The half-life is approximately 60 hours. Abrams[110] logically proposed, on this basis, a once-daily dose but emphasized the necessity of dose titration for each patient.

The common side effects seen with calcium antagonists (hypotension, facial flushing, headache, dizziness, abdominal discomfort, constipation, nausea, rash, weakness, and palpitations) have not been reported in larger initial clinical studies with terodiline, its side effects consisting primarily of those consequent on its anticholinergic action. However, questions have been raised about the occurrence of a rare arrhythmia (torsades de pointes) among patients taking terodiline simultaneously with antidepressants or antiarrhythmic drugs.[116,117] Stewart and colleagues[118] reported a prolongation of the QT and QTc (corrected QT) intervals and a reduction in heart rate among elderly patients taking 12.5 mg terodiline twice a day; these effects were apparent after 1 week but not after 1 day of therapy. These investigators also reported polymorphic ventricular tachycardia in four patients (three older than 80 years of age) receiving the drug. They advised avoidance of the drug in patients with cardiac disease requiring cardioactive drugs, in those with hypokaliemia, and in combination with other drugs that can prolong the QT interval, such as tricyclic antidepressants or antipsychotics. After other reports of apparent cardiac toxicity, the drug was voluntarily withdrawn by the manufacturer pending the results of further safety studies. The studies conducted for approval by the FDA were likewise voluntarily halted by the manufacturer pending the results of further safety studies.

Other calcium-antagonist drugs have not been widely used to treat voiding dysfunction. A bladder-specific membrane calcium channel is not known to exist, and there is no agent that specifically blocks intracellular calcium release only in bladder smooth muscle cells. Available information does not suggest that systemic therapy with calcium antagonists is an effective way to treat DO.

Potassium Channel Openers

Potassium channel openers relax various types of smooth muscle, including the detrusor, by increasing potassium efflux, resulting in membrane hyperpolarization.[8] Hyperpolarization reduces the opening probability of ion channels involved in membrane depolarization, and excitation is reduced. Andersson[119] summarized studies showing that, in isolated human and animal detrusor muscle, potassium channel openers reduced spontaneous contractions and contractions occurring in response to electrical stimulation, carbachol, and low (but not high) external potassium concentrations. There are some suggestions that bladder instability—at least that associated with intravesical obstruction and detrusor hypertrophy—may be secondary to supersensitivity to depolarizing stimuli. Theoretically, then, potassium channel openers might be an attractive alternative for the treatment of DO in such circumstances without inhibiting the normal voluntary contractions necessary for bladder emptying.[120]

Pinacidil is a compound that, in a concentration-dependent fashion, inhibits not only spontaneous myogenic contractions but also contractile responses induced by electrical field stimulation and carbachol in isolated human detrusor[121] and in normal and hypertrophied rat detrusor muscle. However, a preliminary study of this agent in a double-blind, crossover format produced no effects on symptoms in nine patients with DO and bladder outlet obstruction.[122] Nurse and associates[123] reported on the use of cromakalim, another potassium channel opener, in 17 patients who had refractory DO or neurogenic DO or had stopped other drug therapy because of intolerable side effects. Six (37.5%) of 16 patients who completed the study showed a decrease in frequency and an increase in voided volume. Long-term observation was not possible, because the drug was withdrawn owing to reported adverse effects of high doses in animal toxicology studies. Levcromakalim (the pharmacologically active enantiomer of cromakalim) was administered intravenously to six patients with high spinal cord lesions and reflex micturition[124]: other than an increase in the duration of the detrusor contraction, no other urodynamic parameters associated with the neurogenic DO were significantly affected. Levcromakalim resulted in a rapid and significant drop in blood pressure which precluded studies at a higher dose. Overall, potassium channel openers are not at present very specific for the bladder and are more potent in relaxing other tissues—hence, their potential utility in the treatment of hypertension, asthma, and angina. If tissue-selective potassium-activator drugs can be developed, they may prove very useful for the treatment of detrusor instability, irritable bowel syndrome, and epilepsy.[125] Intravesical use has also been suggested[124,125] as a method of potentially eliminating some of the intolerable systemic side effects that limit the clinical utility of these agents.

Side effects of pinacidil have been studied best; they include headache, peripheral edema (in 25% to 50% of patients and dose-related), weight gain, palpitations, dizziness, and rhinitis. Hypertrichosis and symptomatic T-wave changes have also been reported (30%). Fewer data are available on cromakalim, which can produce dose-related headache but rarely edema.[119]

Prostaglandin Inhibitors

Prostaglandins are ubiquitous compounds that have a potential role in the excitatory neurotransmission to the bladder, the development of bladder contractility or tension occurring during filling, the emptying contractile response of bladder smooth muscle to neural stimulation, and even the maintenance of urethral tone during the storage phase of micturition, as well as the release of this tone during the emptying phase. Downie and Karmazyn[126] suggested a different type of contractile influence of prostaglandins on detrusor muscle. They found that mechanical irritation of the epithelium of rabbit bladder increased basal tension and spontaneous activity in response to electrical stimulation and that these responses, related to the intensity of the irritative trauma, were mimicked by prostaglandins. The effect was significantly reduced by pretreatment of the epithelium, but not the muscle, with prostaglandin synthetase inhibitors. Andersson[8] suggested a possible sensitization of sensory afferent nerves by prostaglandins, increasing afferent input at a given degree of bladder filling and contributing to the triggering of IVCs at a small bladder volume. Therefore, there are many mechanisms whereby prostaglandin synthetase inhibitors might decrease bladder contractility in response to various stimuli; however, objective evidence that such effects can occur is scant.

Cardozo and colleagues[127] reported on a double-blind placebo study of the effects of 50 mg flurbiprofen (a prostaglandin synthetase inhibitor) given three times a day on 30 women with DO. They concluded that the drug did not abolish IVCs or abnormal bladder activity but did delay the intravesical pressure rise to a greater degree of distention. Of these patients, 43% experienced side effects—primarily nausea, vomiting, headache, indigestion, gastric distress, constipation, and rash. Cardozo and Stanton[128] reported symptomatic improvement in patients with detrusor instability who were given indomethacin in doses of 50 to 200 mg daily, but this was a short-term study with no cystometric data, and the drug was compared only with bromocriptine. The incidence of side effects was high (19 of 32 patients), although no patient had to stop treatment because of them. Numerous prostaglandin synthetase inhibitors exist, most of which belong in the category of nonsteroidal anti-inflammatory drugs. It should be remembered that these drugs can interfere with platelet function and contribute to excess bleeding in surgical patients; some may also have adverse renal effects.[129]

β-Adrenergic Agonists

The presence of β-adrenoceptors in human bladder muscle has prompted attempts to increase bladder capacity with β-adrenergic stimulation. Such stimulation can cause significant increases in the capacity of animal bladders, which contain a moderate density of β-adrenoceptors.[1] Studies in vitro show a strong dose-related relaxant effect of β_2-agonists on the bladder body of rabbits but little effect on the bladder base or proximal urethra. Terbutaline, in oral doses of 5 mg three times a day, was reported to have a "good clinical effect" in some patients with urgency and urgency incontinence but no significant effect on the bladders of neurologically normal humans without voiding difficulty.[130] Although these results are compatible with those seen in other organ systems (e.g., β-adrenergic stimulation causes no acute change in total lung capacity in normal humans but does favorably affect patients with bronchial asthma), there are few adequate studies of the effects of β-adrenergic stimulation in patients with DO. Lindholm and Lose[131] used 5 mg terbutaline three times a day in eight women with motor urge incontinence and seven with sensory urge incontinence. After 3 months of treatment, 14 patients claimed to have experienced beneficial effects, and 12 became subjectively continent. In six of eight cases, the detrusor became stable on cystometric examination. The volume at first desire to void increased in those patients with originally unstable bladders, from a mean of 200 mL to 302 mL, but the maximum cystometric capacity did not change. Nine patients had transient side effects, including palpitations, tachycardia, or hand tremor, and in three of them the side effects continued but were acceptable to the patient. The drug was discontinued in one patient because of severe adverse symptoms. Gruneberger,[132] in a double-blind study, reported that clenbuterol produced a good therapeutic effect in 15 of 20 patients with motor urge incontinence. Unfavorable results of β-agonist usage for bladder overactivity were published by Castleden and Morgan[133] and by Naglo and associates.[134] As yet there have been no controlled clinical trials on the treatment of OAB with β_3-agonists.

Tricyclic Antidepressants

Many clinicians have found that tricyclic antidepressants, particularly imipramine hydrochloride, are useful for facilitating urine storage, both by decreasing bladder contractility and by increasing outlet resistance. These agents have been the subject of extensive and highly sophisticated pharmacologic investigation to determine the mechanisms of action responsible for their varied effects.[135-137] Most data have been accumulated as a result of trying to explain the antidepressant properties of these agents and consequently involve primarily CNS tissue. Although the results, conclusions, and speculations based on the data are extremely interesting, it should be emphasized that it is essentially unknown whether they apply to, or have relevance for, the lower urinary tract. In varying degrees, all of these agents have at least three major pharmacologic actions: they have central and peripheral anticholinergic effects at some (but not all) sites; they block the active transport system in the presynaptic nerve ending that is responsible for the reuptake of the released amine neurotransmitters noradrenaline and serotonin; and they are sedatives, an action that occurs presumably on a central basis but is perhaps related to antihistaminic properties (at H_1 receptors, although they also antagonize H_2 receptors to some extent). There is also evidence that these agents desensitize at least some α_2- and some β_2-adrenoceptors. Paradoxically, they also have been shown to block some α- and serotonin-1 receptors. Imipramine has prominent systemic anticholinergic effects but only a weak antimuscarinic effect on bladder smooth muscle.[138,139] However, it does have a strong direct inhibitory effect on bladder smooth muscle that is neither anticholinergic nor adrenergic.[136,140,141] This may be the result of a local-anesthetic–like action at the nerve terminals in the adjacent effector membrane, an effect that seems to occur also in cardiac muscle,[142] or it may be caused by an inhibition of the participation of calcium in the excitation-contraction coupling process.[138,140] Akah[143] provided supportive evidence in the rat bladder that desipramine, the active metabolite of imipramine, depresses the response to electrical field stimulation by interfering with calcium movement (perhaps not only extracellular calcium movement but also internal translocation and binding). Direct evidence suggesting that the effect of imipramine on noradrenaline reuptake occurs in lower urinary tract tissue as well as in brain tissue was provided by Foreman and McNulty[144] in the rabbit. In addition, they described a significantly greater but similar effect of tomoxetine in the bladder and urethra in this model. Tomoxetine inhibits noradrenaline reuptake selectively, whereas imipramine has a nonselective effect. This fact suggests a potential new clinical approach to the use of more selective and potent reuptake inhibitors for the treatment of incontinence. In attempting to correlate clinical effects with mechanisms of action, one might also postulate a β-receptor–induced decrease in bladder body contractility if peripheral blockade of noradrenaline reuptake does occur there owing to the increased concentration of β-receptors compared with α-adrenoceptors in that area. An enhanced α-adrenergic effect in the smooth muscle of the bladder base and proximal urethra, where α-receptors outnumber β-receptors, is generally considered the mechanism whereby imipramine increases outlet resistance.

Clinically, imipramine seems to be effective in decreasing bladder contractility and increasing outlet resistance.[145-148] Castleden and colleagues[148] began therapy in elderly patients with DO with a single 25-mg nighttime dose of imipramine, which was increased every third day by 25 mg until the patient was continent or had side effects or a dose of 150 mg was reached. Six of 10 patients became continent; in addition, among those who underwent repeated cystometry, bladder capacity increased by a mean of 105 mL and bladder pressure at capacity decreased by a mean of 18 cm H_2O. Motor unit potential increased by a mean of 30 cm H_2O. Although our subjective impression[146] was that the bladder effects became evident only after days of treatment, some patients in the Castleden series became continent after only 3 to 5 days of therapy. Our usual adult dose for treatment of voiding dysfunction is 25 mg four times a day; less-frequent administration is possible because of the drug's long half-life. Half of that dose is given in elderly patients, in whom the drug half-life may be prolonged. In our experience, the effects of imipramine on the lower urinary tract are often additive to those of atropine-like agents; consequently, a combination of imipramine and an antimuscarinic or an antispasmodic is sometimes especially useful for decreasing bladder contractility.[146] If imipramine is used in conjunction with an atropine-like agent, it should be noted that the anticholinergic side effects of the drugs may be additive.

It has been known for many years that imipramine is relatively effective for the treatment of nocturnal enuresis in children. Doses for this condition range from 10 to 50 mg daily. It is not known whether the mechanisms of drug action in this situation are the same as those for decreasing bladder contractility. Korczyn and Kish[149] presented evidence that the mechanism of the antineuritic effect differs from that of the peripheral anticholinergic effect and the drug's antidepressant effect. The antineuritic effect occurs soon after initial administration, whereas the antidepressant effects usually take 2 to 4 weeks to develop.

Doxepin is another tricyclic antidepressant that has been found (in rabbit-bladder strips in vitro) to be more potent than other tricyclic compounds with respect to antimuscarinic and musculotropic relaxant activity.[142] Lose and colleagues,[150] in a randomized, double-blind, crossover study of women with IVCs and frequency, urgency, or urge incontinence, found that this agent caused a significant decrease in control over nighttime frequency and incontinence episodes, as well as a near-significant decrease in urine loss (by the pad-weighing test) and in the cystometric parameters of first sensation and maximum bladder capacity. The dose of doxepin used was either a single 50-mg bedtime dose or this dose plus an additional 25 mg in the morning. The number of daytime incontinence episodes decreased in both doxepin and placebo groups, and the difference was not statistically significant. Doxepin treatment was preferred by 14 patients, whereas 2 preferred placebo and 3 had no preference. Of the 14 patients who stated a preference for doxepin, 12 claimed that they became continent during treatment and 2 claimed improvement; the 2 patients who preferred placebo also claimed improvement. The AHCPR guidelines[23] combine results for imipramine and doxepin, citing only three randomized controlled trials, with an unknown percentage of women patients. The percentage of cure was listed as 31%, reduction in urge incontinence as ranging from 20% to 88%, and side effects as ranging from zero to 70% (all figures refer to overall percentage minus percentage on placebo).

When the tricyclic antidepressants are used in the generally larger doses employed for antidepressant effects, their most frequent side effects are those attributable to their systemic anticholinergic activity.[135,136] Allergic phenomena, including rash, hepatic dysfunction, obstructive jaundice, and agranulocytosis, may also occur but are rare. CNS side effects may include weakness, fatigue, parkinsonian effects, fine tremors (noted mostly in the upper extremities), a manic or schizophrenic picture, and sedation, probably from an antihistaminic effect. Postural hypotension may also be seen, presumably due to selective blockade (a paradoxical effect) of α_1-adrenoceptors in some vascular smooth muscle. Tricyclic antidepressants may also cause excess sweating of obscure origin and a delay in orgasm or orgasmic impotence, the cause of which is likewise unclear. They may also produce arrhythmias and can interact in deleterious ways with other drugs; therefore, caution must be observed when using these drugs in patients with cardiac disease.[135] Whether cardiotoxicity will prove to be a legitimate concern in patients receiving smaller doses (i.e., smaller than those used for treatment of depression) for lower urinary tract dysfunction remains to be seen, but it is a matter of potential concern. Consultation with a patient's physician or cardiologist is always helpful before such therapy is instituted in questionable situations. The use of imipramine is contraindicated in patients receiving monoamine oxidase inhibitors because severe CNS toxicity can be precipitated, including hyperpyrexia, seizures, and coma. Some potential side effects of antidepressants may be especially significant in the elderly, specifically weakness, fatigue, and postural hypotension. If imipramine or any of the tricyclic antidepressants is to be prescribed for the treatment of voiding dysfunction, the patient should be thoroughly informed about the fact that this is not the usual indication for this drug and that potential side effects exist. Reports of significant side effects (severe abdominal distress, nausea, vomiting, headache, lethargy, and irritability) after abrupt cessation of high doses of imipramine in children suggest that the drug should be discontinued gradually, especially in patients receiving high doses.

Botulinum Toxin

Botulinum toxin (BTX), is a presynaptic inhibitor of acetylcholine release and the release of other neurotransmitters and therefore decreases muscle contractility. It can be administered in the bladder by cystoscopic injection directly into the detrusor muscle. This produces a chemical denervation that is reversible after about 6 months. Of the seven subtypes of botulinum toxin that have been identified, botulinum A toxin (BTX-A) is the most commonly used, with botulinum B toxin (BTX-B) being the next most commonly used.

There have been some open-label and a few double-blind studies reporting its use in the treatment of neurogenic and idiopathic DO. Preliminary studies using BTX-A look promising, but for the use of BTX-B is too early to tell. Schurch[151] evaluated the use of BTX-A in patients with neurogenic DO secondary to spinal cord injury who were on intermittent catheterization. The study was prospective but nonrandomized. Twenty-one patients received 200 to 300 U of BTX-A. At 6 weeks, 17 of 19 patients were completely continent and could decrease or stop oral agents for their DO. The two who did not improve were given the lower dose of BTX-A (200 U). Urodynamics also demonstrated an increase in mean bladder capacity, increased postvoid residual, and a decrease in maximum voiding pressure. In some of the patients, the improvements were still durable out to 36 weeks.

Reitz and colleagues from Europe describe the European experience with BTX-A.[152] This retrospective study examined the data on 200 patients with neurogenic DO. At 12 weeks, there was a significant increase in the mean maximum cystometric bladder capacity, postvoid residual, and compliance. A majority of the patients could reduce or discontinue their anticholinergic medications. Data at 36 weeks revealed continued improvement.

Two studies studied the use of BTX for the treatment of non-neurogenic DO. Rapp and colleagues[153] performed BTX-A intradetrusor injections in 35 patients (29 women and 6 men) with frequency, urgency, and/or urge incontinence. They used 300 U of BTX-A injected transurethrally into 30 different sites within the bladder. There was a significant decrease in the scores recorded by the Incontinence Impact Questionnaire and Urinary Distress Inventory short forms. Overall, 60% of patients reported a slight to complete improvement in symptoms. Improvement was seen for at least 6 months. Dykstra and associates[154] used escalating does of BTX-B in a similar cohort of patients; 14 of 15 patients reported decreased frequency of urination and subjective improvement. BTX does appear to be a promising new therapy for facilitating bladder storage. Further placebo-controlled studies need to be carried out to appreciate its true efficacy and to determine the optimal dosages and locations of injections.

Dimethyl Sulfoxide

Dimethyl sulfoxide (DMSO), a naturally occurring organic compound used as an industrial solvent for many years, has multiple pharmacologic actions (membrane penetration, anti-inflammatory, local analgesic, bacteriostatic, diuretic, cholinesterase inhibitor, collagen solvent, vasodilator) and has been used for the treatment of arthritis and other musculoskeletal disorders. The formulation for human intravesical use is a 50% solution. Sant[155] summarized the pharmacology and clinical usage of DMSO and tabulated good-to-excellent results in 50% to 90% of collected series of patients treated with intravesical instillations for interstitial cystitis. However, DMSO has not been shown to be useful in the treatment of neurogenic or non-neurogenic DO, nor in any patient with urgency or frequency without interstitial cystitis.

Polysynaptic Inhibitors

Baclofen is an agent that decreases outlet resistance secondary to striated sphincter dyssynergia. It is also capable of depressing neurogenic detrusor overactivity resulting from spinal cord injury.[156] Taylor and Bates,[157] in a double-blind crossover study, reported that baclofen was very effective in decreasing both day and night urinary frequency and incontinence in patients with idiopathic DO. Cystometric changes were not recorded, however, and considerable improvement was also obtained in the placebo group. The intrathecal use of baclofen for treatment of DO is a potentially exciting area, and further reports are awaited.

Other Potential Agents

Nitric oxide (NO) is hypothesized to be a mediator of the nonadrenergic, noncholinergic relaxation of the outlet smooth muscle that occurs with bladder contraction.[5] Evidence exists that it is also involved in relaxation of bladder body smooth muscle,[158] and this provides interesting fodder for speculation: Is relaxation impaired in some types of overactivity, and can NO analogues or synthetase stimulators be developed as agents to inhibit detrusor contractility? Glyceryl trinitrate releases NO in vivo and achieves its cardiovascular effects by relaxing vascular smooth muscle. Although the ubiquity of NO might seem to mitigate its potential use in treating bladder overactivity (unless more organ-specific substrates or receptors are found), randomized controlled trials should be conducted.

Soulard and colleagues[159] described the effects of JO1870 on bladder activity in the rat. This non-anticholinergic probable opioid agonist increased bladder capacity and threshold pressure responsible for micturition in a dose-dependent fashion, raising the possibility of the use or development of opioid agonists with selectivity for receptors involved in the micturition reflex.

Constantinou[160,161] described the effects of thiphenamil hydrochloride on the lower urinary tract in healthy female volunteers and in those with detrusor incontinence. This drug was said to be a "synthetic antispasmodic." In a randomized controlled trial, based on diary records from 14 patients with DO, it was reported that voiding frequency per day decreased significantly (from 10.3 to 8.0 times), but placebo values were not given. Daily incontinence episodes decreased in nine analyzable patients, from 2.3 to 1.6 (not significant; placebo values not given), with pad dryness (rated on a scale of 0 to 4) improving from 1.6 to 1.2 (significant, but again no placebo data were given). Objective urodynamic results (in 16 patients) showed no flowmetry changes, no changes in bladder capacity, some increase in first sensation of fullness, and a significant decrease in detrusor voiding pressure (from 46.1 to 31.9 cm H_2O), compared with placebo. The data and interpretation in this article are confusing, especially because the study of healthy volunteers showed no urodynamic differences except an increase in maximum flow rate (from 16.9 to 27.7 mL/sec) at a drug dose of 800 mg. The most that can be said about the clinical use of thiphenamil is that, now a question has been raised, it needs to be addressed by further, "cleaner" studies with internally consistent results.

INCREASING BLADDER CAPACITY BY DECREASING SENSORY (AFFERENT) INPUT

Vanilloids: Capsaicin and Resiniferatoxin

Decreasing afferent input peripherally is the ideal treatment for both sensory urgency and DO in a bladder with relatively normal elastic or viscoelastic properties, in which the sensory afferents constitute the first limb in the abnormal micturition reflex. Maggi has written extensively about this type of treatment, specifically with reference to the properties of capsaicin.[162-164] Capsaicin is an irritant and algogenic compound obtained from hot red peppers that has highly selective effects on a subset of mammalian sensory neurons, including polymodal receptors and warm thermoreceptors.[165] Capsaicin produces pain by selectively activating polymodal nociceptive neurons by membrane depolarization and opening a cation-selective ion channel, which can be blocked by ruthenium red. Repeated administration induces desensitization and inactivation of sensory neurons by several mechanisms. Systemic and topical capsaicin produce a reversible antinociceptive and anti-inflammatory action after an initially undesirable algesic effect. Local or topical application blocks C-fiber conduction and inactivates neuropeptide release from peripheral nerve endings, accounting for local antinociception and reduction of neurogenic inflammation. Resiniferatoxin (RTX) is an analogue of capsaicin and is approximately 1000 times more potent for desensitization than capsaicin,[166] but it is only a few hundred times more potent for excitation.[167] Systemic capsaicin produces antinociception by activating specific receptors on afferent nerve terminals in the spinal cord; spinal neurotransmission is subsequently blocked by a prolonged inactivation of sensory neurotransmitter release. With local administration (intravesical), the potential advantage of capsaicin is a lack of systemic side effects. The actions are highly specific when the drug is applied locally: the compound affects primarily small-diameter nociceptive afferents, leaving the sensations of touch and pressure unchanged, although heat (but not cold) perception may be reduced; motor fibers are not affected. The effects are reversible, although it is not known whether initial levels of sensitivity are regained.

Maggi[164] reviewed the therapeutic potential of capsaicin-like molecules. Capsaicin-sensitive primary afferents (CSPAs) innervate the human bladder, and intravesical instillation of capsaicin into human bladder produces a concentration-dependent decrease in first desire to void, decreased bladder capacity, and a warm burning sensation. Maggi[162] used doses of 0.01, 1.0 and 10 μmol/L, administered in ascending order at intervals of 10 to 15 minutes as constant infusions of 20 mL/min until micturition occurred. Five capsaicin-treated patients with "hypersensitive disorder" reported either a complete disappearance of symptoms (four patients) or marked attenuation of symptoms (one patient), beginning 2 to 3 days after administration and lasting for 4 to 16 days; after that time, the symptoms gradually reappeared but were no worse.[164] Fowler and colleagues[169] found that considerably higher doses (up to 1 to 2 mmol/L for 30 minutes) were necessary to produce an effect in humans[170] however, they reported that bladder control improved within 2 days, and the improvement lasted for 3 to 6 months. Lower doses (0.1 to 100 μmol/L) produced "no long-lasting benefit." In a later study, Fowler and colleagues[171] administered intravesical capsaicin to 14 patients with DO and intractable urinary incontinence, 12 of whom had known spinal cord disease. A single intravesical instillation of 1 or 2 mmol/L capsaicin produced a response in nine patients (all of whom had spinal cord disease), with four of these patients having only a "partial" response and five patients having complete and durable (3 weeks to 6 months) responses, defined as complete continence on intermittent catheterization. Among the nine patients who responded to treatment, mean bladder capacity increased from 106 to 302 mL and maximum detrusor pressure decreased from 54 to 36 cm H_2O. There were no long-term adverse effects from the therapy.

Similar results were noted by Das and colleagues,[172] who treated seven patients with neurogenic bladders with four increasing doses of intravesical capsaicin over a period of several weeks (100 μmol/L, 500 μmol/L, 1 mmol/L, and 2 mmol/L). Only five of seven patients were able to complete the therapy, owing to the discomfort induced by the instillation. Of these five patients, three had symptomatic and urodynamic improvement. Geirsson and associates[173] treated 10 patients with traumatic spinal cord injury and neurogenic bladder with 2 mmol/L intravesical capsaicin; urodynamic improvement (decreased voiding pressure and increased bladder capacity) was noted in 9 of the 10 patients at 6 weeks. Subjective improvement was noted in 4 patients at 2 to 7 months after therapy, 2 of whom became continent. All 10 patients had no improvement or a worsening of symptoms during the first 1 to 2 weeks after instillation. Adverse reactions included severe burning on instillation in those patients with partial spinal lesions, precipitation of autonomic dysreflexia in several other patients, and gross hematuria in four patients. Chandiramani and colleagues[174] were able to reduce significantly the short-term toxicity (triggering of involuntary detrusor contractions) and discomfort of intravesical capsaicin therapy by pretreatment with an instillation of 2% topical lidocaine. Pretreatment with lidocaine did not alter the therapeutic efficacy of the capsaicin.

An efferent function of CSPAs is the release of neurotransmitters from the peripheral endings of these sensory neurons, such as tachykinins and calcitonin gene-related peptide.[162] These neurotransmitters can produce events collectively known as neurogenic inflammation, which can include smooth muscle contractions, increased plasma protein extravasation, vasodilatation, mast cell degranulation, facilitation of transmitter release from nerve terminals, and recruitment of inflammatory cells. This is another reason why intravesical capsaicin could theoretically be useful in treating the pain and related problems of interstitial cystitis and certain types of bladder overactivity that originate in primary afferents.

The peripheral terminals of CSPAs form a dense plexus just below the bladder urothelium, and fibers penetrating the urothelium come into contact with the lumen. This location, combined with their peculiar chemosensitivity, permits CSPAs to detect "backflow" of chemicals across the urothelium, which is thought to occur during conditions leading to breakdown of the "barrier function" of the urothelium.[164] If the "barrier" theory or "leaky urothelium" theory of the pathogenesis of the interstitial cystitis is true for some or many of the patients with this condition, the CSPAs in such patients may be stimulated by urine constituents' leaking back across the urothelium; under these circumstances, a local release of neuropeptides may well contribute to the production of neurogenic inflammation. If this is so, as Maggi suggested,[164] a local treatment leading to desensitization of CSPAs would be doubly advantageous. With capsaicin, however, excitation precedes desensitization, somewhat limiting the potential for therapy in humans. A preferable analogue would produce the latter action while reducing or eliminating the former. Last, Maggi[164] discussed the possible long-term disadvantages of such therapy as related to the potential physiologic roles (trophic or protective) of CSPAs and their secretions in response to stimulation.

RTX has been shown to be beneficial in several studies.[175-179] de Seze and colleagues compared the efficacy and tolerability of nonalcohol capsaicin (1 mmol/L) and RTX (100 nmol/L) in 10% alcohol in a randomized, double-blind, parallel group study in 39 spinal cord–injured patients with neurogenic DO. Follow-up was 3 months. On day 30, similar clinical and urodynamic improvements were found—in 78% and 83% of patients receiving capsaicin and 80% and 60% of those receiving RTX. The benefit remained in two thirds of the two groups after 3 months. There was no difference in side effects between the two groups.

Overall, intravesical capsaicin and RTX treatment may be a promising therapy for DO, and possibly for sensory dysfunction of the lower urinary tract; however, many problems exist. Optimal dosage, method and timing of delivery, and optimum delivery vehicle (diluent) remain unclear. The patients most likely to respond to this therapy are not yet defined, and randomized placebo-controlled studies to determine overall efficacy have not yet been performed. Finally, discomfort and triggering of involuntary bladder activity with instillation and postinstillation gross hematuria may be problematic.

INCREASING OUTLET RESISTANCE

α-Adrenergic Agonists

The bladder neck and proximal urethra contain a preponderance of α-adrenergic receptor sites, which, when stimulated, produce smooth muscle contraction.[1,2,5] The static infusion urethral pressure profile is altered by such stimulation, producing an increase in motor unit potential and maximum urethral closure pressure (MUCP). α-Adrenergic stimulants generally increase outlet resistance to a variable degree but are most often limited by their potential side effects, including blood pressure elevation, anxiety and insomnia due to stimulation of the CNS, headache, tremor, weakness, palpitations, cardiac arrhythmias, and respiratory difficulties. All such agents should be used with caution in patients with hypertension, cardiovascular disease, or hyperthyroidism.[180]

The use of ephedrine to treat SUI was mentioned as early as 1948.[178] Ephedrine is a noncatecholamine sympathomimetic agent that enhances release of noradrenaline from sympathetic neurons and directly stimulates both α- and β-adrenoceptors.[154] The oral adult dosage is 25 to 50 mg four times a day. Some tachyphylaxis develops in response to its peripheral actions, probably as a result of depletion of noradrenaline stores. Pseudoephedrine, a stereoisomer of ephedrine, is used for similar indications and carries similar precautions. The adult dosage is 30 to 60 mg four times a day, and the 30-mg dose form is available in the United States without prescription. Diokno and Taub[181] reported a "good-to-excellent" result in 27 of 38 patients with sphincteric incontinence treated with ephedrine sulphate. Beneficial effects were most often achieved in those with minimal-to-moderate wetting; little benefit was achieved in patients with severe SUI. A dose of 75 to 100 mg norephedrine chloride has been shown to increase motor unit potential and MUCP in women with SUI.[182] At a bladder volume of 300 mL, motor unit potential rose from 82 to 110 cm H_2O, and MUCP from 63 to 93 cm H_2O. The functional profile length did not change significantly. Obrink and Bunne,[183] however, noted that 100 mg norephedrine chloride given twice a day did not improve severe SUI sufficiently to offer it as an alternative to surgical treatment. They further noted in their group of 10 patients that the MUCP was not influenced at rest or with stress at low or moderate bladder volumes. Lose and Lindholm[184] treated 20 women with SUI with norfenefrine, an α-agonist, given as a slow-release tablet: 19 patients reported reduced urinary leakage, and 10 reported no further SUI. MUCP increased in 16 patients during treatment, the mean rise being from 53 to 64 cm H_2O. It is interesting and perplexing that most patients reported an effect only after 4 days of treatment. This delay is difficult to explain on the basis of drug action, unless one postulates a change in the number or sensitivity of α-adrenoceptors.

The group at Kolding Hospital in Denmark has published three other articles of note on the use of norfenefrine for sphincteric incontinence, with interesting results. Forty-four patients with SUI were randomized to treatment with norfenefrine (15 to 30 mg three times a day) versus placebo for 6 weeks.[185] Subjectively, 12 (52%) of 23 of the norfenefrine group reported improvement, as opposed to 7/21 (33%) of the placebo group—a difference that was not significant. Continence was reported by six (26%) norfenefrine patients and three (14%) placebo patients (not significant). Judged by a stress test, seven patients in each group became continent; 11 (48%) of 23 improved both subjectively and objectively in the norfenefrine group, as did 5/21 (24%) of the placebo group ($P = .09$). MUCP increased significantly (from 50 to 55 cm H_2O in the norfenefrine group, but also from 55 to 65 cm H_2O in the placebo group). Although the patients were said to have "genuine SUI," 5 of 12 patients with "urge incontinence" were reported cured with norfenefrine, and 4 of 7 with placebo.

Diernoes and associates[186] reported on the results of a 1-hour pad test in 33 women with either SUI or combined SUI and urgency treated with 30 mg norfenefrine three times a day. Leakage of more than 10 g was required for entry into the study. Subjective improvement was reported by 10 patients (30%). Continence as shown by pad test was found in six patients (18%). Pad tests were graded on a scale of 1 to 4. At 12 weeks, 20 patients (61%) had improved by at least one grade ($P < .05$), but at 3 weeks the number was 13 (39%; not significant).

Lose and colleagues[187] studied 44 women scheduled for operation for SUI who were treated with 15 to 30 mg norfenefrine three times a day versus placebo for 3 to 4.5 months and were then evaluated for outcome after a median observation period of 30 months. The description and categorization of results were somewhat confusing, but the results were interesting. Originally, 23 patients were allocated to the norfenefrine group and 21 to placebo. Results were categorized as follows: cured or much improved with no further treatment wanted; underwent surgery for relief; wanted medical therapy reinstituted; uncertain about what kind of treatment they wanted; used pads or pelvic floor exercises. At the end of a 6-week initial treatment period and re-evaluation, patients whose initial treatment had had no effect at all were crossed over to the other group. It is obvious that a powerful placebo effect occurred, for reasons unknown, and therefore caution must be exercised in the evaluation of all modalities of therapy for sphincteric (and detrusor) incontinence.

Phenylpropanolamine (PPA) hydrochloride shares the pharmacologic properties as ephedrine and is approximately equal in peripheral potency while causing less central stimulation.[188] It is available in tablets of 25 or 50 mg and in 75-mg timed-release capsules and is a component of numerous proprietary mixtures marketed for the treatment of nasal and sinus congestion (usually in combination with an H_1 antihistamine) or as appetite suppressants. Using doses of 50 mg three times a day, Awad and associates[189] found that 11/13 women and 6/7 men with SUI were significantly improved after 4 weeks of therapy. MUCP increased from a mean of 47 to 72 cm H_2O in patients with an empty bladder and from 43 to 58 cm H_2O in patients with a full bladder. Using a capsule containing 50 mg PPA, 8 mg chlorpheniramine (an antihistamine), and 2 mg isopropamide (an antimuscarinic), Stewart and colleagues[190] found that, of 77 women with SUI, 18 were "completely cured" with one sustained-release capsule; 28 patients were "much better," six were "slightly better," and 25 were "no better." In 11 men with SUI after prostatectomy, the numbers in the corresponding categories were 1, 2, 1, and 7. The formulation of Ornade has now been changed, and each capsule of drug contains 75 mg PPA and 12 mg chlorpheniramine. Collste and Lindskog[191] reported on a group of 24 women with SUI who were treated with PPA or placebo with crossover after 2 weeks. Severity of SUI was graded 1 (slight) or 2 (moderate). Average MUCP overall increased significantly with PPA compared with placebo (from 48 to 55 cm H_2O versus 48 to 49 cm H_2O). This was a significant difference in grade 2 but not in grade 1 patients. The average number of leakage episodes per 48 hours was reduced significantly overall for PPA patients but not for placebo patients (5 to 2 versus 5 to 6). This was significant for grade 1 but not for grade 2 patients. Subjectively, 6 of 24 patients thought that both PPA and placebo were ineffective. Among the 18 patients (of 24) who reported a subjective preference, 14 preferred PPA and 4 preferred placebo. Improvements were rated subjectively as good, moderately good, or slight. Improvements obtained with PPA were significant compared with those for placebo for the entire population and for both groups separately. The AHCPR guidelines[23] reported eight randomized controlled trials with PPA 50 mg twice a day for SUI in women. The percentage cure was listed as ranging from zero to 14%, reduction in incontinence from 19% to 60%, side effects from 5% to 33%, and dropouts from zero to 4.3% (all figures refer to overall percentage minus percentage on placebo).

Some authors have emphasized the potential complications of PPA. Mueller[192] reported on a group of 11 patients who had significant neurologic symptoms (acute headache, psychiatric symptoms, or seizures) after taking "look-alike pills" thought to contain amphetamines but actually containing PPA. Baggioni and associates[193] emphasized the possibility of blood pressure elevation, especially in patients with autonomic impairment. Lasagna[194] pointed out that previously reported blood pressure elevations occurred with a product that differed from American PPA and probably contained a different and much more potent isomer. He noted that, although a huge volume of PPA has been consumed in the form of decongestants and anorectic medications, the world literature has reported only a minimum number of possible toxic reactions, most of which involved excessively high doses in combination medications. Liebson and colleagues[195] found no cardiovascular or subjective adverse effects with doses of 25 mg three times a day or with a 75-mg sustained-release preparation in a population of 150 healthy normal volunteers. Blackburn and colleagues,[196] in a larger series of healthy subjects using many over-the-counter formulations, concluded that a statistically significant but clinically unimportant pressor effect existed during the first 6 hours after administration of PPA and that this was greater with sustained-release preparations. Caution should still be exercised in individuals known to be significantly hypertensive and in elderly patients, in whom pharmacokinetic function may be altered.

Midodrine is a long-acting α-adrenergic agonist that is reported to be useful in the treatment of seminal emission and ejaculation disorders after retroperitoneal lymphadenectomy. Treatment with 5 mg twice a day for 4 weeks in 20 patients with SUI produced a cure in 1 and improvement in 14 patients.[197] The MUCP rose by 8.3%, and the planometric index of the continence area on profilometry increased by 9%. The actions of imipramine have already been discussed. On a theoretical basis, an increase in urethral resistance might be expected if, indeed, an enhanced α-adrenergic effect at this level resulted from an inhibition of noradrenaline reuptake. However, as mentioned previously, imipramine also causes α-adrenergic blocking effects, at least in vascular smooth muscle. Many clinicians have noted improvement in patients treated with imipramine primarily for bladder overactivity but who had in addition some component of sphincteric incontinence. Gilja and colleagues[198] reported a study of 30 women with SUI who were treated with 75 mg imipramine daily for 4 weeks: 21 women subjectively reported continence, and the mean MUCP for the group increased from 34.06 to 48.23 cm H_2O.

Although some clinicians have reported spectacular cure and improvement rates with α-adrenergic agonists and agents that produce an α-adrenergic effect in the outlet of patients with sphincteric urinary incontinence, our own experience coincides with those who report that such treatment often produces satisfactory or some improvement in mild cases but rarely total dryness in patients with severe or even moderate SUI. Nevertheless, a clinical trial, when possible, is certainly worthwhile, especially in conjunction with pelvic floor physiotherapy or biofeedback.

β-Adrenergic Antagonists and Agonists

Theoretically, β-adrenergic blocking agents might be expected to "unmask" or potentiate an α-adrenergic effect, thereby increasing urethral resistance. Gleason and colleagues[199] reported success in treating certain patients with SUI with propranolol, using oral doses of 10 mg four times a day; the beneficial effect became manifest only after 4 to 10 weeks of treatment. Cardiac effects occur rather promptly after administration of this drug, but hypotensive effects do not usually appear as rapidly, although it is difficult to explain such a long delay in onset of the therapeutic effect on incontinence on this basis. Kaisary[200] also reported success with propranolol in the treatment of SUI. Although such treatment has been suggested as an alternative to α-agonists in patients with sphincteric incontinence and hypertension, few, if any, subsequent reports of such efficacy have appeared. Others have reported no significant changes in urethral profile pressures in normal women after β-adrenergic blockade.[201] Although 10 mg four times a day is a relatively small dose of propranolol, it should be recalled that the major potential side effects of the drug are related to the therapeutic β-blocking effects. Heart failure may develop, as well as an increase in airway resistance, and asthma is a contraindication to its use. Abrupt discontinuation may precipitate an exacerbation of anginal attacks and rebound hypertension.[188]

β-Adrenergic stimulation is generally conceded to decrease urethral pressure, but β_2-agonists have been reported to increase the contractility of fast-contracting striated muscle fibers (extensor digitorum longus) from guinea pigs and to suppress that of slow-contracting fibers (soleus).[202] Clenbuterol, a selective β_2-agonist, has been reported to potentiate, in a dose-dependent fashion, the field stimulation-induced contraction in isolated periurethral muscle preparation in the rabbit. The potentiation was greater that that produced by isoprenaline and was suppressed by propranolol. Kishimoto and colleagues[203] reported an increase in urethral pressure with clinical use of clenbuterol and speculated on its promise in the treatment of sphincteric incontinence. Although the differential effects on the smooth and striated musculature of the outlet and even on different fiber types of the striated sphincter may be functionally antagonistic, one should not ignore the possibility of an augmentative effect on outlet resistance by a drug such as clenbuterol under certain physiologic conditions. Other β_2-agonists are salbutamol and terbutaline.

Duloxetine

Duloxetine, a combined serotonin- and norepinephrine-reuptake inhibitor, increases sphincteric muscle activity during the filling and storage phase of micturition in the model of the irritated bladder in the cat. This relatively new pharmacologic agent has been used clinically as an antidepressant.[204] In a study of its effects on the lower urinary tract in the cat, Thor and Katofiasc[205] noted that duloxetine significantly increased bladder capacity (probably through a CNS effect) and also enhanced external urethral sphincter activity with no effect on sphincter activity during voiding.

To date, there have been several randomized controlled studies documenting the effects of duloxetine in the treatment of SUI. Dmochowski and colleagues[206] enrolled 683 patients in a double-blind, placebo-controlled study comparing duloxetine 40 mg twice daily to placebo. There was a significantly greater decrease in incontinence episode frequency in the duloxetine group (50%) compared with the placebo group (27%), as well as improvement in quality of life. The improvements with duloxetine were associated with significant increases in the voiding interval (20 minutes versus 2 minutes) compared to placebo. The discontinuation rate was higher in the duloxetine group (24%) than with placebo (4%), and discontinuation was most frequently due to nausea (6.4%), which was usually transient.

Similar results were reported by Millard[207] and van Keerebroek[208] in investigations of the effects of duloxetine in the treatment of SUI outside the United States. At present time, this medication is not indicated for the treatment of SUI in the United States.

Estrogens

Although estrogens were recommended for the treatment of female urinary incontinence as early as 1941,[201] there is still controversy concerning their use and the benefit-risk ratio for this purpose. Numerous clinical studies exist, but there has been little consistency in methodology, many of the studies have been observational, different formulations of estrogens have been tested, and the data can be conflicting. In some cases, raw data seem to have been ignored in favor of statistics; however, as always, there is no lack of opinions.

Significant work has been done on the effects of estrogenic hormones on the lower urinary tract. Hodgson and associates[209] reported that the sensitivity of the rabbit urethra to α-adrenergic stimulation was estrogen dependent. Levin and coworkers[209,210] showed that parenteral estrogen administration can change the autonomic receptor content and the innervation of the lower urinary tract of immature female rabbits, increasing the response to α-adrenergic, muscarinic, and purinergic stimulation in the bladder body, but not in the base, and significantly increasing the number of α-adrenergic and muscarinic receptors in the bladder body but not in the base. Other work[5] showed a decrease in muscarinic receptor density after estradiol treatment of mature female rabbits and either no change or a decreased detrusor response to cholinergic and electrical stimulation. Levin and coworkers[211] concluded that pregnancy induced an increase in the purinergic and a decrease in the cholinergic responses of the rabbit bladder to field stimulation, and Tong and colleagues[212] reported a decrease in the α-adrenergic response of the mid-part and base of the bladder of pregnant as opposed to virgin rabbits. Larsson and associates[213] reported that estrogen treatment of the isolated female rabbit urethra caused an increased sensitivity to noradrenaline. The mechanism was postulated to be related to a more than twofold increase in the α-adrenergic receptor number. Callahan and Creed[214] reported that pretreatment with estrogen of oophorectomized dogs and wallabies did increase sensitivity of urethral strips to α-adrenergic stimulation, but that this did not occur in the rabbit or guinea pig. Bump and Friedman[215] reported that sex hormone replacement with estrogen, but not testosterone, enhanced the urethral sphincter mechanism in the castrated female baboon by effects that were unrelated to skeletal muscle. They added that these effects might be related not just to changes in the urethral smooth musculature but to changes in the urethral mucosa, submucosal vascular plexus, and connective tissue.

Estrogens have been considered in the treatment for SUI because the urethra has four estrogen-sensitive layers that may play a role in maintaining a positive urethral pressure. These layers are the epithelium, the vasculature, the connective tissue, and the musculature.

Two meta-analyses have shed some light on the use of estrogen therapy in the treatment of SUI. In the first, a report by the Hormones and Urogenital Therapy Committee, the use of estrogens to treat all causes of incontinence in postmenopausal women was examined.[216] Of 166 articles reviewed, there were only 6 controlled and 17 uncontrolled series. Although there was a subjective improvement in UI, when an objective parameter (amount of urine loss) was examined, there was no significant change. Maximum urethral closure pressure was also increased in one study. In a second study, by Sultana and Walters,[217] estrogens were found to be not efficacious in the treatment of SUI. The authors did, however, believe estrogens might be useful in the treatment of urgency and urge incontinence. Estrogen alone may not be effective treatment for urinary incontinence, but in combination with other therapies, both pharmacologic and pelvic floor exercises, it may be more efficacious and useful.

Estrogen therapy certainly seems to be capable of facilitating urinary storage in some postmenopausal women. Whether this effect is related just to changes in the autonomic innervation, receptor content, or function of the smooth muscle or to changes in estrogen-binding sites[218] or in the vascular or connective tissue elements of the urethral wall has not been settled. After menopause, urethral pressure parameters normally decrease slightly[219]; although this change is generally conceded to be related in some way to decreased estrogen levels, it is still largely a matter of speculation whether the actual changes occur in smooth muscle, blood circulation, supporting tissues, or the "mucosal seal mechanism." Versi and associates[220] described a positive correlation between skin collagen content (which does decline with declining estrogen status) and parameters of the urethral pressure profile, suggesting that the estrogen effect on the urethra may be predicted, at least in part, by changes in the collagen component.

Beisland and colleagues[221] carried out a randomized, open, comparative, crossover trial in 20 postmenopausal women with urethral sphincteric insufficiency. Both oral PPA, 50 mg twice a day, and estriol vaginal suppositories, 1 mg daily, significantly increased the MUCP and the continence area on profilometry. PPA was clinically more effective than estriol, but not sufficiently so to obtain complete continence. However, with combined treatment, eight patients became completely continent, nine were considerably improved, and only one remained unchanged. Two patients dropped out of the study because of side effects. Bhatia and colleagues[222] used 2 g of conjugated-estrogen vaginal cream daily for 6 weeks in 11 postmenopausal women with SUI; six were cured or improved significantly. Favorable response was correlated with increased closure pressure and increased pressure transmission. Negative effects from estrogen alone on SUI were reported by Walter and colleagues,[223] Hilton and Stanton[224] and Samsioe and associates;[225] however, in each of these studies, urge symptomatology was favorably affected. In a review article, Cardozo[226] concluded that "there is no conclusive evidence that oestrogen even improves, let alone cures, stress incontinence," although it "apparently alleviates urgency, urge incontinence, frequency, nocturia and dysuria".

Kinn and Lindskog[227] described the results of treatment of 36 postmenopausal women with SUI with oral estriol and PPA, alone or in combination, in a double-blind trial after a 4-week run-in period with PPA. Although some of the data are difficult to interpret, the authors concluded that PPA alone and PPA plus estriol raised the intraurethral pressure and reduced urinary loss by 35% (significant) in a standardized physical strain test. Leakage episodes and amounts were significantly reduced by estriol and PPA given separately (28%) or in combination (40%); the authors found no evidence of a synergistic effect but did indicate that an additive effect was present. Walter and colleagues[228] completed a complicated but logical study of 28 postmenopausal women with SUI (out of 38 original subjects). After 4 weeks of a placebo run-in, patients were randomized to oral estriol or PPA alone for 4 weeks and then to combined therapy for 4 weeks. In the group that sequentially received placebo, PPA, and PPA/estriol, the percentages reporting cure or improvement, respectively, were 0% and 13%, 13% and 20%, and 21% and 14%. In the group receiving placebo, estriol, and estriol/PPA, the corresponding percentages were 0% and 0%, 14% and 29%, and 64% and 7%. Objective parameters showed the following: the number of leak episodes per 24 hours in patients treated with PPA first showed a 31% decrease (from ~3 to 2) compared with placebo ($P < .003$). For those treated with estriol first, the change was not significant (~1.5 to 0.8). Combined treatment produced a mean decrease of 48% compared with placebo. There was a greater effect with estriol/PPA than with PPA/estriol. Pad weights (in grams in a 1-hour test) decreased significantly with PPA alone (~27 to 6 g), but there was no difference between PPA and PPA/estriol. Estriol alone significantly decreased pad weights (~47 to 15 g). Although estriol/PPA was not significantly different, there was further numerical loss, from ~15 to 3 g. The overall conclusions were that estriol and PPA are each effective in treating SUI in postmenopausal women and that, on the basis of the subjective data, combined therapy is better than either drug alone. This conclusion was substantiated by a significant decrease in the number of leak episodes among those patients to whom estriol was given before PPA but was not confirmed statistically by pad-weighing tests.

Confusing the data on the potential benefits of estrogen is a recent study by Hendrix and collegues.[229] They reviewed data from 27,347 postmenopausal women participating in the Women's Health Initiative, which was a double blind, randomized, placebo-controlled study of menopausal hormone therapy, to assess the effects of hormonal therapy on stress, urge, and mixed incontinence. Depending on the presence of absence of a uterus, patients were treated with placebo, 0.625 mg/day of conjugated equine estrogen (CEE), or a combination of 0.625 mg/day CEE and 2.5mg/day of medroxyprogesterone acetate (MPA). They evaluated 23,296 women whose urinary incontinence symptoms were known. They found that menopausal hormonal therapy increased all types of urinary incontinence, with SUI being the most common, in women who were continent at baseline after 1 year of use. For those women with urinary incontinence at baseline, frequency worsened with both CEE alone and the combination of CEE and MPA.

Sessions and associates[230] reviewed the benefits and risks of estrogen-replacement therapy. Improvements in vasomotor symptomatology and osteoporosis prevention are well established. There is also substantial evidence of a decreased risk of cardiovascular disease, perhaps because of an effect on the lipid profile. There is little question, however, that unopposed estrogen use in those with an intact uterus increases the risk of endometrial cancer. Progestogen treatment exerts a protective effect, and daily administration of an estrogen and a progestogen provides an attractive alternative because of a lack of withdrawal bleeding (with sequential therapy) and consequent increased patient compliance. Whether progestogen administration adversely affects the results of estrogen treatment of SUI is unknown but must be considered. Progestogens may also cause mastalgia, edema, and bloating. It is concluded, further, that there is no evidence for an increase in thromboembolism or hypertension with estrogen replacement. Transdermal administration of estrogen avoids any theoretical problems associated with the first-pass effect through the liver with oral administration (alteration in clotting factors and increase in renin substrate). The evidence does suggest an association between breast cancer and estrogen replacement therapy, but only for those who have received such therapy for more than 15 years. A preventive role of progestogens in this regard is controversial, as is the dose of estrogen necessary to produce this effect. Grodstein and colleagues[231] looked at the relationship between long-term postmenopausal hormonal replacement therapy and overall mortality in a cohort of nurses over an 18-year period. Although they noted an overall lower risk of death (relative risk, 0.63) for active estrogen users compared with subjects who had never taken hormones, the apparent benefit decreased somewhat (relative risk 0.80) after 10 years of therapy owing to an increased mortality from breast cancer in the hormone-treated group.

As to the type of estrogen preparation preferred, transdermal administration seems to be as effective as oral, and subcutaneous implants appear to produce physiologic serum levels. Percutaneous and intramuscular estrogen seem to produce variable serum levels. Vaginal creams are said to produce variable serum levels but physiologic estradiol/estrone ratios.[230] We agree that "hands on" application to the "affected area" may have a psychological benefit as well, as suggested by Murray.[232] A unique new method for delivering vaginal estrogen involves a silicone ring with an estradiol-loaded core containing 2 mg of 17β-estradiol inserted into the vagina by the patient or the physician. A low, constant dose (5 to 10 g/24 hr) is delivered over a period of 90 days. This mode of administration not only is more acceptable to certain women[233] but also offers a more continuous delivery of estrogen to the affected tissues.[234]

CIRCUMVENTING THE PROBLEM

Antidiuretic Hormone–Like Agents

The synthetic antidiuretic hormone (ADH) peptide analogue desmopressin acetate (DDAVP; 1-desamino-8-D-arginine vasopressin) has been used for the symptomatic relief of refractory nocturnal enuresis in both children and adults.[232,235] The drug can be administered conveniently by intranasal spray at bedtime (in a dose of 10 to 40 μg) and effectively suppresses urine production for 7 to 10 hours. Its clinical long-term safety has been established by continued use in patients with diabetes insipidus. Normal water-deprivation tests, as described by Rew and Rundle,[236] indicate that long-term use does not cause depression of endogenous ADH secretion, at least in patients with nocturnal enuresis. Changes in diuresis during 2 months of treatment in an elderly group of 6 men and 12 women with increased nocturia and decreased ADH secretion were reported by Asplund and Oberg.[237] Nocturia decreased 20% (in milliliters) in men and 34% in women; the number of voids between 20:00 to 08:00 hours decreased from 4.5 to 4.3 in men and from 3.5 to 2.8 in women, but the drug was not given until 20:00 hours. At present, this novel circumventive approach to the treatment of urinary frequency and incontinence has been largely restricted to those with nocturnal enuresis and diabetes insipidus. The fact that the drug seems to be much more effective than simple fluid restriction alone for the former condition is perhaps explained by relatively recent reports suggesting a decreased nocturnal secretion of ADH by such patients.[235] Recently, suggestions have been made that desmopressin might be useful in patients with refractory nocturnal frequency and incontinence who do not belong in the category of primary nocturnal enuresis. Kinn and Larsson[238] reported that micturition frequency "decreased significantly" in 13 patients with multiple sclerosis and urge incontinence who were treated with oral tablets of desmopressin and that less leakage occurred. The actual approximate average change in the number of voids during the 6 hours after drug intake was from 3.2 to 2.5.

A similar circumventive approach is to give a rapidly acting loop diuretic 4 to 6 hours before bedtime. This, of course, assumes that the nocturia is not caused by obstructive uropathy. A randomized, double-blind, crossover study of this approach using bumetanide in a group of 14 general practice patients was reported by Pedersen and Johansen.[239] Control nocturia episodes per week averaged 17.5; with placebo, this decreased to 12, and with bumetanide to 8. Bumetanide was preferred to placebo by 11 of 14 patients.

CONCLUSIONS

There are more pharmacologic therapies available for the treatment of urinary incontinence in women than ever before. The treatments available are limited by their efficacy and their side effects. Continued investigation and a greater understanding of the pathophysiology of urinary incontinence will certainly lead to improvements in treatment of this highly prevalent condition.

References

1. Wein AJ, Levin RM, Barrett DM: Voiding function: Relevant anatomy, physiology, and pharmacology. In Duckett JW, Howards ST, Grayhack JT, Gillenwater JY (eds): Adult and Pediatric Urology, 2nd ed. St Louis, Mosby Year Book, 1991, pp 933-999.
2. Wein AJ, Van Arsdalen KN, Levin RM: Pharmacologic therapy. In Krane RJ, Siroky MB (eds): Clinical Neuro-Urology. Boston, Little Brown, 1991, pp 523-558.
3. Steers WD: Physiology of the urinary bladder. In Walsh PC, Retik AB, Stamey TA, Vaughan ED (eds): Campbell's Urology, 6th ed. Philadelphia, Saunders, 1992, pp 142-169.
4. de Groat WC: Anatomy and physiology of the lower urinary tract. Urol Clin North Am 20:383, 1993.
5. Andersson KE: Pharmacology of lower urinary tract smooth muscles and penile erectile tissues. Pharmacol Rev 45:253, 1993.
6. Jensen D Jr: Pharmacological studies of the uninhibited neurogenic bladder. Acta Neurol Scand 64:145, 1981.
7. Blaivas J, Labib K, Michalik S, et al: Cystometric response to propantheline in detrusor hyperreflexia: Therapeutic implications. J Urol 124:259, 1980.
8. Andersson KE: Current concepts in the treatment of disorders of micturition. Drugs 35:477, 1988.
9. McGuire E, Savastano J: Effect of alpha adrenergic blockade and anticholinergic agents on the decentralized primate bladder. Neurourol Urodyn 4:139, 1985.
10. Andersson KE, Ek A, Hedlund H: Effects of prazosin in isolated human urethra and in patients with lower neuron lesions. Invest Urol 19:3911, 1981.
11. Brading A: Physiology of bladder smooth muscle. In Torrens M, Morrison JFB (eds): The Physiology of the Lower Urinary Tract. New York, Springer Verlag, 1987, pp 161-192.
12. Brading AF: Physiology of the urinary tract smooth muscle. In Webster G, Kirby R, King L, Goldwasser B (eds): Reconstructive Urology. Boston, Blackwell Scientific, 1987, pp 15-26.
13. Bonner TI: The molecular basis of muscarinic receptor diversity. Trends Neurosci 12:148, 1989.
14. Poli E, Monica B, Zappia L, et al: Antimuscarinic activity of telemyepine on isolated human urinary bladder: No role for M-1 receptors. Gen Pharmacol 23:659, 1992.
15. Eglen RM, Watson N: Selective muscarinic receptor agonists and antagonists. Pharmacol Toxicol 78:59, 1996.
16. Levin RM, Ruggieri MR, Wein AJ: Identification of receptor subtypes in the rabbit and human urinary bladder by selective radio-ligand binding. J Urol 139:844, 1988.
17. Levin RM, Ruggieri MR, Lee W, et al: Effect of chronic atropine administration on the rat urinary bladder. J Urol 139:1347, 1988.
18. Nilvebrant L, Andersson KE, Gillberg PG, et al: Tolterodine: A new bladder-selective antimuscarinic agent. Eur J Pharmacol 327:195, 1997.
19. Tobin G, Sjögren C: In vivo and in vitro effects of muscarinic receptor antagonists on contractions and release of [^{3}H] acetylcholine release in the rabbit urinary bladder. Eur J Pharmacol 281:1, 1995.
20. Levin RM, Staskin D, Wein AJ: The muscarinic cholinergic binding kinetics of the human urinary bladder. Neurourol Urodyn 1:221, 1982.
21. Peterson JS, Patton AJ, Noronha-Blob L: Mini-pig urinary bladder function: Comparisons of in vitro anticholinergic responses and in vivo cystometry with drugs indicated for urinary incontinence. J Auton Pharmacol 10:65, 1990.
22. Zorzitto ML, Jewett MA, Fernie GR, et al: Effectiveness of propantheline bromide in the treatment of geriatric patients with detrusor instability. Neurourol Urodyn 5:133, 1986.
23. Urinary Incontinence Guideline Panel: Urinary Incontinence in Adults: Clinical Practice Guidelines (AHCPR Pub. No. 92-0038). Rockville, MD: Agency for Health Care Policy and Research, Public

Health Service, U.S. Department of Health and Human Services, March, 1992.
24. Brown JH: Atropine, scopolamine and related antimuscarinic drugs. In Gilman AG, Rall TW, Nies AS, Taylor P (eds): Goodman and Gilman's The Pharmacological Basis of Therapeutics, 8th ed. New York, Pergamon Press, 1990, pp 150-165.
25. Weiner LB, Baum NH, Suarez GM: New method for management of detrusor instability: Transdermal scopolamine. Urology 28:208, 1986.
26. Cornella JL, Bent AE, Ostergard DR, et al: Prospective study utilizing transdermal scopolamine in detrusor instability. Urology 35:96, 1990.
27. Muskat Y, Bukovsky I, Schneider D, et al: The use of scopolamine in the treatment of detrusor instability. J Urology 156:1989, 1996.
28. Greenstein A, Chen J, Matzkin H: Transdermal scopolamine in prevention of post open prostatectomy bladder contractions Urology 39:215, 1992.
29. Lau W, Szilagyi M: A pharmacological profile of glycopyrrolate: Interactions at the muscarinic acetylcholine receptor. Gen Pharmacol 23:1165, 1992.
30. Nilvebrant L, Gillberg PG, Sparf B: Antimuscarinic potency and bladder selectivity of PNU-200577, a major metabolite of tolterodine. Pharmacol Toxicol 81:169, 1997.
31. Nilvebrant L, Hallen B, Larsson G: A new bladder selective muscarinic receptor antagonist: Preclinical pharmacological and clinical data. Life Sci 60:1129, 1997.
32. Nilvebrant L, Sundquist S, Gillberg PG: Tolterodine is not subtype (m1-m5) selective but exhibits functional bladder selectivity in vivo. Neurourol Urodyn 15:310, 1996.
33. Nilvebrant L, Glas G, Jonsson A, et al: The in vitro pharmacological profile of tolterodine: A new agent for the treatment of urinary urge incontinence. Neurourol Urodyn 13:433, 1994.
34. Stahl MM, Ekstrom B, Sparf B, et al: Urodynamic and other effects of tolterodine: A novel antimuscarinic drug for the treatment of detrusor overactivity. Neurourol Urodyn 14:647, 1995.
35. Jonas U, Hofner K, Madersbacher H, et al: Efficacy and safety of two doses of tolterodine versus placebo in patients with detrusor overactivity and symptoms of frequency, urge incontinence, and urgency: Urodynamic evaluation. The International Study Group. World J Urol 15:144, 1997.
36. Yarker YE, Goa KL, Fitton A: Oxybutynin: A review of its pharmacodynamic and pharmacokinetic properties, and its therapeutic use in detrusor instability. Drugs Aging 6:243, 1995.
37. Rentzhog L, Stanton SL, Cardozo L, et al: Efficacy and safety of tolterodine in patients with detrusor instability: A dose-ranging study. Br J Urol 81:42, 1998.
38. Hills CJ, Winter SA, Balfour JA: Tolterodine. Drugs 55:813, 1998.
39. Clemett D, Jarvis B: Tolterodine: A review of its use in the treatment of overactive bladder. Drugs Aging 18:277, 2001.
40. Appell RA, Sand P, Dmochowski R, et al: Overactive Bladder: Judging Effective Control and Treatment Study Group. Prospective randomized controlled trial of extended-release oxybutynin chloride and tolterodine tartrate in the treatment of overactive bladder: Results of the OBJECT Study. Mayo Clin Proc 76:358, 2001.
41. Diokno AC, Appell RA, Sand PK, et al: OPERA Study Group. Prospective, randomized double-blind study of the efficacy and tolerability of the extended-release formulations of oxybutynin and tolterodine for overactive bladder: Results of the OPERA trial. Mayo Clin Proc 78:687, 2003.
42. Sussman D, Garely A: Treatmenet of overactive bladder with once-daily extended-release tolterodine or oxybutynin: The Antimuscarinic Clinical Effectiveness Trial (ACET). Curr Med Res Opin 18:177, 2002.
43. Zinner NR, Mattiasson A, Stanton SL: Efficacy, safety, and tolerability of extended-release once-daily tolterodine treatment for overactive bladder in older versus younger patients. J Am Geriatr Soc 50:799, 2002.
44. Freeman R, Hill S, Millard R, et al: Reduced perception of urgency in treatment of overactive bladder with extended-releas tolterodine. Obstet Gynecol 102:605, 2003.
45. Haab F, Stewart L, Dwyer P: Darifenacin, an M3 selective receptor antagonist, is an effective and well-tolerated once-daily treatment for overactive bladder. Eur Urol 45:420, 2004.
46. Chapple CR: Darifenacin is well tolerated and provides significant improvement in the symptoms of overactive bladder: A pooled analysis of phase III studies [abstract 487]. J Urol 171(Suppl):130, 2004.
47. Cardozo L, Prescott K, Serdarevic D, et al: Can medication prolong warning time? [abstract 74]. Neurourol Urodyn 22:468, 2003.
48. Chapple CR, Arano P, Bosch JL, et al: Solifenacin appears effective and well tolerated in patients with symptomatic idiopathic detrusor overactivity in placebo- and tolterodine-controlled phase 2 dose-finding study. BJU Int 93:71, 2004.
49. Smith N, Grimes I, Ridge S, et al: YM905 is effective and safe as treatment of overactive bladder in women and men: Results from phase II study [abstract 222]. ICS Proc 138, 2002.
50. Chapple CR, Techberger T, Al-Shukri S, et al: Randomized, double-blind, placebo- and tolterodine-controlled trial of the once-daily antimuscarinic agent solifenacin in patients with symptomatic overactive bladder. BJU Int 93:303, 2004.
51. Cardozo L: Solifenacin succinate improves symptoms of an overactive bladder. Int Urogynecol J Pelvic Floor Dysfunct 14(Suppl):S64, 2003.
52. Gittleman MC, Kaufman J: Solifenacin succinate 10 mg once daily significantly improved symptoms of overactive bladder. Int J Gynecol Obstet 83(Suppl 3), 2003.
53. Thompson I, Lauvetz R: Oxybutynin in bladder spasm, neurogenic bladder and enuresis. Urology 8:452, 1976.
54. Moisey C, Stephenson T, Brendler C: The urodynamic and subjective results of treatment of detrusor instability with oxybutynin chloride. Br J Urol 52:472, 1980.
55. Hehir M, Fitzpatrick JM: Oxybutynin and the prevention of urinary incontinence in spinal bifida. Eur Urol 11:254, 1985.
56. Gajewski J, Awad JA: Oxybutynin versus propantheline in patients with multiple sclerosis and detrusor hyperreflexia. J Urol 135:966, 1986.
57. Holmes DM, Montz FJ, Stanton SL: Oxybutynin versus propantheline in the management of detrusor instability: A patient-regulated variable dose trial. Br J Obstet Gynaecol 96:607-612, 1989.
58. Thuroff J, Bunke B, Ebner A, et al: Randomized double-blind multicenter trial on treatment of frequency, urgency and incontinence related to detrusor hyperactivity: Oxybutynin vs. propantheline vs. placebo. J Urol 145:813, 1991.
59. Zeegers A, Kiesswetter H, Kramer A, et al: Conservative therapy of frequency, urgency and urge incontinence: A double-blind clinical trial of flavoxate, oxybutynin, emepronium and placebo. World J Urol 5:57, 1987.
60. Van Doorn ESC, Zweirs W: Ambulant monitoring to assess the efficacy of oxybutynin chloride in patients with mixed incontinence. Eur Urol 18:49, 1990.
61. Zorzitto ML, Holliday PJ, Jewett MA: Oxybutynin chloride for geriatric urinary dysfunction: A double-blind placebo controlled study. Age Ageing 18:195, 1989.
62. Ouslander JG, Blaustein J, Connor H: Habit training and oxybutynin for incontinence in nursing home patients: A placebo-controlled trial. J Am Geriatr Soc 36:40, 1988.
63. Ouslander JG, Blaustein J, Connor H: Pharmacokinetics and clinical effects of oxybutynin in geriatric patients. J Urol 140:47, 1988.
64. Gupta SK, Sathyan G. Pharmacokinetics of an oral once-a-day controlled-release oxybutynin formulation compared with immediate-release oxybutynin. J Clin Pharmacol 39:289, 1999.
65. Anderson R, Mobley D, Blank B, et al: Once daily controlled versus immediate release oxybutynin chloride for urge urinary incontinence. J Urol 161:1809, 1999.

66. Gleason DM, Susset J, White C, et al., and the Ditropan XL Study Group: Evaluation of a new once daily formulation of oxybutynin for the treatment of urinary urge incontinence. Urology 54:420, 1999.
67. Kato K, Kitada S, Chun A, et al: In vitro intravesical instillation of anticholinergic, antispasmodic and calcium blocking agents (rabbit whole bladder model). J Urol 141:1471, 1989.
68. Mizunaga M, Miyata M, Kaneko S, et al: Intravesical instillation of oxybutynin hydrochloride therapy for patients with a neuropathic bladder. Paraplegia 32:25, 1994.
69. Connor JP, Betrus G, Fleming P, et al: Early cystometrograms can predict the response to intravesical instillation of oxybutynin chloride in myelomeningocele patients. J Urol 151:1045, 1994.
70. Szollar SM, Lee SM: Intravesical oxybutynin for spinal cord injury patients. Spinal Cord 34:284, 1996.
71. Madersbacher H, Jilg G: Control of detrusor hyperreflexia by the intravesical instillation of oxybutynin hydrochloride. Paraplegia 19:84, 1991.
72. Madersbacher H, Knoll M: Intravesical application of oxybutynin: Mode of action in controlling detrusor hyperreflexia. Eur Urol 8:340, 1995.
73. Weese DL, Roskamp DA, Leach GE, et al: Intravesical oxybutynin chloride: Experience with 42 patients. Urology 41:527, 1993.
74. Enzelsberger H, Helmer H, Kurz C:. Intravesical instillation of oxybutynin in women with idiopathic detrusor instability: A randomised trial. Br J Obstet Gynaecol 102:929, 1995.
75. Dmochowski RR, Davila GW, Zinner NR, et al: Efficacy and safety of transdermal oxybutynin in patients with urge and mixed urinary incontinence. J Urol 168:580, 2002.
76. Davila GW, Daugherty CA Sanders SW: A short-term, multicenter, randomized double-blind dose titration study of the efficacy and anticholinergic side effects of transdermal compared to immediate release oral oxybutynin treatment of patients with urge urinary incontinence. J Urol 166:140, 2001.
77. Dmochowski RR, Sand PK, Zinner NR, et al: Comparative efficacy and safety of transdermal oxybutynin and oral tolterodine versus placebo in previously treated patients with urge and mixed urinary incontinence. Urology 62:237, 2003.
78. Downie J, Twiddy D, Awad SA: Antimuscarininc and noncompetitive antagonist properties of dicyclomine hydrochloride in isolated human and rabbit bladder muscle. J Pharmacol Exp Ther 201:662, 1977.
79. Fischer C, Diokno A, Lapides J: The anticholinergic effects of dicyclomine hydrochloride in inhibited neurogenic bladder dysfunction. J Urol 120:328, 1978.
80. Beck RP, Anausch T, King C: Results in testing 210 patients with detrusor overactivity incontinence of urine. Am J Obstet Gynecol 125:593, 1976.
81. Glickman S, Tsokkos N, Shah PJ: Intravesical atropine and suppression of detrusor hypercontractility in the neuropathic bladder: A preliminary study. Paraplegia 33:36, 1995.
82. Awad SA, Bryniak S, Downie JW, et al: The treatment of the uninhibited bladder with dicyclomine. J Urol 114:161, 1977.
83. Ruffman R: A review of flavoxate hydrochloride in the treatment of urge incontinence. J Int Med Res 16:317, 1988.
84. Kimura Y, Sasaki Y, Hamada K, et al: Mechanisms of suppression of the bladder activity by flavoxate. Int J Urol 3:218, 1996.
85. Milani R, Scalambrino S, Milia R, et al: Double-blind crossover comparison of flavoxate and oxybutynin in women affected by urinary urge syndrome. Int Urogynecol J 4:3, 1993.
86. Briggs RS, Castleden CM, Asher MJ: The effect of flavoxate on uninhibited detrusor contractions and urinary incontinence in the elderly. J Urol 123:656, 1980.
87. Benson GS, Sarshik SA, Raezer DM, et al: Bladder muscle contractility: Comparative effects and mechanisms of action of atropine, propantheline, flavoxate and imipramine. Urology 9:31, 1977.
88. Fusgen I, Hauri D: Trospium chloride: An effective option for medical treatment of bladder overactivity. Int J Clin Pharmacol Ther 38:223, 2000.
89. Todorova A, Vonderheid-Guth B, Dimpfel W: Effects of tolterodine, trospium chloride, and oxybutynin on the central nervous system. J Clin Pharmacol 41:636, 2001.
90. Wiedemann A, Fusgen I, Hauri D: New aspects of therapy with trospium chloride for urge incontinence. Eur J Geriatr 3:41, 2002.
91. Stohrer M, Bauer P, Giannetti BM, et al: Effect of trospium chloride on urodynamic parameters in patients with detrusor hyperreflexia due to spinal cord injuries: A multicentre placebo controlled double-blind trial. Urol Int 47:138, 1991.
92. Madersbacher H, Stohrer M, Richter R, et al: Trospium chloride versus oxybutynin: A randomized, double-blind, multicentre trial in the treatment of detrusor hyperreflexia. Br J Urol 75:452, 1995.
93. Allouis S, Laval KU, Eckert R: Trospium chloride (Spasmo-Lyt) in patients with motor urge syndrome (detrusor instability): A double-blind, randomised, multicentre, placebo-controlled study. J Clin Res 1:439, 1998.
94. Cardozo L, Chapple CR, Toozs-Hobson P, et al: Efficacy of trospium chloride in patients with detrusor instability: A placebo-controlled, randomized, double-blind, multicentre clinical trial. BJU Int 85:659, 2000.
95. Junemann KP, Al-Shukri S: Efficacy and tolerability of trospium chloride and tolterodine in 234 patients with urge-syndrome: A double-blind, placebo-controlled multicentre clinical trial. Neurourol Urodyn 19:484, 2000.
96. Halaska M, Ralph G, Wiedemann A, et al: Controlled, double-blind, multicentre clinical trial to investigate long-term tolerability and efficacy of trospium chloride in patients with detrusor instability. World J Urol 20:392, 2003.
97. Zinner N, Gittelman M, Harris R, et al: Trospium chloride improves overactive bladder symptoms: A multicenter phase III trial. J Urol 171:2311, 2004.
98. Rudy D, Cline K, Goldberg K, et al: A multicenter, randomized, placebo-controlled trial of trospium chloride in overactive bladder patients. Neurourol Urodyn 23:600, 2004.
99. Madersbacher H, Murz G. Efficacy, tolerability and safety profile of propiverine in the treatment of the overactive bladder (non-neurogenic and neurogenic). World J Urol 19:324, 2001.
100. Thuroff JW, Chartier-Kastler E, Corcus J, et al: Medical treatment and medical side effects in urinary incontinence in the elderly. World J Urol 16(Suppl):S48, 1998.
101. Stohrer M, Madersbacher H, Richter R, et al: Efficacy and safety of propiverine in SCI patients suffering from detrusor hyperreflexia: A double blind, placebo-controlled clinical trial. Spinal Cord 37:196, 1999.
102. Wehnert J, Sage S: Comparative investigations to the action of Mictonorm (propiverine hydrochloride) and Spasuret (flavoxate hydrochloride) on detrusor veiscae. Z Urol Nephrol 82:259, 1989.
103. Madersbacher H, Halaska M, Voigt R, et al: A placebo-controlled, multicentre study comparing the tolerability and efficacy of propiverine and oxybutynin in patient with urgency and urge incontinence. BJU Int 84:646, 1999.
104. Dorschner W, Stolzenburg JU, Griebenow R, et al: Efficacy and cardiac safety of propiverine in elderly patients: A double-blind, placebo-controlled clinical study. Eur Urol 37:702, 2000.
105. Forman A, Andersson K, Henriksson L, et al: Effects of nifedipine on the smooth muscle of the human urinary tract in vitro and in vivo. Acta Pharmacol Toxicol 43:111, 1978.
106. Husted S, Andersson KE, Sommer L: Anticholinergic and calcium antagonistic effects of terodiline in rabbit urinary bladder. Acta Pharmacol Toxicol 46:20, 1980.
107. Finkbeiner AE: Effect of extracellular calcium and calcium-blocking agents on detrusor contractility: An in vitro study. Neurourol Urodyn 2:245, 1983.
108. Malkowicz SB, Wein AJ, Brendler K, et al: Effect of diltiazem on in vitro rabbit bladder function. Pharmacology 31:24, 1985.

109. Andersson KE, Fovaeus M, Morgan E, et al: Comparative effects of five different calcium channel blockers on the atropine-resistant contraction in electrically stimulated rabbit urinary bladder. Neurourol Urodyn 5:579, 1986.
110. Abrams P: Terodiline in clinical practice. Urology 36(Suppl):60, 1990.
111. Ekman G, Andersson KE, Rud T, et al: A double-blind crossover study of the effects of terodiline in women with unstable bladder. Acta Pharmacol Toxicol 46(Suppl):39, 1980.
112. Peters D: Multicentre Study Group. Terodiline in the treatment of urinary frequency and motor urge incontinence: A controlled multicentre trial. Scand J Urol Nephrol 87(Suppl):21, 1984.
113. Tapp A, Fall M, Norgaard J, et al: Terodiline: A dose titrated, multicenter study of the treatment of idiopathic detrusor instability in women. J Urol 142:1027, 1989.
114. Levin RM, Scheiner S, Zhao Y, et al: The effect of terodiline on hyperreflexia (in vitro) and the in vitro response of isolated strips of rabbit bladder to field stimulation, bethanechol and KCI. Pharmacology 46:346, 1993.
115. Palmer J, Worth P, Exton-Smith A: Flunarizine: A once daily therapy for urinary incontinence. Lancet 2:279, 1981.
116. Veldhuis G, Inman J: Terodiline and torsades de pointes [letter to the editor]. BMJ 303:519, 1991.
117. Connolly MJ, Astridge PS, White EG, et al: Torsades de pointes ventricular tachycardia and terodiline. Lancet 338:344, 1991.
118. Stewart DA, Taylor J, Ghosh S, et al: Terodiline causes polymorphic ventricular tachycardia due to reduced heart rate and prolongation of QT interval. Eur J Clin Pharmacol 42:577, 1992.
119. Andersson KE: Clinical pharmacology of potassium channel openers. Pharmacol Toxicol 70:244, 1992.
120. Malmgren A, Andersson K, Andersson PO, et al: Effects of cromakalim (BRL 34915) and pinacidil on normal and hypertrophied rat detrusor in vitro. J Urol 143:828, 1990.
121. Fovaeus M, Andersson KE, Hedlund H: The action of pinacidil in isolated human bladder. J Urol 141:637, 1989.
122. Hedlund H, Mattiasson A, Andersson KE: Lack of effect of pinacidil on detrusor instability in men with bladder outlet obstruction. J Urol 143:369A, 1990.
123. Nurse DE, Restorick JM, Mundy AR: The effect of cromakalim on the normal and hyper-reflexic human detrusor muscle. Br J Urol 68:27, 1991.
124. Komersova K, Rogerson JW, Conway EL, et al: The effect of Levcromokalim (BRL 38227) on bladder function in patients with high spinal cord lesions. Br J Clin Pharmacol 39:207, 1995.
125. Longman SD, Hamilton TC: Potassium channel activator drugs: Mechanism of action, pharmacological properties, and therapeutic potential. Med Res Rev 12:73, 1992.
126. Downie JW, Karmazyn M: Mechanical trauma to bladder epithelium liberates prostanoids which modulate neurotransmission in rabbit detrusor muscle. J Pharmacol Exp Ther 230:445, 1984.
127. Cardozo LD, Stanton SL, Robinson H, et al: Evaluation of flurbiprofen in detrusor instability. BMJ 2:281, 1980.
128. Cardozo L, Stanton SL: An objective comparison of the effects of parenterally administered drugs in patients suffering from detrusor instability. J Urol 122:58, 1979.
129. Brooks PM, Day RO: Non-steroidal anti-inflammatory drugs: Differences and similarities. N Engl J Med 324:1716, 1991.
130. Norlen L, Sundin T, Waagstein F: Beta-adrenoceptor stimulation of the human urinary bladder in vivo. Acta Pharmacol Toxicol 43:5, 1978.
131. Lindholm P, Lose G: Terbutaline (Bricanyl) in the treatment of female urge incontinence. Urol Int 41:158, 1986.
132. Gruneberger A: Treatment of motor urge incontinence with clenbuterol and flavoxate hydrochloride. Br J Obstet Gynaecol 91:275, 1984.
133. Castleden CM, Morgan B: The effect of beta adrenoceptor agonists on urinary incontinence in the elderly. Br J Clin Pharmacol 10:619, 1980.
134. Naglo AS, Nergardh A, Boreus LO: Influence of atropine and isoprenoline on detrusor hyperactivity in children with neurogenic bladder. Scand J Urol Nephrol 15:97, 1989.
135. Baldesarini RJ: Drugs and the treatment of psychiatric disorders. In Gilman AG, Rall TW, Nies AS, Taylor P (eds): Goodman and Gilman's The Pharmacological Basis of Therapeutics, 8th ed. New York, Pergamon Press, 1990, pp 383-435.
136. Hollister LE: Current antidepressants. Annu Rev Pharmacol Toxicol 26:23, 1986.
137. Richelson E: Antidepressants and brain neurochemistry. Mayo Clin Proc 65:1227, 1990.
138. Olubadewo J: The effect of imipramine on rat detrusor muscle contractility. Arch Int Pharmacodyn Ther 145:84, 1980.
139. Levin RM, Staskin D, Wein AJ: Analysis of the anticholinergic and musculotropic effects of desmethylimipramine on the rabbit urinary bladder. Urol Res 11:259, 1983.
140. Levin RM, Wein AJ: Comparative effects of five tricyclic compounds on the rabbit urinary bladder. Neurourol Urodyn 3:127, 1984.
141. Delaere KJP, Michiels HGE, Debruyne FMJ, et al: Flavoxate hydrochloride in the treatment of detrusor instability. Urol Int 32:377, 1977.
142. Bigger J, Giardino E, Perel JE: Cardiac antiarrhythmic effect of imipramine hydrochloride. N Engl J Med 296:206, 1977.
143. Akah PA: Tricyclic antidepressant inhibition of the electrical evoked responses of the rat urinary bladder strip: Effect of variation in extracellular Ca concentration. Arch Int Pharmacodyn 284:231, 1986.
144. Foreman MM, McNulty AM: Alterations in K(+)-evoked release of 3-H-norepinephrine and contractile responses in urethral and bladder tissues induced by norepinephrine reuptake inhibition. Life Sci 53:193, 1993.
145. Cole A, Fried F: Favorable experiences with imipramine in the treatment of neurogenic bladder. J Urol 107:44, 1972.
146. Raezer DM, Benson GS, Wein AJ: The functional approach to the management of the pediatric neuropathic bladder: A clinical study. J Urol 117:649, 1977.
147. Tulloch AGS, Creed KE: A comparison between propantheline and imipramine on bladder and salivary gland function. Br J Urol 125:218, 1981.
148. Castleden CM, George CF, Renwick AG, et al: Imipramine: A possible alternative to current therapy for urinary incontinence in elderly. J Urol 125:218, 1981.
149. Korczyn AD, Kish I: The mechanism of imipramine in enuresis nocturna. Clin Exp Pharmacol Physiol 6:31, 1979.
150. Lose G, Jorgensen L, Thunedborg P: Doxepin in the treatment of female detrusor overactivity: A randomized double-blind crossover study. J Urol 142:1024, 1989.
151. Schurch B: Botulinum-A toxin for treating detrusor hyper-reflexia in spinal cord injured patients: A new alternative to anticholinergic drugs? Preliminary results. J Urol 164:692, 2000.
152. Reitz A, Stohrer M, Kramer G: European experience of 200 cases treated with botulinum-A toxin injection into the detrusor muscle for urinary incontinence due to neurogenic detrusor overactivity. Eur Urol 45:510, 2004.
153. Rapp D, Lucioni A, Katz E: Use of botulinum-A toxin for the treatment of refractory overactive bladder symptoms an initial experience. Urology 63:1071, 2004.
154. Dykstra D, Enriquez A, Valley M: Treatment of overactive bladder with botulinum toxin type B: A pilot study. Int Urogynecol J Pelvic Floor Dysfunct 14:424, 2003.
155. Sant GR: Intravesical 50% dimethyl sulfoxide (Rimso-50) in treatment of interstitial cystitis. Urology 4(Suppl):17, 1987.
156. Kiesswetter H, Schober W: Lioresal in the treatment of neurogenic bladder dysfunction. Urol Int 30:63, 1975.
157. Taylor MC, Bates CP: A double-blind crossover trial of baclofen: A new treatment for the unstable bladder syndrome. Br J Urol 51:505, 1979.

158. James MJ, Birmingham AT, Hill SJ: Partial mediation by nitric oxide of the relaxation of human isolated detrusor strips in response to electrical field stimulation. Br J Clin Pharmacol 35:366, 1993.
159. Soulard C, Pascaud X, Roman FJ, et al: Pharmacological evaluation of JO-1870—Relation to the potential treatment of urinary bladder incontinence. J Pharmacol Exp Ther 260:1152, 1992.
160. Constantinou CE: Pharmacologic treatment of detrusor incontinence with thiphenamil HCl. Urol Int 48:42, 1992.
161. Constantinou CE: Pharmacologic effect of thiphenamil HCl on lower urinary tract function of healthy asymptomatic volunteers. Urol Int 48:293, 1992.
162. Maggi CA, Barbanti G, Santicioli P, et al: Cystometric evidence that capsaicin-sensitive nerves modulate the afferent branch of micturition reflex in humans. J Urol 142:150, 1989.
163. Maggi CA: Capsaicin and primary afferent neurons: From basic science to human therapy? J Auton Nerv Syst 33:1, 1991.
164. Maggi CA: Therapeutic potential of capsaicin-like molecules: Studies in animals and humans. Life Sci 51:1777, 1992.
165. Dray A: Mechanism of action of capsaicin-like molecules on sensory neurons. Life Sci 51:1759, 1993.
166. Ishizuka O, Mattiasson V, Andersson KE: Urodynamic effects of intravesical resiniferatoxin and capsaicin in conscious rats with and without outflow obstruction. J Urol 154:611, 1995.
167. Szallazi A, Blumgerg PM: Vanilloid receptors: New insights enhance potential as a therapeutic target. Pain 68:195, 1996.
168. Craft RM, Porreca F: Treatment parameters of desensitization to capsaicin. Life Sci 51:1767, 1992.
169. Fowler CJ, Betts C, Christmas T, et al: Botulinum toxin in the treatment of chronic urinary retention in women. Br J Urol 70:387, 1992.
170. Dykstra DD, Sidi AA: Treatment of detrusor-striated sphincter dyssynergia with botulinum A toxin. Arch Phys Med Rehabil 71:24, 1990.
171. Fowler CJ, Beck RO, Gerrard S, et al: Intravesical capsaicin for treatment of detrusor hyperreflexia. J Neurol Neurosurg Psychiatry 57:169, 1994.
172. Das A, Chancellor M, Watanabe T, et al: Intravesical capsaicin in neurologic impaired patients with detrusor hyperreflexia. J Spinal Cord Med 19:190, 1996.
173. Geirsson G, Fall M, Sullivan L: Clinical and urodynamic effects of intravesical capsaicin treatment in patients with chronic traumatic spinal detrusor hyperreflexia. J Urol 154:1825, 1995.
174. Chandiramani VA, Peterson T, Duthie GS, et al: Urodynamic changes during therapeutic intravesical instillations of capsaicin. Br J Urol 77:792, 1996.
175. de Seze M, Wiart L, de Seze MP, et al: Intravesical capsaicin versus resiniferatoxin for the treatment of detrusor hyperreflexia in spinal cord injured patients: A double-blind, randomized, controlled study. J Urol 171:251, 2004.
176. Kim JH, Riva DA, Shenot PJ, et al: Intravesical resiniferatoxin for refractory detrusor hyperreflexia: A multicenter, blinded, randomized, placebo-controlled trial. J Spinal Cord Med 26:358, 2003.
177. Kuo HC: Effectiveness of intravesical resiniferatoxin in treating detrusor hyperreflexia and external sphincter dyssynergia in patients with chronic spinal cord lesions. BJU Int 92:597, 2003.
178. Watanabe T, Yokoyama T, Sasaki K, et al: Intravesical resiniferatoxin for patients with neurogenic detrusor overactivity. Int J Urol 11:200, 2004.
179. Giannantoni A, DiStasi SM, Stephen RL, et al: Intravesical resiniferatoxin versus botulinum-A-toxin injections for neurogenic detrusor overactivity: A prospective randomized study. J Urol 172:240, 2004.
180. Rashbaum M, Mandelbaum CC: Non-operative treatment of urinary incontinence in women. Am J Obstet Gynecol 56:777, 1948.
181. Diokno A, Taub M: Ephedrine in treatment of urinary incontinence. Urology 5:624, 1975.
182. Ek A, Andersson KE, Gullberg B, et al: The effects of long-term treatment with norephedrine on stress incontinence and urethral closure pressure profile. Scand J Urol Nephrol 12:105, 1978.
183. O'Brink A, Bunne G: The effect of alpha adrenergic stimulation in stress incontinence. Urol Int 12:205, 1978.
184. Lose G, Lindholm D: Clinical and urodynamic effects of nofenefrine in women with stress incontinence. Urol Int 39:298, 1994.
185. Lose G, Rix P, Diernoes E, et al: Norfenefrine in the treatment of female stress incontinence. Urol Int 43:11, 1988.
186. Diernoes E, Rix P, Sorenson T, et al: Norfenefrine in the treatment of female urinary stress incontinence assessed by one hour pad weighing test. Urol Int 44:28, 1989.
187. Lose G, Diernoes E, Rix P: Does medical therapy cure female stress incontinence. Urol Int 44:25, 1989.
188. Hoffman BB, Lefkowitz RJ: Catecholamines and sympathomimetic drugs. In Gilman AG, Rall TW, Nies AS, Taylor P (eds): Goodman and Gilman's The Pharmacological Basis of Therapeutics, 8th ed. New York, Pergamon Press, 1990, pp 187-220.
189. Awad SA, Downie J, Kirulita J: Alpha adrenergic agents in urinary disorders of the proximal urethra: I. Stress incontinence. Br J Urol 50:332, 1978.
190. Stewart B, Borowsky L, Montague D: Stress incontinence: conservative therapy with sympathomimetic drugs. J Urol 115:558, 1976.
191. Collste L, Lindskog M: Phenylpropanolamine in treatment of female stress incontinence: Double blind placebo controlled study in 24 patients. Urology 30:398, 1987.
192. Mueller S: Neurological complications of phenylpropanolamine use. Neurology 33:650, 1983.
193. Baggioni I, Onrot J, Stewart CK, et al: The potent pressor effect of phenylpropanolamine in patients with autonomic impairment. JAMA 258:236, 1987.
194. Lasagna L: Phenylpropanolamine and blood pressure. JAMA 253:2491, 1985.
195. Liebson I, Bigelow G, Griffiths RR, et al: Phenylpropanolamine: Effects on subjective and cardiovascular variables at recommended over-the-counter dose levels. J Clin Pharmacol 27:685, 1987.
196. Blackburn GL, Morgan JP, Lavin PT, et al: Determinants of the pressor effect of phenylpropanolamine in healthy subjects. JAMA 261:3267, 1989.
197. Kiesswetter H, Hennrich F, Englisch M: Clinical and pharmacologic therapy of stress incontinence. Urol Int 38:58, 1983.
198. Gilja I, Radej M, Kovacic M, et al: Conservative treatment of female stress incontinence with imipramine. J Urol 132:909, 1984.
199. Gleason D, Reilly R, Bottaccinin M, et al: The urethral continence zone and its relation to stress incontinence. J Urol 112:81, 1974.
200. Kaisary AU: Beta adrenoceptor blockade in the treatment of female stress urinary incontinence. J Urol (Paris) 90:351, 1984.
201. Donker P, Van Der Sluis C: Action of beta adrenergic blocking agents on the urethral pressure profile. Urol Int 31:6, 1976.
202. Fellenius E, Hedberg R, Holmberg E, et al: Functional and metabolic effects of terbutaline and propranolol in fast and slow contracting skeletal muscle in vitro. Acta Physiol Scand 109:89, 1980.
203. Kishimoto T, Morita T, Okamiyo Y: Effect of clenbuterol on contractile response in periurethral striated muscle of rabbits. Tohoku J Exp Med 165:243, 1991.
204. Berk M, du Plessis AD, Birkett M, et al: An open-label study of duloxetine hydrochloride, a mixed serotonin and noradrenaline reuptake inhibitor, in patients with DSM-III-R major depressive disorder. Int Clin Psychopharmacol 12:137, 1997.
205. Thor KB, Katofiasc MA: Effects of duloxetine, a combined serotonin and norepinephrine reuptake inhibitor, on central neural control of lower urinary tract function in the chloralose-anesthetized female cat. J Pharmacol Exp Ther 274:1014, 1995.
206. Dmochowski RR, Miklow JR, Norton PA, et al: Duloxetine versus placebo for the treatment of North American women with stress urinary incontinence. J Urol 170;1259, 2003.

207. Millard RJ, Moore K, Rencken R, et al: Duloxetine versus placebo in the treatment of stress urinary incontinence: A four-continent randomized clinical trial. BJU Int 93:311, 2004.
208. van Kerrebroeck P, Abrams P, Lange R, et al: Duloxetine versus placebo in the treatment of European and Canadian women with stress urinary incontinence. BJOG 111:249, 2004.
209. Hodgson BJ, Dumas S, Bolling DR, et al: Effect of oestrogen on sensitivity of rabbit bladder and urethra to phenylephrine. Invest Urol 16:67, 1978.
210. Levin RM, Shofer FS, Wein AJ: Oestrogen-induced alterations in the autonomic responses of the rabbit urinary bladder. J Pharmacol Exp Ther 215:614, 1980.
211. Levin RM, Zderic SA, Ewalt DH, et al: Effects of pregnancy on muscarinic receptor density and function in the rabbit urinary bladder. Pharmacology 43:69, 1991.
212. Tong Y, Wein AJ, Levin RM: Effects of pregnancy on adrenergic function in the rabbit urinary bladder. Neurourol Urodyn 11:525, 1992.
213. Larsson B, Andersson K, Batra S, et al: Effects of estradiol on norepinephrine-induced contraction, alpha adrenoceptor number and norepinephrine content in the female rabbit urethra. J Pharmacol Exp Ther 229:557, 1984.
214. Callahan SM, Creed KE: The effects of oestrogens on spontaneous activity and responses to phenylephrine of the mammalian urethra. J Physiol 358:35, 1985.
215. Bump RC, Friedman CI: Intraluminal urethral pressure measurements in the female baboon: Effects of hormonal manipulation. J Urol 136:508, 1986.
216. Fantl JA, Cardozo L, McClish DK: Estrogen therapy in the management of urinary incontinence in postmenopausal women: A meta-analysis. First report of the Hormones and Urogenital Therapy Committee. Obstet Gynecol 83:12, 1994.
217. Sultana CJ, Walters MD: Estrogen and urinary incontinence in women. Maturitas 20:129, 1990.
218. Batra SC, Iosif CS: Female urethra: A target for oestrogen action. J Urol 129:418, 1983.
219. Rud T: Urethral pressure profile in continent women from childhood to old age. Acta Obstet Gynecol Scand 59:331, 1980.
220. Versi E, Cardozo L, Buncat L, et al: Correlation of urethral physiology and skin collagen in post menopausal women. Br J Urol Gynaecol 95:147, 1988.
221. Beisland HO, Fossberg E, Moer A, et al: Urethral sphincteric insufficiency in postmenopausal females: Treatment with phenylpropanolamine and estriol separately and in combination. Urol Int 39:211, 1984.
222. Bhatia NN, Bergman A, Karram MM: Effects of oestrogen on urethral function in women with urinary incontinence. Am J Obstet Gynecol 160:176, 1989.
223. Walter S, Wolf H, Barleto H, et al: Urinary incontinence in post menopausal women treated with oestrogens. Urol Int 33:135, 1978.
224. Hilton P, Stanton SL: The use of intravaginal oestrogen cream in genuine stress incontinence. Br J Obstet Gynaecol 90:940, 1983.
225. Samsioe G, Jansson I, Mellström D, et al: Occurrence, nature and treatment of urinary incontinence in a 70- year-old female population. Maturitas 7:335, 1985.
226. Cardozo L: Role of oestrogens in the treatment of female urinary incontinence. J Am Geriatr Soc 38:326, 1990.
227. Kinn AC, Lindskog M: Oestrogens and phenylpropanolamine in combination for stress urinary incontinence in postmenopausal women. Urology 32:273, 1988.
228. Walter S, Kjærgaard B, Lose G, et al: Stress urinary incontinence in postmenopausal women treated with oral oestrogen (estriol) and an alpha-adrenoceptor-stimulating agent (phenylpropanolamine): A randomized double-blind placebo-controlled study. Int Urogynecol J 1:74, 1990.
229. Hendrix SL, Cochrane BB, Nygaard IE, et al: Effects of estrogen with and without progestin on urinary incontinence. JAMA 293:935, 2005.
230. Session DR, Kelly AC, Jewelewicz R: Current concepts in oestrogen replacement therapy in the menopause. Fertil Steril 59:277, 1993.
231. Grodstein F, Stampfer MJ, Colditz GA, et al: Postmenopausal hormone therapy and mortality. N Engl J Med 336:1769, 1997.
232. Murray K: Medical and surgical management of female voiding difficulty. In Drife JO, Hilton P, Stanton SL (eds): Micturition. London, Springer-Verlag, 1990, p 179.
233. Ayton RA, Darling GM, Murkies AI, et al: A comparative study of safety and efficacy of continuous low dose estradiol released from a vaginal ring compared with conjugated equine oestrogen vaginal cream in the treatment of postmenopausal urogenital atrophy. Br J Obstet Gynaecol 103:351, 1996.
234. Johnston A: Estrogens: Pharmacokinetics and pharmacodynamics with special reference to vaginal administration and the new estradiol formulation—Estring. Acta Obstet Gynecol Scand 165:16, 1996.
235. Norgaard JP, Rillig S, Djurhuus JC: Nocturnal enuresis: An approach to treatment based on pathogenesis. J Pediatr 114:705, 1989.
236. Rew DA, Rundle JSH: Assessment of the safety of regular DDAVP therapy on primary nocturnal enuresis. Br J Urol 63:352, 1989.
237. Asplund R, Oberg H: Desmopressin in elderly subjects with increased nocturnal diuresis: A 2 month treatment study. Scand J Urol Nephrol 27:77, 1993.
238. Kinn AC, Larsson PO: Desmopressin: A new principle for symptomatic treatment of urgency and incontinence in patients with multiple sclerosis. Scand J Urol Nephrol 24:109, 1990.
239. Pederson PA, Johansen PB: Prophylactic treatment of adult nocturia with bumetanide. Br J Urol 62:145, 1988.

Chapter 21

PHARMACOLOGIC NEUROMODULATION

Raymond R. Rackley and Patrick J. Shenot

INTRAVESICAL CAPSAICIN AND RESINIFERATOXIN

Anatomy and Function of the Uroepithelium

The internal surface of the urinary bladder is lined with transitional epithelium. Three distinct layers of the uroepithelium have been described.[1] Large umbrella cells form the superficial lining of the bladder urothelium. The permeability barrier of the urothelium is maintained in this stratum by tight junctions that prevent the paracellular passage of urinary solutes across this outer layer into the bloodstream. Umbrella cells are associated with a group of crystalline protein plaques called uroplakins that also contribute to the permeability barrier of the urothelium. Beneath the umbrella cell layer is the intermediate layer of moderately sized cells and a basal layer of small cells.[2] In the bladder, suburothelial afferent fibers form a dense plexus that innervates both the detrusor itself and the basal layer of the urothelium.[3] These afferent fibers are critical for sending sensory input to the central nervous system. The uroepithelium was once thought to serve only as a passive barrier to the contents of the bladder, but there is a growing body of evidence that confirms reciprocal communication between the neuronal system and the uroepithelium. This implies that the uroepithelium may play a significant role in regulating bladder activity via a number of neuron-like properties that modulate bladder sensory function and may represent a potential novel therapeutic target for pharmacologic intervention for bladder dysfunction.

Afferent Innervation of the Urinary Bladder

Normal storage of urine is dependent on spinal reflex mechanisms that activate somatic and sympathetic pathways to the bladder outlet and detrusor muscle as well as tonic inhibitory pathways that suppress parasympathetic excitatory activity leading to detrusor relaxation and bladder filling. Micturition requires efferent nerve input to the bladder from the spinal cord as well as afferent input from the bladder to central nervous system. Sensory information, including the sensations of bladder fullness and pain, is conveyed to the spinal cord via afferent fibers in the pelvic and hypogastric nerves. The most important afferents controlling the micturition process are the small myelinated Aδ fibers, which transmit signals mainly from mechanoreceptors that detect wall tension and bladder fullness, and unmyelinated C fibers, which detect noxious signals and initiate painful sensations.[4-6] At other sites in the body, such as the skin and mucous membranes, C-fiber afferents transmit nociceptive information into the central nervous system and modulate various reflex responses to noxious stimuli such as hot temperatures (see later discussion).

After suprasacral spinal cord injury, there is significant reorganization of micturition reflexes that leads to the emergence of primitive spinal bladder reflexes triggered by C-afferent neurons. Afferent C-fiber activation may also occur in infectious or irritative conditions in the bladder and serve to facilitate or trigger voiding. This may be viewed as a defense mechanism to eliminate bladder irritants or bacteria. Bladder wall C fibers may be responsible for afferent signals that trigger detrusor overactivity (DO). As specific C-fiber neurotoxins, capsaicin and resiniferatoxin (RTX), its ultrapotent analogue, may be used to study and treat lower urinary tract dysfunction.[7,8]

Vanilloid Pharmacology

Current pharmacologic treatment of the overactive bladder relies on partially blocking the efferent parasympathetic innervation to the detrusor with anticholinergic drugs. These drugs often have troublesome side effects and are often used in doses insufficient to provide significant clinical benefit. The afferent pathways of the voiding reflex may be targeted by intravesical instillation of drugs with relative selectivity for sensory nerves. Capsaicin and RTX are potent neurotoxins that desensitize these C-fiber afferent neurons, which may be responsible for signals that trigger DO.

Hot peppers have been eaten and used by humans since prehistorical times.[9] Hogyes, in 1878, reported that the pungent and irritant action of capsicol, an extract of *Capsicum,* is mediated by sensory nerves.[10] Capsaicin and its ultrapotent analogue, RTX, collectively belong to class of neurotoxic agents referred to as vanilloids. RTX is isolated from some species of *Euphorbia,* a cactus-like plant. These compounds are characterized by a terminal homovanilloid moiety that interacts with a specific membrane receptor (Fig. 21-1) The action of vanilloid compounds on sensory neurons is mediated via interaction of the homovanilloid moiety with the vanilloid receptor TRPV1 (transient receptor potential V1 or VR1 receptor), a nonspecific, heat-gated cation channel that mediates the influx of calcium and sodium, resulting in depolarization of nociceptive afferents to initiate a nerve impulse passing through the dorsal root ganglion into the central nervous system.[11,12] Vanilloid receptors are expressed not only by small unmyelinated C fibers but also by uroepithelial cells themselves.

As intracellular calcium levels rise, voltage-sensitive calcium channels are first activated leading initially to local transmitter release, and then inhibited, serving to block the very same response. Noxious temperatures are also sensed via this mechanism, explaining the characteristic sensation of heat that is experienced when eating chili peppers.[13] Therefore, capsaicin mimics the action of physiologic/endogenous stimuli that activates the "nociceptive pathway." At the molecular level, nociception is carried out by ion channels or receptors.

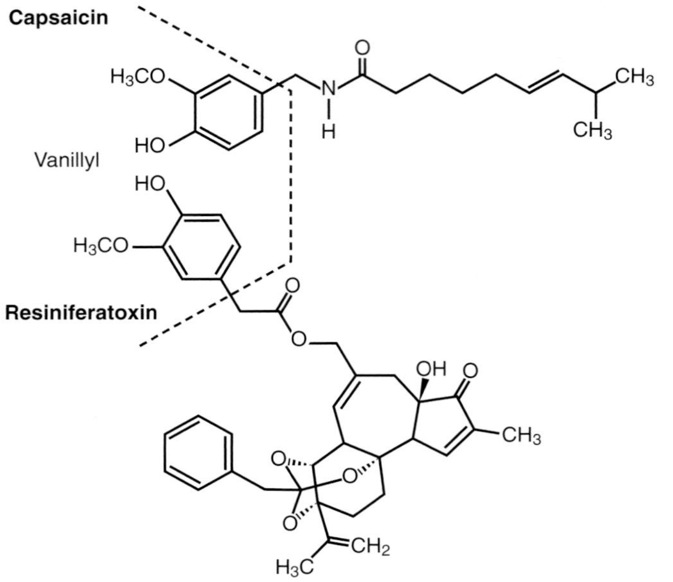

Figure 21-1 Chemical composition of capsaicin and its ultrapotent analogue, resiniferatoxin. These compounds are characterized by a terminal homovanilloid moiety that interacts with a specific membrane receptor.

Both capsaicin and RTX cause initial excitation of sensory neurons with a subsequent lasting refractory state termed desensitization. Jancso discovered that, after a period of initial intense excitation of sensory neurons, animals treated with capsaicin become unresponsive to noxious chemical stimuli and fail to develop inflammation.[14,15] A large number of studies have since confirmed this finding and established capsaicin as an useful agent for the study of sensory neuron function.[16]

Vanilloid Potency

The Scoville heat unit scale is commonly used commercially to compare the potency of pepper strengths. Wilbur Scoville, in 1912, calibrated the potency of peppers by extracting capsicum in alcohol and diluting it until pungency was first detected after placing a drop on his tongue.[17] This technique has since been standardized using high-pressure liquid chromatography (HPLC). In fact, if all known peppers were measured using this technique, their scale of pungency would range from 1 Scoville unit, for the bell pepper, to as much as 300,000 units for the habanero pepper. Pure capsaicin has a Scoville heat unit score of 16 million, and RTX registers at 16 billion Scoville heat units, which is 1000 times the potency of capsaicin (Table 21-1).

Sensitization (Acute Excitatory Effects)

On first contact with capsaicin, afferent neurons are invariably stimulated, and there seems to be no apparent difference whether the drug is applied to the peripheral or central endings or to the cell bodies of sensory neurons. Administration of vanilloids to peripheral nerve endings results in depolarization and discharge of action potentials, which in turn evokes a characteristic burning sensation via stimulation of C-fiber polymodal nociceptors. Acute activation of the sensory neurons via the vanilloid receptor TRPV1 results initially in depolarization and transmitter (peptide) release with eventual neuronal degeneration.[18,19]

Table 21-1 Heat Level Comparisons

Pepper or Derivative	Scoville Value
Sweet Italian bell	0-1
Pepperoncini	100-500
Jalapeno	1000
Cayenne	30,000-50,000
Thai	50,000-100,000
Jamaican hot	100,000-200,000
Habanero	100,000-300,000
Pure capsaicin	16,000,000
Resiniferatoxin (RTX)	16,000,000,000

Desensitization (Secondary Neurotoxic Effects)

After vanilloid-induced stimulation of primary afferent neurons, excitation subsides and the neurons become unresponsive to further applications of drug. Capsaicin desensitization is characterized by long-lasting, reversible suppression of sensory neuron activity.[20] The rate and duration of desensitization is related to the dose and time of exposure to capsaicin and the time interval between consecutive dosings.[7,21]

Although C-fiber neurons have well-described afferent functions, they probably have important efferent functions as well, including local release in the periphery of substance P, neurokinin A, calcitonin gene–related peptides (CGRP), and other neuropeptides that directly and indirectly produce tissue inflammation.[22-25] Desensitization of capsaicin-sensitive nerve fibers is associated with eventual depletion of transmitter neuropeptides.[26,27]

Clinical Results of Intravesical Capsaicin

Hypersensitivity Disorders

Because capsaicin and RTX selectively activate sensory C fibers that convey information about noxious stimuli to the central nervous system, the use of intravesical capsaicin or RTX for interstitial cystitis and other types of sensory or inflammatory bladder conditions is logical.

Maggi and coworkers reported the clinical urologic application of intravesical capsaicin.[28] Intravesical instillation of capsaicin (0.1 to 10 μmol/L) in six patients with bladder hypersensitivity produced a concentration-related reduction of the first desire to void, bladder capacity, and pressure threshold for micturition. All patients reported disappearance or marked attenuation of their symptoms for a few days after capsaicin application. In three other patients, intravesical instillation of the vehicle (0.1% ethanol in saline) alone did not produce significant cystometric changes nor modify the symptomatology, suggesting that capsaicin-sensitive nerves exist in the human bladder. A second series using intravesical capsaicin, a randomized, placebo-controlled trial in patients with bladder hypersensitivity, confirmed the beneficial effect of intravesical instillation of capsaicin on voiding parameters but did not confirm improvement in pain score after capsaicin treatment compared with placebo.[29]

Although intravesical capsaicin has been proposed as a treatment option for interstitial cystitis, its utility has not been widely explored. One small pilot study of intravesical capsaicin in five patients with interstitial cystitis, using criteria of the National

Institute of Diabetes and Digestive and Kidney Diseases (NIDDK), demonstrated subjective improvement in both symptom and pain score in four of them.[30]

Neurogenic Detrusor Overactivity

Fowler and associates reported the first clinical experience with capsaicin in neurologically impaired patients with intractable incontinence due to multiple sclerosis and spinal cord injury.[31,32] After a single intravesical instillation of capsaicin (1 to 2 mmol/L) for 30 minutes, 10 of 14 patients exhibited an improved bladder capacity for up to 9 months without toxicity. Similar findings were noted in small studies in other patients with neurogenic DO.[33,34]

De Ridder and associates described the long-term outcome of intravesical capsaicin instillation in 79 patients with spinal cord disease and treatment-resistant urinary incontinence.[35] Repeated intravesical instillation of intravesical capsaicin (1 to 2 mmol/L in 30% ethanol) was effective, and the benefit persisted for up to 3 to 5 years. In patients with phasic detrusor hyperreflexia, complete continence was achieved in 44%, satisfactory improvement occurred in 36%, and treatment failure was observed in 20%. Clinical benefit from a single instillation lasted 3 to 6 months and was repeated in some patients with similar improvement. There was no clinical or urodynamic improvement in patients treated with the ethanol vehicle alone, and there were no reported long-term complications.

There have been only a few reported randomized, placebo-controlled studies of capsaicin in patients with neurogenic DO. The results of these trials have been mixed. Wiart and colleagues reported that a single intravesical instillation of 1 mmol/L capsaicin resulted in clinical improvement with significant regression of urine leakage episodes and urgency compared with those receiving vehicle (30% ethanol) alone.[36] These findings were supported by a later study in a similar population.[37] A third placebo-controlled crossover study of 12 patients by Petersen and associates showed no benefit for intravesical capsaicin treatment therapy in patients with neurogenic DO.[38]

Resiniferatoxin

RTX is an ultrapotent capsaicin analogue present in the latex of a cactus-like plant, *Euphorbia resinifera*.[19,39] It mimics most biologic characteristics of capsaicin with approximately 1000-fold higher potency and minimal initial acute excitatory effects.[9] There are significant differences in biologic response between RTX and capsaicin. RTX and capsaicin show striking differences in relative potencies to excite and desensitize primary sensory neurons. In most cases, when RTX and capsaicin differ in potency of a particular biologic end point, the response is such that RTX preferentially causes desensitization whereas capsaicin administration leads to profound excitation.[19]

Intravesical RTX in concentrations as low as 100 nmol/L induced full desensitization, whereas a capsaicin concentration of 1 mmol/L was required to induce the same effect.[40-42] In addition, 100 nmol/L RTX solutions were much less irritating to bladder afferents than 1 mmol/L capsaicin solutions. RTX-induced desensitization may occur at concentrations so low that no noxious effect is elicited. Because of its potency and unique property of preferential desensitization, there has been much interest in the application of RTX therapy for patients with interstitial cystitis and DO.

Clinical Results of Intravesical Resiniferatoxin

Interstitial Cystitis

The positive findings of a number of small pilot studies evaluating the efficacy of capsaicin in interstitial cystitis logically led to interest in the use RTX in the treatment of interstitial cystitis, a poorly understood condition. Most of these studies were poorly controlled, but one small, placebo-controlled study did suggest that RTX was effective in the treatment of urinary frequency, urgency, and pelvic pain.[43] A recent, relatively large randomized, double-blind, placebo-controlled trial of a single dose of 0.01 to 0.10 μmol/L RTX found that it was not effective in improving overall symptoms, pain, urgency, frequency, nocturia, or voided volume during 12 weeks of follow-up.[44]

Neurogenic Detrusor Overactivity

The first clinical use of RTX in patients with neurogenic DO was reported by Cruz and colleagues in 1997.[40] They treated seven patients with intravesical instillation of 50 to 100 nmol/L RTX dissolved in 100 mL solution of 10% alcohol. Itching or mild discomfort were the only symptoms evoked in four patients during the first minutes of the treatment. Temporary exacerbation of bladder symptoms, as seen during the first 1 to 2 weeks after capsaicin administration, did not occur. In five of the seven patients, urinary frequency decreased by 33% to 58%, and this effect was detected as soon as the first day after treatment. Three patients were incontinent and became dry on most days. Improvement was sustained for up to 3 months, the longest follow-up period available. Four patients had urodynamic improvement, with a rise in maximum cystometric capacity from 50% to 900% of pretreatment cystometric capacity.

Lazzeri and colleagues reported using intravesical RTX (10 nmol/L) in eight normal patients and seven patients with overactive bladder.[42] RTX did not decrease the volume required to elicit the first desire to void and did not produce warm or burning sensations at the suprapubic or urethral level during infusion in normal subjects. Mean capacity increased significantly in patients with overactive bladder immediately after instillation but was not significantly increased after 4 weeks. There was no significant improvement in bladder capacity in the overall group, but two patients with detrusor hyperreflexia did improve urodynamically in conjunction with clinical improvement in frequency, nocturia, and incontinence episodes.

Although the results of several small studies suggested that intravesical RTX may have a role in the treatment of refractory neurogenic detrusor overactivity, its efficacy has not been conclusively confirmed in any randomized controlled trials.[45-48] RTX has been demonstrated to adsorb to polyethylene, polyvinylchloride, and latex (but not silicone or glass) catheters and containers. These materials were used in some of these studies, possibly leading to lower than expected drug delivery, thereby confounding the results obtained.[49]

A double-blind, randomized, controlled study comparing the efficacy and tolerability of RTX to capsaicin demonstrated significant clinical improvement in approximately two thirds of patients with neurogenic DO for 90 days after treatment with either agent.[50] Patients in the capsaicin arm were treated with capsaicin dissolved in a novel glucidic solvent, whereas the RTX used in this study was diluted in 10% ethanol. There were no significant differences in regard to incidence, nature, or duration of side effects in capsaicin- versus RTX-treated patients, suggesting the importance of considering the role of vehicle solvent when interpreting the efficacy and tolerance of vanilloid instillation.

RTX has also been compared with intravesical injections of botulinum A toxin (BTX-A) into the detrusor muscle in patients with spinal cord injury and refractory DO.[51] With both treatments, there was a significant reduction in mean catheterization and episodes of incontinence and a significant increase in mean first involuntary detrusor contraction and in mean maximum bladder capacity at 6, 12, and 24 months after therapy. Both RTX and BTX-A resulted in beneficial clinical and urodynamic results, with reduction of DO and restoration of urinary continence in most patients. BTX-A injection, however, provided better clinical and urodynamic benefits than intravesical RTX.

Non-neurogenic Detrusor Overactivity

Enthusiasm for intravesical RTX as a treatment for neurogenic DO has led to its investigation as a potential therapy for non-neurogenic detrusor overactivity. RTX instillation may delay or suppress involuntary detrusor contractions and increase mean maximal cystometric capacity for at least 90 days.[52] Relatively modest improvements in clinical symptoms were noted in several studies of patients with non-neurogenic DO in this population.[53-55] To date, there has been no well-controlled randomized trial.

Technique of Intravesical Capsaicin and Resiniferatoxin Administration

Neither capsaicin nor RTX is currently approved for routine clinical intravesical use. Insertion of a small silicone urethral catheter with balloon occlusion of the bladder neck is recommended. Care must be taken to avoid contact with polyethylene, polyvinylchloride, or latex which may result in a diminished effective administered dose. Intravesical lidocaine is commonly instilled before drug administration. Although a 1% to 2% lidocaine solution is most commonly used, there is evidence that 4% lidocaine may improve tolerability.[44]

Capsaicin has typically been used as a 1- to 2-mmol/L solution dissolved in 30% ethanol in saline. RTX is administered as a 0.05- to 0.10-μmol/L solution in 10% ethanol. Both agents are usually left in the bladder for approximately 30 minutes.

Conclusions for Intravesical Capsaicin and Resiniferatoxin

Intravesical instillation of vanilloid agents appears to be a promising therapy for the treatment of neurogenic and non-neurogenic DO. These agents may be used to directly target sensory nerves on the afferent limb of the voiding reflex without systemic side effects. Numerous studies have demonstrated improvement in lower urinary tract symptoms with minimal long-term complications. Despite more than a decade of experience with these neurotoxic agents, however, the true efficacy of these compound has not been clearly defined. RTX, which appears to have efficacy similar to capsaicin but with fewer side effects, holds greater promise as a safe, effective treatment for DO. Prospective randomized, placebo-controlled studies are necessary to truly define the role of intravesical vanilloid therapy in the management of overactive bladder.

BOTULINUM TOXIN

Discovered by Professor Pierre Emile van Ermengem of Ellezelles in 1897, BTX is a neurotoxin produced by the gram-positive, rod-shaped anaerobic bacterium, *Clostridium botulinum*.[56] Although seven immunologically distinct antigenic subtypes of BTX have been isolated (A, B, C1, D, E, F, and G), only types A and B are available for use clinically. BTX-A, known as BOTOX in the United States and DYSPORT in the United Kingdom, is more potent and has a longer duration of action than type B, which is known as MyoBloc in the United States and NeuroBloc in Europe.[57]

BTX exerts its effects by binding to the peripheral cholinergic terminals and inhibiting the release of acetylcholine at the neuromuscular junction. As a result, a flaccid paralysis ensues. There are four steps involved in this process: binding, translocation, cleavage, and inhibition of neurotransmitter release.[57] BTX is made within the bacterial cytosol and is released as a 150-kd polypeptide chain. Proteolytic cleavage results in a heavy chain (100 kd) and a light chain (50 kd), which are linked by heat-labile disulfide bonds. Neither chain can exert neurotoxicity independently. The heavy chain is responsible for binding to the nerve terminal at the neuromuscular junction. The light chain, which is internalized by endocytosis, actively cleaves a specific site on the protein complex responsible for docking and release of vesicles containing neurotransmitters into the neuromuscular junction.[58] By cleaving protein receptors within the nerve terminals, BTX prevents the normal vesicular transport and release of acetylcholine from the motor nerve terminals into the neuromuscular junction.

Based on histologic evidence, recovery of chemodenervation occurs after 3 to 6 months. This is thought to be the result of turnover of the presynaptic molecules and nerve sprouting from the nerve terminal, forming a new functional synapse. Affected nerve terminals do not degenerate, and axonal sprouting and formation of new synaptic contacts can recover function. The time required to recover function after BTX paralysis depends on the subtype of toxin used and the type of nerve terminal.[57] Chemodenervation lasts between 3 and 6 months when BTX is injected near the neuromuscular junction of skeletal muscle and considerably longer (up to 1 year) when it is injected near the autonomic neurons of smooth muscle.[57,58]

Applications in Urology

BTX was first approved by the Food and Drug Administration (FDA) in 1989 for use in people with strabismus and blepharospasm.[56] Since then, its use has been extended to cervical dystonia, cosmesis, hypersecretory disorders, and overactive muscle disorders. Although it is not an FDA-approved use, BTX has been used in urology to treat neurogenic and non-neurogenic DO, detrusor-sphincter dyssynergia (DSD), motor and sensory urgency, and, more recently, chronic pain syndromes.

Detrusor Overactivity

The use of BTX in neurogenic DO was pioneered by Schurch and colleagues in 2000.[59] BTX-A (200 or 300 units) was injected into the trigone of 21 spinal cord–injured patients with DO and urge incontinence managed with clean intermittent catheterization. At 6 weeks, 17 of 19 patients were completely continent. Urodynamic evaluation revealed significant increases in mean filling volume, maximum cystometric capacity, and postvoid residual urine and a decrease in detrusor voiding pressure. In the 11 patients available for follow-up at 16 and 36 weeks, improvements in bladder function and urodynamic parameters persisted. Similarly, significant increases were noted in cystometric bladder capacity, reflex volume, and bladder compliance, and there was a decrease in mean voiding pressures, in a retrospective multicenter European study of 200 patients with neurogenic DO.[60] More recently, Schurch and coworkers compared two different doses of BTX-A in a double-blinded, multicentered, randomized, placebo-controlled study of 59 patients with neurogenic DO.[61] Over 24 weeks, there was a rapid and sustained reduction in the number of incontinence episodes, an increase in maximum cystometric capacity, and a decease in mean detrusor pressure. In a study of 66 patients with neurogenic DO, Grosse and associates examined the effect of repeat detrusor injections of BTX-A. After each BTX-A injection, cystometric capacity and reflex volume increased significantly while the number of reflex contractions decreased significantly from baseline.[62] Repeat injections were as effective as the first injection, indicating no evidence of drug resistance.

Given the benefits of BTX in patients with neurogenic DO, its use has been expanded to patients with idiopathic DO. Dykstra and colleagues conducted a pilot dose-escalation study of BTX-B in 15 women with idiopathic DO. All but one patient reported decreased urgency, decreased frequency, and no incontinence.[63] Although the degree of response was similar for all doses, the duration of response was dose-dependent, with the greatest duration seen at 100-150 units. Rapp and associates looked at the effect of BTX-A on 35 patients with urgency, frequency, and urge incontinence using the Incontinence Impact Questionnaire (IIQ-7) and the Urogenital Distress Inventory (UDI-6).[64] At 3 weeks, the mean IIQ-7 and UDI-6 scores decreased significantly. Overall, 60% of patients experienced improvement in voiding symptoms.

Overactive Bladder without Detrusor Overactivity

In a recent article, Schulte-Baukloh and colleagues examined the effect of 300 units of BTX-A administered by combined bladder and external sphincter injections in women who had overactive bladder symptoms without urodynamic DO.[65] In all cases, the patient's condition was refractory to anticholinergics, biofeedback, and neuromodulation. Significant reductions were noted in daytime frequency, nocturia, and pad use at 3 and 6 months. Maximal bladder capacity increased by 20% at 3 months. Significant improvements were also noted in the UDI-6 and Symptom Impact Index (SII) scores, and no side effects, such as urinary retention, were noted. The authors attributed their low rate of urinary retention to injection of low doses (50 to 75 units) of BTX-A into the external sphincter muscle.

Detrusor Sphincter Dyssynergia

The most widespread application of BTX for urethral conditions is for external sphincter dyssynergia.[58] Dykstra and colleagues, in 1988, were the first to use BTX for treatment of DSD.[66] In a study of 11 patients with spinal cord injuries and DSD, they injected BTX-A into the external urethral sphincter. The majority of patients showed signs of sphincter denervation on electromyography. Urethral pressure profiles and postvoid residual volumes were decreased. The largest series assessing the effect of BTX-A on patients with spinal cord injury and DSD was conducted by Schurch and associates in 1996.[67] Three different protocols, using two different formulations of BTX-A toxin, were studied in 24 patients. Eighty-seven percent of patients (21/24) had improvements in urodynamic parameters regardless of the protocol or formulation used. Complete disappearance of DSD was noted in 8 of 21 patients, while mean maximum urethral pressure during DSD decreased by 48%, mean duration of DSD decreased by 47%, and mean urethral sphincter pressure decreased by 20%. More recently, de Seze and coworkers, in a randomized, double-blinded, lidocaine-controlled study of 13 spinal cord–injured patients with DSD, found that BTX significantly reduced postvoid residuals and maximal urethral pressures at 1, 7, and 30 days when compared with lidocaine.[68]

Urinary Retention and Voiding Dysfunction

Several studies have looked at the role of BTX-A injections into the external urethral sphincter in patients with voiding dysfunction and urinary retention. Phelan and colleagues, in a prospective study of 21 patients with voiding dysfunction, injected 80 to 100 units of BTX-A into the external urethral sphincter.[69] After the BTX-A injection, all but one patient were able to void spontaneously, and all but two discontinued catheterization. Kuo looked at the clinical effects and urodynamic parameters of 50 units of BTX-A in 103 patients with various types of lower urinary tract dysfunction.[70] Overall, 84.5% of patients had decreases in maximum voiding pressure, maximal urethral closure pressure, and postvoid residual. Indwelling urethral catheters and clean intermittent catheterization were discontinued in 87% of patients.

Pelvic Pain, Chronic Prostatic Pain, and Interstitial Cystitis

Although several studies have begun to explore the use of BTX-A in the treatment of pelvic pain, the direct mechanism of action by which BTX produces an antinociceptive effect is unknown. Animal studies have shown that, in addition to blocking acetylcholine release from motor neurons, BTX also inhibits the release of neurotransmitters involved in sensory pathways. BTX has been shown to inhibit the release of substance P and glutamate, neuropeptides involved in sensory and nociceptive pathways.[71] A more recent study looked at the effect of intravesical BTX-A on the release of CGRP in an acetic acid–induced rat bladder pain model. CGRP, a capsaicin-sensitive neuropeptide that has a role in regulation of micturition and mediation of painful bladder sensation, was found to be reduced in animals that received intravesical BTX-A.[72] This finding suggests that BTX inhibits CGRP release, thereby suppressing bladder pain.

Clinically, the literature on BTX in the treatment of pelvic pain syndromes is limited. Zermann and associates performed transurethral perisphinteric injection of BTX-A into 11 men with chronic prostatic pain.[73] Nine of the 11 patients reported subjective pain relief, with an average decrease in pain on a visual analogue scale from 7.2 to 1.6. Postinjection urodynamics showed decreases in functional urethral length, urethral closure pressure, and postvoid residual and increases in peak and average flow rates. Jarvis and coworkers conducted a pilot study evaluating the effect of BTX-A injection into the levator ani of 12 women with chronic pelvic pain and pelvic floor hypertonicity.[74] Under conscious sedation, women were injected with 40 units of BTX-A into the puborectalis and pubococcygeus bilaterally. Pelvic floor manometry showed a 37% reduction in resting pressure at week

4 and a 25% reduction at week 12. Significant improvements were noted in quality of life, dyspareunia, nonmenstrual pelvic pain, and dyschesia, but these changes were not statistically significant.

Three studies have looked at the antinociceptive effect of BTX on patients with interstitial cystitis. The first study, conducted at the Cleveland Clinic Foundation, retrospectively evaluated the effect of two treatment protocols on 10 patients meeting the NIDDK criteria for interstitial cystitis. The first five patients received submucosal injections, and the second five received intravesical instillations. Neither group showed statistically significant changes in subjective or objective outcome measures.[58] In the second study, Smith and colleagues injected the detrusor of 13 female patients with refractory interstitial cystitis.[75] Overall, 69% of patients noted subjective improvement. Statistically significant improvements were noted in the Interstitial Cystitis Symptom Index and the Interstitial Cystitis Problem Index, as well as daytime frequency, nocturia, and pain. On urodynamic testing, statistically significant improvements were noted in first desire to void and maximum cystometric capacity. In the third study, by Kuo, involved eight women and two men with chronic interstitial cystitis; five patients were injected with 100 units of BTX-A suburothelially into 20 sites, and an additional 100 units was injected into the trigone in the other five patients.[76] Therapeutic outcomes, including functional bladder capacity, number of daily urinations, bladder pain, and urodynamic changes, were compared between baseline and 3 months after treatment. The clinical result of suburothelial BTX injection was disappointing. None of the patients was symptom-free, and only a limited improvement in bladder capacity and pain score was achieved in two patients.

Dosage

Although most institutions use between 100 and 300 units of Botox per treatment, the optimal dosage has yet to be established. Recent studies have examined the effects of various dosing regimens in patients with both neurogenic and non-neurogenic DO. For example, Schurch and colleagues conducted a double-blinded, randomized, placebo-controlled study evaluating the efficacy of two doses of BTX-A (200 versus 300 units) in 59 patients with neurogenic urinary incontinence.[61] Both groups demonstrated significant decreases in number of incontinent episodes per week, maximum detrusor pressure during bladder contractions, and number of hyperreflexic detrusor contractions. Both groups experienced significant improvements in Incontinence Quality of Life (I-QOL) total scores which were maintained throughout the 24-week study. There were no statistically significant differences in any of the objective or subjective measures between the patients who received 200 units of BTX and those who received 300 units. Further studies continue to define the optimal dosage of BTX for various treatment conditions.

Injection Techniques

Bladder

For bladder injections, this procedure is typically performed in the outpatient setting. With the patient in the lithotomy position, 100 mL of 2% lidocaine solution is instilled into the bladder and allowed to dwell for 15 to 20 minutes to take effect.[58] In females, a 23-Fr rigid cystoscope with an injection needle (a 23-gauge needle on a 5-Fr injection sheath) is inserted through the urethra. In males, the flexible cystoscope is used along with a flexible injection needle. Depending on the institution and clinical trial, the bladder is typically injected with 100 to 300 units of BTX-A. We typically use one vial of BTX-A that contains 100 units and dilute the dried toxin in 10 mL of injectable saline, yielding a final concentration of 10 units/1 mL. Approximately 30 bladder injections, each ~0.33 mL, are made into the detrusor muscle, avoiding extravasation into the bladder serosa. Injection sites vary depending on whether the trigone-sparing technique is used (Fig. 21-2). If the trigone-sparing technique is used, the 30 injections are distributed between the bladder base and lateral walls, sparing the trigone. If the trigone is injected, six injections, or 20% of the total volume, is made into the trigone. Proponents of trigonal injection argue that patients will have a better clinical response if the BTX is placed in the trigone, an area of greater nerve density. However, opponents argue that trigonal injection could result in distal ureteral paralysis and subsequent ureteral reflux. To date, this theoretical concern has not been observed clinically.

Urethral

The urethra can be injected in one of two ways, cystoscopically or periurethrally.[58] The first method involves localization of the external sphincter using the rigid cystoscope and a 23-gauge needle on a 5-Fr injection sheath. Between 100 and 200 units of BTX-A is injected into the sphincter under direct vision equally

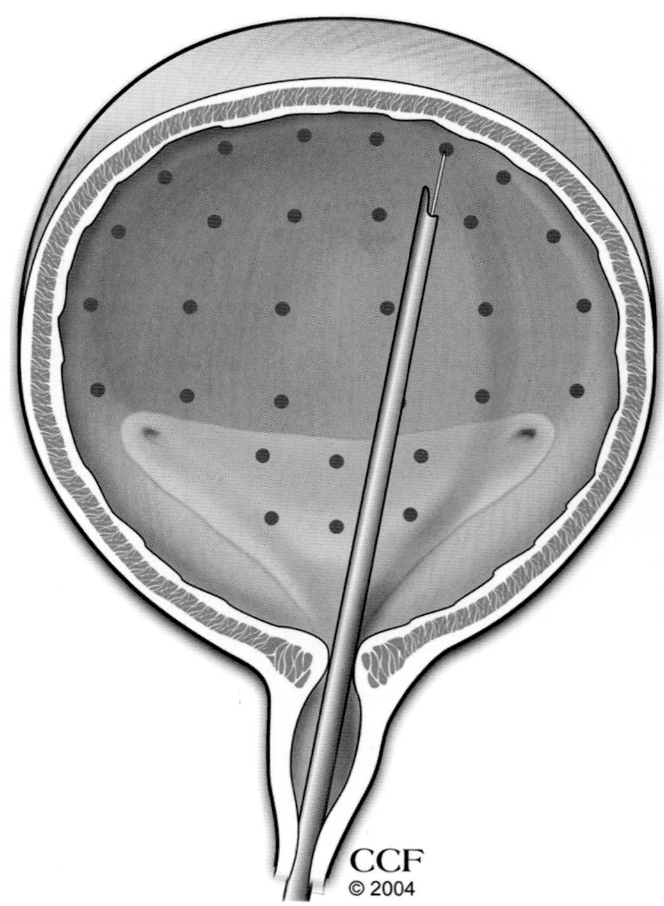

Figure 21-2 Mapping of bladder injections.

at the 3, 6, 9, and 12 o'clock positions. In women, an alternative periurethral technique can be performed easily via a small-gauge spinal needle.

Adverse Events and Contraindications

Side effects of BTX are rare in urologic applications. Not only are the injections localized with little systemic absorption, but the doses used are well below the presumed fatal dose in a 70-kg man.[57] Additionally, patients should be warned about the possibility of urinary retention after BTX treatment, secondary to detrusor hypocontractility. The rates of urinary retention after BTX-A vary from 0% to 50%, depending on injection technique; determining the postvoid residual before injection may aid in determining the proper amount of toxin and method of injection. In a recent study of seven patients, Schulte-Baukloh and colleagues reported no episodes of urinary retention.[65] They attributed this result to injection of the external sphincter muscle with 50 to 75 units of BTX-A after completion of the bladder injections. Kuo recently reported a seven-fold increase in postvoid residual, with 50% of patients requiring temporary clean intermittent catheterization after suburothelial injection of BTX-A.[77] These data suggest that suburothelial injections of BTX-A may have a more profound effect on detrusor contractility or sensation than detrusor injections do.

In nonurological cases, repeated injections of BTX-A caused immune responses in fewer than 5% of patients. Patients undergoing repeated injections are at risk of forming neutralizing antibodies that may interfere with the efficacy of BTX therapy.[58] Therefore, the use of other BTX serotypes which are not known to cause immune reactions, such BTX-C, is being investigated.[57] Currently, new formulations of BTX-A and the timing cycle of repeated injections appear to have eliminated this concern. In patients receiving BTX injections for cervical dystonia, spacing the injection cycles a minimum of 12 weeks apart has drastically reduced the formation of neutralizing antibodies.[58]

Contraindications to BTX injection include preexisting neuromuscular disease, such as myasthenia gravis, Eaton-Lambert syndrome, or amyotrophic lateral sclerosis (Lou Gherig disease).[57,58] BTX should also be avoided in patients who are breastfeeding, pregnant, or using agents that potentiate neuromuscular weakness, such as aminoglycosides. Patients should be informed that some formulations of BTX include stabilizers such as albumin that are derived from human blood; this fact may be of religious or cultural significance to some.

Conclusions for Botulinum Toxin Therapy

BTX therapy is emerging as an alternative therapeutic option in patients with debilitating chronic urologic conditions such as DSD, neurogenic or non-neurogenic DO, and pelvic pain syndromes. Given its low side effect profile and long duration of action (6 to 12 months), BTX offers an attractive alternative to conservative medical therapy and invasive surgery. Limited but growing clinical experience has revealed that temporary chemodenervation with reduction or loss or neuronal activity at the target organ may be achieved with minimal risk. This highly favorable risk-benefit ratio in urology is derived from the clinical ability to effectively treat an end-organ condition with controllable site-specific delivery (e.g., subcutaneous, intramuscular, or instillation) combined with high affinity for toxin uptake by the peripheral nerves. Although many questions remain regarding the optimal use of this minimally invasive option for urologic applications, the opportunity for expanding indications will provide urologists with increasing options for addressing difficult challenges in voiding dysfunction.

References

1. Lewis SA: Everything you wanted to know about the bladder epithelium but were afraid to ask. Am J Physiol Renal Fluid Electrolyte Physiol 278:F867-F874, 2000.
2. Born M, Pahner I, Ahnert-Hilger G, Jons T: The maintenance of the permeability barrier of bladder facet cells requires a continuous fusion of discoid vesicles with the apical plasma membrane. Eur J Cell Biol 82:343-350, 2003.
3. Andersson KE: Bladder activation: Afferent mechanisms. Urology 59(5 Suppl 1):43-50, 2002.
4. de Groat WC, Kawatani M, Hisamitsu T, et al: Mechanisms underlying the recovery of urinary bladder function following spinal cord injury. J Auton Nerv Syst 30:571, 1990.
5. Yoshimura N, Erdman SL, Snider NW, de Groat WC: Effects of spinal cord injury on neurofilament immunoreactivity and capsaicin sensitivity in rat dorsal root ganglion neurons innervating the urinary bladder. Neuroscience 83:633, 1998.
6. Kawatani M, Whitney T, Booth AM, de Groat WC: Excitatory effect of substance P in parasympathetic ganglia of the cat urinary bladder. Am J Physiol 257:R1450, 1989.
7. Maggi CA, Santicioli P, Patacchini R, et al: Regional differences in the motor response to capsaicin in the guinea pig urinary bladder: Relative role of pre- and postjunctional factors related to neuropeptide-containing sensory nerves. Neuroscience 27:675, 1988.
8. Maggi CA: Capsaicin and primary afferent neurons: from basic science to human therapy. J Auto Nerv System 33:1, 1991.
9. Lembeck, F.: Capsicum and capsaicin: past, present and future. Acta Physiol. Hung., 69: 265, 1987.
10. Dasgupta P, Fowler CJ: Chilies: From antiquity to urology. Br J Urol 80:845, 1997.
11. Montell C: Physiology, phylogeny, and functions of the TRP superfamily of cation channels. Science's STKE: Signal Transduction Knowledge Environment 2001(90):RE1, 2001.
12. Vennekens R, Voets T, Bindels RJ, et al: Current understanding of mammalian TRP homologues. Cell Calcium 31:253-264, 2002.
13 Clapham DE: Some like it hot: Spicing up ion channels. Nature 389:783, 1997.
14. Jancso N: Role of the nerve terminals in the mechanism of inflammatory reactions. Bull Millard Fillmore Hosp 7:53, 1960.
15. Jancso N, Jancso GA, Szolcsanyi J: The role of sensory nerve endings in neurogenic inflammation induced in human skin and in the eye and paw of the rat. Br J Pharmacol 33:32, 1968.
16. Holzer P: Capsaicin: Cellular targets, mechanisms of action, and selectivity for thin sensory-neurons. Pharmacol Rev 43:143, 1991.
17. Scoville W: J Am Pharm Assoc 1:453, 1912.
18. Kawatani M, Whitney T, Booth AM, de Groat WC: Excitatory effect of substance P in parasympathetic ganglia of the cat urinary bladder. Am J Physiol 257: R1450, 1989.
19. Szallasi A, Blumberg PM: Vanilloid receptors: New insights enhance potential as therapeutic target. Pain 30:571, 1990.

20. Craft RM, Cohen SM, Porreca F: Long-lasting desensitization of bladder afferents following intravesical resiniferatoxin and capsaicin in the rat. Pain 61:317, 1995.
21. Szolcsanyi J, Jancso-Gabor A, Joo F: Functional and fine structural characteristics of the sensory neuron blocking effect of capsaicin. Naunyn Schmiedebergs Arch Pharmacol 287:157, 1975.
22. Buck SH, Burks TF: The neuropharmacology of capsaicin: Review of some recent observations. Pharmacol Rev 38:179, 1986.
23. Ghatei MA Gu J, Mulderry PK, et al: Calcitonin gene-related peptide (CGRP) in the female rat urogenital tract. Peptides 6:809, 1985.
24. Maggi CA: Therapeutic potential of capsaicin-like molecules: Studies in animals and humans. Life Sci 51:1777, 1992.
25. Sharkey KA, Williams RG, Schultzberg M, Dockray GJ: Sensory substance P-innervation of the urinary bladder: Possible site of action of capsaicin in causing urine retention in rats. Neuorscience 19:861, 1983.
26. Jessell TM, Iversen LL, Cuello AC: Capsaicin-induced depletion of substance P from primary sensory neurons. Brain Res 152:183-188, 1978.
27. Kashiba H, Ueda Y, Senba E: Systemic capsaicin in the adult rat differentially affects gene expression for neuropeptides and neurotrophin receptors in primary sensory neurons. Neuroscience 76:299, 1997.
28. Maggi CA, Barbanti G, Samticioli P, et al: Cystometric evidence that capsaicin-sensitive nerves modulate the afferent branch of micturition reflex of humans. J Urol 142:150, 1989.
29. Lazzeri M, Beneforti P, Benaim G, et al: Intravesical capsaicin for treatment of severe bladder pain: A randomized placebo controlled study. J Urol 156:947, 1996.
30. Flood H, Ireland L, Byrne DS, et al: Intravesical capsaicin for interstitial cystitis. J Urol 157:254A, 1997.
31. Fowler CJ, Jewkes D, McDonard WJ, et al: Intravesical capsaicin for neurogenic bladder dysfunction. Lancet 339:1239, 1992.
32. Fowler CJ, Beck RO, Gerrard S, et al: Intravesical capsaicin for treatment of detrusor hyperreflexia. J Neurol Neurosurg Psychiatry 57:169, 1994.
33. Geirsson G, Fall M, Sullivan L: Clinical and urodynamic effects of intravesical capsaicin treatment in patients with chronic traumatic spinal detrusor hyperreflexia. J Urol 154:1825, 1995.
34. Das AS, Chancellor MB, Watanabe T, et al: Intravesical capsaicin in neurogenic impaired patients with detrusor hyperreflexia. J Spinal Cord Med 19:190, 1996.
35. De Ridder DD, Chandramani V, Dasgupta P, et al: Intravesical capsaicin as a treatment for refractory detrusor hyperreflexia: A dual center study with long term followup. J Urol 158:2087, 1997.
36. Wiart L, Joseph PA, Petit H, et al: The effects of capsaicin on the neurogenic hyperreflexic detrusor: A double blind placebo controlled study in patients with spinal cord disease. Preliminary results. Spinal Cord 36:95, 1998.
37. de Seze M, Wiart L, Joseph PA, et al: Capsaicin and neurogenic detrusor hyperreflexia: A double-blind placebo-controlled study in 20 patients with spinal cord lesions. Neurourol Urodyn 17:513-523, 1998.
38. Petersen T, Nielsen JB, Schroder HD: Intravesical capsaicin in patients with detrusor hyper-reflexia—A placebo-controlled cross-over study. Scand J Urol Nephrol 33:104-110, 1999.
39. Caterina MJ, Schumacher MA, Tominaga M, et al: The capsaicin receptor: A heat-activated ion channel in the pain pathway. Nature 389:816, 1997.
40. Cruz F, Guaraes M, Silva C, Reis M: Suppression of bladder hyperreflexia by intravesical resiniferatoxin. Lancet 350:640, 1997.
41. Lazzeri M, Beneforti P, Turini D: Urodynamic effects of intravesical resiniferatoxin in humans: Preliminary results in stable and unstable detrusor. J Urol 158:2093, 1997.
42. Lazzeri M, Beneforti P, Turini D, et al: Intravesical resiniferatoxin for the treatment of detrusor hyperreflexia refractory to capsaicin. J Urol 159:83A, 1998.
43. Lazzeri M, Beneforti P, Spinelli M, et al: Intravesical resiniferatoxin for the treatment of hypersensitive disorder: A randomized placebo controlled study. J Urol. 164(3 Pt 1):676-679, 2000.
44. Payne CK, Mosbaugh PG, Forrest JB, et al: Frumkin LR. ICOS RTX Study Group (Resiniferatoxin Treatment for Interstitial Cystitis). Intravesical resiniferatoxin for the treatment of interstitial cystitis: A randomized, double-blind, placebo controlled trial. J Urol 173:1590-1594, 2005.
45. Watanabe T, Yokoyama T, Sasaki K, et al: Intravesical resiniferatoxin for patients with neurogenic detrusor overactivity. Int J Urol 11:200-205, 2004.
46. Kim JH, Rivas DA, Shenot PJ, et al: Intravesical resiniferatoxin for refractory detrusor hyperreflexia: A multicenter, blinded, randomized, placebo-controlled trial. J Spinal Cord Med 26:358-363, 2003.
47 Kuo HC: Effectiveness of intravesical resiniferatoxin in treating detrusor hyper-reflexia and external sphincter dyssynergia in patients with chronic spinal cord lesions. BJU Int 92:597-601, 2003.
48. Silva C, Rio ME, Cruz F: Desensitization of bladder sensory fibers by intravesical resiniferatoxin, a capsaicin analog: Long-term results for the treatment of detrusor hyperreflexia. Eur Urol 38:444-452, 2000.
49. Afferon Corporation, Wayne, PA, unpublished data.
50. de Seze M, Wiart L, de Seze MP, et al: Intravesical capsaicin versus resiniferatoxin for the treatment of detrusor hyperreflexia in spinal cord injured patients: A double-blind, randomized, controlled study. J Urol 171:251-255, 2004.
51. Giannantoni A, Mearini E, Di Stasi SM, et al: New therapeutic options for refractory neurogenic detrusor overactivity. Minerva Urol Nefrol 56:79-87, 2004.
52. Silva C, Ribeiro MJ, Cruz F: The effect of intravesical resiniferatoxin in patients with idiopathic detrusor instability suggests that involuntary detrusor contractions are triggered by C-fiber input. J Urol 168:575-579, 2002.
53. Yokoyama T, Nozaki K, Fujita O, et al: Role of C afferent fibers and monitoring of intravesical resiniferatoxin therapy for patients with idiopathic detrusor overactivity. J Urol 172:596-600, 2004.
54. Palma PC, Thiel M, Riccetto CL, et al: Resiniferatoxin for detrusor instability refractory to anticholinergics. Int Braz J Urol 30:53-58, 2004.
55. Kuo HC: Multiple intravesical instillation of low-dose resiniferatoxin is effective in the treatment of detrusor overactivity refractory to anticholinergics. BJU Int 95:1023-1027, 2005.
56. Leippold T, Reitz A, Schurch B: Botulinum toxin as a new therapy option for voiding disorders: Current state of the art. Eur Urol 44:165, 2003.
57. Sahai A, Khan M, Fowler C ,. et al: Botulinum toxin for the treatment of lower urinary tract symptoms: A review. Neurourol Urodyn 24:2, 2005.
58. Frenkl TL, Rackley RR: Injectable neuromodulatory agents: Botulinum toxin therapy. Urol Clin North Am 32:89, 2005.
59. Schurch B, Stohrer M, Kramer G, et al: Botulinum-A toxin for treating detrusor hyperreflexia in spinal cord injured patients: A new alternative to anticholinergic drugs? Preliminary results. J Urol 164:692, 2000.
60. Reitz A, Stohrer M, Kramer G, et al: European experience of 200 cases treated with botulinum-A toxin injections into the detrusor muscle for urinary incontinence due to neurogenic detrusor overactivity. Eur Urol 45:510, 2004.
61. Schurch B, de Seze M, Denys P, et al: Botulinum toxin type A is a safe and effective treatment for neurogenic urinary incontinence: Results of a single treatment, randomized, placebo controlled 6-month study. J Urol 174:196, 2005.
62. Grosse J, Kramer G, Stohrer M: Success of repeat detrusor injections of botulinum a toxin in patients with severe neurogenic detrusor overactivity and incontinence. Eur Urol 47:653, 2005.

63. Dykstra D, Enriquez A, Valley M: Treatment of overactive bladder with botulinum toxin type B: A pilot study. Int Urogynecol J Pelvic Floor Dysfunct 14:424, 2003.
64. Rapp DE, Lucioni A, Katz EE, et al: Use of botulinum-A toxin for the treatment of refractory overactive bladder symptoms: An initial experience. Urology 63:1071, 2004.
65. Schulte-Baukloh H, Weiss C, Stolze T, et al: Botulinum-A toxin detrusor and sphincter injection in treatment of overactive bladder syndrome: Objective outcome and patient satisfaction. Eur Urol 48:984-990, 2005.
66. Dykstra DD, Sidi AA, Scott AB, et al: Effects of botulinum A toxin on detrusor-sphincter dyssynergia in spinal cord injury patients. J Urol 139:919, 1988.
67. Schurch B, Hauri D, Rodic B, et al: Botulinum-A toxin as a treatment of detrusor-sphincter dyssynergia: A prospective study in 24 spinal cord injury patients. J Urol 155:1023, 1996.
68. de Seze M, Petit H, Gallien P, et al: Botulinum a toxin and detrusor sphincter dyssynergia: A double-blind lidocaine-controlled study in 13 patients with spinal cord disease. Eur Urol 42:56, 2002.
69. Phelan MW, Franks M, Somogyi GT, et al: Botulinum toxin urethral sphincter injection to restore bladder emptying in men and women with voiding dysfunction. J Urol 165:1107, 2001.
70. Kuo HC: Botulinum A toxin urethral injection for the treatment of lower urinary tract dysfunction. J Urol 170:1908, 2003.
71. Welch MJ, Purkiss JR, Foster KA: Sensitivity of embryonic rat dorsal root ganglia neurons to Clostridium botulinum neurotoxins. Toxicon 38:245, 2000.
72. Chuang YC, Yoshimura N, Huang CC, et al: Intravesical botulinum toxin A administration produces analgesia against acetic acid induced bladder pain responses in rats. J Urol 172:1529, 2004.
73. Zermann D, Ishigooka M, Schubert J, et al: Perisphincteric injection of botulinum toxin type A. A treatment option for patients with chronic prostatic pain? Eur Urol 38:393, 2000.
74. Jarvis SK, Abbott JA, Lenart MB, et al: Pilot study of botulinum toxin type A in the treatment of chronic pelvic pain associated with spasm of the levator ani muscles. Aust N Z J Obstet Gynaecol 44:46, 2004.
75. Smith CP, Radziszewski P, Borkowski A, et al: Botulinum toxin a has antinociceptive effects in treating interstitial cystitis. Urology 64:871, 2004.
76. Kuo HC: Preliminary results of suburothelial injection of botulinum a toxin in the treatment of chronic interstitial cystitis. Urol Int 75:170-174, 2005.
77. Kuo HC: Clinical effects of suburothelial injection of botulinum A toxin on patients with nonneurogenic detrusor overactivity refractory to anticholinergics. Urology 66:94-98, 2005.

Chapter 22

SACRAL NEUROMODULATION INTERVTIM FOR THE TREATMENT OF OVERACTIVE BLADDER

Steven W. Siegel and Sarah E. Moeller

Urinary incontinence and voiding dysfunction are common conditions affecting the quality of life of millions of men and women. In the case of those with overactive bladder (OAB), anticholinergic medications, behavioral interventions, and pelvic floor reeducation are appropriate initial treatments, but often these are not able to control symptoms comfortably or sufficiently, and other options must be considered. Sacral neuromodulation has gained increased acceptance as a standard of care for these patients.[1] This chapter presents a detailed description of the therapy, including possible mechanism of action, patient selection, surgical technique, troubleshooting, and outcomes assessment for symptoms of OAB, including urge incontinence and urinary frequency and urgency.

HOW SACRAL NEUROMODULATION WORKS

The observation that sacral nerve stimulation (SNS) may reduce or eliminate symptoms of voiding dysfunction implies that the conditions so affected are neuromuscular in nature. A simple concept is that the pathologic state represents an imbalance of reflexes between the bladder, sphincter, and pelvic floor, and that sacral neuromodulation improves or restores the balance. The fact that the same treatment may be effective for symptoms of OAB and retention implies that the therapy is modulating the central nervous system at the level where switching between bladder emptying and storage occurs (Fig. 22-1).[2] This fits with the observations that the impact of neuromodulation may be immediate and that it is usually reversed on therapy withdrawal. Anticholinergic drugs work at the efferent limb of the voiding reflex, inhibiting detrusor activity by receptor blockade. This approach may be ineffective if the underlying disorder represents an upregulation of pelvic visceral afferent input or a destabilization of the switch at the level of the dorsal horn or pons. Sacral neuromodulation is likely to exert its influence via modulation of afferent pathways at multiple possible levels (Box 22-1).[3-20] Because sacral root stimulation evokes a motor movement of the pelvic floor, it is also likely that manipulation of the guarding reflex is an essential mechanism of action. If the guarding behavior is coordinated or decreased, voiding may be facilitated; if it is increased, appropriate storage may be promoted. Symptoms of incontinence or voiding dysfunction may represent an alteration of the pelvic neuromuscular environment that changes pelvic organ function as opposed to a disorder of the organs per se, and neuromodulation is a method of altering the environment to promote normal function.

Indications and Patient Selection

SNS was approved by the U.S. Food and Drug Administration (FDA) for intractable urge incontinence in 1997, and for urgency-frequency and nonobstructive urinary retention in 1999. Later, the labeling was changed to include "overactive bladder" as an appropriate diagnostic category. Patients from these groups are appropriate for SNS if they have chronic symptoms that significantly affect quality of life and if conservative treatments have been unsuccessful.[1,21]

Overactive Bladder

The OAB syndrome represents a mixed group of disorders with a common set of voiding behaviors, including urinary urgency-frequency and urge incontinence. In most instances, the cause is deemed idiopathic. Certainly, a behavioral component or pelvic floor muscle dysfunction is commonly present. There frequently is evidence of pelvic floor muscle spasticity on examination and on urodynamic study. The urodynamic study may or may not demonstrate uninhibited detrusor contractions. There may have been a triggering event, such as a pelvic surgery (e.g., surgery for

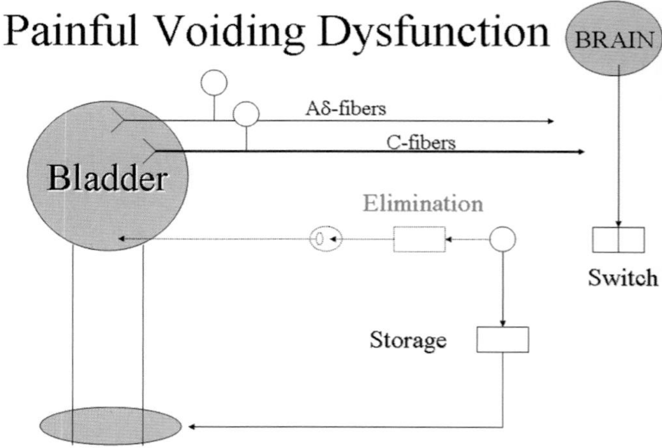

Figure 22-1 Micturition reflex pathways as outlined by de Groat. Note that the Aδ fibers and C fibers provide afferent signaling to the brain as the bladder fills. The brain, in turn, signals spinal pathways, resulting in a "turning off" of the guarding reflex, relaxation of the external urethral sphincter, contraction of the detrusor, and voluntary voiding of urine.

Box 22-1 Possible Mechanisms of Sacral Nerve Stimulation

- Inhibits postganglionic nerve terminals[4-6]
- May inhibit primary afferents presynaptically[7,8]
- May affect pudendal afferents that transmit somatic and visceral neurochemical signaling[9-11]
- Inhibits spinal tract neurons involved in the micturition reflex[12-15]
- May suppress guarding reflexes indirectly by turning off bladder afferent input to internal sphincter sympathetic or external urethral sphincter interneurons[8,16,17]
- May activate bladder efferents to stimulate voiding while simultaneously turning off excitatory pathway to urethra[18-20]

stress incontinence) or trauma. As a rule, patients who are appropriate candidates for SNS are neurologically normal and have no structural abnormality of the bladder (e.g., scarring from radiation therapy, diverticulum).

Neurogenic Disorders

Patients with defined neurologic abnormalities such as multiple sclerosis or partial cord injury may also benefit, but studies in this population of patients have been few. When faced with the alternative of an indwelling catheter or urinary diversion, it may be reasonable to consider a diagnostic trial of SNS. Patients with disorders such as peripheral neuropathy, a cord lesion, multiple sclerosis, parkinsonism, or myelodysplasia are not ideal candidates. Patients with multiple sclerosis, for example, were excluded from the original trials leading to FDA approval of SNS because of the potential for the underlying condition to change.[22] If this were to have occurred, the effectiveness of the therapy might have been called into question by the FDA. However, we know that SNS does help patients who have multiple sclerosis,[23] and, in some cases, it may be the most appropriate option.

Interstitial Cystitis and Pelvic Pain

Interstitial cystitis is not an FDA-approved indication for SNS, but one could define a set of symptoms characteristic of interstitial cystitis as "urinary frequency and urgency with pelvic pain." If a diagnostic label based on objective voiding behaviors is used, patients with interstitial cystitis may readily fit into the approved diagnostic criteria. Although isolated symptoms of pelvic floor muscle dysfunction, pelvic pain, and/or bowel dysfunction are not indications for the therapy, they are commonly present in patients who are otherwise candidates for SNS and frequently improve along with the urinary complaints if the therapy is otherwise successful.[24-29] Patient selection for SNS remains empiric. A key is to think of voiding dysfunctions in terms of voiding behaviors and pelvic floor muscle function, rather than organ-based labels. Patients with intractable urinary frequency, urgency, and urge incontinence should be considered as prime candidates. Evidence of high-tone pelvic floor muscle dysfunction may also be demonstrated on routine physical examination and on diagnostic studies such as pelvic floor electromyography.[30] A successful trial stimulation remains the best indicator for patient selection and should be used as a routine diagnostic test for patients with chronic, life-altering voiding complaints that cannot be adequately resolved by medications or behavioral interventions.

Technique

Brindley and colleagues, Schmidt, and Tanagho were some of the first to describe electrode placement to treat urinary incontinence in humans. Brindley and colleagues treated paraplegic subjects with sacral anterior root stimulation starting in 1976.[31] Thirty of the 50 treated patients reported complete continence, and 26 of the 28 male patients were able to achieve penile erection with sacral root stimulation. Schmidt reported on placement technique for the neurostimulator electrode at the S3 or pudendal nerve level.[32] Pelvic pain symptoms improved by at least 50% in almost half of the patients.[33] In 1990, Tanagho reported that almost 70% of 31 urge-incontinent patients self-rated their symptom improvement as 50% or higher.[34] Since that time, the test stimulation, lead design, and surgical technique have been refined.

Staged Lead Implantation as Initial Trial

It is our preference to perform a staged implantation as the initial therapeutic trial. The benefits of this approach include the ability to place a potentially chronic lead under minimal anesthesia. The design of the chronic lead is useful in correct identification of the anatomic nerve pathway, due to its array of four contact points, which also allows for reprogramming of the site of stimulation during the trial. Use of minimal anesthesia during chronic lead implantation (monitored anesthesia care, or MAC) allows the patient to give sensory feedback during the positioning of the lead, which serves to increase the accuracy of site selection and decrease the risk of uncomfortable sensations with chronic use of the device. We typically conduct the staged lead implantation over a 1-month period, and if there is at least a 50% improvement of the target symptoms to justify the use of an implantable pulse generator (IPG), the patient can depend on the result of the trial phase to accurately predict how the permanent implant will function. It is our impression that this technique results in a lower rate of false-positives, which may occur if there is insufficient time to gauge the response. The more accurate placement of the potentially permanent lead should also result in a higher rate of appropriate patient selection and should decrease the need for later revision surgery.

Preoperative Preparation

The patient should have completed baseline diaries documenting the target voiding dysfunction and/or incontinence. These include specific quantification of urinary frequency, voided volumes per void, degree of urgency, number and severity of incontinence episodes per day, and number and type of pads used per day. We do not ask the patients to do a cleansing bath or shower. Patients are given a preoperative dose of cephazolin (Ancef), or if they are allergic to penicillin, gatifloxacin (Tequin).

Anesthesia

The patient's feedback during lead placement can be essential to the ultimate success of the therapy; therefore, MAC/local anesthesia is most appropriate for lead placement. This also allows for more immediate postoperative programming because of the quicker patient recovery. Developing a routine with the anesthesia team is critical to the ease and success of this procedure. Our anesthesiologists use a cocktail of propofol (Diprivan), fentanyl

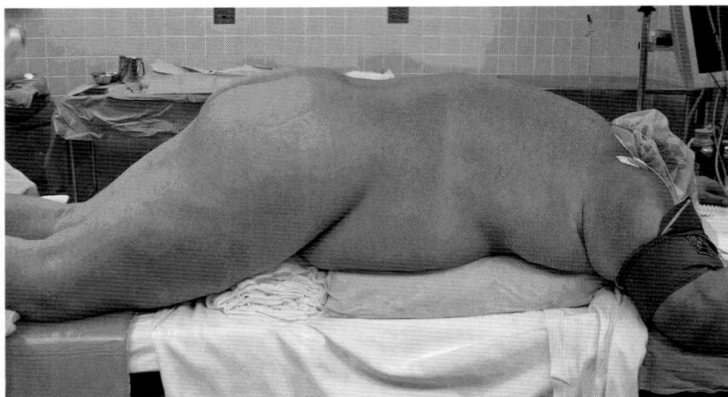

Figure 22-2 The patient is placed on a fluoro-friendly table that allows C-arm access under the pelvis for both anterior-posterior and lateral views. Chest rolls are placed to improve breathing, and a pillow or blanket supports the hips. Access to the feet is maintained out of the sterile field to allow monitoring of responses.

(Sublimaze), and midazolam hydrochloride (Versed). This allows for titration of the level of consciousness during the procedure. There is also a degree of amnesia as a result of the Versed. Some patients are comfortable with remaining alert throughout, whereas others, who may be more pain focused, need a higher level of sedation from the start. In rare instances, a general anesthetic is required due to issues such as sleep apnea or patient choice. If so, it is critical that only short-acting paralyzing agents be used to avoid obscuring pelvic muscle responses turning intraoperative stimulation.

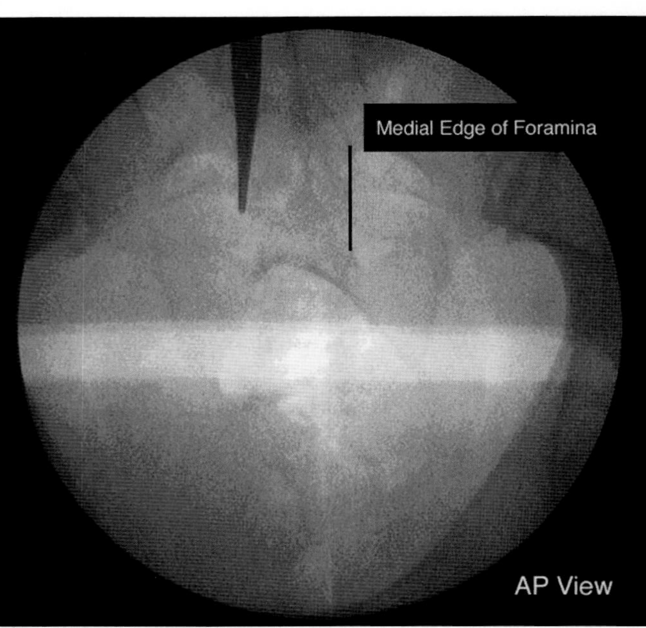

Figure 22-3 An anterior-posterior view is obtained to determine the medial edge of the foramina. A marker is placed on the skin and moved to the edge, where a skin mark is made. The opposite edge is usually two fingerbreaths across from the first mark. All of the foramina line up along the same plane. Once these landmarks have been determined, a cross-table lateral view is used to determine the target foramina for needle placement.

Intraoperative Positioning and Preparation

Patients are placed on a fluoro-friendly table in a prone position (Fig. 22-2). Use of MAC/local anesthesia can aid in allowing the patient to assist in transfer and table positioning. Pillows are helpful under the pelvis and beneath the shins. The hips must be positioned so that a C-arm unit can be passed under the table in order to allow viewing of the sacrum in an anterior-posterior (AP) plane. The feet must remain uncovered to allow for direct observation during the procedure. Two chest rolls are also needed to aid with respiration. The lower back and buttocks are first wiped with alcohol and then painted with DuraPrep (3M) solution. This is allowed to dry completely before the skin is covered with an Ioban (3M). The use of alcohol/DuraPrep/Ioban allows for a quicker and more bactericidal preparation than a prolonged Betadine scrub and paint. When used in this fashion, the Ioban also sticks to the skin very snugly, preventing any direct exposure to the skin other than at the exact site of incision. This is initially placed smoothly over the lower back and sacral area and loosely over the buttocks. After first placement of the Ioban, the cheeks of the buttocks are gently pulled apart and released to allow the covering to dip into the buttocks crease. This provides for excellent visualization of the "bellows" response without risk of field contamination from colonic flora. The buttocks cheeks are not taped apart, because this adds little benefit in discerning a bellows response yet tends to tense-up and humiliate the patient.

Selecting the Appropriate Foramen

As a rule, the target foramen is either the right or left S3 level. In rare instances, S4 is best, and S2 is almost never appropriate for chronic stimulation. If the patient has a lateralizing pain component, that side is usually approached preferentially. If there is no lateralization, and if the surgeon is right-handed, we tend to choose the patient's left side for lead placement and prefer to stand on the patient's right side during the procedure. We therefore preferentially place the IPG in the right upper buttocks, with the lead on the left; this uses up an additional 2 cm of lead length, minimizing potential lead redundancy at the connecting site.

Local Anesthesia

Once the starting point has been estimated, the skin is anesthetized with 0.25% bupivacaine (Marcaine) to create a dime-sized wheal. The skin must exhibit a "peau d'orange" effect to achieve rapid anesthesia, and it is not necessary to infiltrate into the fat below the skin level. It may be necessary to numb the posterior sacral periosteum if the patient exhibits discomfort.

Positioning the Foramen Needle with the Use of Fluoroscopy

Fluoroscopy is needed to identify the target site. Initially, an AP view is obtained to determine the medial edge of the foramina (Fig. 22-3). A skin mark is made at this level on one side, and then, by estimating two fingerbreadths over, the second site is confirmed again with fluoroscopy and marked. An imaginary line parallel to the spine at the level of either mark is where the foramina lineup, and now the S3 level needs to be determined by a cross-table fluoroscopic view. On the cross-table lateral view (Fig. 22-4), the S2 level is readily identified as the point at which the sacroiliac joint fuses, forming a characteristic shadow. The first anterior protrusion or "hillock" from the surface of the sacrum below this shadow is typically S3. Next, a skin marker such as a mosquito clip is positioned in line with the medial edge of the foramina, and a cross-table view is obtained to determine

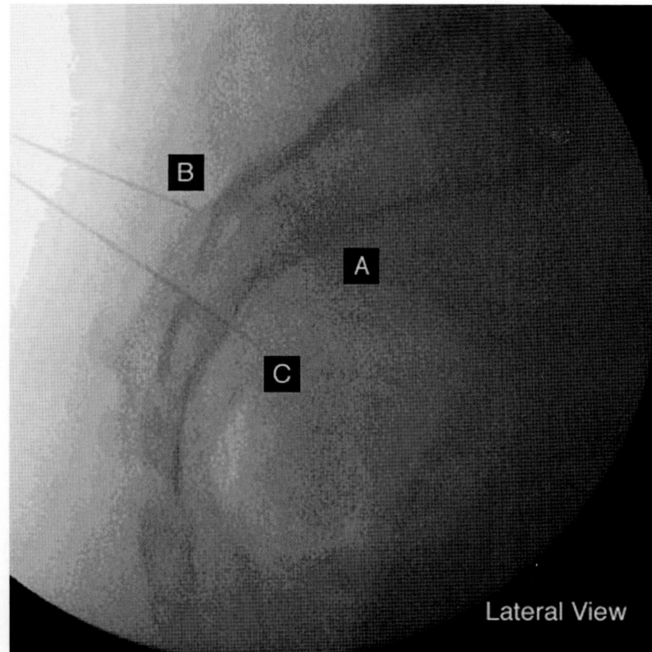

Figure 22-4 The lateral view determines where to aim for needle placement. A skin marker is placed in the line of the foramina determined on the anterior-posterior view. The sacroiliac shadow (A) is usually where S2 is located, and S3 (C) is most often the first hillock below the sacroiliac shadow. Once the target foramen has been identified, it is possible to determine if the needle must be aimed more caudally (B) or more cranially.

the potential course of the foramen needle. It should always be oriented in a cephalocaudal direction, and it should come out as close as possible to the tip of the hillock. Depending on the estimated course of the needle, the marker may need to be moved up or down until appropriately positioned. After the skin is anesthetized and the needle is placed, another fluoroscopic view is obtained to determine whether the needle must be aimed more cranially or more caudally in order to point toward the hillock. The needle is then "walked" up or down along the line of the foramina, which was determined on the AP view, until it drops into the foramen. As the aim of the needle is adjusted up or down, it is important to pull it out and reinsert it, rather than torquing or bending it (see Fig. 22-4). Once the needle enters the foramen, the fluoroscope is used to gauge the depth. We start stimulating just anterior to the bony surface (point C in Fig. 22-4). This is the most consistent location of the sacral nerve ramus relative to the point of introduction. The foramen needle is then stimulated with the screening device to check sacral root responses (Table 22-1).

If responses are not appropriate at this level (i.e., consistent with S2 or S4), the point of introduction at the skin level is re-estimated to aim for the next hillock above or below the initial point of stimulation. If appropriate responses are elicited, the needle is advanced in increments along the relevant length of the permanent electrode (2 cm) to determine whether the foramen needle has paralleled the course of the nerve. If the response is lost on advancement of the needle and retesting, the needle should be pulled back toward the skin and reinserted through the foramen until a more appropriate position has been identified.

Table 22-1 Anticipated Motor and Sensory Responses to Stimulation at S2, S3, and S4 Levels

Level	Motor Responses	Sensory Responses
S2	Bellows (inward movement of intergluteal fold) Clamp (anteroposterior pinching of the perineum or coccyx) Dorsiflexion of the foot, heel rotation, calf cramping	Genital
S3	Bellows Dorsiflexion of the great toe, bottom of the foot	Genital, perineal, anal
S4	Bellows	Anal

Positioning the Tined Lead under Fluoroscopy

Once the course of the nerve has been fathomed using the foramen needle, the tined lead is deployed. A skin nick is made at the foramen needle insertion point, and the metal stylet is placed at the appropriate depth for either the 3- or 5-inch foramen needle. Next, the foramen needle is exchanged for a lead introducer sheath. The tip of the introducer sheath has a radiopaque marker, and the depth of this marker should be about 1 cm proximal to the anterior surface of the bone (Fig. 22-5A). Deploying the lead from this position allows it to release in the fatty plane surrounding the nerve, improving the chance that the lead will "catch the wave" and follow its course (see Fig. 22-5B). It is also very helpful to use the "ball-tipped" stylet, which is an accessory (Medtronic Accessory Kit), because it is softer than the one currently packaged with the lead and is less likely to force the electrode out of the proper plane. The ball-tipped stylet has a slight curve or "hockey stick" appearance to it, and it marries to the lead body at its most external point, allowing the tip to be steered under fluoroscopic guidance (Fig. 22-6).

When deployed properly, the lead should always point caudally to a slight degree (point B in Fig. 22-6) and never cephalad (point A in Fig. 22-6). Additionally, it should flip out laterally. This can be achieved by pointing the hockey stick "down and out" as it first enters the foramen. On the lateral fluoroscopic view, the spaces between the lead contact points (0 to 3) should appear closer together between the more distal sites, indicating that the lead is pointing away as it separates from the anterior surface of the bone. On the posterior-anterior view, the most ideal lead position should course out flat and laterally from the medial aspect of the foramen (Fig. 22-7). We always straddle the bone table with lead sites 3 and 2 (see Fig. 22-6). This allows for a consistent lead depth, prevents premature deployment of the tines, and provides a point of reference in the future. Once a satisfactory trajectory of the lead has been obtained, starting with the most distal contact (point 0), each site is stimulated and the threshold of response is measured. If each site elicits an appropriate response at a relatively low threshold, the position of the nerve has been appropriately paralleled by the lead. If not, the lead should be pulled back under fluoroscopic guidance until the tip is proximal to the end of the introducer sheath, and then reinserted under fluoroscopic control, watching to make sure it takes a different course. It is then retested at each contact point. The goal is to get all four contact points yielding an appropriate response at a similar, relatively low threshold. If this cannot be

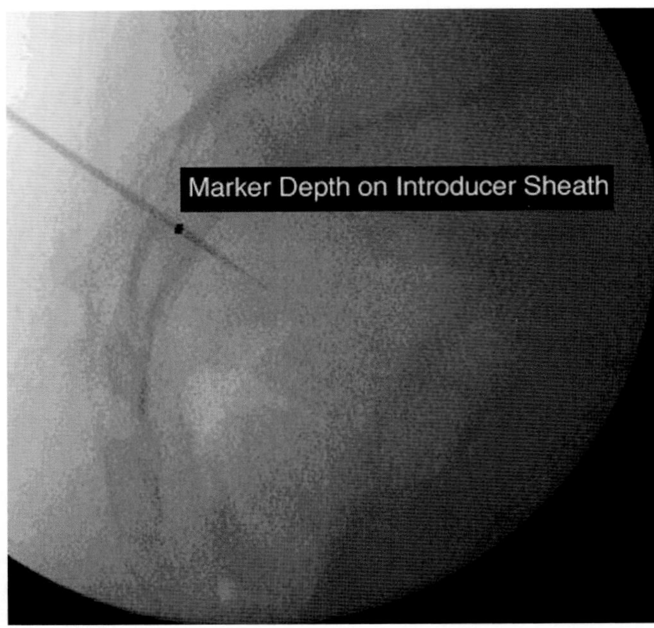

A

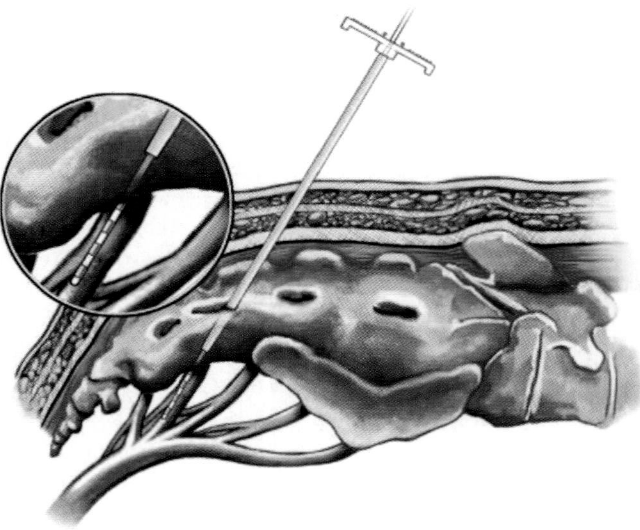

B

Figure 22-5 (A) Once appropriate responses have been determined, the foramen needle is exchanged for the lead introducer sheath. This is placed under fluoroscopic control so that the radiopaque marker remains within the bone table about 1cm posterior to the anterior surface of the sacrum. This allows the lead to be deployed in the fatty plane through which the nerve travels **(B),** and, combined with the use of the ball-tipped stylet, improves the chance that all four contact points will be in line with the nerve.

attained after several repositionings, it may be necessary to bend the lead/stylet to accentuate the hockey stick shape and redeploy it. If this is still unsuccessful, it may be necessary to start again with the foramen needle to map out a different course for the nerve. Once the ideal position has been determined, the tines are deployed by uncoupling the stylet and pulling it back under fluoroscopic guidance, as the position of contacts 3 and 2 are maintained relative to the anterior surface of the sacrum.

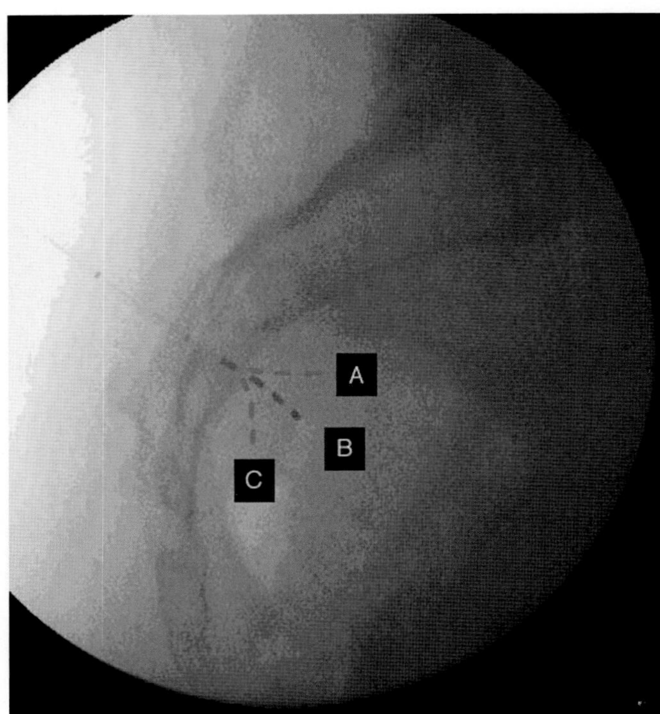

Figure 22-6 Potential positions for lead deployment are shown. Aiming the ball-tipped stylet under fluoroscopic control allows repositioning if needed. Try to aim it down and out to begin with. Point A depicts the lead coursing cephalad, which is inappropriate, and may lead to S2 stimulation at the distal contact points. Position C is too caudal and may lead to S4 stimulation at the distal sites. The proximal contacts (2 and 3) may yield similar responses in all of the deployments. It is unlikely that all four sites would have the same stimulation thresholds in either position A or position C, because the lead is not following the course of a single nerve root. Position B is most ideal. Note how the contact points appear closer together distally, indicating that the lead is headed out laterally along the course of the nerve. All four sites should yield an S3-type response at low thresholds. The lead is deployed with contact sites 2 and 3 straddling the bone table. (Courtesy of Medtronic, Inc.)

Setting Up the Connection between the Lead and Lead Extension

We typically place the connection between the lead and lead extension in the anticipated site for the future IPG (Fig. 22-8). The lateral aspect of the future IPG incision is made at this time (point F on Fig. 22-8). The location is usually on the right side (because of where the surgeon stands), and the future IPG should be lateral to the lateral edge of the sacrum (point A on Fig. 22-8), below the posterior superior iliac crest (point B on Fig. 22-8). These landmarks are outlined with a marking pen, as is the future IPG incision location (point C on Fig. 22-8). Then, the tunneling device is placed from the lateral aspect of this incision across the patient's back to the furthest point away from the connecting incision that the tunneled sheath will allow (point C to point D on Fig. 22-8), minimizing the potential for infection. For the same reason, care should be taken to course the tunnel away from the lead insertion site over the sacrum (point D to point E on Fig. 22-8), so this usually means that the intended IPG incision is on a slant. Once the distance from the connecting incision to the lead extension skin exit point has been estimated, an

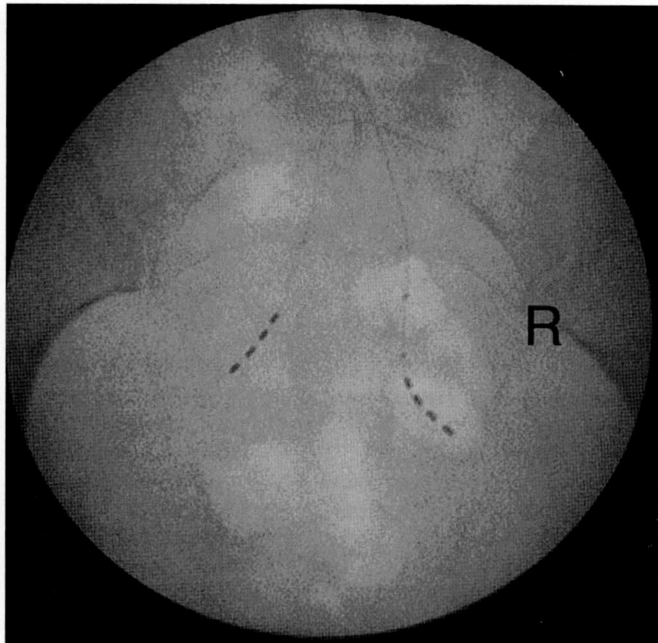

Figure 22-7 Posterior-anterior view of sacrum. The right-sided lead is taking the most appropriate course laterally. This can be achieved by directing the tip of the lead/stylet "down and out" as it is inserted through the introducer sheath. Sometimes, it is helpful to accentuate the curve of the "hockey stick" if initial deployments do not adequately track with the nerve.

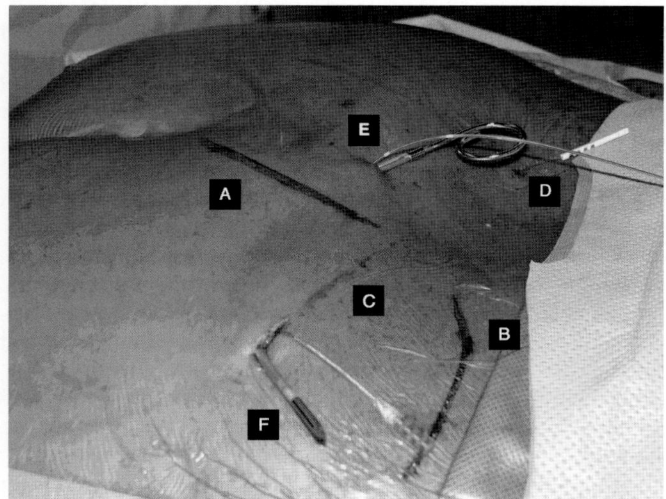

Figure 22-8 The lateral edge of the sacrum (point A) and the posterior superior iliac crest (point B) are marked. The future site of the IPG incision (point C) is marked diagonally so that the implantable pulse generator may be placed in a plane of fat away from bony prominences. The course of the lead extension allows it to exit the skin at a safe distance from the lead (point D). The lead extension is tunneled using an uncurved tunneler, allowing for the maximum tunnel length (point C to point D). The tined lead is tunneled to the lateral aspect of the connecting incision using a curved trocar (point E to point F). This takes up some of the redundant lead length and also allows for the lead to be placed in a predictable position for future reference.

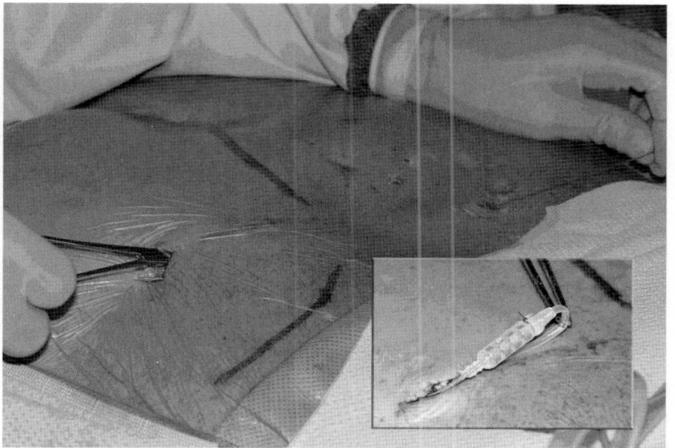

Figure 22-9 The connection hub between the lead and lead extension electrode is placed in the subcutaneous fat underneath the middle portion of the potential implantable pulse generator (IPG) incision (*inset*). This allows for its immediate location during the second-phase procedure. The plastic sheath protecting the lead extension is grasped gently with a hemostat and escorted into the fat in the direction in which it was placed. Once it is in position, the hemostat is spread and released as the lead extension is gently pulled into place. At the next phase, the connecting incision can be reopened to allow for lead removal or extended medially to allow for IPG placement.

anesthetic skin wheal can be made at the lateral aspect of the future IPG incision and at the skin exit point. A 1- to 2-cm incision is made at the connection site, taking care to make it completely through the skin into fat, preventing the lead from getting caught too superficially. The tunneler is then placed about 2 cm deep to the skin from the lateral aspect of the incision, toward the preanesthetized exit point. As long as the tunneler is kept in the fatty tissue beneath the skin, there is little sensation or discomfort during this maneuver, and only the entry and exit points require local anesthesia. The sheath is left in place, and the lead extension can be pushed through it with fingers, or it can be escorted by reinserting the tunneler or the lead introducer stylet if necessary. Next, the lead is tunneled to the lower lateral aspect of the connecting incision. (point F on Fig. 22-8). Care must be taken to be sure the presacral incision is wide (usually 0.75 cm) and deep enough to allow the tunneler to be placed without harming the lead and also to make sure that the lead is in the fat below the skin, to prevent potential infection. We typically curve the tunneling device to cause the lead to sweep down and back up toward the lateral aspect of the connecting incision (point E to point F on Fig. 22-8). This maneuver "uses up" additional length of lead, preventing redundancy at the connection site. Once the lead is coupled to the lead extension, a straight clamp is place on the tip of the plastic sleeve that extents out over the extension, and the lead is escorted in the direction of its pass into the subcutaneous fat just medial to the edge of the incision. The clamp is spread slightly and pulled away as tension is maintained at the lead extension exit site (Fig. 22-9).

This procedure sets up the connection at the medial aspect of the potential IPG site (see Fig. 22-9, insert), where it can readily be found for the next stage. If there is any redundancy of the lead, it is always looped in the fatty tissue inferior to the incision and usually will not be encountered at the next phase unless it is to be removed. The procedure is completed by irrigating with antibiotic solution, achieving final hemostasis, and closing the connecting incision with subcutaneous Vicryl. The skin of both incisions is closed with staples to avoid encountering the knot of a running subcuticular closure in the connecting incision at the time of IPG implantation, because it could not be sterilized. Patients are discharged after programming, and they return in 1 week for staple removal and reprogramming as needed. A 1-month trial period is used routinely. This is helpful in making sure that programming is optimized and for evaluating the veracity of responses in terms of the target symptoms and secondary complaints such as pain and bowel dysfunction.

Completion Phase

We schedule a completion phase procedure 4 weeks after the first stage. The exit site is draped out of the prepared field, with care to leave enough slack to allow pulling of the entire lead extension sleeve into the connecting incision. If symptoms have not been sufficiently improved, the lead is removed under MAC/local anesthesia by infiltrating the connecting incision with 0.25% Marcaine, opening the incision, and discovering the connection hub at the medial margin. It is pulled into the incision, and the lead extension electrode is cut. It will be removed completely at the end of the procedure, once the connecting incision has been closed and dressed. The lead is then pulled sharply from the connecting incision, and it usually comes without resistance. If it is pulled slowly, it tends to elongate and thin out, potentially increasing the risk of lead fracture. There is no risk of nerve injury if the lead is deployed as discussed, because the tines are all outside of the foramen. Finally, the connecting incision is closed loosely with staples to minimize the risk of infection.

Implantation of the Pulse Generator

If there has been a sufficient improvement in the target symptoms to justify IPG implantation, this is done at the completion phase. The incision in marked with a marking pen, extending medially from the 1.5-cm connection incision toward the lead exit point. An area surrounding the intended incision is marked to estimate the space for the IPG and lead extension assembly. The entire area is infiltrated with 0.25% Marcaine, creating a skin wheal over the areas to be surgically dissected. The incision is then made, and hemostasis is carefully maintained to minimize the risk of hematoma formation. The connection between the lead and lead extension is identified; the extension is cut beyond the plastic sleeve, and then it is clamped at the sleeve, allowing the housing to remain as a protection against inadvertent cautery of the lead during creation of the pocket. A subcutaneous pocket is created using cautery and blunt dissection. This should be 2 cm beneath and parallel to the skin, just large enough to comfortably house the IPG and lead assembly. Once hemostasis has been assured, the remaining housing from the previous lead extension is removed from the lead and discarded. The wound is irrigated with antibiotic solution, and the IPG and lead extension are connected to the previously placed lead, taking care to keep the connection clean and dry and to avoid overtightening of the lead extension onto the lead. The device is positioned in the pocket with its noninsulated side (the side with writing) facing up, taking care to tuck the lead and extension behind the device. This step prevents superficial migration of the connection site and also potential lead injury if a revision surgery is ever needed. The incision is closed as described for the first phase.

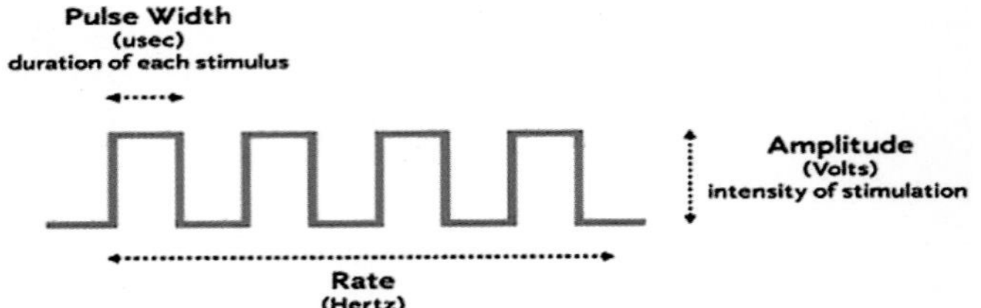

Figure 22-10 Stimulation parameters.

Programming

The goal of programming is to reproduce, with the permanent device, the same results achieved during the trial phase. This goal is greatly aided if the patient has had several weeks to test various bipolar electrode configurations with the external screening device and by the fact that the same electrode is used for the trial and permanent implantation phases when the staged trial is used. We typically do programming before discharge after outpatient placement of the IPG. The settings that were most successful during the trial phase are reproduced with the chronic device. Typical programming parameters for sacral neuromodulation include a rate of stimulation or frequency between 10 and 20 Hz and a pulse width between 180 and 240 μsec (Fig. 22-10). (Note: the manufacturer recommends a rate of 10 to 14 Hz and a pulse width of 180 to 210 μsec.[35]) The sensation of stimulation feels more like a thump at lower rates and like a flutter or buzz at higher rates. Rates of stimulation greater than 30 Hz are thought to be potentially harmful to peripheral nerves; the manufacturer more conservatively recommends not increasing the rate beyond 19 Hz.[36] Increasing the pulse width increases the pulse duration. Pulse widths greater than 270 μsec are not recommended by the manufacturer.[36] The amplitude is variable, determined by patient comfort, and based on the proximity of the lead to the nerve, as determined during lead placement. Ideally, patients should feel paresthesias at thresholds lower than 4 V, which allows for longer battery life. The patient has the ability to increase or decrease the amplitude using the hand-held programmer; in our experience, there is little risk of injury when the patient is allowed to adjust the programmer over the full range of amplitudes. Reprogramming is needed if there is decreased efficacy over time or if the patient experiences diminished or uncomfortable stimulation. Programming is either unipolar or bipolar (Fig. 22-11). A unipolar configuration is any combination of electrodes with at least one negative electrode and with the case positive (case POS, electrode NEG). In a bipolar configuration, the current flows between one negative electrode and one positive electrode (e.g., electrode 1+, 2−, case off). A change in the active (negative) electrode changes the location of the stimulation pattern. For example, deep electrodes (3−) are typically felt more anteriorly, whereas shallow electrodes (0−) are typically felt more posteriorly.

TROUBLESHOOTING

Insufficient Benefit from the First Stage of Implantation

If patients do not document sufficient improvement from baseline symptoms (usually at least 50% improvement in target symptoms), they should not go on to an IPG implantation as a

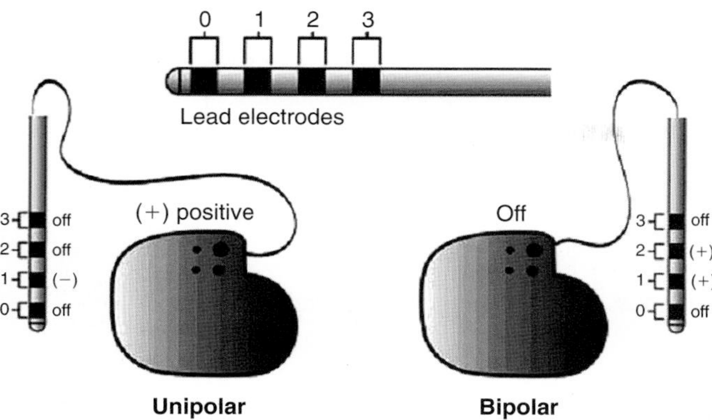

Figure 22-11 Lead electrode array and programming options.

next step. We are looking for a dramatic change in symptoms to justify the completion phase, and if there is only modest or minimal change, it is best to re-evaluate. This may require that a repeat trial phase stimulation be performed at a later date with an attempt to place the electrode on the opposite side or at another level. In our experience, bilateral stimulation has never been an adequate improvement when unilateral stimulation is not sufficiently successful. Because we would ordinarily consider a trial of SNS only in patients for whom both medical management and biofeedback have failed, further treatment options would include pudendal nerve stimulation, intravesical injection of botulinum toxin, or possible augmentation cystoplasty.

Wound Infection

If wound infection occurs, it is necessary to remove all the implanted components. We are unaware of any successful reports of salvage procedures for these devices. If the presacral incision is not fluctuant, it usually does not have to be opened to remove the lead, which can be pulled from the IPG site. It is helpful to remove the capsule that may have formed around the IPG if it has been in place for a sufficient length of time. Wounds usually need to be left open and have to heal by secondary intention. We have had much quicker resolution of wound infections using closed-suction wound systems, and consultation with enterostomal therapy for these services has been a great benefit for our patients. We give a wound infection 3 or more months to resolve completely before considering reimplantation. This would typically be done as a single-stage implantation of both the lead and the device, providing there was a sufficient benefit from the previous implantation and the lead location can be successfully duplicated.

Lack of Efficacy over Time

It is extremely important to be certain of the benefit from the trial phase stimulation. This is why we do a staged implantation as the trial procedure and give the patient a month before we move on to the next phase. Also, placing the lead under conscious sedation reduces the chance that stimulation will be uncomfortable for the patient. The care taken during lead placement—making every effort to identify the course of the nerve, and getting all four contact points in line with it, yielding typical responses at low thresholds—gives maximal flexibility for programming afterward. These steps are all helpful in minimizing the need for a future revision. It is presumed that all combinations of unipolar and bipolar stimulation configurations have been tested. Also, it is helpful to check impedances using the programming device, because this may point to a lead fracture or another problem causing an open circuit (fluid in the connection site). An AP and lateral radiographic study may be helpful in defining a lead displacement or fracture, and having the films available from the original placement is useful for comparison. It may also be helpful to turn the device off completely, letting the patient experience his or her symptoms without the benefit of neuromodulation. This step often demonstrates that the symptoms are indeed controlled to a great degree, although perhaps not completely. If the patient decides that the therapy provides insufficient benefit once both devices have been placed, it may be necessary to do a staged trial at another foramen (most often S3 on the opposite side of the originally implanted lead) and then to compare the result of the implanted system to stimulation with the externalized lead and temporary stimulation device. If there is sufficient improvement, the new lead may be connected to the previously placed IPG as a second-stage completion. If SNS cannot control the symptoms even after revision, it may be reasonable to consider pudendal nerve stimulation (currently off-label) to salvage use of the device.

Pain at the Implantation Site

If there is pain at the IPG site, it can often be improved by programming with bipolar settings. In rare instances, use of an anesthetic patch over the device or performance of a trigger point injection with local anesthesia provides relief. If the device is superficial or if it is over a bony prominence, it may need to be repositioned deeper or more lateral or inferior to the original site. On rare occasions, it is necessary to move the device to the opposite side. If repositioning is done, the previous IPG capsule needs to be excised or sufficiently scarified to minimize the risk of seroma accumulation.

Need for Magnetic Resonance Imaging

As more patients undergo implantation and patients with neurologic conditions are included as candidates for treatment with this option, the likelihood that an occasional patient with an IPG will need a magnetic resonance imaging (MRI) study increases. There is evidence that MRI can be used safely in some patients with the Medtronic InterStim device.[37] These include instances in which the site to be studied is away from the pelvis, such as in the head or upper spine, and a smaller magnet (1.5 tesla) can be used, with an open device if possible. The implanted device must be turned off for the procedure, and the patient must be able to signal to the technician if discomfort develops during the scan. The patient must also be willing to sign a waiver releasing the radiologist from liability if there is damage to the device or other complications after the study.

TREATMENT RESULTS

Treatment of OAB with SNS has been shown to be highly successful and enduring. Siegel and Catanzaro and their colleagues reported on patients who were observed 1.5 to 3 years after sacral neurostimulator implantation. At 3 years, 59% of 41 urinary

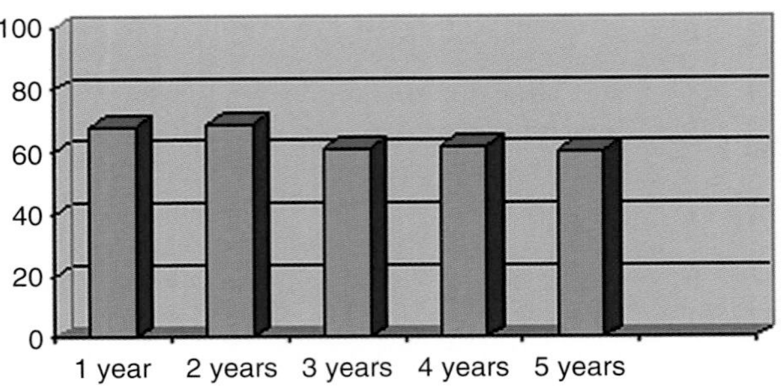

Figure 22-12 Maintained clinical success rates (percentage reporting at least a 50% improvement compared with baseline) in urge-incontinent patients for average number of leaks per day.

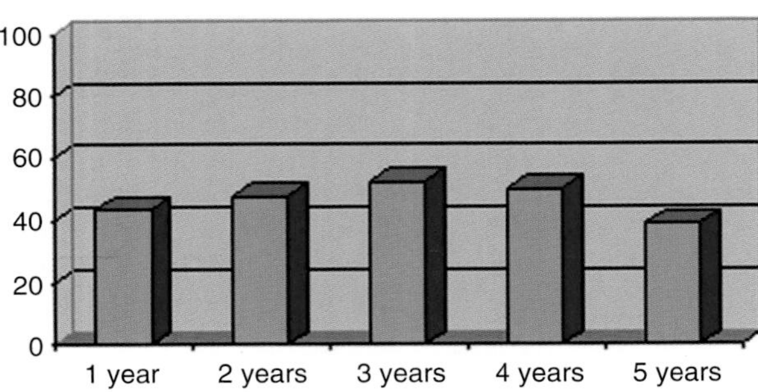

Figure 22-13 The percentage of patients with clinical success in average number of voids per day (at least 50% improvement compared with baseline) is shown for urgency-frequency patients at annual intervals after implantation.

urge-incontinent patients showed 50% or greater improvement in symptoms, including a significant reduction in the number of leakage episodes per day. Forty-six percent of patients reported being completely dry in their voiding diaries. At 2 years after implantation, 56% of the urgency-frequency patients showed at least a 50% reduction in the number of voids per day.[21]

This same cohort of patients was observed in an earlier study wherein patients were randomized to stimulated or nonstimulated groups. All patients who demonstrated a positive response to test stimulation were randomly divided into a stimulation group (25 patients) and a control group (26 patients). The SNS system was implanted into the stimulation group immediately after positive response to test stimulation and after 6 months in the control group. Patients were followed up at 1, 3, and 6 months, and then at 6-month intervals for up to 2 years after implantation. The number of daily voids, the volume voided per void, and the degree of urgency before voiding were assessed. Patients in the stimulation group reported statistically significant ($P < .0001$) improvements in 6-month voiding diary results, including average number of daily voids (from 16.9 ± 9.7 to 9.3 ± 5.1), volume per void (118 ± 74 to 226 ± 124 mL), and degree of urgency (rank of 2.2 ± 0.6 to 1.6 ± 0.9). Patients in the control group showed no significant changes in voiding parameters at 6 months. The stimulation group also reported significant improvements on quality-of-life questionnaires and water cystometry. When the neurostimulators were turned off in the stimulation group at 6 months after implantation, urinary symptoms returned to baseline values, negating the impact of any potential placebo effect. After the stimulators were turned back on, SNS was shown to be effective at 12 and 24 months after implantation.[37]

After FDA approval of electrical neurostimulation for the treatment of OAB, many of these same original (pre-approval) study patients were enrolled into a postmarket study. Additional patients were also enrolled to ensure an adequate sample size. Both groups were monitored for 5 years after implantation to assess the long-term safety and efficacy of SNS for the treatment of urgency and urgency-frequency.[38] Successful clinical treatment of patients was defined as at least 50% improvement in voiding symptoms. The average age of the patients was 45 years, and 90% were female.

Sixty patients who had been diagnosed with urgency were monitored for 5 years after implantation. This group reported significant improvement ($P < .05$) in average number of leaking episodes per day, number of heavy leakage episodes per day, average severity of leakages, and number of pads used per day (compared with baseline values) at every annual visit. By 5 years after implantation, the average number of leakages per day had decreased from 10 to 4 ($P < .0001$), with 60% of patients classified as clinically successful at 5 years (Fig. 22-12). The average number of pads used per day dropped from 5 at baseline to 2 at 5-year follow-up ($P < .0001$), with 68% deemed clinically successful, having at least 50% improvement in the number of pads used per day.

Eighteen patients with urgency-frequency were evaluated at baseline and annually for 5 years after implantation. This group reported an improvement in number of average number of voids per day, from 20 at baseline to 13 at 5-year follow-up ($P = .002$). Clinical success was defined as at least 50% improvement in number of voids per day. At 4 years after implantation, there was a 50% clinical success rate in number of voids per day, and at 5 years the rate was 39% (Fig. 22-13). The average change in degree of urgency per day was also statistically significantly improved ($P < .05$) compared with baseline at each annual visit, with the exception of the 1- and 5-year follow-up visits ($P = .06$ and $P = .10$, respectively). The clinical success rates were 74% at 3 years, 64% at 4 years, and 56% at 5 years after implantation.

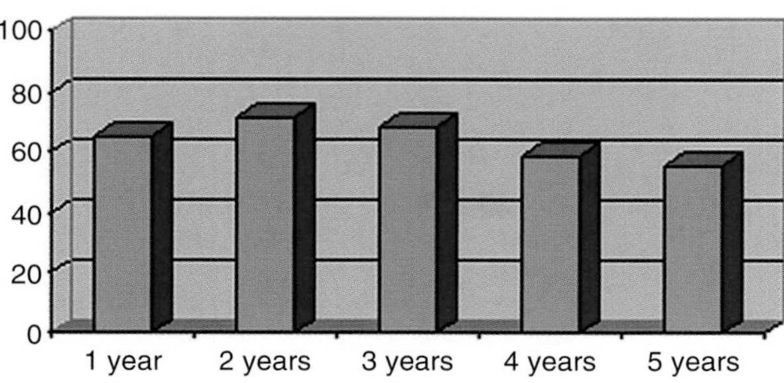

Figure 22-14 The percentage of urgency-frequency patients with clinical success (at least 50% improvement compared with baseline) in average volume per void peaked at 2 years after implantation with 71.4% clinical success. Clinical success was maintained at a reasonably acceptable level (55.6%) at 5 years after implantation.

The volume voided per void was significantly improved at each annual follow-up visit ($P = .004$), with the average volume improving from 101 to 202 mL at 5 years after implantation (Fig. 22-14). Clinical success for this measure (at least 50% improvement) was maintained long-term after SNS implantation. Results were reported as 68% clinical success at 3 years, 59% at 4 years, and 56% at 5 years.

Safety

The long-term safety of SNS has been well characterized. In the same multicenter study[38] 42% of patients required surgical intervention for a device- or therapy-related adverse event that occurred by the time they reached 5 years after implantation. The most common surgical intervention was device explant and replacement (lead, extension, or neurostimulator), which occurred in 24% of patients throughout 5 years of follow-up. If these data are recategorized to include all device- or therapy-related events that did or did not include surgical intervention, the most frequently reported event was new pain or undesirable change in stimulation, occurring in 27% of all patients. Pain at lead or IPG implantation site related to the neurostimulator was the second most common reported event, occurring in 20% of patients. During this study, the tined lead was not used for the testing phase, because it was not approved for use by the FDA until 2002. The use of a tined lead in conjunction with the SNS system can significantly reduce the invasiveness of the procedure as well as the length and depth of the incision required, making it possible to complete the procedure under local anesthesia. The patient remains alert in order to provide sensory feedback that may facilitate more accurate lead placement, leading to fewer revisions and better, more comfortable positioning of the lead.

CONCLUSIONS

SNS for intractable OAB symptoms has emerged as a standard of care and should be considered as an appropriate next step if drugs, behavioral interventions, and pelvic floor rehabilitation have provided insufficient relief. The exact mechanism of action remains unknown, but modulation of afferent nerves at several levels and manipulation of the guarding reflex are key elements in restoring a more normal balance of reflexes among the bladder, sphincter, and pelvic floor muscles. The therapy is most appropriate for OAB patients who are without underlying neuropathology, but it has been successful for a range of problems, including interstitial cystitis, idiopathic nonobstructive urinary retention, neurogenic voiding dysfunction, and fecal incontinence. A key finding on preoperative assessment is evidence of high-tone pelvic floor muscle dysfunction. It is helpful to think of conditions of voiding dysfunction in terms of behaviors, instead of using organ-based labels, and to view the first phase or application of sacral neuromodulation as a test. Urinary diaries are essential to objectively document the target symptoms before, during, and after a therapeutic trial.

We prefer to go directly to a staged lead implantation as the initial trial phase, because it allows a sufficient length of time to evaluate the therapy for a given patient, and the results of the trial using the potentially permanent electrode will most closely predict the outcome once the chronic device has been implanted. Keys to successful lead implantation include performance of the procedure under MAC/local anesthesia, which allows the patient to give sensory feedback during lead placement. Care using fluoroscopy and use of the ball-tipped stylet are essential to identifying the level and course of the appropriate sacral nerve root. It is ideal to have as many contacts as possible yielding the same responses at low thresholds, to give the most flexibility with future programming of the device. The long-term effectiveness of sacral neuromodulation for intractable OAB has been documented, and the therapy continues to undergo further refinements with the hope of improved ease of use and suitability for a host of urologic disorders. Now that the role of neuromodulatory therapies for chronic voiding dysfunction is established, new devices and alternative stimulation targets will emerge, and they will need to be compared to sacral neuromodulation as the gold standard for this treatment modality.

References

1. Abrams P, Blavais JG, Fowler CJ, et al: The role of neuromodulation in the management of urinary urge incontinence. BJU Int 91:355, 2002.
2. de Groat WC: Neuroanatomy and neurophysiology: Innervation of the lower urinary tract. In Raz S (ed): Female Urology, 2nd ed. Saunders, 1996, pp 28-42.
3. Leng WW, Chancellor MB: How sacral nerve stimulation neuromodulation works. Urol Clin North Am 32:11, 2005.
4. Somogyi GT, de Groat WC: Modulation of the release of ^{3}H-norepinephrine from the base and body of the rat urinary bladder by endogenous adrenergic and cholinergic mechanisms. J Pharmacol Exp Ther 255:244, 1990.

5. Somogyi GT, de Groat WC: Evidence for inhibitory nicotinic and facilitatory muscarinic receptors in cholinergic nerve terminals of the rat urinary bladder. J Auton Nerv Syst 37:89, 1992.
6. Somogyi GT, Tanowitz M, de Groat WC: Evidence for facilitatory α_1 adrenoceptors on nerve terminals of the rat urinary bladder. Soc Neurosci Abstr 18:252, 1992.
7. de Groat WC, Araki I, Vizzard MA, et al: Developmental and injury induced plasticity in the micturition reflex pathway. Behav Brain Res 92:127, 1997.
8. de Groat WC, Vizzard MA, Araki I, Roppolo J: Spinal interneurons and preganglionic neurons in sacral autonomic reflex pathways. Prog Brain Res 107:97, 1996.
9. Keast JR, de Groat WC: Immunohistochemical characterization of pelvic neurons which project to the bladder, colon or penis in rats. J Comp Neurol 288:387, 1989.
10. Zoubek JA, Somogyi GT, de Groat WC: A comparison of inhibitory effects of neuropeptide Y on rat urinary bladder, urethra and vas deferens. Am J Physiol 265:R537, 1993.
11. de Groat WC: Spinal cord projections and neuropeptides in visceral afferent neurons. Prog Brain Res 67:165, 1986.
12. de Groat WC, Ryall RW: The identification and antidromic responses of sacral preganglionic parasympathetic neurons. J Physiol (Lond) 196:533, 1968.
13. de Groat WC: Changes in the organization of the micturition reflex pathway of the cat after transection of the spinal cord. Exp Neurol 71:22, 1981.
14. de Groat WC: Nervous control of the urinary bladder of the cat. Brain Res 87:201, 1975.
15. de Groat WC: Mechanisms underlying recurrent inhibition in the sacral parasympathetic outflow to the urinary bladder. J Physiol 257:503, 1976.
16. de Groat WC, Nadelhaft I, Milne RJ, et al: Organization of the sacral parasympathetic reflex pathways to the urinary bladder and large intestine. J Auton Nerv Syst 3:135, 1981.
17. Shaker HS, Hassouna M: Sacral nerve root neuromodulation: An effective treatment for refractory urge incontinence. J Urol 159:1516, 1998.
18. Kruse MN, de Groat WC: Spinal pathways mediate coordinator bladder/urethral sphincter activity during reflex micturition in normal and spinal cord injured neonatal rats. Neurosci Lett 152:141, 1993.
19. Kruse MN, Noto H, Roppolo JR, et al : Pontine control of the urinary bladder and external urethral sphincter in the rat. Brain Res 532:182, 1990.
20. de Groat WC, Theobald RJ: Reflex activation of sympathetic pathways to vesical smooth muscle and parasympathetic ganglia by electrical stimulation of vesical afferents. J Physiol 259:223, 1976.
21. Siegel SW, Catanzaro F, Dijkema HE, et al: Long-term results of a multi-center study on sacral nerve stimulation for treatment of urinary urge incontinence, urgency-frequency, and retention. Urology 56(6 Suppl 1):87, 2000.
22. Personal discussion, sacral nerve stimulation study group and Medtronic, Inc, 1993.
23. Bosch JLHR, Groen J: Sacral nerve neuromodulation in the treatment of patients with refractory motor urge incontinence: Long-term results of a prospective longitudinal study. J Urol 163:1219, 2000.
24. Lukban JC, Whitmore KE, Sant GR: Current management of interstitial cystitis. Urol Clin North Am 29:649, 2002.
25. Everaert K, Devulder J, De Mynck M, et al: The pain cycle: implications for the diagnosis and treatment of pelvic pain syndromes. Int Urogynecol J Pelvic Floor Dysfunct 12:9, 2001.
26. Siegel S, Paszkiewicz E, Kirkpatrick C, et al: Sacral nerve stimulation in patients with chronic intractable pelvic pain. J Urol 166:1742, 2001.
27. Comiter CV: Sacral neuromodulation for the symptomatic treatment of refractory interstitial cystitis: A prospective study. J Urol 169:1369, 2003.
28. Peters KM, Carey JM, Konstandt DB: Sacral neuromodulation for the treatment of refractory interstitial cystitis: Outcomes based on technique. Int Urogynecol J Pelvic Floor Dysfunct 14:223, 2003.
29. Peters KM, Konstadt D: Sacral neuromodulation decreases narcotic requirements in refractory interstitial cystitis. BJU Int 93:777, 2004.
30. Siegel SW: Pelvic neuromodulation: Selecting patients for sacral nerve stimulation. Urol Clin North Am 32:196, 2005.
31. Brindley GS, Polkey CE, Rushton DN, et al : Sacral anterior root stimulators for bladder control in paraplegia: The first 50 cases. J Neurol Neurosurg Psychiatry 49:1104, 1986.
32. Schmidt RA: Application of neurostimulation in urology. Neurourol Urodyn 7:585, 1988.
33. Schmidt RA: Treatment of pelvic pain with neuroprosthesis. J Urol 129:227A, 1988.
34. Tanagho EA: Electrical stimulation. J Am Geriatr Soc 38:352, 1990.
35. Medtronic InterStim Technical Manual, 2002.
36. Elkelini MS, Hassouna MM: Safety of MRI at 1.5 Tesla in patients with implanted sacral nerve neurostimulator. Eur Urol 50:311, 2006.
37. Hassouna MM, Siegel SW, Nyeholt AA, et al: Sacral neuromodulation in the treatment of urgency-frequency symptoms: A multicenter study on efficacy and safety. J Urol 163:1849, 2000.
38. van Kerrebroeck PE, van Voskuilen AC, Heesakkers JP, et al: Five-year results of sacral neuromodulation therapy for urinary voiding dysfunction: Outcomes of a prospective, worldwide clinical study. J Urol 178:2029, 2007.

Chapter 23

POSTERIOR TIBIAL NERVE STIMULATION FOR PELVIC FLOOR DYSFUNCTION

Matthew R. Cooperberg and Marshall L. Stoller

SCOPE OF THE PROBLEM

Pelvic floor dysfunction (PFD) is a highly prevalent functional disorder, affecting both women and men, which may manifest in diverse clinical symptoms including urinary frequency, urgency with or without incontinence, and/or retention, as well as rectal incontinence and pelvic pain. Overactive bladder (OAB), a constellation of symptoms defined by "urgency, with or without urge incontinence, usually with frequency and nocturia,"[1] is one of the most common manifestations of PFD, and it the best-studied epidemiologically. OAB affects approximately 16.5% of adult men and women in population-based studies conducted in both the United States[2] and Europe.[3] Some 9.3% of women and 2.6% of men, respectively, suffer from OAB associated with urge incontinence.[2] These figures translate to an estimated 33 million affected adults in the United States alone, a prevalence similar to that of other major chronic conditions such as hypertension and heart disease.[4] The global costs of treating OAB are estimated at $12 to $17 billion per year, comparable to those attributed to pneumonia, osteoporosis, or arthritis.[2,5]

Pharmaceutical remedies for urinary complaints referable to PFD remain suboptimal due to a high incidence of side effects, relatively modest efficacy, poor patient compliance, and high long-term costs. Surgical procedures described to date do not work well for most cases of PFD featuring a prominent urge component; moreover, surgery may not be a suitable option for the many PFD patients who are elderly and faced with multiple medical comorbidities. Many studies using various measures have found that urge incontinence affects patients' health-related quality of life (QOL) to a greater extent than does stress incontinence[6-8]; nevertheless, in part due to dissatisfaction with treatment alternatives and/or a public perception of unsatisfactory treatment outcomes, OAB often goes unrecognized and undermanaged. In the United States, only 25% of OAB patients surveyed (40% of those with incontinence) had seen a physician for management of bladder symptoms in the past year.[4]

Urologists have long recognized PFD as a root source of diverse voiding complaints, but many patients with concomitant constipation would seek referral for treatment of constipation before a definitive evaluation for voiding dysfunction. Gastroenterologists, in turn, might advise patients to have their urinary problems corrected before offering a definitive opinion and treatment for constipation. Gynecologists faced with a patient with chronic pelvic pain and urinary or fecal continence issues may refer the patient for management of these problems before addressing the pain itself. In many cases, these apparently disparate problems are in fact interrelated manifestations of the common functional problem of PFD.

Recent reports have provided additional evidence for epidemiologic associations among urinary incontinence and other PFD-related complaints such as incontinence of flatus and/or feces and prolapse symptoms.[9] PFD probably also plays a significant role in the pathophysiology of female sexual disorders.[10] In recent years, novel approaches for the treatment of both OAB and other manifestations of PFD have been the subject of growing interest; one of the most promising such approaches is percutaneous neurostimulation as a means of modulation of the sacral outflow tract to the pelvic floor.

PERCUTANEOUS NEUROMODULATION: RATIONALE AND THEORETICAL MECHANISM

Many groups over the past 20 years have focused efforts on stimulation of the S2 through S4 nerve roots at their origin from the sacral cord. Various techniques of central stimulation have been used successfully to treat OAB, pelvic pain, sphincteric incompetence, detrusor hyporeflexia, and idiopathic urinary retention.[11] Central sacral neuromodulation is successful for many patients with PFD[12] and has been shown to improve urinary function by both urodynamic and quality-of-life parameters.[13] This modality, however, has significant drawbacks. Placement of the stimulator is invasive: the system requires trial runs with percutaneous needles placed through the sacral foramina to access the cord for up to 1 week and ultimately requires a general anesthesia for permanent stimulator implantation. Among patients with a successful response to initial lead placement, as many as 20% to 51% do not enjoy similar long-term success with permanent implantation. Moreover, the complication rate varies from 22% to 43%, and up to 50% of patients receiving sacral neurostimulators eventually require reoperation.[14] Lead migration is a late complication that continues to limit the long-term efficacy of the central approach even in contemporary reports.[15]

Various approaches to minimally invasive neuromodulation have been tested, including perineal muscle stimulation for stress urinary incontinence; perineal nerve stimulation via the dorsal nerve of the penis for detrusor hyperreflexia; peripudendal percutaneous neural stimulation; and direct cutaneous stimulation of perineal, perianal, or perivaginal skin for the management of urge incontinence. The proliferation of these novel approaches to minimally invasive neuromodulation of the pelvic floor underscores the limitations of the more invasive central stimulation techniques. One of the most promising new approaches for multiple PFD-related complaints involves percutaneous posterior tibial nerve stimulation (PTNS).

The posterior tibial nerve is a mixed somatic/motor nerve containing fibers originating from spinal roots L4 through S3. These roots comprise the outflow of the sacral nerves, which modulate the somatic and autonomic nervous supply to the pelvic floor, innervating the bladder and urinary sphincter. Initial studies of potential approaches to peripheral neuromodulation of the sacral cord measured skin impedance at various points along the S2 and S3 dermatomes and identified a consistent area of high impedance above the medial malleolus. This area overlies the posterior tibial nerve and corresponds to the *sanyinjiao*, or Sp-6 (spleen-6) acupuncture point. In acupuncture practice, Sp-6 has been targeted for management of a variety of urinary complaints, as well as to stimulate labor and alleviate labor pain; traditional acupuncture at this point previously has been shown to produce transient improvements in urodynamic parameters.[16]

The precise mechanism by which neurostimulation, central or peripheral, exerts its influence on pelvic floor function remains unclear. In particular, conflicting data exist as to whether peripheral neurostimulation exerts a facilitative or inhibitory effect on urinary system neural pathways. Repetitive PTNS exerts a strong inhibitory effect on nociceptive spinothalamic tract neurons in primate studies, especially at high frequencies of stimulation, via activation of myelinated Aδ fibers.[17] Primate data from the University of California at San Francisco (UCSF) demonstrated inhibition and even elimination of uninhibited bladder contractions during PTNS.[18] In a feline model, on the other hand, S2 stimulation induced excitatory bladder effects at lower amperage and complete bladder inhibition at higher intensities.[19] Peripheral afferent nerve stimulation in vivo abolished inappropriate detrusor contractions while leaving the normal micturition reflex intact. The therapeutic effect tended to increase with repetitive weekly treatments over 2 to 3 months.

One theory suggests that posterior PTNS results in improved blood flow to the pelvis. As yet unpublished data from UCSF, for example, found, among a cohort of five men with complete erectile dysfunction, that peripheral neurostimulation yielded an immediate doubling in cavernosal arterial diameter (from a mean of 3.8 mm to 7.5 mm) and velocity (from a mean 11 cm/sec to 20 cm/sec).

Another mechanistic hypothesis suggests that neurostimulation effects a change in the neurochemical environment along the sacral pathways. Chang and colleagues,[20] for example, studied expression of FOS protein, a marker for noxious stimulation of cell growth, in the rat spinal micturition center (L6-S2). Among normal animals, 0 to 4 cells per section at L6 were FOS-positive. After a standardized noxious insult to the rat bladder (1% acetic acid), FOS expression increased to a mean of 76 cells per section. A single 25-minute session of percutaneous neurostimulation at Sp-6 administered 1 hour before acetic acid infusion reduced FOS expression by 73%, to a mean of 20 cells per section.[20]

EARLY EXPERIENCES WITH PERIPHERAL NEUROSTIMULATION

In 1983, McGuire and associates reported their "astonishingly good" results from transcutaneous tibial nerve stimulation (TTNS) applied via an adhesive electrode to 22 patients with a range of urologic diagnoses including detrusor instability, interstitial cystitis, radiation cystitis, and neurogenic bladder. Eight of 11 patients with detrusor instability were judged "dry" after TTNS, as assessed by urodynamics and cystography; two patients with multiple sclerosis were "improved," four of five neurogenic bladder patients were likewise "dry" and one "improved," and four of six cystitis patients experienced some degree of improvement.[21] These early data, although not rigorously collected or reported, certainly indicated the potential utility of peripheral neurostimulation for bladder symptoms.

Based on experience with central neuromodulation both at UCSF[12] and elsewhere, and in the hope of reaching a larger patient population, the Stoller Afferent Nerve Stimulator (SANS) was introduced 4 years later, offering a method for PTNS that would be minimally invasive and less expensive.

The application of PTNS, like that of other neuromodulatory strategies, requires a cooperative patient with a morphologically intact urinary tract, a preserved sacral spinal reflex center, a low degree of peripheral denervation of the pelvic floor striated musculature, and the ability to void spontaneously or via self-catheterization without electrical stimulus.[11] Pretreatment testing mirrors the standard workup for refractory OAB symptoms and includes urinalysis and urine culture, formal urodynamic profiling, and cystoscopy to rule out foreign bodies or anatomic or urothelial abnormalities explaining the symptoms.

For each PTNS session, the patient sits in a frog-leg position, and solid 34-gauge needles are placed bilaterally, three fingerbreadths (6 cm) superior to the medial malleolus. The needles are advanced to a depth of approximately 4 cm, angling posterior to the tibia and about 30 degrees cephalad. The trajectory points toward a potential needle exit anterior to the fibula. A grounding electrode (e.g., an adhesive electrocardiogram pad) is also applied on each side, ipsilaterally overlying the medial calcaneus. Electrical stimulation is typically administered from a battery-powered generator, at an amplitude just beneath the sensory threshold of 0.5 to 10 mA, with a fixed pulse width of 200 μsec and a fixed frequency of 20 Hz. Appropriate needle localization is verified by great toe plantar flexion or fanning of digits 2 through 5 in response to an initial higher amplitude stimulation. If the patient prefers, for increased comfort after the needles are applied, he or she may shift to a more comfortable position (i.e., out of frog-leg position), taking care not to dislodge the needles.

Continued stimulation is applied for 30 minutes, only on the side with the more pronounced response to the test pulse. However, both needles are left in situ during treatment. Sessions are repeated weekly for at least 10 to 12 weeks. Patients complete voiding and pain diaries; if they experience improvement in their symptoms, the frequency of therapy is tapered gradually to every 3 or 4 weeks. Some patients have been treated continuously for up to 10 years with sessions every 4 to 6 weeks, achieving sustained symptomatic relief but consistently experiencing relapse of symptoms when the SANS sessions are stopped for prolonged periods. Patients may experience transient discomfort at the initial skin puncture site, but there is minimal if any pain with needle advancement through the deeper tissues. No patient in our experience has complained of pain during the stimulation session.

In the initial UCSF experience over several years among 98 patients with urinary frequency, incontinence, and pelvic pain treated in weekly sessions for 12 weeks, diurnal frequency episodes fell from 19 to 8 per day, nocturia episodes from 5.5 to 2.5 per night, and pain from 6.9 to 1.9 on a scale of zero to 10. Among the 22 patients complaining primarily of urgency and urge incontinence, 80% had at least a 75% reduction in incontinence, and 45% were completely dry.[22]

RECENT EVIDENCE

PTNS trials reported as of February 2005 are summarized in Table 23-1. Klingler and coworkers were the first European group to report results, having treated 15 OAB patients (11 women) with 12 weekly SANS sessions. They documented follow-up at a mean of 11 months. All patients enjoyed a reduction in pelvic pain (statistically significant reduction in visual analogue scale from a mean of 7.6 to 3.1). Mean diurnal frequency fell from 16.1 to 4.4 episodes, and nocturnal frequency from 8.3 to 1.4 episodes. Seven patients (47%) were considered to have complete responses (≤8 voids/day, ≤2 voids/night, subjective "cure"); three (20%) were improved (8 to 10 voids/day, >2 voids/night, subjective "cure"); and five (33%) failed to respond (>10 voids/day, >2 voids/night, subjective "unchanged"). Significant increases were seen in bladder capacity measurements; maximum flow rate and maximum detrusor pressure decreased somewhat. This study is the only one to date to report cost data. SANS treatment for each patient cost €895 (US$770), compared to €10,290 (US$8849) for implantation of the Medtronic InterStim device.[23]

Three centers in the Netherlands collectively enrolled 49 patients (34 female, 15 male) over a 5-month period; 37 enrollees had OAB, and 12 had nonobstructive retention (detrusor hypocontractility urodynamically confirmed). Patients were treated

Table 23-1 Trials of Percutaneous Tibial Nerve Stimulation

First Author and Ref. No.	Year	Primary Symptoms	*N*	Criteria	Key Findings
Stoller[22]	1998	Frequency, incontinence, pelvic pain	98	Decrease in frequency, pain	Statistically significant improvement in diurnal and nocturnal frequency; 80% of patients had 75% reduction in incontinence
Klingler[23]	2000	OAB	15	Urgency, voiding diary, urodynamics, pelvic pain	>50% reduction in mean pelvic pain score; decrease in mean diurnal and nocturnal frequency from 16 and 4 episodes to 8 and 1 episodes, respectively
Govier[29]	2001	Refractory OAB	53	>25% reduction in diurnal/nocturnal voiding frequency	71% of patients met success criteria ($P < .05$)
Van Balken[24]	2001	OAB, nonobstructive retention	49	Frequency, nocturia, voided volumes, HRQOL	OAB patients: mean 17% reduction in frequency, 38% reduction in nocturia; increased voided volumes; improved HRQOL. Retention patients: modest, nonsignificant improvements in voided volumes and catheterization episodes
Vadoninck[26]	2003	OAB	90	Frequency, incontinence, HRQOL, urodynamics	Decrease in 24-hour frequency from 13 to 10 and in incontinence episodes from 5 to 2 daily; improved bladder capacity but no overall improvement in detrusor instability
Vandoninck[25]	2003	Urge incontinence	35	Incontinence episodes, frequency, nocturia, HRQOL, pad use	Median incontinence episodes per day reduced from 5 to 1; 16 patients completely dry; significant decreases in nocturia and pad use and improvements in HRQOL
Vandoninck[27,28]	2003	Nonobstructive urinary retention	39	Daily catheterizations, residual volume, voided volume, HRQOL	Decrease in mean catheterizations from 2.5 to 2.0 and in residual volume from 241 to 163 mL; improvements in HRQOL, especially incontinence-specific QOL.
Van Balken[34]	2003	Chronic pelvic pain	33	Visual analogue pain scale, HRQOL	≥50% reduction in pain score in 21% of patients, 25%-50% reduction in 18%; improved SF-36 scores
Shafik[36]	2003	Fecal incontinence	32	HRQOL questionnaire, rectometric parameters	Improvement in 78% of patients by fecal incontinence questionnaire
Congregado Ruiz[45]	2004	Frequency/urgency, urge incontinence	51	HRQOL, voiding diaries	Statistically significant improvements in frequency/urgency, HRQOL, and pain

HRQOL, health-related quality of life; OAB, overactive bladder; QOL, quality of life.

with 12 weeks of SANS. The results were positive and statistically significant[24] but considerably more modest than those reported by Klingler and colleagues.[23] Among the OAB cohort, diurnal frequency was reduced by an average of 2.8 episodes, to 16.5 times per day, and nocturnal frequency was reduced by 1 to 2.6 episodes per night. Voided volumes were also increased, and patients reported significant improvements in both general and incontinence-specific health-related QOL. Among the patients with retention, mean voided volumes increased slightly, and number of catheterizations decreased, but these findings were not significant.[24]

The same group later expanded to five sites in the Netherlands and one in Italy and has published three additional papers, focusing, respectively, on urge incontinence,[25] OAB,[26] and nonobstructive retention.[27] A total of 164 patients were treated. Vandoninck and coworkers reported the largest single cohort of patients treated with PTNS to date, accruing 90 consecutive OAB patients (67 female, 23 male) to 12 weekly stimulation sessions. The 24-hour frequency decreased from a mean of 13 to 10 episodes, leakage episodes decreased from a mean of 5 to 2 daily, and mean voided volume increased from 135 to 191 mL (all statistically significant results). Health-related QOL scores also improved significantly. Among 46 patients undergoing urodynamic profiling both before and after PTNS, mean cystometric bladder capacity increased from 243 to 340 mL. The proportion of patients with detrusor instability (70%) did not change, but the volume at which instability was triggered increased from 133 to 210 mL. Also of note, improvement in urodynamic parameters significantly predicted treatment success in terms of subjective improvement.[26]

Thirty-five patients (25 women) with documented urge incontinence received the same 12 weeks of PTNS and had, on average, more dramatic responses. The median baseline number of incontinence episodes was 5 per day. After treatment, this median fell to 1 episode per day, and 16 patients had no leakage episodes. Nocturia likewise decreased from a median of 2 to 1 per night, and pad use declined from a median of 3.5 daily to none. Health-related QOL once again improved. Thirty-one percent of these patients decreased their 24-hour voiding frequency to eight episodes or less. There was a trend toward greater likelihood of subjective improvement with increased stimulation intensity in terms of amperage.[25]

Finally, these authors accrued 39 patients (27 women) with chronic nonobstructive urinary retention to 12 weeks of PTNS. The mean number of catheterizations decreased from 2.5 to 2.0 per day, and the mean catheterized (residual) volume decreased from 241 to 163 mL; the total voided volume increased accordingly. Forty-one percent of patients had a 50% or greater reduction in catheterized volume. Seven patients reduced their catheterization frequency to once daily; two of these patients had no residual urine on frequency-volume charts, but no patient became consistently catheter-free. Once again, both overall and incontinence-specific health-related QOL increased significantly. Contrary to this group's experience with urge-incontinence patients, however, increased amperage in urinary retention patients *decreased* the likelihood of positive subjective success.[27] In a companion paper focusing on urodynamic findings in this cohort, the authors reported that, on multivariate analysis, four pretreatment urodynamic parameters—maximal detrusor pressure, maximal flow rate, bladder voiding efficacy, and bladder contractility index—predicted subjective success on PTNS, with an area under the curve of 0.73.[28]

In the United States, only one experience with PTNS has been reported to date. Govier and associates reported their results from a prospective, multicenter trial at five medical centers, including 53 patients (48 women, mean age 57 years) with OAB refractory to all standard treatments, which they treated with weekly bilateral SANS sessions. Eighty-nine percent of patients completed the 12-session study. Seventy-one percent of patients met the study goal of at least a 25% reduction in diurnal and/or nocturnal urinary frequency, with the mean reductions in diurnal, nocturnal, 24-hour, and excess (>10 episodes/day) frequency being 25%, 21%, 22%, and 70%, respectively (all $P < .05$). On standardized questionnaires administered during the study, study participants reported a mean 35% improvement in urge incontinence episodes, a 30% improvement in pain, and a 20% improvement in incontinence-related QOL (all $P < .05$). The authors did not report longer-term efficacy results. There were no serious adverse events. One patient each experienced moderate pain at the needle site, moderate right foot pain, and stomach discomfort; all of these symptoms resolved spontaneously.[29]

None of these studies examined either survey- or urodynamics-based *acute* effects of PTNS. One paper, however, reported on the acute urodynamic effects of TTNS in 44 patients with OAB. During stimulation, mean first involuntary detrusor contraction occurred at 232 mL of filling, compared with 163 mL at baseline. Maximum cystometric capacity likewise increased, from 221 to 277 mL. Only 50% of these patients had an acute positive response during stimulation in terms of either increased volume at first involuntary detrusor contraction or total cystometric capacity.[30]

PTNS FOR NONURINARY MANIFESTATIONS OF PELVIC FLOOR DYSFUNCTION

To date, PTNS has been studied primarily in patients with OAB, urge incontinence, and detrusor hypocontractility. However, increasing evidence supports the use of this modality for other indications referable to PFD, many of which have been previously validated in studies of central stimulation. Van Balken and coworkers treated 33 patients (22 male) who had chronic pelvic pain with 12 weeks of PTNS. Twenty-one percent of these patients experienced at least 50% improvement in pain as assessed by the visual analogue scale; an additional 18% experienced improvement of 25% to 50%. Among the 14 (42%) subjective responders (i.e., those who requested continued treatment), the mean pain score fell from 5.9 (range, 4.5 to 7.3) to 3.7 (range, 2.7 to 5.2). The authors also reported improvement in several domains of the Medical Outcomes Study Short Form-36 (SF-36), including role physical, physical functioning, pain, change of health, and overall score.[31]

Andrews and Reynard reported a single case of a patient with detrusor hyperreflexia resulting from a T8 spinal cord injury whose bladder capacity doubled, from 150 to 165 mL at baseline to 310 to 320 mL with PTNS.[32] Finally, Shafik and colleagues applied 4 weeks of PTNS treatment using the SANS device every other day to 32 patients (22 women) with fecal incontinence refractory to standard treatments, which was caused either by uninhibited rectal contractions (26 patients) or by anal sphincter relaxation (6 patients). They reported improvement in 78%; after treatment, eight patients relapsed, and six of these responded to repeated PTNS therapy.[33]

Further tangential evidence for the efficacy of PTNS in the management of nonurinary PFD symptoms can be found in small studies of traditional acupuncture and acupressure treatments at the Sp-6 site. Acupuncture at this point has been shown to stimulate labor and to ameliorate labor pains[34]; acupressure has been used for symptoms of acute cystitis, and it was used successfully to alleviate the pain of primary dysmenorrhea in the majority of a cohort of young women.[35] For this latter indication, growing evidence supports the use of transcutaneous neurostimulation at Sp-6 and other sites for greater efficacy.[36]

Box 23-1 Key Advantages of Percutaneous Tibial Nerve Stimulation

- Efficacy is comparable to gold-standard pharmaceutical treatment.
- Nerve stimulation has a minimal side effect profile.
- The approach is cost-effective.
- PTNS does not preclude central neuromodulation or other treatments.

CONCLUSIONS AND FUTURE DIRECTIONS

In a recent review of various techniques of neurostimulation, central and peripheral, for bladder dysfunction, Van Balken and colleagues estimated the overall intent-to-treat success of these modalities at 30% to 50%.[37] Results achieved to date with PTNS should be considered in relation to anticholinergic medications, which constitute the "gold standard" treatment for many of the symptoms related to PFD.

In the largest trial to date of women with OAB, Swift and associates[41] reported on 417 women treated with extended-release tolterodine. They found a 53% reduction in incontinence episodes, from a mean of 3.2 to 1.5 per day, and a 16% drop in 24-hour frequency, from 10.8 to 9.0 voids. These results were statistically significantly better than those realized among the 410 women treated with placebo, whose incontinence episodes and 24-hour frequency fell by 30% and 12%, respectively. The results of Vandoninck and colleagues, described earlier, compare favorably, with a 60% reduction in incontinence episodes and a 23% drop in frequency.[26] The increase in mean voided volume was likewise higher with PTNS (from 135 to 191 mL, for a 41% increase)[26] and with tolterodine (from 141 to 179 mL, for a 26% increase) than with placebo (from 136 to 149 mL, for a 10% increase).[41] Although the PTNS studies were less rigorously designed and less powerful statistically than the larger pharmaceutical trials, it should be stressed that PTNS studies universally have been conducted among patients whose PFD symptoms are refractory to standard therapy, including oral anticholinergic medications; the results of PTNS might therefore be better still among unselected, treatment-naïve cohorts, who have et to be treated with neurostimulation in the context of a published study.

Side effects of treatment are an important further consideration. Twenty-five percent of patients taking extended-release tolterodine complained of dry mouth, 40% of whom had moderate or severe symptoms. There was also a statistically significant increase in abdominal pain with extended-release tolterodine versus placebo (4.3% vs 1.7%).[38] In contrast, no major complications of PTNS have been reported in any of the studies published to date; indeed, even minor complications, such as persistent puncture site bleeding or pain, appear to be consistently rare. Puncture site infection has never been reported. PTNS may also be more cost-effective than chronic oral medication; Klinger reported a cost of $770 for 12 weeks of PTNS and reported sustained improvement in voiding parameters at a mean of 11 months of follow-up.[23] By comparison, 11 months of tolterodine treatment would cost about $1030.[39] Finally, if percutaneous neuromodulation fails, patients may still potentially benefit from central sacral neuromodulation; in pursuing a trial of PTNS, no bridges have been burned with respect to eligibility for or potential success of central stimulation. The principal advantages of PTNS are summarized in Box 23-1.

An implantable device currently under development, named the Urgent-SQ (Cystomedix, Andover, MN), combines the benefits of chronic, at-home therapy—currently offered only by the InterStim sacral stimulator—with the relatively low cost and minimal invasiveness of peripherally targeted neuromodulation. In an ongoing trial, patients with OAB, urge incontinence, and/or functional bladder retention who demonstrate successful responses to percutaneous neuromodulation will receive the Urgent-SQ implant, which consists of a small (<4 cm), round, implantable receiver incorporating an electrode placed under the perineurium of the posterior tibial nerve and a radiofrequency generator that can be worn externally on the lower leg (e.g., under a pant leg). The Urgent-SQ could be implanted with less morbidity than devices targeting the sacral cord; moreover, implantation in the ankle would be less emotionally challenging to patients than a device targeting the perineum or perirectal area, for example. This system would empower the patient to self-administer neurostimulation on an as-needed basis and to increase or decrease the frequency of treatment based on changes in his or her environment. Centrally placed neurostimulators are usually continuously activated, whereas PTNS has to date been administered intermittently. Whether continuous or intermittent stimulation is more effective in the context of a peripheral implantable device is unknown. In either case, however, an implantable device would certainly be expected to reduce the required frequency of physician visits.

A number of caveats must be raised with respect to the literature published to date on peripheral neuromodulation. Patient inclusion and exclusion criteria have been variable, as have been the metrics used to measure responses and the parameters to establish success. Published studies have reported wide variations in degrees of success, even when they used relatively objective measures such as diary-assessed frequency or incontinence episodes. A need clearly exists for randomized, sham-controlled trials using standardized, validated health-related QOL questionnaires in addition to diaries and urodynamic studies. Although urodynamics offers a measure of objectivity, it may not necessarily correlate with the health-related QOL outcomes most relevant to the patient. Sham-controlled trials could certainly be undertaken, with the "control" group treated either with needle placement but no stimulation or with needle placement and stimulation at a location removed somewhat from the properly targeted position; this was done successfully in at least one trial of transcutaneous neurostimulation.[40] Crossover designs would also be useful. Given the extremely good tolerability of PTNS, such trial designs should be ethically acceptable.

Peripheral neuromodulation is a technology still in the relatively early stages of development. How much additional benefit may be realized beyond 12 treatment sessions and the ultimate durability of responses are among the questions about PTNS that have not yet been answered definitively. Although most research in the field has been reported only in the past few years, with few long-term data available, the results to date are exciting. Even if the initial response rates for PTNS are in fact lower than those for central neurostimulation, given the negligible risks and morbidity reported with PTNS, it would seem reasonable to offer this modality to all eligible patients, with those who do not respond remaining candidates for central sacral treatment. The anticipated availability of a peripherally implanted device offers the possibility of patient-controlled, chronic peripheral stimulation, which may produce even greater gains in the treatment of intractable PFD symptoms.

As described earlier, management of symptoms attributed to PFD already accounts for a large fraction of physician visits, with health care expenditures comparable to those of other major chronic ailments. Owing in large part to the aging of the population, demand for PFD management is expected to rise by an additional 45% over the next 30 years.[41] The high prevalence of undiagnosed PFD, discussed earlier, has left a large and growing reservoir of untreated patients, for whom the least invasive successful therapeutic modality would provide the best management. The ultimate standing of neuromodulation will be measured by its success in treating the diverse manifestations of PFD among those countless patients who need better options for improvement of their QOL.[45]

References

1. Abrams P, Cardozo L, Fall M, et al: The standardisation of terminology in lower urinary tract function: Report from the standardisation sub-committee of the International Continence Society. Urology 61:37, 2003.
2. Stewart WF, Van Rooyen JB, Cundiff GW, et al: Prevalence and burden of overactive bladder in the United States. World J Urol 20:327, 2003.
3. Milsom I, Abrams P, Cardozo L, et al: How widespread are the symptoms of an overactive bladder and how are they managed? A population-based prevalence study. BJU Int 87:760, 2001.
4. Tubaro A: Defining overactive bladder: Epidemiology and burden of disease. Urology 64(6 Suppl 1):2, 2004.
5. Hu TW, Wagner TH, Bentkover JD, et al: Estimated economic costs of overactive bladder in the United States. Urology 61:1123, 2003.
6. Coyne KS, Zhou Z, Thompson C, et al: The impact on health-related quality of life of stress, urge and mixed urinary incontinence. BJU Int 92:731, 2003.
7. Hunskaar S, Vinsnes A: The quality of life in women with urinary incontinence as measured by the sickness impact profile. J Am Geriatr Soc 39:378, 1991.
8. Hannestad YS, Rortveit G, Sandvik H, et al: A community-based epidemiological survey of female urinary incontinence: The Norwegian EPINCONT study. Epidemiology of Incontinence in the County of Nord-Trondelag. J Clin Epidemiol 53:1150, 2000.
9. Uustal Fornell E, Wingren G, Kjolhede P: Factors associated with pelvic floor dysfunction with emphasis on urinary and fecal incontinence and genital prolapse: An epidemiological study. Acta Obstet Gynecol Scand 83:383, 2004.
10. Pauls RN, Berman JR: Impact of pelvic floor disorders and prolapse on female sexual function and response. Urol Clin North Am 29:677, 2002.
11. Wein AJ: Neuromuscular dysfunction of the lower urinary tract and its management. In Walsh PC, Retik AB, Vaughan ED, et al (eds): Campbell's Urology, vol 2. Philadelphia, Saunders, 2002.
12. Tanagho EA, Schmidt RA: Electrical stimulation in the clinical management of the neurogenic bladder. J Urol 140:1331, 1988.
13. Cappellano F, Bertapelle P, Spinelli M, et al: Quality of life assessment in patients who undergo sacral neuromodulation implantation for urge incontinence: An additional tool for evaluating outcome. J Urol 166:2277, 2001.
14. Hohenfellner M, Dahms SE, Matzel K, et al: Sacral neuromodulation for treatment of lower urinary tract dysfunction. BJU Int 85(Suppl 3):10, 2000.
15. Kessler TM, Madersbacher H, Kiss G: Bilateral migration of sacral neuromodulation tined leads in a thin patient. J Urol 173:153, 2005.
16. Chang PL: Urodynamic studies in acupuncture for women with frequency, urgency and dysuria. J Urol 140:563, 1988.
17. Chung JM, Lee KH, Hori Y, et al: Factors influencing peripheral nerve stimulation produced inhibition of primate spinothalamic tract cells. Pain 19:277, 1984.
18. Stoller ML, Copeland S, Millard RJ, et al: The efficacy of acupuncture in reversing the unstable bladder in pig-tailed monkeys [abstract 2]. J Urol 137:104A, 1987.
19. Schultz-Lampel D, Jiang C, Lindstrom S, et al: Experimental results on mechanisms of action of electrical neuromodulation in chronic urinary retention. World J Urol 16:301, 1998.
20. Chang CJ, Huang ST, Hsu K, et al: Electroacupuncture decreases c-fos expression in the spinal cord induced by noxious stimulation of the rat bladder. J Urol 160(6 Pt 1):2274, 1998.
21. McGuire EJ, Zhang SC, Horwinski ER, et al: Treatment of motor and sensory detrusor instability by electrical stimulation. J Urol 129:78, 1983.
22. Payne CK: Urinary incontinence: nonsurgical management. In Walsh PC, Retik AB, Vaughan ED, et al (eds): Campbell's Urology, vol 2. Philadelphia, Saunders, 2002.
23. Klingler HC, Pycha A, Schmidbauer J, et al: Use of peripheral neuromodulation of the S3 region for treatment of detrusor overactivity: A urodynamic-based study. Urology 56:766, 2000.
24. van Balken MR, Vandoninck V, Gisolf KW, et al: Posterior tibial nerve stimulation as neuromodulative treatment of lower urinary tract dysfunction. J Urol 166:914, 2001.
25. Vandoninck V, Van Balken MR, Finazzi Agro E, et al: Posterior tibial nerve stimulation in the treatment of urge incontinence. Neurourol Urodyn 22:17, 2003.
26. Vandoninck V, van Balken MR, Finazzi Agro E, et al: Percutaneous tibial nerve stimulation in the treatment of overactive bladder: Urodynamic data. Neurourol Urodyn 22:227, 2003.
27. Vandoninck V, van Balken MR, Finazzi Agr E, et al: Posterior tibial nerve stimulation in the treatment of idiopathic nonobstructive voiding dysfunction. Urology 61:567, 2003.
28. Vandoninck V, van Balken MR, Finazzi Agro E, et al: Posterior tibial nerve stimulation in the treatment of voiding dysfunction: Urodynamic data. Neurourol Urodyn 23:246, 2004.
29. Govier FE, Litwiller S, Nitti V, et al: Percutaneous afferent neuromodulation for the refractory overactive bladder: Results of a multicenter study. J Urol 165:1193, 2001.
30. Amarenco G, Ismael SS, Even-Schneider A, et al: Urodynamic effect of acute transcutaneous posterior tibial nerve stimulation in overactive bladder. J Urol 169:2210, 2003.
31. Bower WF, Moore KH, Adams RD: A pilot study of the home application of transcutaneous neuromodulation in children with urgency or urge incontinence. J Urol 166:2420, 2001.
32. Andrews BJ, Reynard JM: Transcutaneous posterior tibial nerve stimulation for treatment of detrusor hyperreflexia in spinal cord injury. J Urol 170:926, 2003.

33. Shafik A, Ahmed I, El-Sibai O, et al: Percutaneous peripheral neuromodulation in the treatment of fecal incontinence. Eur Surg Res 35:103, 2003.
34. Allais G, Ciochetto D, Airola G, et al: Acupuncture in labor management. Minvera Ginecol 55:503, 2003.
35. Chen HM, Chen CH: Effects of acupressure at the Sanyinjiao point on primary dysmenorrhoea. J Adv Nurs 48:380, 2004.
36. Proctor ML, Smith CA, Farquhar CM, et al: Transcutaneous electrical nerve stimulation and acupuncture for primary dysmenorrhoea. Cochrane Database Syst Rev (1):CD002123, 2002.
37. van Balken MR, Vergunst H, Bemelmans BL: The use of electrical devices for the treatment of bladder dysfunction: A review of methods. J Urol 172:846, 2004.
38. Swift S, Garely A, Dimpfl T, et al: A new once-daily formulation of tolterodine provides superior efficacy and is well tolerated in women with overactive bladder. Int Urogynecol J Pelvic Floor Dysfunct 14:50, 2003.
39. Pricing obtained at http://www.walgreens.com/ Accessed Feb 1, 2005.
40. Bower WF, Moore KH, Adams RD, et al: A urodynamic study of surface neuromodulation versus sham in detrusor instability and sensory urgency. J Urol 160(6 Pt 1):2133, 1998.
41. Luber KM, Boero S, Choe JY: The demographics of pelvic floor disorders: Current observations and future projections. Am J Obstet Gynecol 184:1496, 2001.
42. Congregado Ruiz B, Pena Outeirino XM, Campoy Martinez P, et al: Peripheral afferent nerve stimulation for treatment of lower urinary tract irritative symptoms. Eur Urol 45:65, 2004.

Chapter 24

PUDENDAL NERVE STIMULATION

Richard C. Bennett and Kenneth M. Peters

Pharmacotherapy is the mainstay of treatment for voiding dysfunction, but this modality of treatment has various degrees of effectiveness and is often associated with undesirable side effects. Alternatives to pharmacotherapy include pelvic floor exercises, biofeedback, and neuromodulation. Sacral nerve stimulation has been approved by the U.S. Food and Drug Administration (FDA) since 1997 for treatment of urinary urge incontinence, urgency, frequency, and refractory retention.

Contemporary sacral nerve root stimulation consists of implantation of a tined electrode in the S3 sacral foramen, with subsequent connection to an implantable pulse generator (IPG; InterStim, Medtronic, Minneapolis, MN). Sacral root neuromodulation inhibits the micturition reflex through stimulation of spinal tract neurons and afferent pathways.[1] One limitation of the selection of S3 is that only one of the three afferent pathways inducing the inhibitory reflex is stimulated.

Selection of the pudendal nerve as a site of stimulation provides afferent stimulation of S2, S3, and S4. Afferent pudendal nerve stimulation can inhibit the micturition reflex, abolish uninhibited detrusor contractions, and increase bladder capacity in animals and humans.[2-9] Vodusek and colleagues[5] showed that detrusor contractions at low volumes of bladder filling were reduced or abolished by stimulating the dorsal penile or clitoral nerves transcutaneously in patients with spinal cord lesions. By stimulating the pudendal nerve close to the ischial spine using bipolar electrodes, Vodusek and coworkers[5] later reported electrical stimulation increased the micturition threshold and inhibited detrusor activity.

ANATOMY OF THE PUDENDAL NERVE

The pudendal nerve originates from the S2, S3, and S4 sacral nerve roots. The main trunk of the pudendal nerve takes an extrapelvic course superficial to the coccygeus muscle. The main trunk passes over the ischial spine and enters Alcock's (pudendal) canal. In the upper half of the pudendal canal, the pudendal nerve gives rise to the inferior rectal nerve. The inferior rectal nerve exits the pudendal canal medially and extends motor and sensory branches. Motor branches innervate the levator ani, and the cutaneous branches innervate the perianal skin and the scrotum or labia. The inferior rectal nerve terminates in multiple branches to the external anal sphincter. At the end of the pudendal canal, the pudendal nerve gives rise to two branches, the perineal nerve and the deep dorsal nerve of the clitoris or penis. The deep dorsal nerve continues as a terminal branch to the penis or clitoris. The perineal nerve divides into the scrotal or labial branch and two muscular branches to the bulbocavernosus and the striated urethral sphincter.[10,11] The optimal point of pudendal nerve stimulation is at the level of the ischial spine, proximal to the branch points (Fig. 24-1).

DEVICES AVAILABLE FOR PUDENDAL NERVE STIMULATION

The pudendal nerve can be stimulated on a chronic basis using a tined quadripolar lead (e.g., InterStim) or an implantable microstimulator (Bion, Advanced Bionics, Valencia, CA). Neither of these applications is FDA approved for pudendal stimulation. The development of a tined lead for sacral nerve stimulation allows implantation of the lead without suture fixation (Fig. 24-2). This feature makes it possible to deploy the lead at other sites, such as the pudendal nerve. The advantage is that the lead can be placed at the pudendal nerve by means of a posterior approach, externalized, and tested on an outpatient basis to assess the clinical response. If the patient demonstrates significant improvement in their voiding symptoms, a permanent IPG can be placed in a subcutaneous pocket in the upper buttock.

The Bion microstimulator is a miniature, self-contained, rechargeable, implantable neurostimulator that is designed as a platform technology and is intended to treat a wide variety of disorders through direct electrical stimulation. This device is approved in Europe for commercial use in pudendal nerve stimulation and is in clinical trials in the United States for urinary urge incontinence, urgency or frequency, and chronic headache. The fully integrated microstimulator contains a rechargeable battery, a radio transmitter, an antenna for bidirectional telemetry, a programmable microchip, and stimulating electrode. The implant is 28 mm long and 3.2 mm in diameter, and it has a mass of only 0.7 g (Fig. 24-3).

PATIENT SELECTION

Chronic pudendal neuromodulation is not approved by the FDA for the treatment of voiding dysfunction. With appropriate informed consent, patients suffering from refractory voiding dysfunction, including urinary urgency, frequency, urge incontinence, and nonobstructive urinary retention, could be candidates for pudendal neurostimulation. Patients who had sacral nerve stimulation but did not respond may benefit from pudendal nerve stimulation. Other disease states that may be considered include interstitial cystitis and neurogenic bladder, including cases caused by partial spinal cord injury, multiple sclerosis, Parkinson's disease, and other neurologic disorders.

A complete voiding diary is paramount in the evaluation of the patient considering neuromodulation. The voiding diary evaluates the time of voids, voided volumes, incontinent episodes, urge scores, pain scores, bowel function, and catheterized volumes if in retention. This baseline information allows accurate postoperative evaluation of patient progress. Because these procedures can be done only "on protocol," appropriate Human

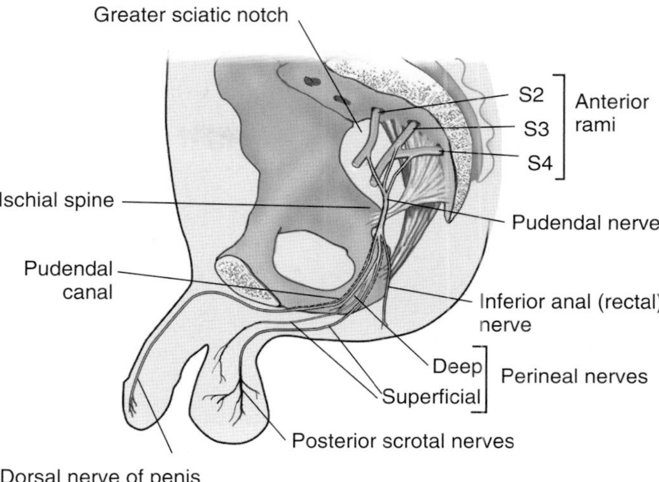

Figure 24-1 Pudendal nerve anatomy.

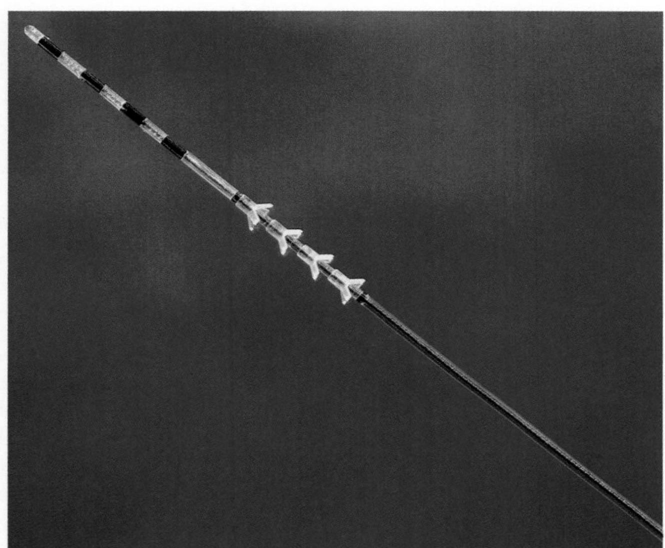

Figure 24-2 Tined quadripolar lead.

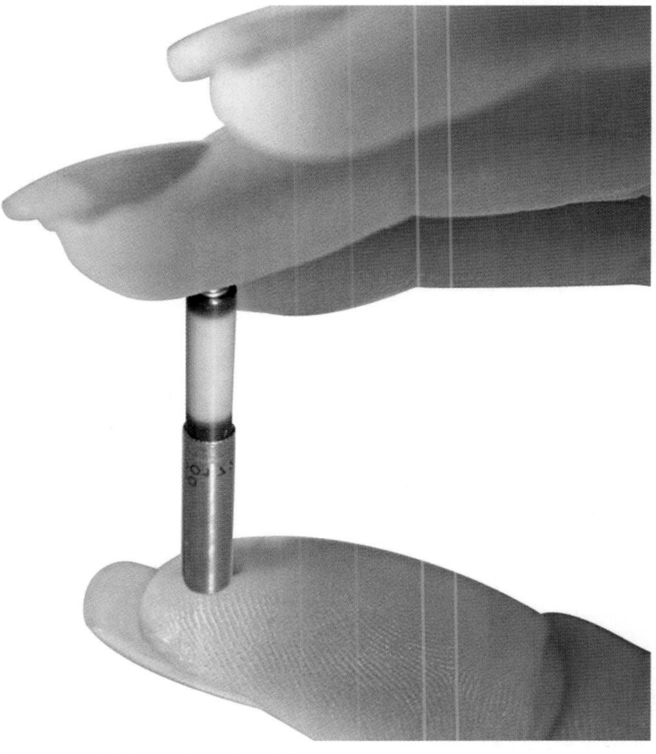

Figure 24-3 Bion microstimulator.

Investigation Committee approval is required, along with the patient's signature on an informed consent form.

PROCEDURE

Using the InterStim Tined Quadripolar Lead

Preoperative Preparation and Patient Positioning

Administer broad-spectrum intravenous antibiotics such as ampicillin and gentamycin. Place the patient in the prone position with appropriate padding and support. Provide light sedation with an agent such as Versed. Perform thorough Betadine preparation of the lower back, buttock, and anus. Place needle or patch electrodes at the external anal sphincter, and connect them to electromyographic device (Fig. 24-4). Use fluoroscopy to image the pelvis in the lateral position to identify the ischial tuberosity and ischial spine (Fig. 24-5).

Identification of the Pudendal Nerve

Palpate the ischial tuberosity posteriorly, and anesthetize the skin 1 cm medial to the tuberosity with 1% lidocaine. Advance a 5.5-inch foramen needle through the skin toward the ischial spine. Stimulate the proximal end of the foramen needle with the standard clip-on stimulating cord (Fig. 24-6). Begin stimulation at 1 Hz, and slowly increase the power from 1 mA to 10 mA while

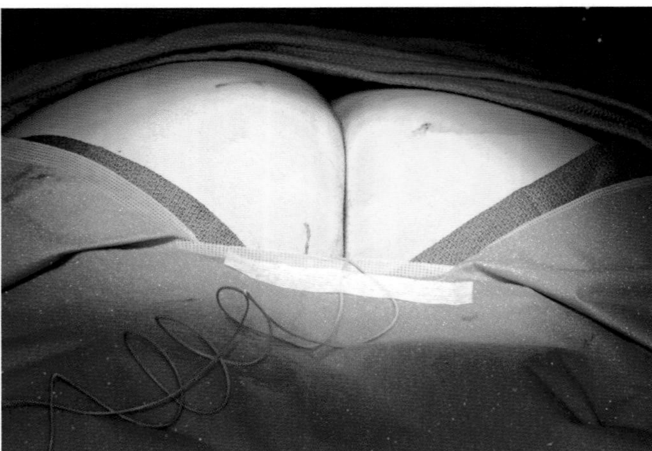

Figure 24-4 Electromyographic electrode at the external anal sphincter.

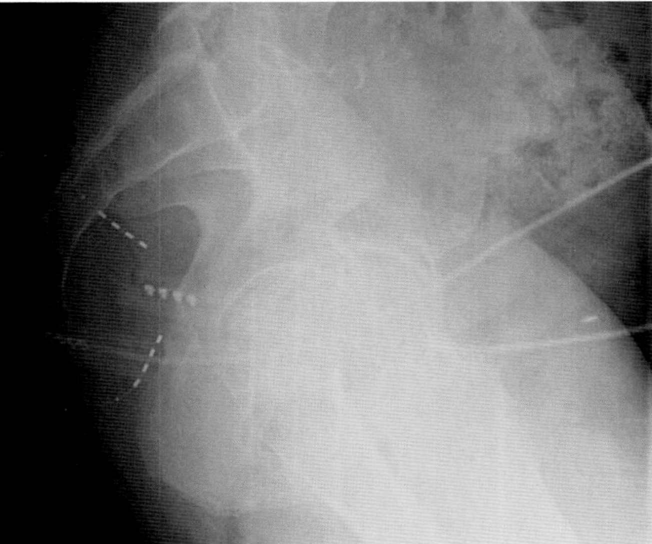

Figure 24-5 Lateral radiograph of the sacral and pudendal quadripolar leads.

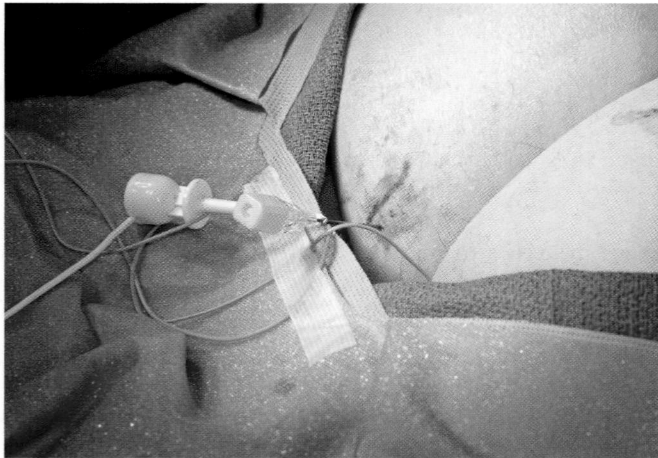

Figure 24-6 Stimulation of the foramen needle near the ischial spine.

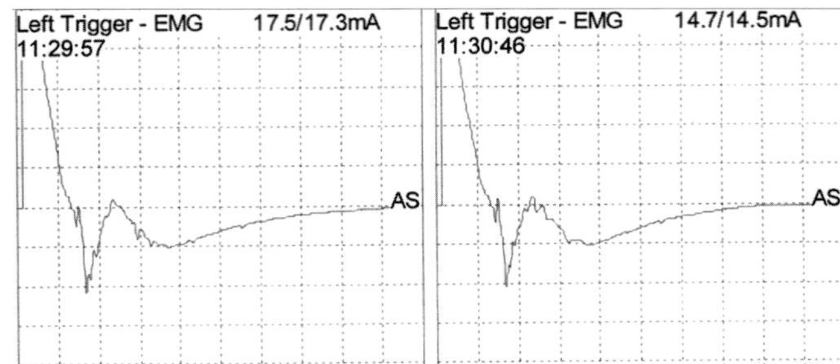

Figure 24-7 Compound muscle action potential, consistent with pudendal nerve stimulation.

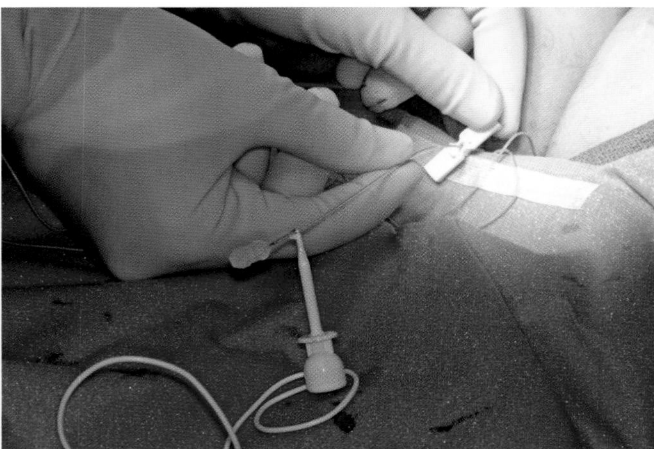

Figure 24-8 A quadripolar lead is advanced through the lead introducer.

examining the anal sphincter and monitoring the electromyographic tracing. The typical motor response is contraction of the external anal sphincter. This should be confirmed as pudendal stimulation by seeing a classic compound muscle action potential (CMAP) consistent with pudendal stimulation (Fig. 24-7). Assess the patient's sensory response. A typical response is comfortable pulsating in the vagina, scrotum, perineum, or rectum. The nerve of the obturator internus sits close to Alcock's canal; be certain there is no leg rotation noted during the acute testing. If leg movement is seen, reposition the needle until only the pudendal stimulation is identified.

Placement of the Quadripolar Tined Lead

After the pudendal nerve is identified, advance the directional guidewire, and remove the foramen needle. Make a small skin nick alongside the wire. Advance the lead introducer over the directional guidewire toward the ischial spine using fluoroscopy. The proximal metal trocar of the lead introducer can be stimulated with the standard stimulation cord. Reconfirm pudendal stimulation, advance the quadripolar lead through the lead introducer, and test each electrode in the standard fashion (Fig. 24-8). The ideal placement is identification of pudendal stimulation on all four electrodes. Deploy the tines by removing the lead introducer.

Externalizing the Percutaneous Extension Lead

The current quadripolar lead is too short to reach the upper buttock where a future IPG will be placed. The lead is tunneled to a 1-cm, midbuttock incision and connected to the temporary percutaneous extension lead. This lead is tunneled out the contralateral side and externalized. A redundant lead is placed in a subcutaneous pocket underneath the skin, and the incision is closed.

Stage I Test

Patients are discharged with the standard Medtronic stimulation box, and stimulation is set to a comfortable sensation for the patient. Voiding diaries are kept for 7 to 14 days, and if a 50% or greater improvement occurs, the lead is connected to an IPG. If no improvement occurs, the lead is explanted.

Implantation of the Implantable Pulse Generator or Removal of the Lead

If the subject does not respond to the stimulation, the midbuttock incision is opened, and the tined lead is removed by gentle traction. If an IPG is to be placed, a standard site is chosen on the upper buttock, and a subcutaneous pocket is created. A 25-cm extension lead is attached to the IPG and tunneled to the midbuttock incision. The tined lead is freed from this incision, and the percutaneous extension lead is removed. The distal end of the 25-cm IPG extension is connected to the proximal end of the tined lead in the standard fashion. The lead and its connector are placed in the subcutaneous pocket of the midbuttock.

Outcomes of Pudendal Stimulation Using a Tined Quadripolar Lead

A direct comparison of the efficacy of pudendal and sacral nerve stimulation has been completed. This was a randomized, single-blinded, single-center trial in which each subject had a sacral lead and a pudendal lead placed as part of an approved protocol. Subjects were randomized to begin stimulation on the sacral or pudendal electrode. In a blinded fashion, each lead was tested for 7 days. Voiding diaries and questionnaires were completed. Subjects rated their percent improvement on each lead and chose the one to be implanted to a permanent generator based on response. Analysis of the data demonstrated the time to place the sacral lead was 25.85 minutes compared with 23.71 minutes for the pudendal lead ($P = .57$). Twenty-four (80%) of 30 of subjects responded and had an IPG implanted, with 19 (79.2%) of 24 choosing pudendal stimulation and 5 (20.8%) of 24 choosing sacral stimulation. The order in which the lead was stimulated had no impact on the final lead implanted. Pudendal nerve stimulation produced significantly higher rates of improvement of symptoms than sacral nerve stimulation: 51% versus 37%, respectively ($P = .02$). On a 7-point scale from markedly worse to markedly better, pudendal nerve stimulation was superior to sacral nerve stimulation for pelvic pain ($P = .024$), urgency ($P = .005$), frequency ($P = .007$), and bowel function ($P = .049$). This preliminary study demonstrated that pudendal nerve stimulation is feasible, safe, and effective using a tined quadripolar lead.[12]

Pudendal Nerve Stimulation Using the Bion Microstimulator

The Bion neurostimulator is placed at Alcock's canal in a minimally invasive fashion through a small incision in the perineum. Its stimulation parameters can be adjusted using a physician programmer, and patients have their own remote control for adjustment of the level of stimulation. The battery is recharged by sitting on a charging pad daily for 20 to 60 minutes, and the battery life is 15 to 20 years.

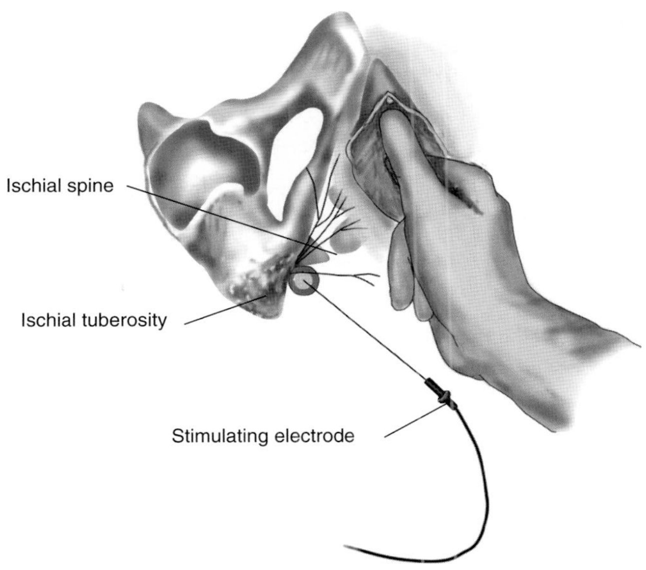

Figure 24-9 Percutaneous screening test.

Percutaneous Screening Test

Before implantation of a permanent Bion, a percutaneous test is performed in the office. The patient is placed in the lithotomy position at a 45-degree angle, and the vagina and perineum are prepared and draped in the normal, sterile fashion. Surface electromyographic electrodes are placed at the anal sphincter. A computerized cystometrogram is performed at a fill rate of 25 mL/min while measuring the volume at first sensation, first urge, maximum cystometric capacity, and first unstable contraction. Next, the ischial tuberosity is palpated and marked with a marking pen. The ischial spine is palpated through the vagina or rectum (i.e., site of Alcock's canal). The skin is anesthetized approximately 1.5 cm medial to the ischial tuberosity. With a finger in the vagina or rectum palpating the ischial spine, a stimulating needle is advanced through the perineum toward the ischial spine while applying electrical stimulation (Fig. 24-9). CMAPs are measured. Muscle contractions are assessed by direct vision and palpation. A good response is contraction of the bulbocavernosus muscle and external anal sphincter. A poor response includes contraction of the obturator internus, leg adductors, or lower extremity muscles. The sensory response is determined, and a pulsating or tingling in the vaginal, vulvar, or anal regions is optimal. Poor responses include leg or foot twitching or pain. After needle placement is confirmed, the pudendal nerve is stimulated for 15 minutes at a pulse frequency of 20 Hz, pulse width of 200 μs, 50% duty cycle, and pulse amplitude up to 10.0 mA. The bladder is emptied with a catheter, and the urodynamic catheter is replaced. The cystometrogram is repeated while stimulation continues. A 50% increase in the volume of first sensation, first urge, cystometric capacity, or at unstable bladder contraction constitutes a positive test result supporting implantation of the permanent Bion device.

Implantation of the Bion

Preoperative, broad-spectrum antibiotics are administered. The patient is brought to the operating room, lightly sedated, and

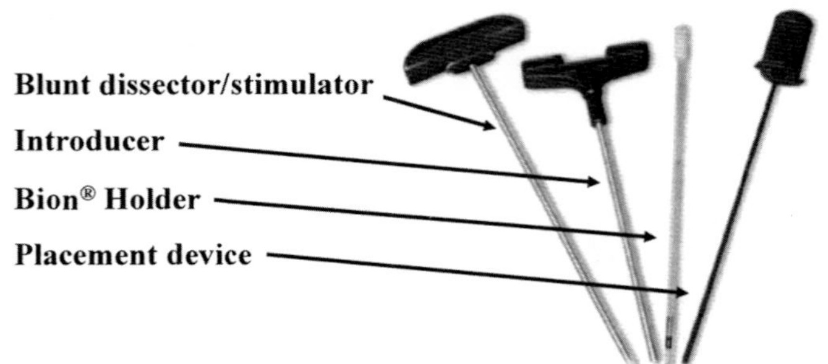

Figure 24-10 Implantation tools. (Courtesy of Advanced Bionics, Valencia, CA)

placed in the lithotomy position. The perineal area is prepared and draped in the normal, sterile fashion. Surface electromyographic electrodes are placed on the outside of the anal sphincter and connected to an electrodiagnostic monitor. The medial aspect of the ischial tuberosity is marked, the skin is infiltrated with 1% lidocaine approximately 1.5 cm medial to the tuberosity, and a 2- to 3-mm incision is made. The Bion implantation tools include a blunt dissector or stimulator, introducer, Bion holder, and placement device (Fig. 24-10). With a finger palpating the ischial spine through the vagina or rectum, the blunt dissector and introducer are inserted together toward the target (Fig. 24-11). Fluoroscopy in the lateral position can help direct the Bion toward the ischial spine. Clinical and electrophysiologic responses facilitate placement as described previously. After the pudendal nerve is confirmed, the blunt dissector is removed, leaving the introducer in place. The Bion in its holder is advanced through the introducer, and the placement tool is advanced through the Bion holder and locked in place by rotating clockwise until it "clicks" into place. The Bion is turned on and activated with a frequency of 20-Hz, pulse width of 200 μs, continuous duty cycle, and amplitude 5 to 10 mA. Sensory, motor, and electrodiagnostic responses are assessed. After the location is optimized, the Bion is delivered by retracting the Bion holder. Retraction is performed by turning the thumbscrew clockwise until it can be turned no further. This deposits the Bion at the site of stimulation. The Bion is deactivated, the introducer is removed, and a Steri-Strip is placed over the skin incision site.

Postoperative Follow-up

One week after implantation, the patient returns to the office for programming of the Bion and for education regarding the system components. The clinician's programmer communicates with the Bion and allows the stimulator to be activated and adjusted.

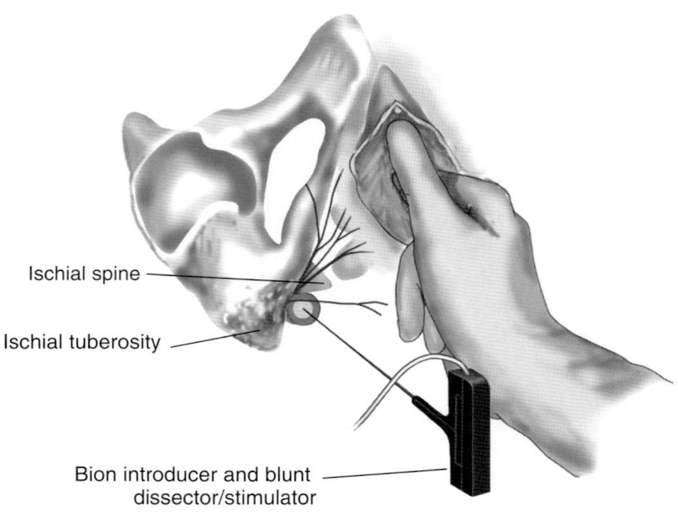

Figure 24-11 Implantation of Bion microstimulator.

Possible adjustments include frequency, pulse width, burst mode, and stimulation limits. The programmer monitors battery life, records the time the device was activated, and gives a history of recharging events. The patients have their own home kit consisting of a remote control, base station or charger, and chair pad used to charge the Bion. The Bion should last 15 to 20 years and can be recharged even if the battery is allowed to completely deplete. The benefit of the Bion is its small size and the minimally invasive approach to implantation. Results of clinical trials will determine its future in treating voiding dysfunction.

CONCLUSIONS

The use of neuromodulation has led to a major advance in our ability to treat patients suffering from voiding dysfunction who have been refractory to standard therapies. In the past, these patients continued to suffer from their disease or underwent irreversible operations such as bladder augmentation or urinary diversion to control their symptoms. Neuromodulation continues to be developed, and the pudendal nerve appears to be a safe and effective area to stimulate. Ongoing studies are assessing the feasibility of placing a tined quadripolar lead or the Bion microstimulator at the pudendal nerve. More patients and longer-term follow-up are needed before this approach is considered standard of care.

References

1. Weil EH, Ruiz-Cerda JL, Erdmans PH, et al: Sacral root neuromodulation in the treatment of refractory urinary urge incontinence: A prospective randomized clinical trial. Eur Urol 37:161-171, 2000.
2. Fall M, Erlandson BE, Carlsson CA, Sundin T: The effect of intravaginal electrical stimulation on the feline urethra and urinary bladder. Neuronal mechanisms. Scand J Urol Nephrol 344(Pt 2, Suppl):19-30, 1978.
3. Lindstrom S, Fall M, Carlsson CA, Erlandson BE: The neurophysiologic basis of bladder inhibition in response to intravaginal electrical stimulation. J Urol 129:405-410, 1983.
4. Light J, Vodusek D, Libby J: Inhibition of detrusor hyperreflexia by a selective electrical stimulation of the pudendal nerve. J Urol 135:198, 1986.
5. Vodusek D, Light J, Libby J: Detrusor inhibition induced by stimulation of pudendal nerve afferents. Neurourol Urodyn 5:381-389, 1986.
6. Erickson B, Bergmann S, Eik-Nes S: Maximal electrostimulation of the pelvic floor in female idiopathic detrusor instability and urge incontinence. Neurourol Urodyn 8:219-230, 1989.
7. Lindstrom S, Sudsuang R: Functionally specific bladder reflexes from pelvic and pudendal nerve branches: An experimental study in the cat. Neurourol Urodyn 8:392-393, 1989.

8. Fall M, Lindstrom S: Electrical stimulation: A physiologic approach to the treatment of urinary incontinence. Urol Clin North Am 18:393-407, 1991.
9. Wheeler J, Walter J: Bladder inhibition by dorsal penile nerve stimulation in spinal cord injured patients. J Urol 147:100-103, 1992.
10. Borirakchanyavat S, Aboseif PR, Tanagho EA, Lue TF: Continence mechanism of the isolated female urethra: An anatomical study of the intrapelvic somatic nerves. J Urol 158:822-826, 1997.
11. Shafik A, Doss S: Surgical anatomy of the somatic terminal innervation to the anal and urethral sphincters: Role in anal and urethral surgery. J Urol 161:85-89, 1999.
12. Peters KM, Konstandt D, Huynh P, Feber K: Sacral vs. pudendal nerve stimulation for voiding dysfunction: A prospective, single blinded, randomized, crossover trail [abstract]. Neurourol Urodyn 24:159-160, 2005.

Chapter 25

DETRUSOR MYOMECTOMY

Linda Ng and Edward J. McGuire

Bladder augmentation has been used in a spectrum of clinical settings in which bladder dysfunction is refractory to more conservative treatment. Enterocystoplasty and gastrocystoplasty offer a reliable improvement in bladder compliance and capacity, decreased rates of upper urinary tract deterioration, and improved quality of life for patients. However, early and late complications related to incorporation of bowel segments in the urinary tract are many, cumulative, and well known. They include bowel contractions leading to incontinence, bowel obstruction, diarrhea syndromes, spontaneous perforation, abundant mucus production leading to stones, chronic bacteriuria, electrolyte imbalances, and the hematuria and dysuria syndrome (if a gastric segment is used).[1-3] Use of bowel segments may also place the patients at risk for future malignancies.[4,5]

Detrusor myomectomy, also known as bladder autoaugmentation, is a simpler, less morbid alternative to enterocystoplasty. Autoaugmentation, as described by Cartwright and Snow[6-8] in 1989, involves excising a portion of the detrusor muscle, allowing the bladder epithelium and lamina propria to form a large-mouthed bladder diverticulum. As the urothelium bulges through the muscular hiatus, bladder capacity is increased, intravesical storage pressures are reduced, and the volume at which a contraction occurs becomes larger. Because only bladder tissue is used in this technique, the risks associated with gastrointestinal segment incorporation into the urinary tract are obviated.

PATIENT SELECTION

In patients with bladder dysfunction, the first line of treatment is anticholinergic medications, α-blocking agents, tricyclic antidepressants, and timed voiding or intermittent catheterization. Surgical intervention is appropriate when patients fail to respond clinically, develop upper tract compromise, or persistent compliance abnormalities. Video urodynamics is performed preoperatively for all patients to evaluate bladder storage and urethral continence function.[9] The cystometric volume at an intravesical pressure of 40 cm H_2O is recorded. In general, enterocystoplasty remains the better procedure for patients with poorly compliant, extremely small-capacity bladders because bladder capacity is increased to a lesser degree after detrusor myomectomy. However, detrusor myomectomy offers many advantages in certain patients in whom bowel complications would exacerbate comorbid conditions, including those who have had prior abdominal surgery, patients with bowel diseases, those with short gut or malabsorption syndromes, and those with prior episodes of peritonitis associated with ventriculoperitoneal shunts. We feel that myomectomy should be the first line of surgical therapy for idiopathic detrusor instability. Bladder autoaugmentation does not preclude a subsequent enterocystoplasty if it is necessary.

PATIENT PREPARATION

Patients with neuropathic lower urinary tract dysfunction require intermittent catheterization after myomectomy. Patients with idiopathic, non-neurogenic bladder contractile incontinence do not require intermittent catheterization after myomectomy. Patients with a low-compliance bladder related to radiation therapy or chemotherapy usually require intermittent catheterization after myomectomy.[9,10] Selected patients are informed that a conventional enterocystoplasty can be performed if detrusor myomectomy is not a technical option intraoperatively. This option is discussed in detail before the operative date so that mechanical and antibiotic bowel preparation can be performed before surgery in these selected patients. Preoperative intravenous antibiotics are also administered.

DETRUSOR MYOMECTOMY TECHNIQUE

The technique employed is modified from the original description by Cartwright and Snow.[6-8] A two-way urethral catheter is placed so that bladder filling and emptying can be readily controlled, and a lower Pfannenstiel incision is made (Fig. 25-1). The rectus muscles are then separated in the midline, the prevesical space is entered (Fig. 25-2), and the dissection is continued until the bladder wall proper is cleared of adventitia (Fig. 25-3). Care is taken to sweep the peritoneum off the bladder dome. The

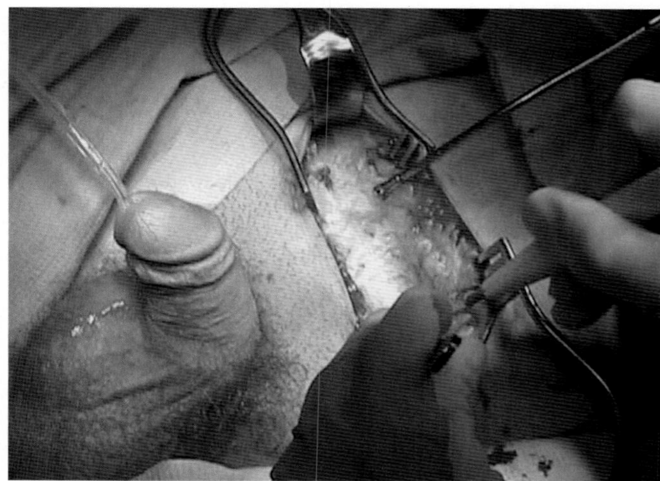

Figure 25-1 A two-way catheter is placed to control bladder filling and emptying. A Pfannenstiel incision is then made. (From McGuire E: Pubovaginal slings. In Hurt MG [ed]: Urogynecologic Surgery. New York, Raven Press, 1992, pp 97-105.)

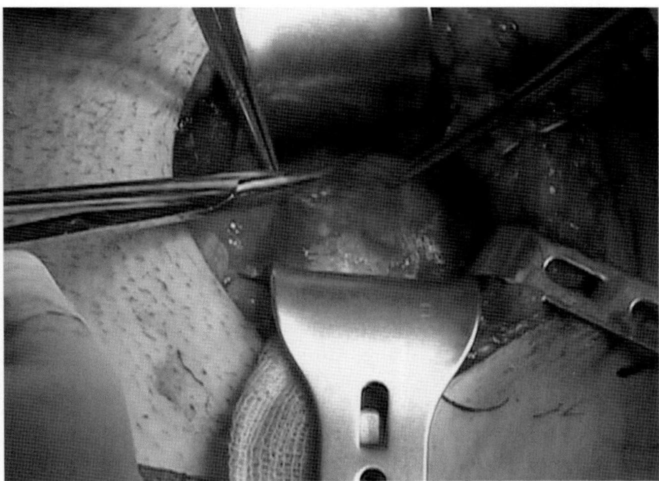

Figure 25-2 The prevesical space is entered after separating the rectus muscles in the midline. (From McGuire E: Pubovaginal slings. In Hurt MG [ed]: Urogynecologic Surgery. New York, Raven Press, 1992, pp 97-105.)

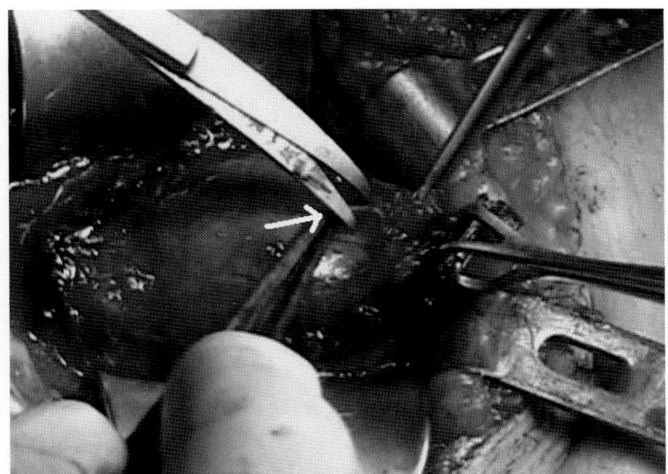

Figure 25-3 The bladder wall proper is cleared of adventitia *(arrow)*. (From McGuire E: Pubovaginal slings. In Hurt MG [ed]: Urogynecologic Surgery. New York, Raven Press, 1992, pp 97-105.)

bladder is then distended, and a no. 15 blade is used to carefully divide the detrusor muscle until the bladder mucosa protrudes from the muscle. A combination of gentle traction and sharp dissection is used to strip the entire detrusor muscle layer covering the dome and anterior wall, denuding the underlying bladder mucosa (Fig. 25-4). During the procedure, changing bladder volumes may help to maximize exposure of the plane of dissection between detrusor and urothelium. If the dissection becomes difficult in a particular area, it is best to move on to an easier adjacent area. Ultimate care is taken to avoid perforation of the bladder mucosa because outcomes are much less satisfactory if this happens. As the procedure progresses, distinct bulging of the mucosal layer should occur. Palpation reveals a loose elastic mucosa surrounded by tense, rather rigid musculature. Autoaugmentation generally involves removing the detrusor from at least

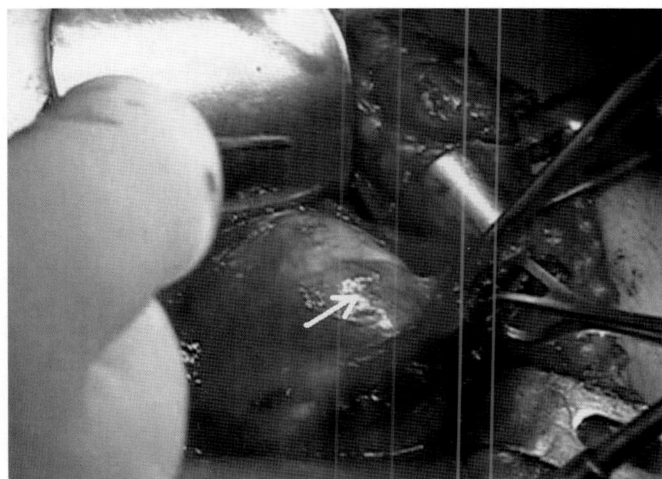

Figure 25-4 The detrusor muscle layer is then stripped, revealing bulging mucosa *(arrow)*. (From McGuire E: Pubovaginal slings. In Hurt MG [ed]: Urogynecologic Surgery. New York, Raven Press, 1992, pp 97-105.)

one third of the bladder. A urethral catheter is left to provide gravity drainage for 1 to 2 days.

POSTOPERATIVE MANAGEMENT

After detrusor myomectomy, the patient is left with an exposed area of thin mucosa that bulges from the bladder with filling. Some surgeons have advocated protection of the mucosal diverticulum with a layer of peritoneum, omentum, or rectus muscle; however, we feel this is unnecessary. Patients who perform intermittent catheterization return to their preoperative routine, and patients on anticholinergic agents maintain their medical regimen. After the diverticulum created by the myomectomy matures, the interval between intermittent catheterization can be increased. Anticholinergic therapy is tapered after follow-up urodynamics reveals improved compliance. Prophylactic antibiotics are used only until removal of the catheter. Patients are seen for follow-up evaluation approximately 3 weeks after detrusor myomectomy. At this time, wound checks are performed, and a thorough interim history is obtained, including the status of "dryness" between intermittent catheterizations or the voiding history. Patients are not evaluated with video urodynamics until 3 months after surgery. An accurate assessment of myomectomy results is feasible at this time.[11,12]

CLINICAL OUTCOME OF DETRUSOR MYOMECTOMY

In the first series of 25 pediatric patients undergoing autoaugmentation in 1989, Snow and Cartwright[6,7] reported an overall good result for 52%, acceptable result for 28%, and poor result for 20%. In most patients, bladder compliance was improved, although bladder capacity changes varied. In one half of their patients, capacity increased by only 0% to 25%. In the other half, capacity increased by 5% to 150%. Fifty-eight percent of incontinent patients became dry, and 63% of patients with preoperative hydronephrosis had improvement in their upper tract status.

Experiences from other institutions have been reported for adult patient populations. Kennelly and asssociates[10] described a series of five adult patients undergoing autoaugmentation. There was an increase in bladder capacity of 40% to 310%, and detrusor compliance improved in all patients. Total continence was achieved in three of five patients, and all were able to extend the interval between catheterizations. Stohrer and colleagues[11] reported their experience in 29 patients with neurogenic and non-neurogenic voiding dysfunction. Their results were generally positive, with increases in bladder capacity, decreased maximal voiding pressure, and improvements in compliance. Outcome was rated subjectively as excellent for 16 patients, good for 8, and improved for 1. In a later study of 50 patients with neurogenic voiding dysfunction, similar efficacy after bladder autoaugmentation was described.[12]

Leng and coworkers[9] compared operative outcomes of 37 patients undergoing detrusor myomectomy with those of 32 patients who had an enterocystoplasty. For comparison, the cases were categorized into six diagnostic subsets: intractable detrusor instability, interstitial cystitis with low-compliance bladder, myelodysplasia, radiation cystitis, neurogenic bladder dysfunction, and other. Preoperative upper tract deterioration was present in 14 patients. Results were stratified for each of the six diagnostic subsets. In 10 patients with idiopathic, overactive bladder incontinence, 8 demonstrated urodynamic improvement, 1 continued to require intermittent catheterization, and 1 failed and went on to augmentation cystoplasty. In the myelodysplasia subgroup, 5 (45%) of 11 patients who underwent detrusor myomectomy exhibited satisfactory urodynamic improvement. This suggests that enterocystoplasty may be superior in some patients with myelodysplasia. MacNeily and associates[13] reported similar findings for 17 patients with myelomeningocele undergoing autoaugmentation. Based on their data, they concluded that short-term reports after autoaugmentation do not appear durable in this patient population. Leng and colleagues[9] reported improved urodynamic findings in three of nine patients with radiation cystitis who underwent myomectomy as a primary procedure. The overall success rate of primary detrusor myomectomy was 73%, with most failures proceeding to enterocystoplasty. Costs for surgery and length of hospitalization are much less for myomectomy than enterocystoplasty. A minor complication rate of 3% was seen in the myomectomy group compared with a major complication rate of 22% for patients treated with primary enterocystoplasties.

Further refinement of the autoaugmentation technique may lead to an improvement in its success rate and a reduced length of operative time, length of hospitalization, and rate of complications. Several investigators have proposed laparoscopic autoaugmentation, but long-term follow-up is still limited.[14-16]

CONCLUSIONS

Since its introduction in 1989, detrusor myomectomy has gained increasing acceptance as a successful method of managing bladder dysfunction. However, patient selection remains key. In particular, patients with idiopathic detrusor instability treated with detrusor myomectomy had equivalent success rates. In other patient subsets, however, it is clear that in regard to increased bladder capacity, myomectomy is still inferior to conventional enterocystoplasty. Overall, myomectomy offers a minimally morbid surgical option for the high-risk surgical candidate who cannot tolerate the rigors of major bowel surgery or its potential complications. The recent trend in laparoscopic bladder augmentation may lead to further success of the technique and improvements in outcome.

References

1. DeKlerk JN, Lambrechts W, Uiljoen I: The bowel as substitute for the bladder. J Urol 121:22, 1979.
2. Hensle TW, Dean GE: Complications of urinary tract reconstruction. Urol Clin North Am 18:755, 1991.
3. Leong CH: Use of the stomach for bladder replacement and urinary diversion. Ann R Coll Surg Engl 60:283, 1978.
4. Filmer RB, Spencer JR: Malignancies in bladder augmentation and intestinal conduits. J Urol 143:671, 1990.
5. Ali-El Dein B, El-Tabey N, Abdel-latif M, et al: Late uro-ileal cancer after incorporation of ileum into the urinary tract. J Urol 167:84, 2002.
6. Cartwright PC, Snow BW: Bladder autoaugmentation: Early clinical experience. J Urol 142:520, 1989.
7. Cartwright PC, Snow BW: Bladder autoaugmentation: Partial detrusor excision to augment the bladder without use of bowel. J Urol 142:1050, 1989.
8. Snow BW, Cartwright PC: Bladder autoaugmentation. Urol Clin North Am 23:323, 1996.
9. Leng WW, Blalock J, Fredrikkson WH, et al: Enteroplasty or detrusor myomectomy? Comparison of indications and outcomes for bladder augmentation. J Urol 16:758, 1999.
10. Kennelly MJ, Gormley EA, McGuire EJ: Early clinical experience with adult bladder autoaugmentation. J Urol 1152:303, 1994.
11. Stohrer M, Kramer A, Goepel M, et al: Bladder autoaugmentation—An alternative for enterocystoplasty. Neurourol Urodyn 14:11, 1995.
12. Stohrer M, Kramer G, Goepel M, et al: Bladder autoaugmentation in adult patients with neurogenic voiding dysfunction. Spinal Cord 35:456, 1997.
13. MacNeily AE, Afshar K, Coleman GU, Johnson HW: Autoaugmentation by detrusor myotomy: Its lack of effectiveness in the management of congenital neuropathic bladder. J Urol 170:1643, 2003.
14. Ehrlich RM, Gershman A: Laparoscopic seromyotomy (autoaugmentation) for nonneurogenic bladder in a child: Initial case report. Urology 42:175, 1993.
15. McDougal EM, Clayman RV, Figenshau RS, Pearle MS: Laparoscopic retropubic autoaugmentation of the bladder. J Urol 153:123, 1995.
16. Braren V, Bishop MR: Laparoscopic bladder autoaugmentation in children. Urol Clin North Am 25:533, 1998.

Chapter 26

BLADDER AUGMENTATION

Linda Ng and Edward J. McGuire

Bladder augmentation has evolved since the initial report in 1899 by Mikulicz,[1] who first described the use of gastrointestinal tract segments for lower urinary tract reconstruction. In large part, this resulted from the introduction of clean intermittent catherization,[2] the poor long-term results associated with the ileal conduit,[3] realization about the importance of detubularization,[4] and the importance of the role of bladder storage pressures in determining upper tract function.[5] Augmentation cystoplasty with various intestinal segments has become an accepted reconstructive option for intractable incontinence and poor bladder compliance in many neuropathic and non-neuropathic disorders.[6] Patient factors then guide individual selection of the augmentation method used.

INDICATIONS

The main indications for bladder augmentation are the presence of upper tract deterioration caused by high detrusor pressures at reduced bladder capacity and incontinence resulting from idiopathic detrusor instability. Compromised bladder capacity may be seen in patients with spina bifida, spinal cord injury, multiple sclerosis, or congenital conditions such as bladder exstrophy and its variants. Less common causes of reduced bladder capacity include chronic, interstitial, or radiation cystitis. Preoperative urodynamic studies should demonstrate a low-capacity, high-pressure bladder that is refractory to optimal medical management and intermittent catherization.[7] When the native urethra is destroyed or cannot be catheterized, a continent catheterizable or an incontinent stoma to the augmented bladder or native bladder can be used. The options for bladder augmentation are intact gastrointestinal segments, seromuscular gastrointestinal segments, augmentation with tissue-engineered urothelium, autoaugmentation, and ureterocystoplasty. Various pros and cons are associated with each of these methods.

AUGMENTATION USING GASTROINTESTINAL SEGMENTS

Augmentation Technique

Enterocystoplasty with ileum or colon is the most commonly used procedure for vesical augmentation. Patients are admitted overnight (i.e., non-neurogenic cases) or 2 days earlier (i.e., neurogenic cases) for a complete mechanical and antibiotic bowel preparation. Intraoperatively, the ileoplasty is fashioned from 25 to 30 cm of ileum at least 15 cm from the ileocecal valve (Fig. 26-1). The segment of chosen bowel on its mesentery should be tested to ensure that it reaches the deep pelvis easily (Fig. 26-2). Using a hand-sewn or stapled technique, an enteroenterostomy is performed. The closed ileal segment is then detubularized at the antimesenteric border, beginning and ending approximately 2 cm from the closed ends (Fig. 26-3). The two adjacent borders of detubularized ileum forming what will be the posterior wall of the ileocystoplasty are then sutured with 2-0 Vicryl (Fig. 26-4). At this point, the bladder is distended with saline, and the overlying peritoneum is stripped from the posterior and superior surfaces (Fig. 26-5). A transverse "smile" incision is then made approximately 3 cm above the ureteral orifices, creating an anteriorly based detrusor flap.[6] The small bowel is sutured to the

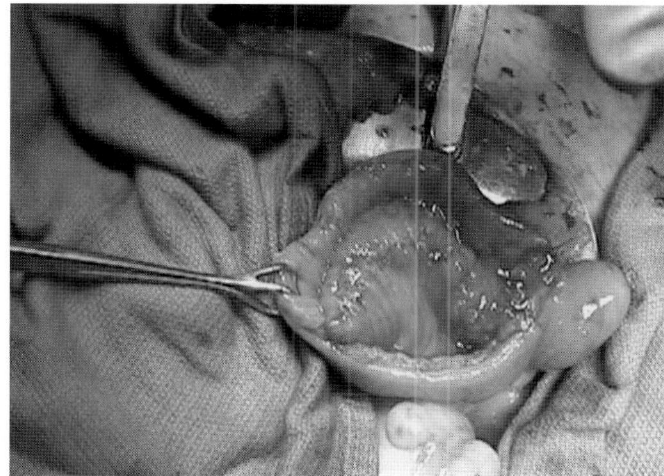

Figure 26-1 The ileoplasty is fashioned from 25 to 30 cm of ileum at least 15 cm from the ileocecal valve.

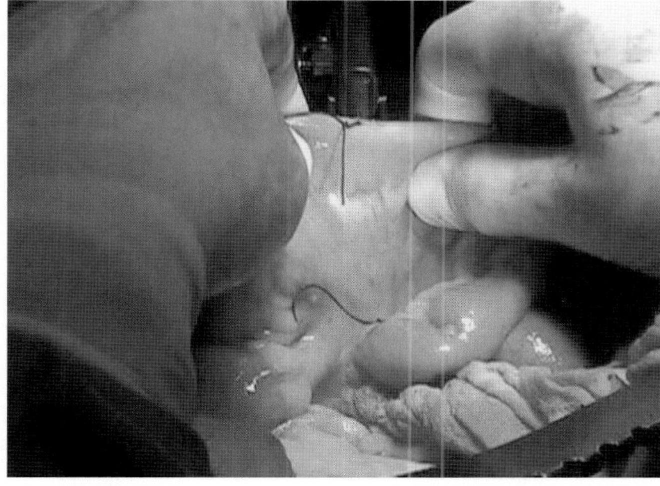

Figure 26-2 The segment of chosen bowel on its mesentery should be tested to ensure that it reaches the deep pelvis easily.

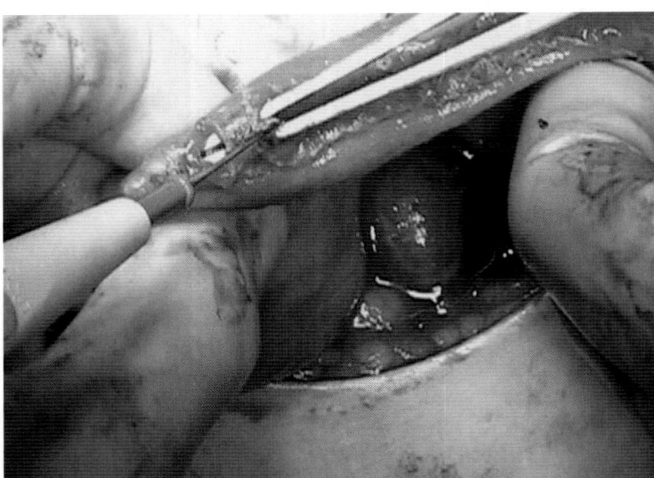

Figure 26-3 The closed ileal segment is detubularized at the antimesenteric border.

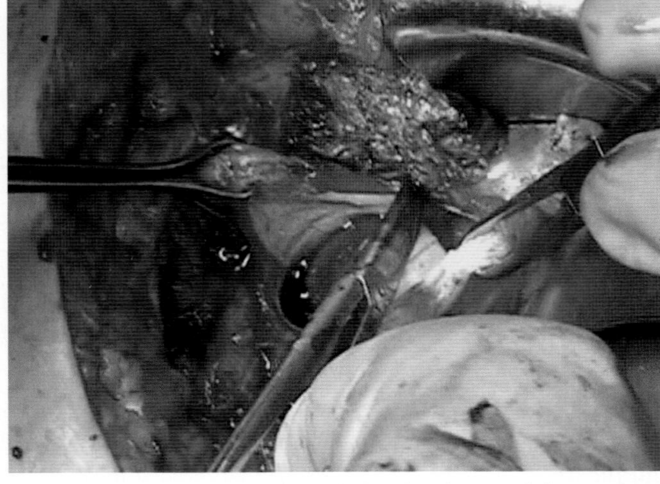

Figure 26-5 The bladder is distended with saline, and the overlying peritoneum is stripped from the posterior and superior surfaces.

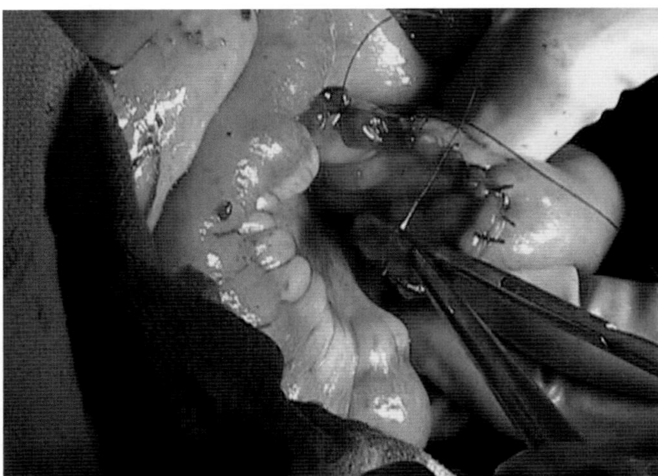

Figure 26-4 The two adjacent borders of detubularized ileum forming what will be the posterior wall of the ileocystoplasty are sutured with 2-0 Vicryl.

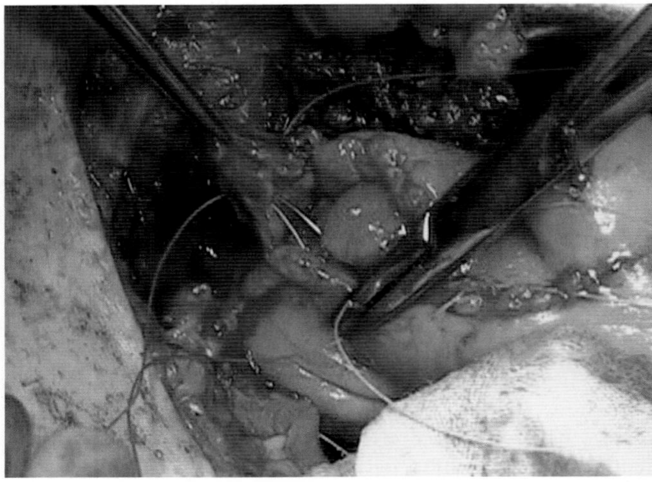

Figure 26-6 The small bowel is sutured to the bladder using a running transluminal suture in the posterior wall and a running suture of 0 Vicryl up both sides so that the anterior flap of bladder is placed between the two anterior walls of the reservoir.

bladder using a running transluminal suture in the posterior wall and then using a running suture of 0 Vicryl up both sides so that the anterior flap of bladder is placed between the two anterior walls of the reservoir (Fig. 26-6). In patients who cannot perform catheterization, the more distal portion of the ileal segment is left longer to bring it to the skin as an incontinent stoma, usually in the right iliac fossa. Patients in whom urethra closure is required need ileocecal augmentation using a reinforced ileocecal valve or the appendix as a continent neourethra for catheterization. Alternatively, if availability or mobility of the ileum is limited, left or right colon can be used. For ileocecocystoplasty, the right colon and ileum are mobilized and prepared as for an Indiana pouch. As first described by Sinaiko in 1956,[8] gastrocystoplasty is a suitable option for patients with cloacal exstrophy or metabolic acidosis from renal insufficiency.[9] Simultaneous pubovaginal slings can also be performed in patients with intrinsic sphincter deficiency, and urethra closure can be carried out in patients with urethral erosion. Overall, whether ileum, colon, or other segments are used, the goal is to ensure a low-pressure, high-volume reservoir with a low incidence of postoperative incontinence.[4,10-12]

Complications of Gastrointestinal Bladder Augmentation

The type of metabolic complications that occurs after an enteric augmentation is directly related to the segment of bowel chosen and the amount of time that the urine spends in contact with the bowel mucosa.[13-15] Because vitamin B_{12} is absorbed from the terminal ileum and is responsible for erythrocyte formation,[16] ileocystoplasty can potentially lead to vitamin B_{12} deficiency and subsequent development of pernicious anemia. The chosen segment of ileum therefore should be selected from an area at least 15 to 20 cm proximal to the ileocecal valve. The interposition of bowel in the urinary tract can also lead to acid-base changes. Hyperchloremic metabolic acidosis can develop with the use of ileum or colon, and hypochloremic metabolic alkalosis can develop if stomach is used.[17] Patients in chronic alkalotic states would therefore do better with an intestinal cystoplasty, and patients with chronic renal insufficiency or metabolic acidosis should be considered for gastrocystoplasty or composite grafts using stomach. Patients considered for gastrocystoplasty should be advised that up to one third of patients, especially those with a sensate bladder (up to 50%), may experience hematuria and dysuria syndrome.[18-20] This has led to recommendations that this procedure not be performed in patients with intact perineal sensation or in incontinent patients because the acidic urine may lead to excoriation of skin.

Studies have shown that alterations in the intestinal epithelium occur in response to urine contact with bowel mucosa. This leads to inflammatory infiltration of the submucosa, producing progressive fibrosis, goblet cell hyperplasia and subsequent loss, reduction or loss of microvilli, and loss of cellular orientation of the bowel epithelium.[21] Alterations in the enteric epithelium may be associated with long-term complications of bladder augmentation: increased risk of stone formation, progressive loss of compliance, and increased risk of spontaneous perforation and neoplasia.[21] Goblet cell hyperplasia leads to enhanced production of mucus. Mucus, permanent sutures, and staples have been identified as potential nidi for stone formation, especially coupled with stagnant urine. Routine bladder irrigation to evacuate mucus and to ensure compete bladder emptying can reduce these risks.[22] The progressive loss of compliance and the increased risk of spontaneous perforation have also been linked to progressive fibrosis of the enteric submucosa.[21] The reported incidence of spontaneous perforation is highest (9.3%) for ileocystoplasty patients, followed by 4.3% for ileocecal cystoplasty, 4.2% for sigmoid cystoplasty, and 2.9% for gastrocystoplasty.[23] Another infrequent complication is chronic postoperative diarrhea. The risk is highest for neuropathic patients in whom the ileocecal valve was used in the augmentation.

Several case reports of adenocarcinoma in patients with bladder augmentations exist.[24,25] Filmer and Spencer[25] reported tumor development in 14 patients with bladder augmentations. Nine of these patients had an ileocystoplasty, two had a cecocystoplasty, and three had a colocystoplasty.[25] The malignancies develop at or near the enterourothelial junction. It has therefore suggested that augmentation patients undergo periodic endoscopic surveillance after 5 to 10 years.

SEROMUSCULAR ENTEROPLASTY

Seromuscular enterocystoplasty or de-epithelialized colocystoplasty has been proposed to decrease the complications associated with cystoplasty using intact gastrointestinal segments.[26] It is hypothesized that removal of the functional enteric epithelium can resolve the risk of metabolic complications and stone formation by allowing re-epithelialization with urothelium. Mucus production and metabolic disturbances were virtually eliminated in one follow-up study on seromuscular colocystoplasty patients.[27] However, regeneration of functional mucosal epithelium or extensive denudation of the submucosa often led to subsequent fibrosis and contracture of the bladder augment.[28-30] The mechanical or chemical means to remove the functional enteric epithelium are also fairly impractical, limiting the widespread use of these techniques.

AUGMENTATION WITH UROTHELIUM

Two other options offered in the search for the ideal material to be used for bladder augmentation include tissue-engineered urothelium and autologous urothelium.[21] The methods used for development of tissue-engineered urothelium involve harvesting uroepithelial cells from the neuropathic or poorly compliant bladder, expanding these cells in culture, and seeding them on an absorbable nonreactive spherical template.[31-33] Concerns exist about whether the physiologic function of tissue-engineered urothelium will be affected by harvesting from hyperreflexic or poorly compliant bladders. Abnormal uroepithelium characteristics such as altered bladder permeability and elevated levels of reactive oxygen species have been associated with cells from neuropathic bladder.[34,35]

Autoaugmentation or detrusor myomectomy is a simpler, less morbid alternative to enterocystoplasty. Autoaugmentation, as described by Cartwright and Snow in 1989,[36,37] involves excising a portion of the detrusor muscle, allowing the bladder epithelium and lamina propria to form a large-mouthed bladder diverticulum. As the urothelium bulges through the muscular hiatus, bladder capacity is increased, intravesical storage pressures are reduced, and the volume at which a contraction occurs becomes larger. Because only bladder tissue is used in this technique, the risks associated with gastrointestinal segment incorporation into the urinary tract are obviated. However, in certain subgroups of neurogenic patients with contracted, poorly compliant bladders, enterocystoplasty remains superior.[38]

URETEROCYSTOPLASTY

The concept of ureterocystoplasty was inspired by patients with the VURD complex: posterior urethral *v*alves, *u*nilateral vesicoureteral reflux, and *r*enal *d*ysplasia of the refluxing renal unit.[21] The refluxing ureter or ureters provided material for bladder augmentation, which was lined by urothelium and free of the complications associated with use of gastrointestinal segments. Unfortunately, the long-term results of ureterocystoplasty have not been favorable. In a multi-institutional study, 64 patients who had undergone ureterocystoplasty at five institutions were evaluated.[39] Only 17 % (12 of 69) of patients had a compliant and continent bladder after ureterocystoplasty; 42% (29 of 69) of patients underwent repeat augmentation using a gastrointestinal segment, with reoperation pending in 26% of the patients.[39]

Current investigations are focused on native urothelial expansion. Using animal models with surgically reduced bladder capacity, isolated urothelial segments are expanded enough to perform bladder augmentation.[40,41] Although promising, no long-term results are available.

LONG-TERM RESULTS OF AUGMENTATION CYSTOPLASTY

Several studies have described the long-term results and complications of augmentation cystoplasty in various groups of patients. In a review of metabolic consequences and long-term complications of enterocystoplasty in children, the investigators show that the use of gastrointestinal segments in the urinary tract is not a perfect solution.[42] They describe short gut syndrome, vitamin B_{12} deficiency, steatorrhea, bone and growth impairment, infection, calculi, spontaneous perforations, and the development of latent tumors. Although the rates and severity of these complications after enterocystoplasty may vary, the study authors state that they may have a profound impact on patients' quality of life.[42]

Blaivas and colleagues[43] published a retrospective study evaluating long-term outcomes for 76 patients undergoing augmentation enterocystoplasty (with or without an abdominal stoma) or continent urinary diversion because of benign disease. Preoperative diagnoses included neurogenic bladder in 41 patients, refractory detrusor overactivity in 9, interstitial cystitis in 7, end-stage bladder disease in 7, radiation cystitis in 3, exstrophy in 3, postoperative urethral obstruction in 3, and low bladder compliance in 3. Sixty-nine percent of the patients considered themselves cured, 20% improved, and 11% failed (all 7 patients with interstitial cystitis failed). Mean bladder capacity increased from 166 to 572 mL, and mean maximal detrusor pressure decreased from 53 to 14 cm H_2O. Long-term complications included stomal stenosis or incontinence in 42% (11 of 26) of patients with stomas; de novo bladder and renal stones in 3% and 1%, respectively; and recurrent bladder stones in 6%. Five patients experienced persistent diarrhea, and 7% of patients had small-bowel obstruction, with surgical exploration required in 6%.[43]

In another study of long-term results and complications using augmentation ileocystoplasty in reconstructive urology, Flood and coworkers[6] reviewed 122 augmentation cystoplasties performed over an 8-year period. The primary urodynamic diagnosis was reduced compliance in 77% of the patients and detrusor hyperreflexia or instability in the remainder of the patients. Preoperative diagnoses included spinal cord injury in 27%, myelodysplasia in 22%, interstitial cystitis in 17%, idiopathic detrusor instability in 11%, radiation cystitis in 7%, Hinman-Allen syndrome in 4%, and miscellaneous causes in 9%. Sixteen patients had a simultaneous fascial sling for urethral incompetence. Mean bladder capacity increased from 108 mL (range, 15 to 500 mL) to 438 mL (range, 200 to 1200 mL). Marked improvement or stability of upper tract function was documented in 99 patients (96%). During the follow-up period, 16% underwent revision of their augmentation; 21% developed bladder stones (30% had recurrent stones); 13% developed urinary incontinence, with one half requiring further treatment; and 11% developed pyelonephritis. Five patients also developed small-bowel obstruction, and in five patients, spontaneous perforation occurred. Overall, the investigators concluded that augmentation cystoplasty has a pivotal role in the treatment of a broad range of lower and upper tract problems, with careful patient selection and close follow-up being the key to successful surgery.[6]

References

1. Mikulicz J: Zur operation der angeboren Blasenspalte. Zentralbl Chir 26:641, 1899.
2. Lapides J, Diokno A, Silber SJ, Lowe BS: Clean, intermittent self-catheterization in the treatment of urinary tract disease. J Urol 107:458, 1972.
3. Pitts WR Jr, Muecke EC: A 20 year experience with ileal conduits. The fate of the kidneys. J Urol 12:154, 1979.
4. Goldwasser B, Webster GD: Augmentation and substitution enterocystoplasty. J Urol 135:215, 1986.
5. McGuire EJ, Woodside JR, Borden TA, Weiss RM: Prognostic value of urodynamic testing in myelodysplastic patients. J Urol 126:205, 1981.
6. Flood HJ, Malhotra SJ, O'Connell HE, et al: Long-term results and complications using augmentation cystoplasty in reconstructive urology. Neurourol Urodyn 14:297, 1995.
7. Schalow EL, Kirsch AJ: Advances in bladder augmentation. Curr Sci 3:125, 2002.
8. Sinaiko ES: Artificial bladder from segment of stomach and study effect of urine on gastric secretion. Surg Gynecol Obstet 102:433, 1956.
9. Leonard MP: Outcome of gastrocystoplasty in tertiary pediatric urology practice. J Urol 164:947, 2000.
10. Light JK, Engelman UN: Reconstruction of the lower urinary tract: Observation of bowel dynamics and the artificial urinary sphincter. J Urol 133:594, 1985.
11. King LR, Webster GD, Bertram RA: Experiences with bladder reconstruction in children. J Urol 138:1002, 1992.
12. Hinman F: Functional classification of conduits for continent diversion. J Urol 144:27, 1990.
13. Duel B, Gonzalez RM, Barthod J: Alternative techniques for augmentation cystoplasty. J Urol 159:998, 1998.
14. Lauvetz R, Monda J, Kramer S, et al: Urinary pH and urea concentration correlate to the bacterial colonization rate in gastric, ileal and myoperitoneal bladder augmentation. J Urol 154:899, 1995.
15. Koch M, McDougal W, Reddy P, et al: Metabolic alterations following continent urinary diversion through colonic segments. J Urol 145:270, 1991
16. Vander AJ: Human Physiology: The Mechanisms of Body Function. New York, McGraw-Hill, 1990.
17. Stampfer DS: Metabolic and nutritional complications. Urol Clin North Am 24:715, 1997.
18. Ngan J, Lau J, Lim S, et al: Long-term results of antral gastrocystoplasty. J Urol 149:731, 1993.
19. Sheldon C, Gilbert A, Wacksman J, et al: Gastrocystoplasty: Technical and metabolic characteristics of the most versatile childhood bladder augmentation modality. J Pediatr Surg 30:283, 1995.
20. Gonsalbez R Jr, Woodard J, Broecker B, et al: The use of stomach in pediatric urinary reconstruction. J Urol 140:428, 1993.
21. Husmann DA, Snodgrass WT: Augmentation cystoplasty: Enteric and urothelial. AUA Update Series 35:282, 2004.
22. Rink RC: Augmentation cystoplasty. In Walsh PC, Retik AB, Vaughan ED Jr, Wein AJ (eds): Campbell's Urology, 7th ed. Philadelphia, WB Saunders, 1998, p 3167.
23. Bauer SB, Hendren WH, Kozakewich H, et al: Perforation of the augmented bladder. J Urol 148(Pt 2):699, 1992.
24. D'Dow J, Pearson J, Bennett M, et al: Mucin gene expression in human urothelium and in intestinal segments transposed into the urinary tract. J Urol 164:1398, 2000.
25. Filmer R, Spencer J: Malignancies in bladder augmentation and intestinal conduits. J Urol 143:671, 1990.
26. Motley RC, Montgomery BT, Zollman PE, et al: Augmentation cystoplasty utilizing de-epithelialized sigmoid colon: A preliminary study. J Urol 143:1257, 1990.
27. Jednak R, Schimke CM, Barroso U Jr, et al: Further experience with seromuscular colocystoplasty lined with urothelium. J Urol 164:2045, 2000.
28. Pippi SJ, Fraga J, Lucib A, et al: Seromuscular enterocystoplasty in dogs. J Urol 144:454, 1990.
29. Lima S, Araujo L, Vilar F, et al: Nonsecretory sigmoid cystoplasty: Experimental and clinical results. J Urol 153:1651, 1995.
30. Gonzalez R, Buson H, Reid C, et al: Seromuscular colocystoplasty lined with urothelium: Experience with 16 patients. Urology 45:24, 1995.
31. Zhang Y, Kropp B, Moore P, et al: Coculture of bladder urothelial and smooth muscle cells on small intestinal submucosa: A potential

application for tissue engineering technology. J Urol 164:928, 2000.
32. Atala A: Tissue engineering for bladder substitution. World J Urol 18:364, 2000.
33. Atala A: Bladder regeneration by tissue engineering. BJU Int 88:765, 2001.
34. Schlager T, Grady R, Mills S, et al: Bladder epithelium is abnormal in patients with neurogenic bladder due to myelomeningocele. Spinal Cord 42:163, 2004.
35. Tarcan T, Siroky M, Krane R: Isoprostane 8-epi PGF2 alpha, a product of oxidative stress, is synthesized in the bladder and causes detrusor smooth muscle contraction. Neurourol Urodyn 19:43, 2000.
36. Cartwright PC, Snow BW: Bladder autoaugmentation: partial detrusor excision to augment the bladder without use of bowel. J Urol 142:1050, 1989.
37. Snow BW, Cartwright PC: Bladder autoaugmentation. Urol Clin North Am 23:323, 1996.
38. Leng WW, Blalock J, Fredrikkson WH, et al: Enteroplasty or detrusor myomectomy? Comparison of indications and outcomes for bladder augmentation. J Urol 16:758, 1999.
39. Husman D, Snodgrass W, Koyle M, et al: Ureterocystoplasty: Indications for a successful augmentation. J Urol 171:376, 2004.
40. Ikeguchi E, Stifelman M, Hensle T: Ureteral tissue expansion for bladder augmentation. J Urol 159:1665, 1998.
41. Satar N, Yoo J, Atala A: Progressive dilatation for bladder tissue expansion. J Urol 162:829, 1999.
42. Gilbert SM, Hensle TW: Metabolic consequences and long-term complications of enterocystoplasty in children: A review. J Urol 173:1080, 2005.
43. Blaivas JG, Weiss JP, Desai P, et al: Long-term followup of augmentation enterocystoplasty and continent diversion in patients with benign disease. J Urol 173:1631, 2005.

Section 5

STRESS INCONTINENCE

Chapter 27

PATHOPHYSIOLOGY OF STRESS INCONTINENCE

Christopher R. Chapple and Francesca Manassero

The lower urinary tract provides continence by storing urine at low pressure until it is socially convenient and appropriate to void. This function is mediated by the presence of an expansible, low-pressure organ, the bladder, and a sphincter-controlled outlet mechanism. The outlet mechanism prevents urinary incontinence during an increase abdominal pressure by means of the sphincter and a complex pelvic support mechanism. Understanding the pathophysiology of stress incontinence at an anatomic level can help to identify specific anatomic defects and direct individualized treatment of patients suffering from incontinence.

THE STRESS CONTINENCE CONTROL SYSTEM

The urethral closure pressure must be greater than the bladder pressure at rest and during increases in abdominal pressure to maintain continence. The anatomic components necessary to meet this goal are a well-vascularized urethral mucosa and submucosa, a well-organized and functioning intrinsic urethral smooth muscle, a properly functioning striated sphincter with intact pudendal innervation (i.e., rhabdosphincter), and a stable, supportive hammock of surrounding muscular and fascial tissues (Fig. 27-1).

Intrinsic urethral function is the product of coaptation and compression along the length of the urethra, from the bladder neck to the proximal and mid-urethra.[1] A robust anatomic support mechanism buttresses a competent bladder neck and functioning urethral mechanics and facilitates appropriate compression and pressure transmission during increases in abdominal pressure affecting the bladder outlet. These functional interactions are complex and remain the subject of ongoing research in terms of understanding mechanisms and developing measures of outlet function. Surgery directed at the bladder outlet continence mechanism at the level of bladder neck or mid-urethra aims to counteract the loss of urethral support by creating a new zone that offers support and acts as a back plate to absorb the transmitted pressure and safeguard the sphincteric configuration.

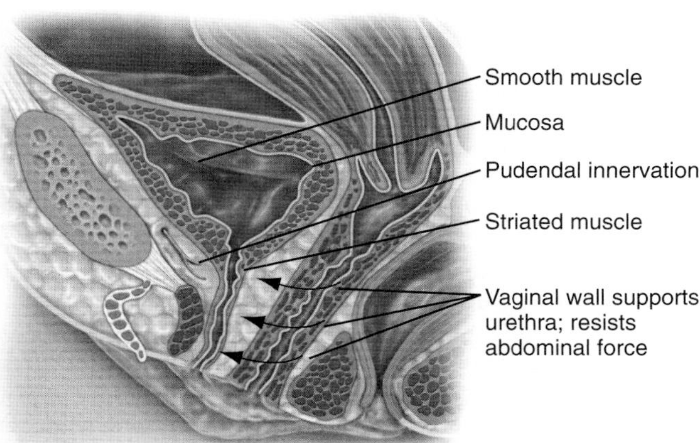

Figure 27-1 Factors that are essential for urogenital diaphragm support and function include pudendal innervation of the urethra, the mucosa and smooth muscle of the urethra, the striated muscle sphincter, and vaginal wall support. (Adapted from Abrams P, Cardozo L, Khoury S, Wein A: Incontinence, 2nd ed. Plymouth, Health Publication, 2002, p 224.)

Urethral Sphincteric Mechanisms

The glandular secretions of the inner mucosa increase the surface tension, promoting its plasticity and increasing its ability to coapt.[2] The abundant middle spongy vascular tissue of the submucosa forms a watertight seal and provides up to 30% of the total closure pressure[3-5]; this vascular cushion, like the other tissues of the urethra, is under the influence of estrogens.[6-8] Estrogenic deficiency in postmenopausal women results in atrophy of this layer, reduces the hermetic seal of the urethra mucosal, and may contribute to the multifactorial cause of stress incontinence. Although there is some consensus among clinicians about the value of estrogen therapy for treating the symptoms of atrophic vaginitis in postmenopausal stress urinary incontinence, there is no evidence to support the use of exogenous estrogen replacement therapy in treating stress incontinence.[9]

The role of smooth muscle in the maintenance of female continence is still uncertain. The U-shaped loop of the detrusor smooth muscle surrounds the proximal urethra and favors its closure by creating a constant tone. Detrusor fibers at the bladder neck are longitudinally oriented, and they extend from the bladder neck to the subcutaneous adipose tissue that surrounds the urethral meatus. The inner longitudinal smooth muscle layer is surrounded by a circular layer that lies inside the outer layer of striated muscle. The smooth muscle layers are present throughout the upper four fifths of the urethra, and their circular disposition suggests that contraction has a role in constricting the lumen. The longitudinal smooth muscle does not seem to have a passive role during the filling; rather, it has been proposed that it acts by shortening and opening the lumen to initiate micturition.[10]

The striated urogenital sphincter consists of two parts, the rhabdosphincter and the compressor urethra and the urethrovaginal sphincter distally.[11] The proximal one third of the urethra is surrounded by a sleeve of circular striated muscle that is continuous with a longer ascending cone, which extends to the vaginal introitus. The rhabdosphincter is composed mainly of type 1 fibers, composed of slow-twitch tissue capable of maintaining constant tonic contractions of the urethral lumen.[12] From manometric and electrophysiologic evaluations, this produces the greatest level of resting pressure and electromyography activity.

This part of the urethra is intrapelvic, immediately posterior to the pubic bone. In the past, it was suggested that when the urethra descended and lost this intra-abdominal position, intra-abdominal forces could no longer constrict it during straining, resulting in stress incontinence. This concept, the *pressure transmission theory*, which was introduced by Enhorning in 1961,[13] evolved into the *hammock theory* of DeLancey[14] (1994), which proposes that the vagina posteriorly offers a back plate against which the urethra is compressed during increases in intra-abdominal pressure. During a sudden increase in intra-abdominal pressure, such as during coughing, a reflex contraction of the pubococcygeus muscle occurs. The vaginal hammock is stretched and stiffened, making it easier for the urethral sphincter to close in a slitwise fashion against this firm back plate. The result and increase in intraurethral pressure, which is thought to be lost in patients suffering from stress incontinence, can be recreated by surgical procedures that stabilize or elevate the sub-urethral vaginal wall.[15-18]

If these postulates are correct, an appropriate contributory factor to female continence is provided by the bladder neck's passive elastic tension, which is important in maintaining urethral closure.[19,20] In the mid-urethra at rest, closure is mostly maintained by the intrinsic striated muscle of the rhabdosphincter; however, the extrinsic striated muscles of pubococcygeus and compressor urethrae may play a significant role in ensuring urethral closure during increases in intra-abdominal pressure. The plasticity of the urethra or its ability to work as a watertight seal is also important in maintaining continence. Approximately one third of the resting urethral pressure is offered by smooth muscle effects, one third by striated muscle effects, and one third by the vascular contribution.[21]

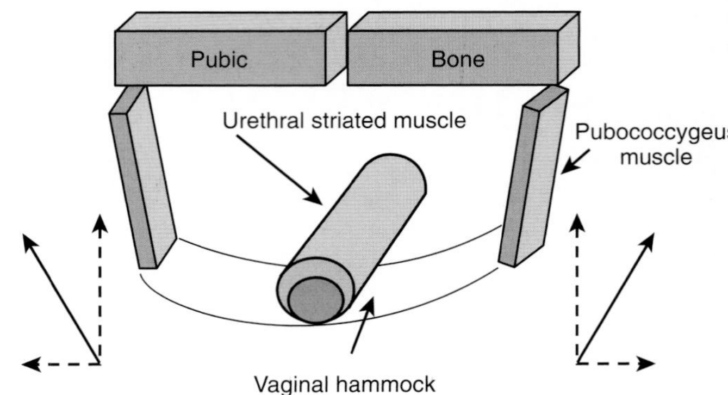

Figure 27-2 Principles of maintenance of continence. During a sudden increase in intra-abdominal pressure, such as during coughing, a reflex contraction of the pubococcygeus muscle occurs. This stretches and stiffens the vaginal hammock, which makes it easier for the urethral sphincter to close in a slitwise fashion. A role for the pubourethral ligamentous support also has been advocated.

Urethral Support Systems

The urethral support mechanism comprises all the structures extrinsic to the urethra that offer a supportive back plate on which the proximal urethra and mid-urethra lie (Fig. 27-2). The anatomic support is derived more from the fascial structures than from the musculature itself. The pubourethral ligament attaches the mid-urethra to the inferior side of the pubic symphysis and prevents downward movement during its rotational descent.[22] It works in conjunction with the pubourethralis muscle, a subdivision of the levator ani muscle that forms a sling around the proximal urethra. Together they form the mid-urethral complex. It has been postulated that elongation of the posterior pubourethral ligaments may be a significant contributory factor to the loss of urethral support seen in stress incontinence. Major fascial support to the urethra also is provided by the urethropelvic ligament, which attaches the urethra to the tendinous arc.[23]

The vesicopelvic fascia or pubocervical fascia, extending between the bladder and the vagina, suspends and attaches the vagina and cervix to the pelvic side wall, to each arcus tendineus fascia pelvis, thereby offering posterior support to the bladder and bladder neck. It has two surfaces: the perivesical fascia on the vaginal side and the endopelvic fascia on the abdominal side. Its upper zone supports the bladder above the cervix, the middle zone supports the trigone, and the lower zone supports the bladder neck. Laxity of the fascia in each of the zones results in uterine prolapse, cystocele, and urethrocele, respectively.[24]

The two arcus tendineus fasciae pelvis are tensile structures located bilaterally on either side of the urethra and vagina. They act like the ropes of a suspension bridge and provide the necessary support needed to hang the urethra on the anterior vaginal wall. They originate as fibrous bands from the pubic bone and broaden out as aponeurotic structures moving dorsally to insert into the ischial spine. The cardinal ligaments and the more medially placed uterosacral ligaments support the uterus and cervix; their relaxation results in uterine prolapse.

The pelvic floor musculature, represented by the levator ani muscles, carries the weight of the pelvic contents and prevents the abdominal pressure from stretching the ligamentous support structures. The levator ani includes the puborectalis muscle, which surrounds the rectum, connecting the pubic bones anteriorly in a U-shaped configuration; the pubococcygeus muscle, which crosses from the pubis to the coccyx; and the iliococcygeus muscle. The iliococcygeus arises laterally from the arcus tendineus levator ani and forms a horizontal sheet that spans the posterior opening of the pelvis, providing a shelf on which the pelvic organs lie. The urethra and vagina pass through an aperture in the levator musculature, the urogenital hiatus. The constant muscle tone,[25] maintained by predominantly type I (slow-twitch) striated muscle fibers, compresses the vagina and urethra anteriorly toward the pubic bone and keeps the hiatus closed.[26]

The pudendal nerve provides somatic innervation to the striated muscle of levator ani and to the striated muscle within the external anal and urethral sphincters. The intrapelvic somatic fibers travel along the anterior vaginal wall from the sacral segments S2 through S4 to provide a somatic nerve supply to the pelvic floor.[27] Neuromuscular injuries have been proposed as an important factor in predisposing to pelvic floor dysfunction. Childbirth and age are considered the two major factors predisposing to pelvic floor denervation.[28] Other factors include pelvic surgery (i.e., rectal and vaginal surgery with extensive pelvic dissection), radiotherapy, and congenital neurologic conditions such as spina bifida and muscular dystrophy.

Support and suspension of the pelvic organs depends on a healthy innervated pelvic floor striated muscle, intact robust con-

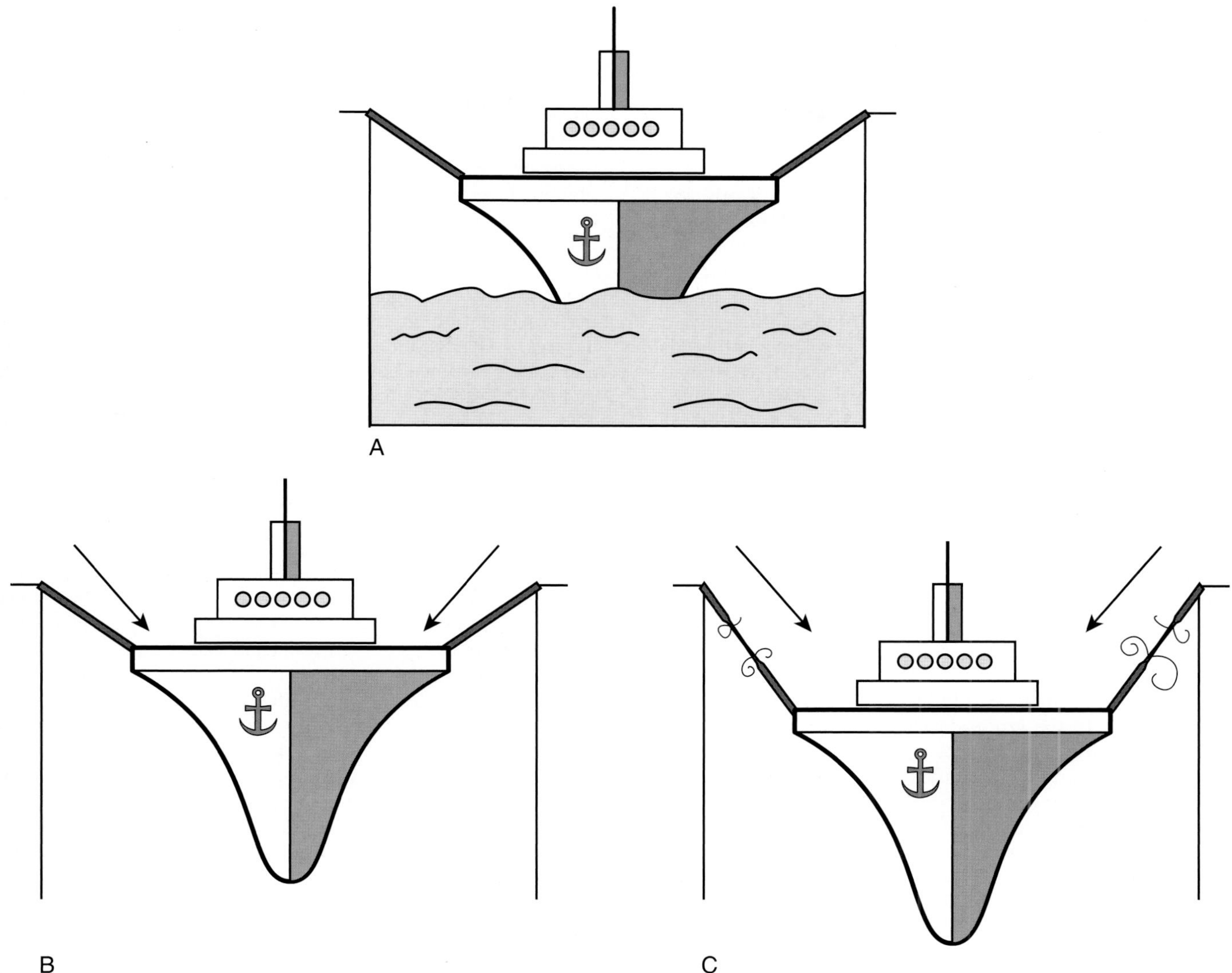

Figure 27-3 In this representation of the pelvic floor support mechanism, water represents the pelvic floor musculature, the guy ropes are the ligaments, and the ship is the pelvic organs **(A)**. If the pelvic muscles are weakened, undue force is applied to the ligaments **(B)**, which weaken and may be damaged **(C)**.

nective tissue, and their attachments to the bony frame of the pelvis. A useful analogy is that described by Peggy Norton, who suggested visualizing the relationships of these factors by considering a ship lying moored in dry dock. The ligaments are represented by the mooring ropes and the pelvic floor musculature by the water on which the ship sits. If the dry dock is emptied, then the influence of the supporting water disappears, leaving all of the tension applied to the mooring robes, which will inevitably weaken and fracture (Fig. 27-3).

The levator ani contains type I fibers that provide resting tone and type II (fast-twitch) fibers that maintain the urethral closure under stress and prevent stretching of the pelvic ligaments. Berglas and Rubin showed that in the nulliparous patients, the lower one third of the vagina is oriented more vertically and the upper two thirds deviate horizontally, thereby maintaining the vaginal axis in an almost horizontal position.[29] This configuration is maintained by the posterior attachments of the cervix with the cardinal and uterosacral ligaments and by the anterior position of the urogenital hiatus. During stressful maneuvers, such as coughing or straining, the levator hiatus shortens anteriorly by the contraction of the pubococcygeus muscles. In the case if genital prolapse, when the levator ani support is lost, the vaginal axis becomes more vertical, the urogenital hiatus broadens, and fascial supports are strained.

EFFECT OF PREGNANCY AND CHILDBIRTH ON THE PELVIC FLOOR

An important pathophysiologic factor is the contribution of pregnancy and childbirth to the development of urinary incontinence in women.[30,31] Epidemiologic studies have reported a prevalence of stress incontinence ranging from 23% to 67 % during pregnancy and 6% to 29% after childbirth. The fear of pelvic floor trauma has been used to justify an increase in the number of indiscriminate and often unnecessary cesarean deliveries.[32]

Our knowledge of pathophysiologic impacts of pregnancy and delivery on lower urinary tract function and the development of urinary incontinence remain scanty and often are somewhat confused.[33] Future works needs to investigate the relative contribution provided by the individual components of pregnancy and delivery. The findings could significantly alter our understanding and treatment of stress incontinence.

It is a widely held view that stress incontinence is principally the consequence of delivery trauma to the pelvic floor. However, many studies have demonstrated that about 40% of nulliparous women experience occasional stress incontinence, which is a significant problem in 5% of them.[34,35] The problem regularly worsens during the first pregnancy, and for the women developing stress incontinence in middle life, pregnancy rather than delivery seems to unmask the problem and worsen it.[36] If incontinence emerges for the first time during pregnancy, it tends to resolve after the puerperium, but it may return in future pregnancies, progressively worsening and becoming a significant problem often many years after the pregnancies.

The prevalence of persistent, clinically important stress incontinence is significantly higher with greater multiparity than in nulliparous women, and it can be related to the number of pregnancies.[37] Women who develop stress incontinence during pregnancy are more likely to experience incontinence later in their life. A study by Viktrup and colleagues[38] of 278 women showed that 30% of them had stress urinary incontinence 5 years after delivery. In the group without stress urinary incontinence during pregnancy or after delivery, the incidence 5 years after delivery was only 19%. In the group developing stress urinary incontinence during the first pregnancy or puerperium with resolution of symptoms within 3 months after delivery, 42% of women had complained of recurrent incontinence 5 years later. In the latter group in which the symptoms of stress urinary incontinence did not resolve 3 months after delivery, the symptoms were still present in 92% 5 years later.[38]

Vaginal delivery has been recognized as being potentially traumatic to the pelvic floor. The first delivery may initiate injury to the continence mechanism as a consequence of direct damage to the pelvic floor muscles or nerves, or both, during the passage of the fetus. The perineal branch of the pudendal nerve courses in Alcock's canal, lateral and anterior to the vagina, making it vulnerable to damage during childbirth.[39] Additional deterioration of the urethral musculature and denervation can occur with aging, producing clinical disability many years after the initial trauma.[40]

The fetal head may dilate and overstretch the vaginal wall or avulse the cardinal and uterosacral ligaments, injuring connective support tissues. Moreover, the presenting part of the fetus during labor may constrict the pelvic structures, resulting in an ischemic injury. Compression of the fetal head against the subpubic urethra or paravaginal attachments may directly injure the urinary tract during labor and delivery. There are many mechanisms by which vaginal delivery can increase the risk of developing stress incontinence.[41]

The contribution of vaginal birth to producing denervation has been clarified by Allen's electromyographic studies, which were performed before and after vaginal birth. Allen and colleagues[42] found that most women have signs of neurologic damage after vaginal birth (but not after cesarean section), as confirmed by an increased motor unit potential, and increasing amounts of damage correlated well with greater evidence of stress urinary incontinence.

Vaginal delivery causes partial denervation of the pelvic floor in most primiparous women, but there is electromyographic evidence of reinnervation after vaginal delivery in 80% of them. The nerve damage is more likely in women with a long, active second stage of labor and heavy babies.

The impaired muscle strength in the days after vaginal deliveries returns to normal within 2 months in most women. In a few of them, severe muscular weakness is associated with urinary and fecal incontinence, a prelude to future problems depending on permanent pelvic floor damage.

Multiparity, a long second stage of labor (>30 minutes), the use of the forceps, high birth weight (>4 kg), and a third-degree perineal tear are important risk factors for pudendal nerve damage.[43] After spontaneous and instrumental deliveries, 21% and 34% of women complained of stress urinary incontinence and 5.5% and 4% reported fecal incontinence, respectively. Only 22% of patients incontinent during pregnancy continued to complain about it after delivery.[44]

Episiotomy, one of the few surgical procedures that does not require the patient's informed consent, is widely performed during delivery despite its doubtful usefulness. It is becoming increasingly accepted that an episiotomy may be more harmful that useful. Supporters of routine episiotomy maintain that it avoids uncontrolled lacerations and extended relaxation of the pelvic floor; the contrary view is that there is no evidence that first- or second-degree perineal tears cause long-term consequences and that episiotomies do not seem to protect against third- and fourth-degree tears, which are associated with unpleasant sequelae. Midline episiotomies cause significantly higher rates of third- and fourth-degree perineal tears than mediolateral episiotomies; they are not helpful in protecting the pelvic floor during delivery and can heavily prejudice anal continence.[45,46] Despite this, midline episiotomy is still widely used, probably because it is believed to improve healing and reduce postpartum pain.

Restrictive episiotomy guidelines have many potential advantages, such as less suturing, more minor complications, and less posterior perineal trauma, but they do not result in any difference in pain therapy and the incidence of severe trauma, and they are associated with an increase risk of anterior perineal trauma.[47,48] The consequences of episiotomy are independent of maternal age, duration of second stage of labor, possible complications, the use of forceps or vacuum extraction during delivery, and baby birth weight.

Regional anesthesia may be used to relieve labor pain, but its correlation with pelvic floor damage remains controversial. Epidural anesthesia, relaxing the pelvic floor, provides a greater control of passage of the fetal head and subsequently reduces perineal lacerations, but a prolonged second stage of labor can enhance the incidence of pudendal nerve damage. Analysis of the relationship between regional anesthesia and pelvic floor injury suggested that the rate of significant damage was higher with epidural anesthesia because of the increase in episiotomies and instrumental deliveries.[49]

In many women with stress incontinence, pelvic floor muscle exercise has been effective in improving it,[50] with no additional benefit accruing from biofeedback.[51] The theoretical basis for physical therapy is that facilitation and strengthening of muscles may improve periurethral muscular efficiency and that training of pelvic floor muscles can improve structural support of the pelvic organs. Morkved and Bo,[52] after a prospective, matched, controlled study evaluating the long-term effect of an immediate postpartum pelvic floor training course, concluded that it is helpful in the prevention and treatment of urinary incontinence and that improvement is still present 1 year after delivery. Miller and coworkers, [53] after studying the characteristics of women "responders" compared with "nonresponders" to pelvic floor electrical stimulation, affirmed that a minimum of 14 weeks was needed to see the first objective improvements (i.e., at least 50% reduction in leakage episodes).

Pelvic floor exercises are not effective in all women. Patient motivation is essential for long-term success, but the quality of the pelvic floor muscles and their innervation are also important. If the muscle is normally innervated and is sufficiently attached to the endopelvic fascia, by contracting her pelvic muscles before and during the stress, a woman is able to reduce the leakage, and the pelvic floor exercises are likely to be an effective therapy. If the pelvic floor muscle is denervated as a result of significant neural damage, it may not be possible to rehabilitate the muscle adequately to make pelvic muscle exercises an effective strategy. If the muscle is totally disconnected from the fascial tissues, any possible contraction may not be effective in supporting the urethra or maintaining its position under strain.[54,55]

ROLE OF CONNECTIVE TISSUE

The bladder is a complex, distensible organ comprising of an inner urothelium and suburothelial layer, an important smooth muscle component (i.e., detrusor muscle) with neurologically controlled tissue, and an outer serosal layer. Connective tissue, composed of collagen, elastin, smooth muscle, fibroblasts, and blood vessels, is present in all of these layers. It has been suggested that collagen has the primary function of tension transfer in most tissues, and it is reasonable to suppose that it plays an equivalent role in the bladder. Types I and III collagen can be found in the detrusor layer, and type IV collagen is in the basement membrane under the urothelial layer and surrounding individual smooth muscle cells. Although the connective tissue is passive in that it does not require energy to function, it plays a unique structural role in providing the bladder wall tissues with resilience and tensile strength. These physical properties are related to the quantity and types of collagen present and its arrangement. Changes in collagen type and content may affect bladder compliance. Collagen is the main constituent of endopelvic fascia, and abnormalities in the quantity, type, and quality of collagen have been observed in women with stress incontinence and in those with genitourinary prolapse.[56-58]

Regulation of collagen synthesis depends on intrinsic factors within individual cell types and on extrinsic factors such as cytokines, growth factors, and mechanical forces. Because progressive alteration of the connective tissue of the bladder or in the pelvis may result in structural weakness, it is important to investigate and define the factors that contribute to abnormal pathophysiology.

It was suggested by Petros and Ulmsten[59] in 1990 in their *integral theory* that stress and urge incontinence may have a common cause, with the anatomic defects related to a primary abnormality of connective tissue failure. With laxity, the anterior vaginal can be a primary etiologic factor, and this may result in the activation of stretch receptors in the bladder neck and proximal urethra, which triggers an inappropriate micturition reflex. These events may produce detrusor overactivity and cause the filling symptoms of the overactive bladder, including urgency, frequency, nocturia, and urgency incontinence. The deficient anterior vaginal wall does not efficiently transmit the closure pressure that would otherwise be generated by proper functioning of the pubourethral ligaments, the vaginal hammock, and the pubococcygeus muscles.

We need to identify the cells responsible for the synthesis of the proteins that contribute to defective connective tissue and to describe the mechanisms by which these cells acquire the altered synthetic phenotype. In some individuals, the changes in connective tissue, which can be associated with the pathogenesis of incontinence, may be related to age or the hormonal milieu.

With increasing age, the ratio of connective tissue to muscle is reduced, and although the formation of collagen cross-links stabilizes the collagen molecules, this also prevents remodeling and flexibility. The hormonal changes during pregnancy can result in abnormal remodeling of collagen, which may be another important factor in the development of incontinence. In every case, the exact cellular mechanisms by which hormones, cytokines, or other peptide factors influence the mechanical properties of connective tissue remain unclear.

Connective tissue plays an important role in the overall physiologic function of the lower urinary tract and pelvic floor. The age-related weakening of connective tissues can influence tissue and organ function, and it is likely that the increased focus on connective tissue changes will in the future provide a better understanding of the pathophysiology and lead to more effective management of stress urinary incontinence and vaginal prolapse.

EFFECT OF URETHRAL POSITION AND FUNCTION ON STRESS URINARY INCONTINENCE

Urethral Hypermobility

The cause of urethral hypermobility (i.e., increased mobility) is thought to be a loss of normal extrinsic support of the urethra because of weakness of the endopelvic fascia and pelvic floor muscles. During stress, the bladder neck and the proximal urethra descend, and there is an incomplete distribution of abdominal pressure to the urethra (i.e., pressure-transmission deficit). The bladder pressure exceeds urethral pressure, and urine leaks. Urethral hypermobility can result from abnormalities of vaginal and pelvic anatomy. It is usually initiated by childbirth, and it is worsened by aging and alterations in hormone levels. Stretching, tearing, and avulsion of the levator muscles result in the urogenital hiatus becoming longer and wider. This change results in chronic anterior displacement of the pelvic organs, with loss of any organ support at rest and especially during straining. Stretching or tearing of the cardinal and uterosacral ligaments may result in anterior displacement of the uterus at rest or during straining, and the resultant stretching of the vaginal wall continues this displacement and causes the loss of the normal superior vaginal sulcus and vaginal folds. The consequence of these forces is a rotational descent of the proximal urethra away from its retropubic position and the eventual development of stress urinary incontinence.

On lateral cystourethrograms, the main anatomic change is loss of the posterior urethrovaginal angle, with the urethra and trigone falling into the same plane.[60-62] Radiographic studies cannot distinguish between lateral or central defects in vaginal wall support because they appear in the same sagittal plane. It is necessary when examining the patient to determine which defect is present and to what extent. Because the proximal urethra rotates out of the focal plane of ultrasonographic probes or magnetic resonance imaging (MRI), coronal images of vaginal relaxation cannot provide adequate anatomic information during leakage.

Despite extensive data about anatomic defects, it is difficult to correlate the influence of these defects, the vaginal position, and the urethral closure mechanism. Not all women with stress incontinence had vaginal prolapse, and prolapse repairs do not always cure the stress incontinence. Conversely, women who redevelop stress incontinence after an apparently successful operation do not always have a recurrence of prolapse.[63] Vaginal support is important for maintaining urinary continence, but intrinsic sphincter deficiency also must be considered.

Intrinsic Sphincter Deficiency

In 1988, Olsson and Blaivas[64] suggested a new classification of stress incontinence, in which for the first time appeared the concept of intrinsic urethral weakness as a cause for incontinence without a vaginal support defect. They called this type III incontinence to differentiate it from types I and II, both of which were associated with movement. This category is often described by the term *intrinsic sphincter deficiency* (ISD),[65] which emphasizes the importance of the intrinsic components of the sphincter acting under the influence of pudendal innervation and comprises the urethral striated and smooth muscle, mucosa, and submucosal layers.

When ISD was proposed as a new type of stress incontinence without vaginal mobility, the diagnostic trend was to evaluate the cause of stress incontinence as a dichotomy caused by hypermobility or ISD. The typical ISD patient was described as having a low urethral closure pressure, a stovepipe (pipe stem) appearance on cystoscopy, and an open or funneled urethra at rest or during minimal effort on radiographic images. Typical causes included ischemia after pelvic or vaginal surgery, multiple previous operations, denervation in neurogenic patients, or radiation damage. These examples of ISD now represent extreme forms and the most severe cases.

Another important aspect is urethral denervation after childbirth and its association with urinary and fecal incontinence.[66,67] Crushing or traction injuries to the pudendal nerve during labor and delivery are a primary cause of sphincteric incompetence. A causal relationship between pudendal nerve injury and stress incontinence has been established in animal studies.[68-70] Because the pudendal nerve innervates the external urethral sphincter, pudendal nerve injury causes denervation and dysfunction of the urethra, resulting in decreased urethral resistance, which is especially evident during stressful physical activities. Stress incontinence is often associated with a decrease in the electrophysiologic function of the pudendal nerve,[71] the striated urethral sphincter,[72] and the pelvic floor muscles.[73,74]

Hypermobility and Intrinsic Sphincter Deficiency: From Dichotomy to Continuum

In the past few years, there has been a gradual change from a dichotomous classification of stress incontinence as hypermobility or ISD. ISD alone is rare, and urethral hypermobility may occur commonly without significant ISD, but usually there is a combination of both. This evolution in our understanding followed development of the concept of Valsalva leak point pressure (VLPP), introduced by McGuire in 1995,[75,76] and the analysis of long-term results of incontinence surgery. During studies of urethral bulking with collagen, researchers documented that continence improvements were not related to changes in urethral closure pressure, but instead corresponded to the level of abdominal pressure required to produce leakage in the absence of intrinsic detrusor contraction. Despite lacking a specific anatomic or theoretical basis and standardization of recording methods or a consensus on how to deal with an associated prolapse, a low VLPP (<60 cm H_2O has been suggested) has been widely considered to be an indicator of ISD, although there is considerable variability in the literature about the extent of correlation between VLPP and outcome. Urethral pressure profilometry has been extensively studied in this context, and a similar lack of correlation with predictive value and outcome appears to exist. For example, a low-pressure urethra may not leak, whereas the high-pressure urethra may, and several studies have failed to show any correlation between the postoperative urethral pressure profile and outcome.[77]

Long-term results of stress incontinence surgery have revealed a higher failure rate for the classic procedures other than slings that seem to ensure the best long-term protection against incontinence recurrence because they offer direct suburethral support.[78] Slings have become the operation of choice for incontinence caused by ISD.

Some degree of ISD may exist in many patients for whom hypermobility is believed to be the only cause of stress incontinence.[79] This understanding clarifies the increasing use of suburethral sling surgery to treat stress incontinence, whereas this procedure formerly was suggested principally for patients with recurrent stress incontinence or severe ISD.[80]

It is necessary to have a unifying hypothesis that can combine all of these observations about hypermobility, ISD, and pudendal denervation. The concept of a continuum of pathologic states offers a model for conducting research and providing treatment for these conditions.

ROLE OF IMAGING AND ULTRASONOGRAPHY

Radiographic studies have given a significant boost to the study of the physiopathology of stress incontinence since the introduction of simple static and dynamic lateral cystograms. MRI and real-time ultrasonography, simultaneously showing what happens during the leakage in terms of movement of the pelvis and the urethra, have suggested spatial and causal relationships between the proximal urethra and vaginal wall movement.

Dynamic fast-scan MRI has been used to visualize all compartments of the female pelvis at rest and under stress.[81] The pubococcygeal line that extends from the inferior border of the pubic symphysis to the last joint of the coccyx represents the level of the pelvic floor and is the reference marker.[82] MRI studies are more qualitative than quantitative, and they give more details about the soft tissues than previous radiographic studies. However, access to dynamic MRI worldwide is confined to a few centers, and MRI remains limited in its ability to delineate precise details of urethral movement. At this time, ultrasonography is still superior for visualizing mobility of the urethra and the vagina.

Suprapubic, translabial, and transperineal sonographic approaches have been used to quantify stress incontinence. With the improving resolution of sonographic probes, the transperineal approach has reached the same diagnostic level as the transrectal approach. In studies with a transrectal probe, funneling of the bladder neck is the typical sonographic sign seen during leakage.

The observed urethral movement and funneling are compatible with the rotational descent described previously. Ultrasonography studies provide more detail than radiographs. Increasing abdominal pressure forces the anterior vaginal wall out of the urogenital hiatus, and the urethra follows it. The anterior portion of the urethra can be slowed and eventually arrested in its movement while the posterior portion continues to rotate out of the pelvis with the vaginal wall.[83,84] This difference in movement seems to result in shearing apart of the walls of the two adjacent structures, resulting in apparent funneling. Suspension procedures at the bladder neck or the mid-urethra may prevent this exaggerated posterior urethral motion. If they can be placed accurately in an intramural position, injection procedures, which depend on urethral coaptation, should have a higher success rate in a patient in whom the shear force associated with anatomic motion is limited.[85]

These anatomic observations, combined with progressive awareness about the role of pudendal innervation in continent and incontinent patients, help to define the relationship between urethral closure and vaginal movement. When intra-abdominal pressure increases, the proximal urethra is subjected to two types of forces that combine to open it. The first is a *shearing force* produced by the asymmetric descent of the anterior and posterior urethral walls below the pubis under stress and the effect of vaginal mobility on urethral closure, which is opposed by counterforces of vaginal support. The second is an *expulsive force*, which is mediated by the transmission of intra-abdominal forces to the bladder and countered by the intrinsic urethral musculature, which depends primarily on intrinsic closure pressure produced by the pudendally innervated rhabdosphincter combined with vaginal support. If these shear and expulsive forces occur simultaneously as intra-abdominal pressure increases and there is a defect in either component, the urethra will reach a point beyond which urethral closure and continence cannot be sustained.

CONCLUSIONS

Two factors govern the predisposition to develop stress urinary incontinence and prolapse. First, after the evolutionary changes in pelvic floor anatomy resulting from the changes to orthograde posture, the pelvic floor had to adapt from its mainly muscular utility (i.e., moving the tail) in four-legged animals to a supportive function in humans. This transition generated a decrease in muscle mass and an increase in connective tissue. Second, the human reproductive process consists of a relatively large fetus with a large bony cranium that must pass through the pelvic floor during the processes of labor and delivery.

The complex causes of stress urinary incontinence and pelvic organ prolapse and the long period over which these problems and their complications develop strongly support the need for prospective studies of the natural history of these processes in the future. An integrated approach to anatomy, radiology, and physiology is essential to a better understanding of the pathophysiology.

The current classification of stress incontinence attempts to incorporate the spectrum of hypermobility and urethral dysfunction. Satisfactory urethral continence depends on many factors (e.g., resting tone, active contraction, external compression, pressure transmission, integrity of configuration), and the focal point appears to be the mid-urethra. Many patients with stress incontinence have some degree of urethral hypermobility and ISD. Some of these patients have primary sphincteric problems, whereas others have an adequately functioning sphincter but significant hypermobility, and the diagnosis for most patients lies between these two extremes.

Repeated episodes of vaginal traction can stretch, tear, or weaken urethral muscles and contribute to a chronically weakened urethra characterized by a low VLPP or low urethral closure pressures, which is suggested to be typical of ISD. However, there is no adequate classification of ISD because most of the measures have limited sensitivity by virtue of their inability to separate the different components of urethral function. Electrophysiologic studies, MRI and, sonography can be used to quantify the morphologic and functional decline in striated sphincter tone, but analysis of the precise etiologic factors is difficult because the pathophysiologic dysfunction develops over many years. Successful operations can restore urethral position but probably do not reverse urethral function, and there are still many questions about whether this is ever possible. In the future, prospective studies taking account of nature and nurture may allow identification of patients who are genetically predetermined to develop these conditions. This information can facilitate the investigation of early, timely interventions to prevent further deterioration of support tissues and urethral closure mechanisms.

References

1. Haab F, Zimmern PE, Leach GE: Female stress incontinence due to intrinsic sphincteric deficiency: Recognition and management. J Urol 156:3-17, 1996.
2. Zinner NR, Sterling AM, Ritter RC: Role of inner urethral softness in urinary continence. Urology 16:115-117, 1980.
3. Raz S, Caine M, Zeigler M: The vascular component in the production of intraurethral pressure. J Urol 108:93-96, 1972.
4. Tulloch AG: The vascular contribution to intraurethral pressure. Br J Urol 46:659-664, 1974.
5. Rud T, Andersson KE, Asmussen M, et al: Factors maintaining the intraurethral pressure in women. Invest Urol 17:343-347, 1980.
6. Caine M, Raz S: The role of female hormones in stress incontinence. Paper presented at the 16th Congress of the International Society of Urology, Amsterdam, 1973.
7. Faber P, Heidenreich J: Treatment of stress incontinence with estrogen in postmenopausal women. Urol Int 32:221-223, 1977.
8. Smith P: Age changes in the female urethra. Br J Urol 44:667-676, 1972.
9. Cardozo L: Role of estrogens in the treatment of female urinary incontinence. J Am Geriatr Soc 38:326-328, 1990.
10. Gosling JA: The structure of the female lower tract and pelvic floor. Urol Clin North Am 12:207-214, 1985.
11. DeLancey JO: Structural aspects of the extrinsic continence mechanism. Obstet Gynecol 72(Pt 1):296-301, 1988.
12. Gosling JA, Dixon JS, Critchley HO, Thompson SA: A comparative study of the human external sphincter and periurethral levator ani muscles. Br J Urol 53:35-41, 1981.

13. Enhorning G: Simultaneous recording of the intravesical an intraurethral pressures. A study on urethral closure in normal and stress incontinent women. Acta Chir Scand 276(Suppl):1-68, 1961.
14. DeLancey JO: Structural support of the urethra as it relates to stress urinary incontinence: The hammock hypothesis. Am J Obstet Gynecol 170:1713-1723, 1994.
15. Bunne G, Obrink A: Influence of pubococcygeal repair on urethral closure pressure at stress. Acta Obstet Gynecol Scand 57:355-359, 1978.
16. Bump RC, Fantl JA, Hurt WG: Dynamic urethral pressure profilometry pressure transmission ratio determinations after continence surgery: understanding the mechanism of success, failure, and complications. Obstet Gynecol 72:870-874, 1988.
17. Van-Geelen JM, Theeuwes AG, Eskes TK, Martin CB Jr: The clinical and urodynamic effects of anterior vaginal repair and Burch colposuspension. Am J Obstet Gynecol 159:137-144, 1988.
18. Penttinen J, Lindholm EL, Kaar K, Kauppila A: Successful colposuspension in stress urinary incontinence reduces bladder neck mobility and increases pressure transmission to the urethra. Arch Gynecol Obstet 244:233-238, 1989.
19. Hilton P, Stanton SL: Urethral pressure measurement by microtransducer: The results in symptom-free women and in those with genuine stress incontinence. Br J Obstet Gynaecol 90:919-933, 1983.
20. Warwick RT, Brown AD: A urodynamic evaluation of urinary incontinence in the female and its treatment. Urol Clin North Am 6:203-216, 1979.
21. Rud T: Urethral pressure profile in continent women from childhood to old age. Acta Obstet Gynecol Scand 59:331-335, 1980.
22. Zacharin RF: The suspensory mechanism of the female urethra. J Anat 97:423-427, 1963.
23. Rovner ES, Ginsberg DA, Raz S: The UCLA surgical approach to sphincteric incontinence in women. World J Urol 15:280-294, 1997.
24. DeLancey JO: Anatomy. In Cardozo L, Staskin D (eds): Textbook of Female Urology and Urogynaecology. London, Isis Medical Media, 2001, pp 11-24.
25. Critchley HO, Dixon JS, Gosling JA: Comparative study of the periurethral and perianal parts of the human levator ani muscle. Urol Int 35:226-232, 1980.
26. DeLancey JO, Hurd WW: Size of the urogenital hiatus in the levator ani muscles in normal women and women with pelvic organ prolapse. Obstet Gynecol 91:364-368, 1998.
27. Borirakchanyavat S, Aboseif SR, Carroll PR, et al: Continence mechanism of the isolated female urethra: An anatomical study of the intrapelvic somatic nerves. J Urol 158(Pt 1):822-826, 1997.
28. Smith AR, Hosker GL, Warrell DW: The role of partial denervation of the pelvic floor in the aetiology of genitourinary prolapse and stress incontinence of urine. A neurophysiological study. Br J Obstet Gynaecol 96:24-28, 1989.
29. Berglas B, Rubin IC: Study of the supportive structures of the uterus by levator myography. Surg Gynaecol Obstet 97:677-692, 1953.
30. Swash M, Snooks SJ, Henry MM: Unifying concept of pelvic floor disorders and incontinence. J R Soc Med 78:906-911, 1985.
31. Beck RP, McCormick S, Nordstrom L: Intraurethral-intravesical cough-pressure spike differences in 267 patients surgically cured of genuine stress incontinence of urine. Obstet Gynecol 72(Pt 1):302-306, 1988.
32. Wall LL, DeLancey JO: The politics of prolapse: A revisionist approach to disorders of the pelvic floor in women. Perspect Biol Med 34:486-496, 1991.
33. Cardozo L, Cutner A: Lower urinary tract symptoms in pregnancy. Br J Urol 80(Suppl 1):14-23, 1997.
34. Francis WJ: Disturbances of bladder function in relation to pregnancy. J Obstet Gynaecol Br Emp 67:353-366, 1960.
35. Hojberg KE, Salvig JD, Winslow NA, et al: Urinary incontinence: Prevalence and risk factors at 16 weeks of gestation. Br J Obstet Gynaecol 106:842-850, 1999.
36. Viktrup L, Lose G, Rolff M, Barfoed K: The symptom of stress incontinence caused by pregnancy or delivery in primiparas. Obstet Gynecol 79:945-949, 1992.
37. Groutz A, Gordon D, Keidar R, et al: Stress urinary incontinence: Prevalence among nulliparous compared with primiparous and grand multiparous premenopausal women. Neurourol Urodyn 18:419-425, 1999.
38. Viktrup L: The risk of lower urinary tract symptoms five years after the first delivery. Neurourol Urodyn 21:2-29, 2002.
39. Swash M: The neurogenic hypothesis of stress incontinence. Ciba Found Symp 151:156-175, 1990.
40. Smith AR, Hosker GL, Warrell DW: The role of pudendal nerve damage in the aetiology of genuine stress incontinence in women. Br J Obstet Gynaecol 96:29-32, 1989.
41. Nichols DH, Randall CL: Vaginal Surgery. Baltimore, Williams & Wilkins, 1989, p 463.
42. Allen RE, Hosker GL, Smith AR, Warrell DW: Pelvic floor damage and childbirth: A neuphysiological study. Br J Obstet Gynaecol 97:770-779, 1990.
43. Snooks SJ, Swash M, Henry MM, Setchell M: Risk factors in childbirth causing damage to the pelvic floor innervation. Int J Colorectal Dis 1:20-24, 1986.
44. Meyer S, Bachelard O, De Grandi P: Do bladder neck mobility and urethral sphincter function differ during pregnancy compared with during the non-pregnant state? Int Urogynecol J Pelvic Floor Dysfunct 9:397-404, 1998.
45. Iosif S, Henriksson L, Ulmsten U: Postpartum incontinence. Urol Int 36:53-58, 1981.
46. Signorello LB, Harlow BL, Chekos AK, Repke JT: Midline episiotomy and anal incontinence: Retrospective cohort study. BMJ 320:86-90, 2000.
47. Angioli R, Gomez-Marin O, Cantuaria G, O'sullivan MJ: Severe perineal lacerations during vaginal delivery: The University of Miami experience. Am J Obstet Gynecol 182:1083-1085, 2000.
48. Carroli G, Belizan J: Episiotomy for vaginal birth. Cochrane Database Syst Rev (2):CD000081, 2000.
49. Robinson JN, Norwitz ER, Cohen AP, et al: Epidural analgesia and third- or fourth-degree lacerations in nulliparas. Obstet Gynecol 94:259-262, 1999.
50. Bo K, Talseth T: Long-term effect of pelvic floor muscle exercise 5 years after cessation of organized training. Obstet Gynecol 87:261-265, 1996.
51. Berghmans L, Hendriks H, Bo K, et al: Conservative treatment of stress urinary incontinence in women: A systematic review of randomized clinical trials. Br J Urol 82:181-91, 1998.
52. Morkved S, Bo K: Effect of postpartum pelvic floor muscle training in prevention and treatment of urinary incontinence: A one-year follow up. BJOG 107:1022-1028, 2000.
53. Miller K, Richardson DA, Siegel SW, et al: Pelvic floor electrical stimulation for genuine stress incontinence: Who will benefit and when? Int Urogynecol J Pelvic Floor Dysfunct 9:265-270, 1998.
54. Miller JM, Ashton-Miller JA, DeLancey JO: A pelvic muscle precontraction can reduce cough-related urine loss in selected women with mild SUI. J Am Geriatr Soc 46:870-874, 1998.
55. DeLancey JO, Ashton-Miller JA: Pathophysiology of adult urinary incontinence. Gastroenterology 126(Suppl 1):S23-S32, 2004.
56. Ulmsten U, Ekman G, Giertz G, Malmstrom A: Different biochemical composition of connective tissue in continent and stress incontinent women. Acta Obstet Gynecol Scand 66:455-457, 1987.
57. Falconer C, Ekman G, Malmstrom A, Ulmsten U: Decreased collagen synthesis in stress-incontinent women. Obstet Gynecol 84:583-586, 1994.
58. Keane DP, Sims TJ, Abrams P, Bailey AJ: Analysis of collagen status in premenopausal nulliparous women with genuine stress incontinence. Br J Obstet Gynecol 104:994-998, 1997.
59. Petros PE, Ulmsten UI: An integral theory of female urinary incontinence. Experimental and clinical considerations. Acta Obstet Gynecol Scand Suppl 153:7-31, 1990.

60. Jeffcoate TN, Roberts H: Observations on stress incontinence of urine. Am J Obstet Gynecol 64:721-738, 1952.
61. Hodgkinson CP: Relationship of female urethra and bladder in urinary stress incontinence. Am J Obstet Gynecol 65:560-573, 1953.
62. Hodgkinson CP: Stress urinary incontinence. Am J Obstet Gynecol 108:1141-1168, 1970.
63. Wall LL, Helms M, Peattie AB, et al: Bladder neck mobility and the outcome of surgery for genuine stress urinary incontinence. A logistic regression analysis of lateral bead-chain cystourethrograms. J Reprod Med 39:429-435, 1994.
64. Blaivas JG, Olsson CA: Stress incontinence: Classification and surgical approach. J Urol 139:727-731, 1988.
65. Abrams P, Cardozo L, Fall M, et al: The standardization of terminology of lower urinary tract function: Report from the Standardisation Sub-committee of the International Continence Society. Neurourol Urodyn 21:167-178, 2002.
66. Snooks SJ, Barnes PR, Swash M: Damage to the innervation of the voluntary anal and periurethral sphincter musculature in incontinence: An electrophysiological study. J Neurol Neurosurg Psychiatry 47:1269-1273, 1984.
67. Snooks SJ, Badenoch DF, Tiptaft RC, Swash M: Perineal nerve damage in genuine stress urinary incontinence. An electrophysiological study. Br J Urol 57:422-426, 1985.
68. Kuo HC: Effects of vaginal trauma and oophorectomy on the continence mechanism in rats. Urol Int 69:36-41, 2002.
69. Kerns JM, Damaser MS, Kane JM, et al: Effects of pudendal nerve injury in the female rat. Neurourol Urodyn 19:53-69, 2000.
70. Sakamoto K, Smith GM, Storer PD, et al: Neuroregeneration and voiding behaviour patterns after pudendal nerve crush in female rats. Neurourol Urodyn 19:311-321, 2000.
71. Ismael S, Amarenco G, Bayle B, Kerdraon J: Postpartum lumbosacral plexopathy limited to autonomic and perineal manifestations: Clinical and electrophysiological study of 19 patients. J Neurol Neurosurg Psychiatry 68:771-773, 2000.
72. Takahashi S, Homma Y, Fujishiro T, et al: Electromyographic study of the striated urethral sphincter in type 3 stress incontinence: Evidence of myogenic-dominant damages. Urology 56:946-950, 2000.
73. Weidner A, Barber MD, Visco AG, et al: Pelvic muscle electromyography of levator ani and external anal sphincter in nulliparous women and women with pelvic floor dysfunction. Am J Obstet Gynecol 183:1390-1399; discussion 1399-1401, 2000.
74. Gunnarsson M, Mattiasson A: Female stress, urge, and mixed urinary incontinence are associated with a chronic and progressive pelvic floor/vaginal neuromuscular disorder: An investigation of 317 healthy and incontinent women using vaginal surface electromyography. Neurourol Urodyn 18:613-621, 1999.
75. McGuire EJ: Diagnosis and treatment of intrinsic sphincter deficiency. Int J Urol 2(Suppl 1):7-10; discussion 16-18, 1995.
76. McGuire EJ, Cespedes RD, O'Connell HE: Leak-point pressures. Urol Clin North Am 23:253-262, 1996.
77. Lemack GE: Urodynamic assessment of patients with stress incontinence: How effective are urethral pressure profilometry and abdominal leak point pressures at case selection and predicting outcome? Curr Opin Urol 14:307-311, 2004.
78. Leach GE, Dmochowski RR, Appell RA, et al: Female Stress Urinary Incontinence Clinical Guidelines Panel summary report on surgical management of female stress urinary incontinence. The American Urological Association. J Urol 158(Pt 1):875-880, 1997.
79. Kayigil O, Iftekhar Ahmed S, Metin A: The coexistence of intrinsic sphincter deficiency with type II stress incontinence. J Urol 162:1365-1366, 1999.
80. Chaikin DC, Rosenthal J, Blaivas JG: Pubovaginal fascial sling for all types of stress urinary incontinence: Long-term analysis. J Urol 160:1312-1316, 1998.
81. Yang A, Mostwin JL, Rosenshein NB, Zerhouni EA: Pelvic floor descent in women: Dynamic evaluation with fast-scan MRI imaging and cinematic display. Radiology 179:25-33, 1991.
82. Fielding JR: Practical MR imaging of female pelvic floor weakness. Radiographics 22:295-304, 2002.
83. Mostwin JL, Yang A, Sanders R, Genadry R: Radiography, sonography and magnetic resonance imaging for stress incontinence. Contributions, uses and limitations. Urol Clin North Am 22:539-549, 1995.
84. Mostwin JL, Genadry R, Saunders R, Yang A: Stress incontinence observed with real time sonography and dynamic fastscan magnetic resonance imaging—Insights into pathophysiology. Scan J Urol Nephrol Suppl 207:94-99, 2001.
85. Plzak L III, Staskin D: Genuine stress incontinence. Theories of etiology and surgical correction. Urol Clin North Am 29:527-535, 2002.

Chapter 28

PELVIC FLOOR REHABILITATION IN THE MANAGEMENT OF URINARY STRESS INCONTINENCE

Alain P. Bourcier

Stress urinary incontinence (SUI) is the complaint of involuntary leakage on effort, exertion, sneezing, or coughing.[1] It results from specific damage to the muscles, fascial structures, and nerves of the pelvic floor.[2] Commonly accepted etiologic factors include perinatal damage, pregnancy, hereditary predisposition, strenuous physical activity, chronic cough, obesity, and aging.[3,4] Many women have difficulty participating in physical exercises and social activities because of urinary leakage. SUI is not a condition that improves over time without treatment,[5,6] and it is remarkable that so few women seek professional care or advice for their symptoms.

The pelvic floor has an important function in relation to lower urinary tract function. The levator ani complex provides anatomic support to the bladder outlet. Parts of the levator collectively play an important role in maintaining the position of the pelvic viscera. Contraction of the attachments of the levator ani to the vagina and external sphincter is responsible for the anterior movement of these viscera toward to the pubis symphysis.[7,8] Urethral support is an important factor in SUI in women, because support in symptomatic women may be inadequate. According to De Lancey and Delmas,[8] the connections of the vagina and urethra to the levator ani muscles and arcus tendineus fasciae pelvis determine the structural stability of the urethra. If the connective tissue fails, the urethral supports cannot stay in their normal alignment, and SUI often occurs. Conversely, if the muscles are damaged, their action in supporting the urethra may be lost. Genuine SUI is defined as an involuntary loss of urine caused by an increase in intra-abdominal pressure that overcomes the resistance of the bladder outlet in the absence of a true bladder contraction. The decrease in bladder outlet or urethral resistance may result from poor anatomic support of the bladder neck (i.e., urethral hypermobility), loss of urethral function (i.e., intrinsic sphincter deficiency), or low urethral closure pressure, alone or in combination with other factors.[9] The anatomic support of the bladder outlet, which is critical to maintaining continence, is provided by constant levator tone in normal females.[10,11]

Physiotherapy for SUI is a widely accepted mode of conservative treatment that involves pelvic floor muscle exercises (PFMEs), with or without biofeedback, electrical stimulation, and weighted vaginal cones and balls. The purpose of pelvic floor re-education is to increase the strength and functional activity of the pelvic floor muscles, which may reduce the problem of SUI.[12] Because conservative therapy seems to have no side effects, it should be the first choice for treating SUI.[13]

PELVIC FLOOR MUSCLE EXERCISES

The main function of the pelvic floor muscles is to provide postural support to the pelvic organs. Consequently, type I (slow-twitch) fibers are predominant. In healthy muscle, these fibers have high endurance and low contraction speed, and they are resistant to fatigue. However, to respond to sudden changes in intra-abdominal pressure, the pelvic floor muscles also contain type II (fast-twitch) fibers that contract strongly and quickly to provide short bursts of activity.

According to Gilpin and associates,[10] within the pelvic floor, the distribution of fiber types is approximately 70% slow-twitch fibers and 30% fast-twitch fibers. These investigators also described a decrease in type II fibers in the periurethral and perianal area in women with symptoms of genitourinary prolapse or urinary stress incontinence. This finding suggests that changes in pelvic floor muscle function are associated with prolapse and incontinence.

During periods of increased intra-abdominal pressure, the pelvic floor muscles are believed to act as a type of platform or hammock, as described by DeLancey.[14] The hammock of muscles under the urethra allows the increased intra-abdominal pressure to compress the urethra against this resistance, preventing urine leakage. Recognizing the role of the endopelvic fascia, Petros and Ulmsten[15] proposed the integral hypothesis based on the view that the pelvic floor is a single functional unit. If a part of the structure (e.g., the pubourethral ligament) is weakened, the hammock loses some of its original function and cannot perform efficiently. The integral theory also suggests that obstruction of the urethra is caused by sphincter activity and compression of the urethra as a result of contraction of the pelvic floor muscles.

Dougherty[16] postulated that the effects of pelvic floor muscle training (PFMT) on the symptoms of stress incontinence are the result of muscle hypertrophy. Muscle hypertrophy accounts for most gains achieved by skeletal muscle; however, Dougherty also suggests that neuromuscular coordination is at least as important as hypertrophy for the successful treatment of stress incontinence. In 1998, Miller and colleagues[17] described a study of older women (mean age, 68 years) who had symptoms of mild to moderate stress incontinence. The intervention group was taught the technique of intentionally contracting the pelvic floor muscles before and during a cough, a method called *the knack*. Within a week, the results showed a significant reduction in urine loss when the women used the knack compared with coughing without precontraction of the pelvic floor.

PFME therapy has proved effective for all three forms of incontinence,[18] and PFMEs are recommended as the first choice of treatment for women with these types of urinary incontinence after remediable conditions have been excluded. In prior studies, up to 70% of patients were cured or improved after therapy,[13] but success rates declined during follow-up as adherence to the program deteriorated.[19-21] An intervention aimed at promoting long-term adherence to PFME therapy seems warranted. Various investigators have pointed out that patient education in physiotherapy, especially the part of encouraging adherence behavior, lacks a systematic behavioral approach.[22] A literature search was conducted to evaluate approaches designed to improve adherence to PFME therapy. In four studies, the PFME program included adherence-promoting strategies: audiocassette tapes to guide exercising at home, telephone calls as reminders, and follow-up visits to provide feedback and reinforcement. One study found that after 6 weeks of training at home, adherence was significantly better in the group that had used an exercise tape, compared with the group without the[23] tape. Surprisingly, in the other three studies, adherence behavior itself was not measured[24] or not related to the adherence-promoting strategies,[25] and the efficacy of these strategies therefore remains unclear.

PFME therapy for stress incontinence focused on the integration of the automatic and subconscious use of the pelvic floor muscles during the daily posture and movement pattern and on the integration of PFMEs in daily life. For urge and mixed incontinence, the therapy focused first on bladder training in which a normal voiding frequency of approximately seven voidings per day is trained. Second, the therapy included the same program as for stress incontinence with the addition of learning to prevent leakage when feeling an urge by contracting the pelvic floor muscles. The therapy included teaching the woman about the anatomy and function of the bladder, the pelvic floor muscles, the continence mechanism, toilet behavior, and the importance of adherence to the advice.

Adherence to PFME therapy was operationalized according to the following behavioral advice:

1. Perform PFMEs regularly. Do 10 slow-twitch contractions (10 to 30 seconds) and 10 fast-twitch contractions (2 to 3 seconds), five times each day, with each contraction followed by relaxation. Increase repetitions in each session to the point of fatigue, and incorporate different starting positions and functional activities into the exercise program. Check contractions with self-palpation.
2. Perform correct toileting and drinking behavior. Sit straight on the toilet and relax the pelvic floor muscles during voiding. Drink 1500 to 2000 mL of water each day. Women with deviant voiding frequency should train the bladder by timing their voidings during the day until a normal frequency of seven voidings per day is reached.
3. Use the knack technique to prevent incontinent wet episodes by contracting the pelvic floor muscles when feeling a sudden urge to void or when coughing, sneezing, or laughing.
4. Automatically and subconsciously use the pelvic floor muscles, especially during moments of abdominal pressure, in the daily posture and movement pattern to prevent leakage.

Most women seem to have learned to adapt their adherence behavior to their symptoms. A similar adaptation pattern was found in the study of Burns and colleagues,[24] who argued that women with mild symptoms may not perceive their incontinence as a problem warranting sustained effort, whereas women with many daily losses recognize it as an ongoing problem and make a persistent effort as a positive response occurs. This structure, coupled with an enthusiastic physiotherapist, seems most important for realizing long-term effects and optimal adherence behavior of organized training.

PELVIC FLOOR MUSCLE TRAINING PROGRAMS

Kegel[26] recommended performing as many as 300 to 400 pelvic floor muscle contractions daily but gave little information about the intensity of each contraction. As described by Bø,[27] the two main principles of strength training for skeletal muscles are overload and specificity. Specificity is particularly important in relation to the pelvic floor muscles because approximately 30% of women have difficulty performing a correct contraction on the first attempt. The pelvic floor is surrounded by many larger groups of muscles, such as the quadriceps and glutei. Women often incorrectly contract these muscle groups when attempting to contract the pelvic floor muscles.

Another common mistake is to produce a Valsalva, or bearing-down, maneuver. Bø[27] also describes the importance of instructor-conducted exercises in establishing the correct action of the pelvic floor muscle and maintaining motivation to continue with the exercise program.

In addition to the muscle group being exercised, specificity concerns the type of training used in relation to the dysfunction and symptoms. For example, in a case of urinary stress incontinence, the function required of the pelvic floor muscles is to assist the urethral closure pressure provided by the urethral sphincter, the resting tone of the levator ani, and mucosal coaptation. This requires a quick, maximum voluntary contraction of the pelvic floor muscles; in this case, the training program must emphasize type II fibers. During contraction of the pelvic floor muscles, motor units are recruited in order of increasing size, with type I fibers recruited at low intensity and type II fibers recruited only at high intensity. The training program therefore must include high-intensity exercises. Type II fibers fatigue rapidly because of the rapid depletion and slow replacement of adenosine triphosphate. For this reason, the exercise program should allow relaxation between contractions. The contribution of type I fibers should not be overlooked; they are responsible for maintaining the postural position of the pelvic floor, from which type II fibers can then function effectively.[28]

Traditionally, PFMEs are practiced in isolation, without activity of the abdominal or hip muscles. However, Sapsford and colleagues[29] describe how this practice has been challenged by a number of physicians, who noticed activity in the rectus abdominis in association with pelvic floor muscle contraction and palpable coactivation of the abdominal muscles during functional activities, such as raising the head and shoulders. Sapsford and colleagues[29] showed that the rectus abdominis, obliquus internus abdominis, obliquus externus abdominis, and transversus abdominis are coactivated with maximal contraction of the pelvic floor muscles. Sapsford and colleagues[29] also showed that the reverse occurs; pubococcygeal electromyographic activity increased in response to isometric contractions of the abdominal muscles. These investigators suggested that this activity could be used for therapeutic effect by encouraging submaximal deep abdominal isometric contractions to enhance pubococcygeal training. The study also considered the effect of altering the position of the lumbar spine during exercise and concluded that a neutral or extended position is preferable.

The functional evaluation of pelvic floor musculature is rife with technologic and cultural challenges. Compared with muscles outside of the pelvis, quantitative and reproducible evaluation of the levator ani kinesiologic function is difficult. The levator ani muscles are attached to the bony surfaces of the pelvis, which hinders the measurement of an isometric contraction in a reproducible manner. These data demonstrate that pelvic floor muscle strength increases with exercise training, which is consistent with previous studies that have determined quantitative increases in perineometry,[17] digital pelvic muscle strength scores,[30,31] and gross vaginal electromyographic activity[24,31] with PFMT. The variations in quantitative alterations reported in these studies no doubt reflects variations in training regimens and recording techniques.

Maximal contractions of skeletal muscle increase strength by a combination of an increase in the efficiency of motor unit activation and hypertrophy of type I (slow-twitch) and type II (fast-twitch) muscle fibers,[32] which lead to an increase in muscle volume. The pelvic floor musculature is uncommon in that it is the only group of voluntary muscles except for the respiratory diaphragm in which type I fibers predominate.[10] The mechanism of efficacy of PFMT is unknown, but it is logical that hypertrophy of the striated levator ani[33] with concomitant increases in kinesiologic function should improve continence by increasing bladder outlet resistance during physical stress and during moments of urgency and inappropriate detrusor activity. Studies of muscles outside of the pelvis in elderly women have demonstrated that strength training preferentially increases the diameter of type I fibers with no alteration in the ratio of fiber types within the muscle. In addition to the absolute strength of a pelvic floor muscle contraction, it is possible that the timing of the contraction can affect leakage during physical stress[17] or urge.

Response to PFMT may in part depend on alterations in neurophysiologic performance of the neuromuscular unit. Studies of muscles outside the pelvis demonstrate that training increases the efficiency of neural activation,[34] and in middle-aged and elderly subjects, increases in muscle strength seem to depend more on increased motor unit activation than on muscle fiber hypertrophy.[35] This type of electromyographic testing has not been used to evaluate pelvic floor muscle response to training. Given that pelvic floor musculature has a high proportion of type I (slow-twitch) muscle fibers, it is likely that improvements in resting pelvic floor muscle tone are important in improving continence during daily activities.

Clinical Studies of Pelvic Floor Muscle Training Programs

Several randomized, controlled trials have demonstrated PFMT to be effective in the treatment of SUI. In experimental studies such as randomized, controlled trials, the investigators seek to change the dependent variable (e.g., urinary leakage) by manipulation of an independent variable (e.g., PFMT) to establish a cause-and-effect relationship.

Few researchers have analyzed the results comparing strength increase or maximal strength with improvement in urinary incontinence after training, and the results of the few published studies are contradictory. Dougherty and colleagues,[36] Hahn and coworkers,[37] and Boyington and associates[38] did not find any correlation between a change in pelvic floor muscle strength and urine loss. However, modifying their analysis, Boyington and colleauges[38] found an association between a decrease in urine loss variables and increases in pelvic floor muscle pressure curve variables.

Conflicting results have been shown in case-control studies measuring pelvic floor muscle strength in continent and incontinent women. Some researchers have shown a significantly higher degree of pelvic floor muscle strength in continent women.[39-41] In other studies, no differences have been demonstrated.[36,42] The conflicting results may reflect small sample sizes, use of unreliable and insensitive outcome measures, and use of unreliable and insensitive methods to measure pelvic floor muscle strength.

We[43] demonstrated that intensive PFME combined with weekly group training was significantly more effective than the same exercises conducted at home. Because all women participating in this study had learned to contract the pelvic floor muscle correctly and had had the same monthly individual follow-up with measurement of pelvic floor muscle strength, development of muscle strength could be analyzed by combining results from responders and nonresponders from both groups. Another justification for analyzing all participants together is that the study is not looking for treatment effect but instead seeks the relationship between pelvic floor muscle strength and other outcomes.

There is no consensus about which outcome measure to choose for assessing cure or how to classify a responder to treatment for incontinence. However, combinations of subjective report and laboratory measurement of the condition have been recommended.[44,45]

In the few published studies in this area,[46] different methods have been used to evaluate pelvic floor muscle function and showed that urine loss decreased as pelvic floor muscle function increased. Boyington and colleagues,[38] measuring vaginal squeeze pressure, did not find a correlation between an increase in muscle strength and improvement in leakage.

To achieve reduction of urinary leakage by PFMT, the training has to be of sufficient intensity, frequency, and duration to cause a significant change in muscle function.[47] The intensity of the contraction is the most important factor in developing muscle strength.[32] To improve the neural adaptation (i.e., recruitment of efficient motor units and frequency of excitation) and hypertrophy, the training period should be at least 5 months.[48] Lack of or insufficient improvement in muscle strength after PFME may explain why some researchers have failed to find significant differences between methods[49,50] or correlation between the independent and dependent variables.[37]

Several studies have demonstrated that more than 30% of incontinent women are unable to contract the pelvic floor muscle correctly.[30,51] Bump and coworkers[51] showed that only 49% of the women able to contract the pelvic floor muscle performed a contraction effective enough to increase urethral pressure.

This may explain who some researchers have failed to find a correlation between increased vaginal pressure and reduction of leakage. Measurement of voluntary contraction in a supine position may not be a valid assessment of automatic co-contraction during an increase in abdominal pressure in an upright position. One study[52] investigated the effect of two approaches to PFMT in stress incontinent women ($N = 128$). It is common practice for women to receive instruction in strength training combined with advice to voluntarily contract the pelvic floor muscles to prevent leakage with increases in intra-abdominal pressure (e.g., cough). The use of a voluntary contraction before an increase intra-abdominal pressure, called the knack, and is based on motor relearning principles.

Randomization to an intervention group by opening sequentially numbered, sealed opaque envelopes took place after clinical history taking, physical examination, baseline measures, and an explanation of the normal anatomy, physiology, and function of the bladder and pelvic floor muscles. Women then received instruction based on motor relearning principles alone or a combination of strengthening and motor relearning. Women trained at home for 20 weeks, with four physiotherapy clinic visits and three phone calls to progress the program and maintain motivation. There were no statistically significant differences in the primary measures of outcome between the strength training plus motor relearning or motor relearning program groups.

The confidence intervals for the difference in leakage episodes and cough test do not rule out clinically important differences. Despite an attempt to design a study of adequate power, a larger trial is needed to address the question of important differences between these two approaches to PFMT. One study[53] was undertaken to determine the degree to which complete loss of the pubococcygeal muscle affected women's ability to volitionally augment their urethral closure pressures by using a volitional pelvic floor muscle contraction (i.e., Kegel effort). The sample consisted of a subset of women who volunteered as healthy controls in a larger study approved by an institutional review board. They were free of urinary leakage or prolapse and had a negative stress test result. Multiplanar, proton-density magnetic resonance images of the pelvis were obtained in all women. A trained observer evaluated each scan to determine pubococcygeal muscle status. Women were selected for analysis if they demonstrated an intact pubococcygeus muscle (n = 28; mean age, 54 years) or absent pubococcygeal muscle (n = 17; mean age, 59 years). Women with parietal defects (e.g., one side only) were excluded. Women were then asked to perform two or three Kegel efforts while the transducer was held at the point of maximal urethral closure pressure. The investigators concluded that women with an absent pubococcygeal muscle are only one half as likely to be able to increase their urethral closure pressure more than 5 cm H_2O and generate 43% less pressure with pelvic muscle contraction compared with women with normal women muscle training.

BIOFEEDBACK THERAPY

As described in the Chapter 19, biofeedback can be defined as the use of monitoring equipment to measure internal physiologic events or various body conditions of which the person is usually unaware. The basic approach is to provide individuals with information about the physiologic activities in their bodies, including their brains. These include sensors (i.e., electromyographic and pressure sensors) for detecting and measuring the activity of anal or urinary sphincters and pelvic floor muscles. Techniques have been also developed to measure activity of urinary stress incontinence. One aim of physical therapy has always been to assist patients by improving physiologic self-regulation within their natural environment.

Pelvic Floor Muscle Biofeedback

Several approaches have been used for measuring pelvic floor muscle activity to provide biofeedback, including urethral, vaginal, or anal feedback using manometry or electromyography. An important technical issue is the quality of the signal source used for feedback. As early as the 1940s, Kegel[28,54] developed and used the perineometer, an instrument that consisted of an intravaginal balloon attached to an external pressure gauge, which registered the pressure exerted by the pubococcygeus muscles. It was the first biofeedback device for PFMT. This method uses manometry (pressure) biofeedback by means of an intravaginal or intrarectal device. An advantage of pressure manometry is that as the patient contracts her pelvic floor muscles, the device produces a resistive pressure that may give additional feedback to the patient. After the vaginal manometry method, electromyography emerged for recording pelvic floor muscle activity. Different signal sources have been used, but electromyographic activity has evolved as the preferred signal source for many types of biofeedback therapy.[55]

Electromyographic activity of pelvic floor muscle contractions has become a common signal source for the treatment of urinary incontinence.[56] Vaginal electromyographic activity is recorded by means of surface electrodes in the vaginal introitus or a vaginal probe with electrodes embedded. The vaginal probe is easy to insert and remove, and it is usually comfortable.

Biofeedback of the urethral or anal sphincter or pelvic floor muscles is used in the management of urinary incontinence and voiding difficulties. The external anal sphincter and the external urethral sphincter have similar innervation through branches of the pudendal nerves. Although there are conflicts in the literature about the issue of correspondence between the anal and urethral sphincters, several studies indicate that these muscles act in concert,[57] and data indicate that training and controlling the anal sphincter results in urinary sphincter activity that corresponds in magnitude.[58] Anal sphincter activity can be measured by pressure balloons located by the external anal sphincter (for manometry) or by surface electrodes placed around the anus at the 10-o'clock and 2-o'clock positions.

Electromyographic activity can be measured by electrodes embedded in a rectal probe. The electromyographic instruments are designed to detect the weak electrical signals generated during muscle contraction. Surface electrodes are electrically conductive pathways in contact with the skin (over abdominal muscles) or mucosa (vaginal or anal tissue). Continuous monitoring of the electromyographic signal is important to ensure that there is no undetected signal interference and that electrode placement provides an appropriate signal. Correct placement of surface electrodes is fundamental to detect and measure a signal accurately. The three common signal sources (bladder pressure, anal sphincter pressure, and vaginal electromyographic activity) are significantly altered by increases in intra-abdominal pressure. Simultaneous measurement of abdominal activity should be done with all biofeedback therapy techniques. Intra-abdominal pressure can be measured easily using an internal rectal balloon. Electromyographic activity of the rectus abdominis muscles can be determined by surface electrodes. The abdominal muscle activity is displayed by means of two active electrodes placed 3 cm apart just below the umbilicus. A ground electrode is placed on a convenient bony prominence, such as the iliac crest.[59-61]

Electromyographic biofeedback training is used to increase the activity of weak muscle groups and to promote relaxation of spastic or tense muscles.[62] In the case of urinary stress incontinence, the function required is to assist the urethral closure pressure provided by the urethral sphincter. This requires a quick, maximal voluntary contraction of the pelvic floor muscles, and the training program must emphasize type II fibers. However, the contribution of type I fibers should not be overlooked. They

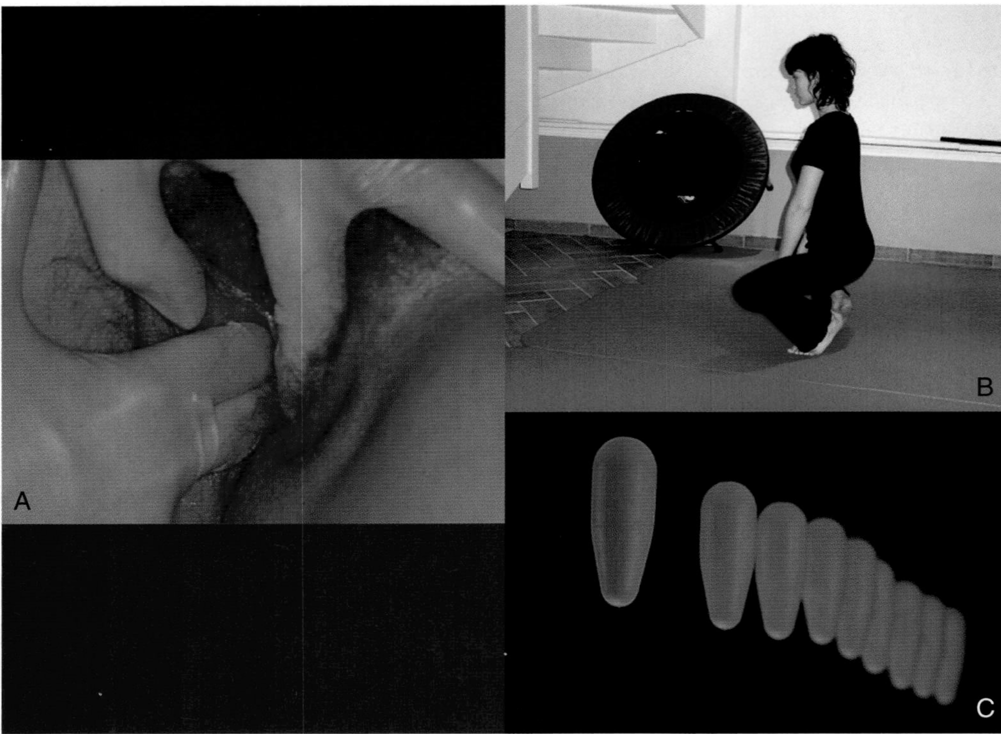

Figure 28-1 Pelvic floor muscle training programs. **A,** Voluntary contractions of the pelvic floor muscles, called the digital perineal technique, are performed with the help of the therapist. **B,** Pelvic floor muscles exercises with coactivation of the abdominal muscles. It is assumed that the activity encourages submaximal deep abdominal contractions that enhance pubococcygeal training. **C,** A set of vaginal cones ranging from 20 to 90 g are inserted into the vagina. When the patient stands and walks around, the vaginal cones tend to drop out of the vaginal, triggering a reflex contraction.

are responsible for maintaining the postural position of the pelvic floor, from which type II fibers can function effectively (Fig. 28-1).

Clinical Practice and Techniques

Using three-channel biofeedback, patients are taught to contract and relax pelvic floor muscles selectively without increasing bladder pressure or intra-abdominal pressure. In our practice,[62-64] my colleagues and I use a microcomputer-based system with a wide range of parameters that allows us to regulate the treatment according to the specific requirements of the patient, especially in daily activities. The system records simultaneous measurements of electromyographic activity of the pelvic floor muscles, rectus abdominis muscles, and other skeletal muscles (e.g., gluteal, adductors).

In clinical practice, I use pelvic floor therapy systems, which include products for home-based and office-based treatments and provide the most comprehensive and advanced platforms for treatment of pelvic floor dysfunction. The available equipment typically ensures effective treatment outcomes for most patients. The most important features are adjustable color and screen configuration, session graphs with summaries of data, audio and visual goal setting, annotated markers, templates, and animation (see Fig. 19-5 and 19-6 in Chapter 19). Using such equipment, it is possible to provide more enjoyable exercise programs (i.e., various levels of difficulty) and to conduct statistical analyses (Fig. 28-2).

Muscle Strengthening

The pelvic floor muscles hold the pelvic organs like a hammock, providing support and stabilization. Normally, when the woman is erect, the levator ani muscles, together with the respective fasciae, contribute to the support of the vaginal canal, urethra, and rectum. In patients with pelvic relaxation, this normal muscular support is lost. The levator ani hiatus is wider, and the levator plate is weakened and relaxed. When the pubococcygeal portions of the levator ani sling contract, they shorten lengthwise, gaining thickness and lessening the pelvic floor aperture transversely, thereby reducing the anteroposterior diameter considerably.[65] A tonic contraction of the levator ani maintains a high position of the vesical neck and may compensate for an increase in intra-abdominal pressure. The levator ani support[66] is provided predominantly by slow-twitch fibers, which are responsible for maintaining static muscle tone. During stressful events, phasic fast-twitch fibers provide a rapid forceful contraction.[67,68] When muscles have weakened, there is little perception of the contraction because the intensity of the proprioceptive feedback to the brain is relative to the amplitude of the muscle contraction. Muscle strength can be improved through a program of PFMEs.

In planning a PFME program, it is important to follow some basic guidelines. Patients should be selected according to grades of the pelvic floor muscles. A trained therapist should be present to give proper instruction about the level of contraction, and the exercise program should be tailored to the individual. Body positions should be modified after several sessions, and types of

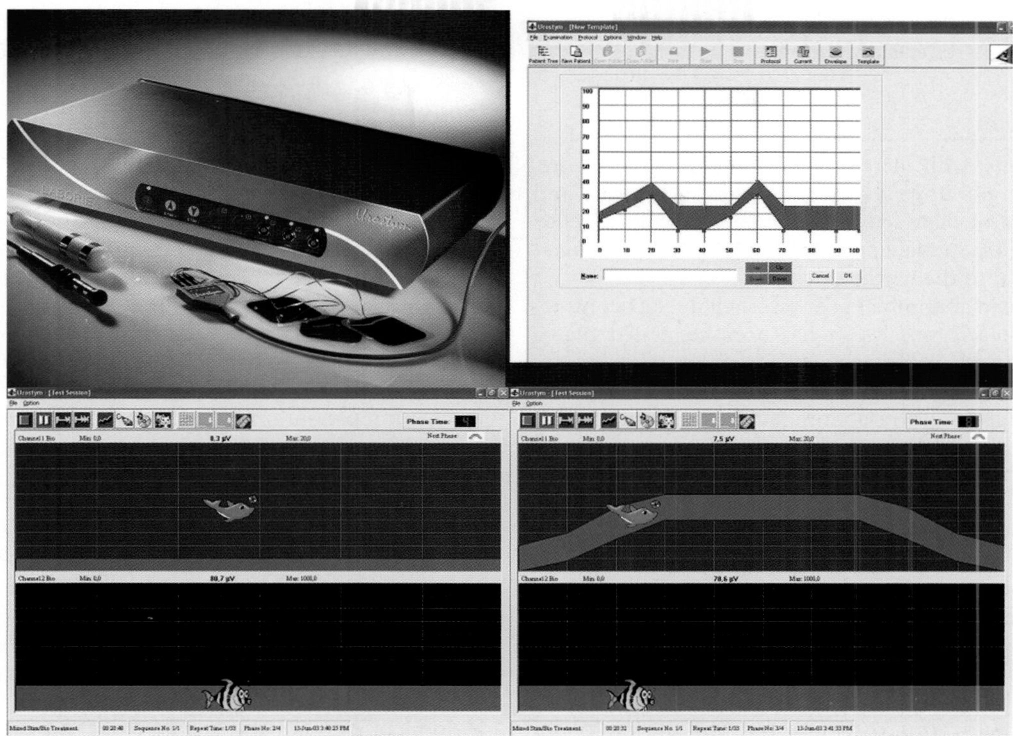

Figure 28-2 A stationary device with a wide range of parameters is used to provide electrical stimulation and biofeedback therapy *(top)*. Using this equipment, it is possible to provide more enjoyable exercise programs, such as the dolphin game *(bottom)*. (Courtesy of Laborie Medical Technologies, Montreal, Canada.)

contraction should be alternated. During exercise sessions, it is important to recruit fast-twitch fibers by fast contractions to develop strength and recruit slow-twitch fibers by slow contractions to increase endurance.[67] Regular strength training increases the number of activated motor units, frequency of excitation, and muscle volume. To induce hypertrophy, both fast- and slow-twitch fibers should be contracted. To achieve these objectives, a successful PFMT program must include rapid forceful contractions, sustained maximal voluntary contractions, and fast contractions superimposed on the end of each prolonged contraction.

Effective strength training relies on specificity (i.e., co-contraction of other groups of muscles such as the glutei and hip adductors should be minimized) and overload (i.e., increasing length and duration of contractions and reduction of rest periods). The only anatomic relationship between the levator ani and the other pelvic floor muscles is provided by the obturator internus. The pubococcygeal segment of the levator ani originates in the tendinous arch, a thickening of the obturator fascia; the iliococcygeus begins at a membranous insertion to the inner surface of the obturator internus at the tendinous arch of the levator ani.[68] This anatomic consideration of the voluntary or reflex contraction of the levator ani and obturator internus is important in setting up the protocol of a PFMT program. This endopelvic connection to the tendinous arch may assist the levator ani in support because it limits the descent of the pelvic organs during increased intra-abdominal pressure. In patients with weakening and stretching of the levator ani, even in those with partial denervation, some muscular components such as the obturator internus may be recruited in the early stages of PFMEs.

If there is a major weakness of the pelvic floor muscles, contraction of the gluteus maximus can produce an overflow of activity into the levator ani. Different exercises may be proposed to such a patient. The *flick contraction* exercise is performed by contracting and relaxing the levator ani as tightly as possible for 1 second. An average of 3 sets of 12 contractions during the session is recommended.

The *hold contraction* exercise is performed by lifting and pulling up the levator ani and holding the contraction for at least 6 seconds. As control improves, the time of this sustained contraction can be extended to 10 or 12 seconds. Patients are instructed to contract their muscles with 3 sets of 8 slow maximal contractions sustained for 6 to 8 seconds each.[27,43] Effective strength training relies on overload (i.e., increasing resistance to, frequency, or duration of muscle contraction). The *intensive contraction* exercise involves the recruitment of levator ani muscles with other groups of muscles in different positions, controlling the levator ani in increments to the point of maximal tension.

The treatment sessions are essentially training sessions that aim to increase the strength and endurance of the pelvic floor muscles. Because biofeedback requires effort, the sessions should not overtax the patient. In general, the initial sessions are shorter than subsequent sessions, and if the patient's performance begins to deteriorate, the session should be interrupted because muscle fatigue leads to muscle compensation. It is thought that PFMT and PFME is most useful if conducted in a variety of positions, including sitting and standing, rather than restricted to the traditional supine positions. Training periods of at least 20 weeks have been recommended, but it is important to assess patients individually to determine the degree of pelvic floor muscle weakness to prevent adverse effects caused by muscle fatigue.

Reflex Contraction

In normal situations, with increased intra-abdominal pressure, the rectum, uterus, and upper vagina are pushed downward and backward. The levator plate tenses and rises because of a reflex muscular contraction. Sudden increases in intra-abdominal pressure are transmitted to the urethra.

Sudden changes in abdominal pressure elicit a reflex contraction of the levator ani muscles. It has been suggested that a strong, fast, well-timed, voluntary pelvic floor muscle contraction[70] can clamp the urethra, preventing urethral descent and leakage during an abrupt intra-abdominal pressure change.[71] It has been claimed that the downward pressure from the abdominal viscera has to be offset by the strength of the urogenital diaphragm and that the forward pressure of the pelvic floor increases the tendency to visceral protrusion. This active element, resulting from a striated muscle effect, allows improved pressure transmission, but it also promotes greater efficiency of the pelvic floor reflex by active means. In pelvic floor disorders, female patients may lose this reflex muscle contraction, and one of the goals of biofeedback therapy is to enable patients to relearn this reflex.[62,72]

The teaching process aims to demonstrate how the levator ani muscles must be contracted before and during increased intra-abdominal pressure, particularly with strenuous effort during heavy physical activity. During the learning process of the reflex contraction (Fig. 28-3), called the *stress strategy* or the *perineal blockage before stress technique*, the levator ani must be contracted before any rise of intra-abdominal pressure.[62,73] At the end of this process, women must be conscious of a constant contraction of the levator ani and can use the technique of perineal blockage before physical stress. This skill of using pelvic floor muscle contraction to prevent stress leakage has also been called the knack.[17,74] In the treatment of SUI, De Lancey[75] posits that a quick, strong pelvic floor muscle contraction can clamp the urethra, increasing urethral pressure and preventing leakage during an abrupt or sustained increase in intra-abdominal pressure. DeLancey[76] also suggests that an effective contraction of the pelvic floor muscle may press the urethra against the pubic symphysis, creating a mechanical pressure rise. The *reflex contraction* is a feed-forward loop because it may precede the bladder pressure rise by 200 to 250 ms.[70]

Use of New Skills in Daily Activities

Urinary stress incontinence and pelvic organ prolapse are primarily related to erect posture. We may assume that erect posture and a constant increase in intra-abdominal pressure alter female urethrovesical function. In the vertical position, the urethra leaves the bladder at the point of maximal combined intra-abdominal pressure and gravity force. We can assume a certain relationship between pelvic floor support and intra-abdominal pressure. A pelvic floor muscle reflex occurs with a sudden

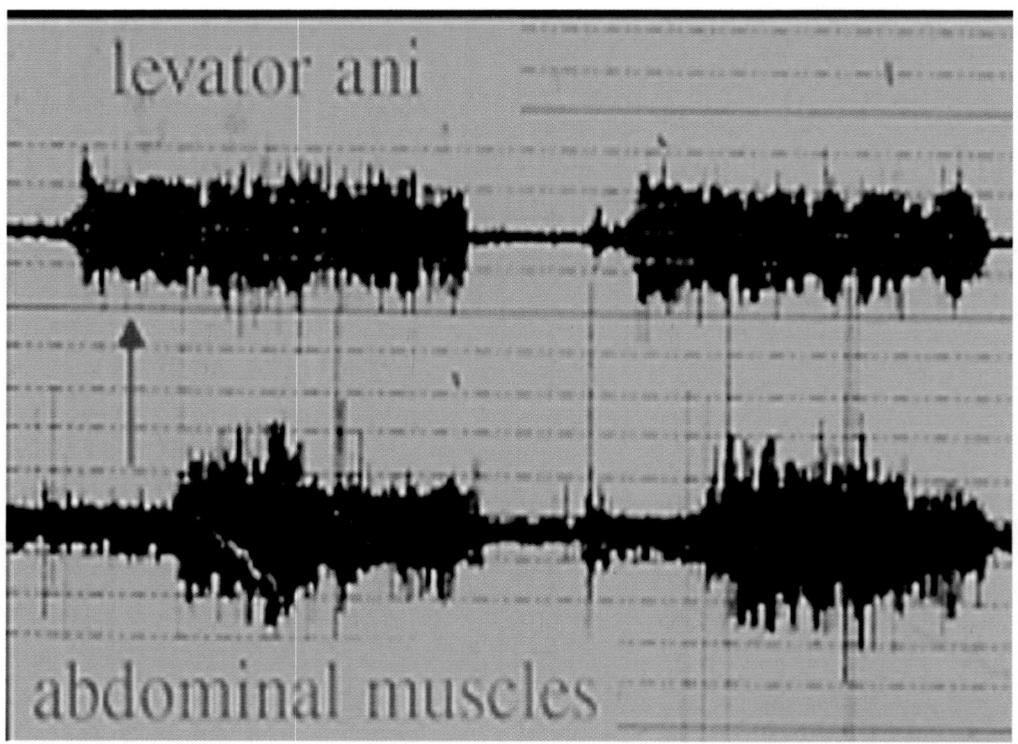

Figure 28-3 Recordings of the levator ani muscles (top) and the transversus abdominis muscles (bottom) during the perineal blockage before stress technique or the knack. During the learning process of the reflex contraction, the levator ani must be contracted before any increase of intra-abdominal pressure.

increase in intra-abdominal pressure. On the basis of this concept, my colleagues and I developed the applied biofeedback technique, referring to electromyographic pattern of the levator ani combined with synergistic and antagonistic muscle activity in a standing position.

The evolution of women's professional and business activities and stressful environments represent high-risk factors for pelvic floor relaxation. The intra-abdominal pressure in the standing position is two or three times greater than that in the supine position. Without a treatment protocol implemented in a standing position, especially with movement, neuromuscular reeducation is pointless. This method is based on the relationship between pelvic floor muscle control and rise in intra-abdominal pressure.

It consists of pelvic floor muscle contraction during the abrupt increase of the intra-abdominal pressure that occurs during standing and exercising.[62,72,77] In our practice,[62,78,79] my colleagues and I use office equipment that allows patients to assume different positions as they learn to use the pelvic floor muscles to prevent incontinence. The trainer helps patients change their reactions by establishing targets and assisting them in developing new habits and modifying their physical activities. The simulation of daily activities is an important stage in which selected "home stress" or a physical task is used to access the patient's ability to perform a real-life activity (Figs. 28-4 and 28-5). The patient usually should start with easy tasks and progressively make the activities more difficult and more functional. It is optimal for patients to be standing when they perform these exercises.

Successful recovery of the ability to perform daily activities without incontinence is most likely when the pelvic floor muscle strength is combined with a refined control of the functional activity. For this purpose, we use equipment,[62,72] including a video monitor connected to a computerized unit, that monitors the electromyographic activity of muscle groups. The patient is asked to perform various tasks that are similar to domestic activities, such as carrying a baby basket or lifting items from the floor. The perineal blockage technique is useful in providing feedback for the active woman during exercise.[62,77,79] In some cases, as soon as the pelvic floor contraction is effective, we request perineal contraction with synergic muscles (i.e., external hip rotators, gluteal muscles, and adductor muscles) and later with antagonist muscles (i.e., rectus abdominis). If the patient has some difficulty in performing these exercises, we suggest that she practice in different positions, such as lying and sitting.

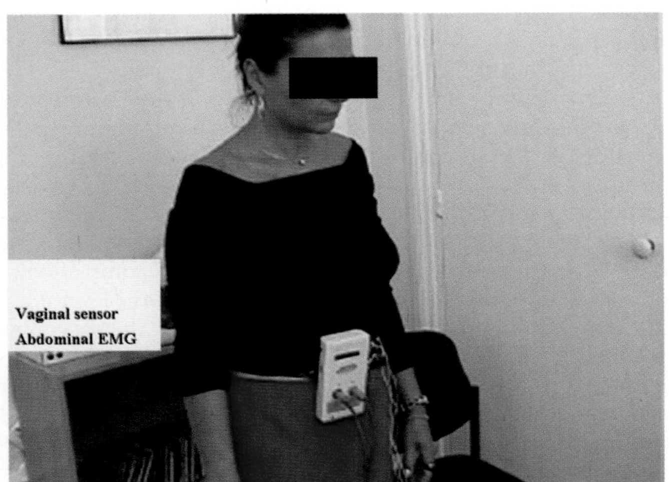

Figure 28-4 To monitor the use of new skills in daily activities, we use infrared telemetry, including a video monitor that allows the patient freedom of movement and activities while she uses the knack technique. All theses programs are conducted in the standing position, and the patient is fully clothed. A light tampon vaginal probe and surface abdominal electrodes are used during the session. (Courtesy of YSY Medical, Nimes, France.)

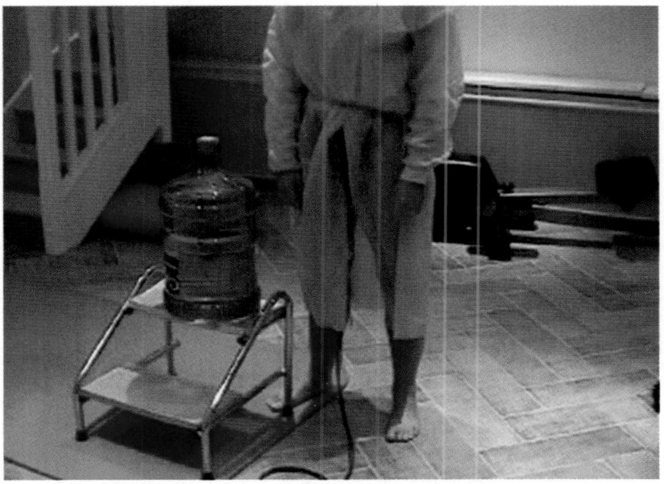

Figure 28-5 Applied biofeedback during physical activities. A short vaginal sensor and electrode wire set for accessory muscles are used for the exercise program. The patient lifts a heavy item while performing the perineal blockage or knack technique.

For sportswomen,[62,64,72,78] my colleagues and I recommend using a treadmill and recently a new device with a mechanized oscillating platform (Huber, Spine Force, LPGS Systems) (Fig. 28-6), which represents the opportunity to combine speed and endurance. The underlying concept is that the circumstances and precipitants of incontinence must be taken into account during treatment sessions to provoke a reflex pelvic floor muscle contraction in response to stress. Accuracy of speed (2.5 to 6 mph) and slope (5% to 12%) is assumed for a precisely controlled workout. The introduction of the treadmill or other sports equipment into our program for sportswomen is one way to allow the patient to perform real physical activities in a medical environment.[62,72,78]

Clinical Results

Many studies have demonstrated that treatment with biofeedback reduces incontinence. The data show that the treatments are safe and effective, and they yield high levels of patient satisfaction. PFMT is commonly implemented using simple verbal feedback given to the patient during palpation of the pelvic floor muscle by the therapist or biofeedback involving vaginal or anal electromyographic probes or pressure sensors. Several trials compared PFMT with biofeedback versus PFMT alone.[79-83] Most of the studies investigated the effect of biofeedback for women with stress incontinence with or without detrusor instability, comparing biofeedback-assisted PFMT with pelvic floor training alone.

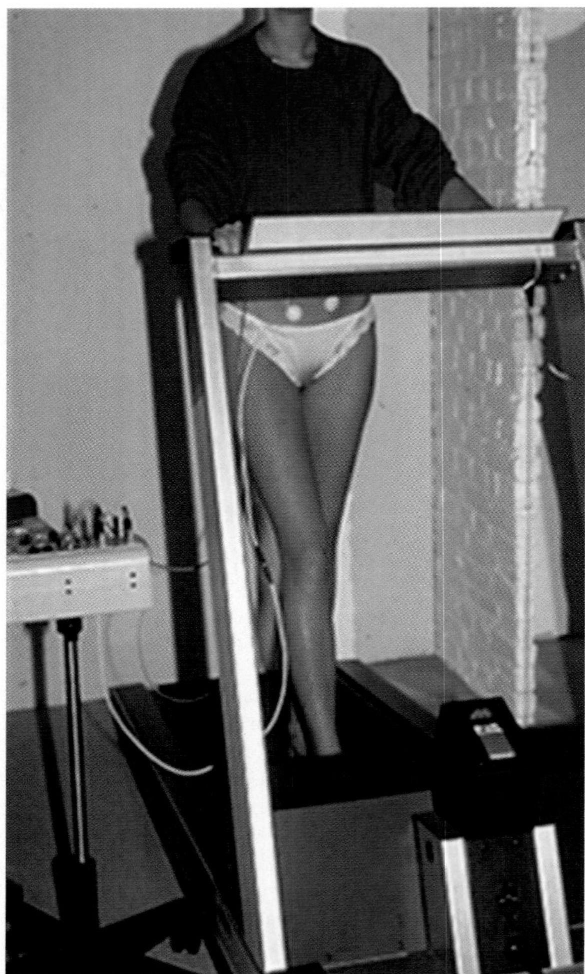

Figure 28-6 Applied biofeedback with a treadmill. The patient jogs for 15 minutes, and parameters are selected according to the type of exercise, strength, and endurance.

Burgio and colleagues[80] treated 24 stress incontinent women, who were between the ages of 29 and 64 years, for 6 weeks. One group received simultaneous bladder, sphincter, and abdominal pressure feedback, and the control group received verbal feedback based on vaginal palpation. All patients in both groups received comprehensive training in 100 trials across four training sessions. Cures or improvement (i.e., at least 50% reduction of incontinence) resulted for 92% of the biofeedback group and 55% of the control patients. The biofeedback group averaged 75.9% reduction in the frequency of incontinence, which was significantly greater than the mean of 51% shown by the verbal feedback group. The investigators concluded that although many patients can succeed without biofeedback, it improves the patient's ability to learn appropriate pelvic floor muscle contractions and increases the likelihood of successful outcome.

Berghmans and colleagues[81] suggested that the group that had biofeedback improved more quickly than the group that used only PFMT at 6 weeks, although there were no significant differences at 12 weeks. This finding has not been confirmed by any other study.[81]

In a controlled clinical trial, Wilson and colleagues[82] compared four groups: PFMT at home, hospital-based PFMT with biofeedback, PFMT with interferential therapy, and PFMT with faradism. They reported greater symptomatic improvement in the group using hospital-based PFMT with biofeedback compared with PFMT at home. In a study by Morkved and colleagues,[83] 94 women with urodynamic stress incontinence were randomized to 6 months of PFMT with a physical therapist, with or without biofeedback at home. Training with home biofeedback resulted in higher rates of objective cure, but the difference between groups was not statistically significant.[83] The researchers found that the value of home biofeedback may be that it motivates many women, and they thought it should be an option in clinical practice.

Using biofeedback, pelvic floor dysfunction, including incontinence, can be brought under conscious awareness, including the contraction and relaxation of skeletal. Although surgery is usually necessary for women who suffer from severe SUI, biofeedback also can be useful for these patients because they can become actively involved in their own treatment and achieve better control of the perineal area.

ELECTRICAL STIMULATION

Basic Principles and Mechanism of Action

Electrical currents are applied therapeutically to stimulate muscle contraction, usually through activation of nerves that supply muscles. Electrical stimulation is an effective treatment for stress incontinence. This technique uses natural pathways and the micturition reflexes, and its efficacy relies on a preserved reflex arc, with complete or partial integrity of the pelvic floor muscle innervation.[84] Based on animal experiments, direct stimulation of afferent or efferent fibers appears to be the most important mechanism to enhance the reflex response. The mechanism of electrical stimulation for stress is urethral closure by contraction of the pelvic floor muscle fibers. Urethral closure occurs by direct stimulation. Closure of the urethra by electrical stimulation of the pudendal nerve is caused mainly by direct stimulation of the pudendal nerve efferent, which supplies the striated paraurethral and pelvic floor muscles and is supported by activation of hypogastric efferents to the smooth paraurethral muscles.[85,86]

Electrical stimulation is commonly used in the treatment of urinary incontinence and pelvic floor dysfunction to improve the function of the urethral sphincteric mechanism, levator ani muscles, and external anal sphincter. These muscles have fast- and slow-twitch fibers. The slow-twitch fibers may be important in developing sustained tone to occlude the urethra, whereas the fast-twitch fibers may be involved in pelvic reflex contraction.

Electrical stimulation may increase the bulk of the levator ani muscles and the proportion of fast-twitch fibers, thereby influencing the ability of muscles to respond to a sudden increase in intra-abdominal pressure. The stimulus may increase the number and strength of slow-twitch fibers, improving resting urethral closure. Threshold intensity varies inversely with fiber diameter. Any pulse configuration can provide nerve activation, and many stimulation waveforms have been used to cause neural excitation.[87,88] These configurations include biphasic capacitively coupled pulses, monophasic square pulses, biphasic square pulses, and monophasic capacitively coupled spike pulses. Short square-wave pulses (200 to 1000 ms) are the most effective. To minimize electrochemical reactions at the electrode-mucosa interface, biphasic or alternating pulses are recommended.[89]

The size and position of the electrodes are of utmost importance to the response. Small electrodes and high charge densities are necessary to avoid tissue damage, which presumably depends on the generation of heat and formation of toxic products through electrochemical reactions. Heat production correlates with the amount of energy delivered and the electrochemical reactions to the electrical charge transferred by each pulse. The use of a low frequency further reduces energy consumption. Bidirectional pulses can reduce electrochemical reactions, and intermittent stimulation helps to avoid harmful effects by decreasing total energy.[90]

The effects of electrical stimulation on urethral closure are optimal with stimulation parameters between 35 and 50 Hz. The sacral afferent nerves, particularly the autonomic nerves of the pelvic organs, are poorly myelinated (Aδ) or unmyelinated (C) fibers, which conduct current at a slow rate of 5 to 20 Hz. Low frequencies (1 to 5 Hz) generate twitch contractions, allowing little sustained tension to develop in the muscle. Slow-twitch muscle fibers have a natural firing rate of 10 to 20 Hz, whereas fast-twitch fibers fire at 30 to 60 Hz. Current frequencies of greater than 40 Hz may cause undue fatigue and should be avoided. In a healthy muscle at frequencies of approximately 30 Hz, muscle contractions usually become fused or tetanized, so that a smooth contraction is apparent. Current frequencies of 10 to 40 Hz that last approximately 250 to 500 ms activate fast and slow motor neurons. At high frequencies, the muscle weakens rapidly because of neuromuscular transmission; at lower frequencies, less fatigue occurs. Chronic stimulation may increase the relative number of slow-twitch fibers, probably by helping to transform fast-twitch fibers to slow units, which can sustain the contraction longer. Stimulation recruits muscle fibers in a less predictable order than that of a voluntary contraction (i.e., type II fibers may be recruited before type I).[91] Long-term electrical stimulation[92,93] induces almost complete transformation of fast-twitch to slow-twitch fibers that have a high-energy capacity. Frequencies of 10 to 60 Hz induce such transformation, which occurs after almost 30 days of electrical stimulation. Most patients have some relapse after 30 days, possibly as a result of the reverse process associated with immobilization or inactivity. During the on time, the stimulation delivers a train of individual pulses of prescribed amplitude, duration, and frequency.

The length of the off time defines the recuperative period for the stimulated muscles.[94] The length of the off time defines the recuperation period for stimulation. The ratio of stimulation time to rest time is called the *duty cycle*. A typical duty cycle is approximately 1 : 2.

The patient's diagnosis and degree of muscle weakness should be considered when identifying a suitable duty cycle for initiation of the electrical stimulation program.[94] In case of weakness or neurologic impairment, a ratio of 1 : 3 may be appropriate.[95] As muscle strength or endurance improves, the ratio of on-to-off time may be decreased. Most commercially available devices allow adjustment of the time that the stimulus takes to reach peak intensity and return to zero intensity. To reduce the problem of discomfort, the amplitude of the stimulus (i.e., intensity) is progressively delivered, allowing the patient to become accustomed to the stimulation as it increases from no perceptible levels to sensory and then to motor thresholds. Most electrical stimulators introduced in the past decade provide constant voltage or constant current that maintains the same current waveform, regardless of changes in impedance. Great individual variations in the stimulus can be tolerated without incurring unpleasant sensations. This difference is related to impedance.

Significant evidence shows denervation of the pelvic floor in women with pelvic floor dysfunction, mainly as a result of vaginal childbirth or other pelvic trauma, surgery, or aging. Pudendal nerve latency is prolonged by vaginal delivery[96,97] and vaginal surgery for prolapse.[98]

Patients with urinary incontinence or pelvic organ prolapse have longer pudendal nerve latency periods than continent control subjects.[99] Histologic evidence of denervation was seen in biopsy specimens taken from the pubococcygeus at surgery for genital prolapse or stress incontinence.[98]

To improve urethral closure, innervation of the pelvic floor must exist. No effect can be expected in patients with complete lower motor neuron lesions. If the muscles are completely denervated, physiotherapy is unlikely to be effective. However, any surviving muscle fibers will be hypertrophied. After denervation injury, such as occurs after pelvic surgery or vaginal childbirth, electrical stimulation may be used to recondition muscle and facilitate sprouting of surviving motor axons. These abnormalities are potentially reversible or at least treatable, because the nerve supply is not completely disrupted.[91] Because electricity has been used to stimulate denervated muscle for many years, electrical stimulation could be used to produce reinnervation or electrical reorganization of the pelvic floor. Although the reason for stimulating denervated muscle appears logical, findings on the efficacy of such treatment are contradictory.

There is no unanimity of opinion about the ultimate degeneration of denervated muscle fibers. When discussing the therapeutic technique, particular attention must be paid to the following requirements:

- The duration of the impulse should be as short as possible but long enough to elicit a contraction.
- The rest period between successive stimuli should be at least four to five times longer than the duration of the stimulus.
- The increase should be as steep as possible to avoid stimulation of intact axons.
- The intensity of the stimulus must be sufficient to achieve a moderately strong contraction, but it should avoid causing the patient unnecessary discomfort.[84]

Stimulation to enhance motor control, whether it is called a facilitation technique or a muscle re-education program, provides a tremendous amount of sensory information to the central nervous system through a variety of sensory modalities and afferent pathways for automatic and conscious processing. Electrical stimulation may improve reinnervation after partial denervation by enhancing sprouting of surviving motor axons.

In summary, therapeutic stimulation is recommended for women with urinary incontinence and pelvic floor dysfunction[84] who underwent unsuccessful PFMT as a first-line treatment. Pelvic floor electrical stimulation offers a nonsurgical approach for treating urinary incontinence. The stimulation increases the urethral resistance by strengthening the pelvic floor muscles. Electrical stimulation must be performed in conjunction with a pelvic floor training program (for stress incontinence) and biofeedback.

Extracorporeal Electromagnetic Stimulation

Pulsed electromagnetic fields, rather than continuous fields, are most commonly used for the stimulation of human tissue. These fields are generated by high-voltage electric currents applied to a surface stimulation coil. At the tissue level, electrical eddy currents are induced by a flow of ions establishing differences in voltage between two spatial points. If the voltage gradient is strong and the change of field is rapid, membrane depolarization occurs, establishing an action potential along adjacent peripheral nerve tissue.[100] In the pelvis, stimulation of the lumbosacral roots initiates this sequence of events, leading to nerve depolarization, stimulation of the motor end plates, and ultimately, pelvic floor muscle contraction.[101] In contrast to electrical stimulation, which directly stimulates the nerve,[102] magnetic stimulation is a vehicle that secondarily generates ion flow and eddy currents to which nerve tissue is particularly sensitive.

Conventional stimulators deliver pulses lasting less than 100 μs at frequencies of 20 to 50 Hz. The depth of magnetic field penetration, or focal length, is proportional to the diameter of the stimulating coil. The spatial distribution of the maximum magnetic field reflects the size and shape of the stimulating coil, usually a hollow-centered doughnut, in contrast to the bull's-eye field that is created by electrical stimulation.[102,103] Magnetic pulses can facilitate the stimulation of autonomic and somatic nerve pathways in the pelvic floor without the use of electrodes.[104]

For therapeutic application, it was first reported that high-frequency or continuous magnetic stimulation of S3, delivering up to 20 pulses/sec, produced clinically useful stimulation of the pelvic floor musculature, increased pressure in the anal canal,[105] and generated contraction of the external sphincter. Extracorporal electromagnetic stimulation does not require any probes, skin preparation, or physical or electrical contact with the skin surface.[102,103]

The patient sits fully clothed on a chair that contains an electromagnet controlled by an external power source (Fig. 28-7). Optimal coil position can be mapped by visual confirmation of toe flexion or abduction of the legs and the sensation of anal contractions. In clinical practice, treatment is typically performed for 6 to 10 weeks, with two sessions weekly. Each session lasts 24 minutes, with 10 minutes at 20 Hz and 10 minutes at 50 Hz and with 4 minutes of rest.

Extracorporal electromagnetic stimulation provides a useful alternative for patients who do not respond to drug therapy, are poor surgical candidates, or lack the agility to manage electrical stimulation devices.[102,103] Electrical stimulation is indicated for patients who are not strongly motivated to perform pelvic floor exercises, for those with weak pelvic floor muscle activity, and for those with contraindications to surgery (e.g., genuine stress incontinence) or medication (e.g., urinary incontinence).

Electrical stimulation is an effective mode of therapy for urinary incontinence and pelvic floor dysfunction. As the use of electrotherapy grows because of advances in technology, it is necessary for health care professionals to carefully analyze innovative applications and demand a demonstration of the efficacy of this therapy.

Clinical Results of Electrical Stimulation

The interpretation of data may be limited because patients often are not classified urodynamically. Sand and colleagues[106] conducted the only placebo-controlled study of electrical stimulation. It showed the unquestionable superiority of the treatment arm. Fifty-two women with genuine stress incontinence were

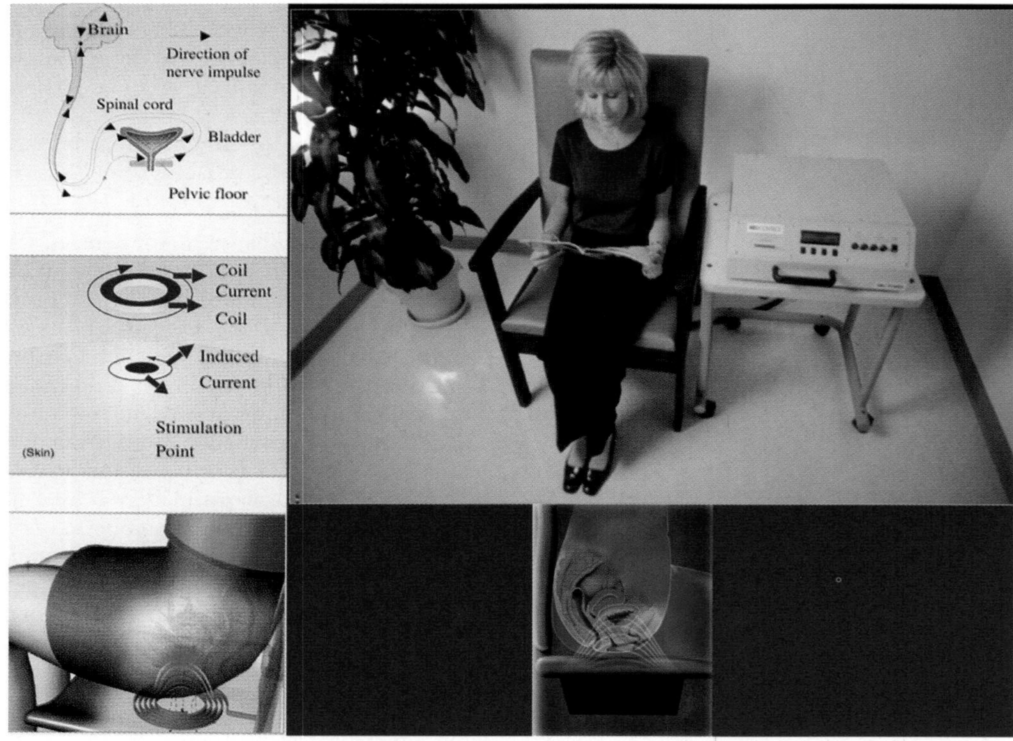

Figure 28-7 Principle of extracorporeal electromagnetic stimulation. The patient sits fully clothed on a chair that contains an electromagnetic controlled by an external power source. The magnetic field activates all of the branches of the pudendal nerves, inducing repetitive contractions of the pelvic floor musculature. (Courtesy of Neotonus Inc., Marietta, GA.)

enrolled (35 in the treatment group; 17 in the placebo group). The treatment group underwent 12 weeks of stimulation twice daily, and current was delivered through a single vaginal electrode. The parameters used were 50 Hz with a pulse width of 0.3 ms. Intensity varied from 0 mA to 100 mA, and the duty cycle was 5 seconds on and 10 seconds off. The placebo group received sham electrical stimulation with output limited to 1 mA. The number of episodes of incontinence decreased significantly in the treatment group, as measured by daily (P = .04) and weekly (P = .009) leakage and by the pad test.

Subjective assessment of frequency of urine loss showed significant improvement in the treatment group. Luber and Wolde-Tsadik[107] performed a prospective, randomized, controlled study to evaluate the effect of electrical stimulation on urinary incontinence. They used a sample of 54 patients who had genuine stress incontinence. Patients in the treatment group (n = 20) underwent treatment for 15 minutes twice daily for 12 weeks with vaginal electrode stimulation at a frequency of 50 Hz and pulse duration of 2 ms. The placebo group (n = 24) underwent sham electrical stimulation with no current in the patient circuit. Subjective cure and improvement rates at 3 months were 25% and 29.2% in the treatment and sham treatment groups, respectively. Rates of objective cure (i.e., negative stress test results on urodynamic studies) were 15% of treatment group and 12% of control group. Subjective cure was improvement in 25% in the treatment group.

Clinic-based electrical stimulation may be useful for women unable to produce a voluntary contraction. However, clinic-based treatment requires that women attend on a regular basis and uses clinic resources and the therapist's time. It has been suggested that home-based electrical stimulation would provide a more cost-effective option.

An interesting study[108] set out to investigate how effective this approach might be in clinical practice. One hundred seventy women, who were diagnosed as having urodynamically proven genuine SUI, were recruited to the study over a 3-year period, and 20 were randomized to have treatment deferred and then went on to receive active stimulation. Having given informed consent, they were randomized to one of four treatment groups: closely supervised conventional pelvic floor exercises, the same exercise program with the use of a portable stimulator, the exercise program and use of an identical but electrically disabled dummy stimulator, or no initial treatment (i.e., control group) Treatment was carried out over a 14-week period and was closely supervised by an experienced research physiotherapist. The control group had no treatment for a 14-week period before entering the active stimulation group. The deferred group showed no statistically significant improvement compared with the other treatment groups.

Symptom scores and quality-of-life scores improved significantly in all treatment groups, but not in the control group. No statistically significant differences between treatment groups were detected. Compliance was assessed as *excellent* if the PFMEs and use of the stimulator were performed daily, *good* if more than three times per week, *poor* if less often than this, and *unrecorded* if not recorded or withdrawn from the study. Compliance with PFMEs was generally good, with three fourths of the women in all groups performing exercises more than three times weekly. Compliance with use of the stimulators was poor, with less than one half of the stimulator groups using the devices regularly. Reasons given for poor compliance with the stimulators included lack of time, lack of privacy, and discomfort caused by the stimulator. The researchers concluded that in a group of women with urodynamically proven genuine SUI, PFMEs under the supervision of an experienced physiotherapist led to significant improvements in pad-test urine loss, symptom scores, and quality-of-life scores. The addition of home electrical stimulation did not improve the results of therapy. Clinic-based electrical stimulation, under supervision, may enhance the results of physiotherapy, but the use of home stimulators is of little benefit and merely increases the cost and complexity of treatment.

Another study reported the women's preferences for treatment of urodynamic stress incontinence by physiotherapy orsurgery.[113] A package was developed for women with urodynamic stress incontinence that had three sequenced sections: a questionnaire eliciting the patient's current knowledge of available treatments, including the origins of the knowledge; three one-page information sheets describing pelvic floor treatment (PFT) by women's health physiotherapists, the tension-free vaginal tape (TVT), and open colposuspension as options for treatment, including success rates and complications; and a questionnaire eliciting hand-written responses about the patient's preferred treatment, the reasons for her choice, and whether she wished to ask questions.

The package was developed by three urogynecologists, two physiotherapists, and a professor of medical sociology. The patients were informed that regardless of their preferences, the final decision about treatment modality would be made jointly between themselves and a doctor after the questionnaire was completed. Based on an estimation that 70% of women choose pelvic floor treatment over surgery and an estimated prevalence of 240 cases of urodynamic stress incontinence per year in the three units, a sample size of 138 was determined. After reading the information sheets, 44 (66%) women chose PFT as their preferred management, followed by the TVT (24%) and colposuspension (9%), with nonsignificant differences among the three units. Nine percent of women attempted to avoid making a choice, requiring encouragement and guidance by the doctor administering the questionnaire. Of the 44 women who chose PFT, 67% cited lack of invasiveness and low risk as the main reasons. Ten percent wanted to avoid a possible cesarean section in the event of a subsequent pregnancy. Of those who chose the TVT, the predominant reasons were failed home pelvic floor exercises (25%), the minimal invasiveness of the TVT (23%), and the early discharge and recovery associated with this procedure (29%) compared with colposuspension. Of those who chose colposuspension, the most common reason (50%) was that it sounded more permanent than the TVT.

Forty-two percent of women said that their physicians did not discuss treatment options. Patients who stated that their physicians discussed only physiotherapy (N = 20) chose this treatment in 80% of cases. In contrast, those whose physicians discussed only surgery (N = 6) chose PFT in only 17% of cases. Similarly, of seven patients who indicated they knew of friends who were happy with their surgical treatment, six chose a surgical option. Among 19 women whose physicians did not discuss treatment and who did not hear about friends' choices, 74% chose PFT, which was not significantly different to the overall PFT. There were 38 (58%) who wanted to ask a question. The most common question was "What does the doctor think is best for me?" (23%). The investigators concluded that making a decision based purely on factual information is difficult for many women. However, when given standardized, unbiased information, 33% of women bypassed PFT and chose surgery, citing failed home pelvic floor training, minimal invasiveness, and fast recovery as the predominant reasons for TVT and the long-lasting effect for colposuspension. Two thirds of women chose PFT, citing low risk as the main reason. These are informed choices based on standardized information sheets, and they may suggest that women choosing surgical options have a speedier course to surgery. Whether in an era of informed choice women choosing surgery should be permitted to bypass PFT is beyond the scope of this study, but it is a matter for debate. The influences on women's preferences are unclear, but it may be that women whose physicians or friends emphasize one treatment are likely to come to urogynecology units with predetermined preferences and are likely to choose that option.

INTRAVAGINAL RESISTANCE DEVICES AND ANTI-INCONTINENCE DEVICES

Many devices—mainly air- or water-inflated balloons or perineometers—operate on the same principle. After the device is inserted into the vagina, the patient is asked to contract the pelvic floor muscles. Rhe device then is pulled out of the vagina with a pulley system that applies gradually increasing force.

Vaginal cones were developed by Plevnik in 1985[114] as a new method to allow patients to train the pelvic floor musculature on a daily basis at home, without the need for a physiotherapist. This simple concept uses a set of cones ranging from 20 to 100 g that are inserted into the vagina. When the patient stands and walks around, the cones tend to slip out of the vaginal ring, giving a sensation of falling out that results in a pelvic floor muscle contraction. After the patient can hold the 20-g cone in the vagina for 20 minutes on two separate occasions, the next heaviest cone is used.

This pelvic floor muscle contraction is carried out through reflex activation of the sensory afferent fibers of the pudendal and pelvic nerves. The activation occurs when vaginal wall mechanical tension receptors are activated and stimulate the pelvic floor muscles by pudendal nerve efferents mediated through an S2-S4 sacral cord reflex. This technique has the advantage of forcing the patient to contract only the pelvic floor muscles and not other groups of muscles, such as the abdominal or gluteal muscles, which are often contracted simultaneously during voluntary pelvic floor exercises. A single trial compared PFMT in combination with cones with PFMT alone and found significant improvement in both groups, with almost identical cure rates (84.5% and 85.5%).[115] PFMT alone seems to be as effective as PFMT combined with biofeedback, intravaginal resistance devices, or electrical stimulation. Many physiotherapists use these other techniques as adjunct treatments for genuine SUI or mixed incontinence.[116]

Devices that are used to manage urinary stress incontinence work by the following mechanisms:

- External urinary collection
- Intravaginal support of the bladder neck
- Blockage of urinary leakage by occlusion at the external meatus or with an intraurethral insert

Indications for anti-incontinence devices include the following:

- Initial or long-term management of urinary incontinence
- As an adjunct to conservative therapy, such as PFMT
- To postpone or avoid surgery
- After other forms of therapy have failed

These devices may allow women to resume a normal level of activity or to participate in sports without the need for surgery. Various degrees of manual dexterity are required, depending on the type of device used. External collecting devices are cumbersome and do not have documented efficacy. Intravaginal devices are familiar to most women because they are similar to sanitary tampons. They are easy to use and can be worn for longer periods without being removed to allow micturition. These features make them practical for everyday use, and they reduce the cost of treatment. Intraurethral devices may be difficult to insert and can cause urethral irritation, urinary tract infection, hematuria, and migration to the bladder. They must be removed to allow voiding, making them expensive for daily use. Various external occlusive devices are available, some of which can be reapplied after voiding and reused for up to 1 week. However, long-term efficacy and safety data have not been reported.

POSTOPERATIVE RECOMMENDATIONS

Changing a person's behavior, environment, or lifestyle can mitigate or reduce symptoms (i.e., urine leakage or incontinence, urgency, frequency, and nocturia), even after anti-incontinence surgery. The main reason for these postoperative recommendations is that most of the causes that lead to urinary stress incontinence remain the same after surgery. Patients can be divided into two categories: those who still have the same lifestyle (group 1) and those who present with high-risk factors for pelvic floor dysfunction (group 2). Group 1 patients present with different conditions, such as smoking, bad dietary habits, obesity, or constipation. Group 2 patients include active women who wish to practice high-impact sports after surgery, Repetitive bouncing can increase abdominal pressure and transmit the impact to the bladder. Because urinary stress incontinence occurs during physical exertion, this condition represents a major problem for women participating in fitness programs or sports activities and is probably a cause of relapse after surgery. Other patients who are at risk after surgery work in a standing position and are obliged to lift heavy loads during the day. This movement may place these women at risk for urine loss due to increased intra-abdominal pressure and an increased gravity load.

Interventions include lifestyle changes (e.g., cessation of smoking, weight reduction, elimination of dietary bladder irritants, adequate fluid intake, bowel regulation, moderation of physical activities, and exercises), toileting programs (e.g., habit training, prompted voiding), and bladder retraining through PFMEs. From our current knowledge about the effect of PFMT, specific training programs should be recommended as the first treatment choice. The perineal blockage technique or the Knack appears to be an adjunctive modality for pelvic floor rehabilitation and can be proposed for active women. The impact of carefully instructed pelvic floor exercises on sports-related incontinence does not have the same beneficial effect as on the normal female population.

CONCLUSIONS

PFMEs and visits to a physiotherapist seem to help to preserve the results of surgery for several years and prevent a relapse of

SUI. Many physicians[13] think that conservative therapy should be the first choice for treatment of SUI.

Electrical stimulation should be used for women not able to contract their pelvic floor muscles. Electrical stimulation applied once each week is not enough when a patient is unable to identify her pelvic floor muscles or if the purpose is to activate motor units and increase pelvic floor muscle function in cases of SUI. Electromyographic biofeedback is very important at the beginning of therapy and in the follow-up period, and it is highly reproducible and reliable in the assessment of pelvic floor muscle activity.[118] It makes it easier for the therapist to teach isolated pelvic floor muscle contraction, facilitates goal setting, and helps the patient to maintain good motivation. It also can detect differences in strength between the right and left pelvic floor muscles.[12] Several methods have been used to stimulate the striated muscles of the pelvic floor, including the levator ani, external urethral sphincter, and external anal sphincter. Correction of continence with electrical stimulation has been achieved with various techniques, with results showing an increased urethral closure.

Many studies demonstrate that PFMEs, biofeedback, and weighted vaginal cones and balls are an effective combination for treatment of female SUI, even in the long term. Electrical stimulation should be used for women who are not able to identify their pelvic floor muscles or if support is needed to back up home exercises. For optimal results, appropriate instruction for using pelvic floor muscles correctly in a standing position, motivation, and follow-up are essential. There is a need for long-term studies to identify optimal therapy modes and common management strategies for female SUI. The conventional first-line treatment for urinary stress incontinence is conservative. However, in an era of informed choice, some women have shown a preference for surgery. Treatment preferences are influenced by their physicians' information, hearsay, and social factors.

References

1. Abrams P, Cardozo L, Fall M: The standardisation of terminology of lower urinary tract function: Report from the Standardisation Subcommittee of the International Continence Society. Neurourol Urodyn 21:167-178, 2002.
2. De Lancey JOL: Stress urinary incontinence: Where are we now, where should we go? Am J Obstet Gynecol 175:311-319, 1996.
3. Iosif S, Ingemarsson I: Prevalence of stress incontinence among women delivered by elective caesarean section. Int J Gynaecol Obstet 20:87-89, 1982.
4. Fantl JA, Newman DK, Colling J: Urinary incontinence in adults: Acute and chronic management. Clinical Practice Guideline, no. 2, 1996 update. Agency for Health Care Policy and Research (AHCPR) publication no. 96-0682. Rockville, MD, U.S. Department of Health and Human Services, Public Health Service, March 1996.
5. Bo K, Hagen R, Kvarstein B: Female stress urinary incontinence and participation in different sports and social activities. Scand J Sports Sci 11:117-121, 1989.
6. Temmel C, Haidinger G, Schmidbauer J: Urinary incontinence in both sexes: Prevalence rates and impact on quality of life and sexual life. Neurourol Urodyn 19:259-271, 2000.
7. DeLancey JO, Starr RA: Histology of the connection between the vagina and levator ani muscles. Implications for urinary tract function. Journal Of reproductive Medicine 35:765-771, 1990.
8. De Lancey JOL, Delmas V: Gross anatomy and functional anatomy of the pelvic floor. In Bourcier AP, McGuire EJ, Abrams P (eds): Pelvic Floor Disorders. Philadelphia, Elsevier-Saunders, 2004, pp 3-7.
9. Staskin D: Lower urinary tract dysfunction in the female. In Bourcier AP, McGuire EJ, Abrams P (eds): Pelvic Floor Disorders. Philadelphia, Elsevier-Saunders, 2004, pp 43-49.
10. Gilpin SA, Gosling JA, Smith ARB, et al: The pathogenesis of genitourinary prolapse and stress incontinence of urine: A histological and histochemical study. Br J Obstet Gynecol 96:15-23, 1989.
11. Deindl F, Vodusek DB, Hesse U, Schüssler B: Activity patterns of puboccogygeal muscles in nulliparous continenent women. A kinesiological EMG study. Br J Urol 73:413, 1994.
12. Knight S, Laycock J: The role of biofeedback in pelvic floor re-education. Physiotherapy 80:145-148, 1994.
13. Berghmans LCM, Hendricks HJM, Bo K: Conservative treatment of stress urinary incontinence in women: A systematic review of randomized clinical trials. Br J Urol 82:181-91, 1998.
14. DeLancey JOL: Structural support of the urethra as it relates to stress urinary incontinence: The hammock hypothesis. Am J Obstet Gynecol 170:1713-1720, 1994.
15. Petros PE, Ulmsten UI: An integral theory and its method for the diagnosis and management of female urinary incontinence. Scand J Urol Nephrol Suppl 153:1-93, 1993.
16. Dougherty MC: Current status of research on pelvic muscle strengthening techniques. J Wound Ostomy Continence Nurs 25:75-83, 1998.
17. Miller JM, Ashton-Miller JA, DeLancey JO: A pelvic muscle precontraction can reduce cough-related urine loss in selected women with mild SUI. J Am Geriatr Soc 46:870-874, 1998.
18. Wilson PJ, Bereghams B, Hagen S, et al: Adult conservative management. In Abrams P, Cardozo L, Khoury S, et al (eds): Health Publications Ltd Paris 11:869-883, 2005.
19. Bo K, Talseth T: Long-term effect of pelvic floor muscle exercise 5 years after cessation of organized training. Obstet Gynecol 87:261-265, 1996.
20. Lagro-Janssen ALM, Breedveldt Boer HP, Van Dongen JJAM: NHG-standard incontinentie voor urine, Nederlands Huisarts Genootschap M46. [Dutch clinical guidelines on urinary incontinence for family physicians]. Huisarts Wet 38:71-80, 1995.
21. Chen HY, Chang WC, Lin WC: Efficacy of pelvic floor rehabilitation for treatment of genuine stress incontinence. J Formos Med Assoc 98:271-276, 1999.
22. Sluijs EM, Van der Zee J, Kok GJ: Differences between physical therapists in attention paid to patient education. Phys Theory Pract 9:103-117, 1993.
23. Gallo ML, Staskin DR: Cues to action: Pelvic floor muscle exercise compliance in women with stress urinary incontinence. Neurourol Urodyn 16:167-177, 1997.
24. Burns PA, Pranikoff K, Nochajski TH, et al: A comparison of effectiveness of biofeedback and pelvic muscle exercise treatment of stress incontinence in older community-dwelling women. J Gerontol 48:M167-M174, 1993.
25. Wyman JF, Fantl JA, McClish DK, et al: Bladder training in older women with urinary incontinence. JAMA 265:609-613, 1991.
26. Kegel AH: Progressive resistance exercise in the functional restoration of the perineal muscles. Am J Obstet Gynecol 56:238-249, 1948.
27. Bø K: Techniques. In Schussler B, Laycock J, Norton P, Stanton S (eds): Pelvic Floor Re-education: Principles and Practice. London, Springer-Verlag, 1994, pp 134-139.
28. Herbert JH: Pelvic Floor muscles exercises. In Bourcier AP, McGuire EJ, Abrams P (eds): Pelvic Floor Disorders. Philadelphia, Elsevier-Saunders, 2004, pp 277-281.
29. Sapsford RR, Hodges PW, Richardson CA, et al: Co-activation of the abdominal and pelvic floor muscles during voluntary exercises. Neurourol Urodyn 20:31-42, 2001.

30. Benvenuti F, Caputo GM, Bandinelli S, et al: Reeducative treatment of female genuine stress incontinence. Am J Phys Med 66:155-168, 1987.
31. Wells TJ, Brink CA, Diokno AC, et al: Pelvic muscle exercises for stress urinary incontinence in elderly women. J Am Geriatr Soc 39:785-791, 1991.
32. DiNubile NA: Strength training. Clin Sports Med 10:33-62, 1991.
33. Bernstein IT: The pelvic floor muscles: Muscle thickness in healthy and urinary-incontinent women measured by perineal ultrasonography with reference to the effect of pelvic floor training. Estrogen receptor studies. Neurourol Urodyn 16:237-275, 1997.
34. Higbie EJ, Cureton KJ, Gordon LW III, Prior BM: Effects of concentric and eccentric training on muscle strength, cross-sectional area, and neural activation. J Appl Physiol 81:2173-2181, 1996.
35. Hakkinen K, Kallinen M, Izquierdo M, et al: Changes in agonist-antagonist EMG, muscle CSA, and force during strength training in middle-aged and older people. J Appl Physiol 84:1341-1349, 1998.
36. Dougherty M, Bishop K, Mooney R: Graded pelvic muscle exercise. Effect on stress urinary incontinence. J Reprod Med 38:684-691, 1993.
37. Hahn I, Naucler J, Sommar S: Urodynamic assessment of pelvic floor training. World J Urol 9:162-166, 1991.
38. Boyington A, Dougherty M, Kasper C: Pelvic muscle exercise effect on pelvic muscle performance in women. Int Urogynecol J 11:212-218, 1995.
39. Lose G: Simultaneous recording of pressure and cross-sectional area in the female urethra: A study of urethral closure function in healthy and stress incontinent women. Neurourol Urodyn 11:54-89, 1992.
40. Hahn I, Milsom I, Ohlson BL: Comparative assessment of pelvic floor function using vaginal cones, vaginal digital palpation and vaginal pressure measurement. Gynecol Obstet Invest 41:269-274, 1996.
41. Morkved S, Salvesen KA, Bo K: Pelvic floor muscle strength and thickness in continent and incontinent nulliparous women. Neurourol Urodyn 21:358-359, 2002.
42. Theofrastous JP, Wyman JF, Bump RC, et al: Relationship between urethral and vaginal pressures during pelvic muscle contraction. Neurourol Urodyn 6553-6558, 1997.
43. Bo K, Hagen RH, Kvarstein B, et al: Pelvic floor muscle exercise for the treatment of female stress urinary incontinence. III. Effects of two different degrees of pelvic floor muscle exercise. Neurourol Urodyn 9:489-502, 1990.
44. Fantl JA, Newman DK, Colling J, et al: Urinary incontinence in adults: Acute and chronic management. 2. Update. Agency for Health Care Policy and Research clinical practice guideline no. 96-0682. Rockville, MD, U.S. Department of Health and Human Services, Public Health Service, 1996.
45. Blaivas JG, Appell RA, Fantl JA, et al: Standards of efficacy for evaluation of treatment outcomes in urinary incontinence: Recommendations of the Urodynamic Society. Neurourol Urodyn 16:147-147, 1997.
46. Taylor K, Henderson J: Effects of biofeedback and urinary stress incontinence in older women. J Geront Nurs 12:25-30, 1986.
47. Bouchard C, Shephard RJ, Stephens T (eds): Physical Activity, Fitness, and Health. Consensus Statement. Champaign, IL, Human Kinetics Publishers, 1993, p 3.
48. American College of Sports Medicine: Position stand: The recommended quantity and quality of exercises for developing and maintaining cardiorespiratory and muscular fitness in healthy adults. Med Sci Sports Ex 22:265-274, 1990.
49. Laycock J, Jerwood D: Does pre-modulated interferential therapy cure genuine stress incontinence? Physiotherapy 79:553-560, 1996.
50. Elser D, Wyman J, McClish D, et al: The effect of bladder training pelvic floor muscle training, or combination training on urodynamic parameters in women with urinary incontinence. Neurourol Urodyn 18:427-436, 1999.
51. Bump R, Hurt WG, Fantl JA: Assessment of Kegel exercise performance after brief verbal instruction. Am J Obstet Gynecol 165:322-329, 1991.
52. Hay-Smith EJC, Herbison GP, Wilson PD: Pelvic floor muscle training for women with symptoms of stress urinary incontinence: A randomsied trial comparing strengthening and motor relearning approaches. Paper presented at the 32nd Annual Meeting of the International Continence Society, Heidelberg, Germany, August 28-30, 2002.
53. Miller JM, Umek WH, De Lancey J, et al: Pubococcygeal muscle integrity and urethral closure pressures during volitional pelvic floor muscle contraction in women without stress incontinence or pelvic organ prolapse. Paper presented at the 33rd Annual Meeting of the International Continence Society, Florence, October 5-9, 2003. Neurourol Urodyn 222:357-548, 2003.
54. Kegel AH: Physiologic therapy for urinary incontinence. JAMA 146:915-917, 1951.
55. Johnson HE, Hockersmith V: Therapeutic electromyography in chronic back pain. In Basmajian JV (ed): Biofeedback: Principles and Practice for Clinicians, 2nd ed. Baltimore, Williams & Wilkins, 1983.
56. O'Donnell PD, Beck C, Eubanks C: Surface electrodes in perineal electromyography. Urol 32:375-379, 1988.
57. Lose G, Tanko A, Colstrup H, Anderssen JT: Urethral sphincter electromyography with vaginal surface electrodes: A comparison with sphincter electromyography recorded via periurethral coaxial, anal sphincter needle, and perineal surface electrodes. J Urol 133:815-818, 1985.
58. Burgio KL, Engel BT, Quilter RE, Arena VC: The relationship between external anal and external urethral sphincter activity in continent women. Neurourol Urodyn 10:555-562, 1991.
59. Burgio KL: Urinary incontinence: Biofeedback therapy. In Benson JT (ed): Female Pelvic Floor Disorders. New York, Norton Medical Books, 1992, pp 210-218.
60. O'Donnell PD, Doyle R: Biofeedback therapy technique for treatment of urinary incontinence. Urology 37:432-436, 1991.
61. Burns PA: Biofeedback therapy. In O'Donnell PD (ed): Urinary Incontinence. St Louis, Mosby–Year Book, 1997, pp 273-277.
62. Bourcier AP, Burgio KL: Biofeedback therapy. In Bourcier AP, McGuire EJ, Abrams P (eds): Pelvic Floor Disorders. Philadelphia, Elsevier-Saunders, 2004, pp 297- 311.
63. Bourcier AP: Pelvic floor rehabilitation. Int Urogynecol J 1:31, 1990.
64. Bourcier AP: Pelvic floor rehabilitation. In Raz S (ed): Female Urology. Philadelphia, WB Saunders, 1996, pp 263-281.
65. Raz S: The anatomy of pelvic floor support and stress incontinence. In Raz S (ed): Atlas of Transvaginal Surgery. Philadelphia, WB Saunders, pp 1-22, 1992.
66. DeLancey JOL: Pubovesical ligaments: A separate structure from the urethral supports (pubo-urethzol ligaments). Neurourol Urodyn 8:53, 1989.
67. Dixon JS, Gosling JA: The role of the pelvic floor in female urinary incontinence. Int Urogynecol J 1:212-217, 1990.
68. Dougherty MC, Bishop KR, Abrams RM, et al: The effect of exercise on the circumvaginal muscles in post partum women. J Nur Midwifery 34:8-14, 1989.
69. De Lancey JOL: Functional anatomy of the female lower urinary tract and pelvic floor. In Block G, Wheland J (eds): Neurobiology of Incontinence. London, John Wiley & Sons, pp 57-76, 1990.
70. Constantinou CE, Govan DE: Contribution and timing of transmitted and generated pressure components in the female urethra. In Zinner NR, Sterling AM (eds): Female Incontinence. New York, Allan Liss, 1981.
71. Bo K: Pelvic floor muscle exercise for the treatment of stress urinary incontinence. Exercise physiology perspective. Int Urol Gynecol J 6:282-291, 1995.

72. Bourcier AP, Juras JC, Jacquetin B: Urinary incontinence in physically active and sportswomen. In Appell RA, Bourcier AP, La Torre F (eds): Pelvic Floor Dysfunction: Investigations and Conservative Treatment. Rome, Casa Editrice Scientifica Internazionale, 1999, pp 9-17.
73. Bourcier AP: Biofeedback and electrical stimulation. In Blaivas J, Karram M (eds): Proceedings of the Second Annual International Seminar on Female Urology and Urogynecology. Yardley, PA, Fusion Medical Education, 2003, pp 26-29.
74. Miller J, Ashton-Miller JA, De Lancey JOL: The knack: Use of precisely timed pelvic muscle contraction can reduce leakage in USI. Proceedings of the International Continence Society, Athens, 1996. Neurourol Urodyn 15:4, 1990.
75. De Lancey JOL: Structural aspects of urethral function in the female. Neurourol Urodyn 7:509-519, 1988.
76. De Lancey JOL: Anatomy and mechanisms of structures around the vesical neck: How vesical neck position might affect its closure. Neurourol Urodyn 7:161-162, 1988.
77. Bourcier AP: Applied biofeedback in pelvic floor reeducation. In Appell RA, Bourcier AP, La Torre F (eds): Pelvic Floor Dysfunction: Investigations and Conservative Treatment. Rome, Casa Editrice Scientifica Internazionale, 1999, pp 241-248.
78. Bo K: Urinary Incontinence pelvic floor dysfunction Exercise and Sport. Sports Medicine 34:451-464, 2004.
79. Castelden CM, Duffin HM, Mitchell EP: The effect of physiotherapy on stress incontinence. Age Ageing 13:235-237, 1984.
80. Burgio KL, Robinson JC, Engel BT: The role of biofeedback in Kegel exercise training for stress urinary incontinence. Am J Obstet Gynecol 154:58-64, 1986.
81. Berghmans LCM, Frederijs CMA, De Bie RA, et al: Efficacy of biofeedback, when included with pelvic floor muscle exercise treatment, for genuine stress incontinence. Neurourol Urodyn 15:37-52, 1996.
82. Wilson PD, Al Samarrai T, Deakin M, et al: An objective assessment of physiotherapy for female genuine stress incontinence. Br J Obstet Gynaecol 94:575-582, 1987.
83. Morkved S, Bo K, Fjortoft T: Effect of adding biofeedback to pelvic floor muscle training to treat urodynamic stress incontinence. Obstet Gynecol 100:730-739, 2002.
84. Bourcier AP, Park TAE: Electrical Stimulation. In Bourcier AP, McGuire EJ, Abrams P (eds): Pelvic Floor Disorders. Philadelphia, Elsevier-Saunders, 2004, pp 281-291.
85. Fall M, Erlandson BE, Carlsson CA, Lindström S: The effect of intravaginal electrical stimulation on the feline urethra and urinary bladder. Scand J Urol Nephrol 44:19-30, 1978.
86. Erlandson BE, Fall M, Carlsson CA, Linder L: Mechanisms for closure of the human urethra during intravaginal electrical stimulation. Scand J Urol Nephrol 44(Suppl):49-54, 1978.
87. Fall M, Lindstrom SHG: Inhibition of overactive bladder by functional electrical stimulation. In Appell RA, Bourcier AP, La Torre F (eds): Pelvic Floor Dysfunction: Investigations and Conservative Treatment. Rome, Casa Editrice Scientifica Internazionale, 1999, pp 267-272.
88. Sundin T, Carlsson CA: Reconstruction of severed dorsal roots innervating the urinary bladder: An experimental study in cats. Studies on the normal afferent pathways in the pelvic and pudendal nerves. Scand J Urol Nephrol 6:176-184, 1972.
89. Plevnik S, Janez J, Vrtacnick P, et al: Short-term electrical stimulation: Home treatment for urinary incontinence. World J Urol 4:24-26, 1986.
90. Crago PE, Peckham PH, Mortimer JT, Van der Meulen JP: The choice of pulse duration for chronic electrical stimulation via surface, nerve and intramuscular electrodes. Ann Biomed Eng 2:252-264, 1974.
91. Mantle J: Physiotherapy for incontinence. In Cardozo L, Staskin D (eds): Textbook of Female Urology and Urogyneacology. London, Isis Medical Media, 2001, pp 351-358.
92. Bazeed MA, Thüroff JW, Schmidt RA: Effect of chronic electrostimulation of the sacral roots on the striated urethral sphincter. J Urol 128:1357-1362, 1982.
93. Eriksen BC, Eik-Nes SH: Long-term electrostimulation of the pelvic floor: Primary therapy in female stress incontinence. Urol Int 44:90-95, 1989.
94. Eriksen BC: Urinary incontinence: Electrical stimulation. In Besnon JT (ed): Female Pelvic Floor Disorders, Investigations and Management. New York, Norton Medical Books, 1992, pp 219-231.
95. Laycock J, Plevnik S, Senn E: Electrical stimulation. In Schüssler B, Laycock J, Norton P, Stanton S (eds): Pelvic Floor Re-education: Principles and Practice. London, Springer-Verlag 1994, pp 143-153.
96. Sultan AH, Kamm MA, Hudson CN: Pudendal nerve damage during labour: Prospective study before and after childbirth. Br J Obstet Gynaecol 101:22-28, 1994.
97. Benson JT, McCellan EJ, Pillai-Allen AV: Bulbocavernosus reflex study in asymptomatic females [abstract]. Int J Urogynecol 4:403, 1993.
98. Smith ARB, Hosker GL, Warrell DW: The role of pudendal nerve damage in the aetiology of genuine stress incontinence in women. Br J Obstet Gynaecol 96:29-32, 1989.
99. Bourcier AP, Mamberti-Dias A, Susset J: Functional electrical stimulation in uro-gynecology. In Appell RA, Bourcier AP, La Torre F (eds): Pelvic Floor Dysfunction: Investigations and Conservative Treatment. Rome, Casa Editrice Scientifica Internazionale, 1999, pp 259-266.
100. Ishikawa N, Suda S, Sasaki T, et al: Development of a non-invasive treatment system for urinary incontinence using a functional continuous magnetic stimulator (FCMS). Med Biol Eng Comput 36:704-710, 1998.
101. Barker AT: An introduction to the basic principles of magnetic nerve stimulation. J Clin Neurophysiol 8:26-37, 1991.
102. Goldberg RP, Galloway NTM, Sand PK: Extracorporeal electromagnetic stimulation therapy. In Bourcier AP, McGuire EJ, Abrams P (eds): Pelvic Floor Disorders. Philadelphia, Elsevier-Saunders, 2004, pp 291-297.
103. Galloway NTM, Appell RA: Extracorporeal magnetic stimulation therapy for urinary incontinence. In Appell RA, Bourcier AP, La Torre F (eds): Pelvic Floor Dysfunction: Investigations and Conservative Treatment. Rome, Casa Editrice Scientifica Internazionale, 1999, pp 291-294.
104. Evans BA: Magnetic stimulation of the peripheral nervous system. J Clin Neurophysiol 8:77-84, 1991.
105. Craggs MD, Sheriff MKM, Shah PJR, et al: Response to multipulse magnetic stimulation of spinal nerve roots mapped over the sacrum in man. J Physiol 483:127, 1995.
106. Sand PK, Richardson DA, Statskin DR, et al: Pelvic floor electrical stimulation in the treatment of genuine stress incontinence: A multicenter, placebo-controlled trial. Am J Obstet Gynecol 173:72-79, 1995.
107. Luber KM, Wolde-Tsadik G: Efficacy of functional electrical stimulation in treating genuine stress incontinence: A randomised clinical trial. Neurourol Urodyn 16:536-540, 1997.
108. Bidmead J, Mantle J, Cardozo L, et al: Home electrical stimulation in additions to conventional pelvic floor exercises: A useful adjunct or expensive distraction. Paper presented at the 32nd Annual Meeting of the International Continence Society, Heidelberg, Germany, August 28-30, 2002.
109. Yamanishi T, Yasuda K, Suda S, Ishikawa N: Effect of functional continuous magnetic stimulation on urethral closure in healthy volunteers. Urol 54:652-655, 1999.
110. Almeida FG, Bruschini H, Strougi M: Urodynamic and clinical evaluation of 91 female patients with urinary incontinence treated with perineal magnetic stimulation: 1 year follow-up. J Urol 171:1571-1575, 2004.
111. Galloway NTM, El-Galley R, Sand PK, et al: Extracorporeal magnetic innervation therapy for stress urinary incontinence. Urology 53:1108-1111, 1999.

112. Sand PK, Appell RA, Bavendam T, et al: Factors influencing success with extracorporeal magnetic innervation (ExMI) treatment of mixed urinary incontinence. Paper presented at the 30th Annual Meeting of the International Continence Society, Tampere, Finland, August 28-31, 2000.
113. Karantanis E, Stanton S, Parsons M, et al: Women's preferences for treatment for stress incontinence physiotherapy or surgery. Paper presented at the 33rd Annual Meeting of the International Continence Society, Florence, October 5-9, 2003. Neurourol Urodyn 22:522-523, 2004.
114. Plevnik S: A new method for testing and strengthening of pelvic floor muscles. In Proceeding of the 15th Annual Meeting of the International Continence Society, September 1985, London. Oxford, UK, Blackwell Science, 1985, pp :267-268.
115. Meyer S, Lose G: Pelvic floor re-education in urogynecology. In Bourcier AP, McGuire EJ, Abrams P (eds): Pelvic Floor Disorders. Philadelphia, Elsevier-Saunders, 2004, pp 331- 340.
116. Pieber D, Zivkovic F, Tamussino G, et al: Pelvic floor exercise alone or with vaginal cones for the treatment of mild to moderate stress urinary incontinence in premenopausal women. Int Urogynecol J 6:14-17, 1995.

Chapter 29

SELECTING THE BEST SURGICAL OPTION FOR THE TREATMENT OF STRESS URINARY INCONTINENCE

Michael Edward Albo

The number of surgical procedures available to treat stress incontinence continues to grow, complicating the process of choosing which procedure should be performed on which patient. The surgeon and patient expect that the procedure chosen will be the one that provides the highest degree of efficacy with the least amount of morbidity. Do certain patients have better outcomes or less morbidity with one surgical treatment or another, and is their evidence to support the decision?

The American Urological Association's guidelines for the surgical treatment of stress urinary incontinence, published in 1997 by Leach and colleagues,[1] were developed from meta-analyses of the incontinence literature through 1996. The report made recommendations for the surgical treatment of stress urinary incontinence (SUI) in an index patient, defined as a woman with uncomplicated SUI who is undergoing her first incontinence surgery and who has no concomitant morbidities. The guidelines state that for short-term efficacy, any of the four classes of procedures evaluated were acceptable but found that the Burch colposuspension and pubovaginal sling had better long-term outcomes.[1] These guidelines predate the arrival of the mid-urethral sling, the development of alternative allogenic and xenograft sling materials, and the use of laparoscopy in the treatment of incontinence, and they are in the process of being updated.

The guidelines may not be relevant for patients who have any of several complicating factors, including women who have undergone multiple incontinence procedures or who have mixed urinary incontinence symptoms, concomitant prolapse, or a host of other medical comorbidities that may affect the efficacy and safety of a given procedure. To achieve the goal of maximal efficacy with minimal morbidity in nonindex women, we must look beyond the guidelines to other criterion. This chapter looks at a number of nonindex patients and reviews the literature supporting the use of one procedure or another for the treatment of stress incontinence. It discusses the reasons for choosing a procedure for certain patients, even when the evidence is not available. It also presents an algorithm for matching procedures with patients.

CHOOSING AN INCONTINENCE PROCEDURE

Several factors influence the choice of a surgical procedure that is most appropriate for a given patient. These factors include the pathophysiology of the incontinence (e.g., sphincter dysfunction or anatomic incontinence), the presence of mixed urinary incontinence symptoms, a history of incontinence surgery, or the need for concomitant prolapse surgery. Specific medical comorbidities, such as such as the patient's age, obesity, estrogen status, preexisting voiding dysfunction, history of pelvic irradiation or neurologic disease, may also play a role in the decision. Clinicians have preferences for one procedure over another based on their training and clinical experience. Patients also have certain values or opinions that can factor into which procedure they are willing to undergo. Some patients are risk averse and seek the operation with the longest track record. Others are willing to forgo long-term data for a newer procedure that offers less short-term morbidity.

Evidence based-medicine is founded on the premise that therapeutic decisions for medical and surgical conditions use five levels of scientific evidence.[2,3] Level 1 evidence is derived from meta-analyses of randomized, clinical trials or a single, good-quality randomized, clinical trial. Level 2 evidence is derived from meta-analyses of prospective cohort studies. Level 3 evidence is gained from good-quality case-control studies, level 4 evidence comes from high-quality case series, and level 5 evidence is derived from expert opinion. Although the ideal is to look for the highest level of evidence, this may not exist for some decisions. When Leach and coworkers[1] performed their meta-analysis in 1996, they remarked on the paucity of level 1 evidence in the incontinence literature. Downs and Black's review[4] of the incontinence literature also highlighted this problem. Since these reviews, there have been efforts to improve the quality of studies in the incontinence field. A number of randomized, clinical trials have assessed outcomes for various procedures performed for the treatment of SUI.[5,6]

Unfortunately, it remains difficult to find adequately powered randomized, clinical trials or cohort studies assessing the differences between two procedures in any of the subgroups of incontinence patients who are thought to be at a higher risk for failure or complications. Most data are from analyses of subgroups within larger series. These are usually retrospective analyses or studies that were not designed to look at those subpopulations, and consequently, they are underpowered to identify significant differences. When we try to compare the results from different studies, we are hindered by the lack of standardized definitions and outcomes measures. Recommendations in the literature for how to treat a given high-risk patient population are based on level 4 and 5 evidence consisting of case-control series and expert opinion. The subsequent discussion looks at the evidence in the literature regarding how these factors may influence the choice of procedure performed.

INTRINSIC URETHRAL DYSFUNCTION

Historically, the presence of intrinsic urethral dysfunction (ISD) has been a critical factor in deciding which procedure to perform for the treatment of SUI. The party line has been that patients with ISD should be identified and treated differently from patients without ISD. This was based on a number of studies suggesting that patients with ISD did not do as well with standard bladder neck suspensions as they did with sling procedures. This concept has become at best controversial and at worst irrelevant in the past few years for a number of reasons. First, there is a lack of agreement on the definition of ISD. It has been defined in a variety of ways, including maximal urethral closure pressure (MUCP) less than 20 cm H_2O, Valsalva leak point pressure (VLPP) less than 60 cm H_2O, or an open bladder neck identified on cystourethrography. Attempts to show correlations between these definitions have been unsuccessful, preventing comparison of studies that used different definitions.[7,8] Second, the measurement tools used to diagnose ISD have been plagued by poor standardization and poor correlation with physiologic parameters. Third, even when similar definitions are used, there are conflicting results with regard to whether and how ISD relates to outcomes of stress incontinence therapy. Weber[9,10] critically assessed MUCP and VLPP as diagnostic tests and found that both fall short with regard to standardization, reproducibility, and predictive value for outcomes. Nevertheless, studies reporting on the difference in outcomes between those with or without ISD have had a significant impact on how patients have been treated in over the past 20 to 30 years. It is useful to look at some of this literature to understand how we got from there to where we are today.

Sand and colleagues[11] published a retrospective analysis in 1987 of patients who had undergone Burch colposuspension and found that those who had an MUCP less than 20 cm H_2O had lower success rates than those with higher MUCPs (82% versus 46%).[11] At the same time, other investigators were reporting good success rates in women with type III incontinence who had undergone pubovaginal sling procedures.[7,12] Subsequent reports documented the long-term success rates of the pubovaginal sling in patients regardless of the presence or absence of ISD defined by VLPP. Chaikin and coworkers[13] reported an overall long-term cure rate of 73% for pubovaginal sling procedures in 251 women with types I, II, or III stress incontinence. Morgan and associates[14] described 247 women who had undergone autologous pubovaginal sling procedures. Continence rates were 91% for type II and 84% for type III incontinence. Hassouna and Ghoniem[15] assessed long-term cure rates with questionnaires in women who had undergone a sling procedure for ISD. They found a 78% cure rate in this population at a mean follow-up of 3 to 4 years. Zaragoza[16] reported 60 consecutive pubovaginal sling procedures in women with type II or type III incontinence and found a 95% continence rate at 2 years. These kind of results, coupled with the belief that there were two distinct types of stress incontinence, led to a widely held view that patients with ISD should undergo pubovaginal sling procedures rather than Burch colposuspension or needle suspension procedures, which should be reserved for women with hypermobility and no ISD.

The data on ISD and its association with outcomes have been less convincing. Culligan and Sand[17] compared the long-term results for modified Burch and pubovaginal sling procedures in women with a low-pressure urethra (MUCP < 20 cm H_2O). Thirty-six women with urodynamic stress incontinence, a low-pressure urethra, urethral hypermobility, and no significant pelvic organ prolapse were randomly assigned to undergo a modified Burch procedure ($n = 19$) or sling placement ($n = 17$). The investigators did not demonstrate any difference between the Burch and pubovaginal sling procedures in subjective cure rates at 3 months (90% versus 100% respectively) or at 6 years of follow-up (93% and 84% respectively). Long-term objective cure rates were also similar for the two groups (84.6% versus 100%). The statistical power of this study was compromised by the unexpectedly high success rates of the Burch colposuspension.[17] Maher and colleagues[18] performed a retrospective review on a subgroup of 45 women (21 Burch and 24 pubovaginal sling procedures) with low preoperative MUCPs from a larger trial comparing outcomes between Burch and pubovaginal sling procedures. Subjective outcomes were based on a visual analogue scale, with patients rating an improvement of 8 or higher on a scale of 1 to 10 considered to be cured and with objective outcome based on the presence of stress incontinence verified by urodynamic study (UDS). The groups were similar in age, body mass index (BMI), parity, presence of hypermobility, and history of previous pelvic surgery. There were no statistically significant differences in outcomes, although there was a trend for higher success rates in the Burch colposuspension group compared with the pubovaginal sling in all categories: subjective (90% versus 71%; $P = .12$), patient-determined visual analogue score (76% versus 67%; $P = .22$), and objective success (67% versus 50%; $P = .26$). Complications were higher in the pubovaginal sling group (5% versus 25%; $P = .06$).[18] One criticism of this paper is that the success rates for slings are lower than has been reported in most sling series. The investigators have suggested that it may reflect that urge incontinence was included in the definition of failure, whereas other studies did not include it. This underscores the need for similar outcome measures to compare results of studies.

Several studies have looked at the success rates of tension-free vaginal tape (TVT) procedures in patients with a so-called bad urethra or ISD. None of these studies provides more than level 3 or 4 evidence, and none compares TVT procedures with other procedures. Some of the studies suggest women fare worse if they have ISD, whereas other studies report no difference. Rezapour and colleagues[19] analyzed data from their series of 400 women who had undergone TVT procedures and identified a subgroup of women with MUCPs less than 20 cm H_2O. This group had a lower cure rate (74%) compared with previously reported cure rates for the general population (85% to 90%). When they performed a multivariate analysis of the bad urethra group, they found the worst cure rates in a subpopulation of women who were older, had an immobile urethra, and had low resting MUCPs.[19] Kulseng-Hanssen[20] demonstrated more severe postoperative incontinence after TVT procedures in women with MUCPs less than 20 cm H_2O. Paick and coworkers[21] performed a retrospective analysis of their data from 221 patients who had undergone TVT procedures. They divided the patients into two groups: VLLP more than 60 ($n = 160$) and VLPP less than 60 ($n = 61$). At the 6-month follow-up, subjective and objective cure rates were 93% and 82% ($P = .013$).[21]

Several investigators have suggested that urodynamically defined ISD does not correlate with TVT outcomes. Fritel and associates[22] compared patients with MUCPs less than 20 cm H_2O to those with MUCP more than 20 cm H_2O who had undergone TVT procedures. They reported objective cure rates of 80% and 85%, respectively. Rodriquez and colleagues[23] analyzed their prospective series of distal polypropylene slings and found no differences in outcomes based on urodynamically defined incontinence.

There is no evidence suggesting that there is a difference in outcomes between the transobturator approach to the mid-urethral sling (TMUS) and the retropubic approach to the mid-urethral sling (RMUS) for patients with ISD. Mellier and associates[24] retrospectively looked at 52 patients with ISD defined by an MUCP less than 30 cm H_2O who had undergone a TMUS procedure ($n = 26$) or a TVT procedure ($n = 26$). They did not see any difference in outcomes.[24] This study is significantly limited by the nonconcurrence of the procedures and a limited telephone response rate of only 75%.[24]

Urethral injections of various bulking agents have been used to treat ISD, and the data confirm the effectiveness in this group. Herschorn and coworkers[25] reported long-term follow-up with collagen that did not differ significantly when subanalyzed for urethral function. Not many studies have compared the overall effectiveness directly with that of standard incontinence procedures. Success rates for collagen are generally lower than those obtained by most series of anti-incontinence surgery, but these results may improve if a longer-lasting bulking agent is developed. Given the significant differences in efficacy and safety between collagen and pubovaginal sling procedures, an adequately designed study to compare the two on multiple levels would be a welcome addition to the literature. With the advent of minimally invasive slings, a randomized, clinical trial comparing urethral injection with mid-urethral sling would also be helpful. Until this is done, the bulking agents are an option for women who do not want surgery or are not candidates for a surgical procedure.

In summary, although it makes sense that a poorly functioning urethra causes more severe incontinence and may be more difficult to repair, there is little evidence demonstrating that one procedure is superior to another in treating this population. The tools used to assess urethral function have not been subjected to adequate analysis with regard to their ability to represent changes in urethral function and how that change correlates with clinical symptoms. To answer the question this chapter poses, whether ISD is a variable that should direct our choice of procedures, we need to compare specific procedures in a standardly defined group of patients with ISD in a properly designed randomized trial.

URETHRAL HYPERMOBILITY

The so-called fixed urethra was associated with severe incontinence and poor urethral function even before the urodynamic definitions for ISD were created. Incontinence in the absence of hypermobility was interpreted as an indicator of poor urethral function. There is controversial evidence regarding the relationship between Burch colposuspension outcomes and the presence or absence of hypermobility. However, there is increasing evidence in the TVT literature suggesting that patients with hypermobility have better outcomes after TVT procedures than those with a fixed urethra.[22,26] Fritel found that success of TVT correlated positively with the amount of preoperative hypermobility. Patients were divided into three groups based on hypermobility defined by cystourethrography: more than 60 degrees, 30 to 60 degrees, and less than 30 degrees. Success rates after TVT procedures were 97% for patients with more than 60 degrees of hypermobility, 86% for patients with 30 to 60 degrees of hypermobility, and 70% for those with less than 30 degrees of hypermobility. The lowest success rates were for women with previous surgery and no urethral hypermobility (68%).[22] There are two theories about this finding. The first is that the mechanism by which TVT cures SUI is urethral kinking during increases in pelvic pressure that occurs due to a downward movement of the urethra against the fixed mesh of the TVT. The second possible explanation is that a fixed urethra needs external compression to increase the resistance. The tension-free sling, by definition, does not place any compression on the urethra. A comparison of mid-urethral sling approaches is needed to investigate whether this is also true of the TMUS procedures.

Transurethral injections were initially indicated only for patients without evidence of hypermobility. Subsequently, a number of studies have shown them to be equally effective in patients with hypermobility.[25]

In summary, although there is no level 1 evidence documenting the superiority of pubovaginal sling or Burch procedures over the mid-urethral sling in patients with immobile urethras, there is level 3 and 4 evidence to suggest that the tension-free mid-urethral sling is less effective in patients with an immobile urethra than it is in patients with evidence of hypermobility.

RECURRENT STRESS INCONTINENCE

Patients who have had a previous anti-incontinence procedure have lower success rates and higher morbidity with subsequent procedures. The reasons include a higher incidence of ISD, increased age of the patients and scarring in the retropubic space. Other confounding variables include the type of procedure the patient had previously undergone. A study looking into complications of TVT after Burch colposuspension is not necessarily going to provide information on the safety and efficacy on performing a TVT after a failed TVT. Comparison of results is difficult given the various outcome measures used in different studies.

The only level 1 evidence that compares two procedures for this subgroup of patients is from a prospective, randomized study comparing the Burch colposuspension with the Lyodura sling in the management of women with recurrent urinary stress incontinence and in whom the only previous continence procedure was anterior repair.[27] Although the objective success rates for the Burch colposuspension (86%) and the pubovaginal sling (92%) were similar, the incidence of detrusor instability and voiding difficulty was significantly greater after sling procedures (29%) compared with Burch colposuspensions (10%). The meta-analyses by Black and Downs[4] identified no difference in outcomes between the Burch and sling procedures when performed as secondary procedures. However, they acknowledged that the number of studies was limited and that all had low power to detect significant differences.[4] Thakar and associates[28] reported on a prospective, cross-sectional, observational study of 56 women who had undergone a secondary Burch colposuspension for recurrent stress incontinence. At 4 years, the median subjective cure rate was 71%, and the objective cure rate was 80%. They did not compare these patients with a cohort of women who were undergoing a primary Burch colposuspension.[28]

Nilsson and Kuuva[29] performed a retrospective review of their TVT series. They reported equivalent outcomes for patients undergoing TVT as primary or secondary procedures. However, they reported twice as many bladder perforations in the secondary group.[29] Rardin and colleagues[30] performed a retrospective, multicenter study of 245 women who had undergone

TVT procedures; 157 patients had primary procedures, and 88 patients had failed previous surgical treatment. At a mean follow-up of 38 weeks, the cure rates were 87% and 85%, respectively. The bladder perforation rates were similar, although overall complication rates were higher in the secondary procedure group (7.6% versus 4.5%).[30] In 2001, Tamussino and coworkers[31] reviewed the data from the Austrian registry for 2795 patients who had undergone TVT procedures. They reported bladder perforation rates twice as high for patients who had previous surgery (4.4% versus 2%).[31] Haab and colleagues[32] found perforation rates of 30% for patients with a history of incontinence surgery and 2.1% for patients with no such history. Because none of these studies included patients who had undergone primary TVT procedures, it remains unclear whether similar results would be obtained for women undergoing repeat TVT procedures.

Several investigators have tried to control for the confounding variables that can affect outcomes of patients undergoing repeat surgical repairs. In a selected group of patients that excluded patients with low VLPPs and concomitant prolapse repairs, Rezapour[33] reported cure rates of 82% for women with recurrent SUI who underwent TVT.

Transurethral injection therapy and the TMUS procedures have the advantage of avoiding the retropubic space, and therefore may prevent bladder injuries in patients at higher risk for complications due to retropubic scarring from previous procedures. Gorton and associates[34] assessed the long-term outcomes of periurethral collagen injections. The number of previous continence operations did not seem to affect the outcome after bulking agents. The transobturator approach has not been adequately evaluated with regard to long-term incontinence outcomes or complications.

In summary, there is no level 1 evidence suggesting that patients with recurrent stress incontinence should undergo one procedure versus another. Most studies suggest lower efficacy or an increased complication rate in this patient population, but few have controlled for the confounding variables potentially responsible for the worse outcomes. The higher morbidity rate among patients who have had previous surgery, especially with regard to bladder perforation with TVT procedures, is reason to further investigate the TMUS procedures. Ultimately, the patient with a history of previous surgery may be a more complicated patient who requires preoperative evaluation aimed at identifying the reason for the failure and defining the type of incontinence causing the patient's symptoms.

MIXED INCONTINENCE

The literature suggests that patients who present with mixed incontinence preoperatively can have both resolution or worsening of their urge-type symptoms after surgical procedures for SUI. Persistent urge incontinence is cited as one of the most common reasons for patient dissatisfaction after surgery for SUI. A number of studies have shown that patients expect their urge symptoms to improve (Mallet VTM, for the Urinary Incontinence Treatment Network, personal communication, 2005). Several studies have looked at risk factors for worsening of urge incontinence and urge symptoms. There have been no randomized, clinical trials to assess whether one procedure is better than another for patients with mixed symptoms. The existing data are limited to level 3 and 4 evidence, and comparisons between studies are hindered by the lack of standardized definitions for urgency and urge incontinence symptoms.

To illustrate the point on how definitions can influence outcome data, we can refer to the two reports by Chaikin and colleagues[13] and Chou and coworkers[35] on patients with mixed urinary incontinence. They reported in 1998 that patients with mixed urinary incontinence do worse than patients with pure SUI after a pubovaginal sling procedure.[13] In 2003, the same investigators, using a slightly different definition for mixed urinary incontinence, reported similar outcomes for patients with mixed incontinence compared with those with pure stress incontinence after pubovaginal sling procedures. They evaluated 131 women, 46 of whom had pure stress incontinence and 52 of whom had mixed urinary incontinence identified by symptoms or on UDS. The 12-month follow-up using the Urinary Incontinence Outcome Score (UIOS) (i.e., 24-hour diary, pad test, and questionnaire) demonstrated no difference in rates of cure or improvement (97% versus 93%).[35] Several investigators have demonstrated a difference in cure rates depending on the type of detrusor overactivity identified on preoperative urodynamics. The latest publication was a report by Schrepferman and colleagues.[36] They looked at 70 patients with mixed urinary incontinence identified by UDS who underwent autologous pubovaginal sling procedures and found that patients with low-pressure involuntary detrusor contractions did better than patients with high-pressure involuntary detrusor contractions and those with sensory urgency (91.3% versus 27.8% and 39.3%).[36]

The TVT literature reports 42% to 100% improvement or cure rates for urgency and urge incontinence. The only comparative trials of TVT procedures with other procedures did not show a difference in outcomes for patients with preoperative mixed urinary incontinence.[6,37,38] The Hilton trial, although not powered to look for a difference in this subgroup, reported similar rates of de novo urge incontinence.[6,38] Rezapour and coworkers[39] retrospectively analyzed a subgroup of 80 patients from their overall TVT series who had urodynamic evidence of preoperative overactivity. At the 4-year follow-up, this group had outcomes similar to those for the group as a whole, with 85% considered cured of incontinence (defined as a 24-hour pad test result of less than 10 g, a negative cough stress test result, and more than 90% improvement in quality of life). No studies have been powered to show a difference between the TMUS and RMUS procedures for patients with mid-urethral slings. Even the TMUS case-controlled series do not have sufficient numbers of patients to assess the difference in outcomes between those with pure SUI and those with mixed urinary incontinence.

Overall, we continue to lack information on the best form of therapy for the mixed urinary incontinence patient population. There are insufficient data to recommend a specific procedure when performing SUI surgery, and we do not know which patients should have surgery at all. Postoperative urge incontinence remains one of the most significant reasons for persistent incontinence and patient dissatisfaction. It reinforces the concept that the distinction is not one that most patients make, even when they are advised on what to expect from SUI surgery. As clinicians, we must take more time to educate the patients about their expectations and continue to evaluate methods for identifying those at the highest risk for failure.

VOIDING DYSFUNCTION

Most incontinence procedures can cause some element of obstruction and can lead to urinary retention or dysfunctional voiding.[40,41] These possibilities prompted concern that women who demonstrate evidence of voiding dysfunction preoperatively may have worsening of their symptoms or end up in urinary retention postoperatively. Investigators have tried to identify specific patient populations at increased risk and whether one procedure may be more likely to cause postoperative voiding problems. Various results are reported in the literature, and they are limited by nonstandardized definitions of voiding dysfunction and different outcome measures for assessing voiding dysfunction. All of the following have been used in creating a definition of voiding dysfunction: patient-reported symptoms, elevated postvoid residual volume, use of a catheter, and any of several UDS parameters, including abnormal flow rate, abnormal flow pattern, high-pressure voiding, absence of detrusor pressure during voiding, electromyographic activity during voiding, and augmentation or substitution of the detrusor pressure with abdominal pressure during voiding. Another significant limitation is the timeframe after surgery during which voiding is assessed or treatment is initiated. Studies vary in defining urinary retention from 2 days to 6 weeks postoperatively.

The American Urological Association guidelines reported a slightly higher risk for obstruction in patients who had undergone sling procedures.[1] Bhatia and Bergman[42] cited a 12-fold increase in urinary retention after Burch procedures for women who had detrusor pressures less than 15 cm H_2O during voiding. Iglesia and associates[43] retrospectively reviewed their series of 50 women who had undergone pubovaginal sling procedures between 1994 and 1996 and compared women who had preoperative Valsalva-induced voiding with a group of women who had non–Valsalva-induced voiding. They defined patients with Valsalva-induced voiding as those who exhibited a more than 10 cm increase in abdominal pressures during a pressure-flow study. They found a lower objective success rate (46% versus 83%; $P = .011$) and longer duration in postoperative catheterization (median, 23 days versus 14 days; $P = .049$) in the 13 Valsalva-induced voiders compared with the 35 non–Valsalva-induced voiders.[4]

Kobak and colleagues[44] demonstrated higher rates of retention or prolonged time to adequate voiding after bladder neck suspension procedures for patients who had preoperative, urodynamically defined evidence of poor detrusor function or Valsalva augmentation during voiding. Miller and associates[45] performed a retrospective review of 73 patients who had undergone pubovaginal sling procedures between 1998 and 2000 in an attempt to identify preoperative, urodynamically defined factors that could predict postoperative voiding dysfunction. They identified four patients with urinary retention and nine who met their criterion for delayed return to voiding. The only predictor of urinary retention was voiding without a detrusor contraction during pressure-flow studies. The risk factor for delay in return to voiding was the postvoid residual volume.[45] Lo[46] assessed symptoms, uroflow, postvoid residual volume, and pressure-flow study results and found no change in the maximal flow rate, postvoid residual volume, or urethral pressure profile for cured or improved patients after TVT procedures. Sokol and colleagues[47] found no association between preoperative subjective or objective voiding parameters and time to adequate voiding after a TVT procedure. Some investigators have theorized that the TMUS procedures may be less obstructive because the sling's position under the urethra is at a less acute angle. This has yet to be confirmed by any level of evidence.

In summary, although any incontinence procedure is potentially obstructing and there may be subpopulations at increased risk for obstruction or voiding dysfunction postoperatively, there is no scientific evidence to support one procedure over the other based on preoperative voiding parameters. More work is required to standardize the definition of voiding dysfunction and the tools used to assess the subjective and objective parameters used to define the problem.

CONCOMITANT SURGICAL PROCEDURES

Incontinence frequently is associated with other pelvic floor dysfunction. The realization that the entire pelvic floor should be assessed when evaluating patients with urinary incontinence has led to significant improvements in treating both disorders. Multiple studies suggest that concomitant surgery does not affect outcomes of patients compared with outcomes for patients not having concomitant surgery. No studies have randomized patients undergoing pelvic floor surgery to one incontinence procedure or another. Cross and coworkers[48] looked at 42 women who underwent pubovaginal sling procedures concomitantly with a grade III and IV cystocele repair. Thirty-six patients returned for a mean follow-up of 12 months, and four required a subsequent procedure for recurrent SUI. In 2003, Lo[46] conducted a literature review and found six publications that provided sufficient detail to assess differences in outcomes for patients undergoing a TVT procedure and concomitant prolapse surgery. Overall, there was little difference in outcomes between the two groups.[46] Meschia and colleagues[49] reported similar cure rates and no increase in morbidity for the patients undergoing a TVT procedure and prolapse repair compared with those undergoing a TVT procedure alone.[49] There is still no agreement on whether the TVT procedure should be performed before or after the prolapse repair is complete or whether it should be done through a separate vaginal incision.

In summary, there is no level 1, 2, or 3 evidence suggesting that one procedure is better than another in women who are undergoing concomitant prolapse repair. Several case-control series suggest it is not a factor in outcomes. This decision more than others is likely to be determined by the clinician's preference. Some clinicians advocate performing a Burch colposuspension in patients who undergo an abdominal prolapse repair because the abdomen is already open. The minimally invasive techniques may lose some of their advantages with regard to length of hospital stay and postoperative discomfort because the prolapse repair usually is the more morbid of the procedures. These recommendations are based solely on physicians' preferences.

CHARACTERISTICS AFFECTING ANTI-INCONTINENCE SURGERY

Age

Increasing age is associated with many of the previously discussed variables that are thought to affect outcomes in stress incontinence surgery. The elderly are known to be at greater risk for morbidity with any surgery. Nevertheless, the choice of procedures for the elderly should be based on the same goals as for the population as a whole: to maximize efficacy and minimize morbidity.

A number of investigators have performed subanalyses of larger series based on patients' ages. Outcomes generally appear to be less favorable and the complications more frequent. Gillon and Stanton[50] reported similar efficacy but longer hospital stay and higher perioperative morbidity in elderly women who underwent Burch procedures. Karantanis and colleagues[51] looked at a group of elderly women (>65 years) who were matched to a younger cohort for BMI, parity, mode of anesthesia, and whether it was a primary or secondary continence procedure. Exclusion criteria included mixed symptoms and concomitant prolapse surgery. The investigators demonstrated lower satisfaction rates for incontinence outcomes in the elderly group. At a median of 12 months, 15 (45%) older versus 24 (73%) younger women had no urinary symptoms ($P = .05$).[51] Other reports are primarily observational and did not match the patients for other variables. Sevestre and associates[52] reported a 70% cure rate for a group of 76 women after a mean of 2 years. Rezapour and colleagues[19] demonstrated that women older than 70 years with a low MUCP and no hypermobility had a lower success rates with TVT procedures than women not fitting these criteria. Two studies have suggested no difference for outcomes in the elderly. Lo and coworkers[26] performed an observational study of 45 older women who had undergone TVT procedures and reported a 90% cure rate with a low rate of morbidity.[42] Carey and associates[53] compared women older than 80 years with those younger than 80 and found no difference in outcomes for procedures using the cadaveric fascia sling. Herschorn and colleagues[25] reported no difference in outcomes of transurethral collagen injections based on age.

In summary, most case-control series of older women demonstrate lower efficacy and higher morbidity, but there is no evidence that this is specific to the type of procedure performed. Age is associated with a higher incidence of other factors affecting the outcome and morbidity of the treatment, and only when a multivariate analysis is performed are we able to determine definitive correlations. If someone is not a candidate for surgical therapy because of comorbidities, it is irrelevant whether a Burch colposuspension is as effective as a TVT procedure. The deciding factor is which procedure the patient can tolerate given her comorbidities.

Body Mass Index

Some studies suggest that obese patients have worse outcomes and higher complication rates with traditional surgical procedures for stress incontinence,[54,55] although others have not found obesity to affect outcomes.[56-61] The transobturator procedures are being promoted as less morbid procedures in obese women because the abdomen can be completely avoided. This idea has not been substantiated. Although there is no level 1 evidence comparing procedures in patients with high BMIs, a number of published studies have looked at the safety and efficacy of the mid-urethral sling in this population.

Chung and colleagues[56] retrospectively compared the efficacy and safety of the TVT and laparoscopic Burch procedures in treating genuine SUI in obese patients. They described 91 consecutive cases of TVT alone or TVT combined with other procedures from April 1999 to March 2000 and 51 consecutive cases of the laparoscopic Burch procedures from January 1998 to February 1999. They found no difference in the outcomes based on BMI.[56] Mukherjee and Constantine[59] compared the subjective cure rates for TVT procedures at 6 months in three groups of women: BMI of 30 or more ($n = 87$), BMI of 25 to 29 ($n = 98$), and BMI less than 25 ($n = 58$). They reported similar cure rates for all three groups.[59] Zivkovic and coworkers[61] retrospectively reviewed the 5-year outcome data from 187 of 291 patients who had undergone various procedures for stress incontinence. Patients were separated into similar groups by BMI: BMI of 30 or more ($n = 42$), BMI of 25 to 29 ($n = 90$), and BMI less than 25 ($n = 55$). They also reported no difference in efficacy among the BMI groups, although they had only 26% power to show a significant difference because of the sample size.[61] Rafii and colleagues[60] reported a series of 187 patients who had undergone TVT procedures and who were separated into the three groups according to BMI: BMI of 30 or more ($n = 86$), BMI of 25 to 29 ($n = 62$), and BMI less than 25 ($n = 39$). No differences were detected in the persistence of stress incontinence or the complication rate. Statistically significant differences were seen in the rate of urge incontinence between first group (3.4%) and the second group (6.4%) and third group (17.9%).[60]

The 2000 review of obesity and stress incontinence therapy by Cummings and Rodning[58] is still relevant. They concluded that "although intuitively and experimentally such procedures are technically more difficult, outcome data reported to date justifies recommending them as the standard of care."[58] In summary, although patients with higher BMIs may have higher overall risks associated with surgery and although the mid-urethral sling procedures may theoretically reduce these risks with less anesthetic and surgical time, there are no data to support selecting a procedure based only on BMI.

Neurogenic Bladder

The therapeutic approach to the neurogenic patient must be based on an understanding of how her neurologic disease plays a role in the symptoms and the role it may play afterward. These patients have the potential for higher morbidity after surgical treatment of SUI, including voiding dysfunction, urinary retention, or de novo urge incontinence. The implications of a lower success rate or higher morbidity on the patient's quality of life are more profound then in the non-neurogenic patient. Preoperative UDS plays a significant role in this group of patients as a plan is developed. They all are at risk for postoperative urinary retention requiring catheterization to empty the bladder. It is therefore important to assess their ability and willingness to do so. Documentation of urodynamic overactivity may make postoperative management of urge symptoms easier.[62] There is no specific evidence to suggest one procedure over another based solely on the presence of neurologic disease. The potential need for intermittent catheterization may reduce the efficacy with collagen. Use the artificial urinary sphincter may be considered in this group of patients.

History of Pelvic Radiation Therapy

Patients who have previously undergone radiation therapy have a number of confounding variables that may affect the outcomes and morbidity of stress incontinence procedures. Irradiated tissue has reduced elasticity and vascularity. The patients are more likely to have an immobile urethra and lower urethral resistance because of atrophy and decrease submucosal vascularity. The use of synthetic material, although not contraindicated, may have a higher rate of complications because of urethral or vaginal wall erosion. The need to add compression to a fixed urethra as describe previously may preclude the use of synthetic material due to the added tension that must be place on the sling. The higher incidence of detrusor overactivity or small-capacity bladder must be assessed before increasing urethral resistance. There are no studies in the literature specifically looking at this challenging group of patients.

Plans for a Future Pregnancy

The usually recommendation from most clinicians is that patients should wait until they completed their childbearing years before undergoing a repair procedure for SUI.[63,64] The TVT product label states that the desire to have children is a contraindication to placement of the TVT. If they have undergone a procedure, they may be advised to undergo a cesarean section as the mode of delivery. A survey of European urogynecologists asked clinicians what type of procedure they would do for a woman who expressed interest in having more children.[63] Seventy-eight percent said they would offer treatment if the patient expressed interest, but 91% would offer cesarean section to women who were continent at the time of delivery. Although most would offer the woman a surgical option, many would not perform a TVT procedure, and most would advise cesarean section as the method of delivery. Urethral injection therapy is also an option in this population. There are few published data to guide the clinician in this area. In all cases, the patient needs to be informed about the potential risks.

HOW AND WHEN TO INCLUDE A NEW PROCEDURE

New procedures are being developed rapidly in this field, but we should remember that there are procedures with documented efficacy and safety that are considered the gold standards in incontinence surgery. Deviation from these established procedures should be based on clearly outlined advantages in achieving better efficacy or less morbidity and demonstrated with high level of evidence. As clinicians, we must remain committed to studying these procedures before widespread use is accepted When that evidence is lacking but clinical experience suggests a benefit exists for our patients, we must demand that the properly designed studies be performed to assess the procedure or product. We must make sure our patients understand what we know about a new procedure when we counsel them about which procedure is best for them.

The fastest-growing procedure for incontinence is the TMUS. Although it addresses an important concern of many clinicians and educators regarding the RMUS—the potential morbidity associated with passing a trocar blindly into the retropubic space—it has not undergone sufficient evaluation to recommend it for widespread use, even in subpopulations of women with SUI. The RMUS sling has produced a significant body of literature over the past 10 years, with more than 250 articles posted on PubMed. It has been compared with one of the gold standards in incontinence surgery, the Burch colposuspension, in a well-designed trial intreating incontinence surgery and found to be equally as effective.[6] Before the TMUS procedure can be considered interchangeable with the RMUS procedure, which has been in use for 8 years and has hundreds of articles published in the international literature on its safety and efficacy, the TMUS procedures must be subjected to a rigorous comparison. This procedure must continue to undergo evaluation in properly designed trials before it can be accepted as a standard option in our surgical armamentarium for the treatment of SUI.

The following algorithm for choosing an incontinence procedure is based on the information provided in this chapter.

Retropubic mid-urethral sling: for the otherwise healthy woman who is bothered by predominant SUI and desires surgical therapy, exhibits hypermobility on examination (i.e., Q-tip resting or straining angle > 30 degrees), has postvoid residual volume of less than 100 mL, with or without the need for concomitant prolapse surgery, regardless of the following urodynamic study parameters: VLPP, detrusor overactivity, or voiding mechanism

Urethral bulking agent: for the poor operative candidate

Transobturator mid-urethral sling (after discussing paucity of data with patient): for those at high risk for retropubic scarring or with a history of multiple procedures

Autologous pubovaginal sling or urethral bulking agent: for those at high risk for erosion, with a history of radiation therapy, with an immobile urethra, or with acute urethral syndrome

Urinary diversion: for a woman with a neurogenic bladder or severely incompetent urethra

Burch colposuspension or mid-urethral sling: for those undergoing simultaneous abdominal prolapse repair

CONCLUSIONS

Despite having many options for treating SUI, we still have insufficient evidence to recommend which procedure will have the greatest efficacy and least morbidity to specific patient populations. To make more evidence-based decisions on which procedure to perform in which patients, we must randomize similar groups of patients to undergo different procedures. Until we have the results of those trials, we must continue to rely on case report series and theoretical reasons for our decisions. Ultimately, the most important tool we have as clinicians is the individualized assessment of and conversation with each patient. This approach includes a thorough history and physical examination that evaluates the neurologic and anatomic condition of the pelvic floor and the patient's comorbidities. These data are combined with our understanding of the mechanism by which a given procedure resolves incontinence to guide the choice of procedure.

References

1. Leach GE, Dmochowski RR, Appell RA, et al: Female stress urinary incontinence clinical guidelines panel summary report on surgical management of female stress urinary incontinence. J Urol 158:875-880, 1997.
2. Canadian Task Force on the Periodic Health Examination: The periodic health exam. Can Med Assoc J 121:1193-1254, 1979.
3. Meakins JL: Innovation in surgery: The rules of evidence. Am J Surg 183:399-405, 2002.
4. Black NA, Downs SH: The effectiveness of surgery for stress incontinence in women: A systematic review. Br J Urol 78:497-510, 1996.
5. Valpas A, Kivela A, Penttnen J, et al: Tension-free vaginal tape and laparoscopic mesh colposuspension in the treatment of stress urinary

incontinence: immediate outcome and complications—A randomized clinical trial. Acta Obstet Gynecol Scand 82:665-671, 2003.
6. Ward K, Hilton P: Prospective multi-center randomized trial of tension-free vaginal tape and colposuspension as primary treatment for stress incontinence. Br Med J 325:789-790, 2002.
7. McGuire EJ, Fitzpatrick CC, Wan J: Clinical assessment of urethral sphincter function. J Urol 1993; 150:1452-1454.
8. Swift SE, Ostergard DR: A comparison of stress leak-point pressure and maximal urethral closure pressure in patients with genuine stress incontinence. Obstet Gynecol 85:704-708, 1995.
9. Weber AM: Is urethral pressure profilometry a useful diagnostic test for stress urinary incontinence? Obstet Gynecol Surv 56:720-735, 2001.
10. Weber AM: Leak-point measurement and stress urinary incontinence: A review. Curr Womens Health Rep 1:45-52, 2001.
11. Sand PK, Bowen LW, Panganiban R, Ostergard DR: The low pressure urethra as a factor in failed retropubic urethropexy. Obstet Gynecol 869:399-402, 1987.
12. Blaivas JG, Jacobs BZ: Pubo-vaginal sling for the treatment of complicated stress urinary incontinence. J Urol 145:1214-1218, 1991.
13. Chaikin DC, Rosenthal J, Blaivas JG: Pubovaginal sling for all types of stress urinary incontinence: Long-term analysis. J Urol 160:1312-1316, 1998.
14. Morgan TO Jr, Westney OL, McGuire EJ: Pubovaginal sling: 4-year outcome analysis and quality of life assessment. J Urol 163:1845-1848, 2000.
15. Hassouna ME, Ghoniem GM: Long-term outcome and quality of life after modified pubovaginal sling for intrinsic sphincter deficiency. Urology 53:287-291, 1999.
16. Zaragoza MR: Expanded indications for the pubovaginal sling: Treatment of type 2 or 3 stress incontinence. J Urol 156:1620-1622, 1996.
17. Culligan PJ, Goldberg RP, Sand PK: A randomized controlled trial comparing a modified Burch procedure and a suburethral sling: Long-term follow-up. Int Urogynecol J 14:229-233, 2003.
18. Maher CF, Dwyer PL, Carey MP, Moran PA: Colposuspension or sling for low urethral pressure stress incontinence? In Urogyncol J 10:384-389, 1999.
19. Rezapour M, Falconer C, Ulmsten U: Tension-free vaginal tape (TVT) in stress incontinent women with intrinsic sphincter deficiency (ISD)—A long-term follow-up. Int Urogynecol J Pelvic Floor Dysfunct 12:S12-S14, 2001.
20. Kulseng-Hanssen S: Success rate of TVT operation in patients with low urethral pressure [abstract]. Neururol Urodyn 20:417, 2001.
21. Paick JS, Ku JH, Shin JW, et al: Tension-free vaginal tape procedure for urinary incontinence with low Valsalva leak-point pressure. J Urol 172:1370-1373, 2004.
22. Fritel X, Zabak K, Pigne A, et al: Predictive value of urethral mobility before suburethral tape procedure for urinary stress incontinence in women. J Urol 168:2472-2475, 2002.
23. Rodriguez LV, De Almeida F, Dorey F, Raz S: Does Valsalva leak point pressure predict outcome after distal polypropylene sling? Role of urodynamics in the sling era. J Urol 172:210-214, 2004.
24. Mellier G, Benayed B, Bretones S, Pasquier JC: Suburethral tape via the obturator route: Is the TOT a simplification of the TVT? Int Urogynecol J 15:227-232, 2004.
25. Herschorn S, Steele DJ, Radomski SB: Follow-up of intraurethral collagen injection for female stress urinary incontinence. J Urol 156:1305-1309, 1996.
26. Lo TS, Huang HJ, Chang CL, et al: Use of intravenous anesthesia for tension-free vaginal tape therapy in elderly women with genuine stress urinary incontinence. Urology 59:349-353, 2002.
27. Enzelsberger H, Kurz C, Seifert M, et al: Surgical treatment of recurrent stress incontinence: Burch versus Lyodura sling operation a prospective study. Geburtshilfe Frauenheilkd 53:467-471, 1993.
28. Thakar R, Stanton S, Prodigalidad L, den Boon J: Secondary colposuspension: Results of a prospective study from a tertiary referral centre. Br J Obstet Gynaecol 109:1115-1120, 2002.
29. Nilsson CG, Kuuva N: The tension-free vaginal tape procedure is successful in the majority of women with indications for surgical treatment of urinary stress incontinence. Br J Obstet Gynaecol 108:414-419, 2001.
30. Rardin CR, Kohli N, Rosenblatt PL, et al: Tension-free vaginal tape: Outcomes among women with primary vs. recurrent stress urinary incontinence. Obstet Gynecol 100:893-897, 2002.
31. Tamussino K, Hanzel E, Kolle D, et al: The Austrian tension-free vaginal tape registry. Int Urogynecol J Pelvic Floor Dysfunct 12(Suppl 2):S28-S29, 2001.
32. Haab F, Traxer O, Ciofu C: Tension-free vaginal tape: Why an unusual concept is so successful. Curr Opin Urol 11:293-297, 2001.
33. Rezapour M: Tension-free vaginal tape (TVT) in women with recurrent stress urinary incontinence—A long term follow-up. Int Urogynecol J Pelvic Floor Dysfunct 12:S9-S11, 2001.
34. Gorton E, Stanton SL, Monga A, et al: Periurethral collagen injections long-term follow-up. Br J Urol 84:966-971, 1999.
35. Chou EC, Flisser AJ, Panagopoulos G, Blaivas JG: Effective treatment for mixed urinary incontinence with a pubovaginal sling. J Urol 170:494-497, 2003.
36. Schrepferman CG, Griebling TL, Nygaard IE, Kreder KJ: Resolution of urge symptoms following sling urethropexy. J Urol 164:1628, 2000.
37. Liapis A, Bakas P, Creatsas G: Burch colposuspension and tension-free vaginal tape in the management of genuine stress incontinence in women. Eur Urol 41:469-473, 2002.
38. Ward K, Hilton P: Prospective multi-center randomized trial of tension-free vaginal tape and colposuspension as primary treatment for stress incontinence: Two-year follow-up. Am J Obstet Gynecol 190:324-331, 2004.
39. Rezapour M, Ulmsten U: Tension-free vaginal tape (TVT) in women with mixed urinary incontinence—A long-term follow-up. Int Urogynecol J Pelvic Floor Dysfunct 12:S15-S18, 2001.
40. Lukacz ES, Luber KM, Nager CW: The effects of the tension-free vaginal tape on voiding function: A prospective evaluation. Into Urogynecol J 15:32-38, 2004.
41. Wall LL, Hewitt JK: Voiding function after Burch colposuspension for stress incontinence. J Reprod Med 41:161-165, 1996.
42. Bhatia NN, Bergman A: Urodynamic predictability of voiding following incontinence surgery. Obstet Gynecol 63:85-91, 1984.
43. Iglesia CB, Shott S, Fenner DE, Brubaker L: Effect of preoperative voiding mechanism on success rate of autologous rectus fascia suburethral sling procedure. Obstet Gynecol 91:577-581, 1998.
44. Kobak W, Walters MD, Piedmont MR: Determinants of urinary retention after three types of incontinence surgery: A multivariable analysis. Obstet Gynecol 97:86-91, 2001.
45. Miller EA, Amundsen CL, Toh KL, et al: Preoperative urodynamic evaluation may predict voiding dysfunction in women undergoing pubovaginal sling. J Urol 169:2234-2237, 2003.
46. Lo TS: Tension-free vaginal tape procedures in women with stress urinary incontinence with and without co-existing genital prolapse. Curr Opin Obstet Gynecol 16:399-404, 2004.
47. Sokol AI, Jelovsek JE, Walters MD, et al: Incidence and predictors of prolonged urinary retention after TVT with and without concurrent prolapse surgery. Am J Obstet Gynecol 192:1537-1543, 2005.
48. Cross CA, Cespedes RD, McGuire EJ: Treatment results using pubovaginal slings in patients with large cystoceles and stress incontinence. J Urol 158:431-434, 1997.
49. Meschia M, Pifarotti P, Bernasconi F, et al: Tension-free vaginal tape: Analysis of outcomes and complications in stress incontinence women. Int Urogynecol J 12(Suppl 2):S24-S27, 2001.
50. Gillon G, Stanton SL: Long-term follow-up of surgery for urinary incontinence in elderly women. Br J Urol 56:478-481, 1984.
51. Karantanis E, Fynes MM, Stanton SL: The tension-free vaginal tape in older women. Br J Obstet Gynaecol 111:837-841, 2004.
52. Sevestre S, Ciofu C, Deval B, et al: Results of the tension-free vaginal tape techniques in the elderly. Eur Urol 44:128-131, 2003.

53. Carey J, Leach G: Transvaginal surgery in the octogenarian using cadaveric fascia for pelvic prolapse and stress incontinence: Minimal one-year results compared to younger patients. Urol 63:665-670, 2004.
54. Dwyer PL, Lee ET, Hay DM: Obesity and urinary incontinence in women. Br J Obstet Gynaecol 95:91-96, 1988.
55. O'Sullivan DC, Chilton CP, Munson KW: Should Stamey colposuspension be our primary surgery for stress incontinence? Br J Urol 75:457-460, 1995.
56. Chung MK, Chung RP: Comparison of laparoscopic Burch and tension-free vaginal tape in treating stress urinary incontinence in obese patients. JSLS 6:17-21, 2002.
57. Cummings JM, Boullier JA, Parra RO: Surgical correction of stress incontinence in morbidly obese women. J Urol 160:754-755, 1998.
58. Cummings JM, Rodning CB: Urinary stress incontinence among obese women: Review of pathophysiology therapy. Int Urogynecol J 11:41-44, 2000.
59. Mukherjee K, Constantine G: Urinary stress incontinence in obese women: Tension-free vaginal tape is the answer. Br J Urol Int 88:881-883, 2001.
60. Rafii A, Darai E, Haab F, et al: Body mass index and outcome of tension-free vaginal tape. Eur Urol 43:288-292, 2003.
61. Zivkovic F, Tamussino K, Pieber D, Haas J: Body mass index and outcome of incontinence surgery. Obstet Gynecol 93:753-756, 1999.
62. Hamid R, Arya M, Patel HRH, Shah PJR: Experience of tension-free vaginal tape for the treatment of stress incontinence in females with neuropathic bladders. Spinal Cord 41:118-121, 2003.
63. Arunkalaivanan A, Barrington J: Questionnaire-based survey on obstetricians' and gynaecologists' attitudes towards the surgical management of urinary incontinence in women during their childbearing years. Eur J Obstet Gynecol Reprod Biol 108:85-93, 2003.
64. Davila GW, Ghoniem GM, Kapoor DS, Contreras-Ortiz O: Pelvis floor dysfunction management practice patterns: A survey of members of the International Urogynecological Association. Int Urogynecol J 13:319-325, 2002.

Chapter 30

OUTCOME MEASURES FOR PELVIC ORGAN PROLAPSE

Lynn Stothers

Developers of outcome measures for pelvic organ prolapse are faced with the difficult task of addressing a wide range of symptoms from the bowel, bladder, and uterus. Historically, instruments were developed that addressed a single organ, but they have progressed to validated tools that include information relating to all three organs. The modern tools should be completed as part of the patient's medical record, along with the physical examination and diagnostic tests. They can be performed before and after medical or surgical treatment. They are an essential part of the clinician's and researcher's tools in partnership with diagnostic tests.

This chapter describes commonly used validated tools developed specifically for women with pelvic organ prolapse and related symptoms. The instruments can be broadly classified as those that quantify and stage prolapse and those that quantify the range of symptoms associated with prolapse. Some scales, such as the Pelvic Organ Prolapse Questionnaire (POP-Q),[1] provide a means of accurately describing the position of the organs relative to one another and the amount of relative descent of each of the organs. Others provide a means of assessing the wide range of urinary tract, bowel, sexual, pain, and quality-of-life symptoms related to prolapse. Some symptom scales are comprehensive measures that try to address all symptoms resulting from bowel, bladder, and uterine prolapse. Others are focused scales that ask detailed questions about a single complex, such as sexual dysfunction.

QUANTIFYING AND STAGING PROLAPSE

Historically, outcome measures for pelvic organ prolapse were single-organ instruments that required supplementation with diagnostic tests for accuracy and reproducibility. For example, the degrees of a cystocele could be staged using a standing-voiding cystourethrogram. To be accurate over time, these scales required repetition of the diagnostic tests to maintain the accuracy of the staging through the patient's treatment and follow-up. More commonly, staging is done by physical examination alone, without the benefit of diagnostic tests. When physical examination of the patient with prolapse is done, the clinician can only speculate about which organs may be included in the prolapse in the descent of the anterior or posterior vaginal wall or the top of the vault. In this situation, the terms *anterior vaginal wall prolapse* and *posterior vaginal wall prolapse* are more appropriate than the terms *cystocele* or *rectocele*.

Researchers and clinicians recognized the need for a more comprehensive staging system that included all the pelvic organs. Although some of the older scales, such as the traditional four-stage classification system,[2] are still in limited use, the POP-Q is the most widely recognized internationally.[3-6]

Pelvic Organ Prolapse Questionnaire

The POP-Q provides a descriptive and quantifying system for the relative position of the organs within the pelvis and enables objective staging of pelvic prolapse. The system, adapted from several classifications by Baden and Walker,[7] was developed by the International Continence Society Committee on Standardisation of Terminology, Subcommittee on Pelvic Organ Prolapse and Pelvic Floor Dysfunction, in collaboration with the American Urogynecologic Society and the Society of Gynecologic Surgeons.[1] The POP-Q system arose from the efforts of the committee to develop a terminology standardization document. The original document was drafted in 1993 and refined in 1994. In 1994, it underwent a 1-year review and trial, during which time several minor revisions were made.

Reproducibility studies for the POP-Q were conducted in six centers in the United States and Europe, documenting interobserver and intraobserver reliability and clinical utility of the system in 240 women.[8-12] Interobserver reliability was studied in 48 women with a mean age of 61 ± 14 years, parity of 3 ± 2, and weight of 74 ± 31 kg. Correlations for each of the nine measurements (r = 0.817, 0.895, 0.522, 0.767, 0.746, 0.747, 0.913, 0.514, and 0.488) were highly significant (P = 0.0008 to <0.0001). Staging and substaging were reported to be highly reproducible (tau_b = 0.702 and 0.652, respectively). In 69% of subjects, the stages identified were identical, and in the remainder, they did not vary by more than one stage among observers. Intraobserver reliability was studied in 25 women. Correlations (r) for the nine measurements were 0.780, 0.934, 0.765, 0.759, 0.859, 0.826, 0.812, 0.659, and 0.431. The position of the subject during measurement was found to affect staging, with upright examinations reflecting greater prolapse. Staging and substaging were reported to be highly reproducible (tau_b = 0.712 and 0.712, respectively). In 64% of subjects, the stages identified were identical, and in the remainder, they did not vary by more than one stage. All variation was increased in the upright position.[12] The standardization studies were done in the English language, and the standardization document was formally adopted by the International Continence Society in October 1995.

The Pelvic Organ Prolapse Questionnaire Descriptive System

The POP-Q descriptive system allows the clinician to quantify precisely a woman's pelvic support without assigning a severity value; to make accurate, site-specific observations of the stability or progression of prolapse over time; and to accurately describe outcome of surgical repair. The system uses six reference points

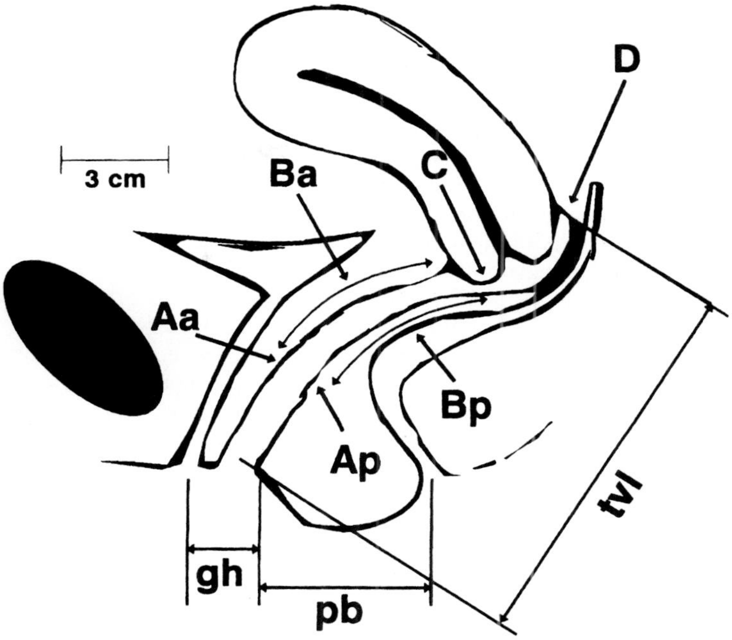

Figure 30-1 Six sites used for pelvic organ support quantitation (points Aa, Ba, C, D, Bp, and AP), genital hiatus (gh), perineal body (pb), and total vaginal length (tvl). (From Bump RC, Mattiasson A, Bo K, et al: The standardization of terminology of female pelvic organ prolapse and pelvic floor dysfunction. Am J Obstet Gynecol 175:10-17, 1996.)

anterior wall Aa	anterior wall Ba	cervix or cuff C
genital hiatus gh	perineal body pb	total vaginal length tvl
posterior wall Ap	posterior wall Bp	posterior fornix D

Figure 30-2 Three-by-three grid for recording a quantitative description of pelvic organ support. (From Bump RC, Mattiasson A, Bo K, et al: The standardization of terminology of female pelvic organ prolapse and pelvic floor dysfunction. Am J Obstet Gynecol 175:10-17, 1996.)

(Fig. 30-1) and a 3 × 3 grid (Fig. 30-2) for recording a quantitative description of pelvic organ support.

The POP-Q descriptive system uses the hymen as the best available fixed point of reference that can be consistently and precisely identified. Six points—two on the anterior vaginal wall, two in the superior vagina, and two on the posterior vaginal wall—are located with reference to the plane of the hymen. The anatomic positions of the six points are recorded as centimeters above or proximal to the hymen (negative number) or centimeters below or distal to the hymen (positive number), with the plane of the hymen recorded as 0.

Points Aa and Ba are located on the anterior vaginal wall. Point Aa (range, −3 to 3 cm relative to the hymen) is located in the midline of the anterior vaginal wall 3 cm proximal to the external urethral meatus. This point corresponds to the approximate location of the urethrovesical crease, a landmark that is obliterated in many patients. Point Ba (−3 cm in the absence of prolapse) represents the most distal or dependent position of any part of the upper anterior vaginal wall from the vaginal cuff or anterior vaginal fornix to point Aa. In women with total posthysterectomy vaginal eversion, point Ba has a positive value equal to the position of the cuff.

Two points on the superior vagina represent the most proximal locations of the lower reproductive tract in a normal position. Point C represents the most distal or dependent edge of the cervix or the leading edge of the vaginal wall cuff (i.e., hysterectomy scar) after total hysterectomy. Point D represents the location of the posterior fornix or pouch of Douglas in a woman who still has a cervix and the level of uterosacral ligament attachment to the proximal posterior cervix. It is helpful in differentiating suspensory failure of the uterosacral–cardinal ligament complex from cervical elongation (symmetric or eccentric), in which the location of point C is significantly more positive than the location of point D. Point D is omitted in the absence of the cervix.

There are two points on the posterior vaginal wall. Point Bp (−4 cm in the absence of prolapse) represents the most distal or dependent position of any part of the upper posterior vaginal wall from the vaginal cuff or posterior vaginal fornix to point Ap. In a woman with total post-hysterectomy vaginal eversion, point Bp has a positive value equal to the position of the cuff. Point Ap (−3 to 3 cm relative to the hymen) is located in the midline of the posterior vaginal wall 3 cm proximal to the hymen.

The numbers in the descriptive system can be recorded in the grid or, more commonly, as a series of numbers (e.g., −2, −2, −6, −7, −3, −3, 10, 3, 2), which represents clinical findings for the six vaginal points relative to the hymen and the total vaginal length (tvl), genital hiatus, and perineal body. The position of the patient during measurement should be documented, because the upright position potentially increases the stage of the descent.

Pelvic Organ Prolapse Questionnaire Staging System

The POP-Q system includes a staging method for quantifying prolapse for the purpose of describing and comparing populations, evaluating symptoms related to prolapse, and assessing and comparing the results of treatment options:

Stage 0: No prolapse is demonstrated. Points Aa, Ap, Ba, and Bp are all at −3 cm, and point C or D is between −tvl and −tvl-2 cm (i.e., the quantitation value for point C or D is less than or equal to tvl-2 cm). Figure 30-3 demonstrates stage 0.

Stage I: The criteria for stage 0 are not met, but the most distal portion of the prolapse is more than 1 cm above the level of the hymen (i.e., its quantitation value is less than −1 cm).

Stage II: The most distal portion of the prolapse is less than or equal to 1 cm proximal to or distal to the plane of the hymen (i.e., its quantitation value is more than or equal to −1 cm but less than or equal to 1 cm).

Stage III: The most distal portion of the prolapse is more than 1 cm below the plane of the hymen but protrudes no further than 2 cm less than the total vaginal length in centimeters (i.e., its quantitation value is more than 1 cm but less than tvl-2 cm). Figure 30-4A demonstrates stage III Ba, and Figure 30-4B demonstrates stage III Bp prolapse.

Stage IV: Essentially, complete eversion of the total length of the lower genital tract is demonstrated. The distal portion of the prolapse protrudes to at least tvl-2 cm (i.e., its quantitation value is more than tvl-2 cm). In most instances, the leading edge of stage IV prolapse is the cervix or vaginal cuff scar. Figure 30-3A demonstrates stage IV C prolapse.

The POP-Q systems provide an excellent means of staging and describing an individual patient's anatomy. However, they do not provide the whole picture of what is happening to the patient unless considered along with symptom scores and a quality-of-life index.

OUTCOME MEASURES FOR PROLAPSE-RELATED SYMPTOMS

Pelvic organ prolapse can involve symptoms from one or more organs, including the uterus or cervix, bowel, and bladder and their supporting anatomic structures. The clinician needs to consider a range of symptoms, from obstructive symptoms to incontinence, sexual dysfunction, and pain, keeping in mind that the alleviation of specific symptoms can be of greater or lesser importance to an individual patient.

Two studies looked at patient-centered and patient-selected goals for pelvic organ prolapse repair.[13,14] The goals of patients in a study by Elkadry and colleagues[13] included improvement or

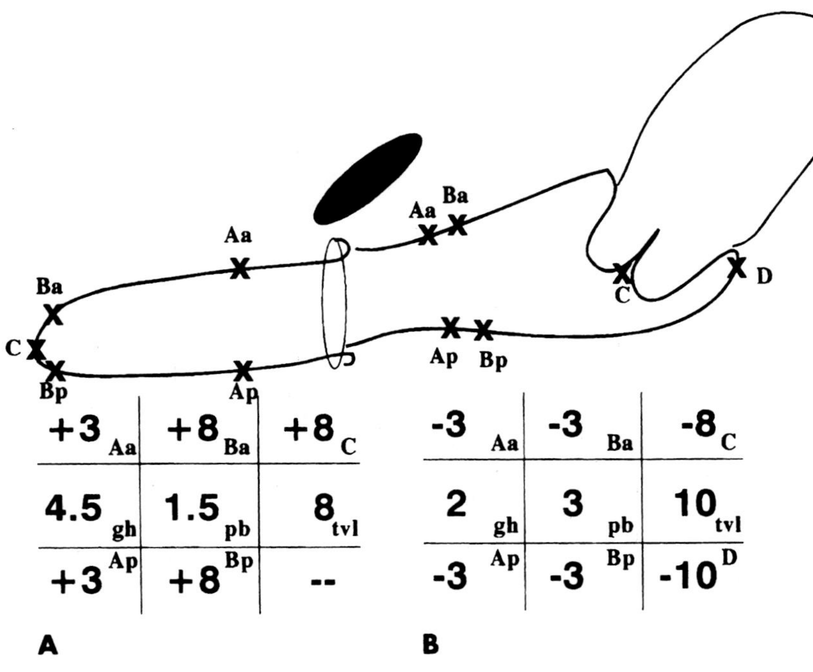

Figure 30-3 A, Grid and line diagram of complete eversion of the vagina. The most distal point of the anterior wall (point BA), the vaginal cuff scar (point C), and the most distal point of the posterior wall (point Bp) are all at the same position (8), and points Aa and Ap are maximally distal (both at 3). Because total vaginal length equals maximum protrusion, this is stage IV prolapse. **B,** Normal support. Points Aa and Ba and points Ap and Bp are all −3 because there is no anterior or posterior wall descent. The lowest point of the cervix is 8 cm above hymen (−8), and the posterior fornix is 2 cm above this (−10). Vaginal length is 10 cm, and the genital hiatus and perineal body measure 2 and 3 cm, respectively. This represents stage 0 support. (From Bump RC, Mattiasson A, Bo K, et al: The standardization of terminology of female pelvic organ prolapse and pelvic floor dysfunction. Am J Obstet Gynecol 175:10-17, 1996.).

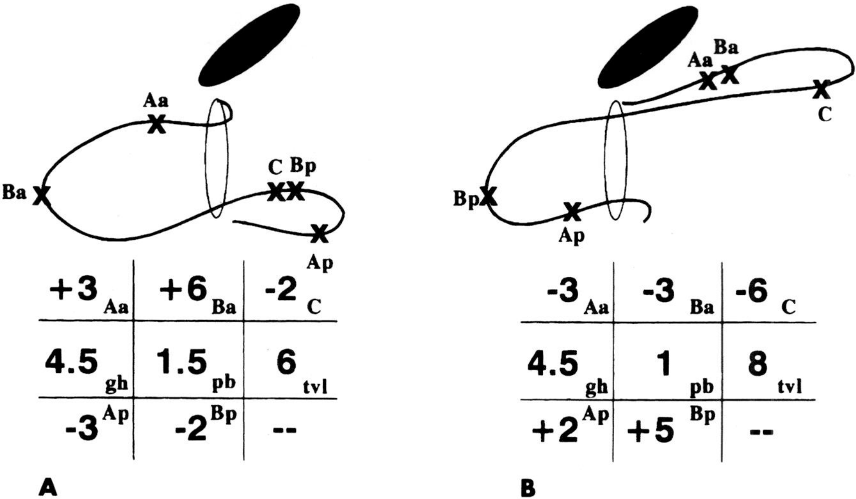

Figure 30-4 **A,** Grid and line diagram of a predominant anterior support defect. The leading point of prolapse is the upper anterior vaginal wall, point Ba (6). There is significant elongation of the bulging anterior wall. Point Aa is maximally distal (3), and the vaginal cuff scar is 2 cm above the hymen (C = –2). The cuff scar has undergone 4 cm of descent because it would be at –6 (total vaginal length) if it were perfectly supported. In this example, the total vaginal length is not the maximum depth of the vagina with an elongated anterior vaginal wall maximally reduced, but rather the depth of the vagina at the cuff with point C reduced to its normal full extent. This represents stage III Ba prolapse. **B,** Predominant posterior support defect. The leading point of prolapse is the upper posterior vaginal wall, point Bp (5). Point Ap is 2 cm distal to the hymen (2), and the vaginal cuff scar is 6 cm above the hymen (–6). The cuff has undergone only 2 cm of descent because it would be at –8 (total vaginal length) if it were perfectly supported. This represents stage III Bp prolapse. (From Bump RC, Mattiasson A, Bo K, et al: The standardization of terminology of female pelvic organ prolapse and pelvic floor dysfunction. Am J Obstet Gynecol 175:10-17, 1996.)

relief of urinary incontinence (58%), pelvic organ prolapse (53%), general health or lifestyle (50%), activity (44%), urgency or frequency (12%), sexual function (11%), and urinary retention (6%). In a study by Hullfish and coworkers,[14] patients identified additional goals, including improvements in bowel symptoms, activity level, social relationships (including sexual activity), self-image, and physical appearance. Elkadry and colleagues[13] found that objective cure, defined as no urodynamic stress incontinence and stage 0 or 1 prolapse, was not related to patient satisfaction, emphasizing the need to evaluate other outcomes.

Several quality-of-life scales have been developed specifically for pelvic organ prolapse conditions. The scales usually cover a broad range of symptoms, such as activities of daily living; urinary, sexual, and bowel function; and pain. In addition to these comprehensive scales, there are more focused scales for urinary symptoms, sexual function, and pain. Incontinence, a symptom frequently associated with pelvic organ prolapse and often evaluated using the stress, emptying, anatomic, protection, and instability (SEAPI) test domains for the score.[15,16]

Quality of Life

Urogenital Distress Inventory and Incontinence Impact Questionnaire

Commonly used, condition-specific, validated quality-of-life measures for pelvic organ prolapse, the Urogenital Distress Inventory (UDI) and the Incontinence Impact Questionnaire (IIQ), were first described by Shumaker and colleagues.[17] The shorter versions, the UDI-6 and the Urge UDI, have also been described.[18,19] FitzGerald and coworkers[20] evaluated the sensitivity of the UDI and IIQ to changes in clinical status after surgery for genuine stress incontinence or pelvic organ prolapse. Of 34 patients surgically treated for pelvic organ prolapse, 31 (90%) were subjectively cured of their prolapse symptoms. Mean IIQ and UDI scores were lower for patients who were subjectively continent.[20] The UDI and IIQ have been used alone or in combination in several studies of outcome after surgical repair for prolapse.[21-23] The two questionnaires can be obtained by contacting the Women's Health Center of Excellence, Wake Forest University Baptist Medical Center, Winston-Salem, NC (http://www.wfubmc.edu/women/whcoe_iiq_udi_instrument.htm).

Pelvic Floor Distress Inventory and Pelvic Floor Impact Questionnaire

The Pelvic Floor Distress Inventory (PFDI) and Pelvic Floor Impact Questionnaire (PFIQ),[24] which incorporate the UDI and IIQ, were developed because of the frequent coexistence and complex interaction of pelvic floor disorders. The PFDI, which assesses symptom distress in women with pelvic floor disorders, has three scales: the UDI, the Colorectal–Anal Distress Inventory, and the Pelvic Organ Prolapse Distress Inventory (Table 30-1). The PFIQ was designed to assess life impact in women with pelvic floor disorders, and it contains the original IIQ and items related to other pelvic floor disorders. The PFDI and PFIQ were shown to be reliable and valid condition-specific, quality-of-life instruments for women with pelvic floor disorders.[24] The instruments are designed for research use and are considered too long to be practical for use in clinical practice (completion time of about 23 minutes in an older population). Short forms have also been validated (Figs. 30-5 and 30-6).

A simpler valid and reliable quality-of-life instrument designed for use in women with pelvic organ prolapse is the Prolapse Quality of Life (P-QOL) questionnaire (Fig. 30-7).[25] In testing the P-QOL questionnaire, 155 symptomatic and 80 asymptomatic women attending gynecology outpatient clinics were asked to complete it. There was a strong correlation between severity according to the P-QOL result and vaginal examination findings

Text continued on page 344

Instructions: Please answer these questions by putting an X in the appropriate box. If you are unsure about how to answer a question, give the best answer you can. While answering these questions, please consider your symptoms over the past 3 months. Thank you for your help.

Name: ______________________________ Date: ____________________

1. Do you usually experience *pressure* in the lower abdomen? ☐No ☐Yes

   If yes, how much does this bother you?
   ☐1 Not at All ☐2 Somewhat ☐3 Moderately ☐4 Quite a bit

2. Do you usually experience *heaviness or dullness* in the pelvic area? ☐No ☐Yes

   If yes, how much does this bother you?
   ☐1 Not at All ☐2 Somewhat ☐3 Moderately ☐4 Quite a bit

3. Do you usually have a bulge or something falling out that you can see or feel in the vaginal area? ☐No ☐Yes

   If yes, how much does this bother you?
   ☐1 Not at All ☐2 Somewhat ☐3 Moderately ☐4 Quite a bit

4. Do you usually have to push on the vagina or around the rectum to have or complete a bowel movement? ☐No ☐Yes

   If yes, how much does this bother you?
   ☐1 Not at All ☐2 Somewhat ☐3 Moderately ☐4 Quite a bit

5. Do you usually experience a feeling of incomplete bladder emptying? ☐No ☐Yes

   If yes, how much does this bother you?
   ☐1 Not at All ☐2 Somewhat ☐3 Moderately ☐4 Quite a bit

6. Do you ever have to push up on a bulge in the vaginal area with your fingers to start or complete urination? ☐No ☐Yes

   If yes, how much does this bother you?
   ☐1 Not at All ☐2 Somewhat ☐3 Moderately ☐4 Quite a bit

7. Do you feel you need to strain too hard to have a bowel movement? ☐No ☐Yes

   If other than never, how much does this bother you?
   ☐1 Not at All ☐2 Somewhat ☐3 Moderately ☐4 Quite a bit

8. Do you feel you have not completely emptied your bowels at the end of a bowel movement? ☐No ☐Yes

   If other than never, how much does this bother you?
   ☐1 Not at All ☐2 Somewhat ☐3 Moderately ☐4 Quite a bit

9. Do you usually lose stool beyond your control if your stool is well formed? ☐No ☐Yes

   If yes, how much does this bother you?
   ☐1 Not at All ☐2 Somewhat ☐3 Moderately ☐4 Quite a bit

10. Do you usually lose stool beyond your control if your stool is loose or liquid? ☐No ☐Yes

    If yes, how much does this bother you?
    ☐1 Not at All ☐2 Somewhat ☐3 Moderately ☐4 Quite a bit

Figure 30-5 The Pelvic Floor Distress Inventory–Short Form 20. (Adapted from the Cleveland Clinic Foundation, Gynecology. Available at http://www.surgery.usc.edu/divisions/Cr/makeanappointment.html/ Accessed July 11, 2005.)

11. Do you usually lose gas from the rectum beyond your control? ☐No ☐Yes

If yes, how much does this bother you?

☐1	☐2	☐3	☐4
Not at All	Somewhat	Moderately	Quite a bit

12. Do you usually have pain when you pass your stool? ☐No ☐Yes

If yes, how much does this bother you?

☐1	☐2	☐3	☐4
Not at All	Somewhat	Moderately	Quite a bit

13. Do you experience a strong sense of urgency and have to rush to the bathroom to have a bowel movement? ☐No ☐Yes

If other than never, how much does this bother you?

☐1	☐2	☐3	☐4
Not at All	Somewhat	Moderately	Quite a bit

14. Does a part of your bowel ever pass through the rectum and bulge outside during or after a bowel movement? ☐No ☐Yes

If yes, how much does this bother you?

☐1	☐2	☐3	☐4
Not at All	Somewhat	Moderately	Quite a bit

15. Do you usually experience frequent urination? ☐No ☐Yes

If yes, how much does this bother you?

☐1	☐2	☐3	☐4
Not at All	Somewhat	Moderately	Quite a bit

16. Do you usually experience urine leakage associated with a feeling of urgency, that is a strong sensation of needing to go to the bathroom? ☐No ☐Yes

If yes, how much does this bother you?

☐1	☐2	☐3	☐4
Not at All	Somewhat	Moderately	Quite a bit

17. Do you usually experience urine leakage related to coughing, sneezing, or laughing? ☐No ☐Yes

If yes, how much does this bother you?

☐1	☐2	☐3	☐4
Not at All	Somewhat	Moderately	Quite a bit

18. Do you usually experience small amounts of urine leakage (that is, drops)? ☐No ☐Yes

If yes, how much does this bother you?

☐1	☐2	☐3	☐4
Not at All	Somewhat	Moderately	Quite a bit

19. Do you usually experience difficulty emptying your bladder? ☐No ☐Yes

If yes, how much does this bother you?

☐1	☐2	☐3	☐4
Not at All	Somewhat	Moderately	Quite a bit

20. Do you usually experience *pain* or *discomfort* in the lower abdomen or genital region? ☐No ☐Yes

If yes, how much does this bother you?

☐1	☐2	☐3	☐4
Not at All	Somewhat	Moderately	Quite a bit

Figure 30-5, cont'd The Pelvic Floor Distress Inventory–Short Form 20. (Adapted from the Cleveland Clinic Foundation, Gynecology. Available at http://www.surgery.usc.edu/divisions/Cr/makeanappointment.html/ Accessed July 11, 2005.)

Instructions: Some women find that bladder, bowel, or vaginal symptoms affect their activities, relationships, and feelings. For each question, place an X in the box next to the response that best describes how much your activities, relationships, or feelings have been affected by your bladder, bowel, or vaginal symptoms or conditions over the past 3 months. Please be sure to mark an answer in all 3 columns for each question. Thank you for your cooperation.

How do symptoms or conditions usually affect your:	***Bladder or urine***	***Bowel or rectum***	***Vagina or pelvis***
1. Ability to do household chores (cooking, housecleaning, laundry)?	☐ Not at all ☐ Somewhat ☐ Moderately ☐ Quite a bit	☐ Not at all ☐ Somewhat ☐ Moderately ☐ Quite a bit	☐ Not at all ☐ Somewhat ☐ Moderately ☐ Quite a bit
2. Ability to do physical activities such as walking, swimming, or other exercise?	☐ Not at all ☐ Somewhat ☐ Moderately ☐ Quite a bit	☐ Not at all ☐ Somewhat ☐ Moderately ☐ Quite a bit	☐ Not at all ☐ Somewhat ☐ Moderately ☐ Quite a bit
3. Entertainment activities such as going to a movie or concert?	☐ Not at all ☐ Somewhat ☐ Moderately ☐ Quite a bit	☐ Not at all ☐ Somewhat ☐ Moderately ☐ Quite a bit	☐ Not at all ☐ Somewhat ☐ Moderately ☐ Quite a bit
4. Ability to travel by car or bus for a distance greater than 30 minutes away from home?	☐ Not at all ☐ Somewhat ☐ Moderately ☐ Quite a bit	☐ Not at all ☐ Somewhat ☐ Moderately ☐ Quite a bit	☐ Not at all ☐ Somewhat ☐ Moderately ☐ Quite a bit
5. Participating in social activities outside your home?	☐ Not at all ☐ Somewhat ☐ Moderately ☐ Quite a bit	☐ Not at all ☐ Somewhat ☐ Moderately ☐ Quite a bit	☐ Not at all ☐ Somewhat ☐ Moderately ☐ Quite a bit
6. Emotional health (nervousness, depression, etc.)?	☐ Not at all ☐ Somewhat ☐ Moderately ☐ Quite a bit	☐ Not at all ☐ Somewhat ☐ Moderately ☐ Quite a bit	☐ Not at all ☐ Somewhat ☐ Moderately ☐ Quite a bit
7. Feeling frustrated?	☐ Not at all ☐ Somewhat ☐ Moderately ☐ Quite a bit	☐ Not at all ☐ Somewhat ☐ Moderately ☐ Quite a bit	☐ Not at all ☐ Somewhat ☐ Moderately ☐ Quite a bit

Figure 30-6 Pelvic Floor Impact Questionnaire–Short Form 7. (Adapted from the Cleveland Clinic Foundation, Gynecology. Available at http://www.surgery.usc.edu/divisions/Cr/makeanappointment.html/ Accessed July 11, 2005.)

Table 30-1 Items in the Scales and Subscales of the Pelvic Floor Distress Inventory and the Pelvic Floor Disorders Impact Questionnaires

Instrument*†	Number of Items	Instrument	Number of Items
Pelvic Floor Distress Inventory	46 total	**Pelvic Floor Disorders Impact Questionnaire**	93 total
Urogenital Distress Inventory	28 total	Urinary Impact Questionnaire	31
Obstructive/discomfort	12	Pelvic Organ Prolapse Impact Questionnaire	31
Irritative	11	Colorectal Impact Questionnaire	31
Stress	5	For each of the above:	
Pelvic Organ Prolapse Distress Inventory	16 total	Travel	6
General	7	Social	11
Anterior	6	Emotional	7
Posterior	3	Physical activity	6
Colorectal-Anal Distress Inventory	17 total		
Obstructive	3		
Incontinence	4		
Pain/irritation	7		
Rectal prolapse	2		

*Some items are used in more than one scale.

†Copies of the questionnaires can be obtained by contacting MD Barber, MHS, 9500 Euclid Avenue A81, Cleveland Clinic Foundation, Cleveland, OH 44145.

From Barber MD, Kuchibhatla MN, et al: Psychometric evaluation of 2 comprehensive condition-specific quality of life instruments for women with pelvic floor disorders. Am J Obstet Gynecol 185:1388-1395, 2001.

Prolapse Quality of Life (P-QOL) Version 4

Name ______________________ Age ________ years Today's date ____________

A prolapse is a bulge coming down the vagina causing discomfort.

PLEASE FILL IN THIS QUESTIONNAIRE EVEN IF YOU FEEL YOU DO NOT HAVE A PROLAPSE.
Please tick one answer to each question.

1. How would you describe your health at present? Very good ☐ Good ☐ Fair ☐ Poor ☐ Very poor ☐
2. How much do you think your prolapse problem affects your life? None ☐ A little ☐ Moderately ☐ A lot ☐

Please indicate with a tick mark if you have any of the following symptoms and how much they affect you.

	Not applicable	None	A little	Moderately	A lot
3. Going to the toilet to pass urine very often.	☐	☐	☐	☐	☐
4. Urgency: a strong desire to pass urine	☐	☐	☐	☐	☐
5. Urge incontinence: urinary leakage associated with a strong desire to pass urine	☐	☐	☐	☐	☐
6. Stress incontinence: urinary leakage associated with coughing	☐	☐	☐	☐	☐
7. Feeling a bulge/lump from or in the vagina	☐	☐	☐	☐	☐
8. Heaviness or dragging feeling as the day goes on from the vagina or the lower abdomen	☐	☐	☐	☐	☐
9. Vaginal bulge interfering with you emptying your bowels	☐	☐	☐	☐	☐
10. Discomfort in the vagina which is worse when standing and relieved by lying down	☐	☐	☐	☐	☐
11. Poor urinary stream	☐	☐	☐	☐	☐
12. Straining to empty your bladder	☐	☐	☐	☐	☐
13. Urine dribbles after emptying your bladder	☐	☐	☐	☐	☐
14. Bowels do not completely empty after opening	☐	☐	☐	☐	☐
15. Constipation: difficulty in emptying	☐	☐	☐	☐	☐
16. Straining to open your bowels	☐	☐	☐	☐	☐
17. Vaginal bulge which gets in the way of sex	☐	☐	☐	☐	☐
18. Lower backache which worsens with vaginal discomfort	☐	☐	☐	☐	☐
19. Do you help empty your bowels with your fingers?	☐	☐	☐	☐	☐
20. How often do you open your bowels?	More than once a day ☐	Once a day ☐	Once every two days ☐	Once every 3 days ☐	Once a week or more ☐

Below are some daily activities that can be affected by your prolapse problem. How much does your prolapse problem affect you? **We would like you to answer every question.** Simply tick the square that applies to you

Role Limitations	None	A little	Moderately	A lot
21. To what extent does your prolapse affect your household tasks (e.g., cleaning, shopping, etc.)?	☐	☐	☐	☐
22. Does your prolapse affect your job or your normal daily activities outside the home?	☐	☐	☐	☐
Physical and Social Limitations				
23. Does your prolapse affect your physical activities (e.g. going for a walk or run, participating in sports or working out)	☐	☐	☐	☐
24. Does your prolapse affect your ability to travel?	☐	☐	☐	☐
25. Does your prolapse limit your social life?	☐	☐	☐	☐
26. Does your prolapse limit your ability to see/visit friends?	☐	☐	☐	☐

Personal Relationships	Not applicable	None	A little	Moderately	A lot
27. Does your prolapse affect your relationship with your partner?	☐	☐	☐	☐	☐
28. Does your prolapse affect your sex life?	☐	☐	☐	☐	☐
29. Does your prolapse affect your family life?	☐	☐	☐	☐	☐

Emotions	None	A little	Moderately	A lot
30. Does your prolapse make you feel depressed?	☐	☐	☐	☐
31. Does your prolapse make you feel anxious or nervous?	☐	☐	☐	☐
32. Does your prolapse make you feel bad about yourself?	☐	☐	☐	☐

Sleep energy	Never	Sometimes	Often	All the Time
Does your prolapse affect your sleep?	☐	☐	☐	☐
Do you feel worn-out/tired?	☐	☐	☐	☐
How often do you use tampons/pads/firm knickers to help your prolapse problem?	☐	☐	☐	☐
How often do you push up the prolapse?	☐	☐	☐	☐
How often do you have pain or discomfort due to the prolapse?	☐	☐	☐	☐
Does the prolapse prevent you from standing?	☐	☐	☐	☐

Thank you. Please check that you have answered all the questions.

Figure 30-7 Prolapse Quality of Life (P-QOL)–Version 4. (Adapted from Digesu GA, Khullar V, Cardozo L, et al: P-QOL: A validated questionnaire to assess the symptoms and quality of life of women with urogenital prolapse. Int Urogynecol J Pelvic Floor Dysfunct 16:176-181, 2005.)

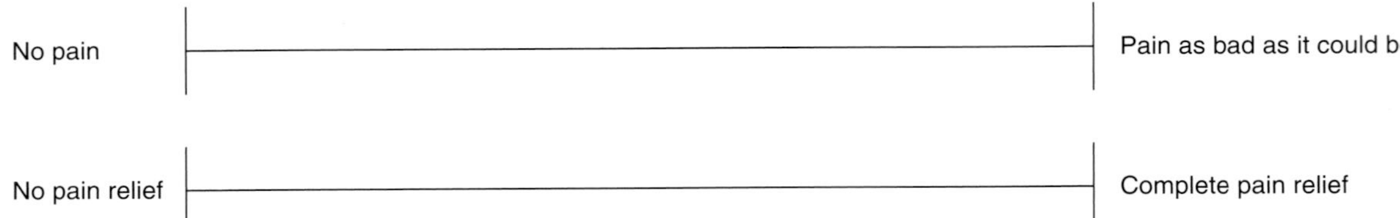

Figure 30-8 The 10-cm visual analogue scales are used for measurement of pain and pain relief. (From Huskisson EC: Measurement of pain. Lancet 2:1127-1131, 1974.)

($P < 0.01$, $r > 0.5$). Total scores for each P-QOL domain were significantly different between symptomatic and asymptomatic women ($P < 0.0001$). Interrater reliability on all items was good (Cronbach's alpha > 0.80). Test-retest reliability showed a highly significant correlation between the total scores for each domain.

Mouritsen and Larsen[26] evaluated patients with pelvic organ prolapse using their own validated questionnaire by relating type and severity of symptoms from the bladder, mechanical, sexual, and bowel domains to bother from the symptoms and to type and grade of prolapse measured. The symptoms from all domains were common and had little relation to the POP-Q value.

Pain

Pain is a recognized symptom related to pelvic organ prolapse. The nature of an individual patient's pain should be evaluated, including vaginal pressure or heaviness, vaginal or perineal pain, sensation or awareness of tissue protrusion from the vagina, low back pain, abdominal pressure or pain, and observation or palpation of a mass.[1] Many standardized tools are available for the evaluation of pain, but none is specific for pelvic organ prolapse. The visual analogue scale (Fig. 30-8) has been shown to be a reliable tool for measuring pain in urogynecologic research.[27,28]

Bowel Dysfunction

There are no isolated scales specifically designed to elicit information about bowel dysfunction associated with pelvic organ prolapse. However, there are useful tools included in more comprehensive scales, including the Pelvic Floor Impact Questionnaire–Long Form (PFIQ-L) (Fig. 30-9) and the PFDI Wexner (Fig. 30-10).[24] These scales include questions related to urgency of bowel movements, frequency of bowel incontinence, and behavioral techniques that women adopt to reduce the impact of bowel dysfunction on quality of life.

Sexual Dysfunction

Pelvic organ prolapse has been strongly associated with sexual complaints in studies of women seeking treatment for pelvic floor disorders. According to a study by Barber and coworkers,[29] pelvic floor symptoms and detrusor instability are more commonly cited as reasons for sexual inactivity than other conditions.

According to Bump and colleagues,[1] some of the sexual function symptoms that should be evaluated include the following areas:

- Is the patient sexually active?
- If she is not sexually active, why?
- Does sexual activity include vaginal coitus?
- What is the frequency of vaginal intercourse?
- Does the patient have pain with coitus?
- Is the patient satisfied with her sexual activity?
- Has there been any change in orgasmic response?
- Is any incontinence experienced during sexual activity?

Several instruments have been designed specifically to address sexual dysfunction related to pelvic organ prolapse, including the long and short versions of the Pelvic Organ Prolapse/Urinary Incontinence Sexual Questionnaire (PISQ).

Pelvic Organ Prolapse/Urinary Incontinence Sexual Questionnaire

The Pelvic Organ Prolapse/Urinary Incontinence Sexual Questionnaire (PISQ-31) is the long or research form of a condition-specific, self-administered, valid, and reliable questionnaire designed to evaluate sexual function in patients with incontinence or uterovaginal prolapse. In the original study by Rogers and associates,[30] factor analysis identified three domains—Behavioral/Emotive, Physical, and Partner-Related—for the 31 questions. There was a strong correlation between sexual function scores and scores on the Sexual History Form-12 (SHF-12) for the questionnaire ($r = -0.74$; $P < 0.001$) and for the Behavioral/Emotive and Partner-Related domains ($r = -0.79$ and -0.5, respectively; $P < 0.001$). The Physical domain was correlated with scores on the IIQ-7 ($r = -0.63$; $P < 0.001$). The PISQ, along with the IIQ, was used in a study of sexual function after surgery for pelvic organ prolapse and showed a decline in sexual function scores after surgery despite improvement in IIQ scores.[21] The questionnaire can be found in the original journal article.[30]

Pelvic Organ Prolapse/Urinary Incontinence Sexual Questionnaire

A shorter version of the PISQ-31, the Pelvic Organ Prolapse/Urinary Incontinence Sexual Questionnaire (PISQ-12) (Fig. 30-11),[31] is less time consuming to complete and therefore more appropriate for clinical use. A data subset from 99 of the original 182 woman surveyed for the PISQ-31 was used, along with data from an additional 46 patients. All subset regression analyses with r greater than 0.92 identified 12 items that predicted PISQ-31 scores. Short-form scores correlated well with long-form scores ($r = 0.75$ to 0.95). Correlations between the short-form score and other tests such as the IIQ-7, SHF-12, and symptom questionnaires scores were similar to correlations between the long-form score and these same tests. Test-retest reliability using data from 20 patients showed moderate to high reliability. A Spanish version of the PISQ-12 also has been validated.[32]

Instructions: Please answer these questions by putting an X in the appropriate box. If you are unsure about how to answer a question, give the best answer you can.

Q1: In general, would you say your health is:
1 ☐ Excellent
2 ☐ Very Good
3 ☐ Good
4 ☐ Fair
5 ☐ Poor

Q2: For each of the items, please indicate how much of the time the issue is a concern of you *due to accidental bowel leakage*. If it is a concern for you for reasons other than accidental bowel leakage then check the box under Not Apply (N/A).

Q2. Due to accident bowel leakage:	Most of the Time	Some of The Time	A little of the Time	None of the Time	N/A
a. I am afraid to go out	1	2	3	4	☐
b. I avoid visiting friends	1	2	3	4	☐
c. I avoid staying overnight away from home	1	2	3	4	☐
d. It is difficult for me to get out and do things like going to a movie or to church	1	2	3	4	☐
e. I cut down on how much I eat before I go out	1	2	3	4	☐
f. Whenever I am away from home, I try to stay near a restroom as much as possible	1	2	3	4	☐
g. It is important to plan my schedule (daily activities) around my bowel pattern	1	2	3	4	☐
h. I avoid traveling	1	2	3	4	☐
i. I worry about not being able to get to the toilet in time	1	2	3	4	☐
j. I feel I have no control over my bowels	1	2	3	4	☐
k. I can't hold my bowel movement long enough to get to the bathroom	1	2	3	4	☐
l. I leak stool without even knowing it	1	2	3	4	☐
m. I try to prevent bowel accidents by staying very near a bathroom	1	2	3	4	☐

Q3: *Due to accidental bowel leakage*, indicate the extent to which you AGREE or DISAGREE with each of the following items. (If it is a concern for you for reasons other than accidental bowel leakage then check the box under Not Apply, N/A).

Q3. Due to accidental bowel leakage:	Strongly Agree	Somewhat Agree	Somewhat Disagree	Strongly Disagree	N/A
a. I feel ashamed	1	2	3	4	☐
b. I can not do many of things I want to do	1	2	3	4	☐
c. I worry about bowel accients	1	2	3	4	☐
d. I feel depressed	1	2	3	4	☐
e. I worry about others smelling stool on me	1	2	3	4	☐
f. I feel like I am not a healthy person	1	2	3	4	☐
g. I enjoy life less	1	2	3	4	☐
h. I have sex less often than I would like to	1	2	3	4	☐
i. I feel different from other people	1	2	3	4	☐
j. The possibility of bowel accidents is always on my mind	1	2	3	4	☐
k. I am afraid to have sex	1	2	3	4	☐
l. I avoid traveling by plane or train	1	2	3	4	☐
m. I avoid going out to eat	1	2	3	4	☐
n. Whenever I go someplace new, I specifically locate where the bathrooms are	1	2	3	4	☐

Q4: During the past month, have you felt so sad, discouraged, hopeless, or had so many problems that you wondered if anything was worthwhile?
1 ☐ Extremely so – to the point that i have just about given up
2 ☐ Very much so
3 ☐ Quite a bit
4 ☐ Some – enough to bother me
5 ☐ A little bit
6 ☐ Not at all

Figure 30-9 Pelvic Floor Impact Questionnaire–Long Version, bowel-related items. (Adapted from the University of Southern California Center for Colorectal and Pelvic Floor Disorders. Available at http://www.surgery.usc.edu/divisions/Cr/makeanappointment.html/ Accessed July 11, 2005.)

Instruction: Please circle the number that describes the status of your fecal incontinence.

Incontinence type	Never	Rarely: *less than once a month.*	Sometimes: *less than once a week but more than once a month.*	Usually: *less than once a day but more than once a week*	Always: *once a day or more*
Solid	0	1	2	3	4
Liquid	0	1	2	3	4
Gas	0	1	2	3	4
Wears pad	0	1	2	3	4
Lifestyle alterations	0	1	2	3	4

Figure 30-10 Pelvic Floor Distress Inventory–Wexner (Adapted from the Cleveland Clinic Foundation, Gynecology. Available at http://www.surgery.usc.edu/divisions/Cr/makeanappointment.html/ Accessed July 11, 2005.)

The Pelvic Organ Prolapse/Urinary Incontinence

Sexual Function Questionnaire (PISQ-12)

Instructions: Following is a list of questions about you and your partner's sex life. All information is strictly confidential. Your confidential answers will be used only to help doctors understand what is important to patients about their sex lives. Please check the box that best answers the question for you. While answering the questions, consider your sexuality over the past *six months*. Thank you for your help.

	Always	Usually	Sometimes	Seldom	Never
1. How often do you feel sexual desire? This feeling may include wanting to have sex, planning to have sex, feeling frustrated due to lack of sex, etc.	☐	☐	☐	☐	☐
2. Do you climax (have an orgasm) while having *sexual intercourse* with your partner?	☐	☐	☐	☐	☐
3. Do you feel sexually excited (turned on) when having sexual activity with your partner?	☐	☐	☐	☐	☐
4. How satisfied are you with the variety of sexual activities in your current sex life?	☐	☐	☐	☐	☐
5. Do you feel pain during sexual intercourse?	☐	☐	☐	☐	☐
6. Are you incontinent of urine (leak urine) with sexual activity?	☐	☐	☐	☐	☐
7. Does fear of incontinence (either stool or urine) restrict your sexual activity?	☐	☐	☐	☐	☐
8. Do you avoid sexual intercourse because of bulging in the vagina (either the bladder, rectum or vagina falling out?)	☐	☐	☐	☐	☐
9. When you have sex with your partner, do you have negative emotional reactions such as fear, disgust, shame or guilt?	☐	☐	☐	☐	☐
10. Does your partner have a problem with *erections* that affects your sexual activity?	☐	☐	☐	☐	☐
11. Does your partner have a problem with premature ejaculation that affects your sexual activity?	☐	☐	☐	☐	☐

12. Compared with orgasms you have had in the past, how intense are the orgasms you have had in the past six months?	Much less intense ☐	Less intense ☐	Same intensity ☐	More intense ☐	Much more intense ☐

Scoring: Scores are calculated by totaling the scores for each question with 0 = never, 4 = always. Reverse scoring is used for items 1, 2, 3, and 4. The short-form questionnaire can be used with up to two missing responses. To handle missing values, the sum is calculated by multiplying the number of items by the mean of the answered items. If there are more than two missing responses, the short form no longer accurately predicts long-form scores. Short-form scores can only be reported as total or on an item basis. Although the short form reflects the content of the three factors in the long form, it is not possible to analyze the data at the factor level. To compare long- and short-form scores, multiply the short-form score by 2.58 (12/31).

Figure 30-11 Pelvic Organ Prolapse/Urinary Incontinence Sexual Function Questionnaire (PISQ-12). (Adapted from Rogers RG, Kammerer-Doak D, Villarreal A, Coates K, Qualls C: A short form of the Pelvic Organ Prolapse/Urinary Incontinence Sexual Questionnaire [PISQ-12)]. Int Urogynecol J 14:164-168, 2003.)

CONCLUSIONS

The most comprehensive clinical picture of a patient with pelvic organ prolapse includes an anatomic assessment using the POP-Q (descriptive and staging) and a comprehensive symptom index. The clinician may choose to supplement these with an in-depth, symptom-specific index to document the patient's perception of the impact of treatment on her symptoms. The benefit of consistent use of a validated, descriptive, and standardized staging index is accurate, ongoing documentation of the success or failure of treatment for the individual patient, regardless of whether management is medical or surgical. It also serves as the foundation for communication among clinicians and researchers.

References

1. Bump RC, Mattiasson A, Bo K, et al: The standardization of terminology of female pelvic organ prolapse and pelvic floor dysfunction. Am J Obstet Gynecol 175:10-17, 1996.
2. Tarnay CM, Dorr CH II: Relaxation of pelvic supports. In DeCherney AH, Nathan L (eds): Current Obstetric and Gynecologic Diagnosis and Treatment, 9th ed. New York, Lange Medical Books/McGraw-Hill, 2003, pp 776-797.
3. Culligan PJ, Blackwell L, Goldsmith LJ, et al: A randomized controlled trial comparing fascia lata and synthetic mesh for sacral colpopexy. Obstet Gynecol 106:29-37, 2005.
4. Digesu GA, Chaliha C, Salvatore S, et al: The relationship of vaginal prolapse severity to symptoms and quality of life. BJOG 112:971-976, 2005.
5. Novara G, Artibani W: Surgery for pelvic organ prolapse: Current status and future perspectives. Curr Opin Urol 15:256-262, 2005.
6. Tan JS, Lukacz ES, Menefee SA, et al, for the San Diego Pelvic Floor Consortium: Predictive value of prolapse symptoms: A large database study. Int Urogynecol J Pelvic Floor Dysfunct 16:203-209; discussion 209, 2005.
7. Baden W, Walker T: Surgical repair of vaginal defects. Philadelphia, JB Lippincott, 1992.
8. Anthanasiou S, Hill S, Gleeson C, et al: Validation of the ICS proposed pelvic organ prolapse descriptive system [abstract]. Neurourol Urodyn 14:414-415, 1995.
9. Schussler B, Peschers U: Standardisation of terminology of female genital prolapse according to the new ICS criteria: Interexaminer reproducibility [abstract]. Neurourol Urodyn 14:437-438, 1995.
10. Montella JM, Cater JR: Comparison of measurements obtained in supine and sitting position in the evaluation of pelvic organ prolapse [abstract]. Proceedings of the Annual Meeting of the American Urogynecologic Society, Oct 12-14, 1995. Seattle, WA. Seattle, American Urogynecologic Society, 1995.
11. Kobak WH, Rosenberg K, Walters MD: Interobserver variation in the assessment of pelvic organ prolapse using the draft International Continence Society and Baden grading systems [abstract]. In Proceedings of the Annual Meeting of the American Urogynecologic Society, Oct 12-14, 1995. Seattle, WA. Seattle, American Urogynecologic Society, 1995.
12. Hall AF, Theofrastous JP, Cundiff GW, et al: Interobserver and intraobserver reliability of the proposed International Continence Society, Society of Gynecologic Surgeons, and American Urogynecologic Society pelvic organ prolapse classification system. Am J Obstet Gynecol 175:1467-1470, 1996.
13. Elkadry EA, Kenton SK, FitzGerald MP: Patient-selected goals: A new perspective on surgical outcome. Am J Obstet Gynecol 189:1551-1558, 2003.
14. Hullfish KL, Bovbjerg VE, Gibson J, Steers WD: Patient-centered goals for pelvic floor dysfunction surgery. What is success, and is it achieved? Am J Obstet Gynecol 187:88-92, 2002.
15. Raz S, Erickson DR: SEAPI-QMM incontinence classification system. Neurourol Urodyn 111:187-192, 1992.
16. Stothers L: Reliability, validity, and gender differences in the quality of life index of the SEAPI-QMM incontinence classification system. Neurourol Urodyn 23:223-228, 2004.
17. Shumaker SA, Wyman JF, Uebersax JS, et al: Health-related quality of life measures for women with urinary incontinence: The Incontinence Impact Questionnaire and the Urogenital Distress Inventory. Qual Life Res 3:291-306, 1994.
18. Uebersax JS, Wyman JF, Shumaker SA, et al: Short forms to assess life quality and symptom distress for urinary incontinence in women. The Incontinence Impact Questionnaire and the Urogenital Distress Inventory. Neurourol Urodyn 14:131-139, 1995.
19. Lubeck DP, Prebil LA, Peebles P, et al: A health related quality of life measure for use in patients with urge urinary incontinence. A validation study. Qual Life Res 8:337-344, 1999.
20. FitzGerald MP, Kenton K, Shott S, Brubaker L: Responsiveness of quality of life measurements to change after reconstructive pelvic surgery. Am J Obstet Gynecol 185:20-24, 2001.
21. Rogers RG, Kammerer-Doak D, Darrow A, et al: Sexual function after surgery for stress urinary incontinence and/or pelvic organ prolapse: A multicenter prospective study. Am J Obstet 191:206-210, 2004.
22. Karram M, Goldwasser S, Kleeman S, et al: High uterosacral vaginal vault suspension with fascial reconstruction for vaginal repair of enterocele and vaginal vault prolapse. Am J Obstet Gynecol 185:1339-1343, 2001.
23. Pang MW, Chan LW, Yip SK: One-year urodynamic outcome and quality of life in patients with concomitant tension-free vaginal tape during pelvic floor reconstruction surgery for genitourinary prolapse and urodynamic stress incontinence. Int Urogynecol J Pelvic Floor Dysfunct 14:256-260, 2003.
24. Barber MD, Kuchibhatla MN, Pieper CF, Bump RC: Psychometric evaluation of 2 comprehensive condition-specific quality of life instruments for women with pelvic floor disorders. Am J Obstet Gynecol 185:1388-1395, 2001.
25. Digesu GA, Khullar V, Cardozo L, et al: P-QOL: A validated questionnaire to assess the symptoms and quality of life of women with urogenital prolapse. Int Urogynecol J Pelvic Floor Dysfunct 16:176-181, 2005.
26. Mouritsen L, Larsen JP: Symptoms, bother and POPQ in women referred with pelvic organ prolapse. Int Urogynecol J 14:122-127, 2003.
27. Lukacz ES, Lawrence JM, Burchette RJ, et al: The use of Visual Analog Scale in urogynecologic research: A psychometric evaluation. Am J Obstet Gynecol 191:165-170, 2004.
28. Barber MD, Visco AG, Wyman JF, et al: Sexual function in women with urinary incontinence and pelvic organ prolapse. Am J Obstet Gynecol 99:281-289, 2002.
29. Rogers RG, Kammerer-Doak D, Villarreal A, et al: A new instrument to measure sexual function in women with urinary incontinence and/or pelvic organ prolapse. Am J Obstet Gynecol 184:552-558, 2001.
30. Rogers RG, Kammerer-Doak D, Villarreal A, et al: A short form of the Pelvic organ Prolapse/Urinary Incontinence Sexual Questionnaire (PISQ-12). Int Urogynecol J 14:164-168, 2003.
31. Romero AA, Hardart A, Kobak W, et al: Validation of a Spanish version of the Pelvic Organ Prolapse Incontinence Sexual Questionnaire. Obstet Gynecol 102:1000-1005, 2003.

Chapter 31

URETHRAL INJECTABLES IN THE MANAGEMENT OF STRESS URINARY INCONTINENCE

Ehab A. Elzayat and Jacques Corcos

HISTORICAL BACKGROUND

Urethral bulking agents have been used for many years to treat intrinsic sphincter deficiency. They are minimally invasive alternatives to operative procedures such as anterior repairs, suspensions, and urethral slings for the management of stress urinary incontinence (SUI). Urethral injection, which can be delivered under local anesthesia as an outpatient procedure, is relatively safe and has few complications. It is an effective treatment for SUI, with complete patient satisfaction comparable to surgery. Urethral injection is cost-effective with less operating time and a shorter hospital stay compared with more invasive surgery.[1,2]

The concept of urethral injectables to increase urethral resistance has been known for 70 years. Murless,[3] in 1938, was the first to report his experience with injection of the sclerosing agent sodium morrhuate into the anterior vaginal wall in 20 patients to induce an inflammatory reaction that compressed the urethra with sclerosis, leading to destruction of the urethral musculature and decreased the compliance of the urethral wall. Quackels,[4] in 1955, injected paraffin wax perineally in two incontinent patients after prostatectomy. Dondren is another sclerosing agent that has been used for urethral injection with some success.[5]

The injection of sclerosing materials such as sodium morrhuate, paraffin, or Dondren causes unacceptable complications, including sloughing of the urethra, urethral stenosis, and pulmonary embolism.[5] Polytetrafluoroethylene (Teflon) was proposed as the first bulking agent by Lopez and colleagues[8] in 1964, and it became popular in the 1970s.[6,7] Since then, several bulking agents have been developed, and new ones are being studied. Nonautologous substances, such as collagen and hyaluronic acid, and autologous substances, such as fat, chondrocytes, and muscle, have been employed clinically or are still under investigation. This chapter reviews the safety and efficacy of available injectable agents for the treatment of female SUI.

MECHANISM OF ACTION OF BULKING AGENTS

The mechanism of continence in urethral injection therapy is uncertain and controversial. Many factors enable normal continence in females, including contraction of the sphincter muscles, musculofascial support of the bladder neck, and a urethra seal mechanism.[8] The functional urethral seal mechanism is probably a major contributor to continence because of its ability to increase urethral resistance and urethral opening pressure during coughing and straining. Common causes for loss of the urethral seal mechanism are scarring from previous operations, birth trauma, estrogen deprivation, or pelvic radiotherapy.[9] Submucosal urethral injection of bulking materials augments bladder neck length and urethral mucosa coaptation and improves the closure mechanism of the urethral sphincter in response to increased intra-abdominal pressure.[10] Some investigators suggest an obstructive mechanism for the action of urethral injectables, as witnessed sometimes by a decrease in the maximum flow rate and heightened voiding maximum detrusor pressure after injection.[11,12] Several laboratories have reported elevation of Valsalva leak point pressure (VLPP) as a result of an increase in functional urethral length.[13-15] Others have found that bulking materials improve the ratio of urethral resistance to abdominal pressure by raising the VLPP but not the detrusor leak point pressure or voiding pressure.[16,17] Monga and Stanton[18] postulated that prevention of bladder neck opening during stress is the mechanism of action of collagen injection, not obstruction.

Cephalad elongation of the urethra caused by bulking agent injection at the bladder neck or proximal urethra probably accounts for increased abdominal pressure transmission in the first quarter of the urethra.[18,19] Placement of the injectable material more distally does not increase the functional length of the urethra or prevent bladder neck opening during episodes of stress. It is suggested that the bulking materials should be placed just distal to the urethral–vesical junction and that the position of the injectable is more important than its quantity for a good bulking effect.[19,20]

INDICATIONS AND CONTRAINDICATIONS

Injectable agents are classically indicated in patients with SUI. Several studies have shown good efficacy for bulking agents, even in the presence of bladder neck mobility. There is a trend to admit some degree of intrinsic sphincter deficiency (ISD) in all cases of SUI. Bulking agent indications then become much broader, and physicians are influenced by other parameters, such as patient preferences, cost, the need for concomitant procedures (e.g., for prolapse), and product availability.[22-25]

An overactive bladder should be treated before undertaking urethral injection. Many physicians believe that untreated bladder instability and low compliance are contraindications to urethral injection; others think that urethral injection can be used to treat the incompetent outlet of an overactive bladder without adverse effects on clinical outcome.[26]

Contraindications to urethral injections are untreated urinary tract infection and hypersensitivity to the injectable materials

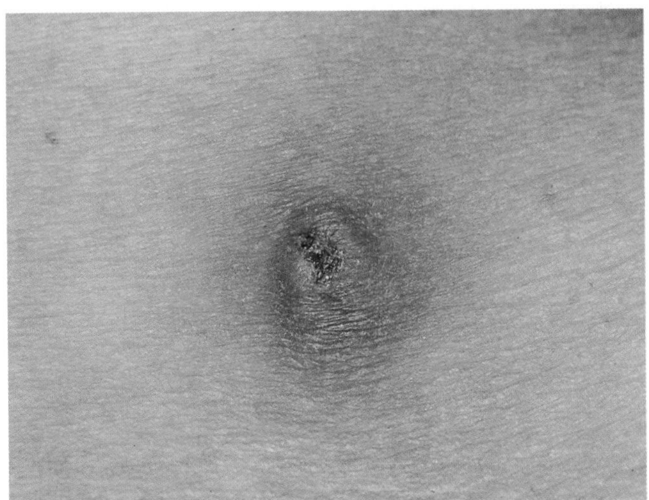

Figure 31-1 Hypersensitive cutaneous reaction after collagen skin testing.

(Fig. 31-1). Extensive scarring of tissue from irradiation or previous surgery or trauma may decrease the retention of injectable material in tissue, leading to a poor outcome.

INJECTION TECHNIQUE

The goal of injection therapy in SUI patients is restoration of the urethral submucosal "cushion" to improve urethral closure pressure during stress episodes without compromising voiding detrusor pressure. The advantages of injection therapy are its minimal invasiveness and technical simplicity, allowing delivery in an outpatient facility under local anesthesia. Urine culture for all patients should be negative, and if collagen is chosen, a skin test to rule out hypersensitivity to collagen must be performed at least 4 weeks before the treatment (see Fig. 31-1). Perioperative antibiotics (e.g., one dose of extended-release quinolone) are usually recommended. After having emptied her bladder, the patient is installed in the lithotomy position, prepared with antiseptic cleaning solution at the level of the external genitalia and urethral meatus, and then draped as usual.

Three injection methods have been proposed: periurethral, transurethral or intraurethral, and antegrade.[27] Only the transurethral technique is still in use.

Periurethral Technique

Injections are usually administered with instillation of transurethral topical anesthetic (i.e., 2% lidocaine jelly) and 3 to 4 mL of 1% lidocaine injected in the periurethral tissues at the 3- and 9-o'clock positions. A 20-gauge needle connected to the syringe of bulking agent is successively inserted slowly at the 3-, 6-, and 9-o'clock positions and advanced into the submucosal tissues (i.e., layer just under the urothelium), approximately 0.5 cm distal to the bladder neck, to raise a urethral bleb. Needle position is controlled by urethroscopy under a 0-degree lens. At each position, the bulking agent should be injected slowly to avoid rupturing the expanding urothelium. The injection is continued until the mucosa appears pale and the lumen is about 30% occluded.[24] To ensure success, visualization of complete coaptation (i.e., bilateral kissing lobes) of the urethral mucosa at the end of the procedure is recommended (Fig. 31-2). For some physicians, this technique can also be done under ultrasonic guidance.[28] In some cases, positioning of the needle can be difficult, leading to repeated mucosal perforations (Fig. 31-3).

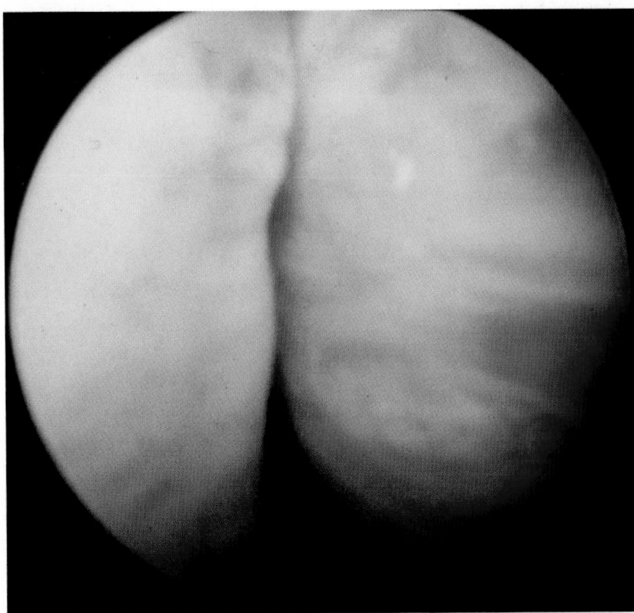

Figure 31-2 Coaptation of the urethra after injection of bulking agents at the 3- and 9-o'clock positions.

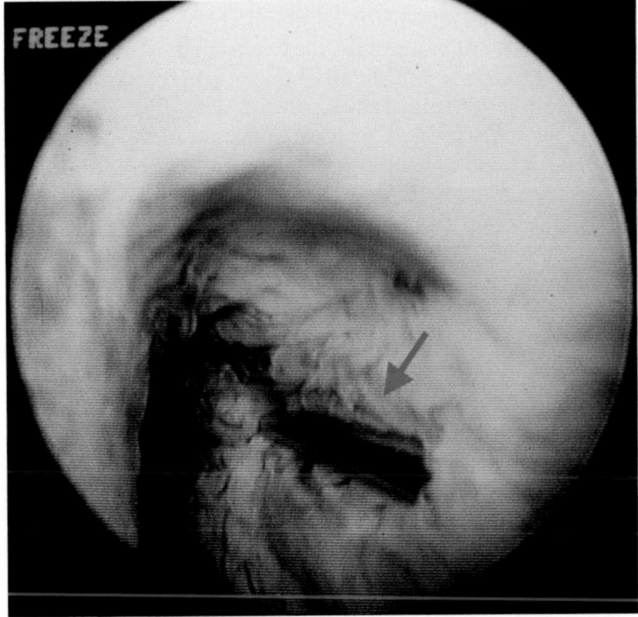

Figure 31-3 Perforation of the mucosa during periurethral injection (*arrow* points to the needle).

Transurethral or Intraurethral Technique

Two transurethral techniques are available: the cystoscopically guided technique and the blind technique. In the first one, needle insertion into the submucosal tissue is achieved under cystoscopic vision with different injection devices. It requires a

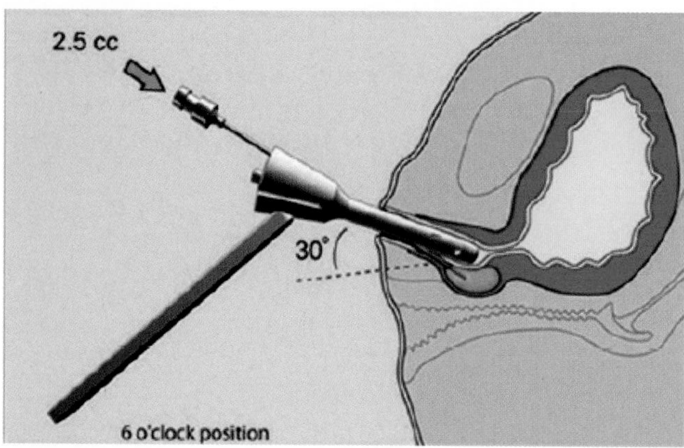

Figure 31-4 Macroplasty injection device.

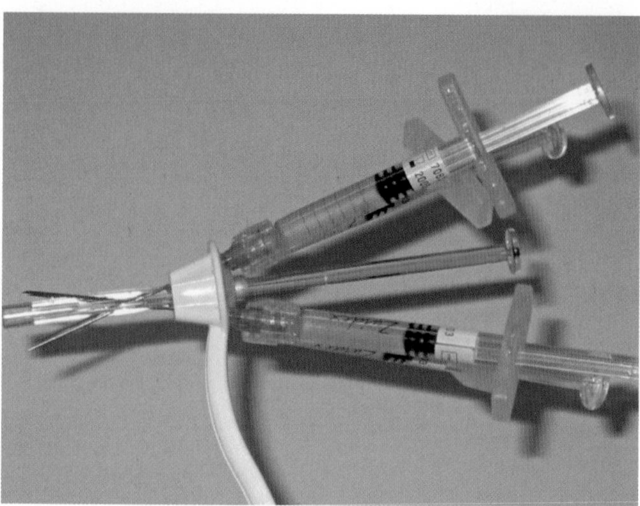

Figure 31-5 Implacer device for Zuidex injection.

cystoscope or a urethrocystoscope with an injection needle (needle size depends on the viscosity of the injectable material) and usually a 0- or 12-degree lens.[29] The needle should be inserted into the submucosal space approximately 0.5 to 1.5 cm distal to the bladder neck at the 3-, 6-, and 9-o'clock positions. The bulking agent is injected slowly until it raises a urethral bleb. Because of the high viscosity of some injectable agents, such as Teflon or silicone microparticles, an injection gun may be necessary (Fig. 31-4). After injection, the physician must avoid advancing the cystoscope beyond the injection site to prevent compression and extrusion of the injectable material.

Faerber and associates[30] compared the intraurethral and periurethral routes and demonstrated significant differences in cure (46% versus 33%) and improvement (50% versus 67%) rates in favor of the intraurethral route. However, Schulz and colleagues[31] compared periurethral and intraurethral injection randomly in 40 women and concluded that both routes of injection were equally effective. In Faerber's report, it was evident that the intraurethral route required much less injectable material (4.7% versus 10.1 mL) for better results. The average number of sessions (1.3) was identical with both approaches. These findings explain why most centers now use only the intra-urethral approach.

The blind transurethral technique uses injection devices that do not require cystoscopic guidance. Henalla and coworkers[32] were the first to apply Macroplastique implantation system to improve and simplify the injection technique (see Fig. 31-4). With this device, the success rate was 74.3%, and the rate of acceptability by surgeons was 95%. The implantation device was developed to control accurate placement of the bulking agent at predefined sites and depth in the female urethra without the need for cystoscopic guidance.[33] The device is advanced into the urethra until urinary drainage is established and then withdrawn 1 cm. The injection needle is inserted into the first deployment site, angling the device in the direction of the injection site to ensure penetration of the mucosa.[34] The device enables consistent bolus placement at a predetermined depth and site. Usually, two to three punctures (at the 4-, 8-, and 12-o'clock positions) are needed for material delivery. If injection treatment fails, transvaginal or transurethral ultrasound can be performed to investigate correct Macroplastique placement. A different version of the device has been introduced by Q-Med AB (Uppsala, Sweden) (Fig. 31-5). The Implacer device has been developed for administration of dextranomer/hyaluronic acid (Dx/HA; Zuidex) without the need for cystoscopic guidance. The Implacer uses four syringes (each containing 0.7 mL of Dx/HA) and 23-guage needles. The device unfolds and fixates the urethral wall to ensure symmetric placement of the injectable agent at four evenly spaced locations around the urethra.

Antegrade Technique

The antegrade technique has been described mainly for incontinence in men after prostatectomy. It is performed through a suprapubic cystostomy and under cystoscopic control. The bulking agent is injected submucosally around the bladder neck until coaptation occurs. The technique can be performed under intravenous sedation, general anesthesia, or spinal anesthesia. It is indicated for patients with a scarred, noncompliant urethra.

POSTOPERATIVE CARE

Patients are usually discharged to their homes after satisfactory voiding. If urinary retention occurs, a small-caliber catheter (14 Fr or smaller) is inserted to empty the bladder. In rare cases of persistent retention, intermittent catheterization with a small-caliber catheter is required until normal micturition resumes.[24] Mechanical pressure to the perineum (e.g., hard seat covers, hard stools, intravaginal sexual intercourse) should be avoided for 2 weeks. If a second injection is necessary, it should be performed after a few weeks to allow healing of the previous implant.[28]

ASSESSMENT OF CLINICAL OUTCOMES

No validated, reproducible, well-accepted instruments have existed for the assessment of outcomes of treatment of urinary incontinence.[35] There is no standard definition of success in studies of anti-incontinence procedures, making it difficult to objectively compare results. Assessment of cure depends on subjective or objective measurements, which are not correlated. In most reported studies, *cure* is defined as the patient being dry by the end of the follow-up period. *Improvement* is defined as rare or minimal leakage and patient satisfaction with the result of the injection.[36]

Table 31-1 Results of Polytetrafluoroethylene Injections

Study	No. of Patients	Follow-up (mo)	Mean No. of Injections	Mean Injection Volume (mL)	Results
Politano,[43] 1982	51	6 (6-16)	1.8	10-15	71% (51% dry, 20% improved)
Lim et al,[48] 1983	28	12	1	11-12	54% (33% improved, 21.4% dry)
Schulman et al,[49] 1983	56	3 (3-24)	1.5	9	86% (16% improved, 70% cured)
Deane et al,[50] 1985	28	13 (3-24)	NS	10	29% improved, 32% dry
Osther and Rohl,[51] 1987	36	3	NS	12	50% good or moderate results
Lockhart et al,[44] 1988	20	NS	1.9	7	50% dry, 35% improved
Vesey et al,[52] 1988	36	9 (3-36)	1-2	7-14	67% (56% dry, 11% improved)
Kiilholma and Makinen,[53] 1991	22	60	NS	7.3	18% (dry or improved)
Beckingham et al,[45] 1992	26	36	1-3	9	27% improved, 7% dry
Lopes et al,[54] 1993	74	31	1.3	19	19% improved, 54.3% dry
Harrison et al,[46] 1993	36	5.1 yr	1-3	7	33% (11% dry, 22% improved)
Herschorn and Glazer,[47] 2000	46	12	2	2.5	30.4% dry, 41.3% improved

NS, not stated.

Initial patient assessment should include a symptom evaluation, patient satisfaction score, quality-of-life questionnaire, leakage gravity index (e.g., pad test, visual scale), physical examination, and urodynamic measurement. Follow-up should monitor the same parameters plus the length of time since the last injection, number of injections performed, volume per injection, and cure criteria (e.g., physical examination, pad usage, pad-weighing tests, urodynamics).[37]

There is a large consensus in favor of a redefinition of outcomes for incontinence treatment. Clinicians and researchers are developing new measures that take into consideration the patient's goals and expectations. We strongly believe that these new paradigms will in the near future replace classic assessments.

INJECTABLE MATERIALS

Ideal bulking agents should be biocompatible, biodegradable, nonmigratory (bulking > 80 μm), nonerosive, noncarcinogenic, nonimmunogenic, permanently bulking, and easily injected.[25] Unfortunately, none of the available bulking agents entirely meets these requirements.

Polytetrafluoroethylene

Polytetrafluoroethylene (PTFE; Teflon, Polytef) was described as a bulking agent by Lopez and colleagues in 1964,[8] and it was popularized by Berg[6] and Politano[7] in 1970. It is a paste consisting of colloidal PTFE micropolymeric, various-sized particles (up to 300 μm, with most being < 50 μm).[8] It is an inert, stable material with a high molecular weight and high viscosity, and it is nonallergenic.

Teflon has several disadvantages that limit its acceptability and prevent it from being approved by the U.S. Food and Drug Administration (FDA) for periurethral injection in the United States. It is difficult to inject because of its density, requiring very high pressure through a large-bore needle. Because of the small size of the particles, PTFE (90% < 40 μm in diameter) can be phagocytosed, resulting in distant migration to the brain, lungs, and lymph nodes.[38,39] Among other major inconveniences, PTFE is not biodegradable, and it carries a risk of granuloma formation at the injection site and at some sites of distant migration.[40] PTFE produces an inflammatory reaction that may lead to urethral fibrosis, periurethral abscess, and urethral diverticulum.[41] The carcinogenic potential of PTFE injection has been suggested but not proved and never reported clinically.[42]

Politano and coworkers[43] first used Teflon for incontinence in men after prostatectomy and later for stress incontinence in women. Their short-term results were promising, with cure and improvement rates of 57% to 85%. However, long-term data have ranged from 18% to 76%.[44-46] The reasons for failure of Teflon injection include the high pressure needed for injection, leading to tissue extrusion, absorption, and migration of Teflon particles, and the inflammatory reactions affecting urethral function.[37] Failures in this series were associated with prior incontinence operations and bladder instability. To minimize the risk of migration, Herschorn and Glazer[47] evaluated the injection of low-volume Teflon, with a success rate of 71.7% (Table 31-1).

Glutaraldehyde Cross-Linked Collagen

Bovine glutaraldehyde cross-linked collagen (Contigen) is the most widely studied bulking agent. It is a well-established injectable material that gained FDA approval in 1993.[24] Periurethral injection of glutaraldehyde cross-linked collagen was first reported by Shortliffe and associates in 1989.[55] Contigen, a highly purified suspension of bovine collagen in normal saline, contains more than 95% type I collagen and less than 5% type III collagen cross-linked with glutaraldehyde. This cross-linking makes collagen more stable and durable, hindering its breakdown by fibroblast-secreted collagenase and enhancing its invasion by fibroblasts and blood vessels with deposition of host collagen, promoting long-term efficacy of the implant.[56] The decreased antigenicity of this mixed collagen is obtained by hydrolysis of the antigenic parts of the molecules, the amino-terminal and carboxyl-terminal segments. Cross-linking also reduces hypersensitivity.

Collagen injection is an easy procedure. It can be delivered periurethrally or transurethrally through a small needle (22 gauge) under local anesthesia. Each syringe contains approximately 2.5 mL of collagen, and some patients may need repeated injections (e.g., two to five injections). If the collagen is placed too deeply, it will be quickly reabsorbed. However, the position and volume of injected collagen are not predictive of clinical outcome, as determined by a magnetic resonance study.[57,58] The advantages of collagen injection include its durable efficacy and safety, with no proven risk of granuloma formation or migration.[59] Considering its price, cost-effectiveness is a concern. Berman and Kreder[60] reported that sling cystourethropexy is more cost-effective than collagen injection in women with type III incontinence. The collagen injection is allergenic in up to 5% of patients, requiring skin tests to rule out hypersensitivity 1 month before injection.[61] There also is some concern regarding the potential for disease transmission from bovine products.[34]

Early results have disclosed subjective cure and improvement rates up to 95% and objective cure rates of 61% to 91%.[36] Herschorn and colleagues[62] reported an early experience with intra-urethral injection of collagen in 31 women, with a mean follow-up of 6 months. The combined cure and improvement rate was 90.3%. Longer-term results of cure and improvement rates vary from 57% to 94% (Table 31-2). In a North American multicenter study, 148 women underwent collagen injection for ISD, with an overall success rate of 78% (45% cured, 33% improved) at 2 years of follow-up.[63] Monga and coworkers[67] achieved a success rate of 86% at 3 months, 77% at 12 months, and 68% at 24 months after urethral injection of collagen in 60 women with SUI. Swami and associates[74] treated 111 patients with periurethral collagen injection for a success rate of 85% at 6 months and 65% at 3 years after injection. There was no difference in maximum urethral closure pressure before and after collagen injection and no predictive factors of success. Some physicians have reported that patients who underwent prior anti-incontinence surgery may have better results than those without previous surgery.[63,65] These findings may be explained by periurethral tissue support and limited mobility by scarring.[63,65] Others have observed no correlation between the degree of urinary incontinence preoperatively and the success rate.[70] Some investigators have obtained higher percentages of injection failure in patients with preoperative detrusor instability.[70,73] The use of collagen in cases of urethral hypermobility has produced results comparable to those without hypermobility.[16,67,69,70,72] Steele and colleagues[82] reported a higher success rate for collagen injection in patients with hypermobility than in those without hypermobility.

Long-term studies have demonstrated continuing success, with a cure rate of 25% to 45% and an improvement rate between 25% and 50%. Corcos and Fournier[78] reported the 4-year follow-up results for 40 women who underwent collagen injection. The cure rate was 30%, and the improvement rate was 40%. One third of these patients required a top-up injection 18 to 24 months after the initial treatment. Gorton and coworkers[79] published their long-term results of collagen injection in 46 women with ISD, showing an overall success rate of 35%.

The morbidity associated with collagen injection is minimal and self-limited. The most common complication is transient urinary retention, urinary tract infection, and transient hematuria. In 337 collagen injection cases, Stothers and associates[83] documented a complication rate of 20%, including de novo urinary urgency in 12.6% of patients. In many patients, the symptoms were irreversible (21% did not respond to anticholinergics) and included hematuria (5%) and urinary retention (1.9%). Delayed reaction at the skin test site occurred in 0.9% (3) of patients and was associated with arthralgia in two cases. Others identified urinary retention (8%,) urinary tract infection (4%), hematuria (2%), and urinary urgency in less than 1%.[84] Rare complications after collagen injection included sterile abscess at the injection site.[85,86] Pulmonary embolism, urethral prolapse, and osteitis pubis have been encountered after urethral collagen injection.[86-88]

Autologous Fat

Autologous fat was first used in plastic surgery to augment soft tissue defects. Periurethral fat injection was introduced in 1989 by Gonzales and colleagues[89,90] to treat ISD. Fat was harvested from lower abdominal subcutaneous tissue by liposuction using a trocar or aspiration syringe under local or general anesthesia. Between 15 and 20 mL of fat was mixed with Ringer's solution or insulin before periurethral or transurethral injection. The advantage of autologous fat is that it is readily available, biocompatible, and inexpensive. Its disadvantages are fat resorption and replacement by fibrous tissues, which necessitate repeated injections. Horl and coworkers[91] employed magnetic resonance imaging to demonstrate a 55% volume loss at 6 months after fat injection but no further volume decline at 9 and 12 months of follow-up. Approximately 50% to 90% of transferred adipose grafts do not survive.[92] Graft survival depends on minimal handling, low suction pressure during liposuction, and large-bore needles for reinjection to minimize injury.[93]

Periurethral fat injection has a reported success rate that is lower than with other injectables (Table 31-3). Palma and associates[97] obtained a success rate of 76% (64% dry and 12% improved) with repeated injections of fat, compared with 69% (31% dry and 38% improved) with a single injection. Haab and associates[76] compared the outcome of fat and collagen injection in 67 women with ISD and achieved cure rates of 13% and 24% for the fat and collagen groups, respectively. Lee and colleagues[99] published the results of a randomized, double-blind, controlled study of fat and saline injection (as a control) and reported success rates of 22% and 20.7% for the fat and saline groups, respectively. They concluded that periurethral fat injection does not appear to be more effective than placebo for treating stress incontinence.

The complications of fat injection include urinary tract infection, urinary retention, hematuria, pain, and hematomas at the site of liposuction. Complications such as urethral pseudolipoma and death due to fat embolism have also been reported.[99-101] These data should exclude fat injection for the treatment of SUI.[37]

Silicone Microimplants

Silicone microimplants (e.g., Macroplastique) are soft, flexible, solid-textured, irregularly shaped implants of heat-vulcanized polydimethylsiloxane (i.e., silicone rubber) suspended in a carrier gel (i.e., polyvinylpyrrolidone). The silicone particles are encapsulated in fibrin, and the nonsilicone carrier gel is absorbed by the reticuloendothelial system and excreted in the urine. The injected particles are organized within 6 to 8 weeks into firm nodules with infiltrated collagen and surrounded by a fibrous sheath that is well developed at 9 months.[102]

Silicone particles are inert, inducing very little local inflammatory reaction. The material is biocompatible, nonbiodegradable, nongenotoxic, noncarcinogenic, and nonteratogenic. The mean particle size ranges from 100 to 300 μm in diameter, limiting the risk of migration, which usually occurs with particles less than 70 μm.[103] Macroplastique can be injected transurethrally or periurethrally under cystoscopic vision or transurethrally with a

Table 31-2 Results of Collagen Injections

Study	No. of Patients	Type of Incontinence	Follow-up (mo)	No. of Injections	Mean Collagen Volume (mL)	Success Rate
Eckford and Abrams,[63] 1991	25	NS	3	NS	1.7	80% (64% dry, 16% improved)
Kieswetter et al,[64] 1992	16	NS	15 (10-22)	8	1	83% (44% cured, 39% improved)
Stricker and Haylen,[65] 1993	50	ISD	11 (1-21)	1.9	14.4	82%(42% cured, 40% improved)
McGuire and Appell,[16] 1994	154	137 ISD 17 HU	>12	NS	NS	HU: 64% (47% cured, 17% improved) ISD: 80% (47% cured, 34% improved)
O'Connell et al,[12] 1995	44	42 ISD 2 HU	Longest: 7 mo	1.5	9.1	63% (45% dry, 18% improved)
Richardson et al,[66] 1995	42	ISD	46 (10-66)	2	28.3	83% (40% cured, 43% improved)
Monga et al,[67] 1995	60	NS	24	3	19	68% (48% cured, 20% improved)
Winters and Appell,[68] 1995	160	ISD	24	NS	NS	78% cured or improved
Moore et al,[69] 1995	10	Type I and III	2	1.5	9.5	80% (20% cured, 60% improved)
Nataluk et al,[14] 1995	12	Type III	2	1.8	12.3	33% cured, 67% improved
Herschorn et al,[70] 1996	187	124 HU 64 ISD 6 neurogenic	22 (4-69)	2.5 (success) 2 (failure)	9.6 (success) 7.8 (failure)	75% (23% cured, 52% improved)
Homma et al,[71] 1996	78	GSI and ISD	24	1.9	23.5	72% (7% cured, 65% improved)
Faerber,[72] 1996	12	Type I	10	1.2	2.2	83% cured, 17% improved
Smith et al,[73] 1997	94	ISD	14	2.1	11.9	67% (38% dry, 29% improved)
Swami et al,[74] 1997	111	NS	38 (24-70)	1.7	12.8	65% (25% cured, 40% improved)
Stanton and Monga,[75] 1997	32	NS	12-24	1.5	17.6	Subjective success rate 69%, objective cured rate 54% at 2 yr post-operation)
Haab et al,[76] 1997	22	ISD	Minimum: 12	1.9	13.5	86% subjective success, 64% objective success
Khullar et al,[19]1997	26	NS	24	1.7	21.6	57% (48% cured, 9% improved)
Cross et al,[77] 1998	103	Type III	18	NS	NS	94% (74% cured, 20% improved)
Corcos and Fournier,[78] 1999	40	8 type I 20 type II 12 type III	50 (47-55)	2.2	9	70% (30% cured, 40% improved)
Gorton et al,[79] 1999	46	GSI	>5 yr	1-3	17	35% subjectively improved
Winters et al,[80] 2000	58	49 ISD 9 GSI (37 HU)	24.4	1.9	14.6	48.3% cured, 31.0% improved, long-term success 60.3%
Groutz et al,[81] 2000	63	NS	12 (1-32)	1-5	3.1	82% (13% cured, 69% improved)
Steele et al,[82] 2000	40	9 HU	8.4	1.9 with HU 1.4 without HU	5.6 with HU 5.3 without HU	71% with HU 32% without HU

GSI, genuine stress incontinence; HU, hypermobile urethras; ISD, intrinsic sphincter deficiency; NS, not stated.

Table 31-3 Results of Autologous Fat Injections

Study	No. of Patients	Follow-up (mo)	No. of Injections	Mean Fat Volume (mL)	Success Rate
Gonzalez de Garibay et al,[89] 1989	12	6	1	10-20	100%
Cervigni and Panei,[94] 1993	14	9.7 (3-19)	NS	21.7	86% (57% cured, 29% improved)
Scotti et al,[95] 1993	10	0.5	1	14-20	60%
Santarosa and Blaivas,[96] 1994	15	12 (1-40)	2.7	5-15	58% cured
Trockman and Leach,[92] 1995	32	6	1.6	21.3	56% (12% cured, 44% improved)
Palma et al,[97] 1997	30	12	12	40	Single injection: 69% Multiple injections: 76%
Haab et al,[76] 1997	45	>7	1.7	20	42% (13% cured, 29% improved)
Su et al,[98] 1998	26	17.4 (12-30)	1	15	65% (50% cured, 15% improved)
Lee et al,[99] 2001	35	3	1-3	30	22% overall success

NS, not stated.

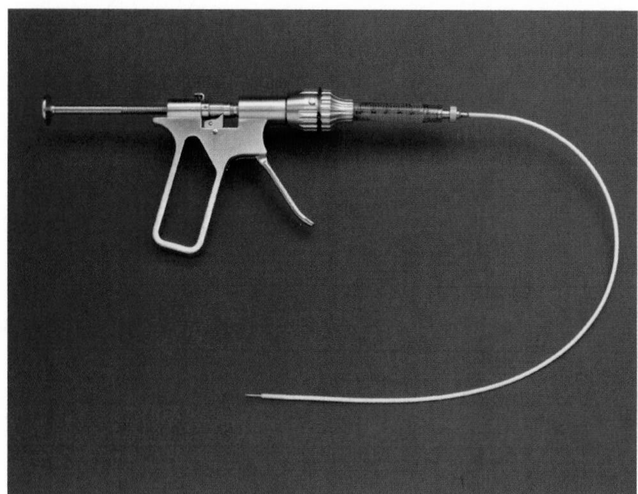

Figure 13-6 Ratchet gun and flexible needle for Macroplastique injection.

special injection system (see Fig. 31-5). The material is viscid, and the needle must be prelubricated with 1 to 2 mL of carrier gel before the vial (2.5 mL) of silicone paste is discharged by means of a high-pressure ratchet gun (Fig. 31-6).

Silicone elastomers have been used since the early 1990s as bulking agents for treating SUI, but they are still not approved for application in the United States. The reported cure rate with silicone ISD varies between 14% and 66.7%. Improvement rates range from 46% to 80%. When ISD is associated with urethral hypermobility, the cure and improvement rates are between 0% and 21.4% and between 0% and 58.9%, respectively.[104]

Sheriff and colleagues[105] reported a success rate of 90% at 1 month after injection, with a time-dependent decrease to 48% at 2 years postoperatively. Other long-term results usually show a lower cure rate and are summarized in Table 31-4.

Reported complications after silicone injection are minimal and self-limited, such as hematuria, dysuria, urinary tract infection (0.9%), and urinary retention (6.8%).[108] There is still concern about small particle migration and granuloma formation, with possible risks of autoimmune reactions associated with silicone injection.[103]

Dextranomer/Hyaluronic Acid Copolymer

Dextranomers are well-known polysaccharides that have been used for topical wound cleaning. HA has been applied in eye surgery and for joint injection.[116] Dx/HA is a copolymer (Zuidex) in a gel of nonanimal, stabilized HA. A high-molecular-weight polysaccharide, HA works as a carrier gel and is resorbed within 2 weeks after injection. Zuidex is a highly viscous solution, nonimmunogenic and biocompatible, with no risk of allergy or granuloma formation. Dx microspheres, the bulking agent, are 80 to 200 μm in diameter and do not fragment, eliminating the risk of distance migration.[117] Dx/HA is biodegraded very slowly by hydrolysis, and it remains at the injected site for up to 4 years. Stenberg and coworkers[118] established that the volume of subcutaneously injected Dx/HA implants decreased by 23% over 12 months in rats. Because the implant consists of 50% microspheres and 50% HA, volume reduction soon after injection should be expected. However, endogenous tissue augmentation is caused by ingrowths of collagen and fibroblasts between the microspheres. Dx/HA has been shown to be well tolerated for endoscopic injection in vesicoureteric reflux (VUR) in children, with efficacy persisting for at least 5 years.[119] It has been approved by the FDA in the United States for VUR and approved in Europe and Canada for the treatment of VUR and SUI.[120]

Initial studies of Dx/HA injection in patients with stress incontinence are promising. Stenberg and associates[121] attained an initial success rate of 85% (cured or improved) for 20 patients with stress incontinence. Long-term follow-up (up to 6.7 years) of their cohort revealed that 57% were still cured or improved without any adverse effects (Table 31-5).[122] Van Kerrebroek and colleagues[123] reported a success rate of 71% among 42 women 1 year after Dx/HA injection. The few adverse effects encountered included a sterile abscess ($n = 1$), urinary tract infection ($n = 5$), hematuria ($n = 4$), urethral disorder ($n = 3$), and decreased urinary flow ($n = 3$). A case of granuloma after Dx/HA injection has been documented.[126] Injection therapy does appear to preclude future surgical interventions, because it does not cause any major tissue changes.[127]

Carbon-Coated Zirconium Beads

Durasphere is a mixture of nonabsorbable, carbon-coated zirconium beads in a water-based carrier gel with β-glucan (i.e., 97%

Table 31-4 Results of Silicone Microimplant Injections

Study	No. of Patients	Follow-up (mo)	No. of Injections	Injected Volume (mL)	Success Rates
Harriss et al,[106] 1996	40	<36	1.2	1-7	73% (33% improved, 40% cured)
Sheriff et al,[105] 1997	34	24	1.1	5	90% at 1 mo, 75% at 3 mo, and 48% at 2 yr
Koelbl et al,[107] 1998	32	12	1.1	3.9	59% cure
Henalla et al,[32] 2000	40	3	1.35	6.8	20% dry, 32.5% improved 41% dry, 33.3% improved with repeated injections
Usman and Henalla,[108] 1998	102	17.6	1	5	71% if they had previous surgery, 66% for primary treatment
Hidar et al,[109] 2000	25	36	1.4	3.7	80% at 6 mo, 60% at 3 yr
Barranger et al,[110] 2000	21	31	1	4	19% dry 29% improved
Radley et al,[111] 2001	60	16-19	1.5	6.7	62.5% cured/improved, 39% objectively cured
Soliman and Evans,[112] 2001	68	19	1	3	35.2% cured, 26.5% improved
Peeker et al,[113] 2002	22	Range: 6-48	1.3	NS	59.1% cured, 18.2% improved
Gurdal et al,[114] 2002	29	29	1	3.5	45% cured
Tamanini et al,[33] 2003	21	12	NS	6.3	76.1% (57.1% cured, 19% improved), 45% objective cure
Tamanini et al,[115] 2004	21	24	NS	6.3	61.9% (47.6% cured, 14.3% improved)

NS, not stated.

Table 31-5 Reported Results of Dextranomer/Hyaluronic Acid Injections

Study	No. of Patients	Follow-up (mo)	No. of Injections	Volume of Injections (mL)	Results
Stenberg et al,[121] 1999	20	3-6	2-4	5.5	85% cure or improvement
Stenberg et al,[122] 2003	20	78	1.6	6.4	57% success, with recurrence in 25%
van Kerrebroeck et al,[120] 2004	42	12	NS	2.8-4	71% subjective improvement at 3 mo, 61% at 12 mo
van Kerrebroek et al,[123] 2004	42	12	NS	2.8-4	75% objective success (24% cured, 51% improved)
Haab et al,[124] 2004	139	6	2.1	NS	67% success rate at 6 mo
van Kerrebroek et al,[125] 2004	20	24		2.8-4	70-90% initial success rate, and 60% at 2 yr

water and 3% glucan). It is safe and has been exploited for many years in heart valve replacements.[37] There is no risk of allergy or distant particle migration because particle size ranges between 250 and 300 μm in diameter. Durasphere is the latest bulking agent approved by the FDA (Table 31-6).

Lightner and coworkers[128] undertook a multicenter, randomized, double-blind study comparing Durasphere ($n = 178$) and collagen ($n = 177$) for the treatment of ISD. At 1 year of follow-up, the success rates were 80.3% and 67.1% for Durasphere and collagen, respectively. The mean number of injections was similar (Durasphere = 1.55, collagen = 1.69), but the injected volume was significantly different (Durasphere = 4.83 mL, collagen = 6.23 mL; $P < .001$). Pannek and associates[129] treated 13 women and 7 men with Durasphere injection and achieved limited success (33% at 1 year after injection). There was distant particle migration in two patients despite the large-size of the Durasphere particles. Chrouser and colleagues[131] studied Durasphere and collagen for the treatment of 43 women with SUI. The initial success rate (63%) was similar in both groups. Longer follow-up (12, 24, and 36 months) showed that Durasphere remained effective in 35%, 33%, and 21% of patients, whereas the collagen efficacy rates were only 33%, 19%, and 9%, respectively. For Chrouser and coworkers[131] the lack of durability of both agents was thought to result from physiologic changes of the bladder neck and urethra with time, altered tissue compliance in response to injection, or poor long-term performance of the agent.

The complication rate with Durasphere is higher than with collagen. Urinary urgency is seen in 24% and 16.9% of patients, respectively. However, resolution of urgency symptoms is greater in the Durasphere group than in the collagen group. Urinary retention is also greater with Durasphere (11.9% versus 3.4%),[128] but it rarely persists to a point at which endoscopic evacuation of Durasphere at the injection site is necessary.[132]

Table 31-6 Reported Results of Durasphere Injection

Study	No. of Patients	Follow-up (mo)	No. of Injections	Volume of Injections (mL)	Results
Lightner et al,[128] 2001	178	11	1.6	4.8	80.3% overall success
Pannek et al,[129] 2001	20	10	NS NS	6	76.9% at 6 mo, 33% at 1 yr
Madjar et al,[130] 2003	46	9.4	1.5	2-3	65.2% (13% cured, 34.7 improved)
Chrouser et al,[131] 2004	56	37	1.6	NS	63% initial success, 33% at 1 yr, 21% at 3 yr

ISD, intrinsic sphincter deficiency; NS, not stated.

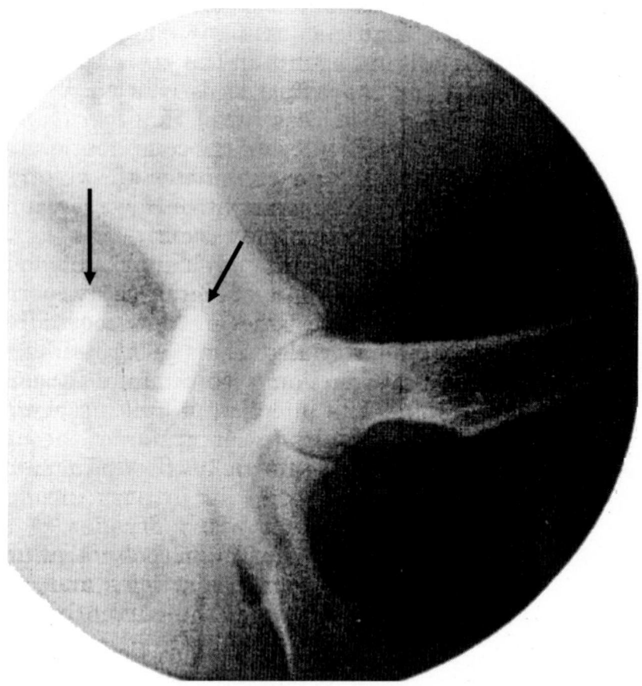

Figure 31-7 Implanted microballoons *(arrows)*.

Microballoon Implantation

Implantable microballoons (UroVIV) are elastomeric silicone capsules with an inflatable volume ranging from 0.2 to 0.9 mL, and they are filled with a poly-*N*-vinyl pyrrolidinone–based, high-water-content, cross-linked hydrogel (Fig. 31-7). In an aqueous environment, the hydrogel remains a gel due to interaction with the hydrophobic domains. The capsule device primarily consists of a membrane and check valve to prevent escape of the solution injected at the time of implantation.[133] A self-detachable, implantable balloon system developed by Atala and coworkers[134] was initially used for the treatment of VUR in children. It was found to be safe, injectable material that was biocompatible and without the risk of migration or local inflammation. It was detectable on plain radiography and ultrasound.

The balloon is injected periurethrally under cystoscopic control. The inflated balloon is approximately 8.5 × 21 mm, and it is usually placed at the 3- and 9-o'clock positions; if necessary, another balloon can be implanted at the 6-o'clock position.[135] Compared with previously described bulking agents, we consider this technique to be complicated, requiring significant training. The injection system is somewhat cumbersome; newer systems with adjustable balloons are being developed.[37]

Pycha and associates[135] treated 19 female SUI patients (6 type I, 4 type II, 9 type III) with microballoon implants (mean, 4.2 balloons), with a 42% cure rate and 36.8% improvement after a mean follow-up of 14.4 months. The procedure failed in all patients with type II SUI, and four patients incurred significant detrusor overactivity. The investigators stated that type III SUI is the ideal indication for microballoon implantation. Mazouni and colleagues[135] recorded an overall success rate of 65% for 59 women 6 months after microballoon injection. Two patients developed urinary retention, balloon migration through the urethral wall occurred in three cases, and three others experienced balloon loss.

Calcium Hydroxylapatite

Calcium hydroxylapatite (CaHA) is a normal constituent of bone and is therefore nonimmunogenic and nontoxic. The bulking substance is a synthetic particle of CaHA with a spherical mean diameter of 100 μm (75 to 125 μm) in an aqueous gel composed of sodium carboxymethylcellulose. Preclinical studies in animal models have confirmed long-term safety and biocompatibility, with minimal inflammation.[137] This material has had previous medical applications in dental restoration and orthopedics.[138] It is radiopaque and can be easily detected by ultrasound, which can aid in its implantation and localization.

The injections are delivered by a 3-ml syringe through a 7-Fr Cook transurethral injection catheter and a 21-gauge needle attached to a ratchet gun. The initial injections are targeted at the 4- and 8-o'clock positions at the bladder neck, and then delivered as needed to provide visual coaptation. Mayer and coworkers[138] described 10 women with ISD who were treated by CaHA injection; the mean volume was 3.9 mL. The average number of injection sites at each treatment was 3.82 (range, 2 to 6 sites). Subjective improvement in pad use 1 year after injection was rated as excellent (no pads) in three patients, good (many fewer pads) in four patients, fair (fewer pads) in two patients, and poor (no change) in one patient. VLPP increased from 39 to 46 cm H_2O at 12 months, with two patients dry on testing. There were no complications except for a higher incidence of transient urinary retention in five patients.

Ethylene Vinyl Alcohol Copolymer

Ethylene vinyl alcohol copolymer (Uryx) is a biocompatible polymer composed of a random mixture of ethylene (hydrophobic) and vinyl alcohol (hydrophilic). It is dissolved in an 8% concentration of anhydrous dimethyl sulfoxide (DMSO). When this mixture comes into contact with aqueous media, DMSO rapidly diffuses away, causing in situ precipitation and solidification of the polymer, with the formation of a spongelike plug that can seal cavities.[139] It has been employed successfully for the embolization of tumors and vascular malformations by selective arterial occlusion in a rabbit model and for brain arteriovenous malformations in clinical cases.[140]

Dmochowski and associates[141] reported the first use of Uryx in women with SUI in a multicenter, randomized, controlled study that compared it with collagen. Two hundred thirty-six women with genuine SUI were randomized and then treated prospectively with Uryx or collagen. The mean total volume injected was 4.6 mL for Uryx and 7.1 mL for collagen. At 1 year, pad tests showed that 68% of Uryx patients were dry, compared with 44% of collagen patients. Significant improvement of incontinence quality-of-life scores at 1 year was achieved in 32% with Uryx and in 20% with collagen. The most common complications of both treatment arms were delayed voiding, dysuria, and frequency. The investigators concluded that the success rate with Uryx was higher compared with collagen and with less injected volume.

Dermal Collagen Implants

Cross-linked collagen fibers can be extracted from intact cadaveric dermal skin specimens. The harvested dermis is separated from the epidermis, pulverized mechanically, and dispersed in solution. The intact fibers are suspended in a buffered phosphate solution at neutral pH.[37,142]

The bulking agent of autologous collagen is recognized as self by the body and therefore should not elicit an immune response. The injected collagen it thought to undergo a breakdown process similar to that occurring in normal scar formation. Natural cross-linking increases implant durability and resists biodegradation by collagenase.[143] Griffiths and Shakespeare[144] undertook a 3-year study of the histologic appearance of glutaraldehyde-treated human fibrous dermal collagen allografts. There was no immune or inflammatory response, and no fibrous capsule was seen. The implants were colonized by host fibroblasts and blood vessels, and collagen resorption was observed.[144]

Permacol is a sterile, tough but flexible, acellular, cross-linked porcine dermal collagen with constituent elastin fibers. It has an acellular architectural organization very close to human tissue and works by supporting fibroblast infiltration and revascularization, so that it gradually becomes permanently incorporated. The disadvantage of this material includes its limited availability and higher viscosity, requiring a large-bore needle. Dermal collagen has been successfully deployed in many ear, nose, and throat procedures, in plastic surgery, in ophthalmology, and in orthopedic and cardiothoracic surgery.[145]

Bano and colleagues[146] studied Macroplastique and porcine dermal collagen (Permacol) in the treatment of 50 women with SUI. At 6 weeks, 64% of Permacol patients were improved (60% were dry) on quantified pad losses compared with 54% of Macroplastique patients (41.6% were dry). These results persisted up to 6 months.

Autologous Chondrocytes

Tissue engineering is an attractive and promising field for treatment approaches to a variety of challenging urologic conditions. Atala and associates[147] are innovators in the application of tissue engineering in urology. In 1994, they reported VUR in a porcine model. Injected chondrocytes can survive in vivo and synthesize new cartilaginous structures according to a template after they are seeded onto preformed biodegradable polymers.[148] The material consists of autologous chondrocytes in a calcium alginate (i.e., natural polysaccharide) gel injected endoscopically through a 22-gauge needle. Chondrocytes isolated from biopsy specimens (approximately 6 × 6 mm) of the external pinna of the patient's ear are expanded in tissue culture media in vitro for 6 weeks and combined with sodium alginate before transfer into five 3-mL syringes for injection.[149] The gel serves as a substrate for injectable delivery and then undergoes hydrolytic biodegradation over time. The newly formed chondrocytes secrete a natural matrix that maintains the volume of the original injection over time and results in new cartilage formation, which is stable, nonantigenic, and nonmigrating.[148]

Autologous chondrocytes have been injected with success and low risk for the treatment of VUR in children.[150] Bent and associates[149] reported 32 patients treated with autologous ear chondrocytes for ISD; 16 patients (50%) were cured, and 10 (31.3%) improved at 12 months. The investigators concluded that endoscopic treatment of ISD with autologous chondrocytes is safe, effective, and durable.

Autologous Myoblasts

Cultured myoblasts can be delivered to the bladder wall (i.e., cellular myoplasty) and urethral sphincter to regenerate, forming new myofibers that build up and improve the urinary sphincter and detrusor contractility.[151] Myoblasts, the mononucleate precursor cells of skeletal muscle, can differentiate to form multinucleated muscle fibers capable of muscle contraction. They fuse to form postmitotic myotubes, which express bioactive protein in a stable fashion for a prolonged period, representing a potentially advantageous method of gene therapy.[152] Age-dependent reduction in the number of striated muscle cells may cause SUI in elderly women and men.[153] Myoblast injection directly into the urethral sphincter to reconstruct the muscle and augment the sphincter may become a possible option in the treatment of ISD. Injectable myoblasts may produce strengthened sphincter contractility by fusing with existing muscle fibers.

Strasser and colleagues[154] performed the first clinical trial of myoblast injection in seven women with SUI. Before injection, skeletal muscle biopsies were taken from the left arm to obtain cultures of autologous myoblasts and fibroblasts. One year after the injection, five of these women remained symptom free. Three-dimensional ultrasound revealed that the thickness of the urethra and rhabdosphincter had increased significantly compared with baseline. Autologous therapy is an exciting field with promising preliminary results for the treatment of SUI.

CONCLUSIONS

Injection therapy for the management of SUI and urethral hypermobility is an attractive alternative to surgery. It is a minimally invasive and easy procedure that can be performed on an outpatient basis. If injectables are well accepted for the frail elderly after the failure of other procedures, and when surgery is contraindicated, their role as the primary treatment of SUI is debatable. Cost-effectiveness must be addressed before promoting a new treatment for SUI, but cost-effectiveness studies are rare or employ questionable methodologies.

Many injectable materials have been shown to be effective with few complications. However, the ideal bulking agent is still to be discovered. It must be biocompatible, biodegradable, nonmigratory, nonallergenic, durable, easy to inject, and cost-effective. All available injectables have a potential for migration, shrinking, or being displaced, requiring multiple injections to achieve or maintain a good result.

Collagen has been the most extensively studied injectable, and it is still the most commonly used. It is reabsorbed with time and warrants preoperative skin testing to check for hypersensitivity. Autologous fat is also reabsorbed, but it has the potential for lethal complications. Durasphere, Zuidex, CaHa, microballoons, and ethylene vinyl alcohol copolymer injections have had initial success in the treatment of SUI, but further long-term and comparative studies of other modalities are required for ensuring safety, efficacy, and cost-effectiveness. Tissue engineering and autologous therapy are promising fields but are in their early developmental phases.

References

1. Oremus M, Collet JP, Shapiro SH, Penrod J, et al: Surgery versus collagen for female stress urinary incontinence: Economic assessment in Ontario and Quebec. Can J Urol 10:1934-1944, 2003.
2. Corcos J, Collet JP, Shapiro S, et al: Surgery vs. collagen for the treatment of female stress urinary incontinence (SUI): Results of a multicentric randomized trial. Abstract presented at the 96th Annual American Urological Association Meeting, June 2-6, 2001.
3. Murless B: The injection treatment of stress urinary incontinence. J Obstet Gynaecol Br Emp 45:67-68, 1938.
4. Quackels R: Deux incontinences après adénonectomie géuries par injection de paraffine dans le périnée. Acta Urol Belg 23:259-262, 1955.
5. Saches H: Die Behandlung der Harninkontinenz mit der Sklerotherapie: Indikationssellung-Ergebnisse-Komplikationen. Urol Int 15:225-244, 1963.
6. Berg S: Polytef augmentation urethroplasty. Correction of surgically incurable urinary incontinence by injection technique. Arch Surg 107:379-381, 1973.
7. Politano VA, Small MP, Harper JM, et al: Periurethral Teflon injection for urinary incontinence. J Urol 111:180-183, 1974.
8. Appell RA: Injection therapy for urinary incontinence. In Walsh J, Retik AB, Vaughan ED Jr, Wein AJ (eds): Campbell's Urology, vol 2, 8th ed. Philadelphia, WB Saunders, 2002, pp 1172-1186.
9. Pineda EB, Hadley HR: Urethral injection treatment for stress urinary incontinence. In Corcos J, Schick E (eds): The Urinary Sphincter. New York, Marcel Dekker, 2001, pp 497-515.
10. Appell RA: Collagen injection therapy for urinary incontinence. Urol Clin North Am 21:177-182, 1994.
11. Appell RA: New developments: Injectables for urethral incompetence in women. Int Urogynecol J 1:117-119, 1990.
12. O'Connell HE, McGuire EJ, Aboseif S, et al: Transurethral collagen therapy in women. J Urol 154:1463-1465, 1995.
13. Bennett JK, Green BG, Foote JE, et al: Collagen injections for intrinsic sphincter deficiency in the neuropathic urethra. Paraplegia 33:697-700, 1995.
14. Nataluk EA, Assimos DG, Kroovand RL: Collagen injections for treatment of urinary incontinence secondary to intrinsic sphincter deficiency. J Endourol 9:403-406, 1995.
15. Wan J, McGuire EJ, Bloom DA, et al: The treatment of urinary incontinence in children using glutaraldehyde cross-linked collagen. J Urol 148:127-130, 1992.
16. McGuire EJ, Appell RA: Transurethral collagen injection for urinary incontinence. Urology 43:413-415, 1994.
17. Bomalaski MD, Bloom DA, McGuire EJ, et al: Glutaraldehyde cross-linked collagen in the treatment of urinary incontinence in children. J Urol 155:699-702, 1996.
18. Monga AK, Stanton SL: Urodynamics: Prediction, outcome and analysis of mechanism for cure of stress incontinence by periurethral collagen. Br J Obstet Gynaecol 104:158-162, 1997.
19. Khullar V, Cardozo LD, Abbott D, et al: GAX collagen in the treatment of urinary incontinence in elderly women: A two year follow up. Br J Obstet Gynaecol 104:96-99, 1997.
20. Benshushan A, Brzezinski A, Shoshani O, et al: Periurethral injection for the treatment of urinary incontinence. Obstet Gynecol Surv 53:383-388, 1998.
21. Gajewski J: Leak point pressure. In Corcos J, Schick E (eds): The Urinary Sphincter. New York, Marcel Dekker, 2001, pp 303-310.
22. McGuire EJ, Fitzpatrick CC, Wan J, et al: Clinical assessment of urethral sphincter function. J Urol 150:1452-1454, 1993.
23. Swift SE, Ostergard DR: A comparison of stress leak-point pressure and maximal urethral closure pressure in patients with genuine stress incontinence. Obstet Gynecol 85:704-708, 1995.
24. Itano NB, Sweat SD, Lightner DJ: The use of bulking agents for stress incontinence. Lesson 5. AUA Update 21:34-39, 2001.
25. McGuire EJ, English SF: Periurethral collagen injection for male and female sphincteric incontinence: Indications, techniques, and result. World J Urol 15:306-309, 1997.
26. Perez LM, Smith EA, Parrott TS, et al: Submucosal bladder neck injection of bovine dermal collagen for stress urinary incontinence in the pediatric population. J Urol 156:633-636, 1996.
27. Defreitas G, Zimmern P: Surgery to improve bladder outlet function. In Corcos J, Schick E (eds): Textbook of Neurogenic Bladder: Adults and Children. London, Martin Dunitz, 2004, pp 565-598.
28. Stenzl A, Strasser H: Submucosal bladder neck injections for management of stress urinary incontinence. Braz J Urol 26:199-207, 2000.
29. Stöhrer M: Surgery to improve reservoir function. In Corcos J, Schick E (eds): Textbook of Neurogenic Bladder: Adults and Children. London, Martin Dunitz, 2004, pp 557-564.
30. Faerber GJ, Belville WD, Ohl DA, et al: Comparison of transurethral versus periurethral collagen injection in women with intrinsic sphincter deficiency. Tech Urol 4:124-127, 1998.
31. Schulz JA, Nager CW, Stanton SL, et al: Bulking agents for stress urinary incontinence: Short-term results and complications in a randomized comparison of periurethral and transurethral injections. Int Urogynecol J Pelvic Floor Dysfunct 15:261-265, 2004.
32. Henalla SM, Hall V, Duckett JR, et al: A multicentre evaluation of a new surgical technique for urethral bulking in the treatment of genuine stress incontinence. Br J Obstet Gynaecol 107:1035-1039. 2000.
33. Tamanini JT, D'Ancona CA, Tadini V, et al: Macroplastique implantation system for the treatment of female stress urinary incontinence. J Urol 169:2229-2233, 2003.
34. van Kerrebroeck P, ter Meulen F, Farrelly E, et al: Treatment of stress urinary incontinence: Recent developments in the role of urethral injection. Urol Res 30:356-362, 2003.
35. Blaivas JG: Outcome measures for urinary incontinence. Urology 51:11-19, 1998.
36. Su TH, Hsu CY, Chen JC: Injection therapy for stress incontinence in women. Int Urogynecol J Pelvic Floor Dysfunct 10:200-206, 1999.
37. Dmochowski RR, Appell RA: Injectable agents in the treatment of stress urinary incontinence in women: Where are we now? Urology 56:32-40, 2000.
38. Claes H, Stroobants D, Van Meerbeek J, et al: Pulmonary migration following periurethral polytetrafluoroethylene injection for urinary incontinence. J Urol 142:821-822, 1989.

39. Dewan PA, Fraundorfer M: Skin migration following periurethral polytetrafluoroethylene injection for urinary incontinence. Aust N Z J Surg 66:57-59, 1996.
40. Malizia AA Jr, Reiman HM, Myers RP, et al: Migration and granulomatous reaction after periurethral injection of polytef (Teflon). JAMA 251:3277-3281, 1984.
41. Kiilholma PJ, Chancellor MB, Makinen J, et al: Complications of Teflon injection for stress urinary incontinence. Neurourol Urodyn 12:131-137, 1993.
42. Dewan PA, Owen AJ, Byard RW: Long-term histological response to subcutaneously injected Polytef and Bioplastique in a rat model. Br J Urol 76:161-164, 1995.
43. Politano VA: Periurethral polytetrafluoroethylene injection for urinary incontinence. J Urol 127:439-442, 1982.
44. Lockhart JL, Walker RD, Vorstman B, et al: Periurethral polytetrafluoroethylene injection following urethral reconstruction in female patients with urinary incontinence. J Urol 140:51-52, 1988.
45. Beckingham IJ, Wemyss-Holden G, Lawrence WT: Long-term follow-up of women treated with perurethral Teflon injections for stress incontinence. Br J Urol 69:580-583, 1992.
46. Harrison SC, Brown C, O'Boyle PJ: Periurethral Teflon for stress urinary incontinence: Medium-term results. Br J Urol 71:25-27, 1993.
47. Herschorn S, Glazer AA: Early experience with small volume periurethral polytetrafluoroethylene for female stress urinary incontinence. J Urol 163:1838-1842, 2000.
48. Lim KB, Ball AJ, Feneley RC: Periurethral Teflon injection: A simple treatment for urinary incontinence. Br J Urol 55:208-210, 1983.
49. Schulman CC, Simon J, Wespes E, et al: Endoscopic injection of Teflon for female urinary incontinence. Eur Urol 9:246-247, 1983.
50. Deane AM, English P, Hehir M, et al: Teflon injection in stress incontinence. Br J Urol 57:78-80, 1985.
51. Osther PJ, Rohl H: Female urinary stress incontinence treated with Teflon injections. Acta Obstet Gynecol Scand 66:333-335, 1987.
52. Vesey SG, Rivett A, O'Boyle PJ: Teflon injection in female stress incontinence. Effect on urethral pressure profile and flow rate. Br J Urol 62:39-41, 1988.
53. Kiilholma P, Makinen J: Disappointing effect of endoscopic Teflon injection for female stress incontinence. Eur Urol 20:197-199, 1991.
54. Lopez AE, Padron OF, Patsias G, et al: Transurethral polytetrafluoroethylene injection in female patients with urinary continence. J Urol 150:856-858, 1993.
55. Shortliffe LM, Freiha FS, Kessler R, et al: Treatment of urinary incontinence by the periurethral implantation of glutaraldehyde cross-linked collagen. J Urol 141:538-541, 1989.
56. Kershen RT, Atala A: New advances in injectable therapies for the treatment of incontinence and vesicoureteral reflux. Urol Clin North Am 26:81-94, 1999.
57. Rivas DA, Chancellor MB, Liu J-B, et al: Endoluminal ultrasonographic and histologic evaluation of periurethral collagen injection. J Endourol 10:61-66, 1996.
58. Carr LK, Herschorn S, Leonhardt C: Magnetic resonance imaging after intraurethral collagen injected for stress urinary incontinence. J Urol 155:1253-1255, 1996.
59. Stegman SJ, Chu S, Bensch K, et al: A light and electron microscopic evaluation of Zyderm collagen and Zyplast implants in aging human facial skin. A pilot study. Arch Dermatol 123:1644-1649, 1987.
60. Berman CJ, Kreder KJ: Comparative cost analysis of collagen injection and fascia lata sling cystourethropexy for the treatment of type III incontinence in women. J Urol 157:122-124, 1997.
61. Stothers L, Goldenberg SL: Delayed hypersensitivity and systemic arthralgia following transurethral collagen injection for stress urinary incontinence. J Urol 159:1507-1509, 1998.
62. Herschorn S, Radomski SB, Steele DJ: Early experience with intraurethral collagen injections for urinary incontinence. J Urol 148:1797-800, 1992.
63. Eckford SD, Abrams P: Para-urethral collagen implantation for female stress incontinence. Br J Urol 68:586-589, 1991.
64. Kieswetter H, Fischer M, Wöber L, et al: Endoscopic implantation of collagen (GAX) for treatment of urinary incontinence. Br J Urol 69:22-25, 1992.
65. Stricker P, Haylen B: Injectable collagen for type 3 female stress incontinence: The first 50 Australian patients. Med J Aust 158:89-91, 1993.
66. Richardson TD, Kennelly MJ, Faerber GJ: Endoscopic injection of glutaraldehyde cross-linked collagen for the treatment of intrinsic sphincter deficiency in women. Urology 46:378-781, 1995.
67. Monga AK, Robinson D, Stanton SL: Periurethral collagen injections for genuine stress incontinence: A 2-year follow-up. Br J Urol 76:156-160, 1995.
68. Winters JC, Appell R: Periurethral injection of collagen in the treatment of intrinsic sphincteric deficiency in the female patient. Urol Clin North Am 22:673-678, 1995.
69. Moore KN, Chetner MP, Metcalfe JB, et al: Periurethral implantation of glutaraldehyde cross-linked collagen (Contigen) in women with type I or III stress incontinence: Quantitative outcome measures. Br J Urol 75:359-363, 1995.
70. Herschorn S, Steele DJ, Radomski SB: Follow-up of intraurethral collagen for female stress urinary incontinence. J Urol 156:1305-1309, 1996.
71. Homma Y, Kawabe K, Kageyama S, et al: Injection of glutaraldehyde cross-linked collagen for urinary incontinence: Two-year efficacy by self-assessment. Int J Urol 3:124-127, 1996.
72. Faerber GJ: Endoscopic collagen injection therapy in elderly women with type I stress urinary incontinence. J Urol 155:512-514, 1996.
73. Smith DN, Appell RA, Winters JC, et al: Collagen injection therapy for female intrinsic sphincteric deficiency. J Urol 157:1275-1278, 1997.
74. Swami S, Batista JE, Abrams P: Collagen for female genuine stress incontinence after a minimum 2-year follow-up. Br J Urol 80:757-761, 1997.
75. Stanton SL, Monga AK: Incontinence in elderly women: Is periurethral collagen an advance? Br J Obstet Gynaecol 104:154-157, 1997.
76. Haab F, Zimmern PE, Leach GE: Urinary stress incontinence due to intrinsic sphincteric deficiency: Experience with fat and collagen periurethral injections. J Urol 157:1283-1286, 1997.
77. Cross CA, English SF, Cespedes RD: A follow-up on transurethral collagen injection therapy for urinary incontinence. J Urol 159:106-108, 1998.
78. Corcos J, Fournier C: Periurethral collagen injection for the treatment of female stress urinary incontinence: 4-year follow-up results. Urology 4:815-818, 1999.
79. Gorton E, Stanton S, Monga A, et al: Periurethral collagen injection: A long-term follow-up study. BJU Int 4:966-971, 1999.
80. Winters JC, Chiverton A, Scarpero HM, et al: Collagen injection therapy in elderly women: Long-term results and patient satisfaction. Urology 55:856-861, 2000.
81. Groutz A, Blaivas JG, Kesler SS, et al: Outcome results of transurethral collagen injection for female stress incontinence: Assessment by urinary incontinence score. J Urol 164:2006-2009, 2000.
82. Steele AC, Kohli N, Karram MM: Periurethral collagen injection for stress incontinence with and without urethral hypermobility. Obstet Gynecol 95:327-331, 2000.
83. Stothers L, Goldenberg SL, Leone EF: Complications of periurethral collagen injection for stress urinary incontinence. J Urol 159:806-807, 1998.
84. Contigen Bard Collagen Implant Product Monograph. Covington, GA, Bard Urological Division, CR Bard, 1999.

85. McLennan MT, Bent AE: Suburethral abscess: A complication of periurethral collagen injection therapy. Obstet Gynecol 92:650-652, 1998.
86. Sweat SD, Lightner DJ: Complications of sterile abscess formation and pulmonary embolism following periurethral bulking agents. J Urol 161:93-96, 1999.
87. Harris RL, Cundiff GW, Coates KW, et al: Urethral prolapse after collagen injection. Am J Obstet Gynecol 178:614-615, 1998.
88. Matthews K, Govier FE: Osteitis pubis after periurethral collagen injection. Urology 49:237-238, 1997.
89. Gonzalex de Garibay S, Morrondo CJ, Jimeno CJM: Endoscopic injection of autologous adipose tissue in treatment of female incontinence. Arch Esp Urol 42:143-146, 1989.
90. Gonzalez Garibay S, Jimeno C, York M, Gomez P, et al: Endoscopic autotransplantation of fat tissue in the treatment of urinary incontinence in the female. J Urol (Paris) 95:363-366, 1989.
91. Horl HW, Feller AM, Biemer E: Technique for liposuction fat reimplantation and long-term volume evaluation by magnetic resonance imaging. Ann Plast Surg 26:248-258, 1991.
92. Trockman BA, Leach GE: Surgical treatment of intrinsic urethral dysfunction: Injectables (fat). Urol Clin North Am 22:665-671, 1995.
93. Herschorn S: Current status of injectable agents for female stress urinary incontinence. Can J Urol 8:1281-1289, 2001.
94. Cervigni M, Panei M: Periurethral autologous fat injection for type III stress urinary incontinence [abstract]. J Urol 149(Pt. 2):403A, 1993.
95. Scotti RP, Zahreddine N, Mendelovici R: Autologous periurethral fat injection for urinary incontinence Int Urogynecol J 4:326-329, 1993.
96. Santarosa RP, Blaivas JG: Periurethral injection of autologous fat for the treatment of sphincteric incontinence. J Urol 151:607-611, 1994.
97. Palma PC, Riccetto CL, Herrmann V, et al: Repeated lipoinjections for stress urinary incontinence. J Endourol 11:67-70, 1997.
98. Su TH, Wang KG, Hsu CY, et al: Periurethral fat injection in the treatment of recurrent genuine stress incontinence. J Urol 159:411-414, 1998.
99. Lee PE, Kung RC, Drutz HP: Periurethral autologous fat injection as treatment for female stress urinary incontinence: A randomized double-blind controlled trial. J Urol 165:153-158, 2001.
100. Palma PC, Riccetto CL, Netto Junior NR: Urethral pseudolipoma: A complication of periurethral lipo-injection for stress urinary incontinence in a woman. J Urol 155:646, 1996.
101. Currie I, Drutz HP, Deck J, et al: Adipose tissue and lipid droplet embolism following periurethral injection of autologous fat: Case report and review of the literature. Int Urogynecol J Pelvic Floor Dysfunct 8:377-380, 1997.
102. Radley SC, Chapple CR, Lee JA: Transurethral implantation of silicone polymer for stress incontinence: Evaluation of a porcine model and mechanism of action in vivo. BJU Int 85:646-650, 2000.
103. Henly DR, Barrett DM, Weiland TL, et al: Particulate silicone for use in periurethral injections: Local tissue effects and search for migration. J Urol 153:2039-2043, 1995.
104. Ter Meulen PH, Berghmans LC, van Kerrebroeck PE: Systematic review: Efficacy of silicone microimplants (Macroplastique) therapy for stress urinary incontinence in adult women. Eur Urol 44:573-582, 2003.
105. Sheriff MK, Foley S, Mcfarlane J, et al: Endoscopic correction of intractable stress incontinence with silicone micro-implants. Eur Urol 32:284-288, 1997.
106. Harriss DR, Iacovou JW, Lemberger RJ: Peri-urethral silicone microimplants (Macroplastique) for the treatment of genuine stress incontinence. Br J Urol 78:722-725, 1996.
107. Koelbl H, Saz V, Doerfler D, et al: Transurethral injection of silicone microimplants for intrinsic urethral sphincter deficiency. Obstet Gynecol 92:332-336, 1998.
108. Usman F, Henalla S: A single transurethral Macroplastique injection as primary treatment for stress incontinence in women. J Obstet Gynaecol 18:56-60, 1998.
109. Hidar S, Attyaoui F, de Leval J: Periurethral injection of silicone microparticles in the treatment of sphincter deficiency urinary incontinence. Prog Urol 10:219-223, 2000.
110. Barranger E, Fritel X, Kadoch O, et al: Results of transurethral injection of silicone micro-implants for females with intrinsic sphincter deficiency. J Urol 164:1619-1622, 2000.
111. Radley SC, Chapple CR, Mitsogiannis IC, et al: Transurethral implantation of Macroplastique for the treatment of female stress urinary incontinence secondary to urethral sphincter deficiency. Eur Urol 39:383-389, 2001.
112. Soliman S, Evans C: Endoscopic Macroplastique injection for the treatment of female stress incontinence: Role and efficacy. Af J Urol 7:45-50, 2001.
113. Peeker R, Edlund C, Wennberg AL, et al: The treatment of sphincter incontinence with periurethral silicone implants (Macroplastique). Scand J Urol Nephrol 36:194-198, 2002.
114. Gurdal M, Tekin A, Erdogan K, et al: Endoscopic silicone injection for female stress incontinence due to intrinsic sphincter deficiency: Impact of coexisting urethral mobility on treatment outcome. Urology 60:1016-1019, 2002.
115. Tamanini JT, D'Ancona CA, Netto NR Jr: Treatment of intrinsic sphincter deficiency using the Macroplastique Implantation System: Two-year follow-up. J Endourol 18:906-911, 2004.
116. Balazs EA: Sodium hyaluronate in viscosurgery. In Balazs EA, Laurent TC (eds): Healon (Sodium Hyaluronate): A Guide to Its Use in Ophthalmic Surgery. Chichester, John Wiley & Sons, 1989, pp 403-404.
117. Stenberg AM, Sundin A, Larsson BS, et al: Lack of distant migration after injection of a 125iodine labeled dextranomer-based implant into the rabbit bladder. J Urol 158:1937-1941, 1997.
118. Stenberg A, Larsson E, Lindholm A, et al: Injectable dextranomer-based implant: Histopathology, volume changes and DNA-analysis. Scand J Urol Nephrol 33:355-361, 1999.
119. Lackgren G, Wahlin N, Skoldenberg E, et al: Long-term followup of children treated with dextranomer/hyaluronic acid copolymer for vesicoureteral reflux. J Urol 166:1887-1892, 2001.
120. van Kerrebroeck P, ter Meulen F, Larsson G, et al: Treatment of stress urinary incontinence using a copolymer system: Impact on quality of life. BJU Int 94:1040-1043, 2004.
121. Stenberg A, Larsson G, Johnson P, et al: DiHA Dextran Copolymer, a new biocompatible material for endoscopic treatment of stress incontinent women. Short term results. Acta Obstet Gynecol Scand 78:436-442, 1999.
122. Stenberg AM, Larsson G, Johnson P: Urethral injection for stress urinary incontinence: Long-term results with dextranomer/hyaluronic acid copolymer. Int Urogynecol J Pelvic Floor Dysfunct 14:335-338, 2003.
123. van Kerrebroeck P, ter Meulen F, Larsson G, et al: Efficacy and safety of a novel system (NASHA/Dx copolymer using the Implacer device) for treatment of stress urinary incontinence. Urology 64:276-281, 2004.
124. Haab F, Fianu-Jonasson A, Dannecker C: Impact of the Zuidex™ system for the treatment of stress urinary incontinence on quality of life: 6 months' results of an open, multicentre study. Abstract presented at the Third International Consultation on Incontinence, Monte Carlo, Monaco, June 26-29, 2004.
125. van Kerrebroeck P, Larsson G, Farrelly E: The Zuidex™ system for the treatment of stress urinary incontinence: 24-month follow-up. Abstract presented at the Third International Consultation on Incontinence, Monte Carlo, Monaco, June 26-29, 2004.
126. Bedir S, Kilciler M, Ozgok Y, et al: Long-term complication due to dextranomer based implant: Granuloma causing urinary obstruction. J Urol 172:247-248, 2004.

127. Fianu-Jonasson A, Edwall L: Stress urinary incontinence: Feasibility of surgery after urethral injection Acta Obstet Gynecol Scand 82:1060, 2003.
128. Lightner D, Calvosa C, Andersen R, et al: A new injectable bulking agent for treatment of stress urinary incontinence: Results of a multicenter, randomized, controlled, double-blind study of Durasphere. Urology 58:12-15, 2001.
129. Pannek J, Brands FH, Senge T: Particle migration after transurethral injection of carbon coated beads for stress urinary incontinence. J Urol 166:1350-1353, 2001.
130. Madjar S, Covington-Nichols C, Secrest CL: New periurethral bulking agent for stress urinary incontinence: Modified technique and early results. J Urol 170:2327-2329, 2003.
131. Chrouser KL, Fick F, Goel A, et al: Carbon coated zirconium beads in beta-glucan gel and bovine glutaraldehyde cross-linked collagen injections for intrinsic sphincter deficiency: Continence and satisfaction after extended followup. J Urol 171:1152-1155, 2004.
132. Hartanto VH, Lightner DJ, Nitti VW: Endoscopic evacuation of Durasphere. Urology 62:135-137, 2003.
133. Yoo JJ, Magliochetti M, Atala A: Detachable self-sealing membrane system for the endoscopic treatment of incontinence. J Urol 158:1045-1048, 1997.
134. Atala A, Peters CA, Retik AB, et al: Endoscopic treatment of vesicoureteral reflux with a self-detachable balloon system. J Urol 148:724-727, 1992.
135. Mazouni C, Bladou F, Karsenty G, et al: Minimally invasive surgery for female urinary incontinence: Experience with periurethral microballoon implantation. J Endourol 18:901-905, 2004.
136. Pycha A, Klingler CH, Haitel A, et al: Implantable microballoons: An attractive alternative in the management of intrinsic sphincter deficiency. Eur Urol 33:469-475, 1998.
137. Drobeck HP, Rothstein SS, Gumaer KI, et al: Histologic observation of soft tissue responses to implanted, multifaceted particles and discs of hydroxylapatite. J Oral Maxillofac Surg 42:143-149, 1984.
138. Mayer R, Lightfoot M, Jung I: Preliminary evaluation of calcium hydroxylapatite as a transurethral bulking agent for stress urinary incontinence. Urology 57:434-438, 2001.
139. Murayama Y, Vinuela F, Ulhoa A, et al: Nonadhesive liquid embolic agent for cerebral arteriovenous malformations: Preliminary histopathological studies in swine rete mirabile. Neurosurgery 43:1164-1175, 1998.
140. Wright KC, Greff RJ, Price RE: Experimental evaluation of cellulose acetate NF and ethylene-vinyl alcohol copolymer for selective arterial embolization. J Vasc Interv Radiol 10:1207-1218, 1999.
141. Dmochowski N, Hershorn S, Corcos J, et al: Multicenter randomized controlled study to evaluate Uryx® urethral bulking agent in treating female stress urinary incontinence. Abstract presented at the 98th Annual American Urological Association Meeting, Chicago, April 26-May 1, 2003.
142. West TB, Alster TS: Autologous human collagen and dermal fibroblasts for soft tissue augmentation. Dermatol Surg 24:510-512, 1998.
143. Cendron M, DeVore DP, Connolly R, et al: The biological behavior of autologous collagen injected into the rabbit bladder. J Urol 154:808-811, 1995.
144. Griffiths RW, Shakespeare PG: Human dermal collagen allografts: A three year histological study. Br J Plast Surg 35:519-523, 1982.
145. Ford CN, Staskowski PA, Bless DM: Autologous collagen vocal fold injection: A preliminary clinical study. Laryngoscope 105:944-948, 1995.
146. Bano F, Barrington JW, Dyer R: Comparison between porcine dermal implant (Permacol) and silicone injection (Macroplastique) for urodynamic stress incontinence. Int Urogynecol J Pelvic Floor Dysfunct 16:147-150; discussion 150, 2005.
147. Atala A, Kim W, Paige KT, et al: Endoscopic treatment of vesicoureteral reflux with a chondrocyte-alginate suspension. J Urol 152:641-643, 1994.
148. Kershen RT, Fefer SD, Atala A: Tissue-engineered therapies for the treatment of urinary incontinence and vesicoureteral reflux. World J Urol 18:51-55, 2000.
149. Bent AE, Tutrone RT, McLennan MT, et al: Treatment of intrinsic sphincter deficiency using autologous ear chondrocytes as a bulking agent. Neurourol Urodyn 20:157-165, 2001.
150. Diamond DA, Caldamone AA: Endoscopic correction of vesicoureteral reflux in children using autologous chondrocytes: Preliminary results. J Urol 162:1185-1188, 1999.
151. Yokoyama T, Huard J, Chancellor MB: Myoblast therapy for stress urinary incontinence and bladder dysfunction. World J Urol 18:56-61, 2000.
152. Chancellor MB, Yokoyama T, Tirney S, et al: Preliminary results of myoblast injection into the urethra and bladder wall: A possible method for the treatment of stress urinary incontinence and impaired detrusor contractility. Neurourol Urodyn 19:279-287, 2000.
153. Strasser H, Ninkovic M, Hess M, et al: Anatomic and functional studies of the male and female urethral sphincter. World J Urol 18:324-329, 2000.
154. Strasser H, Marksteiner R, Margreiter E, et al: Stem cell therapy in treatment of urinary incontinence: First clinical results. Paper presented at the Annual American Urological Association Meeting, San Francisco, May 8-12, 2004.

Chapter 32

ROLE OF NEEDLE SUSPENSIONS

Elizabeth Takacs and Philippe E. Zimmern

Female urinary incontinence (UI) and pelvic organ prolapse (POP) are ubiquitous to the aging female population. A woman has an 11.1% lifetime risk of requiring a single surgery for POP, and one-third of those women will require a repeat procedure.[1] A review of data from the National Hospital Discharge Summary in 1997 and 1998 concluded that 226,000 surgeries for POP[2] and 135,000 for UI[3] were performed, compared with 169,000 total knee replacements and 307,000 cholecystectomies. Twenty-one percent of patients undergo concomitant procedures for POP and UI.[1,2] Both conditions have afflicted women for centuries, but during the past 50 years understanding of the pathophysiology and development of treatment options have progressed.

The bladder neck needle suspension was initially described by Pereyra in 1959[4] for treatment of urethral hypermobility; he initiated the concept of passing a ligature carrier through the retropubic space to transfer sutures placed to suspend or secure the anterior vaginal wall tissue. Today, the role of needle suspensions is decreasing; many practitioners are abandoning the procedure because of its reported low success rate and expansion of the use of the more "minimally invasive" sling procedures.[5,6] One of the most significant advantages of modern-day needle suspensions is the ability to correct urethral hypermobility associated with a cystocele in patients with or without stress urinary incontinence (SUI) by providing support to the urethra, bladder neck, and bladder as a unit without the use of foreign materials.

This chapter briefly reviews the history and evolution of the needle suspensions and looks more in depth at current variations, including indications, technique, complications, and long-term results of the four-corner colposuspension, the anterior vaginal wall suspension, the in situ vaginal wall sling, and the "goalpost" technique. We conclude by debating briefly the pros and cons of using native tissue for these repairs.

HISTORICAL REVIEW OF NEEDLE SUSPENSIONS (1949-1989)

Retropubic bladder neck suspensions were initially described in 1949 by Marshall, Marchetti, and Krantz[7]; the Burch procedure was described in 1961.[8] The goal of these procedures was to fix the bladder neck into a high retropubic position, while returning the urethra to an abdominal position, thus allowing equal transmission of pressures to the bladder and bladder neck/proximal urethral regions. In 1959, Pereyra described "a simplified surgical procedure" to accomplish the same goal (support of the urethra and bladder neck) through a transvaginal approach with a resulting decrease in morbidity.[4]

Pereyra's original procedure described the passage of a trocar needle via a small transverse suprapubic incision blindly through the retropubic space, lateral to the bladder neck, exiting through the anterior vaginal wall. The trocar was passed a total of four times, two times on each side. Pereyra used stainless steel wire; he recognized that the wires were apt to cut through the tissues but served as a temporary support mechanism until scarring and fibrous tissue developed to create a more permanent support. In 1967, Pereyra and Lebherz reported improved urinary continence results when the Pereyra procedure was combined with a Kelly plication.[9] Together, the procedures corrected the anatomic defects that "neither procedure alone could remedy." In his initial description, Pereyra emphasized the need to avoid tension on the sutures, recognizing already that it is scar formation that brings long-term support and good results.

In 1973, Stamey described the endoscopic vesical neck suspension.[10] Similar conceptually to the Pereyra procedure, this technique recommended the use of cystoscopy to observe the needle passage near the bladder neck and introduced a series of specially designed needles for passage of the sutures. A Dacron pledget was used to buttress the periurethral tissues and decrease suture pull-through. The double-pronged ligature carrier was introduced in 1978 by Cobb and Ragde to decrease the number of passages and ensure a consistent fascial bridge.[11]

The Raz bladder neck suspension or modified Pereyra procedure was described in 1981.[12] The key differences were using an inverted U-shaped incision vaginally, to allow dissection lateral to the urethra and bladder neck, entering the retropubic space to allow for adequate mobilization of the bladder and urethra, passing the ligature carrier under fingertip guidance to avoid bladder injury, and placing the anchoring sutures through the full-thickness vaginal wall (excluding epithelium) in addition to the pubocervical fascia (Fig. 32-1). The suspension sutures were secured more laterally in the vaginal wall to decrease the risk of damage or obstruction of the urethra.[13] Because incontinence can occur after an isolated Kelly plication, Raz further modified the Raz bladder neck suspension to concomitantly correct a cystocele and to decrease postoperative incontinence, a procedure known as the "four-corner bladder neck suspension," which is examined in detail later.

In 1987, Gittes and Loughlin proposed a no-incision technique that could be performed under local anesthesia in an outpatient setting.[14] Because the sutures were placed through the full-thickness vaginal mucosa in a helical fashion at the bladder neck level and tied suprapubically under tension, it was believed that the sutures would pull through the vaginal mucosa and form an "autologous pledget" of scar tissue along their retracting path.

The short-term results of all these procedures were very promising, with success rates for subjective cure greater than 90%. As time passed and long-term data became available, it became apparent that it was difficult to reproduce the success of the initial surgeon (Table 32-1).

The morbidity of the needle suspensions was limited and included bleeding from the retropubic space and periurethral

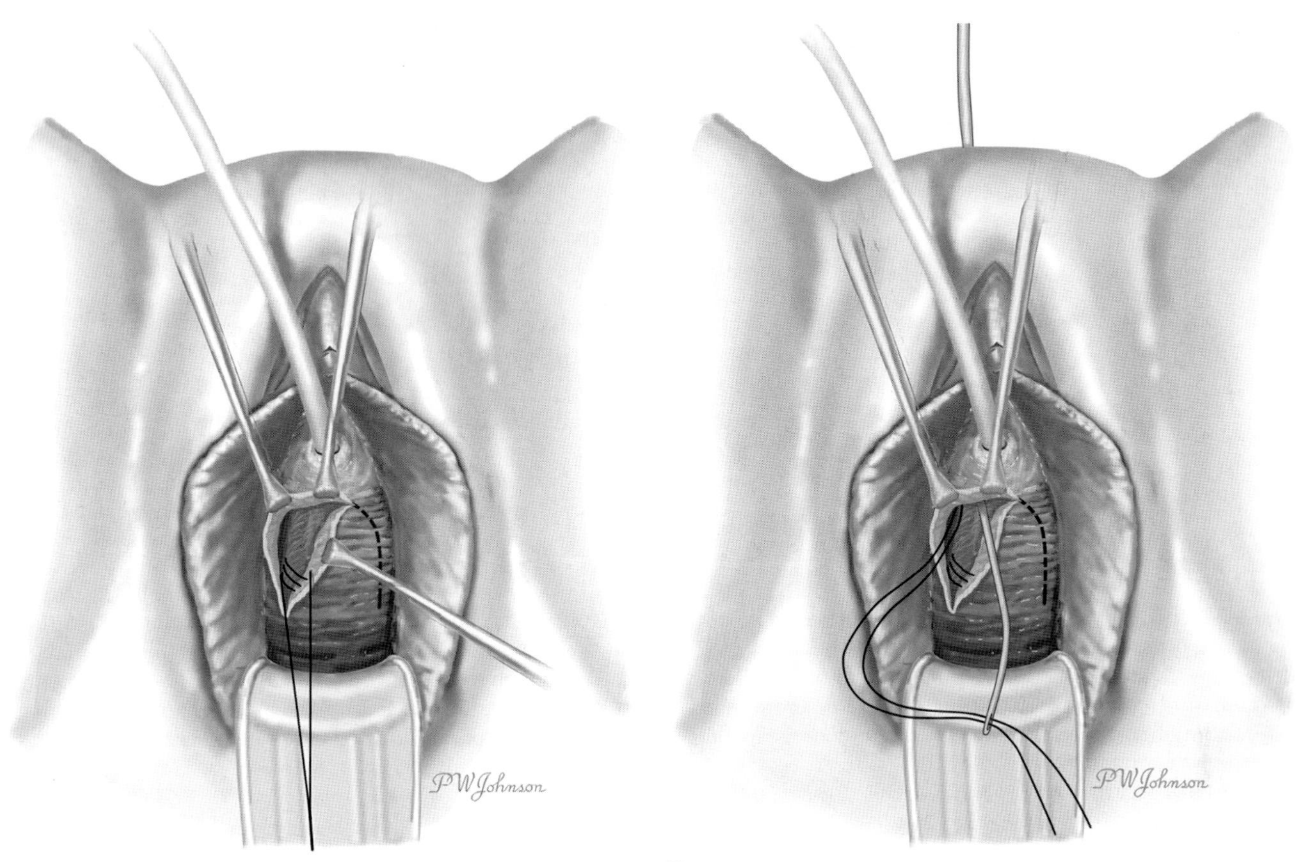

Figure 32-1 Modified Pereyra or Raz bladder neck suspension. **A,** Helical suspension suture placed at the level of the bladder neck provides a narrow anchor point. **B,** Demonstration of the single-prong ligature carrier passed through the retropubic space under fingertip guidance to transfer suspension suture suprapubically. (Adapted from Raz S, Strothers L, Chopra A: Raz techniques for anterior vaginal wall repair. In Raz S (ed): Female Urology, 2nd ed. Philadelphia: W.B. Saunders, 1996; pp. 344-366.)

Table 32-1 Historical Needle Suspensions, Short-term and Longest Follow-up*

First Author and Ref. No.	Year	Follow-up, Mean	Follow-up, Range	*N*	Procedure	% Dry	% Dry + Improved	% De Novo Incontinence
Pereyra[4]	1959	14 mo		31	Pereyra		90	
Pereyra[9]	1967		12-89 mo	172	Pereyra		91.9	
Kursh[15]	1972		0-36 mo	25	Pereyra		<64	
Stamey[10]	1973		0-36 mo		Stamey		68	
Schaeffer[16]	1984		6-48 mo	203	Stamey		91	
Gittes[14]	1987		2-29 mo	38	Gittes		84	
Kondo[17]	1998	8.1 yr	3.2-13.9 yr		Stamey		71.5	12 (combined)
		5.0 yr	1.2-6.8 yr		Gittes		37	
Nigam[18]	2000	8.4 yr	6.3-9.9 yr	34	Stamey	93 at 3 mo, 28 at 9 yr		
		5.3 yr	4.1-6.3 yr	38	Gittes	92 at 3 mo, 14 at 5 yr		
Wennberg[19]	2003	63 mo	28-100 mo	24	Stamey	42	66	37.5
Raz[20]	1992	15 mo	3-95 mo	206	Raz BNS	83	90.3	7.5
Kelly[21]	1991	3.5 yr	2-7.7 yr	114	Raz BNS	51 (no SUI)	76	15.8
Trockman[22]	1995	9.8 yr	5-13 yr	125	Raz BNS	20 (no UI) 49 (no SUI)	71	16

*Short-term, <12 mo; mid-term, 12-60 mo; long-term, >60 mo.
BNS, bladder neck suspension; SUI, stress urinary incontinence; UI, urinary incontinence.

Table 32-2 Historical Evolution of the Needle Suspension into the Contemporary Procedures

Date	Author	Procedure	Novel Feature
1959	Pereyra	Pereyra procedure	Pass trocar through retropubic space
1967	Pereyra, Lebherz	Modified Pereyra	Perform with Kelly plication
1973	Stamey	Stamey endoscopic needle suspension	Pledgets and cystoscopy; Stamey needle
1978	Cobb, Ragde	"Simplified" Stomey endoscopic needle suspension	Double-pronged ligature carrier
1981	Raz	Raz bladder neck suspension	Inverted U-shaped incision giving access to the retropubic space; bilateral helical suspension sutures at the level of the bladder neck
1987	Gittes	Incisionless technique	Secondary scarring of the tracts to hold the repair
1989	Raz	Vaginal wall sling	Use of in situ vaginal wall as sling
1989	Raz, Klutke	Four-corner bladder neck suspension	Concomitant correction of urethral hypermobility and cystocele
1997	Dmochowski, Zimmern	Modified four-corner suspension	Broader anterior vaginal wall anchor for each of the four sutures, leading to the anterior vaginal wall suspension/plate concept

tissues; bladder injury, especially after a prior retropubic anti-incontinence procedure; suture entry into the bladder detected by cystoscopy; failure due to suture pull-through of the anchoring tissues; and rare reports of ilioinguinal nerve entrapment. Urinary retention and the development of de novo urge incontinence were very infrequent.[23]

Based on this overview of the various needle suspensions from 1959 to the late 1980s, it is clear that each new technique improved the preceding one by adding some important modifications that are still in use today (Table 32-2). Avoiding the periurethral tissue, fingertip guidance of the trocar through the retropubic space, and use of cystoscopy are some of the critical steps learned from several decades of vaginal needle suspension procedures.

CONTEMPORARY APPROACHES (1989-2005)

In 1997, the American Urological Association (AUA) Guideline Panel grouped all needle suspensions into one category. Compared to the Burch or the pubovaginal sling procedure, the results at 4 years were globally inferior, but the series were short and had very inhomogeneous methods of reporting and follow-up.[24] More recently, the Cochrane database reviewed the role of needle suspensions for SUI and concluded that, although they were more likely to fail than open retropubic suspensions, the evidence was limited; no conclusions could be drawn when compared to the suburethral sling.[25] Nonetheless, reports still emerge periodically on series from all over the world using the vaginal wall as the support mechanism. Therefore, we review in the following sections four procedures aimed at restoring the support of the anterior vaginal plate, either in its entirety (Four-Corner Bladder Neck Suspension and anterior vaginal wall suspension), beneath the urethra/bladder neck area (vaginal wall sling), or with support of the bladder neck and concomitant anterior colporrhaphy (goalpost technique); we then discuss several other series using similar or slightly modified techniques.

Four-Corner Bladder Neck Suspension (FCBNS)

The FCBNS,[26] initially described by Raz in 1989, was a progression from the original Raz bladder neck suspension and attempted to correct a minimal to moderate cystocele and urethral hypermobility without performing a Kelly plication. Although the Kelly plication and/or anterior colporrhaphy was the standard treatment to repair cystoceles, there was a significant rate of postoperative SUI and cystocele recurrence. For the treatment of SUI, the Kelly plication had a cure rate of 63% to 92% at 1 year and 37% to 54% at 5 years of follow-up.[27,28] Recent randomized studies have also revealed a success rate of 30% to 71% at 1 year for correction of prolapse stage I through IV with this approach.[29-31] The idea of combined correction of a cystocele and urethral hypermobility was a turning point in addressing the vaginal wall as a single unit and not as separate components.

Briefly, the procedure involves creation of an inverted U-shaped anterior vaginal wall incision with the apex midway between the urethral meatus and the bladder neck.[26] The pubocervical fascia is exposed, and the retropubic space is entered and developed laterally. Two pairs of helical nonabsorbable sutures are placed, one pair proximally incorporating the vaginal wall (excluding epithelium), the cardinal ligament, and pubocervical fascia; and the second pair located distally at the level of the bladder neck but avoiding the periurethral tissue (Fig. 32-2). The sutures are transferred suprapubically with a double-pronged Raz ligature carrier. Cystoscopy is performed to confirm no injury to the bladder or ureters and no suture entry. The sutures are then tied to themselves and to the corresponding sutures on the contralateral side, care being taken to avoid tension.

As for many other procedures, the long-term follow-up has not been as promising as the initial short-term reports. Suture pull-through has been a significant criticism. Kilicarslan and colleagues, with a follow-up of 3.8 years, reported a cure rate of 74%; cure was defined as absence of complaints and no evidence of leakage during urodynamic studies.[32] With a mean of 37 months' follow-up and using a standing cystography as an outcome measure, Dmochowski and associates reported a 53% success rate defined as no incontinence and an 83% success rate defined as 0 to 1 incontinent episodes per week.[33] Recurrent cystocele was found in 57%, and 8/33 (24%) of women with their uterus in situ developed symptomatic uterine prolapse postoperatively. Constatini and coworkers reported a success rate of 85% with a mean of 62 months' follow-up.[34] However, in their study, patients underwent concomitant vaginal wall sling if the Valsalva leak point pressure (VLPP) was less than 60 cm H_2O and the FCBNS was performed for correction of POP with or without

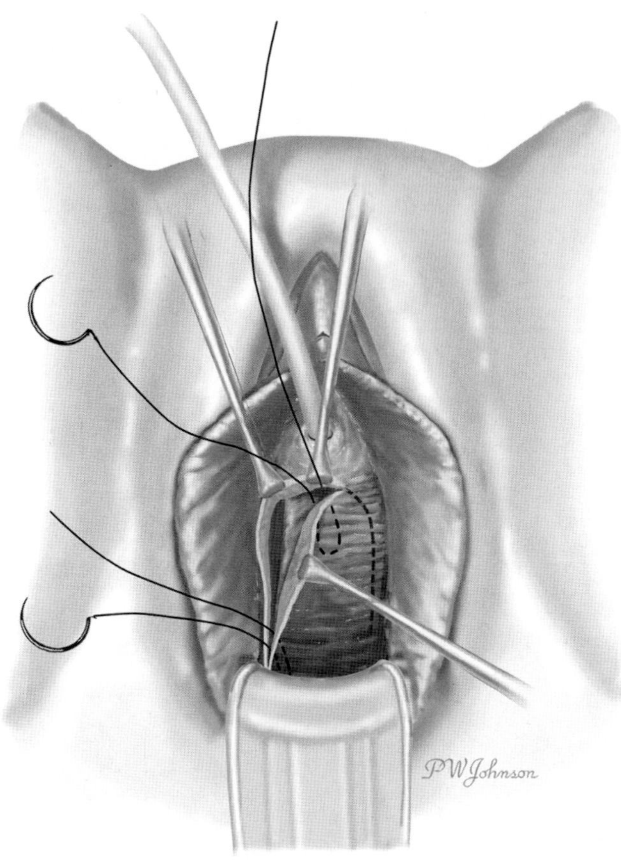

Figure 32-2 Four-corner bladder neck suspension. Placement of two pairs of nonabsorbable sutures incorporating full-thickness vaginal wall minus the epithelium, one pair at the level of the bladder neck and the other at the top of the cystocele. (Adapted from Hadley HR, Zimmern PE, Staskin DR, Raz S: Transvaginal needle bladder neck suspension. Urol Clin North Am 12:291-303, 1985.)

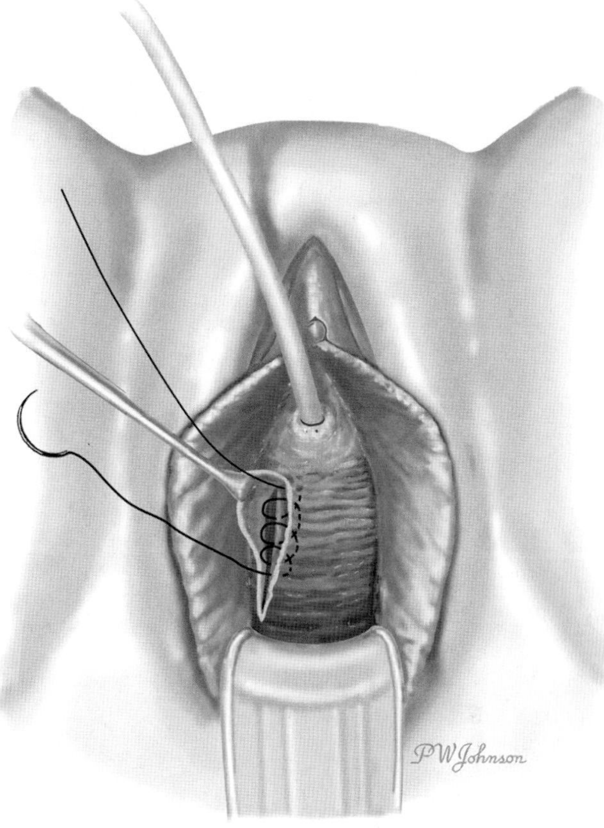

Figure 32-3 Modified four-corner bladder neck suspension. The helical narrow suspension suture is changed to a broad-based suture placement to reduce suture pull-through.

incontinence. For correction of cystocele, 12 of 37 patients with grade 3 cystocele preoperatively failed based on physical examination postoperatively; de novo hysterocele was noted in 4 of 37 patients (10%).

Anterior Vaginal Wall Suspension

The ideal patient for the anterior vaginal wall suspension[35] is a woman who experiences SUI due to urethral hypermobility and has a Baden-Walker grade 1 to 3 cystocele, but no midline defect on physical examination. Cystoceles can be graded not only clinicially but also radiographically. On a voiding cystourethrogram with lateral images, a grade 1 cystocele is defined as 0-2 cm of descent below the inferior margin of the pubic symphysis; grade 2 as 2 to 5 cm of descent; and grade 3 as >5 cm of descent.[36] In women with this lateral detachment, the anterior vaginal wall suspension reestablishes support and prevents the downward mobility of the anterior vaginal wall during straining efforts. This procedure is not intended to correct intrinsic sphincter deficiency. A unique aspect of the anterior vaginal wall suspension is its versatility to correct a cystocele at the time of a sling procedure or urethrolysis.

Conceptually, it is similar to the FCBNS in viewing the bladder, bladder neck, and urethra as a single unit, but the suspension sutures are placed not solely at "four corners" but over the entire length of the vaginal plate, from the bladder neck to the vaginal apex. It is believed that sutures placed broadly allow for greater distribution of pressure, thus decreasing the risk of suture pull-through (Fig. 32-3). This technical change was adopted after studies in a rabbit model done by Bruskewitz and colleagues demonstrated that the cross-sectional area serving as anchor determines the force required for tissue pull-through. These authors reported that suture loops cut through tissue at lower forces and act as a cutting string.[37]

A second important technical difference is the ability to excise redundant vaginal tissue laterally at the site of the primary defect. This maneuver narrows the potential space for lateral cystocele recurrence and recreates the natural lateral sulci present in the vagina. This technical modification resonates with the "pinch test" and "tuck procedure" described by Petros and Ulmsten.[38,39]

After the bladder neck is identified (balloon of Foley catheter) and marked with an ink pen, three marking sutures are placed at the vaginal apex: one in the midline, and then one approximately 1.5 cm lateral to the midline on each side (Figs. 32-4A and 32-5A). An incision is made from approximately 1.5 cm lateral to the bladder neck to the apical marking sutures. This incision is performed on both sides of the vagina, creating a trapezoid-shaped vaginal plate in the center with a width of approximately 3 cm and a length of 4 to 8 cm. A marking pen is used to divide this in situ vaginal wall plate into four equal quadrants (see Figs. 32-4B and 32-5B). A separate no. 1 polypropylene suture is used for each of the four suspension sutures, one suture in each quadrant. The suture is placed in a helical fashion, incorporating large

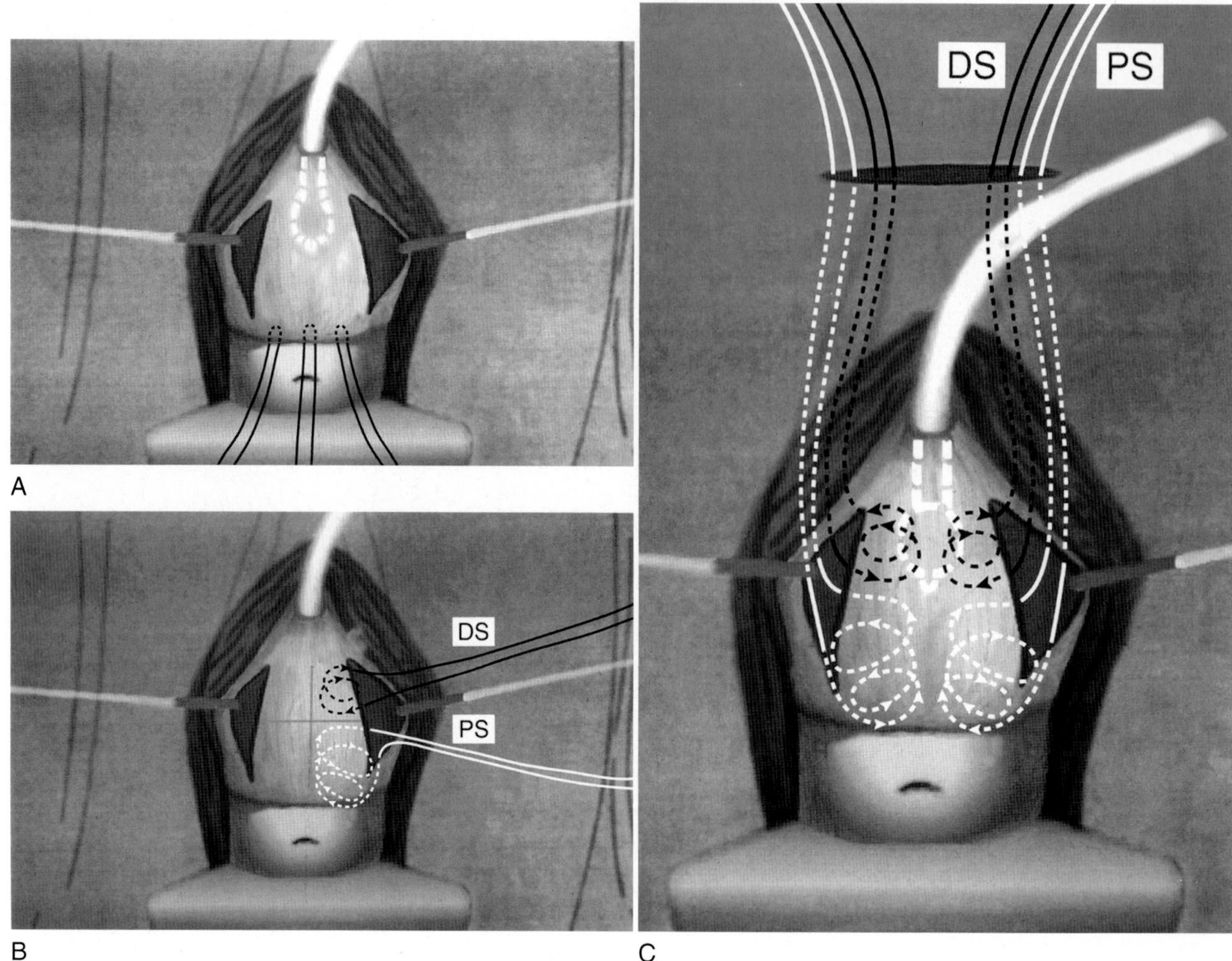

Figure 32-4 Anterior vaginal wall suspension. **A,** Initial setup. Bilateral incisions are created extending from the bladder neck to the vaginal cervix or cuff, with apical marking stitches placed to define the vaginal plate, approximately 3 cm wide and 4 to 8 cm long. **B,** Placement of the suspension sutures. Sutures are helically placed over the entire length of the vaginal plate and approaching the midline. One suture is placed in each of the four quadrants. **C,** Final appearance. Suspension sutures have been placed bilaterally and passed through the retropubic space. Before closure of the vaginal incisions, cystoscopy is performed to confirm no suture entry in the bladder. DS, distal suture; PS, proximal suture. (Adapted from Vasavada SP, Appell RA, Sand PK, Raz S (eds): Female Urology, Urogynecology, and Voiding Dysfunction. New York: Marcel Dekker, 2005.)

segments of vaginal mucosa (minus epithelium) while remaining parallel to the vaginal plate (see Fig. 32-4B). At the proximal portion of the plate, the suture should incorporate the cardinal ligament at the time of hysterectomy or scar at the vaginal cuff.

Once the suspension sutures have been placed, a short suprapubic incision is made one fingerbreadth above the pubic bone to access the tendineus portion of the rectus fascia at its insertion on the pubis. Next, the endopelvic fascia is perforated with blunt and/or sharp dissection, and the retropubic space is easily entered. A double-pronged ligature carrier is passed under fingertip guidance down into the vaginal incision. The two ends of each suture are placed through the eyes of the carrier, which is then withdrawn suprapubically (see Fig. 32-4C). Indigo carmine IV is administered, and a cystoscopy is performed to confirm no bladder or ureteral injury. After the vaginal incisions are closed, the suspension sutures are tied individually with minimal tension, and this is followed by closure of the suprapubic incision (see Fig. 32-5C).

Short and mid-term results for the procedure have been promising. At a mean of 25 months' follow-up, based on questionnaire data, 77% of patients reported that they were cured or improved from their incontinence, and the rate of de novo urge incontinence was reported to be 8%.[40] In an objective study based on voiding cystourethrogram appearance, the lateral height of the cystoceles decreased in a statistically significant fashion postoperatively (Fig. 32-6).[41] Long-term results with 5- to 10-year follow-up will soon be available. From a sexual function perspective, approximately 8% to 13% of middle-aged and elderly women experience dyspareunia.[42,43] Lemack and Zimmern examined the rate of dyspareunia in women undergoing anterior vaginal wall suspension alone or with concomitant posterior repair. Overall, there was no difference between the two groups: 4/22 (18%) of sexually active women reported intercourse as being painful postoperatively, compared with 6/21 (28%) of sexually active patients preoperatively. From these data, it was concluded that the anterior vaginal wall suspension procedure does not adversely affect sexual function.[44]

Cosson and associates, in 2001, described a technique similar to the anterior vaginal wall suspension. In this approach, an in

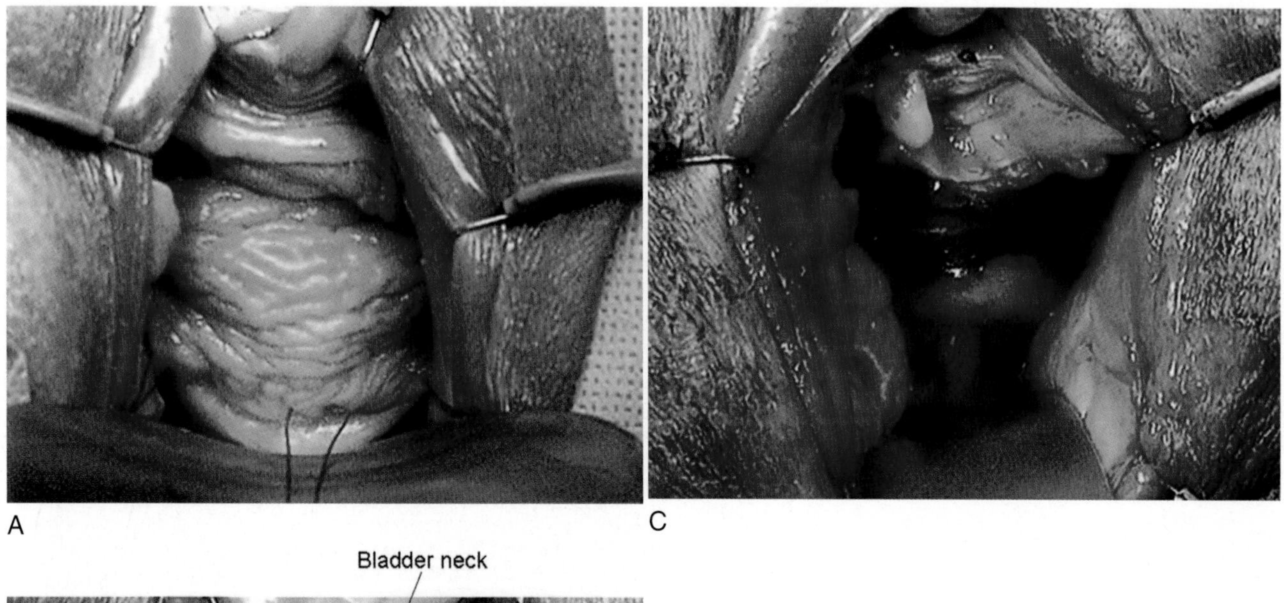

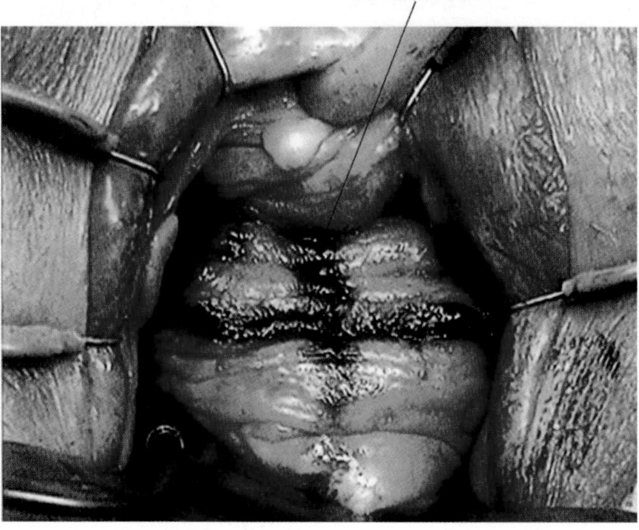

Figure 32-5 Anterior vaginal wall suspension, intraoperative views. **A,** An apical marking stitch has been placed on the midline of the vaginal plate at the level of the vaginal cuff. **B,** The lateral incisions of the vaginal plate have been made, and the plate has been divided into four equal quadrants to guide placement of the four suspension sutures. **C,** The anterior vaginal wall is returned to its normal anatomic position after placement of the suspension sutures and transfer of these sutures suprapubically with a ligature carrier. Note the preserved vaginal depth and no overcorrection of the urethra and bladder base.

situ vaginal patch approximately 4 cm wide and 6 to 8 cm long is created and suspended to the arcus tendineus with three pairs of sutures. The suspended in situ patch is then buried under the anterior colporrhaphy flaps (Fig. 32-7). This approach was performed in 47 patients with grade 3 cystocele, 38% of whom had concomitant UI. A 93% cure rate was achieved for cystocele correction at 16.4 months' follow-up; no result of continence status was reported.[45]

Vaginal Wall Sling

In 1989, Raz also introduced the vaginal wall sling,[46] more to increase outlet resistance than to restore the anatomic support of the urethra. The tension on the vaginal tissue not only increased urethral resistance but created a backboard for improved pressure transmission.

A block A incision is made with the apex just proximal to the urethral meatus and the base extending several centimeters proximal to the bladder neck (Fig. 32-8A). Lateral dissection is performed to mobilize the urethra, but the midline tissue is left intact. A transverse incision is made across the flap at the area of the bladder neck. Proximally, the anterior vaginal wall is further dissected free to raise a vaginal flap. Polypropylene helical sutures are placed in the four corners of the distal vaginal island beneath the urethra. The sutures are transferred by a double-pronged ligature carrier into a previously made small suprapubic incision (see Fig. 32-8B). Cystoscopy is performed to ensure no injury to the bladder or ureters. Next, the proximal vaginal flap is advanced over the "in situ" sling, and the vaginal wall is closed. The suprapubic sutures are then tied and the incisions are closed.

Appell reported modifications of the vaginal wall sling using retropubic or suprapubic bone anchors for suspension, a horizontal mattress suture placed along the lateral edge, and preservation of the endopelvic fascia.[47] Based on these modifications, Goldman and colleagues reported, at 19 months' follow-up, a 79.5% success rate.[48] Mubiayi and associates reported experience with an in situ vaginal sling using a running (nonhelical) suture incorporating the entire lateral edge of the sling.[49] With a mean of 25.1 months' follow-up of the first 75 patients, a 70% rate of

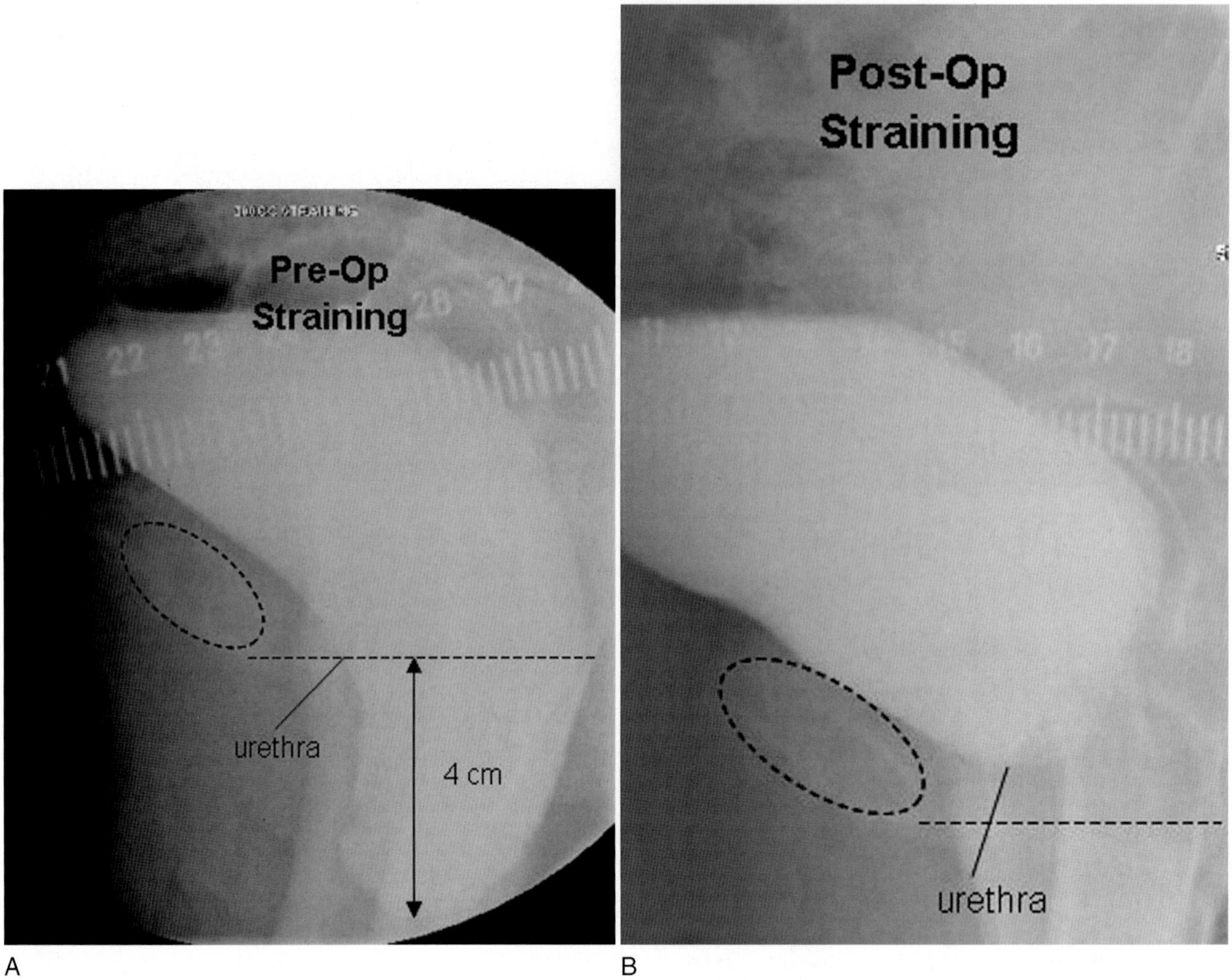

Figure 32-6 Standing cystourethrogram demonstrates the height of a cystocele with straining at maximum bladder capacity on a lateral view. **A,** Preoperatively, a grade 2 cystocele is present. **B,** Six months after an anterior vaginal wall suspension, there is no inferior descent below the level of the pubic symphysis on voiding cystourethrogram.[36]

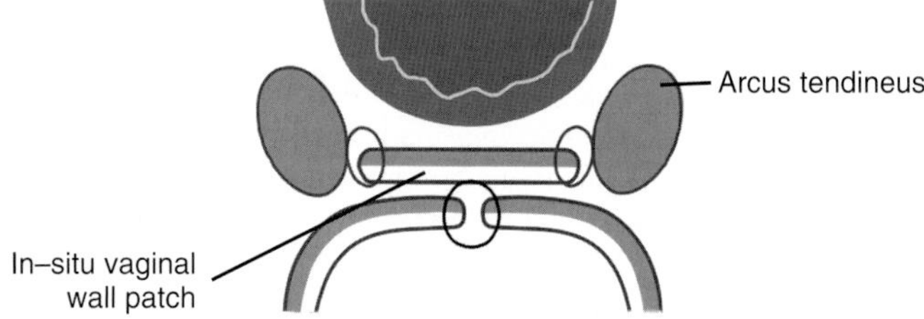

Figure 32-7 Cosson and associates described modification to the anterior vaginal wall suspension. This schematic diagram represents the 4 × 8 cm in situ vaginal patch suspended to the arcus tendineus. The vaginal patch is then covered by anterior colporrhaphy flaps. (Adapted from Cosson M, Collinet P, Occelli B, et al: Cure de cystocele par plastron vaginal. Progres en Urologie 11:340, 2001.)

cure or improvement was achieved. In patients with ISD the rate was 80%. Twenty percent developed de novo urgency or dysuria.

Mikhail and coworkers reported success with several modifications, including a running helical stitch incorporating the entire length of the lateral edge of the sling, bone anchors, denuding of the vaginal patch, and closure over the sling longitudinally rather than by flap advancement.[50] In this study, 53 women with SUI and no ISD underwent a vaginal wall sling with the modifications described, and 31 underwent a concomitant prolapse procedure. Forty-four patients (83%) with a minimum of 5 years of follow-up were reported as being symptomatically dry and without pads; 5.6% reported de novo urgency, and there were no cases of de novo dyspareunia. Serels and colleagues examined the success of combining in situ sling with cystocele repair.[51] Eighteen patients with grade 2 or grade 3 cystocele and SUI with no evidence of ISD on urodynamic studies (VLPP >50 cm H_2O) were evaluated with 6 to 48 months of follow-up. Sixteen patients (89%) were dry postoperatively, 3 (17%) developed de novo urgency, and no patients had recurrence of their prolapse.

The vaginal wall sling appears to afford a mid-term success rate comparable to that of the fascial pubovaginal sling.[52] Two studies, that of Mikhail and colleagues[50] with a minimum follow-up of more than 5 years and that of Kilicarslan and associates[32] with a mean follow-up of 4 years, reported dry rates of 83% and 97%, respectively. However, neither study included patients with ISD based on urodynamic criteria.

Raz cautioned against performing the procedure in sexually active women with a short vagina due to the risk of shortening.

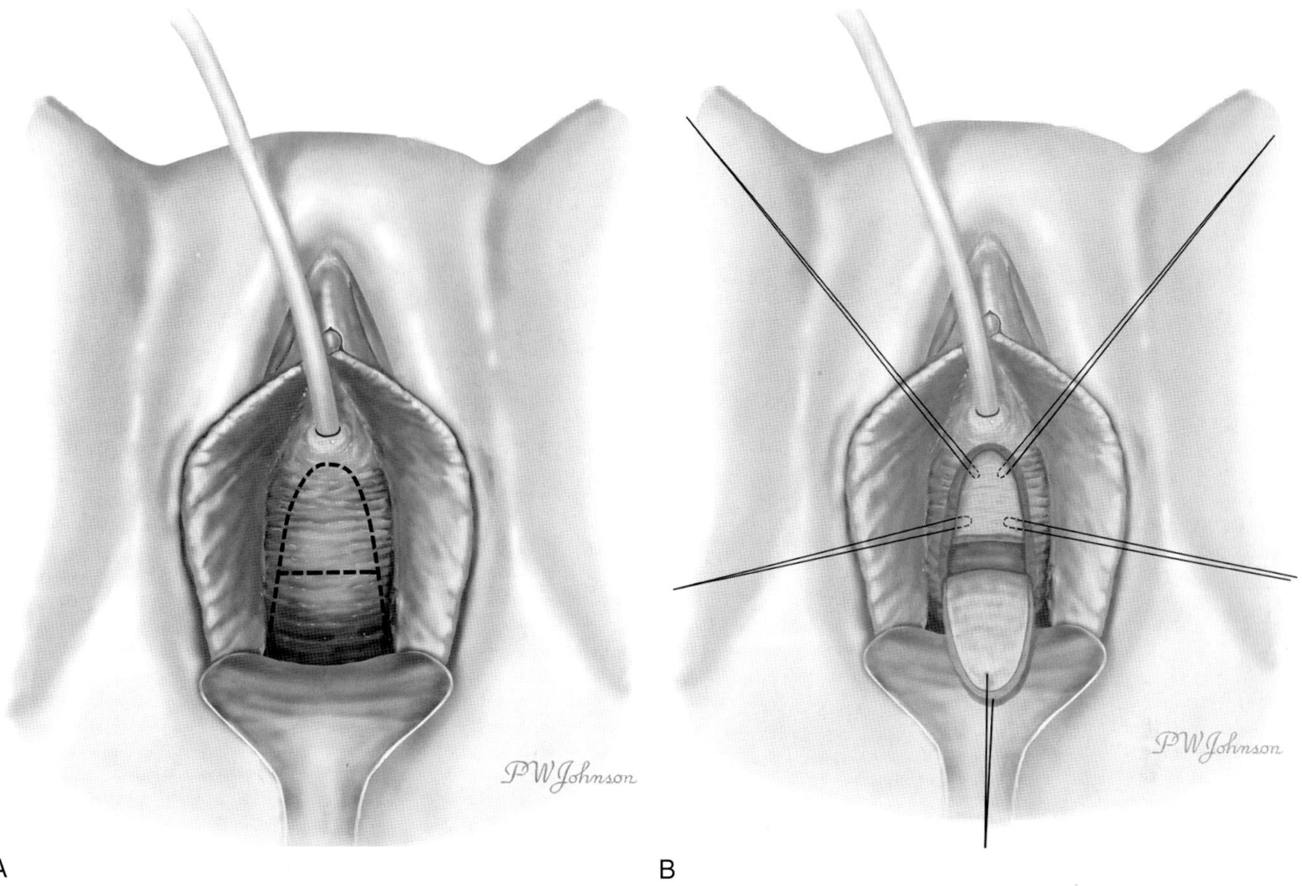

Figure 32-8 Vaginal wall sling. **A,** A "Block A" incision is outlined on the anterior vaginal wall. **B,** Four suspension sutures have been placed with a narrow base anchor. Proximally, a vaginal wall flap has been created and will be advanced over the in situ vaginal sling patch at the end of the procedure. (Adapted from Raz S, Little NA, Juma S. Female Urology. In Walsh PC, Gittes RF, Perlmutter AD, Stamey TA: Compbell's Urology, 6th ed., chap. 75, pp. 2782-2806; 1992. Philadelphia: WB Saunders.)

In older women with significant atrophic vaginitis, adequate tissue strength may be lacking. Additionally, women with significant scarring of the anterior vaginal wall may not be good candidates. In regard to dyspareunia, Mikhail and coworkers, using a longitudinal closure over the flap, reported no de novo dyspareunia in 49 of 51 sexually active patients.[50] Angulo and associates reported a modification using a longitudinal flap placed transversely to avoid the potential of foreshortening the vagina. No sexually active patient had complaints of dyspareunia 6 months postoperatively.[53]

With the technique of the vaginal wall sling, buried epithelium creates a potential for the development of inclusion cysts in the area of the sling. Mubiayi and colleagues reported a 5% (4/75) rate of vaginal mucocele.[49] In the English literature, there have been two further case reports.[54,55]

Goalpost Technique

Raz described his four-defect repair of grade 4 cystocele, a procedure known as the goalpost technique. He used a vaginal wall sling to support the bladder neck and urethra with concomitant reduction of the cystocele by reapproximation of the perivesical fascia and the cardinal ligaments over the midline (Fig. 32-9). Safir and associates reported a 92% (103/112) success rate for cystocele correction and, in patients with preoperative SUI, a cure rate (dry or improved) of 90% (44/49).[57] Leboeuf and colleagues reported a modified procedure wherein Pelvicol mesh was interposed between the reapproximated perivesical fascia and the vaginal wall closure. In this study, 24 patients had the standard four-defect repair, and 19 had Pelvicol interposition. Overall, there was a 93% cure rate of the cystocele. Only 3 of 43 patients had a recurrence, all within the Pelvicol group. For SUI, 22/24 (91.6%) had resolution of their symptoms.[58]

DEBATE: A FUTURE FOR NEEDLE SUSPENSIONS?

[T]he Burch colposuspension was better in controlling stress incontinence but it led to an unacceptable high rate of prolapse recurrence. The anterior colporrhaphy was more effective in restoring vaginal anatomy but it was accompanied by an unacceptable low cure rate of stress incontinence. Neither of the two operations is recommended for women who are suffering from a combination of stress incontinence and advanced cystocele.[59]

As time has progressed, it has become apparent that prolapse and urethral hypermobility are not independent events. The vagina is a dynamic organ, and redistribution of forces may result in herniation in other parts of the vagina. Therefore prolapse disease can be viewed as a global vaginal phenomenon.[60] In recent

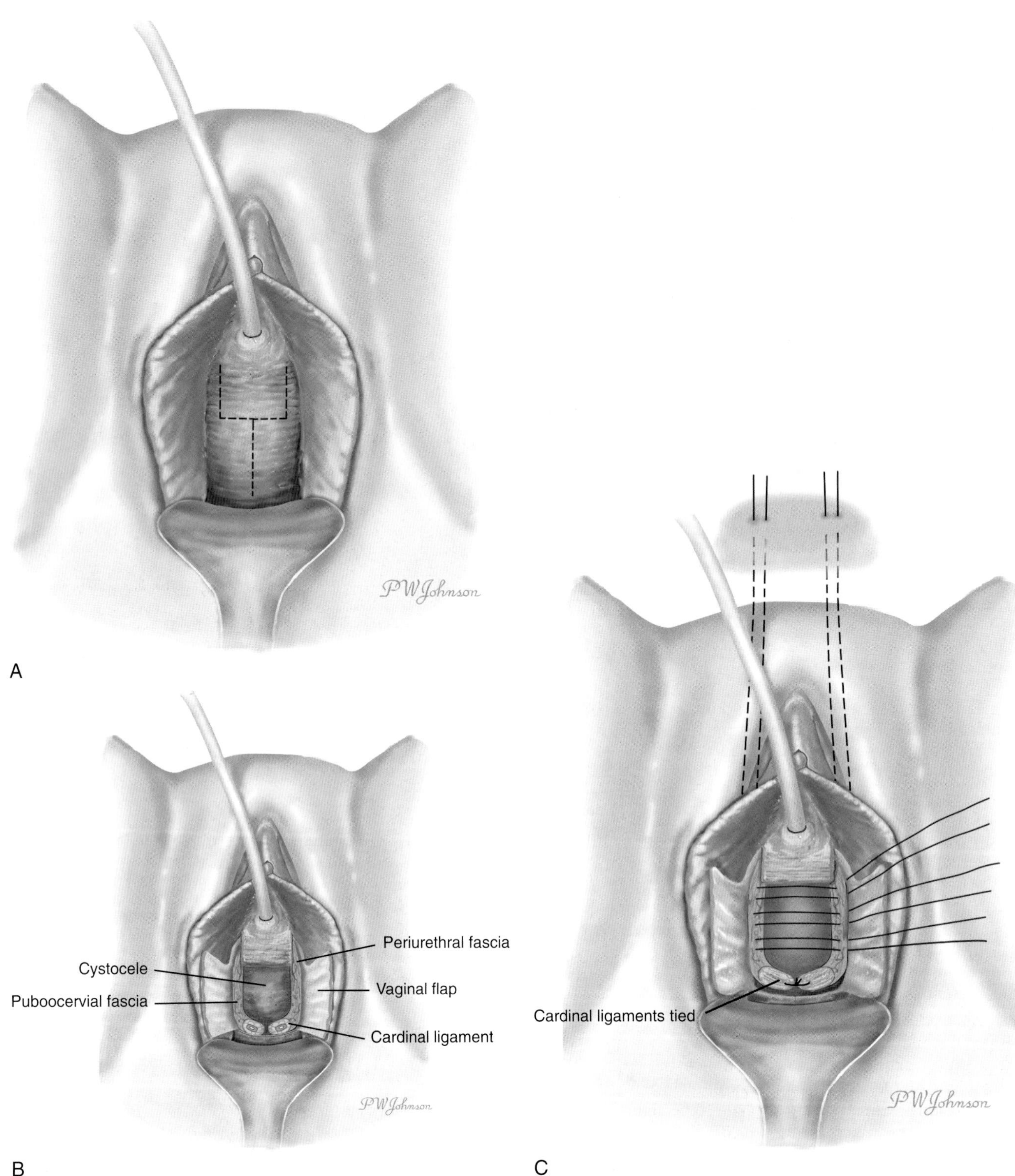

Figure 32-9 Goalpost technique. **A,** Goalpost incision is outlined. The arms extend from the mid-urethra to 1 cm proximal to the bladder neck. The transverse crossbar connects the arms. The post extends from the crossbar (which is 1 cm proximal to the bladder neck and extends to the vaginal cuff). **B,** The vaginal mucosa is dissected off the underlying structures. The mucosa between the arms of the goalpost remains in situ to serve as the vaginal wall sling. **C,** Final appearance, with vaginal wall sling sutures passed through the retropubic space. Sutures are placed transversely to reapproximate the perivesical fascia for correction of the cystocele.

statistics, 18% to 41% of patients undergoing procedures for POP received concomitant anti-incontinence procedures.[2,3]

The paradigm has shifted with regard to the needle suspension procedures. Pereyra first conceptualized needle suspension for the correction of urethral hypermobility and treatment of incontinence; we now have needle suspension procedures that can concomitantly correct cystoceles and SUI secondary to urethral hypermobility. One of the greatest assets of current needle suspension procedures has been the use of native tissue to provide broad support to the anterior vaginal wall as a single unit. Unlike the anterior colporrhaphy, the anterior vaginal wall suspension and the vaginal wall sling do not rely on weakened muscular or fascial attachments but use the actual vaginal mucosa beneath the bladder neck and bladder base to provide the support mechanism. Careful review of more recent literature indicates that experienced vaginal surgeons can attain a good success rate in the correction of cystocele and urethral hypermobility with one simple procedure and with minimal perioperative risks (Table 32-3).

The concept of using a foreign tissue to reinforce the strength of a defective tissue was first applied in general surgery. However, the use of foreign materials such as synthetics, allografts, and xenografts has both real and theoretical beneficial and adverse implications. In the area of vaginal reconstruction and treatment of SUI, surgeons began using foreign materials for midurethral slings a decade ago, and, with increasing practice, this experience has now been extended to reinforce the vaginal mucosa in cystocele repairs and other vaginal compartments.

One can argue for the advantages and disadvantages of every material regarding safety, durability, and effectiveness (Table 32-4). This is beyond the scope of this chapter, but it is fair to state that, for the transvaginal repair of SUI with

Table 32-3 Midterm Incontinence Results of Contemporary Needle Suspension Procedures, Alone and with Associated Anterior Compartment Prolapse

First Author and Ref. No.	Year	Follow-up, Mean (mo)	Follow-up, Range (mo)	*N*	Procedure	% Cystocele Correction	% Dry	% Dry + Improved	% Subjective Cure	% De Novo Incontinence
Raz[46]	1989		10-28	26	VWS				88	23
Juma[61]	1992	23.9	7-52	65	VWS		90.7	94.4		14.8
Kaplan[62]	1996	21.4	6-51	43	PVS		95		89	14
				36	VWS		97		94	8
Serels[51]	1999		12-48	18	VWS + AC	No comment	89		89	17
Goldman[48]	2000	19	13-28	39	VWS				79.5	
					Group 1: VLPP >50				93	
					Group 2: VLPP <50				40	
Kaplan[60]	2000	39.8	4-77	373	VWS		93 at 1 yr (*n* = 341) 95 at 5 yr (*n* = 114)		93	8
Angulo[53]	2001	42	12-83	41	VWS modified + AC	93		88		7
Mikhail[50]	2003	67	63-98	53	VWS + other			83		5.6
Kilicarslan[32]	2003	43.2		20	Burch		70			0
		45.6		29	FCBNS		74			
		49		39	VWS		97			
Raz[26]	1989	24	6-60	107	FCBNS	98		94		5
Dmochowski[33]	1997	37	15-80	47	FCBNS		53	83	92	2
Costantini[34]	2003	62	36-83	37	FCBNS (VWS if VLPP <60)		85			
Safir[57]	1999	21	6-42	112	Goalpost	92		90		7
Leboeuf[58]	2004	15	6-48	43	Goalpost	93			91.6	11.7
Lemack[39]	2000	25	Minimum 12	61	AVWS				77	3

AC, anterior colporrhaphy; AVWS, anterior vaginal wall suspension; FCBNS, four-corner bladder neck suspension; PVS, pubovaginal sling; VLPP, Valsalva leak point pressure; VWS, vaginal wall sling.

Table 32-4 Advantages and Disadvantages of Use of Native Tissue in Anterior Vaginal Wall Reconstruction

Topic	Advantages	Disadvantages
Goal	FCBNS and AVWS: Anterior vaginal wall support VWS: Sling effect	Does not correct ISD Does not provide support to the upper anterior vaginal wall
Technique	Low cost Simple and versatile Short OR time No change in vaginal length	Basic training in vaginal surgery
Recovery	Minimal discomfort and narcotic use	Longer convalescence recommended than for midurethral sling
Safety	Low morbidity (bladder injury, transfusion) Low rate of de novo urge incontinence and rare voiding dysfunction	
Results	Effective for anatomic correction of urethral hypermobility and cystocele	No long term data (>5 years) Concern in young patients

AVWS, anterior vaginal wall suspension; FCBNS, four-corner bladder neck suspension; ISD, intrinsic sphincter deficiency; VWS, vaginal wall sling.

concomitant cystocele, an ideal mesh material has not yet been identified. In the case of synthetics, additional issues currently debated are related to surgical technique, how and where to anchor the mesh material, mesh shrinkage, changes in sexual function, and challenges posed by removal of the mesh material if erosion, infection, or pain forces a reoperation.[63-67]

As with any surgical procedure, there will always be failures. Failure of a procedure can be attributed to technical factors, tissue factors, and, perhaps most importantly, patient selection. We now understand the process of detachment of the anterior vaginal wall from its lateral pelvic support resulting in SUI and a lateral defect cystocele, possibly progressing to a more advanced stage with a central defect,[68,69] and we better understand the intrinsic "flaws" of many of the early needle suspension procedures. Today, we realize that repetitive stitch placement in the same plane will create a point of weakness resulting in suture pull-through, that tension on the tissues leading to overcorrection should be avoided, and that broad-based plates are better than narrow flaps. We also better understand that satisfactory results depend on retropubic scar formation induced by the dissection of the retropubic space (as in a Burch procedure) and has little to do with the variable atrophic appearance of the vaginal tissue. We have also recognized that all patients with SUI are not equal; there is an important subgroup that has ISD. In this group of patients, stabilization of the anterior vaginal wall to eliminate urethral hypermobility is unlikely to correct their incontinence.

It is well known that we lack good scientific data to compare the outcomes of different surgical procedures and that the definition of success is not uniform across studies. The Cochrane report exemplified this in its statement: "[B]ladder neck needle suspension surgery is probably not as good as open abdominal retropubic suspension. . . . However, the reliability of the evidence was limited by poor quality and small trials. . . . There was not enough information to comment on comparisons with suburethral sling operations."[25] These observations spurred interest for several randomized control trials on incontinence and prolapse repair,[21-23,70] including multicenter study sponsored by the National Institutes of Health to compare the Burch procedure versus rectus fascia sling in women with stress-predominant incontinence.[71]

CONCLUSION

Despite the shortfalls of the literature, it appears that the current role of the needle suspension procedures is their applicability to patients with anterior vaginal wall mobility resulting in cystocele and/or SUI. The safety, simplicity, and minimal morbidity of these procedures need to be weighed against the long-term concern of using native tissue for repair. Recently, the trend has been to enhance the traditional anterior colporrhaphy with the interposition of a variety of mesh materials, but very little is known about the results and complications of these newer materials. Both the Cochrane and International Consultation on Incontinence (ICI) groups reviewing existing data cautioned that these materials should be used only in the context of well-designed randomized controlled trials on properly consented patients.[72] Ongoing studies on the biomechanical properties of the human anterior vaginal wall may shed light on the changes of the vaginal wall with aging and help in designing an ideal biocompatible material suited to an individual patient.[73]

References

1. Olsen AL, Smith VJ, Bergstrom JO, et al: Epidemiology of surgically managed pelvic organ prolapse and urinary incontinence. Obstet Gynecol 89:501, 1997.
2. Brown JS, Waetjen LE, Subak LL, et al: Pelvic organ prolapse surgery in the United States, 1997. Am J Obstet Gynecol 186:712, 2002.
3. Waetjen LE, Subak LL, Shen H, et al: Stress urinary incontinence surgery in the United States. Obstet Gynecol 101:671, 2003.
4. Pereyra AJ: A simplified surgical procedure for the correction of stress incontinence in women. West J Surg Obstet Gynecol 67:223, 1959.
5. Gee WF, Holtgrewe HL, Albertsen PC, et al: Practice trends of American urologists in the treatment of impotence, incontinence, and infertility. J Urol 156:1778, 1996.
6. Kim HL, Gerber GS, Patel RV, et al: Practice patterns in the treatment of female urinary incontinence: A postal and internet survey. Urology 57:45, 2001.

7. Marshall VF, Marchetti AA, Krantz KE: The correction of stress incontinence by simple vesicourethral suspension. Surg Gynecol Obstet 88:509, 1949.
8. Burch JC: Urethrovaginal fixation to Cooper's ligament for correction of stress incontinence, cystocele, and prolapse. Am J Obstet Gynecol 81:281, 1961.
9. Pereyra AJ, Lebherz TB: Combined urethrovesical suspension and vaginourethroplasty for correction of urinary stress incontinence. Obstet Gynecol 30:537, 1967.
10. Stamey TA: Endoscopic suspension of the vesical neck for urinary continence. Surg Gynecol Obstet 136:547, 1973.
11. Cobb OE, Ragde H: Correction of female stress incontinence. J Urol 120:418, 1978.
12. Raz S: Modified bladder neck suspension for female stress incontinence. Urology 17:82, 1981.
13. Hadley HR, Zimmern PE, Staskin DR, Raz S: Transvaginal needle bladder neck suspension. Urol Clin North Am 12:291, 1985.
14. Gittes RF, Loughlin KR: No-incision pubovaginal suspension for stress incontinence. J Urol 138:568, 1987.
15. Kursh ED, Wainstein M, Persky L: The Pereyra procedure and urinary stress incontinence. J Urol 108:591, 1972.
16. Schaeffer AJ, Stamey TA: Endoscopic suspension of vesical neck for urinary incontinence. Urology 23:484, 1984.
17. Kondo A, Kato K, Gotoh M, et al: The Stamey and Gittes procedures: Long-term followup in relation to incontinence types and patient age. J Urol 160:756, 1998.
18. Nigam AK, Otite U, Badenoch DF: Endoscopic bladder neck suspension revisited: Long-term results of Stamey and Gittes procedures. Eur Urol 38:677, 2000.
19. Wennberg A, Edlund C, Fall M, Peeker R: Stamey's abdominovaginal needle colposuspension for the correction of female genuine stress urinary incontinence. Scand J Urol Nephrol 37:419, 2003.
20. Raz S, Sussman EM, Erickson DB, et al: The Raz bladder neck suspension: Results in 206 patients. J Urol 148:845, 1992.
21. Kelly MJ, Roskamp D, Knielsen K, et al: Symptom analysis of patients undergoing modified Pereyra bladder neck suspension for stress urinary incontinence. Urology 37:213, 1991.
22. Trockman BA, Leach GE, Hamilton J, et al: Modified Pereyra bladder neck suspension: 10-Year mean followup using outcomes analysis in 125 patients. J Urol 154:1841, 1995.
23. McGuire EJ, Savastano JA: Stress incontinence and detrusor instability/urge incontinence. Neurourol Urodyn 4:313, 1985.
24. Leach GE, Dmochowski RR, Appell RA, et al: Female stress urinary incontinence clinical guidelines panel summary report on surgical management of female stress urinary incontinence. J Urol 158:875, 1997.
25. Glazener CM, Cooper K: Bladder neck needle suspension for urinary incontinence in women. Cochrane Database Syst Rev 2004;2: CD003636.
26. Raz S, Klutke CG, Golomb J: Four-corner bladder and urethral suspension for moderate cystocele. J Urol 142:712, 1989.
27. Bergman A, Elia G: Three surgical procedures for genuine stress incontinence: Five-year follow-up of a prospective randomized study. Am J Obstet Gynecol 173:66, 1995.
28. Thaweekul Y, Bunyavejchevin S, Wisawasukmongchol W, Santingamkun A: Long term results of anterior colporrhaphy with Kelly plication for the treatment of stress urinary incontinence. J Med Assoc Thai 87:357, 2004.
29. Weber AM, Walters, MD, Piedmonte MR, Ballard LA: Anterior colporrhaphy: A randomized trial of three surgical techniques. Am J Obstet Gynecol 185:1299, 2001.
30. Sand PK, Koduri S, Lobel RW, et al: Prospective randomized trial of polyglactin 910 mesh to prevent recurrence of cystoceles and rectoceles. Am J Obstet Gynecol 184:1357, 2001.
31. Gandhi S, Goldberg RP, Kwon C, et al: A prospective randomized trial using solvent dehydrated fascia lata for the prevention of recurrent anterior vaginal wall prolapse. Am J Obstet Gynecol 192:1649, 2005.
32. Kilicarslan H, Guvenal T, Ayan S, et al: Comparison of outcomes of three different surgical techniques performed for stress urinary incontinence. Int J Urol 10:126, 2003.
33. Dmochowski RR, Zimmern PE, Ganabthi LS, Leach GE: Role of the four-corner bladder neck suspension to correct stress incontinence with a mild to moderate cystocele. Urology 49:35, 1997.
34. Constatini E, Pajoncini C, Zucchi A, et al: Four-corner colposuspension: Clinical and functional results. Int Urogynecol J Pelvic Floor Dysfunction 14:113, 2003.
35. Wilson TS, Zimmern PE: Anterior vaginal wall suspension. In Vasavada SP, Appell RA, Sand PK, Raz S (eds): Female Urology, Urogynecology, and Voiding Dysfunction. New York: Marcel Dekker, 2005.
36. Zimmern PE: The role of voiding cystourethrography in the evaluation of the female lower urinary tract. Probl Urol 5:23, 1991.
37. Bruskewitz RC, Nielsen KT, Graversen PH, et al: Bladder neck suspension material investigated in a rabbit model. J Urol 142:1361, 1989.
38. Petros PE, Ulmsten UI: Pinch test for the diagnosis of stress urinary incontinence. Acta Obstet Gynecol Scand 69(Suppl 153):33, 1990.
39. Petros PE, Ulmsten UI: The tuck procedure: A simplified vaginal repair for treatment of female urinary incontinence. Acta Obstet Gynecol Scand 69(Suppl 153):41, 1990.
40. Lemack GE, Zimmern PE: Questionnaire-based outcome after anterior vaginal wall suspension for stress urinary incontinence [abstract]. J Urol 163(4 suppl): 73, abstract no. 321, 2000.
41. Showalter PR, Zimmern PE, Roehrborn CG, Lemack GE: Standing cystourethrogram: An outcome measure after anti-incontinence procedures and cystocele repair in women. Urology 58:33, 2001.
42. Osborn M, Hawton K, Gath D: Sexual dysfunction among middle aged women in the community. BMJ 296:959, 1988.
43. Diokno AC, Brown MB, Herzog AR: Sexual function in the elderly. Arch Intern Med 150:197, 1990.
44. Lemack GE, Zimmern PE: Sexual function after vaginal surgery for stress incontinence: Results of a mailed questionnaire. Urology 56:223, 2000.
45. Cosson M, Collinet P, Occelli B, et al: Cure de cystocele par plastron vaginal. Progres en Urologie 11:340, 2001.
46. Raz S, Siegel AL, Short JL, Synder JA: Vaginal wall sling. J Urol 141:43, 1989.
47. Appell RA: In situ vaginal wall sling. Urology 56:499, 2000.
48. Goldman HB, Rackley RR, Appell RA: The in situ anterior vaginal wall sling: Predictors of success. J Urol 166:2259, 2001.
49. Mubiayi N, Lucot J, Narducci F, et al: Cure chirurgicale de l'incontinence urinaire d'effort par fronde de tissue vaginal: Technique, resultats, indications. Progres in Urologie 12:60, 2002.
50. Mikhail MS, Rosa H, Packer P, et al: A modified vaginal wall patch sling technique as a first-line surgical approach for genuine stress incontinence with urethral hypermobility: Long-term follow up. Int Urogynecol J Pelvic Floor Dysfunct 15:132, 2004.
51. Serels SR, Rackley RR, Appell RA: In situ slings with concurrent cystocele repair. Tech Urol 5:129, 1999.
52. Kaplan SA, Santarosa RP, Te AE: Comparison of fascial and vaginal wall slings in the management of intrinsic sphincter deficiency. Urology 47:885, 1996.
53. Angulo JC, Lera R, Esteban M, Hontoria JM: Vaginal wall transverse flap sling for repair of severe cystocele and cystourethrocele with associated stress incontinence. Braz J Urol 27:386, 2001.
54. Woodman PJ, Davis GD: The relationship of the in-situ advancing vaginal wall sling to vaginal epithelial inclusion cyst. Int Urogynecol J Pelvic Floor Dysfunct 11:124, 2000.
55. Baldwin DD, Hadley HR: Epithelial inclusion cyst formation after free vaginal wall swing sling procedure for stress urinary incontinence. J Urol 157:952,1997.
56. Raz S, Stothers L, Chopra A: Raz techniques for anterior vaginal wall repair. In Raz S (ed): Female Urology, 2nd ed. Philadelphia: Saunders, 1996.

57. Safir MH, Gousse AE, Rovner ES, et al: Four-defect repair of grade 4 cystocele. J Urol 161:587, 1999.
58. Leboeuf L, Miles RA, Kim SS, Gousse AE: Grade 4 cystocele repair using four-defect repair and porcine xenograft acellular matrix (Pelvicol): Outcome measures using SEAPI. Urology 64:282, 2004.
59. Colombo M, Vitobello D, Proietti F, Milani R: Randomized comparison of Burch colposuspension versus anterior colporrhaphy in women with stress urinary incontinence and anterior vaginal wall prolapse. BJOG 107:544, 2000.
60. Shull BL: Pelvic organ prolapse: Anterior, superior, and posterior vaginal segment defects. Am J Obstet Gynecol 181:6, 1999.
61. Juma S, Little NA, Raz S: Vaginal wall sling: Four years later. Urology 39:424, 1992.
62. Kaplan SA, Te AE, Young GPH, et al: Prospective analysis of 373 consecutive women with stress urinary incontinence treated with a vaginal wall sling: The Columbia–Cornell University experience. J Urol 164:1623, 2000.
63. Cervigni M, Natale F: The use of synthetics in the treatment of pelvic organ prolapse. Curr Opin Urol 11:429, 2001.
64. Bukkapatnam R, Shah S, Raz S, Rodriguez L: Anterior vaginal wall surgery in elderly patients: Outcomes and assessment. Urology 65:1104, 2005.
65. Cervigni M, Natale F, Weir J, et al: Prospective randomized trial of two new materials for the correction of anterior compartment prolapse: Pelvicol and Prolene soft [abstract]. Neurourol Urodyn 24:585, 2005.
66. Balmforth J, Cardozo L: Prospective multicentre observational trial of composite polyglactin/polypropylene mesh (Vypro mesh) for reconstruction of recurrent anterior vaginal wall prolapse [abstract]. Neurourol Urodyn 24:588, 2005.
67. Cosson M, Caquant F, Collinet P, et al: Prolift mesh (Gynecare) for pelvic organ prolapse surgical treatment using the TVM group technique: A retrospective study of 687 patients [abstract]. Neurourol Urodyn 24:590, 2005.
68. Mostwin JL: Current concepts of female pelvic anatomy and physiology. Urol Clin North Am 18:175, 1991.
69. Rosenblum N, Eilber KS, Rodriguez LV, Raz S: Anatomy of pelvic support. In Vasavada SP, Appell RA, Sand PK, Raz S (eds): Female Urology, Urogynecology, and Voiding Dysfunction. New York: Marcel Dekker, 2005.
70. Hilton P: Trials of surgery for stress incontinence: Thoughts on the "Humpty Dumpty principle." BJOG 109:1081, 2002.
71. Urinary Incontinence Treatment Network (UITN) Continence Treatment Centers. National Institute of Diabetes & Digestive & Kidney Diseases. Available at: http://www.niddk.nih.gov/patient/uitn/uitn.htm (accessed July 13, 2007).
72. Brubaker L, et al: Surgery for pelvic organ prolapse. In Abrams P, Cardozo L, Khoury S, Wein A (eds): Brubaker L, Bump R, Fynes M, et al: Surgery for pelvic organ prolapse. In Abrams P, Cardozo L, Khoury S, Wein A (eds): Incontinence: 3rd International Consultation on Incontinence, vol. 2, chap. 21. Paris: Health Publications, Ltd., 2005; pp 1373-1401.
73. Weber AM, Buchsbaum GM, Chen B, et al: Basic science and translational research in female pelvic floor disorders: Proceedings of an NIH-sponsored meeting. Neurourol Urodyn 23:288, 2004.

Chapter 33

VAGINAL WALL SLING

Rodney A. Appell

There are a plethora of surgical procedures for the treatment of female stress urinary incontinence (SUI). More than 200 procedures currently exist, and the list is still growing. Sincere attempts to overcome imperfect results and to avoid complications, as well as pressures from industry and patients, have all taken part in this evolution, or perhaps revolution, with innovative, creative attempts over the last decade aimed at performing less invasive surgery for SUI, to decrease morbidity, hospital stay, postoperative discomfort, and perhaps even the cost of surgery. There are nonlaparoscopic procedures available for SUI that are minimally invasive and share many of these qualities just described; in the carefully chosen patient, they provide a reasonable surgical option for the treatment of SUI. This chapter reviews the surgical techniques and results of vaginal wall slings.

Surgical procedures in this category are really modifications of transvaginal suspensions that were designed to support the proximal urethra and bladder neck into a high retropubic position transvaginally, presumably in a less invasive way than with retropubic suspensions. A midline or inverted U-shaped incision was created at the anterior vaginal wall. The periurethral ligaments and, in some procedures, the deep part of the vaginal epithelium were included in a helical suture. The suture was then transferred, using a long needle passer, to a small suprapubic incision. This step was then repeated on the contralateral side. Tying the sutures in the suprapubic area resulted in suspension of the bladder neck and the proximal urethra into a high retropubic position. Variations on these themes included modifications by Pereyra in 1959,[1] Stamey in 1973[2] and 1981,[3] and Gittes in 1987.[4] These variations differed in the shape of the vaginal incision (midline, T-shaped, inverted U), the way the needle was passed (direct finger guidance or blindly), the anchoring tissue, and the use of cystoscopy (to rule out injury or to confirm suture placement). As a group, these procedures have been less efficacious than retropubic suspensions or sling procedures. They carry a success rate of 67% with 4 or more years of follow-up.[5] A possible explanation for their lesser efficacy may include pull-through of the sutures through the supporting anchoring structures and eventual failure of the supporting mechanism at the level of the bladder neck and proximal urethra. Future applications for these procedures seem to be limited unless they can be used in conjunction with the "sling concept."

MINIMALLY INVASIVE SLING PROCEDURES

Sling procedures have been used for almost a century in efforts to correct SUI and are constantly evolving. In recent years, several observations have helped direct innovations. In the past, SUI was separated into urethral hypermobility (type I and II) and intrinsic sphincter deficiency or ISD (type III). Now it is believed that, if SUI is present, there must be some component of sphincteric deficiency. Sling procedures were originally designed for the treatment of the ISD type of urinary SUI and for recurrent SUI when prior surgical treatments had failed. Now, however, sling procedures are used also in the treatment of primary SUI.

If a sling procedure is chosen, there are many technical options available for placement and choice of sling material: in situ vaginal wall, free vaginal wall graft, synthetic material, cadaveric fascia lata, autologous rectus fascia, and autologous fascia lata. Despite the success of synthetic slings placed at the mid-urethra, there are many patients and surgeons for whom the placement of a foreign body through the vagina is not acceptable. For such patients, and especially for those with abdominal (Valsalva) leak point pressure (VLLP) greater than 50 cm H_2O, an acceptable alternative is an in situ vaginal wall sling.[6] Through the use of the vaginal wall, the time and morbidity of the sling procedure can be decreased, and the use of any foreign material is avoided. Furthermore, regardless of the sling material, preservation of the endopelvic fascia may help to prevent recurrent paravaginal defects may decrease the operative morbidity by reducing the surgical dissection and adverse side effects such as detrusor instability. The sling should then be fixed in position and tied without tension.

PREOPERATIVE ASSESSMENT

Every patient undergoes a careful pelvic examination, measurement of postvoid residual volume, and a supine stress test. Patients with mixed incontinence or an elevated postvoid residual volume always undergo urodynamic testing. Patients with pure SUI, on the other hand, should have urodynamic testing with determination of VLLP to help determine whether the type of sling material to be used is in question. Cystoscopy can be reserved preoperatively for the patient with complaints of significant urgency. Any pelvic organ prolapse noted on physical examination should be addressed at the time of the proposed incontinence surgery.

METHOD: IN SITU VAGINAL WALL SLING WITH PRESERVATION OF THE ENDOPELVIC FASCIA

An incision is created in the anterior vaginal wall in the shape of an "A." The island of the "A" is used as the in situ sling. The proximal end of the island is at the bladder neck, and the distal end is at the mid-urethra. The anterior vaginal wall tissue lateral to the in situ sling is mobilized to the inferior pubic rami just to the level of the endopelvic fascia. The legs of the "A" are then further dissected so as to create a flap to cover the in situ sling (Fig. 33-1).

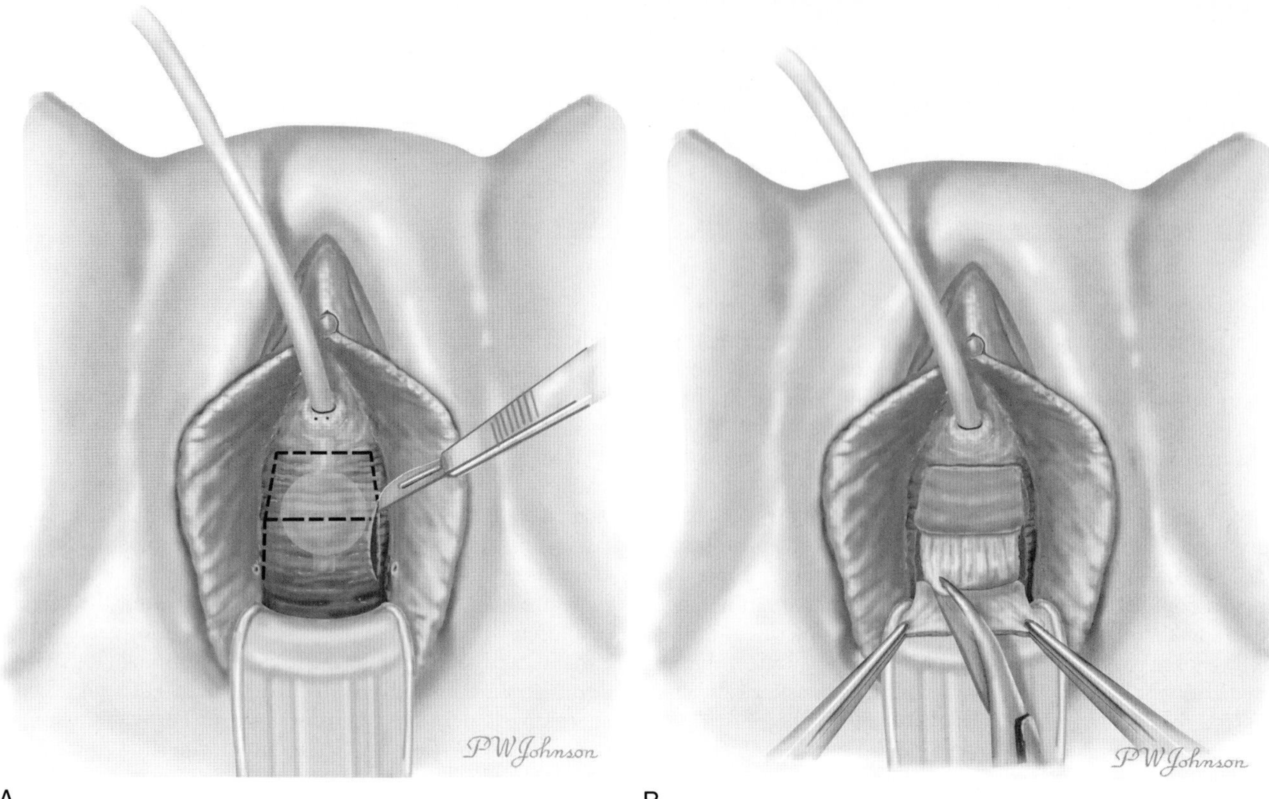

Figure 33-1 A, Incision line for formation of the in situ sling. **B,** Dissection of vaginal flap for ultimate closure.

A suprapubic incision is then made, and a heavy, nonabsorbable suture is fixed into position. Classically, the fixation may take place in one of three ways. The suture can be anchored using bone anchors into both pubic tubercles, or it can be anchored by taking a no. 6 free Mayo needle and driving it through the fascial leaf overlying the insertion of the rectus fascia behind the pubic bone or into the pubic bone itself.[7,8] One end of the suture is then passed from the suprapubic site into the vaginal lumen via the lateral sling incision, using a 15- or 30-degree Stamey-type needle. The suture is then loaded onto the no. 6 free Mayo needle and placed through the in situ sling as well as the pubocervical fascia, using a horizontal mattress or U-stitch suture. The Stamey-type needle delivers the suture back to the suprapubic wound (Figs. 32-2 and 33-3). Cystoscopy is then performed with a 70-degree lens to evaluate for efflux of urine from the ureteral orifices and bladder perforation.

The vaginal wall is closed with a running locking 2-0 polyglycolic acid suture. At this point, the catheter and vaginal retractors are removed (Fig. 33-4). A wink sign (i.e., a tugging up of the bladder neck when pressure is applied to pull on the sling sutures) is noticed, and the sutures are tied over a clamp or Hegar dilator that is approximately 5 to 7 mm in diameter or over the forefinger of the surgical assistant. The catheter is replaced, and gentle traction is applied to the bladder neck to allow the suprapubic knots to lie correctly. A vaginal pack with estrogen cream is then applied.

The use of transvaginal bone anchors and vaginal wall to correct SUI has also been reported.[9,10] In these studies, two vaginal wall screws on either side of the urethra were placed through the

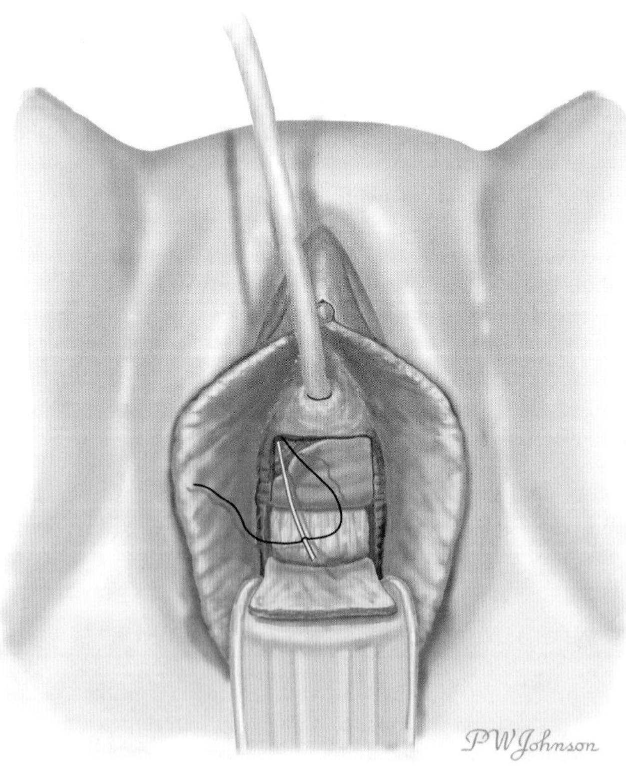

Figure 33-2 Stabilization of bladder neck: placement of vaginal sutures.

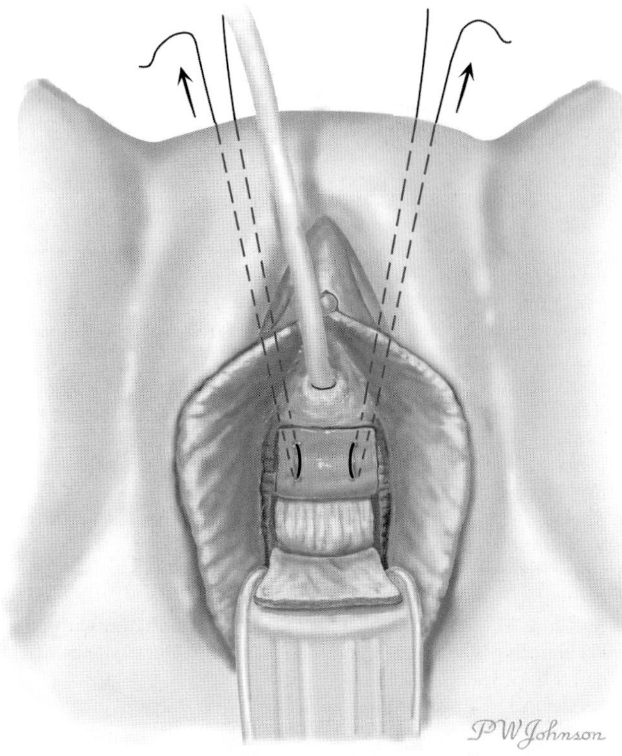

Figure 33-3 Stabilization of bladder neck: transfer of sutures to suprapubic site.

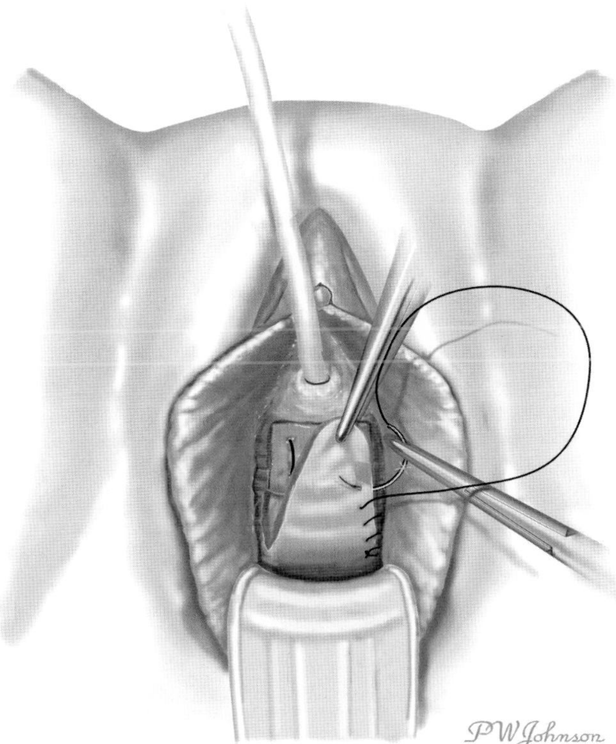

Figure 33-4 Closure of vaginal incision.

vaginal wall itself, for a total of four bone anchors. The bone anchors were driven into the pubic bone on either side of the symphysis. They were placed approximately 2 cm from the urethra, and each pair of ipsilateral sutures was approximately 1 to 2 cm apart. On each side, one of the sutures was passed through its defect created in the vaginal wall to the ipsilateral suture vaginal wall defect, a distance of approximately 1 to 2 cm. The ipsilateral sutures were then tied to each other, and the knot was buried in the vaginal wall.

RESULTS

The Cleveland Clinic Foundation reported on a series of patients using the in situ sling technique.[11] In this series, 20 patients with a mean age of 55 years were monitored for a mean of 26 months (range, 24 to 29 months). Follow-up consisted of a questionnaire and physical examination with provocative pad test. Ninety-five percent of the patients were cured. One patient had recurrent SUI. Three patients had a delay in voiding until 3 weeks after the procedure. There were two patients with de novo instability in whom the problem resolved within 2 months. Raz and colleagues[12] had previously reported success in 77% of patients, and in a follow-up study 4 years later, Juma and associates[13] reported a success rate of 94.4% in a series of 65 patients. Kaplan and colleagues[14] performed a comparison of rectus fascia and vaginal wall slings. The satisfaction and success rates were similar, and the group that underwent the vaginal wall sling had a shorter operative time and shorter hospital stay.

The procedure has few complications reported to date. The disadvantages are thought to be the fact that the vaginal tissue used is weak[6] and that there may be a risk of epithelial inclusion cyst formation.[15]

The group from Israel has published results on their transvaginal bone anchoring techniques.[9,10] The most recently published study evaluated 61 patients with a mean follow-up of at least 12 months (range, 12 to 30 months). In this study, the cure rate was reported as 82%.[9] An earlier study of 50 patients with a 12-month mean follow-up showed a cure rate of 82% and a mean operative time of 28 minutes.[10] There were no instances of urinary retention or osteitis pubis noted. However, three patients did report transient dyspareunia, and three patients were found to have suture material in their bladder which required removal. There was no mention of preprocedure urgency or of de novo urgency or urge incontinence.

POSTOPERATIVE MANAGEMENT

All patients stay in the hospital for up to 23 hours. The vaginal packing and catheter are then removed before the patient is discharged.

COMMENT

The pubovaginal sling, when used in conjunction with preservation of the endopelvic fascia, can cure SUI. It is known that entry into the retropubic space may increase the risk of bleeding, neurovascular damage, and injury to adjacent structures.[15-18] In a study by Kohle and colleagues,[19] there was a greater incidence of recurrent cystocele formation and paravaginal defects after Raz needle suspension procedures that involved detachment of the endopelvic fascia from its insertion on the arcus tendineus.

The in situ sling, in the carefully chosen patient, is an excellent way to correct SUI. The currently available data seem to support the use of bone fixation with preservation of the endopelvic fascia without a need to enter the space of Retzius, although there is a lack of comparative studies to confirm this statement. However, it is clear that this technique can reduce morbidity and provide a more stable point of fixation for the sling. The procedure provides an appropriate alternative sling for those patients and/or physicians who reject the idea of foreign body slings through the vagina.

References

1. Pereyra A: A simplified surgical procedure for the correction of stress urinary incontinence in women. West J Surg 67:223, 1959.
2. Stamey TA: Endoscopic suspension of the vesical neck for urinary incontinence. Surg Gynecol Obstet 136:547, 1973.
3. Raz S: Modified bladder neck suspension for female stress incontinence. Urology 17:82, 1981.
4. Gittes RF, Loughlin KR: No-incision pubovaginal suspension for stress incontinence. J Urol 138:568, 1987.
5. Leach GE, Dmochowski RR, Appell RA, et al: Female stress urinary incontinence clinical guidelines panel summary report on surgical management of female stress urinary incontinence. J Urol 158:875-880, 1997.
6. Appell RA, Goldman H, Rackley RR: Efficacy and predictors of success for the in situ anterior vaginal wall sling with bone anchors. J Urol 159(Suppl):44, 1998.
7. Appell RA, Rackley RR, Dmochowski RR: Vesica percutaneous bladder neck stabilization. J Endourol 10:221-225, 1996.
8. Leach GE: Bone fixation technique for transvaginal needle suspensions. Urology 31:388-390, 1988.
9. Levin S. Bennet AE, Levin D, et al: Minimally invasive surgical treatment of female stress urinary incontinence. Int Urogynecol J 9:405-408, 1998.
10. Nativ O, Levin S, Madjar S, et al: Incisionless per vagina bone anchor cystourethropexy for the treatment of female stress incontinences: Experience with the first 50 patients. J Urol 158:1742-1744, 1997.
11. Vasavada SP, Rackley RR, Appell RA: In situ vaginal wall sling formation with preservation of the endopelvic fascia for treatment of stress urinary incontinence.. Int Urogynecol J 9:379-384, 1998.
12. Raz S, Siegel AL, Short JL, et al: Vaginal wall sling. J Urol 141:43-46, 1989.
13. Juma S, Little NA, Raz S: Vaginal wall sling: Four years later. Urology 39:424-428, 1992.
14. Kaplan SA, Santarosa RP, Te AE: Comparison of fascial and vaginal wall slings. Urology 47:885-889, 1996.
15. Choe JM, Battino BS: Antimicrobial mesh versus vaginal sling: A comparative outcome analysis. J Urol 163:1829-1834, 2000.
16. McGuire EJ, Bennett CJ, Konnak JA, et al: Experience with pubovaginal slings for urinary incontinence at the University of Michigan. J Urol 138:525-529, 1987.
17. Kreder KJ: Complications associated with female incontinence surgery. AUA Update Series 12, 1993.
18. Benson JT, McClellan E: The effect of vaginal dissection on the pudendal nerve. Obstet Gynecol 82:387-389, 1993.
19. Kohle N, Sze EH, Roat TW, Karram MM: Incidence of recurrent cystocele after colporrhaphy with and without concomitant transvaginal needle suspension. Am J Obstet Gynecol 175:1476-1480, 1996.

Chapter 34

FREE VAGINAL WALL SLING

Dmitry U. Pushkar

Pubovaginal sling procedures are the main surgical operations used to correct stress urinary incontinence (SUI). These procedures provide for a tape insertion underneath the urethra or bladder neck. The American Urological Association guidelines panel studied the long-term efficacy of all anti-incontinence procedures and found that pubovaginal slings were among the most versatile and successful.[1-14]

Until the end of the 1990s in most cases autologous tissues were used to create a tape. However, by the late 1990s specialists began to make use of synthetic materials, mainly in the form of Prolene tapes.[9,13]

This chapter covers several aspects of the free vaginal wall sling procedure. At the same time, it touches on the technical particularities of the full-thickness, nonisolated vaginal wall flap, based on the bladder neck area. This procedure was first described in 1996 by the French group from Nice.[11] The patient is placed in the lithotomy position with access to the suprapubic area, and an 18-Fr Foley catheter is inserted. After the vaginal cavity is exposed a U-shaped incision is made to create a rectangular flap based superiorly in the bladder neck (Fig. 34-1). During vaginal dissection, it is preferable to create a thin flap to preserve perivesical tissue for cystocele repair. After flap mobilization, the cystocele is repaired with a running double-layer 3-0 monofilament polyglyconate suture (Fig. 34-2). The rectangular vaginal flap is then rolled to form a tube and secured at each end with two 2-0 polypropylene sutures. Before being rolled, the vaginal flap must be de-epithelialized with a scalpel to prevent postoperative cyst formation. Then, the vaginal tube is positioned in the bladder neck and sutured to periurethral tissues or suspended subcutaneously with two 2-0 polypropylene sutures (Fig. 34-3). Cystoscopy is performed to rule out urethral or bladder perforation and confirm bladder neck suspension. Posterior colporrhaphy is performed, and a povidone-iodine–impregnated vaginal gauze is inserted; it is removed the following day. Normally, the Foley catheter is withdrawn after 48 hours.

It is still questionable whether the vaginal wall sling procedure should remain in the surgical armamentarium. We believe that this textbook would not be complete without coverage of this procedure.

The desire to make use of autologous vaginal tissue for the treatment of SUI first surfaced at the beginning of the 20th century. This was motivated by patients experiencing a combination of incontinence and cystocele, which provided for the enlargement of the vaginal wall, with subsequent preparation of a viable vaginal flap. Previously, full-size flaps had been employed, which led to a high rate of morbidity.

The application of monofilament polypropylene materials, such as Prolene sutures, allowed for further minimization of the procedures, with shorter flap creation. These sutures were used for a wide variety of suspensions. The flap itself had to meet several requirements. The primary requirement was that the flap must be long enough to support the bladder neck, and it must be viable, providing for full thickness of the vaginal wall.

It remains to be asked whether the classification of type 1, 2, or 3 SUI is still useful. Sling procedures were in the past reserved for correction of ISD. Today, it has been shown that most female patients with SUI have some kind of ISD. In our department, we have edged away from a standard classification of SUI and now pay particular attention to the anatomy of the patient. We believe that SUI associated with either cystocele, rectocele, or pelvic floor dysfunction clearly calls for a change in accepted "textbook" treatment planning.

Why do patients choose free vaginal wall sling procedures? What are the long-term functional results of these procedures? What is the purpose of the patient-doctor conversation, and

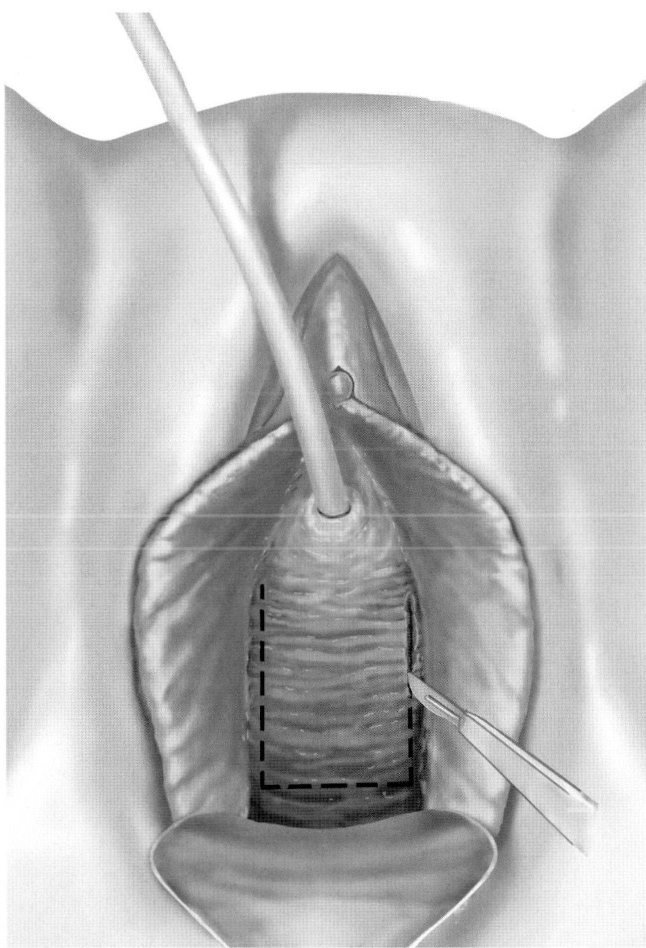

Figure 34-1 A U-shaped incision is performed to create a rectangular vaginal flap based on the bladder neck area.

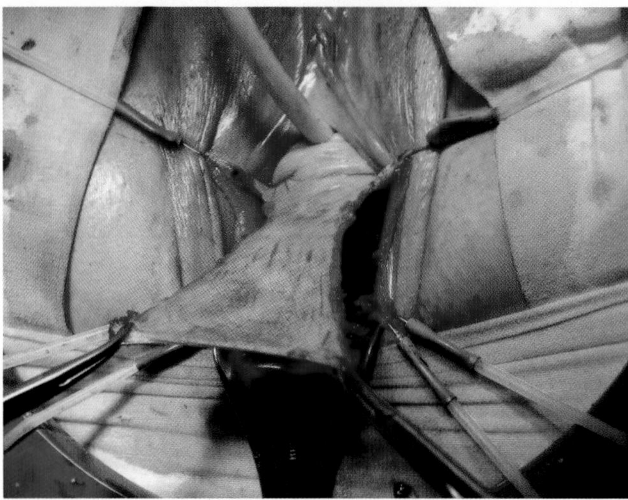

Figure 34-2 A full-thickness rectangular flap based on the bladder neck area is created from the anterior vaginal wall. This flap may be kept and used as a fixed flap based on the bladder neck suspended by two 1-0 Prolene sutures in the suprapubic area. Cystocele is repaired. This flap may also be isolated if a free vaginal wall sling by isolated flap is preferred.

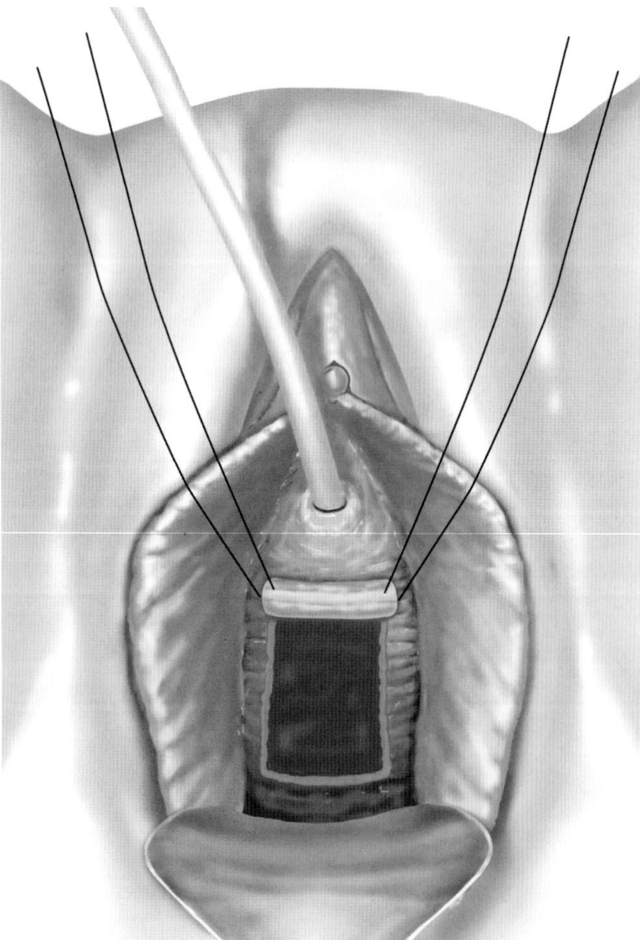

Figure 34-3 A vaginal flap is rolled to form a tube and is secured at each end with two 1-0 Prolene sutures, with subsequent passage and attachment of these sutures suprapubicly.

should we convince our patients to proceed with this type of surgery? Should the free vaginal wall procedure remain in the surgical armamentarium? Finally, should we make any comparison with synthetic tapes or other tension-free vaginal tape (TVT)-like procedures?

RATIONALE

The free vaginal wall procedure may have the following applications:

1. Mild to moderate SUI in elderly patients with cystocele
2. Patients unwilling to use any synthetic materials
3. Young patients with mild SUI, who are rarely scheduled for surgery. There is a lack of long-term follow-up of synthetic materials. These patients may develop recurrence in the distant future, which can dictate the use of synthetic materials such as TVT.
4. Patient desire to have a minimal operation with use of autologous tissue and no abdominal scar.

PREOPERATIVE CONSIDERATIONS

Preoperative considerations currently include the following requirements:

1. Mild to moderate SUI
2. Symptoms confirmed by signs is always preferable, which means demonstrable involuntary urine loss during physical examination while coughing or sneezing
3. No signs of vaginal atrophy
4. No signs of detrusor instability—cystometry must be performed if detrusor instability is suspected
5. Cystocele provides enlarged vaginal wall to create viable flap; surgeon may decide whether flap can be created from posterior part if rectocele is present
6. Urinary tract infection excluded
7. Cystoscopy, which is routinely performed in our department
8. Ultrasound examination, also a usual part of preoperative assessment
9. Informed consent and strong will of the patient to undergo surgery

SURGICAL TECHNIQUE

We believe that several flap sizes may be used. The choice depends on the surgeon's experience and preference. For example, if the surgeon has substantial experience in using full-size slings, he or she may opt for a longer vaginal wall flap. If the patient's anatomy does not allow for the creation of such a long flap, the operation may nonetheless still be performed. Our patient experience has shown an average flap size of 1.5 to 3.5 cm. An isolated vaginal flap may be formed from either the anterior or the posterior vaginal wall. Rectocele facilitates a vaginal flap formation from the posterior part of the vaginal wall (Fig. 34-4). After the flap has been prepared, the next step of the procedure is cystocele repair, using conventional techniques with several layers of absorbable sutures. Because a lack of vaginal mucosa may occur after the flap formation, care must be taken to restore the

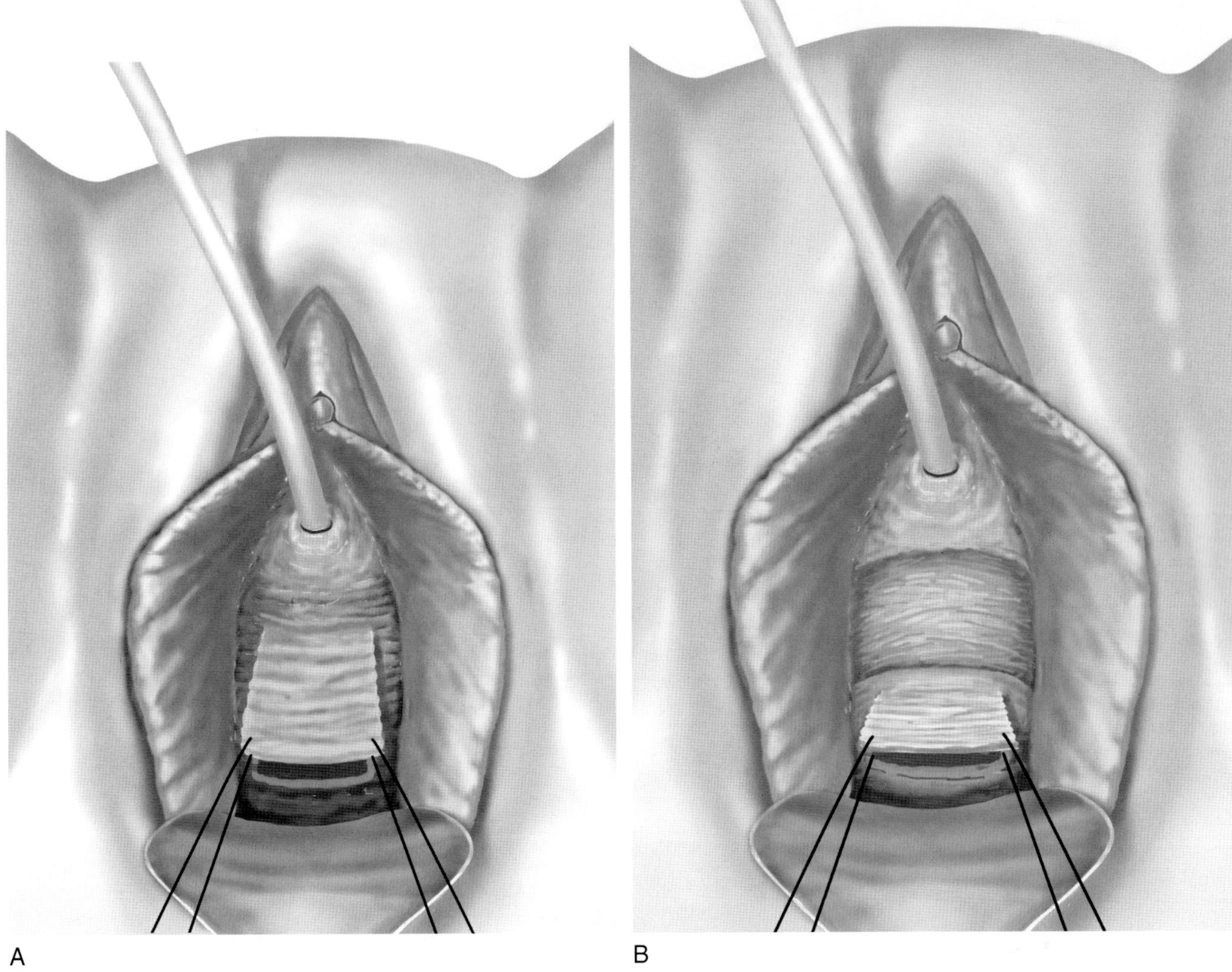

Figure 34-4 Isolated flaps may be formed from either the anterior **(A)** or the posterior **(B)** vaginal wall.

cystocele well, in order to provide a tension-free closure of the vaginal wall. Normally, we use Monocryl 3/0, providing several layers of sutures. Recently, we have tried to avoid extensive mobilization of the perivesical tissues.

On each corner of the flap, four Prolene 1-0 sutures are attached and the flap is placed in an antibiotic solution (Fig. 34-5). The flap will be positioned in such a way that the vaginal mucosa is exposed. We have now decided to lengthen the vaginal incision, in order to locate the vaginal flap around the midurethra (Fig. 34-6). This allows us to avoid the creation of perivesical tunnels. Previously, we used Pereyra ligature carriers to pass Prolene sutures from the vagina to the suprapubic area. Now, we opt for a different approach, which provides for passage of the suture from the vagina to the suprapubic area with the use of special vaginal needles, called tunnelers (Fig. 34-7).

In cases where the flap is taken from the posterior vaginal wall, rectocele repair should be performed. If there is no cystocele or rectocele, the flap should always be taken from the anterior vaginal wall and positioned in the midurethral area.

Cystoscopy must be performed on all patients to exclude bladder perforation. A 70-degree cystoscopic lens should be used. We do not inject indigo carmine intravenously. If a bladder perforation should occur, we extract the suture and insert it again in a more lateral position. In such cases, we leave a Foley catheter in place for 72 hours. Otherwise, in normal cases, the Foley catheter is removed on the morning after surgery. Vaginal closure with either running or interrupted absorbable sutures is a final step of the procedure (Fig. 34-8). Vaginal packing is routinely used after this procedure and is removed the next day.

Antibiotic therapy is administered to all patients intraoperatively and during the course of the three following days.

The average hospital stay for patients experiencing noncomplicated cases is 2.1 days. For those patients who have undergone simultaneous rectocele or cystocele repair, 4.2 days is the average stay.

RESULTS

Free vaginal wall sling procedures have been performed in our department since 1989. A total of 189 patients, with a mean age of 67.3 years (range, 31 to 87 years) have undergone free vaginal wall sling procedures. The mean operative time was 43.1 minutes. The vast majority of patients had flaps taken from the anterior

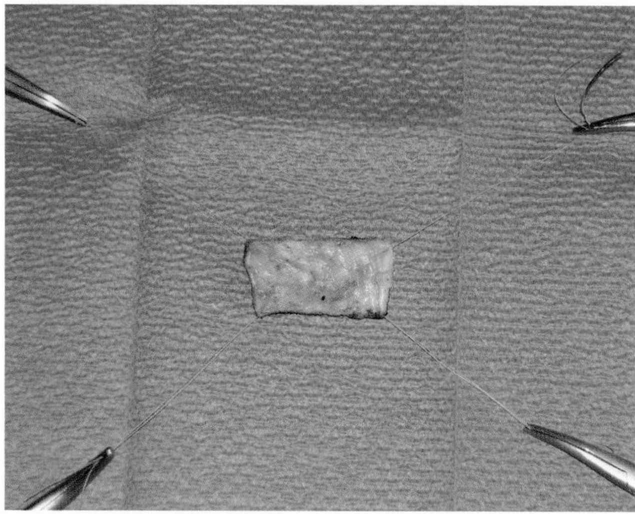

A

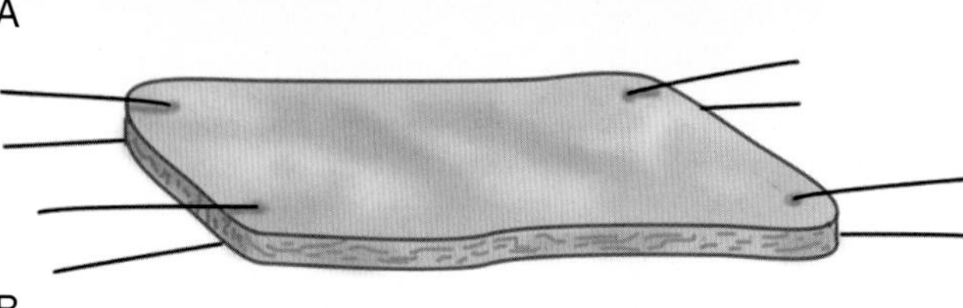

B

Figure 34-5 **A,** An isolated full-thickness vaginal wall flap is formed. **B,** The four 1-0 Prolene sutures are attached on each corner of the flap.

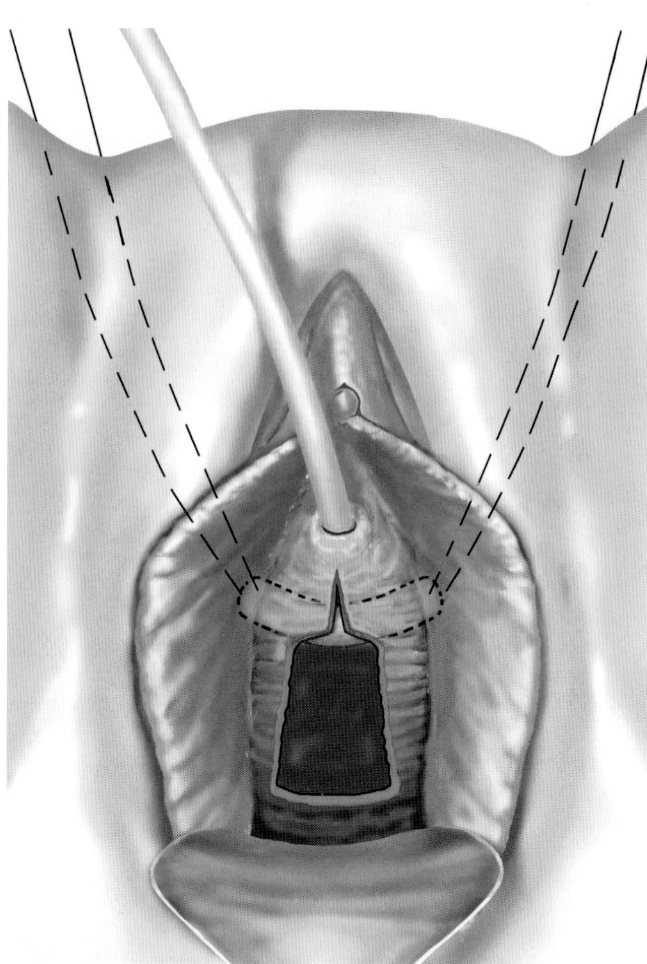

Figure 34-6 The vaginal incision is lengthened to locate the vaginal flap around the mid-urethra. A vaginal flap is secured by two 1-0 Prolene sutures with subsequent attachment of these sutures suprapubicly.

vaginal wall. We were able to conduct follow-up studies of 109 (57.7%) of these patients after a mean of 9.7 years. Other patients were unavailable for follow-up.

Eighty-six percent of the patients undergoing free vaginal wall sling procedures showed good results after a 6-month follow-up (i.e., no signs of SUI or other voiding disorders). Sixty-seven (61.5%) of the 109 patients showed good results after a mean of 9.7 years with no anatomic problems. Retrospectively, it was observed that those patients with mild to moderate SUI showed better results. There was no correlation between grade of cystocele and continence restoration. Patients applying to us during the follow-up with recurrent SUI after 1999 underwent TVT procedures. When performing TVT procedures on these patients, we did not observe any technical difficulties.

SURGICAL TIPS AND TRICKS AND POSSIBLE INTRAOPERATIVE COMPLICATIONS

A careful vaginal examination, once the surgical procedure has started and the patient is under anesthesia (we use spinal anesthesia for most patients), helps to determine the flap location and create a final surgical plan.

In most cases, we employ a hydropreparation of the vaginal wall, which facilitates flap creation.

Careful mobilization of the perivesical tissues toward the pelvic wall permits a proper repair of the cystocele and minimizes tension on the vaginal wall during vaginal closure. Usually, it should not be a problem to close the vaginal wall during the final step of the procedure if the tissues were properly mobilized.

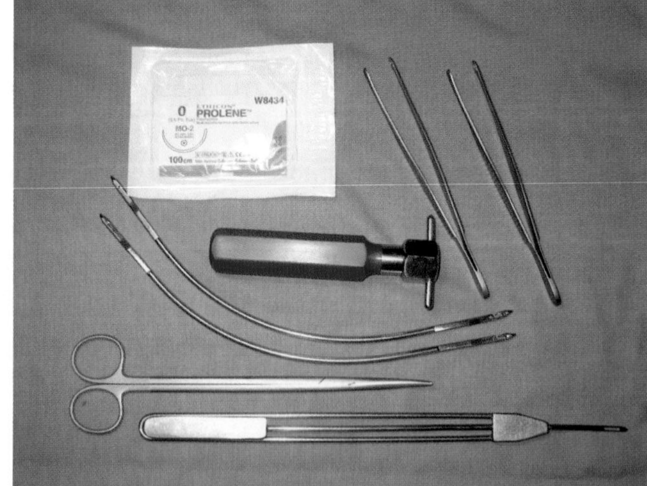

Figure 34-7 The main surgical instruments and suture material used to perform a vaginal wall sling procedure. It should be noticed that either Pereyra ligature carrier or a vaginal tunneler with handles may be used for Prolene suture passage. A Metzenbaum dissecting scissors is used to mobilize perivesical tissues and to create a periurethral space. Russ. modell forceps are helpful to facilitate tissue traction.

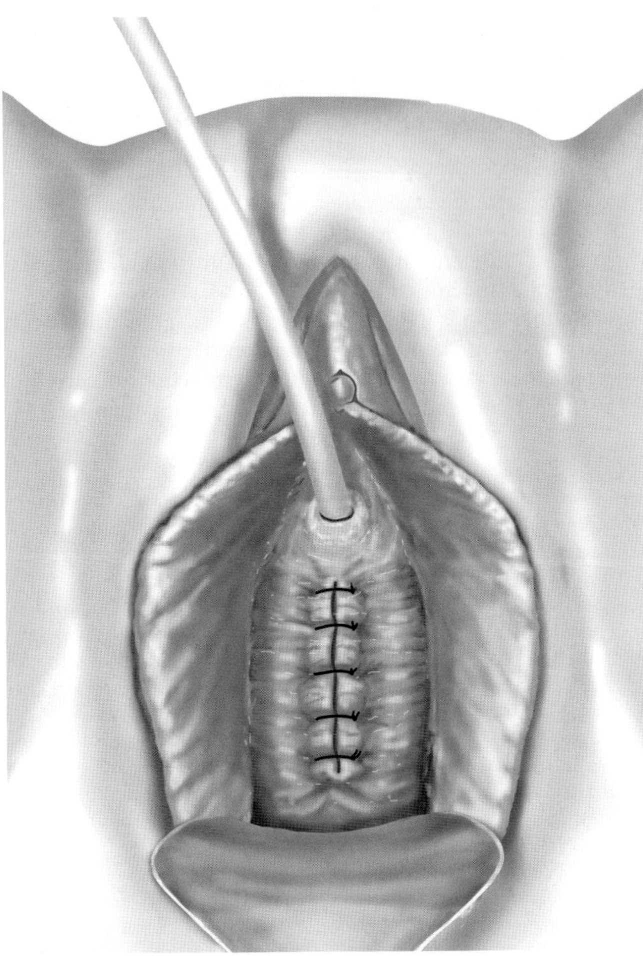

Figure 34-8 A vaginal wall closure is the final step of the procedure.

Nowadays, both a vaginal and suprapubic needle passage may be used, because several tunnelers have been introduced on the market.[13] Pereyra ligature carriers are the standard applicator used to pass sutures from the vaginal to suprapubic area, tying them over the rectus fascia. Passing needles from the vagina suprapubically can facilitate the procedure, avoiding extra mobilization of the periurethral areas and preserving the bladder neck.

Bleeding from the perivesical venous systems can be massive. It stops once the vaginal wall restoration has been completed. We usually employ mattress sutures to provide additional hemostasis.

Bladder perforation is a rare complication and should be discovered once a cystoscopy is performed. If a needle should be found penetrating inside the bladder, one must reinsert the needle, with a prolonged Foley placement for an additional 48 hours.

In rare cases, if a newly created flap appears to be nonviable, the surgeon should consider a new operative plan. In such cases, we normally use a different tissue for the flap (i.e., the patient's skin taken from the abdominal wall). Notwithstanding that this is a rare condition, the patient must be aware beforehand that this is a possible outcome of the procedure and that the treatment plan might have to be changed if the vaginal tissue is not viable enough.[11]

A vaginal hysterectomy may be easily performed, if necessary, before flap creation. In this case, the flap is created in the same fashion.

EARLY POSTOPERATIVE COMPLICATIONS (0 TO 48 HOURS)

Early postoperative complications may include inability to void, pain, SUI, and hematoma formation.

We differentiate inability to void after surgery from typical bladder outlet obstruction, which has been described after several sling procedures. We believe that anatomic changes are the main cause for bladder outlet obstruction. In our experience, 11 patients (5.8%) demonstrated an inability to void after the procedure, which was resolved after a simple catheterization.

Pain in the suprapubic or groin area is rarely noted, and it usually disappears after secondary medical treatment with nonsteroidal anti-inflammatory medications. Two patients in our series experienced severe pain, which lasted more than 3 months.

Immediate recurrence of SUI after the procedure has not been noted.

Perivesical hematoma formation is a rare complication if a Pererya ligature carrier is used. Two patients in our series developed large hematomas with associated fever, which required percutaneous drain placement. In the case of smaller hematomas, careful follow-up is important. Abdominal ultrasound postoperatively is used for the residual volume assessment, facilitating hematoma evaluation.

LONG-TERM POSTOPERATIVE COMPLICATIONS AND OPERATIVE RESULTS

Long-term follow-up data were obtained from 109 (57.7%) of 189 patients who underwent free vaginal wall sling procedures. The mean follow-up time was 9.7 years. For various reasons, the remainder of patients were not available for subsequent evaluation.

We did not observe any de novo voiding dysfunctions at 3 or 6 months after the procedure. After 6 months, de novo detrusor instability was observed in 6% of the patients, which is slightly lower than after other procedures.

We began to analyze results 6 months after completion of the individual procedures. Good results included no sign of SUI and no voiding dysfunctions. Those patients who were well acquainted with the operative procedure and involved in the decision-making process had better functional results, with faster voiding restoration. Good results were noted in 86% of the patients 6 months after the procedure.

Currently, we do not have regular annual data, and therefore we may report only that 67/109 patients (61.5%) had good results with no signs of incontinence or anatomic abnormalities.

Retrospectively, it should be noted that earlier recurrences of SUI occurred in patients with severe SUI symptoms, whereas patients with mild to moderate SUI had better results, with later or no recurrences of SUI. It should also be emphasized that no correlation between SUI recurrence and the degree of cystocele was found.

Patients with SUI recurrence who applied to us after 1999 underwent TVT procedures. We did not experience any technical difficulties doing TVT procedures on patients who had previously had vaginal wall sling operations.

CONCLUSIONS

The use of autologous tissues in SUI surgery in female patients should remain in the surgical armamentarium for specialists dealing with patients suffering from SUI. Currently, this procedure should be reserved for patients who choose autologous tissues instead of synthetics for their treatment. At the same time, cystocele provides extra tissue for the flap creation—mainly for elderly patients with mild to moderate SUI .

It should be emphasized that patients with mild to moderate SUI and cystocele showed better results, with no sign of involuntary loss of urine or new voiding dysfunctions.

The success rate of 61.5% for such a procedure, although lower than that of the TVT procedure, has a longer follow-up study period.[15] The TVT procedure can still be easily performed in case of recurrence of SUI after the vaginal wall sling.

The vaginal wall sling leads to a lower rate of complications, which in any case are easier to manage. This should be emphasized in patient-doctor consultations.

Abdominal ultrasound is an easy tool to evaluate patients postoperatively for hematoma formation. Hematomas may be managed conservatively. New voiding dysfunctions occurred in 6% of the patients and were mainly of a transitory nature.

References

1. Blaivas JC, Olsson CA: Stress incontinence: Classification and surgical approach. J Urol 139:727-731, 1988.
2. Horbach NS, Blanco JS, Ostergard DR, et al: A suburethral sling procedure with polytetrafluoroethylene for the treatment of genuine stress incontinence in patients with low urethral closure pressure. Obstet Gynecol 71:648-652, 1988.
3. Iosif CS: Sling operation for urinary incontinence. Acta Obstet Gynecol Scand 64:187-190, 1985.
4. Juma S, Little NA, Raz S: Vaginal wall sling: Four years later. Urology 39:424-428, 1992.
5. McGuire EJ, Bennett CJ, Konnak JA, et al: Experience with pubovaginal slings for urinary incontinence at the University of Michigan. J Urol 138:525-526, 1987.
6. Raz S, Siegel AL, Short JL, Snyder JA: Vaginal wall sling. J Urol 141:43-46, 1989.
7. Aldridge AH: Transplantation of fascia for relief of urinary stress incontinence. Am J Obstet Gynecol 44:398-411, 1942.
8. Blaivas JG, Jacobs BZ: Pubovaginal fascial sling for the treatment of complicated stress urinary incontinence. J Urol 145:1214-1218, 1991.
9. Morgan JE, Farrow GA, Stewart FE: Marlex sling operation for the treatment of recurrent stress urinary incontinence: A 16 year review. Am J Obstet Gynecol 151:224-226, 1985.
10. Bourcier AP, McGuire EJ, Abrams P: Pelvic Floor Disorders. Philadelphia: Elsevier Saunders, 2004, pp 414-420.
11. Benizri EJ, Volpe P, Pushkar DU, et al: A new vaginal procedure for cystocele repair and treatment of stress urinary incontinence. J Urol 156:1623-1625, 1996.
12. Staskin DR, Hadley HR, Leach GE, et al: Anatomy of vaginal surgery. Semin Urol 4:2-6, 1986.
13. Niknejad K, Plzak LS 3rd, Staskin DR, Loughlin KR: Autologous and synthetic urethral slings for female incontinence. Urol Clin North Am 29:597-611, 2002.
14. The Female Stress Urinary Incontinence Clinical Guidelines Panel: Report on the Surgical Management of the Female Stress Urinary Incontinence. Baltimore: American Urological Association, 1997.
15. Nilsson CG, Falconer C, Rezapour M: Seven-year follow-up of the tension-free vaginal tape procedures for the treatment of urinary incontinence. Obstet Gynecol 104:1259-1262, 2004.

Chapter 35

COLPOCYSTOURETHROPEXY

Emil A. Tanagho

Genuine stress urinary incontinence (SUI) is a specific entity directly related to an anatomic abnormality that results in impaired efficiency of the urethral sphincteric mechanism, allowing loss of urine with increased intra-abdominal pressure. Owing to recent advances in urodynamic studies and the appreciation of the pathophysiology of true SUI, the treatment of this problem has become better understood; consequently, the purpose of surgical repair and the means of achieving it can be clearly defined.

SURGICAL PRINCIPLES

In pure SUI, the sphincteric mechanism, with its striated somatic component and its smooth sphincteric element, is essentially normal. It is loss of the normal anatomic position or normal anatomic support, or both, that weakens the functional efficiency of this sphincteric unit. Accordingly, restoration of normal position and support of the vesicourethral segment usually reestablishes normal sphincteric function.

From this basic principle, it is clear that a suprapubic approach is both more effective than an anterior vaginal repair and longer lasting in terms of restoring the position and support of the sphincteric unit. Trying to push the urethrovesical junction into a normal retropubic position from below is obviously less sound than achieving the same result from above. The latter is the logical approach for placing the urethra and the urethrovesical segment in a secure, well-supported, normal anatomic position.

Preoperative demonstration of the presence of the anatomic abnormality is essential to the evaluation of the patient, because, in the absence of any anatomic variance, there is no reason for a surgical repair primarily intended to restore normal anatomy and support.

A lateral cystogram obtained with a radiopaque, soft red Robinson catheter permits visualization of the vesicourethral segment and its anatomic relationships. Two exposures with the patient in the absolute lateral position, first relaxed and then with maximum straining (Figs. 35-1 and 35-2), will demonstrate the extent of mobility and thus the effectiveness of the support to the vesicourethral segment. This study permits evaluation of both the normal resting position and the extent of mobility. If the resting position is abnormal (lower than normal), if the mobility of the vesicourethral segment is excessive (Fig. 35-3), or if both conditions are present, the lateral cystogram will confirm the anatomic basis for the existing and clinically established fact of SUI. It must be emphasized that this cystographic study does not permit the diagnosis of SUI but demonstrates the presence of the basic anatomic abnormality responsible for genuine SUI.

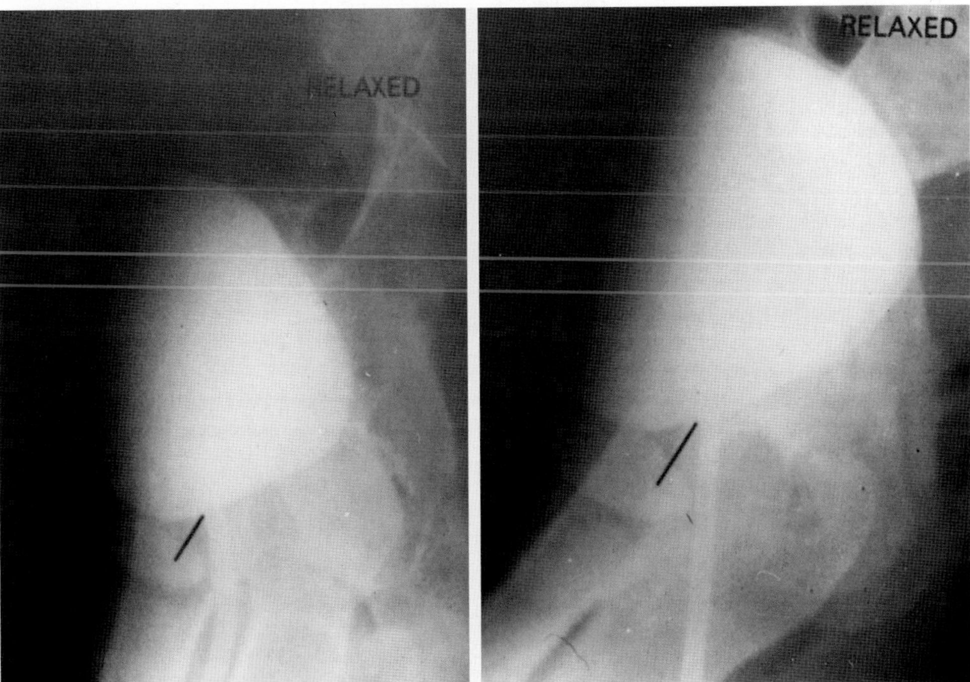

Figure 35-1 Cystogram (two views) shows the relationship between the vesicourethral segment and the pubic bone in the relaxed state. The perpendicular line from the vesicourethral point over the long axis of the pubic bone meets the pubic bone opposite its lower third.

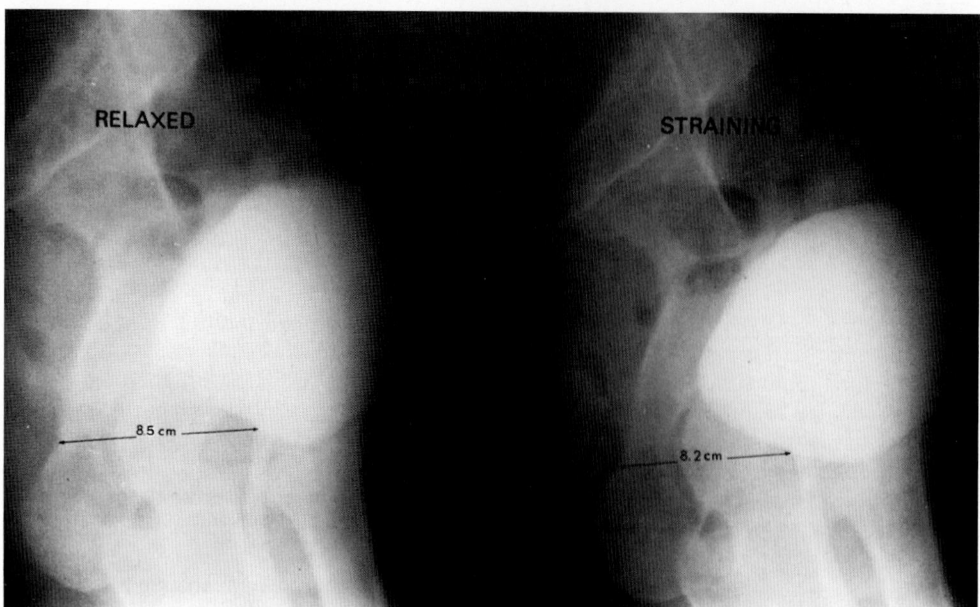

Figure 35-2 Lateral cystogram shows the patient in the relaxed state (*left*), then straining (*right*). Note the extent of mobility of the vesicourethral segment in relation to any bony point. Normally, movement is less than 1.5 cm in any direction.

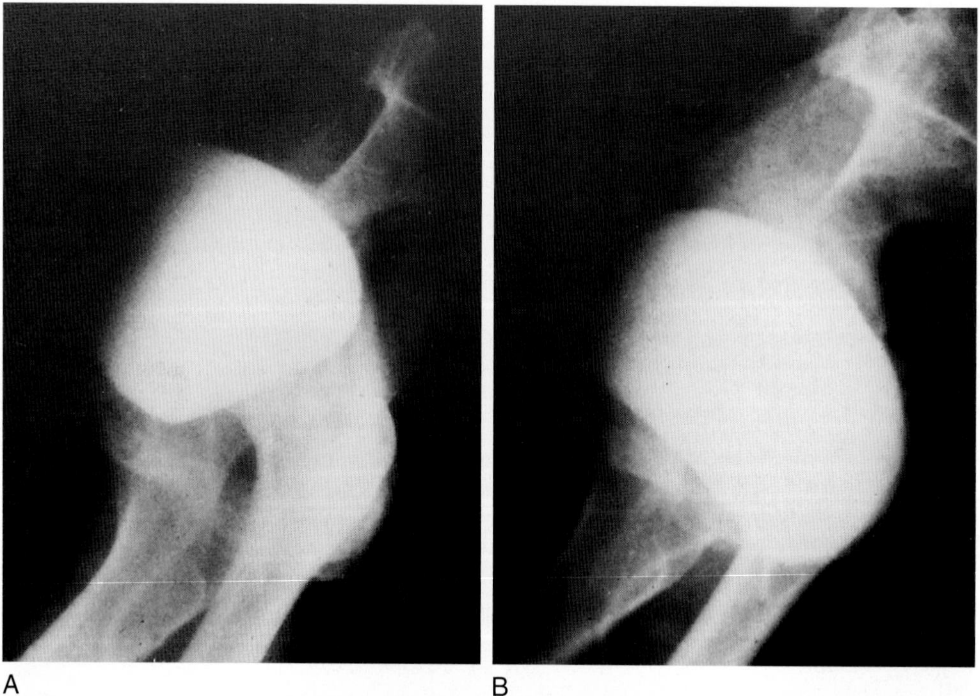

Figure 35-3 Lateral cystourethrogram of a patient with urinary stress incontinence, in the relaxed position **(A)** and with straining **(B).** Note the excessive drop of the vesicourethral segment and an increase in intra-abdominal pressure associated with straining. This is the classic anatomic abnormality of urinary stress incontinence.

Surgical repair should attempt to restore normal position and support without compression or obstruction. SUI is encountered frequently in multiparous women after middle age as a result of pelvic floor weakness, which might have begun earlier in life but has progressed and become manifest. As mentioned earlier, the intrinsic sphincteric mechanism is essentially normal. However, because of the laxity of the pelvic floor and the weakness of the normal mechanism of support to the vesicourethral segment, the latter tends to lie abnormally low and exhibits excessive mobility with increased intra-abdominal pressure (see Fig. 35-3) or with assumption of the upright position. The intrinsic sphincteric mechanism can be restored to normal function once this anatomic abnormality is corrected, without any need to plicate, constrict, or otherwise directly interfere with the sphincteric unit itself.

It is imperative to avoid the creation of any obstruction or damage to the delicate intrinsic sphincteric muscular element. If this principle is adhered to, the sphincter will regain and maintain its effectiveness, and the repair will be permanent. In my opinion, the suprapubic approach is the best way to achieve this goal.

SURGICAL TECHNIQUE

The patient is supine, with the lower limbs stretched and supported in a slightly abducted position. The footpiece of the operating table is dropped down to permit easy access to the vagina, which is properly prepared and draped into the sterile field. A 22- or 24-Fr 5-mL Foley catheter is passed and kept in the sterile field.

The retropubic space is exposed through a suprapubic transverse or midline incision. In making this incision, one should stay close to the back of the pubic bone, dropping the anterior bladder wall, the urethra (easily palpated with the Foley catheter in place), and the anterior vaginal wall downward. This step is easy in patients who have had no previous surgical intervention in this area but is otherwise extremely difficult, and it is of critical importance. In the latter situation, adhesions are usually dense, and the anterior bladder wall frequently is found displaced downward and adherent to the back of the pubic bone. Unless the anterior bladder wall is freed and pulled upward, it will not be possible to expose the urethra and the urethrovesical junction.

Virginal Cases

Once the retropubic space is entered and the urethra is dropped downward with the anterior vaginal wall, no dissection should be done in the midline over the urethra. Whatever amount of tissue is covering it should be left undisturbed. In this way, the delicate musculature of the urethra is protected from any possibility of surgical trauma. Attention should be directed to the anterior vaginal wall on each side of the urethra—again, easily identified with the catheter in it. Most of the overlying fat should be dissected and cleared away to permit future firm adherence to any tissue brought into contact with it. This area is extremely vascular because it has a rich, thin-walled venous plexus which should be avoided as much as possible. As this region is cleared, the vesicourethral junction becomes more apparent. This step can be facilitated by palpating the Foley balloon or, even better, by partially distending the bladder and defining the rounded lower margin of the anterior bladder wall as it meets the anterior vaginal wall. No dissection should be done at the vesicourethral junction itself, because at that point all the detrusor muscle fibers are moving downward to encircle the urethra, and every effort should be made to protect them from trauma. More laterally, however, the inferior margin of the bladder is identified and mobilized upward. The extent of this mobilization depends on the extent of downward displacement, and on occasion very little is needed. Placing fingers in the vagina facilitates this dissection and also is essential to determine the extent of the needed mobilization and freeing of the anterior vaginal wall.

Repeat Cases

The dissection in repeat cases is most difficult, particularly if three or four previous attempts at repair have failed. Nevertheless, it is in such circumstances that the dissection must be impeccable if good results are to be achieved. Unless the urethrovaginal wall is adequately exposed, all adhesions are severed, and the lower margin of the bladder, together with the vesicourethral junction, is permitted to slide upward, proper positioning and support will not be obtained. Utmost care must be taken not to lacerate or damage the urethral or vesical musculature. If identification of the lower margin of the bladder is difficult, one should open the bladder and, with a finger inside the cavity, define its limits for easier dissection and mobilization.

Sutures

Once mobilization is completed and judged adequate (as determined by inserting two fingers in the vagina and lifting the anterior vaginal wall upward and forward, thus revealing adequate mobility and bringing the vesicourethral segment to a normal position), it is time to place the sutures. I prefer absorbable suture material and use no. 1 Maxon or Vicryl on an atraumatic tapered needle. Positioning of sutures is a most important step in the procedure, second only to proper mobilization. The sutures should be placed as far laterally in the anterior vaginal wall as is technically possible. I apply two sutures on each side. The distal suture is placed first, opposite the mid-urethra. The proximal suture is the most essential and is placed just below the reflection of the anterior bladder wall at the level of the vesicourethral junction, yet far laterally from it (Fig. 35-4).

In placing these sutures, one should take a good bite in the vaginal wall parallel to the urethra, taking full thickness but sparing the mucosa and being guided by the vaginal finger at the appropriate selected sites. A double-bite or figure-eight suture is preferable. All four sutures are placed in the vagina and left with their needles attached before being placed anteriorly. As noted previously, this area is extremely vascular, and visible vessels should be avoided if at all possible. If excessive bleeding occurs, it can be controlled by under-running with figure-of-eight

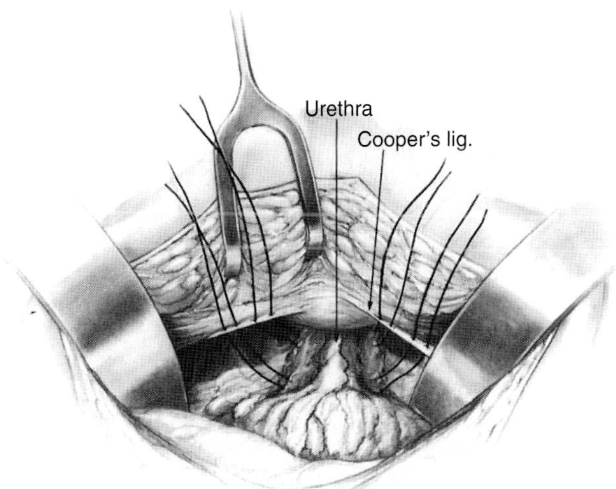

Figure 35-4 Placement of the sutures in the anterior vaginal wall. They are placed lateral to the vesicourethral segment, and there are two on each side. The lower ones are opposite the midurethral segment, and the upper ones are exactly at the level of the vesicourethral junction. Sutures are then passed through Cooper's ligament. (Adapted from Tanagho EA: Colpocystourethropexy: The way we do it. J Urol 116:751, 1976.)

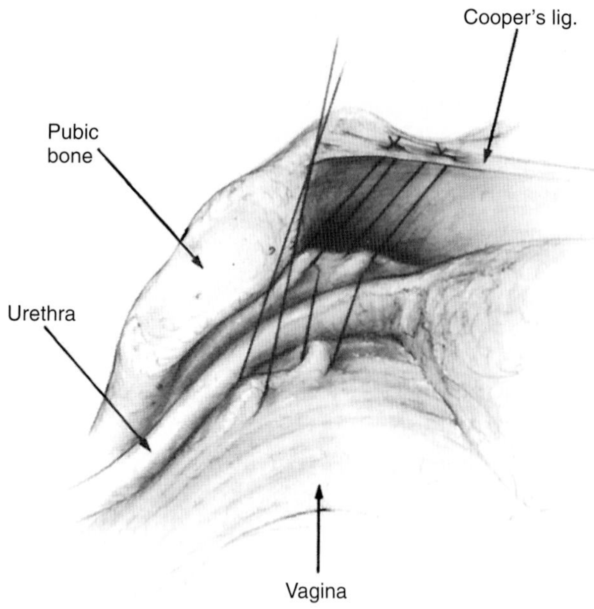

Figure 35-5 Lateral view of the sutures as placed in Figure 35-4 with one side tied. Note that the vaginal wall did not meet Cooper's ligament and that there is free suture between the two. (Adapted from Tanagho EA: Colpocystourethropexy: The way we do it. J Urol 116:751, 1976.)

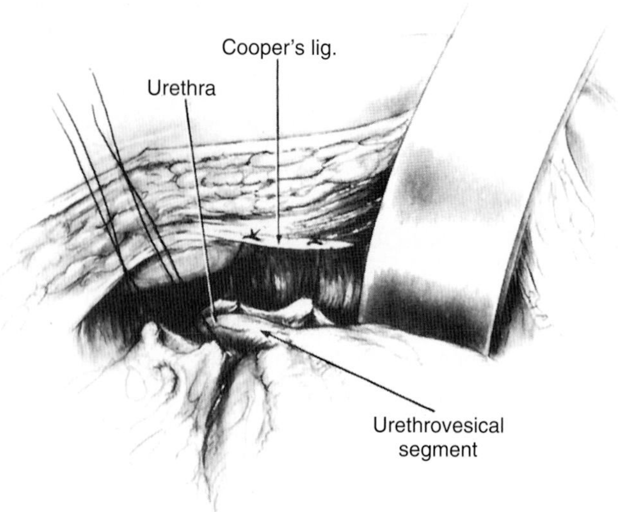

Figure 35-6 Same as Figure 35-5 except at a different projection; this view shows the vesicourethral segment well supported by the vaginal wall behind it. Note that the urethra is free in the retropubic space without being compressed against the pubic bone.

sutures. Less severe bleeding usually stops once these fixation sutures are finally tied.

The vaginal sutures are then attached to Cooper's ligament. They are not placed in the midline of the symphysis but are pulled straight upward to Cooper's ligament. With the needle that was left attached to the vaginal suture, a deep bite is taken in the ligament. A Mayo needle is threaded to the free end of the vaginal suture and passed superficially in Cooper's ligament. When this suture is tied, it is tied around the main thickness of the ligament. The distal two sutures are placed first, followed by the two proximal sutures, which are placed in the same ligament but slightly lateral (Fig. 35-5). Once all the sutures are placed, with the operator's fingers in the vagina lifting it upward and forward, the assistant ties the distal sutures and then the proximal ones. In tying the sutures, one does not have to be concerned about whether the vaginal wall site of the suture meets Cooper's ligament, and one should not overdo the tension on the vaginal wall. The suture is approximated as close as the supporting fingers in the vagina feel it to be safe. There should be no tension on the sutures beyond that governed by the fingers lifting the vaginal wall. Free suture material between the two points is of no disadvantage (Fig. 35-6). After the two sutures are tied, the vaginal fingers will appreciate immediately how much the vaginal wall is lifted upward and forward, carrying with it the vesicourethral segment. However, the latter is still free in the retropubic space. One should be able to insert two fingers easily between the pubic bone and the urethra. The urethra is in no way compressed against the bone. Its continuing fixation and support are dependent on fibrosis and scarring of opposed tissues rather than on the suture material's holding it in place. Absorbable sutures are meant to last only long enough for tissue fixation to take place.

Closed drainage of the retropubic space lateral to the sutures is established, and the wound is closed. The catheter is then changed to a 16-Fr 5-mL Foley and left indwelling for 5 days. The patient is restricted to bed for about the same period.

Voiding after removal of the catheter is usually free, without problems of urinary retention or residual urine. If for any unexpected reason the patient has to strain to void, the catheter is replaced for a few more days. This replacement is rarely necessary and has been used only in cases of atonic bladder that did not demonstrate any detrusor activity in the preoperative physiologic studies. Postoperative activity is restricted for 3 to 4 months and is then gradually built up to the normal individual level.

PRECAUTIONS

The following precautions should be kept in mind:

1. Make every effort to avoid direct dissection of the delicate urethral sphincteric muscular element throughout the entire length of the urethra as well as close to the vesicourethral junction.
2. Avoid by any means creating any compression or obstruction of the urethra while placing the sutures (Fig. 35-7).
3. Keep in mind that healing and permanent support will be achieved by the adherence and fibrosis that occurs and not by the sutures placed at the time of surgery. Accordingly, absorbable suture material is usually advised. Nonabsorbable suture, no matter how far from the bladder, not infrequently finds its way toward the lumen of the urinary tract.

The preexisting funneling of the internal meatus and vesiculation of the proximal urethral segment are a result of the downward and posterior sagging of the vesical neck as well as its poor support. This need not be corrected surgically, because the vesical neck will regain tonus and normal configuration once the normal support and position are restored. The posterior urethrovesical angle is not in itself a critical factor in maintaining continence or losing it. It is usually corrected spontaneously with the proper suspension and support of the vesicourethral segment, so no special effort to should be made to create a posterior angle. At the end of the procedure, the retropubic space should be relatively free, and there should be an adequate space for the urethra

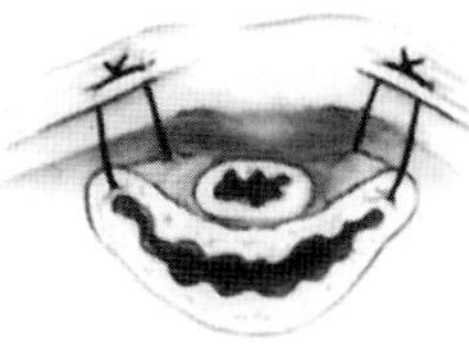

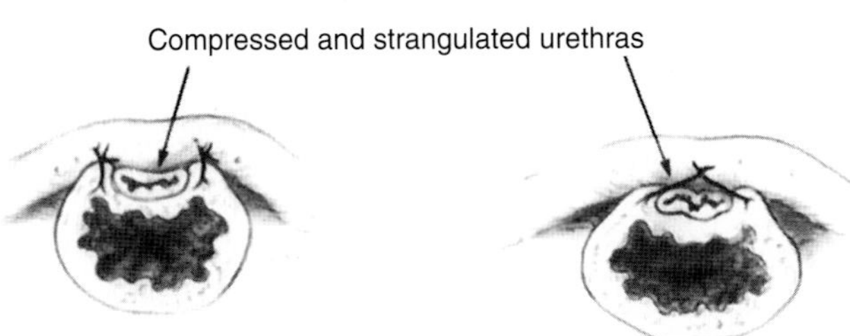

Figure 35-7 Effect of the suspension in the technique described in the text. Top drawing shows the urethra free in a widely opened retropubic space; drawings below show other techniques, in which the urethra can be compressed and strangulated between the bone and the vaginal wall. (Adapted from Tanagho EA: Colpocystourethropexy: The way we do it. J Urol 116:751, 1976.)

to move without being compressed against the pubic bone. There is no need to fix the anterior bladder wall itself; once the entire vesicourethral segment is supported in a normal position, the rest of the bladder will follow suit. Pulling the anterior bladder wall close to the bladder neck (toward the anterior abdominal wall) will probably defeat the free mobility and ability of the muscular tonus to occlude the internal meatus and keep it open.

CONCLUSIONS

The technique described here has been uniformly successful, and highly so in repeat cases, regardless of the number of previous failures, as long as the urodynamic studies showed an element of active sphincteric musculature. Physiologic studies have confirmed the fact that the only failures were those in which severe intrinsic damage had been inflicted previously on the sphincteric mechanism by surgical repairs that had traumatized and scarred the urethral musculature. The extent of the damage is usually dependent on the techniques used initially. Excessive scarring and fibrosis create a rigid drain pipe that, whatever amount of support or elevation is provided, will never function as an active sphincter unit. There is no remedy possible in these cases except creation of obstruction by compression or slings. What was learned from these cases led to adoption of the technique described, by which one can avoid any close dissection toward the vesicourethral segment, thus sparing its delicate musculature from any surgical damage. From experience, I believe that adherence to these principles will result in the highest rate of success and the longest-lasting repairs.

References

1. Balmforth J, Cardozo LD: Trends toward less invasive treatment of female stress urinary incontinence. Urology 62(4 Suppl 1):52, 2003.
2. Bergman A, Koonings PP, Ballard CA: Proposed management of low urethral pressure type of genuine stress urinary incontinence. Gynecol Obstet Invest 27:155, 1989.
3. Bidmead J, Cardozo L: Genuine stress incontinence: Colpocystourethropexy versus sling procedures. Curr Opin Obstet Gynecol 12:421, 2000.
4. Bidmead J, Cardozo L: Retropubic urethropexy (Burch colposuspension). Int Urogynecol J Pelvic Floor Dysfunct 12:262, 2001.
5. Bombieri L: Is there a role for colposuspension? Br J Obstet Gynaecol 111(Suppl 1):44, 2004.
6. Brieger G, Korda A: The effect of obesity on the outcome of successful surgery for genuine stress incontinence. Aust N Z J Obstet Gynecol 32:71, 1992.
7. Burch JC: Urethrovaginal fixation to Cooper's ligament for correction of stress incontinence, cystocele, and prolapse. Am J Obstet Gynecol 81:281, 1961.
8. Burch JC: Urethrovaginal fixation to Cooper's ligament in the treatment of cystocele and stress incontinence. Prog Gynecol 4:591, 1963.
9. Carey MP, Dwyer PL: Position and mobility of the urethrovesical junction in continent and in stress incontinent women before and after successful surgery. Aust N Z J Obstet Gynecol 31:279, 1991.
10. Demirci F, Petri E: Perioperative complications of Burch colposuspension. Int Urogynecol J Pelvic Floor Dysfunct 11:170, 2000.
11. Drouin J, Tessier J, Bertrand PE, Schick E: Burch colposuspension: Long-term results and review of published reports. Urology 54:808-814, 1999.
12. Durfee RB: The anterior vaginal suspension operation: A report of 110 cases. Am J Obstet Gynecol 92:610, 1965.
13. Eriksen BC, Hagen B, Eik-Nes SH, et al: Long-term effectiveness of the Burch colposuspension in female urinary stress incontinence. Acta Obstet Gynecol Scand 69:45, 1990.
14. Fecheco-Mena M, Cedano-Gomez R: Treatment of stress incontinence by vaginopubic urethropexy. Urology 5:536, 1975.
15. Ferriani RA, Silva de Sa MF, Dias de Moura M, et al: Ureteral blockage as a complication of Burch colposuspension: Report of 6 cases. Gynecol Obstet Invest 29:239, 1990.
16. Green TH Jr: Development of a plan for the diagnosis and treatment of urinary stress incontinence. Am J Obstet Gynecol 83:632, 1962.
17. Hilton P, Mayne CJ: The Stamey endoscopic bladder neck suspension: A clinical and urodynamic investigation, including actuarial follow-up over four years. Br J Obstet Gynecol 98:1141, 1991.
18. Hutch JA: A modification of the Marshall-Marchetti-Krantz operation. J Urol 99:607, 1968.
19. Imparato E, Aspesi G, Rovetta E, Pretsi M: Surgical management and prevention of vaginal vault prolapse. Surg Gynecol Obstet 175:233, 1992.
20. Jeffcoate TNA, Roberts H: Effects of urethrocystopexy for stress incontinence. Surg Gynecol Obstet 98:743, 1954.
21. Kelly HA: Incontinence of urine in women. Urol Cutan Rev 17:291, 1913.
22. Kiilholma P, Makinen J, Chancellor MB, et al: Modified Burch colposuspension for stress urinary incontinence in females. Surg Gynecol Obstet 176:111, 1993.
23. Korda A, Ferry J, Hunter P: Colposuspension for the treatment of female urinary incontinence. Aust N Z J Obstet Gynecol 29:146, 1989.
24. Langer R, Golan A, Arad D, et al: Effects of induced menopause on Burch colposuspension for urinary stress incontinence. J Reprod Med 37:956, 1992.

25. Langer R, Golan A, Ron-El R, et al: Colposuspension for urinary stress incontinence in premenopausal and postmenopausal women. Surg Gynecol Obstet 171:13, 1990.
26. Lapides J: Simplified operation for stress incontinence. J Urol 105:262, 1971.
27. Lapides J: Operative technique for stress urinary incontinence. Urology 3:657, 1974.
28. Lee RA, Symmonds RE: Repeat Marshall-Marchetti procedure for recurrent stress urinary incontinence. Am J Obstet Gynecol 122:219, 1975.
29. Lim PH, Brown AD, Chisholm GD: The Burch colposuspension operation for stress urinary incontinence. Singapore Med J 31:242, 1990.
30. Marchetti AA, Marshall VF, Shultis LD: Simple vesicourethral suspension: A survey. Am J Obstet Gynecol 74:57, 1957.
31. Marshall VF, Segaul RM: Experience with suprapubic vesicourethral suspension after previous failure to correct stress incontinence in women. J Urol 100:647, 1968.
32. Miklos JR, Kohli N: Laparoscopic paravaginal repair plus Burch colposuspension: Review and descriptive technique. Urology 56(6 Suppl 1):64, 2000.
33. Miller NF: The surgical treatment of urinary incontinence in the female. JAMA 98:628, 1932.
34. Moehrer B, Carey M, Wilson D: Laparoscopic colposuspension: A systematic review. Br J Obstet Gynaecol 110:230, 2003.
35. Murnaghan GF: Colposuspension in the management of stress incontinence. Br J Urol 47:236, 1975.
36. Nygaard IE, Heit M: Stress urinary incontinence. Obstet Gynecol 104:607, 2004.
37. Penttinen J, Kaar K, Kauppila A: Colposuspension and transvaginal bladder neck suspension in the treatment of stress incontinence. Gynecol Obstet Invest 28:101, 1989.
38. Pereyra AJ: A simplified surgical procedure for the correction of stress incontinence in women. West J Surg Obstet Gynecol 67:223, 1959.
39. Pereyra AJ, Lebherz TB: Combined urethrovesical suspension and vaginourethroplasty for correction of urinary stress incontinence. Obstet Gynecol 30:537, 1967.
40. Read CD: Stress incontinence of urine with special reference to failure of cure following vaginal operative procedure. Am J Obstet Gynecol 59:1260, 1950.
41. Rosenzweig BA, Bhatia NN, Nelson AL: Dynamic urethral pressure profilometry pressure transmission ratio: What do the numbers really mean? Obstet Gynecol 77:586, 1991.
42. Stamey TA: Endoscopic suspension of the vesical neck for urinary incontinence. Surg Gynecol Obstet 136:547, 1973.
43. Symmonds RE: The suprapubic approach to anterior vaginal relaxation and urinary stress incontinence. Clin Obstet Gynecol 15:1107, 1972.
44. Tanagho EA: Simplified cystography in stress urinary incontinence. Br J Urol 46:295, 1974.
45. Tanagho EA: Anatomy and physiology of the urethra. In Caldwell KPS (ed): Urinary Incontinence. New York: Grune & Stratton, 1975, p 27.
46. Tanagho EA: Genuine stress incontinence, the retropubic procedure: A physiologic approach to repair. In Ostergard DR (ed): Gynecologic Urology and Urodynamics. Baltimore: Waverly Press, 1980, p 285.
47. Tanagho EA: The effect of hysterectomy and periurethral surgery on urethrovesical junction. In Ostergard DR (ed): Gynecologic Urology and Urodynamics. Baltimore: Waverly Press, 1980, p 293.
48. Tanagho EA: Bladder neck reconstruction for total urinary incontinence: Ten years' experience. J Urol 125:321, 1981.
49. Tanagho EA: Urinary incontinence management: Neourethra repair. Dialog Pediatr Urol 4:5, 1981.
50. Tanagho EA: Colpocystourethropexy. AUA Update 12, 1993, p 27.
51. Tanagho EA: Managing urinary incontinence: The role of the gynecologist. Int Urogynecol J Pelvic Floor Dysfunct 5:1, 1994.
52. Tanagho EA: Urinary incontinence [editorial]. J Urol 152:1471, 1994.
53. Tanagho EA: Urinary stress incontinence: Surgical treatment. Int Urogynecol J Pelvic Floor Dysfunct 9:1, 1998.
54. Tanagho EA, Miller ER: Functional considerations of urethral sphincteric dynamics. J Urol 109:273, 1973.
55. Thunedborg P, Fischer-Rasmussen W, Jensen SB: Stress urinary incontinence and posterior bladder suspension defects: Results of vaginal repair versus Burch colposuspension. Acta Obstet Gynecol Scand 69:55, 1990.
56. Vierhout ME, Mulder AF: De novo detrusor instability after Burch colposuspension. Acta Obstet Gynecol Scan 71:414, 1992.
57. Wheelahan JB: Long-term results of colposuspension. Br J Urol 65:329, 1990.
58. Wiskind AK, Creighton SM, Stanton SL: The incidence of genital prolapse after the Burch colposuspension. Am J Obstet Gynecol 167:399, 1992.

Chapter 36

AUTOLOGOUS FASCIAL SLINGS

Edward J. McGuire and Linda Ng

HISTORICAL BACKGROUND

Slings are relatively old procedures; they have in use sporadically since the turn of the last century.[1] Since the 1960s, slings have been used mainly to treat recurrent stress urinary incontinence (SUI) after one or more failed operative procedures and in reconstructive surgery on the urethra.[2-4] These applications of the sling technique developed because operative failure was common for traditional SUI procedures. Anterior repairs failed at least 50% of the time, a rate which led to adoption of the retropubic suspension as the standard operation for SUI. Although retropubic operations had better outcomes than anterior repairs, they also had high late failure rates.[5]

Autologous fascial slings used to treat incontinence that persists or develops after a prior retropubic or needle suspension operative procedure have relatively good outcomes.[6] Because good results were obtained in these cases and in other complex urethral reconstructive procedures performed with autologous slings, surgeons began using slings as a primary procedure for most patients with SUI. The introduction of slings made from synthetic materials was based on the realization that a sling provided superior support for the urethra. Early experience with synthetic slings was not good, but recent changes in materials used for slings have led to vastly improved results and dramatic decreases in the complications related to synthetic materials.

Uncomplicated primary SUI associated with urethral mobility can be very successfully treated with synthetic slings.[7-9] Some authors have suggested that synthetic material slings can be used for severe intrinsic sphincter deficiency (ISD) and even for neuropathic urethral dysfunction.[10,11] On the other hand, autologous fascial slings have an excellent record in reconstructive urethral surgery and in neuropathic urethral dysfunction, in which proximal urethral failure leads to severe incontinence.[12-14] In these cases, compression of the urethra by the sling is a requirement to reestablish urethral continence function. Synthetic materials do not allow much tension to be applied, because they tend to erode into the urethra if used in that manner. There are data suggesting that patients with ISD, defined by videourodynamics, do not do as well with synthetic material slings.[15]

SPECIFIC INDICATIONS FOR AUTOLOGOUS PUBOVAGINAL SLINGS

Neuropathic Urethral Dysfunction

Neuropathic conditions are not always associated with urethral dysfunction, but specific neural conditions are associated with total absence, or loss of, proximal urethral function and severe SUI.[16-18] Prototypical proximal urethral failure occurs in myelodysplasia affecting the lumbosacral area; in sacral agenesis; after injury to the T12-L1 spinal cord segments, where the sympathetic nerve supply to the urethra originates; and after peripheral pelvic neural injury, for example that sustained during extirpative surgery on the rectum or uterus. It can also occur in patients with pelvic fracture. All of these urethral conditions are associated with a neural lesion which almost always also produces decentralization of the bladder. The bladder is thus *areflexic,* but it is not *flaccid* by any means. The decentralized bladder reacts to volume increments, although the pressure developed is controlled by the magnitude of the outlet resistance associated with residual urethral closing function. That is, in an untreated situation, the bladder gains pressure related to incremental volume until the urethra leaks. Although the bladder can develop dangerously high pressures if the distal sphincter urethral resistance is high, proximal urethral function from the bladder outlet to the distal sphincter mechanism is simply lost. There is no function, reflex or static, in the proximal urethra. The urethra is open and stays that way (Fig. 36-1). This condition is associated with very low abdominal pressure–driven leakage from the urethra (Fig. 36-2). Leakage occurs with movement, transfers, coughing and straining, and the upright position.

Patients with proximal urethral and bladder decentralization *after pelvic surgery* preserve partial reflex and full volitional function of the distal sphincter. Partial preservation of reflex activity of the distal sphincter refers to the fact that sphincteric activity

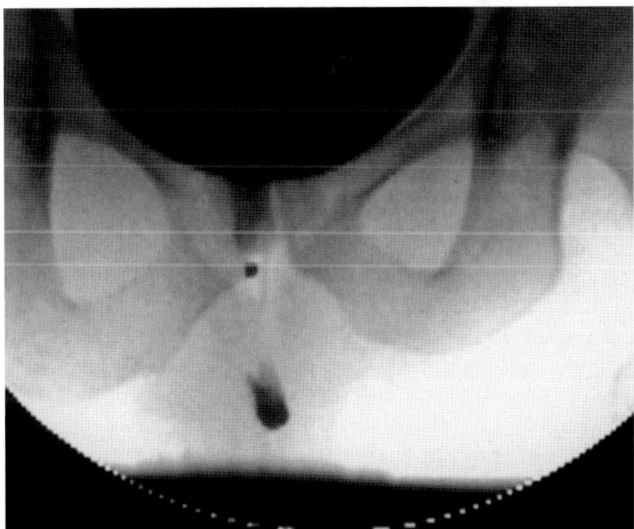

Figure 36-1 Upright cystourethrogram taken during a videourodynamics study from an 18-year-old male patient with a T12-L1 spinal cord injury. The patient has severe stress incontinence despite excellent bladder storage function and frequent intermittent catheterization. The patient is straining at the time of the exposure. Note the open proximal urethra and the leakage with stress at a total vesical pressure of 34 cm H_2O.

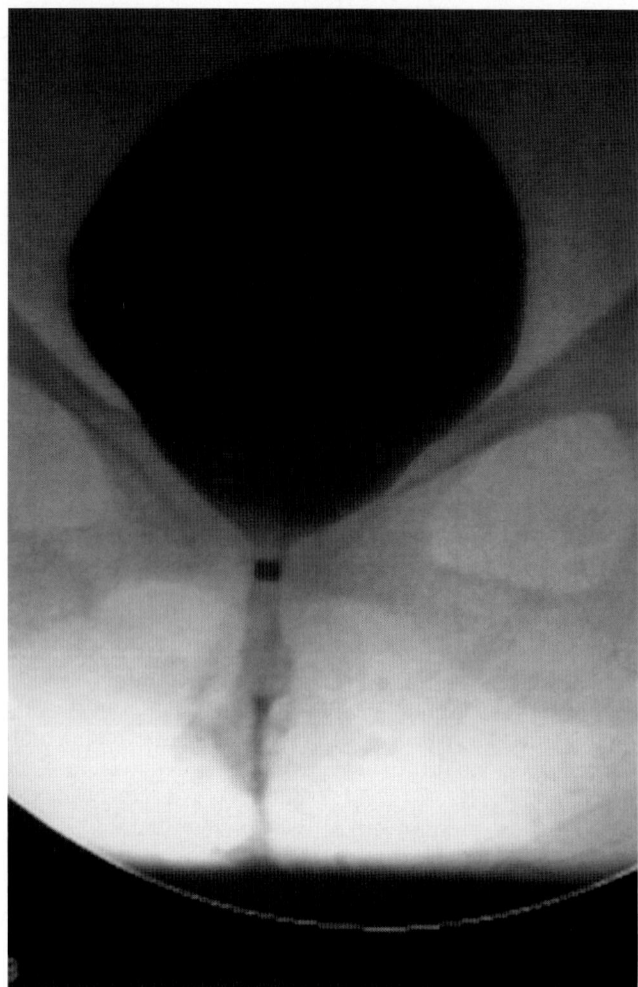

Figure 36-2 Upright cystourethrogram taken during a videourodynamics study from an 18-year-old female patient with a lumbosacral myelomeningocele. The proximal urethra is open and nonfunctional, and the Valsalva leak point pressure is 52 cm H_2O. The image was taken at the onset of leakage associated with straining.

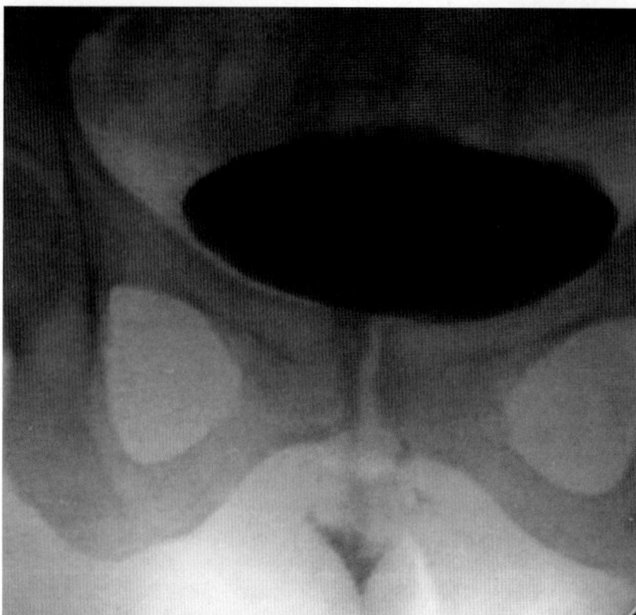

Figure 36-3 Videourodynamic study from a 34-year-old woman after a complicated urethral diverticulectomy. Leakage is gross and continuous. The urethra functions so poorly that there in no hold up of contrast in the urethra at all, only continuous leakage. There is an urethrovaginal fistula as well. The Valsalva leak point pressure in not measurable and is close to 0.

is no longer linked to detrusor behavior. There is no neural network to support that activity. Thus, relatively fixed urethral resistance is offered by the distal sphincter to detrusor pressure generated by incremental bladder volume. The latter is the result of constant urine production. Distal urethral closure does not mean that the urethra is stress competent, and severe SUI in men and women is the rule in these cases. Nevertheless, the distal sphincter closing function does require a certain detrusor pressure to induce leakage, and that can be a problem. This same situation occurs in the other causes of neuropathic urethral dysfunction, such as myelodysplasia and T12 spinal cord injury, although distal sphincter function is less well preserved in these cases.

A concrete risk of upper tract damage is related to the detrusor pressure at leakage.[18] Although any urethral resistance results in changes in detrusor storage behavior, this is dangerous if the outlet resistance approaches 40 cm H_2O. That degree of outlet resistance leads to high ambient storage pressures that overwhelm ureteral peristaltic function. One example of this are the problems that developed in children with myelodysplasia treated with a bladder neck artificial sphincter. The device effectively raised both the detrusor and abdominal leak point pressure and was associated with upper tract deterioration.[19] Similar problems were associated with the Kropp urethral reimplantation procedure in children with myelodysplasia.[20]

The problem here is to gain closure of the proximal urethra without increasing the detrusor leak point pressure. Slings—either the standard posterior vector force sling, the fascial urethral wrap, or the crossover sling—increase the Valsalva leak point pressure substantively but change the detrusor leak point pressure either very slightly or not at all.[4] Therefore, these are safe procedures.

Acquired Urethral Incompetence

Severe loss of proximal urethra function can occur after erosion of synthetic slings into the urethra, after urethral diverticulectomy, or in association with other types of urethral trauma, including surgery (Figs. 36-3 and 36-4). Acquired loss of proximal urethral function is associated with a very low abdominal leak point pressure but usually with little or no urethral mobility on an upright videourodynamic study. Erosion into the urethra after placement of synthetic slings or of donor fascia slings suspended with bone anchors can be associated with urethrovaginal fistulas that are difficult to recognize in the face of severe constant urethral urinary loss.

Very severe urethral dysfunction is also associated with chronic indwelling catheters, especially in patients with neurogenic conditions, in whom complete loss of closing function often occurs. In addition, complete or partial urethral erosion is associated with chronic catheterization (Fig. 36-5). These conditions are not effectively treated by synthetic material slings. Anterior urethral

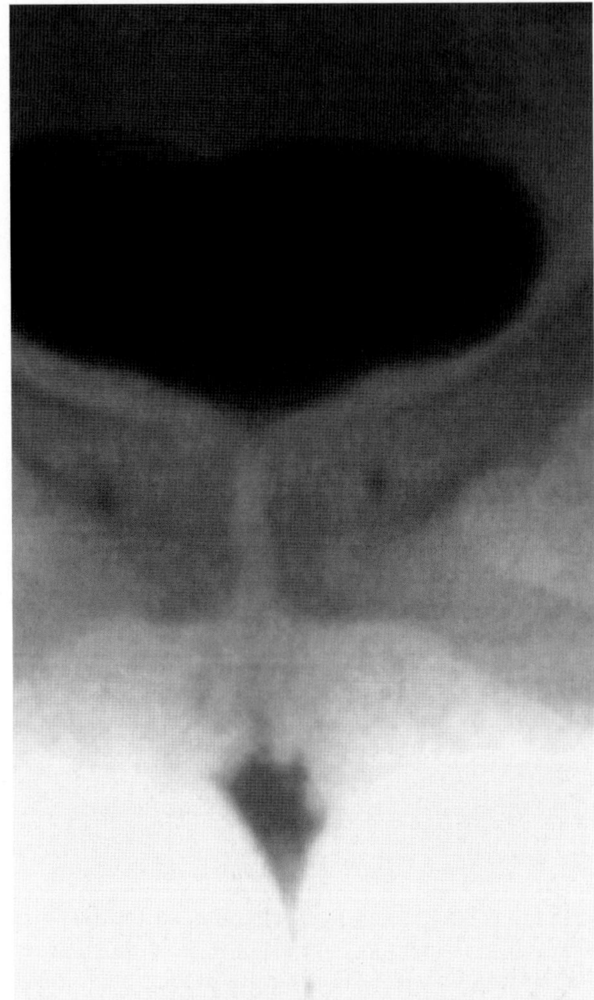

Figure 36-4 Image taken during a video study from a 42-year-old woman with severe continuous incontinence after a bone anchor cadaveric sling. There is continuous low-pressure leakage. The urethra is poorly functional, but the major problem is a high fistula involving the bladder neck and proximal urethra. The Valsalva leak point pressure cannot be accurately determined.

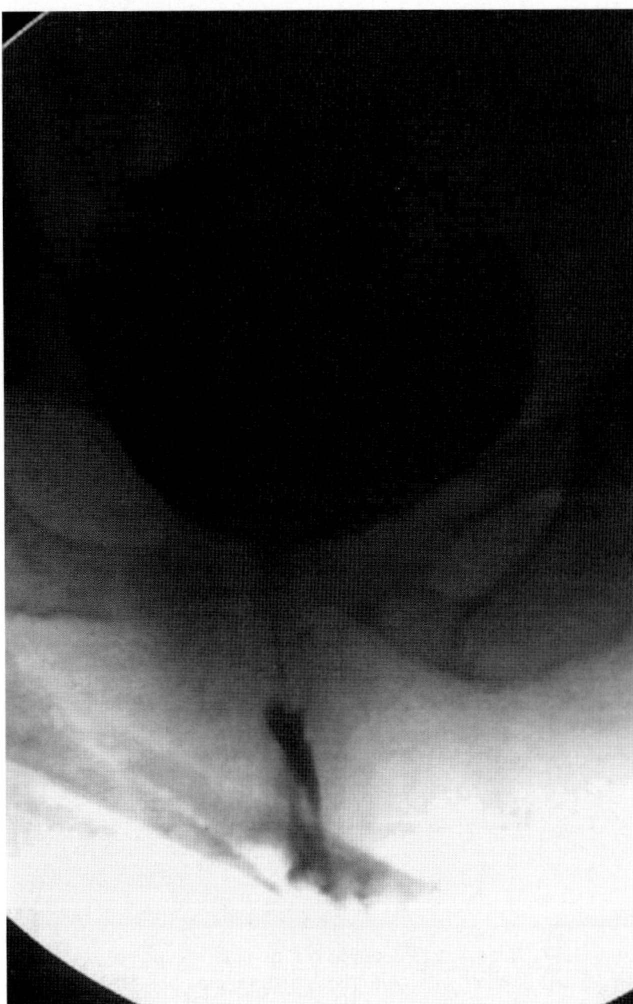

Figure 36-5 Image taken during a videourodynamics study from a 72-year-old woman with a spinal cord injury treated for incontinence with a Foley catheter. There is no urethral function at all. The Valsalva leak point pressure is essentially 0.

erosion almost always destroys the bladder neck, in which case no sling procedure will be effective (Fig. 36-6).

Radiation therapy for cervical and other uterine malignancy can be associated with the late development of loss of reflex bladder function and severe ISD. Often, bladder compliance is very poor, and the urethra is fixed and immobile but poorly functioning. If bladder dysfunction can be controlled with the combination of an anticholinergic medication, a tricyclic antidepressant, and an α-adrenergic blocking agent (for their effects on compliance) and the patient accepts intermittent catheterization, then a sling can be done to gain urethral competence. If the low-compliance bladder is not controlled before the sling procedure, the increase in urethral resistance associated with the sling leads only to more leakage at a higher detrusor pressure—not a good situation. In some cases, bladder function after prolonged catheter usage or late after radiation therapy is so poor that an augmentation cystoplasty must be done at the same time as the sling (Fig. 36-7).

Pelvic fractures can seriously disturb urethral support and function. Wide diastasis of the symphysis, associated with violent

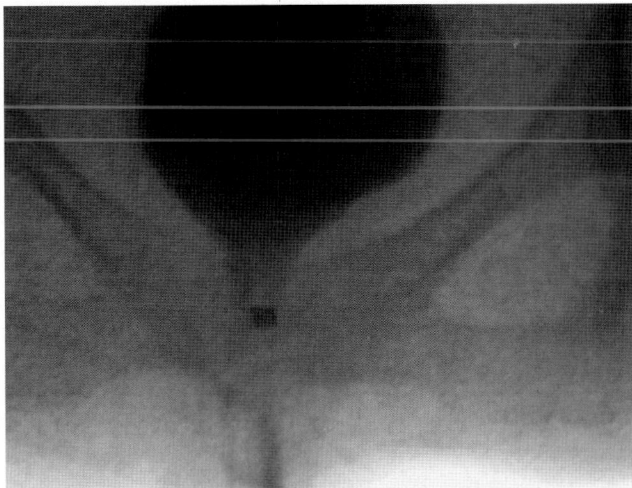

Figure 36-6 Upright video image from a 52-year-old woman with a neurogenic bladder treated for 5 years with a Foley catheter. There is no urethral function, and the posterior urethra is eroded into the vagina. The Valsalva leak point pressure is 0.

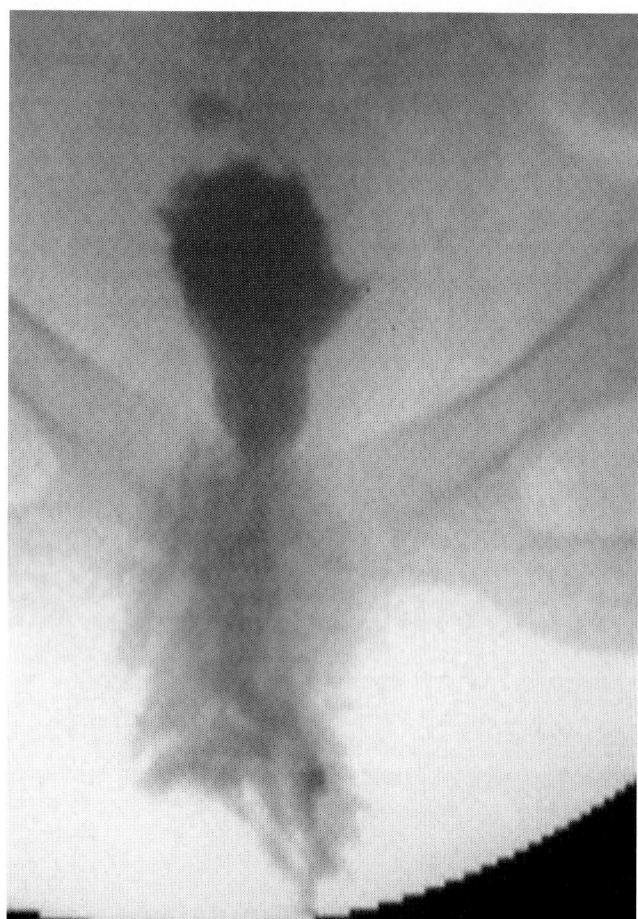

Figure 36-7 Video image taken at 50 mL bladder volume from a 73-year-old woman with continuous incontinence. She had cobalt 60 irradiation for carcinoma of the cervix in the late 1960s. There is very low bladder compliance and very gross leakage. Most of the leakage is related to the bladder dysfunction, but that was determined only after the low-compliance bladder was treated.

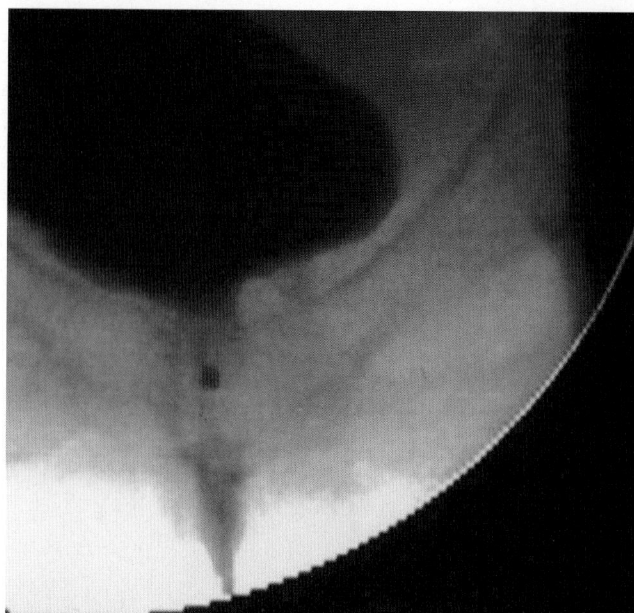

Figure 36-8 Very poor urethral function and gross leakage associated with a pelvic fracture. The urethra is not very mobile, but there is gross leakage at very low pressures.

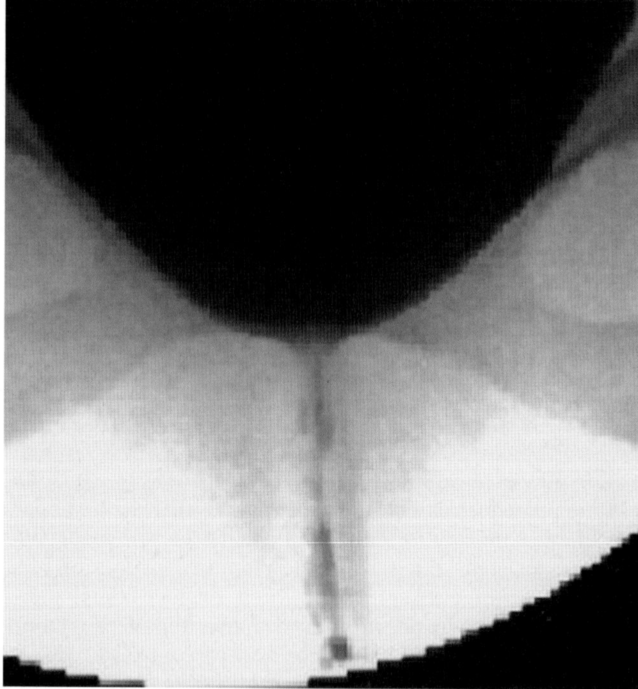

Figure 36-9 Low-pressure leakage with straining during a videourodynamics study. The Valsalva leak point pressure is 34 cm H_2O. The patient is 27 years old and developed stress incontinence after a difficult labor and delivery. The incontinence did not improve with time.

pelvic trauma, disrupts the levator muscle attachments to the arcus and bony pelvis and thus the support of the vagina, urethra, and bladder (Fig. 36-8). Very severe SUI is often present in association with a lack of urethral and bladder support. Autologous fascial slings can work here, but the challenge is to find some solid tissue on which to anchor the sling, because the lower abdominal muscle and fascia often are poorly functional, widely separated, or simply gone in the suprapubic area.

Severe SUI that develops immediately after labor and delivery is often associated with profound loss of proximal urethral function (Fig. 36-9). This condition does not resolve with time. Abdominal leak point pressures are very low, and the urethra may or may not be mobile. Crossover slings work in these cases (see later discussion), but, if the urethra is very mobile, a standard posterior vector force sling may be a better option. Crossover slings provide good compression but are less effective at urethral support than a standard sling.

Severe SUI can follow cystectomy and orthotopic neobladder construction. No urethral function, as demonstrated on a videourodynamics study, is often compounded by poor reservoir storage function in the short term. Often, the severe, constant incontinence is treated by catheter drainage which exacerbates the reservoir storage problem even after a continent urethra is reestablished with a crossover sling (Fig. 36-10).

Erosion of any kind of sling into the urethra mandates total removal. After that procedure, severe SUI is almost always present (Fig. 36-11). There may also be an urethrovaginal fistula. These

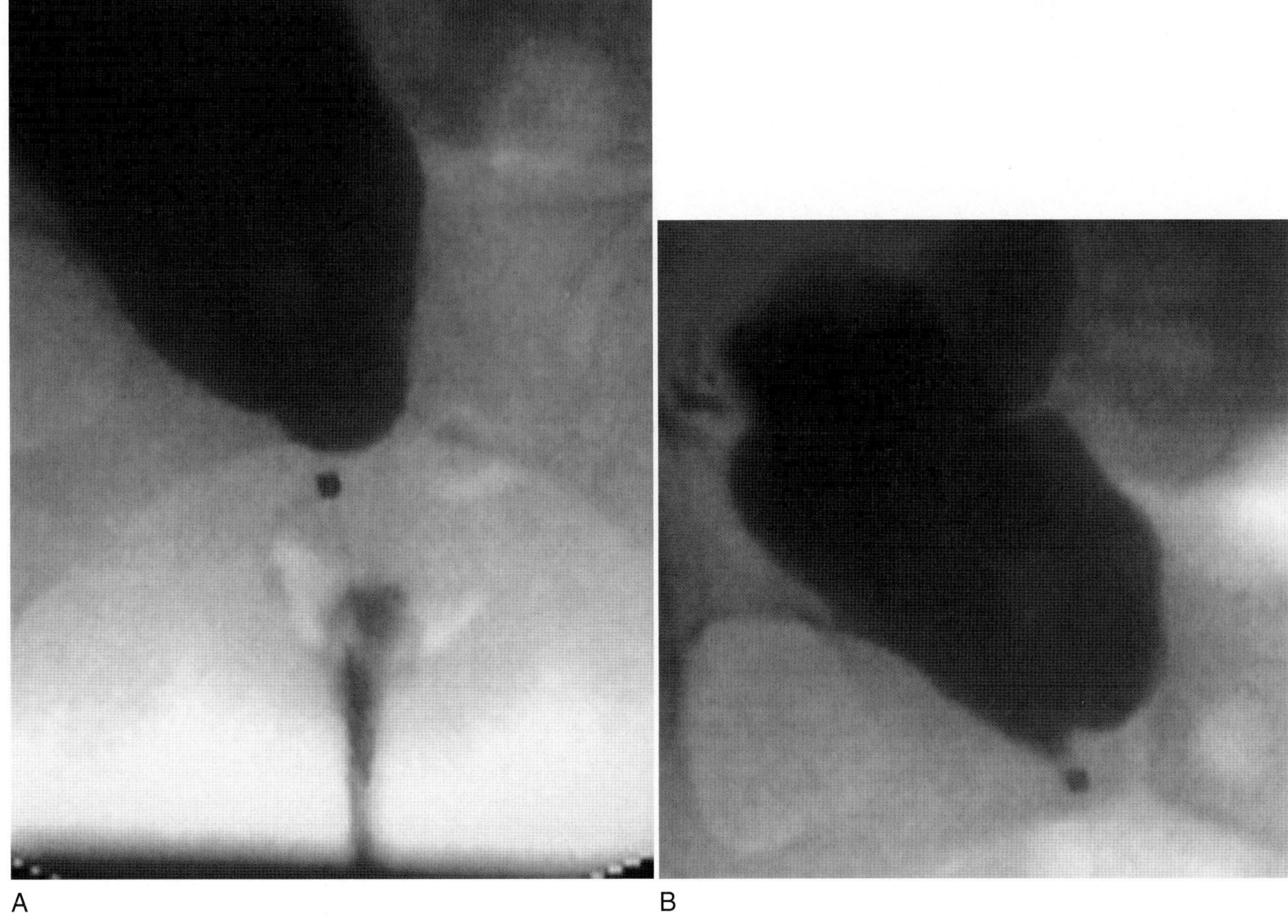

Figure 36-10 A, Upright cystogram made during a video study from a 63-year-old woman with severe incontinence after a cystectomy and neobladder construction. She had continuous incontinence despite placement of a suprapubic catheter to achieve better drainage. Reservoir storage behavior is poor, with sustained pressures in excess of 60 cm H_2O, but there is very little functional urethra, and there is severe stress incontinence as well. **B,** After removal of the suprapubic tube, medical therapy to achieve better reservoir storage function, and a sling procedure, there is no stress incontinence, and reservoir function continues to improve. The patient does intermittent catheterization and is troubled now only by nocturnal incontinence. At the time of this exposure, the total vesical pressure with straining was 124 cm H_2O.

are complex reconstructive cases, and a crossover sling, in conjunction with closure of the fistula and reinforced with a Martius flap, is required to correct the problem.

More Common Expressions of Stress Incontinence

SUI associated with little or no urethral mobility and a low Valsalva leak point pressure is an indication for a sling of some kind (Fig. 36-12). We typically use autologous fascia for this condition, but other natural materials work just as well.

Recurrent or persistent SUI after a prior retropubic operation or sling procedure, where the urethra is well supported but leaks at a low pressure, is a relative indication for an autologous fascial sling, because compression of the urethra is usually required to regain continence. It may be advantageous in those cases in which a prior sling procedure has been done to use a crossover sling. These slings provide compression with fewer tendencies to cause retention. A midline approach to the retropubic space can be used to avoid the scarring related to prior surgery lateral to the urethra. This is a different situation than that encountered after a Burch-type retropubic suspension, in which there is scarring and fixation of the bladder to the symphysis. An approach to the retropubic space lateral to each rectus muscle is the best route to avoid scarring associated with the prior procedure. Bone anchor fascial or donor dermal slings create a dense band along the posterior surface of the symphysis, usually well lateral to the midline, so that a midline approach between the rectus muscles is generally the best route.

In primary SUI conditions associated with urethral hypermobility and urethral mobility, autologous fascia can be used, but other materials work very well and may be less troublesome in terms of retention and pain. Sling patients usually are discharged on the first postoperative day, but most patients receiving synthetic slings are discharged on the day of surgery; most of the latter group will not require intermittent catheterization, whereas most autologous sling patients will.

The primary advantages of autologous fascia are nonreactivity, a lack of influence of growth on sling function when used in adolescents and children, and tissue tolerance for considerable applied tension. Spontaneous erosion of autologous fascia slings has been described but is rare.[21] In my experience, this occurs only in association with traumatic catheterization in which the

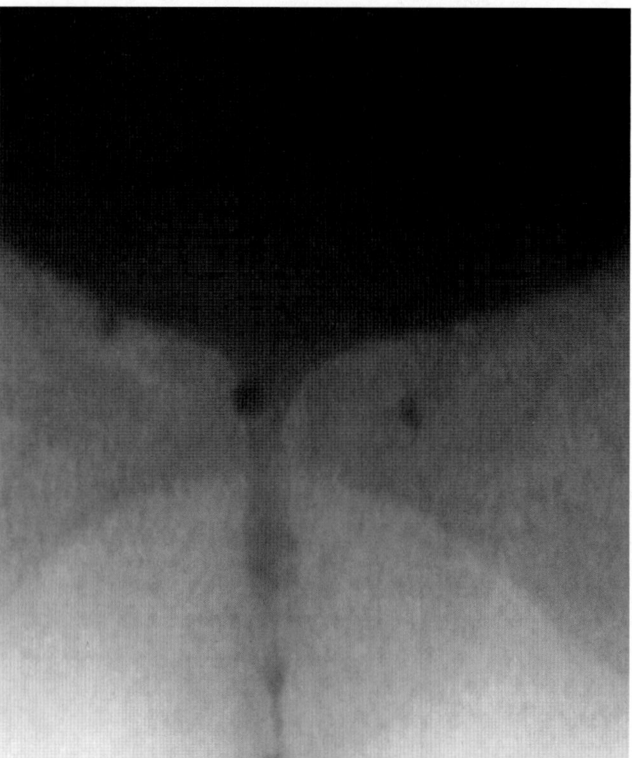

Figure 36-11 Severe stress incontinence after a prior sling-type procedure. The Valsalva leak point pressure is 54 cm H_2O. The proximal urethra is open at rest. This image was made during straining.

catheter tip actually penetrates the urethra, exposing the sling. A short period of catheter drainage assures healing without sling resection or removal.

OPERATIVE PROCEDURE

Preoperative antibiotic prophylaxis is started 1 hour before the patient enters the operating room. The nursing staff teaches the patient self-catheterization well before the procedure. The choice of anesthetic is usually left to the patient and the anesthesia staff. Either spinal or general anesthesia with an endotracheal tube or a laryngeal mask is satisfactory. The procedure takes about 35 minutes unless there are problems. Problems include obesity, prior surgery on the bladder or urethra, pelvic fracture, neobladder construction, and fistula formation, among other things.

Positioning

We use Yellowfin stirrups and place the patient in lithotomy position. For the primary part of the operation, we lower the stirrups to provide better access to the retropubic space.

Suprapubic Approach

A transverse suprapubic incision is made just above the symphysis. The dissection is carried to the rectus fascia, which is opened. The fascia is mobilized off the rectus muscles, and the sling is taken from the inferior leaf of rectus fascia (Fig. 36-13). The sling measures 6 to 9 cm long; about 1.5 cm wide in the center; and about 0.7 cm wide at either end. The sling is oversutured at each

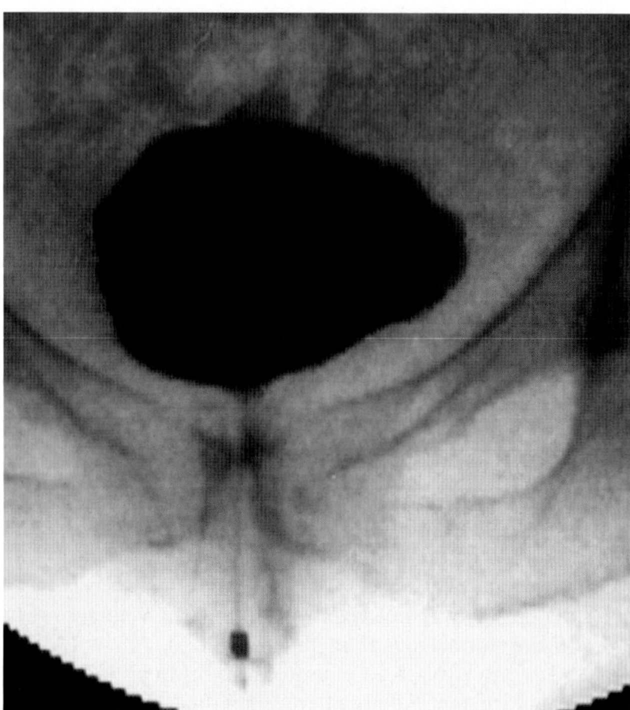

Figure 36-12 Valsalva leak point pressure from a 45-year-old woman 1 year after a cadaveric sling procedure. There is gross leakage at a vesical pressure of 13 cm H_2O during straining. There is a small urethrovaginal fistula as well.

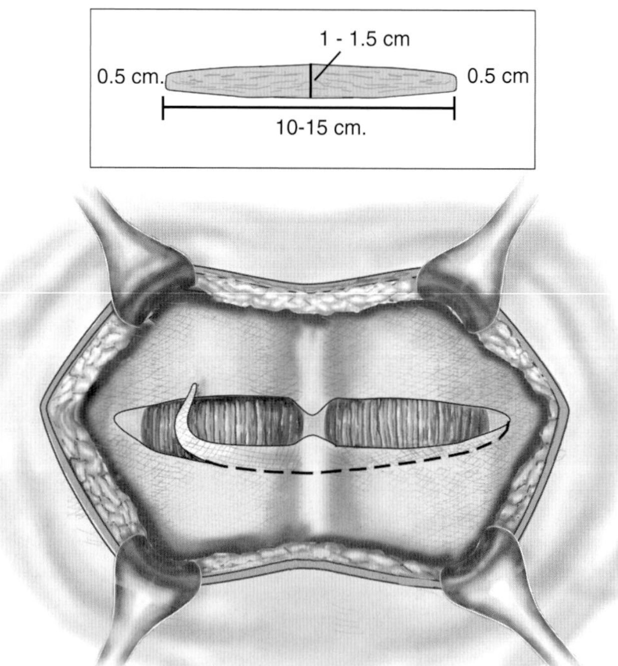

Figure 36-13 The sling is harvested from the lower leaf of the fascial incision. The fascial incision runs to the lateral border of the recti muscles. (Adapted from Hurt WG [ed]: Urogynecologic Surgery. New York: Raven Press, 1992.)

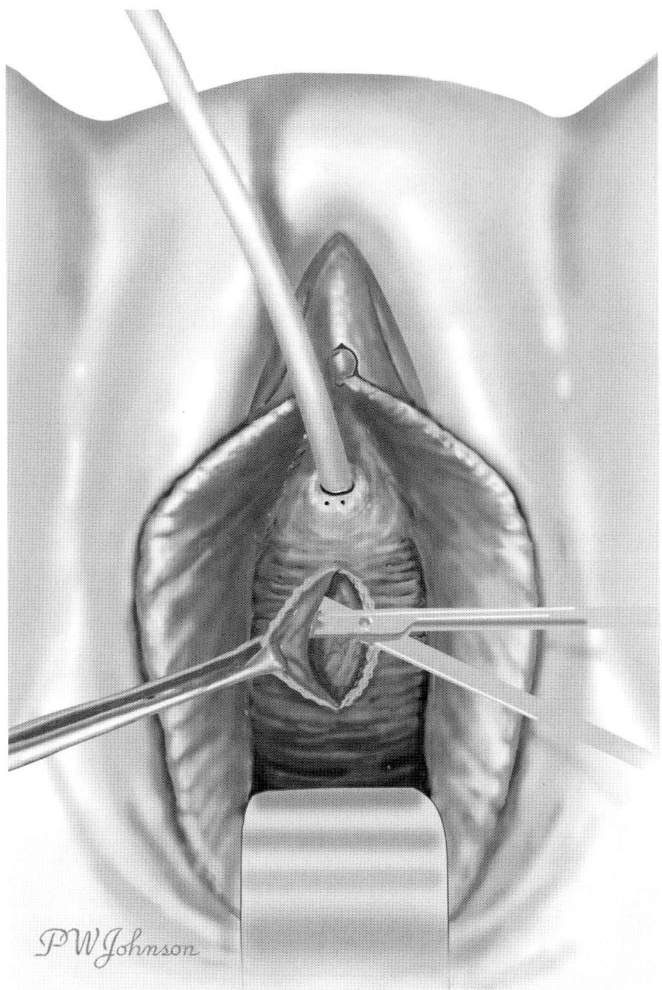

Figure 36-14 Entering the retropubic space from below. The scissors are kept flat and parallel with the perineum. (Adapted from Hurt WG [ed]: Urogynecologic Surgery. New York: Raven Press, 1992.)

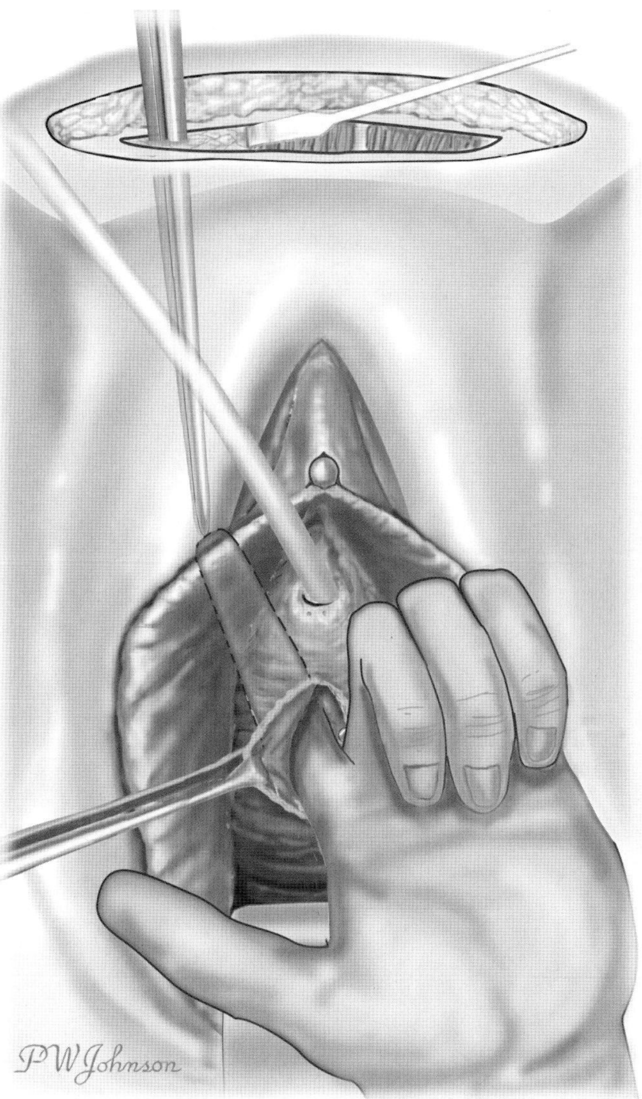

Figure 36-15 Passing the clamp down the tunnel. (Adapted from Hurt WG [ed]: Urogynecologic Surgery. New York: Raven Press, 1992.)

end with 1-0 polyglactin suture material. Several bites are taken, and the sutures are tied down, but the ends are left full length. The sling is placed in saline solution.

Depending on the circumstances, one of two approaches to the retropubic space is used. If there has been prior surgery in the midline area of the retropubic space (e.g., a Burch urethropexy, one of the needle suspensions), a lateral approach is used. Just lateral to the insertion of the rectus muscle on the symphysis, the transverses abdominis fascia is opened sharply, and blunt, gentle, finger dissection used to develop the retropubic space down to the endopelvic fascia on either side of the urethra. This can be difficult but usually is not. If our procedure follows a synthetic sling, a cadaveric fascial sling, or other type of sling procedure in which retropubic bone anchors have been used, an approach between the rectus muscles is safer and stays away from the scarring and other problems related to the prior operations. The rectus muscles are gently separated, and the bladder is pushed gently posteriorly off the symphysis right down to the urethra.

At this point, the abdominal wound is covered, the legs are flexed more at the hip, and a vaginal retractor is placed. A 16-Fr Foley catheter is used to aid the dissection and keep the bladder empty. An inverted U-shaped vaginal incision is made, and the vagina is carefully dissected off the periurethral fascia. The periurethral fascia should not be entered, because doing so causes brisk bleeding. The dissection is continued until the upper two thirds of the urethra is visible. Starting in the superior corner of the U incision, an entry plane is made with dissecting scissors lateral to the urethra into the retropubic space (Fig. 36-14). This requires only very gentle dissection. The entry point through the tissue lateral to the urethra into the free retropubic space is kept small. Under bimanual control, an instrument (a Crawford clamp, a Bard Ligature Carrier, or the like) is passed from above down into the vagina (Fig. 36-15). It is most important to keep the instrument tip on the symphysis during passage.

The sling sutures are then grasped and passed up into the abdomen (Fig. 36-16). After the tension of the sling is checked, the sling sutures are passed through the lower fascial leaf and tied (Fig. 36-17). If passage from above is difficult or the operator senses that the bladder is in the path of the instrument, then passage from the vagina upward into the suprapubic incision is safer. Under vision, the instrument is placed in the dissection

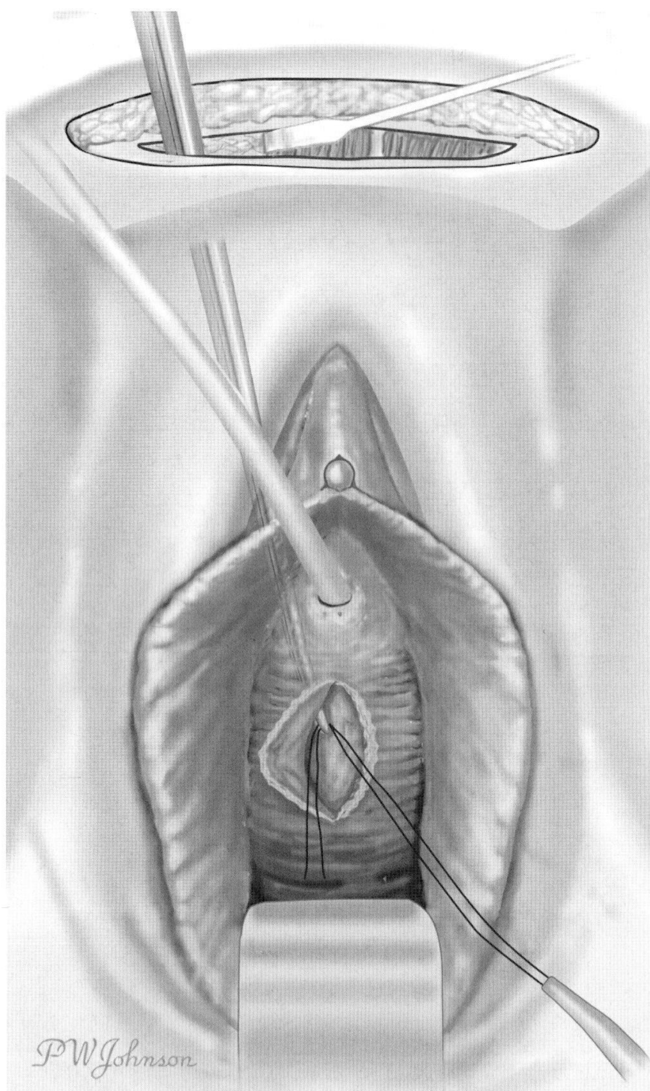

Figure 36-16 Grasping the sling sutures before passing them up into the abdomen. (Adapted from Hurt WG [ed]: Urogynecologic Surgery. New York: Raven Press, 1992.)

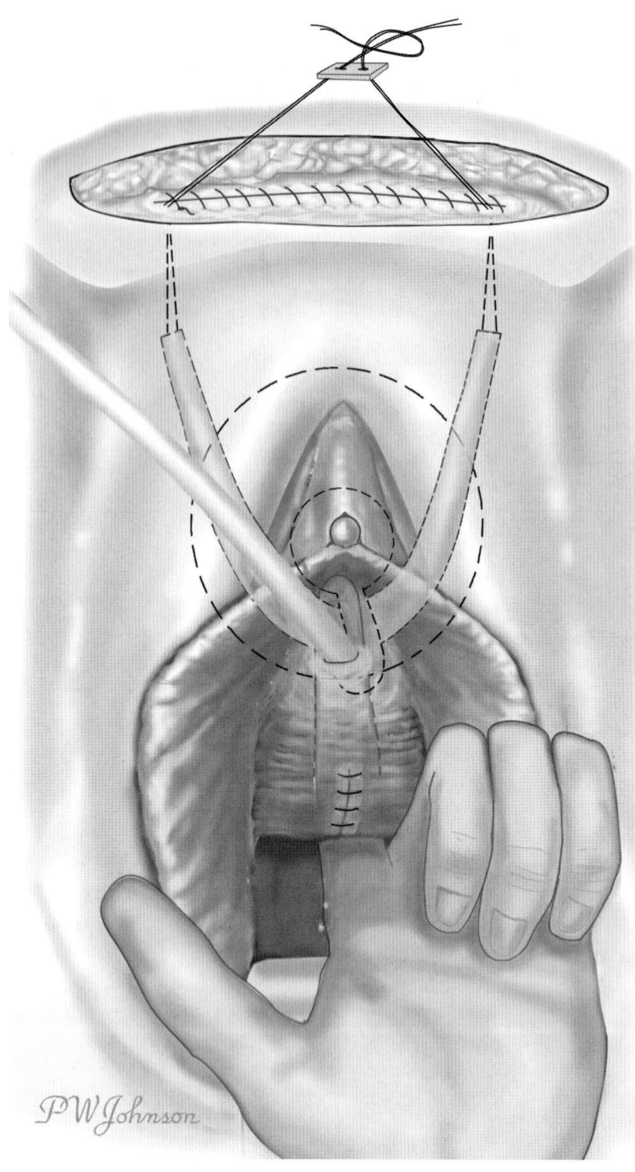

Figure 36-17 Checking the tension of the sling. The sling sutures are passed through the lower fascial leaf and tied. The fascial incision should be closed before the knot is tied. (Adapted from Hurt WG [ed]: Urogynecologic Surgery. New York: Raven Press, 1992.)

plane lateral to the urethra and advanced to the endopelvic fascia and held there. The vaginal retractor must be removed at this point, so that the proper angle of the instrument can be achieved. The instrument should be in a periosteal plane on the posterior surface of the symphysis at all times. The angle upward is steep to achieve this plane, and the vaginal retractor is always in the way. The technique is a little cumbersome, in that the sling has to be pulled down from above after the first passage and then loaded on the instrument for transfer to the contralateral side, but in cases where there is no free retropubic space, it is safe. We use this technique, for example, when doing slings in women with incontinence related to urethral dysfunction after cystectomy and neobladder construction in whom there is no free retropubic space at all in any plane lateral or medial.

References

1. Goebell R: Zur Operativen der Angeborenen Incontenencia Vesicae. Atschr Gynak Urol 2:87, 1910.
2. Deval B, El Houari Y, Rafii A: Pubovaginal and suburethral slings: A review. J Gynecol Obstet Biol Reproduct 31:131, 2002.
3. McGuire E, Lytton B: Pubovaginal sling procedure for stress incontinence: 1978. J Urol 167:1120, 2002.
4. Morgan TO, Westney OL, McGuire E: Pubovaginal sling: 4 Year outcome analysis and quality of life assessment. J Urol 163:1845, 2000.
5. Cugudda A, Jerome C, Crivellaro S, et al: Long term results of Burch culposuspension and anterior culpoperinealorraphy in the treatment of stress urinary incontinence and cystocele. Ann Urol 36:76, 2002.

6. Zaragoza MR: Expanded indications for the pubovaginal sling: Treatment of type 2 or 3 stress urinary incontinence. J Urol 156:1620, 1996.
7. Gunnesmann A, Heleis W, Pohl J, et al: The transobturator tape (TOT): A minimally invasive procedure for the treatment of female stress incontinence. Urology 43:1106, 2004.
8. Allahdin S, McKinley CA, Mahmood JA: Tension free vaginal tape: A procedure for all ages. Acta Obstet Gynecol Scand 83:937, 2004.
9. Rodriguez LV, Raz S: Prospective analysis of patients treated with distal urethral polypropylene sling for symptoms of stress urinary incontinence: Surgical outcome and satisfaction by patient driven questionnaire. J Urol 170:857, 2003.
10. Liapas A, Blkas P, Salamalekis E, et al: Tension free vaginal tape in woman with low urethral closing pressure. Eur J Obstet Gynecol Reproduct Biol 116:67, 2004.
11. Hamid R, Khastgir J, Arya, M, et al: Experience of tension free vaginal tape for the treatment of stress incontinence in females with neuropathic bladder. Spinal Cord 41:118, 2003.
12. Flisser AJ, Blaivas JG: Outcome of urethral reconstruction surgery in a series of 74 women. J Urol 169:2248, 2003.
13. Sweirzewski JS 3d, McGuire EJ: Pubovaginal sling for treatment of female stress incontinence complicated by urethral diverticulum. J Urol 149:1012, 1993.
14. Leng WW, McGuire EJ: Reconstructive surgery for urinary incontinence. Urol Clin North Am 26:61, 1999.
15. Paick JS, Ku JH, Shin JW, et al: Tension free vaginal tape procedure for urinary incontinence associated with a low Valsalva leak point pressure. J Urol 172:1370, 2004.
16. McGuire EJ: Urodynamic evaluation after abdominal perineal resection and lumbar intervertebral disc herniation. Urology 16:63, 1975.
17. McGuire EJ, Woodside JR, Bordon TA, et al: Prognostic value of urodynamic testing in myelodysplastic patients. J Urol 166:1372, 2001.
18. Flood HD, Malhotra SJ, O'Connell HE, et al: Long term results and complications using augmentation cystoplasty in reconstructive urology. Neurourol Urodyn 14:297, 1995.
19. Belman AB, Kaplan GW: Experience with the Kropp anti-incontinence procedure. J Urol 141:1160, 1989.
20. Murrary KH, Nurse DE, Mundy AR: Detrusor behavior following implantation of the Brantley Scott artificial urinary sphincter for neuropathic incontinence. Br J Urol 61:122, 1988.
21. Austin PF, Westney OL, Leng WW, et al: Advantages of rectus fascial slings for stress incontinence in children with neuropathic bladders. J Urol 165:2369, 2001.

Chapter 37

USE OF CADAVERIC FASCIA FOR PUBOVAGINAL SLINGS

Neil D. Sherman and George D. Webster

The pubovaginal sling (PVS) is a popular and successful treatment for female stress urinary incontinence whether due to urethral hypermobility or intrinsic sphincter deficiency. There are many variations for this procedure, and techniques have changed since it was first introduced in 1907[1] and then later resurrected by McGuire and Lytton.[2] Over the last two decades, there have been many modifications in technique, and even the supposed underlying principle of function has changed. Historically, the mechanism by which the PVS was thought to work was to provide support and prevent urethral descent during increases in intra-abdominal pressure and to provide a backstop against which urethral compression would occur. The "new era" slings, positioned at the mid-urethra, are suggested to function by providing a point of support about which distortional "obstruction" occurs during stress.

Other variables aside, the debate about the most appropriate material for sling construction remains heated. There are proponents for each of the various alternatives, which include autologous, allograft, xenograft, and synthetic materials. Although current literature emphasizes the minimally invasive approach using synthetic materials, it is important that surgeons performing this procedure be versed in other options, because the individual patient may have an indication or contraindication for use of any one of these materials.

The ideal graft material would be durable, inexpensive, and readily available; could be obtained without the need for harvesting with its associated morbidity; and would not be susceptible to infection, immune reaction/rejection, or erosion. Unfortunately, no material meets all of these criteria. Historically, the autologous PVS was fashioned from the fascia lata or, less commonly, from the abdominal wall fascia, and it is with these that other nonautologous alternatives should be compared.

This chapter concentrates on the use of one of these alternatives, the human cadaveric (allograft) fascia.

PATIENT SELECTION

The specific criteria for those patients who are candidates for PVS placement are well described elsewhere in the text. Essentially, all patients undergo a thorough urogynecologic history and physical examination before any form of surgical intervention. We require a positive stress test during physical examination or demonstration of stress incontinence during urodynamic study, in addition to the patient's history, before acknowledging the existence of stress urinary incontinence. We also use a 3-day bladder diary, a 24-hour pad weight study, and videourodynamic evaluation before proceeding with surgery. If pelvic organ prolapse is present, we routinely repair it simultaneously.

GRAFT SELECTION

Of the various factors that may influence the selection of graft material it is probably true to say that the major influence comes from physician philosophy and patient preference, each of which may be uninformed.

Cadaveric Fascia

The successful use of cadaveric fascia has been described in the orthopedic and ophthalmologic literature for many years,[3,4] and the use of allograft fascia for PVS surgery was first reported in 1994.[5] Currently in the United States, more than 90,000 soft tissue allografts are used annually.[6] These tissues are harvested, processed, preserved, and distributed by certified tissue banks that comply with the policies of the American Association of Tissue Banks.

The benefits of allograft fascia over autologous fascia include shorter operative time and hospital stay, lower morbidity, and less postoperative pain.[7-10] Potentially, the cadaveric fascia might also be superior to the patient's own fascia, because the latter may be collagen deficient, which may be a cause for the original support deficiency. It has been reported that the theoretical mechanism of action of the allograft fascia is to serve as a scaffold for the in-growth of host tissues, ultimately leading to replacement of the allograft collagen with host collagen.[11] However, in many cases in our experience with exploration years after the original surgery, these grafts usually have maintained their integrity and show little evidence of "incorporation" by the host.

PROCESSING OF FASCIA

The preparation of cadaveric fascia is a multistep process. It begins with the medical and social screening of a potential donor, using information provided by the potential donor's family and physician. Next comes testing of the potential donor's blood with tests approved by the U.S. Food and Drug Administration (FDA) to rule out AIDS, hepatitis B and C, human immunodeficiency virus (HIV) types 1 and 2, and syphilis.[12]

After completion of the screening step, the fascia is harvested with aseptic technique and processed to remove all cells and DNA, thus further decreasing the risk of disease transmission while maintaining the native collagen/protein framework. Ideally, the fascia should be harvested from within 2 cm of the iliotibial band, because only this location has the integrity for graft strength and durability. Processing and decellularization techniques vary, but all maintain a common theme that requires incubation in

70% isopropyl alcohol or other bactericidal and antiviral solutions to remove any viruses.

The tissue is then dehydrated via deep-freezing (lyophilization) or with organic solvents. The fascia may then undergo gamma irradiation. Radiation dosage is not standardized, and it is suggested that doses greater than 25,000 Gy (2.5 Mrads) may increase tissue weakening.[13]

Despite these preparation techniques, intact genetic material has still been found in final allografts.[14,15] Whether this isolated DNA has the ability to replicate or to transmit infectious material remains to be seen. Explanations for failure of disease transmission include an unclear mode of pathogen transmission, an unidentified pathogen, and a window of time before a donor seroconverts with positive antibody (e.g., HIV testing).[14] Of course, the donors may simply have been free of transmissible disease.

Fitzgerald and colleagues showed that allografts retain donor antigens after processing but that ultimately host antigens replace donor antigens after implantation.[16] Because donors and recipients are not cross-matched, and graft rejection does not appear to be a problem, the identification of donor antigens in a graft is of questionable clinical significance.

Effect of Preparation on Fascia Strength

Tissue banks differ in the method used for graft preparation, and researchers have attempted to determine which process is associated with improved outcomes. However, outcomes are influenced by many other patient variables that are rarely included when these analyses are considered. Not surprisingly, therefore, the results have been conflicting. Sutaria and Staskin compared freeze-dried, freeze-dried/gamma-irradiated, and solvent-dehydrated/gamma-irradiated fascias and found no statistical differences in maximum load and thickness-adjusted maximum load.[17] However, Lemer and coworkers found that freeze-dried allograft had inferior mechanical properties compared with autologous fascia or solvent-dehydrated fascia.[18] Hinton and associates compared solvent-dehydrated/gamma-irradiated fascia with freeze-dried/nonirradiated fascia and found a higher stiffness, higher maximum load to failure, and higher maximum load per unit width of graft with the former.[19]

The cause of the potential differences in various fascia preparations is unclear and also is of questionable significance. A possible explanation for the difference between freeze-dried and solvent-dried fascia is that ice crystal formation during the freeze-drying process may weaken the collagen structure in the fascia.[18] Of note, the forces generated in studies measuring fascial strength are usually much greater than the physiologic forces created at the bladder neck and proximal urethra. This raises the issue that ex vivo strength is not the only variable necessary for success with an allograft fascia PVS. Lin and colleagues attempted to confirmed this suspicion, showing that, with the patient in a horizontal and mild tilt position, the tension placed on the sling was far less than that necessary to break the fascia.[20] Finally, but most importantly, the variability of fascial thickness is not addressed in any of these studies.

Risk of Disease Transmission

The prevention of disease transmission focuses on the areas of screening and sterilization. Since 1985, when the American Association of Tissue Banks began requiring the screening of prospective donors and testing of tissue for viruses, there have been no documented cases of HIV transmission.[21] Other extensive reviews have not identified a single case of disease originating from transplanted allograft fascia.[22]

However, there remains concern about the transmission of prions, the causative agent of Creutzfeldt-Jakob disease (CJD) and other forms of spongioencephalopathies. It is estimated that, with current methods of processing, the theoretical risk of a patient's developing CJD from an allograft is 1 in 3,500,000. This is significantly lower than the 1 in 10,000 to 1 in 100,000, overall risk in the general population of "naturally" acquiring the disease.[23]

Current FDA guidelines contain recommendations to exclude donors of tissue (musculoskeletal, ocular, integumental) who are diagnosed or have risk factors for tissue spongioencephalopathies, specifically classic CJD. However, current FDA regulations for human tissue do not address tissue spongioencephalopathies.[24] In an FDA guidance to industry on screening and testing donors of human tissue intended for transplantation, the agency recommends that the donor medical history screening interview should include questions to defer potential donors with a diagnosis or a known family history (blood relative) of CJD and those who have received human pituitary growth hormone or dura mater transplants.[24] Additionally, in 2002, the FDA updated a policy that would defer from blood donation anyone who spent three months or more cumulatively in the United Kingdom between 1980 and 1996.[25] This was done to help reduce the possible risk of transmission of CJD by blood and blood products. There have been no reports of transmission of CJD through transplantation of human tissues.[26]

Intraoperative Fascia Preparation

Intraoperative preparation varies with each specific tissue bank recommendation. Common among all fascias is reconstitution by soaking in room-temperature saline for at least 20 minutes before placement. Additionally, the fascia must be folded over and figure-of-eight or horizontal mattress sutures used to prevent sutures' "pulling through" the longitudinally arranged collagen fibers.[17,27] The fascia should be pulled/distracted to confirm adequate tensile strength.[28]

Ideally, the fascia should be of sufficient length (at least 12 to 14 cm) to pass under the urethra and through the endopelvic fascia bilaterally. This allows the ends of the sling to scar into the retropubic space, thus improving its fixation.[29]

SURGICAL TECHNIQUE

Surgery is performed under spinal or general anesthesia with the patient in the lithotomy position. Sequential compression hose and padded leg stirrups improve the safety of this position, especially if surgery is prolonged. After surgical preparation, a 16-Fr urethral catheter is inserted, and the balloon is used to identify the location of the bladder neck, which is marked on the vaginal epithelium with a marking pen. A midline vaginal wall epithelial incision or bilateral incisions centered at the bladder neck allow the vaginal epithelium to be dissected from the underlying pubocervical fascia. We prefer the latter technique, because it allows for creation of a tunnel for the sling beneath the bladder neck (Fig. 37-1), helping to prevent cephalad or caudal migration when the sling is tensioned.

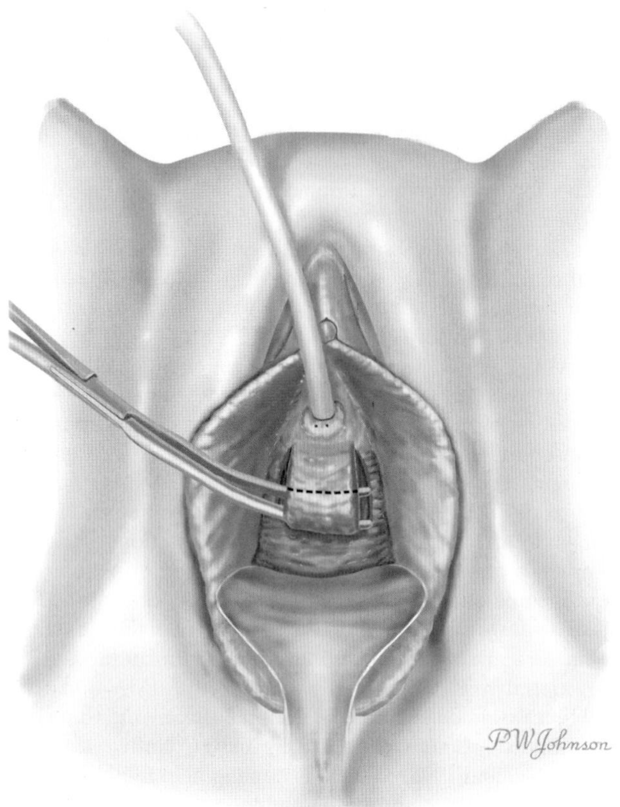

Figure 37-1 Sharp dissection of the subepithelial tunnel beneath the bladder neck for later passage of the sling.

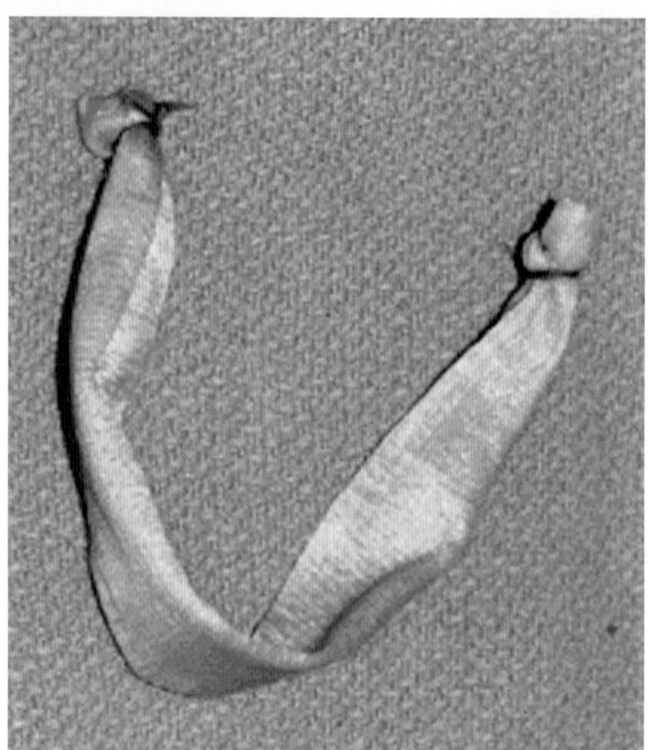

Figure 37-2 Transfixion binding of the sling ends with 0-0 Vicryl prevents "pull out" of the suture.

If repair of a central defect cystocele is also required, a midline vaginal incision from the mid-urethra to the vaginal cuff is always used. With the bladder empty, the urethropelvic ligament is perforated bilaterally with scissors. The location of the hiatus should be at its lateral attachment to the inferior ramus and at the level of the bladder neck. The hiatus allows access to the retropubic space, which may then be dissected digitally, freeing the bladder from the symphysis pubis to create a space for the sling to traverse the retropubic space through the endopelvic fascia.

A 2-cm transverse midline abdominal skin incision is made down to the superior surface of the symphysis pubis. A double-pronged Pereyra ligature carrier (Cook Urological Inc., Spencer, IN) is then passed through the rectus fascia directly behind the pubic symphysis and lateral to the proximal urethra, with the needle tips emerging through the vaginal wall hiatus. This needle is digitally guided along its course from the rectus fascia to the vaginal hiatus by keeping the needle on the tip of a finger passed through the vaginal wall hiatus.

The ends of the allograft sling are transfixed and bound with a 0-0 Vicryl suture (polyglactin suture material; Ethicon Inc., Johnson & Johnson, Somerville, NJ) (Fig. 37-2). A 1-0 Prolene suture (polypropylene suture material; Ethicon Inc.) is placed through the bound ends (see Fig. 37-2). The free ends of the Prolene suture are attached to the ligature carrier and transferred across the retropubic space and out through the suprapubic incision. The opposite end of the sling is passed through the previously dissected tunnel and across the opposite retropubic space in a similar fashion. Sling tension is adjusted according to the requirements of the individual case, but usually, if there is sufficient urethral hypermobility, it is held away from the bladder neck (Fig. 37-3) as the Prolene suture on each side of the sling is tied first over the rectus fascia and then the right side is tied to the left. Indigo carmine may then be given intravenously and cystoscopy performed to exclude bladder or ureteral injury and to confirm correct sling placement and tension. Visualization of free urine flow with the Crede maneuver and a full bladder confirms that the sling has not been made too tight. The vaginal incisions are then closed with 4-0 absorbable suture. A vaginal pack and suprapubic tube are usually unnecessary.

WHAT HAPPENS TO THE FASCIA IN FAILED CASES

Results using allograft fascia are mixed, and some authors have suggested that failure of allografts, as opposed to autologous fascia, may due to problems with the material itself.[30] In hope of determining the validity of this belief, studies have been performed on cadaveric fascia in animal models and on fascia identified during re-explorations.

Dora and colleagues used a rabbit model to show that human cadaveric fascia tensile strength decreased up to 80% and stiffness decreased by 90% at 12 weeks; autologous fascia and polypropylene mesh did not have significant change in tensile strength or stiffness over the same time period.[31] In a rat model, Kim and associates found that cadaveric fascia decreased in toughness over 4 months.[32] Walter and coworkers also showed a decrease in tensile strength of the fascia after it was implanted in a rabbit vagina model for 12 weeks.[33] The clinical implications of these findings remain unclear.

Multiple authors have commented on the appearance of cadaveric fascia slings at the time of re-exploration. Fitzgerald explored 12 women who had received irradiated, freeze-dried grafts and found graft tissue in only 7 of them. The grafts showed an immune reaction and areas of disorganized remodeling and

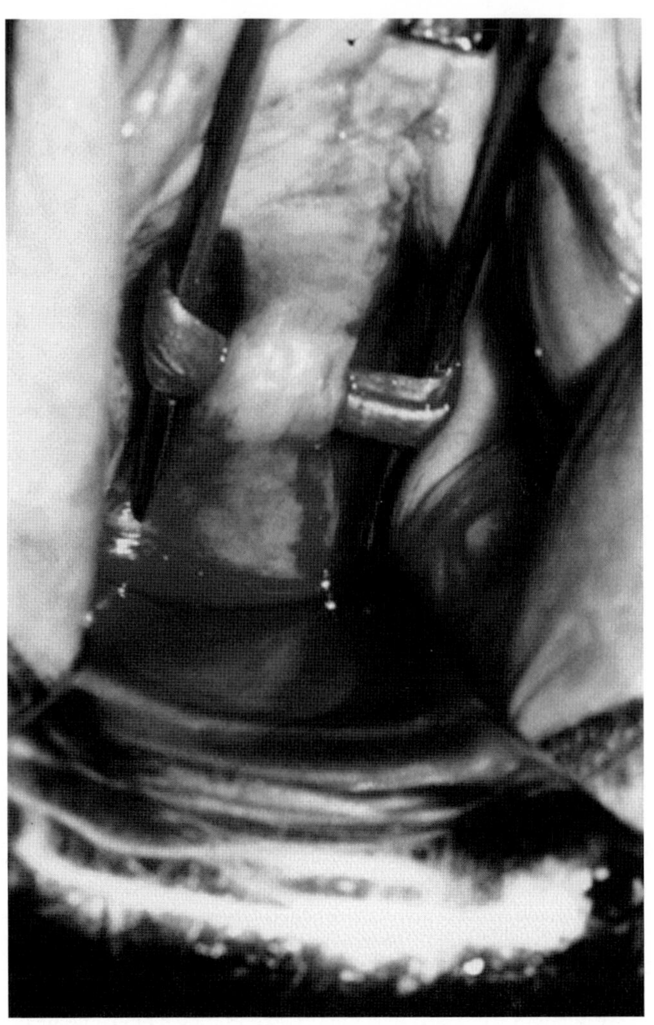

Figure 37-3 The sling is held away from the bladder neck as the sutures are being tied.

graft degeneration. It is unclear whether this is a normal host response, because none of the patients who experienced success underwent reoperation.[10]

Huang and associates reoperated on one patient after cadaveric fascia PVS and found the graft to be very friable. Histologic examination showed loosely packed fibroblasts with wavy collagen fibers and focal areas of edema and degenerative changes.[30]

Blander and Zimmern explored five "failed" cadaveric fascial slings and, on microscopic examination of the removed cadaveric fascia, found collagen with almost complete absence of cellularity and no evidence of capillary in-growth or rejection.[34]

Ultimately, the explanation for failure of some allografts remains unclear. Possibilities are many and include a persistent level of antigenicity,[35] an unsuitable environment for the allograft,[30] contamination by vaginal flora, host-versus-graft reaction, and undue stress on the graft.[36]

RESULTS

During the middle to late 1990s, the enthusiasm for cadaveric fascial slings increased as allograft tissue became more widely available. The shortened operative time and decreased morbidity (due to the lack of a donor site) combined with longer-term follow-up increased the frequency with which the procedure was performed. Although minimally invasive techniques with synthetic material have increased in popularity over the last few years, it is important for the pelvic surgeon to maintain cadaveric fascia placement in the surgical armamentarium.

The outcomes for allograft fascia vary among authors (Table 37-1). Huang and associates showed a failure rate of 28% with recurrent incontinence within 6 months of surgery.[30] Fitzgerald and colleagues identified a greater than 20% material failure rate for freeze-dried, irradiated fascia.[36] In contrast, Amundsen and other showed an 87% satisfaction rate for freeze-dried, non irradiated fascia.[27] Elliot and Boone evaluated their experience with

Table 37-1 Outcomes of Cadaveric Fascia Pubovaginal Slings

First Author and Ref. No.	Processing Method	*N*	Follow-up, Mean (mo)	% Improved (0-2 pads/day)	% Cure (0 pads/day)
Handa[5]	Freeze-dried, −IR	16	12	85	79
Wright[7]	Freeze-dried, −IR	59	12	98	N.A.
Amundsen[27]	Freeze-dried, +IR	104	19	84	63
Elliot[29]	Solvent-dehydrated, +IR	26	15	92	77
Fitzgerald[36]	Freeze-dried, +IR	35	6	83	69
Walsh[37]	Freeze-dried	31	13.5	N/A	93.5
Richter[38]	Freeze dried −IR	102	35	90	N/A
McBride[39]	Freeze-dried −IR	26	35	91	43
Almeida[40]	Freeze dried + IR	30	36	28	40
Brown[41]	Freeze-dried, ?IR	121	12	83	74
Bodell[42]	Solvent-dehydrated, −IR	186	16.4	76	27
Vereecken[43]	Freeze-dried	8	24	N/A	100
Flynn[44]	Freeze-dried, +IR	63	29	N/A	87
Chien[45]	N/A	83	27.4	N/A	90.1
Fitzgerald[46]	Freeze-dried, +IR	27	12	48	N/A
Carbone[47]	Freeze-dried, +IR	154	10.6	62	60
Soergel[48]	Freeze-dried, +/−IR	12	6	N/A	33
Ellerkmann[49]	Solvent-dehydrated, −IR	32	N/A	N/A	90.5
Simsiman[50]	N/A	80	29	N/A	66

IR, gamma irradiation.

cadaveric fascia and found a 96% satisfaction rate with a mean follow-up of 15 months.[29] Walsh and coworkers showed complete resolution of stress urinary incontinence in 93% of patients at a mean follow-up of 13.5 months.[37]

CONCLUSIONS

Allograft fascia for PVS offers decreased morbidity and operative time, compared with autologous fascia, while limiting the risk of erosion and infection seen with synthetic material. Although appropriate screening has essentially removed the risk of disease transmission, the technique to process the fascia remains variable. With success rates similar to those seen with autologous fascia, allograft fascia offers the surgeon another material available for the treatment of stress urinary incontinence in women. Further investigations are needed to determine the most durable method of preparation.

References

1. Giordano D: Vingtieme Congres Francais de Chirurgie. Paris, 1907, p 506.
2. McGuire EJ, Lytton B: Pubovaginal sling procedure for stress incontinence. J Urol 119:82-84, 1978.
3. Bedrossian EH Jr: Banked fascia lata as an orbital floor implant. Ophthal Plast Reconstr Surg 9:66-70, 1993.
4. Noyes FR, Barber-Westin SD: Reconstruction of the anterior cruciate ligament with human allograft: Comparison of early and later results. J Bone Joint Surg Am 78:524-537, 1996.
5. Handa VL, Jensen JK, Germain MM, et al: Banked human fascia lata for the suburethral sling procedure: A preliminary report. Obstet Gynecol 88:1045-1049, 1996.
6. American Association of Tissue Banks (AATB): Annual Registration Survey, McClean, VA: AATB, 2003.
7. Wright EJ, Iselin CE, Carr LK, Webster GD: Pubovaginal sling using cadaveric allograft fascia for the treatment of intrinsic sphincter deficiency. J Urol 160:759-762, 1998.
8. Singla AK: The use of cadaveric fascia lata in the treatment of stress urinary incontinence in women. BJU Int 85:264-269, 2000.
9. Flynn BJ, Marinkovic SP, Yap WT: Risks and benefits of using allograft fascia late for pubovaginal slings [abstract]. J Urol 161:1195, 1999.
10. Fitzgerald MP, Mollenhauer J, Bitterman P, Brubaker L: Functional failure of fascia lata allografts. Am J Obstet Gynecol 181:1339-1346, 1999.
11. Walter AJ, Morse AN, Leslie KO, et al: Histologic evaluation of human cadaveric fascia lata in a rabbit vagina model. Int Urogynecol J Pelvic Floor Dysfunct 17:136-142, 2006. Epub 2005 June 23.
12. Food and Drug Administration: The FDA intra-agency guidelines for human tissue intended for transplantation. Federal Register 58:65514, 1993.
13. Ghoniem GM: Allograft sling material: Is it the state of the art? Int Urogynecol J 11:69-70, 2000.
14. Hathaway JK, Choe JM: Intact genetic material is present in commercially processed cadaver allografts used for pubovaginal slings. J Urol 168:140-143, 2002.
15. Sadhukhan P, Rackley RR, Bandyopadhyay S, et al: Extraction of cellular genetic material from human fascia lata allografts. In Programs and Abstracts of the American Urological Association Annual Meeting, May 1999, Dallas, Texas, Abstract 396.
16. Fitzgerald MP, Mollenhauer J, Brubaker L: The antigenicity of fascia lata allografts. BJU Int 86:826-828, 2000.
17. Sutaria PM, Staskin DR: A comparison of fascial "pull through" strength using four different suture fixation techniques [abstract]. J Urol 161:79, 1999.
18. Lemer ML, Chaikin DC, Blaivas JG: Tissue strength analysis of autologous and cadaveric allografts for the pubovaginal sling. Neurourol Urodyn 18:497-503, 1999.
19. Hinton R, Jinnah RH, Johnson C, et al: A biomechanical analysis of solvent-dehydrated and freeze-dried human fascia lata allografts: A preliminary report. Am J Sports Med 20:607-612, 1992.
20. Lin AT, Wang SJ, Chen KK, Chang LS: In vivo tension sustained by fascial sling in pubovaginal sling surgery for female stress urinary incontinence. J Urol 173:894-897, 2005.
21. Simonds RJ, Hulmder SD, Hurwitz RL, et al: Transmission of human immunodeficiency virus from seronegative organ and tissue donors. N Engl J Med 326:726-728, 1992.
22. Parizek J, Mericka P, Husek Z, et al: Detailed evaluation of 2959 allogenic and xenogenic dense connective tissue grafts (fascia lata, pericardium, and dura mater) used in the course of 20 years for duraplasty in neurosurgery. Acta Neurochir (Wien) 139:827-838, 1997.
23. Prusiner SB: Prions. Proc Natl Acad Sci U S A 95:13363-13383, 1998.
24. FDA Guidance for Industry: Screening and Testing of Donors of Human Tissue Intended for Transplantation. Federal Register 62:40429, 1997.
25. FDA: Guidance for Industry: Revised Preventive Measures to Reduce the Possible Risk of Transmission of Creutzfeldt-Jakob Disease (CJD) and Variant Creutzfeldt-Jakob Disease (vCJD) by Blood & Blood Products, 2002. http://www.fda.gov/cber/gdlns/cjdvcjd.htm
26. Draft Issue Summaries: Transmissible Spongiform Encephalopathies Advisory Committee Meeting, January 18-19, 2001, Issue 2.
27. Amundsen CL, Visco AG, Ruiz H, Webster GD: Outcome in 104 pubovaginal slings using freeze-dried allograft fascia lata from a single tissue bank. Urology 56(Suppl 6A):2-8, 2000.
28. Chaiken DC, Blaivas JG: Weakened cadaveric fascial sling: An unexpected cause of failure. J Urol 160:2151, 1998.
29. Elliot DS, Boone TB: Is fascia lata allograft material trustworthy for pubovaginal sling repair. Urology 56:772-776, 2000.
30. Huang YH, Lin ATL, Chen KK, et al: High failure rate using allograft fascia lata in pubovaginal sling surgery for female stress urinary incontinence. Urology 58:943-946, 2001.
31. Dora CD, Dimarco DS, Zobitz, ME, Elliot DS: Time dependent variations in biomechanical properties of cadaveric fascia, porcine dermis, porcine small intestine submucosa, polypropylene mesh and autologous fascia in the rabbit model: Implications for sling surgery. J Urol 171:1970-1973, 2004.
32. Kim HL, LaBarbera MC, Patel RV: Comparison of cadaveric and autologous fascia using an in vivo model. Urology 58:800-804, 2001.
33. Walter AJ, Morse AN, Leslie KO, et al: Changes in tensile strength of cadaveric human fascia lata after implantation in a rabbit vagina model. J Urol 169:1907-1910, 2003.
34. Blander DS, Zimmern PE: Cadaveric fascia lata sling: Analysis of five recent adverse outcomes. Urology 56:596-599, 2000.
35. Rodrigo JJ, Jackson DW, Simon TM, et al: The immune response to freeze-dried bond-tendon-gone ACL allografts in humans. Am J Knee Surg 6:47-53, 1993.
36. Fitzgerald MP, Mollenhauer J, Brubaker L: Failure of allograft suburethral slings. BJU Int 84:785-788, 1999.
37. Walsh IK, Nambirajan T, Donellan SM, et al: Cadaveric fascia lata pubovaginal slings: Early results of safety, efficacy and patient satisfaction. BJU Int 90:415-419, 2002.

38. Richter HE, Burgio KL, Holley RL, et al: Cadaveric fascia lata sling for stress urinary incontinence: A prospective quality-of-life analysis. Am J Obstet Gynecol 189:1590-1595, 2003.
39. McBride AW, Ellerkmann RM, Bent AE, Melick CF: Comparison of long-term outcomes of autologous fascia lata slings with Suspend Tutoplast fascia lata allograft slings for stress incontinence. Am J Obstet Gynecol 192:1677-1681, 2005.
40. Almeida SHM, Gregorio E, Grando JPS, et al: Pubovaginal sling using cadaveric allograft fascia for the treatment of female urinary incontinence. Transplant Proc 36:995-996, 2004.
41. Brown SL, Govier FE: Cadaveric versus autologous fascia lata for the pubovaginal sling: surgical outcome and patient satisfaction. J Urol 164:1633-1637, 2000.
42. Bodell DM, Leach GE: Update on the results of the cadaveric transvaginal sling (CATS) [abstract 308]. J Urol 167(Suppl):78, 2002.
43. Vereecken RL, Lechat A: Cadaver fascia lata sling in the treatment of intrinsic sphincter weakness. Urol Int 67:232-234, 2001.
44. Flynn BJ, Yap WT: Pubovaginal sling using allograft fascia versus autograft fascia for all types of stress urinary incontinence: 2-Year minimum follow-up. J Urol 167:608-612, 2002.
45. Chien GW, Tawadroas M, Kaptein JS, et al: Surgical treatment for stress urinary incontinence with urethral hypermobility: What is the best approach? World J Urol 20:234-239, 2002.
46. Fitzgerald MP, Edwards SR, Fenner D: Medium-term follow-up on use of freeze-dried, irradiated donor fascia for sacrocolpopexy and sling procedures. Int Urogynecol J Pelvic Floor Dysfunct 15:238-242, 2004.
47. Carbone JM, Kavaler E, Hu JC, Raz S: Pubovaginal sling using cadaveric fascia and bone anchors: Disappointing early results. J Urol 165:1605-1611, 2001.
48. Soergel TM, Shott S, Heit M: Poor surgical outcomes after fascia lata allograft slings. Int Urogynecol J Pelvic Floor Dysfunct 12:247-253, 2001.
49. Ellerkmann RM, McBride AW, Bent AE, Melick CF: Comparison of long-term outcomes of autologous fascia lata slings to Suspend Tutoplast fascia lata allograft slings for stress incontinence. Oral poster 38. 2004 Joint Scientific Meeting of The American Urogynecologic Society and The Society of Gynecologic Surgeons, San Diego, 2004.
50. Simsiman AJ, Powell CR, Stratford R, Menefee SA: Failure rates for porcine dermal and cadaveric fascial slings as compared to autologous tissue for treatment of urodynamic stress incontinence. 31st Annual Scientific Meeting of The Society of Gynecologic Surgeons, Rancho Mirage, CA, 2005.

Chapter 38

FASCIA LATA SLING

Neil T. Dwyer and Karl J. Kreder

Pubovaginal sling cystourethropexy is considered one of the gold standards of female stress urinary incontinence (SUI) surgery. The bladder neck sling can be performed using autologous, allograft, or synthetic material. The two autologous methods use either rectus or fascia lata fascia. This chapter summarizes the literature on the indications, surgical technique, and outcomes of using fascia lata to treat female SUI.

HISTORY

The autologous sling used to affect the urethra as a method of urinary control was first mentioned in 1907 by Von Giordano, who described the use of gracilis muscle to wrap around the urethra.[1] The pyramidalis muscle was used to suture behind the urethra by Goebell in 1910.[2] Squier referred to the use of the levator ani muscles to augment bladder outlet resistance.[3] In 1942, Aldridge described the use of bilateral strips of rectus fascia passed inferiorly through the rectus abdominis muscles to support the urethra posteriorly.[4] In 1978, McGuire and Lytton described using an autologous fascial sling in 52 patients with SUI.[5] Forty-two of the patients had had previous corrective incontinence surgery. Postoperative urethral pressure measurements showed urethral pressure increase but no occlusion. Fifty patients had a successful outcome, and there were 2 failures. These results were further confirmed by Blaivas and Jacobs in 1991, when they observed 67 patients who had undergone a pubovaginal fascia sling repair and reported that 82% were completely dry and 9% were dramatically improved.[6]

The fascia lata sling was first described by Price in 1933.[7] Beck and colleagues examined the use of fascia lata as a suburethral sling for the treatment of recurrent urinary incontinence.[8-10] They first described the use of the fascia lata sling in 1974[8] and in 1988 reported their results in 170 patients.[10] They used the fascia lata suburethral sling after failed primary incontinence surgery in 69 cases and after multiple failed prior anti-incontinence repairs in 101 cases. The overall success was reported at 98.2%.[10]

Cadaveric fascia lata (CFL) has been used to repair tissue defects for a number of years, but its first use for incontinence surgery was reported in 1996.[11] Handa and colleagues used CFL in 16 patients, 14 with genuine SUI and 2 who had a previously placed synthetic graft that became infected. Eighty-eight percent were subjectively improved, and 79% of the patients with genuine SUI were objectively improved.[11]

The use of xenograft material for sling surgery has been reported as well. In 2002, a pilot study examined the use of bovine pericardium placed as a suburethral sling in 22 females.[12] At 20 months, 21 of 22 patients were cured with no incidences of erosion or rejection. Another study recently looked at the use of processed porcine small intestine submucosa (SIS) as a pubovaginal sling in 152 female patients with SUI.[13] In this 4-year series, there was a 93.4% cure rate, with three additional patients demonstrating marked improvement. There was no erosion, infection, or rejection in the group.

Synthetic materials have been used for incontinence since 1961, with the use of nylon strips fashioned into a suburethral sling.[14] Numerous materials have been tried since then, including Silastic,[15] Gore-Tex,[16] Mersilene,[17] Marlex,[18] Prolene,[19] and Vicryl.[20]

INDICATIONS

The indication for the use of a fascia lata sling can be stated simply as SUI. At first, fascia lata slings and suburethral slings were recommended for complicated SUI such as previous SUI corrective surgery and intrinsic sphincter dysfunction (ISD). Type 2 SUI was usually treated with a needle suspension or colposuspension, such as a Burch procedure. This stemmed from the progression in the development of various surgeries for the correction of SUI.

ISD has been associated with multiple etiologies. The presence of previous SUI corrective surgeries is a risk factor. A neurologic insult to the sacral area may result in compromise of the bladder's innervation and ISD. This insult could come from damage to the nerve roots as they leave the spine or via major pelvic surgery such as a radical hysterectomy. In addition, patients with diabetic neuropathy may also have peripheral neurologic problems interfering with sphincteric function. Patients who have undergone previous radiation treatment are at risk of developing ISD-based SUI.[21] Another possible cause of ISD is estrogen deficiency: as women age, lower levels of estrogen may predispose to ISD.[22] Horbach and Ostergard examined 263 consecutive patients with urodynamic studies for urinary leakage.[23] In this population, 132 women had ISD, defined as urethral closure pressure lower than 20 cm H_2O, and the only independent risk factor for ISD was age greater than 50 years.

ISD is classically diagnosed using video urodynamics, which shows an open bladder neck at rest. In addition, a low Valsalva (abdominal) leak-point pressure (VLPP) is seen (<60 cm H_2O) in patients with ISD. Incontinent women with a VLPP greater than 90 cm H_2O usually have type 2 SUI according to fluoroscopic assessment.[24] There is also correlation between worsening SUI subjective symptoms and a lower VLPP.[25] Urethral pressure profilometry has been used to define SUI in women. Weber performed an extensive review of published articles using urethral pressure profilometry and found the technique to be nonstandardized and poorly reproducible.[26]

The recommendations from the American Urological Association clinical guidelines panel summary report published in 1997 suggested that the standard patient should be informed about the four major surgical correction categories: retropubic suspension, transvaginal suspensions, anterior repairs, and sling surgeries.[27] According to the panel, the patient should understand that retropubic suspensions and sling surgeries carry a higher complication rate along with their higher rate of longer-term cure. The panel suggested categorizing patients as having urethral hypermobility, ISD, or both, although they acknowledged that there was no standardized method to make this diagnosis. These recommendations decreased the popularity and use of needle suspensions and anterior repairs as treatment options for women with SUI. In May 2007 the Urinary Incontinence Treatment Network, led by Albo and colleagues, published a large randomized study to examine the differences between a Burch colposuspension and an autologous fascial sling.[28] Six hundred fifty-five women were randomized to either the Burch or a fascial sling and followed for 24 months with standardized assessments. Seventy-nine percent of the women completed the assessments. Success rates were higher for the women who underwent the sling procedure versus the women who had a Burch (47% vs. 38%, $p = 0.01$). Specific to stress incontinence, there was a 66% success rate in the sling group whereas the Burch group had a 49% success rate. Complications were higher in the sling group, with more urinary tract infections, voiding difficulty, and postoperative urge incontinence. Performance of prolapse repair with the stress incontinence surgery did not affect the outcomes between the groups.

This study demonstrates a significantly higher success rate with an autologous fascial sling versus a Burch colposuspension at only 24 months. The increased complications need to be considered in the decision-making process as well.

The recommendation to apply a particular surgery depending on the type or degree of SUI was suggested by Sand and associates in 1987.[29] They found a 54% failure rate in patients who underwent a Burch procedure and who had a mean urethral closure pressure (MUCP) lower than 20 cm H_2O, whereas the patients with a MUCP greater than 20 cm H_2O had an 18% failure rate. Koonings and coworkers compared 19 women with SUI and low urethral pressure to 106 patients with SUI and a normal urethral pressure.[30] The patients underwent a modified Pereyra procedure or a Burch colposuspension. The women with low urethral pressure preoperatively had a higher failure rate, regardless of the surgical procedure used, compared to patients with normal urethral pressure profilometry. These data suggest the limitations of colposuspension and needle suspensions but do not limit the indication of the pubovaginal sling.

Several studies have examined the use of pubovaginal slings in groups of female patients with type 2, type 3, or a combination of both SUI types. Kreder and Austin examined 28 female patients with SUI.[31] Eleven had ISD alone, and 16 had a combination of urethral hypermobility and ISD. The diagnostic definitions were obtained with the use of multichannel video urodynamics. ISD existed if the VLPP was lower than 60 cm H_2O and the bladder neck was open at rest. Urethral hypermobility was defined via a pelvic examination with the patient performing a Valsalva maneuver and a cough. Overall, the patients in the sling group (17 with rectus fascia and 11 with fascia lata) had a 70% dry rate at an average of 22 months. The patients with ISD alone did poorly, with a 55% dry rate, whereas the patients with combination type 2/3 SUI had an 81% dry rate. One patient in the ISD group had a complete surgical failure.

In another study, by Zaragoza, 60 consecutive female patients with SUI were examined with multichannel video urodynamics.[32] ISD was defined in 22 patients, who had a VLPP lower than 60 cm H_2O (mean, 42 cm H_2O), and 38 patients diagnosed with type 2 SUI had a mean VLPP of 95 cm H_2O. At an average of 25.1 months after a rectus fascia pubovaginal sling procedure, 95% of the patients were completely continent. The three failures were due to urgency incontinence, which was present in all three patients preoperatively. The success rate was almost identical between the patients diagnosed with type 2 and those with type 3 SUI.

Finally, Cross and colleagues examined a large group of female patients diagnosed with SUI, all treated with a rectus fascia pubovaginal sling.[33] There were 134 patients who were contacted at an average of 22 months after surgery, and their initial diagnosis was type 2 SUI (45 patients), type 3 SUI (73 patients), or a combination of both (16 patients). The overall dry rate was 93%, as confirmed by video urodynamics: 96% of the type 2 patients, 89% of the type 3 patients, and 100% of the type 2/3 patients.

All three of these studies included patients who had had prior SUI surgery, patients with concomitant procedures, and patients with simple SUI (pure SUI, plus or minus urge urinary incontinence). These studies demonstrated the ability to use the pubovaginal sling in women with type 2 and/or type 3 SUI.

CHOICE OF FASCIA LATA SLING AND SOURCE

Autologous rectus and fascia lata are commonly used for pubovaginal slings as well as allogenic fascia. The advantage of autologous material is the lack of potential disease transmission and low erosion rates. Fascia lata offers advantages over rectus fascia such as greater tensile strength and lack of abdominal wall hernias related to graft harvest; moreover, it is rare that the patient's past surgical history would interfere with harvesting of a long strip of fascia lata.[34] The harvesting of autologous fascia adds operative time and possible morbidity to sling surgery, compared with synthetic and allograft fascia sources.

Allograft fascia lata is from a cadaveric source and has been used in sling surgery since 1996.[35] There is a theoretical advantage for the use of CFL compared with a synthetic source in that there is a lower risk of erosion, whereas the disadvantage is a chance of disease transmission.[36] Choe and Bell examined 16 allograft sources of tissue, including 8 freeze-dried gamma-irradiated CFL allografts.[37] Fourteen of the allografts contained DNA material, as determined from standardized DNA extraction techniques. FitzGerald and colleagues found donor antigens still present in CFL prepared via the freeze-dried and the Tutoplast techniques.[38] Hathaway and Choe took four commercially available human cadaveric allografts and subjected 10 of each type to DNA extraction. Thirty-nine (97.5%) of the allografts contained DNA with variable amounts.[39] The significance of the presence of DNA and antigens in the allograft material is unknown. The risk of contracting Creutzfeldt-Jacob disease from allograft material is approximately 1 in 3.5 million,[40] and the risk of human immunodeficiency virus (HIV) transmission is estimated to be 1 in 8 million.[41]

CFL is mainly made via two techniques: solvent dehydration with gamma irradiation (Tutoplast) or freeze-drying (tissue banks and FasLata). Both of these preparations require 15 to 30 minutes to rehydrate in saline before implantation.[36] A study by Lemer and associates examined the tensile strength of two types of CFL (solvent-dehydrated and freeze-dried), autologous rectus fascia, and cadaveric dermal grafts.[42] They found no significant difference between solvent-dried fascia lata, dermal graft, and autologous rectus fascia. Freeze-dried fascia lata had a significantly lower maximum-load-to-failure rate than either of the other types tested. In contrast, Sutaria and Staskin examined the tensile strength after three methods of CFL preservation (freeze-dried/gamma-irradiated, freeze-dried, and solvent-dehydrated/gamma irradiated).[43] They found no significant difference in the tensile strength among the three CFL preparations. Choe and colleagues studied the biomechanical properties of full-strip slings and patch-suture slings using autologous tissue, cadaveric tissues, and synthetic materials.[44] For the full-strip slings, cadaveric tissues (including CFL) had the best tensile strength, followed by synthetics and then autologous tissue. In the analysis of patch-suture slings, the synthetic material was the strongest, followed by CFL and then autologous rectus fascia. Dora and coworkers examined the biomechanical properties of several sling materials in a time-dependent fashion.[45] They placed the materials in rabbit models and tested them before implantation and again at 12 weeks. The tensile strength of polypropylene mesh and autologous fascia remained consistent with baseline. CFL and porcine xenografts decreased in tensile strength by 60% to 89%. Walter and colleagues further reviewed the change in tensile strength of three lots of freeze-dried CFL after implanting it into a rabbit model.[46] They demonstrated significant preimplantation variability in the tensile strength of the CFL. At 12 weeks, the samples were explanted and retested and showed a 90% decrease in tensile strength. The significance of variations in tensile strength among the various sling materials has not been shown to be clinically significant. Based on the earlier failure of some sling materials, the presence of tensile strength variations and degradation may play a role in long-term clinical success.

Table 38-1 Outcomes of Cadaveric Fascia Lata Sling in Women with Stress Urinary Incontinence

First Author and Ref. No.	Year	*N*	Follow-up, Mean (mo)	Method of Follow-up	% Cured/ Improved	% Failure	CFL Preparation Method	Comments
Elliott[68]	2000	26	12-20 (15)	Subjective	77/15	7.6	Solvent-dehydrated	4 patients had no leakage preoperatively (3 with occult SUI)
Brown[64]	2000	104	(12)	Subjective	74/19	7	Freeze-dried	19% improved used 1-3 pads/day; 26% used ≥1 pads/day
Soergel[69]	2001	12	(3)	UDS	33.3	66.6	Freeze-dried	Cure was no SUI (could have detrusor instability)
Huang[70]	2001	18	6.9-11.6 (9.2)	Subjective	72.7	27.8	Solvent-dehydrated	Failed within 3-6 mo
Carbone[71]	2001	154	6-16 (10.4)	Subjective	60/2	37.9	Solvent-dehydrated/ freeze-dried	Bone-anchored CFL: 16.9% reoperation rate for SUI failure
Flynn[62]	2002	63	26-32 (29)	Subjective	71/13	16	Freeze-dried	29% used ≥1 pads/day
Chien[72]	2002	83	(27.4)	Subjective	90.1	9.9	Freeze-dried	Cured/improved = 0-1 pads/day
Walsh[73]	2002	31	12-14 (13.5)	Subjective	93.5	6	Freeze-dried	85% reported satisfaction at 1 yr
Richter[74]	2003	100	12-48 (35)	Subjective	~30/79.7		Freeze-dried	Two-thirds had some leakage at 12 mo
Amundsen,[40] Wright[47]	1998, 2000	91	3-37 (19.4)	Subjective	62.6/21	25.2	Freeze-dried	34.7% of failures due to urge leakage; failure defined as ≥1 pads/day
FitzGerald[38,75]	1999, 2004	27	0.5-51 (median, 12)	UDS and Subjective	48 (subjectively)	41	Freeze-dried	37% reoperation rate for SUI failure; some failed by 2 wk

CFL, cadaveric fascia lata; SUI, stress urinary incontinence; UDS, urodynamic studies.

CADAVERIC FASCIA LATA OUTCOMES

Using CFL for pubovaginal slings offers the advantage of decreased operative time and less patient morbidity.[47] The results from performing the procedure are less favorable than with their autologous counterparts. Table 38-1 displays the results of several series of patients undergoing CFL sling cystourethropexy. Overall, the follow-up periods were short and most studies used subjective assessment methods with varying definitions of postsurgical success. Numerous studies showed high failure rates using CFL slings, with postsurgical SUI rates ranging from 6% to 66.6% as early as 3 months postoperatively.

O'Reilly and Govier examined eight patients who had recurrence of SUI after CFL sling placement.[48] Five of the eight patients underwent urodynamic studies, which demonstrated ISD with lower VLPPs than the patients had had preoperatively. No other reason for failure was identified.

Carey and Leach examined the use of CFL for treatment of SUI and pelvic organ prolapse in patients at least 80 years old.[49] Thirty-one patients were followed up with a questionnaire at a mean of 21.4 months postoperatively. Fifty-five percent of the patients reported a 70% improvement in SUI symptoms, and 90% had no symptoms of pelvic organ prolapse recurrence. This compared similarly with the patients who were younger than 80 years of age. The moderate success in the elderly may be an acceptable use of CFL slings to decrease the morbidity of harvesting autologous fascia.

SURGICAL TECHNIQUE

Preoperatively, patients are evaluated with a complete history, physical examination, urine analysis, multichannel urodynamic studies, and necessary ancillary tests according to their medical history. All patients receive perioperative intravenous antibiotics and compressive stockings, and mechanical antiembolism devices are applied.

Fascia Lata Harvest

Once the patient is anesthetized, the lower limbs are positioned for fascia lata harvesting. Usually, we use the right side and preoperatively mark the patient accordingly, but either lower extremity may be used, depending on patient or surgeon preference or the presence of previous surgery. The stockings and antiembolism device are placed below the patient's patella on the right side. The right knee is elevated and supported with a 1-L bag of intravenous fluid or a suitable alternative pad or cushion. The extremity is internally rotated at the right hip and secured using 3-inch tape across the leg below the operative site. The operative site is prepped and draped as to expose the whole anterolateral aspect of the right thigh from the greater trochanter to distal to the patella. The anterior superior iliac spine (greater trochanter) and lateral femoral condyle are identified and marked. These landmarks identify the proximal and distal attachments of the fascia lata.

A 3-cm longitudinal incision is marked beginning just above the patella over the iliotibial band (Fig. 38-1). Dissection is carefully performed to the level of the fascia lata. At this point, two parallel incisions are made longitudinally in the fascia lata, approximately 2 cm apart. The autologous fascia lata is bluntly lifted off the underlying muscle and clamped as far distally as possible with a right angle clamp (3 to 4 cm) and transected to allow one free end. The free distal end of the fascia lata is secured with a 1-0 Prolene suture, and the proximal fascia lata is lifted off the muscle belly with the use of a thin malleable retractor. The retractor is passed superficial and deep to the fascia lata to separate it from both the adipose tissue and muscle fibers. Now the free distal end is placed under tension, and a Crawford fascial stripper (Fig. 38-2) is used to extend the fascial incisions proximally (Fig. 38-3). The Crawford fascial stripper is used to mobilize as much fascia lata as possible and divide it proximally before it is removed. Immediate compression is applied to the thigh to constrict any perforating vessels. The fascial strip is usually 20 × 2 cm in dimension, and a second 1-0 Prolene suture is attached to the proximal end of the fascia lata strip. While compression is maintained on the thigh, the fascia lata is immediately

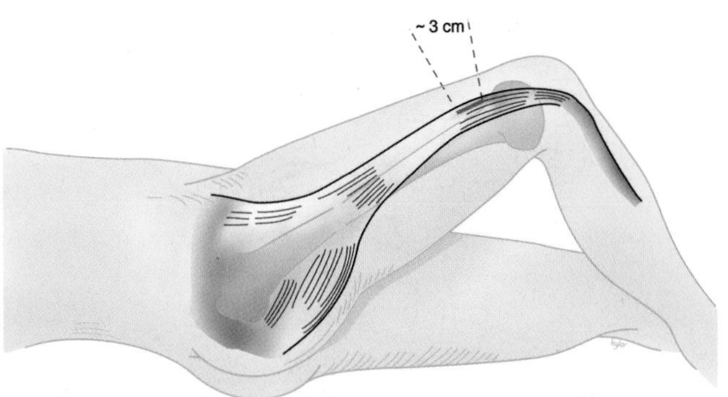

Figure 38-1 Patient's lower extremity in position for autologous fascia lata harvest. The incision is illustrated. (From Latini JM, Lux MM, Kreder KJ: Efficacy and morbidity of autologous fascia lata sling cystourethropexy. J Urol 2004; 171:1180-1184.)

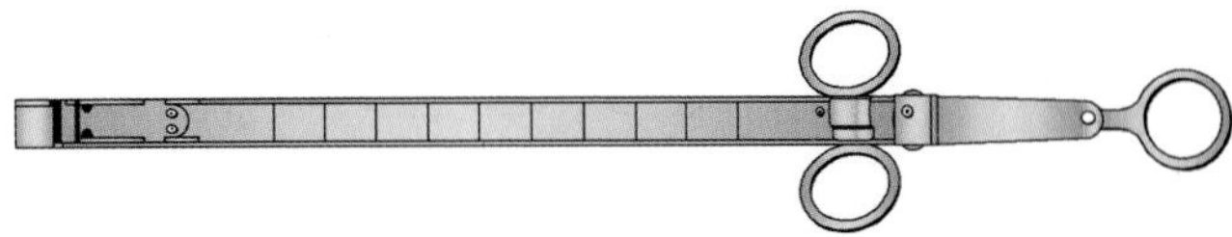

Figure 38-2 Crawford fascial stripper. (From Latini JM, Lux MM, Kreder KJ: Efficacy and morbidity of autologous fascia lata sling cystourethropexy. J Urol 2004; 171:1180-1184.)

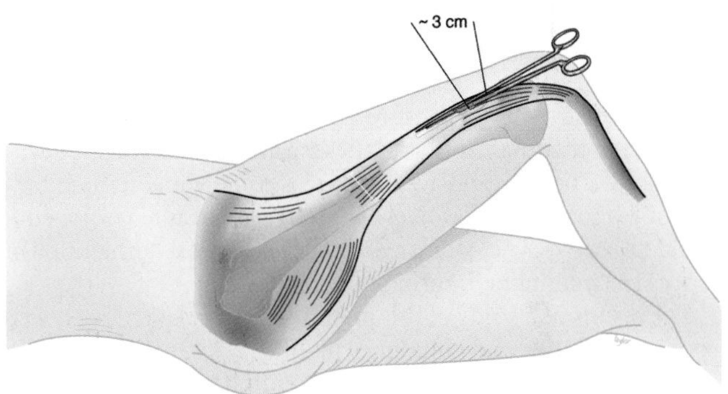

Figure 38-3 Incising the fascia lata medially and laterally, along the line of the fibers, using the Crawford fascial stripper. A 1.5 cm by 18- to 22-cm piece of fascia lata can be harvested using the technique. (From Latini JM, Lux MM, Kreder KJ: Efficacy and morbidity of autologous fascia lata sling cystourethropexy. J Urol 2004; 171:1180-1184.)

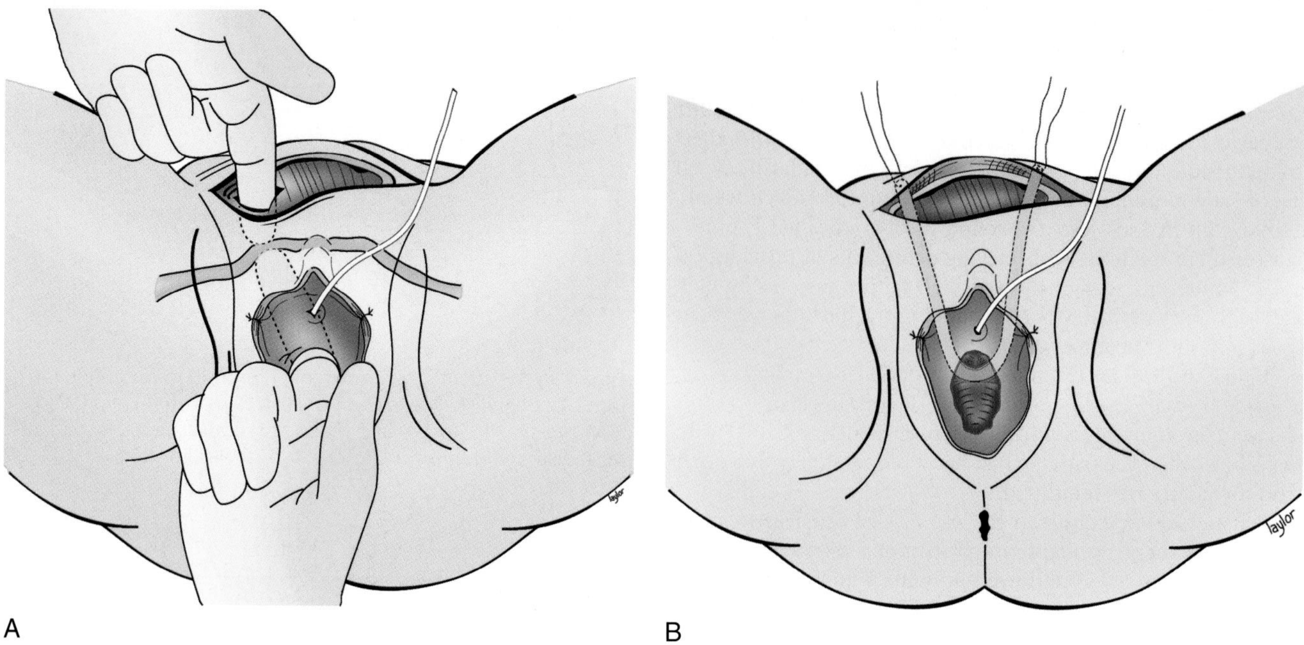

Figure 38-4 Sling cystourethropexy. **A,** Preparing to place the fascia lata autograft. **B,** Fascia lata autograft in position before the sutures are tied. (From Latini JM, Lux MM, Kreder KJ: Efficacy and morbidity of autologous fascia lata sling cystourethropexy. J Urol 2004; 171:1180-1184.)

placed in a basin of sterile saline until it is required for sling placement. The wound is irrigated and closed in three layers with no attempt to close the fascia lata. Before closure, the area is carefully checked to ensure that there is no evidence of arterial bleeders. Once the thigh closure is complete, a compressive wrap is applied to the thigh, and the stocking and antiembolism device is replaced. The compressive bandage is usually maintained for a total of 8 hours postoperatively, and the patient is encouraged to ambulate early. The stockings and mechanical antiembolism devices are maintained during the hospital stay.

The results of a study of this method of fascia lata harvest were reported by Latini and colleagues in 2004.[50] At an average of 4.4 years, 63 patients returned surveys, and charts were reviewed. Postoperatively, 47% of patients reported being able to walk pain-free immediately, and this number increased to 93% by postoperative day 7. One patient reported a hematoma which was treated conservatively. There were no infections, thrombotic events, or delays in hospital discharge related to the harvest site. Foley and Adamson obtain the fascia lata graft similarly, but with a Moseley fasciatome.[51] Of their 16 patients there were no immediate complications, and at 3 months the patients were uniformly satisfied with the cosmetic result.

Walter and coworkers described a different method of obtaining the fascia lata graft using two incisions.[52] The first was similar to the incision we use, described earlier, and the second was made 20 cm superiorly. The fascia was mobilized with long Metzenbaum scissors, and the final dimensions were 24 to 27 cm by 3 cm. Eleven percent of their 71 patients experienced an objective complication, but all were short-term. One patient required drainage of a hematoma, two had a seroma (treated conservatively), and five patients developed incisional cellulitis requiring oral antibiotics. They were able to monitor the patients for an average of 25 months, and 55 of 71 patients responded to a questionnaire. Of the responding patients, 45% listed 36 separate complaints related to the fascia lata harvest. Only 8% were rated as clinically significant, and their complaints included discomfort for two patients and unacceptable cosmesis for the third patient. The authors noted that all patients younger than 60 years of age had at least one subjective complaint, whereas the patients with no complaints had an average age of 70 years. These data suggest higher rates of complication and patient dissatisfaction with fascia lata harvest when a fasciatome is not used. Perhaps the improved technical capabilities of a fasciatome allow for a speedier recovery with fewer long-term sequelae.

Sling Placement

Once the fascia lata strip has been obtained and the thigh incision has been closed, attention is turned to the sling placement. The patient is repositioned into the dorsal lithotomy position, and the lower abdomen and vagina are prepared and draped in the standard fashion for a sling cystourethropexy. The method described for placement of the sling is a modification of the methods described by Beck and colleagues[8-10] and by McGuire and Lytton.[5] Initially, a small, transverse, lower abdominal incision is created, and dissection is carried down to the rectus abdominis fascia just superior to the symphysis pubis. A Foley catheter and a weighted vaginal speculum are placed. Silk stay sutures may be used to open the labia minor if they are redundant. The vaginal mucosa is incised longitudinally on either side of the urethra at the level of the bladder neck. A tunnel is then created in the retropubic space on either side of the urethra, using sharp and blunt dissection. This tunnel is dissected to the level of the posterior rectus abdominis fascia (Fig. 38-4A). A space is created between the urethra and the vaginal mucosa, and the fascia lata graft is placed in position posterior to the urethra. A tonsil clamp is then used to pierce the rectus abdominis fascia just lateral to the midline. The clamp is passed by fingertip guidance through the previously created retropubic tunnel to the vagina. The ends of the 1-0 Prolene sutures at one end of the sling are then grasped with the clamp and brought out through the abdominal incision. The procedure is repeated on the contralateral side (see Fig. 38-4B). The two sides of the sling are tied above the rectus fascia via the 1-0 Prolene. The knot is placed without any tension on the graft, which is allowed to act as a hammock underneath the urethra. Cystoscopy is performed to ensure that no iatrogenic bladder or ureteral injuries have occurred. The abdominal and vaginal incisions are closed with absorbable sutures, and a saline-soaked vaginal pack is placed. A new Foley catheter is placed to provide postoperative bladder drainage. The vaginal pack is removed on postoperative day 1, and the catheter is removed on day 7 for a voiding trial. The patient is instructed to perform postvoid self-catheterization until residual urine volumes are consistently less than 100 mL.

Suture Techniques

Intuitively, there are a number of methods to secure the fascia sling. Initially, the fascial sling was secured directly to the rectus fascia on each side. Subsequently, Govier and associates described a technique where they obtained a piece of fascia lata long enough (24 to 28 cm) to tie the two ends of the sling together over the rectus fascia without anchoring the sling directly to the rectus fascia.[53] In an attempt to improve urethral coaptation, Pérez and colleagues described securing the ends of the fascial graft to Cooper's ligament with or without crossing the ends of the graft across the midline.[54] To further enhance urethral coaptation, Ghoniem described wrapping the sling around the urethra at the level of the bladder neck in patients with myelomeningocele.[55] Once the sling is in place, several methods of securing it at the level of the bladder neck have been described. Suturing the midportion of the sling to the periurethral fascia was described by Gormley and associates.[56] A more complex method was described by Govier and coworkers, who used three interrupted absorbable sutures to tack the sling to the bladder and urethra.[53] The use of a submucosal tunnel appears to limit the need to secure the sling at the urethra.

Sling Tension

Since the introduction of the sling, there have been problems with overcorrection of the urethral axis causing obstructive symptoms or urinary obstruction.[57,58] Most surgeons performing suburethral sling surgery would agree that proper sling placement using a tension-free technique is vital for an acceptable surgical outcome. Excessive sling tension has been identified as a significant risk factor for persistent postoperative urinary retention.[57,58] The technique we prefer takes the ends of the graft, which are brought up to the rectus abdominis fascia, allowed to settle into position by gentle traction on the Foley catheter, and secured above the rectus abdominis fascia as previously described. The urethra is carefully inspected after this procedure to ensure that it is in an anatomic position without evidence of overcorrection.

Numerous methods of adjusting sling tension intraoperatively have been reported. An intraoperative urethral manometry to create an intraurethral pressure of 50 to 90 cm H_2O at the sling site was used by Beck and colleagues.[10] Endoscopic observation with direct visualization of mucosal "soft" coaptation was described by McGuire and colleagues as a method to adjust sling tension.[59] Alternatively, Govier described adjusting the sling tension until one finger could be placed between the suture and the anterior abdominal wall.[53] Rovner and coworkers used a cystoscope sheath placed transurethrally to maintain the urethral position while the sling was secured above the rectus abdominis fascia.[60] Nguyen and coauthors described the use of a cotton swab placed at the urethrovesical junction and maintained at an angle between 0 and 10 degrees to the horizontal plane while the suspension sutures were tied down.[61]

CLINICAL OUTCOMES

The results of the CFL sling have been discussed (see Table 38-1). The autologous fascia lata sling has been reported dating back to 1933.[7] Table 38-2 details some of the series of patients who have been examined. The cure rate from the autologous fascia lata sling ranges from 50% to 93%, and the improved rate represents another 2.3% to 27% of patients. Most of the studies had a failure rate of less than 10%, but one was as high as 27%. Only 3 of 13 studies used urodynamic studies to define cure; the remaining 10 studies used subjective data in the form of standardized and author-initiated questionnaires. The variability in assessment methods creates difficulty when comparing results from various studies. Overall, the successful trend of the autologous fascial sling is obvious. The autologous fascial sling has a higher success rate than its cadaveric counterpart.

COMPLICATIONS

After a pubovaginal sling placement, the complications specific to the surgery are urinary retention, de novo urgency, and urge incontinence.

Latini and colleagues used autologous fascia lata and surveyed 63 patients at an average of 4.4 years after surgery.[50] Postoperatively, 93% of the patients walked pain-free by 7 days, and there were no harvest site complications.

The rate of development of de novo urgency after pubovaginal sling placement has been reported to be from 10.8% to 28%.[31,62,63] Flynn and Yap studied the outcomes of 134 women who underwent placement of a pubovaginal sling (63 CFL and 71 autologous fascia lata).[62] The follow-up was a mean of 29 months in the CFL group and 44 months in the autologous fascia lata group. The CFL group had recurrence of the SUI in 13% and urge urinary incontinence (UUI) in 24%, with half of these being de novo cases. The autologous fascia lata group had recurrence of SUI in 10% and a 16% rate of UUI, with only 2 of 11 cases being de novo in origin. Two patients had a bladder perforation which healed uneventfully after a week of catheter drainage. Overall, there were 23 urinary tract infections and 4 abdominal wound infections, with slightly more of each in the autograft group. The allograft group had one case of prolonged retention that resolved at 56 days; the autograft group had three cases, two of which resolved at 45 and 90 days. The last patient in the autograft group required vaginal urethrolysis. Brown and Govier had a median postoperative catheterization of 9 days in their 104 patients who underwent a CFL pubovaginal sling.[64] Their 46 patients in the autograft group had a median catheterization of 14 days. There were two cases of prolonged retention in the CFL group and three cases in the autograft group, with one of the latter requiring urethrolysis.

Miller and associates attempted to predict who is at risk for development of urinary retention after pubovaginal sling placement.[65] Urodynamics and clinical evaluation were performed in 73 women before and after sling surgery. The average time to efficient voiding was 3.9 days. Twenty-one women voided preoperatively without a detrusor contraction, and 4 went into postsurgery retention. The remaining women who had a preoperative detrusor contraction of at least 12 cm H_2O did not develop postoperative retention. This study demonstrated that

Table 38-2 Outcomes of Autologous Fascia Lata Sling in Women with Stress Urinary Incontinence

First Author and Ref. No.	Year	*N*	Follow-up in Months, Range (Mean)	Method of Follow-up	% Cured/ Improved	% Failure	Fascial Source	Comments
Low[76]	1969	36	24-84 (12)	Subjective	86/9	5	FL	—
Addison[77]	1985	97		UDS and subjective	86.7/8	5	FL	94 procedures were performed secondarily
Beck[10]	1988	170	1.5-264 (24)	UDS and subjective	92.4/2.3	5	FL	Recommend reserve FL sling surgery for postsurgical SUI
Karram[78]	1990	10	12-24	UDS	90/10	Nil	FL	Used patch FL sling (5 × 7 cm)
Golomb[79]	1997	20	12-53 (30.7)	Subjective	90/10	Nil	RF/FL	5% voiding dysfunction postoperatively
Haab[63]	1997	37	24-60 (48.2)	Subjective	73 (combined)	27	RF/FL	62.1% with DI, 10.8% de novo DI
Breen[80]	1997	60	6-42	Subjective	90 (combined)	10	FL	13.4% slings needed to be released for urinary retention
Govier,[53] Brown[64]	1997, 2000	30	(44)	Subjective	73/27	Nil	FL	Improved defined as 1-3 pads/day; 1997 study found 10% failure rate
Petrou[81]	2001	14	5-41 (17)	Subjective	50/7	Nil	RF/FL	Used Blavis-Groutz score to measure outcomes
Flynn[62]	2002	71	30-58 (44)	Subjective	77/13	10	RF/FL	16% total UUI, 5% de novo UUI
Kreder,[31] Latini[50]	1996, 2004	63	9.6-111.6 (52.8)	Subjective	85 (combined)	15	FL	Success = 75% improvement over preoperative SUI symptoms

DI, detrusor instability; FL, fascia lata; RF, rectus fascia; SUI, stress urinary incontinence; UDS, urodynamic studies; UUI, urge urinary incontinence.

the absence of a preoperative detrusor contraction is a risk factor for retention after pubovaginal sling placement.

Amundsen and associates reported finding 9 cases of urethral erosion in a population of 57 women referred for urethrolysis.[66] Six of the 9 patients had had fascia lata used for their sling (5 CFL, 1 autologous fascia lata). All were treated with transvaginal lysis, and in no case did SUI recur. Kammerer-Doak and colleagues reported 5 of 22 patients with CFL for pubovaginal sling developing vaginal erosion at a mean of 36.8 days after the procedure.[67] They also noted 3 of 11 cases of vaginal erosion after abdominal sacrocolpopexy. The only risk factor identified for erosion was the development of a postsurgical febrile episode.

CONCLUSIONS

Fascia lata cystourethropexy is an appropriate choice for patients who require surgery for treatment of SUI. The success rate of the CFL sling ranges from 30% to 93.5%, and the failure rate can be from 6% to 66.6%. The autologous fascia lata sling has a higher success rate, from 50% to 93%, with a more acceptable failure rate of about 10%. Overall, the procedures are safe, with the autologous fascia lata causing more short-term patient morbidity than the CFL, which may be acceptable considering its improved outcomes.

References

1. Von Giordano D: Vingtieme Congres Français de Chirurgie. Proceedings, 1907, p 506.
2. Goebell R: Zur operativen beseitigung der angelborenen incontinenz vesicae. Zeitschr Gynakol Urol 2:187, 1910.
3. Squier JB: Postoperative urinary incontinence. Med Rec 79:868, 1911.
4. Aldridge AA: Transplantation of fascia for relief of urinary stress incontinence. Am J Obstet Gynecol 44:398-411, 1942.
5. McGuire EJ, Lytton B: Pubovaginal sling procedure for stress incontinence. J Urol 119:82-84, 1978.
6. Blaivas JG, Jacobs BZ: Pubovaginal sling for the treatment of complicated stress urinary incontinence. J Urol 145:1214-1218, 1991.
7. Price PB: Plastic operation for incontinence of urine and of faeces. Arch Surg 26:1043-1053, 1933.
8. Beck RP, Grove D, Arnusch D, Harvey J: Recurrent urinary stress incontinence treated by the fascia lata sling procedure. Am J Obstet Gynecol 120:613-621, 1974.
9. Beck RP, Lai AR: Results in treating 88 cases of recurrent urinary stress incontinence with the Oxford fascia lata sling procedure. Am J Obstet Gynecol 142:649-651, 1982.

10. Beck RP, McCormick S, Nordstrom L: The fascia lata sling procedure for treating recurrent genuine stress incontinence of urine. Obstet Gynecol 72:699-703, 1988.
11. Handa VL, Jensen JK, Germain MM, Ostergard DR: Banked human fascia lata for the suburethral sling procedure: A preliminary report. Obstet Gynecol 88:1045-1049, 1996.
12. Pelosi MA II, Pelosi MA III, Pelekanos M: The YAMA UroPatch sling for treatment of female stress urinary incontinence: A pilot study. J Laparoendosc Adv Surg Tech A 12:27-33, 2002.
13. Rutner AB, Levine SR, Schmaelzle JF: Processed porcine small intestine submucosa as a graft material for pubovaginal slings: Durability and results. Urology 62:805-809, 2003.
14. Zoedler D: [On surgical management of stress incontinence in women.] Z Urol 54:355-358, 1961.
15. Korda A, Peat B, Hunter P: Experience with Silastic slings for female urinary incontinence. Aust N Z J Obstet Gynecol 29:150-154, 1989.
16. Barbalias GA, Liatsikos EN, Athanasopolous A: Gore-Tex sling urethral suspension in type III female urinary incontinence: Clinical results and urodynamic changes. Int Urogynecol J Pelvic Floor Dysfunct 8:344-350, 1997.
17. Guner H, Yildiz A, Erdem A, et al: Surgical treatment of urinary stress incontinence by a suburethral sling procedure using a Mersilene mesh graft. Gynecol Obstet Invest 37:52-55, 1994.
18. Morgan JE, Farrow GA, Stewart FE: The Marlex sling operation for the treatment of recurrent stress urinary incontinence: A 16-year review. Am J Obstet Gynecol 151:224-226, 1985.
19. Morgan JE, Heritz DM, Stewart FE, et al: The polypropylene pubovaginal sling for the treatment of recurrent stress urinary incontinence. J Urol 154:1013-1014, 1995.
20. Fianu S, Soderberg G: Absorbable polyglactin mesh for retropubic sling operations in female urinary stress incontinence. Gynecol Obstet Invest 16:45-50, 1983.
21. Haab F, Zimmern PE, Leach GE: Female stress urinary incontinence due to intrinsic sphincter deficiency: Recognition and management. J Urol 156:3-17, 1996.
22. Elia G, Berman A: Estrogen effects on the urethra: Beneficial effects in women with genuine stress urinary incontinence. Obstet Gynecol Surv 48:509-517, 1993.
23. Horbach NS, Ostergard DR: Predicting intrinsic urethral sphincter dysfunction in women with stress urinary incontinence. Obstet Gynecol 84:188-192, 1994.
24. McGuire EJ, Fitzpatrick CC, Wan J, et al: Clinical assessment of urethral sphincter function. J Urol 150:1452-1454, 1993.
25. Nitti VW, Coombs AJ: Correlation of Valsalva leak point pressure with subjective degree of stress urinary incontinence. J Urol 155:281-285, 1996.
26. Weber AM: Is urethral profilometry a useful diagnostic test for stress urinary incontinence? Obstet Gynecol Surv 56:720-735, 2001.
27. Leach GE, Dmochowski RR, Appell RA, et al: Female Stress Urinary Incontinence Clinical Guidelines Panel summary report on surgical management of female stress urinary incontinence. The American Urological Association. J Urol 158:875-880, 1997.
28. Albo MR, Richter HE, Brubaker L, et al: Urinary Incontinence Treatment Network. Burch colposuspension versus fascial sling to reduce urinary stress incontinence. N Engl J Med 356:2143-2155, 2007.
29. Sand PK, Bowen LW, Panganiban R, Ostergard DR: The low pressure urethra as a factor in failed retropubic urethropexy. Obstet Gynecol 69:399-402, 1987.
30. Koonings PP, Bergman A, Ballard CA: Low urethral pressure and stress urinary incontinence in women: Risk factor for failed retropubic surgical procedure. Urology 36:245-248, 1990.
31. Kreder KJ, Austin JC: Treatment of stress urinary incontinence in women with urethral hypermobility and intrinsic sphincter deficiency. J Urol 156:1995-1998, 1996.
32. Zaragoza MR: Expanded indications for the pubovaginal sling: Treatment of type 2 or 3 stress incontinence. J Urol 156:1620-1622, 1996.
33. Cross CA, Cespedes RD, McGuire EJ: Our experience with pubovaginal slings in patients with stress urinary incontinence. J Urol 159:1195-1198, 1998.
34. Leach G, Sirls L: Pubovaginal sling procedures. Atlas Urol Clin North Am 2:61-72, 1994.
35. Handa VL, Jensen JK, Germain MM, Ostergard DR: Banked human fascia lata for the suburethral sling procedure: A preliminary report. Obstet Gynecol 88:1045-1049, 1996.
36. Gomelsky A, Scarpero HM, Dmochowski RR: Sling surgery for stress urinary incontinence in the female: What surgery, which material? AUA Update Series, Lesson 34, Volume 22. Houston: American Urological Association, 2003.
37. Choe JM, Bell T: Genetic material is present in cadaveric dermis and cadaveric fascia lata. J Urol 166:122-124, 2001.
38. FitzGerald MP, Mollenhauer J, Brubaker L: Failure of allograft suburethral slings. BJU Int 84:785-788, 1999.
39. Hathaway JK, Choe JM: Intact genetic material is present in commercially processed cadaver allografts used for pubovaginal slings. J Urol 168:1040-1043, 2002.
40. Amundsen CL, Visco AG, Ruiz H, Webster GD: Outcome in 104 pubovaginal slings using freeze-dried allograft fascia lata from a single tissue bank. Urology 56(6 Suppl 1):2-8, 2000.
41. Buck BE, Malinin TI: Human bone and tissue allografts: preparation and safety. Clin Orthop 303:8-17, 1994.
42. Lemer ML, Chaikin DC, Blaivas JG: Tissue strength analysis of autologous and cadaveric allografts for the pubovaginal sling. Neurourol Urodyn 18:497-503, 1999.
43. Sutaria PM, Staskin DR: Tensile strength of cadaveric fascia lata allograft is not affected by current methods of tissue preparation [abstract 1194]. J Urol 161(4 Suppl):310, 1999.
44. Choe JM, Kothandapani R, James L, Bowling D: Autologous, cadaveric, and synthetic materials used in sling surgery: Comparative biomechanical analysis. Urology 58:482-486, 2001.
45. Dora CD, Dimarco DS, Zobitz ME, Elliott DS: Time dependent variations in biomechanical properties of cadaveric fascia, porcine dermis, porcine small intestine submucosa, polypropylene mesh and autologous fascia in the rabbit model: Implications for sling surgery. J Urol 171:1970-1973, 2004.
46. Walter AJ, Morse AN, Leslie KO, et al: Changes in tensile strength of cadaveric human fascia lata after implantation in a rabbit vagina model. J Urol 169:1907-1910, 2003.
47. Wright EJ, Iselin CE, Carr LK, Webster GD: Pubovaginal sling using cadaveric allograft fascia for the treatment of intrinsic sphincter deficiency. J Urol 160:759-762, 1998.
48. O'Reilly KJ, Govier FE: Intermediate term failure of pubovaginal slings using cadaveric fascia lata: A case series. J Urol 167:1356-1358, 2002.
49. Carey JM, Leach GE: Transvaginal surgery in the octogenarian using cadaveric fascia for pelvic prolapse and stress incontinence: Minimal one-year results compared to younger patients. Urology 63:665-670, 2004.
50. Latini JM, Lux MM, Kreder KJ: Efficacy and morbidity of autologous fascia lata sling cystourethropexy. J Urol 171:1180-1184, 2004.
51. Foley SJ, Adamson AS: Minimally invasive harvesting of fascia lata for use in the pubovaginal sling procedure. BJU Int 88:293-294, 2001.
52. Walter AJ, Hentz JG, Magrina JF, Cornella JL: harvesting autologous fascia lata for pelvic reconstructive surgery: Techniques and morbidity. Am J Obstet Gynecol 185:1354-1359, 2001.
53. Govier FE, Gibbons RP, Correa RJ, et al: Pubovaginal slings using fascia lata for the treatment of intrinsic sphincter deficiency. J Urol 157:117-121, 1997.
54. Pérez LM, Smith EA, Broecker BH, et al: Outcome of sling cystourethropexy in the pediatric population: A critical review. J Urol 156:642-646, 1996.
55. Ghoniem GM: Bladder neck wrap: A modified fascial sling in the treatment of incontinence in myelomeningocele patients. Eur Urol 25:340-342, 1994.

56. Gormley EA, Bloom DA, McGuire EJ, Ritchey ML: Pubovaginal slings for the management of urinary incontinence in female adolescents. J Urol 152:822-827, 1994.
57. Kreder KJ, Webster GD: Evaluation and management of incontinence after implantation of the artificial urinary sphincter. Urol Clin North Am 18:375-381, 1991.
58. Carr LK, Webster GD: Voiding dysfunction following incontinence surgery: Diagnosis and treatment with retropubic or vaginal urethrolysis. J Urol 157:821-823, 1997.
59. McGuire EJ, Bennett CJ, Konnak JA, et al: Experience with pubovaginal slings for urinary incontinence at the University of Michigan. J Urol 138:525-526, 1987.
60. Rovner ES, Ginsberg DA, Raz S: A method for intraoperative adjustment of sling tension: prevention of outlet obstruction during vaginal wall sling. Urology 50:273-276, 1997.
61. Nguyen A, Mahoney S, Minor L, Ghoneim G: A simple objective method of adjusting sling tension. J Urol 162:1674-1676, 1999.
62. Flynn BJ, Yap WT: Pubovaginal sling using allograft fascia lata versus autograft fascia lata for all types of stress urinary incontinence: 2-Year minimum followup. J Urol 167:608-612, 2002.
63. Haab F, Trockman BA, Zimmern PE, Leach GE: Results of pubovaginal sling for the treatment of intrinsic sphincteric deficiency determined by questionnaire analysis. J Urol 158:1738-1741, 1997.
64. Brown SL, Govier FE. Cadaveric versus autologous fascia lata for the pubovaginal sling: Surgical outcome and patient satisfaction. J Urol 164:1633-1637, 2000.
65. Miller EA, Amundsen CL, Toh KL, et al: Preoperative urodynamic evaluation may predict voiding dysfunction in women undergoing pubovaginal sling. J Urol 169:2234-2237, 2003.
66. Amundsen CL, Flynn BJ, Webster GD: Urethral erosion after synthetic and nonsynthetic pubovaginal slings: Differences in management and continence outcome. J Urol 170:134-137, 2003.
67. Kammerer-Doak DN, Rogers RG, Bellar B: Vaginal erosion of cadaveric fascia lata following abdominal sacrocolpopexy and suburethral sling urethropexy. Int Urogynecol J Pelvic Floor Dysfunct 13:106-109, 2002.
68. Elliott DS, Boone TB: Is fascia lata allograft material trustworthy for pubovaginal sling? Urology 56:772-776, 2000.
69. Soergel TM, Shott S, Heit M: Poor surgical outcomes after fascia lata allograft slings. Int Urogynecol J 12:247-253, 2001.
70. Huang Y-H, Lin ATL, Chen K-K, et al: High failure rate using allograft fascia lata in pubovaginal sling surgery for female stress urinary incontinence. Urology 58:943-946, 2001.
71. Carbone JM, Kavaler E, Hu JC, Raz S: Pubovaginal sling using cadaveric fascia and bone anchors: Disappointing early results. J Urol 165:1605-1611, 2001.
72. Chien GW, Tawadroas M, Kaptein JS, et al: Surgical treatment for stress urinary incontinence with urethral hypermobility: What is the best approach? World J Urol 20:234-239, 2002.
73. Walsh IK, Nambirajan T, Donellan SM, et al: Cadaveric fascia lata pubovaginal slings: Early results on safety, efficacy and patient satisfaction. BJU Int 90:415-419, 2002.
74. Richter HE, Burgio KL, Holley RL, et al: Cadaveric fascia lata sling for stress urinary incontinence: A prospective quality-of-life analysis. Am J Obstet Gynecol 189:1590-1596, 2003.
75. FitzGerald MP, Edwards SR, Fenner D: Medium-term follow-up on use of freeze-dried, irradiated donor fascia for sacrocolpopexy and sling procedures. Int Urogynecol J 15:238-242, 2004.
76. Low JA: Management of severe anatomic deficiencies of urethral sphincter function by a combined procedure with a fascia lata sling. Am J Obstet Gynecol 105:149-155, 1969.
77. Addison WA, Haygood V, Parker RT: Recurrent stress urinary incontinence. Obstet Gynecol Ann 14:253-265, 1985.
78. Karram MM, Bhatia NN: Patch procedure: modified transvaginal fascia lata sling for recurrent or severe stress urinary incontinence. Obstet Gynecol 75:461-463, 1990.
79. Golomb J, Shenfeld O, Shelhav A, Ramon J: Suspended pubovaginal fascial sling for the correction of complicated stress urinary incontinence. Eur Urol 32:170-174, 1997.
80. Breen JM, Geer BE, May GE: The fascia lata suburethral sling for treating recurrent stress urinary stress incontinence. Am J Obstet Gynecol 177:1363-1366, 1997.
81. Petrou SP, Frank I: Complications and initial continence rates after a repeat pubovaginal sling procedure for recurrent stress urinary incontinence. J Urol 165:1979-1981, 2001.

Chapter 39

TENSION-FREE VAGINAL TAPE

John J. Klutke and Carl G. Klutke

Correction of female stress urinary incontinence (SUI) with the use of tension-free vaginal tape (TVT) was described in its present form in 1996.[1] Its unique features included intentional placement of support at the mid-urethra (previous surgical correction of SUI aimed to suspend the proximal urethra) and the use of a stress test to guide the surgeon in determining the degree of outlet resistance created. The biologically inactive nature of Prolene was recognized, and a Prolene mesh strip was placed to support the mid-urethra. The mesh was held in place by contact with adjacent tissue and was not separately fixed in place.

Ulmsten and colleagues recognized that correction of SUI carried a risk of interference with normal voiding.[2] TVT was designed to surgically correct support of the urethra at the level of the mid-urethra, the area where the pubourethral ligaments insert on the urethra. Ulmsten believed that the proximal urethra, the site of initiation of voiding, should be left in its normal, anatomically mobile state. The procedure was also designed to avoid excessive tension on the urethra by including a check mechanism in which mesh placement was adjusted based on a cough stress test. In order to do this, the patient had to remain awake and as close as possible to her normal state, eliciting the SUI.

The procedure was introduced in the United States in November of 1998. It soon became enormously popular with gynecologists and urologists alike, and within 5 years it became the most commonly performed procedure for SUI. With this remarkable change in practice came reports of TVT-associated complications. Shortly after introduction of the TVT procedure into mainstream practice, bowel and large vessel injury were reported.[3,4] In some cases, complications resulting from TVT placement had fatal consequences. Such serious complications are exceedingly rare with TVT. Nonetheless, introduction of the procedure into mainstream use brought to light unique challenges inherent in training surgeons to perform it properly and the need to develop an effective credentialing instrument. Furthermore, it was recognized that serious adverse events can occur even when an expert performs the procedure.

TECHNIQUE

Figures 39-1 and 39-2 illustrate the technique used in the TVT procedure. Use of a vaginal incision (see Fig. 39-1) as opposed to an abdominal incision (see Fig. 39-2) as the starting point for trocar passage is a defining feature for the procedure and verifies accurate placement of support at the mid-urethra. Although the direction of trocar passage has been hypothesized to increase the potential for bladder injury, three randomized comparisons of TVT to conventional sling operations with blind "up to down" mesh introduction showed no difference in the incidence of inadvertent bladder puncture.[5-8]

The procedure can and should be performed with the patient under local anesthesia and conscious sedation. Data have shown higher rates of voiding dysfunction and lower success rates with procedure deviations in which the cough stress test is not used.[9,10] The cough stress test with spinal anesthesia is misleading because of paralysis of the pelvic floor. The TVT procedure is pain free when performed properly and with adequate levels of local anesthetic.[11] In the absence of comparative studies with sufficient power to discern small differences in outcome when deviations from the original technique are used, it is our opinion that the TVT procedure should be performed as described by Ulmsten and colleagues,[1] using the cough stress test to guide placement.

Figure 39-3 illustrates passage of the introducing trocars. This step is a coordinated motor task without visual input. In other words, placement of the device is "blind." The tactual and kinesthetic cues involved in passing the trocar through the body are subtle. Bladder perforation is a relatively common complication, and cystoscopy is a required part of the procedure. Whether the procedure is performed by an expert or an amateur, unrecognized bowel injury is a possibility.

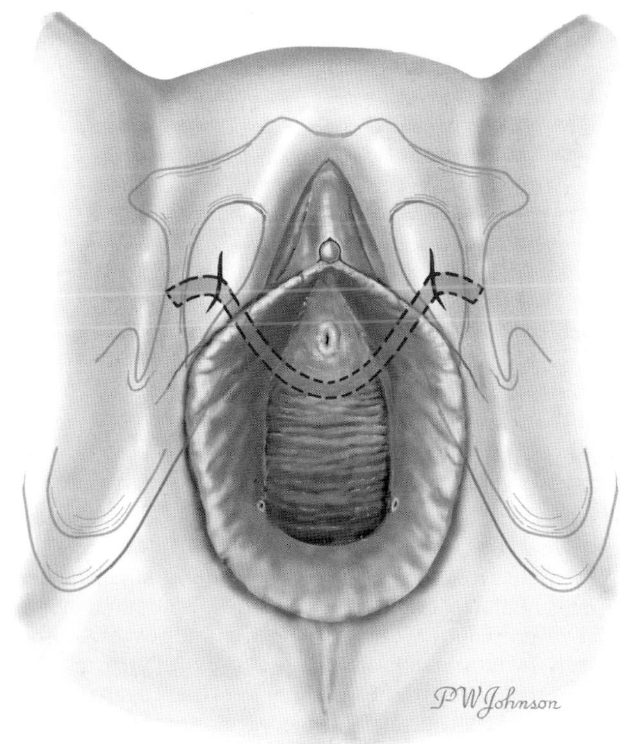

Figure 39-1 Tension-free vaginal tape procedure: vaginal incision.

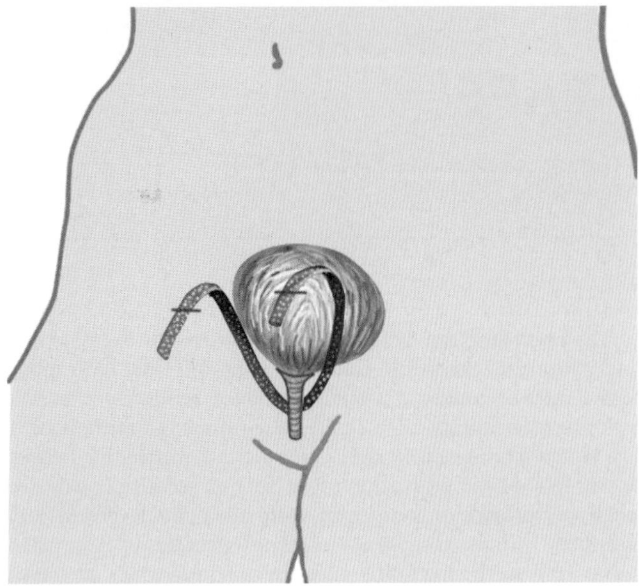

Figure 39-2 Tension-free vaginal tape procedure: abdominal incision.

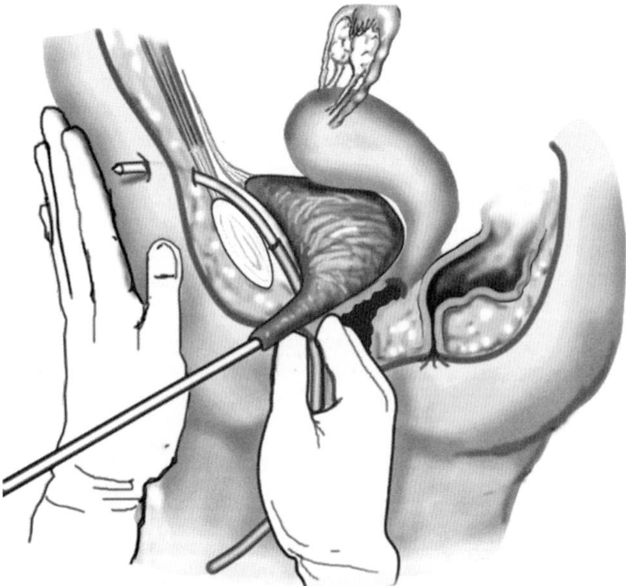

Figure 39-3 Blind passage of the introducing trocars.

PROOF OF CONCEPT

The published clinical experience with TVT is extensive and supports Ulmsten's promise of a simple, minimally invasive and highly effective solution to incontinence. Four studies have demonstrated minimal or no alteration in proximal urethral mobility after TVT procedure.[12-15] In a comparative study of colposuspension and TVT, Atherton and Stanton demonstrated that both procedures resulted in decreased mobility of the proximal urethra, but that statistically greater change was present after colposuspension.[16] It is apparent that cure of SUI is possible without affecting proximal urethral mobility.[12]

Urodynamic studies of voiding after the TVT procedure show conflicting results. Increased urethral resistance is demonstrated in two studies, but not in two others.[17-20] In a comparative study, Wang and Chen reported increased urethral resistance and decreased flow rates after colposuspension.[19] There was no difference in these measurements after TVT. Both increased and unchanged pressure transmission at the mid-urethra after TVT have been reported.[20-22] Conflicting measurements of urodynamic parameters after TVT may reflect small sample size in some of the studies or variable operator experience with the technique. They may also have resulted from the use of spinal anesthesia in two of the studies.[19,20] This is a deviation from the original technique, and with motor block of the pelvic floor affecting the cough stress test, it is conceivable that the degree of tension placed on the sling could be affected as well.

The rationale for performing TVT is to avoid overcorrection of anatomy and its systemic consequences. In a randomized comparative trial of TVT and colposuspension, significantly more women underwent corrective surgery for prolapse in the colposuspension group during the 2-year follow-up period.[23] Colposuspension, but not TVT, appeared to be causative in the development of the prolapse. There was a statistically significant increased incidence of voiding dysfunction in the colposuspension group at the 2-year follow-up. These findings highlight the importance of minimizing the changes induced in the system to restore continence, to minimize subsequent vulnerability to prolapse or the development of voiding dysfunction.

CONNECTIVE TISSUE RESPONSE

With the present widespread use of synthetic material in reconstructive pelvic surgical procedures, the potential for vaginal healing complications warrants close attention. Mesh or suture introduced in the vagina is, ideally, biologically inert and restores structural support by stimulating connective tissue growth with minimal inflammatory response. Clearly, different materials vary in the host reaction that is elicited when they are implanted in the body. Biologically active materials should be avoided.

Polypropylene mesh placed near the bladder in rabbits is well accepted by the host without exaggerated inflammation.[24] The material is also well accepted in humans, with fibrosis but little inflammatory response to mesh placed in paraurethral tissue.[25] Pore size, dimension, and weave of the mesh may also play a role in the host reaction, but they have less impact than the bioactivity of the material itself.

Comparison of bioactivity of Prolene versus Mersilene (polyester) has been made in humans. During the development of the TVT procedure, a high incidence of rejection of urethral slings made of Mersilene, but not slings made of polypropylene, was noted. Given this observation, Falconer and associates correlated clinical outcome with slings of both materials with biochemical measurements of connective tissue taken by biopsy near the site of sling placement.[26] Histologic differences were apparent, with greater tissue inflammatory reaction recorded in the Mersilene group. Greater collagen was also present in the Mersilene group, suggesting an increased host response.

The best indicator of the biologic inactivity of Prolene mesh in humans has been the clinical experience that has accrued since introduction of the TVT procedure. Vaginal healing complications have been rare with the TVT technique. In a large analysis of complications associated with the TVT procedure, the incidence of vaginal mesh extrusion was 0.7 %.[27] Most of these complications are better termed exposures than erosions, because the technique allows for placement of the polypropylene mesh in the tissue without excessive tension, or hang, on the capillary bed of the surrounding tissue.

Several authors have described conservative management of vaginal mesh exposure (i.e., excision of the exposed fragment and closure).[21,28-31] Complete excision of mesh, technically a very difficult procedure with the potential for excessive blood loss and dissection injury to the urethra and bladder, appears to be unnecessary in most cases.

EFFICACY

Efficacy was initially reported in 1998. Ulmsten and colleagues evaluated 131 consecutive cases performed at six centers.[32] All of the procedures were performed with the patient under local anesthesia. Outcome was determined by subjective and objective testing and was reported for the 1-year follow-up visit. Ninety-one percent of the study subjects were cured. The incidence of voiding dysfunction was minimal, with only one subject requiring catheterization for longer than 10 days.

Two other prospective studies were published in 1998. Nilsson reported cure in all of 31 consecutive patients who underwent the TVT procedure for SUI.[33] The procedure was performed with the patient under local anesthesia. Only one patient required catheterization for longer than 24 hours after the operation. Wang and Lo reported objective cure in 83% of 70 subjects after the TVT procedure for SUI.[34] In most cases, the surgery was performed with the patient under epidural anesthesia. Although still low, the incidence of voiding dysfunction was greater than in the other two studies, and the authors cited the choice of anesthesia as a potential explanation.

Soulie and colleagues,[35] Meschia and colleages,[28] Nilsson and Kuuva,[36] and Olson and Kroon[37] published other prospective studies. This brought the total number of subjects studied prospectively to 900. Although these initial studies were observational and reported short-term follow-up, they suggested high rates of efficacy with minimal voiding dysfunction, supporting the unique concepts that the TVT procedure introduced.

Ulmsten and coworkers, reported a study with 3-year follow-up in 1999, showed stable results that were comparable to those of previous studies.[38] Data with longer follow-up were available in 2001. Ninety consecutive patients were monitored for 5 years, with subjective and objective success rates reported to be 85%.[39] In other studies with long-term follow-up, Ulmsten's group reported cure in 82% of 34 women who underwent TVT for recurrent SUI, 74% of 49 women who had ISD, and 85% of 80 women who had mixed urinary incontinence.[40-42] Mid-term and long-term follow-up data are summarized in Table 39-1. Kuuva and Nilsson[43] and Jomaa[44] reported stable cure rates for TVT at 7-year follow-up.

Ward and Hilton reported a prospective randomized comparison of TVT to colposuspension in women with Genuine Stress Urinary Incontinence (GSUI).[21,23] Exclusion criteria were detrusor instability, voiding problems, prolapse requiring treatment, and previous surgery for incontinence or prolapse. A total of 344 subjects were recruited. Two years after surgery, objective cure rates for SUI were 63% for the TVT procedure group and 51% for the colposuspension group. These rates initially seem low in comparison to those typically reported for anti-incontinence operations in general, and it is important to consider the study design in interpreting the data. First, the study outcome was based on intent to treat, and those subjects who withdrew or were lost to follow-up were considered failures. Second, the criteria used to define cure in the study were stricter than those usually used: Only those subjects with less than 1 g of change in perineal pad weight after a 1-hour pad test were defined as cured. When cure was based purely on urodynamic findings, common practice in the urogynecology literature, TVT and colposuspension cured 89% and 85% of the subjects, respectively. These results suggest that, in a large group of randomly assigned patients, TVT was effective and appeared to be as effective as colposuspension in the treatment of SUI.

Operative complications were also described in the Ward and Hilton study.[23] In the initial 6-month follow-up report, the rate of operative complication was higher for the TVT procedure. The

Table 39-1 Outcome after Tension-Free Vaginal Tape Procedure: Mid-term and Long-term Follow-up

Investigators and Ref. No.	Year	*N*	Follow-up, Mean (yr)	% Cured
Ulmsten et al.[38]	1999	50	3	86
Olsson and Kroon[37]	1999	51	3	90 (objective)
Nilsson and Kuuva[36]	2001	85	4	85 (objective)
Nilsson et al.[39]	2001	90	5	85 (subjective) 85 (objective)
Rezapour and Ulmsten[40]	2001	34*	4	82 (objective)
Rezapour et al.[41]	2001	49†	4	74 (objective)
Rezapour and Ulmsten[42]	2001	80‡	4	85 (objective)
Villet et al.[29]	2002	124	3	89 (objective) 95 (subjective)
Kuuva and Nilsson[55]	2003	51*	2-5	80 (subjective) 90 (objective)
Total		564		84

*Recurrent stress incontinence.
†Intrinsic sphincter deficiency.
‡Mixed urinary incontinence.

Table 39-2 Complications Associated with Tension-Free Vaginal Tape

Complication	Tamussino et al (2001)[53] (*N* = 2795)	Kuuva and Nilsson (2002)[52] (*N* = 1455)	Ethicon, Inc. Complaint Reporting Statement[54] (*N* = 700,000)
Bladder perforation	Not reported	4.00%	Not reported
Major vascular injury	0.68%	0.07%	49 cases (0.007%)
Vaginal healing defect	Not reported	0.70%	Not reported
Nerve injury	0	0.07%	7 cases (0.001%)
Tape division or displacement for retention	1.00%	0.20%	Not reported
Bowel perforation	0.036%	0	35 cases (0.005%)
Urethral erosion	0	0	30 cases (0.004%)
Urinary tract infection	17%	14.10%	Not reported
De novo detrusor overactivity	Not reported	1%	Not reported

most frequent complications, bladder and vagina penetration, were not serious (Table 39-2). Fifteen bladder perforations occurred in the TVT group and 3 in the colposuspension group. None of these complications led to further adverse effects. Estimated blood loss was greater during colposuspension, although there was one serious hemorrhage in the TVT group. Postoperative complications, especially voiding dysfunction, occurred most commonly after colposuspension. Significantly more women in the colposuspension group required a subsequent prolapse operation.

Other comparative studies have been published.[5-8,45-48] Although these studies reported on smaller numbers of patients and had limited power to determine differences in outcome, they suggested equal results for TVT compared with colposuspension, laparoscopic colposuspension, and sling procedures.

BLADDER PERFORATION

A wide range for incidence of bladder perforation has been reported in prospective studies. In the hands of experts, the incidence of perforation is small, 1% or less. Others have encountered the complication more frequently, with a range of incidence from 4.4% to 71% reported in the literature.[49] Previous surgery has been cited as a contributing factor, but most perforations occurred in patients without scarring or distortion of the anatomy. Although proper patient selection plays a role in avoiding perforation, operator experience may be a more important factor.[50] Bladder perforation can be assumed to be due to improper trocar passage. This mechanism, taken as an error pathway, could also explain inadvertent bowel or vessel perforation. Bladder perforation does not have permanent implications for the individual patient, but it can be viewed as a sentinel event for operator error during introduction. It may therefore be related to the genesis of other complications resulting from operator error, which may have more serious implications for the patient.

Delayed penetration of the bladder or urethra has been reported.[51] This may represent delayed recognition or true migration of the tape. Urinary tract fistulas have also been reported.[52]

OTHER COMPLICATIONS

Two national registry databases are available that report complications associated with the TVT procedure.[52,53] It appears that the incidence of most complications with TVT is low relative to colposuspension and sling procedures. Gynecare company data are also available and provide an estimate of the incidence of serious complications.[54] Reporting complications to the company is voluntary, and the incidence determined is likely an underestimation. Based on 700,000 TVT procedures performed worldwide, there were 49 cases of vascular injury, an incidence of 0.007%. There were 35 cases of bowel injury (0.005%). Seven deaths were reported as of December 31, 2004, all related to vascular or bowel injury.

CONCLUSIONS

The emergence of the TVT procedure may represent the most significant development in incontinence treatment in the last 50 years. There is ample scientific data supporting its use. The procedure is highly effective and has long-lasting, if not permanent, results. Studies indicate that the procedure is safe when performed by well-trained individuals who have experience in pelvic anatomy. Nevertheless, there are troubling issues related to this blind procedure that is meant to be a mainstream solution to an extremely prevalent disorder. Complications are possible and can be fatal. The genesis of these complications is complex and includes operator error. Conventional prospective outcome studies, so useful in determining how well TVT works, explain very little about how it can go wrong. Clearly, there remains much work to be done in the area of anti-incontinence surgery.

References

1. Ulmsten U, Henriksson L, Johnson P, Varhos G: An ambulatory surgical procedure under local anesthesia for treatment of female urinary incontinence. Int Urogynecol J 7:81-86, 1996.
2. Petros P, Ulmsten U: An integral theory of female urinary incontinence: Experimental and clinical considerations. Acta Obstet Gynecol Scand (Suppl 153):5-93, 1993.
3. Brink DM: Bowel injury following insertion of tension-free vaginal tape. S Afr Med J 90:45-42, 2000.
4. Primicerio M, DeMatteis G, Montanino Oliva M, et al: Use of the TVT (tension-free vaginal tape) in the treatment of female urinary stress incontinence: Preliminary results. Minerva Ginecol 51:355-358, 1999.

5. Deval B, Levardon M, Samain E, et al: A French multicenter clinical trial of SPARC for stress urinary incontinence. Eur Urol 44:254-259, 2003.
6. Tseng L, Wang A, Lin Y, et al: Randomized comparison of the suprapubic arc sling procedure vs tension-free vaginal taping for stress incontinent women. Int Urogynecol J Pelvic Floor Dysfunct. 16:230-235, 2005. Epub 2004 Oct 27.
7. Andonian S, Chen T, St-Denis B, Corcos J: Randomized clinical trial comparing suprapubic arch sling (SPARC) and tension-free vaginal tape (TVT): One-year results. Eur Urol 47:537-541, 2005.
8. Lim YN, Muller R, Corstiaans A, et al: Suburethral slingplast evaluation study in North Queensland, Australia: The SUSPEND trial. Aust N Z J Obstet Gynaecol 45:52-59, 2005.
9. Wang AC, Lo TS: Tension-free vaginal tape: A minimally invasive solution to stress urinary incontinence in women. J Reprod Med 43:429-434, 1998.
10. Murphy M, Culligan PJ, Arce CM, et al: Is the cough-stress test necessary when placing the tension-free vaginal tape? Obstet Gynecol 105:319-324, 2005.
11. Schatz H, Henriksson L: Pain during the TVT procedure performed under local anesthesia. Int Urogynecol J Pelvic Floor Dysfunct 14:347-349, 2003.
12. Klutke JJ, Carlin B, Klutke C: The tension-free vaginal tape procedure: Correction of stress incontinence with minimal alteration in proximal urethral mobility. Urology 55:512-514, 2000.
13. Lukacz ES, Luber KM, Nager CW: The effects of the tension-free vaginal tape on proximal urethral position: A prospective, longitudinal evaluation. Int Urogynecol J Pelvic Floor Dysfunct 14:179-184, 2003.
14. Lo TS, Wang A, Horng SG, et al: Ultrasonographic and urodynamic evaluation after tension-free vaginal tape procedure (TVT). Acta Obstet Gynecol Scand 80:65-70, 2001.
15. Halaska M, Otcenasek M, Havel R, et al: Suspension of the lower third of the urethra in out-patient practice: Minimally invasive treatment of stress incontinence of urine—Technique and experience. Ces Gynek 1:4-9, 2000.
16. Atherton M, Stanton S: A comparison of bladder neck movement and elevation after tension-free vaginal tape and colposuspension. Br J Obstet Gynaecol 107:1366-1370, 2000.
17. Sander P, Moller LMA, Rudnicki PM, Lose G: Does tension free vaginal tape procedure (TVT) affect the voiding phase? Pressure-flow studies before and 1 year after surgery. BJU Int 89:694-698, 2002.
18. Gateau T, Faramarzi-Roques R, Le Normand L, et al: Clinical and urodynamic repercussions after TVT procedure and how to diminish patient complaints. Eur Urol 44:372-376, 2003.
19. Wang AC, Chen MC: Comparison of tension-free vaginal taping versus modified Burch colposuspension on urethral obstruction: A randomized controlled trial. Neurourol Urodyn 22:185-190, 2003.
20. Lin L, Sheu B, Lin H: Sequential assessment of urodynamic findings before and after tension-free vaginal tape (TVT) operation for female genuine stress incontinence. Eur Urol 45:362-366, 2004.
21. Ward KL, Hilton P, on behalf of the UK and Ireland TVT Trial Group: Prospective multicentre randomised trial of tension-free vaginal tape and colposuspension as primary treatment for stress incontinence. BMJ 325:67-70, 2002.
22. Mutone N, Mastropietro M, Brizendine E, Hale D: Effect of tension-free vaginal tape procedure on urodynamic continence indices. Obstet Gynecol 98:638-645, 2001.
23. Ward KL, Hilton P, on behalf of the UK and Ireland TVT Trial Group: A prospective multicenter randomized trial of tension-free vaginal tape and colposuspension for primary urodynamic stress incontinence: Two-year follow-up. Am J Obstet Gynecol 190:324-331, 2004.
24. Rabah DM, Spiess PE, Begin LR, Corcos J: Tissue reaction of the rabbit urinary bladder to tension-free vaginal tape and porcine small intestinal submucosa. BJU Int 90:601-606, 2002.
25. O'Sullivan S, Avery N, Bailey A, Keane D: The effect of surgery on the collagen metabolism of paraurethral tissue in women with genuine stress incontinence. Int Urogynecol J Pelvic Floor Dysfunct 11(Suppl 1):O10, 2000.
26. Falconer C, Soderberg M, Blomgren B, Ulmsten U: Influence of different sling materials on connective tissue metabolism in stress urinary incontinent women. Int Urogynecol J Pelvic Floor Dysfunct 12(Suppl 2):S19-S23, 2001.
27. Kuuva N, Nilsson CG: A nationwide analysis of complications associated with the tension-free vaginal tape (TVT) procedure. Acta Obstet Gynecol Scand 81:72-77, 2002.
28. Meschia M, Buonaguidi A, Amicarelli F, et al: Multicenter study on the effectiveness of tension free vaginal tape (TVT) in the treatment of stress urinary incontinence. Minerva Ginecol 52:375-379, 2000.
29. Villet R, Atallah D, Cotelle-Bernede O, et al: Treatment of stress urinary incontinence with tension-free vaginal tape (TVT): Mid-term results of a prospective study of 124 cases. Prog Urol 12:70-76, 2002.
30. Kobashi KC, Govier FE: Management of vaginal erosion of polypropylene mesh slings. J Urol 169:2242-2243, 2003.
31. Abouassaly R, Steinberg JR, Lemieux M, et al: Complications of tension-free vaginal tape surgery: A multi-institutional review. BJU Int 94:110-113, 2004.
32. Ulmsten U, Falconer C, Johnson P, et al: A multicenter study of tension-free vaginal tape for surgical treatment of stress urinary incontinence. Int Urogynecol J 9:210-213, 1998.
33. Nilsson CG: The tension free vaginal tape procedure (TVT) for treatment of female urinary incontinence: A minimally invasive surgical procedure. Acta Obstet Gynecol Scand 77(Suppl 168):34-37, 1998.
34. Wang AC, Lo TS: Tension-free vaginal tape: A minimally invasive solution to stress urinary incontinence in women. J Reprod Med 43:429-434, 1998.
35. Soulie M, Cuvillier X, Benaissa A, et al: The tension-free transvaginal tape procedure in the treatment of female urinary stress incontinence: A French prospective multi-centre study. Eur Urol 39:709-715, 2001.
36. Nilsson CG, Kuuva N: The tension-free vaginal tape procedure is successful in the majority of women with indications for surgical treatment of stress urinary incontinence Br J Obstet Gynaecol 108:414-419, 2001.
37. Olsson I, Kroon U-B: A three-year postoperative evaluation of tension-free vaginal tape. Gynecol Obstet Invest 48:267-269, 1999.
38. Ulmsten U, Johnson P, Rezapour M: A three-year follow up of tension free vaginal tape for surgical treatment of female stress urinary incontinence. Br J Obstet Gynecol 106:345-350, 1999.
39. Nilsson CG, Kuuva N, Falconer C, et al: Long-term results of the tension-free vaginal tape (TVT) procedure for surgical treatment of female stress urinary incontinence. Int Urogynecol J 12(Suppl 2): S5-S8, 2001.
40. Rezapour M, Ulmsten U: Tension-free vaginal tape (TVT) in stress incontinent women with intrinsic sphincter deficiency (ISD): A long-term follow-up. Int Urogynecol J 12(Suppl 2):S9-S11, 2001.
41. Rezapour M, Falconer C, Ulmsten U: Tension-free vaginal tape (TVT) in stress incontinent women with intrinsic sphincter deficiency (ISD): A long-term follow-up. Int Urogynecol J 12(Suppl 2): S12-S14, 2001.
42. Rezapour M, Ulmsten U: Tension-free vaginal tape in women with mixed urinary incontinence: A long-term follow-up. Int Urogynecol J 12(Suppl 2):S15-S18, 2001.
43. Nilsson CG, Rezapour M, Falconer C: Seven years follow-up of the tension-free vaginal tape procedure. Int Urogynecol J 14(Suppl 1): S35, 2003.
44. Jomaa M: A seven-year follow up of tension free vaginal tape (TVT) for surgical treatment of female stress urinary incontinence under local anaesthesia. Int Urogynecol J Pelvic Floor Dysfunct 14(Suppl 1):S69-S70, 2003.

45. Liapis A, Bakas P, Creatsas G: Burch colposuspension and tension-free vaginal tape in the management of genuine stress incontinence in women. Eur Urol 41:469-473, 2002.
46. Valpas A, Kivela A, Penttinen J, et al: Tension-free vaginal tape and laparoscopic mesh colposuspension in the treatment of stress urinary incontinence: Immediate outcome and complications—A randomized clinical trial. Acta Obstet Gynecol Scand 82:665-671, 2003.
47. Liang C, Soong Y: Tension-free vaginal tape versus laparoscopic bladder neck suspension for stress urinary incontinence. Chang Gung Med J 25:360-366, 2002.
48. Paraiso MF, Walters M, Karram M, Barber M: Laparoscopic Burch colposuspension versus the tension-free vaginal tape procedure: A randomized clinical trial. Obstet Gynecol Surv 60:166-167, 2005.
49. Atherton MJ, Stanton SL: The tension-free vaginal tape reviewed: An evidence-based review from inception to current status. BJOG 111:1-13, 2004.
50. Lebret T, Lugagne PM, Herve JM, et al: Evaluation of the tension-free vaginal tape procedure: Its safety and efficacy in the treatment of female stress urinary incontinence during the learning phase. Eur Urol 40:543-547, 2001.
51. But I, Bratus D, Faganelj M: Prolene tape in the bladder wall after TVT procedure: Intramural tape placement or secondary tape migration? Int Urogynecol J Pelvic Floor Dysfunct 16:75-76, 2005.
52. Kuuva N, Nilsson CG: A nationwide analysis of complications associated with the tension-free vaginal tape (TVT) procedure. Acta Obstet Gynecol Scand 81:72-77, 2002.
53. Tamussino KF, Hanzal E, Kolle D, et al; Austrian Urogynaecology Working Group: Tension-free vaginal tape operation: Results of the Austrian registry. Obstet Gynecol 98:732-736, 2001.
54. Complaint Reporting Statement: Reported complication rate as of December 2004, based on 700,000 procedures. Provided by Ethicon, Inc.

Chapter 40

MIDURETHRAL TO DISTAL URETHRAL SLINGS

Peter R. Petros

MIDURETHRAL TO DISTAL URETHRAL SLINGS

The first part of this chapter addresses the anatomic basis for the midurethral sling operations, and the second part describes the surgical techniques themselves.

Short History of Midurethral Slings

The first prototype midurethral sling, the "intravaginal slingplasty" operation, was performed in 1986. This operation[1,2] was based on the anatomic work of Robert Zacharin[3] and the observation that an implanted plastic fiber causes a controlled deposition of collagen. It was reasoned that a tape placed at the site of the pubourethral ligament, *without tension,* would create a scar tissue reaction and strengthen the weakened ligament. It was also reasoned that a midurethral tape placement without abdominal attachment would eliminate most of the postoperative pain and urinary retention associated with sling and colposuspension procedures. These hypotheses were proven in the prototype intravaginal slingplasty operations. The one remaining problem, a high rate of foreign body reaction to Mersilene, was resolved by using polypropylene.[2]

Structural Anatomy

Without ligamentous support, the bladder, urethra, and vagina have no shape, strength, or function. Fibroligamentous attachments connect urethra and bladder base to the vaginal membrane (Fig. 40-1), so any laxity of the underlying vagina may influence the urethra and bladder base. Stress urinary incontinence (SUI) is a mechanical process.[1] To better understand the pathogenesis and treatment of SUI, it is useful to examine how ligaments, fascia, and muscle forces all combine to give shape, strength, and function to the vagina. All the component structures in Figure 40-2 are interconnected, and all have a role in the functioning of the system. It follows that more than one damaged structure may need to be repaired for optimal restoration of a particular function.

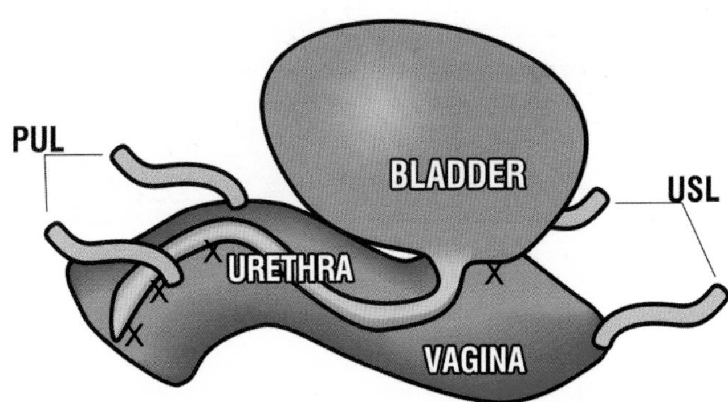

Figure 40-1 Unsupported organs have no strength, structure, or function. *X* indicates fibroligamentous attachments of distal urethra and bladder base to the vagina. The proximal urethra is not attached. *PUL,* pubourethral ligament; *USL,* uterosacral ligament.

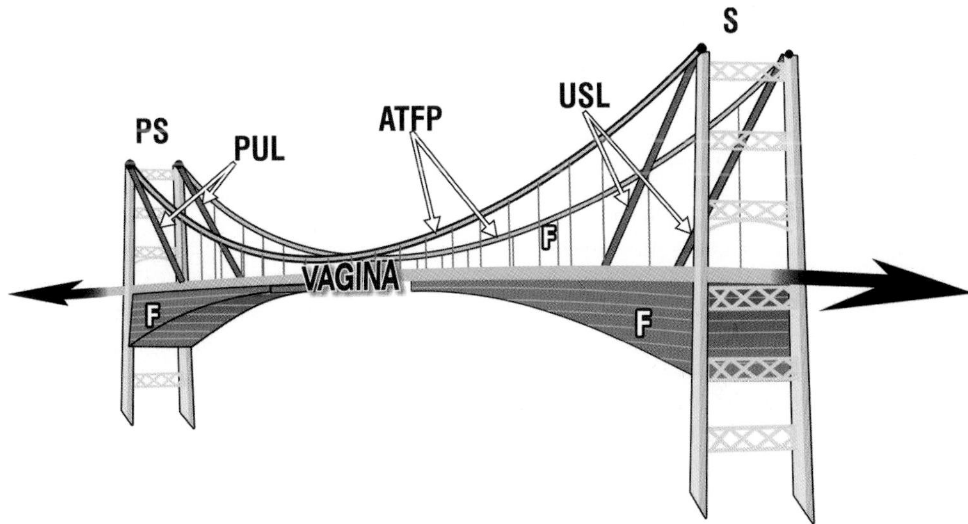

Figure 40-2 The suspension bridge analogy. The vagina is suspended anteriorly by the pubourethral ligament *(PUL),* posteriorly by the uterosacral ligament *(USL),* superiorly by arcus tendineus fascia pelvis *(ATFP),* and by attached fascia *(f).* Muscle forces *(arrows)* stretch the vaginal membrane against the suspensory ligaments to create shape and strength. *PS,* pubic symphysis; *S,* sacrum.

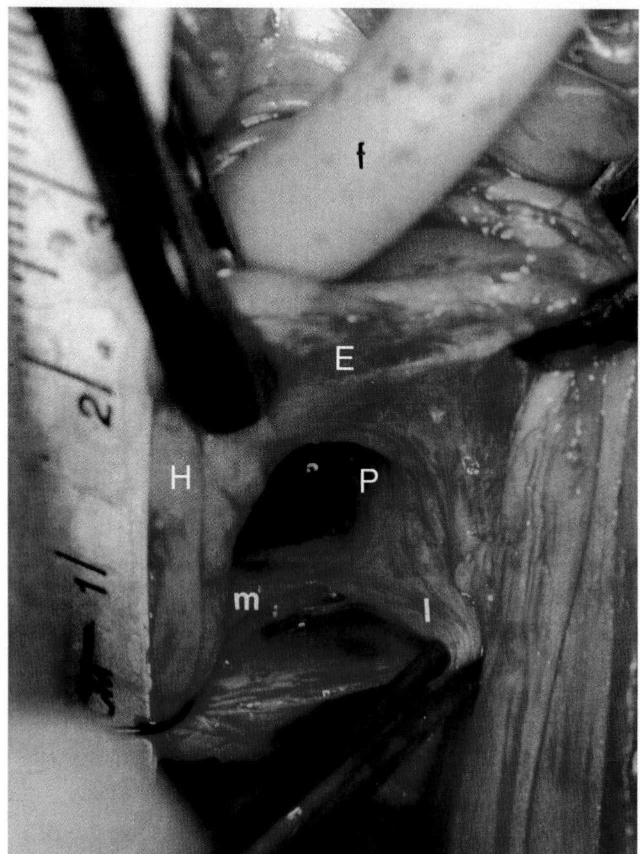

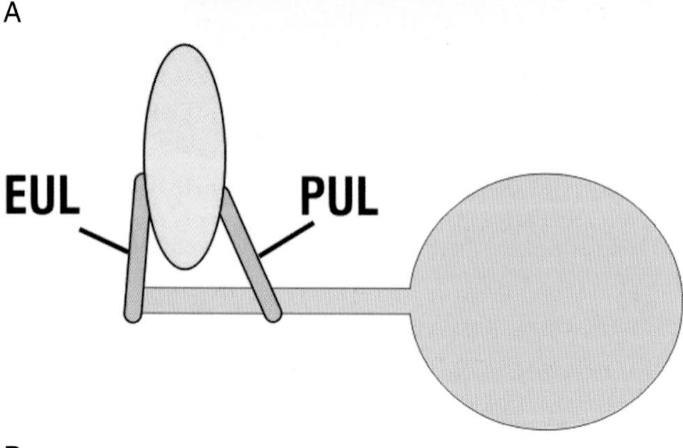

Figure 40-3 **A,** Suspensory ligaments of the distal urethra: view into the vagina, left paraurethral incision. The labels *m* and *l* indicate the medial and lateral branches of the pubourethral ligament, *P*. *E*, external urethral ligament; *f*, Foley catheter; *H*, hammock. **B,** Schematic sagittal view. *EUL*, external urethral ligament; *PUL*, pubourethral ligament.

Anatomy of the Urethra's Attachments

Figure 40-3 is a live anatomic study[4] of the structures involved in urethral closure. They are, in order of importance, the pubourethral ligament (P), the suburethral vaginal hammock (H), and the external urethral ligaments (E). The external ligament E attaches the external urethral meatus to the anterior surface of the pubic bone. The pubourethral ligament P descends from the posterior surface of the pubic bone.[3] Its medial part (m) attaches to the middle part of the urethra, and its lateral part (l) to the pubococcygeus muscle and, by extension, to the vagina.

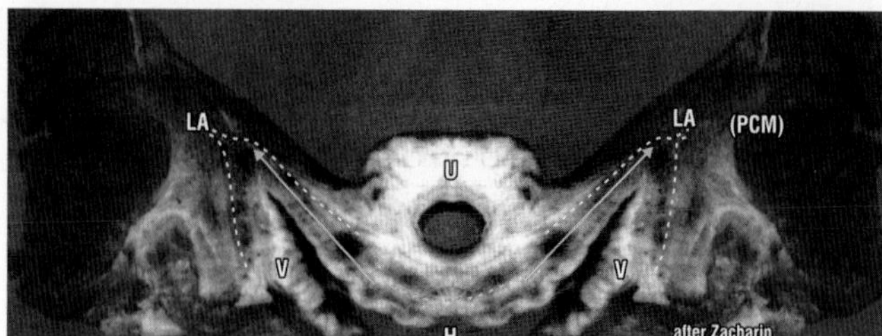

Figure 40-4 Anatomy of the vaginal hammock. Coronal section, cadaveric study. *Arrows* show direction of muscle forces. *H*, suburethral vaginal hammock; *LA*, levator ani also known as; pubococcygeus muscle *PCM*; *U*, urethra; *V*, vagina.

In 1963, Robert Zacharin demonstrated that the vaginal hammock is inserted into the lateral closure muscles (Fig. 40-4). This anatomy is consistent with dynamic video radiographic studies and ultrasound observations (Figs. 40-5 and 40-6).

Dynamic Anatomy of Urethral Closure

Abdominal ultrasound[5] (see Fig. 40-5B) demonstrates the contribution of the hammock and external ligament (E) to urethral closure. Closure occurs from behind, presumably by forward stretching of the hammock (H) against (E) by contraction of the pubococcygeus muscle (PCM).

Importance of Midurethral Anchoring for Closure and Micturition

The importance of a midurethral anchoring point is evident on the sequence of radiographs in Figure 40-6. During straining (see Fig. 40-6B, *arrow*), the distal urethra is pulled forward against the pubourethral ligament (PUL) for "urethral closure."[1] The proximal urethra is stretched backward and downward against the PUL (*arrows*) for "bladder neck closure."[1] During micturition (see Fig. 40-6C, *arrows*), the forward muscle force appears to relax, allowing the posterior urethral wall to be pulled open by the backward/downward muscle forces, right down to the PUL anchoring point. This opening vastly reduces the intraurethral resistance, facilitating the expulsion of urine. A surgical attachment at the bladder neck (Burch, fascial sling) may forcibly restrain the urethra from being stretched open during micturition, so that the detrusor has to expel urine through a narrower channel with a much higher resistance. The patient perceives this symptomatically as a slow flow, stopping and starting, incomplete emptying, and so on. From these radiographs it can be deduced that, whatever the operation performed for SUI, anchoring at or near the mid-urethra without excessive tension is an important factor in preventing postoperative urinary retention.

Clinical Anatomy: "Simulated Operations"

The individual contribution of the PUL, hammock, and the external urethral ligament (EUL) to urethral closure can be demonstrated directly by the office technique of "simulated operations." This technique also directly tests the theory underlying this work[1] for truth or falsity. A patient with known urine loss on coughing is tested with a full bladder in the supine position.[7]

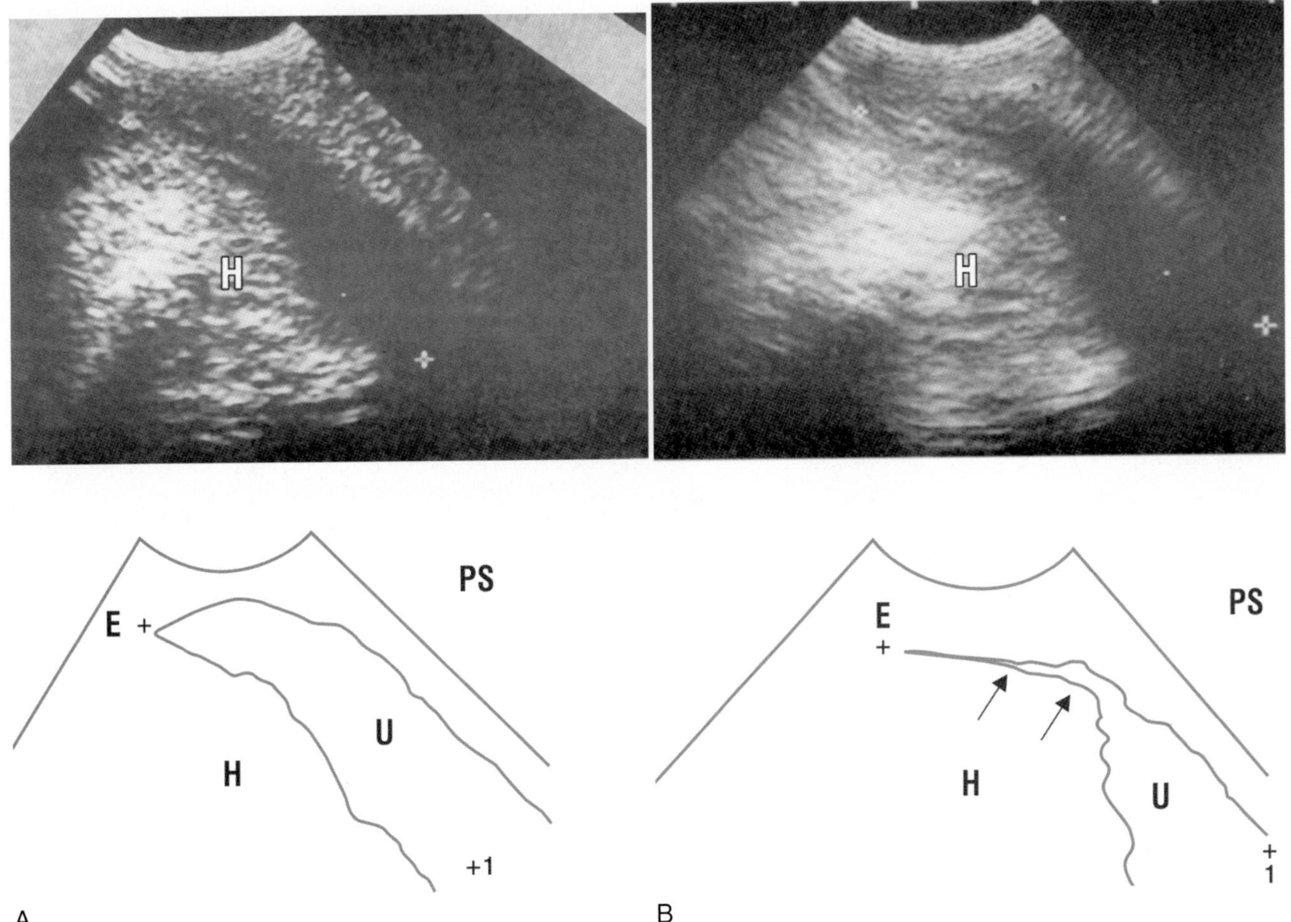

Figure 40-5 A, Abdominal ultrasound image and schematic diagram of distal urethra at rest. *E,* external urethral ligament attaching external meatus to the anterior surface of pubic bone; *H,* suburethral vaginal hammock; *PS,* pubic symphysis; *U,* urethral cavity. **B,** Same patient, image while straining. Note how the hammock is closed from behind *(arrows)*. The ligament *E* needs to be firmly anchored for optimal action of the closure forces. (From Petros PE, Ulmsten U: An integral theory of female urinary incontinence. Acta Obstet Gynecol Scand 69[Suppl 153]:7-31, 1990.)

Pressing upward on the anterior vaginal wall at the level of midurethra with a hemostat during coughing (Fig. 40-7) provides a temporary anchoring mechanism and mimics a midurethral sling. This maneuver immediately reduces urine loss in approximately 70% to 80% of patients.[7] Taking a fold of the hammock with a second hemostat ("pinch test")[8] usually restores complete continence in the remaining 20% to 30% of patients.[7] Anchoring the external urethral meatus may decrease urine loss in approximately 10% of patients. The synergistic actions of these structures can be demonstrated by anchoring one and then two structures simultaneously.

Anatomic Basis for Simulated Operations

During closure, the backward muscle forces (see Fig. 40-7, *arrows*) stretch the vaginal membrane and the trigone backward against the PUL. This action tensions the urethral tube and the vaginal hammock.[7] The forward force, the anterior portion of pubococcygeus (PCM), then stretches the vaginal hammock (H) forward to close the urethra from behind. Finally, the downward force, the longitudinal muscle of the anus (LMA), rotates the vagina and bladder base in a plane around the PUL to close off the bladder neck and proximal urethra. A weak PUL cannot sufficiently anchor the two backward forces (see Fig. 40-7), so the urethra is forcibly pulled from the closed (C) to the open (O) position during effort (Fig. 40-8). This is the clinical condition of SUI. It follows that a competent PUL is very important for stress continence control.

Figure 40-8 demonstrates the sequence of events in a patient with SUI. The anterior (a) and posterior (p) walls of the vagina are pulled backward and downward during straining (see Fig. 40-8B), opening out the outflow tract and causing urine loss (i.e., SUI). Midurethral anchoring (see Fig. 40-8C) restored normal bladder neck anatomy and continence in this patient. The sequence of events in Figure 40-8 indicates that the mechanism for causation of SUI is active opening out of the outflow tract by muscle forces, secondary to a lax midurethral anchoring point (see Fig. 40-7).

SURGERY

Five approaches to the tension-free midurethral sling are presented here: midline vaginal, suprapubic, paraurethral, transobturator, and subpubic. All work the same way anatomically.

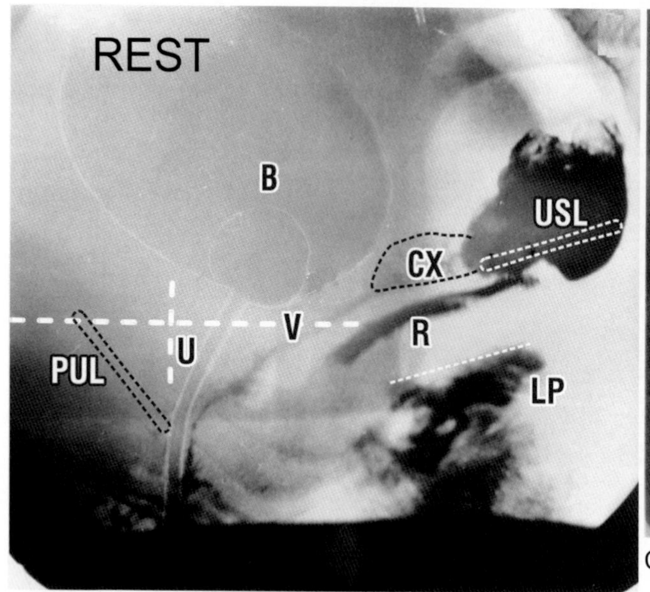

A

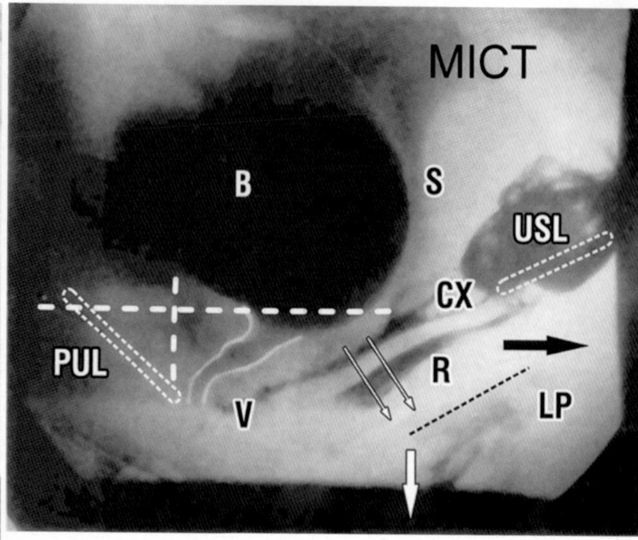

C

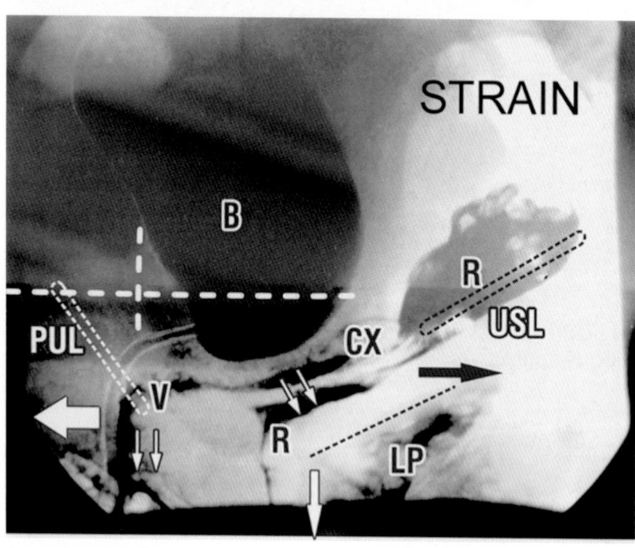

B

Figure 40-6 Role of the pubourethral ligament *(PUL)* during straining and micturition: radiographs taken at rest **(A)**, on straining **(B)**, and with micturition **(C)** in the same patient. The pubourethral ligament *(PUL)* is a critical anchoring point for the muscle forces *(large arrows)* in both straining and micturition. During straining, three muscle forces *(arrows)* act against the *PUL*. On micturition, the forward force relaxes; the backward/downward vectors *(diagonal arrows)* pull against *PUL* to open out the urethra and bladder neck. The white broken lines are drawn against fixed bony points. Note the downward angulation of the levator plate *(LP)* in **B** and **C.** *B*, bladder; *CX*, cervix; *R*, rectum; *U*, urethra; *USL*, uterosacral ligament; *V*, vagina.

Surgical Anatomy: Importance of Repairing the Whole System

Surgery is about restoration of anatomy. Based on the anatomic evidence presented, reconstruction of all damaged structures contributing to urethral closure is recommended: a midurethral tape (obligatory), hammock repair (obligatory), and, if it is lax, repair of the EUL. The midurethral sling is the most important component[7] of the closure mechanism. However, each structure contributes differently within each patient. The differential contribution to SUI of the EUL, hammock, and PUL can be estimated by performing a simulated operation (see Fig. 40-7), supporting each structure in turn while asking the patient to cough. In patients with intrinsic sphincter defect, or ISD (maximal urethral closure pressure <20 cm H_2O), it is advisable to repair all damaged structures so as to achieve optimal urethral closure. Using the paraurethral approach in a group of 11 patients with ISD, a cure rate of greater than 90% was achieved by repairing both the sling and the hammock.[9] A sling repair without hammock tightening achieved a 74% cure rate.[10]

Midline Vaginal Approach

An 18-french catheter in the urethra is used as a splint to lessen the possibility of urethral perforation (Fig. 40-9). Place the vaginal epithelium under stretch. Make a full-thickness incision in the midline from meatus to mid-urethra. Dissect between vagina and urethra laterally with scissors. Proceed with perforation of the diaphragm with scissors between the periosteum and subpubic ligaments, creating a space sufficient for entry of the delivery instrument.

Making a hole in the perineal membrane is the most critical step, no matter which delivery instrument is used, because it confers built-in safety to what is, essentially, a blind procedure. The hole prevents excessive thrust and allows perfect control of

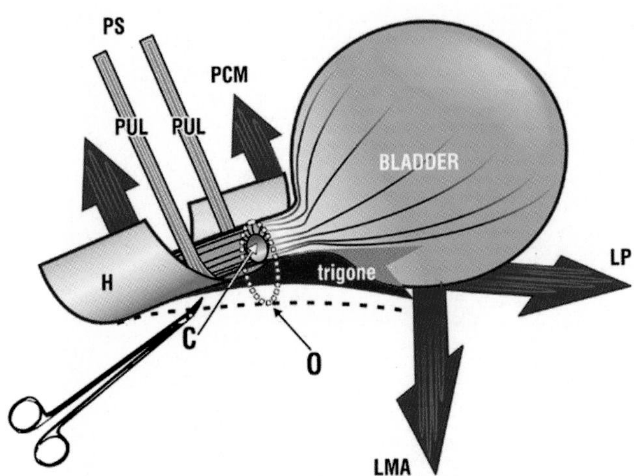

Figure 40-7 The mechanism of a "simulated operation." The hemostat mimics the anchoring effect of a normal pubourethral ligament *(PUL)*. This allows levator plate *(LP)* and longitudinal muscle of the anus *(LMA)* forces *(arrows)* to rotate and close the proximal urethra and the pubococcygeus muscle *(PCM)* to stretch the vaginal hammock *(H)* to close the distal urethra. The urethral cavity converts from the open position, *O*, to the closed position, *C*. *PS*, public symphysis.

the instrument at all times, helping avoid the major complications of this procedure, damage to the bladder and major vessels. Furthermore, if the subpubic venous sinuses are breached, this can be identified, because the bleeding flows out through the hole. The bleeding can be controlled by applying digital pressure for 3 minutes against the pubic bone from below.

Once the tip of the delivery instrument has entered the diaphragm, move the delta wing handle so it is horizontal. This is another critical step, because the external iliac vessels may be only 1.5 to 2 cm lateral to the exit point of the delivery instrument. The instrument can only move upward if the delta wing is horizontal. No pressure is applied against the posterior part of symphysis pubis. Use fingertip pressure only to gently roll the tip of the instrument over the posterior surface of the pubic bone. This vastly reduces the incidence of bladder perforation. A resistance is met at the level of the rectus sheath. At this point, sufficient pressure is applied to "pop through" the tip. The insert is left in situ, and the procedure is repeated on the contralateral side. With both inserts now in situ, the bladder is filled with 500 mL of saline, and a cystoscopy is performed. A volume of 500 mL is required to distend the bladder sufficiently to ensure that there are no bladder folds obscuring the tape should perforation occur. Care is taken to search especially around the air bubble at the 11 and 1 o'clock positions, the most common perforation sites.

If a nonelastic tape is used, a no. 7 Hegar dilator is inserted to splint the urethra, and the tapes are pulled up one by one. Sufficient tension is exerted to ensure that the tape has no folds. At all times during this step, downward pressure is exerted on the dilator to minimize urethral constriction. At this point, the tape is directly inspected for excessive tightness. The tape should be touching the urethra without indenting it. If there is indentation, loosen the tape. The tape is left tension-free, and is not sutured in any way to the abdominal muscles.

If an elastic tape is used, a space should be left between the tape and the urethra to allow for postoperative retraction. Otherwise, the technique is similar.

Hammock Tightening

It is recommended that hammock tightening be performed with all the techniques described in this chapter. With a no. 18 French Foley catheter in situ and using the tip of a short needle, the fascial tissue is firmly penetrated on both sides from the inside with a horizontal mattress suture so that the fascial tissue is brought toward the midline (see Fig. 40-9). It is essential to avoid contact with the tape during suturing. By taking the needle into the lower end of EUL, it is possible to tighten EUL and hammock using only one suture. If longer-term sutures are used, they need to be deeply anchored and cut onto the knot, otherwise they may surface and cause problems during intercourse.

External Urethral Ligament Shortening

It is recommended that EUL shortening be performed with all the techniques described here, if the EUL is loose. With a no. 18 Foley catheter in situ, and using a 1-0 or 2-0 suture on a small needle, sutures are inserted into the ligament vaginal fascia, contralateral EUL and tied. A stronger repair can be made by incising each EUL downward almost to the bone, inserting a 0.5-cm length of tape, and suturing the incision sufficiently tightly to prevent its later extrusion. The EULs are not approximated with this technique.

Paraurethral Approach

The paraurethral approach was first used in the Goebell-Frangenheim-Stoeckel sling in the early 1900s. It allows a more anatomically accurate restoration in that the hammock can be reattached to the closure muscles (Fig. 40-10). It is especially indicated if the vaginal sulcus is shallow. It has built-in safety, because the direction of instrument insertion is always upward. Its disadvantages are that it requires two incisions. Also, a tunnel has to be made in the tissue between vaginal epithelium and urethra, something that may be difficult to accomplish in patients with a deep paraurethral sulcus.

Two full-thickness longitudinal incisions are made in the lateral vaginal sulcus, extending from just below the level of the external urethral meatus to the level of the mid-urethra (see Fig. 40-10). A Foley catheter identifies the bladder neck.

A suburethral tunnel (TU in Fig. 40-10) is created between vagina and urethra at the level of the mid-urethra. The tape is inserted into the tunnel and brought through the anterior abdominal wall with the delivery instrument. Cystoscopy is performed. The tapes are pulled up one side at a time and adjusted for tension over a no. 7 Hegar dilator.

Transobturator Approach

The transobturator approach is not strictly anatomic, because the PULs descend vertically. The entry point is from the medial border of the obturator foramen, at the level of the clitoris. This anatomy explains instances of bladder perforation with this method, suggesting that it may be prudent to perform cystoscopic examination after placement of the tape. The tape is horizontally disposed, so care needs to be taken that it sits at the mid-urethra. The transobturator approach avoids small bowel and major vessel perforation. Potential disadvantages are damage to the obturator nerve or vessels or to the urethra.

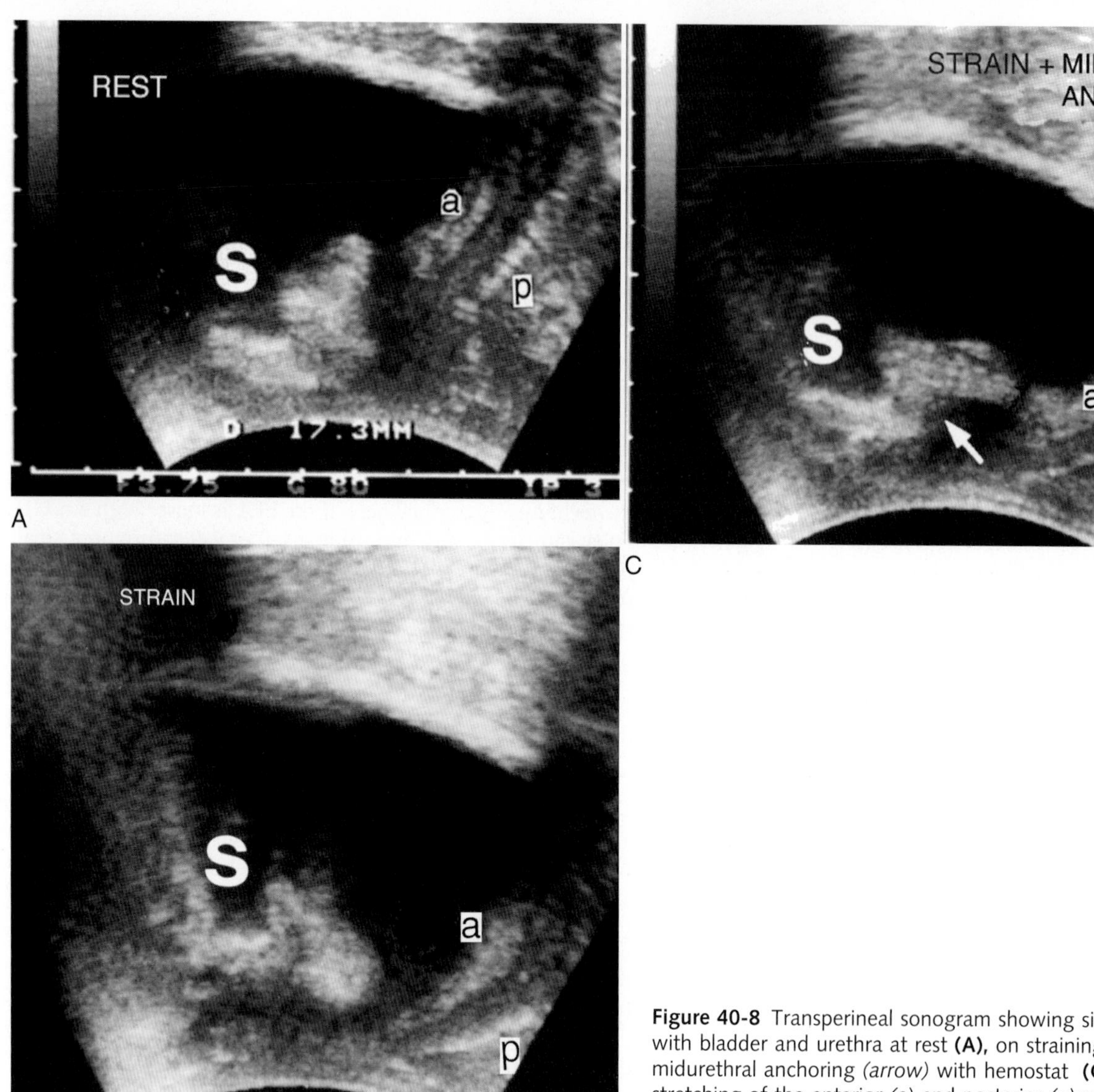

Figure 40-8 Transperineal sonogram showing simulated operation with bladder and urethra at rest **(A)**, on straining **(B)**, and after midurethral anchoring *(arrow)* with hemostat **(C)**. Note backward stretching of the anterior *(a)* and posterior *(p)* vaginal walls on straining and their apparent tensioning after midurethral anchoring. S = symphysis pubis.

Suprapubic Approach

Anatomically, the suprapubic approach is similar to the midline vaginal approach, except that entry of the application instrument is from above downward.

Potential Intraoperative and Postoperative Problems of the Suburethral Tension-Free Tape Slings

It is emphasized that inserting a suburethral sling with a delivery instrument is a blind procedure. The small bowel in the prevesical pouch, the bladder, the external iliac vessels, and the obturator nerves and vessels all lie within 2 cm of the track taken by the instrument. Creating a hole in the pelvic diaphragm directly below the bone and orienting the delivery instrument so that it can move only upward greatly reduce (but do not eliminate) the possibility of major complications.

Difficulty with Passage of the Delivery Instrument

Often, the subpubic ligaments are strong. Dissect a space with scissors. Avoid excessive pressure on the delta wing handle, because this may make the point dig into the soft cartilage of the symphysis and obstruct upward movement. Always ensure that the delta wing is horizontal on re-entry.

Retropubic Fibrosis from Previous Incontinence Surgery

Use dissecting scissors to create a plane of dissection between periosteum and scar tissue. Continue for 2.5 to 3 cm. This creates a plane between bone and scar tissue. If resistance continues, reinsert scissors and continue further dissection upward. Reinsert the delivery instrument. On rare occasions, it is only possible to insert one side of the sling. In such circumstances, attach the other side deep into the pubococcygeus muscles.

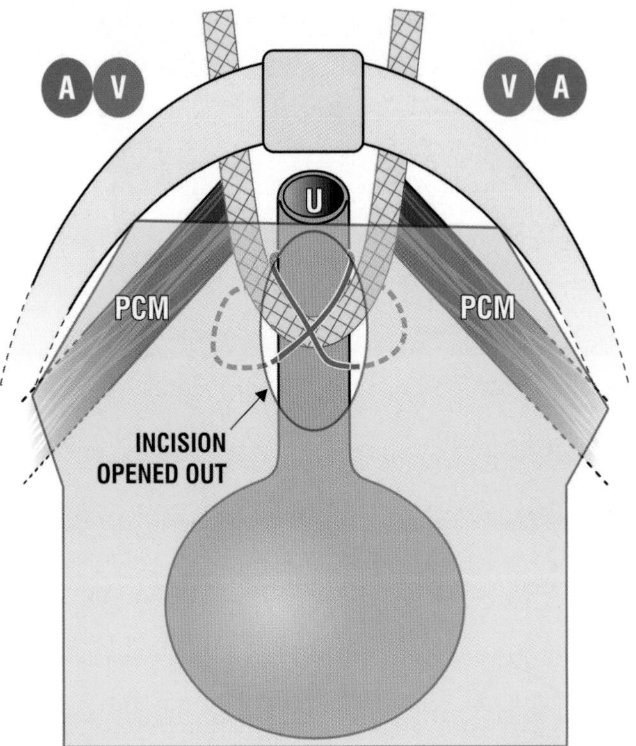

Figure 40-9 Midline approach. The perspective is looking into the anterior vaginal wall. A midline incision is made. Hammock tightening supports the tape from below. *A*, external iliac artery; *PCM*, pubococcygeus muscle; *U*, ureter; *V*, external iliac vein.

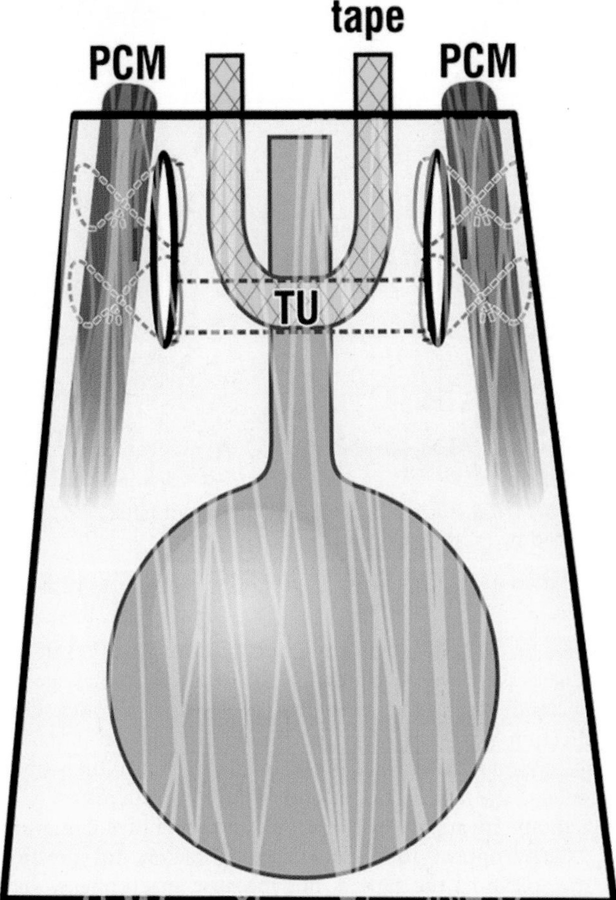

Figure 40-10 Paraurethral approach. Paraurethral vaginal skin incisions are made. The tape is passed through a tunnel *(TU)* between the incisions. The perspective is looking directly into the vagina. *PCM*, anterior portion of pubococcygeus muscle.

Scarring in the Rectus Sheath

Because of a previous abdominal operation, the surgeon may occasionally need to cut down onto the rectus sheath with a scalpel.

Bleeding

There are venous sinuses immediately below the pubic bone As soon as the tape has been inserted, apply digital pressure for 2 to 3 minutes. If there is overt bleeding, insert a hemostatic gel along the tape from below and reapply digital pressure until the bleeding ceases.

Bladder Perforation

Bladder perforation may occur in the superolateral surface, usually between 11 and 12 o'clock. If this occurs, remove the tape and reinsert it. Use a cystoscope with a sheath, and fill the bladder with 500 mL of fluid. Sometimes, there is no bleeding with perforation. The only sign of perforation may be the finding of a low bladder volume at the end of the operation due to extraperitoneal loss. If bladder perforation is suspected and cannot be identified, inject 1 ampoule of methylene blue into 100 to 200 mL of saline, fill the bladder, and look for suprapubic staining at the abdominal exit of tape.

Urethral Constriction by the Tape

Failure to pass any urine at all within 48 hours usually indicates a tape obstruction that needs to be surgically relieved. In the few cases that have occurred in my experience, microscopic loops were used to identify the shiny fibrils of the tape, which is always under tension. The tape retracts immediately when touched (cut) gently with a sharp blade. Constriction can generally be avoided by pressing downward against an intraurethral no. 7 Hegar dilator when tightening anon-elastic tape, or leaving a space if elastic.

Tape Rejection

This technology works by creating a foreign body reaction in the form of scar tissue to reinforce a damaged ligament. An excessive reaction is uncommon and may manifest as a purulent discharge. The pus is sterile and nonthreatening. A more common problem is tape slippage and surfacing into the vagina. This is also mostly benign, because the tape by that time is encased in a fibrous tissue cylinder. Almost invariably, the patient is afebrile, with a normal white blood cell count and a lack of bacterial growth on vaginal swabs.[6] To remove a partly rejected (surfaced) tape, place scissors on each side of the extruded tape, press upward against the vagina, and cut the tape. If there is significant infiltration of tissue into the tape, a segment may need to be excised and the vagina sutured.

Tape Infection

A virulent organism such as streptococcus may cause a bacterial infection. Unlike a foreign body reaction, this is potentially serious, and the patient may present with pyrexia, swelling, and erythema at the site of the tape. Under no circumstances should

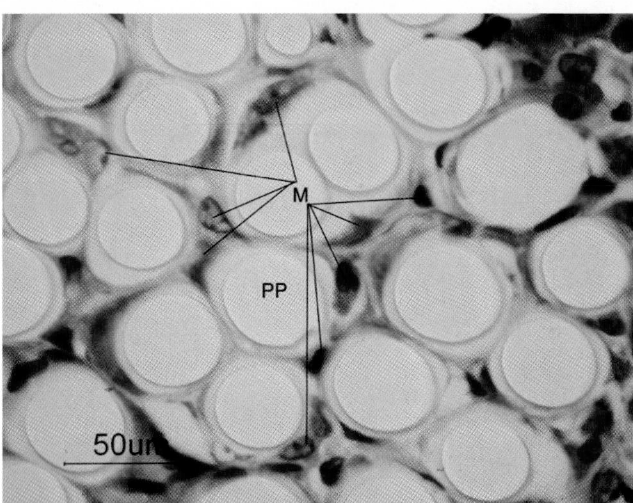

Figure 40-11 Rat study at 2 weeks. Multifilament fibrils *(PP)* are surrounded by macrophages *(M)*.

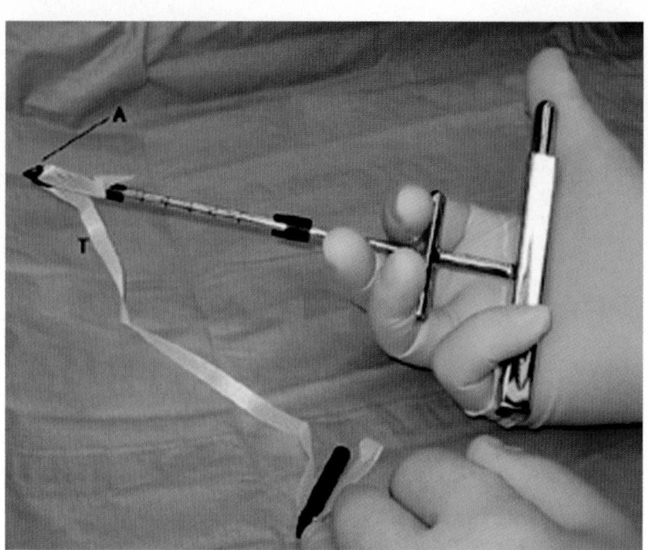

Figure 40-12 The tissue fixation system *(TFS)*. *A*, soft tissue anchor; *T*, tape.

the sinus be excised, because attempts to do so may result in a pelvic abscess or even bacteremia. The best way to manage this complication is to take a swab and treat with antibiotics. Once the infection has settled, the tape should be removed in part or completely *from the vagina.* In the operating room, the sinus is located, and the tape is grasped and removed by pulling on it. An infected tape invariably just slips out. Intraoperative hematoma and obesity appear to be predisposing factors to infection, but the weave of the tape is not, because macrophages have been demonstrated to surround the fibrils as early as 2 weeks[11] (Fig. 40-11).

Subpubic Approach: A Promising Direct-Vision "Micro" Technique

Although minimal morbidity is the norm, all midurethral sling operations, without exception, have a potential for major, even fatal complications, such as small bowel injury, obturator nerve injury, and external iliac and obturator vessel injury.[12] Ostergard[12] attributed such complications to the blind nature of these procedures. The growing list of serious complications[12] was the motivating factor behind the development of a safer delivery instrument, the tissue fixation system (TFS). The TFS consists of a polypropylene tape with two soft tissue anchors at each end (Fig. 40-12).

The anchors sit inside a plastic saddle and are ejected 0.5 cm into the tissues below the pubic bone by a stainless steel applicator. The TFS anchor works like a grappling hook, anchoring into the soft tissues below the pubic symphysis. The base of the anchor incorporates a one-way system for tightening of the tape. This is a crucial part of the TFS system, because muscle forces need an adequately firm ligament for the optimal contraction required to effect watertight urethral closure.

The TFS is performed under direct vision, so it avoids viscus, nerve, and major vessel injuries. It vastly decreases operating time (mean, 5 to 6 minutes). The operation is identical to the first part of a midline midurethral sling operation. A full-thickness midline incision is made into the vagina from just below the external urethral meatus to the mid-urethra. The vagina is dissected off the urethra with dissecting scissors, and the dissection is carried

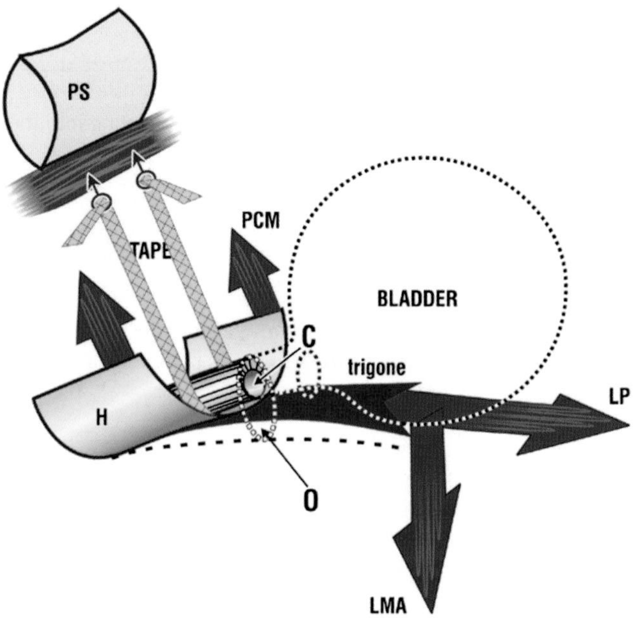

Figure 40-13 Subpubic midurethral sling. The tape reinforces the pubourethral ligament, restoring contractility of all three muscle forces *(arrows)*, so that the urethral tube is restored from the open *(O)* to the closed *(C)* position during effort. *H*, hammock; *LMA*, longitudinal muscle of the anus; *LP*, levator plate; *PCM*, pubococcygeus muscle; *PS*, pubic symphysis.

down just below the pubic bone. The TFS applicator is placed into the space and triggered so that the TFS anchor enters the perineal membrane (Fig. 40-13). The procedure is repeated on the contralateral side. The tape is tensioned just sufficiently for it to fit snugly on the urethra without indenting it over an 18-gauge Foley catheter. Both ends of the tape are cut 1.5 cm from the TFS anchor, and the hammock and EUL are tightened as described earlier. No cystoscopy is required. Intraoperative bleeding is minimal.

Results ($N = 35$) at 9 months[13] and at 3 years are promising >80% cure (Petros PEP and Richardson PA, unpublished data).

All patients to date were discharged within 24 hours of surgery, with no postoperative urinary retention. No opiates were needed postoperatively for the anterior sling operations. No significant complications were encountered. Surgical cure for both SUI and ISD was equivalent to that previously described for tension-free tape slings.[2,9] The main potential disadvantage of the TFS is that the operation will not work unless the anchor grips into the target tissue. The cause of failure may be poor tissues or surgeon error in placement; both were encountered in the first group of patients. Half of the sling was found surrounded by a granuloma in one patient, and the operation failed in another four patients without tape surfacing. The operation was successfully repeated in four of the five patients. In another patient with a "frozen" retropubic space, subpubic anchoring was not possible, and the anchor required more lateral anchoring.

CONCLUSIONS

The importance of a midurethral sling for continence control is now well accepted. Future challenges are the application of less invasive methods, how to more accurately assess the other connective tissue structures contributing to continence control, and how best to repair them.

References

1. Petros PE, Ulmsten U: An integral theory and its method for the diagnosis and management of female urinary incontinence. Scand J Urol Nephrol (Suppl 153)69:1-93, 1993.
2. Ulmsten U, Henriksson L, Johnson P, Varhos G: An ambulatory surgical procedure under local anesthesia for treatment of female urinary incontinence. Int Urogynecol J Pelvic Floor Dysfunct 9:210-213, 1996.
3. Zacharin RF: The suspensory mechanism of the female urethra. J Anat 97:423-427, 1963.
4. Petros PE: The pubourethral ligaments: An anatomical and histological study in the live patient. Int J Urogynecol 9:154-157, 1998.
5. Petros PE, Ulmsten U: An integral theory of female urinary incontinence. Acta Obstet Gynecol Scand 69(Suppl 153), 7-31, 1990.
6. Petros PEP: The Female Pelvic Floor: Function, Dysfunction and Management, according to the Integral Theory. Heidelberg: Springer, 2004, pp 14-138.
7. Petros PE, Von Konsky B: Anchoring the midurethra restores bladder neck anatomy and continence. Lancet 354:997-998, 1999.
8. Petros PE, Ulmsten U: Pinch test for diagnosis of stress urinary incontinence. Acta Obstet Gynecol Scand 69(Suppl 153), 33-35, 990.
9. Petros PE: New ambulatory surgical methods using an anatomical classification of urinary dysfunction improve stress, urge, and abnormal emptying. Int J Urogynecol 8:270-278, 1997.
10. Rezapour M, Falconer C, Ulmsten U: Tension-free vaginal tape (TVT) in stress incontinence women with intrinsic sphincter deficiency: A long-term follow-up. Int Urogynecol J Pelvic Floor Dysfunct 12(Suppl2):S12-S14, 2001.
11. Papadimitriou J, Petros PEP: Histological studies of monofilament and multifilament polypropylene mesh implants demonstrate equivalent penetration of macrophages between fibrils. Hernia 9:75-78, 2005. Epub 2004 Nov 19.
12. Ostergard DR: The epochs and ethics of incontinence surgery: Is the direction forward or backwards? [editorial]. Int Urogynecol J 13:1-3, 2002.
13. Petros PEP, Richardson PA, The midurethral TFS sling—a 'micro method' for cure of stress incontinence—a preliminary report ANZJOG 45:372-375, 2005.

Chapter 41

DISTAL URETHRAL POLYPROPYLENE SLING

Nasim Zabihi, M. Grey Maher, and Larissa V. Rodríguez

The sling procedure, first described in 1907 by Von Giordano, has been used for the treatment of female stress urinary incontinence (SUI) for almost 100 years.[1] This procedure was reintroduced in 1978 by McGuire and Lytton, who used autologous rectus fascia suspended under the bladder neck for the treatment of intrinsic sphincter deficiency.[2] In the past 25 years, a significant number of surgical procedures have been devised for the treatment of SUI, including multiple sling variations. A meta-analysis of various surgical techniques used in the treatment of SUI revealed that slings have similar durability to retropubic suspensions and are more efficacious than transvaginal suspensions and anterior repairs.[3] In the past decade, slings have gained popularity, because new surgical techniques, sling materials, and anchoring methods have led to decreased surgical morbidity and convalescence time while providing good durability and ease of placement.

Given this widespread popularity, many new procedures, materials, and packaged kits have emerged. Most sling procedures can be categorized by location of the sling (proximal urethra and bladder neck versus middle to distal urethra), choice of sling material (autologous graft, xenograft, cadaveric graft, or synthetic material), anchoring method, sling length, and degree of penetration into the retropubic space. This chapter discusses mid-distal urethral slings and describes the surgical technique and clinical outcomes of the distal urethral polypropylene sling (DUPS) procedure.

MID-DISTAL TO DISTAL SUBURETHRAL SLINGS

Slings were classically reserved for the treatment of SUI in the absence of urethral hypermobility. Although the exact mechanism by which slings restore continence remains elusive, the introduction and success of the mid-distal to distal slings have expanded understanding of the urethral support and continence mechanism. Klutke and colleagues demonstrated that anatomic correction of bladder neck hypermobility was not necessary to cure SUI.[4] The tension-free vaginal tape (TVT), introduced in 1996, has been shown to be an effective treatment for SUI.[4-18] Studies have demonstrated the TVT procedure to be as effective as open colposuspension, with documented cure rates of 81% and an improvement rate of 94%.[19] Given the success of the TVT and based on the same anatomic principle and mechanism of action, other procedures such as SPARC (American Medical Systems, USA), Safyre (Promedon, Argentina), SABRE (Mentor Corporation, USA), and the transobturator tape (TOT; Mentor), among others, have been described for the treatment of SUI. All of these procedures involve the placement of a synthetic sling at the level of the mid-distal to distal urethra and are available as commercially packaged kits that include placement needles or passers and prefabricated slings. The primary difference is the approach to placement (i.e., from the suprapubic area to the vagina or from the vagina to the suprapubic area), sling length, passage through the retropubic region or not, and variations in the hardware necessary for placement. The special equipment requirements along with the high cost of the packaged kits make it difficult to use these devices in many parts of the world. Additionally, many of these techniques are done blindly without finger guidance, which can lead to high rates of bladder perforation and rare but major complications such as bowel or major vessel injuries resulting in severe morbidity.[20-22]

DUPS uses the same anatomic location and therapeutic principles as the other mid-distal slings described mentioned earlier, and it has been shown to be effective in the treatment of SUI.[23,24] However, it has a lower risk of major injuries, because the sling is placed under tactile guidance through the retropubic space. The sling used is a 10 × 1 cm, short piece of soft, loosely woven mesh with large pores attached to absorbable sutures. Although the sutures traverse the retropubic space, the mesh itself traverses only 2 to 3 cm on each side into the retropubic space, because the presence of a small segment of mesh in the retropubic space is an important factor to cure SUI. Most of the other slings are self-fixating to the abdominal wall or the obturator muscle; DUPS uses a short segment of mesh attached to absorbable sutures for temporary support of the mesh until it becomes incorporated. This avoids complications such as infection or inguinal pain secondary to nerve entrapment from the suprapubic fixation while providing adequate attachment and fixation to the retropubic space. Additionally, these mesh properties lessen the chance of complications such as mesh erosion into the urethra. DUPS is a simple, quick, and inexpensive procedure with a lower risk of major complications compared with other slings.

SURGICAL TECHNIQUE

The patient is placed in high dorsal lithotomy position. The lower abdomen and genitalia are prepared and draped in sterile fashion, the labia are retracted laterally with stay sutures, and the bladder is emptied with a 16-Fr urethral Foley catheter. A weighted vaginal speculum is used for exposure. An Allis clamp is used to grasp the anterior vaginal wall just proximal to the meatus. Two oblique lateral incisions are made in the anterior vaginal wall (Fig. 41-1). Another Allis clamp is placed at the distal end of each of the oblique incisions, and the dissection is carried out laterally over the glistening periurethral fascia toward the ipsilateral shoulder. The retropubic space is entered at the level of the mid-

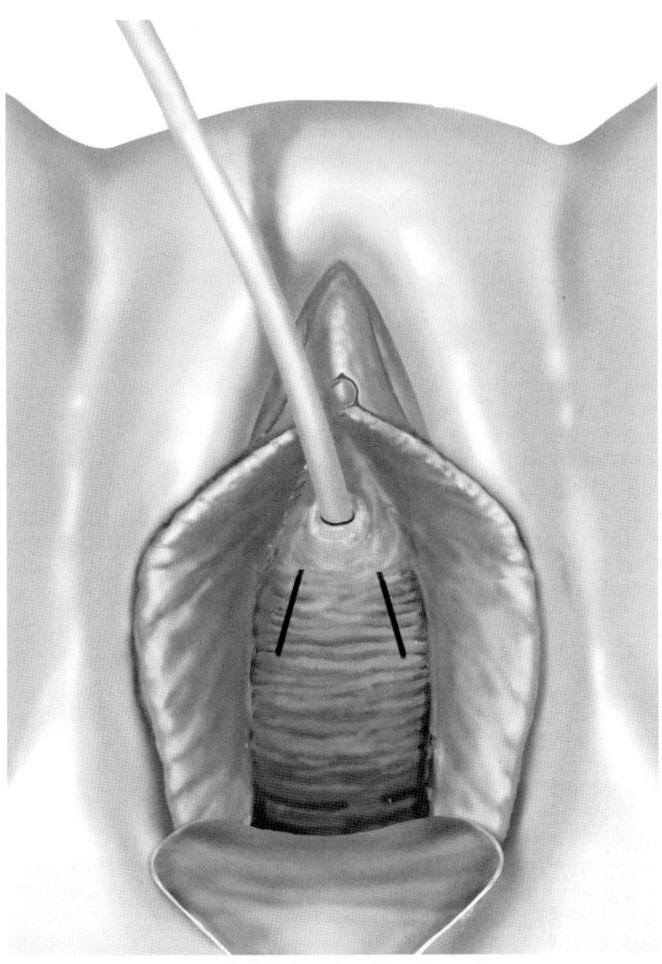

Figure 41-1 Two oblique lateral incisions are made in the anterior vaginal wall.

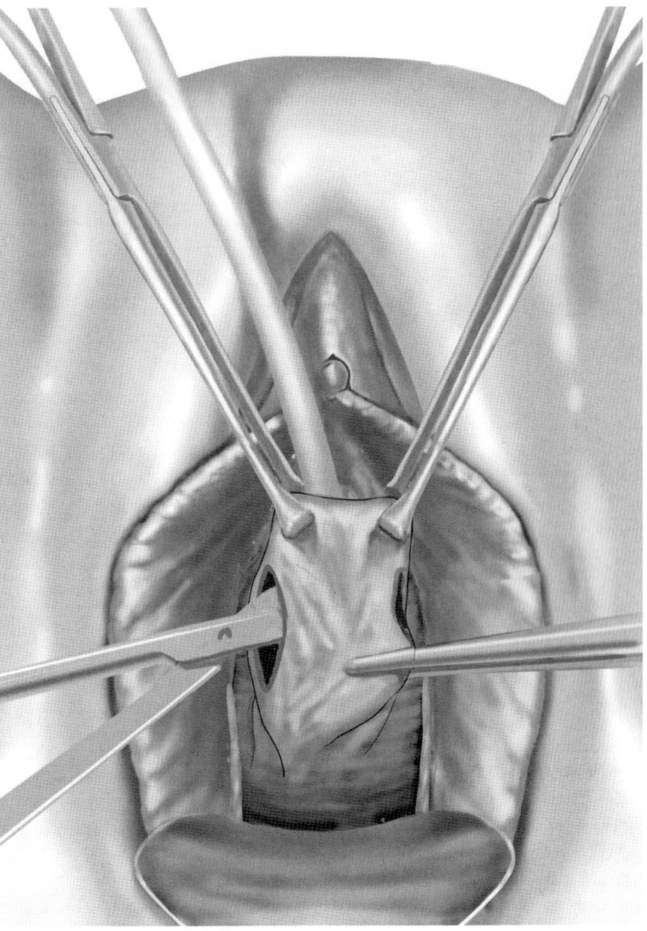

Figure 41-2 The retropubic space is entered at the level of the mid to distal urethra using curved scissors.

distal to distal urethra, using curved scissors directed parallel to the urethra just under the pubic bone (Fig. 41-2).

A fine right angle clamp is then used to create a suburethral tunnel in the anterior vaginal wall, 1.5 cm from the urethral meatus (Fig. 41-3). The sling, which is a 1 × 10 cm, thinly woven, soft polypropylene (Ethicon, Inc., NJ) mesh with 1-0 polyglactin (Vicryl) sutures placed at each end, is then transferred underneath the suburethral tunnel (Fig. 41-4). The next step is to transfer the ligature attached to the sling through the retropubic space.

One fingerbreadth cephalad to the symphysis pubis, a small puncture wound is made with a no. 15 scalpel. A double-pronged needle (Cook Urological, Spencer, IN) is passed under finger guidance through the fascia and retropubic space to the level of the oblique vaginal incision (Fig. 41-5). This prevents vascular and bowel injuries, because the needle is transferred under direct control just posterior to the pubic bone. The polyglactin sutures previously placed at the edge of the soft polypropylene mesh are transferred to the suprapubic incision. This maneuver is done bilaterally, and cystoscopy is performed to rule out bladder or urethral perforations.

To ensure a tension-free sling, one Allis clamp is placed through each vaginal incision, and the mesh is grasped and held firmly in the horizontal plane (Fig. 41-6) while the assistant ties the polyglactin sutures suprapubically, 1 mm below the skin level and not immediately above the fascia. The vaginal incisions are closed with 3-0 polyglactin running stitch, and the suprapubic puncture wound is closed with a with 4-0 polyglactin subcuticular stitch. A vaginal pack and dressing are applied.

In the recovery room, 2 hours after the procedure, the vaginal pack and the Foley catheter are removed and the patient is discharged home. If the surgeon prefers to keep the bladder drained, the patient can be sent home with the urethral catheter, or a suprapubic tube (SPT) can be placed at the beginning of the case. We place an SPT only if concomitant extensive vaginal reconstruction or hysterectomy has been performed. If a suprapubic tube is left in place, it is capped before discharge, and the patient is instructed to record her postvoid residuals; it is removed once the residuals are less than 50 mL.

SURGICAL OUTCOMES

A total of 840 patients have undergone the DUPS procedure at the University of California, Los Angeles Medical Center. The procedure is durable with equivalent 1-year and 5-year outcomes.[24,25] The original cohort, which included 69 patients, was monitored for 5 years. This cohort represented a complex

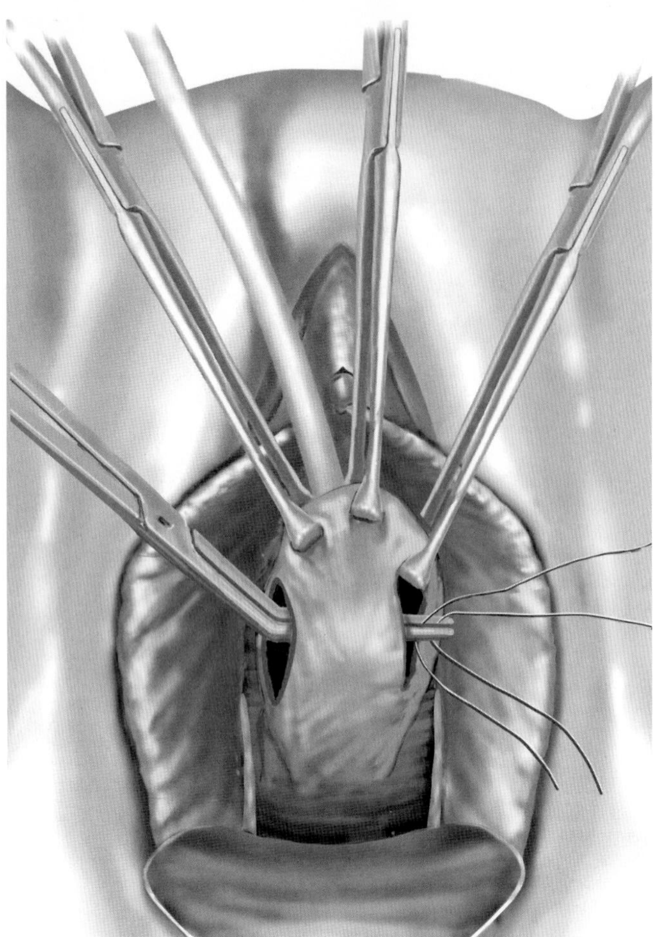

Figure 41-3 Suburethral tunnel is created in the anterior vaginal wall using a fine tipped right angle clamp.

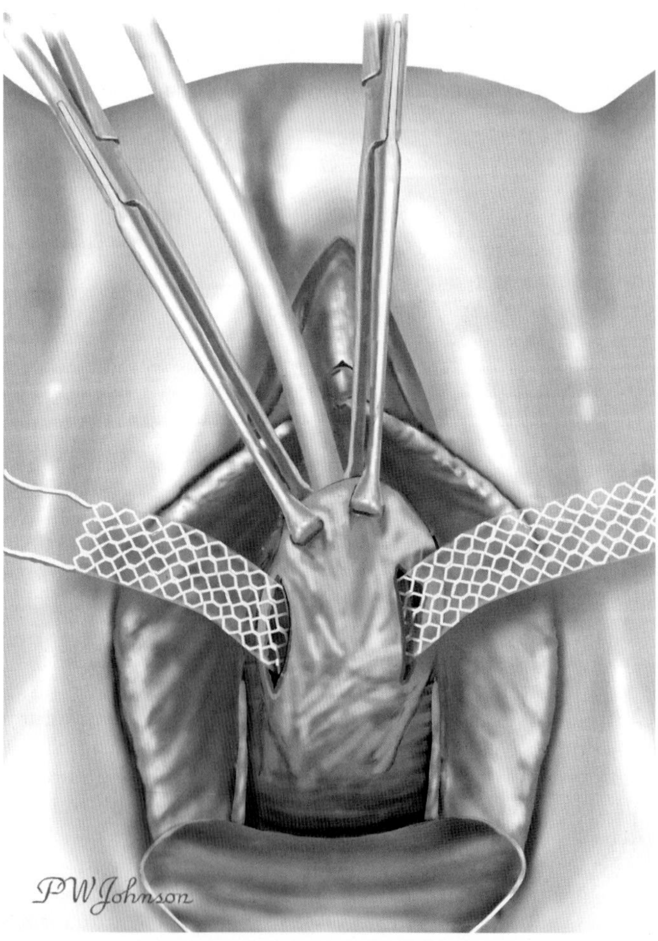

Figure 41-4 The mesh is transferred under the previously created tunnel.

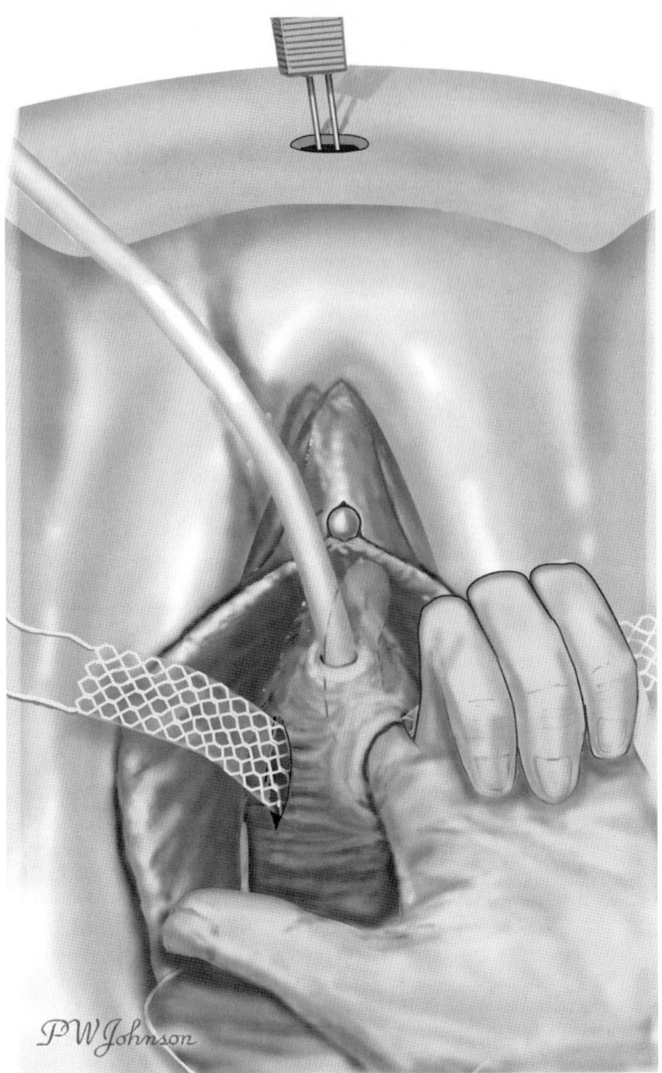

Figure 41-5 A double-pronged needle is passed under finger guidance from the suprapubic stab wound, through the retropubic space, to the level of the oblique vaginal incision.

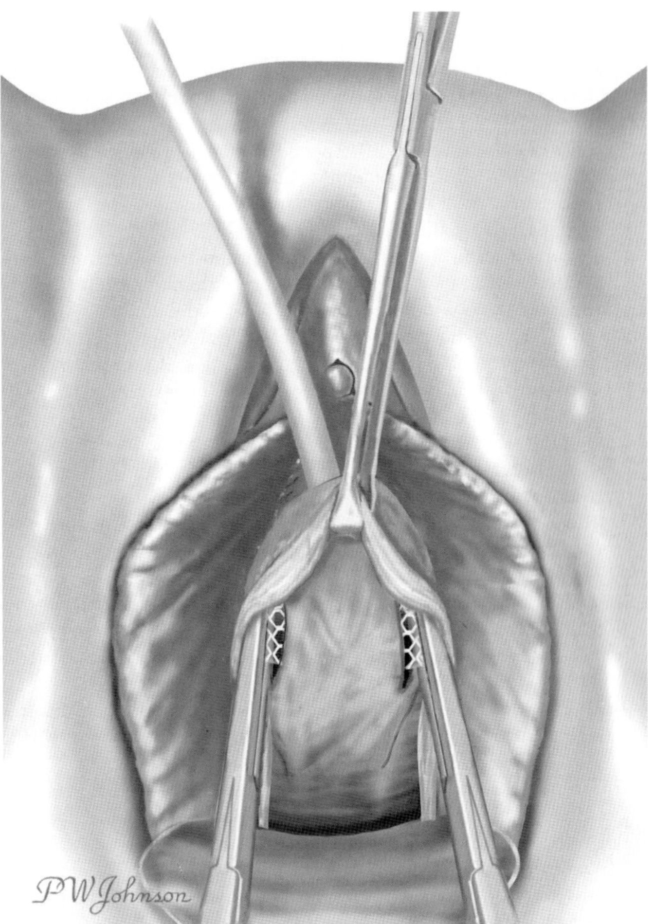

Figure 41-6 Allis clamps are used to hold the sling in the horizontal plane.

group of patients, as expected in a tertiary referral center: 52% percent had prior failed anti-incontinence therapy, 36% underwent concomitant prolapse surgery, and 54% suffered from mixed urinary incontinence. There were no intraoperative complications.

To report their outcomes, the authors used patient self-assessment questionnaires to eliminate physician bias, because studies have shown that evaluation of treatment outcomes using patient self-assessment tools demonstrates lower cure rates compared with physician assessments and that objective cure rates and clinical outcomes do not always translate to patient satisfaction.[26-29] Patients completed a symptom questionnaire and the short form of the Urogenital Distress Inventory (UDI-6).[30,31] They also answered a global quality-of-life question related to urinary symptoms and recorded the quantity of pads used per day. Seventy-two percent of the patients denied any symptoms, 74% denied any bother from SUI, and 93% reported that they had SUI less than once per week and were rarely bothered by symptoms of SUI. The average pad usage decreased by 74% ($P < .05$), and 56% reported wearing no pads at all. Patients, on average, reported a symptom improvement of 81% after surgery, and 62% of patients reported a 90% or greater improvement. At a minimum follow-up of 5 years, none of the patients had permanent retention or had undergone removal of the sling material for pain, infection, or mesh erosion.[32]

A multicenter randomized trial documented objective cure rates of 63% for TVT and 51% for colposuspension.[33] The cure rates of DUPS at 72% are similar but slightly better than those of other sling procedures when the assessment is done by subjective, patient-driven questionnaires.[33,34]

CONCLUSIONS

The DUPS is an effective, safe, simple and inexpensive procedure for the treatment of SUI. It offers effective therapy while eliminating the prohibitive cost and equipment requirements associated with the use of other prepackaged slings.

References

1. Von Giordano D: Twentieth Congress. Franc de chir, 1907, p. 506.
2. McGuire EJ, Lytton B: Pubovaginal sling procedure for stress incontinence. J Urol 119:82-84, 1978.
3. Leach GE, Dmochowski RR, Appell RA, et al: Female Stress Urinary Incontinence Clinical Guidelines Panel summary report on surgical management of female stress urinary incontinence. The American Urological Association. J Urol 158(3 Pt 1):875-880, 1997.
4. Klutke JJ, Carlin BI, Klutke CG: The tension-free vaginal tape procedure: Correction of stress incontinence with minimal alteration in proximal urethral mobility. Urology 55:512-514, 2000.
5. Lebret T, Lugagne PM, Herve JM, et al: Evaluation of tension-free vaginal tape procedure: Its safety and efficacy in the treatment of female stress urinary incontinence during the learning phase. Eur Urol 40:543-547, 2001.
6. Klutke JJ, Klutke CG, Bergman J, Elia G: Urodynamics changes in voiding after anti-incontinence surgery: An insight into the mechanism of cure. Urology 54:1003-1007, 1999.
7. Jeffry L, Deval B, Birsan A, et al: Objective and subjective cure rates after tension-free vaginal tape for treatment of urinary incontinence. Urology 58:702-706, 2001.
8. Haab F, Sananes S, Amarenco G, et al: Results of the tension-free vaginal tape procedure for the treatment of type II stress urinary incontinence at a minimum followup of 1 year. J Urol 165:159-162, 2001.
9. Brophy MM, Klutke JJ, Klutke CG: A review of the tension-free vaginal tape procedure: Outcomes, complications, and theories. Curr Urol Rep 2:364-369, 2001.
10. Carlin BI, Klutke JJ, Klutke CG: The tension-free vaginal tape procedure for the treatment of stress incontinence in the female patient. Urology 56(6 Suppl 1):28-31, 2000.
11. Azam U, Frazer MI, Kozman EL, et al: The tension-free vaginal tape procedure in women with previous failed stress incontinence surgery. J Urol 166:554-556, 2001.
12. Ulmsten U, Henriksson L, Johnson P, Varhos G: An ambulatory surgical procedure under local anesthesia for treatment of female urinary incontinence. Int Urogynecol J Pelvic Floor Dysfunct 7:81-85, discussion 85-86, 1996.
13. Rezapour M, Falconer C, Ulmsten U: Tension-free vaginal tape (TVT) in stress incontinent women with intrinsic sphincter deficiency (ISD): A long-term follow-up. Int Urogynecol J Pelvic Floor Dysfunct 12(Suppl 2):S12-S14, 2001.
14. Rezapour M, Ulmsten U: Tension-free vaginal tape (TVT) in women with recurrent stress urinary incontinence: A long-term follow up. Int Urogynecol J Pelvic Floor Dysfunct 12(Suppl 2):S9-S11, 2001.
15. Nilsson CG, Kuuva N, Falconer C, et al: Long-term results of the tension-free vaginal tape (TVT) procedure for surgical treatment of female stress urinary incontinence. Int Urogynecol J Pelvic Floor Dysfunct 12(Suppl 2):S5-S8, 2001.
16. Nilsson CG, Kuuva N: The tension-free vaginal tape procedure is successful in the majority of women with indications for surgical treatment of urinary stress incontinence. BJOG 108:414-419, 2001.
17. Niemczyk P, Klutke JJ, Carlin BI, Klutke CG: United States experience with tension-free vaginal tape procedure for urinary stress incontinence: Assessment of safety and tolerability. Tech Urol 7:261-265, 2001.
18. Moran PA, Ward KL, Johnson D, et al: Tension-free vaginal tape for primary genuine stress incontinence: A two-centre follow-up study. BJU Int 86:39-42, 2000.
19. Smith AR: Surgery for urinary incontinence in women. In Abrams P (ed): Incontinence Management. Paris, Health Publication Ltd, 2005, pp 1307-1319.
20. Kuuva N, Nilsson CG: A nationwide analysis of complications associated with the tension-free vaginal tape (TVT) procedure. Acta Obstet Gynecol Scand 81:72-77, 2002.
21. Madjar S, Tchetgen MB, Van Antwerp A, et al: Urethral erosion of tension-free vaginal tape. Urology 59:601, 2002.
22. Klutke C, Siegel S, Carlin B, et al: Urinary retention after tension-free vaginal tape procedure: Incidence and treatment. Urology 58:697-701, 2001.
23. Rodriguez LV, Raz S: Polypropylene sling for the treatment of stress urinary incontinence. Urology 58:783-785, 2001.
24. Rodriguez LV, Berman J, Raz S: Polypropylene sling for treatment of stress urinary incontinence: An alternative to tension-free vaginal tape. Tech Urol 7:87-89, 2001.
25. Rutman M, Itano N, Dng D, et al: Long-term durability of the distal urethral polypropylene sling procedure for stress urinary incontinence: Minimum 5-year followup of surgical outcome and satisfaction determined by patient reported questionnaires. J Urol 175:610-613, 2006.
26. Eisen SV: Assessment of subjective distress by patients' self-report versus structured interview. Psychol Rep 76:35-39, 1995.
27. Deval B, Jeffry L, Al Najjar F, et al: Determinants of patient dissatisfaction after a tension-free vaginal tape procedure for urinary incontinence. J Urol 167:2093-2097, 2002.
28. Korman HJ, Sirls LT, Kirkemo AK: Success rate of modified Pereyra bladder neck suspension determined by outcomes analysis. J Urol 152(5 Pt 1):1453-1457, 1994.
29. Sirls LT, Keoleian CM, KormanHJ, Kirkemo AK: The effect of study methodology on reported success rates of the modified Pereyra bladder neck suspension. J Urol 154:1732-1735, 1995.
30. Uebersax JS, Wyman JF, Shumaker SA, et al: Short forms to assess life quality and symptom distress for urinary incontinence in women: The Incontinence Impact Questionnaire and the Urogenital Distress Inventory. Continence Program for Women Research Group. Neurourol Urodyn 14:131-139, 1995.
31. Shumaker SA, Wyman JF, Uebersax JS, et al: Health-related quality of life measures for women with urinary incontinence: The Incontinence Impact Questionnaire and the Urogenital Distress Inventory. Continence Program in Women (CPW) Research Group. Qual Life Res 3:291-306, 1994.
32. Gilja I, Deban R, Bokarica P, et al: [A new approach to the transvaginal needle suspension technique after Raz technique and long-term results.] Urologe A 45:202-208, 2006.
33. Ward KL, Hilton P: A prospective multicenter randomized trial of tension-free vaginal tape and colposuspension for primary urodynamic stress incontinence: Two-year follow-up. Am J Obstet Gynecol 190:324-331, 2004.
34. Amundsen CL, Visco AG, Ruiz H, Webster GD: Outcome in 104 pubovaginal slings using freeze-dried allograft fascia lata from a single tissue bank. Urology 56(6 Suppl 1):2-8, 2000.

Chapter 42

THE SPARC SLING SYSTEM

David R. Staskin and Renuka Tyagi

The SPARC Sling System (American Medical Systems, Minnetonka, MN) is a minimally invasive pubovaginal sling procedure using a loosely knitted, self-fixating, 1-cm wide, 4-0 polypropylene mesh, which is placed at the level of the midurethra by passing the suspension needle via a suprapubic-to-vaginal approach.[1-3] The placement of pubovaginal slings in the treatment of genuine stress urinary incontinence has historically been effective, with excellent long-term outcomes.[4] This variation of surgical technique results from the drive to decrease surgical morbidity associated with autologous fascia harvesting; it also minimizes the risk of intraoperative complications from minimally invasive sling placement without affecting surgical outcomes (Fig. 42-1).[5-12]

MECHANISM OF ACTION

Continence results from multiple factors: resting urethral tone, active sphincter contraction, external compression, pressure transmission, and integrity of anatomic configuration. The

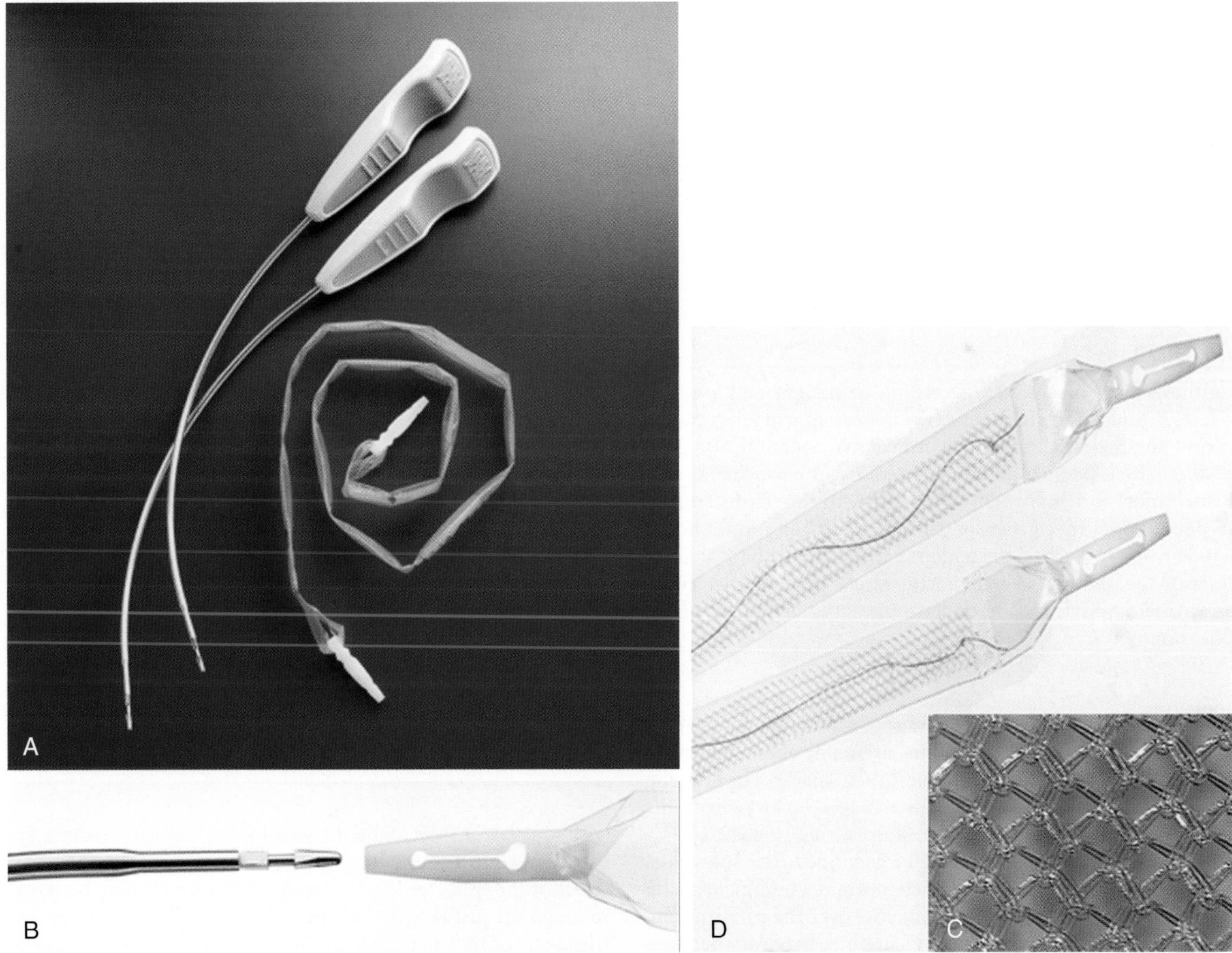

Figure 42-1 (A) Suspension needles: disposable ergonomic, 0.118 inches diameter, 8.2 inches long, and noncutting. (B) Connector-dilators: create the sling tract and enable the suspension needles to be of small diameter, minimizing trauma; do not require sling attachment and tract formation until the needle position has been confirmed; permit untwisting of the mesh after attachment. (C) Mesh sling: biocompatible 4-0 loosely knitted polypropylene. (D) Plastic sheath: permits smooth placement of self-fixating mesh.

success of midurethral sling techniques has prompted a re-evaluation of the pathophysiology of genuine stress urinary incontinence and the paradigm for its surgical correction. The mechanism of action for midurethral slings is presumed to be mimicking of the support provided by the pubourethral ligaments and suburethral fascial support.[13]

The importance of urethral stabilization from rotational motion has generally been accepted and was introduced as the "integral theory" based on data collected during radiologic evaluation of micturition.[14] This correlated with structures documented on anatomic dissection and was dubbed an "anatomic hammock."[15] The importance of urethral configuration suggests that midurethral support prevents separation of the posterior urethral wall from the anterior urethral wall during rotational motion around the inferior portion of the pubic ramus, which appears integral to continence.[16] Suburethral support and stability, in conjunction with urethral coaptation, appears to be the critical factor in the restoration of continence, and elevation of the bladder neck may no longer be a prerequisite.

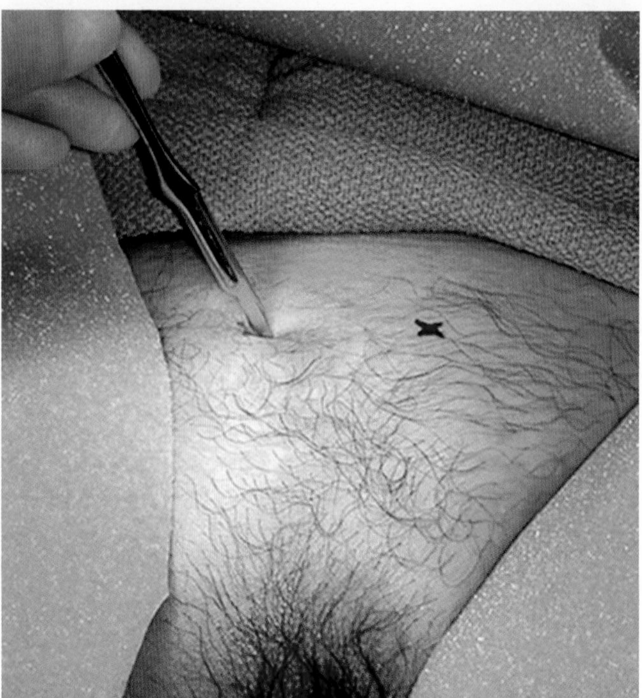

Figure 42-2 Suprapubic transverse stab incisions placed 1.5 cm from the midline at the upper margin of the pubic symphysis.

SURGICAL TECHNIQUE

Positioning

A standard or modified lithotomy position may be elected based on surgical preference and concomitant procedures, with a supine pelvis-inclined (Trendelenburg) position recommended. Adequate distal vaginal exposure for a 1.5-cm midurethral incision is required; however, vaginal retraction sutures or a complex retractor is usually not required for sling placement alone. A weighted speculum and placement of a Foley catheter (14 to 18 Fr) through the urethra to completely drain the bladder is preferred.

Anesthesia

Anesthesia may be selected according to patient and surgeon preference and may include any of the following: general, regional, or local anesthesia with/without intravenous sedation. If a local anesthetic is elected, it should be noted that the primary source of discomfort for the patient is contact with the periosteum of the pubic bone during needle passage. Local injections should include two approaches: the abdominal surface, with local anesthesia of the abdominal skin, rectus fascia, and muscle; and a paravaginal approach, to anesthetize the inferior border of the pubic ramus.

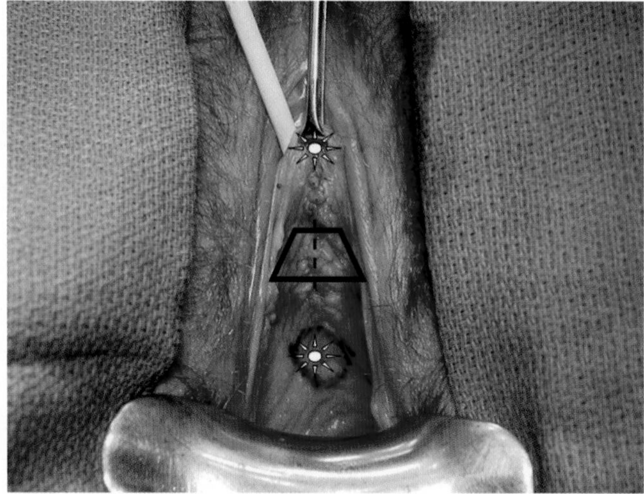

Figure 42-3 The vaginal mucosal incision is placed at the level of the mid-urethra, as demonstrated in this image by the "starburst" marks over the urethral meatus and bladder neck. The incision may vary in total length between 1.5 and 3 cm.

Incisions

Two parallel, 15-blade stab incisions are made above the pubic symphysis 1.5 cm from the midline (3 cm apart). The surgeon should avoid incisions lateral to this area to keep away from the ilioinguinal nerve exiting from the external ring (Fig. 42-2).

Next, the bladder neck should be identified, the submeatal fold may be elevated using an Allis clamp, and a midline incision is performed through the vaginal mucosa over the mid-urethra. This incision, centered over the mid-urethra, may vary between 1.5 and 3 cm (Fig. 42-3). If the procedure is performed without local anesthetic, a saline injection at the level of the mid-urethra, extending laterally, may be elected to aid in development of the plane of dissection between the vaginal epithelium and the periurethral fascia. Metzenbaum scissors are used to create a submucosal tunnel to the inferior border of the pubic ramus at the level of the mid-urethra bilaterally. The tunnels may be narrow enough for just the needle and connector dilator to traverse the distance, or they may be wide enough to accommodate insertion of a fingertip. With the "narrow tunnel" approach, the fingertip is placed in the paravaginal fornix, outside the incision, in order to palpate needle perforation through the endopelvic fascia (recommended).

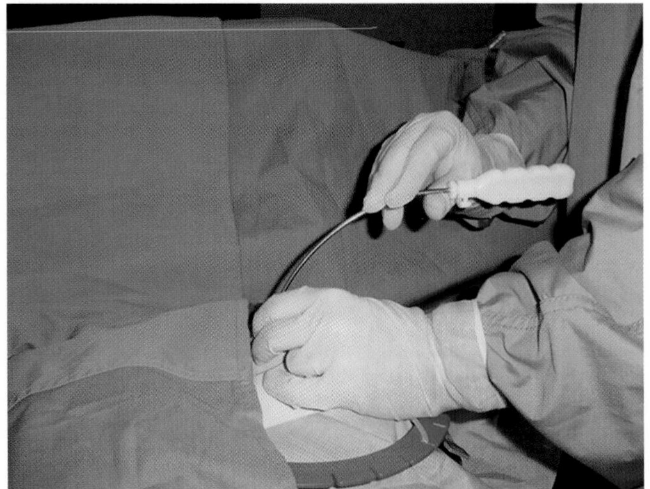

Figure 42-4 Initial placement of the SPARC needle through the suprapubic incision directly onto the pubic symphysis with the handle directed toward the surgeon. Throughout passage of the needle, the surgeon's hands remain on the needle shaft, and the needle handle is used only as a visual reference point.

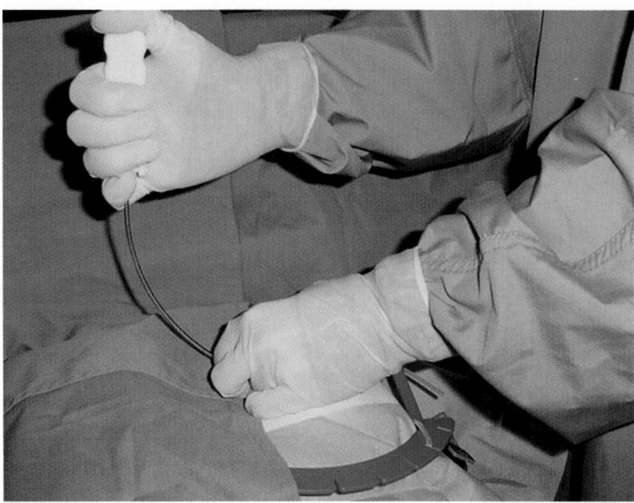

Figure 42-5 Perforation of the rectus fascia above the pubic symphysis by the needle is followed by immediate 90-degree rotation of the needle. The handle of the needle is now directed toward the ceiling, and the needle is advanced along the posterior surface of the pubic bone.

Needle Passage

Effective needle passage is divided into two phases: entrance into and traversing of the retropubic space first, followed by perforation of the endopelvic and periurethral fascia. Needle passage may be described in five steps:

1. *Approach to the anterior surface of pubic symphysis:* Holding the needle itself with the fingertips of both hands, pass the needle from the stab incisions above the pubic symphysis directly down on the bone. During this maneuver, the needle handle is pointed toward the surgeon (Fig. 42-4).
2. *Perforation of the rectus fascia and rotation around the superior surface of the pubic symphysis:* Slide the tip of the needle along the superior surface of the bone and then direct it downward to perforate the rectus fascia and muscle. Grasping the needle itself near the end with the fingertips rather than the handle permits more control of the straight portion of the curved needle. After fascial perforation, the needle handle should rotate to 90 degrees (up toward the ceiling) as the needle is advanced, to keep the tip of the needle on the posterior surface of the pubic bone (Fig. 42-5).
3. *Traversing the retropubic space:* Guide the needle inferiorly, with the handle rotated 10 degrees medially—"walking downward along the bone," again with the fingertips, until the endopelvic fascia is encountered (Fig. 42-6).
4. *Palpation of the needletip at the endopelvic fascia:* Grasp the handle of the needle; palpate the needletip with the alternate index finger beneath the vaginal wall and guide it to the desired point of perforation. Locate the needlepoint beneath the vaginal wall with the finger and guide it to the perforation point. The perforation point is as lateral as possible against the inferior border of the pubic ramus, at the level of the mid-urethra (Fig. 42-7).
5. *Perforation of the endopelvic/periurethral fascia and exposure of the needletip through the vaginal incision:* To perforate the fascia, push the needle through the endopelvic and periurethral fascia without placing the finger within the vaginal incision (recommended) or by placing a fingertip in the incision. Once the needle perforates the fascia and can be felt beneath the epithelial layer, it can be guided through the dissected tunnel. Be sure the needle has perforated the fascia before directing it medially. If necessary, allow needlepoint perforation of the vaginal epithelium, withdraw the needle, and then guide it out of the incision. Failure to completely perforate the fascia before medial direction of the needle out of the incision decreases the distance between the perforation point and the urethra (Fig. 42-8).

The following guidelines are suggested to avoid intraoperative complications during needle passage.

1. To avoid perforation of the bladder, keep the tip of the needle on the superior, then posterior portion of the symphysis pubis *at all times.*
2. To avoid urethral trauma, pass the needle directly against the surface of the inferior portion of the pubic ramus at the level of the mid-urethra onto the lateral tip of the index finger, while deviating the urethral catheter medially with the superior surface of the finger.
3. Major vessel injury should be avoided by adhering to the surface of the pubic bone. The inferior epigastric artery and vein and the endopelvic veins are subject to inadvertent trauma with any needle passage. The iliac and obturator veins are not in the direction of needle passage or the force vector of perforation with suprapubic needle passage, in contrast to the situation with periurethral fascia or endopelvic fascia perforation from the vaginal approach.
4. Small and large bowel injury should similarly be avoided by maintaining the needletip against the pubic bone during passage. Bowel should not be adherent to the pubic bone *except* in the case of prior abdominal surgery that entered the retropubic space or the presence of a lower abdominal incisional or inguinal hernia.

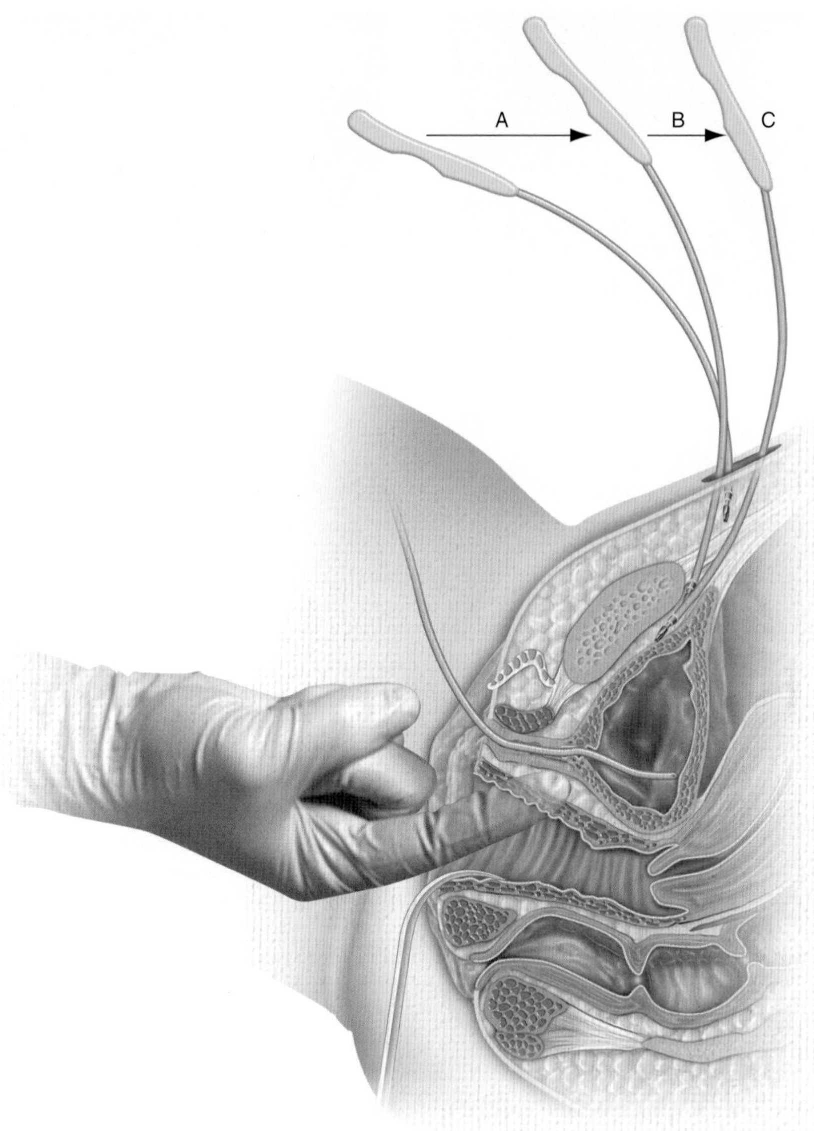

Figure 42-6 Retropubic advancement of the needle is performed with the needletip against the posterior surface of the pubic bone and the handle rotated 10 degrees medially. The needle is advanced inferiorly until the tip is palpable with a finger in the vagina.

Cystoscopy

After both needles have been passed, cystoscopy is performed with a minimum of 350 mL in the bladder to ensure that the needles are not in a bladder fold or "mucosal pinch." Needle perforation, if present, is often noted at 10 or 2 o'clock near the bladder neck, and additional care should be taken to view the urethra on scope insertion and/or removal. The bladder may be left distended on removal of the scope.

Sling Attachment and Transfer

Sling attachment and transfer is performed as follows:

1. The plastic sheath containing the sling material may be irrigated with sterile saline or water before attachment to aid in smooth removal of the plastic.
2. The sling is positioned for attachment to the needles by facing the markings toward the surgeon. The center of the sling is clearly marked with arrows radiating from the center (Fig. 42-9).
3. The connectors are attached to the needletips using gentle pressure until a "snap" is felt and heard.
4. The surgeon confirms that the sling is correctly positioned flat and with the markings on the outside of the mesh. The connectors can be twisted on the needletips to adjust the sling position.
5. The needles are directed into the retropubic space by placing the index finger at the tip of the connector and pushing the connector-needle up into the retropubic space. This "pushing" maneuver minimizes disruption of the periurethral and endopelvic fascia. The surgeon should avoid pulling the handle of the needle until the white connector has been "pushed" back into the retropubic space through the endopelvic fascia.

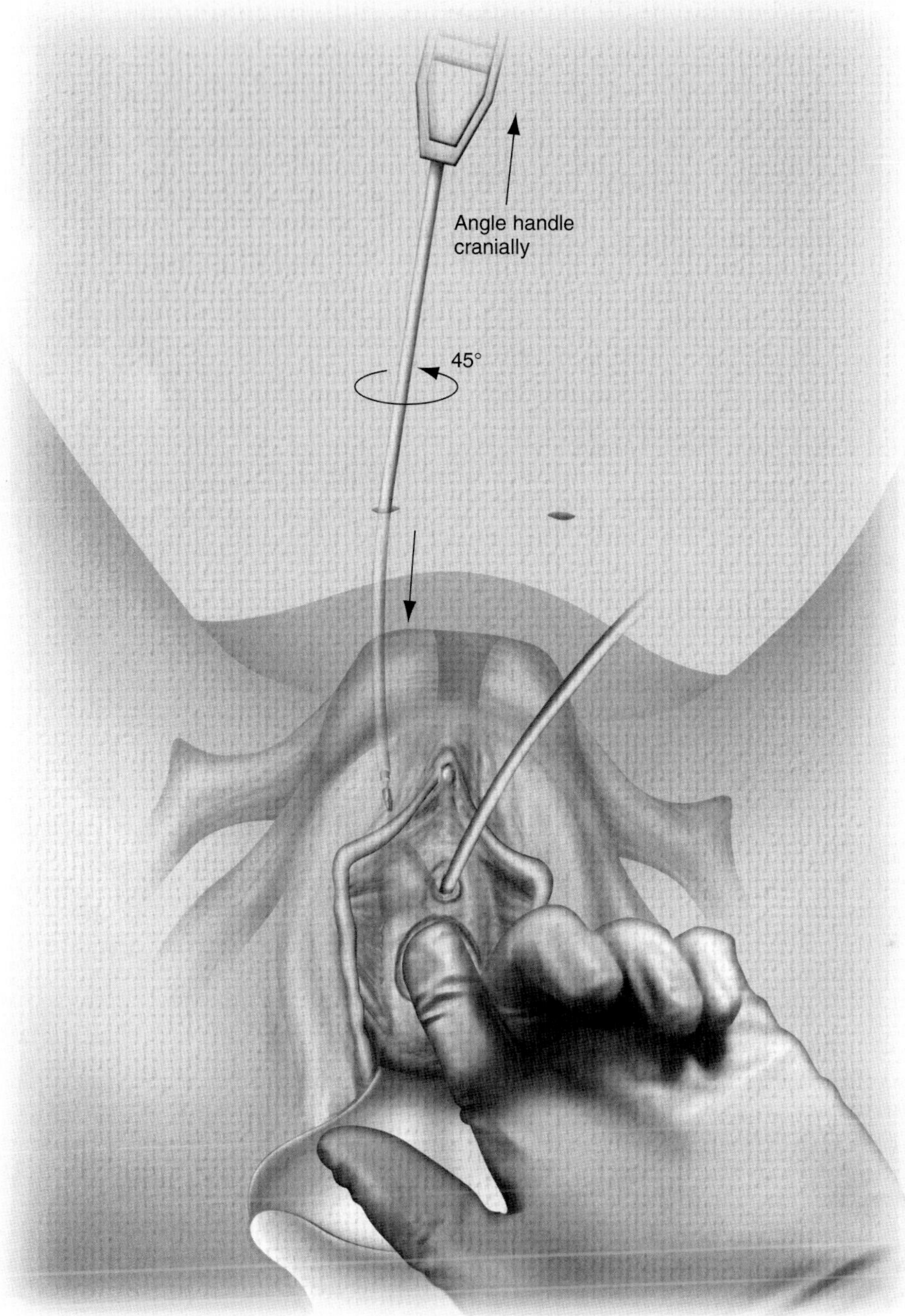

Figure 42-7 Perforation of the endopelvic fascia under guidance of the finger in the vagina. The needletip is palpated with a finger in the vagina that is concurrently displacing the urethra medially. The needle is positioned on the lateral edge of the finger and then advanced through the endopelvic/periurethral fascia.

6. The needle handle is used to complete retrograde removal of the suspension needle. Gentle traction on the needle at the level of the skin permits complete needle removal with minimal dilation at the skin level. The sling is pulled through the skin incision for several centimeters on each side.
7. Before adjusting sling tension, the plastic sheath should be re-examined at the vaginal incision for leakage from the bladder. If there is any suspicion of leakage, a repeat cystoscopy should be performed. If the sling is identified within the bladder, it should be cut closely below the white dilator-connector, withdrawn within the plastic sheath, and repositioned with an alternative "free suspension needle" by suturing the plastic to the needletip. The Foley catheter is now replaced for drainage of the bladder.

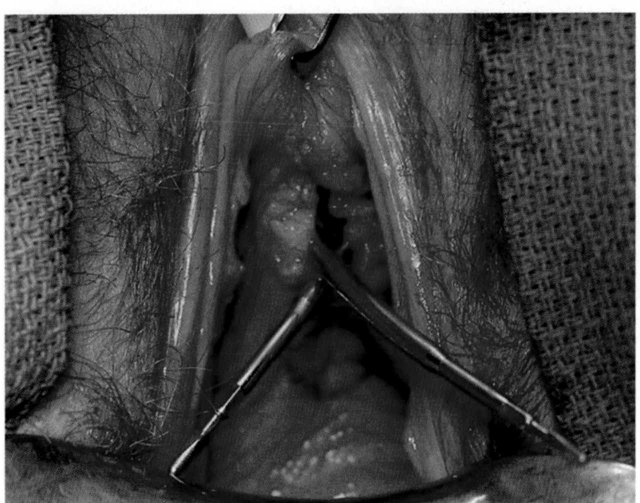

Figure 42-8 Vaginal exposure of the needletip. The needles are guided through the previously dissected submucosal tunnels and out the vaginal incision, either with a fingertip within the tunnel or with palpation through the mucosa.

Sling Tensioning and Fixation

The sling tension is adjusted by pulling the sling up through the suprapubic incisions against a spacer placed in the vaginal loop, or, based on individual surgeon preference, against a large scissor or dilator (e.g., no. 8 Hagar). Optimal sling tension is demonstrated when slight movement of the instrument within the mesh loop initially occurs.

The sling and plastic sheath are cut at the level of the "blue dots" below the dilator-connectors (Fig. 42-10). Hemostats are placed on each of the cut plastic sheaths, using care to avoid the mesh (Fig. 42-11). The suburethral spacer is stabilized with one hand as the plastic sheath on each side is removed with the other. The mesh is then cut below the skin level, with gentle traction on the ends to allow retraction of the mesh beneath the skin level (Fig. 42-12).

Closure

Steri-Strips are applied to the suprapubic incisions, and the vaginal incision is closed using a running 2-0 absorbable suture.

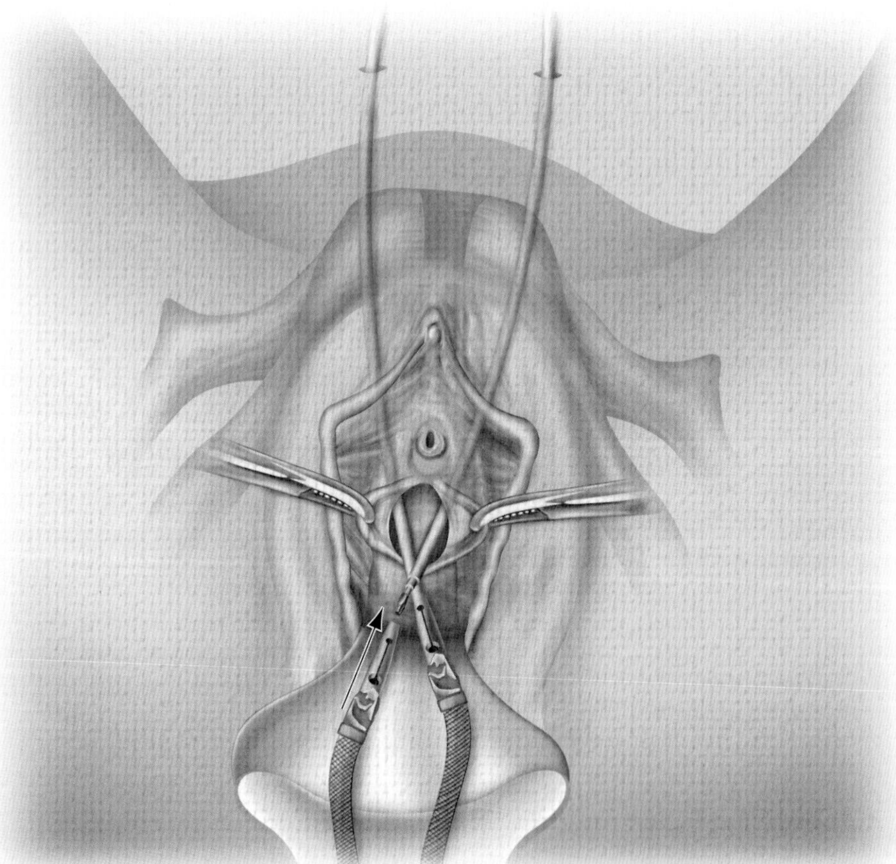

Figure 42-9 Sling attachment. The sling connectors are positioned adjacent to the needletip with the sling markings adjacent to the connector and in the center of the sling facing toward the surgeon. Gentle pressure is applied to the connectors until they "snap" onto the needletips.

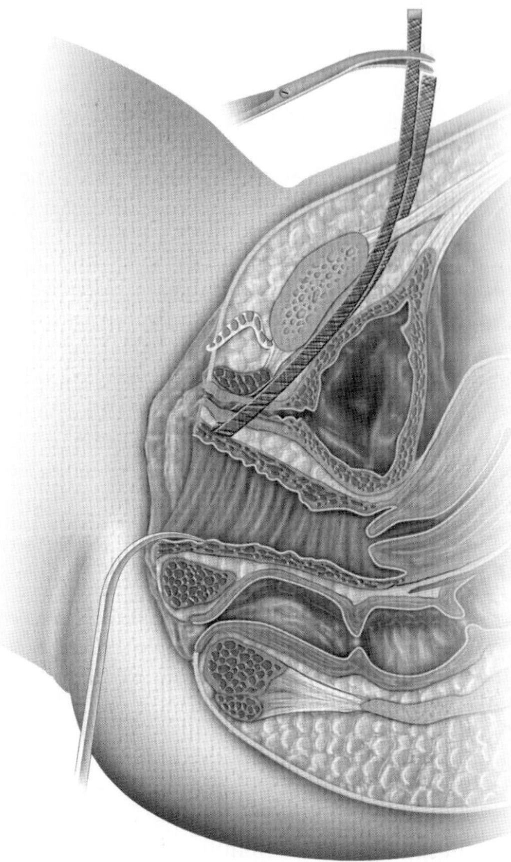

Figure 42-10 Cutting of the plastic sheath. The plastic sheath and sling material are cut below the blue dots to allow for removal of the sheath.

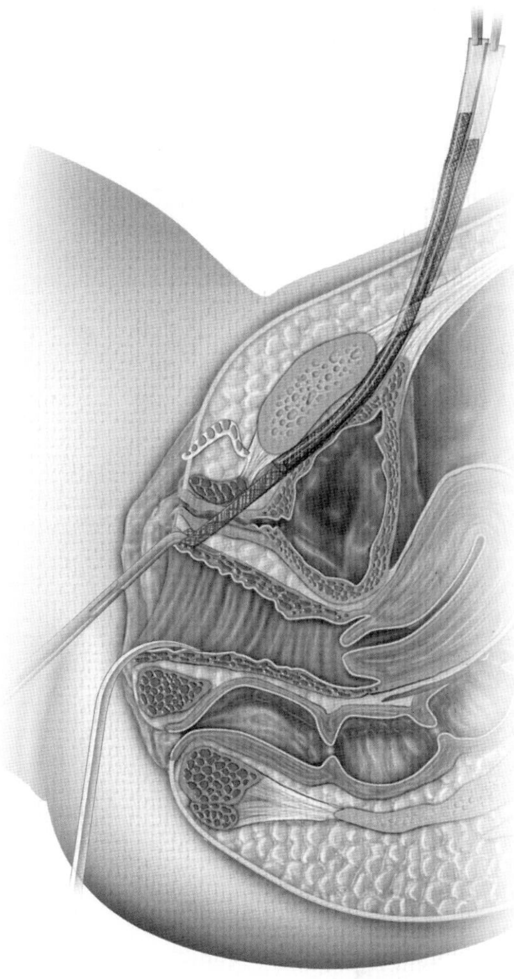

Figure 42-11 Sheath removal. Hemostats grasp the plastic sheath alone and are used to remove the sheath. The spacer should be stabilized as the plastic is removed.

CONCOMITANT PROCEDURES

If additional pelvic organ prolapse repair procedures are planned, apical and anterior vaginal repairs may be completed before placement of the SPARC sling. In particular, if a cystocele repair is planned, it should be performed with repair of the bladder base but *not* the bladder neck area. A Kelly repair is not recommended, because it may elevate bladder neck support and may disrupt the pressure transmission to the mid-urethra by altering bladder neck motion with reference to the sling. In addition, use of a separate incision, if possible, for placement of the SPARC sling avoids extension of a hematoma or drainage from the cystocele repair and prevents resultant disruption of the incision over the sling.

POSTOPERATIVE CARE

The patient is sent to the recovery room with a Foley catheter in place. It is important, especially after an epidural or spinal anesthesia, that the patient be fully ambulatory and free of any residual anesthetic before the voiding trial, to avoid iatrogenic anesthetic retention.

The active voiding trial is performed as follows:

1. Fill the bladder via the Foley catheter to 300 mL or until full, and remove the catheter.
2. Measure the void. A void of greater than 200 mL (two-thirds of capacity) or a residual measured by ultrasound of less than 100 mL (one-third of capacity) is considered adequate for discharge.
3. If the residual is greater than 100 mL, the patient is rechecked after an additional void. The patient may be discharged with a leg bag and the voiding trial repeated in the office the next day.

Managing Postoperative Retention

The SPARC procedure results in placement of the sling below the mid-urethra with no tension and minimal disruption of normal proximal urethral mobility. This change in sling placement has resulted in a substantial decrease in urinary retention, similar to other minimally invasive pubovaginal slings.[17]

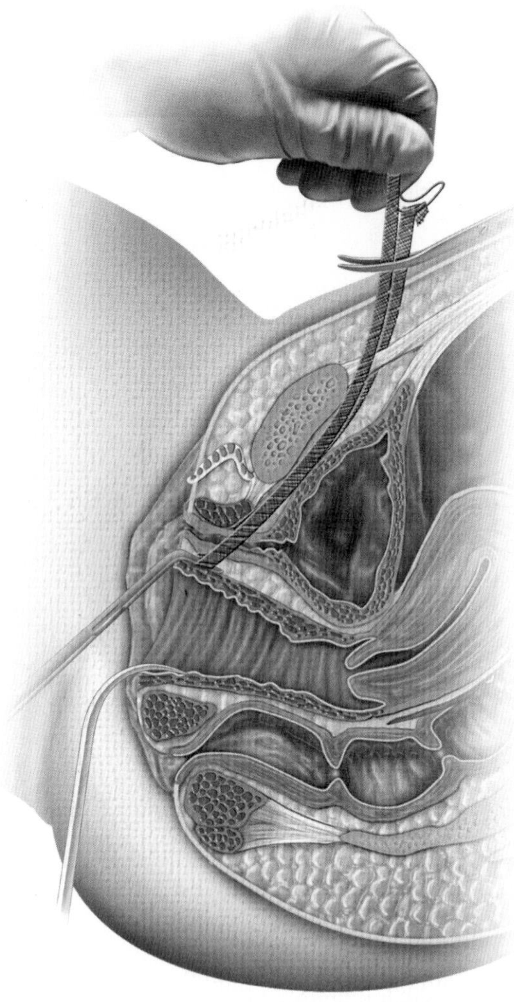

Figure 42-12 Excess mesh is cut below skin level at the suprapubic incisions. Gentle traction on the mesh allows the ends to retract beneath the skin.

Loosening of the SPARC sling may be initiated intraoperatively if the sling is tensioned too tightly during removal of the plastic sheath, or postoperatively if the patient presents with urinary retention or symptomatic impaired voiding. The tensioning suture within the sling mesh provides a restraint to sling stretching during loosening of the sling tension. The sling can be loosened by placing a right angle beneath the sling and then pulling the sling down with a right angle clamp or with a 1-0 Prolene suture that has been placed around the sling. Postoperative sling adjustment should done within 2 to 3 weeks after implantation, because local tissue in-growth and biodegradation of the tensioning suture soon begin to affect the ability to "move" the sling. Pulling on the sling will result in a "pop" and slight patient discomfort at the suprapubic site, indicating that the sling has moved at the rectus fascia layer.

Late postoperative retention that does not improve with conservative management or early adjustment of sling tensioning may be addressed with urethrolysis. A midline urethrolysis may be performed if there has been no significant tissue in-growth into the sling. If significant in-growth exists, a lateral approach is recommended to avoid urethral injury. After identification of the sling, a nerve hook or right angle clamp may be used to mobilize the sling and hold it on tension. The sling may be transected with scissors, after which the sling tension is adjusted.

Managing Postoperative Sling Extrusion

The disadvantages of synthetic mesh graft includes the risks of infection, rejection, extrusion, and erosion. Erosion should refer to the entrance (or placement) of the sling within the urinary tract (the bladder or urethra), whereas extrusion refers to the migration or exposure of the sling material into the vagina. Extrusion of sling mesh into the vagina can be managed immediately in the postoperative period by thorough antibiotic irrigation and wound closure. Delayed closure may involve mobilization of the vaginal edges. Observation and conservative management until the vaginal wall completely heals over the sling mesh may be elected for late extrusion. If the vaginal wall heals "through the mesh," the exposed portion of the mesh should be excised, with the vaginal wall closed primarily or left to heal secondarily.

Complication rates with artificial materials may be underreported, because erosion can occur relatively late, at 1 to 4 years postoperatively. In fact, the American Urological Association Female Stress Urinary Incontinence Clinical Guidelines Panel recommended 5-year follow-up as a true test of time for such continence procedures. Initial success with a novel graft material must therefore be judged cautiously until long-term results are available. Given the fact that the midurethral polypropylene slings are made of loosely knitted mesh and are placed under no tension, the incidence of significant problems appears to be lower than previously anticipated, in the region of 1% to 6%.[17-18]

References

1. SPARC Sling System. Patent 6,612,977, Appl. No. 917443. Minnetonka, MN: American Medical Systems, Inc., September 2, 2003.
2. Deval B, Lavardon M, Samain E, et al: A French multicenter clinical trial of SPARC for stress urinary incontinence. Eur Urol 44:254-259, 2003.
3. Staskin DR, Tyagi R: The SPARC sling system. Atlas Urol Clin 12:185-195, 2004.
4. Leach G, Dmochowski RR, Appell RA, et al: Female Stress Urinary Incontinence Clinical Guidelines Panel summary report on surgical management of female stress urinary incontinence. The American Urological Association. J Urol 158:875-880, 1997.
5. Beck RP, McCormick S, Nordstrom L: The fascia lata sling procedure. Obstet Gynecol 72:699-703, 1988.
6. Hilton P: A clinical and urodynamic study comparing the Stamey bladder neck suspension and suburethral sling procedures in the treatment of genuine stress incontinence. Br J Obstet Gynecol 96:213-220, 1989.
7. Niknejad K, Plzak LS 3rd, Staskin DR, Loughlin KR: Autologous and synthetic urethral slings for female incontinence. Urol Clin North Am 29:597-611, 2002.
8. Staskin DR, Plzak L: Synthetic slings: Pros and cons. Curr Urol Rep 3:414-417, 2002.
9. Ghoniem GM, Shaaban A: Sub-urethral slings for treatment of stress urinary incontinence. Int Urogynecol J 5:228-239, 1994.
10. Morgan JE, Heritz DM, Stewart FE, et al: The polypropylene pubovaginal sling. J Urol 154:1013-1015, 1995.

11. Jarvis GJ: Surgery for genuine stress incontinence. Br J Obstet Gynecol 101:371-374, 1994.
12. Kersey J: The gauze hammock sling operation in the treatment of stress incontinence. Br J Obstet Gynaecol 90:945-949, 1983.
13. Petros PE, Ulmsten U: An anatomical classification: A new paradigm for management of urinary dysfunction in the female. Int Urogynecol J Pelvic Floor Dysfunct 10:29-35, 1999.
14. Petros P, Ulmsten U: An integral theory on female urinary incontinence. Acta Obstet Gynecol Scand 69(Suppl):153, 1990.
15. Delancey JOL: Structural support of the urethra as it relates to stress incontinence: The hammock hypothesis. Am J Obstet Gynecol 170:1713, 1994.
16. Plzak L, Staskin D: Genuine stress incontinence: Theories of etiology and surgical correction. Urol Clin North Am 29:527-535, 2002.
17. Tseng LH, Wang AC, Lin YH, et al: Randomized comparison of the suprapubic arc sling procedure vs tension-free vaginal taping for stress incontinent women. Int Urogynecol J Pelvic Floor Dysfunct 16:230-235, 2005. Epub 2004 Oct 27.
18. Kobashi KC, Govier FE: Perioperative complications: The first 140 polypropylene pubovaginal slings. J Urol 170:1918-1921, 2003.

Chapter 43

PERCUTANEOUS VAGINAL TAPE SLING PROCEDURE

Sandip P. Vasavada and Raymond R. Rackley

The classification of stress urinary incontinence (SUI) has evolved from fundamental anatomic findings to a more physiologic description of urinary leakage secondary to increases in abdominal pressure. Although considered by some as controversial, intrinsic sphincter deficiency (ISD) often coexists in the setting of urethral hypermobility. Conventional management has largely been with bladder neck sling placement. Recent changes to the etiologies of SUI have led to changes in these beliefs.[1] Currently, it appears that the degree of ISD and the degree of anatomic displacement of urethral support determine the fundamental basis for selection of surgical treatment options.

There exists a strong interest in maintaining a simple, effective, and minimally invasive approach to the management of SUI that may, in fact, address almost all types of incontinence. To this end, the tension-free vaginal tape (TVT; Gynecare, Johnson & Johnson, Somerville, NJ) was devised in the mid 1990s as an alternative to other synthetic and biological mesh placements suburethrally. Data that are now becoming available reveal that success (depending on how measured) is quite good and durable.[2-4] Accordingly, the advent of the TVT procedure and its accordant success has yielded the development of the percutaneous vaginal tape (PVT), which allows placement of a synthetic polypropylene mesh tape suburethrally in an antegrade fashion.[5] The technique is similar to TVT in that it places a synthetic sling below the mid-urethra in a tension-free fashion, but it uses the widely available generic polypropylene mesh and Stamey needle passers for antegrade passage. The mesh itself can be tailored to size, offering the surgeon flexibility in the management of more severe types of incontinence or complex situations or anatomy.

This chapter describes the methods used for successful sling placement at the level of the mid-urethra of a synthetic tape in an antegrade fashion (PVT, using a percutaneous ligature carrier). This technique allows the surgeon an opportunity to reliably cure SUI without the significant added costs that other commercially available devices may have. This technique has recently been studied in a noninferiority testing fashion and compared with the "gold standard" midurethral mesh sling, the TVT.

PATIENT SELECTION

When the procedure for TVT was introduced, all female patients with SUI who had maximized their nonsurgical treatment were considered candidates for this procedure.[2,3] As with all anti-incontinence procedures, relative contraindications included an active urinary tract infection and anticoagulation therapy. Although no procedure is 100% effective, recent studies on the outcomes of patients undergoing the TVT procedure provide an opportunity to make some basic selection criteria for ensuring a high rate of successful outcomes.[2-4] As described in the following paragraphs, there may be potential patient selection limitations for midurethral slings that are not inherent in the traditional pubovaginal sling placed at the proximal urethra and bladder neck.

In general, moderate to severe obesity is not a contraindication; obese patients appear to have minimal operative and postoperative complications with the TVT procedure.[6] Successful outcomes are achieved when the TVT procedure is performed in patients undergoing concomitant pelvic organ prolapse repairs. Major complications of vascular injury and bowel injury leading to death are unique to the TVT procedure as secondary consequences of blindly passing large trocars in a retrograde, retropubic fashion. Although major vascular bleeding and possibly bowel injuries have been rarely reported with other anti-incontinence procedures, the inability to reliably prevent these complications from occurring at all has been the major reason for surgeons' opting to place the midurethral sling using small, percutaneous ligature carriers in an antegrade, retropubic fashion.[5,7] By this method, the ligature carrier can be safely guided along the posterior aspect of the symphysis pubis, thereby decreasing risks for vascular or bowel injury.

Because the sling material for PVT and TVT are placed at the mid-urethra, continence is provided by midurethral kinking or "knee kinking" of the urethra during active movement of the urethra with Valsalva or stress maneuvers. This has several important implications in regard to patient selection. First, although several reports have shown that correction of the hypermobile proximal urethra and bladder neck demonstrated by magnetic resonance imaging (MRI) and Q-tip testing is not required for a successful outcome, successful outcome appears to be dependent on a hypermobile urethra that induces ISD.[8] The midurethral placement of the sling is at the fulcrum of the mobile urethra and does not affect displacement of the urethra and bladder neck as defined by Q-tip testing. However, for the sling to provide a continence mechanism, the urethra must be actively "bent" over the midurethral sling, in order to prevent urinary leakage during stress maneuvers. Therefore, patients with a mobile urethra demonstrating significant hypermobility (>30 degrees) with SUI in the absence of a bladder contraction would seemingly have the highest probability for a successful outcome.

Alternatively, patients with severe ISD at rest with or without hypermobility are more likely to have less favorable outcomes. Severe ISD is indicative of an open bladder neck at rest and is not affected by a midurethral sling that is placed tension-free without causing an increase in urethral resistance at rest. Even in cases of severe ISD and a hypermobile urethra, leakage may occur with an open bladder neck before any urethral movement begins to

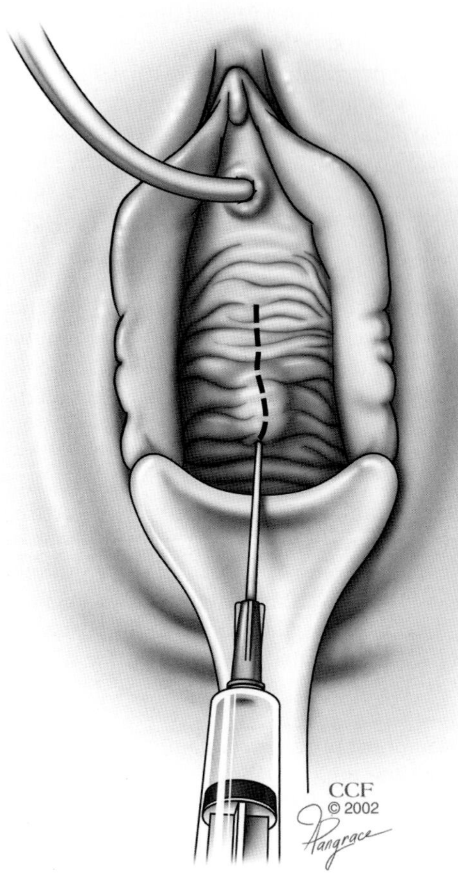

Figure 43-1 Marking of a midline anterior vaginal wall incision over the mid-urethra. (Courtesy of the Cleveland Clinic Foundation, copyright 2002.)

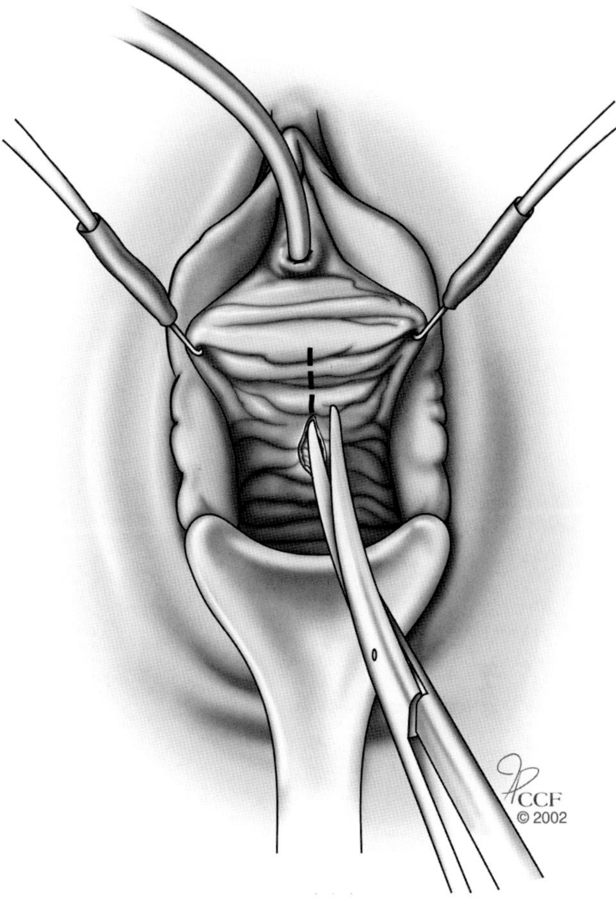

Figure 43-2 Development of a suburethral anterior vaginal wall pocket. (Courtesy of the Cleveland Clinic Foundation, copyright 2002.)

provide coaptation by "kinking" of the midurethral sling. No prospective reports have been published on preoperative leak point pressures before TVT placement and postoperative leak point pressures on failed cases of TVT.

OPERATIVE TECHNIQUE OF PERCUTANEOUS VAGINAL TAPE PLACEMENT

Midurethral Sling

Obtain vaginal exposure via the dorsal lithotomy position. Use a marking pen to draw the abdominal percutaneous puncture and midurethral vaginal wall incision sites. Place a 16-Fr urethral catheter into the bladder (Fig. 43-1).

Vaginal Incision

Use a scalpel to make a midline anterior vaginal wall incision at the level of the mid-urethra. Develop a pocket of space at the level of the mid-urethra between the vaginal wall and underlying urethral and paraurethral tissue by dissecting the vaginal wall tissue off laterally with the curved Mayo scissors from the 1.5- to 2.0-cm midline incision to the lateral anterior vaginal sulcus. No true entry into the retropubic space is required (Fig. 43-2). When the pocket of space is completed laterally to the junction of the inferior aspect of the pubic ramus and the urethropelvic complex (Fig. 43-3), one can proceed with antegrade passage of the needle carrier.

Before the percutaneous ligature carrier is passed (Fig. 43-4), the bladder should be emptied of all fluid. The patient's position on the operating table should result in placement of the symphysis pubis in a near-vertical plane; this usually means keeping the patient's torso and head in a level horizontal position or slightly in a Trendelenburg position.

Small (5 mm) puncture sites using the no. 15 scalpel blade through the abdominal skin overlying the top of symphysis should be made on either side of a finger placed in the midline. This maneuver allows easier manipulation of the ligature carrier for the antegrade approach by avoiding any resistance at the skin level. It also provides a visual location for avoiding perforation of the skin and rectus fascia too laterally for both approaches, which could lead to the reported complication of ilioinguinal nerve or inferior epigastric vascular damage. Attention to staying on the posterior or back side of the symphysis is required to prevent entering the rectus muscle and fascia too far cephalad from its insertion on the symphysis. Furthermore, passage anterior to the symphysis is not recommended at the present time with this approach. By taking the time to create the pocket of space at the level of the mid-urethra and to identify the correct anatomic structures (urethra medially, arcus tendineous levator ani laterally, and the inferior aspect of the pubic ramus and

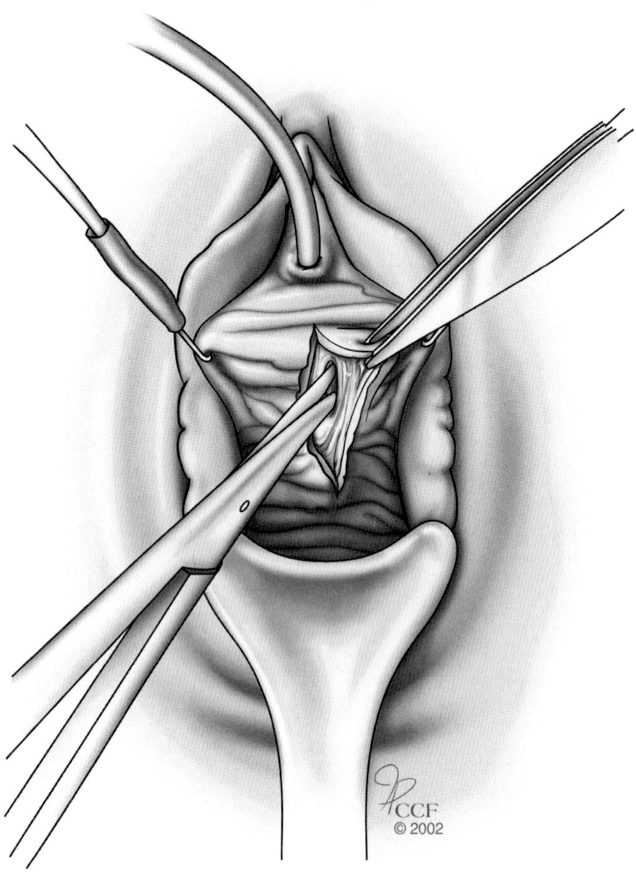

Figure 43-3 Suburethral pocket opened to confluence of endopelvic and periurethral fascia. (Courtesy of the Cleveland Clinic Foundation, copyright 2002.)

urethropelvic complex anteriorly), one facilitates the safest movement of the Stamey needles in a vertical direction that minimizes the likelihood of urethral or bladder injury.

When using the percutaneous ligature carrier, we fashion the free sling from a large sheet of polypropylene mesh (PML, Ethicon, Somerville, NJ) to approximately the same size as supplied in the TVT kit (1.2 mm wide by 30 cm long). Using 1-0 Ethibond suture, we simply weave suspending sutures into each end of the Prolene sling for placement into the ligature carrier.

Cystoscopy is performed to inspect for foreign body material within the urinary tract, and it is best to do this inspection when the ligature carrier for PVT is still within the retropubic space. Inspection must take place with a full bladder and use of the 30- and 70-degree lenses. If the ligature carrier has been placed through the bladder, simply extract the device and try again. No further precautions need be taken postoperatively in cases of bladder entry, as long as the entry is recognized and corrected. Unlike bladder perforations, trocar injury of the urethra rarely occurs. It is not advisable to proceed with placement of a synthetic graft next to a healing urethral injury with limited surrounding intervening tissues, because doing so might result in erosion and infection of the graft material. Instead, terminate the procedure and return at a later date to repeat the surgery.

Positioning the Sling

After completion of the procedure on both sides, the next step is to set the midurethral sling to stabilize, not suspend, the urethra. The sutures placed into the sling are passed into the Stamey needle passer, and the sling and sutures are transferred into the retropubic position. Although the tension-free vaginal tape contains no surrounding plastic sheath, it is easily manipulated through the surrounding tissues and can be set into place (Figs. 43-5 and 43-6).

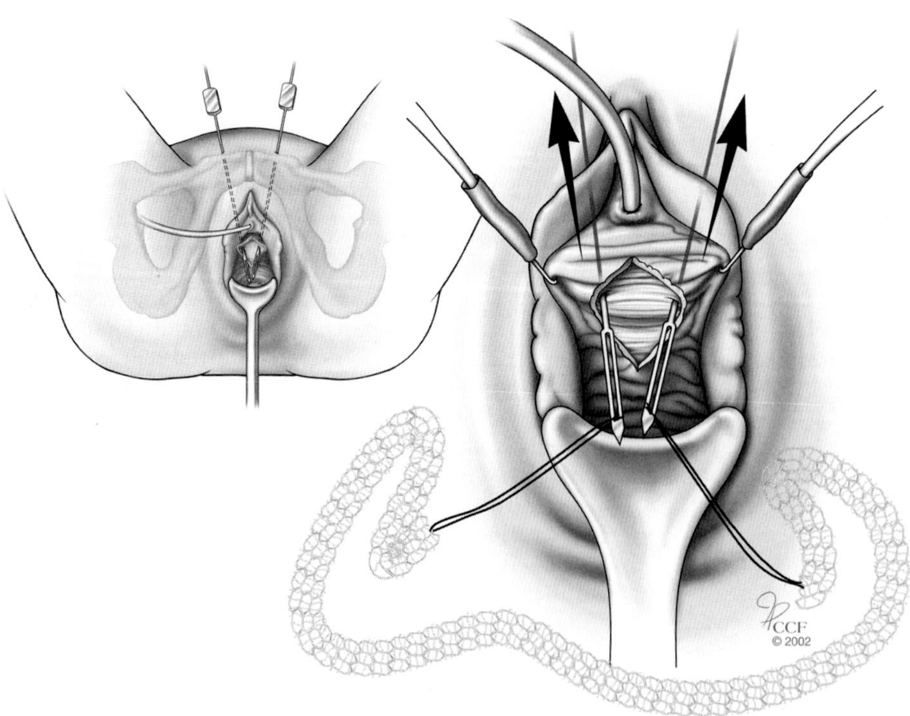

Figure 43-4 Antegrade passage of a ligature carrier through the retropubic space in a percutaneous vaginal tape procedure. (Courtesy of the Cleveland Clinic Foundation, copyright 2002.)

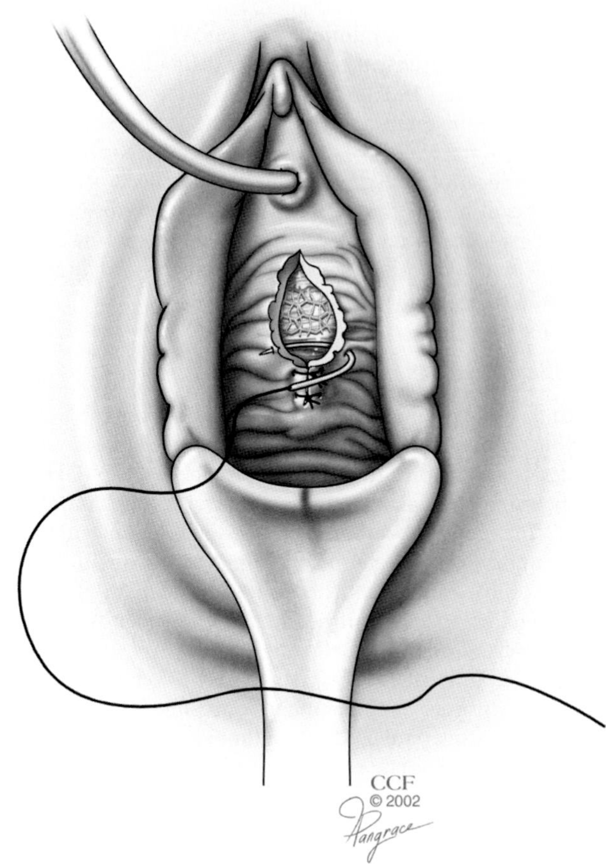

Figure 43-5 Ensuring a loose position of the synthetic sling at the mid-urethra. A curved Mayo scissor tips or open Kelly clamp is used to ensure a "tension free" placement. (Courtesy of the Cleveland Clinic Foundation, copyright 2002.)

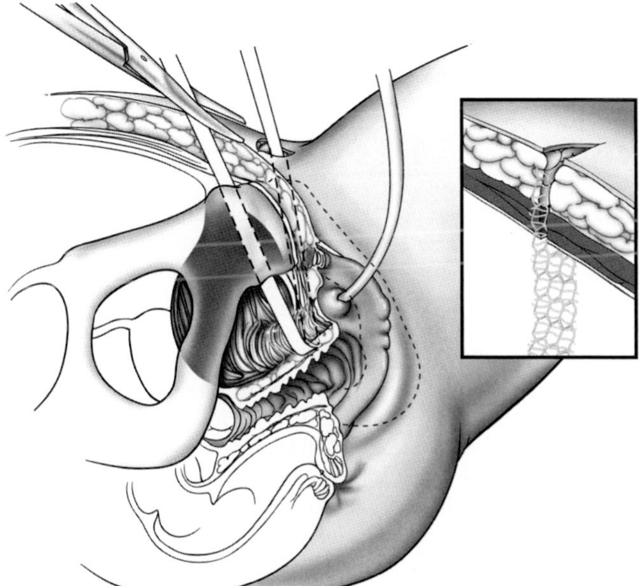

Figure 43-6 Lateral or sagittal view of percutaneous vaginal tape sling in place before the excess tape is cut suprapubically. (Courtesy of the Cleveland Clinic Foundation, copyright 2002.)

We prefer to place the tips of the curved Mayo scissor between the urethra and the sling to ensure ample looseness of the sling material. We have not found the intraoperative cough/stress test for determination of sling tension useful in patients undergoing the PVT, because many patients with documented SUI never leak in the supine or lithotomy position. Therefore, we typically verify that the sling is "tension free" with the placement of open Mayo scissors or a Kelly clamp between the sling and the periurethral tissue.

Once proper positioning of the sling is achieved, the remaining excess sling material at the abdominal skin site for the PVT is cut below the level of the skin. The vaginal incision site is irrigated with copious amounts of an antibiotic or iodine solution, and the incision closed with a running absorbable suture. The skin edges of the abdominal puncture site are approximated with skin adhesive closures. A vaginal pack and urethral catheter are placed for patients remaining in the hospital overnight; otherwise, the bladder is drained and a urethral catheter and vaginal pack are not usually placed in patients planned for same-day discharge from the recovery room.

POSTOPERATIVE CARE

Many surgeons who perform the TVT or PVT procedure with the patient under local anesthesia and sedation without concomitant prolapse repairs have opted to send patients home the same day without a catheter if a voiding trial is successfully completed. If the patient cannot void immediately after the procedure in the recovery room or the bladder was perforated during the procedure, catheter drainage for a brief period of 1 to 2 days may be required, with a voiding trial completed on an outpatient basis. After the procedure, patients are given an oral cephalosporin for several days, as well as oral medications for pain control.

RESULTS

We recently sought to evaluate whether the PVT was inferior to the established gold standard midurethral synthetic sling (TVT). All women who attended the Urology Outpatient Clinic at our institute complaining of SUI that was objectively (by office supine stress test) or urodynamically demonstrated and in whom midurethral sling surgery (TVT or PVT) was indicated were invited to participate and given an explanation of the study. Those who agreed to participate were given the informed consent document to read, understand, and sign. Patients were nonrandomly allocated into either the TVT or the PVT group according to the type of sling procedure typically performed by the treating surgeon. Nine different surgeons participated in this Institutional Review Board–approved study.

Patients who had previously failed anti-incontinence procedures, women with mixed incontinence, and those with SUI associated with pelvic organ prolapse were included in this study. Exclusion criteria were Valsalva-induced detrusor instability, neurogenic lower urinary tract dysfunction, and voiding dysfunction defined urodynamically as a voiding pressure greater than 50 cm H_2O, maximum flow rate lower than 15 mL/sec, or residual urine volume greater than 100 mL.

Evaluation of Effectiveness

Patients' perception of their symptoms and quality of life were assessed by asking them to complete three validated questionnaires before the operation: the Patient Global Subjective Score (Global, a visual analogue scale), the Incontinence Impact Questionnaire–Short form (IIQ-7), and the Urogenital Distress Inventory–Short form (UDI-6). One year after the operation, changes in the patients' symptoms, their quality of life, and treatment outcome were reassessed by mailing four questionnaires for the patients to complete and return: the three previously mentioned instruments and the Anti-Incontinence Surgery Response Score (AISRS), a postoperative-only scoring system. Patients were also asked to complete a 24-hour voiding diary and a 24-hour pad test as components of the AISRS; instructions for both were sent to patients by mail.

Evaluation of Safety

Safety of the procedure was assessed by recording intraoperative complications, such as bleeding necessitating blood transfusion and bladder perforation, and the following postoperative complications: erosion of sling material into the genitourinary tract; infection, whether at the surgical wound (abdominal or vaginal) or in the sling; de novo urgency; and bladder outlet obstruction. Outlet obstruction is defined by any of the following criteria: history of new-onset irritative symptoms (frequency, urgency, or urge incontinence) or obstructive symptoms (hesitancy, intermittency, weak stream, or sense of incomplete evacuation of the bladder); postoperative postvoid residue (PVR) equal to or greater than 100 mL; or urodynamic criteria of Chassagne and colleagues[9] (i.e., maximum flow rate of ≤15 mL/sec and detrusor pressure at maximum flow rate of >20 cm H_2O).

Operative Techniques

The TVT procedure was carried out according to the technique described by Ulmsten and associates,[3] and the PVT was performed according to the technique we described earlier.[5] All patients were sent home on the same day without a catheter if a voiding trial was successful. If a patient could not void or the bladder was perforated during the procedure, catheter drainage for 1 to 2 days was required, and a voiding trial was completed on an outpatient basis.

Outcome Measures

The primary outcome measure was the AISRS.[10] Patient responses were classified as cure, good, fair, poor, or failure according to the AISRS. For example, the patient was considered cured if she scored 0—that is, she had no stress or urge urinary incontinence episodes, she considered herself to be cured, and the total weight gain of the pad on her postoperative 24-hour pad test was less than 8 g.[10,11] Secondary outcome measures were Global, IIQ-7, and UDI-6.

Our sample size was based on testing the noninferiority of PVT to TVT on the primary outcome measure of being cured (score of 0) on the AISRS. We used a noninferiority "delta" of 10%, defined as the smallest true difference in the distribution of the AISRS such that PVT would still be considered noninferior to TVT. Assuming a 90% cure rate for both groups, we needed 226 total patients (113 patients in each group) to have 80% power to conclude noninferiority of PVT. With our recruited sample size of 191 patients, we had about 75% power to show noninferiority under these assumptions. In our data analysis of the AISRS, we conservatively used a smaller delta of 5% than we had planned for in the AISRS analysis.

In regard to the safety analysis, with our sample size of 191 we had little power (31%) to show noninferiority on any of the binary complication outcomes using an equivalency delta of 5%. Nonsignificant results for complications are therefore not interpreted as evidence of no difference between the groups.

Sample size calculations were made using the sample size software Unify POW, a macro for the SAS system.[12]

Statistical Analysis

PVT and TVT groups were compared on baseline variables including demographics, medical history, diagnosis, surgical variables, and incontinence questionnaires (IIQ, UDI, and Global), using chi-square tests for binary variables and either *t* tests or Wilcoxon rank-sum tests for ordinal or continuous variables, as appropriate. We also compared those with and without complete follow-up data for the AISRS, the UDI, and the IIQ on baseline factors to determine whether responders and nonresponders were similar at baseline.

One-tailed noninferiority tests of PVT versus TVT were made for the primary and secondary outcomes, using both univariate and multivariate methods, although all conclusions were based on the multivariate results. We adjusted for as many baseline covariates as possible in attempts to negate any assignment bias or baseline differences (due to nonrandomization). The usual tests for superiority of either PVT or TVT were done as well.

Tests for superiority of PVT or TVT were also performed. In the univariate case, we used chi-square tests for the AISRS and either two-tailed *t* tests or Wilcoxon rank-sum tests for ordinal outcomes. In multivariate analysis, we used the usual tests for significance from the logistic regression and cumulative logic regression analyses described earlier. For the change in Global score, we used cumulative logic regression to adjust for the covariates, and we reported the estimated odds ratio for having a higher change in TVT versus PVT.

RESULTS

A total of 278 women met the study criteria and, with input from their physician, chose to be treated with either TVT or PVT. Seventy-seven patients (27.7%) did not fully complete the questionnaires and were excluded from analysis (51 in the TVT group and 26 in the PVT group); 49 of these 77 patients were not willing to complete the follow-up even when contacted by telephone, and 28 were lost to follow-up because we were not able to contact them. The remaining 191 patients (72.3%) responded and followed our protocol; 99 (51.8%) of them underwent TVT, and 92 (48.2%) underwent the PVT procedure. Of the 191 patients, 107 (56%) were compliant to perform the entire study protocol, including the three domains of the AISRS (questionnaire, 24-hour voiding diary, and 24-hour pad test) and the three questionnaires of the secondary outcome measures; 84 patients (44%) refused to perform both the 24-hour pad test and the 24-hour voiding diary, whereas 60 patients (31%) refused to perform the 24-hour pad test only.

Table 43-1 Effectiveness of TVT versus PVT Based on AISRS Score*

	% Cured			*Superiority*		*Noninferiority*
Analysis	**TVT (*N* = 84)**	**PVT (*N* = 85)**	**Chi-Square P Value**	**% Cured (95% CI), TVT minus PVT**	**OR (95% CI), TVT vs PVT (Ref = PVT)**	**P Value†**
Univariate	33 (39.3%)	48 (56.5%)	.025	−17.2 (−29.6 to −4.7)	0.50 (0.27 to 0.92)	.002
Adjusted for covariates‡	33 (38.6%)	48 (55.4)	.060	−16.8 (−32.6 to 0.67)§	0.51 (0.26 to 1.03)	.003§,¶

*Association between AISRS "cured" (yes/no) and procedure (TVT or PVT) while adjusting for all preoperative baseline covariates. "Cured" was defined as a score of 0 on the AISRS.
†One-tailed test with noninferiority delta (or buffer) of .05.
‡Logistic regression adjusting for prolapse (*P* = .22), previous operation (*P* = .31), stress incontinence vs mixed incontinence (*P* = .24), age (OR = 0.68 per 10 yr, *P* = .008), and follow-up months (*P* = .08).
§Covariate-adjusted CI and noninferiority P value based on 1000 bootstrap resamples.
¶One-tailed upper limit for CI on difference in predicted percent success was −3.3%, well less than the +5% noninferiority delta (*P* = .003).
AISRS, Anti-Incontinence Surgery Response Score; CI, confidence interval; OR, odds ratio; PVT, percutaneous vaginal tape; TVT, tension-free vaginal tape.

AISRS: Primary Outcome Assessment

Multivariate analysis showed the noninferiority of PVT to TVT in the proportion cured (*P* = .002) after adjusting for baseline covariates and follow-up months, but PVT was not found to be superior to TVT (*P* = .06). We used a logistic regression model to assess the association between AISRS cured (yes/no) and procedure (TVT or PVT) while adjusting for all preoperative baseline covariates, including associated prolapse, previous operation (yes/no), preoperative diagnosis of stress incontinence versus mixed incontinence, age, and duration of postoperative follow-up in months (Table 43-1). Of the preoperative covariates assessed, only age was significantly associated with the outcome (*P* = .008). Higher age was associated with lower odds of success (odds ratio, 0.68; 95% confidence interval [CI], 0.52 to 0.90). The covariate-adjusted noninferiority test, using a delta of 5%, was significant (*P* = .022), so we concluded that PVT is not inferior to TVT (i.e., at least not 5% worse) on the AISRS cure score. Using bootstrap resampling, we also obtained a one-tailed upper limit estimate for the difference between PVT and TVT on the predicted probability of being cured after adjusting for covariates. This estimated upper limit was −3.3% (PVT 3.3% better), which is 8.3% lower (i.e., better in favor of PVT) than the +5% tolerance we had set.

Our naïve (i.e., unadjusted) univariate analysis revealed that PVT had a higher proportion "cured" in the test for superiority (chi-square *P* = .025), with the 95% CI ranging from 0.05 to 0.30 better than TVT (see Table 43-1). The estimated odds ratio from logistic regression indicated that TVT patients were only about half as likely to be cured as PVT patients. The univariate noninferiority test was then, of course, significant as well (*P* = .002), meaning that there was evidence to reject the null hypothesis and conclude that PVT is not inferior to TVT based on the AISRS.

Secondary Outcome Measures

Table 43-2 compares PVT and TVT on change from baseline to last follow-up on the secondary outcome measures. Univariate and multivariate results for superiority and noninferiority tests are given, along with estimated 95% CIs for the difference (TVT minus PVT) in mean or median change. In testing for the superiority of either TVT or PVT, we found no significant differences between treatment groups (Table 43-3), evidenced by zero being included within the confidence limits for each score and P values greater than .05.

In univariate analysis, PVT was shown to be noninferior to TVT for both IIQ and UDI (using three-point and two-point buffers, respectively) in change from baseline, but not for change in global assessment (one-point buffer).

In multivariate analysis adjusting for all available covariates, noninferiority of PVT was found only in the change in IIQ score (*P* = .038). The covariate-adjusted one-tailed upper 95% confidence limit for the change in IIQ was 2.8 (favoring TVT); this is significant because it is lower than the prespecified delta of 3.0. The adjusted one-tailed upper limit for UDI is above the prespecified delta (and therefore nonsignificant). We used cumulative logic regression for the Global assessment, because the data were far from normally distributed and linear regression was not appropriate. The odds of having a higher change score after PVT was an estimated 1.4 (95% CI, 0.69 to 2.7) times higher that for TVT. This method did not allow assessment of noninferiority of the Global assessment, but the odds ratio CI is quite wide and does not suggest noninferiority.

For each of IIQ (*P* = .005), UDI (*P* < .001), and Global (*P* = .005) scores, higher or increasing age was significantly associated with less improvement in the score (negative correlation). For both the IIQ and the UDI, patients with stress incontinence patients had significantly more improvement than did patients with mixed incontinence; the adjusted mean (and standard error) for the difference in score between these two groups was 4.7 (1.6) for the IIQ and 3.4 (0.89) for the UDI. None of the other covariates was significant at the .05 level, but they were retained in the multivariate models to improve the inference regarding PVT and TVT.

Nine surgeons performed the procedures, but we were not able to make a meaningful adjustment for surgeon because most surgeons did either PVT or TVT surgery exclusively. For example, the PVT procedures were done by one of two surgeons who respectively performed 68% and 26% of the PVTs (together, 94.5%) but only 13% of the TVT procedures. Likewise, 77% of the TVT procedures were done by one of three surgeons, and two of them performed only one PVT surgery each.

Analysis of domain no. 2 of the UDI-6 (*Do you experience urinary leakage related to the feeling of urgency? If yes, how much*

Table 43-2 Effectiveness of TVT versus PVT Based on Secondary Outcomes*

			Superiority		Noninferiority		
Outcome	**TVT**	**PVT**	**P Value**	**Difference between TVT-PVT (95% CI)**	**Buffer**	**One-tailed Upper CL**	**One-tailed P Value**
IIQ-7							
Sum Preop	17.8 (6.6)	16.1 (7.7)					
Sum Postop	5.1 (6.5)	3.6 (6.6)					
Change	12.7 (8.6)†	12.5 (10.2)	.91‡	0.18 (−3.0, 3.4)	§	2.9	.044
Adjusting for covariates	—	—	.88¶	−0.20 (−3.8, 3.3)	§	2.8	.038
UDI-6							
Sum Preop	11.3 (3.8)	11.6 (3.7)					
Sum Postop	3.6 (3.7)	4.3 (4.5)					
Change	7.7 (4.7)¶	7.3 (5.8)	.66‡	0.41(−1.4, 2.2)	¶¶	1.9	.044
Adjusting for covariates	—	—	.70§	0.38 (−1.6, 2.3)	¶¶	2.01	.10
Global							
Preop	10.0 (8.0, 10.0)	10.0 (8.0, 10.0)					
Postop	1.0 (0.0, 3.0)	1.0 (0.0, 3.0)					
Change	8.0 (5.0, 10.0)**	7.0 (5.0, 9.0)	.35††	0.26 (−2, 2)‡‡	‡	¶¶	.10 5
Adjusting for covariates	—	—	.37§§	1.4 (0.69, 2.7)§§		N/A	N/A

*Change (mean or median) from baseline to last follow-up on the Incontinence Impact Questionnaire–Short form (IIQ-7), the Urogenital Distress Inventory–Short form (UDI-6), and the Patient Global Subjective Score (Global).
†*N* = 68 TVT, 65 PVT.
‡Student's *t* test, mean (standard deviation).
§Multiple linear regression adjusting for prolapse (*P* = .51), previous operation (*P* = .57), SI vs MI (*P* < .001), age (*P* < .001), and follow-up months (*P* = .79).
¶¶Multiple linear regression adjusting for prolapse (*P* = .67), previous operation (*P* = .40), SI vs MI (*P* = .005), age (*P* = .008), and follow-up months (*P* = .62).
¶*N* = 65 TVT, 63 PVT.
***N* = 63 TVT, 65 PVT.
††Wilcoxon rank-sum test, median (25th percentile, 75th percentile).
‡‡Univariate confidence interval for difference in medians and noninferiority P value based on 1000 bootstrap resamples of difference in medians.
§§Odds ratio (95% CI) from cumulative logic regression adjusting for previous operation (*P* = .21), SI vs MI (*P* = .10), age (*P* = .005), and follow-up months (*P* = .61). Interpretation: odds for higher level of improvement in PVT vs TVT.
CI, confidence interval; CL, confidence limit; MI, mixed incontinence; PVT, percutaneous vaginal tape; SI, stress incontinence; TVT, tension-free vaginal tape.

Table 43-3 Comparison of Treatment Groups on Baseline Variables

Preoperative Variable	TVT	PVT	*P* Value*
Prolapse, *n*	33 (33.3%)	29 (31.5%)	.79
Previous anti-incontinence operation, *n*	19 (20.4%)	21 (23.6%)	.48
Preoperative diagnosis (SI vs MI), *n*	44 (44.4%)	52 (56.5%)	.095
Low ALPP (defined urodynamically as <60 cm H_2O), *n*	11 (19.3%)	6 (15.8%)	.66
Age (yr)†	59 (50, 73)	54 (46, 65)	.005‡
ALPP (cm H_2O)†	90 (64, 113)	100 (63, 120)	.49‡
Follow-up (mo)†	16 (13, 23)	12.5 (12, 14)	<.001‡

*Chi-square test unless otherwise noted.
†Median (25th percentile, 75th percentile).
‡Wilcoxon rank-sum test.
ALPP, abdominal leak point pressure; MI, mixed incontinence; PVT, percutaneous vaginal tape; SI, stress incontinence; TVT, tension-free vaginal tape.

Table 43-4 Comparison of TVT and PVT on Complications

Complication	Total No. of Patients	TVT	PVT	Chi-Square *P* Value
Bladder perforation, *n*	4	0 (0%)	4 (4%)	0.10
Obstruction	25	12 (12.1%)	13 (14.1%)	0.68
Urethrolysis	15	5 (5.1%)	10 (10.9%)	0.14
CIC	10	7 (7.1%)	3 (3.3%)	0.24
Persistent UTI	5	4	1	
Vaginal pain	1	0	1	
New-onset prolapse	2	2	0	
Recurrent prolapse	1	1	0	

CIC, clean intermittent catheterization; PVT, percutaneous vaginal tape; TVT, tension-free vaginal tape; UTI, urinary tract infection.

does it bother you?) showed that, for the combined TVT and PVT groups, 65% of patients decreased their score (65%), 30% stayed with the same degree of urge, 7 patients (5%) had de novo urge after the midurethral sling procedure. There was no difference between TVT and PVT on the change categories ($P = .72$, Wilcoxon test). In both groups, there was a large postprocedure increase in the proportion of patients with a score of zero.

Complications

The overall incidence of complications in the combined groups was 20% (38 patients). A summary of procedure-related complications is shown in Table 43-4. There was no difference between treatment groups in the proportion of patients with any specific complication. Median blood loss in both groups was comparable: 50 mL for the TVT group, 68 mL for the PVT group, with no significant difference ($P = .65$). According to our definition, a total of 25 women (13%) met the criteria of bladder outlet obstruction, 12 in the TVT group (12%) and 13 in the PVT group (14%) ($P = .68$). A total of 15 patients underwent urethrolysis to relieve obstruction (5 after TVT and 10 after PVT), with no significant difference between the two procedures in rate of urethrolysis. In the remaining 10 patients, obstruction was managed by clean intermittent catheterization and was relieved within 3 months with no need for any further intervention ($P = .18$).

DISCUSSION

Preliminary reports and the experience at our own institution suggest that the techniques of midurethral synthetic sling placement of TVT and PVT are reproducible, easy to master, and minimally invasive with respect to tissue handling. The combination of these advantages provides the opportunity to perform these procedures under local anesthesia with sedation when applicable, to minimize the time of postoperative bladder drainage, and to shorten the time of convalescence.

Although no absolute contraindications for using these procedures to treat SUI have been established based on a review of the current literature, midurethral sling procedures such as TVT or PVT should be performed with caution on patients with severe ISD without hypermobility (a low leak point pressure of ≤60 cm H_2O) until more available data are available.

Complications exist with all anti-incontinence procedures, and there is a growing database of information on adverse events unique to these procedures that will place proper perspective on their respective incidences. We have tried to outline the anatomic considerations when performing these procedures as well as suggestions for the technical methodology that should minimize patient morbidity, avoid patient mortality, and produce the highest rate of durable success.

As with all surgical endeavors associated with reconstructive surgery, modifications of the best procedures continue to evolve. Although the TVT procedure appears to be the most recent step toward this goal, modifications such as the PVT procedure will surely continue to evolve the technique of midurethral sling formation. At present, PVT does not appear to be inferior to TVT based on our retrospective review. A prospective study may confirm this finding, but this more economical way of viewing the data may allow us to draw some of the same inferences.

CONCLUSION

While the long-term results of minimally invasive synthetic sling procedures are maturing, enthusiasm for considering the TVT and PVT procedures stems from the incorporation of techniques acquired from traditional sling procedures. Learning to stabilize the urethra and bladder neck instead of performing suspension sling procedures has greatly reduced the rate of urinary obstruction and the concomitant morbidity of urgency and urge incontinence in contemporary reports of all sling procedures, proximal or midurethral.

Because of the reduced tension placed on synthetic slings that are made of a mesh material with large interstices instead of tightly woven and impermeable, less potential for graft erosion is currently being reported. With future studies reporting the preoperative urodynamic profile of the patients undergoing these unique procedures, better inclusion and exclusion criteria for performing these procedures will be established. Furthermore, cost-effective solutions to midurethral sling placement may allow expanded use of these techniques around the world.

References

1. Ulmsten U, Petros P: Intravaginal slingplasty (IVS): An ambulatory surgical procedure for treatment of female urinary incontinence. Scand J Urol Nephrol 29:75, 1995.
2. Constantine GHP: The use of tension free vaginal tape (TVT) in complex cases of incontinence: Effect on quality of life. Int Urogynecol J Pelvic Floor Dysfunct 11(Suppl 1):S95, 2000.
3. Ulmsten U, Falconer C, Johnson P, et al: A multicenter study of tension-free vaginal tape (TVT) for surgical treatment of stress urinary incontinence. Int Urogynecol J Pelvic Floor Dysfunct 9:210, 1998.
4. Ward K, Hilton P: Prospective multicentre randomised trial of tension-free vaginal tape and colposuspension as primary treatment for stress incontinence. BMJ 325:67, 2002.
5. Rackley RR, Abdelmalak JB, Tchetgen MB, et al: Tension-free vaginal tape and percutaneous vaginal tape sling procedures. Tech Urol 7:90, 2001.
6. Chung MK, Bradley AB, Chung RP: TVT for treatment of urinary incontinence in obese women. Presented at the 21st American Urogynecologic Society Meeting, Hilton Head, South Carolina, October 26-28, 2000.
7. Brink DM: Bowel injury following insertion of tension-free vaginal tape [letter]. S Afr Med J 90:450-452, 2000.
8. Klutke JJ, Carlin BI, Klutke CG: The tension-free vaginal tape procedure: Correction of stress incontinence with minimal alteration in proximal urethral mobility. Urology 55:512, 2000.
9. Chassagne S, Bernier PA, Haab F, et al: Proposed cutoff values to define bladder outlet obstruction in women. Urology 51:408, 1998.
10. Groutz A, Blaivas JG, Rosenthal JE: A simplified urinary incontinence score for the evaluation of treatment outcomes. Neurourol Urodyn 19:127, 2000.
11. Singh M, Bushman W, Clemens JQ: Do pad tests and voiding diaries affect patient willingness to participate in studies of incontinence treatment outcomes? J Urol 171:316, 2004.
12. O'Brien RG: A tour of Unify POW: A SAS macro for sample-size analysis. In Proceedings of the 23rd SAS Users Group International Conference. Cary NC: SAS Institute, 1998, pp 1346-1355.

Chapter 44

TRANSOBTURATOR APPROACH TO MIDURETHRAL SLING

Carl G. Klutke and John J. Klutke

Surgery for stress urinary incontinence has changed rapidly in the past decade. This change was preceded and to some extent catalyzed by critical appraisal of anti-incontinence surgery as an empirical therapy that, at best, provides a compensatory abnormality to restore continence. Implicit in this view is the acceptance that surgery has the potential to upset the balance of neurologic and anatomic factors that govern the bladder and its outlet. The rationale for recent innovation has been to limit the detrimental effect on this balance that can result from surgical therapy.

A few specific concepts have been introduced to limit the impact of surgery on normal function. It is recognized that mobility of the proximal urethra is normal and, in fact, important for the initiation of voiding. Surgery should avoid interference with the mobility of this structure if possible. The use of a cough stress test can minimize the potential to cause voiding disturbance by providing a physiologic feedback to guide the surgeon in applying outlet resistance. The notion of surgical wounding and its effect on the nervous system, a concept that has been explored in the anesthesia literature, has been applied in the arena of anti-incontinence surgery, leading to the employment of local anesthesia as a means of pre-emptive block to reduce negative neurologic consequences.

It is appropriate to attribute much of the recent improvement in surgical therapy of incontinence to the work of Ulf Ulmsten. Ulmsten's original thinking and his insistence on scrutinizing the concepts that he formulated with rigorous scientific methodology are laudable, and his work represents a milestone in the evolution of surgical practice.[1-3] His tension-free vaginal tape (TVT) procedure has become the "gold standard" for anti-incontinence surgery. Improvement in technique will need to incorporate its innovative features.

The improvement offered by the transobturator sling (TOT) over other midurethral slings is a reduction in the incidence of penetration injuries during sling introduction. Although complications associated with the TVT procedure are uncommon, stress incontinence is an exceedingly common condition. Now, with experience with TVT totaling hundreds of thousands of women, it has become apparent that serious complications can result from the procedure and from the other retropubic sling procedures that copy it. Injury to the colon, small bowel, ureter, urethra, bladder vasculature, tube, and ovary have been associated with the procedure, as have erosions of the sling material into the vagina, bladder, and urethra.[4-6] Bleeding, hematoma, abscess formation, retention, and voiding dysfunction can occur. The most feared of these complications is bowel perforation. If this occurs during blind sling introduction, its recognition is not immediate, yet it is potentially fatal, especially if diagnosis is delayed. The extent to which this particular complication is related to human error is probably irrelevant. The fact is that TVT is a blind procedure, with needle passage occurring in proximity to the bowel. Bowel perforation is to some extent related to the technique involved in retropubic midurethral sling placement, and even experienced surgeons can encounter it.

Limitations are also inherent in the therapeutic effect that the procedure offers. Connective tissue abnormalities are recognizable in women with incontinence, but surgery does not restore the connective tissue to its predisease state. Midurethral slings result in a dense, collagen-rich structure in the anterior vagina, rather like a ligament. Such a structure is not normally present in the vagina. Although the procedures are effective, they do not correct the underlying defect responsible for stress incontinence, which remains unknown. Although improvement of outcome may be possible with modification of the basic theme of the midurethral sling procedure, all approaches currently share this theoretical limitation.

DESCRIPTION

In the continuing effort to evaluate and improve surgical therapy for incontinence, the TOT approach has recently reached mainstream clinical practice.[7] It is a type of midurethral sling that incorporates midurethral placement, the use of local anesthesia, and a cough stress test (Fig. 44-1). No technique is without surgical risk, but TOT seems to offer less risk than retropubic midurethral sling procedures do. TOT logically avoids the potential for bowel or large vessel injury, because it avoids blind retropubic needle passage.

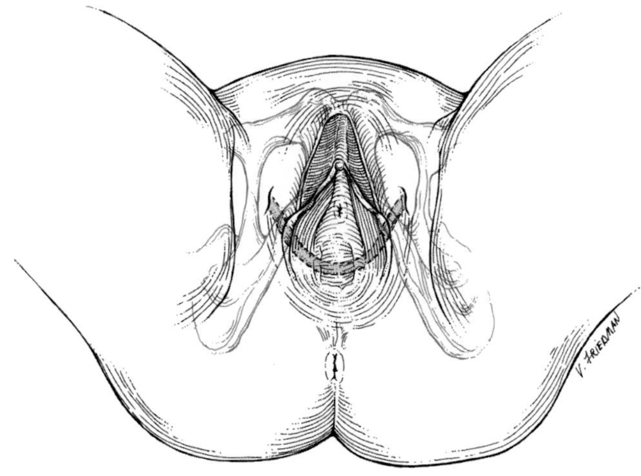

Figure 44-1 Axial view of transobturator, suburethral sling.

In most respects, the TOT and retropubic TVT procedures are identical. Both use an identical hammock-like strip of polypropylene placed beneath the mid-urethra to support it from above. The main difference is in technique: with TOT placement, the introducer needle remains superficial to the urogenital diaphragm. Because the introducer needle is not allowed to pass through the retropubic space, the risk that the needle tip could cause injury to bladder, bowel, or blood vessels is lessened. The TOT sling and its instruments have been approved by the U.S. Food and Drug Administration for the treatment of stress urinary incontinence in females. This chapter discusses anatomy pertinent to TOT route, the technique itself, and the published literature supporting its use.

ANATOMY

The fact that the obturator foramen is unfamiliar to most urologists has to do with its lack of urologic surgical applications and not with any inherent danger of dissection in the area. Most urologists consider this part of the pelvis to be an end point, not a gateway, and are unfamiliar with its anatomy. The obturator foramen is not without common surgical applications, however. Access to the obturator vessels through the obturator foramen for vascular bypass, for instance, is a classic approach for relief of vascular insufficiency in the lower extremity.[8] Veterinary surgeons predate urologists in the treatment of stress incontinence in female dogs via this approach.[9] The advantages of TOT sling placement now makes a complete understanding of the anatomy of the obturator foramen relevant to the urologist as well.

The obturator foramen is an oval opening in the anterior ventral bony pelvis formed by the confluence of the pubic and ischial bones. The obturator membrane is a thin fibrous sheet which almost completely closes the obturator foramen. Its fibers are arranged in interlacing bundles, mainly transverse in direction; the uppermost bundle is attached to the obturator tubercles and completes the obturator canal for passage of the obturator vessels and nerve in its lateral aspect. Both obturator muscles are continuous with this membrane: the obturator internus padding the inner aspect and the obturator externus its outer surface.[10]

The obturator nerve arises from the ventral divisions of the second, third, and fourth lumbar nerves. It descends through the fibers of the psoas major and emerges from its medial border. It runs along the lateral wall of the pelvis above and in front of the obturator vessels to the upper lateral part of the obturator foramen. Here it enters the thigh to innervate the muscles of adduction. The obturator artery and vein that supply and drain the muscles of the medial thigh course together with the nerve through the foramen laterally. The anatomic location of the nerve and vessels in the upper outer part of the obturator foramen allows for safe passage of introduced trocars along the medial aspect of the foramen.[11]

The obturator foramen, its membrane, the obturator internus muscle, and its surrounding fascia lie external to the endopelvic fascial lining of the pelvis and the peritoneal cavity. Normal passage of the introducing needle during the TOT sling procedure avoids both spaces. Anatomic studies in cadavers have demonstrated that, when properly positioned, the TOT sling travels in a horizontal plane across the origin of the adductor muscles and through the inferior margin of the obturator foramen. The sling then passes through the internal obturator muscle, above the pedicle of the internal pudendal artery, through the levator ani muscle, past the tendinous arc of the pelvic fascia, and beneath the middle third of the urethra.[12] There are no major blood vessels or viscera along this route. Kocjancic and colleagues demonstrated that properly placed TOT tape lies 2 cm away from the urethra and 4 to 5 cm from the obturator nerve and vessels in the obturator foramen. The angle formed between the tape and the urethra is approximately 15 degrees, which does not place extra anatomic strain on the urethra.[13] Despite the theoretical increased safety of this approach, improper placement of the needle device increases the risk of vesical and/or vaginal perforation.

TECHNIQUE

This section describes our technique for placement of a TOT sling. It is not meant as a definitive description, nor is it intended to supplant surgical training in the operating room by an experienced teacher.

Preoperative Assessment

The TOT sling, like all midurethral slings, is primarily indicated for patients with stress incontinence with urethral mobility. Documentation of stress incontinence, either on an office cough stress test or by formal cystometry, is the first step toward a satisfactory outcome. Our own preference is to perform a urodynamic study, because this not only provides an accepted, objective documentation of the incontinence but also gives an indication of other aspects of bladder behavior, such as tone (compliance), reflex excitability, and sensation, which may indicate the need for additional therapy in other areas. A vaginal examination or cotton swab test is important to identify a fixed or nonmobile urethra, which may result in failure for midurethral slings.

Contraindications to the TOT sling procedure include the following:

- Pure urge incontinence
- Fixed urethra
- Underlying bleeding diathesis
- Anticoagulant medication
- Anesthetic contraindications (to local anesthesia with intravenous sedation)
- Hip deformity precluding dorsolithotomy position

The patient should be given a thorough explanation of the procedure with a full review of the potential risks and potential complications, specifically including the possibility of blood loss; infection; injury to bladder, urethra. or vagina; tape exposure; failure; and general risks. A fully informed consent, documented in the chart, will help to alleviate problems later on.

Anesthetic Considerations

The TOT sling procedure can be performed with the patient under local anesthesia with intravenous sedation, spinal anesthesia, or general anesthesia. It is our strong preference to use local anesthesia if possible. This approach is less morbid from an anesthetic standpoint, and, more importantly, it is the only way to ensure an adequate stress test. Properly placed, the local anesthetic does not paralyze the musculature of the pelvic floor and ensures that biofeedback will accurately determine the degree of resistance necessary at the bladder outlet. Local anesthetic injected into the areas of the pelvis through which the sling will pass also creates tissue "hydrodissection," which allows easier passage of the needle. Finally, the administration of local anesthetic is a "trial run" of the needle passage and gives the surgeon a better feel for the anatomy of individual patient's pelvis. A long-acting local anesthetic with or without epinephrine is recommended.

If local anesthesia with intravenous sedation is chosen, close communication between surgeon and anesthetist is required. Although TOT sling placement is a short procedure, it requires deeper sedation for some segments (local anesthetic injection and actual needle passage) and minimal sedation for some segments (resistance adjustment and completion of the procedure). For this reason, it is imperative that both the operating surgeon and the anesthetist be acquainted with the steps of the operation and that the surgeon keep the anesthetist apprised of its progress. Our typical intravenous sedation regimen includes 2 mg versed administered while the patient is in the holding area, 2 mg fentanyl administered in the operating room, and a Diprivan titrated infusion before local anesthetic administration.

Preparation

Because the surgery is focused on the vagina and perineum only, patients are positioned in the high dorsolithotomy position, and a full vaginal and perineal preparation is performed. The surgeon positions the table to height preference, and the anesthesiologist confirms adequate sedation before local anesthetic administration.

Local anesthesia is injected with the intent of anesthetizing all areas of soft tissue involved in dissection and ultimate placement of the sling. We use a long-acting local agent such as 0.25% Ropivacaine or Marcaine and plan on giving 40 to 45 mL in total for the procedure. Needles used for this purpose include a 25-gauge 1.5-inch needle for skin and vaginal epithelium, and a 20-gauge spinal needle for deeper infiltration. Infiltration sites ultimately include the skin over perineal incision sites, the anterior vaginal wall, and the intervening soft tissue.

Confirmation of Landmarks, Incisions, and Dissection

A number of visual and palpable landmarks must be recognized for proper placement of the tape. The adductor muscle tendons, inferior pubic ramus, external urethral meatus, clitoris, bladder neck, inguinal-gluteal folds, and, in nonobese patients, the obturator foramen itself can be either seen or palpated in the course of planning the incision sites. Two sets of incisions are then made: a 1-inch, sagittal vaginal incision placed midway between the bladder neck and the external urethral meatus, and two perineal skin stabs overlying the left and right medial obturator foramina at the level of the clitoris one fingerbreadth lateral to the inguinal-gluteal fold. It is important to incise the vagina deep to the vaginal epithelial layer, to avoid problems of wound healing later on.

Having made the incision in the vagina overlying the midurethra, the surgeon must identify the tissue plane between urethra and vagina and develop this plane laterally to allow digital palpation of the medial edge of the ischiopubic ramus. Once the plane is developed, the 20-gauge spinal needle is used to administer local anesthetic into the soft tissue between the perineal stab incisions and the vaginal incision.

Needle Passage

The goal of needle passage is to place the sling from mid-urethra to perineum while avoiding damage to the bladder, bladder neck, and urethra; penetration of the vaginal epithelial layer; and injury to the obturator nerves and vessels. Whether this is accomplished by an "outside-in" approach or an "inside-out" approach at this stage of procedural evolution is largely a matter of personal preference. We have been most comfortable with passage of the needle from the perineal stab incisions, through the obturator foramen, and then, under fingertip guidance, out the vaginal incision. After the needle is through the vaginal incision site, the sling is attached and withdrawn through the perineal stab, and the same procedure is carried out on the other side with the other end of the sling.

Once the sling is in place, cystoscopy is used to confirm that the urethra and bladder are intact and were not penetrated during sling placement. Whether cystoscopy is required in all cases of TOT sling placement is a matter of conjecture at present, but reports of bladder and urethral injury exist, and we recommend the use of a zero-degree 17-Fr cystoscope for complete visualization of urethra and bladder neck in all cases in which the possibility of injury cannot otherwise be ruled out.

Cough Test

If local anesthesia and intravenous sedation have been employed, a cough test can be performed to guide tensioning of the TOT sling. The bladder is filled with normal saline to the volume at which leakage was previously demonstrated. The patient is placed in a reverse Trendelenburg position, and the weighted vaginal speculum, instruments, and retractors are removed from the vagina. The surgeon and anesthesiologist should assess the awake status of the patient and confirm a strenuous cough effort. With leakage per urethra as a starting point, we adjust tension on the sling by pulling the free ends incrementally until leakage ceases. The overall goal is to place as little resistance at the outlet of the bladder by the tape as is necessary to stop leakage with cough.

Completion of Procedure

Once proper tensioning is complete, excess tape is excised flush with the perineal skin, with care taken to avoid injuring the surrounding skin. Closure of the vaginal incisions with absorbable suture, such as 2-0 polyglycolic acid, is accomplished. Noting that vaginal exposure due to improper wound healing of the vaginal incision is one of the more common complications, we recommend careful placement of interrupted sutures, making sure that no sling is involved with the closure. The perineal stabs can be closed with Steri-Strips. Finally, before the patient is transported to the recovery room, the surgeon must confirm hemostasis and estimate blood loss.

Recovery Room Check

In the recovery room, confirmation of complete bladder emptying must be documented. If a cough test in the operating room was performed, the volume instilled should also be emptied. Uncommonly, short-term catheter drainage may be required. Discharge instructions, including limitation of strenuous activity and abstinence from sexual activity for at least 6 weeks from the date of surgery, should be given and documented. Patients are given postoperative prescriptions including analgesics, short-term antibiotics, and stool softeners to avoid postoperative constipation.

COMPLICATIONS

The most common reported complication of TOT urethral sling placement is de novo urge urinary incontinence, which has been reported in 2% to 7% of patients.[14-16] Short-term urinary obstructive symptoms have been reported in 1% to 3%.[14-16] Short-term obstruction can be managed by intermittent or indwelling catheterization; however if symptoms persist longer than 1 week, we recommend early sling loosening.[17] Other reported complications include pain; dyspareunia (<1%); bladder neck laceration (<1%); perforation of the bladder, vagina, or urethra (1%); and delayed erosion of the sling into the vagina or urethra (1% to 3%).[18-21] Significant injury to major blood vessels or bowel has not been reported. There has been no reported mortality.

CLINICAL OUTCOMES

Because the TOT approach is relatively new, only short-term efficacy for the treatment of stress incontinence has been demonstrated. Subjective cure and improvement rates of 83% to 93% and 5.4% to 9.4%, respectively, have been reported with follow-up ranging from 3 months to 1 year.[16,21] Aside from these subjective reports, at least one study has demonstrated significant improvement in urinary pad usage, sexual function, and overall quality of life after TOT sling placement.[19] The TOT sling was evaluated in patients who had previously undergone anti-incontinence surgery and was found to provide with cure rates of 79% and improvement rates of 9.2%.[21] The procedure has been demonstrated to be equally efficacious in obese and nonobese patients and in women older than 70 years.[22,23] TOT sling concomitant with pelvic organ prolapse repair has also been evaluated, with results showing 87.2% cure and 7.7% improvement in stress incontinence symptoms at a mean follow-up of 12 months.[24]

CONCLUSION

The TOT approach to suburethral sling placement is an exciting modification in the management of stress urinary incontinence in women. Like the TVT procedure, the TOT approach is a minimally invasive procedure with good short-term efficacy but has the added benefit of avoiding deep penetration of the pelvis. Additional prospective studies with longer follow-up are needed before the TOT sling can replace the gold standard TVT.

References

1. Petros P, Ulmsten U: An integral theory of female urinary incontinence: Experimental and clinical considerations. Acta Obstet Gynecol Scand 69(Suppl 153), 7-31, 1990.
2. Ulmsten U, Henriksson L, Johnson P, Varhos G: An ambulatory surgical procedure under local anesthesia for treatment of female urinary incontinence. Int Urogynecol J Pelvic Floor Dysfunct 7:81-85, 1996.
3. Ulmsten U, Johnson P, Rezapour M: A 3 year follow-up of TVT for surgical treatment of female urinary stress incontinence. BJOG 106:345-350, 1990.
4. De Tayrac R, Deffieux X, Droupy S, et al: A prospective randomized trial comparing tension-free vaginal tape and transobturator suburethral tape for surgical treatment of stress urinary incontinence. Am J Obstet Gynecol 190:602-608, 2004.
5. Tamussino KF, Hanzal E, Kolle D, et al: Tension-free vaginal tape operation: Results of the Austrian registry. Obstet Gynecol 98(5 Pt 1):732-736, 2001.
6. Castillo OA, Bodden E, Olivaries RA, Urena RD: Intestinal perforation: An infrequent complication during insertion of tension-free vaginal tape. J Urol 172:1364, 2004.
7. Delorme E: Transobturator urethral suspension: mini-invasive procedure in the treatment of stress urinary incontinence in women. Prog Urol 11:1306-1313, 2001.
8. Patel A, Taylor SM, Langan EM, et al: Obturator bypass: A classic approach for the treatment of contemporary groin infection. Am Surg 68:653-658, 2002.
9. Nickel RF, Wiegand U, van den Brom WE: Evaluation of a transpelvic sling procedure with and without colposuspension for treatment of female dogs with refractory urethral sphincter mechanism incompetence. Vet Surg (2):94-104, 1998.
10. Gray H: Gray's Anatomy, 24th ed. Philadelphia: Lea & Febiger, 1942.
11. Moore K: Clinically Oriented Anatomy, 3rd ed. Philadelphia: William and Wilkins, 1992.
12. Delmas V, Ortuno F, et al: Anatomical Structures by a Sling Crossed to Treat Urinary Incontinence in the Female. 25th Congress of the International French Society of Urodynamics, 2002.
13. Kocjancic E, Costa P, Wagner L, et al: Safety and efficacy of trans obturator tape in the treatment of stress urinary incontinence [abstract 116]. International Continence Society Meeting, Paris 2004.
14. Delorme E, Droupy S, de Tayrac R, Delmas V: Tranobturator tape: A new minimally invasive procedure to treat female urinary incontinence. Eur Urol 45:203-207, 2004.
15. Boccon-Gibod L, Grise P, de Tayrac R, et al: Trans-obturator tape for the treatment of female stress urinary incontinence: A multicentric prospective study [abstract 311]. Annual Meeting of the International Continence Society, Paris 2004.
16. Mellier G, Moore R, Jacquetin B: A meta-analysis of the intraoperative safety and effectiveness of the transobturator hammock seen in results of two prospective studies in 9 countries with 204 patients. ICS/IUGA Joint Meeting, Paris 2004.
17. Klutke C, Siegel S, et al: Urinary retention after tension-free vaginal tape procedure: Incidence and treatment. Urology 58:697-701, 2001.
18. Jacquetin B, DeBodinance P, et al: Six-month data from the transobturator hammock procedure for female stress urinary incontinence: A prospective study in 8 countries. ICS/IUGA Joint Meeting, 2004.
19. Cindolo L, Salzano L, et al: Tension-free transobturator approach for female stress urinary incontinence. Minerva Urol Nefrol 55:89-98, 2003.
20. Minaglia S, Ozel B, Klutke C, et al: Bladder injury during transobturator sling. Urology 64:376-377, 2004.
21. Costa P, Grise P, et al: Surgical treatment of female stress urinary incontinence with trans obturator tape (T.O.T.®): Short term results of a prospective multicenter study. Eur Urol 46:102-106, Paris 2004.
22. Droupy S, DeTayrac R, et al: Outcome of obese female patients treated by T.O.T® for stress urinary incontinence [abstract 705]. Annual Meeting of the International Continence Society, Paris 2004.
23. Vincent D, Philippe G, et al: T.O.T.®: Clinical outcome in elderly female patients with stress urinary incontinence [abstract 705]. Annual Meeting of the International Continence Society, Paris 2004.
24. De Tayrac R, Deffieux X, et al: A prospective randomized trial comparing tension-free vaginal tape and transobturator suburethral tape for surgical treatment of stress urinary incontinence. Am J Obstet Gynecol 190:602-608, 2004.

Chapter 45

CADAVERIC FASCIAL SLING USING BONE ANCHORS

Sarah A. Rueff and Gary E. Leach

Transvaginal slings are now considered the primary procedure of choice for female stress urinary incontinence (SUI).[1] Although historically female SUI was thought to be caused by either urethral hypermobility or intrinsic sphincter deficiency (ISD), it is now accepted that all patients with SUI have some component of ISD. Therefore, regardless of the cause, a sling procedure may be the first line of treatment recommended. We first began performing the cadaveric transvaginal sling (CaTS) procedure with bone anchors in 1998. Early results showed patient outcome and continence rates to be comparable to those obtained with other techniques and sling materials.[2]

PREOPERATIVE EVALUATION

A thorough preoperative evaluation is essential before intervention for SUI. Gynecologic history should include number of vaginal deliveries and prior anti-incontinence procedures. Micturition history should include type of incontinence present, type and number of pads used, and a measure of degree of "bother" via questionnaire analysis. The stress-related leakage, emptying ability, anatomy, protection, inhibition (SEAPI) incontinence score is a subjective assessment of patient symptoms and impact on quality of life (Table 45-1).[3] Physical examination should focus on assessment and documentation of degree of urethral hypermobility. A thorough examination of the anterior and posterior vaginal wall and the uterus or vaginal cuff should be performed with the patient both supine and standing. Associated pelvic organ prolapse should be repaired simultaneously with the sling procedure. Patients who have undergone prior anti-incontinence procedures may have urethral fixation secondary to scarring at the bladder neck and will require urethrolysis at the time of sling placement. A focused neurologic examination should document any deficits with further evaluation as indicated. Preoperatively, urodynamic evaluation is performed in all patients to confirm SUI and document abdominal leak point pressure. In addition, urodynamic evaluation excludes underlying bladder dysfunction, such as detrusor overactivity or poor compliance, and evaluates the patient's ability to empty the bladder.

CADAVERIC FASCIA

The use of autologous fascia for transvaginal sling, using either rectus fascia from the anterior abdominal wall or fascia lata from the lateral thigh, has been previously described.[4,5] Fascia lata is known to be universally strong regardless of patient age or medical condition. When compared, fascia lata has reproducibly three to four times greater tensile strength than rectus fascia.[6] Rectus fascia can become attenuated and scarred as a result of cesarean section, abdominal hysterectomy, or other abdominal procedures. However, harvesting fascia inevitably increases operative time, morbidity of the procedure, postoperative pain, and length of hospital stay. For that reason, cadaveric fascia lata (CFL) has become a popular choice for sling material.

Our fascia of choice is a non-frozen CFL, Tutoplast (Mentor Corporation, Santa Barbara, CA). Tutoplast preparation involves a five-step process that includes solvent-dehydration and gamma-irradiation. The process is summarized as follows:

1. *Screening:* The U.S. Food and Drug Administration serologically screens potential donors and rejects those with a medical or social history that places them at risk of infectious disease or malignancy. The fascia is then inspected and must meet stringent cleanliness, structure, quality, and size standards.
2. *Processing:* The first step in the cleaning process involves osmotic treatment with various concentrations of saline solution in order to destroy bacteria and viruses and remove most of the antigens from the tissue.

Table 45-1 SEAPI Incontinence Score

Stress-related leakage ("S")	0 = No urine loss 1 = Loss with strenuous activity 2 = Loss with moderate activity 3 = Loss with minimal activity
Emptying ability ("E")	0 = No obstructive symptoms 1 = Minimal symptoms 2 = Significant symptoms 3 = Only dribbles or retention
Anatomy ("A")	0 = No descent with strain 1 = Descent, not to introitus 2 = Through introitus with strain 3 = Through introitus at rest
Protection ("P")	0 = Never used 1 = Certain occasions 2 = Daily, occasional accidents 3 = Continually, frequent accidents or constant leakage
Inhibition ("I")	0 = No urge symptoms 1 = Rare urge urinary incontinence (UUI) 2 = UUI once/week 3 = UUI at least once/day

From Raz S, Erickson DR: SEAPI QNM incontinence classification system. Neurourol Urodyn 11:187-199, 1992.

3. *Denaturization:* The second step of the cleaning process involves treatment with NaOH and H_2O_2 that removes the remainder of antigens and destroys prions (Creutz Feldt-Jakob Disease) and viruses (hepatitis, HIV). Limited exposure to NaOH allows this to be accomplished without significant alteration of the collagenous structure.
4. *Preservation:* Extraction of water from the tissue is accomplished via organic solvents, resulting in preservation of a dense collagenous structure without a chemical residue.
5. *Gamma irradiation:* The tissue is cut to various sizes, packaged, and sterilized with gamma irradiation. Radiation is limited to less than 25,000 Gy (2.5 Mrad) to limit weakening of the fascia.

The strength and quality of solvent-dehydrated CFL have been compared to those of freeze-dried CFL, another commercially available preparation. Solvent-dehydrated CFL was found to have significantly greater stiffness, maximum load to failure, and maximum load per unit of graft.[7]

Many authors have published their outcomes using either the solvent-dehydrated or the freeze-dried CFL, and their results have confirmed a difference in the tissue quality. Boone published results on 26 women who underwent pubovaginal sling with solvent-dehydrated CFL (Tutoplast) for SUI.[8] Minimum follow-up was 12 months. The outcome revealed that 25 (96%) of the 26 patients were "significantly" improved: 77% wore no pads postoperatively, and an additional 15% wore no more than 1 pad per day. No patients required an additional operation for incontinence.

On the other hand, Raz's group published results on 154 consecutive patients with SUI who underwent pubovaginal sling placement using freeze-dried CFL.[9] With an average time to follow-up of 10.6 months, 58 (38%) of the 154 patients had recurrent SUI and 26 (17%) required a second operation for SUI. With an average time to reoperation of 9 months, the authors noted that the fascia was either absent, fragmented, or attenuated. Brubaker's associates reported similar results.[10] Thirty-two patients underwent pubovaginal sling placement with freeze-dried CFL and were available for short-term follow-up. Although 22 (69%) of the 32 patients were objectively dry, the remaining 10 (31%) had recurrent SUI by 6 months' follow-up. Eight patients underwent reoperation for SUI, and in 7 (87.5%) of them little or no fascia remained at the urethrovesical junction. Fascial strands that were present were sent for histologic analysis and showed evidence of autolysis and degeneration.

As is evident, all commercially available CFL preparations are not the same. The method used to prepare the tissue ultimately affects its tensile strength and surgical results with its use. We prefer to use the nonfrozen cadaveric fascia to avoid the synthetic sling materials that have been associated with higher rates of erosion and/or infection.[11,12]

BONE ANCHORS

The incorporation of bone fixation in the treatment of SUI was first described with the Marshall-Marchetti-Krantz vesicourethropexy.[13] Since that time, a number of techniques have been described that involve fixation of suspension sutures directly to the pubic bone, which avoids the risk of nerve entrapment that can occur with attachment to the rectus fascia. Leach described a technique using a needle to place the suspension sutures into the pubic bone,[14] and Benderev later incorporated the use of bone anchors for suture placement.[15] Nativ and colleagues were the first to employ transvaginal bone anchors using a handheld drill in 1997.[16] Their procedure allowed cystourethropexy to be performed entirely transvaginally and was subsequently modified into a sling procedure.

The advantages of transvaginal bone anchor fixation are many. Because the procedure is performed completely transvaginally, no abdominal incisions are required, and postoperative pain is decreased. Suture placement via bone anchors does not require needle or suture passage through the retropubic space and therefore reduces the risks of bleeding and bladder perforation. There has been speculation that perforation of the endopelvic fascia during sling placement may increase the risk of postoperative vaginal prolapse and recurrent SUI.[17] The CaTS procedure, described later, does not involve perforation of the endopelvic fascia and minimizes the potential risks of postoperative prolapse or sling failure.

The risk of osseous complications associated with the use of transvaginal bone anchors appears to be less than that reported with suprapubic anchor fixation. Frederick and coworkers published a review of the osseous complications within their prospective cohort of patients in addition to those of 15 other published reports. Among a total of 1228 patients, the incidence of osteitis pubis was 2 (0.16%), and the incidence of osteomyelitis was 1 (0.08%).[18] A prior review published by Rackley and colleagues in 2001 reported no osseous complications among 314 patients who had undergone transvaginal bone anchor with sling placement, compared to a 0.86% incidence associated with suprapubic placement of bone anchors.[19] The incidence of osseous complications with the Marshall-Marchetti-Krantz retropubic urethropexy has been reported to be 0.76%.[20]

PREOPERATIVE PREPARATION

Before cadaveric transvaginal sling with bone anchors (CaTS) procedure is performed, the urine is confirmed to be sterile. Patients are taught self-catheterization preoperatively. In the event that a patient is unable to learn self-catheterization or has documented incomplete emptying preoperatively, consideration of placing a suprapubic tube intraoperatively should be made. Preferably, patients with vaginal wall atrophy should use estrogen vaginal cream for 4 to 6 weeks before surgery. Patients are instructed to use one-third of an applicator of estrogen three times a week to improve the quality of tissue and postoperative healing properties. A povidone-iodine vaginal douche is performed on the night before and on the morning of surgery. Perioperative antibiotics are given. We prefer to use a first-generation cephalosporin, ampicillin, or vancomycin (if the patient is allergic to penicillin) combined with an aminoglycoside.

Transvaginal repair of associated pelvic prolapse is performed with the CaTS procedure. A thorough discussion of the risks and complications of sling surgery is undertaken before repair. Patients are counseled regarding the possibility of prolonged or permanent urinary retention, recurrent SUI, and persistent or de novo urgency symptoms that may require treatment in the future.

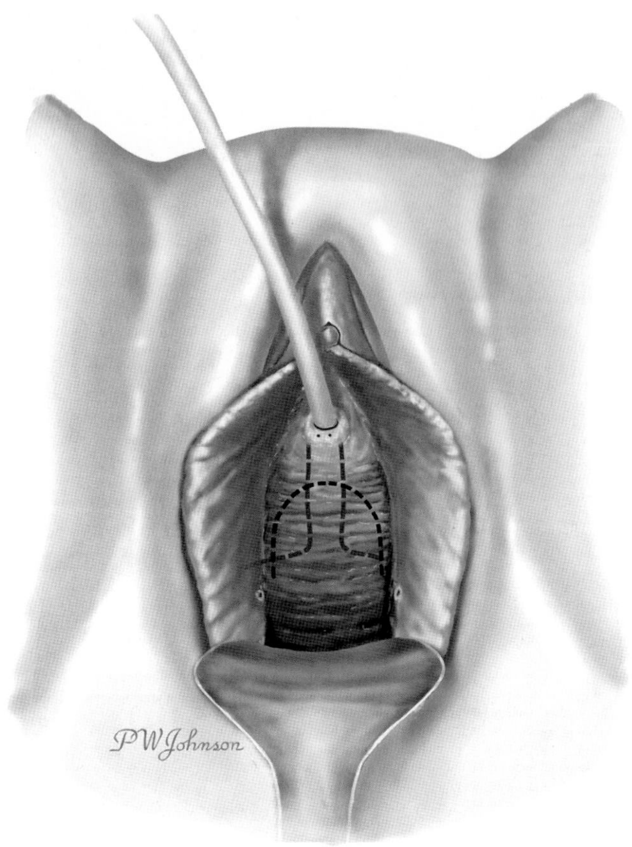

Figure 45-1 An inverted U-shaped incision is made from the mid-urethra to the bladder neck.

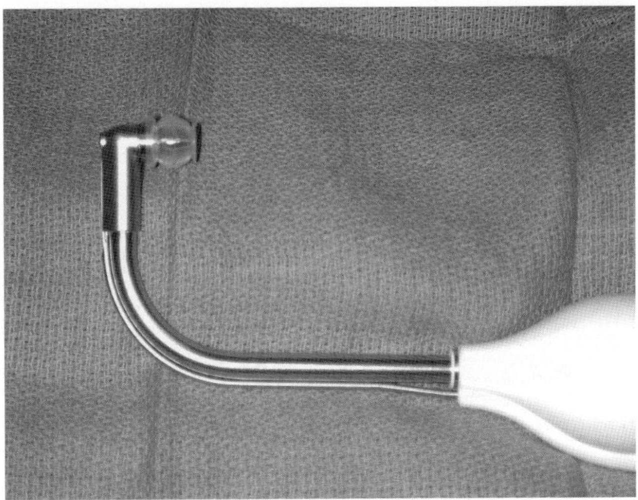

Figure 45-2 Transvaginal drill for bone anchor placement changes tone to signify firm placement into the bone.

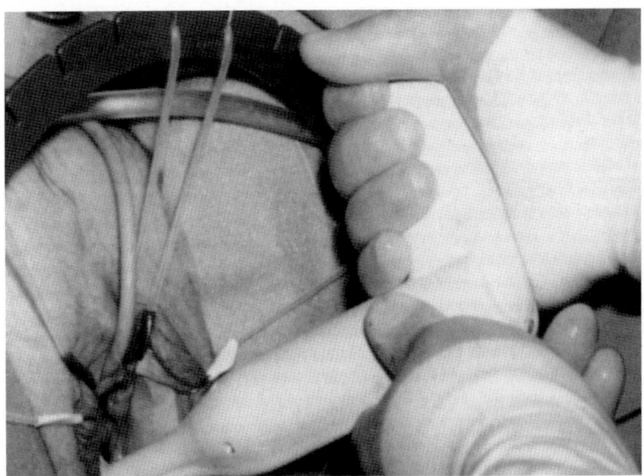

Figure 45-3 The drill positioned on the undersurface of the pubic bone for bone anchor placement.

OPERATIVE PROCEDURE

The procedure is performed with the patient in the dorsal lithotomy position. A Foley catheter is placed, and a Scott retractor (Lonestar, Houston, TX) is secured to the medial buttocks with towel clamps. The anterior vaginal wall is infiltrated with saline, and the Foley balloon is palpated at the bladder neck. An inverted U-shaped incision is made from the mid-urethra to the bladder neck (Fig. 45-1). The flap is mobilized proximally to the bladder neck, but not further, to prevent proximal migration of the sling. Lateral dissection at the bladder neck is performed to clear the undersurface of the pubic bone for bone anchor placement. Perforation of the endopelvic fascia is not necessary, so the risk of significant bleeding and bladder injury is reduced. Patients with significant scarring or urethral fixation due to prior surgeries may require urethrolysis before sling placement. Releasing the urethra from surrounding scar tissue allows the sling to provide adequate compression after placement.[21]

Our preference for bone anchor placement is the InFast drill system (American Medical Systems, Inc. Minneapolis, MN), which changes tone to signify firm placement into the bone (Fig. 45-2). Before placement of the bone anchors, the bladder is placed on drainage, and the bladder and bladder neck are retracted medially. A polypropylene suture with its anchor attached are threaded onto the drill, and the drill is positioned flush with the undersurface of the bone (Fig. 45-3). The drill is activated until a change in tone is audible; then it is removed, and the suture is firmly pulled to confirm anchor placement. The process is repeated on the opposite side.

The CaTS procedure is performed using a 2 cm × 7 cm piece of nonfrozen CFL presoaked in antibiotic solution. The edge of the fascia is folded over to allow cross-hatching of the fibers and to minimize the chance of suture pull-through.[22] An 18-gauge needle is used to allow atraumatic passage of the suture through the folded edge (Fig. 45-4). The bladder neck suture is placed more medially than the distal suture in order to keep the fascia tight against the bladder neck (Fig. 45-5). One side of the sling is secured in place up to the pubic bone. The distal edge of the sling is secured in place using a 2-0 absorbable suture to prevent the sling from rolling toward the bladder neck. The free edge of the fascia is folded over, and the appropriate position of the contralateral sutures is determined (Fig. 45-6). The fascia should lie firmly against the urethra without excessive tension. In our experience, the use of a right angle clamp placed between the urethra and the sling while deciding proper tension can result in the sling's being tied too loosely. Once the proper position is

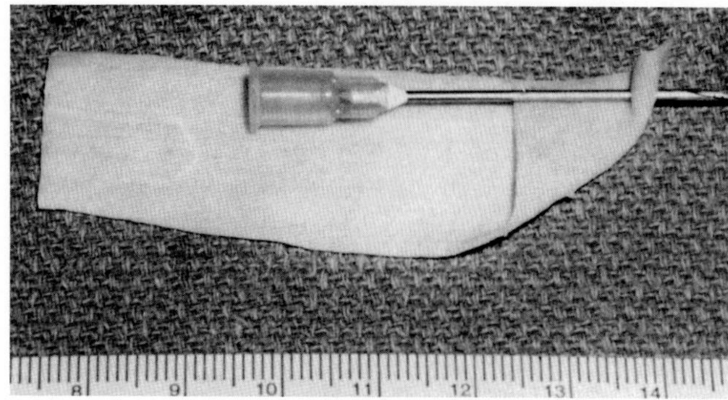

Figure 45-4 An 18-gauge needle is used for atraumatic passage of the suture through the fascia. The edge of the fascia is folded over to minimize suture pull-through.

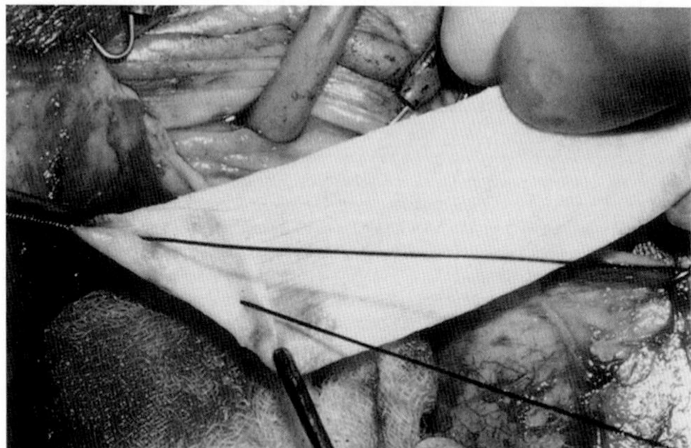

Figure 45-5 The proximal suture is passed more medial to the distal suture to place the sling snugly against the bladder neck.

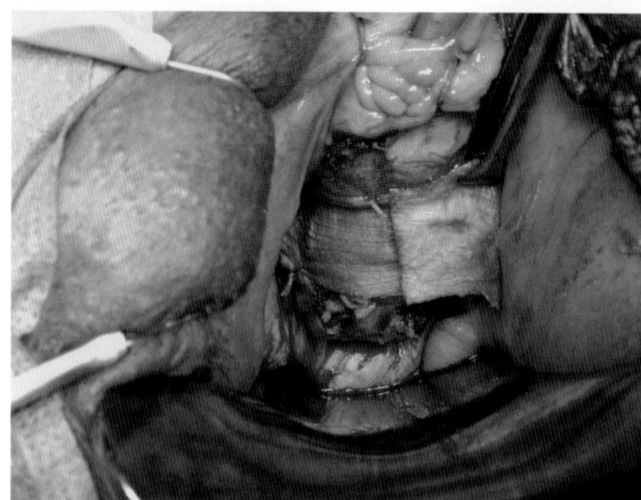

Figure 45-6 The distal edge of the sling is secured in place with 2-0 absorbable suture to prevent it from rolling toward the bladder neck. The free edge is folded over to determine proper tension and position of the contralateral sutures.

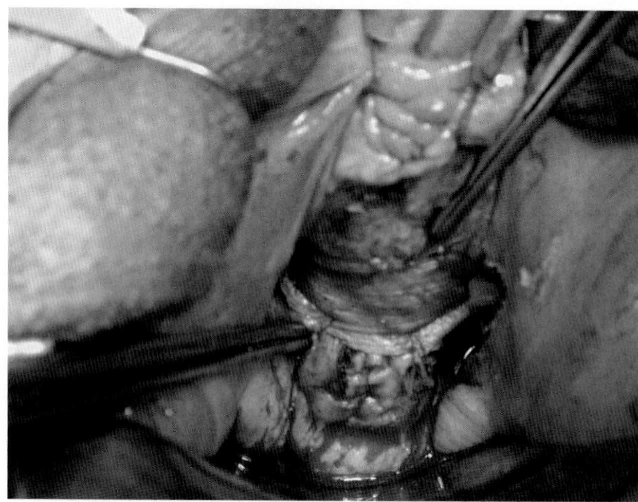

Figure 45-7 Final sling position at the mid-urethra with sutures tied and appropriate amount of tension.

determined, the sutures are passed through the fascia and tied firmly against the pubic bone (Fig. 45-7). Before the procedure is completed, cystoscopy is performed with both a 70-degree lens to rule out bladder injury and a 0-degree lens to rule out urethral injury. Irrigation with antibiotic solution is performed throughout the procedure. The vaginal incision is closed with 2-0 absorbable suture. A Betadine-soaked vaginal pack and Foley catheter are left in place.

POSTOPERATIVE CARE

The vaginal packing and Foley catheter are removed on the morning of the first postoperative day. Fluid intake is restricted to 1500 mL/day. A voiding trial is administered, and a residual urine measurement is obtained via intermittent catheterization. Eighty percent of patients void to completion immediately after surgery. If residual urine is greater than 100 mL, the patient is reinstructed on self-catheterization. If a suprapubic tube was placed intraoperatively, residuals are checked in this manner. Patients are continued on intravenous antibiotics for 24 hours postoperatively and then begun on oral antibiotic (cephalexin or fluoroquinolone) for 1 week to minimize the risk of osteitis pubis or a wound infection. Patients are routinely discharged on postoperative day 1 with oral analgesics and stool softeners in addition to antibiotics. Patients with elevated postvoid residuals are instructed to continue to monitor at home via self-catheterization or suprapubic tube until residuals are consistently less than 100 mL. In the event that a patient is unable to learn or is uncomfortable performing self-catheterization, she can be discharged with a Foley catheter and return for a trial of voiding in the office. At the time of discharge, patients are instructed to do no heavy lifting or straining and to observe pelvic rest (i.e., no intercourse, no tampons) for 6 weeks postoperatively.

Patients are seen for follow-up at 1 week, 6 weeks, 6 months, 12 months, and yearly thereafter. Evaluation should consist of urinalysis, postvoid residual urine measurement, and physical examination, as well as determination of subjective SEAPI scores. Patients are also administered a confidential, validated continence and satisfaction questionnaire every 6 to 12 months postoperatively, the results of which are entered into a prospective patient database.

RESULTS

The CaTS procedure has been performed on a total of 484 patients aged 23 to 90 years old (mean, 63.7 years). Of these, 414 (85.5%) have had a minimum questionnaire follow-up of 6 months (range, 6 to 78 months; mean, 30.2 months). Distribution of follow-up data is presented in Figure 45-8. According to the confidential patient-driven questionnaire, 89 (22%) of 414 patients reported 100% improvement in their incontinence symptoms; 195 (47%) reported greater than 80% improvement, and 279 (67%) reported 50% improvement or better. Mean SEAPI scores were significantly decreased from 5.5 preoperatively to 2.7 postoperatively ($P < .001$). Overall, 241 (58%) of 414 patients were more than 80% satisfied with the procedure on a visual analogue scale (mean satisfaction, 68%; median, 90%). Two hundred ninety-five patients (72%) would have the surgery again, and 292 (71%) would recommend the surgery to a friend.

One hundred thirty patients (31%) reported less than 50% improvement in incontinence symptoms and were considered "failures." Thirty-three (8%) complained of recurrent SUI, 56 (13.5%) complained of mixed urinary incontinence, 14 (3.4%) complained of urge urinary incontinence, and 27 (6.5%) were unsure regarding the type of incontinence responsible for their dissatisfaction. Recently, we evaluated multiple preoperative variables in an attempt to determine risk factors for failure (Table 45-2). The variables considered were

1. Preoperative urinary urgency
2. Preoperative urge urinary incontinence
3. Detrusor overactivity on preoperative urodynamic evaluation
4. Abdominal leak point pressure less than 50 cm H_2O
5. History of prior anti-incontinence procedure
6. Presence of cystocele requiring concurrent repair

The presence of preoperative urge urinary incontinence was the only considered variable associated with an increased risk of failure ($P < .01$). Conversely, the presence of a concurrent cystocele was found to be associated with a significant decrease in failure ($P < .05$), perhaps due to a redistribution of the forces at the mid-urethra and bladder neck over the entire anterior vaginal wall. Time to failure is shown in Figure 45-9. Notably, 100 (77%) of the 130 failures occurred after 12 months' follow-up.

Of 209 patients who complained of urinary urgency preoperatively, 71 (34%) experienced persistent urge symptoms postoperatively. Of 205 patients without preoperative urinary urgency, 20 (10%) developed de novo urge symptoms. Prolonged urinary retention (>30 days) occurred in 7 patients, 1 of whom required urethrolysis. Osteitis pubis occurred in 2 patients and was

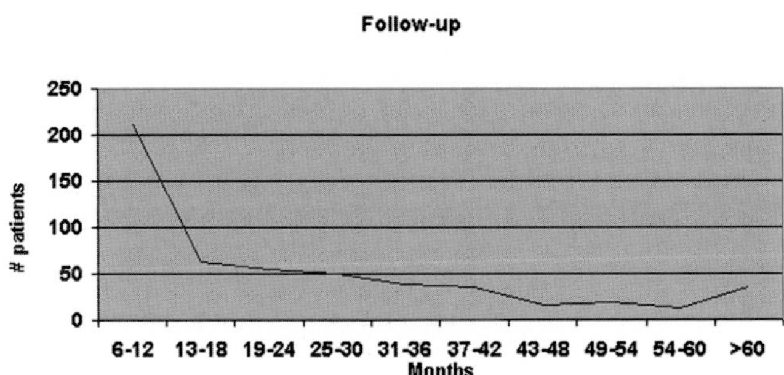

Figure 45-8 Distribution of questionnaire follow-up for the cadaveric transvaginal sling (CaTS) procedure.

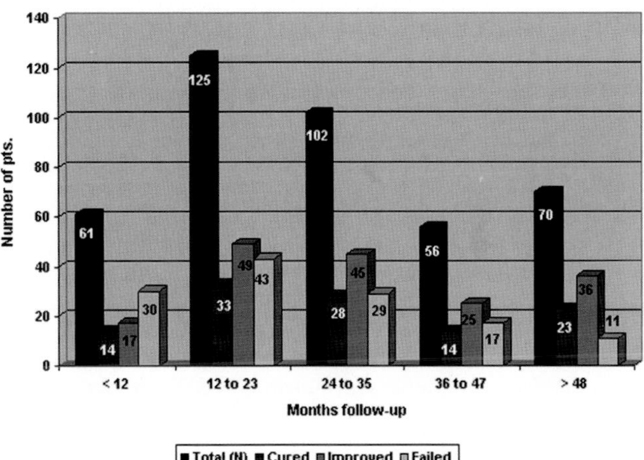

Figure 45-9 Time to failure after the cadaveric transvaginal sling (CaTS) procedure.

Table 45-2 Relation of Preoperative Variables to Failure of the Cadaveric Transvaginal Sling Procedure

			Failure Rate		
Preoperative Variable	**Present**	**Absent**	**Present**	**Absent**	**P Value**
Urinary urgency	197	133	54/197 (27%)	31/133 (23%)	.44
Urge incontinence	124	206	44/124 (35%)	41/206 (20%)	<.01
Leak point pressure <50 cm H_2O	84	246	24/84 (29%)	61/246 (25%)	.56
Detrusor overactivity	72	258	22/72 (31%)	63/258 (24%)	.29
Concurrent cystocele	232	98	52/232 (22%)	33/98 (34%)	.04
Prior anti-incontinence procedure	71	259	20/71 (28%)	65/259 (25%)	.65

managed conservatively with nonsteroidal medications. Wound separation occurred in 9 patients, but all eventually healed secondarily with conservative management. There have been no mortalities associated with the CaTS procedure.

CONCLUSION

Transvaginal slings are considered first-line treatment for SUI. The choice of nonfrozen CFL avoids the need to harvest the patient's own fascia intraoperatively and consequently reduces operative time, postoperative pain, and length of hospital stay. Whereas early results with the CaTS procedure were very encouraging and comparable to those obtained with other materials and techniques of placement, long-term results have been less durable, with failure rates approaching 30%. To improve continence results, we are currently exploring other materials and approaches for sling placement. The CaTS procedure remains an excellent option for patients who wish to avoid the use of synthetic materials. Familiarity with this technique is recommended as part of the armamentarium of a surgeon's transvaginal sling procedures.

References

1. Leach GE, Dmochowski RR, Appell RA, et al: Female stress urinary incontinence clinical guidelines panel summary report on surgical management of female stress urinary incontinence. J Urol 158:875-880, 1997.
2. Walsh IK, Nambirajan T, Donellan SM, et al: Cadaveric fascia lata pubovaginal slings: Early results on safety, efficacy and patient satisfaction. BJU Int 90:415-419, 2002.
3. Raz S, Erickson DR: SEAPI QNM incontinence classification system. Neurourol Urodyn 11:187-199, 1992.
4. McGuire EJ, Gormley EA: Abdominal fascial slings. In Raz S (ed): Female Urology. Philadelphia: WB Saunders, 1996.
5. Sirls LT, Leach GE: Use of fascia lata for pubovaginal sling. In Raz S (ed): Female Urology. Philadelphia: WB Saunders, 1996.
6. Crawford JS: Nature of fascia lata and its fate after transplantation. Am J Ophthalmol 67:900-907, 1969.
7. Jinnah RH, Johnson C, Warden K, Clarke HJ: A biochemical analysis of solvent-dehydrated and freeze dried human fascia lata allografts: A preliminary report. Am J Sports Med 20:607-612, 1992.
8. Eliot DS, Boone TB: Is fascia lata allograft material trustworthy for pubovaginal sling repair? Urology 56:772-776, 2000.
9. Carbone JM, Kavaler E, Raz S: Pubovaginal sling using cadaveric fascia and bone anchors: Disappointing early results. J Urol 165:1605-1611, 2001.
10. Fitzgerald MP, Mollenhauer J, Brubaker L: Failure of allograft suburethral slings. BJU 84:785-788, 1999.
11. Kobashi KC, Dmochowski R, Mee SL, et al: Erosion of woven polyester pubovaginal sling. J Urol 162:2070-2072, 1999.
12. Ducket JR, Constantine G: Complications of silicone sling insertion for stress urinary incontinence. J Urol 163:1835-1836, 2000.
13. Marshall VF, Marchetti AA, Krantz DE: The correction of stress incontinence by simple vesicourethral suspension. Surg Gynecol Obstet 88:509-513, 1949.
14. Leach GE: Bone fixation technique for transvaginal needle suspension. Urology 31:388-390, 1988.
15. Benderev T: Anchor fixation and other modifications of endoscopic bladder neck suspension. Urology 40:409-418, 1992.
16. Nativ O, Lavine S, Madjar S: Incisionless vaginal bone anchor cystourethropexy for the treatment of female stress urinary incontinence: Experience with the first 59 patients. J Urol 158:1742-1744, 1997.
17. Kohle N, Sze EHM, Roat TW: Incidence of recurrent cystocele after transvaginal needle suspension procedures with and without concurrent anterior colporrhaphy. Am J Obstet Gynecol 175:1476-1480, 1996.
18. Frederick RW, Carey JM, Leach GE: Osseous complications after transvaginal bone anchor fixation in female pelvic reconstructive surgery: Result from single largest prospective series and literature review. Urology 64:669-674, 2004.
19. Rackley RR, Abdelmalak JB, Madjar S: Bone anchor infections in pelvic reconstructive procedures: A literature review series and case reports. J Urol 165:1975-1978, 2001.
20. Kammerer-Doak DN, Cornella JL, Magrina JF: Osteitis pubis after Marshall-Marchetti-Krantz urethropexy: A pubic osteomyelitis. Am J Obstet Gynecol 179:586-590, 1998.
21. Carey JM, Chon JK, Leach GE: Urethrolysis with martius labial fat pad graft for iatrogenic bladder outlet obstruction. Urology 61:21-25, 1993.
22. Sutaria PM, Staskin DR: A comparison of fascial "pull-through" strength using four different suture fixation techniques [abstract]. J Urol 161:79, 1999.
23. Rueff S, Leach GE: Preoperative evaluation of multiple variables as predictors of outcome following cadaveric transvaginal sling. J Urol (in press).

Chapter 46

RADIOFREQUENCY TREATMENT FOR THE MANAGEMENT OF GENUINE STRESS URINARY INCONTINENCE

Emily E. Cole and Roger R. Dmochowski

Genuine stress incontinence (SUI) affects a substantial and increasing proportion of the female population.[1-4] It is well accepted that SUI is often associated with substantial quality-of-life disruption and desire on the part of the sufferer for improvement in or resolution of attendant symptomatic bother. A recent outcomes analysis suggested that women seeking therapy for genuine SUI would accept symptom improvement as an important and positive outcome aspect even if cure were not obtained.[5] The referral and usage trends for surgical interventions such as colposuspensions and suburethral slings suggest that, for women with less advanced symptoms, factors including patient fear or reluctance about surgical morbidity rates, recovery times, and other lifestyle concerns cause these procedures to be employed in a relatively small percentage of the overall affected population.[2,6,7] In addition, despite minimal invasiveness and positive safety profiles, nonsurgical modalities have in many cases been plagued with unfavorable compliance rates and chronic treatment requirements, as well as questionable effectiveness and durability.[8,9]

For the large population of less symptomatically bothered patients who desire treatment for their condition, the application of radiofrequency (RF) energy to the endopelvic fascia has been proposed as a new category of less invasive, first-line surgical intervention. In other disciplines, RF microremodeling has been shown to be well suited for the treatment of disorders characterized by the inappropriate passage of luminal contents through a dysfunctional anatomic and/or physiologic barrier, for example in fecal incontinence[10] and gastroesophageal reflux disease.[11] The RF energy procedure aims to treat genuine SUI by correcting the laxity and elasticity of the fascial "hammock"[12] supporting the urethra and bladder neck via thermally induced tissue shrinkage and contraction.[13] Specific heating of the endopelvic fascia denatures collagen fibers, causing acute contraction (shrinkage) of the treated tissue while also stimulating a fibrotic response.[14] In subsequent weeks, collagen in-growth and scar tissue formation further shrink and stabilize the endopelvic fascia, reducing its compliance to intra-abdominal pressure increases and stabilizing the position of the bladder neck.[15] This summary introduces the theoretical principles behind RF treatment of genuine SUI and reviews available literature describing approaches and results of currently available RF modalities.

THEORETICAL PRINCIPLES

The pathophysiology of genuine SUI is generally attributed to loss of passive support of the urethra due to tissue injury, stretching, or loss of stability, and/or lack of functioning neurologic control of the muscles of the pelvic floor and urethra.[12,16-18] Passive support weakness may provide inadequate support to the urethra, resulting in urethral hypermobility and poor urethral compression during stress events and periods of increased physical activity, leading to urine leakage.[19-21] A compounding effect of passive support failure is displacement of the urethra, which results in unequal distribution of sudden intra-abdominal pressure to the bladder and urethra, with the bladder pressure overcoming the pressure within the descended urethra, thereby further contributing to episodes of uncontrolled urine loss.

Developers of RF treatment hypothesized that if the collagen-rich endopelvic fascia in women with genuine SUI could be shrunk, and thus stabilized, through a direct application of controlled heat, these non-neurologic continence mechanisms could be positively affected and continence restored. It was envisioned that this could be accomplished via a minimally invasive approach with a very low associated risk of surgical complications.

ENERGY-TISSUE INTERACTIONS

The ability of heat to effect shrinkage of collagen-containing tissue is a function of several characteristics of the collagen molecule, which is triple-helical and fibrillar in structure. The intramolecular hydrogen bonds, or cross-links, that maintain the triple-helical configuration are thermally labile, whereas the intermolecular bonds that maintain the fibrillar structure are thermally stable. Heat in the range of 60°C to 80°C will disrupt the intramolecular cross-links, causing the helix to unwind, while the heat-stable fibrillar structure remains intact. This results in shrinkage on the longitudinal axis along with swelling of the fibrils.[13]

The clinical use of RF energy to achieve tissue shrinkage via collagen denaturation is well documented in the literature.[13,22-25] In this context, RF energy is applied to the tissue via direct contact with electrodes, and tissue heating occurs as the tissue resists the flow of the RF current. Heat conducts from high to low temperature regions in the tissue, creating a three-dimensional thermal effect. This thermal effect is specific to the amount of RF energy delivered, the tissue resistance, and the electrode configuration.

These concepts were modeled after studies demonstrating tissue shrinkage via RF energy. Hecht and colleagues described the use of monopolar RF energy to treat bovine joint capsular tissue in vivo.[13] They found that the application of RF energy was followed by tissue reaction and concomitant degradation of collagen with the ensuing build-up of new collagen over a 12-week period, resulting in remodeling of the joint capsular tissue. The primary treatment effect was heat-induced tissue shrinkage associated with the denaturation of collagen; maximal shrinkage occurred at temperatures ranging from 60°C to 80°C. Post-treatment histologic evaluation revealed that thermal effects were localized to the region of RF energy application. Subsequent evaluations showed a tissue healing response characterized by fibroblast and capillary proliferation that ultimately resulted in complete tissue healing at 12 weeks. Chen and associates performed a series of experiments on fresh bovine heart tendons.[26] The tissue was mounted in a tension-free holder, and the amount of shrinkage was measured as a function of time and temperature. The study showed that maximal tissue shrinkage occurred only if the thermal treatment time and temperature exceeded a certain threshold. Notably, a temperature of 70°C effected near-maximal shrinkage when applied for a minimum of 30 seconds. Temperatures lower than 70°C demonstrated significantly diminished capacity for effective shrinkage regardless of the duration of the heat application. This information was used to develop an RF energy treatment algorithm for shrinking the endopelvic fascia to restore continence in women with genuine SUI.

TREATMENT METHODOLOGY

Based on the theoretical and experimental information described, a commercially available RF bladder neck suspension procedure was developed. The SURx Transvaginal System (SURx System, CooperSurigcal, Inc. Trumbull, CT) is composed of a small bipolar RF generator and a sterile, single-use applicator that allows application of RF energy to the tissue. The applicator has a handle, a trigger, and a 270-degree rotational tip with microbipolar electrodes and a saline drip at the distal end of the probe. Additionally, there is a thermistor located between the electrodes for accurate monitoring of treatment tissue temperatures.

The specific treatment area for the RF procedure is an area of the endopelvic fascia located at least 1 cm lateral to the mid-urethra on each side. The targeted treatment area can be assessed laparoscopically or transvaginally, with both approaches facilitating treatment of the same tissue (on the superior or inferior surface, respectively).

All patients should be carefully screened preoperatively with a comprehensive history and physical examination, voiding diary, and urodynamics if possible. Patients should demonstrate objective SUI and should have evidence of urethral hypermobility on physical examination. Most transvaginal RF procedures can be performed in an outpatient setting with general or regional anesthesia.

The patient is placed in the dorsal lithotomy position, a Foley catheter is placed, the bladder is actively emptied, and the balloon is inflated. Hydrodissection of the vaginal wall is recommended, using an appropriate dilute vasoconstrictive solution (20 U vasopressin in 50 mL injectable saline or epinephrine at a 1:200,000 dilution in injectable saline) to minimize excess bleeding. A 2- to 3-cm incision is made 1 cm lateral to the urethra centered at the level of the mid-urethra. This incision is carried through the full thickness of the vaginal mucosa, and further dissection is performed to expose a 1.5 × 2 cm area of the inferior aspect of the endopelvic fascia. Care must be taken not to disrupt the underlying fascial layer. It is recommended that the treatment area be kept as dry as possible with continuous suction, because this may affect eventual outcomes.

After dissection, the tip of the applicator is applied to the underlying endopelvic fascia with enough pressure to cause deflection of the tissue. The SURx RF system is used to deliver a minimum of 70°C to the target tissue for a minimum of 30 seconds to achieve the desired shrinkage and associated therapeutic effect. The system uses low-power (15 W) bipolar RF energy to produce a volume of treated tissue meeting the 70/30 criteria (≥70°C for at least 30 seconds) for effecting shrinkage, as described by Chen and associates.[26] The RF energy is activated, and application of RF energy is accomplished by drawing the RF device tip over the fascia in a slow, sweeping manner along the longitudinal axis, making sure that both tines of the applicator tip are equally in contact with the tissue until all exposed endopelvic fascia has been treated. Care must be taken to remain 1 cm lateral to the urethra at all times during the procedure. Treatment of one side should be concluded based on aural feedback from the RF generator indicating that adequate thermal effect has been imparted to the underlying tissue on the basis of changes in recorded treatment impedance. Thermal effect within the tissue can be confirmed by visualizing blanching and shrinkage. The procedure is then repeated on the contralateral side.

After delivery of the RF energy, the incisions are irrigated and closed, and the Foley catheter may be removed. The patient is transferred to the recovery suite until the anesthesia effects are no longer present and spontaneous voiding has occurred (usually 2 to 4 hours). Based on clinical judgment, patients may be discharged home on the day of treatment.

The technique for the laparoscopic approach is similar. Laparoscopic ports should be placed according to surgeon preference to facilitate access to the pelvis. A combination of blunt and sharp dissection may be used to expose the endopelvic fascia. Treatment can be delivered to the superior aspect of the endopelvic fascia in a manner similar to that described for the transvaginal approach. Care should be taken to remain 1 cm lateral to the urethra, which can be confirmed by locating the Foley catheter so that it traverses the urethra and bladder neck. Treatment is typically applied to the fascia from this point at approximately the level of the mid-urethra to the beginning of the arcus tendineous.

RESULTS

Initially, two prospective investigational device exemption (IDE)-approved clinical trials were conducted to demonstrate the safety and comment on the efficacy of the RF procedure.[27,28] A total of 214 patients with genuine SUI were enrolled at 16 U.S. study sites; 94 (44%) underwent a laparoscopic approach, and 120 (56%) underwent the transvaginal approach. Once access to the endopelvic fascia was gained, treatment was carried out bilaterally as previously described. Clinical efficacy at 12-month follow-up was assessed for both groups. Diagnosis of genuine SUI was based on patient history and objective demonstration of leakage during physical examination. All women had urethral hypermobility as determined by an abnormal cotton swab test (>30 degrees). Detrusor overactivity was excluded by cystometry. Patients who were taking antidepressants or α-adrenergic or anticholinergic medications, as well as those with grade III or IV anterior prolapse or other vaginal support defects, were excluded from analysis. Patients included in the study had had previous unsuccessful outcomes after at least 3 months of conservative, noninvasive therapies such as Kegel exercises or electrical stimu-

Table 46-1 Clinical Efficacy of Radiofrequency Treatment

	Laparoscopic Group			*Transvaginal Group*		
Parameter	**Baseline**	**1 Year**	**Long-term**	**Baseline**	**1 Year**	**Long-term**
No. patients	94	85	61	120	96	73
Negative Valsalva test	0%	79%	71%	0%	76%	66%
Patient quality-of-life assessment	%	88%	79%	%	74%	73%
Patient uses ≤1 pad per day	%	85%	60%	%	72%	58%

Table 46-2 Summary of Reported Complications (% of Patients) after Radiofrequency Treatment

Complication	Laparoscopic Group	Transvaginal Group
Bladder	2	0
Cardiovascular	0	0
Pulmonary	0	0
Additional surgery	0	0
Transfusion	0	0
Retention >4 wk	0	0
Urinary tract infection	2	0
Sexual dysfunction	0	0
Postoperative urgency	1	1

lation of the pelvic floor. No patient was receiving any active incontinence therapy. Cure was described as a negative Valsalva test on physical examination and improvement was defined as decreased daily episodes or pad use. Results are shown in Table 46-1. There were no reported device-related events during the study time, and an excellent safety profile was demonstrated (Table 46-2). On further data assessment, two treatment parameters emerged that had a significant impact on procedure efficacy: the relative dryness of the surgical field (excessive fluid in the surgical field was noted to cause energy dissipation and resultant superficial, insufficient treatment) and the continuity of thermal delivery to the treatment area (numerous intermittent energy applications as a result of multiple "on/off" cycles resulted in inadequate thermal effect in the targeted tissues).

Additional follow-up of the original patient cohort was undertaken using the same measurement criteria. The average long-term follow-up was 38 ± 3.51 months in the laparoscopic group and 30 ± 3.29 months in the transvaginal group. An actuarial survival analysis of objective and subjective outcomes from the 6-month evaluation out to 30 ± 3.3 months is shown in Figure 46-1.[29]

FUTURE DIRECTIONS

Recently, the RF concept has been explored further, and a transurethral modality for the delivery of RF energy has been described. Appell and coworkers described a system introduced by Novasys (Novasys Medical, Inc., Newark, CA) that consists of a 21-Fr transurethral RF microremodeling probe connected to an RF generator.[30] An intravenous line carrying sterile, room-temperature water is routed through a pump on the RF generator to the probe, providing irrigation to the mucosa overlying the submucosal treatment sites during RF delivery. The system is monopolar, and a standard return electrode ("grounding pad") is placed on the patient and connected to the RF generator.

Cystoscopic visualization is not required. After transurethral passage into the bladder lumen, a balloon on the probe tip is insufflated and then palpably anchored within the bladder outlet, identical to positioning a Foley catheter. Four 23-gauge needle electrodes are simultaneously deployed, and the needletips are advanced through the mucosa and into the submucosa (Fig. 46-2). RF is delivered to the four needles for 60 seconds, micro-remodeling four submucosal tissue targets. A series of rotational maneuvers between periods of RF delivery should place the four needles in nine different positions (for a total of 9 minutes of RF delivery). This treatment resulted in the microremodeling of 36 microscopic, submucosal, circumferential targets ranging from the bladder neck cranially, to the middle aspect of the proximal urethra caudally.[30]

This pilot study randomized 110 women to an RF treatment group and 63 to a sham treatment group. Improvement of 10 points or greater on the Incontinence Quality of Life (I-QOL) score—a magnitude of improvement with a demonstrated responsiveness to patient satisfaction with treatment and to 25% or greater reduction in both incontinence episode frequency and stress pad weight—served as a subjective outcome measurement. Change in mean leak point pressure (LPP) served as an objective outcome measurement. Adverse events were recorded for each group. The 12-month RF safety profile was identical to that of the sham group (Table 46-3). Seventy-four percent of the patients with moderate to severe genuine SUI experienced at least 10 points of I-QOL score improvement after RF remodeling, compared with 50% of those who underwent sham treatment (P = .03). Twenty-two percent of women with mild genuine SUI who received RF treatment reported improvement, compared with 35% of those who received sham treatment (P = .2). Women who underwent RF treatment demonstrated an increase in mean LPP at 12 months (13.2 ±39.2 cm H_2O), whereas women in the sham treatment group demonstrated a reduction in mean LPP at 12 months (−2.0 ± 33.8 cm H_2O) (P = .02).[30]

SUMMARY

Tissue responses induced by RF thermal energy are well described and reproducible.[12,13] Acute effects include denaturation of collagen fibers, which results in loss of collagen fibril integrity. At 1 week, a more generalized granulation response is seen, and by 21 days after treatment, fibroplasia and fibrosis response are predominant. By 6 weeks after treatment, the expected fibrotic healing response continues to progress, and inflammatory cellu-

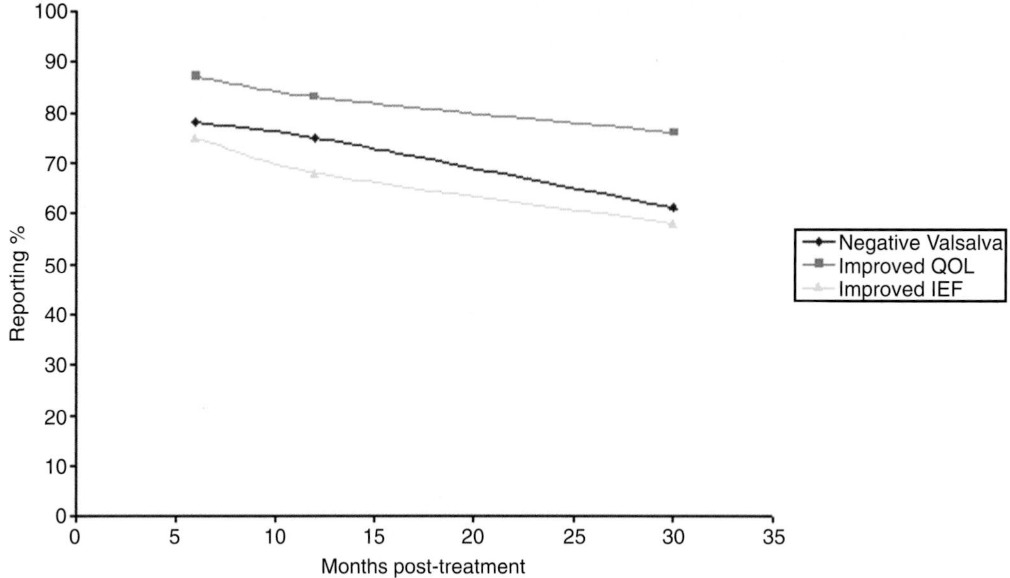

Figure 46-1 Actuarial survival analysis of objective and subjective outcome measures. IEF, Incontinence episode frequency; QOL, quality of life.

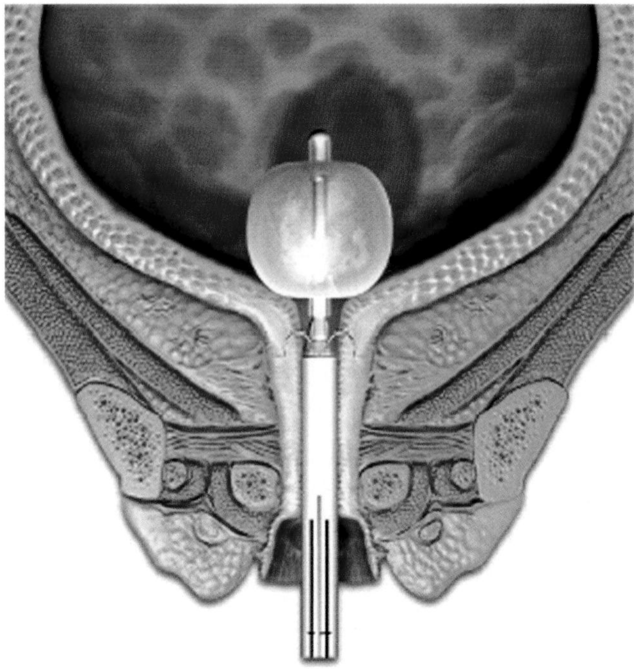

Figure 46-2 Novasys® radio frequency device position at bladder neck with RF probes deployed into urethra. Transurethral approach.

lar components are minimal.[15] The final histologic result is fibrotic tissue that replaces the elastic endopelvic fascia. This process shortens, stiffens, and thickens the fascia, increasing support of the bladder neck, and changes the collagen structure of the tissue. RF thermal tissue treatment has been used in dermatology, in orthopedics, and for treatment of varicose veins.[28] The contractile response to RF energy has also been applied to the treatment of tissue within joints to shorten and strengthen tendineous ligamentous attachments.[27]

The endopelvic fascia may demonstrate loss of integrity that usually is caused by pregnancy and childbirth.[31,32] However, other women, such as athletes, can also suffer from genuine SUI.[33] Loss of integrity of the pelvic floor is manifested by bladder descensus with resultant urethral hypermobility during stress events, such as coughing or other activities that increase abdominal pressures. Accepted treatments that stabilize the bladder neck include retropubic suspension and pubovaginal sling; however, these procedures are associated with known complication risks. Early studies indicate that the RF procedure offers a safe and effective means to impart shrinkage of the endopelvic fascia, replacing elastic tissue with inelastic tissue. This shrinkage decreases the elasticity of the endopelvic fascia and stabilizes the proximal urethra and bladder neck, recapitulating the suburethral tissue used as a backboard for urethral closure.

The need to balance procedure "tolerability" issues with expectations for objectively measured efficacy has been explored and validated in recent discourse[31-33] and has parti cular applicability when addressing the population with mild to moderate SUI. For this large patient group, the risks and considerations associated with more invasive procedures may be viewed differently than they would by those with a more advanced disease state. Issues such as the need for a Foley catheter or self-catheterization postoperatively, even for a brief time after surgery, become salient for the patient who is considering treatment for mild to moderate SUI. Likewise, most of these patients may be unwilling to assume the restrictions on future pregnancy that are inherent to sling and suspension procedures. Heightened sensitivity to the risks of viral or prion transmission with the use of biomaterials may also more significantly influence patient preference in cases of mild to moderate SUI.

Several aspects of the RF thermal energy approach may not be explicitly apparent to the patient but may contribute to the overall favorable risk profile of the procedure and warrant consideration by the physician. The shallow incision and dissection used in this procedure provides a therapeutic option for genuine SUI that does not involve the blind passage of needle or trocar devices, thereby minimizing the potential for injury to the bladder, bowel, and major vessels. Further, the use of thermally induced shrinkage to tighten the periurethral tissue inherently avoids the use of implanted materials to provide structural

Table 46-3 12-Month Adverse Event Profile for Transurethral Approach*

Adverse Event	Treatment Arm (*N* = 110) (%)	Sham Treatment Arm (*N* = 63) (%)	P Value
Dysuria	10 (9.1)	1 (1.6)	.06
Hematuria	1 (0.9)	0 (0)	1.0
Urinary retention	1 (0.9)	0 (0)	1.0
Urinary tract infection	5 (4.5)	3 (4.8)	1.0
Hesitancy	0 (0)	1 (1.6)	.4
Asymptomatic detrusor overactivity	2 (1.8)	4 (6.3)	.2
Dry overactive bladder	8 (7.3)	2 (3.2)	.3
Wet overactive bladder	11 (10.0)	6 (9.5)	1.0

*Figures indicate number and percentage of patients in each group.
From Appell RA, Juma S, Wells WG, et al: Transurethral radiofrequency energy collagen micro-remodeling for the treatment of female stress urinary incontinence. Neurourol Urodyn 25:331-336, 2006.

support, thereby eliminating the concerns of proper sling placement and the potential for foreign material erosion in the near or long term.

More comprehensive studies with longer-term follow-up are needed to determine the true efficacy of this relatively new treatment modality; however, the RF tissue shrinkage procedure provides a compelling risk-to-benefit profile that is of particular relevance to physicians treating mild to moderate genuine SUI. The avoidance of permanently implanted foreign materials and the corresponding positive impact on procedure morbidity and patient lifestyle distinguish it as a uniquely conservative first-line surgical intervention for this patient group.

References

1. Hannestad YS, Rortveit G, Sandvik H, et al: A community based epidemiological survey of female urinary incontinence: The Norwegian EPINCONT study. J Clin Epidemiol 53:1150-1157, 2000.
2. Luber KM: The definition, prevalence, and risk factors for stress urinary incontinence. Rev Urol 6(Suppl 3):S3-S9, 2004.
3. Luber KM, Boero S, Choe JY: The demographics of pelvic floor disorders: Current observations and future projections. Am J Obstet Gynecol 184:1496-1501, 2001.
4. Hampel C, Weinhold N, Eggersmann C, et al: Definition of overactive bladder and epidemiology of urinary incontinence. Urology 50(Suppl 6A):4-14, 1997.
5. Elkadry EA, Kenton KS, Fitzgerald MP, et al: Patient selected goals: A new perspective on surgical outcome. Am J Obstet Gynecol 189:1551-1558, 2003.
6. Kinchen KS, Burgio K, Diokno AC, et al: Factors associated with women's decisions to seek treatment for urinary incontinence. J Women's Health 12:687-698, 2003.
7. Norton PA, MacDonald LD, Sedgwick PM, et al: Distress and delay associated with urinary incontinence, frequency, and urgency in women. BMJ 297:1187-1189, 1988.
8. Cammu H, Van Nylen M, Amy JJ: A 10-year follow-up after Kegel pelvic floor muscle exercises for genuine stress incontinence. BJU Int 85:655-658, 2000.
9. Goode PS, Burgio KL, Locher JL, et al: Effect of behavioral training with or without pelvic floor electrical stimulation on stress incontinence in women: A randomized controlled trial. JAMA 290:345-352, 2003.
10. Takahashi T, Garcia-Osogobio S, Valdovinos MA, et al: Extended two-year results of radio-frequency energy delivery for the treatment of fecal incontinence (the Secca procedure). Dis Colon Rectum 46:711-715, 2003.
11. Fanelli RD, Gersin KS, Bakhsh A: The Stretta procedure: Effective endoluminal therapy for GERD. Surg Technol Int 11:129-134, 2003.
12. DeLancey JO: Structural support of the urethra as it relates to stress urinary incontinence: The hammock hypothesis. Am J Obstet Gynecol 170:1713-1720, 1994.
13. Hecht P, Hayashi K, Lu Y, et al: Monopolar radiofrequency energy effects on joint capsular tissue: Potential treatment for joint instability. An in-vivo mechanical, morphological, and biochemical study using an ovine model. Am J Sports Med 27:761-771, 1999.
14. Galen DL: Histologic results of a new treatment for stress urinary incontinence without implantable materials. Obstet Gynecol 95:530-533, 2000.
15. Fulmer BR, Sakamoto K, Turk TM, et al: Acute and long-term outcomes of RF BNS. J Urol 167:141-144, 2002.
16. Smith A, Hosker GL Warrell DW: The role of partial denervation of the pelvic floor in the aetiology of genito-urinary prolapse and stress incontinence of urine: A neurophysical study. Br J Obstet Gynaecol 96:24-28, 1989.
17. Allen R, Hosker GL, Smith AR, et al: Pelvic floor damage and childbirth: A neurophysiologic study. Br J Obstet Gynaecol 97:770-779, 1990.
18. Keane DP, Sims TJ, Abrams P, et al: Analysis of collagen status in premenopausal nulliparous women with genuine stress incontinence. Br J Obstet Gynaecol 104:994-998,1997.
19. Norton P: Pelvic floor disorders: The role of fascia and ligaments. Clin Obstet Gynecol 36:929-939, 1993.
20. Aronson M, Bates SM, Jacoby AF, et al: Periurethral and paravaginal anatomy: An endovaginal magnetic resonance imaging study. Am J Obstet Gynecol 173:1702-1710, 1995.
21. Richardson A: Cystocele: Paravaginal repair. In Benson J (ed): Female Pelvic Floor Disorders. New York, Norton Medical Books, 1992, p 280.
22. Osmond C, Hecht P, Hayashi K, et al: Comparative effects of laser and radio frequency energy on joint capsule. Clin Orthop 286:299, 2000.
23. Hecht P, Hayashi K, Cooley AJ, et al: The thermal effect of monopolar radio frequency energy on the properties of joint capsule: An in-vivo histologic study using a sheep model. Am J Sports Med 26:808, 1998.
24. Lopez MJ, Hayashi K, Fanton GS, et al: The effect of radio frequency energy on the ultrastructure of joint capsular collagen. Arthroscopy 14:495, 1998.
25. Allain JC, Le Lous M, Cohen S, et al: Isometric tensions developed during the hydrothermal swelling of rat skin. Connect Tissue Res 7:127-132, 1980.
26. Chen SS, Wright NT, Humphrey JD: Heat-induced changes in the mechanics of a collagenous tissue: Isothermal free shrinkage. J Biomech Eng 119:372-378, 1997.

27. Dmochowski RR, Avon M, Ross J, et al: Transvaginal radio frequency treatment of the endopelvic fascia: A prospective evaluation for the treatment of genuine stress urinary incontinence. J Urol 169:1028-1032, 2003.
28. Ross J, Galen D, Abbott K, et al: A prospective multisite study of radiofrequency bipolar energy for treatment of genuine stress incontinence. J Am Assoc Gynecol Laparosc 9:493-499, 2002.
29. Dmochowski RR, Ross JW, Levy BS, et al. (Unpublished data, 2005). Three-year cure and improvement rates of a transvaginal radio frequency procedure for genuine stress incontinence.
30. Appell RA, Juma S, Wells WG, et al. (Unpublished data, 2005). Transurethral radiofrequency energy collagen micro-remodeling for the treatment of female stress urinary incontinence.
31. Tincello DG, Alfirevic Z: Important clinical outcomes in urogynecology: Views of patients, nurses and medical staff. Int Urogynecol J Pelvic Floor Dysfunct 13:96-98, 2002.
32. Hullfish KL, Bovbjerg VE, Gibson J, et al: Patient-centered goals for pelvic floor dysfunction surgery: What is success, and is it achieved? Am J Obstet Gynecol 187:88-92, 2002.
33. Robinson D, Anders K, Cardozo L, et al: What women want: Their interpretation of the concept of cure. Neurourol Urodyn 21:429-430, 2002.

Chapter 47

SURGERY FOR REFRACTORY URINARY INCONTINENCE: SPIRAL SLING

Arthur Mourtzinos, M. Grey Maher, Shlomo Raz, and Larissa V. Rodríguez

Treatment of stress urinary incontinence (SUI) caused by urethral hypermobility or intrinsic sphincter deficiency with urethral sling procedures may yield success rates of up to 80% to 90%, depending on the definition of success.[1-5] In a minority of patients, however, there is persistence or worse incontinence after surgical therapy. Female patients with urethral incompetence and severe incontinence due to multiple failed surgeries, neurologic injury, or congenital anomalies represent a unique surgical challenge. Patients with neurologic conditions may have sacral arc lesions with paralysis of the skeletal musculature and an open urethra. Other patients who have failed multiple sling and anti-incontinence procedures may have severe symptoms of SUI and an open urethra with a low Valsalva leak point pressure (VLPP). These patients often have an incompetent, difficult to compress urethra, most likely resulting from a combination of urethral denervation and violation of the periurethral fascia, as well as their underlying risk factors for SUI.[6] These patients have low chances of cure after repeat anti-incontinence surgery, and they are more likely to suffer from complications including retention.[7] In this patient population, a routine sling procedure providing only posterior support will not typically yield an appropriate response. Management options include placement of a "tight" pubovaginal sling, with the intent of putting the patient in urinary retention, or constructing an artificial urinary sphincter (AUS). Many of these patients are often forced to undergo bladder neck closure with continent catheterizable augmentation.

This chapter describes a transvaginal sling procedure in adult women that encircles the urethra, providing circumferential coaptation. The spiral sling is a salvage procedure for a small, yet severely affected group of female patients with a totally incompetent urethra. The procedure was initially described in patients with congenital or neurologic diseases.[8] It has more recently been described in patients with multiple failed surgeries for SUI.[9] In our experience, it provides better outcomes and fewer complications than the AUS.

In addition, we discuss the AUS as a treatment option for the female patient with urinary incontinence. The AUS is an effective alternative to the urethral sling for the treatment of urinary incontinence caused by primary urethral sphincter insufficiency (type III SUI).[10] The AUS is a synthetic device that includes an internal cuff made of silicone rubber with Dacron reinforcement and is designed to provide a uniform circumferential compression on the urethra. Continence or cuff inflation is maintained by continuous pressure in the cuff, which is modulated by the pressure balloon, which in turn is usually positioned in the prevesical space. The patient manipulates a labially placed pump to open the cuff before voiding. The American Medical System (Minnetonka, MN) AS-800 is the currently used model; it may be implanted via a transvaginal,[10,11] transabdominal,[12] or laparoscopic transperitoneal approach.[13] In this chapter, we limit our discussion to the transvaginal approach.

EVALUATION OF THE PATIENT

The preoperative evaluation should include a standard history and physical examination, radiographic evaluation, and videourodynamic studies. Multiple prior anti-incontinence operations, radical pelvic surgeries, orthopedic conditions, or neurologic disorders (myelomeningocele, sacral cord tumor, or peripheral neuropathy) are important historical data. A thorough neurologic examination of the lower extremities and perineum may elucidate abnormal sensory and motor responses in the lower lumbar and sacral cord segments. A formal pelvic examination may reveal evidence of a urethral diverticulum, abscess, or mesh erosion in patients with a history of an anti-incontinence or vaginal prolapse procedures.

Complex videourodynamic study and cystourethroscopy should be performed to rule out any definitive evidence of voiding dysfunction, detrusor overactivity, intrinsic sphincter deficiency, or abnormal urethral and bladder pathology. Radiographic evaluation may include a standing voiding cystourethrogram with resting and straining views. In many tertiary centers, videourodynamic testing is done with the patient in the sitting position. Cystourethroscopy can also assess bladder trabeculation and rule out the presence of any urethral pathology.

The patient's clinical history of incontinence is important in the overall assessment; these patients typically have incontinence of nonresistance due to an incompetent urethra. When selecting patients for surgery, we do not rely solely on a low VLPP. A patient with clinically significant incontinence (incontinence of nonresistance) may not always have a low VLPP.

THE SPIRAL SLING

Surgical Technique

A 1 × 15 cm, thinly woven polypropylene (Ethicon, Inc., Somerville, NJ) mesh is prepared, and a 1-0 polyglactin suture is applied at each end. The patient is positioned and prepared in a similar manner as for the AUS (described later). A 16-Fr Foley catheter is inserted per urethra, and the bladder is emptied. A weighted speculum is then placed into the vagina for exposure.

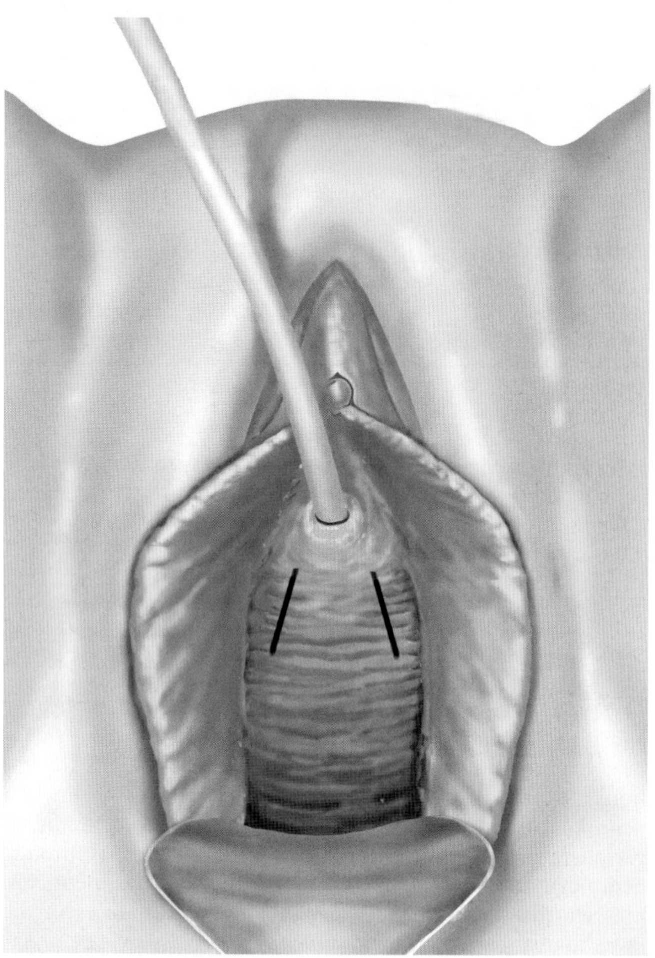

Figure 47-1 Two oblique lateral incisions are made in the anterior vaginal wall.

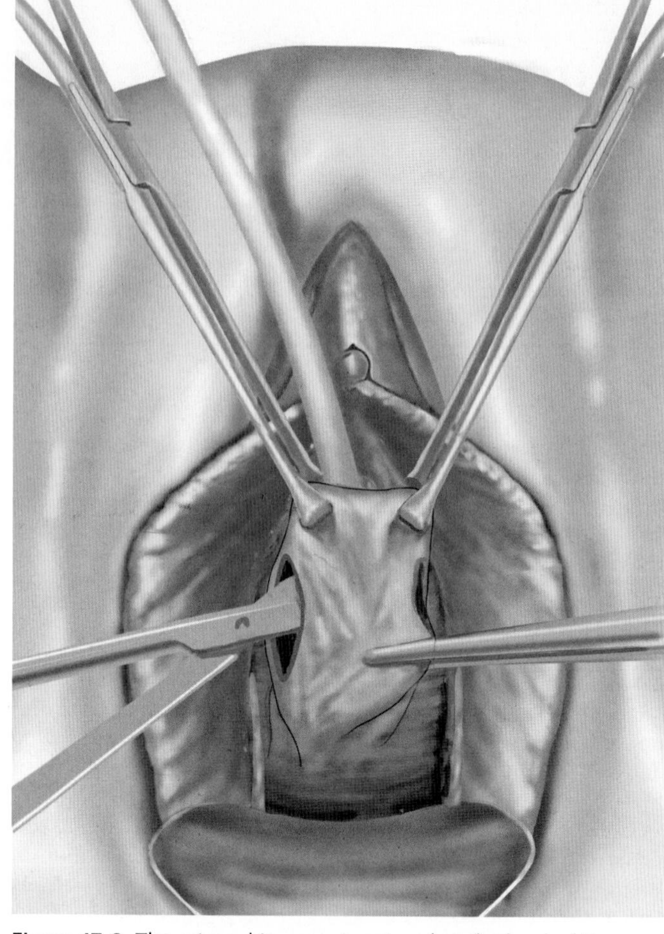

Figure 47-2 The retropubic space is entered at the level of the mid-urethra to distal urethra using curved scissors.

An Allis clamp is used to grasp the anterior vaginal wall just proximal to the meatus. Two parallel distal oblique incisions are made in the anterior vaginal wall (Fig. 47-1). One additional Allis clamp is placed at the distal portion of each of the oblique incisions to aid in the exposure. The dissection is carried out laterally, over the glistening periurethral fascia, toward the ipsilateral shoulder. The retropubic space is entered, and a complete urethrolysis is performed by detaching the urethropelvic ligaments from the arcus tendineous fascia pelvis and freeing all retropubic adhesions (Fig. 47-2). The urethral dissection is started in the midurethral area just proximal to the pubourethral ligaments and carried proximally to free the rest of the urethra and the bladder neck. The dissection is maintained close to the periosteum of the pubic bone to avoid injuries to the dorsal venous complex, bladder, and urethra. The dorsal aspect of the urethra is freed from the pubis. A suburethral tunnel is created in the anterior vaginal wall, 1.5 cm from the urethral meatus, with a fine, right angle clamp connecting the two oblique incisions (Fig. 47-3A).

A Derra clamp is used to pass the 1 × 15 cm soft polypropylene mesh dorsally, between the urethra and the pubis. The ends of the mesh are crossed ventrally through the previously made vaginal tunnel with a right angle clamp. This maneuver creates a complete circle of mesh around the urethra. A suprapubic puncture is made just above the symphysis. A double-pronged needle (Cook Urological, Inc., Spencer, IN) is passed under finger control through the fascia and retropubic space to the level of the oblique vaginal incision. The previously placed 1-0 polyglactin sutures from the polypropylene mesh are transferred to the suprapubic incision. This is repeated on the contralateral side. Cystoscopy is performed to rule out bladder or urethral perforation.

To ensure securing of the sling under no tension, one Allis clamp is placed through each vaginal incision to firmly hold the sling in place in a horizontal plane while the assistant ties the sutures suprapubically under no tension. The suture knots are located approximately 3 to 4 mm below the skin. The retropubic space is irrigated with Betadine solution. The vaginal incisions are closed with 3-0 polyglactin sutures. The suprapubic incision is closed with a 4-0 polyglactin subcuticular stitch. A vaginal pack and suprapubic dressing are applied. Drainage of the bladder is accomplished with either a suprapubic catheter, a urethral catheter, or clean intermittent catheterization taught to the patient preoperatively.

Postoperatively, the vaginal pack is removed in the recovery room approximately 2 hours after completion of the procedure. Patients can be sent home on the day of the procedure if they are tolerating oral intake and their pain is under adequate control, or they may be admitted for 24-hour observation. Patients with a urethral catheter may be instructed to return to the office for a

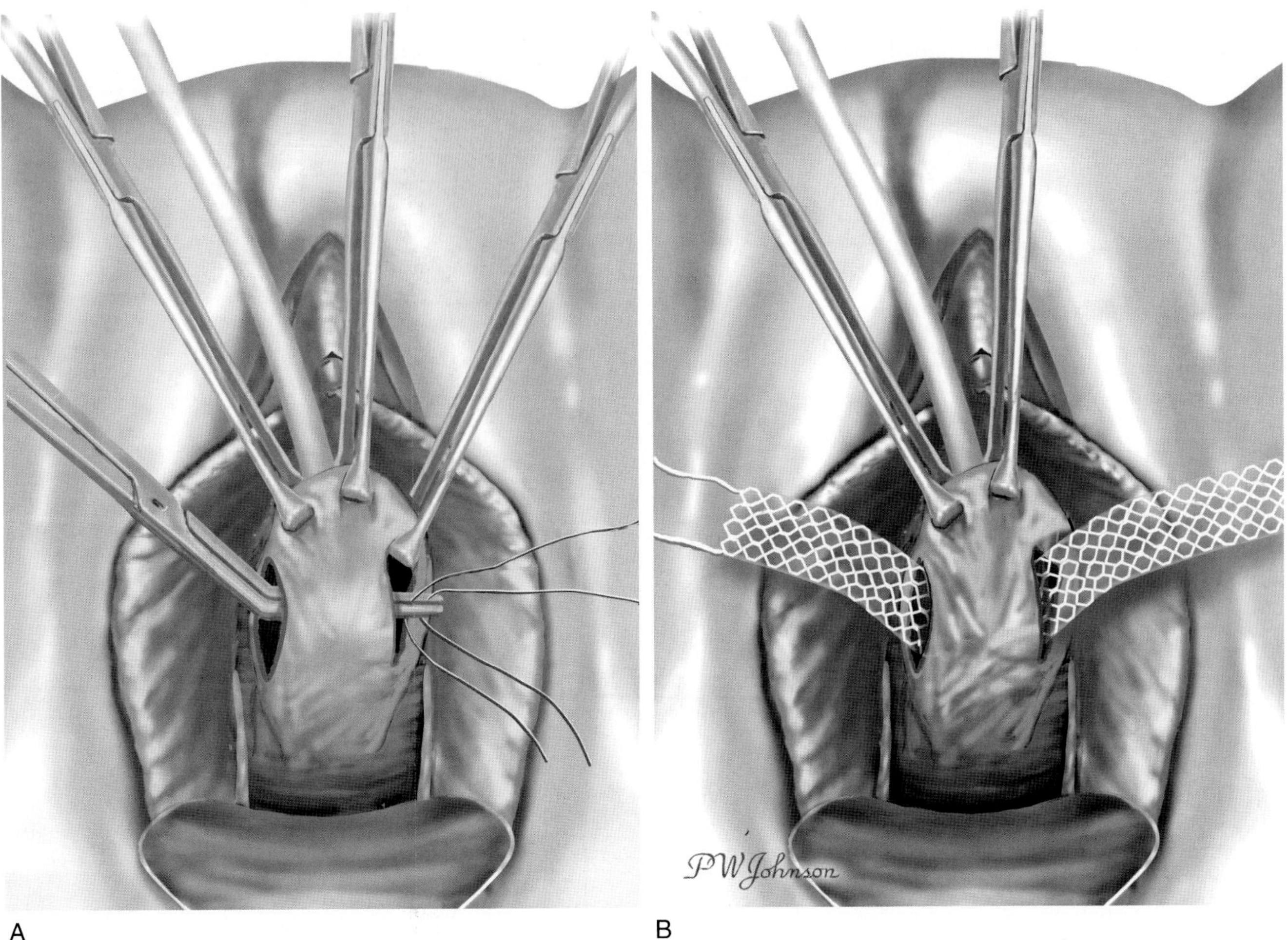

Figure 47-3 The mesh is transferred under the previously created tunnel.

voiding trial in 5 to 7 days. In those with a suprapubic tube, the catheter is capped and the patient is instructed to void every 3 hours and record the postvoid residual volume. The suprapubic tube is left in place for at least 1 week and is removed once post-void residuals are less than 50 mL. The patients are discharged home with empiric antibiotic coverage for 5 days.

Discussion

Between August 1999 and February 2006, 93 patients underwent placement of a spiral sling.[8] Patients with congenital or neurologic diseases were initially the candidates for this procedure. Since March 2002, however, the technique was expanded to include those patients with multiple failed surgeries for SUI and an incompetent "lead pipe" urethra. The initial results of the spiral sling procedure in 47 patients with congenital and neurologic anomalies were recently reported in the literature.[8] Of the 47 patients, 7 were lost to follow-up. The mean age of the remaining 40 patients was 59.0 years (range, 23 to 86 years). This represented a complex cohort of patients, with 98% having failed a prior anti-incontinence surgery. The patients had undergone a mean of 2.6 previous anti-incontinence surgeries and used an average of 6 pads per day. There were two patients who had previous augmentation cystoplasty and were performing intermittent self-catheterization but had significant SUI between catheterizations. All patients were considered candidates for urethral closure and continent diversion as a salvage procedure.[8]

In this group of 40 patients, the average follow-up was 12 months (range, 6 to 37 months). There were no intraoperative complications. The de novo urge incontinence rate was 7.4%. Of the 27 patients with preoperative urge incontinence, 9 (33%) had resolution of their symptoms with the procedure. One of the patients had persistent refractory urge urinary incontinence and subsequently underwent a sacral neuromodulation procedure. No patient experienced de novo retention after the spiral sling. The four patients who were performing intermittent self-catheterization preoperatively continued to do so after the procedure. There were no urethral or vaginal erosions. Overall, three patients underwent eventual bladder neck closure and continent augmentation and were considered failures.[8]

Patients were evaluated with self-assessment questionnaires. Questionnaires consisted of a validated short form of the Urogenital Distress Inventory (UDI-6), a standardized symptom questionnaire that assessed the presence or absence and frequency of symptoms, and a urinary symptom-specific global quality of life (QOL) questionnaire validated for the evaluation of patients with benign prostatic hyperplasia.[4,14] Forty patients were included in the analysis with a minimum of 6 months follow-up; 65% reported never having symptoms of SUI, and 87% reported symptoms of SUI never or less than once per week.

On the UDI-6 questionnaire, 68% reported never being bothered by symptoms of SUI, and 95% reported never or rarely being bothered by SUI. The mean number of pads decreased from 6.0 preoperatively to 0.9 postoperatively ($P < .005$). Seventy-eight percent of patients reported greater than 90% improvement. Overall, patients reported a mean improvement in symptoms of 87% after surgery (on a scale of zero to 100%).[8]

The technique was recently described in 46 non-neurogenic patients with multiple failed surgeries for SUI.[9] The mean age of the study population was 62 years, and the mean follow-up was 15 months (range, 6 to 45 months). All patients had failed a prior anti-incontinence surgery. There were no intraoperative complications, and, postoperatively, there were no cases of permanent urinary retention requiring transvaginal urethrolysis. On patient-driven subjective assessment, 49% of patients reported never experiencing SUI, and 72% experienced no or rare episodes of SUI. Overall, patients reported a mean improvement of 84%, with a decrease in daily pad use from 5.5 to 1.0. In addition, there was no statistically significant difference between preoperative and postoperative symptoms of incomplete bladder emptying ($P > .05$).

A review of the literature for alternatives to bladder neck closure revealed no existing circumferential sling procedure in the adult population. Mingin and colleagues described a transabdominal technique of a urethral sling using rectus muscle wrapped around the urethra for pediatric patients with congenital urethral incompetence.[15] Of the 37 patients reported, 92% remained dry between catheterizations. The pediatric population is unlike our target population, because these adult patients had undergone approximately three anti-incontinence surgeries with subsequent scarring and more difficult coaptation. The mechanism of cure of the transvaginal spiral sling is not completely understood. It most likely supports the midurethral segment while preventing urethral descent and improving pressure transmission to the urethra. In addition, unlike a routine sling procedure, the spiral sling also provides circumferential coaptation to the urethra at the time of increased intra-abdominal pressures.

ARTIFICIAL URINARY SPHINCTER: TRANSVAGINAL APPROACH

The AUS is no longer commonly performed worldwide for SUI in the female population. The need for multiple revisions, the short length of the female urethra as compared to that of the male, and the difficulty encountered in placing an AUS in patients with multiple prior operations has limited its use. In this section, we discuss the transvaginal insertion technique and surgical outcomes.

Surgical Technique

The AUS is composed of three parts: the inflatable cuff, the pressure-regulating balloon or reservoir, and the pump (Fig. 47-4). The cuff is placed circumferentially around the bladder neck, the reservoir is positioned in the prevesical space, and the pump is put in the labia majora. When the pump is squeezed, fluid moves from the cuff to the balloon reservoir. This decompression of the cuff opens the bladder neck and allows the patient to void. After 1 to 2 minutes, the reservoir automatically reinflates the cuff, which then reestablishes urethral coaptation and continence.

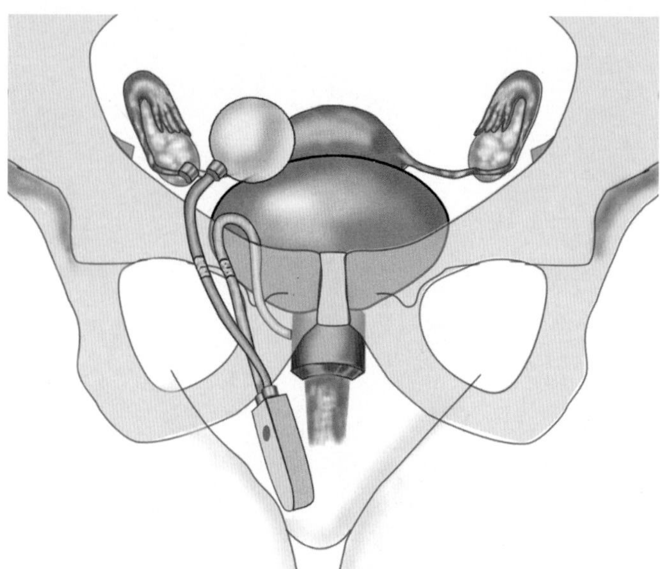

Figure 47-4 The AS-800 artificial urinary sphincter in the female.

The advantage of the transvaginal technique is that it allows dissection of the urethrovaginal plane under direct vision. Preoperative parenteral antibiotics (gentamicin and vancomycin) are given before the operation. The patient is placed in high dorsal lithotomy position with the knee and hip at 90 degrees of flexion. The lower abdomen and genitalia are prepared and draped in the usual sterile surgical fashion. The labia are retracted laterally with stay sutures. A 14-Fr Foley catheter is inserted per urethra, and the bladder is emptied. A weighted speculum is then placed into the vagina for exposure.

A vertical incision is made in the anterior vaginal wall between the mid-urethra and proximal bladder neck. A plane under the vaginal wall is created on each side of the incision with sharp dissection. The scissors are first pointed laterally to the pubic ramus and then upward, toward the ipsilateral shoulder of the patient (Fig. 47-5). If the patient has not had a previous bladder neck operation, blunt finger dissection may be performed to separate the endopelvic fascia from its lateral attachments to the pubic ramus. Using this combination of sharp and blunt dissection, the retropubic space is then entered lateral to the bladder neck.

Attention is next directed to the anterior aspect of the proximal urethra or bladder neck to free its attachments from the overlying pubic symphysis. To achieve this, a combination of sharp and blunt dissection is used. Overly aggressive dissection may lead to an unintentional cystotomy or urethral injury. If the dissection of the anterior side of the urethra proves to be difficult due to dense scarring from previous retropubic operations, a separate suprameatal incision above the external meatus may be used. After the proximal urethra has been freed circumferentially, a Derra clamp is passed around the urethra from left to right. The cuff-measuring tape is grasped and passed around the urethra (Fig. 47-6), and the circumference of the urethra is measured. If the circumference is equivocal, it is best to choose a slightly larger size. Using a curved clamp, the appropriate size AUS cuff is placed around the proximal urethra (Fig. 47-7). If the pump is to be inserted into the right labium majoris, the cuff is withdrawn from right to left. The opposite is true if the pump is placed on the left side. After the cuff is locked in place, it is rotated 180 degrees so that the hard-locking button lies on the anterior

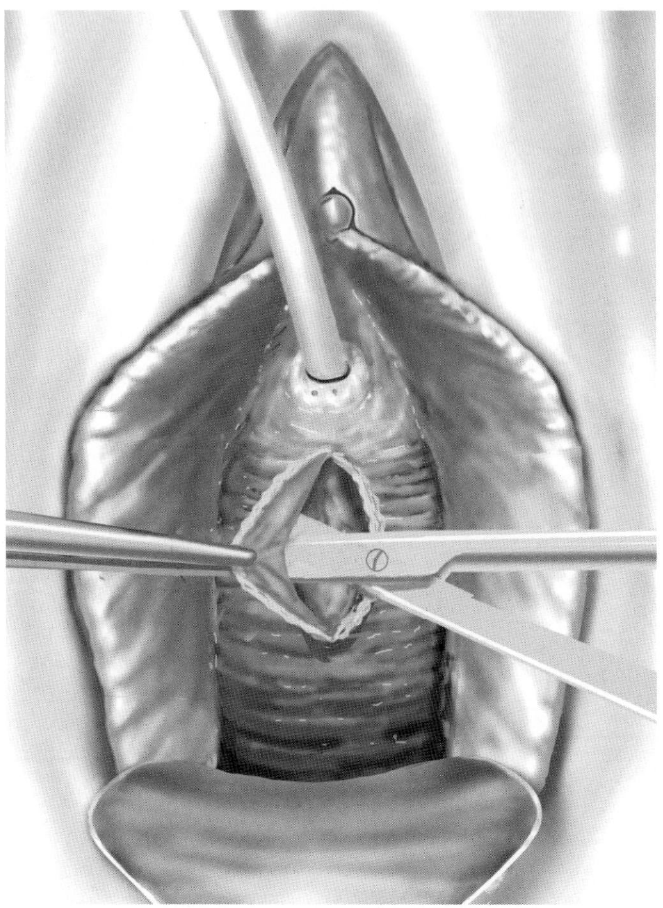

Figure 47-5 Using a combination of sharp and blunt dissection, the retropubic space is entered lateral to the bladder neck.

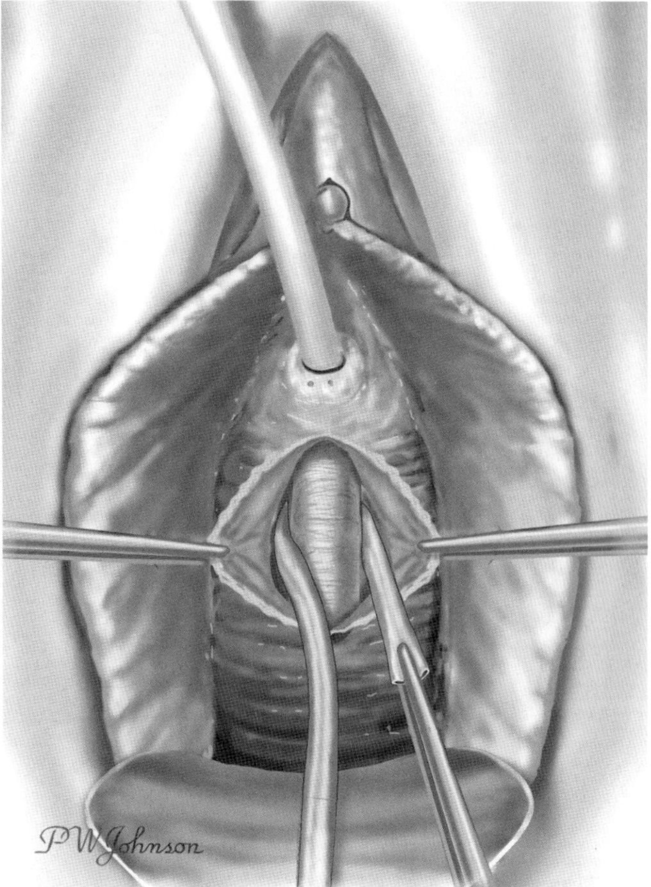

Figure 47-6 A Penrose drain is placed around the bladder neck to demonstrate the completed circumferential dissection.

aspect of the urethra, away from the anterior vaginal wall (Fig. 47-8).

On the side where the pump and balloon are to be placed, a 4-cm transverse suprapubic incision is made and carried down to the fascia. The anterior rectus sheath is incised transversely, the prevesical space is developed bluntly adjacent to the bladder, and the reservoir is inserted into the prevesical space. In females, the 51- to 60-cm H_2O pressure balloon reservoir is routinely used. The fascial incision is closed with a running 1-0 delayed absorbable suture. The cuff tubing is attached to the tubing passer and then withdrawn up to the suprapubic incision. From the suprapubic incision, a subcutaneous tunnel is created through which the pump will be inserted into the labium majoris. The pump is passed to the level of the urethra with the deactivation button facing anteriorly. A Babcock clamp is used to secure the pump in position.

The reservoir is filled with 22 mL of a solution composed of Hypaque and normal saline according to the instructions specified by the manufacturer. The tubings are trimmed to the appropriate lengths and then irrigated to remove any air or debris from the system. A straight Quick Connector is placed between the pump and the balloon reservoir. A right angle Quick Connector attaches the pump to the cuff. The AUS is cycled several times to ensure proper functioning of the system and then left in the deactivated position. Both wounds are irrigated copiously with Betadine solution and closed in multiple layers with delayed absorbable sutures to ensure good coverage of the prosthesis with healthy overlying tissue.

A vaginal packing with Clomycin ointment is placed and then is removed 2 hours postoperatively. The Foley catheter is removed just before discharge. The patient usually voids without difficulty after removal of the Foley catheter. If the patient is stable and pain is adequately controlled, she is discharged home on the same day. A prescription for a 2-week course of oral antibiotics (Keflex) and pain medication is given to each patient. The patient returns to the office in 6 weeks for activation of the AUS.

Discussion

The AUS in the female population differs from the suburethral sling in that it does not provide a backboard or urethral support; it attempts to mimic the sphincter mechanism of the urethra with circumferential compression.[16] The few published reports of the AUS implanted through the transvaginal approach described favorable outcomes. Appell reported a continence rate of greater than 90% in 19 patients with a follow-up of 3 years.[10] Three patients required revisions for inadequate cuff compression and connector leak. Abbassian described a similar transvaginal technique in four patients, all of whom were dry at 14 months' follow-up.[17] Costa and colleagues evaluated the efficacy of the AS-800 system in women using a modified surgical procedure through an abdominal approach. Of the 190 patients with working devices, continence was achieved in 88.7% and 81.8% of those with non-neurogenic and neurogenic bladders, respectively, at a mean follow-up of 3.9 years.[18]

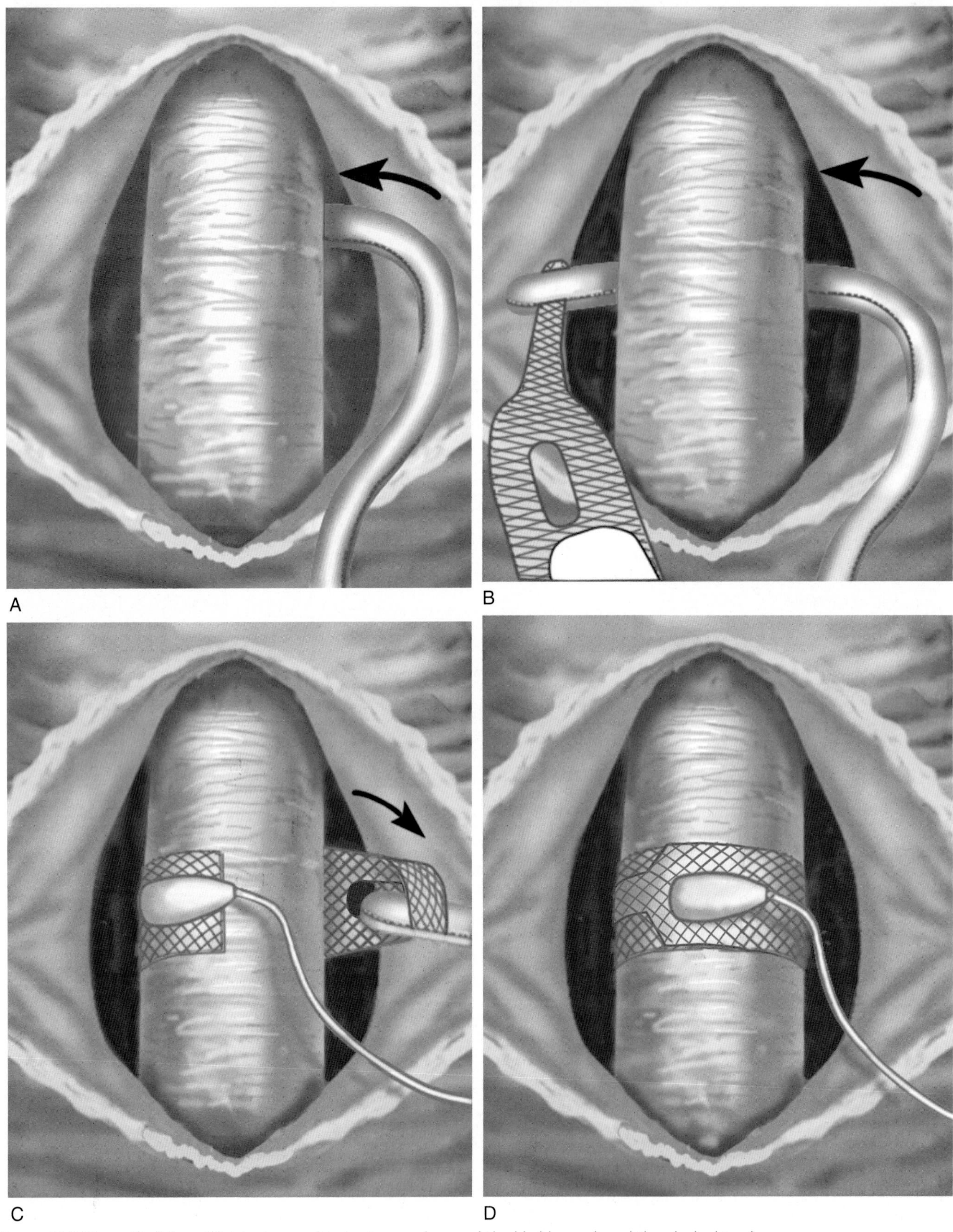

Figure 47-7 The cuff of the artificial urinary sphincter is passed around the bladder neck and then locked in place.

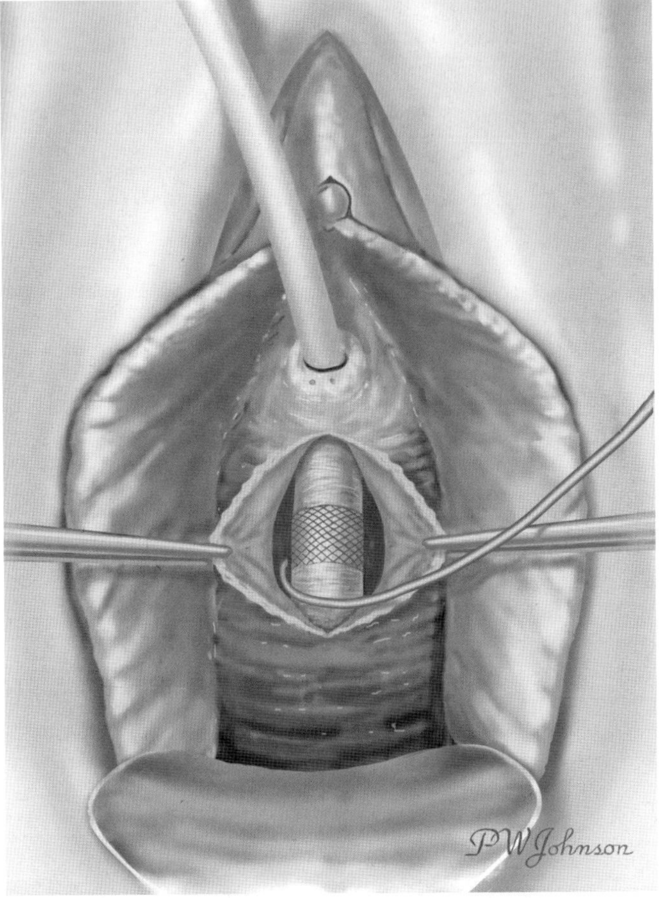

Figure 47-8 The cuff is rotated so that the hard-locking button lies anterior to the urethra, away from the anterior vaginal wall.

One major disadvantage of the AUS is the risk of erosion of the device. Device erosion has been attributed to poor circulation, low-grade infection, technical difficulties, and shifting of the cuff.[17] With the introduction of a newly improved cuff design and in situ activation-deactivation control assembly in the AS-800 model in 1983, the incidence of mechanical malfunction dramatically decreased.[11] However, the risk of revision surgery still remained high. Thomas and associates reported 12-year follow-up in 68 patients who underwent placement of an AS-800 model AUS. Despite an 81% continence rate, 46% required removal or replacement for erosion or infection.[19] They concluded by recommending an AUS for patients with SUI after failure of one anti-stress incontinence operation and not as a last resort.

CONCLUSIONS

The AUS is a viable alternative treatment modality for the female patient with a nonmobile, well supported urethra and a history of unsuccessful anti-incontinence operations. The advantage of the transvaginal approach for placement of the AUS is that it offers the surgeon the ability to dissect through the urethrovaginal plane under direct vision. However, many patients require revision surgery due to malfunction, erosion, or infection of the device.

The spiral sling is an effective salvage transvaginal procedure that may be considered for a small subset of female patients with nonfunctional urethra as a last resort before urethral closure procedures. This includes patients with urethral incompetence caused by neurologic disease, congenital anomalies, or iatrogenic injury from multiple failed anti-incontinence surgeries. The initial outcomes look promising, but longer follow-up will better define its role in refractory female incontinence and demonstrate the durability of the spiral sling.

References

1. Liapis A, Bakas P, Creatsas G: Burch colposuspension and tension-free vaginal tape in the management of stress urinary incontinence in women. Eur Urol 41:469, 2002.
2. Nilsson CG, Falconer C, Rezapour M: Seven-year follow-up of the tension-free vaginal tape procedure for treatment of urinary incontinence. Obstet Gynecol 104:1259, 2004.
3. Nilsson CG, Kuuva N, Falconer C, et al: Long-term results of the tension-free vaginal tape (TVT) procedure for surgical treatment of female stress urinary incontinence. Int Urogynecol J Pelvic Floor Dysfunct 12(Suppl 2):S5, 2001.
4. Rodriguez LV, Raz S: Prospective analysis of patients treated with a distal urethral polypropylene sling for symptoms of stress urinary incontinence: Surgical outcome and satisfaction determined by patient driven questionnaires. J Urol 170:857, 2003.
5. Ward KL, Hilton P: A prospective multicenter randomized trial of tension-free vaginal tape and colposuspension for primary urodynamic stress incontinence: Two-year follow-up. Am J Obstet Gynecol 190:324, 2004.
6. Bump RC, Norton PA: Epidemiology and natural history of pelvic floor dysfunction. Obstet Gynecol Clin North Am 25:723, 1998.
7. Petrou SP, Frank I: Complications and initial continence rates after a repeat pubovaginal sling procedure for recurrent stress urinary incontinence. J Urol 165:1979, 2001.
8. Rutman M, Deng D, Shah S, et al: The spiral sling salvage anti-incontinence surgery for female patients with a non-functional urethra: Technique and initial results. J Urol 175:1794-1798; discussion 1798-1799, 2006.
9. Mourtzinos A, Maher MG, Raz S, Rodriguez LV: The spiral sling salvage anti-incontinence surgery for the female patient with refractory stress urinary incontinence: Surgical outcome and satisfaction determined by patient driven questionnaires. (In press.)
10. Appell RA: Techniques and results in the implantation of the artificial urinary sphincter in women with type III stress urinary incontinence by a vaginal approach. Neurourol Urodyn 7:613, 1988.
11. Webster GD, Perez LM, Khoury JM, Timmons SL: Management of type III stress urinary incontinence using artificial urinary sphincter. Urology 39:499, 1992.
12. Parulkar BG, Barrett DM: Application of the AS-800 artificial sphincter for intractable urinary incontinence in females. Surg Gynecol Obstet 171:131, 1990.
13. Ngninkeu BN, van Heugen G, di Gregorio M, et al: Laparoscopic artificial urinary sphincter in women for type III incontinence: preliminary results. Eur Urol 47:793, 2005.
14. Uebersax JS, Wyman JF, Shumaker SA, et al: Short forms to assess life quality and symptom distress for urinary incontinence in women: The Incontinence Impact Questionnaire and the Urogenital Distress Inventory. Continence Program for Women Research Group. Neurourol Urodyn 14:131, 1995.

15. Mingin GC, Youngren K, Stock JA, Hanna MK: The rectus myofascial wrap in the management of urethral sphincter incompetence. BJU Int 90:550, 2002.
16. Light JK, Scott FB: Management of urinary incontinence in women with the artificial urinary sphincter. J Urol 134:476, 1985.
17. Abbassian A: A new operation for insertion of the artificial urinary sphincter. J Urol 140:512, 1988.
18. Costa P, Mottet N, Rabut B, et al: The use of an artificial urinary sphincter in women with type III incontinence and a negative Marshall test. J Urol 165:1172, 2001.
19. Thomas K, Venn SN, Mundy AR: Outcome of the artificial urinary sphincter in female patients. J Urol 167:1720, 2002.

Chapter 48

MIXED URINARY INCONTINENCE

Karen E. Smith and Edward J. McGuire

DEFINITION AND PREVALENCE

The term mixed urinary incontinence (MUI) has been defined by the International Continence Society as a condition characterized by symptoms of both stress and urge incontinence, or a combination of leakage associated with urgency as well as with exertion.[1] However, this is a term that can apply both to a combination of incontinence symptoms and to a combination of urodynamic findings in the same individual.

Studies have reported variable prevalence estimates for MUI symptomatology, ranging historically from 30% to 50%.[2] According to the more recent National Overactive Bladder Evaluation (NOBLE) study, which relied on census data from the year 2000, approximately one third (34.4%) of the 14.8 million women with urinary incontinence were defined as having MUI.[3] Mixed symptoms appear to be more prevalent in clinical-based than in population-based epidemiologic studies.[4] Sandvik and colleagues[5] summarized eight articles and demonstrated that as many as 61% of incontinent women reported MUI. In contrast, Hampel and associates[6] reported that 29% of women with incontinence had MUI, based on the average prevalence from 21 epidemiologic studies.

It is well recognized that incontinence symptoms poorly predict the true etiology of an individual patient's incontinence. Several studies have demonstrated that mixed symptoms are much more common than mixed conditions.[7] Cardozo and Stanton[8] reported that, of those patients presenting with MUI symptoms, more than 50% had only stress urinary incontinence (SUI) and approximately 40% had only detrusor instability as seen on urodynamics. Sandvik and colleagues[5] found that, of the 46% of patients presenting with MUI symptoms, only 44% were diagnosed with a mixed condition. This trend was also demonstrated by a sample of 950 incontinent women evaluated at Duke University: 52% presented with mixed symptoms, but only 14% had mixed conditions.[9]

Several studies have attempted to define MUI using findings seen on urodynamics, namely the coexistence of SUI and detrusor overactivity. Prevalence of MUI in urodynamic studies ranges from 36% to 56% of patients. However, the characteristics of these groups have often not been clearly defined, and therefore these studies have comprised patients with many different pathologic processes, most likely including those with abnormal compliance.[10] Furthermore, 50% of patients with motor urge incontinence can have a normal cystometrogram (CMG),[11,12] whereas normal patients can exhibit uninhibited bladder contractions of unknown significance on CMG. Therefore, the true prevalence of MUI as defined by urodynamics is difficult to estimate.

The condition known as MUI has historically lacked a unified definition. The symptom complex itself has not been well defined. Specifically, there are those with both urge and stress incontinence, often referred to as overactive bladder (OAB) or wet OAB, and those with stress incontinence plus urge symptoms but without urge incontinence, called dry OAB.[13] Furthermore, because some studies have been based on symptoms and others have been based on urodynamic findings, meaningful comparison of the results of different studies is often difficult. Given the lack of a strict universal definition, as well as the limitations of any urodynamic study, the quoted prevalence of MUI is probably inaccurate, and the true prevalence is almost impossible to determine.

IMPLICATIONS OF MIXED URINARY INCONTINENCE

Several studies have shown that women with MUI symptoms typically report more severe incontinence than do women with either SUI or urinary urge incontinence (UUI) alone. In the Norwegian Epidemiology of Incontinence in the County of Nord-Trondelag (EPINCONT) study,[14] "severe incontinence," as defined by validated instruments, was seen in 38% of women with MUI, compared with 28% of those with UUI and 17% of those with SUI. Furthermore, more women with MUI (47%) were bothered by their incontinence, compared to women with UUI (36%) or SUI (24%). Bump and coworkers[4] conducted a secondary analysis of data from the duloxetine study group and found that the 171 women (31%) with baseline MUI complained of more severe urinary incontinence than did those with SUI.

The negative personal impact of MUI on patients with this condition appears to be significant. Coyne and associates[15] sought to examine the impact of urinary incontinence on health-related quality of life (HRQOL). A case-control study of 171 incontinent women showed that respondents with UUI or MUI reported not only significantly greater ratings of urinary urge intensity and more incontinence episodes, but also significantly worse HRQOL, compared to patients with isolated SUI.

ETIOLOGY

Before being able to critically evaluate the theories proposed to explain the etiology of MUI, it is important to note the following facts, some of which may seem counterintuitive. First, of those women with SUI who also complain of urgency, frequency, and/or urge incontinence, 50% to 75% of them are cured of their urge symptomatology by surgery for SUI.[16-23] Furthermore, overall cure rates are poor for those patients with MUI treated with anticholinergics alone.[19,24] Several theories have addressed the potential causes of mixed symptomatology, although not all of them can reconcile these facts.

One theory is that MUI is the result of a patient's having two separate conditions. The greater perceived severity of MUI is attributed to the additive effects of the two conditions being more severe and bothersome than the effect of a single condition.[4] However, this would not explain the poor response rates of anticholinergics in these patients or the fact that surgery may cure most of these symptoms.

An alternative explanation is that mixed symptoms are a result of more severe incontinence rather than the presence of two conditions.[4] As stated previously, women with more severe incontinence are more likely to report mixed symptoms. In the study by Bump and associates,[4] as the severity of incontinence improved during treatment, mixed symptoms resolved. Furthermore, in patients with severe SUI, the bladder may never completely fill, thereby leading to an essentially defunctionalized bladder and concomitant urge symptomatology. Severity of incontinence causing a mixed symptom complex is perhaps a reason for resolution of these symptoms once a successful anti-incontinence surgery is completed.

Others suggest that these symptoms may be the result of a behavioral adaptation in the woman with SUI. For instance, the patient may empty her bladder more frequently in an attempt to reduce stress-induced leakage and therefore induce symptoms of frequency and urgency.[25] These symptoms may represent a false interpretation of impending stress-induced leakage. The patient rushes to the toilet to protect herself from stress-induced leakage at the perception of the first or normal desire, which may result in a learned behavior that the patient develops and reinforces over time. These patients are seen as having SUI with "pseudo-urgency syndrome."[26]

Other theories have lent support to an actual link between SUI and detrusor overactivity. One such theory is that, in patients with SUI, traction on or stretching of the pelvic nerves as a result of poor pelvic floor support and severe urethral hypermobility causes this symptom complex.[19] When the bladder neck is stabilized to prevent this stretching, both SUI and UUI are corrected. A solid experimental background has suggested a link between the pelvic floor, pudendal innervation, and detrusor inhibition. Artibani[27] suggested that decreased inhibition from the pelvic floor or the urethra, caused by pelvic floor or urethral deficiency, can lead to increased efferent activity and subsequent detrusor overactivity. In his opinion, the best support for this hypothesis is given by the positive clinical results of pelvic floor electrical stimulation and rehabilitation.

Mahoney and colleagues[28] proposed that "micturition reflex instability" may result from malfunction of the detrusor reflex or instability of the pudendal nucleus, which innervates the pelvic floor muscles and external sphincter. He proposed that detrusor instability is the result of hyperexcitability of the sacral micturition reflex center, due to either its underinhibition or overfacilitation. Pathologic relaxation and weakness of the striated muscles of the pelvic floor and perineum can result in underactivity of the perineodetrusor inhibitory reflex, causing underinhibition of the sacral micturition reflex center, and may predispose a patient to detrusor instability.

Other scientists, who support a correlation between urethral afferents and the micturition reflex, suggest that it is rather urine entering the proximal urethra that stimulates the urethral afferents and therefore the voiding reflex.[29] It is widely held that urethral relaxation occurs in the initial phase of micturition. In the healthy adult, urine enters the urethra only during micturition. However, urine is present in the urethra in patients with SUI because of poor pelvic support and/or sphincteric deficiency. It is proposed that the entry of urine into the proximal urethra could act as a stimulus to potentiate or even initiate a detrusor contraction.[29]

Urethral instability, as seen as fluctuations in urethral pressure, is evidenced in women with detrusor instability. In one study, urethral instability was reported to have occurred in 42% of patients with detrusor instability and was associated with the sequence of urethral relaxation before an unprovoked contraction.[30] In a report by Low,[31] bladder and urethral pressures were simultaneously measured during bladder filling in 77 women with idiopathic detrusor instability. Low found that 85% of patients developed urethral relaxation 5 seconds before detrusor contraction. He concluded that the involuntary detrusor contractions were preceded by a fall in urethral pressure, similar to that observed in normal voiding. Hindmarsh and coworkers[32] also demonstrated urethral relaxation preceding detrusor contractions in a series of patients with detrusor instability, not only supporting the concept that urethral instability can be associated with unstable bladder contractions but also suggesting that detrusor instability may be initiated from the bladder outlet region or proximal urethra.

Mahony and colleagues[33] described two urethrodetrusor reflexes that could increase the excitability of the micturition reflex and trigger a detrusor contraction when activated by urine flow across urethral mucosa. The theory that urine or fluid in the posterior urethra could result in a detrusor contraction has been supported by several animal models. As early as 1931, Barrington[34] reported that running water through the urethra or distending the proximal urethra in the cat caused contraction of the detrusor. Also using the cat model, Kiruluta and colleagues[35] noted that urethral perfusion triggered spontaneous bladder contractions of such intensity that bladder filling was not possible. More recently, Jung and associates[29] sought experimental support for the hypothesis that stimulation of urethral afferent nerves can induce reflex detrusor contractions. By measuring urethral perfusion pressure and isovolumetric bladder pressure with catheters inserted through the bladder dome of female rats, they demonstrated that fluid passing though the urethra can result in activation of the mechanosensitive urethral afferents, which can in turn increase the excitability of the micturition reflex.

Therefore, in patients with SUI, leakage of urine into the proximal urethra may stimulate urethral afferents and facilitate the voiding reflex. This would imply that SUI can induce and/or increase detrusor instability. There is little direct support for this theory in humans,[4,36] and some believe that the effect may be species specific. However, the fact that this phenomenon has not been demonstrated convincingly in humans may be a result of study design. For example, although Sutherst and Brown[36] did not detect such facilitatory reflexes in the human, they believed that the transurethral catheter might have interfered with the activation of afferent receptors that respond to flow through the urethra. Furthermore, not all women with MUI symptoms have both urodynamically proven SUI and detrusor instability. Absence of urodynamic "proof" may be a result of an inhibitory effect of the patient during the study.

In short, it is likely that women with MUI symptoms have SUI as their primary problem and that detrusor overactivity results secondarily when urethrodetrusor facilitative reflexes are activated, either because an incompetent bladder neck allows urine to enter into the proximal urethra during physical activity or because of traction on the pelvic nerves due to a weakened pelvic floor.

IMPORTANCE OF URODYNAMICS

An accurate diagnosis is essential for effective treatment of the incontinent patient. Although a detailed history is important, symptoms alone are often a poor guide to a final diagnosis. The urologist is therefore encouraged to rely on a combination of symptoms, physical findings, and objective testing. In addition to a routine evaluation, secondary testing in patients with mixed symptomatology should include urine cytology and cystourethroscopy to rule out pathologic conditions of the bladder, especially carcinoma in situ.

Urodynamic evaluation is integral in determining the true underlying etiology of a patient's incontinence, especially in the patient with mixed symptomatology. Videourodynamic evaluation, which combines the use of fluoroscopy with measurement of bladder and urethral pressures, allows simultaneous evaluation of structure and function and is the preferred method.[37]

The most important reason to perform videourodynamic studies in a patient with MUI is to rule out poor bladder compliance. A high-pressure or poorly compliant bladder poses significant risk to ureteral and renal function. It can be caused by a number of conditions, including neurologic conditions, prolonged catheter drainage, radiation therapy, prior pelvic or urethral surgery, interstitial cystitis, and obstructive uropathy. If there is suspicion of altered bladder compliance in any incontinent patient, that patient should undergo urodynamic testing to determine the condition of the bladder's storage function. Poor compliance adversely influences the outcome of any procedure done to increase bladder outlet resistance and could create a situation in which the upper tracts are at risk from high bladder pressures. Fortunately, urodynamic testing is accurate and sensitive in the diagnosis of poor compliance.

CONSERVATIVE THERAPY

Anticholinergics

There is a paucity of data specifically addressing anticholinergic therapy in patients with MUI, and the results have historically been less than optimal. In patients with MUI, anticholinergic therapy has been associated with significant resolution of the urge component symptoms in only 50% to 60% of patients, while not improving the stress component.[19,26] Patients report poor satisfaction because of poor response, side effects, and need for continuous treatment.[26] Poor response has been thought to be secondary to the fact that the SUI component is not addressed with medical therapy.[26]

More recently, Kreder and colleagues[38] compared the efficacy of Tolterodine in those with urge-predominant MUI versus UUI in a single-blind, multicenter trial. They found a 67% and 75% decrease in incontinence episodes in the MUI and UUI groups, respectively, with a "dry rate" of 39% and 44% in the two groups, respectively. There were no significant intergroup differences in success rates. The Mixed Incontinence Effective Research Investigating Tolterodine (MERIT) study, a multinational, double-blind, placebo-controlled trial, examined the efficacy of antimuscarinic therapy in patients with urge-predominant MUI.[39] In total, 854 patients MUI were studied, with 634 (74.5%) reporting UUI as their initial symptom. After 8 weeks of treatment, 76% in the drug group reported improvement, compared with 53% in the placebo group. There was no difference in response of those who experienced UUI as their initial symptom compared with those who noted SUI first in this study.

Several studies have directly compared surgery to drug therapy for patients with MUI. Karram and Bhatia treated 52 patients with MUI with either Burch colposuspension or medical therapy. They found no significant difference in cure rate between the two groups, and their recommendation was primary medical treatment for patients with MUI.[18] A more recent prospective, randomized study by Osman compared patients with MUI and a normal CMG undergoing surgery to those undergoing treatment with anticholinergic therapy.[26] One third of patients received a 6-month course of an anticholinergic, whereas the remaining patients underwent surgery for SUI. In the surgery group, patients underwent either a Burch colposuspension or pubovaginal sling placement, depending on their Valsalva leak point pressure. A group of 20 patients with pure SUI were also used as a control. No patient in the drug group became dry. In contrast, among those who underwent surgery for SUI, 87% in the Burch group and 83% in the pubovagainal sling group were both stress and urge continent after surgery. After therapy, persistent UUI was seen in 43% of patients who received anticholinergic therapy compared to 13% and 12% of those in the Burch and sling groups, respectively.

Behavioral Therapy, Biofeedback, and Pelvic Floor Rehabilitation

Behavioral therapies such as timed voiding, avoidance of bladder irritants, and bladder retraining have been used with some success in patients with both SUI and UUI. Additionally, pelvic floor electrical stimulation or biofeedback has been used successfully in both UUI and SUI, with excellent success rates and high levels of patient satisfaction.[40] Several studies have investigated the response of pelvic floor stimulation in patients with MUI specifically. Sand[41] found a greater than 50% improvement in approximately 38% of subjects, with 8% being completely dry after 8 weeks of treatment. In this study, symptoms of urgency, frequency, and stress incontinence improved significantly, whereas symptoms of UUI remained relatively stable. Bent and colleagues[42] reported a 52% success rate in patients with MUI, whereas Caputo and associates[43] reported a 70% response rate in these patients. Siegel and coworkers[40] studied patients with both UUI and MUI undergoing 20 weeks of pelvic floor electrical stimulation, either daily or every other day. Treatment resulted in significantly lower urge and stress leakage, with decrease in urge episodes and total number of voids and improvement in quality-of-life measures. Overall, 72% of patients were satisfied with their therapy.

When compared directly to drug therapy, electrical stimulation has been shown to have better results and higher patient satisfaction. Goode[44] studied 197 women with UUI or MUI in a randomized controlled trial comparing biofeedback-assisted behavioral treatment with anticholinergics and placebo. The biofeedback group demonstrated the best results, with an 80% decrease in incontinence episodes, 78% of patients being "completely satisfied", and 97% wanting to continue treatment. A modified crossover trial was conducted, which showed that combination treatment is more effective than monotherapy with either drug or biofeedback alone, a finding supported by other studies.[40,41,45]

In short, treatment of patients with MUI can be challenging and should be tailored to the individual. In those patients with

MUI, it is wise to direct treatment at the dominant symptom first. When in doubt, it is most reasonable to proceed with conservative treatment of the urge component before consideration of surgical therapy for SUI.[2] In that small proportion of patients whose symptoms may be improved enough with drug therapy alone, surgery may be prevented.

SURGICAL TREATMENT

As stated previously, as many as 75% of women with MUI are cured of their urge component by surgery aimed at correcting their SUI. These encouraging results were demonstrated in several studies and seem to hold regardless of the actual procedure performed. Improvement of urge symptoms by providing support for the bladder neck can be seen in studies in which support was achieved by temporary, nonsurgical means. For example, Kondo and coworkers reported that, in a group of 20 women with symptoms of MUI, 85% had an improvement of 50% or better with the use of a bladder-neck support prosthesis.[46]

To date, few studies have specifically addressed the resolution of urge symptomatology in MUI patients undergoing a Burch colposuspension. Scotti and colleagues[47] evaluated 46 patients with both mixed symptoms and urodynamically diagnosed genuine SUI and detrusor instability who underwent a Burch colposuspension. The study demonstrated an overall resolution of urge incontinence in 56.5% of patients. More recently, Osman[26] demonstrated resolution of urge incontinence in 87% of patients with MUI and a normal CMG who had undergone a Burch colposuspension. Langer and colleagues[48] evaluated 127 women who underwent a Burch colposuspension, of whom 33% had preoperative urge incontinence and 55% had urgency. Only 9% of the patients with preoperative urge incontinence still had this complaint at 1 year after surgery, whereas 25% of those patients with preoperative urgency still complained of this postoperatively at 1 year.

Serels and colleagues[19] evaluated 36 patients with urodynamically diagnosed Valsalva-induced detrusor instability who underwent various types of pubovaginal sling procedures, including in situ vaginal wall sling, free swing vaginal wall slings, rectus fascia slings, cadaveric fascia slings, and synthetic slings. Preoperatively, 21 patients (58%) had MUI. Cure of SUI was achieved in 92% of these patients, and 75% demonstrated resolution of their urge incontinence.

McGuire and Lyton[16] and Fulford and colleagues[20] both reported resolution of urge symptomatology in 69% of patients after pubovaginal sling, and 74% of patients in a study by Morgan and associates[21] had resolution. Osman[26] reported resolution of urge incontinence in 83% of their patients who had undergone a pubovaginal sling procedure.

The tension-free vaginal tape (TVT) procedure is a relatively new suburethral sling procedure, first described in 1996. To date, few studies have evaluated the effect of the TVT on patients with MUI. Segal and colleagues[49] reviewed outcomes of 98 patients with pure SUI and MUI who underwent a TVT procedure. After TVT, 63.1% of those with preoperative UUI had resolution; 57.3% of those with preoperative urgency, frequency, and nocturia had resolution of symptoms; and 57.7% of those who used anticholinergics preoperatively no longer needed to do so.

The transobturator (TOT) tape procedure was first described in 2001 by Delorme as the newest minimally invasive suburethral sling procedure. Long-term studies are not available at this point. However, in his original article published in 2004, Delorme[50] described outcomes of 32 incontinent patients who underwent TOT, 18 of whom had MUI, with a minimum of 1 year follow-up. Among the 18 patients with preoperative MUI, 10 (55%) had either resolution or improvement in their urge component, 7 (39%) had no change in their symptoms, and 1 (5%) reported worsening of urge symptoms. There are currently no studies examining the use of collagen injections specifically in patients with MUI.

Voiding Dysfunction after Anti-incontinence Surgery

Up to 40% of patients develop voiding dysfunction after anti-incontinence surgery.[51] There is no good method to identify with certainty preoperatively who will have persistent, worsened, or new-onset symptoms.[25,49] Voiding disorders addressed here include urethral obstruction, de novo urgency and urge incontinence, and persistent or worsening urgency in patients with preoperative urge symptoms.

Urethral obstruction is an uncommon but disturbing complication of anti-incontinence surgery, the incidence of which is reported to be 1% to 11% in the literature.[52,53] Patients with voiding dysfunction due to urethral obstruction usually present with new-onset urgency or urge incontinence and incomplete bladder emptying, which is suggested by an elevated postvoid residual volume. A complete workup is warranted but may be inconclusive, because obstruction may be present even in the face of normal emptying. It can be difficult in certain cases to differentiate among obstructive symptoms, new urge symptoms, and worsening of urge symptoms in the patient with preoperative MUI.

De novo urge syndrome implies the development of new symptoms of frequency, nocturia, urgency, and/or urge incontinence after surgery for SUI. Most series report that 7% to 15% of patients develop de novo urge symptoms,[12] with some reporting this phenomenon in up to 30% of patients after anti-incontinence surgery.[49,54] Specifically, de novo detrusor overactivity has been cited to occur in 5% to 32% of patients after a retropubic suspension, in 11% after a needle suspension, and in 3% to 24% after pubovaginal sling procedures,[53] with a few studies citing irritative bladder symptoms in up to 50% of those undergoing suburethral sling procedures.[49] De novo detrusor overactivity is seen in 6% to 15%[49] of patients undergoing a TVT. Segal and colleagues[49] reviewed outcomes of 98 patients with pure SUI or MUI who underwent a TVT procedure. Postoperatively, de novo urge incontinence symptoms developed in 9.1% and de novo urgency in 4.3%. In a recent study by Nilsson and associates,[55] which looked at 7-year follow-up data on patients undergoing TVT, de novo urge symptoms were present in 6.3% of patients. The two studies published on outcomes of TOT to date cited de novo urgency occurring in 2 (14%) of patients, in Delorme's study,[50] and in 0.8% of patients, in a more recent study by Spinosa and colleagues.[56] It has been suggested that de novo irritative voiding symptoms may be more bothersome to the patient than the original SUI.

Persistent or worsening urge symptomatology in patients with preoperative urge symptomatology can also occur. Historically, it is estimated that 25% of patients who had these symptoms preoperatively still have them postoperatively.[12] However, the prevalence of this symptom may be even higher than previously thought. A meta-analysis of several hundred articles in the literature was done by the Female Stress Urinary Incontinence Clinical

Guidelines Panel,[53] which looked at probability estimates for treatment complications, including the presence of urinary urgency, after surgery for SUI. They found that, for retropubic suspensions, 66% of patients with urgency and detrusor instability preoperatively had persistent postoperative urgency, whereas 36% of patients with urgency and no detrusor instability preoperatively had persistent postoperative urgency. For sling procedures, 46% of patients with urgency and detrusor instability preoperatively had persistent postoperative urgency, compared with 34% of patients with urgency and no detrusor instability preoperatively. In general, if urgency and detrusor instability are present preoperatively, there is a significant risk that these symptoms will persist postoperatively, and the prevalence may be higher than previously thought. It is also clear that patients with persistent UUI after pubovaginal sling placement have the lowest degree of satisfaction with the procedure.[21]

Etiology

Many have questioned the exact causes of de novo urge/UUI and persistent urge symptomatology after anti-incontinence surgery, and several different theories exist.

Some have suggested that de novo urge/UUI and/or worsening of urge symptoms may be caused by obstruction.[57] The question of whether normal voiding physiology and function are altered by surgery has been the subject of much debate. The potential physiologic changes in voiding function that might occur after a particular outlet-enhancing procedure are not entirely understood. Some studies suggest that successful anti-incontinence procedures can normally result in an increase in urethral resistance during voiding, suggesting obstruction,[58-60] but others have not demonstrated this phenomenon.[61,62] Because some patients with postoperative de novo UUI are indeed clinically obstructed, one must maintain a high index of suspicion for obstruction in any patient with de novo urge syndrome after surgery.

Osman[26] suggested that the pathogenesis of preoperative urge symptomatology may not be the same as that of persistent or residual symptoms after surgery, and that persistent symptoms may be related to outlet obstruction. In their study, those patients who had persistent symptoms of UUI after surgery had a significant decrease in their maximum flow rate on uroflowmetry, a finding that was not seen in those who were cured of their UUI. They concluded that residual urgency after surgery may be caused by iatrogenic relative obstruction.

Another possibility for the development of new postoperative urge symptoms is that the symptoms may have actually been present preoperatively. Patients may have had prior MUI symptoms, with symptoms of urge and/or UUI that were minimized preoperatively by their stress component. Once the SUI was corrected, urge symptoms may have become more prominent and bothersome.

Others argue that patients with SUI, who may have denervation of the pelvic floor, suffer more injury to the autonomic nerves of the bladder, bladder neck, and urethra from dissection during anti-incontinence surgery.[61] Further denervation is thought to cause detrusor supersensitivity and overactivity. There is some evidence against this, however. For instance, the TVT is placed without tension at the level of the mid-urethra, with no significant dissection in this area. It should therefore result in a lower rate of voiding dysfunction. However, as previously stated, up to 15% of patients undergoing TVT develop de novo urge symptoms, suggesting that there is an alternate explanation for these symptoms. Also, the Ingleman-Sundberg procedure, a relatively underused surgical therapy for severe, intractable motor urge incontinence, consists of transvaginal dissection of the perivesical fascia from the area of the trigone, including purposeful division of the terminal branches of the pelvic nerves. In a study by Westney and associates,[63] long-term cure or improvement was seen in 68% of patients who underwent this procedure.

In patients with severe intrinsic sphincteric deficiency and resultant bladder defunctionalization, the sudden ability to store urine may cause new symptoms of urgency. Furthermore, symptoms in the immediate postoperative period may be due in part to surgically induced inflammation and edema. In most of these cases, symptoms resolve with nonsurgical measures, such as anticholinergic medications and timed voiding. In Serels' study[19] of patients undergoing pubovaginal sling procedures, 5 (24%) of 21 patients had persistent UUI postoperatively, and an additional 8 had persistent urgency. All patients with urge and UUI were improved or cured with anticholinergics. In a study by Cross and colleagues,[22] of the 26 patients (19%) with de novo urgency/UUI, all but 4 had resolution of their symptoms within 3 months. These 4 patients (3%) with persistent UUI had ultimate resolution of symptoms with medication and timed voiding.

Finally, some argue that urge symptoms may not resolve after surgery because the repair aimed at fixing their SUI incontinence has failed. Fulford and colleagues,[20] who reported persistent urge in 31% of their patients, attributed these symptoms to failure to achieve bladder neck closure at rest.

CONTROVERSIES CONCERNING PREDICTORS OF POOR OUTCOMES

As previously stated, the postoperative course of urge symptomatology in patients with MUI is unpredictable. Several studies over the years have attempted to describe preoperative predictors of poor outcomes. We address here the more common controversies surrounding surgical therapy in patients with MUI.

Does the Presence of an Urge Component Predict Failure of an Anti-incontinence Procedure?

In several studies in the 1970s, an unexpectedly high incidence of detrusor instability was found in women who failed surgical procedures for SUI.[64] Other studies tended to confirm these early findings, and a general feeling that detrusor instability was the major reason for failure of these operations to cure SUI emerged. For example, in a study by Karram and Bhatia[18] of patients with MUI undergoing Burch colposuspension, all failures in the surgical group were thought to be due to persistent detrusor instability. The authors recommended medical over surgical therapy for patients with MUI. This in turn led to efforts to treat detrusor control problems in women presenting with symptomatic SUI with conservative measures, which, as previously stated, did not yield very promising results.

This finding was not supported by later studies. Columbo and colleagues[65] studied 44 women with MUI who underwent a Burch colposuspension, compared with matched controls with pure SUI. At 2 years, the cure rate for SUI was 75%, compared with 95% in the control group; however, there were no obvious findings on urodynamics that could explain this discrepancy. In fact, most failures were due to inadequate urethral support. The authors did not find any preoperative CMG parameter that predicted outcome in their study. Alcalay and associates[66] studied late outcomes after colposuspension operations and noted that detrusor instability identified preoperatively had no influence on outcome at 10 to 20 years.

In a recent study by Chou and coworkers,[67] which compared patients with pure SUI and MUI undergoing pubovaginal sling placement, cure rates for SUI were similar, with 97% in SUI group and 93% in the MUI group being cured. However, those patients with MUI who failed or who were merely improved had greater urgency and UUI episodes preoperatively. Univariate analysis of MUI cases showed that the higher the number of urgency or UUI episodes preoperatively, the more likely it was that the pubovaginal sling would fail.

So, the literature has been divided on this topic. As previously discussed, definitions of MUI have varied widely, with some studies using strict urodynamic definitions for MUI. We know that as many as 50% of patients with UUI do not demonstrate an unstable detrusor contraction on CMG, leading us to assume with relative certainty that patients with symptoms of UUI and a negative CMG have the same condition as those with a positive CMG. This creates an obvious bias and obscures the true effect of MUI on outcomes, because we are not able to prove with any certainty which patients may have been selected to be in the "wrong" group. In short, we do not believe that presence of a positive CMG has a bearing on the success of a procedure done for SUI, and therefore its presence should not be used as a factor to exclude patients from surgical treatment.

What Factors Predict Persistent Urgency/Urge Incontinence or Resolution of Symptoms?

To date, published series designed to identify risk factors for persistent postoperative urgency have been contradictory. In short, currently no consistent preoperative risk factor has been identified that predicts either resolution or persistence of urge symptomatology.

There has been historical controversy surrounding the question of whether preoperative UUI is a predictor of persistent urge symptoms in patients with MUI who undergo surgery for SUI. Furthermore, it had been suggested that the presence of urodynamically proven detrusor instability predicts persistent symptoms. In a study by Chaikin and colleagues,[68] the presence of UUI preoperatively was a risk factor for persistent UUI after 10 years of follow-up in 41% of patients who underwent a pubovaginal sling procedure.

Some studies have suggested that high pressure motor urge, or detrusor instability as seen on urodynamics, compared to low pressure motor urge, is a risk factor for persistent urge and/or UUI. These results were seen in patients who underwent anterior vaginal repair in a study by Jorgensen and associates[69] and in patients treated with retropubic bladder neck suspensions in a study by Lockhart and colleagues.[70] This finding was also demonstrated in a series of patients who underwent pubovaginal slings by Schrepferman and associates.[71]

Several others also did not find any preoperative or clinical variable predictive of outcome and disputed the use of preoperative urodynamics to predict resolution of urge/UUI postoperatively. McGuire and Savastano[72] demonstrated that women with demonstrable detrusor instability did no better or worse than those with detrusor instability diagnosed only by history. Demarco and colleagues[73] also noted that CMG had no predictive value in determining postoperative outcome in patients who underwent pubovaginal sling procedures.

Other studies have focused on the predominant symptom or timing of symptoms in patients with preoperative MUI in predicting persistence of urge symptoms postoperatively. Studies have demonstrated that, if the stress symptoms predominate and SUI is objectively demonstrated, surgical repair alleviates urge symptoms in most patients.[2] However, if urge symptoms predominate, or if the degree of SUI seems minimal in comparison with the severity of the urge symptoms, repair of the SUI may not be helpful at all and may even intensify the patient's symptoms.[74] Scotti and coworkers[47] studied 46 women with both symptoms and urodynamic findings of MUI who underwent Burch colposuspension. They found that UUI resolved with surgery in 78.6% of those in whom the stress component preceded the urge component by history, compared with only 22.2% of those in whom the urge component preceded the stress component.

What Factors Predict Development of De Novo Urgency/ Urge Incontinence?

Others have attempted to predict preoperatively who may develop de novo urge/UUI. The presence of isolated detrusor instability on preoperative urodynamics has not been shown to predict development of de novo urgency.[75] In a study by Morgan and colleague[21] of 247 patients who underwent pubovaginal sling placement, there was no variable that predicted the development of de novo urgency with or without incontinence. Overall, no preoperative urodynamic parameter has been found to significantly correlate with development of new urge/UUI.

EVALUATION OF POSTOPERATIVE VOIDING DYSFUNCTION

When evaluating a patient with de novo or worsening urge/UUI symptoms, it is imperative to rule out urinary retention. This can be done with a simple postvoid residual volume measurement. Once retention has been ruled out, it is suggested to wait at least 6 weeks before undertaking a complete formal evaluation, because residual symptoms may be a normal consequence of the healing process. Most cases resolve with nonsurgical measures, such as anticholinergic medications and timed voiding.

A careful history is important, because urge symptomatology may have been present preoperatively but downplayed due to severe SUI symptoms. A temporal relationship between the onset of symptoms and the anti-incontinence procedure is integral to diagnosing urethral obstruction but may be less clear in a patient with preoperative urge symptoms, as in the patient with MUI. Information on whether retention was present postoperatively and for how long may suggest an obstructive picture. Obstructive symptoms, such as a slow, dribbling stream, straining to void, needing to lean over or back to void, hesitancy, intermittency, and sensation of incomplete emptying, are often present along with irritative symptoms.

As previously stated, an elevated postvoid residual volume, routinely accepted as a value greater than 60 mL, is suggestive of obstruction or instrinsic detrusor dysfunction in a patient with evidence of complete bladder emptying preoperatively. A urine culture is done to rule out infection, a common cause of irritative symptoms. A 3-day voiding diary may be helpful as well.

On pelvic examination, the anterior vaginal wall is examined specifically for the appearance of the bladder neck and proximal urethra. Urethral tethering and fixation to the underside of the pubis is detected visually by the appearance of a fixed horizontal groove on the anterior vaginal wall in the region of the bladder neck. Direct palpation of the urethra and bladder neck to assess mobility and degree of scar is important, as is evaluation for pelvic prolapse. A large cystocele, for example, can exert traction on the pelvic nerves, resulting in de novo urge symptoms and UUI. Additionally, a cystoscopy may be done to rule out a foreign body (e.g., a suture) or occult neoplasm.

If urge symptoms and/or UUI persist, urodynamics with fluoroscopy should be done. The development of altered compliance is very unusual, but if this condition occurs, the possibility of an original occult detrusor component should be considered. It is also important to observe the bladder neck during a Valsalva maneuver to rule out hypersuspension or an anatomic point of obstruction.

Others have relied on pressure-flow studies to evaluate for obstruction, because obstruction can occur even in the presence of normal emptying. This is often difficult to prove, because there are no strict urodynamic criteria to define urethral obstruction in female patients. However, several studies have stated that a detrusor pressure greater than 30 to 40 cm H_2O and peak flow rate of less than 15 mL/second suggests obstruction in women. Carr and Webster[76] demonstrated that only 22% of patients in their series of women undergoing urethrolysis met these obstructive parameters, but 56% of patients met these criteria in a study by Nitti and Raz.[77] Nevertheless, 75% of patients treated with urethrolysis responded with good results. Some believe that obstruction can be recognized by the observation of a sustained, high-pressure detrusor contraction resulting in a reduced-amplitude flow rate.[78] Preoperative pressure-flow data can be useful, because a direct comparison can be made.

We recommend relying on a multimodal approach, using a combination of symptoms, physical examination, fluoroscopic and/or pressure-flow data, and a high degree of clinical suspicion.

TREATMENT OF REFRACTORY POSTOPERATIVE URGE SYMPTOMS AND DYSFUNCTIONAL VOIDING

In the absence of obstruction, we recommend conservative therapy with timed voiding, limited consumption of bladder irritants, anticholinergics, and biofeedback, especially in patients with dysfunctional voiding.

Cases in which conservative treatment has failed are obviously more difficult to treat. Botox injection into the detrusor muscle has been used for refractory urge symptoms.[78] Injection of Xylocaine and steroids periurethrally has been used to treat external sphincter spasticity and dysfunctional voiding.[78] Botox injection into the external sphincter has resulted in significant subjective improvement in voiding in 67% of patients after a single dose.[79] Smith and associates[80] demonstrated the efficacy of this treatment for functional urethral obstruction and detrusor acontractility after pubovaginal sling surgery. Finally, neuromodulation has also been used with some success.[78]

CONCLUSION

MUI is a common yet poorly understood entity that is surrounded by controversy, inconsistent definitions, and many differing opinions. Several potential etiologies exist, none of which has been proven definitively. However, it is likely that the cause is multifactorial, and perhaps different among patients presenting with similar symptoms. Given that a large proportion of patients are cured of their urge component by surgery aimed at correcting their SUI, we believe that the etiologies in those cases are related to severity of incontinence, facilitation of the urethrodetrusor reflex due to urine entering the proximal urethra, and/or traction on the pelvic nerves due to laxity of the pelvic floor. However, other patients may respond to more conservative therapy, namely anticholinergic medications and biofeedback, suggesting a potential alternative etiology in these cases.

It is still unknown which patients with MUI will respond to surgery and whose symptoms will remain unchanged or even intensify. It is well documented that patients with persistent urge symptoms after surgery have less satisfaction with the procedure, even if they are cured of their SUI. Patients with MUI who undergo definitive surgical therapy for their SUI need extensive counseling preoperatively to prepare them for potential adverse outcomes. Because of this, we recommend a brief trial of conservative therapy in certain patients with urge-predominant MUI, because some will improve and may not require surgery.

In short, tailoring treatment to fit the individual patient can often result in successful resolution of both the urge and the stress components in this very challenging group of patients.

Disclaimer

The opinions or assertions contained herein are the private views of the authors and are not to be construed as reflecting the views of the Department of the Army or the Department of Defense.

References

1. Abrams P, Blaivas JG, Stanton S, Andersen JT: The standardization of terminology of lower urinary tract function. Neurourol Urodyn 7:403-426, 1988.
2. Blaivas JG, Groutz A: Urinary incontinence: Pathophysiology, evaluation, and management overview. In Walsh PC, Retik AB, Vaughan ED, Wein AJ (eds): Campbell's Urology, 8th ed. Philadelphia: Saunders, 2002, pp 1027-1052.
3. Stewart WF, Van Rooyen JB, Cundiff GW, et al: Prevalence and burden of overactive bladder in the United States. World J Urol 20:327-336, 2003.
4. Bump RC, Norton PA, Zinner NR, Yalcin I, and Duloxetine Urinary Incontinence Study Group: Mixed urinary incontinence symptoms: Urodynamic findings, incontinence severity, and treatment response. Obstet Gynecol 102:76-83, 2003.
5. Sandvik H, Hunskaar S, Vanvik A, et al: Diagnostic classification of female urinary incontinence: An epidemiological survey corrected for validity. J Clin Epidemiol 48:339-343, 1995.
6. Hampel C, Wienhold D, Benken N, et al: Definition of overactive bladder and epidemiology of urinary incontinence. Urology 50(6A):4-14, 1997.

7. McGuire EJ: Mixed symptomotology. BJU Int 85(3L):47-52, 2000.
8. Cardozo LD, Stanton SL: Genuine stress incontinence and detrusor instability: A review of 200 patients. Br J Obstet Gynecol 87:184-190, 1980.
9. Weidner AC, Myers AG, Visco AG, et al: Which women with stress incontinence require urodynamics? Am J Obstet Gynecol 184:200-227, 2001.
10. Chaliha C, Khullar V: Mixed incontinence. Urology 63(3A):51-57, 2004.
11. McGuire EJ: Applying advances in neurourology to clinical practice. Stress urinary incontinence: Novel treatment approaches in the new millennium. Contemp Urol (Suppl):14-16, Sept 2002.
12. McGuire EJ, Clemens JQ: Pubovaginal slings. In Walsh PC, Retik AB, Vaughan ED, Wein AJ (eds): Campbell's Urology, 8th ed. Philadelphia: Saunders, 2002, pp 1151-1171.
13. Wein JA: Urological survey: Voiding function and dysfunction, bladder physiology and pharmacology, and female urology. J Urol 173:2054-2059, 2005.
14. Hannestad YS, Rortveit G, Sandvik H, Hunskaar S: A community-based epidemiological survey of female urinary incontinence: The Norwegian EPINCONT study. J Clin Epidemiol 53:1150-1157, 2000.
15. Coyne KS, Zhou Z, Thompson C, Versi E: The impact on health-related quality of life of stress, urge and mixed urinary incontinence. BJU Int 92:731-735, 2003.
16. McGuire EJ, Lyton G: Pubovaginal sling procedure for stress incontinence. J Urol 119:82, 1978.
17. McGuire EJ: Bladder instability in stress incontinence. Neurourol Urodyn 7:563-567, 1988.
18. Karram MM, Bhatia NN: Management of coexistent stress and urge urinary incontinence. Obstet Gynecol 73:4-7, 1989.
19. Serels SR, Rackley RR, Appell RA: Surgical treatment for stress urinary incontinence associated with Valsalva induced detrusor instability. J Urol 163:884-887, 2000.
20. Fulford SCV, Flynn R, Barrington J, et al: An assessment of the surgical outcome and urodynamic effects of the pubovaginal sling for stress incontinence and the associated urge syndrome. J Urol 162:135-137, 1999.
21. Morgan TO, Westney OL, McGuire EJ: Pubovaginal sling: Four-year outcome analysis and quality of life assessment. J Urol 163:1845-1848, 2000.
22. Cross CA, Cespedes RD, McGuire EJ: Our experience with pubovaginal slings in patients with stress incontinence. J Urol 159:1195-1198, 1998.
23. Blaivas JG, Jacobs BZ: Pubovaginal fascial sling for the treatment of complicated stress urinary incontinence. J Urol 145:1214, 1991.
24. McGuire EJ: Idiopathic bladder instability. In Kursh ED, McGuire EJ (eds): Female Urology. Philadelphia: Lippincott, 1994, pp 95-101.
25. Teleman PM, Lidfeldt J, Nerbrand C, et al: the WHILA study group: Overactive bladder: prevalence, risk factors and relation to stress incontinence in middle-aged women. BJOG 111:600-604, 2004.
26. Osman T: Stress incontinence surgery for patients presenting with mixed incontinence and a normal cystometrogram. BJU Int 92:964-968, 2003.
27. Artibani W: Diagnosis and significance of idiopathic overactive bladder. Urology 50(Suppl 6A):25-32, 1997.
28. Mahoney DT, Laferte RO, Blais DJ: Incontinence of urine due to instability of micturition reflexes. Part I: Detrusor reflex instability. Urology 15:229-239, 1980.
29. Jung SY, Fraser MO, Ozawa H, et al: Urethral afferent nerve activity affects the micturition reflexes: Implication for the relationship between stress incontinence and detrusor instability. J Urol 162:204-212, 1999.
30. Wise BG, Cardoza LD, Cutner A, et al: Prevalence and significance of urethral instability in women with detrusor instability. Br J Urol 26:72, 1993.
31. Low JA: Urethral behavior during the involuntary detrusor contraction. Am J Obstet Gynecol 32:128, 1977.
32. Hindmarsh JR, Gosling PT, Deane AM: Bladder instability: Is the primary defect in the urethra? Br J Urol 55:648-651, 1983.
33. Mahoney DT, Laferte RO, Blais DJ: Integral storage and voiding reflexes: Neurophysiologic concept of continence and micturition. Urology 9:95-105, 1977.
34. Barrington FSF: The component reflexes of micturition in the cat: Parts I and II. Brain 54:177, 1931.
35. Kiruluta HG, Downie JW, Awad SA: The continence mechanisms: The effect of bladder filling on the urethra. Invest Urol 18:460, 1981.
36. Sutherst JR, Brown M: The effect on the bladder pressure of sudden entry of fluid into the posterior urethra. Br J Urol 50:406-409, 1978.
37. McGuire EJ, Cespedes RD, Cross CA, O'Connell HE: Videourodynamic studies. Urol Clin North Am 23:309-321, 1996.
38. Kreder KJ, Brubaker L, Mainprize T: Tolterodine is equally effective in patients with mixed incontinence and those with urge incontinence alone. BJU Int 92:418-421, 2003.
39. Khullar V, Hill S, Laval KU, et al: Treatment of urge-predominant mixed urinary incontinence with tolterodine extended release: A randomized, placebo-controlled trial. Urology 64:269-274, 2004.
40. Siegel SW, Richardson DA, Miller KL, et al: Pelvic floor electrical stimulation for the treatment of urge and mixed urinary incontinence in women. Urology 50:934-940, 1997.
41. Sand PK: Pelvic floor stimulation in the treatment of mixed incontinence complicated by a low-pressure urethra. Obstet Gynecol 88:757-760, 1996.
42. Bent AE, Sand PK, Ostergard DR, Brubaker L: Transvaginal electrical stimulation in the treatment of genuine stress urinary incontinence and detrusor instability. Int Urogynecol J 4:9-13, 1993.
43. Caputo RM, Benson ST, McClellan E: Intravaginal maximal electrical stimulation in the treatment of urinary incontinence. J Reprod Med 38:667-671, 1993.
44. Goode PS: Behavioral and drug therapy for urinary incontinence. Urology 63(3 Suppl 1):58-64, 2004.
45. Davila GW, Bernier F: Multimodality pelvic physiotherapy treatment of urinary incontinence in adult women. Int Urogynecol J 6:187-194, 1995.
46. Kondo A, Yokoyama E, Koshiba K, et al: Bladder neck support prosthesis: A non-operative treatment for stress or mixed urinary incontinence. J Urol 157:824-827, 1997.
47. Scotti RJ, Angell G, Flora R, Greston WM: Antecedent history as a predictor of surgical cure of urgency symptoms in mixed incontinence. Obstet Gynecol 91:51-54, 1998.
48. Langer R, Lipshitz Y, Halperin R, et al: Long-term (10-15 years) follow-up after Burch colposuspension for urinary stress incontinence. Int Urogynecol J Pelvic Floor Dysfunct 12:1290-1291, 2001.
49. Segal JL, Vassallo B, Kleeman S, et al: Prevalence of persistent and de novo overactive bladder symptoms after the tension-free vaginal tape. Obstet Gynecol 104:1263-1269, 2004.
50. Delorme E, Droupy S, Tayrac R, Delmas V: Transobturator tape (Uratape): A new minimally-invasive procedure to treat female urinary incontinence. Eur Urol 45:203-207, 2004.
51. Richter HE, Varner RE, Sanders E, et al: Effects of pubovaginal sling procedure on patients with urethral hypermobility and intrinsic sphincteric deficiency: Would they do it again? Am J Obstet Gynecol 184:14, 2001.
52. Wright EJ, Carr LK, Webster GD: Pubovaginal sling using cadaveric allograft fascia for the treatment of intrinsic sphincteric deficiency. J Urol 63:1182, 1998.
53. Leach GE, Dmochowski RR, Appell RA, et al: Female Stress Urinary Incontinence Clinical Guidelines Panel summary report on surgical management of female stress urinary incontinence. J Urol 158:875-880, 1997.

54. Iglesia CB, Shott S, Fenner DE, Brubaker L: Effect of preoperative voiding mechanism on success rate of autologous rectus fascia suburethral sling procedure. Obstet Gynecol 91:577-581, 1998.
55. Nilsson CG, Falconer C, Rezapour M: Seven-year follow-up of the tension-free vaginal tape procedure for treatment of urinary incontinence. Obstet Gynecol 104:1259-1262, 2004.
56. Spinosa JP, Dubuis PY: Suburethral sling inserted by the transobturator route in the treatment of female stress urinary incontinence: Preliminary results in 117 cases. Eur J Obstet Gynecol Reprod Biol 123:212-217, 2005. Epub 2005 Jul 15.
57. Pope AJ, Shaw PJR, Coptcoat MJ, et al: Changes in bladder function following a surgical alteration in outflow resistance. Neurourol Urodyn 9:503-508, 1990.
58. Klutke JJ, Klutke CG, Bergman J, Elia G: Urodynamics changes in voiding after anti-incontinence surgery: An insight into the mechanism of cure. Urology 54:1003-1007, 1999.
59. Blair G, Tessier J, Bertrand PE, et al: Retropubic cystourethropexy: Is it an obstructive procedure? J Urol 158:553-538, 1997.
60. Sandler P, Moller LM, Rudnicki PM, et al: Does the tension-free vaginal tape procedure affect the voiding phase? Pressure-flow studies before and 1 year after surgery. BJU Int 89:694-698, 2000.
61. Kuo HC: Videourodynamic results after pubovaginal sling procedure for stress urinary incontinence. Urology 54:802-807, 1999.
62. Monga AK, Stanton SL: Urodynamics: Prediction, outcome, and analysis of mechanism for cure of stress incontinence by periurethral collagen. Br J Obstet Gynecol 104:158-162, 1997.
63. Westney OL, Lee JT, McGuire EJ, et al: Long-term results of Ingelman-Sundberg denervation procedure for urge incontinence refractory to medical therapy. J Urol 168:1044-1047, 2002.
64. Arnold EP, Webster JR, Loose H, et al: Urodynamics of female incontinence: Factors influencing the results of surgery. Am J Obstet Gynecol 117:805-813, 1973.
65. Columbo M, Zanetta G, Vitobello D, Milani R: The Burch colposuspension for women with and without detrusor overactivity. BJOG 103:255-260, 1996.
66. Alcalay M, Monga A, Stanton SL: Burch colposuspension: A 10-20 year follow up. Br J Obstet Gynaecol 102:740-745, 1995.
67. Chou ECL, Flisser AJ, Panagopoulos G, Blaivas JG: Effective treatment for mixed urinary incontinence with a pubovaginal sling. J Urol 170:494-497, 2003.
68. Chaikin DC, Rosenthal J, Blaivas JG: Pubovaginal fascial sling for all types of stress urinary incontinence: Long-term analysis. J Urol 160:1312-1316, 1998.
69. Jorgensen L, Lose G, Molsted-Pedersen L: Vaginal repair in female motor urge incontinence. Eur Urol 13:382, 1987.
70. Lockhart JL, Vorstman B, Politano VA: Anti-incontinence surgery in females with detrusor instability. Neurourol Urodyn 3:201, 1984.
71. Schrepferman CG, Griebling TL ,Nygaard IE, Kreder KJ: Resolution of urge symptoms following sling cystourethropexy. J Urol 164:1628-1631, 2000.
72. McGuire EJ, Savastano JA: Stress incontinence and detrusor instability/urge incontinence. Neurourol Urodyn 4:313-316, 1985.
73. Demarco E, Heritz DM, Blaivas JG: Can we predict which patients will have urge incontinence following pubovaginal sling? [abstract 770]. J Urol 151:420A, 1994.
74. Meyhoff HH, Walter S, Gerstenberg TC, et al: Incontinence surgery in female motor urge incontinence. Acta Obstet Gynecol Scand 62:365-368, 1983.
75. Miller EA, Amundsen CL, Toh KL, et al: Preoperative urodynamic evaluation may predict voiding dysfunction in women undergoing pubovaginal sling. J Urol 169:2234-2237, 2003.
76. Carr LK, Webster GD: Voiding dysfunction following incontinence surgery: Diagnosis and treatment with retropubic or vaginal urethrolysis. J Urol 157:821, 1997.
77. Nitti VW, Raz S: Obstruction following anti-incontinence procedures: Diagnosis and treatment with transvaginal urethrolysis. J Urol 152:93, 1994.
78. Kershen RT, Appell RA: Voiding dysfunction after anti-incontinence surgery in women. Issues in Incontinence Spring/Summer:1-10, 2003.
79. Phelan MW, Franks M, Somogyi GT, et al: Botulinum toxin urethral sphincter injection to restore bladder emptying in men and women with voiding dysfunction. J Urol 165:1107-1110, 2001.
80. Smith CP, O'Leary M, Erickson J, et al: Botulinum toxin urethral sphincter injection resolves urinary retention after pubovaginal sling operation. Int Urogynecol J 13:55-56, 2002.

Chapter 49

COMPLICATIONS OF INCONTINENCE PROCEDURES IN WOMEN

Chad Huckabay and Victor W. Nitti

Stress urinary incontinence (SUI) is a common problem that affects millions of women in the United States. Various treatments exist, including physiotherapy, medications, devices, periurethral bulking agents, and more definitive surgeries. In contrast to less invasive therapies, surgery for SUI is associated with relatively high success rates. However, it also has potentially higher risks of morbidity and, rarely, mortality. Typically, surgery for SUI involves restoring support to the bladder neck, proximal urethra, or mid-urethra. Traditionally, anti-incontinence procedures have been broadly categorized as anterior repairs, transvaginal needle suspensions, retropubic suspensions, and sling procedures. More recently, midurethral synthetic slings, done in a minimally invasive fashion, have become the most popular procedures to treat SUI.

In addition to procedure-specific complications, there are a number of complications that are common to all types of incontinence surgery. Although complication rates vary, they have been reported to approach 50%. This chapter discusses the types of complications encountered when performing the various procedures with respect to their temporal occurrence (intraoperative, sequelae of intraoperative complications, then early and late postoperative problems). To better avoid complications, the surgeon should know how to thoroughly evaluate SUI in each individual patient. Careful preoperative planning is crucial, as is knowledge of specific surgical techniques. These factors inherent to avoiding complications are discussed elsewhere in this text. In this chapter, we focus specifically on the complications themselves.

INTRAOPERATIVE COMPLICATIONS

Bleeding

A thorough history should uncover any bleeding diathesis. Significant bleeding is infrequent in either transabdominal or transvaginal approaches, occurring in 0.6% to 10% of cases.[1] In one study,[2] of 117 women who underwent Marshall-Marchetti-Krantz (MMK) cystourethropexy, 20 lost more than 500 mL of blood and 5 lost more than 1200 mL. Intraoperative bleeding during transabdominal approaches most commonly occurs in the retropubic space, owing to its rich network of venous complexes. If bleeding cannot be controlled by suture ligating, packing may be used.

During transvaginal procedures, bleeding commonly occurs at two points. The first is during the dissection of the vaginal wall off of the periurethral fascia. If this dissection is too deep, bleeding can be encountered. It is important to carry out dissection just above the glistening white surface of the fascia. This can be more difficult in cases of previous surgery, and greater care should be taken to ensure that the proper plane is dissected. The second point at which bleeding may occur is with perforation of the endopelvic fascia. This bleeding can be difficult to control, because the vessels responsible may not be directly visible. We have found that the best way to control this bleeding is to place the sling (or suspension sutures) and transfer them to the suprapubic region expeditiously. Also, a vaginal packing placed after closure of the vaginal wall helps to tamponade bleeding. The retropubic space is a contained space, and bleeding is usually self-limited. If vaginal packing is ineffective, a Foley catheter balloon has been reported to achieve transvaginal tamponade.[3,4] Rarely, embolization may be done. Recently, Zorn and colleagues reported successful embolization of massive retropubic hemorrhage from a branch of the obturator artery injured during placement of a tension-free vaginal tape sling (TVT).[5]

With the widespread use of TVT and other midurethral slings, surgeons should be aware of problems related to bleeding specific to this procedure. Nilsson and Kuuva reported a retropubic hematoma rate of 3.3% and an additional 3.3% of patients with blood loss of greater than 200 mL.[6] Flock and associates reported that a pelvic hematoma larger than 300 mL and requiring surgical intervention was found in 1.2% of patients.[7] In 7 cases (2.1%), increased intraoperative blood loss (250 to 400 mL) was managed by cauterization, compression, or tamponade.[7] Others have reported hemorrhage rates of 0.9% to 2.5% with TVT.[8-10] In the Austrian registry of 2795 TVT procedures, 0.7% of the patients required laparotomy for bleeding control or evacuation of hematomas.[11] Kuuva and Nilssons[12] reported an incidence of 0.1% for injury to major vessels and nerves in their cohort of 1455 patients.

For the TVT procedure, the trocars are usually placed blindly, and knowledge of pelvic anatomy is crucial in avoiding disastrous complications. Deviation of curved trocars laterally can cause injury to the external iliac vein[13] or artery[14] and to the obturator neurovascular bundle. Cephalad displacement of the TVT trocar can cause injury not only to bowel but also to the iliac vessels more proximally. Patient movement during a TVT procedure peformed with local anesthesia can directly cause deviation from the intended path of the trocar. Anatomic dissections and cadaver studies have shown that the TVT trocars pass an average 4.9 cm from the external iliacs and 3.2 cm from the obturator vessels.[15] With the transobturator (TOT) approach to placement of the TVT, the device passed on average 1.1 ± 0.4 cm from the most medial branch of the obturator vessels. The mean distance to the obturator nerve was 2.5 ± 0.7 cm.[16] Currently, 30 cases of major blood vessel injury have been reported, including 2 fatalities.[17] No significant bleeding complications have been reported with the TVT placed in a transobturator route. In most cases, bleeding after TVT procedures is self-limited and no specific intervention, other than perhaps transfusion, is required. However, in cases of large blood loss, open exploration or embolization may be necessary.[5,11]

Bladder and Urethral Injuries

Historically, injuries to the bladder and urethra occurred as a result of perforation during dissection or inadvertent placement of a suture or needle through the bladder or urethra. Today, most injuries to the urinary tract, and to the bladder specifically, are secondary to trocar injury at the time of minimally invasive midurethral sling placement. Cystoscopy during incontinence surgery is critical to rule out such injuries.

If injury to the bladder, bladder neck, or urethra occurs as a result of needle or trocar passage or suture placement, it is usually recognized during cystoscopy, after suspension sutures or pubovaginal slings have been transferred. In our experience, this occurs more commonly in cases in which the needle is passed "blindly" rather than under direct finger guidance. If the injuries are small and are not associated with tearing, the sutures or instruments can simply be removed and replaced. The small perforation should heal with several days of catheter drainage. Larger injuries should be repaired with absorbable suture, and urethral tears should be treated with at least 5 to 7 days of catheter drainage. If a urethral injury occurs, absorbable suture may close the defect, depending on size and location. For TVT and similar devices, the trocar should be removed and another pass of the trocar should be performed. Bladder injury due to intravesical trocar passage may be treated with 48 to 72 hours of continuous bladder drainage with a Foley catheter. Bladder perforation from the TVT trocars occurs in 1.1% to 25% of TVT cases.[12,18-22] The higher rates of bladder perforations occur in cases of previous failed anti-incontinence surgeries causing retropubic scarification. There may be a propensity for bladder perforations to occur opposite the side of the surgeon's dominant hand.[23]

It is paramount to find intravesical TVT sling material during the initial placement, because secondary postoperative detection may require significant retropubic surgery. It is important to fill the bladder with at least 250 mL of irrigant or to near bladder capacity, because folds of mucosa may otherwise hide the tape. The 70-degree lens shows the anterolateral bladder wall, and the 0- and 12-degree lenses show the urethra optimally. Buchsbaum and colleagues[24] reported on bladder injuries identified not by cystoscopy but by having high fluid/irrigant leakage from trocar or incision sites. Shobieri and coworkers[25] reported a series of occult bladder injuries with TVT seen not on initial cystoscopy but only after removal and retrieval of trocars on second cystoscopy. In the TOT passage of synthetic midurethal tapes, case reports exist, and one series reported a 0.5% incidence of bladder perforations; hence, we recommend cystoscopy in this procedure as well.[26,27] Using an inside-to-outside technique of TOT trocar passage, de Leval[28] reported no instances of bladder perforation or visceral injuries in a series of 107 patients. The technique clearly holds promise, and further randomized studies to determine efficacy and complications of this technique should be performed.

Injuries occurring during transvaginal procedures that are closer to the bladder neck should be repaired primarily. These commonly occur when the vaginal dissection is done deep to the periurethral fascia and the surgeon attempts to perforate into the retropubic space. These injuries tend to be larger than trocar or needle perforations, and primary closure is usually recommended. If such an injury is found, a two-layer closure with absorbable sutures (e.g., polyglycolic acid) can usually be accomplished transvaginally. A drain can be placed in the retropubic space percutaneously from the suprapubic area, in much the same way that the suspension needle is passed, but this is rarely needed. Infrequently, a retropubic approach must be taken to ensure proper closure of a massive injury. If there is a history of prior pelvic radiation therapy in a patient who has sustained a bladder injury, tissue interposition (i.e., omentum, labial fat pat) is recommended.[29,30]

If an injury at or near the bladder neck occurs, we usually recommend against placing a synthetic sling in such cases, because the risk of erosion is probably increased. However, we have successfully placed autologous fascial slings in under such circumstances.

For retropubic procedures, bladder repair is usually easy, as long as the injury is recognized. If an injury is suspected but cannot be found, the bladder can be filled with methylene blue or other irrigant to better identify leakage. Cystoscopy also may be instrumental. We prefer a primary two-layer closure with absorbable sutures. Depending on the size of the injury and the quality of the closure, a drain may be placed for several days, but usually this is not necessary in the absence of infection. In any case, the bladder should remain on catheter drainage for 5 to 7 days.

Ureteral Injuries

Injuries to the ureters are much less common than bladder and urethral injuries. They may be encountered in retropubic operations (e.g., MMK, Burch) as well as transvaginal procedures (needle suspensions and pubovaginal slings), and they usually occur near the ureterovesical junction.[31] Rosen and colleagues,[32] in a review article, reported 19 ureteral injuries in the literature secondary to Burch colposuspension (Table 49-1). It is important to emphasize that there may also be a risk of ureteral kinking with overcorrection, as described in the original article.[33] Erikson and associates reported a 1% rate if unrecognized ureteral obstruction.[34] Perforating injuries can be managed by removing the suture and stenting the ureter. If the injury is severe, ureteral reimplantation may be necessary. Ureteral injuries should be suspected if, on cystoscopy during anti-incontinence procedures, no efflux is seen from the ureteral orifices. If a delayed diagnosis of ureteral obstruction or laceration is made postoperatively, the patient may present with unexplained flank pain, fever, or drainage. An intravenous urogram, retrograde ureteropyelography, or computed tomographic urogram will usually delineate the injury. Immediate retrograde ureteral stenting is recommended. If this

Table 49-1 Ureteral Injury or Kinking with Burch Colposuspension

Authors and Ref. No.	*N*	Ureteral Injury/Kinking (%)
Klutke et al.[152]	97	0
Harris et al.[153]	60	6.7
Eriksen et al.[3]	75	1.3
Galloway et al.[154]	50	2
Korda et al.[155]	174	1.1
Petri[156]	1500	0.2

is not possible, stenting can be performed in an antegrade fashion. If this fails, open repair with removal of suture and sometimes ureteroneocystostomy are necessary. Ureteral injuries are uncommon with transvaginal procedures and usually involve the inclusion of the ureter in the suspension sutures. If this is recognized intraoperatively (when indigo carmine is not seen excreted from the ureter), the suspension sutures should be removed. It may be helpful to place a stent before replacing the suspension suture, but this is rarely needed. If such an injury is discovered after surgery, during the postoperative period, it is handled in the same fashion as described previously. We know of no cases of ureteral injuries associated with TVT.

Other Injuries

If the peritoneum is inadvertently incised during either approach, it should be closed with an absorbable suture. Bowel injuries are rare but can occur with transfer of sutures or slings and with TVT and similar procedures. They may also occur with placement of a suprapubic tube. A small bowel laceration and small perforations of the colon below the peritoneal reflection can usually be closed primarily. However, perforations of the colon above the peritoneal reflection in unprepared bowel may require proximal colostomy if significant spillage occurs intraperitoneally. Bowel injuries have not been reported with the TOT procedure. The traditional TVT trocars passed retropubically may cause bowel injury when the trocars do not "shave" the posterior aspect of the pubis and are directed more cephalad. The risk of bowel perforation is small, but several cases have been reported.[8,35-38] Patients with prior transperitoneal pelvic surgeries are at highest risk. Peyrat recommended preoperative computed tomography in women with a history of multiple abdominal and retropubic surgeries, which increase the risk of bowel adhesion to the pubis.[39] Patients typically present with abdominal pain, peritoneal signs, or leakage of feculent material from suprapubic incision sites. High suspicion levels for bowel injury should be maintained for those patients complaining of abdominal pain after TVT. A small bowel obstruction caused by intraperitoneal TVT performed with concomitant vaginal hysterectomy for prolapse was reported.[40]

Sequelae of Intraoperative Injuries

Fistula

A fistula may develop after a surgical injury to the urinary tract. Unrecognized bladder or urethral injury may lead to a vesicovaginal or a urethrovaginal fistula, respectively (Fig. 49-1). If intraoperative cystoscopy is routinely used as described by Stamey,[41] urethral and bladder injuries should be recognized, thereby decreasing the risk of subsequent fistula formation. Some instances of unrecognized injuries missed by cystoscopy may be detected when fluid leakage is more than expected from incision sites. Methylene blue or sterile infant formula may also be instilled into the bladder to aid detection. Kuuva and Nilsson, in a nationwide analysis of complications associated with TVT in 1455 patients, found only one case for an incidence of 0.7/1000 of vesicovaginal fistula.[12]

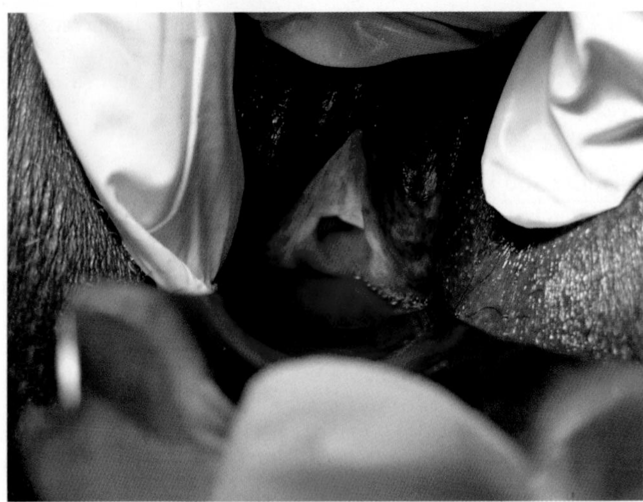

Figure 49-1 Urethrovaginal fistula after major urethral injury during anti-incontinence procedure.

Nerve Injury

Three types of nerve injury may occur during incontinence surgery. The first is a result of intraoperative positioning. The most common nerve injured is the common peroneal nerve; injury is caused by direct compression of the nerve against the leg support while the patient is in the dorsal lithotomy position. A femoral nerve palsy may result from hyperflexion of the hip wherein the thigh is brought too cephalad and in a prolonged position may cause postoperative weakness of the thigh extensor muscles. A second type of nerve injury involves direct trauma to the nerve during surgery. Intraoperative events may pose injurious risk to the ilioinguinal nerve as it travels in the vicinity of suprapubic transverse incisions, needles, slings, and trocar passages. Geis and Dietl first reported ilioinguinal nerve entrapment by TVT.[42] Local anesthetic injections along the nerve can aid in diagnosis and treatment without the need for TVT removal. Patients present with lower abdominal wall pain radiating into the groin, labia majora, or upper inner thigh. Certainly, the obturator nerve is at risk in placement of midurethral synthetic slings (e.g., TVT, TOT).[21,43,44] A third type of nerve injury involves disruption of the innervation of the urethra and surrounding structures. Some evidence suggests that vaginal dissection may affect this innervation. Zivkovic and colleagues[45] showed that vaginal dissection, especially during endoscopic bladder neck suspension, can worsen preexisting perineal neuropathy in patients with SUI. Vaginal innervation seems to be concentrated on the anterior vagina[46] and may be affected by anti-incontinence operations. Modification of innervation of the anterior vaginal wall could account for postoperative discomfort with intercourse.[47] It is unknown whether alterations in neuroanatomy are responsible for some cases of sexual dysfunction after anti-incontinence procedures. Mazouni and associates[48] reported that 25.6% of patients who were monitored prospectively with questionnaires had some deterioration of sexual function after TVT placement. Glavind and Tetsche[49] found that 23% of previously sexually active women reported improved sexual life. Maaita and colleagues[50] reported no change in sexual function after TVT procedures. Only prospective studies using validated symptom questionnaires will delineate the impact of TVT and incontinence treatment on sexual functioning.

Table 49-2 Postoperative Retention with Tension-Free Vaginal Tape Procedures

Authors and Ref. No.	*N*	No. Patients with Retention (%)	No. with Resolution
Karram et al.[10]	350	17 (4.9)	11
Hung et al.[158]	23	2 (8.7)	0
Tsivian et al.[68]	200	14 (7)	0
de Tayrac et al.[159]	31	8 (25.8)	8
Levin et al.[67]	313	8 (2.5)	7
Abouassaly et al.[9]	241	47 (19.5)	37
Paick et al.[157]	247	38 (13.9)	33

EARLY POSTOPERATIVE COMPLICATIONS

Voiding Dysfunction

Immediate postoperative urinary retention is the most common type of voiding dysfunction encountered after any anti-incontinence procedure (Table 49-2). Kelly and colleagues[51] reported acute urinary retention requiring catheterization in 41% of 114 women who underwent modified Pereyra bladder neck suspension. Twenty-seven percent of women undergoing MMK cystourethropexy had postoperative urinary retention, according to Parnell and associates.[52] Yalcin and coworkers[53] noted that 3.2% of patients had temporary voiding dysfunction after TVT. In most of these patients, urinary retention (complete or partial) is transient, secondary to postoperative edema of the bladder neck and urethra, and resolves with catheter drainage. The estimated probability of temporary urinary retention lasting longer than 4 weeks is 5% for retropubic and transvaginal suspensions and 8% for sling procedures.[54]

Various options for drainage are available, including suprapubic tube drainage. Occasionally, a suprapubic tube is placed intraoperatively in anticipation of immediate postoperative urinary retention. This is kept in place until normal emptying resumes (usually 1 to 4 weeks). Suprapubic tube placement is less common with midurethral synthetic slings, because most patients void within 24 hours after surgery. Intermittent catheterization or an indwelling urethral catheter may also be used. It has been our experience that normal emptying occurs a bit sooner after retropubic procedures compared with transvaginal suspensions or traditional pubovaginal slings. Permanent retention is much less common (see later discussion).

Irritative or storage symptoms, including frequency, urgency, and urge incontinence, are also common after incontinence surgery. Usually, this is not a problem in the immediate postoperative period, if the patient is well prepared. It is important to be sure that the patient is emptying well; if not, intermittent catheterization should be considered. In the patient who is emptying well, a trial of anticholinergic drugs can be used. Sometimes, however, it is only time that will cure this problem. Postoperative voiding symptoms are likely to persist for up to 4 weeks. Patients with preoperative urgency are more likely to have continued urgency postoperatively (13% to 68% for pubovaginal slings and 22% to 79% for retropubic suspensions) than those with no preoperative urgency (3% to 45% and 0% to 33%, respectively).[54]

Infection

Urinary tract infections (UTIs) in the immediate postoperative period are uncommon, provided that preoperative urine cultures are negative and perioperative antibiotics are employed. If patients present with acute symptoms of a UTI, including increased irritative symptoms, during the first few months after surgery, urine culture should be obtained, and if it is positive the patient should be treated with appropriate antibiotics. Debodinance and colleagues[55] found an incidence of UTI of 4.5% in a series of 800 patients having anti-incontinence procedures, of whom 281 had TVT. UTI rates are usually related to length of catheterization. Rarely, a patient develops recurrent postoperative UTI despite complete emptying of the bladder. In these cases, cystoscopy should be performed to rule out suture or sling erosion (see later discussion). However, in our experience, there are a small number of patients who develop recurrent UTI after incontinence surgery with no obvious cause.

The incidence of wound infections varies from 2% to 16%.[56-58] The wound infection rate after TVT was 0.4% in a single series.[9] Predisposing factors are no different than those for any other surgery and include obesity, diabetes, immunocompromise, and reoperation. The vagina is a contaminated space; therefore, we routinely cleanse the vagina with a Hibiclens or povidone sponge before the surgical preparation to minimize infection. Perioperative antibiotics are important in the prevention of infection. We routinely use ampicillin and gentamicin perioperatively for the prevention of infection. An oral cephalosporin or quinolone is used for 7 days postoperatively.

Pelvic infections and abscess are rare occurrences. Appropriate management should include broad-spectrum antibiotics and usually surgical drainage (vaginal or abdominal) depending on size. Neuman managed two infected hematomas after TVT with ultrasound-guided aspiration and antibiotics, avoiding open surgery and removal of TVT material.[59] One case of necrotizing fasciitis with massive debridement after TVT has been reported, but it is questionable whether this was primarily related to the TVT or whether seeding or contamination of incision sites from a distal infected extremity occurred.[60]

DELAYED OR LATE POSTOPERATIVE COMPLICATIONS

Pain

After needle suspension, some patients experience a chronic suprapubic pain that may radiate down the medial aspect of the inner thigh or cause a pulling sensation. This is thought to occur because of entrapment of the sensory branches of the ilioinguinal nerve or the genital branches of the genitofemoral nerve as the suspension sutures are tied to the rectus fascia.[61] This complication was noted in as many as 8% to 16% of patients in early series.[62] The passage of needles and trocars closer to the midline and adjacent to the pubic bone should reduce the risk of this complications. Hilton and associates[63] reported two cases of chronic vaginal and pelvic pain of unknown etiology in patients who were eventually found to have eroded intraurethral/bladder neck TVT. We also have seen patients with pain out of proportion to physical examination findings who were subsequently found to have urethrally eroded TVT.

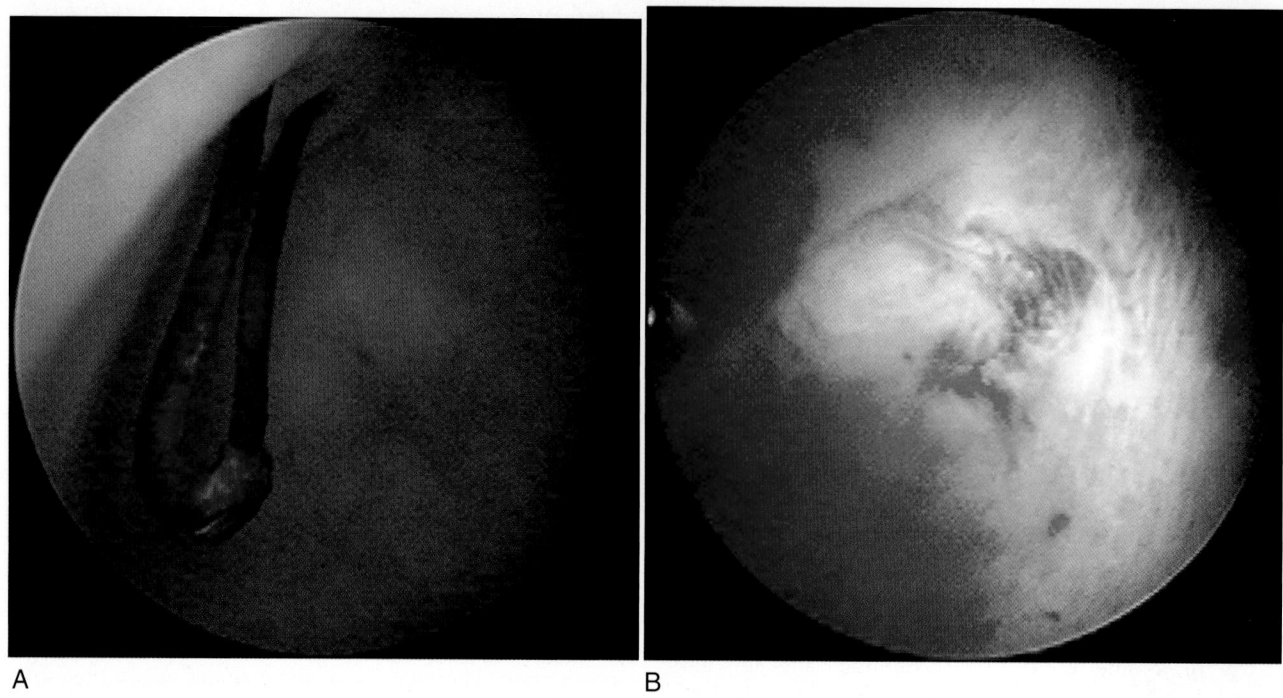

Figure 49-2 A, Intravesical Burch colposuspension suture with small calculus. B, After holmium:YAG ablation of suture and calculus.

Table 49-3 Urethral Erosion/Vaginal Extrusion of Synthetic Slings

Authors and Ref. No.	Sling	*N*	Urethral Erosion (*n*)	Vaginal Extrusion (*n*)	Total Erosion (*n* [%])
Karram et al.[10]	TVT	350	1	2	3 (0.9)
Levin et al.[67]	TVT	313	0	4	4 (1.3)
Tsivian et al.[68]	TVT	200	1	5	6 (3)
Kuuva & Nilsson[12]	TVT	1455	0	0	0 (0)
Kobashi & Govier[69]	Polypropylene	90	0	4	4 (4.4)
Rodriquez & Raz[66]	Polypropylene	301	0	1	1 (0.33)
Abouassaly et al.[9]	TVT	241	0	2	2 (0.008)
Paick et al.[157]	TVT	247	0	0	0 (0)

TVT, tension-free vaginal tape.

Suture Erosion

Rarely, a patient presents with postoperative irritative symptoms and/or recurrent UTI secondary to a permanent suture that has "eroded" into the bladder (Fig. 49-2A). These sutures, or slings in the case of TVT,[64] may act as a nidus for stone formation. It is more likely that this phenomenon occurs due to unrecognized placement of sutures into or through the bladder rather than an actual erosion. Most of the time, suture erosion can be treated endoscopically by cutting the suture, which often retracts through the bladder wall, or by using the holmium:yttrium-aluminum-garnet (YAG) laser to ablate the suture and/or stone (see Fig. 49-2B).[65]

Infection and Erosion of Sling Material

Vaginal Extrusion

The exposure of synthetic material uncovered by vaginal epithelium is more properly termed vaginal *extrusion* rather than vaginal *erosion* (Fig. 49-3; Table 49-3). Vaginal extrusion is uncommon. Possible reasons for this complication are subclinical infection, inadequate vaginal incision closure, impaired wound healing, and tape/sling rejection. For the TVT, local vaginal flaps around the extruded site can be created and advanced over the exposed tape. Alternatively, the exposed tape can be excised, with vaginal flaps used to close the defect. A small area may be observed and treated with local estrogen cream, allowing re-epithelialization. Vaginal extrusion rates for TVT and polypropylene slings have varied from 0% to 4.4%.[10,12,66-69] Other materials, such as polyester multifilament (Mersilene), silicone, polytetrafluoroethylene (Gore-Tex, Teflon), or even multifilament polypropylene, have higher extrusion and infection rates.[70] Pore size less than 10 μm increases the risk of infection, because bacteria may enter the interstices but macrophages and neutrophils larger than 10 μm cannot penetrate the pores of the mesh to fight infection. Monofilament polypropylene also may have better incorporation into surrounding tissues, because its pores allow passage of fibrocytes.

Infected type I mesh can usually be removed partially or in the segment involved. TVT is a macroporous type I mesh with

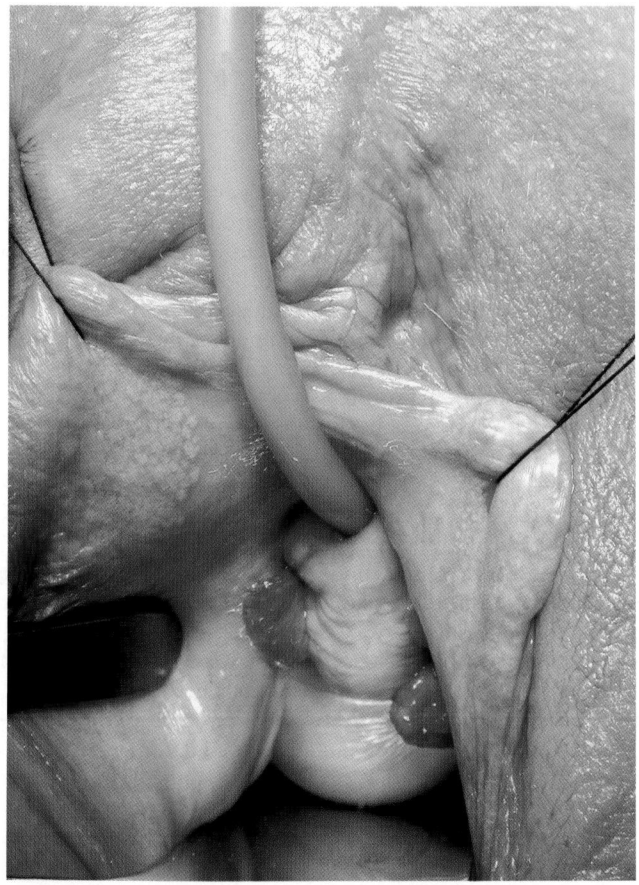

Figure 49-3 Vaginal extrusion of synthetic tape material and bone anchors used to fix the sling. Note primarily the existence of granulation tissue. Granulation tissue in the vagina often is associated with underlying foreign body extrusion through the vaginal epithelium, although the foreign body itself may be obscured.

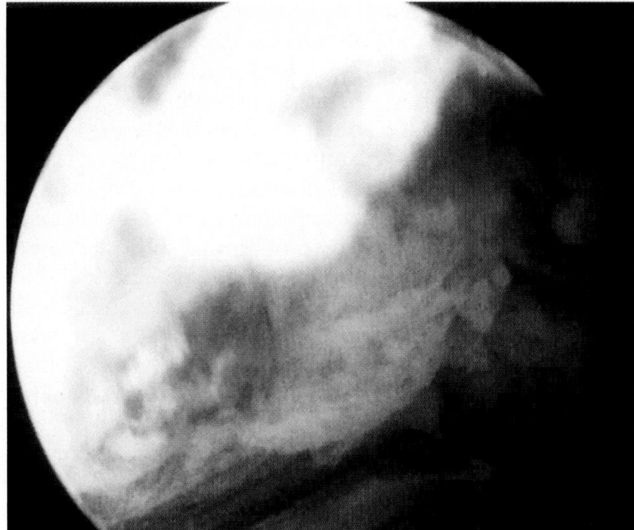

Figure 49-4 Intravesical tension-free vaginal tape found on cystoscopy for recurrent urinary tract infections. Pain in the suprapubic or vaginal/perineal area may also be a presentation of intravesical or intraurethral suburethral sling placement.

pores larger than 75 μm that allow bacteria, macrophages, and fibroblasts to enter the pores.[71] An exception is when type I mesh has been anchored to tissue using permanent multifilament sutures that harbor infection. Types II and III mesh usually have to be removed entirely if they become infected. Type III mesh has microporous portions that allow sequestration of bacteria but not macrophages.[72] TVT extrusion in the lateral vaginal fornices may result from improper placement of the sling during the TOT technique when the vaginal epithelium is inadvertently punctured with the trocar.

Urethral Erosions

Urethral erosion is quite uncommon. Leach and coworkers[54] reported an erosion rate of 0.003% with autologous slings and 0.02% with synthetic slings. It most likely results from dissection too close to the urethra with thinning and devascularization of tissues, placement of the sling between the urethra and periurethral fascia, excessive tension, or direct urethral injury including perforation that is missed. If the periurethral fascia is disrupted beneath the urethra, then it is best to repair the periurethral fascia before placement of the suburethral sling. In the use of trocars, more caution should be used when passing trocars toward the urethra rather than away, because the surgeon usually has less precise control of the distal aspect of the trocar. Small (seemingly inconsequential) movements of the proximal aspect of trocars translate to much larger ranges of movement in the distal trocar. Finger guidance is very helpful when trocars are passed toward the urethra.

A high index of suspicion must be maintained, because the presentation of urethral erosion can be quite delayed and of variable symptomatology. Patients may have dysuria, irritative or obstructive symptoms, recurrent incontinence, pain, vaginal discharge, UTIs, hematuria, pyuria, or other symptoms and signs. Slings can be removed endoscopically by cutting each end of the eroded material.[73,74] We prefer an open approach via transvaginal suburethral incision in which all eroded material is removed from the urethral wall. Repair of the urethra with absorbable suture should be performed, and a catheter should be left in place for 5 to 10 days, depending of the extent of the injury. In severe cases, local flaps may be necessary to cover the repair and prevent fistulization.

For intravesical synthetic sling erosions or placements, the holmium:YAG laser may ablate the intravesical portion of the sling. For more complicated cases, an open retropubic approach may be needed for complete excision (Fig. 49-4).

Osteitis Pubis and Osteomyelitis

Osteitis pubis is a noninfectious inflammation of the periosteum overlying the symphysis pubis that usually occurs 1 to 8 weeks after the inciting event. It manifests with symptoms and signs of suprapubic pain and tenderness, adductor spasm, elevated erythrocyte sedimentation rate, and a "waddling" gait. It has been historically associated with the MMK cystourethropexy, and its incidence ranges from 1% to 10%, depending on the series.[52,75,76] Plain film radiography is usually diagnostic; however, on occasion, a bone scan may be necessary to demonstrate increased activity in the area of the pubis. With osteitis pubis, there may be a delay in radiographic appearance after clinical symptoms of 3 to 4 weeks. Although the symptoms are disabling, they usually resolve over time with conservative management consisting of bed rest and anti-inflammatory agents.

Several modifications of the needle suspension and bladder neck sling that involve anchoring of the suspension/sling to bone have been described.[77-80] The theoretical advantages of bone anchoring have not been proven in randomized, controlled studies. Goldberg and colleagues[81] reported that three (1.3%) of their patients who underwent suprapubic bone-anchored bladder neck suspension later developed osteomyelitis requiring debridement, removal of bone anchors, and long-term intravenous antibiotics. Others have reported cases of osteomyelitis after various incontinence procedures using bone anchoring devices.[82-85] Both osteitis pubis and osteomyelitis may be characterized by the absence of fever, symmetric bony destruction of the symphysis, pelvic pain and gait disturbances, a delayed onset of symptoms, and failure to improve with antibiotics alone. In a literature review, Frederick and coworkers[86] found the incidence of osteitis pubis and osteomyelitis to be 0.16% and 0.08%, respectively, after transvaginal bone anchor fixation. It is unknown whether removal of bone anchors is helpful, and this is not absolutely indicated unless associated infection exists.

Chronic Voiding Dysfunction and Retention

The true incidence of iatrogenic voiding dysfunction after anti-incontinence surgery is unknown and varies among the different types of procedures. In a large series of 503 patients that compared Burch colposuspension to Stamey endoscopic needle suspension, voiding dysfunction was noted to be the most frequent complication (12.1%).[87] Voiding dysfunction after incontinence surgery is usually the result of obstruction, detrusor overactivity, or detrusor failure. In general, this complication, especially when it includes de novo urgency, is the most common complication after any anti-incontinence surgery.

Obstruction and Incomplete Emptying

A potential complication of all procedures to correct SUI is iatrogenic outlet obstruction leading to voiding dysfunction. This may cause urinary retention (partial or complete), obstructive voiding symptoms, or storage symptoms such as frequency, urgency, and urge incontinence.

The true incidence of voiding dysfunction and iatrogenic obstruction after incontinence surgery is unknown and is probably underestimated. Estimates of 2.5% to 24% have been reported for various procedures.[88-92] In a 1997 review, urinary retention lasting longer than 4 weeks occurred in 3 to 7% of retropubic suspensions, 4 to 8% of transvaginal suspensions, and 6 to 11% of slings. For the same procedures, urinary retention longer than 4 weeks occurred in 3% to 7%, 4% to 8%, and 6% to 11%, respectively. The incidence of permanent retention for all three procedures was thought to be less than 5%.[54] Chaikin and colleagues found postoperative de novo urge incontinence in 3%, persistent urge incontinence in 23%, and unexpected permanent urinary retention in 2% of patients undergoing pubovaginal sling procedures.[93] For the same procedure, Morgan and colleagues reported de novo urgency in 23% and de novo urge incontinence in 7%; five women had retention after 3 months requiring urethrolysis. Interestingly, they reported a 74% resolution of urge incontinence (although concomitant anterior colporrhaphy may have contributed, $P = .07$) and return to normal voiding in 92% at 1 month postoperatively.[94] Reported rates of urinary retention after TVT placement have ranged from 1.4% to 9%.[8,12,95-99] Others have described rates of voiding dysfunction after TVT as being 2% to 4%.[100]

Dunn and colleagues recently performed an extensive literature review to determine the incidence of "voiding dysfunction" after incontinence procedures.[17] They searched the Medline data base from 1966 to 2001 for various procedures. All available reports were retrospective collections, case reports, or case cohort series. Rates of voiding dysfunction varied from 4% to 22% after Burch colposuspension, 5% to 20% after MMK urethropexy, 4% to 10% after pubovaginal sling, 5% to 7% after needle suspension, and 2% to 4% after TVT. Although it cannot be said that all patients with voiding dysfunction in these series were obstructed, it can be inferred that a number were.

In patients with preexisting urgency symptoms, postoperative urgency occurs more frequently. The large review sponsored by the American Urological Association in 1997 suggested that postoperative urgency occurred in 36% to 66% of patients undergoing retropubic suspensions, in 54% after transvaginal procedures and 34% to 46% after slings.[54]

The rate of true "obstruction" may be underestimated, because irritative and obstructive symptoms tend to be overlooked in the face of normal emptying.

Whether a procedure causes an obstruction is largely based on technical factors such as suture placement or sling tension. Sutures too medial, close to the urethra, can cause urethral deviation or periurethral scarring. In addition, if sutures are tied too tightly overcorrection and "hypersuspension" of the bladder neck may result, kinking it shut. Even when properly performed, certain procedures designed to correct anatomic incontinence will cause an increase in urethral resistance. In a prospective interval analysis of patients undergoing endoscopic bladder neck suspension, Coptcoat and associates showed a ninefold increase in urethral resistance at two months after suspension in a small group of 7 patients.[101] A sling, whether at the bladder neck or at the mid-urethra, can certainly cause obstruction if it is too tight. There is no precise way to determine tension, but available techniques have kept obstruction rates reasonably low, although not zero.

The key to a diagnosis of obstruction in women is a high index of suspicion and thorough evaluation. Many women void by relaxing pelvic floor muscles, and some may augment voiding by straining. Even a slight degree of increased outlet resistance with "relative obstruction" can cause considerable voiding dysfunction. The diagnosis of obstruction after anti-incontinence procedures can be inferred if a patient remains in urinary retention despite having had normal emptying before surgery. A history of normal voiding and emptying before surgery is one of the most important factors in deciding on treatment. A review of preoperative urodynamic testing can be helpful. If such studies are not available or if the patient empties well but has irritative or obstructive symptoms, then a repeat evaluation is necessary.

No universally accepted urodynamic criteria for the diagnosis of female bladder outlet obstruction exists, and this is even more true for obstruction after SUI surgery.

Sometimes obstruction is obvious (high-pressure/low-flow voiding dynamics), but many women who are obstructed after SUI surgery do not demonstrate such voiding dynamics on urodynamic studies. Carr and Webster performed fluorourodynamic studies on all patients but eventually offered urethrolysis even to women with normal study findings when a clear temporal relationship between surgery for incontinence and the onset of voiding symptoms could be demonstrated.[102] Nitti and Raz performed video urodynamics on all patients and reported that voiding dynamics had little effect on the outcome of surgery, and, in fact, all four women who failed to generate a detrusor contraction during urodynamics voided successful after urethrolysis.[103]Foster and McGuire had similar findings.[104]We no longer believe that a complete urodynamic evaluation is necessary for those with retention or high postvoid residual volumes, provided that they had normal emptying preoperatively.[103] A patient with incomplete emptying who emptied adequately before SUI surgery should not be excluded from urethrolysis, even if hypocontractility or failure to generate a detrusor contraction occurs. Occasionally, unanticipated urodynamic findings are seen, such as learned voiding dysfunction. The utility of urodynamics may be considered as follows. First, for the patient in retention, urodynamics can provide valuable information (such as detrusor overactivity or significantly impaired compliance, the latter being an absolute indication for intervention) and can confirm a diagnosis of obstruction but should not exclude the patient from urethrolysis, even if there is no contraction or impaired contractility. Urodynamics may also identify learned voiding dysfunction. Second, for the patient with storage symptoms with normal emptying, urodynamics can diagnose obstruction and, equally as important, rule out obstruction. It can help to provide a specific diagnosis that is useful in directing therapy, especially if obstruction can be ruled out.

Endoscopic evaluation of the urethra may show scarring, narrowing, occlusion, kinking, or deviation. These finding are especially helpful in cases in which urodynamic findings are equivocal. The urethra and bladder should be carefully inspected for eroded sutures, sling material, or the presence of a fistula. This is facilitated by the use of a rigid scope with a 0- to 30-degree lens and little or no beak to allow for complete distention of the urethra. In cases in which intervention is anticipated, endoscopy should be done routinely, either before surgery or at the time of surgery before incision. Radiographic imaging may be done independent of videourodynamics. A standing cystogram in the anterior-posterior, oblique, and lateral positions, with and without straining, assesses the degree of bladder and urethral prolapse and displacement or distortion of the bladder. A voiding cystourethrogram can assess the bladder, bladder neck, and urethra during voiding to determine narrowing, kinking, or deviation. Although imaging is not mandatory, it can be extremely useful in equivocal cases.

When discussing intervention for obstruction after incontinence procedures, it is important to distinguish between midurethral synthetic slings, such as TVT, and other procedures, such as traditional pubovaginal sling, retropubic suspension, and needle suspension, because the timing and type of intervention vary. With midurethral synthetic slings, intervention is usually done sooner and is less invasive. With other procedures, longer periods of postoperative obstruction and retention are common, and intervention is usually deferred for weeks to months.

No consistent preoperative parameters, such as urethrolysis or sling incision, predict success or failure of intervention. Several studies failed to show any correlation between urodynamic findings and the likelihood of successful voiding after urethrolysis.[103-105] Without dispute, those women who have retention and increased postvoid residuals after incontinence surgery (but who had normal emptying preoperatively) are good candidates for urethrolysis. The patient's history of new voiding difficulties may be one of the most significant indicators of obstruction, independent of any other findings.

For traditional pubovaginal sling, needle suspension, and retropubic suspension procedures, most of the literature on intervention concerns patients at least 3 months out from surgery. Disappointed, uncomfortable patients with retention or significant irritative symptoms may be hard to convince that waiting is suitable. Therefore, there has been a trend to more early intervention perhaps at 1 to 2 months, especially for patients with significant retention requiring catheterization. Some patients may choose to continue intermittent catheterization indefinitely, especially if they have had marked improvement of very severe incontinence.

One can also attempt to cut suspension sutures from above in cases of obstruction after transvaginal needle suspensions. One or both sutures may be cut. In cases of pubovaginal sling, the sling may be cut in the midline after a vaginal incision has been made. However, sometimes obstruction can be effectively treated only with a formal urethrolysis. With synthetic midurethral slings such as the TVT, it has been our practice to intervene early, often within 7 to 10 days for patients in retention. In the early postoperative period, these slings can often be loosened or cut with the use of local anesthesia, occasionally in an office setting.

Techniques for Treating Postoperative Obstruction

For the synthetic midurethral slings, sling loosening techniques, urethral dilation, and sling incision alone can be performed within a shorter postoperative period before significant scarring occurs. Of note, we rarely perform sling loosening procedures and do not advocate urethral dilation.

Synthetic Midurethral Sling Loosening or Lysis

For those patients with retention within approximately 2 weeks after placement of a TVT sling, an office procedure may be used. After infiltration with local anesthetic, the previous incision is opened (usually by removal of the suture used to close the incision), and the sling is found by direct inspection or palpation. A right angle clamp is placed around the tape. During the early postoperative period (up to about 10 days), the tape may be pulled down or loosened. After longer periods of time, it is usually necessary to cut the tape. We have found this technique to be effective in relieving obstruction and the recurrence of SUI to be small. For those surgeons who are uncomfortable doing this in an office setting and for anxious patients, the same procedure may be done in the operating room. In cases of obstruction beyond 2 weeks, the lysis of the TVT sling is best performed in the operating theater, and in more chronic cases this is imperative. Scarring and patient discomfort are factors to consider, because more extensive dissection may be needed to identify and cut the sling. It is imperative to identify the sling, which may be more difficult if it has rolled onto itself in a band, and then transect the sling (Figs. 49-5 and 49-6). The suburethral portion of the sling may also be excised at the surgeon's discretion. Simply cutting or loosening a midurethral synthetic sling has yielded excellent results.[10,95,97,106] Klutke and colleagues reported resolution of obstruction in all 17 of their patients, and recurrent SUI in 1 patient.[95] Rardin and associates found that impaired bladder emptying resolved in 100% of 23 patients, with 61% remaining continent, 26% having partial recurrence, and 13% having complete recurrence of SUI.[97]

Transvaginal Pubovaginal Sling Incision

Intervention for obstruction caused by pubovaginal slings is usually done after a longer period of time than with midurethral

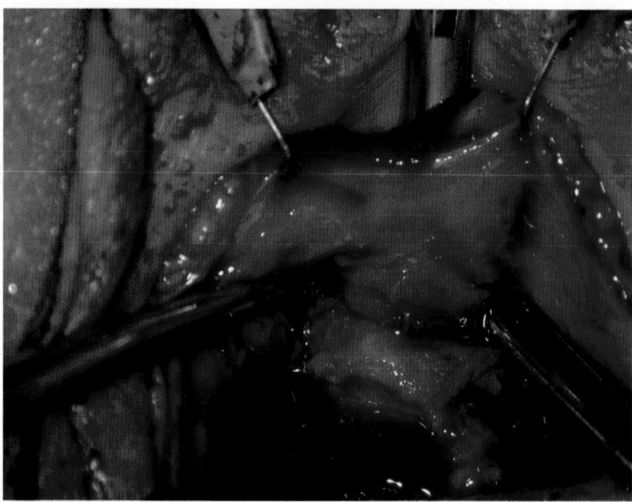

Figure 49-5 Obstructing tension-free vaginal tape (TVT) has twisted into a 2-mm band. A right angle clamp can be placed between the TVT and the periurethral fascia, and the TVT can be isolated and cut.

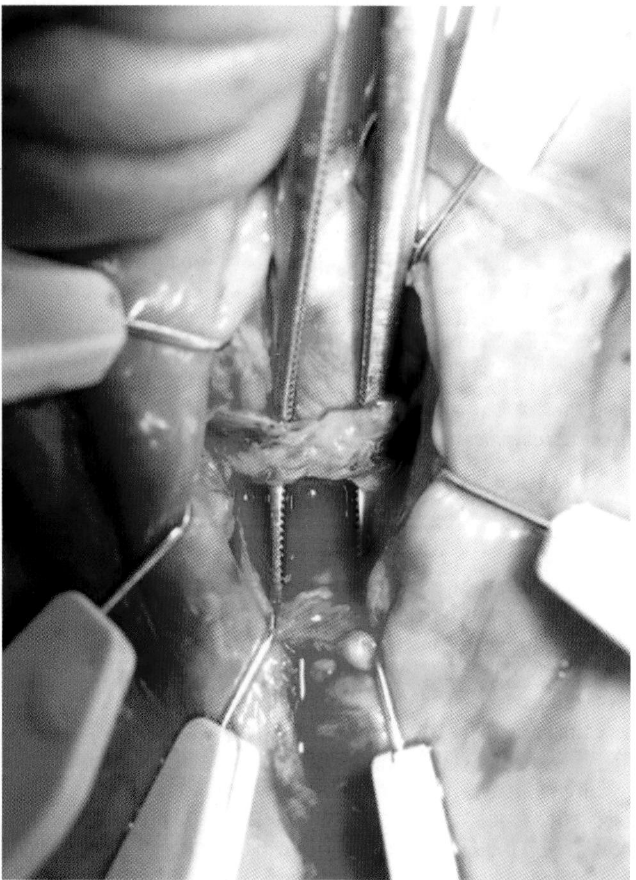

Figure 49-6 Obstructing tension-free vaginal tape. Note fibrous incorporation of sling material. After the sling is cut in the midline, a distinct "pop" and retraction of sling material occurs. Simultaneous dropping of the urethra occurs as well.

synthetic slings; the dissection is usually more extensive, so general or regional anesthesia is required. Transvaginal incision of the pubovaginal sling alone (autologous, allograft, xenograft, or synthetic) may effectively eliminate obstruction with similar results to formal urethrolysis. We, along with others, use a simple sling incision as first-line treatment.[107-110] We believe that this procedure, rather than formal urethrolysis, may limit morbidity, potential injury to soft tissue or nerve, and fibrosis from surgical dissection. Commonly, the sling is encased in scar. Initial painstaking dissection may be aided by placing a cystoscope or Walther sound in the urethra with cephalad deflection of the working end, both to bring the bladder neck down and to palpate the ridge caused by the sling. Allis clamps placed on each side (or on one side) of the sling with downward traction may facilitate dissection (Fig. 49-7). If scarification is dense, not allowing identification of the sling in the midline, it can be isolated lateral to the midline, off of the urethra. If the sling cannot be clearly cut, then formal urethrolysis should be performed (Table 49-4).

Transvaginal Urethrolysis

Because sling incision alone is commonly performed today, we offer repeat formal transvaginal urethrolysis to these patients if obstruction remains. We prefer transvaginal urethrolysis, as originally described by Leach and Raz,[111] as a primary operation (rather than retropubic urethrolysis), because it is easier, is less morbid with quicker recovery times, and is highly effective.

We begin with intraoperative cystoscopy, even if cystoscopy was previously performed clinically. We exclude foreign bodies, sutures, stones, and erosion of suture or sling. Sagittal rotation of the scope with simultaneous anterior vaginal palpation is useful. Leach and Raz (1984) originally described the most commonly used transvaginal procedure (Fig. 49-8).[111]

Carey and colleagues reported the use of a Martius labial fat pad flap with transvaginal urethrolysis with success in 87% of patients.[112] The Martius flap may decrease the risk of recurrent fibrosis and provide some urethral support; with any future surgery, a sling may be placed outside the fat pad, thus decreasing the risk of urethral injury. We reserve it for selected cases (e.g., repeat urethrolysis, extensive fibrosis). We usually divide the robust fat pad flap midway along its longitudinal axis and wrap the flap around the urethra, effectively supporting the undersurface and retropubic surface of the urethra.

If a vaginal approach is not feasible due to the patient's anatomy, or if the surgeon prefers, urethrolysis can be performed via a retropubic approach. We advocate an approach similar to that described by Webster and Kreder.[105] They reported excellent results with a retropubic takedown in which all adhesions from the prior cystourethropexy are sharply incised and complete mobility of the anterior vaginal wall is restored. The procedure is completed by performing an obturator shelf repair to prevent rotational decent and placing an omental pedicle to fill the retropubic dead space and prevent further scarring. In this case, careful sharp dissection is done to completely free the urethra from the undersurface of the pubic bone.

Urethrolysis may also be performed by a suprameatal approach, making a small inverted U-shaped incision above the urethral meatus and dissecting the urethra dorsally. This is usually done without any other major dissection or resuspension. A Martius labial fat pad flap can be interposed.

Regardless of the technique chosen, when formal urethrolysis is performed, we recommend a complete freeing of the urethra

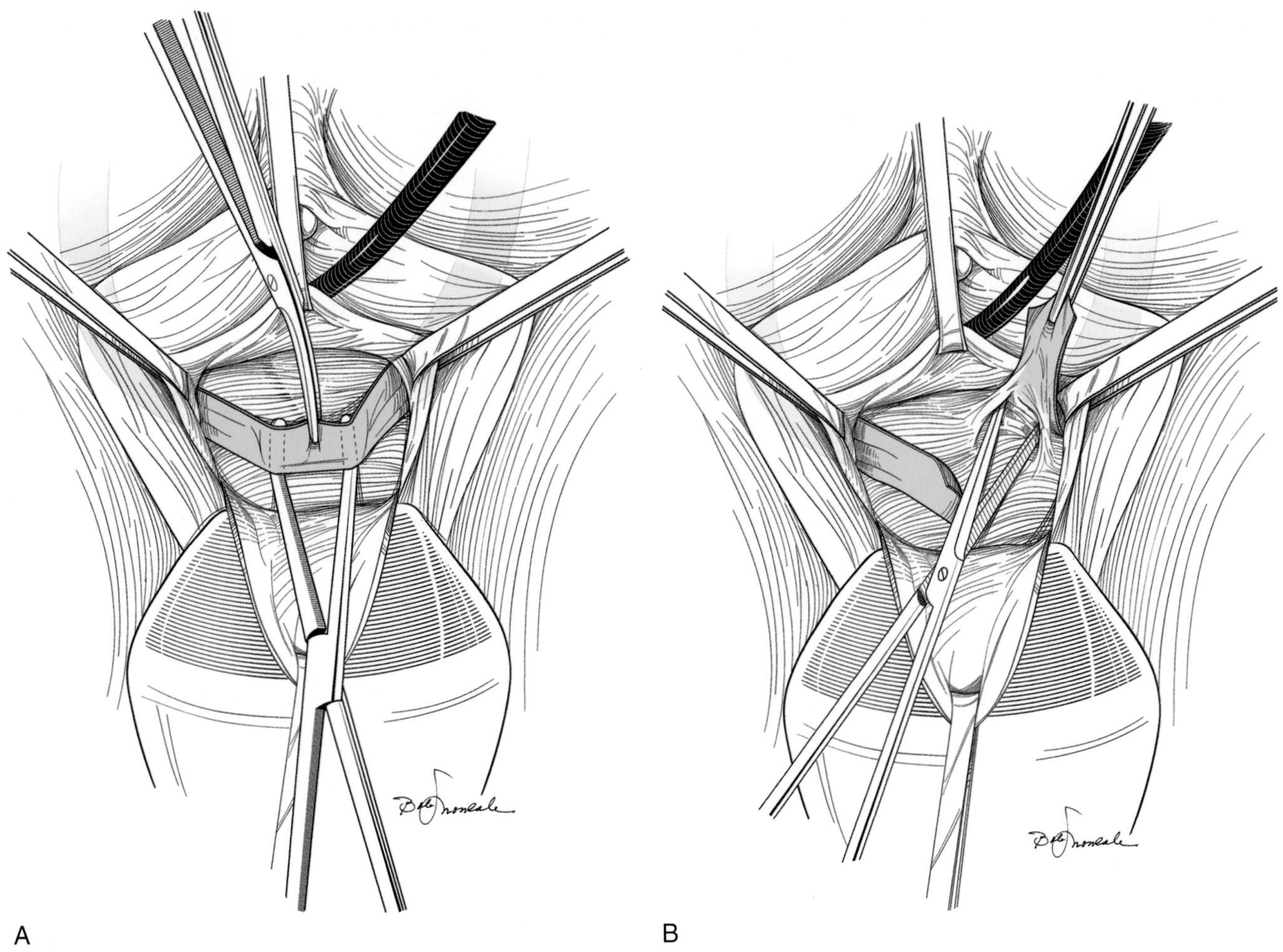

Figure 49-7 **A,** After an inverted U or midline incision and wide dissection of flaps, the sling is isolated in the midline and incised. A right angle clamp may be placed between the sling and the periurethral fascia to avoid injury to the urethra. **B,** The sling is freed from the undersurface of the urethra toward the endopelvic fascia. Ends may be excised or left in situ. Release of the sling causes a distinct drop in the urethra, with increased mobility of the urethral sound/cystoscope. Without retropubic space entry, we preserve lateral support and do not free it from the posterior pubic bone. (From Nitti VW, Carlson KV, Blaivas JG, Dmochowski RR: Early results of pubovaginal sling lysis by midline sling incision. Urology 59:47-52, 2002.)

in the retropubic space, because it is often quite adherent to the pubic bone.

In selected cases (e.g., extensive mobilization or SUI coexisting with obstruction), it may be desirable to resupport the urethra at the time of urethrolysis. Resuspension or sling may be done. Currently, our practice is to consider this only if the patient had SUI before urethrolysis or if support structures were severely compromised during urethrolysis. We rarely find this to be the case. Resuspension does increase the risk of persistent obstruction, and because most patients are distraught about obstruction, we believe it is best to take care of this problem and deal with recurrent SUI at a later time should it occur. Patients may be salvaged with transurethral collagen injections if SUI recurs. Goldman and colleagues reported a 66% response rate to collagen in women with recurrent SUI after transvaginal urethrolysis.[113] Additionally, the option of other procedures for SUI at a later date exists.

Urethrolysis is 65% to 93% effective for relieving iatrogenic obstruction.[102-105,109,113-116]

In patients who fail to void satisfactorily after urethrolysis, repeat urodynamics does not give conclusive information as to the cause of the failure.[103] Explanations include poor contractility insufficient to overcome even the reduced outlet resistance and persistent obstruction. In some patients, this continued obstruction is the result of intrinsic damage to the urethra from surgery and is not caused by periurethral fibrosis and scarring. In such cases, urethrolysis will not relieve the obstruction. It is possible that some failures "reobstruct" after a complete urethrolysis.

Chronic Irritative Symptoms and Urge Incontinence

After any anti-incontinence procedure, irritative voiding symptoms (frequency, urgency, urge incontinence) can persist or develop de novo. Irritative symptoms are more likely to be present postoperatively if they were present preoperatively. In the study by Kelly and colleagues, both preoperative and postoperative symptom analyses were obtained in 114 women who

Table 49-4 Summary of Series on Urethrolysis and Sling Incision/Loosening for the Treatment of Obstruction after Incontinence Surgery

Author and Ref. No.	*N*	Type of Urethrolysis	Success (%)*	Recurrent SUI (%)†
Zimmern et al.[160]	13	Transvaginal	92	N/A
Foster & McGuire[104]	48	Transvaginal	53	0
Nitti & Raz[103]	42	Transvaginal	71	0
Cross et al.[114]	39	Transvaginal	72	3
Goldman et al.[113]	32	Transvaginal	84	19
Carey et al.[112]	23	Transvaginal with Martius flap	87	16
Petrou et al.[116]	32	Suprameatal	67	3
Webster & Kreder[105]	15	Retropubic	93	13
Petrou & Young[115]	12	Retropubic	83	25
Carr & Webster[102]	54	Mixed	78	14
Amundsen et al.[107]	32	Transvaginal and sling incision	94 (retention) 67 (urge sx)	9
Nitti et al.[109]	19	Sling incision	84	17
Goldman[108]	14	Sling incision	93	21
Klutke et al.[95]	17	TVT incision and/or loosening	100	6
Rardin et al.[97]	23	TVT incision	100 (retention) 30 (urge sx cured) 70 (urge sx improved)	39 (two-thirds less SUI than before TVT)

*Success is usually defined as cure or significant improvement in presenting symptoms (resumption of normal bladder emptying for patients in retention; resolution of symptoms for patients with obstructive symptoms or frequency, urgency, or urge incontinence). In some series, success for specific symptoms is noted.

†Recurrent SUI is defined as the percentage of patients without SUI before urethrolysis who experienced SUI after urethrolysis.

N/A, not applicable; SUI, stress urinary incontinence; sx, symptoms; TVT, tension-free vaginal tape.

underwent modified Pereyra bladder neck suspension.[51] If urgency symptoms were present postoperatively, there was a statistically significant correlation with a poor objective and subjective outcome. In the large review sponsored by the American Urological Association, persistent postoperative urgency occurred in 36% to 66% of women undergoing retropubic suspension, 54% of those with transvaginal procedures, and 34% to 46% of those with slings.[54] (The higher percentage reflects patients with documented detrusor overactivity, and the lower percentage reflects patients who had preoperative urgency without overactivity.) Among patients who had no urgency and no detrusor overactivity preoperatively, de novo urgency occurred in 8% to 16% of those with retropubic suspensions, 3% to 10% of those with transvaginal suspensions, and 3% to 11% of those with slings (all ranges represent 95% confidence intervals).[54] No major statistical differences existed between the various procedures regarding postoperative urgency rates.

If irritative symptoms are present chronically after incontinence surgery, it is important to rule out obstruction as a cause. If obstruction exists, consideration may be given to sling lysis or urethrolysis. Chronic irritative symptoms not associated with obstruction are often difficult to manage. Anticholinergics, biofeedback, behavioral modification, or neuromodulation may be used. Age may play a role, because Allahdin and coworkers[117] found a higher rate of postoperative urgency in a group of patients aged 70 to 90 years. They found rates of urgency up to 60%, with 44% de novo urgency in this older group.[118] Occasionally, postoperative dysfunctional voiding is discovered, and this is effectively treated with biofeedback and patient education about changes in the lower urinary tract after surgery. In refractory cases, augmentation cystoplasty may be considered. In cases of de novo or worsened symptoms, consideration may be given to urethrolysis, although there are no data to support its success in patients without obstruction.

Conversely, some have improved overactive bladder symptoms after anti-incontinence procedures. After TVT, Segal and colleagues reported resolution of urgency in 63.1% of patients with preoperative mixed incontinence symptoms.[119]

COMPLICATIONS OF LAPAROSCOPIC SUSPENSIONS

Previously reported trials of laparoscopic colposuspension have had success rates of 40% to 100%.[120-126] However, these trials were nonrandomized, they had short follow-up times, and a number of factors, including patient selection and severity of incontinence, were not clearly defined.

Su, TH and coauthors[127] published results of a prospective trial comparing conventional colposuspension to laparoscopic colposuspension in 92 patients with 1 year follow-up. Although the reported success rates were significantly lower in the laparoscopic group (80.4% versus 95.6%), blood loss, hospital stay, and complication rates (17.4% versus 10.8%) were higher in the traditional colposuspension group. Moehrer and colleagues[128] found, in comparing laparoscopic with open colposuspension, that perioperative complications (including UTIs, dysuria, hematuria, voiding difficulties, wound infections, and retropubic hematoma) were slightly more frequent, but not significantly so, with the laparoscopic approach. The incidence of bladder injuries was higher with the laparoscopic technique.[128]

In randomized trials of laparoscopic colposuspension and TVT, Valpas and associates[129] found no difference in cure rates at 6 weeks' follow-up, but the TVT procedure was associated with

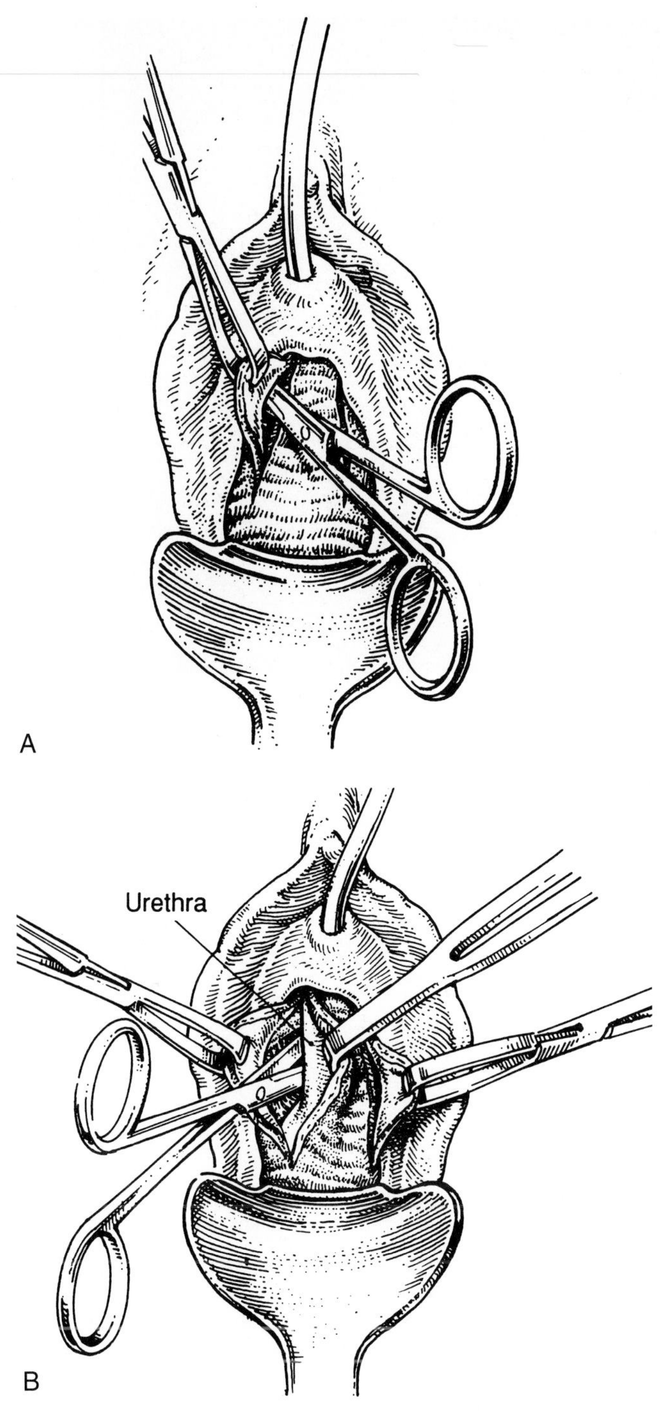

Figure 49-8 Transvaginal urethrolysis. **A,** An inverted U-shaped anterior vaginal wall incision is made after subepithelial injection of local anesthetic with epinephrine. The apex of the "U" is midway between the bladder neck and the urethral meatus. If a midline incision is made, it should extend from the mid-urethra to 2 cm behind the bladder neck. Sharp dissection is performed laterally beneath the vaginal epithelium on each side to the level of the pubic bone. The endopelvic fascia is perforated sharply at the level of the urethra on each side. The retropubic space is entered. **B,** Vaginal epithelial flaps are reflected laterally, and the "glistening" periurethral fascia is exposed. With sharp and blunt dissection, the urethra is mobilized laterally and circumferentially from the distal one third to the bladder neck. Attachments to the undersurface of the pubic bone are excised or swept down with the index finger retropubically. After initial mobilization, we place a long-nose right angle clamp around the urethra (ventrally or cephalad) under direct vision and pull through a Penrose drain. Downward traction on the Penrose further aids visualization and sharp dissection of all retropubic attachments. The index finger then may be placed completely around the urethra and against the posterior pubic bone. (From Nitti VW, Raz S: Obstruction following anti-incontinence procedures: Diagnosis and treatment with transvaginal urethrolysis J Urol 152:93-98, 1994.)

less analgesic use, shorter hospital stay, and faster return to normal voiding. Persson and colleagues[130] found no difference in cure rates at 1 year follow-up. In a separate trial of 33 patients randomized to undergo a laparoscopic Burch procedure, there were two cases of intravesical sutures, one bowel injury, three conversions to laparotomy because of adhesions, four patients with postoperative hematocrits lower than 28%, one ileus, and one pulmonary embolism.[131] A systematic review found laparoscopic colposuspension to have a 9% higher risk of failure after up to 18 months of follow-up.[128] Complications of laparoscopic surgery for SUI are similar to those of open surgery. Bladder injury is the most common intraoperative complication and can be repaired laparoscopically.

Complications of the Artificial Urinary Sphincter

The current artificial urinary sphincter (AUS) device, the AS-800 (American Medical Systems, Minneapolis, MN), may be placed by a retropubic or transvaginal approach.[132-135] The abdominal approach has been supported, but dissection through the urethrovaginal septum may be difficult due to extensive scarring. In 1988, Appell described vaginal placement of the artificial urinary sphincter and reported a 100% success rate in 34 women with no increase in device infection or erosion rate.[133]

Although continence rates with the AUS are favorable (60% to 100%), the advent of periurethral bulking agents and modifications in sling surgery has created a limited role in women with intrinsic sphincter dysfunction. Mark and Webster compared the results of the AUS with those of the pubovaginal sling in 77 patients with intrinsic sphincter dysfunction.[136] Both procedures were favorable, with success rates of 84% and 91%, respectively. Complications associated with AUS implantation include erosion, infection, device failure, and intraoperative injury to the urethra, bladder, and/or vagina. Inadvertent injury to these organs should not necessarily preclude implantation of the device[137] but may affect the explantation rate.[137,138] In the series of Costa and associates,[138] 51 of 206 patients had intraoperative injuries, and 14 required explantation of the device at a median of 11 months after implantation. Risk factors for explantation include age, type and number of prior surgeries, elapsed time between last procedure and AUS insertion, and perioperative injury. Risk of erosion has decreased since the introduction of a modified cuff, but concerns of late urethral atrophy still exist. The reoperation rate for revision was reported to be 9% to 22% over a 2.5- to 3-year period.[133,135] Unlike in men, where infection is usually localized to the perineum and superficial abdominal wall, in women an infected device could result in a pelvic abscess requiring drainage.[135]

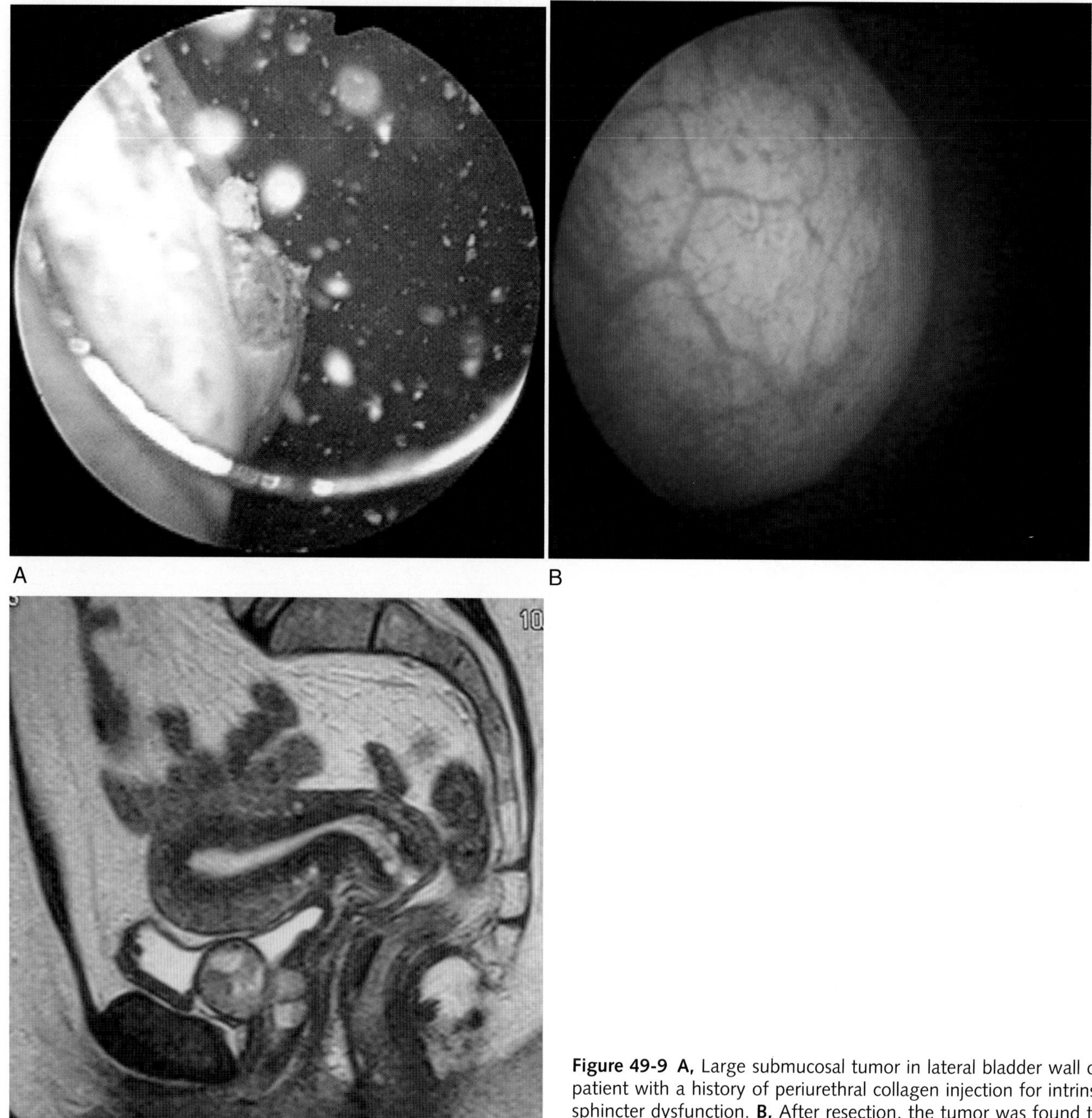

Figure 49-9 A, Large submucosal tumor in lateral bladder wall of a patient with a history of periurethral collagen injection for intrinsic sphincter dysfunction. **B,** After resection, the tumor was found to be a collagenoma from previous collagen displacement of periurethral injection. **C,** Magnetic resonance image showing bladder neck collagenoma causing obstruction.

Complications of Periurethral Bulking Agents

Periurethral bulking agents are placed submucosally, usually by injection, into the intrinsically damaged urethra and serve to increase coaptation and raise urethral resistance to increases in abdominal pressure (Fig. 49-9). Bulking agents can be delivered by a transurethral or a periurethral route.[139] Polytetrafluoroethylene (PTFE) paste, introduced in the 1970s, was the first bulking agent used.[140] There has been documented evidence of PTFE particle migration.[141] This has led to concerns regarding the safety of this procedure and has limited its use in the United States. Glutaraldehyde cross-linked (GAX) collagen is the most widely used agent.[142-144] GAX collagen (Contigen, C.R. Bard Inc., Covington, GA) is a highly purified 35% suspension of bovine collagen in a phosphate buffer containing at least 95% type I collagen and 1% to 5% type III collagen. Due to a 1% to 4% reported incidence of allergic reaction to GAX collagen, all patients are skin-tested 1 month before planned treatment. Some patients have experienced delayed hypersensitivity reactions despite preoperative skin testing.[145]

The U.S. Food and Drug Administration approved the bulking agent Durasphere (Advanced UroScience, St. Paul, MN), which consists of nonabsorbable pyrolytic carbon-coated zirconium oxide beads suspended in a water-based carrier gel. Target bead size ranges from 251 to 300 μm, which is greater than the 80-μm threshold for particle sizes associated with migration in tissue.[145] The pyrolytic carbon is nonreactive, has no associated antigenicity, and does not require preoperative skin testing. Complications associated with Durasphere are similar to those associated with collagen. The incidences of acute urinary retention and urgency may be higher with Durasphere (24.7% versus 16.9%, respectively) than with bovine collagen (11.9% and 3.4%, respectively).[146] Although Durasphere is reported to be nonmigratory,[146] Pannek and colleagues observed migration into local and distant lymph nodes, but this has unknown clinical significance.[147]

Complications associated with injection of periurethral bulking agents are rare and usually self-limited. The most common is transient urinary retention lasting 24 to 48 hours. Most series report transient retention rates of 1% to 10%.[142-144,148,149] One series reported a rate of 60%.[150] Retention beyond 48 hours is unusual. One series reported that 6% of patients had transient retention of 2 weeks.[150] Our own experience is that difficulty in emptying occurs in about 1% of patients and almost always resolves within 24 hours. Transient hematuria has been reported in 2% to 16% of cases.[142,148] Transient irritative voiding symptoms, including urge incontinence, may occur in 8% to 10% of patients.[149,150] The incidence of UTI is similarly low (0% to 12%).[148-151] Complications reported with periurethral bulking agents resolve quickly and are usually minor.

CONCLUSION

Pelvic floor surgeons treat SUI with a variety of effective procedures. Performing a thorough evaluation before treatment achieves the best short- and long-term results. Use of the appropriate surgical procedure for an individual patient lessens the likelihood of complications and morbidity. However, complications are unavoidable with surgical procedures. Patients should be informed of common potential complications, and their treatment, before surgery. A well-informed patient, one who understands a range of treatments and surgeries as well as their success and complication rates, will be the most satisfied patient.

References

1. Chaliha C, Stanton SL: Complications of surgery for genuine stress incontinence. Br J Obstet Gynaecol 106:1238, 1999.
2. Benson RC: Retropubic vesicourethropexy: Success or failure? Obstet Gynecol 35:665, 1970.
3. Katske FA, Raz S: Use of Foley catheter to obtain transvaginal tamponade. Urology (May):18, 1987.
4. Aungst M, Wagner M: Foley balloon to tamponade bleeding in the retropubic space. Obstet Gynecol 102:1037, 2003.
5. Zorn KC, Daigle S, Belzile F, et al: Embolization of a massive retropubic hemorrhage following a tension-free vaginal tape (TVT) procedure: Case report and literature review. Can J Urol 12:2560, 2005.
6. Nilsson CG, Kuuva N: The tension-free vaginal tape procedure is successful in the majority of women with indications for surgical treatment of urinary stress incontinence. BJOG 108:414, 2001.
7. Flock F, Reich A, Muche R, et al: Hemorrhagic complications associated with tension-free vaginal tape procedure. Obstet Gynecol 104:989, 2004.
8. Tamussino KF, Hanzal E, Kolle D, et al: Tension-free vaginal tape operation: Results of the Austrian registry. Obstet Gynecol 98:732, 2001.
9. Abouassaly R, Steinberg JR, Lemieux M, et al: Complications of tension-free vaginal tape surgery: A multi-institutional review. BJU Int 94:110, 2004.
10. Karram MM, Segal JL, Vassallo BJ, et al: Complications and untoward effects of the tension-free vaginal tape procedure. Obstet Gynecol 101:929, 2003.
11. Tamussino K, Hanzal E, Kolle D, et al: The Austrian tension-free vaginal tape registry. Int Urogynecol J Pelvic Floor Dysfunct 12(Suppl 2):S28, 2001.
12. Kuuva N, Nilsson CG: A nationwide analysis of complications associated with the tension-free vaginal tape (TVT) procedure. Acta Obstet Gynecol Scand 81:72, 2002.
13. Primicerio M, De Matteis G, Montanino Oliva M, et al: [Use of the TVT (tension-free vaginal tape) in the treatment of female urinary stress incontinence: Preliminary results.] Minerva Ginecol 51:355, 1999.
14. Zilbert AW, Farrell SA: External iliac artery laceration during tension-free vaginal tape procedure. Int Urogynecol J Pelvic Floor Dysfunct 12:141, 2001.
15. Muir TW, Tulikangas PK, Fidela Paraiso M, et al: The relationship of tension-free vaginal tape insertion and the vascular anatomy. Obstet Gynecol 101:933, 2003.
16. Whiteside JL, Walters MD: Anatomy of the obturator region: relations to a trans-obturator sling. Int Urogynecol J Pelvic Floor Dysfunct 15:223, 2004.
17. Dunn JS, Jr, Bent AE, Ellerkman RM, et al: Voiding dysfunction after surgery for stress incontinence: literature review and survey results. Int Urogynecol J Pelvic Floor Dysfunct, 15:25, 2004.
18. Gordon D, Groutz A, Lessing J: [PVT—tension-free vaginal tape—a new minimally invasive surgical technique for female stress incontinence: Preliminary results.] Harefuah 137:433, 1999.
19. Nilsson CG, Kuuva N, Falconer C, et al: Long-term results of the tension-free vaginal tape (TVT) procedure for surgical treatment of female stress urinary incontinence. Int Urogynecol J Pelvic Floor Dysfunct 12(Suppl 2):S5, 2001.
20. Lebret T, Lugagne PM, Herve JM, et al: Evaluation of tension-free vaginal tape procedure: Its safety and efficacy in the treatment of female stress urinary incontinence during the learning phase. Eur Urol 40:543, 2001.
21. Meschia M, Pifarotti P, Bernasconi F, et al: Tension-free vaginal tape: Analysis of outcomes and complications in 404 stress incontinent women. Int Urogynecol J Pelvic Floor Dysfunct 12(Suppl 2): S24, 2001.
22. Azam U, Frazer MI, Kozman EL, et al: The tension-free vaginal tape procedure in women with previous failed stress incontinence surgery. J Urol 166:554, 2001.
23. Jeffry L, Deval B, Birsan A, et al: Objective and subjective cure rates after tension-free vaginal tape for treatment of urinary incontinence. Urology 58:702, 2001.
24. Buchsbaum GM, Moll C, Duecy EE: True occult bladder perforation during placement of tension-free vaginal tape. Int Urogynecol J Pelvic Floor Dysfunct 15:432, 2004.
25. Abbas Shobeiri S, Garely AD, Chesson RR, et al: Recognition of occult bladder injury during the tension-free vaginal tape procedure. Obstet Gynecol 99:1067, 2002.
26. Krauth JS, Rasoamiaramanana H, Barletta H, et al: Sub-urethral tape treatment of female urinary incontinence—Morbidity assessment of the trans-obturator route and a new tape (I-STOP): A multi-centre experiment involving 604 cases. Eur Urol 47:102, 2005.

27. Hermieu JF, Messas A, Delmas V, et al: [Bladder injury after TVT transobturator.] Prog Urol 13:115, 2003.
28. de Leval J: Novel surgical technique for the treatment of female stress urinary incontinence: Transobturator vaginal tape inside-out. Eur Urol 44:724, 2003.
29. Tancer ML: Urologic injuries: Bladder and urethra. In Schaefer G, Greber E (eds): Complications in Obstetric and Gynecologic Surgery. New York: Harper and Row, 1981.
30. Kreder KJ: Female urethral diverticulum and urethral fistulae. In Webster GD, Kirby B, Goldwasser B, et al. (eds): Reconstructive Urology. Oxford: Blackwell Publishers, 1993.
31. Persky L, Guerriere K: Complications of Marshall-Marchetti-Krantz urethropexy. Urology 8:469, 1976.
32. Rosen DM, Korda AR, Waugh RC: Ureteric injury at Burch colposuspension: Four case reports and literature review. Aust N Z J Obstet Gynaecol 36:354, 1996.
33. Burch JC: Urethrovaginal fixation to Cooper's ligament for correction of stress incontinence, cystocele, and prolapse. Am J Obstet Gynecol 81:281, 1961.
34. Eriksen BC, Hagen B, Eik-Nes SH, et al: Long-term effectiveness of the Burch colposuspension in female urinary stress incontinence. Acta Obstet Gynecol Scand 69:45, 1990.
35. Meschia M, Busacca M, Pifarotti P, et al: Bowel perforation during insertion of tension-free vaginal tape (TVT). Int Urogynecol J Pelvic Floor Dysfunct 13:263, 2002.
36. Leboeuf L, Tellez CA, Ead D, et al: Complication of bowel perforation during insertion of tension-free vaginal tape. J Urol 170:1310; discussion 1310, 2003.
37. Castillo OA, Bodden E, Olivares RA, et al: Intestinal perforation: An infrequent complication during insertion of tension-free vaginal tape. J Urol 172:1364, 2004.
38. Brink DM: Bowel injury following insertion of tension-free vaginal tape. S Afr Med J 90:450, 2000.
39. Peyrat L, Boutin JM, Bruyere F, et al: Intestinal perforation as a complication of tension-free vaginal tape procedure for urinary incontinence. Eur Urol 39:603, 2001.
40. Leboeuf L, Mendez LE, Gousse AE: Small bowel obstruction associated with tension-free vaginal tape. Urology 63:1182, 2004.
41. Stamey TA: Endoscopic suspension of the vesical neck for urinary incontinence in females: Report on 203 consecutive patients. Ann Surg 192:465, 1980.
42. Geis K, Dietl J: Ilioinguinal nerve entrapment after tension-free vaginal tape (TVT) procedure. Int Urogynecol J Pelvic Floor Dysfunct 13:136, 2002.
43. Chmel R: [Surgical procedure using the tension-free vaginal tape: A safe method for treatment of stress incontinence?] Ceska Gynekol 68:143, 2003.
44. Sergent F, Sebban A, Verspyck E, et al: [Pre- and postoperative complications of TVT (tension-free vaginal tape).] Prog Urol 13:648, 2003.
45. Zivkovic F, Tamussino K, Ralph G, et al: Long-term effects of vaginal dissection on the innervation of the striated urethral sphincter. Obstet Gynecol 87:257, 1996.
46. Hilliges M, Falconer C, Ekman-Ordeberg G, et al: Innervation of the human vaginal mucosa as revealed by PGP 9.5 immunohistochemistry. Acta Anat (Basel) 153:119, 1995.
47. Lemack GE, Zimmern PE: Sexual function after vaginal surgery for stress incontinence: Results of a mailed questionnaire. Urology 56:223, 2000.
48. Mazouni C, Karsenty G, Bretelle F, et al: Urinary complications and sexual function after the tension-free vaginal tape procedure. Acta Obstet Gynecol Scand 83:955, 2004.
49. Glavind K, Tetsche MS: Sexual function in women before and after suburethral sling operation for stress urinary incontinence: A retrospective questionnaire study. Acta Obstet Gynecol Scand 83:965, 2004.
50. Maaita M, Bhaumik J, Davies AE: Sexual function after using tension-free vaginal tape for the surgical treatment of genuine stress incontinence. BJU Int 90:540, 2002.
51. Kelly MJ, Knielsen K, Bruskewitz R, et al: Symptom analysis of patients undergoing modified Pereyra bladder neck suspension for stress urinary incontinence: Pre- and postoperative findings. Urology 37:213, 1991.
52. Parnell JP 2nd, Marshall VF, Vaughan ED Jr: Management of recurrent urinary stress incontinence by the Marshall-Marchetti-Krantz vesicourethropexy. J Urol 132:912, 1984.
53. Yalcin O, Isikoglu M, Beji NK: Results of TVT operations alone and combined with other vaginal surgical procedures. Arch Gynecol Obstet 269:96, 2004.
54. Leach GE, Dmochowski RR, Appell RA, et al: Female Stress Urinary Incontinence Clinical Guidelines Panel summary report on surgical management of female stress urinary incontinence. The American Urological Association. J Urol 158:875, 1997.
55. Debodinance P, Delporte P, Engrand JB, et al: [Complications of urinary incontinence surgery: 800 Procedures.] J Gynecol Obstet Biol Reprod (Paris) 31:649, 2002.
56. Kirby RS, Whiteway JE: Assessment of the results of Stamey bladder neck suspension. Br J Urol 63:21, 1989.
57. Lee RA, Symmonds RE, Goldstein RA: Surgical complications and results of modified Marshall-Marchetti-Krantz procedure for urinary incontinence. Obstet Gynecol 53:447, 1979.
58. Morgan JE: The suprapubic approach to primary stress urinary incontinence. Am J Obstet Gynecol 115:316, 1973.
59. Neuman M: Infected hematoma following tension-free vaginal tape implantation. J Urol 168:2549, 2002.
60. Johnson DW, ElHajj M, OBrien-Best EL, et al: Necrotizing fasciitis after tension-free vaginal tape (TVT) placement. Int Urogynecol J Pelvic Floor Dysfunct 14:291, 2003.
61. Kelly MJ, Zimmern PE, Leach GE: Complications of bladder neck suspension procedures. Urol Clin North Am 18:339, 1991.
62. Diaz DL, Fox BM, Walzak MP, et al: Endoscopic vesicourethropexy: Experience and complications. Urology 24:321, 1984.
63. Hilton P, Mohammed KA, Ward K: Postural perineal pain associated with perforation of the lower urinary tract due to insertion of a tension-free vaginal tape. BJOG 110:79, 2003.
64. Irer B, Aslan G, Cimen S, et al: Development of vesical calculi following tension-free vaginal tape procedure. Int Urogynecol J Pelvic Floor Dysfunct 16:245, 2005.
65. Bagley DH, Schultz E, Conlin MJ: Laser division of intraluminal sutures. J Endourol 12:355, 1998.
66. Rodriguez LV, Raz S: Prospective analysis of patients treated with a distal urethral polypropylene sling for symptoms of stress urinary incontinence: Surgical outcome and satisfaction determined by patient driven questionnaires. J Urol 170:857, 2003.
67. Levin I, Groutz A, Gold R, et al: Surgical complications and medium-term outcome results of tension-free vaginal tape: A prospective study of 313 consecutive patients. Neurourol Urodyn 23:7, 2004.
68. Tsivian A, Kessler O, Mogutin B, et al: Tape related complications of the tension-free vaginal tape procedure. J Urol 171:762, 2004.
69. Kobashi KC, Govier FE: Management of vaginal erosion of polypropylene mesh slings. J Urol 169:2242, 2003.
70. Bafghi A, Benizri EI, Trastour C, et al: Multifilament polypropylene mesh for urinary incontinence: 10 Cases of infections requiring removal of the sling. BJOG 112:376, 2005.
71. Glavind K, Sander P: Erosion, defective healing and extrusion after tension-free urethropexy for the treatment of stress urinary incontinence. Int Urogynecol J Pelvic Floor Dysfunct 15:179, 2004.
72. Amid PK: Classification of biomaterials and their related complications in abdominal wall hernia surgery. Hernia 1:15, 1997.
73. Morgan JE, Farrow GA, Stewart FE: The Marlex sling operation for the treatment of recurrent stress urinary incontinence: A 16-year review. Am J Obstet Gynecol 151:224, 1985.

74. McLennan MT: Transurethral resection of transvaginal tape. Int Urogynecol J Pelvic Floor Dysfunct 15:360, 2004.
75. McDuffie RW Jr, Litin RB, Blundon KE: Urethrovesical suspension (Marshall-Marchetti-Krantz): Experience with 204 cases. Am J Surg 141:297, 1981.
76. Riggs JA: Retropubic cystourethropexy: A review of two operative procedures with long-term follow-up. Obstet Gynecol 68:98, 1986.
77. Leach GE: Bone fixation technique for transvaginal needle suspension. Urology 31:388, 1988.
78. Appell RA, Rackley RR, Dmochowski RR: Vesica percutaneous bladder neck stabilization. J Endourol 10:221, 1996.
79. Nativ O, Levine S, Madjar S, et al: Incisionless per vaginal bone anchor cystourethropexy for the treatment of female stress incontinence: Experience with the first 50 patients. J Urol 158:1742, 1997.
80. Benderev TV: A modified percutaneous outpatient bladder neck suspension system. J Urol 152:2316, 1994.
81. Goldberg RP, Tchetgen MB, Sand PK, et al: Incidence of pubic osteomyelitis after bladder neck suspension using bone anchors. Urology 63:704, 2004.
82. FitzGerald MP, Gitelis S, Brubaker L: Pubic osteomyelitis and granuloma after bone anchor placement. Int Urogynecol J Pelvic Floor Dysfunct 10:346, 1999.
83. Enzler M, Agins HJ, Kogan M, et al: Osteomyelitis of the pubis following suspension of the neck of the bladder with use of bone anchors: A report of four cases. J Bone Joint Surg Am 81:1736, 1999.
84. Matkov TG, Hejna MJ, Coogan CL: Osteomyelitis as a complication of vesica percutaneous bladder neck suspension. J Urol 160:1427, 1998.
85. Franks ME, Lavelle JP, Yokoyama T, et al: Metastatic osteomyelitis after pubovaginal sling using bone anchors. Urology 56:330, 2000.
86. Frederick RW, Carey JM, Leach GE: Osseous complications after transvaginal bone anchor fixation in female pelvic reconstructive surgery: Report from single largest prospective series and literature review. Urology 64:669, 2004.
87. Wang AC: Burch colposuspension vs. Stamey bladder neck suspension: A comparison of complications with special emphasis on detrusor instability and voiding dysfunction. J Reprod Med 41:529, 1996.
88. Juma S, Sdrales L: Etiology of urinary retention after bladder neck suspension [abstract]. J Urol 149:400A, 1993.
89. Spencer JR, O'Conor VJ Jr, Schaeffer AJ: A comparison of endoscopic suspension of the vesical neck with suprapubic vesicourethropexy for treatment of stress urinary incontinence. J Urol 137:411, 1987.
90. Rost A, Fiedler U, Fester C: Comparative analysis of the results of suspension-urethroplasty according to Marshall-Marchetti-Krantz and of urethrovesicopexy with adhesive. Urol Int 34:167, 1979.
91. Mundy AR: A trial comparing the Stamey bladder neck suspension procedure with colposuspension for the treatment of stress incontinence. Br J Urol 55:687, 1983.
92. Cardozo LD, Stanton SL, Williams JE: Detrusor instability following surgery for genuine stress incontinence. Br J Urol 51:204, 1979.
93. Chaikin DC, Rosenthal J, Blaivas JG: Pubovaginal fascial sling for all types of stress urinary incontinence: Long-term analysis. J Urol 160:1312, 1998.
94. Morgan TO Jr, Westney OL, McGuire EJ: Pubovaginal sling: 4-Year outcome analysis and quality of life assessment. J Urol 163:1845, 2000.
95. Klutke C, Siegel S, Carlin B, et al: Urinary retention after tension-free vaginal tape procedure: Incidence and treatment. Urology 58:697, 2001.
96. Niemczyk P, Klutke JJ, Carlin BI, et al: United States experience with tension-free vaginal tape procedure for urinary stress incontinence: Assessment of safety and tolerability. Tech Urol 7:261, 2001.
97. Rardin CR, Rosenblatt PL, Kohli N, et al: Release of tension-free vaginal tape for the treatment of refractory postoperative voiding dysfunction. Obstet Gynecol 100:898, 2002.
98. Sander P, Moller LM, Rudnicki PM, et al: Does the tension-free vaginal tape procedure affect the voiding phase? Pressure-flow studies before and 1 year after surgery. BJU Int 89:694, 2002.
99. Moran PA, Ward KL, Johnson D, et al: Tension-free vaginal tape for primary genuine stress incontinence: A two-centre follow-up study. BJU Int 86:39, 2000.
100. Rackley RR, Abdelmalak JB, Tchetgen MB, et al: Tension-free vaginal tape and percutaneous vaginal tape sling procedures. Tech Urol 7:90, 2001.
101. Coptcoat MJ, Shah PJ, Cumming J, et al: How does bladder function change in the early period after surgical alteration in outflow resistance? Preliminary communication. J R Soc Med 80:753, 1987.
102. Carr LK, Webster GD: Voiding dysfunction following incontinence surgery: Diagnosis and treatment with retropubic or vaginal urethrolysis. J Urol 157:821, 1997.
103. Nitti VW, Raz S: Obstruction following anti-incontinence procedures: Diagnosis and treatment with transvaginal urethrolysis. J Urol 152:93, 1994.
104. Foster HE, McGuire EJ: Management of urethral obstruction with transvaginal urethrolysis. J Urol 150:1448, 1993.
105. Webster GD, Kreder KJ: Voiding dysfunction following cystourethropexy: Its evaluation and management. J Urol 144:670, 1990.
106. Croak AJ, Schulte V, Peron S, et al: Transvaginal tape lysis for urinary obstruction after tension-free vaginal tape placement. J Urol 169:2238, 2003.
107. Amundsen CL, Guralnick ML, Webster GD: Variations in strategy for the treatment of urethral obstruction after a pubovaginal sling procedure. J Urol 164:434, 2000.
108. Goldman HB: Simple sling incision for the treatment of iatrogenic urethral obstruction. Urology 62:714, 2003.
109. Nitti VW, Carlson KV, Blaivas JG, et al: Early results of pubovaginal sling lysis by midline sling incision. Urology 59:47, 2002.
110. Kusuda L: Simple release of pubovaginal sling. Urology 57:358, 2001.
111. Leach GE, Raz S: Modified Pereyra bladder neck suspension after previously failed anti-incontinence surgery: Surgical technique and results with long-term follow-up. Urology 23:359, 1984.
112. Carey JM, Chon JK, Leach GE: Urethrolysis with Martius labial fat pad graft for iatrogenic bladder outlet obstruction. Urology 61:21, 2003.
113. Goldman HB, Rackley RR, Appell RA: The efficacy of urethrolysis without re-suspension for iatrogenic urethral obstruction. J Urol 161:196, 1999.
114. Cross CA, Cespedes RD, English SF, et al: Transvaginal urethrolysis for urethral obstruction after anti-incontinence surgery. J Urol 159:1199, 1998.
115. Petrou SP, Young PR: Rate of recurrent stress urinary incontinence after retropubic urethrolysis. J Urol 167:613, 2002.
116. Petrou SP, Brown JA, Blaivas JG: Suprameatal transvaginal urethrolysis. J Urol 161:1268, 1999.
117. Allahdin S, McKinley CA, Mahmood TA, et al: Vaginal wall erosion of the tension-free vaginal tape procedure: An unusual complication. J Obstet Gynaecol 23:443, 2003.
118. Allahdin S, McKinley CA, Mahmood TA: Tension free vaginal tape: A procedure for all ages. Acta Obstet Gynecol Scand 83:937, 2004.
119. Segal JL, Vassallo B, Kleeman S, et al: Prevalence of persistent and de novo overactive bladder symptoms after the tension-free vaginal tape. Obstet Gynecol 104:1263, 2004.

120. Vancaillie TG, Schuessler W: Laparoscopic bladderneck suspension. J Laparoendosc Surg 1:169, 1991.
121. McDougall EM, Klutke CG, Cornell T: Comparison of transvaginal versus laparoscopic bladder neck suspension for stress urinary incontinence. Urology 45:641, 1995.
122. Radomski SB, Herschorn S: Laparoscopic Burch bladder neck suspension: early results. J Urol 155:515, 1996.
123. Liu CY: Laparoscopic retropubic colposuspension (Burch procedure). A review of 58 cases. J Reprod Med 38:526, 1993.
124. Langebrekke A, Dahlstrom B, Eraker R, et al: The laparoscopic Burch procedure: A preliminary report. Acta Obstet Gynecol Scand 74:153, 1995.
125. Das S, Palmer JK: Laparoscopic colpo-suspension. J Urol 154:1119, 1995.
126. Polascik TJ, Moore RG, Rosenberg MT, et al: Comparison of laparoscopic and open retropubic urethropexy for treatment of stress urinary incontinence. Urology 45:647, 1995.
127. Su TH, Wang KG, Hsu CY, et al: Prospective comparison of laparoscopic and traditional colposuspensions in the treatment of genuine stress incontinence. Acta Obstet Gynecol Scand 76:576, 1997.
128. Moehrer B, Carey M, Wilson D: Laparoscopic colposuspension: A systematic review. BJOG 110:230, 2003.
129. Valpas A, Kivela A, Penttinen J, et al: Tension-free vaginal tape and laparoscopic mesh colposuspension for stress urinary incontinence. Obstet Gynecol 104:42, 2004.
130. Persson J, Teleman P, Eten-Bergquist C, et al: Cost-analyzes based on a prospective, randomized study comparing laparoscopic colposuspension with a tension-free vaginal tape procedure. Acta Obstet Gynecol Scand 81:1066, 2002.
131. Paraiso MF, Walters MD, Karram MM, et al: Laparoscopic Burch colposuspension versus tension-free vaginal tape: A randomized trial. Obstet Gynecol 104:1249, 2004.
132. Hadley HR: The artificial sphincter in the female. Probl Urol 5:123, 1991.
133. Appell RA: Techniques and results in the implantation of the artificial urinary sphincter in women with type III stress urinary incontinence by a vaginal approach. Neurourol Urodyn 7:613, 1988.
134. Abbassian A: A new operation for insertion of the artificial urinary sphincter. J Urol 140:512, 1988.
135. Diokno AC, Hollander JB, Alderson TP: Artificial urinary sphincter for recurrent female urinary incontinence: indications and results. J Urol, 138: 778, 1987.
136. Mark SD, Webster GD: Stress urinary incontinence due primarily to intrinsic sphincteric deficiency: Experience with artificial urinary sphincter and sling cystourethropexy. J Urol 151:769, 1994.
137. Petrou SP, Elliott DS, Barrett DM: Artificial urethral sphincter for incontinence. Urology 56:353, 2000.
138. Costa P, Mottet N, Rabut B, et al: The use of an artificial urinary sphincter in women with type III incontinence and a negative Marshall test. J Urol 165:1172, 2001.
139. Appell RA, Winters JC: Intraurethral injections. In O'Donnell PA (ed): Urinary Incontinence. St. Louis: Mosby, 1997, pp 228-234.
140. Politano VA: Periurethral polytetrafluoroethylene injection for urinary incontinence. J Urol 127:439, 1982.
141. Malizia AA Jr, Reiman HM, Myers RP, et al: Migration and granulomatous reaction after periurethral injection of polytef (Teflon). JAMA 251:3277, 1984.
142. Faerber GJ: Endoscopic collagen injection therapy in elderly women with type I stress urinary incontinence. J Urol 155:512, 1996.
143. Appell RA: Collagen injection therapy for urinary incontinence. Urol Clin North Am 21:177, 1994.
144. Herschorn S, Steele DJ, Radomski SB: Followup of intraurethral collagen for female stress urinary incontinence. J Urol 156:1305, 1996.
145. Dmochowski RR, Appell RA: Injectable agents in the treatment of stress urinary incontinence in women: Where are we now? Urology 56:32, 2000.
146. Lightner D, Calvosa C, Andersen R, et al: A new injectable bulking agent for treatment of stress urinary incontinence: Results of a multicenter, randomized, controlled, double-blind study of Durasphere. Urology 58:12, 2001.
147. Pannek J, Brands FH, Senge T: Particle migration after transurethral injection of carbon coated beads for stress urinary incontinence. J Urol 166:1350, 2001.
148. O'Connell HE, McGuire EJ, Aboseif S, et al: Transurethral collagen therapy in women. J Urol 154:1463, 1995.
149. Stricker P, Haylen B: Injectable collagen for type 3 female stress incontinence: The first 50 Australian patients. Med J Aust 158:89, 1993.
150. Haab F, Zimmern PE, Leach GE: Urinary stress incontinence due to intrinsic sphincteric deficiency: Experience with fat and collagen periurethral injections. J Urol 157:1283, 1997.
151. Santarosa RP, Blaivas JG: Periurethral injection of autologous fat for the treatment of sphincteric incontinence. J Urol 151:607, 1994.
152. Klutke JJ, Klutke CG, Hsieh G: Bladder injury during the Burch retropubic urethropexy: Is routine cystoscopy necessary? Tech Urol 4:145, 1998.
153. Harris RL, Cundiff GW, Theofrastous JP, et al: The value of intraoperative cystoscopy in urogynecologic and reconstructive pelvic surgery. Am J Obstet Gynecol 177:1367, 1997.
154. Galloway NT, Davies N, Stephenson TP: The complications of colposuspension. Br J Urol 60:122, 1987.
155. Korda A, Ferry J, Hunter P: Colposuspension for the treatment of female urinary incontinence. Aust N Z J Obstet Gynaecol 29:146, 1989.
156. Petri E: Treatment of incontinence, prolapse and related conditions. In: Cardoo L, Staskin (eds): The Textbook of Female Urology and Urogynecology. Oxford: Isis Medical Media, 1999.
157. Paick JS, Ku JH, Shin JW, et al: Complications associated with the tension-free vaginal tape procedure: The Korean experience. Int Urogynecol J Pelvic Floor Dysfunct 16:215-219, 2004. Epub 2004 Oct 26.
158. Hung MJ, Liu FS, Shen PS, et al: Analysis of two sling procedures using polypropylene mesh for treatment of stress urinary incontinence. Int J Gynaecol Obstet 84:133, 2004.
159. deTayrac R, Deffieux X, Droupy S, et al: A prospective randomized trial comparing tension-free vaginal tape and transobturator suburethral tape for surgical treatment of stress urinary incontinence. Am J Obstet Gynecol 190:602, 2004.
160. Zimmern PE, Hadley HR, Leach GE, et al: Female urethral obstruction after Marshall-Marchetti-Krantz operation. J Urol 138:517, 1987.

Section 6

FEMALE SEXUAL FUNCTION AND DYSFUNCTION

Chapter 50

FEMALE SEXUAL FUNCTION AND DYSFUNCTION

Irwin Goldstein

Why is there a chapter concerning women's sexual function and dysfunction in a textbook entitled *Female Urology*? The answer should be obvious. Urologists and gynecologists who practice "female urology" will encounter women with sexual health concerns.[1,2]

A woman's general health is a fundamental human right. If this is accepted, then urologic health and gynecologic health are fundamental human rights. If this is accepted, then sexual health should be a fundamental human right. If sexual health is a woman's fundamental human right, then health care providers need to be educated on the fundamentals of women's sexual health care delivery.[3,4]

The goal of a female urologic practice must be to maximize "female urology" health care delivery to all women, and this includes maximizing sexual health care delivery to women. Currently, there are limited numbers of female urology health care professionals offering comprehensive psychological and biologic sexual health care for women.

It is the objective of this chapter to help the interested female urologist to achieve the goal of maximizing sexual health care delivery to all their women patients. The aim is to provide relevant, evidence-based clinical information to help diagnose and treat specific biologic-based sexual health pathophysiologies. It is neither logical nor rational to continue to focus sexual health care delivery primarily on males with sexual health concerns, as is currently occurring in medicine.

It is not within the realm of this chapter to thoroughly discuss psychological management of sexual health issues in women. Even though health care professionals need to be holistic in managing female (and male) sexual dysfunction, the goals of this chapter are to educate the biologic-focused health care professional on how to identify the pathologies associated with the sexual health concerns and to provide evidence-based safe and effective biologic management strategies. A clinical, biologic-based paradigm is presented at the end of the chapter, founded on results derive d from emerging basic science and evidence-based data drawn from clinical research.

Ideally, state-of-the-art sexual health care for afflicted women and couples will be directed from medical school–based sexual medicine centers that are devoted to the study, diagnosis, and treatment of men and women with sexual disorders. These facilities will be composed of multidisciplinary groups, including female urologists. Cases in such multidisciplinary centers would be managed by a team of allied health care professionals, mental health care professionals, and physical therapists, under the direction of sexual medicine physicians who may be board-certified in urology or female urology.

SEXUAL HEALTH

According to the World Health Organization,[3] sexual health "refers to a state of physical, emotional, mental, and social well-being related to sexuality." All women have the right to a "positive and respectful approach to sexuality and sexual relationships, having pleasurable and safe sexual experiences, free of coercion, discrimination and violence." Moreover, "For sexual health to be attained and maintained, the sexual rights of all persons must be respected, protected and fulfilled."[3]

The World Association of Sexual Health has stated[4] that women (and men) have the right to sexual equity—the freedom from all forms of discrimination regardless of sex, gender, sexual orientation, age, race, social class, religion, or physical and emotional disability." Women (and men) also have the right to sexual pleasure—sexual pleasure is a source of physical, psychological, intellectual, and spiritual well-being.

What are the Barriers to Providing Women's Sexual Health Care in the Female Urology Practice

Physicians in general and female urologists in particular face a challenge in finding the time and opportunity to discuss their women patient's sexual health concerns, especially with the increasing and growing demands for other health care issues, including the significant financial pressures of providing "managed care." Additionally, most physicians have limited training in the diagnosis and treatment of sexual health concerns. Currently, American medical schools devote on average less than 10 hours to sexual medicine education.[5] Independent of the physicians, patients are also often unwilling or too uncomfortable to initiate a discussion about their own sexual problems.[6]

Sexual medicine issues are complex, and it is often difficult to separate psychological issues and interpersonal relationship concerns from biologic disorders.[7] There are only limited evidence-based data available for diagnosis and management. Sexual health concerns are, in general, secondary to mind, body, and relationship issues that are interrelated in unique and individual ways and molded with distinct couple dynamics to cause the particular sexual problem.[7] Psychological factors include previous sexual trauma and abuse, sexual neuroses, sexual inhibitions or idiosyncracies, and interpersonal relationship issues.[8] Biologic factors may involve such pertinent aspects as aging; exposure to vascular risk factors; urologic conditions such as interstitial cystitis, previous radical cystecomy, and recurrent urinary tract infections; gynecologic conditions such as endometriosis, previous hyster-

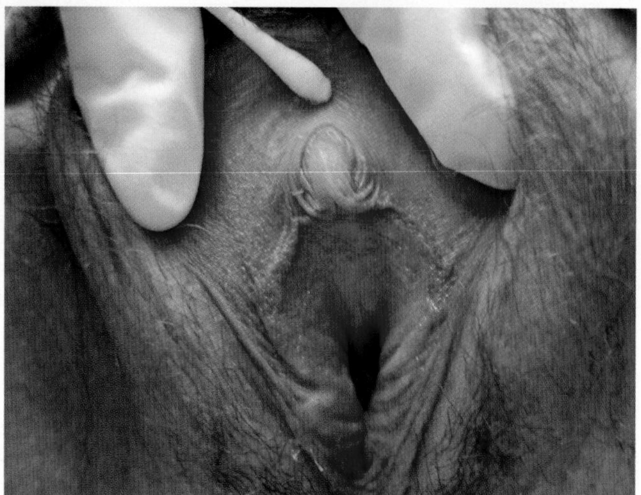

Figure 50-1 Examination of the genitalia exposed to a normal hormonal milieu reveals a well-defined and robust clitoral glans and corona, bilateral frenular tissue, bilateral labia minora, shiny vaginal lubricating material, and vaginal rugae. The clitoral prepuce is retracted.

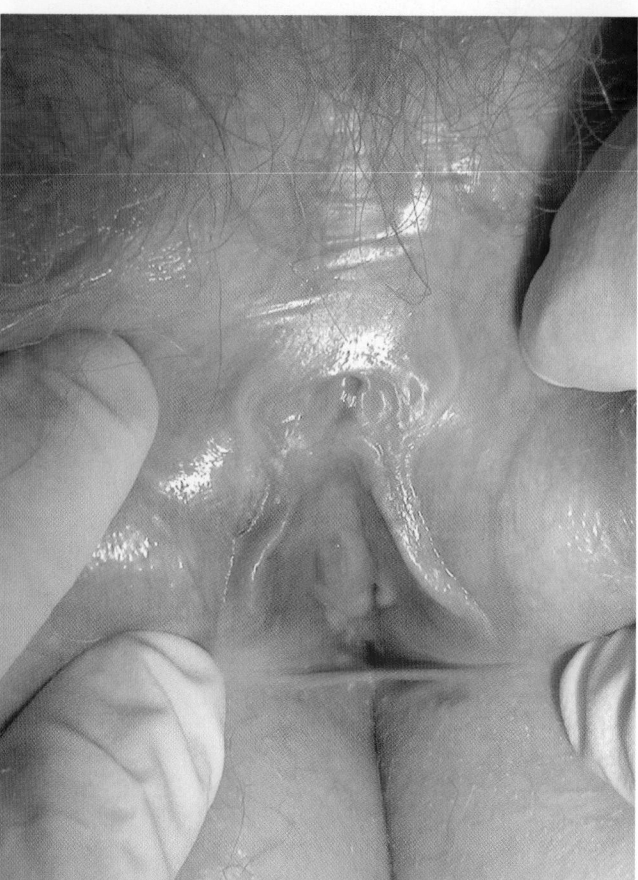

Figure 50-2 Examination of the genitalia exposed to an abnormally low hormonal milieu reveals an atrophied, poorly defined clitoral glans. The corona and bilateral frenular tissue are not visible. The clitoral prepuce is phimotic, the vaginal rugae are absent, and the vestibular tissue appear erythematous.

ectomy, childbirth, infertility issues, and sexually transmitted infections; inflammation; abnormal immunologic conditions; abnormal hormonal states (Figs. 50-1 and 50-2); tumors; mechanical compartment syndromes; blunt or penetrating traumatic injury; tissue weakness with organ prolapse; and others. Sexual health problems may also stem from the contribution of the male partner in women's sexual health.[1,7,8]

Why Should Female Urology Practice Expand to Include Women's Sexual Heath Care

Female urologists offer urogynecologic health care to women, and this should include comprehensive sexual health care. Over the last 30 years, urologic specialists have led the many advances realized in the biologic-based knowledge in sexual medicine.[9] Furthermore, urologists have revolutionized the therapeutic armamentarium for contemporary management of biologic-focused men's sexual health care.[9] Practically, female urologists are in a unique position to understand that female peripheral sexual organs are an essential component of the anatomy and physiology of the peripheral genitalia and pelvic floor constituents.

Many population-based studies have revealed a high prevalence of sexual health concerns in women of all ages.[2,8,10-15] A woman's sexual problems can cause significant personal distress in approximately 25% of those with sexual health concerns, including a diminution of self-worth and self-esteem, a reduction in life satisfaction, and a decline in the quality of her relationship with her partner.[10-15] Many investigations have shown that a satisfying sex life is important to most women throughout most of their lives.[16] As life expectancy increases, there are increasing numbers of aging women.[17] Sexual health concerns are more common among aging women than among younger women.[10-15] The number of postmenopausal women worldwide in the year 2000 was 569 million; that number is projected to grow to 967 million by 2020 and to 1.2 billion by 2030.[17] As a result of the controversy concerning hormone therapy that followed the release of the Women's Health Initiative findings in 2002[18] millions of menopausal women altered and or discontinued hormone therapy practices, and this directly influenced many women's subsequent vaginal physiology and sexual interest states.[19] As the decline in estrogen production begins in transition to menopause, sexual dysfunction becomes common, often interfering with women's interest in, and satisfaction with, sexual activity.

It is important to note the existence of the International Society for the Study of Women's Sexual Health (ISSWSH), an international, multidisciplinary, academic, clinical, and scientific organization. The purposes of ISSWSH are to provide opportunities for communication among scholars, researchers, and practitioners about women's sexual health; to support the highest standards of ethics and professionalism in research, education, and clinical practice relative to women's sexual health; and to provide the public with accurate information about women's sexual health. Interested health care professionals should visit the organization's web site, (http://www.isswsh.org) for more information. More detailed information about ISSWSH and the management of women's sexual health concerns may be found in the multidisciplinary textbook written primarily by ISSWSH members entitled, *Women's Sexual Function and Dysfunction: Study, Diagnosis and Treatment.*[20]

EPIDEMIOLOGY AND CLASSIFICATION

There are limited population-based epidemiologic studies of women with sexual health concerns.[2,8,10-15] Based on current published information, the following is the most contemporary, internationally consensed classification system.[21]

Women's sexual interest/desire disorder: Absent or diminished feelings of sexual interest or desire, absent sexual thoughts or fantasies and a lack of responsive desire. Motivations (here defined as reasons/incentives) for attempting to become sexually aroused are scarce or absent. The lack of interest is considered to be beyond a normative lessening with life cycle and relationship duration.

Subjective sexual arousal disorder: Absence of or markedly diminished feelings of sexual arousal (sexual excitement and sexual pleasure) from any type of sexual stimulation. Vaginal lubrication or other signs of physical response still occur.

Genital sexual arousal disorder: Complaints of absent or impaired genital sexual arousal. Self-reports may include minimal vulval swelling or vaginal lubrication from any type of sexual stimulation and reduced sexual sensations from caressing genitalia. Subjective sexual excitement still occurs from nongenital sexual stimuli.

Combined genital and subjective arousal disorder: Absence of, or markedly diminished feelings of, sexual arousal (sexual excitement and sexual pleasure) from any type of sexual stimulation as well as complaints of absent or impaired genital sexual arousal (vulval swelling, lubrication).

Persistent sexual arousal disorder: Spontaneous, intrusive and unwanted genital arousal (e.g., tingling, throbbing, pulsating) in the absence of sexual interest and desire. Any awareness of subjective arousal is typically but not invariably unpleasant. The arousal is unrelieved by one or more orgasms and the feelings of arousal persist for hours or days.

Women's orgasmic disorder: Despite the self-report of high sexual arousal/excitement, there is either lack of orgasm, markedly diminished intensity of orgasmic sensations or marked delay of orgasm from any kind of stimulation.

Dyspareunia: Persistent or recurrent pain with attempted or complete vaginal entry and/or penile vaginal intercourse.

Vaginismus: Persistent difficulties to allow vaginal entry of a penis, a finger, and/or any object, despite the woman's expressed wish to do so. There is variable involuntary pelvic muscle contraction, (phobic) avoidance and anticipation/fear/experience of pain. Structural or other physical abnormalities must be ruled out/addressed.

Sexual aversion disorder: Extreme anxiety and/or disgust at the anticipation of/or attempt to have any sexual activity.

Laumann and associates, in a U.S. population-based study of more than 1700 women, observed that more than 40% reported sexual health concerns.[15] In that investigation, the most common sexual health concern was lack of sexual desire, followed by inability to achieve orgasm, lack of pleasure from sex, and pain during sex. Poor health, emotional problems or stress, decline in social status, and having ever been forced sexually were among the factors associated with low desire, arousal disorder, and sexual pain. A worldwide survey of more than 27,000 men and women aged 40 to 80 years assessed the relevance of sex and the prevalence of sexual dysfunction.[22] In that survey, women's sexual health concerns were classified into five subcategories: lack of interest in sex, inability to achieve orgasm, lubrication difficulties (dryness), sex not pleasurable, and pain during sexual intercourse (dyspareunia). The percentage of women who reported having at least one sexual health concern on a frequent or persistent basis was 39%. The percentage of women who reported having only one of the five sexual health concerns ranged from 10% for "dyspareunia" to 21% for "lack of interest in sex."[8,22]

Contemporary international prevalence data concerning women's sexual health problems, are represented in Table 50-1.[2,8,10-15,22]

Table 50-1 Estimated International Prevalence of Women's Sexual Health Concerns from Various Studies

Concern	Current Prevalence (%)	1-Year Prevalence (%)	Lifetime Prevalence (%)
Problems with sexual desire or sexual interest	7		31
Problems with excitement or pleasure		23	20
Lubrication difficulties or vaginal dryness		20	19-23
Infrequent orgasm or difficulties in reaching orgasm			4-41
Inability to experience orgasm			
For several months	16*		
For 2 months or longer	18†		
More than 50% of the time	25†		
Pain during or after sex	3-48		17-19 (population-based) 10-20 (clinic-based)
Any problem with desire, arousal, orgasm, or pain	33-35‡		
Any current sexual problem	45§		
Any sexual problem	43		

*Estimate is from a single population-based study.
†Both estimates are from a single population-based study.
‡Estimates are from two population-based surveys using similar instruments.
§Estimate (1-month prevalence) is from a single national study.
Data from references 2, 8, 10-15, 22.

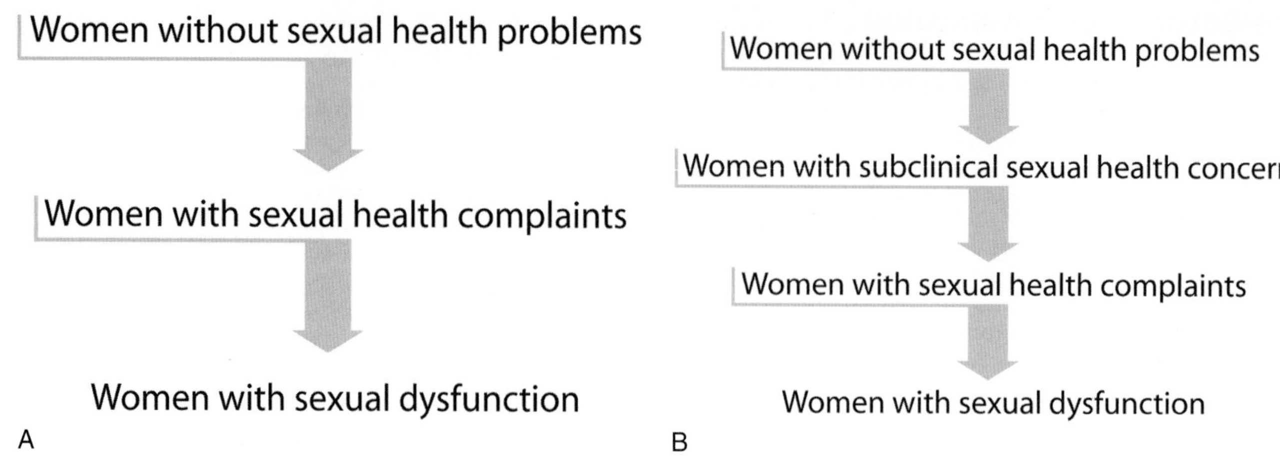

Figure 50-3 A, It is proposed that, in the clinical spectrum of women's sexual function/dysfunction, there is an as yet undefined continuum of conditions that gradually blend into each other such that it is difficult to say where one stage becomes the next. In the continuum hypothesis of women's sexual health complaints, there are women without sexual health problems, women with specific conditions of frank sexual dysfunction, and an intermediate group including women with sexual health complaints. **B,** In the continuum hypothesis of women's sexual health complaints, the intermediate stage may begin in some asymptomatic women with a recognizable subclinical stage in which abnormal testing or laboratory values may be a harbinger that precedes overt symptoms and distress.

The Continuum Hypothesis for Women's Sexual Health Concerns

In various medical conditions, there are those individuals who are free of a specific condition and there are those, at the opposite end of the spectrum, who are afflicted with the overt clinical manifestations of the condition. The same must hold true for women's sexual health conditions. There likely is an as yet undefined continuum whereby women without sexual health problems ultimately develop the condition of frank sexual dysfunction. A continuum may be considered as a continuous series of events that blend into each other so gradually and seamlessly that it is impossible to say where one stage becomes the next.

One hypothesis is that women without the condition first develop an intermediate stage involving complaints of problems with sexual desire, arousal, lubrication, sensation, orgasm, and pain without any accompanying personal distress.[23] The pathophysiology is most likely multifactorial and may be secondary to medical conditions such as hormonal milieu changes or vascular disease; psychological conditions such as depression; medications that may contribute to symptoms, such selective serotonin reuptake inhibitors and antipsychotics; or any other social or relationship issues that may play a role, such as a history of sexual abuse or partner-related issues. Ultimately, when personal distress results as a consequence of the persistence or intensity of the sexual symptoms, the problem is considered to have evolved into frank sexual dysfunction (Fig. 50-3A).[23,24]

Consistent with the hypothesis that sexual health concerns exist in a continuum, one may then introduce the additional concept of an earlier intermediate stage. The idea of a subclinical stage of women's sexual health concerns, one that occurs before the onset of overt symptoms but is recognized clinically by abnormal questionnaire results and/or laboratory values, comes from recent prospective, multi-institutional studies.[25,26] With the goal of defining androgen levels in a premenopausal population, prospective candidates underwent an initial interview to identify those "free of sexual health problems." Women who met inclusion and exclusion criteria subsequently underwent determination of androgen levels and completion of a validated sexual function questionnaire on which low scores indicated poor sexual function. A subgroup of women from that study, who perceived themselves as having no deficits in sexual function and presented to take part in the study as the control population, were found to have scores on the validated sexual function questionnaire consistent with sexual health problems. These abnormal findings precluded their inclusion in the control group. We subsequently attempted to better characterize the women in this group by recording androgen levels. In these asymptomatic women with low validated sexual function questionnaire scores, androgen levels were found to be virtually indistinguishable from those of women with symptomatic sexual dysfunction and significantly lower than those of women who denied sexual concerns and scored higher on the validated sexual function questionnaire.

The concept of a subclinical stage of a medical condition is well established in the literature. For example, subclinical hypothyroidism[27] is considered to exist when there is an abnormally elevated thyroid-stimulating hormone level in a patient who has not yet manifested obvious or evident symptoms of hypothyroidism (e.g., fatigue, depression, osteoporosis, weight gain). Other scenarios of subclinical medical conditions are well described, such as impaired glucose tolerance, elevated liver function tests,[28] or abnormal electrocardiogram associated with early coronary atherosclerosis.[29] The term *subclinical* refers to those situations in which abnormal testing or laboratory values may be a harbinger that precedes overt symptoms of the condition.

There is a previously undefined population of women who claim an absence of sexual health problems on initial clinical interview but who are found to have validated psychometric questionnaire scores consistent with the presence of sexual health concerns and androgen levels comparable to those seen with androgen insufficiency. It is hypothesized that the development and progression of women's sexual health problems follows a continuum. In this continuum hypothesis, women without sexual health complaints may progress first through a subclinical stage, followed by a symptomatic stage, and subsequently develop frank sexual dysfunction when the sexual problem becomes clinically meaningful and is associated with personal distress (see Fig. 50-3B). Future research studies are needed to assess the relevance of these intermediate stages of women's sexual health, in general, and the subclinical state of female sexual dysfunction, specifically. In particular, it would be of interest to investigate the role of any prophylactic management strategies, psychological and biologic, that may halt the development of future overt clinical symptoms and/or frank sexual dysfunction.

PHYSIOLOGY AND PATHOPHYSIOLOGY

Effect of the Male Partner who has Erectile Dysfunction

Whereas substantial investigation has taken place on the effects of selective phosphodiesterase type 5 (PDE5) inhibitors in men with erectile dysfunction (ED), little attention has been given to the sexual responses of their female partners. A typical inclusion criterion in the trials of such drugs was the existence of a stable heterosexual relationship. Participation of the woman was voluntary and was limited to assessments of treatment satisfaction. The female partners of men with ED were thought to unconditionally support their partners' sexual treatment. The issues relating to the perspective of the woman, her well-being, quality of life, sexual function and sexual satisfaction, in relation to either existing or successfully treated ED, were not taken into consideration.

Couples share their sexual dysfunctions. Women with men who have ED may have their own sexual function adversely affected. What are the scientific data available concerning changes in sexual function among those women whose partners have ED? Blumel and colleagues examined a sample of 534 otherwise healthy women who had ceased sexual activity with their male partners. It was noted that, in the cohort younger than 45 years of age, ED was the most frequently cited reason for cessation of the woman's sexual activity.[30]

Initial studies were, however, obtained with data from the man's perspective. Past research in this area involved inquiries addressed to men with ED about the effect of their sexual problem on their women partners. One study showed significant improvement in the marital interaction score when men with ED used a selective PDE5 inhibitor.[31]

Contemporary research has finally begun to address the issue from the woman's perspective. Data from several investigations are derived from the woman herself, as her own study subject. Cayan and colleagues performed a prospective study assessing the sexual function of women with men who had ED.[32] The study involved 38 such women, as well as a control group of 49 women whose male partner did not have ED. Women's sexual functions, including sexual arousal, lubrication, orgasm, satisfaction, pain, and total score, were significantly diminished among women with men who had ED. Among those women whose male partners received treatment (penile prosthesis insertion, oral PDE5 inhibitor treatment) for their ED, significant improvements in sexual arousal, lubrication, orgasm, satisfaction, and pain in the women were identified.

Montorsi and Althof investigated thoughts and views on intercourse satisfaction in 930 women whose male partners were taking a selective PDE5 inhibitor to manage ED.[33] These women had significantly higher intercourse satisfaction than did women whose men were using a placebo.

Chevret and coworkers developed and validated the Index of Sexual Life to measure sexual function of women in relationships with men with ED.[34] Such women were found to have significantly diminished sexual drive and sexual satisfaction compared to women whose male partners did not have ED.

Oberg and colleagues examined data from a nationally representative Swedish cross-sectional population investigation of sexual life, attitudes, and behavior.[11] A total of 926 women, aged 18 to 65 years, were sexually active in a steady heterosexual relationship during the 12 months before the investigation. Data from women who claimed personally distressing sexual dysfunctions quite often, almost all the time, or all the time were compared with data from women who had no sexually dysfunctional distress. Women reporting distress due to low sexual interest or orgasmic dysfunction were very likely to have a partner with an ED (odds ratios, 47.6 and 20.0, respectively).

In the Female Experience of Men's Attitudes to Life Events and Sexuality study,[35] data were analyzed from 283 women in eight countries whose male partners had ED. They were asked questions comparing their sexual activity, sexual function, and beliefs about sexuality before and since their partner had experienced difficulties with erection. Data were stratified by the man's self-reported degree of ED (mild, moderate, or severe). Women whose partners had ED reported a lower frequency of sexual activity currently, compared with before their partner developed erectile difficulties. Significantly fewer women reported that they experienced sexual desire, sexual arousal, orgasm, or sexual satisfaction ("almost always" or "most times") currently, compared with before their partner developed erectile difficulties. There was a significant correlation between the reduction in the woman's frequency of orgasm, and her reduction in sexual satisfaction, and the degree of her partner's self-reported ED. Women had the lowest frequency of orgasm and the lowest satisfaction with the sexual experience when their partners had severe ED.

Scientific data were obtained from a double-blind, multicenter, 3-month, randomized trial involving men with ED who had been in a stable heterosexual couple relationship for at least 6 months.[36,37] In this trial, women whose male partner had ED were asked at initial screening to complete the validated Female Sexual Function Inventory. Significant improvement in the woman's sexual function and sexual satisfaction were observed after their partner was treated with a selective PDE5 inhibitor, vardenafil (Fig. 50-4) versus placebo.

Effect of the Male Partner Who Has Premature Ejaculation

Because premature ejaculation is the most common male sexual dysfunction, affecting approximately 25% of men, it is likely that many women will experience a sexual relationship with a man with premature ejaculation.[38] Premature ejaculation is objectively determined using a stopwatch to record intravaginal ejaculatory latency time, defined as the time between vaginal intromission and intravaginal ejaculation. It has been suggested that an intravaginal ejaculatory latency time of 2 minutes or less may serve as a criterion for defining premature ejaculation.[39]

Women with men who have premature ejaculation may have significant distress, interpersonal difficulties, and dissatisfaction with sexual intercourse.[40] The woman's distress is a common

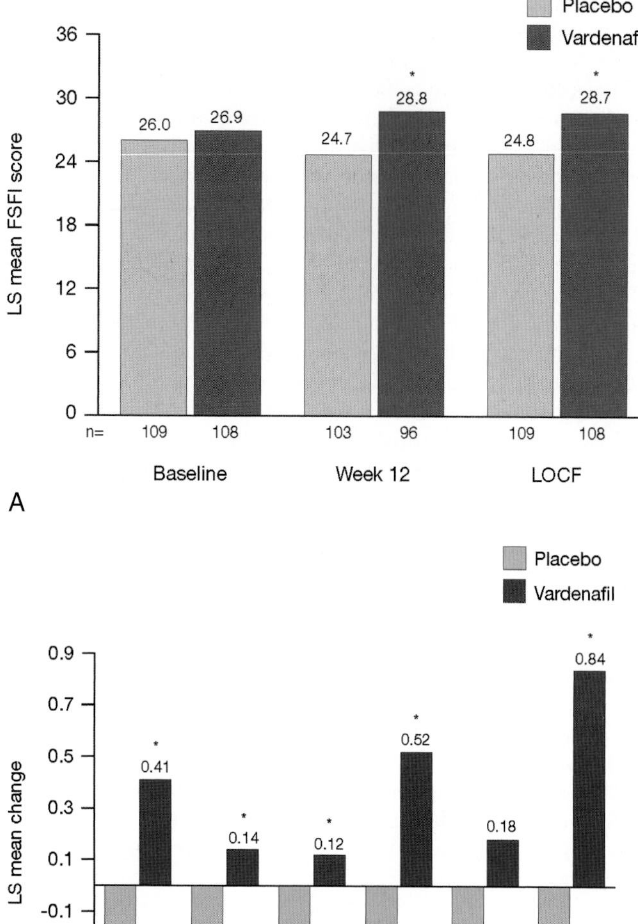

Figure 50-4 **A,** At baseline, there was no difference in total Female Sexual Function Index (FSFI) scores of untreated woman whose partners with erectile dysfunction were assigned to placebo versus treatment with vardenafil, a selective phosphodiesterase type 5 (PDE5) inhibitor. At 3 months or last observation carried forward (LOCF), the total FSFI score fell if the woman's partner was assigned to placebo and increased if he was assigned to PDE5 inhibitor treatment. The total FSFI scores were significantly different (*asterisk*) between placebo and active groups by Week 12 and at LOCF. **B,** At 3 months, those untreated women whose male partners with erectile dysfunction received the active PDE5 inhibitor vardenafil had significant increases in all domains of the FSFI except for sexual pain; those whose partners received placebo had significant decreases in all domains of the FSFI except for sexual pain.

reason for the man to consult a clinician about premature ejaculation.

Byers and Grenier investigated the effect of premature ejaculation on the sexual function of 152 couples.[41] Concerning the couple's perceptions of whether the premature ejaculation was a problem, reports of women and men were only moderately correlated. For both the women and the men, having more premature ejaculation characteristics was related to lower sexual satisfaction. The results suggested that, for most couples, the premature or early timing of ejaculation adversely affects sexual satisfaction.

Patrick and colleagues[40] carefully selected patients with and without premature ejaculation based on stopwatch testing. The mean intravaginal ejaculatory latency time was 1.8 minutes in the 207 men with premature ejaculation. This was significantly lower than the time (7.3 minutes) in the 1380 men without premature ejaculation. Women whose male partner had premature ejaculation had significantly decreased satisfaction with sexual intercourse and significiantly increased interpersonal difficulty and distress, compared to women whose partner did not have premature ejaculation ($P < .0001$). They also reported "poor" or "very poor" satisfaction with sexual intercourse (28% versus 2%) and gave worse ratings ("quite a bit" or "extremely") for personal distress (44% versus 3%) and interpersonal difficulty (25% versus 2%), compared to women whose partner did not have premature ejaculation ($P < .0001$).

Changes in the Female Genitalia with Aging

The structure and function of a woman's genitalia are highly dependent on the sex steroid hormonal milieu.[1,19,42-46] As a woman ages or a young woman is exposed to medicines that interfere with the hormonal milieu (e.g., oral contraceptives, tamoxifene), her supply of sex steroid hormones (estradiol, testosterone, and progesterone) diminishes significantly.[1,19]

Of importance, not all women have absent estradiol synthesis in the menopause. During menopause, ovarian estradiol production ceases in all women. However, estrogen continues to be synthesized in the periphery (e.g., skin, adipose tissue, bone, muscle) in postmenopausal women through conversion of androstenedione to estrone and testosterone to estradiol, but the amount of estradiol synthesized depends, in part, on the enzymatic activity of aromatase.

Estrogens and androgens are required for genital tissue structure and function.[19] These hormones act on estrogen and androgen receptors, respectively, which exist in high numbers in genital tissues, including the epithelial/endothelial cells and smooth muscle cells of the vagina, vulva, vestibule, labia, and urethra. Diminished estrogen production for natural or iatrogenic reasons renders women's genital tissues highly susceptible to atrophy (see Figs. 50-1 and 50-2). Physical examination[7,47] of the postmenopausal woman's genitalia shows clitoral atrophy, phimosis, and nearly absent labia minora (Fig. 50-5). The appearance of a woman's labia minora mirrors her level of estradiol, because these labia are exquisitely sensitive to estradiol. The urogenital area termed the vestibule is very important in female sexual function because it contains organs that are sensitive to both estrogen and androgen. For example, the clitoral tissues and prepuce are androgen sensitive. The minor vestibular glands (Fig. 50-6), which are located in the labial-hymenal junction, are embryologically derived from the glands of Littre, which are also androgen dependent. The glands of Littre are located on the anterior surface of the urethra.

A host of structural changes and cellular dysfunctions occur in women's genital tissues as a result of estrogen deficiency.[7,48-51] For example, estrogen deficiency specifically in the vagina leads to vaginal atrophy. One consequence is an alteration in the normally acidic vaginal pH that discourages the growth of pathogenic bacteria. The change to an alkaline pH value in the atrophic

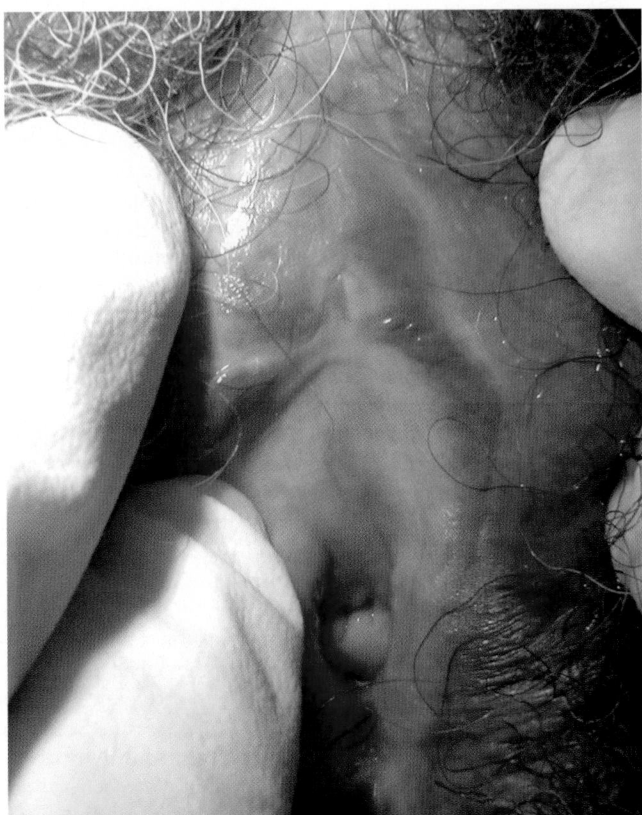

Figure 50-5 This is a photograph of a postmenopausal woman with clitoral atrophy, phimosis, and nearly absent labia minora.

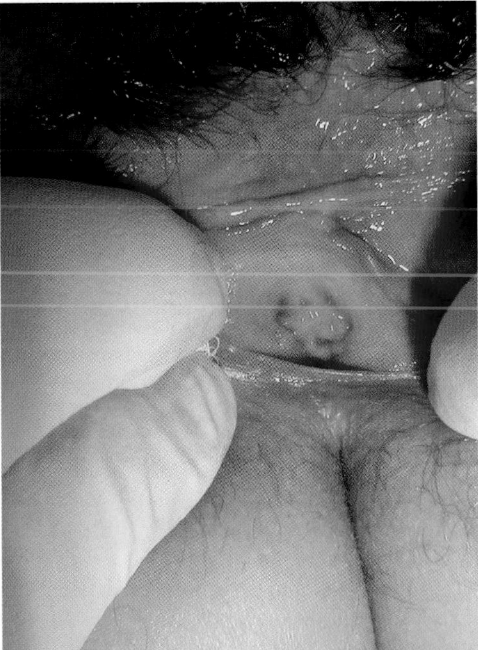

Figure 50-6 This is a photograph of a premenopausal woman with bilateral erythema overlying the minor vestibular glands at the labial-hymenal junction. Note also the clitoral atrophy, phimosis, and nearly absent labia minora.

vagina leads to a shift in the vaginal flora, increasing the likelihood of discharge and odor. In an estrogen-rich environment, glycogen from sloughed epithelial cells is hydrolyzed into glucose and then metabolized to lactic acid by normal vaginal flora. In postmenopausal women, however, epithelial thinning reduces the available glycogen.

In addition to vaginal atrophy and a reduction in organ size, other signs of a decline in sex hormones in women include vaginal dryness, absent secretions or lubrication, pale or inflamed tissue, petechiae, epithelial/mucosal thinning, organ prolapse, changes in external genitalia, decreased tissue elasticity, and loss of smooth muscle. Symptoms of women's sexual health concerns that the clinician may elicit when taking a history in a menopausal woman are include dyspareunia, vaginismus, coital anorgasmia, vaginal and/or urinary tract infections (pH imbalance), and overactive bladder/incontinence.[7,48-52]

Effects of Sex Steroid Hormones on the Vagina

The human vagina consists of three layers of tissue: the epithelium (composed of squamous cells), the lamina propria, and the muscularis (inner circular and outer longitudinal smooth muscle). The epithelium undergoes mild changes during the menstrual cycle. The lamina propria is replete with tiny blood vessels that become engorged with blood during sexual arousal, leading to lubrication. The smooth muscle of the muscularis enables the vagina to dilate and lengthen during penile penetration. Relaxation of that muscle leads to arousal. These three layers of tissue may function in an interrelated way (Fig. 50-7). It is hypothesized that the blood vessels in the lamina propria that allow for lubrication are dependent on growth factors, and that the growth factors are derived from the muscularis. Postmenopausal atrophy of vaginal tissues may be caused by decreased synthesis these growth factors that results in diminished number of critical blood vessels in the lamina propria.

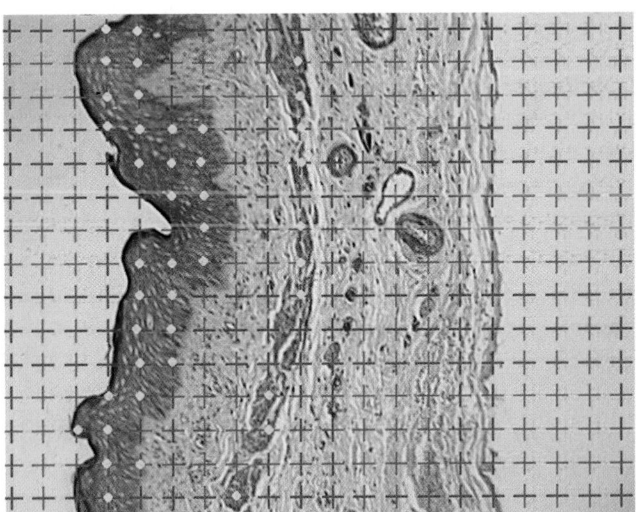

Figure 50-7 A grid overlies a histologic section of animal vagina illustrating the epithelium (*left side of section*), the lamina propria (*middle*) and the vaginal muscularis (*right side*). The grid is used to objectively measure the structural changes in the various vaginal layers in response to oophorectomy and then replacement by various doses and combinations of sex steroid hormones.

Controlled studies employing a rat model of vaginal atrophy demonstrated the effects of various dosages of estrogen, progestin, testosterone, and combinations of these hormones on physiologic and anatomic outcome parameters.[52] These measures included organ wet weight, vaginal blood flow, epithelial height, muscularis thickness, and vaginal innervation. In each study, the effects on the vagina of of the hormones being tested were compared between rats that had undergone sham ovariectomies and rats that had actually had both ovaries removed. The hormones (or saline) were delivered through a pump inserted into the back of the neck of each animal. A Doppler probe inserted into the vagina was used to record blood flow after electrical stimulation of a nerve next to the vagina. All animals were then killed, and vaginal tissue was removed for biochemical or histologic studies. Removal of the ovaries was found to reduce the wet weight of the uterus, which rose again with administration of estrogen, because the uterus is a very estrogen-sensitive organ, much more so than the vagina.

Increased vaginal blood flow is an indicator of sexual arousal. Genital swelling and lubrication are responses to increased clitoral and vaginal perfusion; increased length and diameter of the vaginal canal and clitoral corpora cavernosa; engorgement of the vagina wall, clitoris, labia majora, and labia minora; and transudation of lubricating fluid from the vaginal epithelium. In the animal studies just described, blood flow to the vagina was greatly reduced in the oophorectomized rats compared with the intact rats. Contrary to what one might expect, subphysiologic doses of estradiol increased vaginal blood flow in oophorectomized rats more than either physiologic or supraphysiologic doses.[52] Ovariectomy deprived the rats of estradiol, causing the vaginal epithelium to thin down to a single layer. Subphysiologic doses of estradiol increased the thickness of the vaginal epithelium most, because the oophorectomized rats had more estrogen ERα receptors in the epithelium than the intact animals did. A small amount of estradiol delivered to tissue with many estrogen ERα receptors produced a huge response. Thus, estradiol regulates estrogen receptors through a negative feedback system. The more estradiol that is available, the fewer estrogen receptors there are. The muscularis, the muscle that enables the vagina to lengthen and widen during sexual arousal, also atrophies without estrogen. In postmenopausal women who do not take hormone therapy, the vaginal epithelium, lamina propria blood vessels, and muscularis all decrease. Like the epithelium, the muscularis responds to estradiol by increasing in thickness.[52]

Role of the Pelvic Floor in Women's Sexual Function

Female urologists are familiar with the diagnosis and treatment of disorders of the female pelvic floor, especially bladder/urethra and sexual dysfunction. Normal function of the pelvic floor musculature is essential in maintaining appropriate sexual function. Both "low-tone pelvic floor dysfunction" and "high-tone pelvic floor muscle dysfunction" can be closely associated with women's sexual health concerns.[53-57] Hypotonus of the pelvic floor muscles, resulting from childbirth, trauma, and/or aging, is related to urinary incontinence during orgasm, vaginal laxity, and/or thrusting dyspareunia secondary to pelvic organ prolapse. Hypertonus of the pelvic floor caused by childbirth, postural stressors, microtrauma, infection, adhesions, or surgical trauma and can contribute to symptoms of urinary retention, reduced force of stream, dysuria, urgency, penetrative dyspareunia, and/or vaginismus.[53-61]

The assessment of tone in the pelvic floor is determined by the woman's ability to isolate, contract, and relax the pelvic floor muscles. During a pelvic examination, a digital examination is used to assess pelvic floor tone; light pressure is exerted on the lateral walls of the vagina while the woman is asked to squeeze on the examining finger and to elevate the pelvic floor without simultaneously contracting the abdominal, gluteal, or adductor muscle groups. If the patient is not able to produce sufficient muscle strength to compress the finger or is not able to sustain that pressure for several seconds, she may be exhibiting a low-tone pelvic floor dysfunction pattern. Conversely, if the woman experiences muscle tenderness or pain when pressure is applied to the lateral vaginal wall or during an attempted squeeze against resistance, she may be exhibiting a high-tone pelvic floor dysfunction pattern. A perineometer or an electromyography probe designed to measure muscle activity can verify these physical examination findings.[53-61]

Hypersensitivity disorders involving the genitourinary tract represent a spectrum of symptoms and conditions that include chronic bacterial cystitis, urgency and frequency syndrome, sensory urgency, urethral syndrome, interstitial cystitis, vulvar pain, vaginal pain, perineal pain, and pelvic pain. Hypersensitivity disorders, associated with hypertonus of the pelvic floor musculature, account for some of the concerns of female patients who present for evaluation of sexual health concerns. Sexuality is adversely affected for most women with hypersensitivity disorders of the bladder, bowel, or vulva or high-tone pelvic floor dysfunction. Those that are able to tolerate coitus often suffer a flare of their symptoms for days as a result of sexual activity, and this becomes a negative reinforcement for future sexual activity.[53-61]

Weakness and laxity of the pelvic floor muscles represent a spectrum of symptoms and conditions that include pelvic organ prolapse with or without urinary or fecal incontinence. Risk factors include age, heredity, vaginal birth trauma, previous pelvic/vaginal surgery, history of radiation therapy, menopausal status, lifestyle factors such as strenuous lifting, and chronic medical conditions including obstructive pulmonary disease, obesity, and constipation. Stress incontinence that occurs with increased intra-abdominal pressure and maneuvers such as sneezing, coughing, and straining is related to abnormalities in urethral closure and poor pelvic muscle support. Sexuality is often adversely affected for women with severe low-tone pelvic floor dysfunction, especially for those with severe incontinence and prolapse in whom symptoms are a source of anxiety and interfere with the overall sense of sexual satisfaction. Women who experience incontinence during intercourse express concern about feeling undesirable, fearing embarrassment, and possibly infecting themselves or their partner.[53-61]

Urethritis, Recurrent Urinary Tract Infections, and Interstitial Cystitis

It is very common for women, especially during transition and in menopause, to complain of irritative voiding symptoms, especially burning, frequency, urgency, and nocturia, which significantly interfere with sexual activity.[62-65] In such women, the vulvovaginal and urinary irritative and burning symptoms are often poorly defined. Patient and physician confusion in this area occurs because the differential diagnosis of irritation and burning in the perineum, especially after coitus, involves multiple different urologic and gynecologic conditions. Urologic conditions that do not involve the urethral meatus include, for example, recurrent urethritis, recurrent urinary tract infections, urethral diverticula, irritable bladder, cystocele, ureteral stones, and endometriosis of the ureter and/or bladder. Irritative symptoms that occur during voiding, especially after coitus, may also be associated with inflammatory gynecologic conditions. In such situations, the contact of voided urine against the inflamed vestibular, vulvar, and/or vaginal tissues can result in significant perineal burning and stinging. Vaginal yeast infections, vulvar dermatitis conditions, and uterine prolapse with or without rectocele are common gynecologic pathophysiologies. In many cases, expert urologic and gynecologic consultations are required to confirm the multiple diagnoses in the individual patient so that varied specific focused treatments may be initiated.[62-65]

One rare genital sexual pain condition, called "interstitial cystitis," is confusing and ill-defined; it is associated with severe urogenital and pelvic pain, urgency, frequency, nocturia, and dyspareunia.[53,66] The pathophysiology of interstitial cystitis is unknown but appears be unrelated to any recognized bacterial pathophysiology. Interstitial cystitis symptoms, including the dyspareunia, often increase with the menses, increase during bladder filling, and decrease with bladder emptying. There is no definitive diagnostic test for interstitial cystitis. History, physical examination, urinalysis, urine culture, and maintenance of a voiding log are mandatory. Specific patient questionnaires are often useful. Other specific testing procedures include potassium sensitivity testing and cystoscopy with or without hydrodistention. Because it relates to the dyspareunia and genital sexual pain component associated with interstitial cystitis, treatment of the underlying condition is important.[53,66]

Dermatologic Conditions

Lichen sclerosis is a chronic genital dermatitis condition that is associated with varying intensity of symptoms including vulvar itch and/or burning and various degrees of vulvar scarring leading to narrowing of the introitus and dyspareunia.[61-64,66] There is a wide variation in presentation symptoms. In some women, especially those not sexually active, there can be minimal symptoms and the patient may be unaware of the condition of lichen sclerosis for years. Alternatively, the burning and itching symptoms can be so intense as to severely interfere with sexual activity, day-to-day activities, and even sleep. If the scarring of lichen sclerosis involves the perianal area, the patient may also complain of perianal fissuring and painful defecation. The diagnosis of lichen sclerosis is suspected by physical examination showing white color genital, vulvar, and vestibular tissue with paleness, loss of pigmentation, and a characteristic "cigarette paper" wrinkling (Fig. 50-8). Classically, the genital tissue changes do not involve the inside of the vagina, and if they involve the perianal area, there is a traditional "figure of eight" extension. The lichen sclerosis condition commonly involves the vestibule with associated labia minora atrophy and the vaginal introitus with loss of elasticity and narrowing.

Lichen planus[67] is another chronic genital dermatitis condition that is probably pathophysiologically related to various immunologic disorders. The presenting symptoms vary widely, most likely due to the varied pathophysiologies. Lichen planus may occur secondary to use of drugs such as antihypertensives, diuretics, oral hypoglycemics, and nonsteroidal anti-inflammatory agents, which may rarely induce a lichen planus–like eruption. One type of lichen planus is primarily associated with itching and does not result in scarring. Another type is erosive and destructive. Overall, patient complaints may include severe vulvar itching, pain, burning, and irritation. Dyspareunia[61-64,66,67] occurs in sexually active women secondary to vaginal introital scarring. Some types of lichen planus, unlike lichen sclerosis, may involve the vaginal mucosa. If there is vaginal involvement, a purulent, malodorous discharge may be noted. Findings on physical examination of women with lichen planus vary widely. The pruritic type of lichen planus is associated with a purple color and multiple papules and plaques on the vulva and vestibule. The erosive type is associated with vestibular ulcers, scarring, and atrophy of the clitoris and labia minora; destruction of the vagina has been reported. A biopsy and dermatopathologic review may be needed to establish the diagnosis of lichen planus.[67]

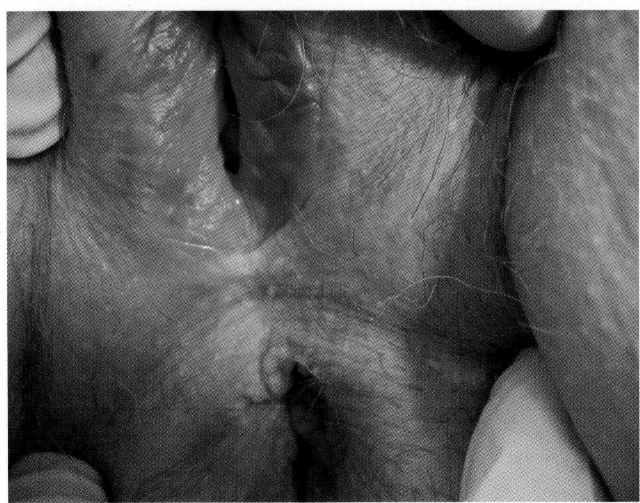

Figure 50-8 This is a photograph of a postmenopausal woman with lichen sclerosis that reveals white color perineal and perinanal tissue with characteristic "cigarette paper" wrinkling. There are also classic signs of vaginal atrophy with fusion of the labia minora to the labia majora.

Genital Sexual Pain Disorders

Generalized vulvodynia[59,61,62,68,69] refers to a diffuse, constant, burning pain anywhere on the vulva, from mons to anus, which is hyperpathic and greatly out of proportion to the stimulus. Afflicted patients have a constant or sporadic awareness of the vulva with widespread sensation that "everything hurts," vulvar soreness, rawness, constant irritation, various paresthesias, aching, and/or stinging. Generalized vulvodynia may be considered primary if it occurs with the first penetrative sexual encounter or with a tampon or speculum examination. Generalized vulvodynia may be considered secondary if it occurs after previous nonpainful vaginal penetrations. The diagnosis of generalized vulvodynia[59,61,62,68,69] is made by ruling out, on physical examination and laboratory testing, such diagnoses as candida vaginitis and chronic genital dermatitis conditions. Q-tip testing shows all vulvar areas positive for pain and/or tenderness. The treatment of any genital sexual pain disorder involves a multidisciplinary team approach, and this is especially true for the disabling condition of generalized vulvodynia.

Vulvar vestibulitis syndrome is another genital sexual pain disorder. On history, there is severe pain on vestibular touch or attempted vaginal entry. On physical examination, there is ery-

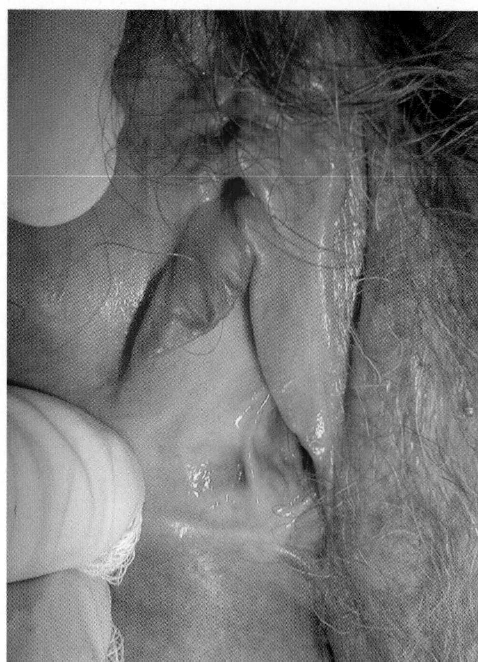

Figure 50-9 This is a photograph of a premenopausal woman with vulvar vestibulitis syndrome involving minor vestibular glands at the 6- to 7-o'clock position. Cotton swab testing revealed extreme sensitivity and burning to touch.

thema of various degrees within the vestibule. During Q-tip testing, there is tenderness to pressure that is "localized" within the vulvar vestibule. Often, the tender localized region is along the labial-hymenal junction associated with the presence of minor vestibular glands (Fig. 50-9). Vulvar vestibulitis syndrome[59,61,62,68,69] is one of the most likely causes of dyspareunia, especially in women younger than 50 years of age. Afflicted patients with vulvar vestibulitis syndrome complain of severe pain during sexual activity, often described as raw, red burning, feeling like sandpaper, or feeling like burnt tissue being rubbed. Most women experience the pain in the vulvar region with initial penetration. There is another group of women who do not experience pain during initial penetration but experience severe pain on deep penetration when the man's perineum comes into contact with the woman's. In this latter group, physicians are misguided to the cervix, when the site of the pain trigger is really within the vulvar region. With vulvar vestibulitis syndrome, genital sexual pain may also be experienced with the use of tampons, during speculum examination, when wearing tight pants, or during straddling while bicycling or horseback riding. Although there is no known pathophysiology, there are several possible pathophysiologic factors, including exposure to human papillomavirus, exposure to the irritant oxalate, abnormal immunologic conditions, psychopathology, and an abnormal sex steroid hormonal milieu.

DIAGNOSIS OF WOMEN'S SEXUAL HEALTH CONCERNS

History

There are limited consensus management paradigms for the diagnosis of women with sexual health complaints. The cornerstone of the physical-based diagnosis of sexual dysfunction is a history and physical examination performed by the biologically focused health care professional. Specifically, obtaining a careful history is crucial, because this aspect of the diagnosis establishes impressions and forms the basis of emphasis on physical examination.[7,47]

The history of a woman with sexual health concerns includes sexual, medical, and psychosocial aspects, in order to characterize the many physical and psychological factors that often contribute to the sexual health difficulty. It is advised that women with sexual health concerns undergo a separate and concomitant psychological interview by a psychologically focused health care professional to broaden the psychosocial information derived during the interview process.[7,47]

Sexual History

The sexual history should begin with the patient describing the sexual problem. The following questions may be used to help obtain maximal descriptive information.

What is the sexual problem?

When did the sexual problem manifest? How long have you had the sexual problem? Does the sexual problem happen all the time?

Does the sexual problem occur during partner-related sexual activity? Does the sexual problem occur during self-stimulation? In which situations is the sexual problem minimized? In which situations is the sexual problem maximized?

Did you ever experience full capabilities for sexual interest, sexual arousal, and sexual orgasm? How many years were you at peak sexual function? What is your current sexual functioning in terms of interest, arousal, and orgasm compared to when you were at peak sexual function?

Is the sexual problem associated with any degree of discomfort, tenderness, soreness, or pain? If so, can you localize the site of the pain on a schematic diagram of a woman's genitalia?

What tests have you already had in the evaluation of your sexual health concern? What treatments have you already received, and what have been the outcomes of the various treatments?

How does the sexual problem affect you? How is your partner affected by the sexual problem? Does the sexual problem cause you to withdraw from partner-related sexual activity, from self-stimulated sexual activity, or from the relationship?

How would you feel if the sexual problem were cured?

It is relevant to inquire after the sexual health of the partner. For women with a male partner, there may exist male sexual dysfunctions such as ED, early ejaculation, or an anatomic concern (e.g., Peyronie's disease). Data on the importance of the male partner to the sexual function of the woman are expanding exponentially. Current knowledge indicates that, in a committed heterosexual relationship, the male partner's sexual performance is linked to the female partner's sexual function and sexual satisfaction. Therefore, if the male partner has some form of sexual dysfunction, such as ED, the woman's desire, arousal, ease of achieving orgasm, and satisfaction are reduced. This information is critical to obtain during history-taking.

The use of validated, reliable, standardized self-rated questionnaires[70-73] is a very helpful clinical starting point to assist in identification of the presence or absence of a sexual problem and which of the disorders of desire, arousal, orgasm, and/or sexual pain are involved. Such self-report measures are valuable screening tools that are easy to administer and score and have normative values for populations of women with and without sexual dysfunction. Common self-rated questionnaires include the Female Sexual Function Index and the Sexual Function Questionnaire. As in all areas of clinical medicine, the use of screening tools for clinical diagnosis has recognized limitations. The determination of particular psychological contributors or confounds, contextual conditions, and other features and characteristics that cause individual women their unique sexual concerns requires more traditional assessment through structured history and physical examination.

Medical History

The medical history should include focused questions on any accompanying medical/surgical illnesses or use of medications. Topics of importance in the medical history include

1. Chronic medical illnesses such as diabetes, anemia, or renal failure
2. Neurologic illnesses such as spinal cord injury, multiple sclerosis, or lumbosacral disc disease
3. Endocrinologic illnesses such as hypogonadism, hyperprolactinemia, or thyroid disorders
4. Atherosclerotic vascular risk factor exposure such as hypercholesterolemia, hypertension, diabetes, smoking, or family history
5. Nonhormonal medication or recreational drug use such as antihypertensives, selective serotonin-reuptake inhibitor (SSRI) antidepressants, over-the-counter drugs, street drugs, alcohol, or cocaine
6. Hormonal medication use such as combined oral contraceptives, infertility drugs, or leuprolide acetate
7. Pelvic/perineal/genital trauma such as pelvic fracture or bicycling injury
8. Gynecologic history such as childbirth, abortions, episiotomy, abnormal Papanicolaou (PAP) smears, sexually transmitted diseases, pelvic inflammatory disorder, endometriosis, fibroids, hysterectomy with or without oophorectomy, or menopause
9. Urologic history such as incontinence, frequent urinary tract infections, interstitial cystitis, or pelvic surgeries
10. Surgical history such as laminectomy, colon/anal surgery, or vascular bypass surgery
11. Psychiatric history such as depression, panic, or anxiety

Because sex steroid hormones are critical for genital structure and function, the medical history should routinely probe and evaluate for symptoms of estrogen deficiency, such as vaginal dryness, vaginal bleeding with minimal sexual contact, pain and soreness after sexual activity, hot flashes, and night sweats. Symptoms of androgen deficiency include fatigue, lack of energy, diminished skeletal muscle strength, depressed mood, falling asleep after meals, decreased athletic performance, and lack of interest in sexual activity.

Psychosocial History

The psychosocial history should assess such issues as social factors, past sexual beliefs, past sexual abuse and trauma, emotional concerns, and interpersonal relationship matters. Any past history of mood or psychiatric disorders should be identified.

There are multiple caveats to history taking in women with sexual health concerns. One is that the health care professional should consider history taking as having more significance than the first diagnostic step toward resolution of the sexual problem. The fact is that history taking may be viewed as actually the beginning of treatment for women with sexual health concerns. Women often feel empowered after this detailed discussion about their sexual health, because they have taken the first step in overcoming their past failures to take action in this area. It is not uncommon for the discussion with the health care provider to become a model of what is possible in conversations about sexual health. Many patients then are able to initiate a sexual health conversation with their partner, a close friend, or a family member.

The second caveat is that the health care professional should be cognizant that, whereas the women may have a specific sexual health complaint (e.g., lack of interest), there may be additional and more complex mind, body, and relationship issues in the overall pathophysiology. For example, a woman may experience sexual pain during intercourse. She may be so psychologically distracted by the discomfort, throbbing, stinging, aching, soreness, burning, and/or tenderness that physiologic desire, arousal, and orgasm responses during sexual stimulation are not able to manifest. This woman may present to the health care provider with a primary sexual complaint, such as lack of interest or orgasm, but a more detailed history and physical examination may yield the concomitant long-standing genital sexual pain problem.

Physical Examination

The physical examination for a woman with sexual health concerns should be tailored to the sexual medicine complaint obtained on history taking. For example, if during history taking genital itching is found to be a major sexual health problem, a careful assessment would follow for the presence of a genital dermatitis condition. If a woman with sexual health problems is younger than 50 years of age and has sexual pain, a careful physical examination should evaluate for the presence or absence of vulvar vestibulitis syndrome/vestibular adenitis. Similar complaints of sexual pain in a woman older than 50 years of age should lead to assessment for the presence of vaginal atrophy with dryness, loss of rugae, mucosal thinning, pale hue, and lack of shiny vaginal secretions. The physical examination should be performed ideally without menses and without intercourse or douching for 24 hours before the examination. If dysfunction occurs at a specific time, such as midcycle dyspareunia, the physical examination should be scheduled at the time of the sexual problem. Such scheduling may require two visits: one for history taking and one for the physical examination.[7,47]

The genitally focused examination should be considered routine in the diagnosis of women's sexual health problems, but its personal character demands that a rational explanation exist for its inclusion in the diagnostic process. A focused peripheral genital examination is recommended in women with sexual dysfunction for complaints of dyspareunia, vaginismus, genital or combined arousal disorder, orgasmic disorder, pelvic trauma history, and any disease affecting genital health such as herpes or lichen sclerosis. For women with suspected neurologic disorders, the examiner may also assess for anal and vaginal tone, voluntary tightening of anus, and bulbocavernosal reflexes.

It is particularly important that the patient with sexual dysfunction have full communication with the health care provider and have final authority during the physical examination to terminate at any time, to ask questions, to control who is in attendance, and to understand the extent of the assessment. It is vital that the patient be aware of the purpose of the examination. Inclusion of the sexual partner, with permission of the patient, is advantageous and provides needed patient support. Allowing the patient (and the partner) to observe any pathology via mirrors or digital photography is often therapeutic. It allows them, for the first time in many cases, an illustration and connection of a detected physical abnormality with the sexual health problem. If there exists a genital sexual pain history, the patient should point with her finger to the locations of the discomfort during the physical examination.

Independent of the gender of the examining health care provider, it is strongly recommended that a female chaperone health care provider be present in the examination room. The following equipment should be available: examination table, hospital gown, bed sheet, disposable absorbing chucks, patient covering sheet, surgical loupes or magnifying glass, examination light source, examination gloves, gauze, lubricant, Q-tips, speculum, pH paper, glass slides, saline, and microscope. The patient should wear a hospital gown, and a sheet should cover her lower torso. The patient should be placed in the lithotomy position, equipment for magnified vision and a carefully focused light source should be arranged, and the examining health care provider should be seated comfortably.

The first part of the examination involves inspection. If appropriate, lubricant should be placed on the vulva. Gauze can be grasped between thumb and index finger and used to retract the labia majora for a full inspection of the vestibular contents. Two gloved fingers are placed on either side of the clitoral shaft, and, with an upward force in the cephalic direction, the prepuce is retracted to gain full exposure of the glans clitoris, corona, and right and left frenula emanating at 5- and 7-o'clock from the posterior portion of the glans clitoris (Fig. 50-10). With the use of gauze to retract the labia minora, the labial-hymenal junction is identified. A Q-tip cotton swab test is performed, with gentle pressure applied on the minor vestibular glands, to document the quality of the discomfort or pain. The Q-tip cotton swab may also be placed at multiple locations in the vulva and vestibule. Palpation is next performed, using a single-digit examination. This procedure occurs before speculum insertion or bimanual searches for vaginismus. Single-digit palpation is achieved by gently placing a finger into the vaginal opening and depressing the bulbocavernosus muscle. The test is positive if there is hypertonicity and pain.

The goals of the physical examination for a woman with sexual health concerns are to confirm normal architecture, to detect any existing pathology or abnormalities, to educate the woman about normal anatomy and physiology, and, if pain is a feature, to reproduce and localize the pain to potential tender areas of the vulva, vagina, or pelvis or hypertonicity of the pelvic floor.

A bimanual examination and evaluation of the pelvic floor may be performed subsequently if indicated. Two fingers are placed against the lateral walls, and the levators and underlying obturator are assessed for tenderness or taut bands. In addition, a bimanual examination can evaluate the integrity of the fornices, bladder, urethral bases, and pelvic organs. A rectovaginal examination and speculum examination can be performed if indicated. For the speculum examination, a warm, lubricated speculum is used. The vaginal wall is examined for estrogen milieu integrity, inflammation of the walls, and any vaginal lesions.

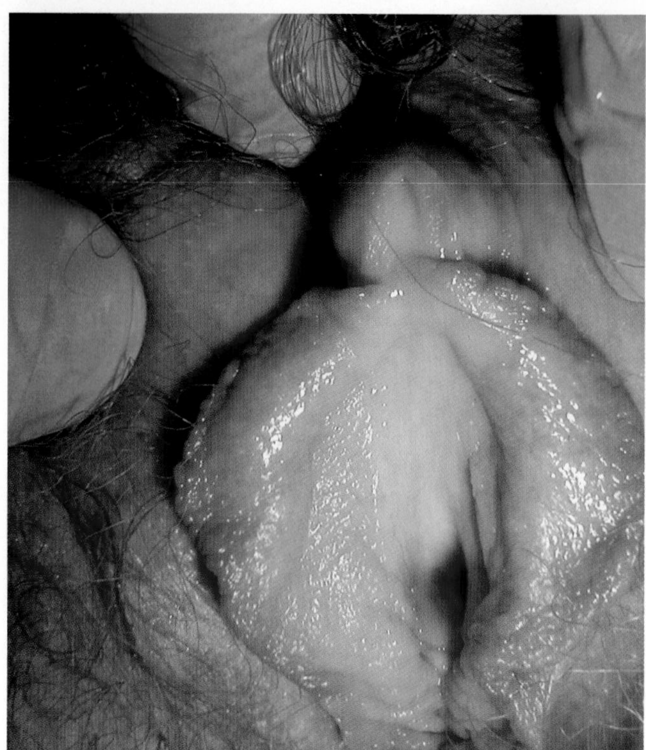

A

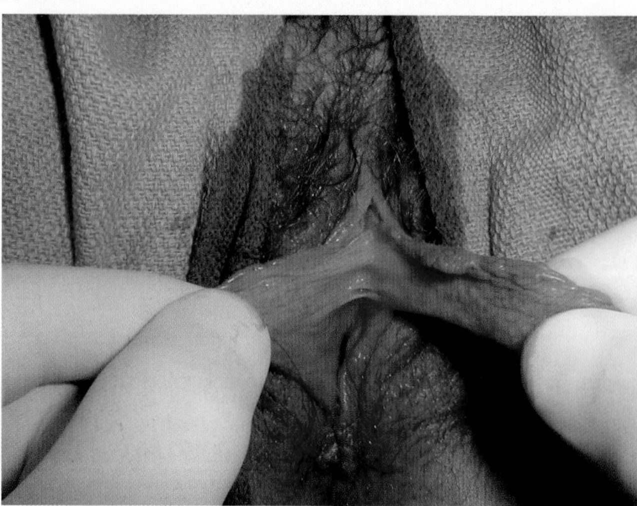

B

Figure 50-10 A, This is a photograph of a premenopausal woman with clitoral phimosis and a prepucial cyst. This woman experienced discomfort in the clitoral region during sexual activity. **B,** This is an intraoperative photograph of a woman who developed labial redundancy after her third childbirth. The woman complained that the excessive labia occasionally entered the vaginal canal during sexual activity and lead to dyspareunia.

The health care physician should also perform a complete physical examination, to rule out other comorbid conditions (e.g., thyrod goiter) that might be causing sexual dysfunction. A general physical examination is highly recommended in women with chronic illnesses and as part of good medical care, including evaluation of blood pressure, heart rate measurement, and a detailed breast examination.[7,47]

Laboratory Testing

There are no consensus recommended routine laboratory tests for the evaluation of women with sexual health concerns about desire, arousal, and orgasm. Blood testing should be dictated by clinical suspicion, especially the results of the history and physical examination. If appropriate, the health care clinician may assess multiple androgen and estrogen values, such as dehydroepiandrosterone sulphate (DHEAS), androstenedione, total testosterone, free testosterone, sex hormone binding globulin (SHBG), dihydrotestosterone, estradiol, and estrone. Pituitary function may be evaluated by measuring luteinizing hormone (LH), follicle-stimulating hormone (FSH), and prolactin. Thyroid-stimulating hormone (TSH) should be measured to exclude subclinical thyroid disease.[25,26,74,75]

There are many problems with the determination of serum hormone levels. The normal ranges of testosterone concentration values for women of different age groups without sexual dysfunction are not well defined. Testosterone levels reach a nadir during the early follicular phase, with small but less significant variation across the rest of the cycle. Testosterone assays are not uniformly sensitive or reliable enough to accurately measure testosterone at the low serum concentrations typically found in women. Free testosterone is clinically more important than total testosterone in sexual function, because most testosterone is bound to SHBG, and only a small amount of total testosterone is biologically available. The measurement of SHBG is not controversial and is relatively simple to perform with good reproducibility. Equilibrium dialysis is a highly sensitive assay for free testosterone; however, this method is not feasible for clinical practice. Measurement of free testosterone by analogue assays is unreliable. Free androgen may also be calculated using the free androgen index, which is defined as total testosterone divided by SHBG (both measured in nanomols per liter). Calculated free testosterone may be determined and takes into account total testosterone, SHBG, and albumin. A calculator for free testosterone is available online at http://www.issam.ch/freetesto.htm.[25,26,74,75]

DHEAS is commonly measured because the half-life is much longer than that of dehydroepiandrosterone (DHEA), resulting in more stable levels. The immunoassay for DHEAS sulphate is relatively robust and simple to perform. DHEAS does not vary in concentration over the phases of the menstrual cycle. Many investigators have shown consistent decline curves for DHEAS with aging.

Although there is a lack of clinical consensus as to the value, specificity, and sensitivity of individual hormone blood tests, there are evidence-based, placebo-controlled, double-blind data supporting the efficacy of exogenous sex steroid hormone treatment in women with sexual health concerns. The prudent physician may wish to discuss with the patient the strategy of serial blood test surveillance testing to address safety concerns during such treatment.

A most common and controversial question concerns the "normal range" for sex steroid blood test values in women with sexual health problems. Guay and colleagues examined androgen values in women who were "without sexual dysfunction" as determined by a validated Sexual Function Questionnaire. Androgen concentrations were highest in women aged 20 to 29 years, decreased at approximately age 30, and remained relatively constant thereafter. The free androgen index in women without sexual dysfunction was approximately 3.7 for women aged 20 to 29 years and 2.0 for women between the ages of 30 and 39 years.[25,26,74,75]

Serum levels of sex steroids can measure only deficiency or excess. Sex steroid hormone actions are quite complex and involve critical enzymes and hormone receptors that also determine tissue exposure, tissue sensitivity, and tissue responsiveness, independent of the blood concentrations. For example, there are interindividual variations in the amount and activity of critical enzymes such as 5α-reductase and aromatase, as well as variations in individual sex steroid hormone receptor sequencing. More research is needed regarding the blood testing of sex steroid hormones in women with sexual health concerns.

TREATMENT

This goal of this section to discuss the biologically focused management of sexual health issues in women. The ideal management of sexual health concerns is holistic, engaging both psychological and biologic strategies.

Hormonal

Sex steroid hormones are critical for sexual structure and function.[19,25,26,45,74,75] A number of studies have demonstrated that hormone therapy using systemic or local preparations improves sexual desire, arousal, orgasm, and frequency of sexual activity. There is no single hormonal intervention that will be effective in all women with desire, arousal, or orgasm sexual health concerns that are secondary, in part, to sex steroid hormone deficiency states.

Studies have consistently reported that androgen sex steroid hormone values decline gradually and estradiol values decline abruptly in menopausal women. Hormone insufficiency states may also be caused by a number of clinical conditions and medications, including the use of oral contraceptive therapy.

The use of systemic testosterone or systemic and/or local estrogen with or without systemic progesterone must be individualized to each patient's desires, wishes, requirements, and expectations.[21] Systemic hormone therapy can successfully improve hot flushes, night sweats, and sleep disturbances that can otherwise markedly diminish afflicted women's body image and mood. Local hormone therapy can successfully improve vaginal lubrication dryness and dyspareunia. Alleviation of hormone deficiency–induced symptoms through the use of systemic and/or localized sex steroid hormones can increase quality of life, desire, arousal, and orgasmic function. Although not yet specifically approved for clinical use in women with sexual health concerns, sex steroid hormones may eventually provide a safe and effective treatment option. However, more research is indicated.

The following paragraphs describe a clinical paradigm currently used in our outpatient sexual health clinic for the evidence-based, biologically focused treatment of women with desire, arousal, and orgasm sexual health concerns. As discussed previously, treatment is holistic and is based on the history, physical examination, and laboratory test results.

Phase 1

It is important to emphasize that no single type of hormonal intervention or regimen is effective in all women with desire, arousal, or orgasm sexual health concerns. Women who seek treatment may have symptoms of sexual health problems due in part to the onset of natural menopause or menopause induced by chemotherapy or surgery. Or, they may be younger women whose labia minora have begun to atrophy because of the adverse effects of oral contraceptives on the sex steroid hormonal milieu. Treatmets for infertility or endometriosis may also disturb the sex steroid hormone milieu.

The hormonal abnormalities that are identified determine which of the following four biologic treatment options are offered to women in Phase 1. Based on blood test results, systemic androgen treatment may be achieved with DHEA alone, systemic testosterone alone, or a combination of both. Based on the history and physical examination, local estrogen treatment may be achieved with vestibular estradiol alone, intravaginal estradiol alone, or a combination.

Systemic androgens (DHEA and/or testosterone) have been shown to improve mood, energy, stimulation, sensation, arousal, and orgasm.[76-78] Limited clinical trials have examined the effects of DHEA therapy on sexual function in women. Baulieu and colleagues administered DHEA (50 mg) or placebo to 140 women between the ages of 60 and 79 years for 12 months. DHEA treatment produced approximately a doubling of serum total testosterone concentration and also significantly increased skin hydration and bone density. Libidinal interest was increased after 6 months of treatment, and sexual activity and sexual satisfaction were increased after 12 months.[76-78]

Testosterone has been used to treat women with sexual dysfunction for more than 50 years.[79] Transdermal patches or gels, which are more consistently absorbed and avoid first-pass metabolism in the liver, are currently being studied for their safety and efficacy in reducing sexual symptoms associated with testosterone insufficiency.[80.81] Recently, transdermal testosterone patches were compared with placebo in estrogenized women who had undergone oophorectomy and hysterectomy.[80] The study results showed that the 300-μg testosterone patch was significantly more effective than the 150-μg patch or placebo in improving frequency of sexual activity, pleasure, and fantasy during a 12-week period. Typically, testosterone is used in gel form (Food and Drug Administration–approved delivery system for men) and is applied to the back of the calf. One tenth of the dose used in men is appropriate for initial therapy in women.

One benefit of administering DHEA and testosterone is that a certain percentage of these hormones will aromatize to an estrogen, thus relieving hot flashes and night sweats without the administration of systemic estrogen.

Local estrogen, whether it is prescribed in the form of vaginal estradiol or a vestibular cream, improves perfusion, lubrication, tissue tone, and elasticity and restores the normal pH and vaginal health.[48,82,83] Vaginal estradiol also relieves dyspareunia, atrophic vaginitis, and vaginismus. Some systemic absorption occurs with all local estrogens, but less so than with oral therapy. Daily application of a film of vestibular estrogen is recommended as well, because it promotes the health of the frenulum (the most sensitive part of the external genitalia), labia minora, urethral meatus, hymenal tissue, and vestibular glands.

Women with sexual dysfunction who are placed on Phase 1 treatment need to undergo surveillance blood tests after 3 months of therapy to monitor the levels of estradiol, progesterone, DHEA, testosterone, androstenedione, dihydrotestosterone, FSH, LH, prolactin, and TSH as indicated.

Women with desire, arousal, or orgasm sexual health concerns whose symptoms of distress are not resolved satisfactorily with phase 1 treatments may consider progressing to phase 2 treatments.

Phase 2

In phase 2, women receive systemic estrogen and/or systemic testosterone. Several clinical trials have shown that the distressing symptoms of vaginal atrophy associated with low estrogen states are ameliorated after estrogen therapy. Low doses of systemic bioidentical nonsynthetic 17-β estradiol reduced vaginal atrophy compared with placebo in healthy menopausal women.[84] Systemic estrogen therapy can also successfully improve hot flushes, night sweats, and sleep disturbances that negatively affect body image, mood, and sexual desire. All efforts are made to keep serum estradiol levels between 30 and 50 pg/mL. Risks of systemic estrogen use include breast cancer, heart attack, and stroke. The concept of maintaining estradiol values at low levels is to reduce the side effect risk while achieving a minimum efficacious dose.

In women with an intact uterus, systemic estrogen should always be opposed by a progestogen. All efforts are made to use a bioidentical nonsynthetic progesterone and to keep values in the range of 1 pg/mL.

Phase 3

In phase 3, attention is given to the possible role of dopamine agonists in facilitating desire and orgasm sexual responses. Sexual motivation is encouraged, sustained, and ended by a number of central nervous system neurotransmitter and receptor changes induced, in part, by the actions of sex steroids, androgens, estrogens, progestins, and the central neurotransmitter dopamine.[85,86] The activation of dopamine receptors may be a key intermediary in the stimulation of incentive sexual motivation and sexual reward. These neurotransmitter and receptor changes, in turn, activate central sexual arousal and desire. Contemporary animal research has revealed that dopamine neurotransmitter systems may play a critical intermediary role in the central regulation of sexual arousal and excitation, mood, and incentive-related sexual behavior—and in particular, in the motivational responses to conditioned external stimuli. In summary, the complex central neurochemical actions of steroid hormones stimulate sensory awareness, central sexual arousal, mood, and reward and relate them to an individual's relevant sexual experiences involving a partner, a place, and an action.

Bupropion may have a beneficial effect on women with hypoactive sexual desire disorder. In a placebo-controlled trial, bupropion produced an increase in desire and frequency of sexual activity compared with placebo.[85,86] However, frequency was correlated to total testosterone level at baseline and during treatment. A traditional starting dose is 100 mg bupropion per day taken in the morning.

Vasodilators

Basic science studies investigating the physiology of sexual function using female animal models support the role of nitric oxide–cyclic guanosine monophosphate–PDE5 pathways in the peripheral arousal physiology of the clitoral corpus cavernosum,[88,89] corpus spongiosum, vaginal epithelium, and vaginal lamina propria.

There have been several clinical studies on selective PDE5 inhibitors over the last few years, conducted with either premenopausal or postmenopausal women with arousal sexual health concerns as well as healthy women without sexual dysfunction. Many studies did not take into account the hormonal milieu of the subjects in the inclusion and exclusion criteria. An important point in treating women with arousal sexual health concerns is that an adequate sex steroid (androgen and estrogen) hormonal milieu is critical for benefits from selective PDE5 inhibitor treatment.[19] Several studies did assess the safety and efficacy of selective PDE5 inhibitors in subjects with a normal hormonal milieu.

A double-blind, crossover, placebo-controlled safety and efficacy study with a selective PDE5 inhibitor was performed in premenopausal women with normal ovulatory cycles and normal levels of steroid hormones who were affected by female sexual arousal disorder without hypoactive sexual desire disorder. Subjects were observed to benefit from treatment with the active selective PDE5 inhibitor versus placebo, showing improvement in sexual arousal, orgasm, frequency, and enjoyment of sexual intercourse.[90]

A double-blind, placebo-controlled safety and efficacy study with a selective PDE5 inhibitor was performed in postmenopausal women with female sexual arousal disorder who had adequate serum estradiol and free testosterone values. Women with female sexual arousal disorder without hypoactive sexual desire disorder assigned the active drug had a significantly greater improvement in sexual arousal, orgasm, intercourse, and overall satisfaction with sexual life compared with placebo. No efficacy was shown for women with concomitant hypoactive sexual desire disorder.[91]

Another study was performed using selective PDE5 inhibitors in women with psychotropic-induced sexual dysfunction. Women who had normal premorbid sexual function and who had developed sexual dysfunction, particularly anorgasmia with or without other sexual disturbances (i.e., loss of libido), lubrication difficulties, or uncomfortable or painful intercourse, were treated with a selective PDE5 inhibitor. The subjects showed improvement of the presenting condition, usually depression, anxiety, or both, and experienced sexual side effects continuously for more than 4 weeks. Patients took selective PDE5 inhibitors and reported a complete or very significant reversal of their sexual dysfunction. This included return of effective duration and intensity of adequate arousal, lubrication, and orgasmic function.[92]

SEXUAL PAIN MANAGEMENT

Medical Therapy for Genital Sexual Pain Disorders

Biologic pathophysiologies resulting in woman's sexual health problems associated with sexual pain may occur in the clitoris, urethra, bladder, vulva, vestibule, vagina, and pelvic floor muscles. It is not within the scope of this chapter to detail all the management of genital sexual pain disorders. If the reader is interested, one option would be to refer to the reference text book entitled *Women's Sexual Function and Dysfunction: Study, Diagnosis and Treatment.*[20]

Clitoris, Prepuce, and Frenulae

In women with focused clitoral pain, clitoral itching, or clitoral burning, careful inspection of the glans clitoris should be performed. Failure to visualize the whole glans clitoris with the corona is consistent with some degree (mild, moderate, or severe) of prepucial phimosis, based on the elasticity of the prepuce and its ability to retract on examination.[93] Because it can create a closed compartment, phimosis is often the underlying pathology in clitoral glans balanitis associated with recurrent fungal infections. Initial treatment may be conservative with topical estrogen and/or testosterone creams to determine whether the prepuce can be made more elastic and retractile.[94] Topical antifungal agents such as nystatin or oral antifungal agents such as fluconazole[95] may be considered. Infections can also be related to herpesvirus infection, and appropriate treatment can be administered (e.g., acyclovir). If conservative treatment fails due to the phimotic prepuce, surgical management by dorsal slit procedure should be considered.

Urethral Meatus

Gentle retraction of the labia minora should provide a full view of the urethral meatus. Prolapse of the urethral mucosa out the urethral lumen is highly associated with estrogen deficiency states such as natural menopause, surgical menopause due to bilateral oophorectomy, or deficiency caused by chemotherapy for malignancy. Clinical symptoms include urgency, frequency, and discomfort on urination; also, spotting of blood may be observed on the toilet paper after wiping following voiding. The abnormal voiding history is often accompanied by a unique sexual history. Women with urethral prolapse often have the ability to have full sexual pleasure and satisfaction during self-stimulation of the clitoris, but with a partner or with a mechanical device she experiences pain, urgency to urinate, and/or inability to have orgasm secondary to distracting pain. Conservative treatment options include topical or systemic estrogens, although the risks and benefits of estrogen treatment need to be fully discussed.[64,69]

Vulva and Vestibule

Genital sexual pain in the vulva and vestibule may be related to various specific disorders. Generalized vulvodynia[69] refers to genital sexual pain with a nonlocalized, persistent, irritating pain anywhere on the vulva, from mons to anus, that is very sensitive and greatly out of proportion to the stimulus. The treatment of any genital sexual pain disorder involves a multidisciplinary team approach, and this is especially true for the disabling condition of generalized vulvodynia. Patient management includes education and support, especially regarding avoidance of contacts and practice of healthy vulvar hygiene, pelvic floor physical therapy treatment, management of concomitant depression, and management of any associated neurologic, dermatologic, gynecologic, orthopedic, or urologic conditions. Medical management includes amitriptyline and/or gabapentin.

Vulvar vestibulitis syndrome is one of the most common causes of dyspareunia, especially in premenopausal women.[96,97] The treatment of vulvar vestibulitis syndrome also begins with conservative measures including education, support, counseling, physical therapy, and/or biofeedback. Elimination of the pain trigger should be performed. Topical estrogen and topical xylocaine creams or ointments should be considered. Systemic medications include tricyclic antidepressants or gabapentin. Correction of the sex steroid hormonal milieu should be considered. Unlike generalized vulvodynia, in women with vulvar vestibulitis syndrome, if medical management fails surgery (e.g., vestibulectomy) can be considered.

The symptoms of atrophic vaginitis include vaginal dryness, dyspareunia, stinging, bleeding, and dysuria.[98] On physical examination, women with atrophic vaginitis have vaginal mucosal changes. The classic healthy-appearing vagina has a pink hue with vaginal folds and rugae that, when touched with a Q-tip,

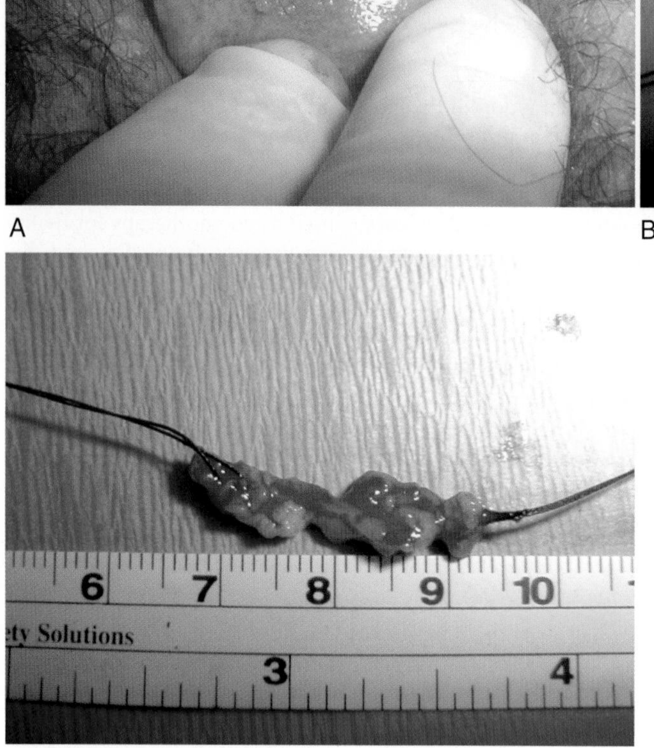

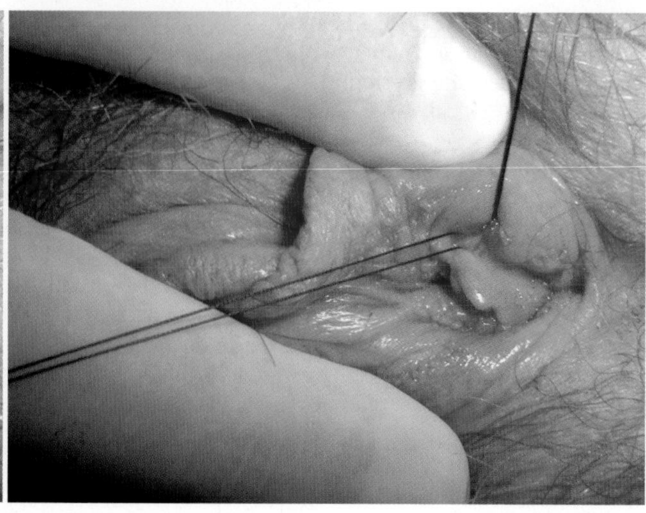

Figure 50-11 Modified vestibulectomy for vulvar vestibulitis syndrome. **A,** Intraoperative photograph. The tip of the surgical instrument has entered into the ostia of the minor vestibular gland. **B,** Intraoperative photograph. Tagging sutures have been placed into the ostia of the minor vestibular glands prior to local excision. **C,** This surgical excision specimen was 2.5 cm long and 0.5 cm deep and wide.

reveal a shiny lubricating substance and, when rubbed with a Q-tip, do not bleed. In atrophic vaginitis, the vagina transforms to an unhealthy pale complexion, with a lack of vaginal folds and rugae, a lack of lubricating substance on the surface, and bleeding ot the tissue with minimal contact. On wet mount, the microscopic examination reveals parabasal cells, increased white blood cells, and absent background flora of lactobacilli. The vaginal pH is elevated to 6.0 to 7.0. Conservative treatment involves the use of local topical vestibular and/or intravaginal estrogen. There are multiple products on the market, including intravaginal rings, intravaginal pills, and creams. There are also multiple estrogen alternatives, such as soy, although there are limited double-blind placebo-controlled safety and efficacy trials with these products.

Disorders of the female pelvic floor, especially those involving bladder/urethra and sexual dysfunction, are common. Conservative therapies for hypersensitivity disorders of the pelvic floor are aimed at muscle reeducation. A pelvic floor rehabilitation program aimed at facilitating sexual comfort and pleasure for patients can be designed. Massage of the pelvic floor can be performed to elongate shortened muscles and decrease high-tone spasm. Conservative therapies for low-tone pelvic floor dysfunction are also aimed at muscle reeducation. Pelvic floor muscle-strengthening exercises, augmented with biofeedback and/or electrical stimulation to the pelvic floor, can be initiated. If this and other conservative treatment options fail, surgical procedures, including sling and tension-free vaginal tape placement, provide cure rates as high as 95% when performed in appropriate candidates.[55,56,59]

Surgical Therapy for Genital Sexual Pain Disorders

Surgical Treatment for Vulvar Vestibulitis Syndrome

Surgical intervention for management of vulvar vestibulitis syndrome is offered to those for whom initial conservative medical, psychological, and/or physical therapy treatment has failed. Surgery is based on the hypothesis that the pathophysiology of vulvar vestibulitis syndrome is associated with inflamed, irritated, and hypersensitive vestibular glandular tissue and related increased nerve density in the vestibular mucosa. Surgical success is, therefore, based on excision of this abnormal glandular and nerve tissue in the vestibule.[99,100]

In women with vulvar vestibulitis syndrome, the first surgical and reconstructive procedure consisted of excision of a semicir-

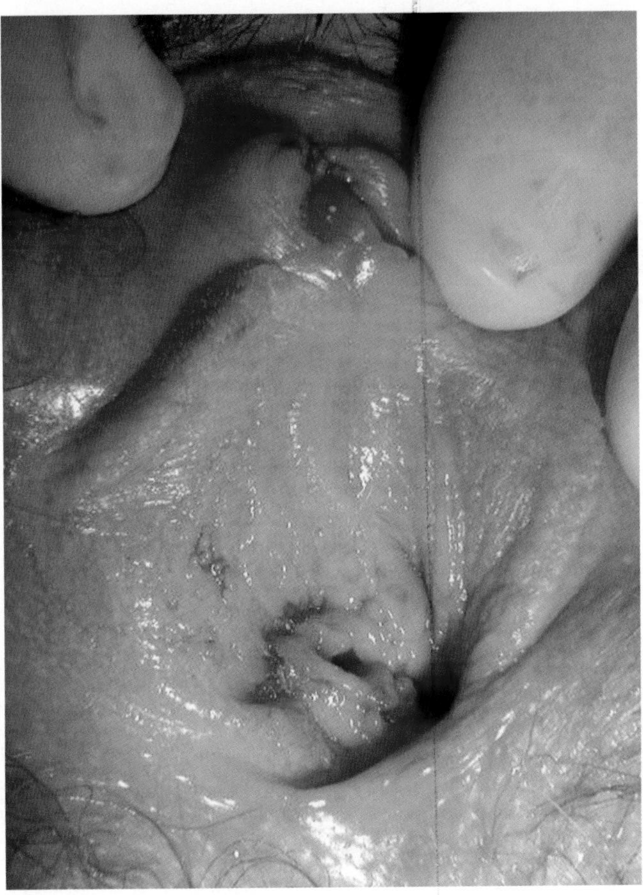

D

Figure 50-11 D, Intraoperative photograph of a woman undergoing modified vestibulectomy for vulvar vestibulitis syndrome and dorsal slit for clitoral phimosis. Interrupted 4-0 chromic sutures have been used to reestablish vestibular tissue integrity.

cular segment of perineal skin, the mucosa of the posterior vulvar vestibule, and the posterior hymenal ring. The reconstruction consisted of undermining 3 cm of the vaginal mucosa and approximating this directly to the perineum. Subsequently, variations and modifications have evolved. Specifically, in contemporary vulvar vestibulectomy procedures, the posterior incision extends only to the posterior fourchette and does not include excisions of perineal skin. A "complete vulvar vestibulectomy" includes excision of the vestibular mucosa adjacent to the urethral meatus/Skene's glands region anteriorly, and excision of vestibular mucosa laterally and posteriorly, with reconstruction including the posterior vaginal flap advancement. A "modified vulvar vestibulectomy" limits the excision of vestibular mucosa to the posterior vestibule. Both procedures are usually performed with the patient under general or regional anesthesia. During vestibulectomy, the vaginal advancement may cover the ostia of the Bartholin glands; however, the risk of postoperative Bartholin gland cysts is only 1%. A vestibuloplasty or excision of vestibular adenitis consists only of excision of localized painful areas of vestibular mucosa without vaginal advancement and can be performed with local anesthesia. Most surgeons choose the procedure based on the individual needs and symptoms of the patient. The complications of surgery for vulvar vestibulitis syndrome increase with the invasiveness of the procedure performed. Specifically, complications include bleeding, infection, increased pain, hematoma, wound dehiscence, vaginal stenosis, scar tissue formation, and Bartholin duct cyst formation. As always with surgery, the risks of these complications can be reduced with appropriate surgical techniques. Various closure techniques have been described to minimize the risks of postoperative complications. Specifically, the vaginal advancement flap should be anchored by multiple subcutaneous mattress sutures of 3-0 Vicryl placed in an anterior-posterior direction and should be approximated to the perineum with interrupted stitches of 4-0 Vicryl (Fig. 50-11).[99,100]

Other Surgical Procedures

Distressing and disabling clitoral pain may occur secondary to phimosis of the clitoral prepuce and recurrent fungal balanitis of the clitoral glans or frenula. If conservative treatment fails, a dorsal slit procedure of the prepuce may be indicated to relieve the closed compartment that is perpetuating the recurrent fungal clitoral glans infection.[93]

Distressing and disabling vestibular pain, urinary urgency and frequency, and genital sexual pain may occur secondary to urethral prolapse. If conservative treatments fail, surgical excision of the prolapsed urethral mucosa may be indicated.[55]

Distressing vulvar or vestibular discomfort may occur secondary to a Bartholin's cyst. If conservative treatments fail, marsupialization of the cyst may be indicated to enable drainage of the highly viscous and mucinous cyst fluid.[101]

CONCLUSIONS

It is entirely appropriate to have a detailed chapter on women's sexual health concerns in a textbook on female urology. Increasing numbers of health care professionals manage sexual health concerns as part of their goal to maximize the all health care delivery to each patient.

The basic premise of biologically focused management of women's sexual health concerns is that physiologic processes can be altered by pathology. Understanding how specific medical conditions modulate a woman's sexual health requires much investment in basic science investigation. From the perspective of biologically focused clinicians, the essential principle guiding medical decision-making is identification of the underlying pathophysiology of the sexual dysfunction. If the biologic basis of the sexual health concern can be diagnosed, management may be successfully directed to the source pathophysiology. Two of the many challenges facing health care professionals today are improving their ability to accurately diagnose sexual health concerns in women and ensuring that they offer women the best available, evidence-based treatment options. To achieve these goals, biologically focused clinicians need to be familiar with evidence-based, state-of-the-art data and current biologically focused management strategies.

References

1. Nappi R, Salonia A, Traish AM, et al: Clinical biologic pathophysiologies of women's sexual dysfunction. J Sex Med 2:4-25, 2005.
2. Salonia A, Zanni G, Nappi R, et al: Sexual dysfunction is common in women with lower urinary incontinence: Results of a cross-sectional study. Eur Urol 45:642-648, 2004.
3. World Health Organization. Department of Reproductive Health and Research (RHR). Gender and Reproductive Rights. Available at: http://www.who.int/reproductive-health/gender/sexual_health.html (accessed August 6, 2007).
4. World Association of Sexual Health. Declaration of Sexual Rights. Available at: http://www.tc.umn.edu/~colem001/was/wdeclara.htm (accessed August 6, 2007)
5. Solursh DS, Ernst JL, Lewis RW, et al: The human sexuality education of physicians in North American medical schools. Int J Impot Res 15(Suppl 5):S41-S45, 2003.
6. Marwick C: Survey says patients expect little physician help on sex. JAMA 281:2173-2174, 1999.
7. Basson R, Althof S, Davis S, et al: Summary of the recommendations on sexual dysfunctions in women. J Sex Med 1:24-34, 2004.
8. Lewis RW, Fugl-Meyer KS, Bosch R, et al: Epidemiology/risk factors of sexual dysfunction. J Sex Med 1:35-39, 2004.
9. Lue TF, Giuliano F, Montorsi F, et al: Summary of the recommendations on sexual dysfunctions in men. J Sex Med 1:6-23, 2004.
10. Laumann EO, Paik A, Rosen RC: Sexual dysfunction in the United States: Prevalence and predictors. In Laumann EO, Michael RT (eds): Sex, Love, and Health in America: Private Choices and Public Policies. Chicago: University of Chicago Press, 2001.
11. Öberg K, Fugl-Meyer SK: On Swedish women's distressing sexual dysfunctions: Some concomitant conditions and life satisfaction. J Sex Med 2:169-180, 2005.
12. Basson R, Brotto LA, Laan E, et al: Assessment and management of women's sexual dysfunctions: Problematic desire and arousal. J Sex Med 2:291-300, 2005.
13. Weijmar Schultz W, Basson R, Binik Y, et al: Women's sexual pain and its management. J Sex Med 2:301-316, 2005.
14. Hayes R, Dennerstein L: The impact of aging on sexual function and sexual dysfunction in women: A review of population based studies. J Sex Med 2:317-330, 2005.
15. Laumann EO, Paik A, Rosen RC: Sexual dysfunction in the United States: Prevalence and predictors. JAMA 281:537-544, 1999.
16. National Council on the Aging. Press Room: News Archive. Half of older Americans report they are sexually active; 4 in 10 want more sex, says new survey (September 28, 1998). Available at: http://www.ncoa.org/content.cfm?sectionID=105&detail=128 (accessed August 6, 2007).
17. Menopause—One Woman's Story, Every Woman's Story: A Resource for Making Healthy Choices. NIH Publication No. 01-3886. Gaithersburg, MD: National Institute on Aging, U.S. Department of Health and Human Services, 2001.
18. Bossouw JE, Anderson GL, Prentice RL; Writing Group for the Women's Health Initiative Investigators: Risks and benefits of estrogen plus progestin in healthy postmenopausal women: Principal results from the Women's Health Initiative randomized controlled trial. JAMA 288:321-333, 2002.
19. Giraldi A, Marson L, Nappi R, et al: Physiology of female sexual function: Animal models. J Sex Med 1:237-253, 2004.
20. Goldstein I, Meston C, Davis S, Traish AM (eds): Women's Sexual Function and Dysfunction: Study, Diagnosis and Treatment. London: Taylor and Francis, 2005.
21. Basson R, Leiblum S, Brotto L, et al: Revised definitions of women's sexual dysfunction. J Sex Med 1:40-48, 2004.
22. Nicolosi A, Laumann EO, Glasser DB, et al: Sexual behavior and sexual problems after age 40: The Global Study of Sexual Attitudes and Behaviors. Urology 64:991-997, 2004.
23. Derogatis LR, Rosen R, Leiblum S, et al: The Female Sexual Distress Scale (FSDS): Initial validation of a standardized scale for assessment of sexually related personal distress in women. J Sex Marital Ther 28:317-330, 2002.
24. Basson R, Berman J, Burnett A, et al: Report of the International Consensus Development Conference on female sexual dysfunction: Definitions and classifications. J Urol 163:888-893, 2000.
25. Guay A, Munarriz R, Jacobson J, et al: Serum androgen levels in healthy premenopausal women with and without sexual dysfunction: Part A. Serum androgen levels in women aged 20-49 years with no complaints of sexual dysfunction. Int J Impot Res 16:112-120, 2004.
26. Guay A, Jacobson J, Munarriz R, et al: Serum androgen levels in healthy premenopausal women with and without sexual dysfunction: Part B. Reduced serum androgen levels in healthy premenopausal women with complaints of sexual dysfunction. Int J Impot Res 16:121-129, 2004.
27. Khalife WI, Tang YD, Kuzman JA, et al: Treatment of sub-clinical hypothyroidism reverses ischemia and prevents myocyte loss and progressive LV dysfunction in hamsters with dilated cardiomyopathy. Am J Physiol Heart Circ Physiol 289:H2409-H2415, 2005. Epub 2005 Jul 15.
28. de Ledinghen V, Combes M, Trouette H, et al: Should a liver biopsy be done in patients with subclinical chronically elevated transaminases? Eur J Gastroenterol Hepatol 16:879-883, 2004.
29. Schmermund A, Mohlenkamp S, Berenbein S, et al: Population-based assessment of subclinical coronary atherosclerosis using electron-beam computed tomography. Atherosclerosis 185:177-182, 2005. Epub 2005 Jul 11.
30. Blumel JE, Castelo-Branco C, Cancelo MJ, et al: Impairment of sexual activity in middle-aged women in Chile. Menopause 11:78-81, 2004.
31. Paige NM, Hays RD, Litwin MS, et al: Improvement in emotional well-being and relationships of users of sildenafil. J Urol 166:1774-1778, 2001.
32. Cayan S, Bozlu M, Canpolat B, Akbay E. The assessment of sexual functions in women with male partners complaining of erectile dysfunction: Does treatment of male sexual dysfunction improve female partner's sexual functions? J Sex Marital Ther 30:333-341, 2004.
33. Montorsi F, Althof SE: Partner responses to sildenafil citrate (Viagra): Treatment of erectile dysfunction. Urology 63:762-767, 2004.
34. Chevret M, Jaudinot E, Sullivan K, et al: Quality of sexual life and satisfaction in female partners of men with ED: Psychometric validation of the Index of Sexual Life (ISL) questionnaire. J Sex Marital Ther 30:141-155, 2004.
35. Fisher WA, Rosen RC, Eardley I, et al: Sexual experience of female partners of men with erectile dysfunction: The Female Experience of Men's Attitudes to Life Events and Sexuality (FEMALES) study. J Sex Med 2:675-684, 2005.
36. Fisher WA, Rosen RC, Mollen M, et al: Improving the sexual quality of life of couples affected by erectile dysfunction: A double-blind, randomized, placebo-controlled trial of vardenafil. J Sex Med 2:699-708, 2005.
37. Goldstein I, Fisher WA, Sand M, et al: Women's sexual function improves when partners are administered vardenafil for erectile dysfunction: A prospective, randomized, double-blind placebo-controlled trial. J Sex Med 2:819-832, 2005.
38. Rowland DL, Perelman MA, Althof S, et al: Self-reported premature ejaculation and aspects of sexual functioning and satisfaction. J Sex Med 1:225-232, 2004.
39. Rowland DL, Cooper SE, Schneider M: Defining premature ejaculation for experimental and clinical investigations. Arch Sex Behav 30:235-253, 2001.

40. Patrick D, Althof S, Ho K-F, et al: Premature ejaculation: An observational study of men and their partners. J Sex Med 2:358-367, 2005.
41. Byers ES, Grenier G: Premature or rapid ejaculation: Heterosexual couples' perceptions of men's ejaculatory behavior. Arch Sex Behav 32:261-270, 2003.
42. Bixo M, Backstrom T, Winblad B, Andersson A: Estradiol and testosterone in specific regions of the human female brain in different endocrine states. J Steroid Biochem Mol Biol 55:297-303, 1995.
43. Roselli CE, Resko JA: Aromatase activity in the rat brain: Hormone regulation and sex differences. J Steroid Biochem Mol Biol 44:499-508, 1993.
44. McEwen BS: Estrogen action throughout the brain. Recent Prog Horm Res 57:357-384, 2002.
45. Bachmann G, Bancroft J, Braunstein G, et al: Female androgen insufficiency: The Princeton consensus statement on definition, classification, and assessment. Fertil Steril 77:660-665, 2002.
46. Traish AM, Huang YH, Min K, et al: Binding characteristics of [3H]delta(5)-androstene-3beta,17beta-diol to a nuclear protein in the rabbit vagina. Steroids 69:71-78, 2004.
47. Hatzichristou D, Rosen RC, Broderick G, et al: Clinical evaluation and management strategy for sexual dysfunction in men and women. J Sex Med 1:49-57, 2004.
48. Bachmann GA, Leiblum SR: The impact of hormones on menopausal sexuality: A literature review. Menopause 11:120-130, 2004.
49. Reynolds RF, Obermeyer CM: Age at natural menopause in Spain and the United States: Results from the DAMES project. Am J Hum Biol 17:331-340, 2005.
50. Kovalevsky G: Hormones and female sexual dysfunction in postmenopasual women. Menopausal Medicine 12:1-5, 2004.
51. Freedman MA: Quality of life and menopause: The role of estrogen. J Women's Health 11:703-718, 2002.
52. Pessina MA, Hoyt RF, Goldstein I, Traish AM: Differential effects of estradiol, progesterone, and testosterone on vaginal structural integrity. Endocrinology 147:61-69, 2006. Epub 2005 Oct 6.
53. Lukban JC, Whitmore KE: Pelvic floor muscle re-education: Treatment of the overactive bladder and painful bladder syndrome. Clin Obstet Gynecol 45:273-280, 2000.
54. Fitzgerald MP, Kotarinos R: Rehabilitation of the short pelvic floor. Int Urogynecol J 14:269-275, 2003.
55. Weber A,Walters M, Peidmonte M: Sexual function and vaginal anatomy in women before and after surgery for pelvic organ prolapse and incontinence. Am J Obstet Gynecol 182:1610-1615, 2000.
56. Glazer CMA, Herbison GP, Wilson PD, et al: Conservative management of persistent postnatal urinary and fecal incontinence. BMJ 323:593-599, 2001.
57. Reissing ED, Binik YM, Khalife S, et al: Vaginal spasm, pain, and behavior: An empirical investigation of the diagnosis of vaginismus. Arch Sex Behav 33:5-17, 2004.
58. Glazer H, Romanzi L, Polaneczky M: Pelvic floor muscle surface electromyography: Reliability and clinical predictive validity. J Reprod Med 44:779-782, 1999.
59. Bergeron S, Binik YM, Khalife S, et al: A randomized comparison of group cognitive-behavioral therapy, surface electromyographic biofeedback, and vestibulectomy in the treatment of dyspareunia resulting from vulvar vestibulitis. Pain 91:297-306, 2001.
60. Shafik A, El-Sibai O: Study of the pelvic floor muscles in vaginismus: A concept of pathogenesis. Eur J Obstet Gynecol Reprod Biol 105:67-70, 2002.
61. Stewart EG: Developments in vulvovaginal care. Curr Opin Obstet Gynecol 14:483-488, 2002.
62. Haefner HK: Current evaluation and management of vulvovaginitis. Clin Obstet Gynecol 42:184-195, 1999.
63. Anderson MR, Klink K, Cohrssen A: Evaluation of vaginal complaints. JAMA 291:1368-1379, 2004.
64. Harlow BL, Wise LA, Stewart EG: Prevalence and predictors of chronic genital discomfort. Am J Obstet Gynecol 185:545-550, 2001.
65. Stewart EG, Berger BM: Parallel pathologies? Vulvar vestibulitis and interstitial cystitis. J Reprod Med 42:131-134, 1997.
66. Bracco GL, Carli P, Sonni L, et al: Clinical and histologic effects of topical treatments of vulval lichen sclerosus: A critical evaluation. J Reprod Med 38:37-40, 1993.
67. Lewis FM, Shah M, Harrington CI: Vulval involvement in lichen planus: A study of 37 women. Br J Dermatol 135:89-91, 1996.
68. Bergeron S, Brown C, Lord MJ, et al: Physical therapy for vulvar vestibulitis syndrome: A retrospective study. Sex Marital Ther 28:183-192, 2002.
69. Harlow BL, Stewart EG: A population-based assessment of chronic unexplained vulvar pain: Have we underestimated the prevalence of vulvodynia? J Am Med Women's Assoc 58:82-88, 2003.
70. Rosen R, Brown C, Heiman J, et al: The Female Sexual Function Index (FSFI): A multidimensional self-report instrument for the assessment of female sexual function. J Sex Marital Ther 26:191-208, 2000.
71. Meston CM: Validation of the Female Sexual Function Index (FSFI) in women with female orgasmic disorder and in women with hypoactive sexual desire disorder. J Sex Marital Ther 29:39-46, 2003.
72. Wiegel M, Meston C, Rosen RC: The Female Sexual Function Index (FSFI): Cross-validation and development of clinical cutoff scores. J Sex Marital Ther 31:1-20, 2005.
73. Quirk FH, Heiman JR, Rosen RC, et al: Development of a sexual function questionnaire for clinical trials of female sexual dysfunction. J Womens Health Gend Based Med 11:277-289, 2002.
74. Davis SR, Guay AT, Shifren JL, Mazer NA: Endocrine aspects of female sexual dysfunction. J Sex Med 1:82-86, 2004.
75. Guay A, Davis SR: Testosterone insufficiency in women: Fact or fiction. World J Urol 20:106-110, 2002.
76. Baulieu E-E: Dehydroepiandrosterone (DHEA): A fountain of youth? J Clin Endocrinol Metab 81:3147-3151, 1996.
77. Baulieu E-E, Thomas G, Legrain S, et al: Dehydroepiandrosterone (DHEA), DHEA sulfate, and aging: Contribution of the DHEA Study to a sociobiomedical issue. Proc Natl Acad Sci U S A 97:4279-4284, 2000.
78. Arlt W, Callies F, Van Vlijmen JC, et al: Dehydroepiandrosterone replacement in women with adrenal insufficiency. N Eng J Med 341:1013-1020, 1999.
79. Loeser A: Subcutaneous implantation of female and male hormone in tablet from in women. BMJ 1:479-482, 1940.
80. Shifren JL, Braustein GD, Simon JA, et al: Transdermal testosterone treatment in women with impaired sexual function and oophorectomy. N Engl J Med 343:682-688, 2000.
81. Lobo RA, Rosen RC, Yang HM, et al: Comparative effects of oral esterified estrogens with and without methyltestosterone on endocrine profiles and dimensions of sexual function in postmenopausal women with hypoactive sexual desire. Fertil Steril 79:1341-1352, 2003.
82. Buckler H, Al-Azzawi F; The UK VR Multicentre Trial Group: The effect of a novel vaginal ring delivering oestradiol acetate on climacteric symptoms in postmenopausal women. BJOG 110: 753-759, 2003.
83. Barentsen R, van de Weijer PHM, Schram JHN: Continuous low dose estradiol released from a vaginal ring versus estriol vaginal cream for urogenital atrophy. Eur J Obstet Gynecol Reprod Biol 71:73-80, 1997.
84. Rioux JE, Devlin C, Gelfand MM, et al: 17beta-Estradiol vaginal tablet versus conjugated equine estrogen vaginal cream to relieve menopausal atrophic vaginitis. Menopause 7:156-161, 2000.
85. Giuliano F, Allard J: Dopamine and male sexual function. Eur Urol 40:601-608, 2001.
86. Clayton AH, Warnock JK, Kornstein SG, et al: A placebo-controlled trial of bupropion SR as an antidote for selective

serotonin reuptake inhibitor-induced sexual dysfunction. J Clin Psychiatry 65:62-67, 2004.
87. Segraves RT, Clayton A, Croft H, et al: Bupropion sustained release for the treatment of hypoactive sexual desire disorder in premenopausal women. J Clin Psychopharmacol 24:339-342, 2004.
88. Park K, Moreland RB, Goldstein I, et al: Sildenafil inhibits phosphodiesterase type 5 in human clitoral corpus cavernousum smooth muscle. Biochem Biophys Res Commun 249:612-617, 2008.
89. Burnett AL, Calvin DC, Silver RI, et al: Immunohistochemical description of nitric oxide syntheses isoforms in human clitoris. J Urol 158:75-78, 1997.
90. Caruso S, Intelisano G, Lupo L, Agnello C: Premenopausal women affected by sexual arousal disorder treated with sildenafil: A double-blind, crossover, placebo-controlled study. Br J Obstet Gynaecol 108:623-628, 2001.
91. Berman JR, Berman LA, Toler SM, et al: Safety and efficacy of sildenafil citrate for the treatment of female sexual arousal disorder: A double-blind, placebo controlled study. J Urol 170:2333-2338, 2003.
92. Nurnberg HG, Lauriello J, Hensley PL, et al: Sildenafil for sexual dysfunction in women taking antidepressants. Am J Psychiatry 156:1664, 1999.
93. Munarriz R, Talakoub L, Kuohung W, et al: The prevalence of phimosis of the clitoris in women presenting to the sexual dysfunction clinic: Lack of correlation to disorders of desire, arousal and orgasm. J Sex Marital Ther 28(Suppl 1):181-185, 2002.
94. Crandall C: Vaginal estrogen preparations: A review of safety and efficacy for vaginal atrophy. J Womens Health (Larchmt) 11:857-877, 2002.
95. Sobel JD, Kapernick PS, Zervos M, et al: Treatment of complicated Candida vaginitis: Comparison of single and sequential doses of fluconazole. Am J Obstet Gynecol 185:363-369, 2001.
96. Bergeron S, Binik YM, Khalife S, et al: Vulvar vestibulitis syndrome: Reliability of diagnosis and evaluation of current diagnostic criteria. Obstet Gynecol 98:45-51, 2001.
97. Friedrich EG: Vulvar vestibulitis syndrome. J Reprod Med 32:110-114, 1987.
98. Utian WH, Shoupe D, Bachmann G, et al: Relief of vasomotor symptoms and vaginal atrophy with lower doses of conjugated equine estrogens and medroxyprogesterone acetate. Fertil Steril 75:1065-1079, 2001.
99. Kehoe S, Luesley D: Vulvar vestibulitis treated by modified vestibulectomy. Int J Gynaecol Obstet 64:147-152, 1999.
100. Gaunt G, Good A, Stanhope CR: Vestibulectomy for vulvar vestibulitis. J Reprod Med 48:591-595, 2003.
101. Omole F, Simmons BJ, Hacker Y: Management of Bartholin's duct cyst and gland abscess. Am Fam Physician J 68:135-140, 2003.

Section 7

FEMALE ORGAN PROLAPSE

Chapter 51

EPIDEMIOLOGY OF PELVIC ORGAN PROLAPSE

Firouz Daneshgari and Courtenay K. Moore

EPIDEMIOLOGY

Although pelvic organ prolapse (POP) is one of the most common indications for gynecologic surgery, little is known about the epidemiology of the condition.[1] Caring for women with pelvic floor disorders has become an increasingly important component of women's health. An analysis of U.S. procedure codes for prolapse surgery estimates that more than a half-million procedures are performed annually accounting for more than 1 billion US health care dollars.[2] It is estimated that women have an 11% lifetime risk of undergoing a single operation for POP and urinary incontinence by age 80 years.[3] Studies have shown that 50% of parous women lose pelvic floor support, with resulting prolapse.[3] Yet, of these women, only 10% to 20% seek medical care. The Oxford Family Planning Association study monitored more than 17,000 women aged 25 to 39 years for 26 years.[4] Whereas the annual incidence of hospital admission for the diagnosis of prolapse was 0.204%, the annual incidence of surgery for prolapse was only 0.162%.[4] This highlights the fact that only a fraction of women with POP seek medical attention. Therefore, incidence and prevalence rates based on surgical intervention significantly underestimate the magnitude of POP.

Given the difficulties in determining the number of women affected by POP, there has been little agreement on the resources needed to serve this population. It is estimated that the proportion of the U.S. population between the ages of 30 and 89 years will grow by 22% over the next 30 years (Fig. 51-1).[5,6] One of the most dramatic features of this population change is the large increase in the number of Americans older than 50 years of age. The population of women aged 50 years and older is expected to increase by 72%. Luber and colleagues found that women aged 60 years and older are far more likely to seek medical care for pelvic floor disorders than their younger cohorts.[6] They estimated that, over the next 30 years, the demand for services to care for female pelvic floor disorders will increase at twice the rate of growth of the general population (Fig. 51-2). Therefore, at a time when the general population is projected to increase by 22%, there will be a 45% increase in the demand for care for pelvic floor disorders.[6]

One of the reasons that the demographics of POP are so poorly understood is that its prevalence varies widely in different populations, ranging from 30% to 93%. Differences in prevalence and incidence rates may be explained by varying diagnostic criteria, different examination techniques, and the sensitivity of these techniques. Before 1995, one of the main problems in studying the epidemiology of POP was the absence of a standardized tool for evaluating the degree or stage of POP. In 1996, an international committee comprised of members from the International Continence Society (ICS), the American Urogynecologic Society, and the Society of Gynecologic Surgeons met to develop an objective, site-specific system to describe, quantify, and stage female POP.[7] The result was the Pelvic Organ Prolapse Quantification system (POPQ). The creation of this classification system was a major advance in the study of POP, allowing researchers to report findings in a standardized fashion. The POPQ has demonstrated good reliability as well as intraexaminer and interexaminer reproducibility.[8]

A second reason for lack of understanding of the epidemiology of POP is that there have been no epidemiologic studies of

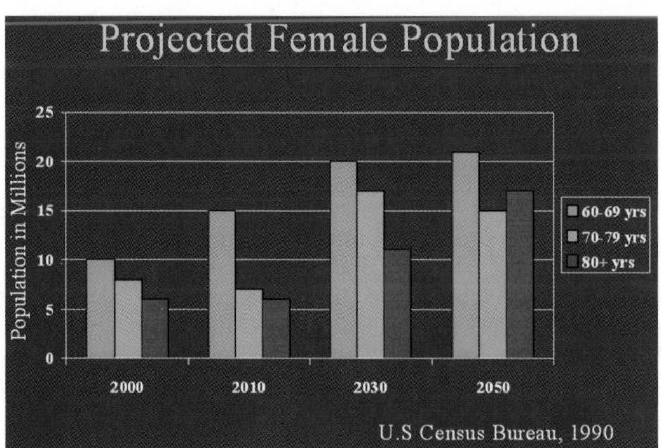

Figure 51-1 Projected U.S. female population.

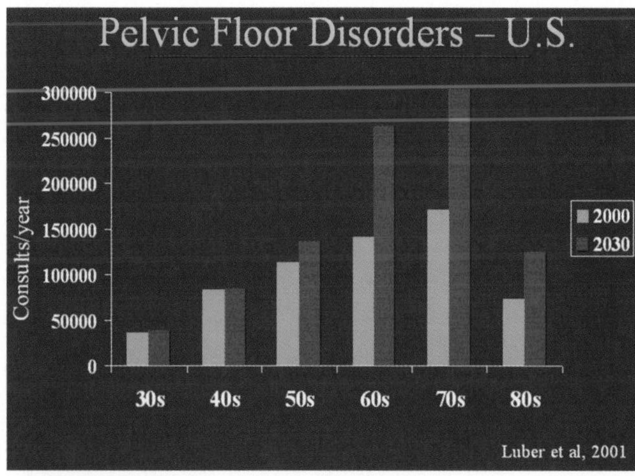

Figure 51-2 Estimated increase in pelvic floor disorders among women aged 30 to 80 years. (From Luber KM, Boero S, Choe JY: The demographics of pelvic floor disorders: Current observations and future projections. Am J Obstet Gynecol 184:1496, 2001.)

POP in community-based populations.[9] Instead, most studies are based on small, mainly white clinical populations or surgical databases. An additional limitation in understanding the epidemiology of POP is inherent to the condition itself. Studies on POP are wrought with difficulties. Complying with the ICS definition of POP requires an invasive examination that limits the feasibility of large community-based studies. Furthermore, symptoms associated with POP have not been shown to correspond to the severity of prolapse. This inconsistency limits the use of symptoms in the epidemiologic definition of prolapse.

Finally, lack of understanding of the distribution of normal versus abnormal female pelvic organ mobility and support remains another limitation. In a study of young nulligravid women, Dietz and coworkers found a wide range of pelvic organ mobility, concluding that the "range of 'normality' in pelvic organ mobility is wider than previously assumed."[10] In 2000, Swift performed an observational study on the distribution of pelvic organ support of women seen at outpatient gynecology clinics for routine gynecologic care. The distribution of POP was a bell-shaped curve, with most subjects having stage 1 or 2 prolapse.[11] The overall distribution was as follows: stage 0, 6.4%; stage 1, 43.3%; stage 2, 47.7%; and stage 3, 2.6%.[11] The Pelvic Organ Support Study (POSST), a multicenter, cross-sectional observational study of 1004 women undergoing annual gynecologic examinations, found a similar distribution. The prevalence of POP quantification stages was as follows: stage 0, 24%; stage 1, 38%; stage 2, 35%; and stage 3, 2%.[12]

PREVALENCE

The *prevalence* of a disease refers to the number of affected persons present in the population at a specific time divided by the number of persons in the population at that time.[13] Prevalence also describes the probability of experiencing a symptom or having a condition or a disease within a defined population at a defined time.[9] This is important in establishing the distribution of a condition in the population and projecting the need for future health and medical services.

The data on prevalence of POP is limited and highly variable. Many estimates of the prevalence of POP define prolapse based on symptoms alone or a nonvalidated genital examination, not on the POPQ. To date, only two studies have used the ICS definition of POP. The first, done by Swift in 2000, found that 94% of women aged 18 to 82 years had stage 1 POP or greater; when only women with stage 2 or greater were considered, the prevalence fell to 51%.[11] A second study, also done by Swift and colleagues, found that 22% of women aged 18 to 83 years seeking routine gynecologic care had POP, which was detected on routine examination.[12]

Two other studies have looked at the prevalence of POP using physical examination; however, these studies used nonvalidated genital examination classification systems. Hendrix and associates looked at the prevalence of POP in women aged 50 to 79 years who were enrolled in the Women's Health Initiative Hormone Replacement Therapy Clinical Trial. Forty-one percent of women with a uterus had some form of prolapse (34.3% cystocele, 14.2% uterine prolapse, 18.6% rectocele), compared to 38% of the women without a uterus (32.9% cystocele, 18.3% rectocele).[14] In the second study, Samuelsson and colleagues examined Swedish women aged 20 to 59 years and found the overall prevalence of genital prolapse to be 30.8%.[15] In comparison, the prevalence studies of POP based on symptoms alone tend to report lower rates of POP, ranging from 7% to 25%.[16-18] This discrepancy in prevalence rates highlights the lack of correlation between POPQ and prolapse symptoms.

INCIDENCE

The *incidence* of a disease is the number of new cases of a disease that occur during a specified period of time in a population at risk of developing the disease or the probability of developing the condition under study during a defined time period.[13] Studies of the incidence of POP come primarily from surgical databases (Table 51-1). Cases are identified by the International Classification of Diseases (ICD) diagnosis and procedures codes. In the United States, the annual incidence of surgery for POP ranges from 1.5 to 4.9 cases per 1000 women.[3,19,20] Olsen and coworkers looked at the incidence of POP surgery in a managed care setting. They found that the age-specific incidence of surgically managed POP increased with age (Fig. 51-3); with the overall lifetime risk of a woman's undergoing at least one operation for POP being 11.1%.[3]

In 1997, Brown and associates[20] calculated the incidence of surgery for POP from the National Hospital Discharge Survey and National Census records of 225,964 women to be 22.7 per 10,000 women. The rate of prolapse surgery increased with age, peaking at age 60 to 69 years with a rate of 42.1 per 10,000 women. Interestingly, rates for surgery varied significantly by region. Women living in the South had the highest overall rate of surgery for POP (29.3 per 10,000), whereas women living in the Northeast had the lowest overall rate of surgical intervention (16.1 per 10,000; see Fig. 51-1).

Boyles and colleagues[19] looked at the trends in surgery performed for POP from 1979 to 1997 using data from the National Hospital Discharge Survey. During this period, 3,734,000 procedures were performed for POP. The number of POP procedures decreased significantly from 226,000 in 1979 to 205,000 in 1997. The age-adjusted rate of POP procedures decreased from 2.2 per 1000 women in 1979 to 1.3 per 1000 from 1988 to 1992. This number rose slightly to the rate of 1.5 per 1000 in 1997. Overall, the absolute number of prolapse procedures in women younger than 50 years of age decreased from 135,000 in 1979 to 80,000 in 1997. However, the number of prolapse procedures in women older than 50 years rose from 91,000 in 1979 to 125,000 in 1997. Therefore, the age-adjusted rate of prolapse surgery from 1979 to 1997 in women younger than 50 years of age decreased from 1.9 to 0.8 per 1000 women, but it did not change in women older than 50 years.

RISK FACTORS

POP is a common disorder, accounting for more than a half-million surgical procedures and more than 1 billion health care dollars annually.[2] The ratio of procedures performed for POP to those performed for urinary incontinence is 2 : 1.[1] Despite its commonality, little is know about the pathophysiology of POP. Like urinary incontinence, POP seems to be multifactorial. Age, gender, and parity are established risk factors for POP, and many other factors have been suggested but not rigorously proven. Without identifying the risk factors of POP, efforts at prevention are fruitless and therapy can only be empiric.[21]

Table 51-1 Summary of Epidemiology of Pelvic Organ Prolapse (POP) Studies

Study	Design/Study Population	No. Patients	Classification of POP	Results
Hendrix	USA. Cross-sectional study of healthy, postmenopausal women enrolled in Women's Health Initiative Hormone Replacement Clinical Trial	27,342	Nonvalidated gynecologic examination (not POPQ)	Risk of POP increases with age, parity, obesity. Risk of POP varies among ethnic groups: lowest among African Americans, highest among Hispanics
Progetto	Italy. Cross-sectional study of women attending menopausal clinics	21,449	Examination using Baden Walker	Risk of uterine prolapse increased with age, BMI, vaginal deliveries
Swift	USA. Case-control study	368 controls 87 cases	POPQ examination	Factors predictive of severe POP: age, weight largest vaginal delivery, hysterectomy, previous prolapse surgery
Brown	USA. National Hospital Discharge Survey	300,000	Surgical procedure and discharge diagnosis codes	Surgery for POP among Caucasians was three times greater than for African Americans. Regional differences: South highest, Northeast lowest rate of surgery for POP
Mant	UK. Cohort from Oxford Family Planning Study	17,032	Hospital in-patient admission with diagnosis of prolapse (ICD codes)	Risk of POP increased with age, parity, weight, hysterectomy
Moalli	USA. Case-control study. Cases selected from patients who underwent surgery for POP ± UI. Controls patients seen in gynecology for routine examination	80 cases 176 controls	Nonvalidated examination	Development of POP associated with: younger age at first delivery, higher BMI, forceps delivery, prior gynecologic surgery
Nygaard	USA. Cohort of healthy, postmenopausal women enrolled in Women's Health Initiative Hormone Replacement Clinical Trial	270	POPQ examination	Risk of POP increased with less education, higher vaginal parity, larger babies

BMI, body mass index; ICD, International Classification of Diseases; POPQ, Pelvic Organ Prolapse Quantification system.

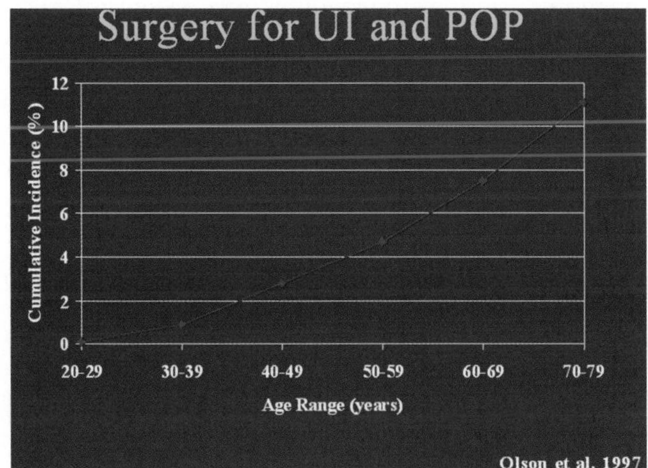

Figure 51-3 Lifetime risk of undergoing surgery for urinary incontinence (UI) and pelvic organ prolapse (POP). (From Olsen AL, Smith VJ, Bergstrom JO, et al: Epidemiology of surgically managed pelvic organ prolapse and urinary incontinence. Obstet Gynecol 89:501, 1997.)

Age

Studies have shown a rise in the incidence and prevalence of POP with age. In a cross-sectional analysis of women enrolled in the Women's Health Initiative Hormone Replacement Therapy Clinical Trial, Hendrix and colleagues found that the risk of developing uterine prolapse, rectocele, and cystocele increased with advancing age.[14] Women aged 60 to 69 years had an odds ratio (OR) of 1.16 for uterine prolapse compared to women aged 50 to 59 years; for women aged 70 to 79 years, the OR was 1.36. Similarly, the ORs for both cystocele and rectocele increased with advancing age. In another cross-sectional study of Italian women, a similar rise in uterine prolapse with age was noted. Compared with women aged 51 years or younger, women aged 52 to 55 years and those aged 56 years or older had ORs for uterine prolapse of 1.3 and 1.7, respectively.[22] Swift and coworkers found that the OR of POP increased by 1.38 per 10-year period.[12] Among women with severe prolapse (stage 3 or 4), the odds of having severe prolapse increased 12% with each year of advancing age.[23]

Surgery for POP is uncommon in patients younger than 30 years of age and in those older than 80 years. Surgical rates of

POP increase with age, peaking in the sixth decade.[20] Brown and coworkers found that, whereas African American women have a lower risk of developing POP than white women, the mean age at which African American women undergo surgery for POP is younger than that for their white counterparts (49.3 versus 54.3 years).[20]

Race

U.S. data suggest a protective effect of African American race compared to white race for POP.[9] Brown found there to be large racial difference in the rates of POP surgery. Compared with African American women, white women have a much higher rate of surgery for POP (6.4 versus 19.6 per 10,000). Hendrix and coworkers[14] also found that, compared with white and Hispanic women, African American women had the lowest rate of uterine prolapse, cystocele, and rectocele. Hispanic women were found to have the highest rate of uterine prolapse and an increased risk for cystocele but not rectocele. American Indian women, although a small sample size, had lower risks than white women for all types of pelvic floor relaxation. Asian women had the greatest risk of all women for cystocle and rectocele. Swift and colleagues found similar results for Hispanic race (OR = 4.29), but black race was not protective (OR = 1.20).[12]

Parity

Multiple studies have shown a positive association between parity and POP. In the Oxford Family Planning Association study, parity was the strongest risk factor for the development of POP, with an adjusted relative risk of 10.85.[4] Although the risk increased with increasing parity, the rate of increase slowed after two deliveries. Hendrix and associates[14] also found an increase in the risk of uterine prolapse, cystocele, and rectocele with increasing parity. Similarly, the Progetto Study showed an OR of 2.6 when comparing nulliparity to a parity of 1 and an OR of 3.0 when comparing nulliparity to a parity of 3 or greater.[22] Nygaard and associates, in a multivariate analysis of 270 women, found that those women who had had no vaginal deliveries had a marked reduction in risk of POP compared with parous women.[24] Higher vaginal parity was associated with the development of stage 2 or greater POP (OR = 1.61).[24]

Moalli and coauthors, in a case-control study, found an increased likelihood of pelvic floor surgery among women who underwent spontaneous vaginal delivery compared with cesarean section. Compared with cesarean delivery, vaginal delivery was associated with an OR of 2.9 for POP surgery.[25] Forceps delivery carried the greatest risk of pelvic floor surgery, with an OR of 5.4.[25] Swift and coworkers identified not only gravidity, parity, and number of vaginal deliveries as risk factors for POP, but also the weight of vaginally delivered infants.[12]

Obesity

Both moderate and severe obesity are associated with increased risks of POP. Hendrix and associates found overweight women (body mass index [BMI] = 25 to 30 kg/m^2) to have an increased risk for the occurrence of uterine prolapse of 31%; for rectocele, 38%; and for cystocele, 39%. Obese women (BMI >30 kg/m^2) also had increased risks 40%, 75%, and 57%, respectively. Women with a waist circumference of 88 cm or greater had a 17% increased risk of cystocele and rectocele. In the Progetto Italia Study, the risk of uterine prolapse increased with increasing BMI. In comparison with women with BMI less than 23.8, women with a BMI of 23.8 to 27.2 had an OR of 1.4, and those with a BMI greater than 27.2 had an OR of 1.6. Other studies have found similar associations between BMI and POP.[12]

Bowel Dysfunction

Chronic constipation with repeated defecatory straining has been linked to POP because of pelvic floor denervation and pudendal neuropathy. In a British case-control study, straining with bowel movements and constipation (fewer than two bowel movements per week) as a young adult were significantly more common in women with uterovaginal prolapse than in controls.[26] Women with uterovaginal prolapse were also noted to have prolonged pudendal nerve terminal motor latency compared with controls, suggesting pudendal neuropathy as a factor involved in the pathogenesis of POP.[26]

Menopause and Gynecologic Factors

Hormonal Status

Swift and colleagues, in 2001, found that postmenopausal women who were not taking hormone replacement therapy (HRT) had a higher rate of prolapse than premenopausal or postmenopausal women taking HRT.[23] Moalli and associates also found that women not taking HRT were at a greater risk of developing POP. Menopausal women who took HRT for 5 or more years had a 90% decreased risk of surgery for POP.[25]

Gynecologic Surgery

Several studies have shown that gynecologic surgery, notably hysterectomy and previous prolapse surgery, predispose women to POP. Swift and colleagues, in their study on severe POP, found a previous history of prolapse surgery or hysterectomy to be among the strongest etiologic predictors of severe POP.[23] The odds of having severe POP increased by more than 200% in patients with a previous history of hysterectomy and by 500% in women with a previous history of prolapse surgery (Fig. 51-4).[24] Mant and colleagues found that women who had a hysterectomy for prolapse were 5.5 times more likely to have a surgery for POP than women whose hysterectomy had been done for other reasons.[4] The cumulative risk of repair after hysterectomy increased in a linear fashion, rising from 1% at 3 years to 5% at 15 years.[4]

Lifestyle

Chronic Obstructive Pulmonary Disease and Smoking

Chronic illnesses such as chronic obstructive pulmonary disease (COPD) are often cited as conditions that appear to predispose women to POP because of the increased stress and stain on the pelvic floor. However, the data are mixed and inconclusive.[3,11,12,17,24] Similarly, the data regarding the effect of smoking on POP are also controversial at his time.[4,12,15,24,27]

High-Impact Activity and Manual Labor

Strenuous high-impact exercise and heavy physical labor have been implicated in female pelvic floor disorders. In 1996, Davis reported three cases of severe POP after the rigors of airborne training in young nulliparous soldiers who had previously

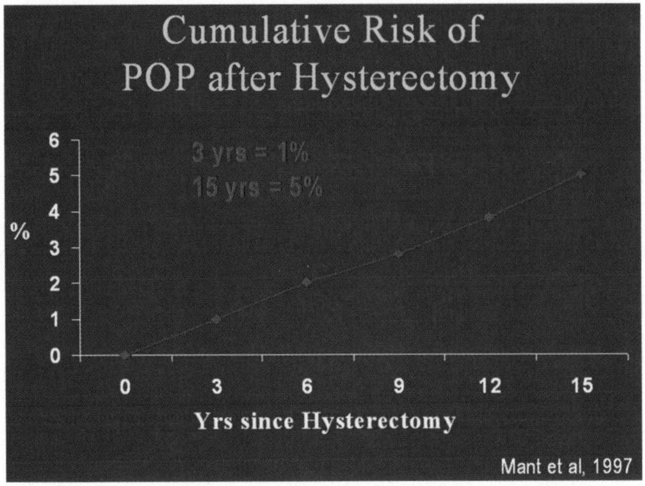

Figure 51-4 Lifetime risk of pelvic organ prolapse (POP) after hysterectomy. (From Mant J, Painter R, Vessey M: Epidemiology of genital prolapse: Observations from the Oxford Family Planning Association Study. Br J Obstet Gynaecol 104:579, 1997.)

undergone laparoscopic uterine nerve ablation.[28] The Danish National Registry of Hospitalized Patients also looked at the effect of heavy physical activity (heavy lifting) on surgery for POP. The risk of surgery for POP in 28,000 nursing assistants aged 20 to 69 years was compared with the risk in 1.6 million age-matched controls. The OR for POP surgery for nursing assistants compared with controls was 1.6.[1] In a case-control study, Italian housewives were found to be at an increased risk of POP when compared with professional/managerial women (OR = 3.1).[27] On univariate analysis, Swift and colleagues also found an increased risk of POP among laborers versus nonlaborers. However, labor did not remain statistically significant in the multivariate logistic regression analysis.[12] Nygaard and associates reported no overall association with employment history, current exercise, or past history of strenuous exercise among women in the United States; however, women with a history of past heavy, manual labor were more likely to have uterine prolapse than those who did not engage in heavy, manual labor.[24]

Genetics and Collagen

In a Finnish study, the familial incidence of genital prolapse was 30%.[29] The risk of POP was higher among women who had a mother or sister with POP. Compared with women whose relatives did not have POP, the OR for these women was 3.2 if their mother had POP and 2.4 if a sister had POP.[27]

It has been suggested that genetic or intrinsic differences in connective tissues may predispose individuals toward urinary incontinence or POP. Ehlers-Danlos syndrome is a connective tissue disorder involving collagen gene defects. Several studies have suggested that women with Ehlers-Danlos syndrome are at an increased risk of POP given these collagen defects. Carley and coworkers looked at women with Ehlers-Danlos syndrome and found that 75% of them had POP.[30] McIntosh and associates also found that women with Ehlers-Danlos syndrome had a higher prevalence of POP than the general population.[31]

It has also been suggested that women with clinical joint hypermobility (a sign of connective tissue laxity) have a higher prevalence of cystocele, rectocele, and uterine prolapse than women with normal joint hypermobitily.[32] Al-Rawi and Al-Rawi found that 66% of Iraqi women with POP had clinical joint hypermobility, compared with 18% of controls.[33]

The results on collagen content of vaginal and pelvic tissues in women with prolapse are variable, given inconsistent data. The data vary based on biopsy site, biochemical tests used for analysis, and heterogeneity of the populations studied.[34] Chen and coworkers found women with POP to have an increased rate of collagen breakdown compared with controls.[35] Similarly, Wong and associates found women with POP to have a significantly decreased amount of cervical collagen compared with controls.[36]

SUMMARY

POP is a common condition among women, with an estimated 11% lifetime risk of undergoing surgery by age 80 years. Yet despite its commonality and its significant cost to the health care system, little is truly known about the epidemiology of POP. Lack of standardized definitions, differing physical examination techniques, difficulty in recruitment, embarrassment surrounding the condition, and coexistence with other pelvic floor disorders have all hindered understanding of POP. Although the POPQ system has facilitated standardization, scientific communication, and epidemiologic and clinical studies of POP, understanding of the epidemiology of POP is still rudimentary. Age, race, parity, obesity, menopause, bowel dysfunction, pelvic surgeries, genetic factors, and lifestyle choices appear to contribute to POP, but further epidemiologic and clinical studies are needed to identify the modifiable risk factors to prevent POP.

References

1. Bump RC, Norton PA: Epidemiology and natural history of pelvic floor dysfunction. Obstet Gynecol Clin North Am 25:723, 1998.
2. Handa VL, Garrett E, Hendrix S, et al: Progression and remission of pelvic organ prolapse: A longitudinal study of menopausal women. Am J Obstet Gynecol 190:27, 2004.
3. Olsen AL, Smith VJ, Bergstrom JO, et al: Epidemiology of surgically managed pelvic organ prolapse and urinary incontinence. Obstet Gynecol 89:501, 1997.
4. Mant J, Painter R, Vessey M: Epidemiology of genital prolapse: Observations from the Oxford Family Planning Association Study. Br J Obstet Gynaecol 104:579, 1997.
5. Bureau USC: U.S. Population Projections by Age and Sex 2000-2050. Washington, DC: U.S. Department of Commerce, 1990.
6. Luber KM, Boero S, Choe JY: The demographics of pelvic floor disorders: Current observations and future projections. Am J Obstet Gynecol 184:1496, 2001.
7. Bump RC, Mattiasson A, Bo K, et al: The standardization of terminology of female pelvic organ prolapse and pelvic floor dysfunction. Am J Obstet Gynecol 175:10, 1996.
8. Hall AF, Theofrastous JP, Cundiff GW, et al: Interobserver and intraobserver reliability of the proposed International Continence Society, Society of Gynecologic Surgeons, and American Urogynecologic Society pelvic organ prolapse classification system. Am J Obstet Gynecol 175:1467, 1996.
9. Hunskaar S: Epidemiology of Urinary and Faecal Incontinence and Pelvic Organ Prolapse, 3rd ed. Plymouth, MA: Health Publication Ltd., 2005, pp. 3-59.

10. Dietz HP, Eldridge A, Grace M, et al: Pelvic organ descent in young nulligravid women. Am J Obstet Gynecol 191:95, 2004.
11. Swift SE: The distribution of pelvic organ support in a population of female subjects seen for routine gynecologic health care. Am J Obstet Gynecol 183:277, 2000.
12. Swift S, Woodman P, O'Boyle A, et al: Pelvic Organ Support Study (POSST): The distribution, clinical definition, and epidemiologic condition of pelvic organ support defects. Am J Obstet Gynecol 192:795, 2005.
13. Gordis L: Epidemiology, 3rd ed. Philadelphia: Elsevier, 2004, p. 335.
14. Hendrix SL, Clark A, Nygaard I, et al: Pelvic organ prolapse in the Women's Health Initiative: Gravity and gravidity. Am J Obstet Gynecol 186:1160, 2002.
15. Samuelsson EC, Arne Victor FT, Tibblin G, et al: Signs of genital prolapse in a Swedish population of women 20 to 59 years of age and possible related factors. Am J Obstet Gynecol 180:299, 1999.
16. Kumari S, Walia I, Singh A: Self-reported uterine prolapse in a resettlement colony of north India. J Midwifery Womens Health 45:343, 2000.
17. Uustal Fornell E, Wingren G, Kjolhede P: Factors associated with pelvic floor dysfunction with emphasis on urinary and fecal incontinence and genital prolapse: An epidemiological study. Acta Obstet Gynecol Scand 83:383, 2004.
18. MacLennan AH, Taylor AW, Wilson DH, et al: The prevalence of pelvic floor disorders and their relationship to gender, age, parity and mode of delivery. BJOG 107:1460, 2000.
19. Boyles SH, Weber AM, Meyn L: Procedures for pelvic organ prolapse in the United States, 1979-1997. Am J Obstet Gynecol 188:108, 2003.
20. Brown JS, Waetjen LE, Subak LL, et al: Pelvic organ prolapse surgery in the United States, 1997. Am J Obstet Gynecol 186:712, 2002.
21. Weber AM, Buchsbaum GM, Chen B, et al: Basic science and translational research in female pelvic floor disorders: Proceedings of an NIH-sponsored meeting. Neurourol Urodyn 23:288, 2004.
22. Risk factors for genital prolapse in non-hysterectomized women around menopause: Results from a large cross-sectional study in menopausal clinics in Italy. Progetto Menopausa Italia Study Group. Eur J Obstet Gynecol Reprod Biol 93:135, 2000.
23. Swift SE, Pound T, Dias JK: Case-control study of etiologic factors in the development of severe pelvic organ prolapse. Int Urogynecol J Pelvic Floor Dysfunct 12:187, 2001.
24. Nygaard I, Bradley C, Brandt D: Pelvic organ prolapse in older women: Prevalence and risk factors. Obstet Gynecol 104:489, 2004.
25. Moalli PA, Jones Ivy S, Meyn LA, et al: Risk factors associated with pelvic floor disorders in women undergoing surgical repair. Obstet Gynecol 101:869, 2003.
26. Spence-Jones C, Kamm MA, Henry MM, et al: Bowel dysfunction: A pathogenic factor in uterovaginal prolapse and urinary stress incontinence. Br J Obstet Gynaecol 101:147, 1994.
27. Chiaffarino F, Chatenoud L, Dindelli M, et al: Reproductive factors, family history, occupation and risk of urogenital prolapse. Eur J Obstet Gynecol Reprod Biol 82:63, 1999.
28. Davis GD: Uterine prolapse after laparoscopic uterosacral transection in nulliparous airborne trainees: A report of three cases. J Reprod Med 41:279, 1996.
29. Rinne KM, Kirkinen PP: What predisposes young women to genital prolapse? Eur J Obstet Gynecol Reprod Biol 84:23, 1999.
30. Carley ME, Schaffer J: Urinary incontinence and pelvic organ prolapse in women with Marfan or Ehlers Danlos syndrome. Am J Obstet Gynecol 182:1021, 2000.
31. McIntosh LJ, Stanitski DF, Mallett VT, et al: Ehlers-Danlos syndrome: Relationship between joint hypermobility, urinary incontinence, and pelvic floor prolapse. Gynecol Obstet Invest 41:135, 1996.
32. Norton PA, Baker JE, Sharp HC, et al: Genitourinary prolapse and joint hypermobility in women. Obstet Gynecol 85:225, 1995.
33. Al-Rawi ZS, Al-Rawi ZT: Joint hypermobility in women with genital prolapse. Lancet 1:1439, 1982.
34. Goh JT: Biomechanical and biochemical assessments for pelvic organ prolapse. Curr Opin Obstet Gynecol 15:391, 2003.
35. Chen BH, Wen Y, Li H, et al: Collagen metabolism and turnover in women with stress urinary incontinence and pelvic prolapse. Int Urogynecol J Pelvic Floor Dysfunct 13:80, 2002.
36. Wong MY, Harmanli OH, Agar M, et al: Collagen content of nonsupport tissue in pelvic organ prolapse and stress urinary incontinence. Am J Obstet Gynecol 189:1597, 2003.

Chapter 52

PREGNANCY, CHILDBIRTH, AND PELVIC FLOOR INJURY

Asnat Groutz

Pregnancy and childbirth have long been considered risk factors in the genesis of pelvic floor disorders. Mechanical and hormonal changes that occur during pregnancy, as well as the mechanical strain of labor and delivery, may all cause partial denervation of the pelvic floor and direct injury to pelvic muscles and connective tissue. These injuries may further lead to the development of stress urinary incontinence, anal incontinence, pelvic organ prolapse, and/or voiding dysfunction. Although many studies have shown some correlations between various obstetric risk factors and the development of these symptoms, there is no consensus regarding the impact and relative contribution of the various parameters. Moreover, the etiology of pelvic floor disorders is multifactorial. Additional risk factors, other than pregnancy and childbirth, include heredity, collagen abnormalities, obesity, and aging. Reliable antenatal models for the identification of women at risk are not yet available. Further studies are required to establish such risk models and the manner in which labor should be managed to minimize potential childbirth-induced pelvic floor injuries.

PHYSIOLOGY

Functional Changes

The physiology of the lower urinary tract during normal pregnancy has not been thoroughly investigated. Furthermore, significant hemodynamic changes may directly affect urinary tract function throughout the course of pregnancy. Total blood volume increases by up to 40%, and cardiac output is increased by 30% to 50% by the third trimester of pregnancy. Simultaneously, systemic vascular resistance is reduced due to progesterone-induced smooth muscle relaxation. Glomerular filtration rate and renal plasma flow consequently increase by 40% to 50%, and 60% to 80%, respectively.[1] These changes result in increased urine output and, with the pressure effect of the gravid uterus on the bladder, may cause urinary frequency, urgency, and nocturia. Up to 80% of women experience urinary frequency during pregnancy, and the symptom usually appears early (i.e., in the first trimester) and tends to worsen as pregnancy progresses.[2-5]

Anatomic Changes

Early radiologic and endoscopic studies showed that the bladder is pressed by the gravid uterus and pushed upward and anteriorly.[2,6,7] More recent studies investigated the mobility of the bladder neck and pelvic floor during pregnancy. Peschers and colleagues[8] reported that bladder neck position at rest is changed at the end of pregnancy, compared with the position in nulligravidas. This finding suggests that mechanical pressure of the fetal head and uterus and/or hormonal and connective tissue changes may alter the bladder neck position during pregnancy. Similarly, Wijma and associates[9] used perineal ultrasound to study a cohort of 117 pregnant nulliparous and 27 nonpregnant nulliparous women. The angle of the urethrovesical junction at rest and the displacement/pressure coefficient during coughing showed a significant increase during pregnancy. King and Freeman,[10] also using perineal ultrasound, found that women with stress urinary incontinence at 10 to 14 weeks postpartum had significantly greater bladder neck mobility antenatally than those who were continent postpartum. There were no significant differences in obstetric parameters between the postpartum continent and incontinent groups. The authors suggested that collagen susceptibility to changes during pregnancy, measured by changes in bladder neck mobility, could predict postpartum incontinence. Dietz and colleagues[11] investigated pelvic organ mobility in 28 pregnant women, seen at 10 to 17 weeks and again at 32 to 39 weeks of gestation, and 88 nonpregnant controls. Pregnant women showed greater bladder and urethral mobility. The effect was already noticeable in the first trimester, but it was significantly augmented later in pregnancy. Because similar changes were also noted in elbow hyperextension, the authors speculated that pregnancy may adversely affect connective tissue biomechanics. This speculation is further supported by earlier data suggesting that, compared with nonpregnant women, connective tissue in pregnant women contains less collagen and has less tensile strength, greater extensibility under low pressure, and loss of recoil after overstretching.[12]

Urodynamic Observations

Only a few urodynamic studies have been performed on pregnant women. Van Geelen and coworkers[13] assessed the urethral pressure profile during pregnancy and after delivery in 42 nulliparas. Lower values of urethral pressure profile parameters were observed in almost all women who experienced stress urinary incontinence during pregnancy and/or after delivery. The investigators concluded that "inherent weakness of the urethral sphincter mechanism plays a key role in the pathogenesis of stress incontinence."[13] Other urodynamic studies revealed decreased cystometric parameters during pregnancy. Chaliha and colleagues[14] studied 286 nulliparous women during the third trimester of pregnancy, 161 of whom returned for postpartum urdynamic evaluation. The mean urodynamic values in the third trimester and after delivery were lower than the reported normal limits of the nonpregnant population. Antenatally, the prevalence of urodynamically proven stress incontinence was 9% and that of detrusor instability was 8%; after delivery, these values were 5% and 7%, respectively. Similarly, Nel and associates[15] studied 66 pregnant women, 40 of whom returned for postpartum urodynamic evaluation. A strong desire to void, urgency, maximum cystometric capacity, and maximum and average flow rates were all significantly decreased during pregnancy. Urodynamically proven stress incontinence was present in 12% of the pregnant subjects, and detrusor instability in 23%.

The cystometric capacity of the bladder during pregnancy has been studied by several investigators, but findings are contradictory. An early study by Muellner[16] found that bladder capacity gradually increased from 12 to 32 weeks of gestation, reaching an average capacity of 1300 mL, and was associated with bladder hypotonia. This finding was confirmed by another small urodynamic study[17] but doubted later by Francis,[2] who found a reduced bladder capacity in the third trimester. Francis[2] also found increased detrusor irritability in late pregnancy, rather than bladder hypotonia. More recent studies have confirmed these latter observations.[14,15]

PATHOPHYSIOLOGY

Labor and delivery have long been known to be the major causes of pelvic floor injury. However, it is unknown whether the insult begins during pregnancy, before the active process of labor and delivery, and whether delivery by elective cesarean section, with no trial of labor, provides any protective effect. Major injury mechanisms include partial denervation of the pelvic floor and direct injury to the pelvic soft tissues.

Neurologic Damage

Electromyography (EMG) and pudendal nerve terminal motor latency (PNTML) measurements are considered to be useful in detecting denervation of the pelvic floor. Prolonged PNTML is obtained when large myelinated nerve axons have been damaged. Snooks and colleagues[18,19] used electrophysiologic techniques to study 71 women at 48 to 72 hours after delivery and again, in 70% of these women, 2 months later. An increased PNTML was found in 42% of the women 48 to 72 hours after vaginal delivery, but not in any of those who delivered by cesarean section. Multiparity, forceps delivery, increased duration of the second stage of labor (defined as the interval between full cervical dilatation and the delivery of the newborn), third degree perineal tear and high birth weight were all found to be associated with increased risk of pudendal neuropathy. However, by 2 months postpartum, the PNTML had returned to normal in 60% of the women, implying that the denervation injury is usually reversible. Fourteen multiparas of the original cohort underwent repeated neurophysiologic studies 5 years after delivery.[20] Five of these 14 women complained of stress urinary incontinence and were found to have marked pudendal neuropathy. The investigators concluded that childbirth-associated pudendal neuropathy may persist and worsen with time.

Allen and colleagues[21] studied the innervation of the pelvic floor muscles before and 2 months after delivery in 96 nulliparas. Using motor unit potential duration as a sign of reinnervation in response to denervation injury, they found evidence of partial denervation of the pelvic floor with consequent reinnervation in 80% of the women after vaginal delivery. It was unclear whether the EMG changes were due to stretching of the pudendal nerve or to direct pressure of the fetal head on the nerve branches. Furthermore, evidence of partial denervation was also found in women who had undergone cesarean section during labor. This finding suggests that the denervation process may start during the first stage of labor, before delivery. Women who had a long (>56.7 min) active second stage of labor (defined as the stage of active pushing) and heavier (>3.41 kg) babies showed the most EMG evidence of nerve damage. The investigators concluded that vaginal delivery causes partial denervation of the pelvic floor in the majority of women delivering their first baby. For most women, the degree of denervation is slight, but in some there is severe damage that may be associated with loss of sphincteric control. Of the original study cohort of 96 women, 77 (80%) were available for 7-year and 65 (68%) for 15-year follow up.[22] The motor unit potential durations were found to be increased significantly after delivery, and again at 7 and 15 years; however, no correlation was found between this EMG finding and the symptom of stress incontinence. The investigators concluded that the absence of an adequate marker for pelvic floor denervation makes it difficult to determine the role of denervation/reinnervation after the first delivery in the etiology of stress urinary incontinence.

Muscular Damage

Relative weakness of the pelvic floor muscles after vaginal delivery was confirmed in several clinical studies. Insult may be secondary to nerve damage, local ischemia, muscle distention, or direct tearing of muscle fibers. Peschers and associates[23] demonstrated that pelvic muscle strength was significantly reduced 3 to 8 days after vaginal delivery but not after cesarean section. In most women, muscle strength was restored to antepartum values 6 to 10 weeks postpartum. However, Sampselle and coauthors[24] reported that recovery of levator ani contractility could take as long as 6 months after delivery.

Advanced imaging techniques have enabled visualization of the pelvic floor structures before and after labor and delivery. Sultan and colleagues[25] used endosonography to assess antenatal and postnatal anal sphincter anatomy. At 6 to 8 weeks postpartum, 35% of the 79 primiparous women studied had occult disruption of the internal or external anal sphincter. None had such sphincter defects before delivery. Of 48 multiparous women, 40% had a sphincter defect before delivery and 44% thereafter. None of the 23 women who underwent cesarean section had a new sphincter defect after delivery. Further analysis revealed that forceps delivery was significantly associated with anatomic damage.

Magnetic resonance imaging (MRI) has been used to detect anatomic and chemical changes, as well as to localize specific injury sites. DeLancey and coworkers[26] used MRI to explore the appearance of the levator ani muscle after vaginal delivery. The study population consisted of 80 nulliparous and 160 primiparous women. The primiparas were all examined 9 to 12 months after vaginal delivery. As many as 20% of the primiparas were found to have levator ani defects on MRI. Most defects were identified in the pubovisceral portion of the levator ani (consists of the pubococcygeus, puborectalis, and puboperineus muscles), and some were in the iliococcygeal portion of the muscle. No levator ani muscle defects were identified in nulliparous women. Moreover, stress-incontinent women were twice as likely to have levator ani defects than continent women. More recently, Lien and colleagues[27] used MRI to create a three-dimensional computer model of the levator ani muscle. This model was used to quantify levator ani muscle stretch during the second stage of labor. The investigators found that the medialmost pubococcygeus muscle is at greater risk for stretch-related injury than any other levator ani muscle during the second stage of labor. Tissue stretch ratios were also proportional to fetal head size.

Connective Tissue Damage

Normally, the endopelvic fascia and the anterior vaginal wall form a hammock-like layer in which the bladder and vesical neck rest. During increased intra-abdominal pressure, the urethra is compressed against this supporting hammock, and continence is maintained. Simultaneous contraction of the levator ani and the urethral sphincter muscles must also occur to support the vesical neck and to occlude the urethra.[28] Indirect evidence of the effects of childbirth on this coordinated support mechanism was obtained by sonogram measurements of the vesical neck position before and after delivery. Both transperineal and transvaginal ultrasound were used to facilitate visualization of the vesical neck at rest; then, with the Valsalva maneuver, the relative descent was measured. Several studies showed lower vesical neck position in women who delivered vaginally, compared with those who underwent elective cesarean section and with nulliparous women. Likewise, mobility of the vesical neck during the Valsalva maneuver was found to increase after vaginal delivery. However, it is less clear whether this increased vesical neck mobility is also associated with long-term pelvic floor disorders.[8,10,29-31]

OBSTETRIC RISK FACTORS

Parity, prolonged labor, instrument-assisted delivery, and increased birth weight have always been considered predisposing factors for pelvic floor injury and subsequent development of long-term pelvic floor dysfunction. However, clear scientific data regarding various obstetric parameters, as well as the possible protective effects of cesarean section, are inconsistent. These conflicting data stress the need for further investigation of the role of pregnancy and delivery in the development of pelvic floor disorders.

Parity

Several investigators reported a positive correlation between parity and stress urinary incontinence.[32-35] However, data concerning a possible linear correlation versus a certain threshold of parity for the development of urinary incontinence are subject to controversy. Foldspang and colleagues[36] found the prevalence of urinary incontinence in women aged 30 to 44 years to be correlated with parity. However, in women aged 45 years or older, only three or more deliveries were associated with an increased risk of incontinence. Thomas and associates,[37] in a postal questionnaire study of more than 7000 women, reported an increased prevalence of urinary incontinence in women with four or more children. Nulliparous women had a lower prevalence of urinary incontinence than did those who had been delivered of one, two, or three babies, but within the parity range of one to three there were no differences in prevalence. Similarly, Wilson and coworkers[38] reported that the odds ratio for postpartum urinary incontinence increased significantly after four deliveries.

The association between parity and urinary incontinence was also investigated by two large epidemiologic studies, the Norwegian Epidemiology of Incontinence in the County of Nord-Trondelag (EPINCONT) study[39] and the Nurses' Health Study.[40] The EPINCONT study was a large survey performed in one county in Norway during the years 1995-1997. The association between parity and urinary incontinence was analyzed in an unselected sample of 27,900 women who answered a detailed questionnaire. Overall, urinary incontinence was reported by 25% of participants. Parity was associated only with stress and mixed types of incontinence, the first delivery being the most significant. The association was strongest in the age group 20 to 34 years, with relative risks of 2.2 and 3.3 for primiparas and grand multiparas, respectively. A weaker association was found in the age group 35 to 64 years (relative risks, 1.4 and 2.0, respectively), and no association was found among women older than 65 years of age. The investigators concluded that all effects of parity seem to disappear in later years. The Nurses' Health Study comprised 83,168 women aged 50 to 75 years. Overall, urinary incontinence was reported by 34% of participants. Similar to the EPINCONT study results, parity was associated with increased prevalence of urinary incontinence; however, the association was weaker among women aged 60 years or older. Results of these two large epidemiologic studies suggest that additional factors, other than childbirth, become more significant in older women, thereby minimizing the effects of parity per se.

Birth Weight

The importance of specific labor parameters and their etiologic role in the development of pelvic floor disorders remains controversial. Dimpfl and associates[41] found a similar incidence of postpartum stress urinary incontinence among mothers whose neonates weighed 3500 g or more and those with infants weighing less than 3500 g. Viktrup and coworkers[42] reported increased birth weights in infants of mothers who developed stress urinary incontinence after delivery, although statistical significance was not reached. Our group[34] found that the prevalence of postpartum stress incontinence among grand multiparas who had given birth to at least one baby weighing more than 4000 g was significantly higher than in those who had not (29.4% versus 16.7%, respectively). Similarly, Persson and colleagues[35] found that the risk of later surgery for stress incontinence after vaginal delivery correlated with the weight of a woman's largest infant.

The effect of various obstetric parameters and urinary incontinence in later life was also investigated in the Norwegian EPINCONT study.[43] The investigators analyzed data from 11,397 women who had delivered vaginally only and who had no more than five children. Nine obstetric parameters were investigated: birth weight, gestational age, head circumference, functional delivery disorders, injuries/tears, breech, forceps, vacuum deliveries, and epidural anesthesia. Statistically significant associations were found between any incontinence and birth weight of 4000 g or more and between stress urinary incontinence and high birth weight; however, odds ratios were relatively weak (1.1 and 1.2, respectively).

Dysfunctional Labor

Early electrophysiologic studies showed that prolonged second stage of labor can cause partial denervation of the pelvic floor.[18,19,21] However, clinical studies have presented conflicting data regarding the association between duration of labor and the later risk of sphincteric incontinence.[44-48] The EPINCONT study grouped various disorders, among which were labor duration of more than 24 hours, cervical dystocia, uterine atonia, and attenuation of contraction, into one category entitled "functional delivery disorders."[43] Statistically significant association was observed between this general category and moderate or severe urinary incontinence; however, the odds ratio (1.3) was relatively weak. No further analysis was undertaken to examine specific parameters, such as duration of the second stage of labor, within this category.

Instrument-Assisted Delivery

Results regarding the possible role of instrument-assisted vaginal delivery (i.e., vacuum or forceps) in the development of pelvic floor disorders are also conflicting. Dimpfl and colleagues[41] found a higher incidence of incontinence after instrumental-assisted vaginal delivery. However, other studies did not confirm this finding.[38,49,50] Sultan and coworkers[25] used endosonography to assess antenatal and postnatal anal anatomy. Forceps delivery was found to be significantly associated with anatomic damage: sphincter defects developed in 8 of the 10 primiparas who underwent forceps delivery, but not in any of the 5 who had underwent vacuum extraction. In another study of 43 patients who had undergone an instrumental delivery, Sultan's group[50] reported that 81% of forceps deliveries were associated with sonographic anal sphincter damage, compared with 24% of vacuum deliveries. Several other studies also demonstrated an increased risk of pelvic floor injury after forceps compared with vacuum deliveries.[52-55] However, one study reported a higher rate of vacuum rather than forceps deliveries in patients with postpartum fecal incontinence.[56] Differences between obstetricians in their primary choice of instrument delivery (vacuum versus forceps), as well as their clinical skills and experience, may explain some of these results. Furthermore, it is possible that the main cause of pelvic floor damage during instrument deliveries is the obstetric indication for such an intervention, namely a prolonged second stage, rather than the type of instrument used per se. Therefore, avoidance of instrumental intervention may facilitate prolonged distention of the vagina by the fetal head, causing greater damage to the pelvic floor.[57] This speculation may be supported by the recent EPINCONT findings suggesting a tendency for these procedures to protect against urinary incontinence, particularly for vacuum delivery.[43]

Cesarean Section

Several studies have examined the association between delivery by cesarean section and urinary incontinence. Persson and colleagues,[35] in a large population-based study of 1942 women, studied risk factors for stress urinary incontinence as represented by a history of anti-incontinence surgery. No association was found between anti-incontinence surgery and pregnancy per se. Vaginal delivery was found to be associated with increased risk for anti-incontinence surgery, compared with elective cesarean section. Moreover, the odds ratio for anti-incontinence surgery was similarly decreased for nulliparas and for primiparas delivered by elective cesarean section. Wilson and associates[38] studied the prevalence of urinary incontinence at 3 months after delivery in a heterogeneous group of 1505 primiparous and multiparous women. They found a significantly lower prevalence of urinary incontinence after cesarean section, in particular among primiparas with no previous history of incontinence, compared to normal vaginal delivery. However, the difference between cesarean sections performed before labor and those performed during labor was nonsignificant. A follow-up study, performed 5 to 7 years later,[58] confirmed the lack of difference between elective and emergency cesarean sections; however, no differentiation was made between the various indications for emergency cesarean section. Farrell and colleagues[59] studied the association between the mode of first delivery and prevalence of urinary incontinence at 6 months postpartum. Vaginal delivery was associated with a higher prevalence of urinary incontinence (relative risk, 2.8) compared with cesarean section. No significant difference was found between cesarean sections performed before and during labor. The authors concluded that cesarean section at any stage of labor reduced postpartum urinary incontinence. Rortveit and coworkers[60] investigated the association between childbirth and urinary incontinence in a large community-based cohort of 15,307 women who were younger than 65 years of age and were either nulliparous, had undergone only cesarean deliveries, or had had only vaginal deliveries. This analysis was part of the EPINCONT study described earlier. The prevalence of stress urinary incontinence was 4.7% in the nulliparous group, 6.9% in the cesarean section group, and 12.2% in the vaginal delivery group. Further classification of cesarean sections into elective versus nonelective, performed in a subgroup of 239 primiparas, failed to reveal a statistically significant difference. However, as in all other aforementioned studies, nonelective cesarean sections were analyzed as one group, with no further differentiation among cesarean sections for obstructed labor, fetal distress, maternal indications, and other obstetric conditions.

Grouping all cesarean section deliveries into one category may be associated with an overestimation bias, because it is possible that, in cases of cesarean section performed for obstructed labor, pelvic floor injury is already too extensive to be prevented by surgical intervention. To investigate this possibility, our group recently studied the prevalence of stress urinary incontinence 1 year postpartum according to the mode of delivery: spontaneous vaginal delivery versus elective cesarean section versus cesarean section performed for obstructed labor.[61] Our results showed a similar prevalence of stress urinary incontinence 1 year after delivery among primiparas who underwent spontaneous vaginal delivery and those who had undergone cesarean section for obstructed labor (10.3% and 12%, respectively; $P = .7$). Conversely, elective cesarean section, with no trial of labor, was associated with a significantly lower prevalence of postpartum stress incontinence (3.4%; $P = .02$). This low prevalence of stress urinary incontinence among primiparas who had elective cesarean sections was similar to that reported for nulliparous women.[34,60]

Whether prevention of pelvic floor injury should be an indication for elective cesarean section is controversial[62] and involves medical, financial, and ethical aspects. It should be borne in mind that cesarean section may expose women to greater morbidity and mortality. Furthermore, the etiology of stress urinary incontinence is multifactorial. Additional risk factors, other than mode of delivery, include heredity, collagen abnormalities, aging, obesity, and parity. Specific labor plans should therefore be based on overall judgment, taking into consideration personal clinical status and risk factors.

CLINICAL PRESENTATIONS

Stress Urinary Incontinence

Stress urinary incontinence is an exceedingly common symptom during pregnancy and the puerperium. Viktrup and associates[42] interviewed 305 primiparas in regard to stress urinary incontinence before and during pregnancy and after delivery. Of these, 4% had stress urinary incontinence before pregnancy, 32% during pregnancy, and 7% after delivery. Among those women who reported stress incontinence during pregnancy, fewer than 5% remained symptomatic 12 months after delivery. Of those who developed the condition after delivery, 24% remained symptomatic at 12 months. These observations suggest that pregnancy-associated stress incontinence resolves after delivery in most women. The question of greater interest is whether women with pregnancy-associated stress incontinence are at increased risk for incontinence in later life. Of the original study cohort of 305 primiparous women reported by Viktrup and colleagues,[42] 278 (91%) were available for a 5-year follow-up.[63] The overall prevalence of stress urinary incontinence at 5 years postpartum was 30%. Among those women with pregnancy-associated stress incontinence but full remission at 3 months postpartum, symptoms recurred 5 years later in 42%. Up to 92% of those with stress incontinence at 3 months postpartum developed stress incontinence 5 years later. The investigators concluded that first pregnancy and delivery are important in the development of long-lasting stress incontinence and that the use of vacuum delivery and episiotomy seems to increase the risk.

Schytt and colleagues[64] studied the prevalence and predictors of stress incontinence 1 year after childbirth. The study cohort comprised 2390 Swedish women who completed questionnaires during pregnancy and again at 2 months and 1 year after delivery. One year postpartum, 22% of the women were stress-incontinent, but only 2% considered it a major problem. The strongest predictor for stress incontinence at 1 year, in primiparas as well as multiparas, was urinary incontinence during pregnancy and at 4 to 8 weeks after delivery. Of those who had urinary incontinence during the third trimester, 31% to 41% were stress-incontinent 1 year after delivery. Of those who had urinary incontinence 4 to 8 weeks after delivery, 44% to 59% were stress incontinent 1 year postpartum. Other predictors unrelated to parity were obesity and constipation during pregnancy and after delivery. Several other investigators found that, regardless of the mode of first delivery, new onset of stress urinary incontinence during pregnancy is associated with increased risk of long-lasting stress urinary incontinence[5,34,35,38,61,65] These observations suggest that the etiology of stress incontinence is more complicated than previously estimated and that the onset of incontinence is also related to the pregnant status, rather than to obstetric trauma per se.

Anal Incontinence

The true prevalence of anal incontinence is unknown and most probably has been underestimated. Although anal incontinence is more common among elderly patients, many young female patients are also affected. Previous studies reported that 3% to 7% of women experienced anal incontinence several months after delivery.[45,56,66] Pollack and colleagues[67] studied the prevalence of anal incontinence in primiparous women 5 years after their first delivery. The study population included 242 women who completed questionnaires before pregnancy and at 5 months, 9 months, and 5 years after delivery. Among women with no visible sphincter tears at their first delivery, 25% reported anal incontinence at 9 months and 32% at 5 years. Among those with sphincter tears, 44% reported anal incontinence at 9 months and 53% at 5 years. The majority of symptomatic women had infrequent incontinence to flatus, whereas frank fecal incontinence was rare. Risk factors for anal incontinence at 5 years were age, sphincter tear, and subsequent childbirth.

The reported incidence of anal sphincter tears after first delivery and subsequent childbirth varies widely. Moreover, sphincter tears may be overt (third- or fourth- degree tears), diagnosed and repaired immediately after delivery, or occult, identified by endoanal ultrasonography after childbirth. The incidence of overt sphincter injury is estimated to be 0.5% to 3.3% in centers where mediolateral episiotomy is practiced or higher, 11% to 28%, in centers where midline episiotomies are used.[68-70] Women with third- and fourth-degree sphincter tears are more likely to develop anal incontinence. Fornell and associates[71] compared 51 women with and 31 women without anal sphincter injury and found that as many as 40% of the affected women reported fecal incontinence 6 months after delivery. Twenty-six of the original study group and 6 of the original controls were objectively and subjectively re-examined 10 years later.[72] Incontinence to flatus and liquid stool was more severe in the study group than in controls. Subjective and objective anal function after sphincter injury was found to deteriorate over time and with subsequent vaginal deliveries. Moreover, 7 of the original 51 women underwent second repair of the sphincter defect (5 before the follow-up study, and 2 more afterward by referral for secondary repair due to fecal incontinence). The investigators indicated that fecal incontinence must be considered a strong marker for unsatisfactory results of primary repair. In view of the disappointing results obtained with secondary repairs, preventive measures and optimal primary repair are strongly recommended.

A relatively high incidence of occult sphincter injury was reported after apparently uneventful vaginal deliveries. Sultan and associates[25] used endosonography to assess antenatal and postnatal anal anatomy. No sphincter defects were demonstrated antenatally among 79 primiparous patients studied. However, at 6 to 8 weeks postpartum, 35% had occult disruption of the internal or external anal sphincter. Of the 48 multiparous women, 40% had a sphincter defect prenatally and 44% postnatally. None of the 23 women who underwent cesarean section had a new sphincter defect after delivery. When the women studied 6 weeks after delivery, anal incontinence or fecal urgency was found in 13% of the primiparas and 23% of the multiparas who delivered vaginally. A strong association was observed between sphincter defects and the development of bowel symptoms. In another study of 43 patients who had had instrumental deliveries, Sultan and colleagues[51] reported that 81% of forceps deliveries were associated with sonographic anal sphincter damage, compared with 24% of vacuum deliveries. A recent meta-analysis of five studies, with overall 717 women who underwent endoanal ultrasonography after childbirth, revealed a 26.9% incidence of anal sphincter defects in primiparous women and an 8.5% incidence of new sphincter defects in multiparous women. About one third of women with occult anal sphincter defects were symptomatic after delivery.[73]

Pelvic Organ Prolapse

Pelvic organ prolapse is very common and is seen in up to 50% of parous women.[74] Hendrix and associates[75] studied the prevalence of pelvic organ prolapse among 27,342 women (the Women's Health Initiative Study). Among the 16,616 women with a uterus, the rate of uterine prolapse was 14.2%; the rate of cystocele was 34.3%, and the rate of rectocele was 18.6%. Among the 10,727 women who had undergone hysterectomy, prevalence of cystocele was 32.9% and that of rectocele was 18.3%. In 1997, the rate of pelvic organ prolapse surgery in the United States was 22.7 per 10,000 women, making prolapse one of the most common surgical indications in women.[76] Similarly, the lifetime risk of surgery for prolapse by age 80 years was estimated to be 11%.[77]

Pregnancy and childbirth are major risk factors for pelvic organ prolapse. Both the levator ani muscle and the endopelvic fascia are important in maintaining the pelvic organs in their normal anatomic position. Both may be injured during pregnancy and delivery, thus predisposing to the later development of pelvic organ prolapse. Sze and colleagues[78] found that some degree of pelvic organ prolapse existed in their subjects during the third trimester of pregnancy and that the prevalence of prolapse at 6 weeks after delivery was similar in women who underwent vaginal delivery and those who had emergency cesarean section. Similarly, O'Boyle and associates[79] found that nulliparous pregnant women were more likely to have pelvic organ prolapse than their nulliparous, nonpregnant controls. These findings imply that the prolapse process begins during pregnancy and early labor. The risk is further increased after vaginal deliveries. Mant and colleagues[80] studied a cohort of 17,000 British women. Parity was the strongest variable related to surgery for pelvic organ prolapse. Samuelsson and coworkers[81] studied a cohort of 487 Swedish women. The risk for pelvic organ prolapse was found to increase with parity and age. Parity and obesity were also strongly associated with increased risk for pelvic organ prolapse in the large Women's Health Initiative Study.[75] Women who had had at least one child were twice as likely to have pelvic organ prolapse as were nulliparous controls, after adjusting for age, ethnicity, body mass index, and other factors.

Richardson and colleagues[82] documented breaks in the endopelvic fascia in women with pelvic organ prolapse and stress urinary incontinence. These breaks are considered to be secondary to obstetric trauma. The anatomic injury may be further complicated by childbirth-associated denervation injury. Evidence of such denervation has been detected in up to 50% of women with symptomatic pelvic organ prolapse.[83-85] However, one should bear in mind that, as with sphincteric incontinence, the etiology of pelvic organ prolapse is complex and multifactorial. Possible risk factors, other than pregnancy and childbirth, include connective tissue abnormalities, aging, hysterectomy, menopause, and factors associated with chronically raised intra-abdominal pressure.[86]

Voiding Difficulties

Data regarding the correlation between obstetric parameters and voiding phase disorders are scarce and controversial. Conceptually, voiding phase dysfunction may be result from bladder and/or urethral causes. Bladder causes include detrusor contraction of inadequate magnitude and/or duration to effect bladder emptying (detrusor underactivity) and the absence of detrusor contraction (detrusor areflexia). Urethral causes consist of bladder outlet obstruction due to urethral overactivity (functional obstruction) or anatomic pathologies (mechanical obstruction). These mechanisms may all be responsible for abnormal voiding during the puerperium. Mechanical bladder outlet obstruction may develop secondary to local hematoma or edema, functional obstruction may be secondary to pain, and detrusor underactivity may be the end result of pelvic floor denervation or neglected bladder overdistention.

Most previously published studies used postvoid residual urine volume, measured by either ultrasound or transurethral catheterization, to detect postpartum voiding dysfunction. Andolf and colleagues[87] investigated residual urinary volumes on the third postpartum day in 539 women who delivered vaginally. Eight women (1.5%) had a residual volume exceeding 150 mL. Retention was more common after instrument delivery or epidural analgesia. Yip and associates[88,89] reported a 4.9% incidence of acute, symptomatic postpartum urinary retention among 691 women who delivered vaginally. An additional 9.7% of patients had no urinary symptoms, but their postvoid residual urinary volume on the first postpartum day was 150 mL or greater (up to 1000 mL). A significant correlation was found between the duration of the first and second stages of labor and postpartum residual urinary volume. We recently reported that approximately half of 277 consecutive women complained of significant voiding difficulties in the immediate postpartum period. The main risk factors included prolonged first and second stages of labor, vacuum extraction, and birth weight 3800 g or greater.[90]

Most cases of early postpartum voiding difficulties resolve spontaneously within few days. Persistent postpartum urinary retention, beyond the early puerperium, is uncommon. In a study of 8402 consecutive, unselected parturients delivered in a university-affiliated maternity hospital over a 1-year period, only 4 patients (0.05%) developed persistent postpartum urinary retention.[91] Risk factors for persistent postpartum urinary retention included vaginal delivery after cesarean section, prolonged second stage of labor, epidural analgesia, and delayed diagnosis and intervention. Urodynamic evaluation, performed in two of these patients 1 month after removal of the suprapubic catheter, revealed stress incontinence in one and detrusor overactivity in the other. Similarly, Carley and colleagues[92] reported a 0.45% prevalence rate of clinically overt postpartum urinary retention among 11,332 vaginally delivered women. Urinary retention was found to be highly associated with instrument-assisted delivery and epidural analgesia. Most affected women resumed spontaneous voiding within 72 hours, but 13 women (0.1%) developed persistent postpartum urinary retention. These two studies indicate that persistent postpartum urinary retention is rare in modern obstetric practice but may be associated with long-term bladder dysfunction. Early diagnosis of postpartum voiding dysfunction and adequate intervention are therefore required to prevent irreversible bladder damage.

SUMMARY

Pregnancy and childbirth are associated with anatomic and neuromuscular injuries of the pelvic floor. These injuries predispose for various pelvic organ disorders that may manifest during pregnancy and after delivery or develop in later years. Cesarean section appears to be protective, especially if undertaken electively, with no trial of labor. Whether the prevention of pelvic floor injury should be an indication for elective cesarean section is controversial. It should be borne in mind that cesarean section may expose women to greater morbidity and mortality, and that the etiology of pelvic organ disorders is multifactorial. Additional risk factors, other than pregnancy and childbirth, include heredity, collagen abnormalities, obesity, and aging. Better understanding of pathophysiologic mechanisms associated with pelvic floor dysfunction may provide the possibility of using appropriate preventive measures other than elective cesarean section. Furthermore, as new therapies emerge, it is likely that different pathophysiologies will be treated differently. Exploring these processes and quantifying subjective and objective findings remains a clinical challenge.

References

1. Dafnis E, Sabatini S: The effect of pregnancy on renal function: physiology and pathophysiology. Am J Med Sci 303:184-205, 1992.
2. Francis WJA: Disturbances of bladder function in relation to pregnancy. J Obstet Gynaecol Br Empire 67:353-366, 1960.
3. Stanton SL, Kerr-Wilson R, Harris GV: The incidence of urological symptoms in normal pregnancy. Br J Obstet Gynaecol 87:897-900, 1980.
4. Cutner A, Carey A, Cardozo LD: Lower urinary tract symptoms in early pregnancy. J Obstet Gynecol 12:75-78, 1992.
5. Thorp JM Jr, Norton PA, Wall LL, et al: Urinary incontinence in pregnancy and the puerperium: A prospective study. Am J Obstet Gynecol 181:266-273, 1999.
6. Hundley JM Jr, Siegel IA, Hachtel FW, Dumler JC: Some physiological and pathological observations on the urinary tract during pregnancy. Sur Gynecol Obstet 66:360-379, 1938.
7. Malpas P, Jeffcoate TNA, Lister UM: The displacement of the bladder and urethra during labor. J Obstet Gynaecol Br Empire 56:949-960, 1949.
8. Peschers U, Schaer G, Anthuber C, et al: Changes in vesical neck mobility following vaginal delivery. Obstet Gynecol 88:1001-1006, 1996.
9. Wijma J, Weis Potters AE, de Wolf BT, et al: Anatomical and functional changes in the lower urinary tract during pregnancy. Br J Obstet Gynaecol 108:726-732, 2001.
10. King JK, Freeman RM: Is antenatal bladder mobility a risk factor for postpartum stress incontinence? Br J Obstet Gynaecol 105:1300-1307, 1998.
11. Dietz HP, Eldridge A, Grace M, Clarke B: Does pregnancy affect pelvic organ mobility? Aust N Z J Obstet Gynecol 44:517-520, 2004.
12. Lavin JM, Smith ARB, Anderson J, et al: The effect of the first pregnancy on the connective tissue of the rectus sheath. Neurourol Urodyn 16:381-382, 1997.
13. Van Geelen JM, Lemmens WA, Eskes TK, Martin CB Jr: The urethral pressure profile in pregnancy and after delivery in health nulliparous women. Am J Obstet Gynecol 144:636-649, 1982.
14. Chaliha C, Bland JM, Monga A, et al: Pregnancy and delivery: A urodynamic viewpoint. Br J Obstet Gynaecol 107:1354-1359, 2000.
15. Nel JT, Diedericks A, Joubert G, Arndt K: A prospective clinical and urodynamic study of bladder function during and after pregnancy. Int Urogynecol J 12:21-26, 2001.
16. Muellner SR: Physiological bladder changes during pregnancy and the puerperium. J Urol 41:691-695, 1939.
17. Youssef AF: Cystometric studies in gynecology and obstetrics. Obstet Gynecol 8:181-188, 1956.
18. Snooks SJ, Swash M, Setchell M, Henry MM: Injury to innervation of pelvic floor sphincter musculature in childbirth. Lancet 2:546-550, 1984.
19. Snooks SJ, Swash M, Henry MM, Setchell M: Risk factors in childbirth causing damage to the pelvic floor innervation. Int J Colorectal Dis 1:20-24, 1986.
20. Snooks SJ, Swash M, Mathers SE, Henry MM: Effect of vaginal delivery on the pelvic floor: A 5-tear follow-up. Br J Surg 77:1358-1360, 1990.
21. Allen RE, Hosker GL, Smith ARB, Warrell DW: Pelvic floor damage and childbirth: A neurophysiological study. Br J Obstet Gynaecol 97:770-779, 1990.
22. Dolan LM, Hosker GL, Mallett VT, et al: Stress incontinence and pelvic floor neurophysiology 15 years after the first delivery. Br J Obstet Gynaecol 110:1107-1114, 2003.
23. Peschers UM, Shaer GN, DeLancey JO, Schuessler B: Levator ani function before and after childbirth. Br J Obstet Gynaecol 104:1004-1008, 1997.
24. Sampselle CM, Miller JM, Mims BL, et al: Pelvic muscle exercise reduces transient incontinence during pregnancy and after birth. Obstet Gynecol 91:406-412, 1998.
25. Sultan AH, Kamm MA, Bartram CI, Hudson CN: Anal-sphincter disruption during vaginal delivery. N Engl J Med 329:1905-1911, 1993.
26. DeLancey JO, Kearney R, Chou Q, et al: The appearance of levator ani muscle abnormalities in magnetic resonance images after vaginal delivery. Obstet Gynecol 101:46-53, 2003.
27. Lien KC, Mooney B, DeLancey JOL, Ashton-Miller JA: Levator ani muscle stretch induced by simulated vaginal birth. Obstet Gynecol 103:31-40, 2004.
28. DeLancey JOL: Stress urinary incontinence: Where are we now, where should we go? Am J Obstet Gynecol 175:311-319, 1996.
29. Wijma J, Weis Potters AE, De Wolf BTHM, et al: Anatomical and functional changes in the lower urinary tract following spontaneous vaginal delivery. Br J Obstet Gynaecol 110:658-663, 2003.
30. Meyer S, Schreyer A, DeGrandi P, Hohlfeld P: The effects of birth on urinary continence mechanisms and other pelvic-floor characteristics. Obstet Gynecol 92:613-618, 1998.
31. Dietz HP, Steensma AB: Which women are most affected by delivery-related changes in pelvic organ mobility? Eur J Obstet Gynecol Reprod Biol 111:15-18, 2003.
32. Jolleys JV: Reported prevalence of urinary incontinence in women in a general practice. BMJ 296:1300-1302, 1988.
33. Milsom I, Ekelund P, Molander U, et al: The influence of age, parity, oral contraception, hysterectomy and menopause on the prevalence of urinary incontinence in women. J Urol 149:1459-1462, 1993.
34. Groutz A, Gordon D, Keidar R, et al: Stress urinary incontinence: Prevalence among nulliparous compared with primiparous and grand mulitiparous premenopausal women. Neurourol Urodyn 18:419-425, 1999.
35. Persson J, Wolner-Hanssen P, Rydhstroem H: Obstetric risk factors for stress urinary incontinence: A population-based study. Obstet Gynecol 96:440-445, 2000.
36. Foldspang A, Mommsen S, Lam GW, Elvin L: Parity as a correlate of adult female urinary incontinence prevalence. J Epidemiol Community Health 46:595-600, 1992.
37. Thomas TM, Plymat KR, Blannin J, Meade TW: Prevalence of urinary incontinence. BMJ 281:1243-1245, 1980.
38. Wilson PD, Herbison RM, Herbison GP: Obstetric practice and the prevalence of urinary incontinence three months after delivery. Br J Obstet Gynaecol 103:154-161, 1996.
39. Rortveit G, Hannestad YS, Daltveit AK, Hunskaar S: Age- and type-dependent effects of parity on urinary incontinence: The Norwegian EPINCONT study. Obstet Gynecol 98:1004-1010, 2001.
40. Grodstein F, Fretts R, Lifford K, Curhan G: Association of age, race, and obstetric history with urinary symptoms among women in the Nurses' Health Study. Am J Obstet Gynecol 189:428-434, 2003.
41. Dimpfl T, Hesse U, Schussler B: Incidence and cause of postpartum urinary incontinence. Eur J Obstet Gynecol Reprod Biol 43:23-33, 1992.
42. Viktrup L, Lose G, Rolff M, Barfoed K: The symptom of stress incontinence caused by pregnancy or delivery in primiparas. Obstet Gynecol 79:945-949, 1992.

43. Rortveit G, Daltveit AK, Hannestad YS, Hunskaar S: Vaginal delivery parameters and urinary incontinence: The Norwegian EPINCONT study. Am J Obstet Gynecol 189:1268-1274, 2003.
44. Thom DH, Van den Eeden SK, Brown JS: Evaluation of parturition and other reproductive variables as risk factors for urinary incontinence in later life. Obstet Gynecol 90:983-989, 1997.
45. Groutz A, Fait G, Lessing JB, et al: Incidence and obstetric risk factors of postpartum anal incontinence. Scand J Gastroenterol 34:315-318, 1999.
46. Varma A, Gunn J, Lindow SW, Duthie GS: Do routinely measured delivery variables predict anal sphincter outcome? Dis Colon Restum 42:1261-1264, 1999.
47. Abramowitz L, Sobhani I, Ganansia R, et al: Are sphincter defects the cause of anal incontinence after vaginal delivery? Dis Colon Restum 43:590-596, 2000.
48. Van Kessel K, Reed S, Newton K, et al: The second stage of labor and stress urinary incontinence. Am J Obstet Gynecol 184:1571-1575, 2001.
49. Foldspang A, Mommsen S, Djurhuus JC: Prevalent urinary incontinence as a correlate of pregnancy, vaginal childbirth, and obstetric techniques. Am J Public Health 89:209-212, 1999.
50. Meyer S, Holfeld P, Achtari C, et al: Birth trauma: Short and long term effects of forceps delivery compared with spontaneous delivery on various pelvic floor parameters. Br J Obstet Gynaecol 107:1360-1365, 2000.
51. Sultan AH, Kamm MA, Hudson CN, et al: Anal sphincter trauma during instrumental delivery: A comparison between forceps and vacuum extraction. Int J Gynaecol Obstet 43:263-70, 1993.
52. Johanson RB, Rice C, Doyle M, et al: A randomized prospective study comparing the new vacuum extractor policy with forceps delivery. Br J Obstet Gynaecol 100:524-530, 1993.
53. Sultan AH, Kamm MA, Hudson CN, Bartram CI: Third degree obstetric anal sphincter tears: Risk factors and outcome of primary repair. BMJ 308:887-891, 1994.
54. Bofill JA, Rust OA, Schorr SJ, et al: A randomized prospective trial of the obstetric forceps versus the M-cup vacuum extractor. Am J Obstet Gynecol 175:1325-1330, 1996.
55. Arya LA, Jackson ND, Myers DL, Verma A: Risk of new-onset urinary incontinence after forceps and vacuum delivery in primiparous women. Am J Obstet Gynecol 185:1318-1323, 2001.
56. MacArthur C, Bick DE, Keighley MRB: Faecal incontinence after childbirth. Br J Obstet Gynaecol 104:46-50, 1997.
57. DeLancey JOL: Childbirth, continence, and the pelvic floor. N Engl J Med 329:1956-1957, 1993.
58. Wilson PD, Herbison P, Glazener C, et al: Obstetric practice and urinary incontinence 5-7 years after delivery [abstract]. Neurourol Urodyn 21:289-291, 2002.
59. Farrell SA, Allen VM, Baskett TF: Parturition and urinary incontinence in primiparas. Obstet Gynecol 97:350-356, 2001.
60. Rortveit G, Daltveit AK, Hannestad YS, Hunskaar S: Urinary incontinence after vaginal delivery or cesarean section. N Engl J Med 348:900-907, 2003.
61. Groutz A, Rimon E, Peled S, et al: Cesarean section: Does it really prevent the development of postpartum stress urinary incontinence? A prospective study of 363 women one year after their first delivery. Neurourol Urodyn 23:2-6, 2004.
62. Bewley S, Cockburn J. Commentary: The unfacts of "request" caesarean section. Br J Obstet Gynaecol 109:597-605, 2002.
63. Viktrup L, Lose G: The risk of stress incontinence 5 years after first delivery. Am J Obstet Gynecol 185:82-87, 2001.
64. Schytt E, Lindmark G, Waldenstrom U: Symptoms of stress incontinence 1 year after childbirth: Prevalence and predictors in a national Swedish sample. Acta Obstet Gynecol Scand 83:928-936, 2004.
65. Pregazzi R, Sartore A, Troiano L, et al: Postpartum urinary symptoms: Prevalence and risk factors. Eur J Obstet Gynecol Reprod Biol 103:179-182, 2002.
66. Sleep S, Grant A: Pelvic floor exercises in postnatal care. Br J Midwifery 3:158-164, 1987.
67. Pollack J, Nordenstam J, Brismar S, et al: Anal incontinence after vaginal delivery: A five-year prospective cohort study. Obstet Gynecol 104:1397-1402, 2004.
68. Coats PM, Chan KK, Wilkins M, Beard RJ: A comparison between midline and mediolateral episiotomies. Br J Obstet Gynaecol 87:408-412, 1980.
69. Samuelsson E, Ladfors L, Wennerholm UB, et al: Anal sphincter tears: Prospective study of obstetric risk factors. Br J Obstet Gynaecol 107:926-931, 2000.
70. Fenner DE, Genberg B, Brahma P, et al: Fecal and urinary incontinence after vaginal delivery and sphincter disruption in an obstetrics unit in the United States. Am J Obstet Gynecol 189:1543-1550, 2003.
71. Fornell E, Berg G, Hallbook O, et al: Clinical consequences of anal sphincter rupture during vaginal delicery. J Am Coll Surg 183:553-558, 1996.
72. Fornell EU, Matthiesen L, Sjodahl R, Berg G: Obstetric anal sphincter injury ten years after: Subjective and objective long term effects. Br J Obstet Gynaecol 112:312-316, 2005.
73. Oberwalder M, Connor J, Wexner SD: Meta-analysis to detrmine the incidence of obstetric anal sphincter damage. Br J Surg 90:1333-1337, 2003.
74. Beck RP, McCormick S, Nordstrom L:. A 25-year experience with 519 anterior colporrhaphy procedures. Obstet Gynecol 78:1011-1018, 1991.
75. Hendrix SL, Clark A, Nygaard I, et al: Pelvic organ prolapse in the Women's Health Initiative: Gravity and gravidity. Am J Obstet Gynecol 186:1160-1166, 2002.
76. Brown JS, Waetjen LE, Subak LL, et al: Pelvic organ prolapse surgery in the United States, 1997. Am J Obstet Gynecol 186:712-716, 2002.
77. Olsen AL, Smith VJ, Bergstrom JO, et al: Epidemiology of surgically managed pelvic organ prolapse and urinary incontinence. Obstet Gynecol 89:501-505, 1997.
78. Sze EH, Sherard GB, Dolezal JM: Pregnancy, labor, delivery and pelvic organ prolapse. Obstet Gynecol 100:981-986, 2002.
79. O'Boyle AL, Woodman PJ, O'Boyle JD, et al: Pelvic organ support in nulliparous pregnant and non-pregnant women: A case control study. Am J Obstet Gynecol 187:99-102, 2002.
80. Mant J, Painter R, Vessey M: Epidemiology of genital prolapse: Observations from the Oxford Family Planning Association study. Br J Obstet Gynaecol 104:579-585, 1997.
81. Samuelsson EC, Victor FTA, Tibblin G, Svardsudd KF: Sings of genital prolapse in a Swedish population of women 20 to 59 years of age and possible related factors. Am J Obstet Gynecol 180:299-305, 1999.
82. Richardson AC, Lyon WB, Williams NL: A new look at pelvic relaxation. Am J Obstet Gynecol 126:568-571, 1976.
83. Sharf B, Zilberman A, Sharf M, Mitrani A: Electromyogram of pelvic floor muscles in genital prolapse. Int J Gynaecol Obstet 14:2-4, 1976.
84. Gilpin SA, Gosling JA, Smith ARB, Warrell DW: The pathogenesis of genitourinary prolapse and stress incontinence of urine: A histological and histochemical study. Br J Obstet Gynaecol 96:15-23, 1989.
85. Smith ARB, Hosker GL, Warrell DW: The role of partial denervation of the pelvic floor in the aetiology of genitourinary prolapse and stress incontinence of urine: A neurophysiological study. Br J Obstet Gynaecol 96:24-28, 1989.
86. Maher C, Baessler K, Glazener CMA, et al: Surgical management of pelvic organ prolapse in women. Cochrane Database Syst Rev (4): CD004014, 2004.
87. Andolf E, Iosif CS, Jorgensen C, Rydhstorm H: Insidious urinary retention after vaginal delivery: Prevalence and symptoms at follow-up in a population-based study. Gynecol Obstet Invest 38:51-53, 1994.
88. Yip SK, Brieger G, Hin LY, Chung T: Urinary retention in the postpartum period: The relationship between obstetric factors and the

post-partum post-void residual bladder volume. Acta Obstet Gynecol Scand 76:667-672, 1997.

89. Yip SK, Hin LY, Chung TKH: Effect of the duration of labor on postpartum postvoid residual bladder volume. Gynecol Obstet Invest 45:177-180, 1998.
90. Groutz A, Hadi E, Wolf Y, et al: Early postpartum voiding dysfunction: Incidence and correlation with obstetric parameters. J Reprod Med 49:960-964, 2004.
91. Groutz A, Gordon D, Wolman I, et al: Persistent postpartum urinary retention: prevalence, obstetric risk factors and management. J Reprod Med 46:44-48, 2000.
92. Carley ME, Carley JM, Vasdev G, et al: Factors that are associated with clinically overt postpartum urinary retention after vaginal delivery. Am J Obstet Gynecol 187:430-433, 2002.

Chapter 53

FUNCTIONAL ANATOMY AND PATHOPHYSIOLOGY OF PELVIC ORGAN PROLAPSE

Yvonne Hsu and John O.L. DeLancey

Pelvic floor disorders, including pelvic organ prolapse and urinary incontinence, are debilitating conditions that result in surgery in one of nine women.[1] In the United States, the National Center for Health Statistics estimates that 400,000 operations are performed for pelvic floor dysfunction each year, with 300,000 of these occurring in the inpatient setting.[2,3] This is six to eight times more operations than radical prostatectomies performed each year. Although there is wide recognition of urinary incontinence, pelvic organ prolapse is responsible for twice as many operations, yet its causes are largely unknown. Prolapse arises because of injuries and deterioration of the muscles, nerves, and connective tissues that support and control normal pelvic function. This chapter addresses the *functional* anatomy of the pelvic floor in women and specifically focuses on how the pelvic organs are supported by the surrounding muscle and fasciae. It also considers the pathophysiology of pelvic organ prolapse as it relates to changes in these structures.

SUPPORT OF THE PELVIC ORGANS: CONCEPTUAL OVERVIEW

The pelvic organs rely on their connective tissue attachments to the pelvic walls and on support from the levator ani muscles, which are under neuronal control from the peripheral and central nervous systems. In this chapter, the term *pelvic floor* is used broadly to include all of the structures that support the pelvic cavity rather than just the levator ani group of muscles.

The pelvic floor consists of several components lying between the peritoneum and the vulvar skin. From above downward, these are the peritoneum, pelvic viscera and endopelvic fascia, levator ani muscles, perineal membrane, and superficial genital muscles. The support for all these structures comes from connections to the bony pelvis and its attached muscles. The pelvic organs are often thought of as being supported by the pelvic floor, but they are actually a part of it. The pelvic viscera play an important role in forming the pelvic floor through their connections with structures such as the cardinal and uterosacral ligaments.

In 1934, Bonney pointed out that the vagina is in the same relationship to the abdominal cavity as the in-turned finger of a surgical glove is to the rest of the glove (Fig. 53-1).[4] If the pressure in the glove is increased, it forces the finger to protrude downwards in the same way that increases in abdominal pressure force the vagina to prolapse. Figure 53-2 provides a schematic illustration of this prolapse phenomenon. In Figure 53-2C, the lower end of the vagina is held closed by the pelvic floor muscles, which prevents prolapse by constricting the base of the invaginated finger. Figure 53-2D shows suspension of the vagina to the pelvic walls. Figure 53-2E demonstrates that spatial relationships are important in the flap-valve closure, in which the suspending fibers hold the vagina in a position against the supporting walls of the pelvis; increases in pressure force the vagina against the wall, thereby pinning it in place. Vaginal support is a combination of constriction, suspension, and structural geometry.

The female pelvis can naturally be divided into anterior and posterior compartments (Fig. 53-3). The genital tract (vagina and uterus) divides these two compartments through lateral connections to the pelvic sidewall and suspension at its apex. The levator ani muscles form the bottom of the pelvis. The organs are attached to the levator ani muscles when they pass through the urogenital hiatus and are supported by these connections.

Functional Anatomy and Prolapse

The pelvic organ support system is multifaceted and includes the endopelvic fascia, the perineal membrane, and the levator ani muscles, which are controlled by the central and peripheral nervous system. The supports of the uterus and vagina are different in different regions (Fig. 53-4).[5] The cervix (when present) and the upper third of the vagina (level I) have relatively long suspensory fibers that are *vertically* oriented in the standing position, whereas the midportion of the vagina (level II) has a more direct attachment *laterally* to the pelvic wall (Fig. 53-5). In the most caudal region (level III), the vagina is attached directly to the structures that surround it. At this level, the levator ani muscles and the perineal membrane have important supportive functions.

In the upper part of the genital tract, a connective tissue complex attaches all the pelvic viscera to the pelvic sidewall. This endopelvic fascia forms a continuous, sheet-like mesentery, extending from the uterine artery at its cephalic margin to the point at which the vagina fuses with the levator ani muscles below. The fascial region that attaches to the uterus is called the parametrium, and that which attaches to the vagina is the paracolpium. Level I is composed of both parametrium and paracolpium. The uterosacral and cardinal ligaments together form the parametrium and support the uterus and upper third of the vagina. The paracolpium portion of level I consists of a relatively long sheet of tissue that suspends the superior aspect of the vagina by attaching it to the pelvic wall. This is true whether or not the cervix is present. The uterosacral ligaments are important components of this support. At level II, the paracolpium changes configuration and forms more direct lateral attachments of the

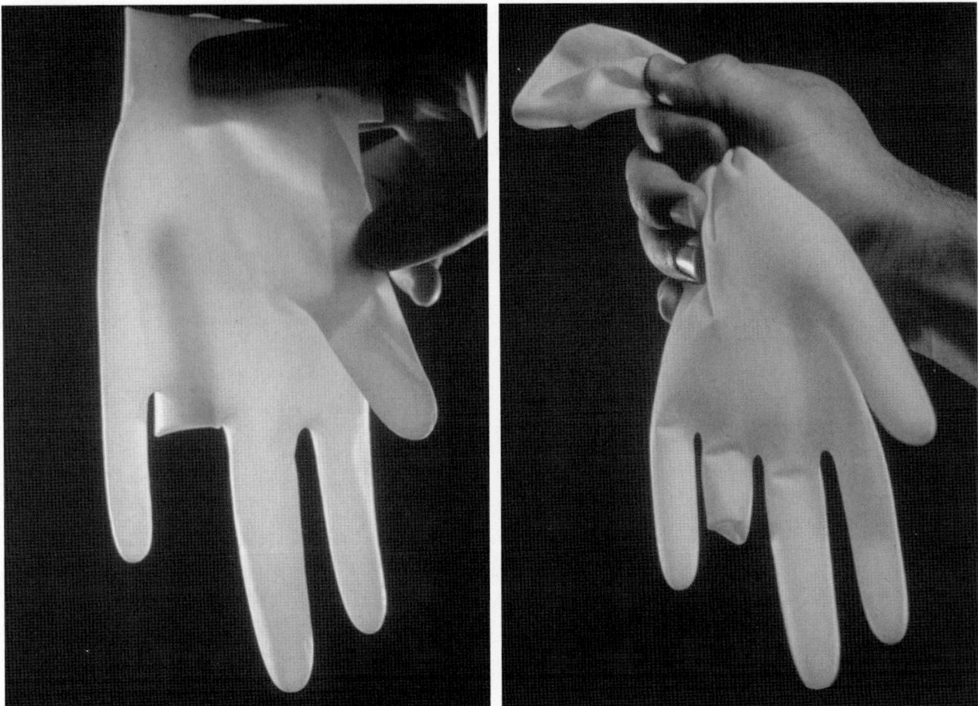

Figure 53-1 Bonney's analogy of vaginal prolapse. The vagina is in the same relationship to the abdominal cavity as the in-turned finger of a surgical glove is to the rest of the glove *(left)*. The eversion of an intussuscepted surgical glove finger by increasing pressure within the glove is analogous to prolapse of the vagina *(right)*. (© 2002 DeLancey; with permission.)

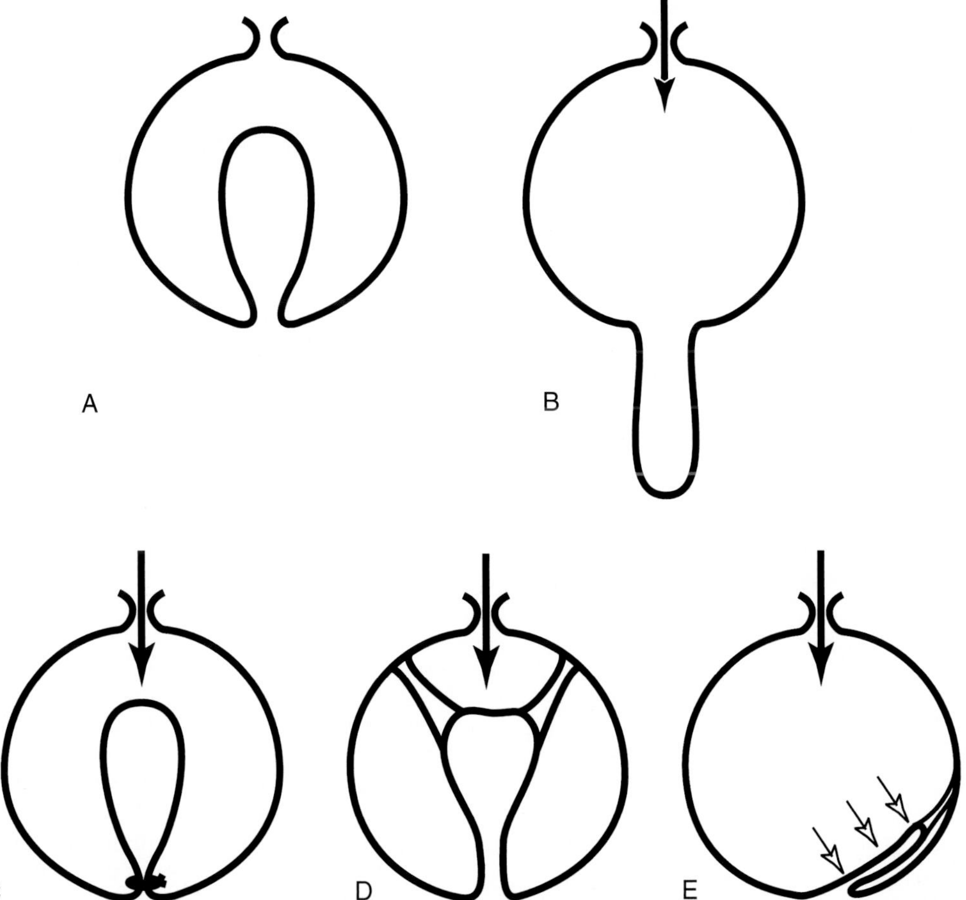

Figure 53-2 Diagrammatic display of vaginal support. **A,** Invaginated area in a surrounding compartment. **B,** The prolapse opens when the pressure *(arrow)* is increased. **C,** Closing the bottom of the vagina prevents prolapse by constriction. **D,** Ligament suspension. **E,** With flap-valve closure, suspending fibers hold the vagina in a position against the wall, allowing increases in pressure to pin it in place. (© 2002 DeLancey; with permission.)

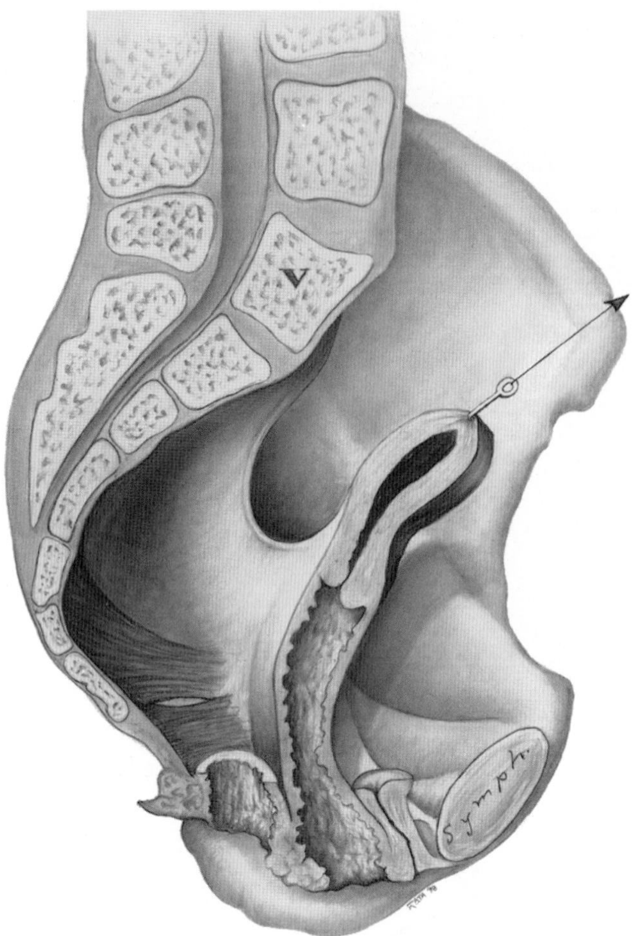

Figure 53-3 Compartments of the pelvis. The vagina, connected laterally to the pelvic walls, divides the pelvis into an anterior and posterior compartment. (© 1998 DELANCEY.)

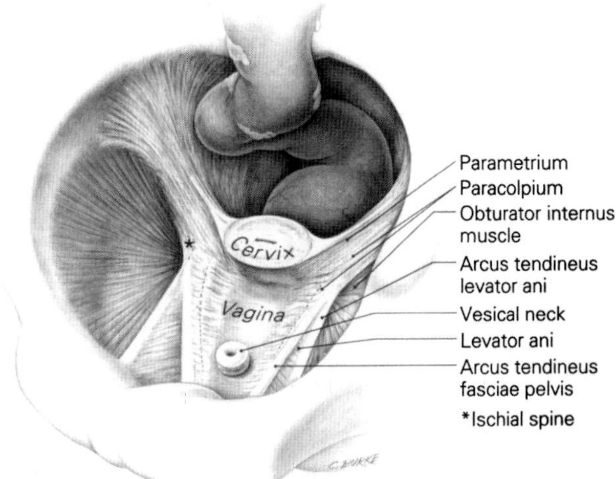

Figure 53-4 Attachments of the cervix and vagina to the pelvic walls, demonstrating different regions of support with the uterus in situ. Note that the uterine corpus and the bladder have been removed. (© 2002 DeLancey; with permission.)

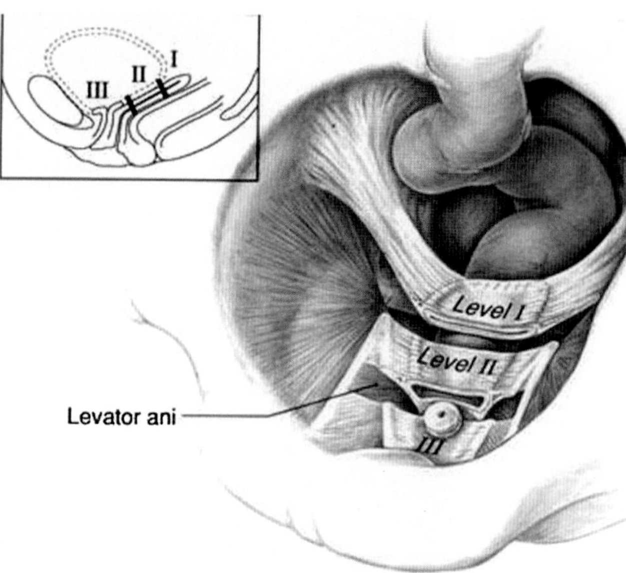

Figure 53-5 Levels of vaginal support after hysterectomy. In *level I* (suspension), the paracolpium suspends the vagina from the lateral pelvic walls. Fibers of *level I* extend both vertically and also posteriorly toward the sacrum. In *level II* (attachment), the vagina is attached to the arcus tendineus fascia pelvis and the superior fascia of levator ani. Sagittal view (*inset*) shows the three regions of support. (© 2002 DeLancey; with permission.)

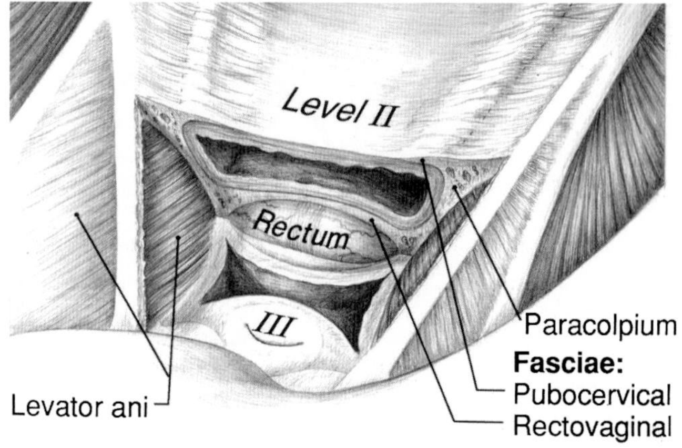

Figure 53-6 Close-up diagram of the lower margin of *level II* vaginal support system after a wedge of vagina has been removed (*inset*). Note how the anterior vaginal wall, through its connections to the arcus tendineus fascia pelvis, forms a supportive layer clinically referred to as the pubocervical fascia. (© 2002 DeLancey; with permission.)

midportion of the vagina to the pelvic walls (Fig. 53-6). These lateral attachments have functional significance: they stretch the vagina transversely between the bladder and the rectum. In the distal vagina (level III), the vaginal wall is directly attached to surrounding structures without any intervening paracolpium. The vagina fuses anteriorly with the urethra, posteriorly with the perineal body, and laterally with the levator ani muscles.

Damage to level I support can result in uterine or vaginal prolapse of the apical segment. Damage to the level II and III portions of vaginal support results in anterior and posterior vaginal wall prolapse. The varying combinations of these defects

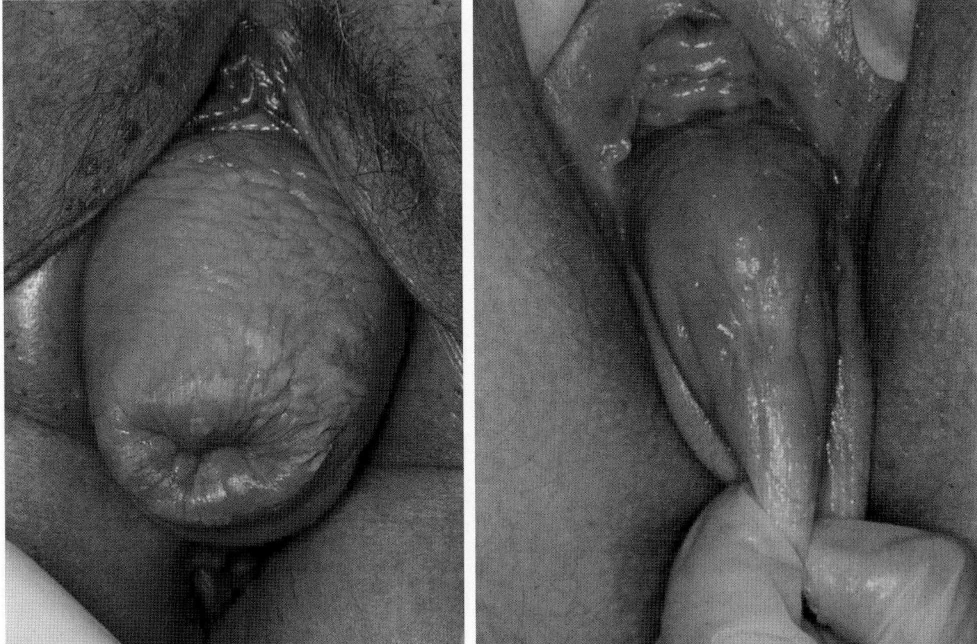

Figure 53-7 Uterine prolapse, showing the cervix protruding from the vaginal opening *(left)* and vaginal prolapse where the puckered scar indicates where the cervix used to be *(right)*. (© 2002 DeLancey; with permission.)

are responsible for the diversity of clinically encountered problems and are discussed in the following sections.

Apical Segment

In level I, the cardinal and uterosacral ligaments attach the cervix and the upper third of the vagina to the pelvic walls.[6,7] Neither is a true ligament in the sense of a skeletal ligament that is composed of dense regular connective tissue similar to knee ligaments. Rather, they are "visceral ligaments" that are similar to bowel mesentery. They are made of blood vessels, nerves, smooth muscle, and adipose tissue intermingled with irregular connective tissue. They have a supportive function in limiting the excursion of the pelvic organs, much as the mesentery of the small bowel limits the movement of the intestine. When these structures are placed on tension, they form condensations that surgeons refer to as ligaments.

The uterosacral ligaments are bands of tissue that run under the rectovaginal peritoneum; they are composed of smooth muscle, loose and dense connective tissue, blood vessels, nerves, and lymphatics.[6] They originate from the posterolateral aspect of the cervix at the level of the internal cervical os and from the lateral vaginal fornix.[6] Although macroscopic investigation showed insertion of the ligament to the levator ani, the coccygeus, and the presacral fascia,[8] examination by magnetic resonance imaging (MRI) showed that the uterosacral ligaments overlie the sacrospinous ligament and coccygeus in 82% of the cases and overlie the sacrum in only 7% of the cases.[9] The difference between the appearance of these structures on MRI and on dissection may have to do with the tension placed on the structures during dissection and require further research to clarify.

The cardinal ligament is a mass of retroperitoneal areolar connective tissue in which blood vessels predominate; it also contains nerves and lymphatic channels.[7] It has a configuration similar to that of "chicken wire" or fishing net in its natural state, but when placed under tension it assumes the appearance of a strong cable as the fibers align along the lines of tension.[7] It originates from the pelvic sidewall and inserts on the uterus, cervix, and upper third of the vagina. Both the uterosacral and cardinal tissues are critical components of level I support and provide support for the vaginal apex after hysterectomy (see Figs. 53-5 and 53-6). The cardinal ligaments are oriented in a relatively vertical axis (in the standing posture), whereas the uterosacral ligaments are more dorsal in their orientation.

The nature of uterine support (Fig. 53-7) can be understood when the cervix is pulled downward with a tenaculum during dilation and curettage. After a certain amount of descent, the level I supports become tight and arrests further cervical descent. Similarly, downward descent of the vaginal apex after hysterectomy is resisted by the paracolpium. Damage to the upper suspensory fibers of the paracolpium (cardinal and uterosacral ligaments) allows uterine or apical segment prolapse (Fig. 53-8).

Although descriptions of uterine support often imply that the uterus is suspended by the cardinal/uterosacral complex, much like a light suspended by a wire from the ceiling, this is not the case. The suspensory ligaments hold the uterus in position over the levator muscles, which in turn reduce the tension on the ligaments and protect them from excessive tension. This concept is discussed later, in the section on interactions between muscles and ligaments.

Anterior Compartment

Anterior compartment support depends on the connections of the vagina and periurethral tissues to the muscles and fascia of the pelvic wall via the arcus tendineus fascia pelvis (Fig. 53-9). On both sides of the pelvis, the arcus tendineus fascia pelvis is a

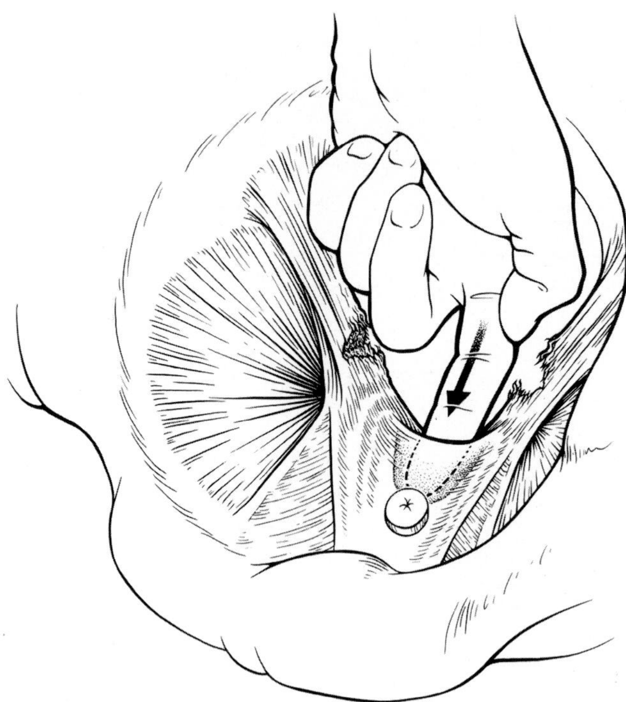

Figure 53-8 Damage to the suspensory ligaments (tears) can lead to eversion of the vaginal apex when subjected to downward forces *(arrow)*. (© 2002 DeLancey; with permission.)

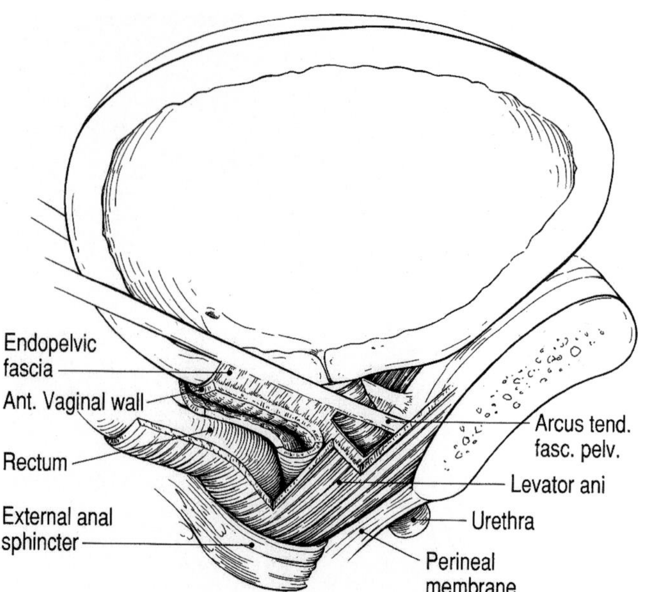

Figure 53-9 Lateral view in the standing position of the pelvic floor structures related to urethral support. The cut is just lateral to the midline. Note that windows have been cut in the levator ani muscles, vagina, and endopelvic fascia so that the urethra and anterior vaginal walls can be seen. (© 2002 DeLancey; with permission; redrawn after © 1994 DeLancey).

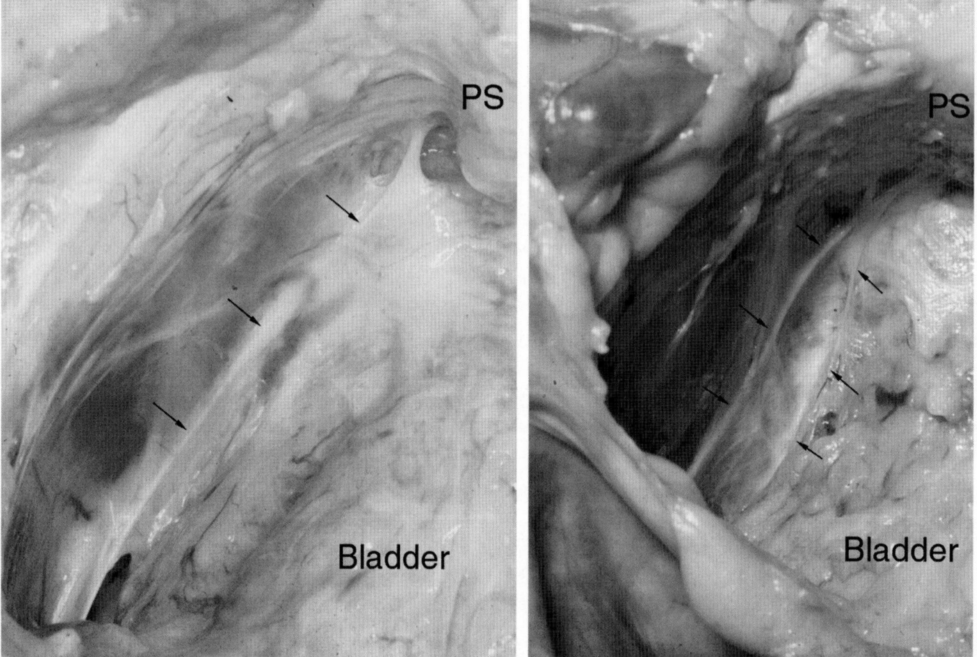

Figure 53-10 *Left,* Attachment of the arcus tendineus pelvis to the pubic bone, the arcus tendineus pelvis *(black arrows)*. *Right,* A paravaginal defect wherein the cervical fascia has separated from the arcus tendineus *(black arrows* point to the sides of the split). PS, pubic symphysis. (© 2002 DeLancey; with permission.)

band of connective tissue attached at one end to the lower sixth of the pubic bone, 1 cm lateral to the midline, and at the other end to the ischium, just above the spine.

The anterior wall fascial attachments to the arcus tendineus fascia pelvis have been called the paravaginal fascial attachments by Richardson.[10] Lateral detachment of the paravaginal fascial connections from the pelvic wall is associated with stress incontinence and anterior prolapse (Fig. 53-10). Further details of the structural mechanics of anterior wall support are provided later. In addition, the upper portions of the anterior vaginal wall are

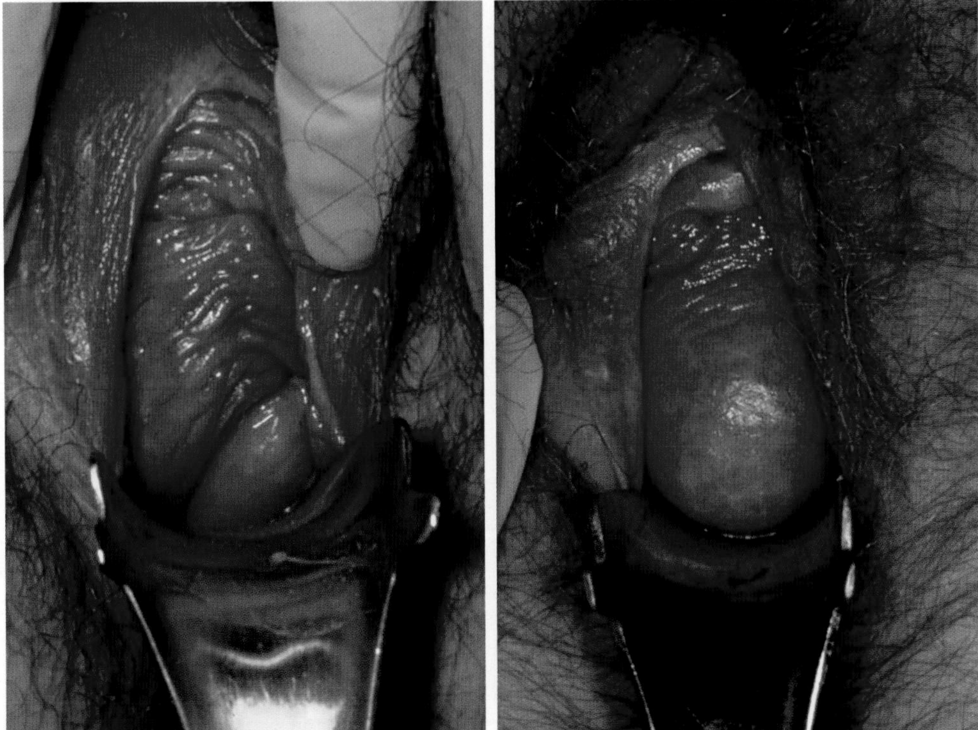

Figure 53-11 *Left,* Displacement "cystocele": the intact anterior vaginal wall has prolapsed downward due to paravaginal defect. Note that the right side of the patient's vagina and cervix has descended more than the left because of a larger defect on that side. *Right,* Distention "cystocele": the anterior vaginal wall fascia has failed, and the bladder is distending the mucosa. (© 2002 DeLancey; with permission.)

affected by the suspensory actions of level I. If the cardinal and uterosacral ligaments fail, the upper vaginal wall prolapses downward while the lower vagina (levels II and III) remains supported.

Anterior vaginal wall prolapse can occur either because of lateral detachment of the anterior vaginal wall at the pelvic side wall, referred to as a displacement "cystocele," or as a central failure of the vaginal wall itself that results in distention "cystocele" (Fig. 53-11). Although various grading schemes have been described for anterior vaginal prolapse, they are often focused on the degree of prolapse rather than the anatomic perturbation that results in descent; therefore, it is important to describe anterior prolapse with regard to the location of the fascial failure (lateral detachment versus central failure). At present, although a number of investigators have described techniques to distinguish central from lateral detachment, validation of these techniques remains elusive.

Cystocele caused by defects of the midline fascia is easy to understand, but understanding how lateral detachment results in cystocele is not as obvious. The fact that lateral detachment is associated with cystourethrocele was first established by Richardson and colleagues[10] (see Fig. 53-10). A study of 71 women with anterior compartment prolapse showed that paravaginal defect usually results from a detachment of the arcus tendineus fascia pelvis from the ischial spine, and rarely from the pubic bone.[11] A visual analogy is that of a swinging trapezoid (Fig. 53-12). The mechanical effect of this detachment allows the trapezoid to rotate downward. When this happens, the anterior vaginal wall protrudes through the introitus. Upward support of the trapezoid is also provided by the cardinal and uterosacral ligaments in level I. For this reason, resuspension of the vaginal apex at the time of surgery, in addition to paravaginal or anterior colporrhaphy, helps to return the anterior wall to a more normal position.

Anatomically, the term *endopelvic fascia* refers to the areolar connective tissue surrounding the vagina. It continues down the length of the vagina as loose areolar tissue surrounding the pelvic viscera (Fig. 53-13). The term "fascia" is often used by surgeons to refer to the strong tissue that they sew together during anterior repairs. This has led to confusion and misunderstanding of the anatomy. Histologic examination has shown that the vagina is made up of three layers: epithelium, muscularis, and adventitia (Fig. 53-14).[12-14] The adventitial layer is loose areolar connective tissue made up of collagen and elastin. These layers form the vaginal tube. The tissue that surgeons plicate during repairs is not what an anatomist would refer to as endopelvic fascia; rather, it is the vaginal muscularis and the adventitial layer of the vaginal tube. Also, many basic science studies that are addressed later in this chapter have used biopsies from the vaginal tube and not from the endopelvic fascia that connects the vaginal wall to the pelvic sidewalls.

Perineal Membrane (Urogenital Diaphragm)

Spanning the anterior part of the pelvic outlet, below the levator ani muscles, there is a dense triangular membrane called the perineal membrane. The term *perineal membrane* replaces the old term, urogenital diaphragm, reflecting the fact that this layer is not a single muscle layer with a double layer of fascia (i.e., a "diaphragm") but rather a set of connective tissues that surround the urethra.[15] The orientation consists of a single connective tissue membrane, with muscle lying immediately above. The

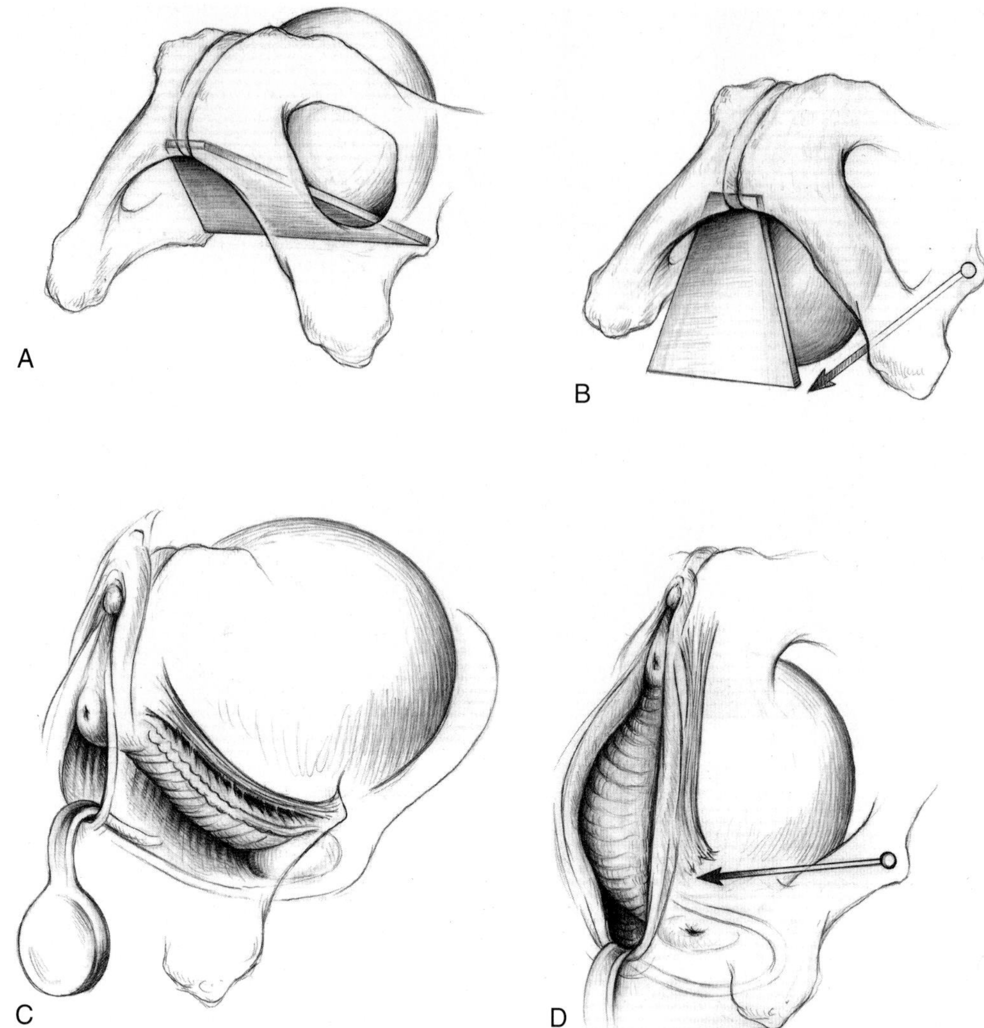

Figure 53-12 Conceptual diagram showing the mechanical effect of detachment of the arcus tendineus fascia pelvis from the ischial spine. **A,** Trapezoidal plane of the pubocervical fascia. The attachments to the pubis and the ischial spines are intact. **B,** The connection to the spine has been lost, allowing the fascial plane to swing downward. **C,** Normal anterior vaginal wall as seen with a weighted speculum in place. **D,** The effect of dorsal detachment of the arcus from the ischial spine. (© 2002 DeLancey; with permission.)

perineal membrane lies at the level of the hymen and attaches the urethra, vagina, and perineal body to the ischiopubic rami (Fig. 53-15). The compressor urethrae and urethrovaginal sphincter muscles are associated with the cranial surface of the perineal membrane.

Posterior Compartment and Perineal Membrane

The posterior vagina is supported by connections between the vagina, the bony pelvis, and the levator ani muscles.[16] The lower third of the vagina is fused with the perineal body (level III), (Fig. 53-16) which connects the perineal membranes on either side. The midposterior vagina (level II) is connected to the inside of the levator ani muscles by sheets of endopelvic fascia (Fig. 53-17). These connections prevent vaginal descent during increases in abdominal pressure. The most medial aspects of these paired sheets are the rectal pillars. In its upper third, the posterior vagina is connected laterally by the paracolpium of level I. Separate systems for anterior and posterior vaginal support do not exist at level I.

The fibers of the perineal membrane connect through the perineal body, thereby providing a layer that resists downward descent of the rectum. If this attachment becomes broken, then the resistance to downward descent is lost (see Fig. 53-16B). This situation is somewhat like an incisional hernia seen after disruption of a vertical incision, in which the bowel protrudes through a defect between the rectus abdominus muscles if the hernia is due to a defect in the rectus sheath. In the same way, protrusion of the rectum between the levator ani muscles can be seen if a disruption of the perineal body and connections of the perineal membrane occurs (Fig. 53-18). Reattachment of the separated structures during perineorrhphy corrects this defect and is a mainstay of reconstructive surgery. Because the levator ani muscles are intimately connected with the cranial surface of the perineal membranes, this reattachment also restores the muscles to a more normal position under the pelvic organs, in a location where they can provide support.

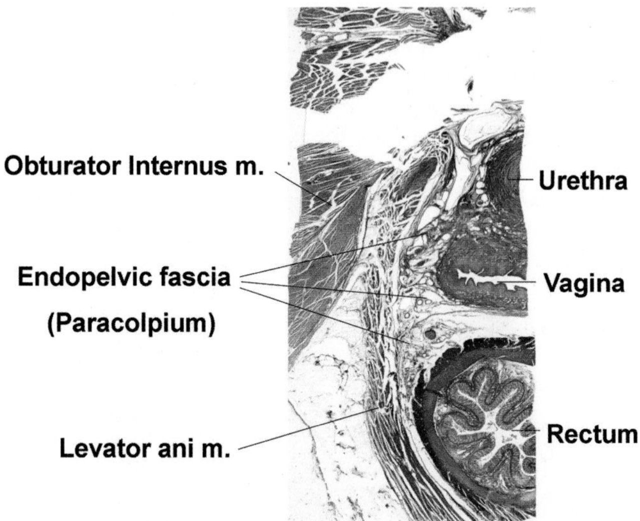

Figure 53-13 Histiologic cross-section of pelvis at the level of the mid-urethra. (From the collection of Dr. Thomas E Oelrich. © 2005 DeLancey; with permission.)

Levator Ani Muscles

Below and surrounding the pelvic organs are the levator ani muscles (Fig. 53-19).[17] When these muscles and their covering fascia are considered together, the combined structures are referred to as the *pelvic diaphragm* (not to be confused with the so-called urogenital diaphragm, discussed in the previous section).

There are three components of the levator ani muscle. The iliococcygeal portion forms a thin, relatively flat, horizontal shelf that spans the potential gap from one pelvic sidewall to the other. The pubovisceral muscle (also known as the pubococcygeus muscle) attaches the pelvic organs to the pubic bone, and the puborectal muscle forms a sling behind the rectum. The origins and insertions of these muscles as well as their characteristic anatomic relations are shown in Table 53-1 and Figure 53-19.[18]

The opening between the levator ani muscles through which the urethra, vagina, and rectum pass is the levator hiatus. The portion of the levator hiatus that lies ventral to the perineal body

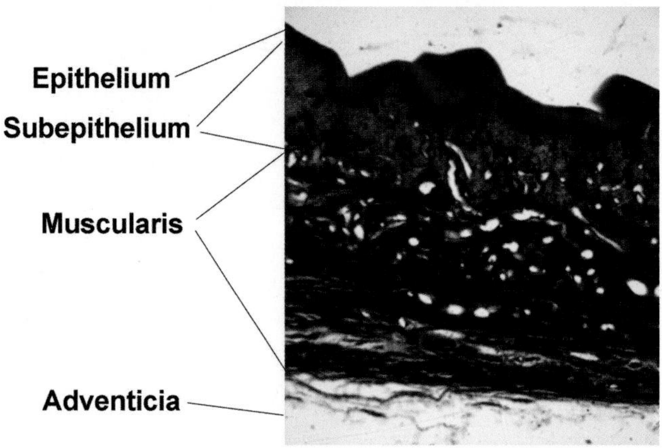

Figure 53-14 Higher magnification of a section of vaginal wall. Note the lack of a fascial layer. The endopelvic fascia is not seen at this magnification. (© 2005 DeLancey; with permission.)

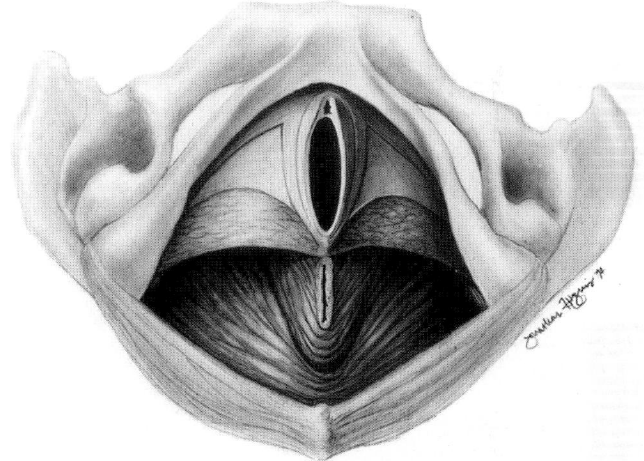

Figure 53-15 Position of the perineal membrane and its associated components of the striated urogenital sphincter, the compressor urethrae, and the urethrovaginal sphincter (© DeLancey; with permission.)

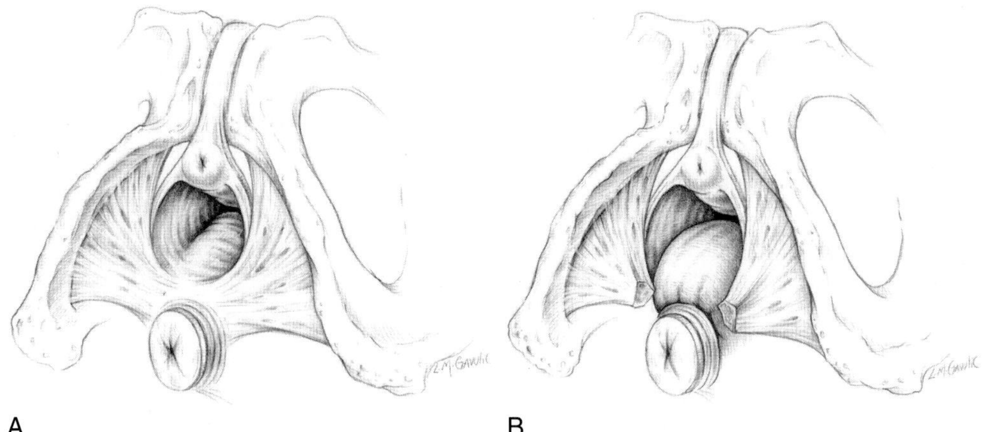

Figure 53-16 **A,** The perineal membrane spans the arch between the ischiopubic rami, with each side attached to the other through their connection in the perineal body. **B,** Note that separation of the fibers in this area leaves the rectum unsupported and results in a low posterior prolapse. (© 1999 DeLancey; with permission.)

is referred to as the urogenital hiatus, and it is through this opening that prolapse of the vagina, uterus, urethra, and bladder occurs. The urogenital hiatus is bounded anteriorly by the pubic bones, laterally by levator ani muscles, and posteriorly by the perineal body and external anal sphincter. The baseline tonic activity of the levator ani muscle keeps the hiatus closed by compressing the urethra, vagina, and rectum against the pubic bone, pulling the pelvic floor and organs in a cephalic direction.[19] This continuous muscle action closes the lumen of the vagina, much as the anal sphincter closes the anus. This constant action eliminates any opening within the pelvic floor through which prolapse could occur and forms a relatively horizontal shelf on which the pelvic organs are supported.[20] Damage to the levators resulting from nerve or connective tissue injury leaves the urogenital hiatus open and results in prolapse.

Endopelvic Fascia and Levator Ani Interactions

The interaction between the levator ani muscles and the endopelvic fascia is one of the most important biomechanical features of pelvic organ support. As long as the muscles maintain their constant tone closing the pelvic floor, the ligaments of the endopelvic fascia have very little tension on them even with increases in abdominal pressure. If the muscles become damaged so that the pelvic floor sags downward, the organs are pushed through the urogenital hiatus. Once they have fallen below the level of the hymenal ring, they are unsupported by the levator ani muscles, and the ligaments must carry the entire load. Although the endopelvic fascia can sustain these loads for short periods, if the pelvic muscles do not close the urogenital hiatus, the connective tissue

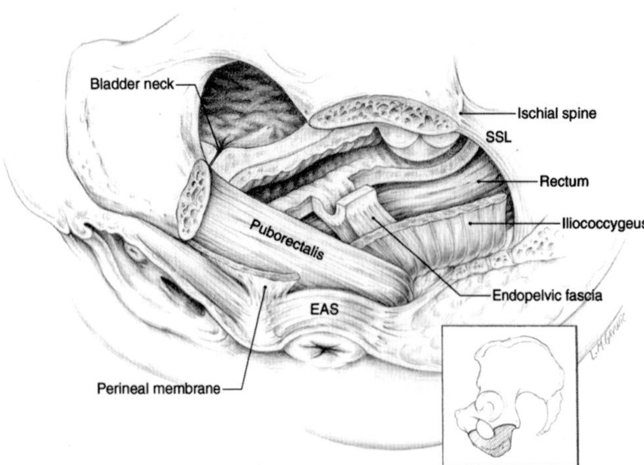

Figure 53-17 Lateral view of the pelvis showing the relationships of the puborectalis, iliococcygeus, and pelvic floor structures after removal of the ischium below the spine and sacrospinous ligament (SSL). EAS, external anal sphincter. The bladder and vagina have been cut in the midline, with the rectum left intact. Note how the endopelvic fascial "pillars" hold the vaginal wall dorsally, preventing its downward protrusion. (© 1999 DeLancey; with permission.)

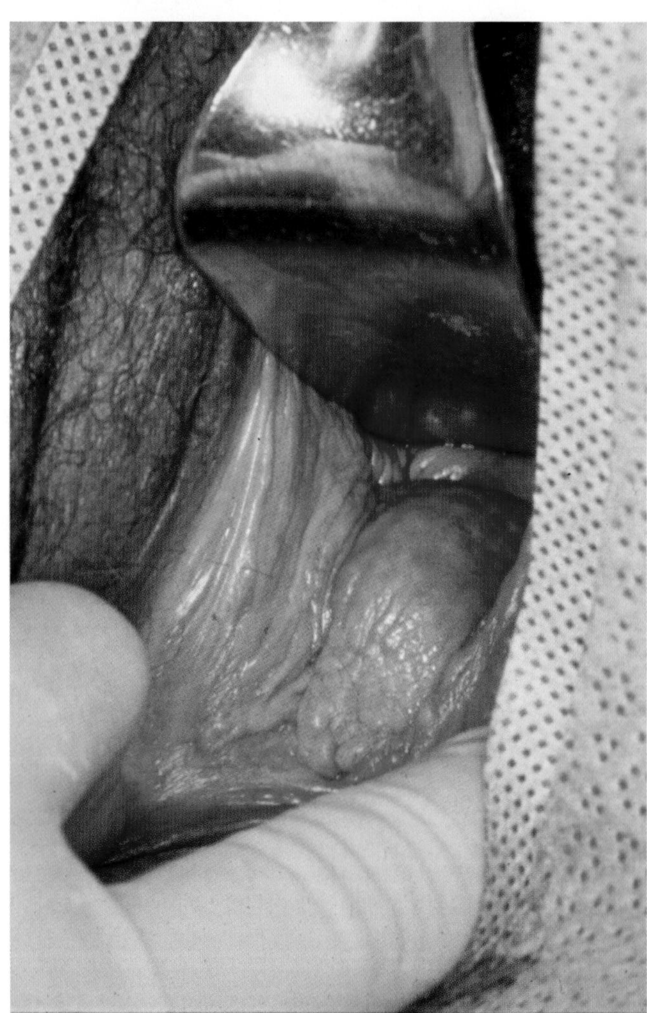

Figure 53-18 Posterior prolapse due to separation of the perineal body. Note the end of the hymenal ring that lies laterally on the side of the vagina, no longer united with its companion on the other side. (© DeLancey; with permission.)

Table 53-1 International Standardized Terminology: Divisions of the Levator Ani Muscles

Nomina Terminologica	Origin	Insertion
Puboviseral muscle (pubococcygeus)		
Puboperinealis (PPM)	Pubis	Perineal body
Pubovaginalis (PVM)	Pubis	Vaginal wall at the level of the mid-urethra
Puboanalis (PAM)	Pubis	Intersphincteric groove between internal and external anal sphincter to end in the anal skin
Puborectalis (PRM)	Pubis	Forms sling behind the rectum
Iliococcygeus (ICM)	Tendinous arch of the leavtor ani	The two sides fuse in the iliococcygeal raphe

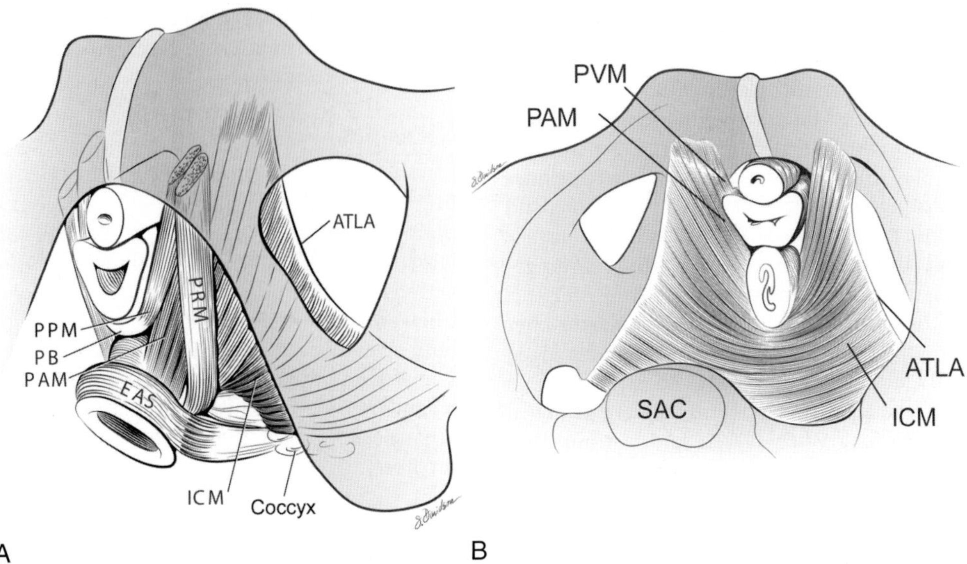

Figure 53-19 A, Schematic view of the levator ani muscles from below after the vulvar structures and perineal membrane have been removed, showing the arcus tendinius levator ani *(ATLA)*; external anal sphincter *(EAS)*; puboanal muscle *(PAM)*; perinal body *(PB)* uniting the two ends of the puboperineal muscle *(PPM)*; iliococcygeal muscle *(ICM)*; and puborectal muscle *(PRM)*. Note that the urethra and vagina have been transected just above the hymenal ring. **B,** The levator ani muscle seen from above, looking over the sacral promontory *(SAC)*, showing the pubovaginal muscle *(PVM)*. The urethra, vagina, and rectum have been transected just above the pelvic floor. (The internal obturator muscles have been removed to clarify levator muscle origins.) (© 2003 DeLancey; with permission.)

eventually fails, resulting in prolapse. The support of the vagina has been likened to a ship in its berth, floating on the water and attached by ropes on either side to a dock.[21] The ship is analogous to the vagina, the ropes to the ligaments, and the water to the supportive layer formed by the pelvic muscles. The ropes' function to hold the ship (pelvic organs) in the center of its berth as it rests on the water (pelvic muscles). However, if the water level were to fall far enough that the ropes would be required to hold the entire weight of the ship, the ropes would all break.

Once the pelvic musculature becomes damaged and no longer holds the organs in place, the ligaments are subjected to excessive forces. These forces may be enough to cause ligament failure over the course of time. A woman who sustains an injury to her pelvic floor muscles when she is young must depend to a greater extent on strength of her ligaments to prevent pelvic organ prolapse over the subsequent years of her life. An woman with injured muscles may have strong connective tissue that compensates and therefore may never develop prolapse, whereas another woman, who has the same degree of muscular damage but was born with weaker connective tissue, may experience prolapse as she ages.

In addition, the interaction between the pelvic floor muscles and the endopelvic fascia is responsible for maintaining the flap-valve configuration in the pelvic floor that lessens ligament tension because of the supportive nature of the levator plate (see Fig. 53-2E). The flap-valve requires the dorsal traction of the uterosacral ligaments, and to some extent the cardinal ligaments, to hold the cervix back in the hollow of the sacrum. It also requires the ventral pull of the pubovisceral portions of the levator ani muscle to swing the levator plate more horizontally to close the urogenital hiatus. It is this interaction between the two forces that is so critical in maintaining the normal structural relationships that lessen the tension on ligaments and muscles.

Nerves

There are two main nerves that supply the pelvic floor relative to pelvic organ prolapse. One is the pudendal nerve, which supplies the urethral and anal sphincters and perineal muscles, and the other is the nerve to the levator ani, which innervates the major musculature that supports the pelvic floor. These are distinct nerves with differing origins, courses, and insertions. The nerve to the levator originates from S3 to S5 foramina, runs inside the pelvis on the cranial surface of the levator ani muscle, and provides the innervation to all the subdivisions of the muscle.[22] The pudendal nerve originates from S2 to S4 foramina and runs through Alcock's canal, which is caudal to the levator ani muscles. The pudendal nerve has three branches—the clitoral, perineal, and inferior hemorrhoidal—which innervate the clitoris, the perineal musculature and inner perineal skin, and the external anal sphincter, respectively.[22]

PATHOPHYSIOLOGY

The previous section described how different structures work together to provide pelvic organ support; this section explores the current scientific literature regarding possible causes of structural failure leading to prolapse. The discussion has been divided based on the components that are thought to be important in pelvic support: connective tissue supports and vaginal wall, levator ani muscles, and nerves. At the end of each component section, we discuss the challenges and questions that confront future research. In addition to the three components, we also briefly discuss the pathophysiologic effects of vaginal delivery, because of its special importance in the natural history of prolapse. Finally, we have devoted a section to biomechanical research on prolapse, an area of increasing clinical and research interest.

Connective Tissue Supports and Vaginal Wall

The adventitial layer of the vagina, referred to as the endopelvic fascia, is composed of collagen and elastin that separates the muscular wall of the vagina and the paravaginal tissues. Investigators have studied the biology of pelvic connective tissue. Its structural support comes from its composition, which includes collagen and elastin arranged in different fiber orientations and embedded in a dynamic ground substance. Much of the distensibility of collagen and connective tissues comes from rearrangement of the fibers. A collagen fiber by itself is relatively inelastic, able to stretch only 4% longitudinally, whereas an elastin fiber can stretch up to 70%.[23] Therefore, if the fibers were arranged longitudinally, the tissue would not be able to stretch much before rupture. Instead, collagen and elastin fibers are arranged in different directions, so that, when placed under strain, they can stretch much more before being subject to rupture. An analogy can be made in comparing a cotton ball to a cotton dress shirt. When you pull on a cotton ball, there is a great deal of stretch that occurs until all the individual fibers become aligned in the same direction. After fiber alignment occurs, there is little stretch before rupture as the mechanical properties of the individual fiber come into play. In a cotton dress shirt, the individual fibers are already in alignment, and not much stretch can occur before rupture.

Several studies have explored whether differences in the vaginal tissues of women with prolapse and normal support explain the pathophysiology of prolapse. Researchers have focused on collagen, elastin, smooth muscle, and hormone receptors as the major factors in vaginal support.

Collagen

Collagen provides much of the tensile strength for the endopelvic fascia and vaginal epithelium. Over the years, collagen studies have yielded varying, and at times conflicting, results. Women with prolapse had just as much if not greater rates of collagen synthesis than women without prolapse in earlier histochemical studies using fibroblast cultures.[24] In contrast, Jackson and colleagues found that women with prolapse had a 25% reduction in total collagen compared to controls.[25] Types I and III are the most common collagen fibers in vaginal tissues. Type I fibers are the more abundant, and type III contributes more of the elastic properties of the tissue.[26] Liapis and associates found a modest reduction in collagen type III in women with prolapse and a more significant decrease in women with stress incontinence, suggesting that an altered ratio could lead to pelvic floor dysfunction.[26] However, other researchers found no difference in the collagen ratios.[25]

Recently, attention has turned toward collagen metabolism and turnover as markers of prolapse. There does seem to be consistent evidence that collagen metabolism is significantly altered in the pelvic tissues of women with prolapse. Collagen fibers are stabilized by intermolecular covalent cross-links. The formation of cross-links and glycation lead to maturation and inhibit turnover. Degradation depends on the activity of proteinases secreted from connective tissue cells.[25] Whereas women with prolapse have collagen with more cross-links and other signs of maturation, they also have increased synthesis of new collagen, which is degraded in preference to older material because it has fewer cross-links.[25] Chen and cowrkers found increased expression of matrix metalloproteinase messenger RNA, which is responsible for collagen breakdown, and decreased expression of inhibitors of metalloproteinases in women with stress incontinence and prolapse.[27]

Elastin

Elastin provides much of the elastic properties of the pelvic connective tissue.[23] Compared with collagen, fewer studies have examined the role of elastin in the development of prolapse. Jackson and colleagues did not find a difference in elastin content between premenopausal women with prolapse and controls.[25] Chen and coworkers examined elastolytic activity in women with both stress incontinence and prolapse compared with controls. They found little difference in elastolyic activity but a decrease in α_1-antitrypsin, an inhibitor of elastin turnover, in women with prolapse, suggesting that there may be higher elastin turnover in prolapse.[28]

Smooth Muscle

Smooth muscle is another important aspect of the endopelvic fascia, because it is a major component of the vaginal wall. Smooth muscle analysis of anterior vaginal wall sections from the urethrovesical junction of fresh cadavers showed quantifiable variations in thickness and densities.[29] Morphometric analysis of the anterior and posterior vaginal walls showed decreased fraction of smooth muscle in the muscularis of women with pelvic organ prolapse compared with controls.[30,31] Other markers suggest that women with prolapse have less smooth muscle contractility and force maintenance.[32]

Hormone Receptors

It has long been assumed that pelvic floor dysfunction is related to changes in menopause and is influenced by hormones. Untangling loss of hormonal action from age-related changes is extremely difficult. In blinded, randomized, placebo-controlled studies, two selective estrogen receptor modulators (SERMs), idoxifene and levormeloxifene, were thought to be associated with an increased incidence of pelvic organ prolapse in postmenopausal women participating in clinical trials of osteoporosis.[33] In contrast, neither amoxifen nor toremifene, two clinically available SERMs, was associated with pelvic floor relaxation.[34,35] More recently, there has been evidence that raloxifene reduces the likelihood or need for prolapse surgery by 50%.[36] Paradoxically, Vardy and coauthors suggested that there was an increase in prolapse in women receiving raloxifene and tamoxifen, but the status of support in the population was not given, and most changes were small (1 cm), with only one individual having a change in prolapse stage.[37] This finding might be a result of minor differences in vaginal pliability and might not reflect structural changes, such as connective tissue rupture and muscle damage, that go with actual prolapse.

Several studies have looked at the presence or absence of hormone receptors in tissues that are involved in pelvic organ support.[38,39] Other studies have examined the effects of estrogen on biologic markers such as collagen.[40-42] Estrogen receptors are present throughout the body, and yet there are important differential effects. For example, endometrium is highly sensitive to fluctuations in estrogen, but skin is much less responsive. Any supposition that hormones play a major role in pelvic organ prolapse must be based on human studies that actually prove differences in prolapse occurring in those with and without hormonal supplementation or administration of hormonal antagonists.

Challenges

There has been a significant body of basic science research regarding the components of the vaginal wall (vaginal tube). However, relatively little has been done to investigate the connections of the vagina to the pelvic walls (e.g., endopelvic fascia). Most of the studies reviewed used either partial- or full-thickness vaginal biopsies. It is difficult to make any assumptions about the endopelvic fascia, because it is not included in samples of the vaginal wall (see Fig. 53-13). Therefore, the question of whether it is the connection between the vagina to the pelvic sidewall that fails, as suggested by Richardson,[10] or whether it is the vaginal wall itself that is involved in prolapse remains scientifically unresolved. Also, although some of the differences found in women with prolapse suggest that biochemical changes in the connective tissue may play an important role in prolapse, these studies were unable to explain the sequence of prolapse progression. In other words, we are left to wonder whether the alterations in connective tissue led to the prolapse or were a response to the mechanical effects of prolapse.

Levator Ani

MRI has been established as a technique for examination of the levator ani muscle.[43,44] Using MRI, visible levator ani defects are beginning to be linked to the development of prolapse. Up to 20% of primiparous women have a visible defect in the levator ani muscle, probably as a result of birth injury.[45] Also, computer-generated birth models using MRI have found that the medial puboviseral muscle is at greatest risk for stretch-induced injury.[46] A few investigations have found that the levator ani mucles of women with prolapse have different morphologic characteristics than those of controls.[47-49] The changes in morphoglogy are beginning to be quantified. Investigators have found that women with prolapse have smaller overall levator volume,[47,48] larger levator symphysis gap, and wider levator hiatus.[49] Aside from these MRI findings, histologic evidence of muscle damage has been found as well[50] and is associated with operative failure.[51]

Challenges

Quantification of levator ani differences or defects in prolapse have so far been limited to measurements of volume or thickness.[47,48,52] The maximal force that a muscle generates depends on the cross-sectional area of the muscle perpendicular to its fiber direction.[53] Measurement of this force is challenging because of the complex shape of the levator ani muscles, with different sections having differing fiber directions. Continued advances in imaging may make it possible to relate levator ani appearance to function.

Nerves

A unifying neurogenic hypothesis has been well established as a contributor to pelvic floor dysfunction. Although there is a significant body of literature regarding neurogenic causes of fecal incontinence and urinary incontinence, there is comparatively little exploring the relation between nerve damage and prolapse. Prospective study of perineal descent on defecography and pudendal nerve terminal motor latency failed to show any relationship between pudendal nerve damage and increased degree of perineal descent.[54] Two studies in which patients with prolapse were included did not show a difference in pudendal nerve terminal motor latencies in patients with prolapse.[55,56] However, electromyographic studies of women with pelvic floor dysfunction, including prolapse and incontinence, found changes consistent with motor unit loss or failure of central activation.[57] More electromyographic and nerve studies are needed to tie neurogenic injury and pelvic organ prolapse.

Vaginal Birth

Although it is clear that incontinence and prolapse increase with age,[1] there is no time during a woman's life when these structures are more vulnerable than during childbirth. Vaginal delivery confers a fourfold to 11-fold higher risk of prolapse that increases with parity.[58] Increased descent of vaginal wall points after vaginal delivery has been found in studies using a combined method of clinical examination and functional cine-MRI.[59] Two studies suggested that pregnancy alone may be a risk factor for worsening prolapse; however, both of these studies used definitions of prolapse that many would consider clinically normal.[60,61]

Biomechanics

Biologic specimens exhibit a mixture of elastic, viscous, and plastic properties. Elasticity is the ability of a tissue to return to its original shape after loading. Viscosity refers to the elongation of the tissue over time. Plasticity is the residual deformation that remains after loading is complete. There is a paucity of biomechanical studies of pelvic organ supports. Previous biomechanical research was performed using constant elongation to induce failure or rupture.[62-64] This does not provide accurate information about the physiologic function of the tissue, because it does not account for the viscoelastic and plastic properties of connective tissues. Ettema and colleagues proposed a more accurate way of measuring the elastic properties of vaginal tissue, using a slow-rate, linear elongation method.[65] This method is able to discriminate small changes in a tissue's elastic properties at lower stress levels and therefore is functionally more meaningful. Using this method, Goh and coworkers compared the biomechanical properties of premenopausal and postmenopausal women with prolapse and found little difference between the groups.[66]

CONCLUSION

Understanding the functional anatomy of prolapse lays the necessary groundwork for understanding the mechanisms of pelvic organ prolapse. When the components of pelvic support and how they relate to each other have been identified, we will be able to understand how disruptions result in failure. Compared to stress incontinence, prolapse has received relatively little scientific attention. Although basic science research concerning the vaginal connective tissue and levator ani muscles has been performed, little has been done on other vital structures, such as the endopelvic fascia. In addition, investigations into the biomechanical processes of prolapse are lacking. Although this chapter provides an overview of existing knowledge on pelvic organ prolapse, it also looks ahead to the many unanswered scientific questions.

References

1. Olsen AL, Smith VJ, Bergstrom JO, et al: Epidemiology of surgically managed pelvic organ prolapse and urinary incontinence. Obstet Gynecol 89:501-506, 1997.
2. Boyles SH, Weber AM, Meyn L: Procedures for pelvic organ prolapse in the United States, 1979-1997. Am J Obstet Gynecol 188:108-115, 2003.
3. Boyles SH, Weber AM, Meyn L: Procedures for urinary incontinence in the United States, 1979-1997. Am J Obstet Gynecol 189:70-75, 2003.
4. Bonney V: The principles that should underlie all operations for prolapse. Obstet Gynaecol Br Empire 41:669, 1934.
5. DeLancey JO: Anatomic aspects of vaginal eversion after hysterectomy. Am J Obstet Gynecol 166(6 Pt 1):1717-1724; discussion 1724-1728, 1992.
6. Campbell RM: The anatomy and histology of the sacrouterine ligaments. Am J Obstet Gynecol 59:1, 1950.
7. Range RL, Woodburne RT: The gross and microscopic anatomy of the transverse cervical ligaments. Am J Obstet Gynecol 90:460, 1964.
8. Blaisdell FE: The anatomy of the sacro-uterine ligaments. Anat Record 12:1-42, 1917.
9. Umek WH, Morgan DM, Ashton-Miller JA, DeLancey JO: Quantitative analysis of uterosacral ligament origin and insertion points by magnetic resonance imaging. Obstet Gynecol 103:447-451, 2004.
10. Richardson AC, Edmonds PB, Williams NL: Treatment of stress urinary incontinence due to paravaginal fascial defect. Obstet Gynecol 57:357, 1981.
11. DeLancey JOL: Fascial and muscular abnormalities in women with urethral hypermobility and anterior vaginal wall prolapse. Am J Obstet Gynecol 187:93-98, 2002.
12. Ricci JV, Thom CH: The myth of a surgically useful fascia in vaginal plastic reconstructions. Q Rev Surg Obstet Gynecol 11:253-261, 1954.
13. Gitsch E, Palmrich AH: Operative Anatomie. Berlin: De Gruyter; 1977.
14. Weber AM, Walters MD: Anterior vaginal prolapse: Review of anatomy and techniques of surgical repair. Obstet Gynecol 89:311-317, 1990.
15. Oelrich TM: The striated urogenital sphincter muscle in the female. Anat Rec 205:223, 1983.
16. DeLancey JO: Structural support of the urethra as it relates to stress urinary incontinence: The hammock hypothesis. [Comment.] Am J Obstet Gynecol 170:1713, 1994.
17. Lawson JO: Pelvic anatomy: I. Pelvic floor muscles. Ann R Coll Surg Engl 54:244, 1974.
18. Kearney R, Sawhney R, DeLancey JO: Levator ani muscle anatomy evaluated by origin-insertion pairs. Obstet Gynecol 104:168-173, 2004.
19. Taverner D: An electromyographic study of the normal function of the external anal sphincter and pelvic diaphragm. Dis Colon Rectum 2:153, 1959.
20. Nichols DH, Milley PS, Randall CL: Significance of restoration of normal vaginal depth and axis. Obstet Gynecol 36:251, 1970.
21. Paramore RH: The uterus as a floating organ. In Paramore RH (ed): The Statics of the Female Pelvic Viscera. London: HK Lewis and Company, 1918, p. 12.
22. Barber MD, Bremer RE, Thor KB, et al: Innervation of the female levator ani muscles. Am J Obstet Gynecol 187:64-71, 2002.
23. Goh JT: Biomechanical and biochemical assessments for pelvic organ prolapse. Curr Opin Obstet Gynecol 15:391-394, 2003.
24. Makinen J, Kahari VM, Soderstrom KO, et al: Collagen synthesis in the vaginal connective tissue of patients with and without uterine prolapse. Eur J Obstet Gynecol Reprod Biol 24:319-325, 1987.
25. Jackson SR, Avery NC, Tarlton JF, et al: Changes in metabolism of collagen in genitourinary prolapse. Lancet 347:1658-1661, 1996.
26. Liapis A, Bakas P, Pafiti A, et al: Changes of collagen type III in female patients with genuine stress incontinence and pelvic floor prolapse. Eur J Obstet Gynecol Reprod Biol 97:76-79, 2001.
27. Chen BH, Wen Y, Li H, Polan ML: Collagen metabolism and turnover in women with stress urinary incontinence and pelvic prolapse. Int Urogynecol J Pelvic Floor Dysfunct 13:80-87, 2002.
28. Chen B, Wen Y, Polan ML: Elastolytic activity in women with stress urinary incontinence and pelvic organ prolapse. Neurourol Urodyn 23:119-126, 2004.
29. Morgan DM, Iyengar J, DeLancey JO: A technique to evaluate the thickness and density of nonvascular smooth muscle in the suburethral fibromuscular layer. Am J Obstet Gynecol 188:1183-1185, 2003.
30. Boreham MK, Wai CY, Miller RT, et al: Morphometric analysis of smooth muscle in the anterior vaginal wall of women with pelvic organ prolapse. Am J Obstet Gynecol 187:56-63, 2002.
31. Boreham MK, Wai CY, Miller RT, et al: Morphometric properties of the posterior vaginal wall in women with pelvic organ prolapse. Am J Obstet Gynecol 187:1501-1508; discussion 1508-1509, 2002.
32. Boreham MK, Miller RT, Schaffer JI, Word RA: Smooth muscle myosin heavy chain and caldesmon expression in the anterior vaginal wall of women with and without pelvic organ prolapse. Am J Obstet Gynecol 185:944-952, 2001.
33. Silfen SL, Ciaccia AV, Bryant HU: Selective estrogen receptor modulators: Tissue specificity and differential uterine effects. Climacteric 2:268-283, 1999.
34. Fisher B, Costantino JP, Wickerham DL, et al: Tamoxifen for prevention of breast cancer: Report of the National Surgical Adjuvant Breast and Bowel Project P-1 Study. J Natl Cancer Inst 90:1371-1388, 1998.
35. Maenpaa JU, Ala-Fossi SL: Toremifene in postmenopausal breast cancer: Efficacy, safety and cost. Drugs Aging 11:261-270, 1997.
36. Goldstein SR, Neven P, Zhou L, et al: Raloxifene effect on frequency of surgery for pelvic floor relaxation. Obstet Gynecol 98:91-96, 2001.
37. Vardy MD, Lindsay R, Scotti RJ, et al: Short-term urogenital effects of raloxifene, tamoxifen, and estrogen. Am J Obstet Gynecol 189:81-88, 2003.
38. Fu X, Rezapour M, Wu X, et al: Expression of estrogen receptor-alpha and -beta in anterior vaginal walls of genuine stress incontinent women. Int Urogynecol J Pelvic Floor Dysfunct 14:276-281, 2003.
39. Ewies AA, Thompson J, Al-Azzawi F: Changes in gonadal steroid receptors in the cardinal ligaments of prolapsed uteri: immunohistomorphometric data. Hum Reprod 19:1622-1628, 2004. Epub 2004 May 13.
40. Jackson S, James M, Abrams P: The effect of oestradiol on vaginal collagen metabolism in postmenopausal women with genuine stress incontinence. BJOG 109:339-344, 2002.
41. Chen B, Wen Y, Wang H, Polan ML: Differences in estrogen modulation of tissue inhibitor of matrix metalloproteinase-1 and matrix metalloproteinase-1 expression in cultured fibroblasts from continent and incontinent women. Am J Obstet Gynecol 189:59-65, 2003.
42. Moalli PA, Talarico LC, Sung VW, et al: Impact of menopause on collagen subtypes in the arcus tendineous fasciae pelvis. Am J Obstet Gynecol 190:620-627, 2004.
43. Tunn R, DeLancey JO, Quint EE: Visibility of pelvic organ support system structures in magnetic resonance images without an endovaginal coil. Am J Obstet Gynecol 184:1156-1163, 2001.
44. Singh K, Reid WM, Berger LA: Magnetic resonance imaging of normal levator ani anatomy and function. Obstet Gynecol 99:433-438, 2002.
45. DeLancey JO, Kearney R, Chou Q, et al: The appearance of levator ani muscle abnormalities in magnetic resonance images after vaginal delivery. Obstet Gynecol 101:46-53, 2003.

46. Lien KC, Mooney B, DeLancey JO, Ashton-Miller JA: Levator ani muscle stretch induced by simulated vaginal birth. Obstet Gynecol 103:31-40, 2004.
47. Hoyte L, Schierlitz L, Zou K, et al: Two- and 3-dimensional MRI comparison of levator ani structure, volume, and integrity in women with stress incontinence and prolapse. Am J Obstet Gynecol 185:11-19, 2001.
48. Hoyte L, Fielding JR, Versi E, et al: Variations in levator ani volume and geometry in women: the application of MR based 3D reconstruction in evaluating pelvic floor dysfunction. Arch Esp Urol 54:532-539, 2001.
49. Singh K, Jakab M, Reid WM, et al: Three-dimensional magnetic resonance imaging assessment of levator ani morphologic features in different grades of prolapse. Am J Obstet Gynecol 188:910-915, 2003.
50. Koelbl H, Saz V, Doerfler D, et al: Transurethral injection of silicone microimplants for intrinsic urethral sphincter deficiency. Obstet Gynecol 92:332-336, 1998.
51. Hanzal E, Berger E, Koelbl H: Levator ani muscle morphology and recurrent genuine stress incontinence. Obstet Gynecol 81:426, 1993.
52. Hoyte L, Jakab M, Warfield SK, et al: Levator ani thickness variations in symptomatic and asymptomatic women using magnetic resonance-based 3-dimensional color mapping. Am J Obstet Gynecol 191:856-861, 2004.
53. Ikai M, Fukunaga T: Calculation of muscle strength per unit cross-sectional area of human muscle by means of ultrasonic measurement. Int Z Angew Physiol 26:26-32, 1968.
54. Jorge JM, Wexner SD, Ehrenpreis ED, et al: Does perineal descent correlate with pudendal neuropathy? Dis Colon Rectum 36:475-483, 1993.
55. Beevors MA, Lubowski DZ, King DW, Carlton MA: Pudendal nerve function in women with symptomatic utero-vaginal prolapse. Int J Colorectal Dis 6:24-28, 1991.
56. Bakas P, Liapis A, Karandreas A, Creatsas G: Pudendal nerve terminal motor latency in women with genuine stress incontinence and prolapse. Gynecol Obstet Invest 51:187-190, 2001.
57. Weidner AC, Barber MD, Visco AG, et al: Pelvic muscle electromyography of levator ani and external anal sphincter in nulliparous women and women with pelvic floor dysfunction. Am J Obstet Gynecol 183:1390-1399; discussion 1399-1401, 2000.
58. Mant J, Painter R, Vessey M: Epidemiology of genital prolapse: Observations from the Oxford Family Planning Association Study. Br J Obstet Gynaecol 104:579-585, 1997.
59. Dannecker C, Lienemann A, Fischer T, Anthuber C: Influence of spontaneous and instrumental vaginal delivery on objective measures of pelvic organ support: Assessment with the pelvic organ prolapse quantification (POPQ) technique and functional cine magnetic resonance imaging. Eur J Obstet Gynecol Reprod Biol 115:32-38, 2004.
60. Sze EH, Sherard GB 3rd, Dolezal JM: Pregnancy, labor, delivery, and pelvic organ prolapse. Obstet Gynecol 100(5 Pt 1):981-986, 2002.
61. O'Boyle AL, Woodman PJ, O'Boyle JD, et al: Pelvic organ support in nulliparous pregnant and nonpregnant women: A case control study. Am J Obstet Gynecol 187:99-102, 2002.
62. Kondo A, Narushima M, Yoshikawa Y, Hayashi H: Pelvic fascia strength in women with stress urinary incontinence in comparison with those who are continent. Neurourol Urodyn 13:507-513, 1994.
63. Reay Jones NH, Healy JC, King LJ, et al: Pelvic connective tissue resilience decreases with vaginal delivery, menopause and uterine prolapse. Br J Surg 90:466-472, 2003.
64. Cosson M, Lambaudie E, Boukerrou M, et al: A biomechanical study of the strength of vaginal tissues: Results on 16 post-menopausal patients presenting with genital prolapse. Eur J Obstet Gynecol Reprod Biol 112:201-205, 2004.
65. Ettema GJC, Goh JTW, Forwood MR: A new method to measure elastic properties of plastic-viscoelastic connective tissue. Med Eng Physics 20:308-314, 1998.
66. Goh JT: Biomechanical properties of prolapsed vaginal tissue in pre- and postmenopausal women. Int Urogynecol J 13:76-79, 2002.

Chapter 54

PELVIC ORGAN PROLAPSE: CLINICAL DIAGNOSIS AND PRESENTATION

Chi Chiung Grace Chen and Mark D. Walters

Pelvic organ prolapse (POP) is a heterogeneous condition in which weaknesses of the pelvic floor musculature and connective tissue result in herniation of pelvic organs into the vaginal lumen. In more severe cases, this herniation can protrude through the vaginal introitus and beyond the hymenal ring. Organs that may potentially herniate into the vaginal canal include the bladder with or without involvement of the urethra, resulting in cystourethroceles and cystoceles, respectively. Patients may have uterine prolapse, or, after hysterectomy, the vaginal cuff may herniate resulting in apical vaginal prolapse. The rectum, small bowel, and sigmoid colon may also herniate, resulting in rectoceles, enteroceles, and sigmoidoceles, respectively. This chapter focuses on the definition, diagnosis, and classification of POP.

DEFINITION AND EPIDEMIOLOGY

It is estimated that more than 300,000 surgeries are performed to correct POP annually, at a cost of greater than $1 billion.[1] Furthermore, the number of patients seeking care for these disorders is expected to increase by 45% in the future.[2] Despite this high prevalence, POP is a poorly understood condition, and many of the accepted definitions are based on expert opinion and consensus rather than epidemiologic or clinical data. The American College of Obstetrics and Gynecology (ACOG) defines POP as the protrusion of pelvic organs into the vaginal canal.[3] More specifically, in a terminology workshop convened by the National Institutes of Health (NIH) for researchers in female pelvic floor disorders, POP was defined as the descent of vaginal segments to within 1 cm of the hymen or lower.[4] POP encompasses anterior and posterior vaginal prolapse as well as apical or uterine prolapse. Terms such as "cystocele" and "rectocele" are intentionally not used because they imply an unrealistic certainty as to the specific organs behind the vaginal wall at the time of physical examination.

It is important to note that, although most clinicians can recognize the extremes of normal support versus severe prolapse, most cannot objectively state at what point vaginal laxity becomes pathologic and requires intervention. There are limited data concerning the normal distribution of POP in the population and the correlations between symptoms and physical findings. In a study of 497 women, Swift demonstrated that the distribution of prolapse in a population exhibited a bell-shaped curve, with most women having stage I or II prolapse by the Pelvic Organ Prolapse Quantification (POPQ) classification system (discussed later) and only 3% having stage III prolapse.[5] This signifies that, at baseline, most women have some degree of pelvic relaxation. However, these women are typically asymptomatic and develop symptoms only as their prolapse increases in severity.[6] Therefore, even if POP is found on physical examination by the definition given, it may not be clinically relevant and may not require intervention if the patient is asymptomatic.

HISTORY

Although it has been shown previously that patients' histories cannot be used alone to differentiate or diagnose different types of urinary incontinence,[7,8] less is known about the reliability of patients' symptoms for diagnosing POP. Patients with POP may present with a plethora of symptoms relating to voiding, defecatory, and sexual dysfunction as well as symptoms directly associated with the prolapse, such as vaginal pressure and discomfort. Despite the few studies specifically addressing the association between reported symptoms and POP, the consensus in the literature seems to be that the severity of the prolapse is not necessarily associated with increased visceral symptomatology.

Vaginal prolapse in any compartment—anterior, apical, or posterior—can manifest as vaginal fullness, pain, and/or protruding mass. In a recent study by Tan and associates, the feeling of "a bulge or that something is falling outside the vagina" had a positive predictive value of 81% for POP, and the lack of this symptom had a negative predictive value of 76%.[9] Not surprisingly, increased degree of prolapse, especially beyond the hymen, is associated with increased pelvic discomfort and visualization of a protrusion.[10]

Stress urinary incontinence and voiding difficulties can occur in association with anterior and apical vaginal prolapse. However, women with advanced degrees of prolapse may not have overt symptoms of stress incontinence, because the prolapse may cause a mechanical obstruction of the urethra, leading to a higher urethral closure pressure and thereby preventing urinary leakage.[11] Instead, these women may require vaginal pressure or manual replacement of the prolapse in order to accomplish voiding. They are therefore at risk for incomplete bladder emptying and recurrent or persistent urinary tract infections, and for the development of de novo stress incontinence after the prolapse is repaired. Patients who require digital assistance to void in general have more advanced degrees of prolapse.[12]

In addition to difficulty voiding, other urinary symptoms such as urgency, frequency, and urge incontinence, are found in women with POP.[13] However, it is not clear whether the severity of prolapse is associated with more irritative voiding symptoms or bladder pain.[10,12]

POP, especially in the apical and posterior compartments, can be associated with defecatory dysfunction, such as pain with defecation, the need for manual assistance with defecation, and anal incontinence of flatus, liquid or solid stool. These patients often have outlet-type constipation secondary to the trapping of stool within the rectal hernia, necessitating splinting or application of manual pressure in the vagina, rectum, or perineum to reduce the hernia and aid in defecation. Although defecatory dysfunction remains the area that is least understood in patients with POP, clinical and radiographic studies have shown that the severity of prolapse is not strongly correlated with increased symptomatology.[9,10,12,14]

Although women with isolated posterior prolapse (e.g., rectocele, enterocele, perineal body defect) may also have the sensation of vaginal bulge and pressure, these women are often asymptomatic and the prolapse is recognized only on physical examination. Once a posterior vaginal defect is identified, questions regarding defecatory dysfunction must be elicited.

Although the relationship between sexual function and POP is not clearly defined, questions regarding sexual dysfunction must be included in the evaluation of any patient with POP. Patients may report symptoms of dyspareunia, decreased libido and orgasm, and increased embarrassment with altered anatomy that affects body image. Some studies have reported that prolapse adversely affects sexual functioning, with subsequent improvement in sexual function after repair of prolapse.[15-17] However, other studies have shown little correlation between the extent of prolapse and sexual dysfunction.[12] It is important to note that the evaluation of sexual function may be especially difficult in this patient population because the hindrances to sexual function may include factors other than POP, such as partner limitations and functional deficits.

PHYSICAL EXAMINATION

The physical examination for POP should be conducted with the patient in dorsal lithotomy position, as for a routine pelvic examination. If physical findings do not correspond to symptoms, or if the maximum extent of the prolapse cannot be confirmed, the woman can be reexamined in the standing position.

Initially, the external genitalia are inspected; if no displacement is apparent, the labia are gently spread to expose the vestibule and hymen. The integrity of the perineal body is evaluated, and the extent of all prolapsed parts is assessed. A retractor, a Sims speculum, or the posterior blade of a bivalve speculum may be used to depress the posterior vagina to aid in visualizing the anterior vagina, and vice versa for the posterior vagina. Because most patients with POP are postmenopausal, the vaginal mucosa should be examined for atrophy and thinning, which may affect management. Healthy, estrogenized tissue without significant evidence of prolapse, is well perfused and exhibits rugations and physiologic moisture. Atrophic vaginal tissue appears pale and thin, is without rugation, and can be friable.

After the resting vaginal examination, the patient is instructed to perform a Valsalva maneuver or to cough vigorously. During this maneuver, the order of descent of the pelvic organs is noted, as is the relationship of the pelvic organs at the peak of increased intra-abdominal pressure. A rectovaginal examination is also required to fully evaluate prolapse of the posterior vaginal wall and perineal body. Digital assessment of the contents of the rectovaginal septum during straining examination can differentiate between a "traction" enterocele (in which the posterior cul-de-sac is pulled down by the prolapsing cervix or vaginal cuff but is not distended by intestines) and a "pulsion" enterocele (in which the intestinal contents of the enterocele distend the rectovaginal septum and produce a protruding mass). Other clinical observations and tests to help delineate POP include cotton swab (Q-tip) testing for the measurement of urethral axis mobility; measurement of perineal descent; measurement of the transverse diameter of the genital hiatus or of the protruding prolapse; measurement of vaginal volume; description and measurement of posterior prolapse; and examination techniques differentiating among various types of defects (e.g., central versus paravaginal defects of the anterior vaginal wall). Inspection should also be made of the anal sphincter because fecal incontinence is often associated with posterior vaginal support defects. Grossly, women with a torn external sphincter may have scarring or a "dovetail" sign on the perineal body.

Anterior vaginal wall descent usually represents bladder descent with or without concomitant urethral hypermobility. However, in 1.6% of women with anterior vaginal prolapse, an anterior enterocele can mimic a cystocele on physical examination.[18] Furthermore, lateral paravaginal defects, identified as detachment of the lateral vaginal sulci, may be distinguished from central defects, seen as a midline protrusion with preservation of the lateral sulci. This is done with the use of a curved forceps placed in the anterolateral vaginal sulcus and directed toward the ischial spine. Bulging of the anterior vaginal wall in the midline between the forcep blades implies a midline defect; blunting or descent of the vaginal fornices on either side with straining suggests lateral paravaginal defects. However, researchers have shown that the physical examination technique used to detect paravaginal defects is not particularly reliable or accurate. In a study by Barber and colleagues of 117 women with prolapse, the sensitivity of clinical examination to detect paravaginal defects was good (92%), yet the specificity was poor (52%).[19] Despite a high prevalence of paravaginal defects, the positive predictive value was only 61%. Fewer than two thirds of the women believed to have a paravaginal defect on physical examination were confirmed to possess the same at surgery. Another study by Whiteside and associates, demonstrated poor reproducibility of clinical examination to detect anterior vaginal wall defects.[20] Therefore, the clinical value of determining the location of midline, apical, and lateral paravaginal defects remains unknown.

In regard to posterior defects, it has previously been demonstrated that preoperative clinical examinations do not always accurately differentiate between rectoceles and enteroceles.[21,22] Some investigators have advocated performing imaging studies to further delineate the exact nature of the posterior wall prolapse. Traditionally, most clinicians believe they are able to detect the presence or absence of these defects without anatomically localizing them. However, little is known regarding the accuracy or utility of clinical examinations in evaluating the anatomic locations of posterior vaginal defects. Burrows and colleagues found that clinical examinations often did not accurately predict the specific location of defects in the rectovaginal septum subsequently found intraoperatively.[23] Clinical findings corresponded with intraoperative observations in 59% of patients and differed in 41%; sensitivities and positive predicative values of clinical examinations were less than 40% for all posterior defects. However, what remains unclear is the clinical consequence of not detecting these defects preoperatively.

Clinical evaluation for POP also should include a lumbosacral neurologic evaluation consisting of strength, sensory, and reflex examinations. First, the strength of the pelvic floor musculature is assessed by palpating the levator ani muscle complex in the posterior vaginal wall approximately 2 to 4 cm cephalad to the hymen. The patient is then asked to squeeze around the examiner's fingers. Weakness in this muscle can be a result of neurologic deficits or direct trauma during childbirth. Internal and external anal sphincter tone is assessed by placing a finger in the rectum and noting the initial resistance to entry and then the resistance after the patient maximally squeezes her anal sphincter. Sensory function is assessed with the use of pinprick and light-touch of the mons pubis, perineum/perianal area, and labia majora. Cystometry and anal manometry can be used to evaluate the visceral sensation of the bladder and rectum, respectively. Lastly, anal and bulbocavernosus reflexes can be elicited by lightly stroking the perianal skin and observing or palpating the contraction of the anal sphincter, and by lightly tapping the clitoris and observing the contraction of the bulbocavernosus muscle and/or anal sphincter.

CLASSIFICATION OF PELVIC ORGAN PROLAPSE

Presently, there are two widely accepted classification systems for assessing the severity of POP: the Baden-Walker "half-way" vaginal profile and the POPQ, which was established by the International Continence Society (ICS) in 1996.[24] The purpose of any classification system is to facilitate understanding of the etiology and pathophysiology of disease, to establish and standardize treatment and research guidelines, and to aid precision and avoid confusion among practitioners.

For many years, POP has been described using criteria modified from the Baden-Walker "half-way" vaginal profile.[25-27] This grading system is simple to use; it is widely understood among gynecologic surgeons and has been found to have reasonable inter-examiner reliability for all segments of the vagina and for uterine support.[28] The most dependent position of the pelvic organs during maximum straining or standing is used and graded as normal or first-, second-, or third-degree prolapse. First-degree prolapse refers to vaginal segments that descend halfway (but not to) the hymen; second-degree is descent to the hymen; and third-degree is prolapse beyond the hymen. A rectovaginal examination can also be used to better delineate the severity of rectoceles. This classification system, although popular, is slowly being replaced by the more precise and standardized POPQ system.

In the POPQ system, the pelvic organ anatomy is described during physical examination of the external genitalia and vaginal canal.[24] Segments of the lower reproductive tract replace the terms cystocele, enterocele, rectocele, and urethrovesical junction, because these terms imply an unrealistic certainty as to the structures on the other side of the vaginal bulge, particularly in women who have had previous prolapse surgery. The examiner sees and describes the maximum protrusion noted by the patient during her daily activities. The details of the examination, including criteria for the end point of the examination and full development of the prolapse, should be specified. Suggested criteria for demonstration of maximum prolapse include any or all of the following: any protrusion of the vaginal wall that has become tight during straining by the patient; traction on the prolapse causes no further descent; the subject confirms that the size of the prolapse and the extent of the protrusion seen by the examiner are as extensive as the most severe protrusion she has had (a small hand-held mirror to visualize the protrusion may be helpful); and a standing/straining examination confirms that the full extent of the prolapse was observed in the other positions.

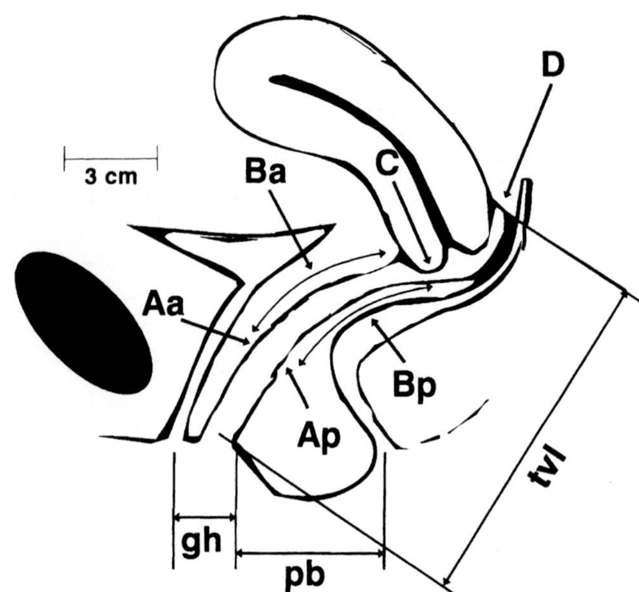

Figure 54-1 Six sites (points Aa, Ba, C, D, Bp, and Ap), genital hiatus (gh), perineal body (pb), and total vaginal length (tvl) are used for pelvic organ support quantitation. (From Bump RC, Mattiasson A, Bø K, et al: The standardization of terminology of female pelvic organ prolapse and pelvic floor dysfunction. Am J Obstet Gynecol 175:10, 1996.)

Details about patient position, types of vaginal specula or retractors, type and intensity of straining used to develop the prolapse maximally, and fullness of the bladder should be stated.

This descriptive system contains a series of site-specific measurements of the woman's pelvic organ support. It can be easily learned and taught by means of a video tutorial.[29] Prolapse in each segment is evaluated and measured relative to the hymen (not introitus), which is a fixed anatomic landmark that can be identified consistently and precisely. The anatomic position of the six defined points for measurement should be in centimeters above or proximal to the hymen (negative number) or centimeters below or distal to the hymen (positive number), with the plane of the hymen being defined as zero. For example, a cervix that protrudes 3 cm distal to (beyond) the hymen should be described as +3 cm.

Six points (two on the anterior vaginal wall, two in the superior vagina, and two on the posterior vaginal wall) are located with reference to the plane of the hymen (Fig. 54-1). In describing the anterior vaginal wall, the term *anterior vaginal wall prolapse* is preferable to *cystocele* or *anterior enterocele* unless the organs involved are identified by ancillary tests. There are two anterior sites:

Point Aa: A point located in the midline of the anterior vaginal wall 3 cm proximal to the external urethral meatus, corresponding to the proximal location of the urethrovesical crease. By definition, the range of position of point Aa relative to the hymen is −3 to +3 cm.

Point Ba: A point that represents the most distal (i.e., most dependent) position of any part of the upper anterior vaginal wall from the vaginal cuff or anterior vaginal fornix to point Aa. By definition, point Ba is at −3 cm in the absence of prolapse and would have a positive value equal to the position of the cuff in women with total posthysterectomy vaginal eversion.

Two points are on the superior vagina. These points represent the most proximal locations of the normally positioned lower reproductive tract.

Point C: A point that represents either the most distal (i.e., most dependent) edge of the cervix or the leading edge of the vaginal cuff (hysterectomy scar) after total hysterectomy.

Point D: A point that represents a location of the posterior fornix in a woman who still has a cervix. It represents the level of uterosacral ligament attachment to the proximal posterior cervix. It is included as a point of measurement to differentiate suspensory failure of the uterosacral—cardinal ligament complex from cervical elongation. Point D is omitted in the absence of the cervix.

Two points are located on the posterior vaginal wall. Analogous to anterior prolapse, posterior prolapse should be discussed in terms of segments of the vaginal wall rather than the organs that lie behind it. Thus, the term *posterior vaginal wall prolapse* is preferable to *rectocele* or *enterocele* unless the organs involved are identified by ancillary tests. If small bowel appears to be present in the rectovaginal space, the examiner should comment on this fact and clearly describe the basis for this clinical impression (e.g., by observation of peristaltic activity in the distended posterior vagina or palpation of loops of small bowel between an examining finger in the rectum and one in the vagina).

Point Ap: A point located in the midline of the posterior vaginal wall 3 cm proximal to the hymen. By definition, the range of position of point Ap relative to the hymen is −3 to +3 cm.

Point Bp: A point that represents the most distal (i.e., most dependent) position of any part or the upper posterior vaginal wall from the vaginal cuff or posterior vaginal fornix to point Ap. By definition, point Bp is at −3 cm in the absence of prolapse and would have a positive value equal to the position of the cuff in a woman with total posthysterectomy vaginal eversion.

Other landmarks include the genital hiatus, which is measured from the middle of the external urethral meatus to the posterior midline hymen. The perineal body is measured from the posterior margin of the genital hiatus to the midanal opening. The total vaginal length is the greatest depth of the vagina in centimeters when point C or D is reduced to its full normal position. The points and measurements are presented in Figure 54-1.

The positions of points Aa, Ba, Ap, Bp, C, and (if applicable) D with reference to the hymen are measured and recorded. Positions are expressed as centimeters proximal to (above) the hymen (negative number) or centimeters distal to (below) the hymen (positive number), with the plane of the hymen defined as zero. Measurements may be recorded as a simple line of numbers (e.g., −3, −3, −7, −9, −3, −3, 9, 2, and 2 for points Aa, Ba, C, D, Bp, Ap, total vaginal length, genital hiatus, and perineal body, respectively). Alternatively, a 3 × 3 grid can be used to concisely organize the measurements, as shown in Figure 54-2, or a line diagram of a configuration can be drawn, as shown in Figures 54-3 and 54-4. Figure 54-3 is a grid and line diagram contrasting measurements that indicate normal support with those of complete posthysterectomy vaginal eversion. Figure 54-4 is a grid and line diagram representing predominant anterior and posterior vaginal wall prolapse with partial apical descent.

anterior wall **Aa**	anterior wall **Ba**	cervix or cuff **C**
genital hiatus **gh**	perineal body **pb**	total vaginal length **tvl**
posterior wall **Ap**	posterior wall **Bp**	posterior fornix **D**

Figure 54-2 Three-by-three grid for recording quantitative description of pelvic organ support. (From Bump RC, Mattiasson A, Bø K, et al: The standardization of terminology of female pelvic organ prolapse and pelvic floor dysfunction. Am J Obstet Gynecol 175:10, 1996.)

The profile for quantifying prolapse provides a precise description of anatomy for individual patients. An ordinal staging system of pelvic organ prolapse is suggested using these measurements and can be useful for the description of populations and for research comparisons. Stages are assigned according to the most severe portion of the prolapse when the full extent of the protrusion has been demonstrated. For a stage to be assigned to an individual subject, it is essential that her quantitative description be completed first. The five stages of pelvic organ support (0 through IV) are described in Table 54-1. Because precise characterization of pelvic floor muscle strength and description of functional symptoms are of vital importance, the reader is referred to the ICS committee document for further details.[24]

Studies have demonstrated excellent interexaminer and intraexaminer reliability for the POPQ system in quantifying POP.[28,30] Steele and associates showed that the system can be taught effectively to residents and medical students using a 17-minute video.[29] Furthermore, the measurements can be obtained quickly by both experienced and nonexperienced clinicians (2.1 and 3.7 minutes, respectively).[30] The POPQ system does not take into account lateral defects and perineal body prolapse, but these can be added in descriptive terms. Despite its limitations, the POPQ system is currently the classification system used in most research studies and NIH trials, and it is gaining popularity in clinic practice.

DIAGNOSTIC TESTS

After a careful history and physical examination, few diagnostic tests are needed to further evaluate patients with POP if there is no concomitant voiding or defecatory dysfunction. For example, hydronephrosis does occur in a small proportion of women with prolapse, but even if it is identified, it usually does not change management in the women for whom surgical repair is planned.

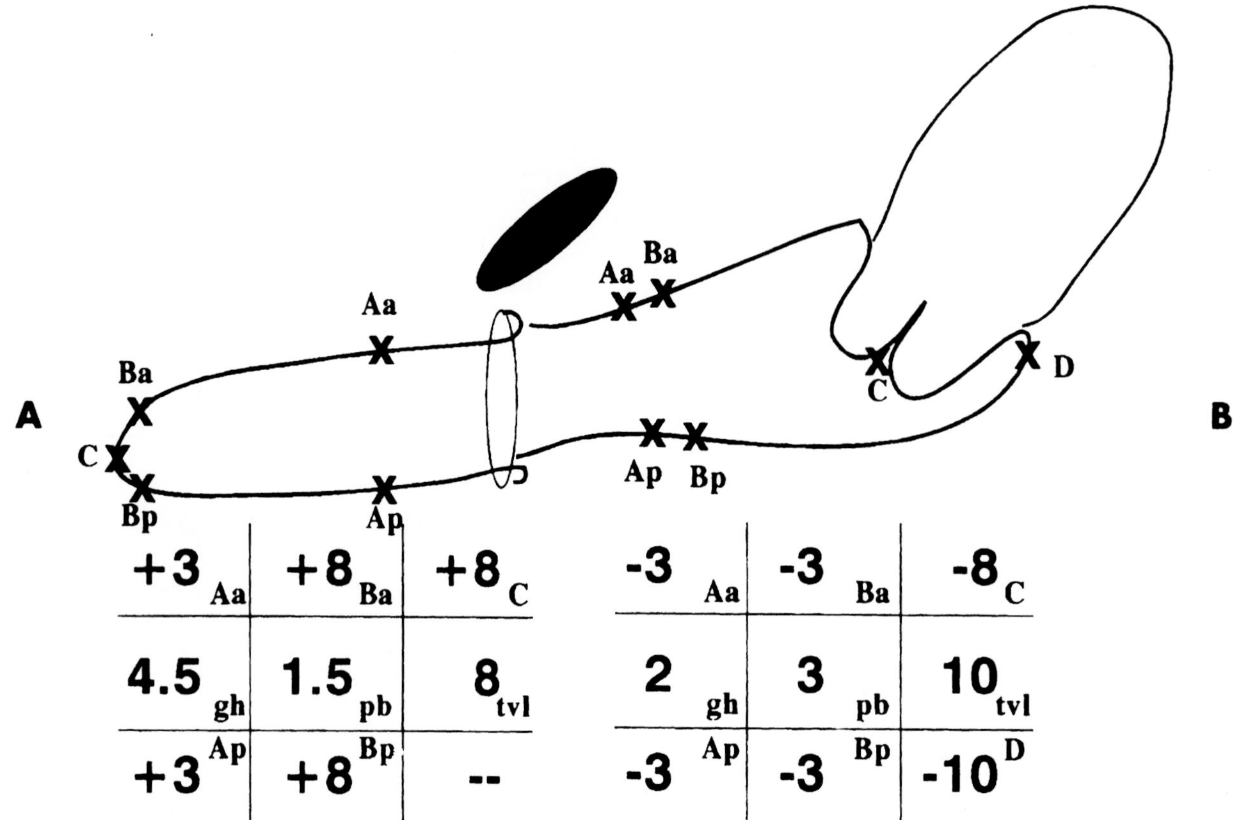

Figure 54-3 A, Grid and line diagram of complete eversion of vagina. The most distal point of the anterior wall (point Ba), vaginal cuff scar (point C), and the most distal point of the posterior wall (point Bp) are all at same position (+8), and points Aa and Ap are maximally distal (both at +3). Because total vaginal length equals maximum protrusion, this is stage IV prolapse. **B,** Normal support. Points Aa and Ba and points Ap and Bp are all –3 because there is no anterior or posterior wall descent. The lowest point of the cervix is 8 cm above the hymen (–8), and the posterior fornix is 2 cm above this (–10). The vaginal length is 10 cm, the genital hiatus is 2 cm, and the perineal body measures 3 cm. This represents stage 0 prolapse. (From Bump RC, Mattiasson A, Bø K, et al: The standardization of terminology of female pelvic organ prolapse and pelvic floor dysfunction. Am J Obstet Gynecol 175:10, 1996.)

Table 54-1 Stages of Pelvic Organ Prolapse

Stage	Description
0	No prolapse is demonstrated. Points Aa, Ap, Ba, and Bp are all at –3 cm, and either point C or point D is between –TVL cm and –(TVL–2) cm; that is, the quantitation value for point C or D is ≤–[TVL–2] cm. In **Fig. 54-3, B** represents stage 0.
I	The criteria for stage 0 are not met, but the most distal portion of the prolapse is >1 cm above the level of the hymen (i.e., its quantitation value is <–1 cm).
II	The most distal portion of the prolapse is ≤1 cm proximal to or distal to the plane of the hymen (i.e., its quantitation value is ≥–1 cm but ≤+1 cm).
III	The most distal portion of the prolapse is >1 cm below (distal to) the plane of the hymen but protrudes no further than 2 cm less than the TVL (i.e., its quantitation value is >+1 cm but <+[TVL–2] cm). In **Fig. 54-4, A** represents stage III anterior and **B** represents stage III posterior prolapse.
IV	Essentially complete eversion of the total length of the lower genital tract is demonstrated. The distal portion of the prolapse protrudes to at least (TVL–2) cm (i.e., its quantitation value is ≥+[TVL–2] cm). In most instances, the leading edge of stage IV prolapse is the cervix or vaginal cuff scar. In **Fig. 54-3, A** represents stage IV C prolapse.

TVL, total vaginal length.
From Bump RC, Mattiasson A, Bo K, et al: The standardization of terminology of female pelvic organ prolapse and pelvic floor dysfunction. Am J Obstet Gynecol 175:10, 1996.

Therefore, routine imaging of the kidneys and ureters is not necessary.

Because patients with anterior, apical, or posterior prolapse may have voiding dysfunction due to obstruction of the urethra, the completeness of bladder emptying should be assessed with timed and measured voids followed by either catheterization or bladder ultrasound to measure postvoid residual urine volumes. Kinking of the urethra may also obscure any indication of urinary incontinence that may be present.[11,31] Therefore, it is important to assess for evidence of incontinence after reduction of the prolapse. This can be done with a pessary, vaginal packing, or ring forceps at the time of the office bladder filling or urodynamic

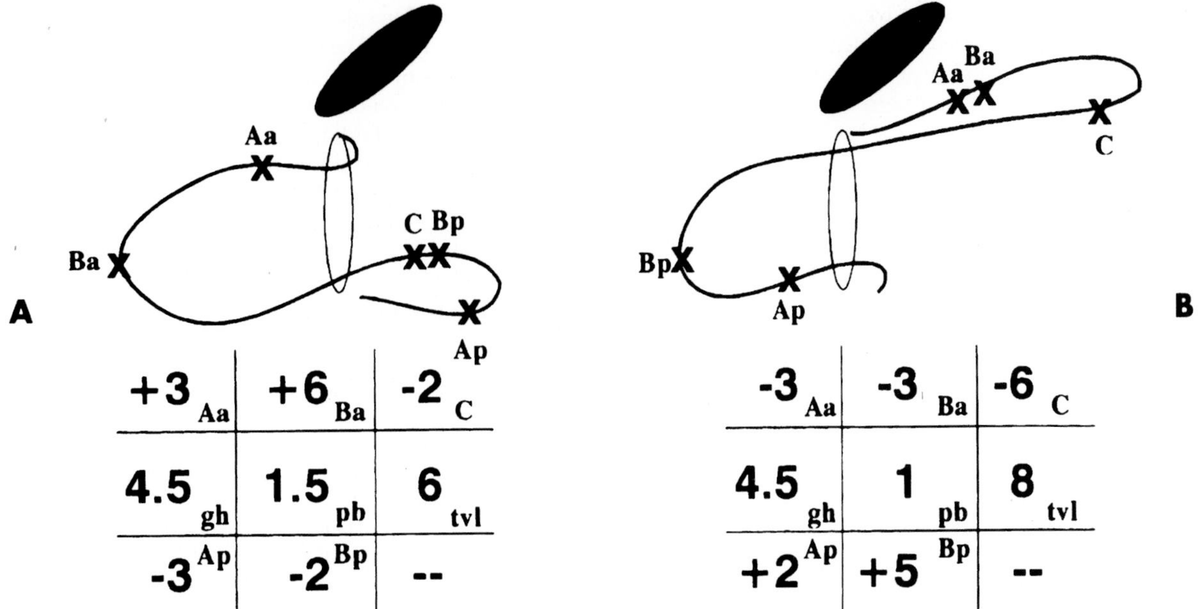

+3 Aa	+6 Ba	-2 C
4.5 gh	1.5 pb	6 tvl
-3 Ap	-2 Bp	--

-3 Aa	-3 Ba	-6 C
4.5 gh	1 pb	8 tvl
+2 Ap	+5 Bp	--

Figure 54-4 A, Grid and line diagram of predominant anterior support defect. The leading point of prolapse is the upper anterior vaginal wall, point Ba (+6). There is significant elongation of the bulging anterior wall. Point Aa is maximally distal (+3), and the vaginal cuff scar is 2 cm above the hymen (C = –2). The cuff scar has undergone 4 cm of descent, because it would be at –6 (total vaginal length) if it were perfectly supported. In this example, total vaginal length is measure not as the maximum depth with the elongated anterior vaginal wall maximally reduced but rather as the depth of the vagina at cuff with point C reduced to its normal full extent, as specified in the text. This represents stage III anterior prolapse. **B,** Predominant posterior support defect. The leading point of prolapse is the upper posterior vaginal wall, point Bp (+5). Point Ap is 2 cm distal to the hymen (+2), and the vaginal cuff scar is 6 cm above the hymen (–6). The cuff has undergone only 2 cm of descent, because it would be at –8 (total vaginal length) if it were perfectly supported. This represents stage III posterior prolapse. (From Bump RC, Mattiasson A, Bø K, et al: The standardization of terminology of female pelvic organ prolapse and pelvic floor dysfunction. Am J Obstet Gynecol 175:10, 1996.)

testing. If urinary leakage occurs with coughing or Valsalva maneuvers after reduction of the prolapse, the urethral sphincter is probably incompetent, even if the patient is normally continent. This can occur in up to half of women with stage III or IV prolapse. In this situation, the surgeon should choose a sling procedure in conjunction with the prolapse repair.[32] If sphincteric incompetence is not present even after reduction of the prolapse, an anti-incontinence procedure may not be indicated.

As discussed in previous sections, preoperative clinical assessments of specific support defects involved in POP often do not correspond to subsequent intraoperative findings. Therefore, some investigators have advocated using imaging procedures such as ultrasonography, contrast radiography, and magnetic resonance imaging (MRI) to further describe the exact nature of the support defects before attempting surgical repairs. For example, some practioners have used contrast ultrasonography to evaluate for paravaginal defects by placing a water-filled condom in the vaginal canal to better delineate the paravaginal spaces.[33] Others have used MRI to better characterize the soft tissue and viscera of the pelvis.[34] However, there is a lack of standardized radiologic criteria for diagnosing POP. Therefore, the clinical utility of imaging studies remains unknown, and they are currently used mostly for research purposes.

Similar to patients with POP who are without voiding dysfunction, patients with POP who are without symptoms of defecatory dysfunction generally do not warrant ancillary bowel testing. For example, although defecating proctography can provide additional information regarding rectal emptying, studies have demonstrated that it is no more sensitive at detecting rectoceles than physical examination alone.[35] However, patients with concomitant defecatory dysfunction or motility disorders do merit further evaluation.

In patients with defecatory dysfunction, it is necessary to differentiate between those with colonic motility disorders and those with pelvic outlet symptoms. Useful ancillary tests include anoscopy and proctosigmoidoscopy to evaluate for prolapsing hemorrhoids and intrarectal prolapse. Motility disorders can be assessed with colonic transit studies, which involve a series of radiographs that document the passage of ingested radiopaque markers. Depending on the specific protocol used, passage of less than 80% of the ingested markers could indicate the presence of a motility disorder, whereas collection of markers in the sigmoid colon could indicate the presence of an outlet obstruction.[36]

In patients with apical and posterior vaginal prolapse who also complain of difficult or incomplete bowel emptying, it is important to evaluate for pelvic floor dyssynergia. During the physical examination, patients with pelvic floor dyssynergia often have hypercontracted and tender puborectalis muscles that may not relax on command. Tests for diagnosing pelvic floor dyssynergia include electromyography and the balloon expulsion test, which demonstrates a paradoxical contraction of the puborectalis muscle during defecation. Defecating proctography, which involves dynamic and still images of patients at rest, during defecation, and while contracting the anal sphincter, can also be used for diagnosis. Defecography has the added advantage of providing radiographic evidence of the specific organ that is herniating into the posterior vaginal wall, and it is the gold standard for measuring perineal descent.[37]

Dynamic MRI defecography can also be used to provide information regarding defecation and anatomic soft tissue defects. It has the advantages of being noninvasive and not requiring ionizing radiation, and it is unrivaled in its depictions of pelvic soft tissue. However, the clinical utility of this costly imaging modality is debatable, because it has not been shown to alter clinical decision-making.[38]

CONCLUSIONS

POP is a heterogeneous group of conditions that has wide medical and social implications for the current aging female population. Many fundamental concepts such as epidemiology, natural disease progression, and associations with urinary, bowel, and sexual dysfunction have yet to be fully established and are consequently areas of active research. In this chapter, we have discussed the basic evaluation of patients with POP, from pertinent history to physical findings, classification systems, and ancillary studies. We have also addressed some of the controversies inherent in this emerging field. Because this is an area of active research, we did not attempt to provide an all-encompassing view of POP. Rather, we have provided a foundation from which the reader can extrapolate for patient care as well as for understanding of the current literature.

References

1. Subak LL, Waetjen LE, van den Eeden S, et al: Cost of pelvic organ prolapse surgery in the United States. Obstet Gynecol 98:646-651, 2001.
2. Luber KM, Boero S, Choe JY: The demographics of pelvic floor disorders: Current observations and future projections. Am J Obstet Gynecol 184:1496-1501, 2001.
3. American College of Obstetricians and Gynecologists: Pelvic Organ Prolapse. Technical Bulletin No. 214. Washington DC: The College, 1995.
4. Weber AM, Abrams P, Brubaker L, et al: The standardization of terminology for researchers in female pelvic floor disorders. Int Urogynecol J 12:178-186, 2001.
5. Swift SE: The distribution of pelvic organ support in a population of women presenting for routine gynecologic healthcare. Am J Obstet Gynecol 183:277-285, 2000.
6. Swift S, Woodman P, O'Boyle A, et al: Pelvic organ support study (POSST): The distribution, clinical definition, and epidemiologic condition of pelvic organ support defects. Am J Obstet Gynecol 192:795-806, 2005.
7. Jensen JK, Nielsen FR Jr, Ostergard DR: The role of patient history in the diagnosis of urinary incontinence. Obstet Gynecol 83:904-910, 1994.
8. Melville JL, Miller EA, Fialkow MF, et al: Relationship between patient report and physician assessment of urinary incontinence severity. Am J Obstet Gynecol 189:76-80, 2003.
9. Tan JS, Lukacz ES, Menefee SA, et al: Predictive value of prolapse symptoms: A large database study. Int Urogynecol J 16:203-209, 2005.
10. Ellerkmann RM, Cundiff GW, Melick CF, et al: Correlation of symptoms with location and severity of pelvic organ prolapse. Am J Obstet Gynecol 185:1332-1338, 2001.
11. Bump RC, Fantl JA, Hurt WG: The mechanism of urinary continence in women with severe uterovaginal prolapse: Results of barrier studies. Obstet Gynecol 72:291-295, 1988.
12. Burrows LJ, Meyn LA, Walters MD, Weber AM: Pelvic symptoms in women with pelvic organ prolapse. Am J Obstet Gynecol 104:982-988, 2004.
13. Romanzi LJ, Chaiken DC, Blaivis JG: The effect of genital prolapse on voiding. J Urol 161:581-586, 1999.
14. Kelvin FM, Maglinte DD, Hornback JA: Dynamic cystoproctography of female pelvic floor defects and their interrelationships. Am J Radiol 169:769-774, 1997.
15. Barber MD, Visco AG, Wyman JF, et al: Sexual function in women with urinary incontinence and pelvic organ prolapse. Continence Program for Women Research Group. Obstet Gynecol 99:281-289, 2002.
16. Rogers RG, Villarreal A, Kammerer-Doak D, et al: Sexual function in women with and without urinary incontinence and/or pelvic organ prolapse. Int Urogynecol J 12:361-365, 2001.
17. Weber AM, Walters MD, Piedmonte MR: Sexual function and vaginal anatomy in women before and after surgery for pelvic organ prolapse and urinary incontinence. Am J Obstet Gynecol 182:1610-1615, 2000.
18. Tulikangas PK, Lukban JC, Walters MD: Anterior enterocele: A report of three cases. Int Urogynecol J 15:350-352, 2004.
19. Barber MD, Cundiff GW, Weidner AC, et al: Accuracy of clinical assessment of paravaginal defects in women with anterior vaginal wall prolapse. Am J Obstet Gyneol 181:87-90, 1999.
20. Whiteside JL, Barber MD, Paraiso MF, et al: Clinical evaluation of anterior vaginal wall support defects: Interexaminer and intraexaminer reliability. Am J Obstet Gynecol 191:100-104, 2004.
21. Kenton K, Shott S, Brubaker L: Vaginal topography does not correlate well with visceral position in women with pelvic organ prolapse. Int Urogynecol J 8:336-339, 1997.
22. Kelvin FM, Hale DS, Maglinte DD, et al: Female pelvic organ prolapse: Diagnostic contribution of dynamic cystoproctography and comparison with physical examination. Am J Roentgenol 173:31-37, 1999.
23. Burrows LJ, Sewell C, Leffler KS, Cundiff GW: The accuracy of clinical evaluation of posterior vaginal wall defects. Int Urogynecol J 14:160-163, 2003.
24. Bump RC, Mattiasson A, Bø K, et al: The standardization of terminology of female pelvic organ prolapse and pelvic floor dysfunction. Am J Obstet Gynecol 175:10-17, 1996.
25. Beecham CT: Classification of vaginal relaxation. Am J Obstet Gynecol 136:957-958, 1980.
26. Baden WF, Walker TA, Lindsey JH: The vaginal profile. Tex Med 64:56-58, 1968.
27. Baden WF, Walker TA: Genesis of the vaginal profile: A correlated classification of vaginal relaxation. Clin Obstet Gynecol 15:1048-1054, 1972.
28. Kobak WH, Rosenberger K, Walters MD: Interobserver variation in the assessment of pelvic organ prolapse. Int Urogynecol J 175:1467-1471, 1996.
29. Steele A. Mallipeddi P, Welgoss J, et al: Teaching the Pelvic Organ Prolapse Quantification system. Am J Obstet Gynecol 179:1458-1464, 1998.
30. Hall AF, Theofrastous JP, Cundiff GC, et al: Interobserver and intraobserver reliability of the proposed International Continence Society, Society of Gynecologic Surgeons, and the American Urogynecologic Society pelvic organ prolapse classification system. Am J Obstet Gynecol 175:1467-1469, 1996.
31. Myers DL, Lasala CA, Hogan JW, Rosenblatt PL: The effect of posterior wall support defects on urodynamic indices in stress urinary incontinence. Obstet Gynecol 91:710-714, 1998.
32. Meschia M, Pifarotti P, Spennacchio M, et al: A randomized comparison of tension-free vaginal tape and endopelvic fascia plication in women with genital prolapse and occult stress urinary incontinence. Am J Obstet Gynecol 190:609-613, 2004.
33. Ostrzenski A, Osborne NG, Ostrzenska K: Method for diagnosing paravaginal defects using contrast ultrasonographic technique. J Ultrasound Med 16:673-677, 1997.

34. Aronson MP, Bates SM, Jacoby AF, et al: Periurethral and paravaginal anatomy: An endovaginal magnetic resonance imaging study. Am J Obstet Gynecol 173:1702-1710, 1995.
35. Siproudhis L, Robert A, Vilotte J, et al: How accurate is clinical examination in diagnosing and quantifying pelvirectal disorders? A prospective study in a group of 50 patients complaining of defecatory difficulties. Dis Colon Rectum 36:430-438, 1993.
36. Cundiff GW, Fenner D: Evaluation and treatment of women with rectocele: Focus on associated defecatory and sexual dysfunction. Obstet Gynecol 104:1403-1421, 2004.
37. Kelvin FM, Maglinte DD: Dynamic evaluation of female pelvic organ prolapse by extended proctography. Radiol Clin North Am 41:395-407, 2003.
38. Matsuoka H, Wexner SD, Desai MB: A comparison between dynamic pelvic magnetic resonance imaging and videoproctography in patients with constipation. Dis Colon Rectum 30:199-222, 2001.

Chapter 55

IMAGING IN THE DIAGNOSIS OF PELVIC ORGAN PROLAPSE

Steven S. Raman and Lousine Boyadzhyan

Pelvic organ prolapse and pelvic floor relaxation are two related and often coexistent conditions. *Prolapse* refers to an abnormal and noticeable protrusion of bladder, urethra, vagina, or rectum through fascial and hiatal defects typically involving the perineum. Pelvic floor *relaxation,* which typically accompanies prolapse, refers to a weakening of the suspensory fascia, ligaments, and muscles of the pelvic sling. Patients typically do not present with an isolated organ defect; instead, these often complex disorders typically comprise a combination of abnormalities such as a rectocele, an enterocele, or a cystocele. These disorders often occur in middle-aged to elderly women. Symptoms may include urinary incontinence, pain, pressure, perineal herniation, and bulging. On physical examination, findings are often equivocal, because the pelvic anatomy may be distorted due to prior pelvic surgery or severe abnormalities. Clinicians rely on a combination of imaging modalities and functional testing (e.g., urodynamics, anorectal manometry) to help describe the anatomic and functional defects.[1,2] Currently, both fluoroscopy and magnetic resonance imaging (MRI) are widely used and complementary techniques to evaluate disorders of the bladder, vagina, and rectum.[3]

IMAGING MODALITIES FOR EVALUATION OF PELVIC FLOOR DISORDERS

Fluoroscopy

Fluoroscopic evaluation of either voiding or defecation may be performed with the patient in the upright position after opacification with contrast material (Fig. 55-1). Some believe that the upright position most closely resembles the physiologic condition reproducing symptoms, and it has been used as a natural extension of the physical examination.[4] Disorders of the posterior pelvic compartment, which typically include constipation and incomplete defecation, may be studied by instilling a barium paste into the rectum and performing a dynamic fluoroscopic evacuation proctogram or defecogram. Similarly, the bladder may be instilled with a water-soluble iodinated contrast agent during dynamic evaluation of filling and voiding by the traditional voiding cystourethrogram (VCUG). Also, the vagina may be similarly studied by dynamic vaginography.[5] With the "four-contrast" defecogram (in which the bowel, rectum, vagina, and bladder are opacified), the relationships among these compartments may be studied simultaneously.[1]

Defecography

Defecography, or evacuation proctography, is a simple radiologic technique that is used to image the rectal voiding process of a barium-based paste enema. During the examination, the patient sits on a special defecography radiolucent commode while fluoroscopic images are recorded in the lateral projection. Although exact protocols vary, in general, one obtains views at rest, at maximal contraction of the voluntary anal sphincter and pelvic floor musculature without actual defecation, while coughing, while emptying the rectum as completely as possible, and while straining maximally after the evacuation is complete (Figs. 55-2 and 55-3).[5] In addition to using barium-based enemas, many urogenital imagers also administer an oral barium suspension with Gastrografin 30 to 60 minutes before the examination to opacify the bowel and thus facilitate the identification of enteroceles. One can also use contrast gel injected into the vaginal apex and look for rectovaginal separation on the images as an indication of an enterocele.[6] The recording process varies from obtaining spot films to videotaping the entire process during so-called dynamic proctography.

The most essential part of the examination is the assessment of evacuation rate and completeness.[7] Defecography yields both morphologic and functional information, because it provides imaging of the rectal configuration throughout all of the phases of evacuation and allows assessment of whether the latter process is normal or prolonged.[6] Such factors of pelvic floor function as rectal emptying and volume, anal sphincter competency, and perineal and pelvic floor musculature can be evaluated with this technique. It is possible to identify the prolapsed organs, to evaluate the morphology of the bladder neck, and to identify the axis of the bladder and the vagina. However, defecography does not assess fine mucosal abnormalities.[6]

There is an important caveat that pertains to the interpretation of defecographic findings by clinicians. Given that there is a rather wide overlap between standard defecographic measurements and findings among normal asymptomatic patients and those with significant symptomatology, radiographic findings obtained during defecography are not to be used as reliable diagnostic criteria of pelvic floor abnormalities.[8-10] They must be combined with clinical measurements and subjective symptoms reported by the patient for interpretation. Many experts agree that defecography alone is of limited value in clinical decision-making and should be interpreted with the results of complementary testing such as anorectal manometry and pelvic MRI.[6]

Colpocystodefecography

Colpocystodefectography (CCD) or dynamic cystoproctography (DCP) combines voiding cystography, vaginal opacification, and defecography (discussed in the previous section). The imaging study itself is very similar to that described for defecography. The patient is either upright or seated in a special defecography stool-chair, depending on the phase of the examination, with the images being taken during the static and the dynamic phases of

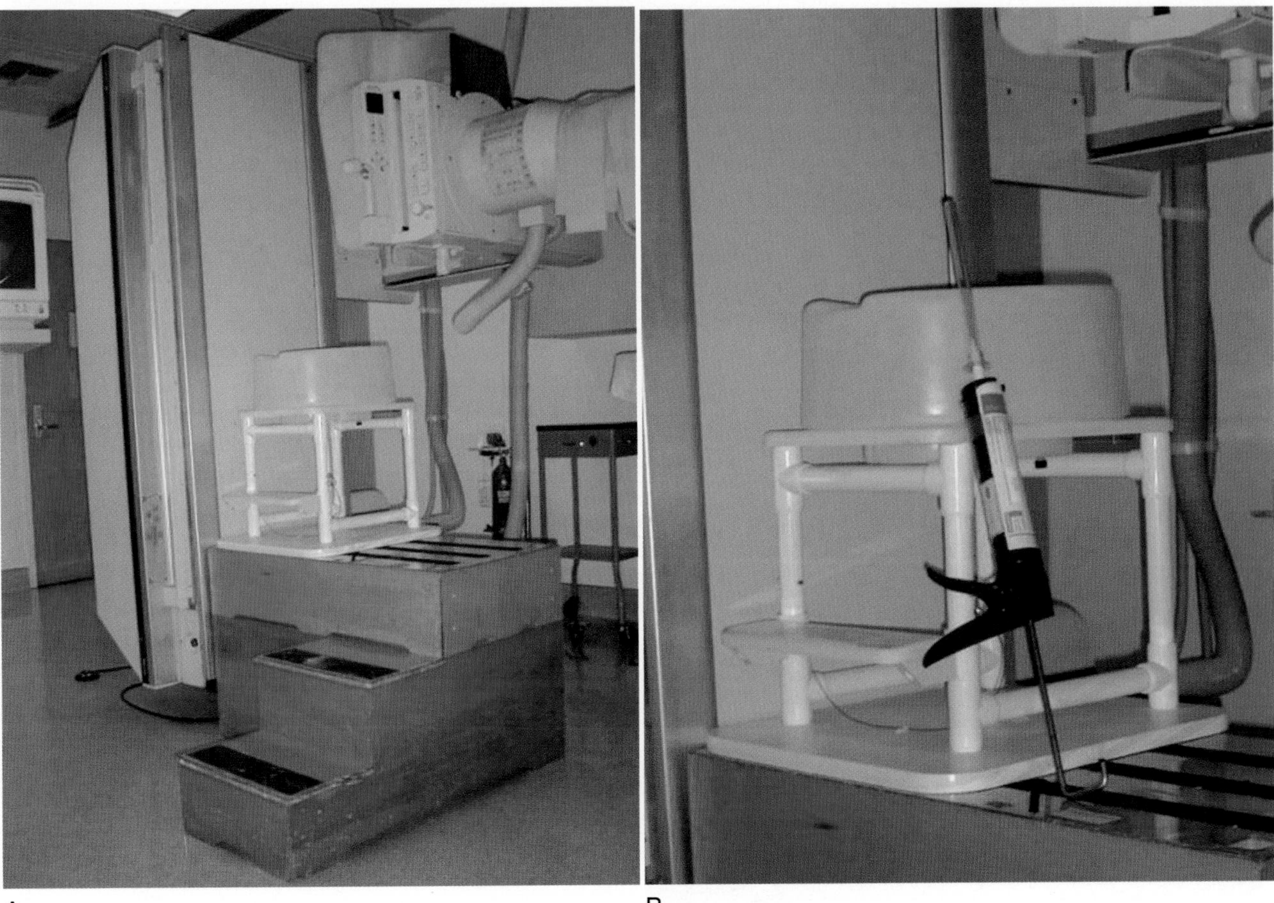

A B

Figure 55-1 Defecography or evacuation proctography suite **(A)** and commode **(B)** used to image patients during various phases of defecation or micturition in lateral projection.

the examination. During the former phase, the patient is either resting, performing a Valsalva maneuver, or maximally contracting her anal sphincter; the latter phase of the study involves micturition and defecation.[11] Therefore, information obtained during a single CCD study is a combination of voiding cystography and defecography.

CCD has been shown to be more sensitive than physical examination in the detection of various forms of female pelvic organ prolapse, and it was developed to complement the physical examination.[12] It has the advantage of examining the patient under the force of gravity in either upright or seated position, thus revealing pelvic floor weakness during physiologic activities as well as rest. However, it does include exposure of the patient to the effects of ionizing radiation, and it puts a time-constraint on both the examiner and the examinee. In addition, it is a rather intrusive technique and requires a great deal of cooperation from the patient as well as patience from the examiner.

Ultrasonography

Ultrasonography is popular because it is an inexpensive, noninvasive imaging technique that does not involve the use of ionizing radiation. It is currently best reserved for evaluation of pelvic organs and bladder volume. The main disadvantages of this technique are its operator dependence and suboptimal ability for comprehensive visualization of tissue planes.[5] Because of these drawbacks, pelvic floor prolapse has been graded by physical examination far more often than by either transvaginal, transrectal, or transperineal ultrasound.[4]

Endoanal Approach

Endoanal ultrasound is used to assess the anorectal junction in patients with incontinence, because other approaches such as abdominal, perineal, or transvaginal scanning are not capable of visualizing the anal sphincter muscles as adequately as the endoanal approach.[13] Although the anal sphincter and even, to a certain extent, upper anal canal defects can be visualized, there is a very wide range of normal findings owing to differences in methodology and reproducibility of measurements with fibers that lie oblique to the plane of the imaging probe.[5] Positioning of the patient is also important and somewhat gender specific. Whereas in men the left lateral position is adequate, female patients should be imaged either prone or in lithotomy position so as to not disturb the anterior anatomy and to increase the diagnostic accuracy of the study.[14] In general, series of images are taken at several levels of depth as the probe is being withdrawn from the anal canal, with detailed examination of any abnormality encountered along the way.

Transvaginal Approach

Female anatomy is unique in that it allows a transvaginal approach to imaging of anal sphincter abnormalities. It is possible to obtain

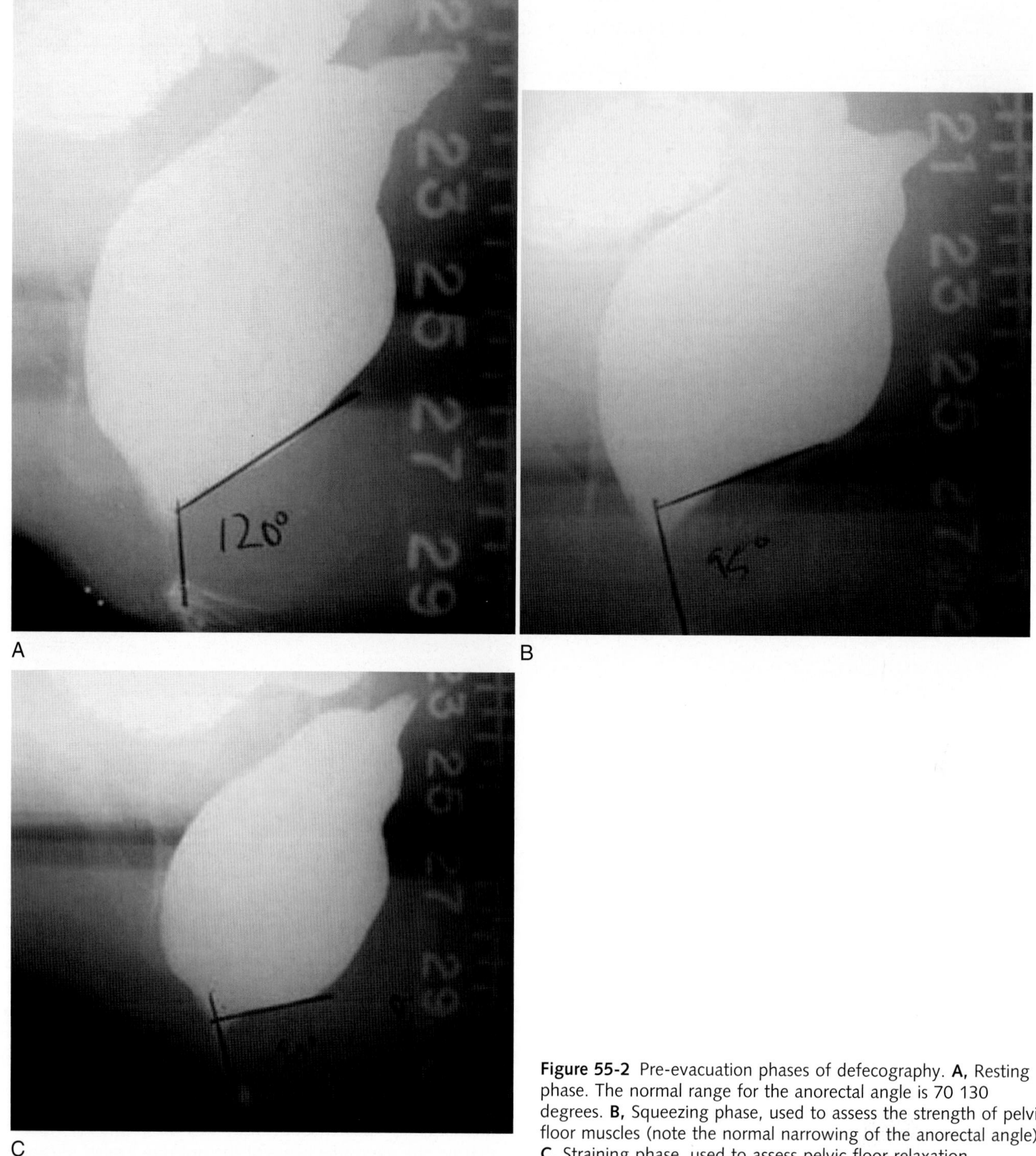

Figure 55-2 Pre-evacuation phases of defecography. **A,** Resting phase. The normal range for the anorectal angle is 70 130 degrees. **B,** Squeezing phase, used to assess the strength of pelvic floor muscles (note the normal narrowing of the anorectal angle). **C,** Straining phase, used to assess pelvic floor relaxation.

a unique view of the sphincter in its closed state during this study when the probe placed in the distal vagina/perineum is angled backward. Perineal body thickness, the subepithelial thickness, anal cushions, and sphincter damage can be assessed.[15] However, even though the transvaginal approach allows for assessment of the anal sphincters, the endoanal approach is superior for defining the extent of sphincter tears and confirming their intactness throughout their length.[13,15] In addition to assessing the anal sphincter, transvaginal sonography allows assessment of the urethra and bladder in supine or sitting positions as well as during dynamic studies in the assessment of urinary continence mechanisms.[16] In some cases of enteroceles, it is possible to visualize bowel loops extending down into the rectovaginal space during this examination.[17]

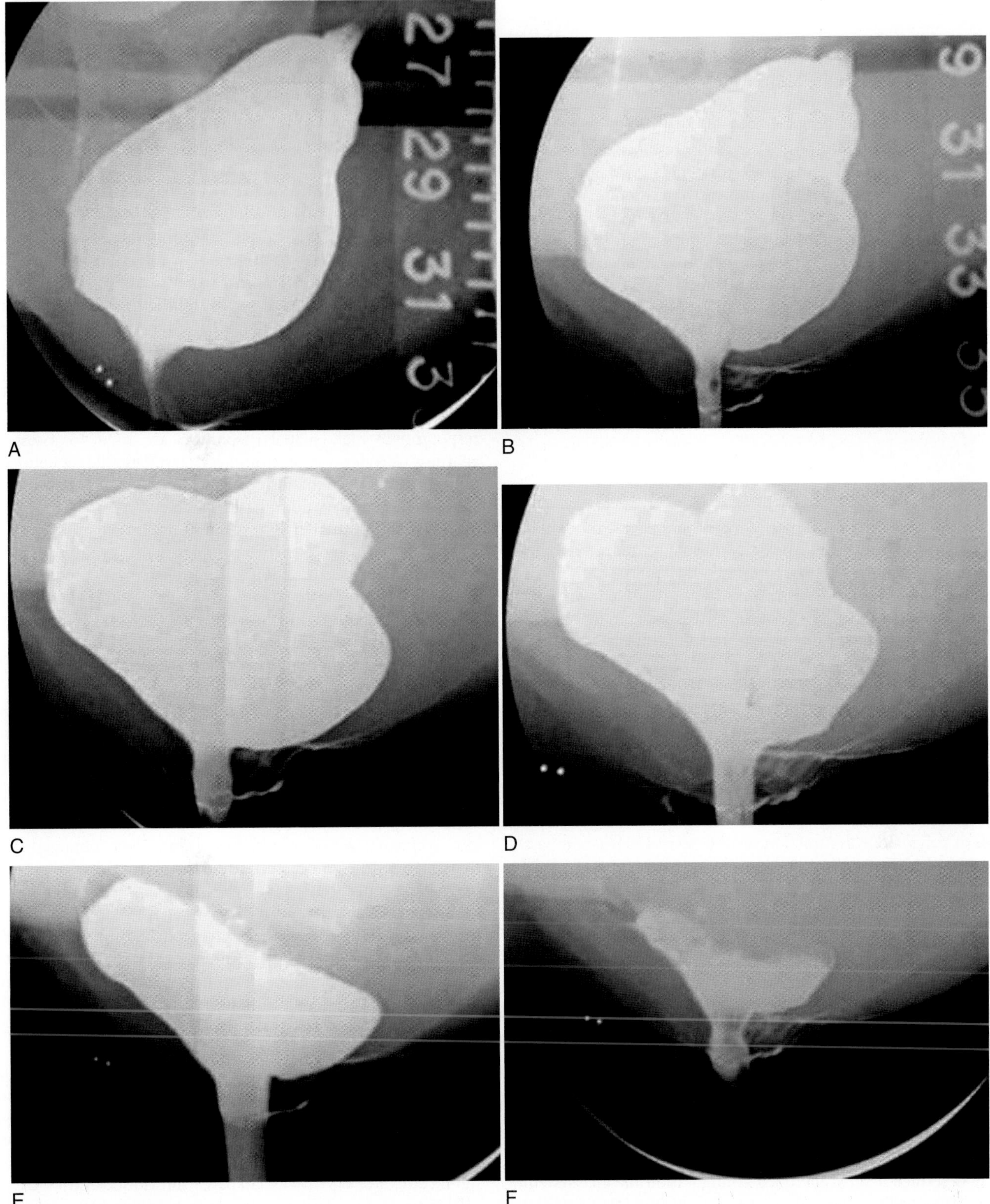

Figure 55-3 **A** through **F**, Dynamic phases of defecography, in which the patient is asked to initiate evacuation rapidly. The latest images **(E, F)** show near-complete evacuation.

Perineal Approach

In the perineal approach, the pelvic floor is imaged while the ultrasound probe is placed on the perineum. It is also possible to obtain good images of the bladder neck and pubic symphysis at rest and during Valsalva maneuvers in the sagittal plane with the probe placed over the vulva. Although the relationship of dynamic transperineal ultrasound to other, more established imaging modalities remains to be fully assessed, it has a great potential as a simple, cheap, and relatively noninvasive technique. With the perineal approach the position of the bladder neck, the puborectalis, and the anorectal angle can be measured. In addition, during straining phases, it is sometimes possible to visualize rectoceles, cystoceles, enteroceles, and rectal intussusceptions.[15] Some investigators recommend using rectal and vaginal opacification with ultrasound coupling gel during dynamic transperineal ultrasound studies. With the patient in the left lateral position and a full bladder, movement of the pelvic floor muscles is observed in the sagittal and coronal planes during straining and squeezing.[18]

Magnetic Resonance Imaging

MRI offers a myriad of advantages over other imaging modalities: lack of ionizing radiation, ease of performance, reproducibility, excellent depiction of pelvic floor soft tissues, multiplanar imaging, and, perhaps most important, its dynamic rapid acquisition capabilities.[19-23] Because MRI is capable of superior differentiation between soft tissues and fluid-filled viscera, the musculofascial support structures of the pelvic organs can be visualized.[24] By using different imaging systems, it is possible to tailor the imaging examination to the needs of the patient and the clinician. Whereas endoanal coils yield the highest-resolution images of the anal sphincter, with somewhat limited visualization of other pelvic floor structures, a body coil permits greater flexibility during the examination, because it results in a more global view of the perineum and the pelvic floor.[5] In addition, most cases of pelvic floor dysfunction involve several pelvic compartments, and MRI is an invaluable technique because it is ideally suited for simultaneous multicompartmental anatomic assessment during a given imaging study.[2,25]

The patient's prone position inside the magnet during the study is the only obvious disadvantage of using MRI, because it naturally eliminates the gravity component from the pelvic prolapse, which may be more pronounced while standing or sitting.[26] However, practically speaking, most clinical physical examinations by urologists and gynecologists are performed with the patient in the prone position. In addition, at least one study designed to compare MRI findings in the upright and supine positions found no significant differences, although the small sample size of this study could have contributed to the statistical insignificance reported by the authors.[25,27] More important, this study described a vertically open-configuration magnet system, which, albeit with artifacts, demonstrated the potential feasibility of eventually being able to conduct dynamic MRI studies with patients in upright and seated positions.[27]

Yet another group described dynamic magnetic resonance defecography with a superconducting open-configuration magnet system with the patients studied in the sitting position. The authors showed that magnetic resonance defecography is superior to fluoroscopic defecography and is a superb method for the detection of clinically relevant pelvic floor pathology.[26] Once again, this study used a small number of patients, so the findings remain to be further confirmed by larger trials. Because open MRI configuration systems still remain in the experimental stages and are not widely available, clinicians should be well aware of this potential drawback of MRI and rely on the entire clinical picture, complemented with other studies and physical examination findings, in making their final decisions. Another potential disadvantage of MRI is its unsuitability for claustrophobic patients and those with cardiac pacemakers.[24]

Given the numerous advantages of MRI in the study of pelvic organ prolapse and pelvic floor relaxation, there is a rather wide spectrum of methods used by several investigators, as opposed to a single optimal protocol. Some patients may be imaged at rest, whereas others are studied while straining or during dynamic voiding or evacuation in the MRI scanner. In addition, MRI studies have been done without contrast material, with catheters to identify the urethra, with vaginal and rectal markers, and with vaginal, urethral, rectal, and bladder contrast material.[19,28] In general, whereas classic T2-weighted static sequences with correspondingly high spatial resolution are used to assess the anatomy (e.g., levator ani trophicity), fast dynamic sequences are used to study morphologic changes during rest and contraction, straining, and evacuation phases.[4,25] The entire imaging study is usually accomplished in 20 to 25 minutes. Information obtained about peritoneal and digestive compartments is especially useful, because it allows evaluation of complex multicompartmental cases of pelvic prolapse in which physical examination appears grossly inadequate. MRI is also very useful in the assessment of postsurgical recurrences.[25]

The development of dynamic rapid T2 sequences (e.g., single-shot fast spin-echo [SSFSE], half-Fourier acquisition turbo spin-echo [HASTE], true fast imaging with steady-state precision [True FISP]) allows acquisition of superb anatomic detail during brief periods of breath-holds. Of note, no patient preparation or instrumentation is needed to complete these studies. In fact, the ureters, bladder, uterus, vagina, rectum, bowel, ovaries, and even abnormally dilated ureters may be visualized without the use of any contrast agents. More important, data obtained from dynamic MRI are more accurate than physical examination in diagnosing enteroceles, cystoceles, vaginal vault prolapse, and uterine hypermobility.[24] From a surgical point of view, MRI clearly identifies the ovaries, which greatly aids in the decision to perform oophorectomy at the time of hysterectomy if certain abnormalities are present during the preoperative imaging workup of patients. In addition, one is able to visualize other important pelvic pathology, such as uterine leiomyomas, ureteral dilatation, and other pelvic masses.[29]

Opponents of MRI bring up the issue of the costliness of this diagnostic modality. Some investigators concluded in their studies of the economic aspects of MRI that there is a paucity of evidence in the literature to guide such decisions. Yet others have reported that dynamic MRI of the pelvis may be designed to be significantly less expensive than pelvic ultrasound and VCUG. An MRI time of 15 minutes or less may help decrease cost.[4] Most likely, it is these latter factors that will eventually lead to greater cost-effectiveness of MRI for pelvic floor disorders across numerous medical centers in the country.

Data Analysis Using Magnetic Resonance Imaging Data

Results of the MRI are analyzed with respect to pelvic organ position at rest and during contraction and straining phases relative to anatomic landmarks.[29] The latter are in turn divided into fixed and mobile landmarks. The so-called pubococcygeal line (PCL) comprises the fixed landmark, and although there are slight variations among various investigators as to the exact manner of its delineation, it essentially extends from the inferior aspect of the pubis to the sacrococcygeal joint. Mobile landmarks consist of the bladder neck, urethra, uterine cervix (or vaginal vault in cases of hysterectomy), the lowest point of the peritoneum, and the rectoanal junction for the posterior compartment. By measuring the distance between the mobile landmarks and the PCL during the straining phases of the study, one is able to comment on the presence and degree of corresponding pelvic floor prolapse and the organs involved.[25,29]

A rather simple and objective grading system, called the HMO system, has been proposed to quantify pelvic floor relaxation and prolapse and to differentiate between organ prolapse and pelvic floor descent by using MRI images.[24,29] These two terms are often are used synonymously, but they are not interchangeable and should be differentiated. Pelvic floor relaxation is composed of hiatal enlargement and pelvic floor descent, two entities defined clearly by the HMO classification system (Fig. 55-4). The so-called H-line (Levator hiatus width) measures the width of the levator hiatus and refers to the distance from the pubis to the posterior anal canal; it represents the hiatal enlargement. The M-line (muscular pelvic floor relaxation) represents the descent of the levator plate from the PCL and measures the muscular pelvic floor relaxation. With significant pelvic floor relaxation, one is able to demonstrate levator hiatal widening and levator plate descent, as indicated by corresponding increases in the H and M lines on MRI data (Fig. 55-5).

Whereas the H and M measurements are used to demonstrate pelvic floor descent, the so-called O-component of the HMO system gives a grading to the visceral (organ) prolapse. For all of the pelvic organs involved (i.e., cystocele, urethrocele, rectocele, enterocele, or uterine descent), the prolapse is defined as the degree of visceral descent beyond the H-line.[24,29] By obtaining these measurements on dynamic MRI obtained with very fast MRI sequences, one can readily differentiate between pelvic organ descent and pelvic floor prolapse and grade the degree of

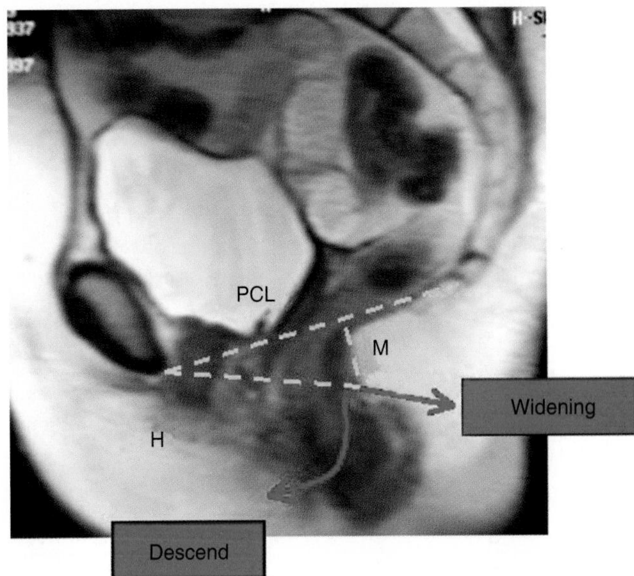

Figure 55-4 Reference lines drawn on a resting sagittal magnetic resonance image demonstrating two components of pelvic floor prolapse (descend and widening) in the HMO classification system. Descent is measured by descent of the H-line relative to the pubococcygeal line (PCL) and thus an increasing M, whereas widening is seen by increase in the anteroposterior dimension of the hiatus and thus lengthening of the H line. See text for details.

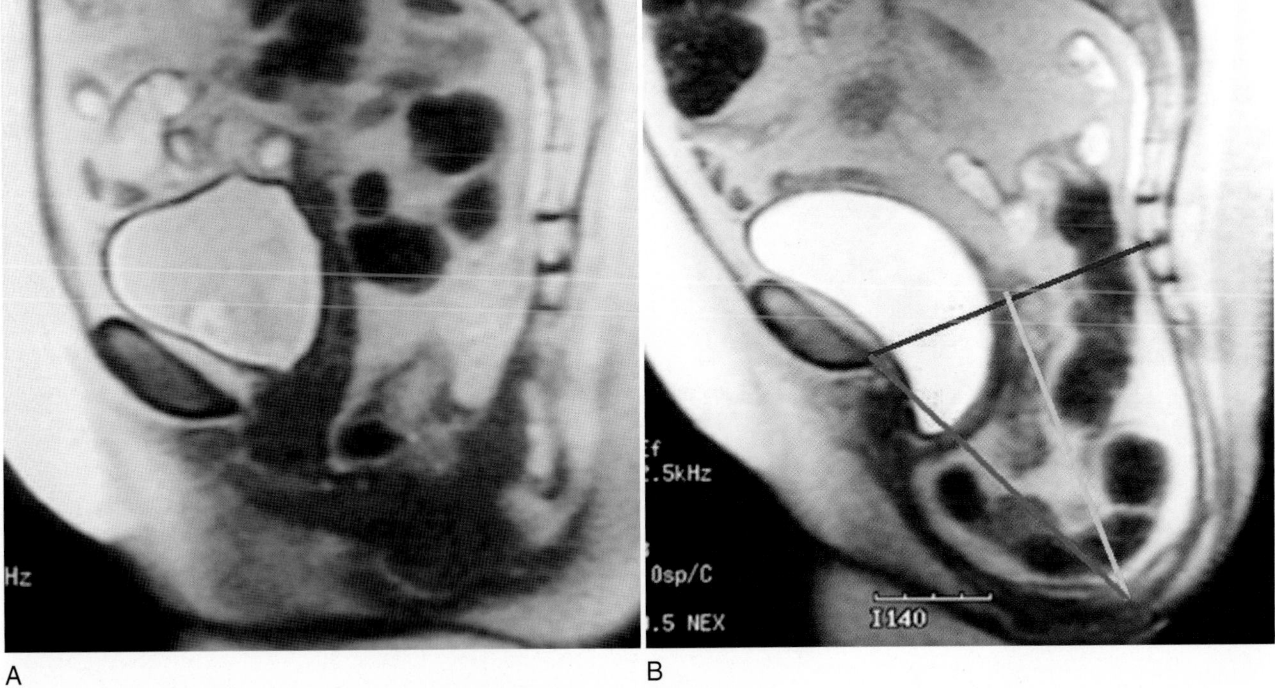

Figure 55-5 **A,** Resting phase magnetic resonance image (MRI). **B,** A severe perineal hernia is appreciated on the MRI in the dynamic phase. The reference lines are drawn on the image to illustrate the accompanying pelvic floor prolapse, with a tremendous increase in the M-line (*yellow*).

pelvic floor abnormalities (Tables 55-1 and 55-2). In addition to being rather simple and reproducible, the HMO grading system allows better definition and understanding of the pathology involved by enabling differentiation between pelvic organ descent and pelvic organ prolapse.[29]

Table 55-1 Proposed Pelvic Organ Prolapse Grading System Using Dynamic Magnetic Resonance Imaging Data

Grade	Organ Location
0 (no prolapse)	Above H-line
1 (mild, small)	0-2 cm below H-line
2 (moderate)	2-4 cm below H-line
3 (severe, large)	>4 cm below H-line
4 (procidentia)	Only for cystourethrocele

From Barbaric ZL, Marumoto AK, Raz S: Magnetic resonance imaging of the perineum and pelvic floor. Topics Magn Res Imaging 12:83-92, 2001.

Table 55-2 Proposed Pelvic Floor Descent (Length of the M-Line) Grading System Using Dynamic Magnetic Resonance Imaging Data

Grade	Pelvic Floor Descent (cm)
0 (normal)	0-2
1 (mild)	2-4
2 (moderate)	4-6
3 (severe)	>6

From Barbaric ZL, Marumoto AK, Raz S: Magnetic resonance imaging of the perineum and pelvic floor. Topics Magn Res Imaging 12:83-92, 2001.

Regardless of the exact classification system used to interpret the MRI data, the standard radiologic report includes information on the presence of any incidental lesions (ovarian, uterine, gastrointestinal tract); the morphology of the levator ani muscles; pelvic organ position at rest, during contraction, and during maximum straining; the degree of prolapse; and any coexisting masked prolapse in addition to the main prominent prolapse.[25] According to current studies, MRI appears to be at least equivalent to physical examination for prolapse detection in the anterior pelvic compartments such as the bladder and uterus, and it is superior to the clinical examination in cases of posterior compartment prolapse such as peritoneal and gastrointestinal organs.[30-33] Yet another advantage of MRI over some of the other methods, such as conventional defecography, is lower interobserver variability in the interpretation of the imaging studies.[28]

Three-dimensional Magnetic Resonance Imaging

Three-dimensional MRI represents an advanced method of presentation and interpretation of data obtained during MRI studies (Fig. 55-6). It has been gaining popularity among investigators in the field, because it enables volumetric analysis of the data and demonstrates with remarkable clarity the spatial relationships among the anatomic structures of interest.[34] For instance, this method has been applied to better define the levator ani morphology and to demonstrate, not only qualitatively but also quantitatively, the pathologic changes involved in various grades of pelvic prolapse.[35-37] Although these findings have not been applied to clinical practice as yet, they could potentially be important in generating treatment plans for patients, predicting the course of progression of prolapse severity, and even predicting the likelihood of recurrence after corrective surgery.[34]

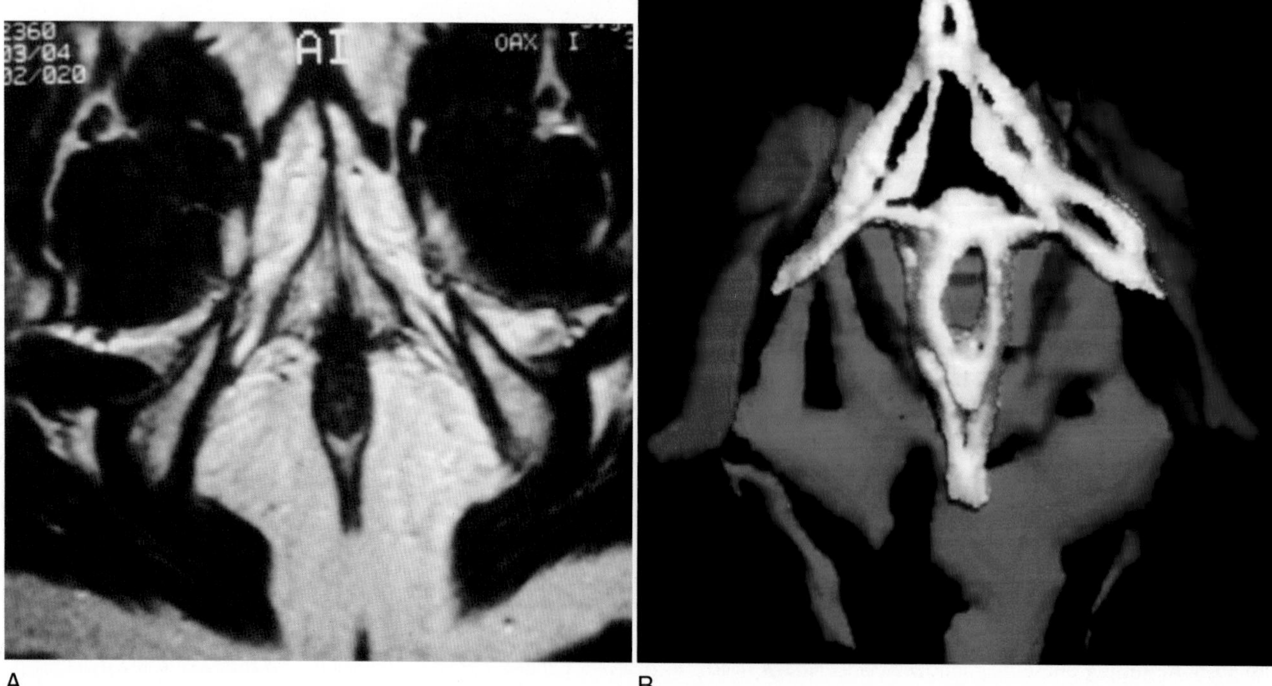

Figure 55-6 Image of perineum shown in conventional magnetic resonance imaging **(A)** and in three-dimensional reconstruction **(B)**.

Computed Tomography

Computed tomography (CT) scanning allows multiplanar visualization of anatomy and becomes especially useful for patients who are unable to tolerate MRI due to the presence of medical devices such as pacemakers, general debilitation, or claustrophobia. However, even though CT is a well-established axial imaging modality, it has limited application in the field of female pelvic prolapse simply because of anatomic limitations. The urogenital diaphragm and levator ani are mostly situated in the axial plane, they are best assessed by coronal imaging. However, with traditional CT, one is able to obtain coronal images only by reformatting the axial images, resulting in loss of spatial resolution during the process and inevitable degradation of the image quality.[5] Because of these factors, very little attention has been paid in the field of radiology to CT scanning as a possible imaging modality for female pelvic floor dysfunction.

A preliminary study using a small number of patients explored the use of CT scanning in the diagnosis of prolapse of female pelvic organs and commented on its potential role in patients intolerant of MRI.[38] Despite the fact that the soft tissue contrast on CT if far inferior to that of MRI, it was possible to identify the bladder, uterus, small bowel, peritoneal fat, and rectum, as well as changes in position with straining, if CT was performed adequately. Another possible advantage of CT scanning is its ability to assess the contour of the levator ani muscles and obtain pelvic images in multiple planes. Both modalities image the patient while supine, thus introducing the possibility of suboptimal results in this nonphysiologic position, especially if the patient's straining is suboptimal.[38] With further evolution of CT technology, such as availability of multiple-detector-row CT scanners and lower image acquisition times, it might be possible to obtain dynamic images almost in real time. In addition, the possibility of acquiring thinner slices will potentially lead to decreased artifacts during volume rendering. However, as with fluoroscopy, radiation exposure will always remain a major concern with CT scanning.

CLINICAL APPLICATIONS

Cystoceles

In an ideal world, imaging studies used in the evaluation of cystoceles should yield information on the presence or absence of urinary retention, ureteral obstruction, urethral hypermobility, and other forms of pelvic floor prolapse, as well as evaluation for stress urinary incontinence, in the least invasive manner to the patient.[3] Radiographically, a cystocele usually appears during the maximal straining phase of the imaging study as descent of the normally horizontal bladder base below the inferior margin of the pubic symphysis and as a concave impression on the superior aspect of the vagina.[5] Traditionally, a VCUG and videourodynamics with the patient standing in both straining and relaxed states have been performed as part of the workup for cystoceles. Although these studies are helpful in the evaluation of cystocele severity, postvoid residual volume, stress urinary incontinence, and urethral hypermobility, they fail to comment on the presence of related pelvic floor dysfunction.[3] Because of this drawback of the technique, fluoroscopic cystocolpoproctography or dynamic contrast roentgenography with pelvic organ opacification have been used to determine the presence of related pelvic floor prolapse. However, these studies fail to detect up to 20 % of enteroceles, are time-consuming, and expose the patient to ionizing radiation.[1,11,30-32,39,40]

Even though ultrasonography does not have the drawback of radiation exposure to the patient, it fails to provide optimal visualization of soft tissue planes and is extremely operator dependent.[41]

MRI lacks most of these shortcomings and has numerous advantages previously mentioned.[4,19,24] Studies have shown a very high degree of correlation between dynamic MRI and lateral cystourethrography.[42] The only possible disadvantage of MRI is the fact that, because it is performed with the patient in the supine position, the physiologic effect of gravity cannot be studied.[3] With dynamic MRI, one is able to both quantitate the degree of a cystocele present and diagnose any coexisting pelvic floor descent (Figs. 55-7 and 55-8).

Enteroceles

Before the introduction of MRI to the study of female pelvic prolapse, defecography was the primary modality in the diagnostic workup of enteroceles (Figs. 55-9 and 55-10). In order to visualize the small bowel loops between the rectum and the vagina, indicative of an enterocele, the patient is asked to strain repeatedly after evacuation. Very often, opacification of the vagina is also necessary to better visualize the pathology.[5] In some cases, voiding cystograms were performed to rule out a cystocele. Later, fluoroscopic cystocolpoproctography or dynamic contrast roentgenography gained popularity. These studies involve opacification of the bladder, vagina, small bowel, and rectum in order to visualize pelvic prolapse. Even though triphasic opacification is more time-consuming, it has been shown to improve recognition of enteroceles during the examination.

In addition to performing the imaging study with all organs opacified at the same time, one can also choose to opacify each organ individually before each straining phase.[1,31,32,39] The diagnosis of an enterocele is made by comparing the images obtained during the straining phase of the study with those recorded during relaxation. Here, an increase in the distance between the vagina and the rectum, which are delineated by the contrast material, is suggestive of an enterocele. Occasionally, physiologic bowel gas bubbles in the contents of this herniated small bowel may be seen to further identify it as such.[30] Unfortunately, in addition to being rather time-consuming and invasive, defecography and cystocolpoproctography fail to detect enteroceles in up to 20% of cases.[3,11,30,40]

Before the introduction of MRI into the field, many considered multiphasic cystocolpoproctography to be the best-suited imaging modality for detection of female organ prolapse (Fig. 55-11). However, many experts now believe that dynamic MRI is a superior radiographic technique in the diagnosis of enteroceles and that the invasiveness of organ opacification is not justified in the light of the very minimal yield of additional information, if any.[3,4,30,32] Studies have shown repeatedly that MRI is far more sensitive than physical examination and dynamic cystocolpoproctography in the diagnosis of enteroceles.[4,30] The diagnosis of an enterocele on an MRI study is made by measuring the distance between the lowest point of the peritoneal borderline and the H (hiatal) anteroposterior reference line obtained during the dynamic (straining) phases of the study. In fact, magnetic resonance colpocystorectography, which utilizes sonography gel to opacify the vagina and the rectum, is the only method available

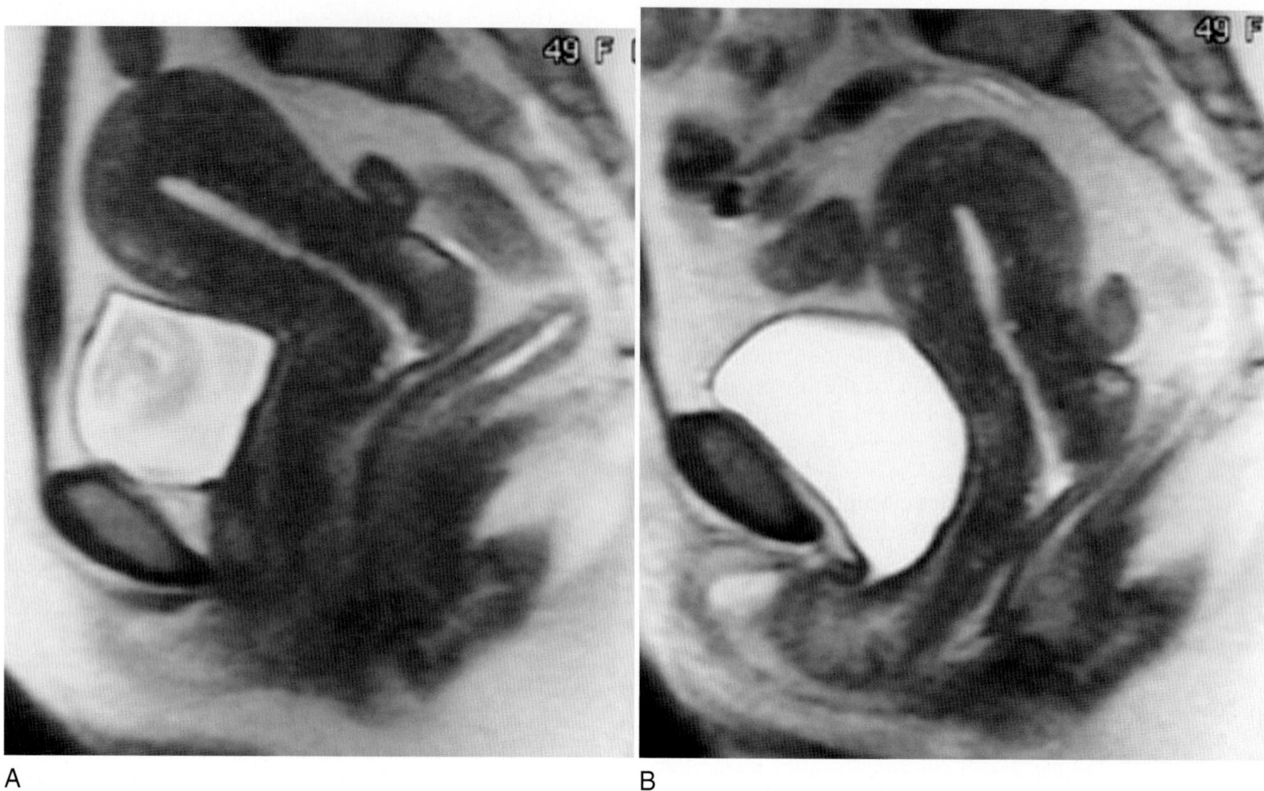

Figure 55-7 Magnetic resonance images showing a cystocele in resting position **(A)** and with pelvic floor descent appreciated on straining **(B).**

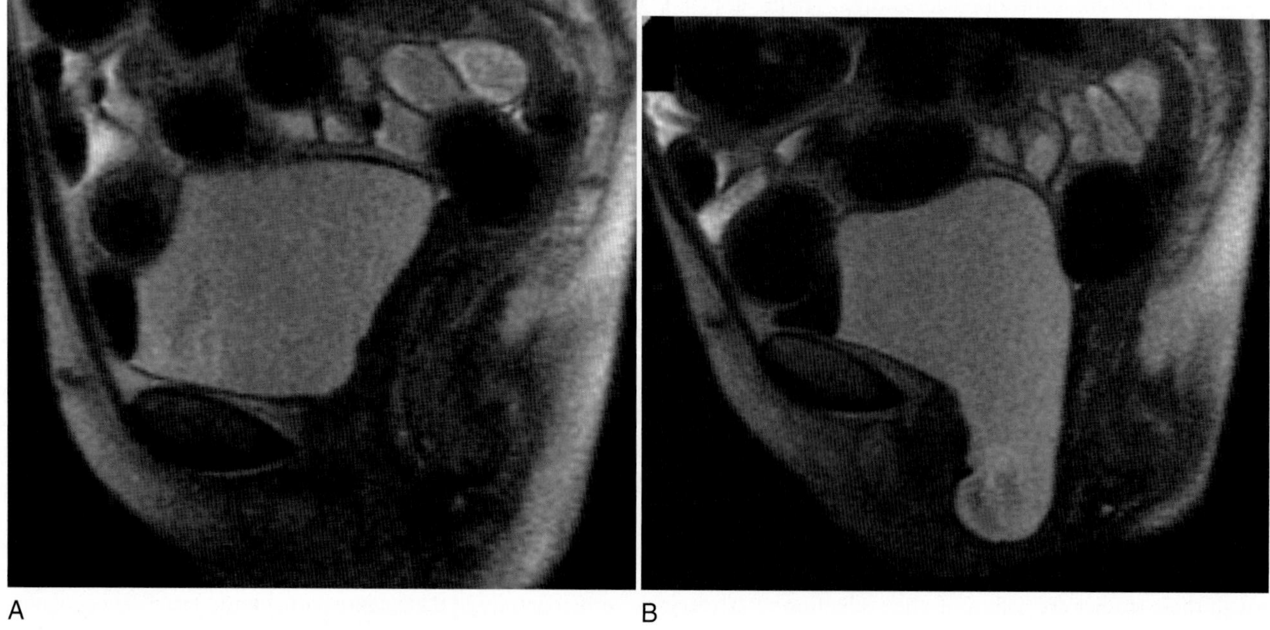

Figure 55-8 Magnetic resonance images in resting **(A)** and dynamic **(B)** phases, demonstrating pelvic floor prolapse and severe cystocele in a 52-year-old woman with complaints of vaginal prolapse and frequency.

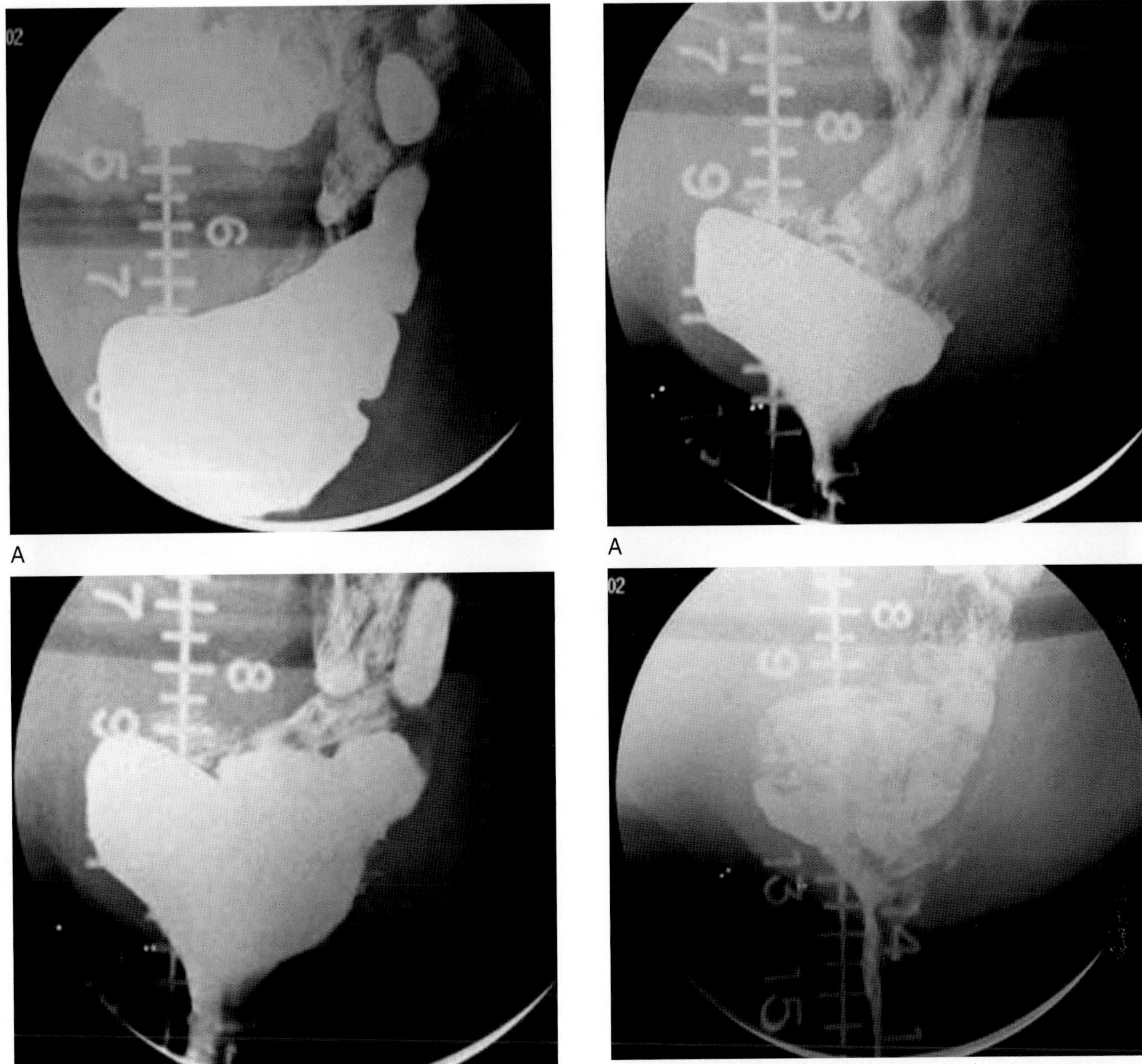

Figure 55-9 A and **B**, Enteroceles shown on dynamic evacuation proctography images.

Figure 55-10 A and **B**, Enterocele with pelvic floor prolapse demonstrated on dynamic defecography study.

that can precisely visualize the parietal peritoneum, thus allowing one to make the diagnosis of an enterocele with utmost confidence.[30] An isolated enterocele can be differentiated from one present as part of a combined organ prolapse, and any other coexisting conditions can be diagnosed as well (Fig. 55-12). More importantly, MRI enables the differentiation of contents of enteroceles, revealing such entities as mesenteric fat, rectosigmoidoceles, and small and large bowel. In fact, by taking into account the axial turbo spin echo sequences, often one is able to differentiate sigmoid colon from small bowel loops. On the contrary, hernias containing mostly fluid and components of the mesenteric tissue give a homogenous intense signal on the T2-weighted images. In addition, this method of visualization of the herniated contents does not require prior additional measures (e.g., small bowel opacification) to be taken.

Many urologists find MRI particularly useful in differentiating high rectoceles from enteroceles, which is an important distinction as far as safe and efficient surgical planning is concerned.[3-4,30] Because it does not expose patients to ionizing radiation, MRI also has the advantage of no time pressure constraints and gives patients more flexibility and control during repeated phases of straining which often needed to visualize pelvic floor defects.

For completeness, comments should be made about the utility of ultrasonography and defecoperitoneography in the diagnosis

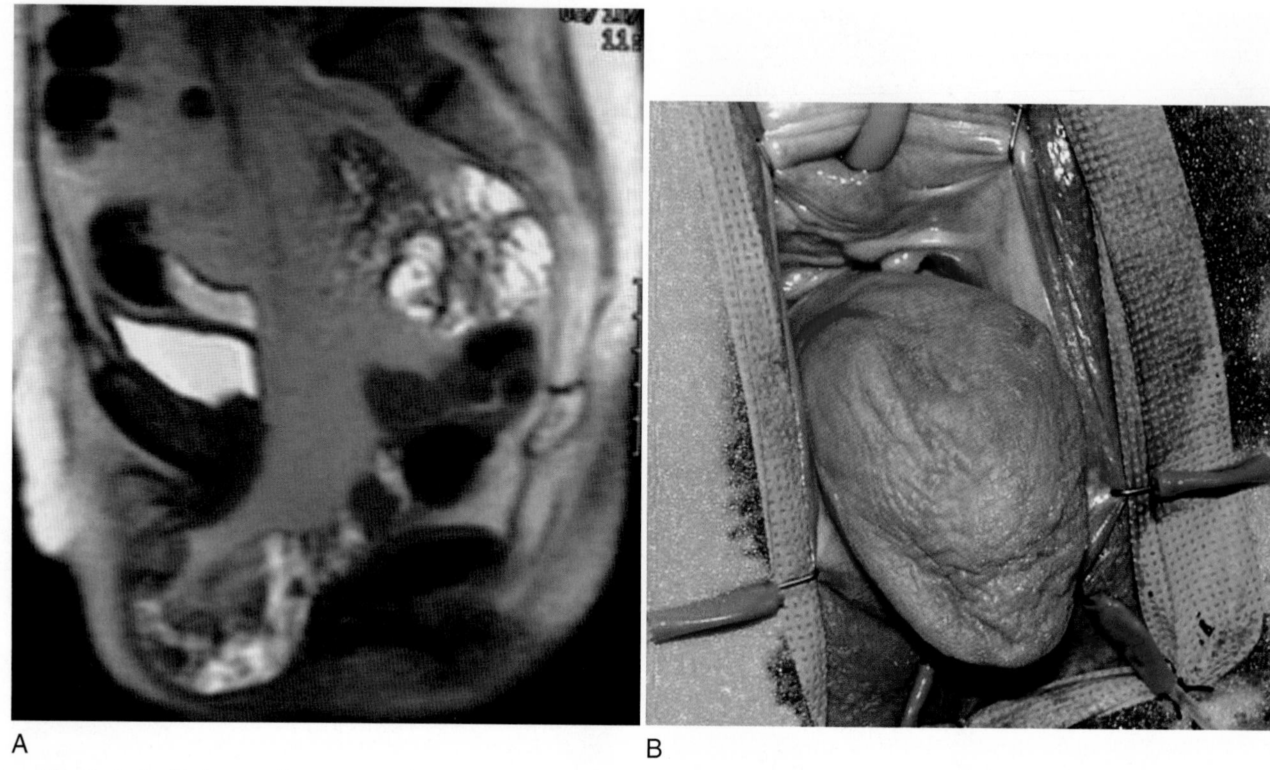

Figure 55-11 A, Sagittal magnetic resonance image showing an enterocele on dynamic phase. B, Corresponding operating room findings.

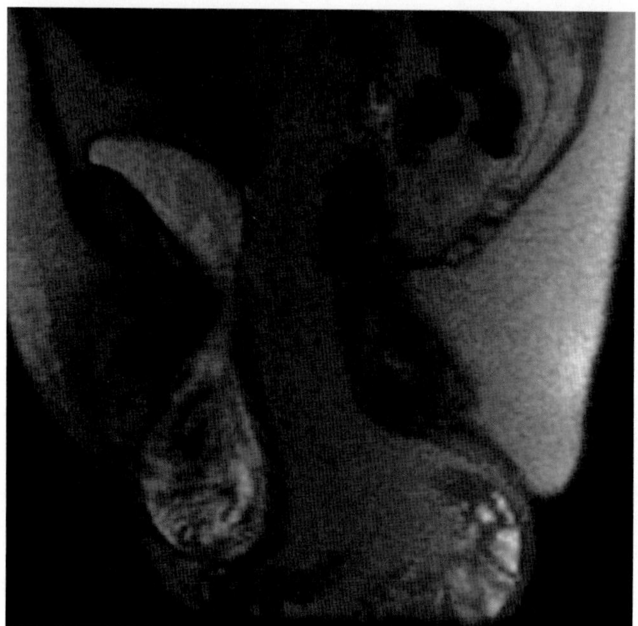

Figure 55-12 Large cystocele and an enterocele in a patient with chronic frequency, nocturia, urgency, urge incontinence, and history of urine leaks with standing appreciated on a dynamic sagittal magnetic resonance image.

of enteroceles. It is possible to indirectly visualize the intestinal loops in the herniated sack as a dorsal attenuation with endovaginal sonography. However, this examination is rather difficult, because it requires a firm and stable contact between the ultrasound probe and the vaginal wall, even during repeated straining phases of the examination.[17]

Defecoperitoneography is a combination of a small-bowel enteroclysm, evacuation proctography, and intra-abdominal puncture.[43,44] Even though magnetic resonance colpocystorectography is comparable to defecoperitoneography in its time-consuming aspects, the latter is a much more invasive procedure associated with several rather morbid complications (e.g., perforation).[45] In addition, defecoperiotoneography misses many cases of enteroceles, because the radiation dose with this technique forbids more than one round of straining, and several rounds of repeated straining and defecation are often required to induce and visualize organ prolapse during a given study.[30,46] Therefore, MRI is a superior technique in the diagnosis of enteroceles or peritoneoceles, because it is highly specific, sensitive, versatile, noninvasive, radiation-free, and relatively safe.

Rectoceles

Because physical examination has a wide range of sensitivities for diagnosis of rectoceles and is unreliable in differentiating enteroceles from high rectoceles, imaging modalities are very helpful in the diagnostic workup of suspected rectoceles.[3] Defecography has

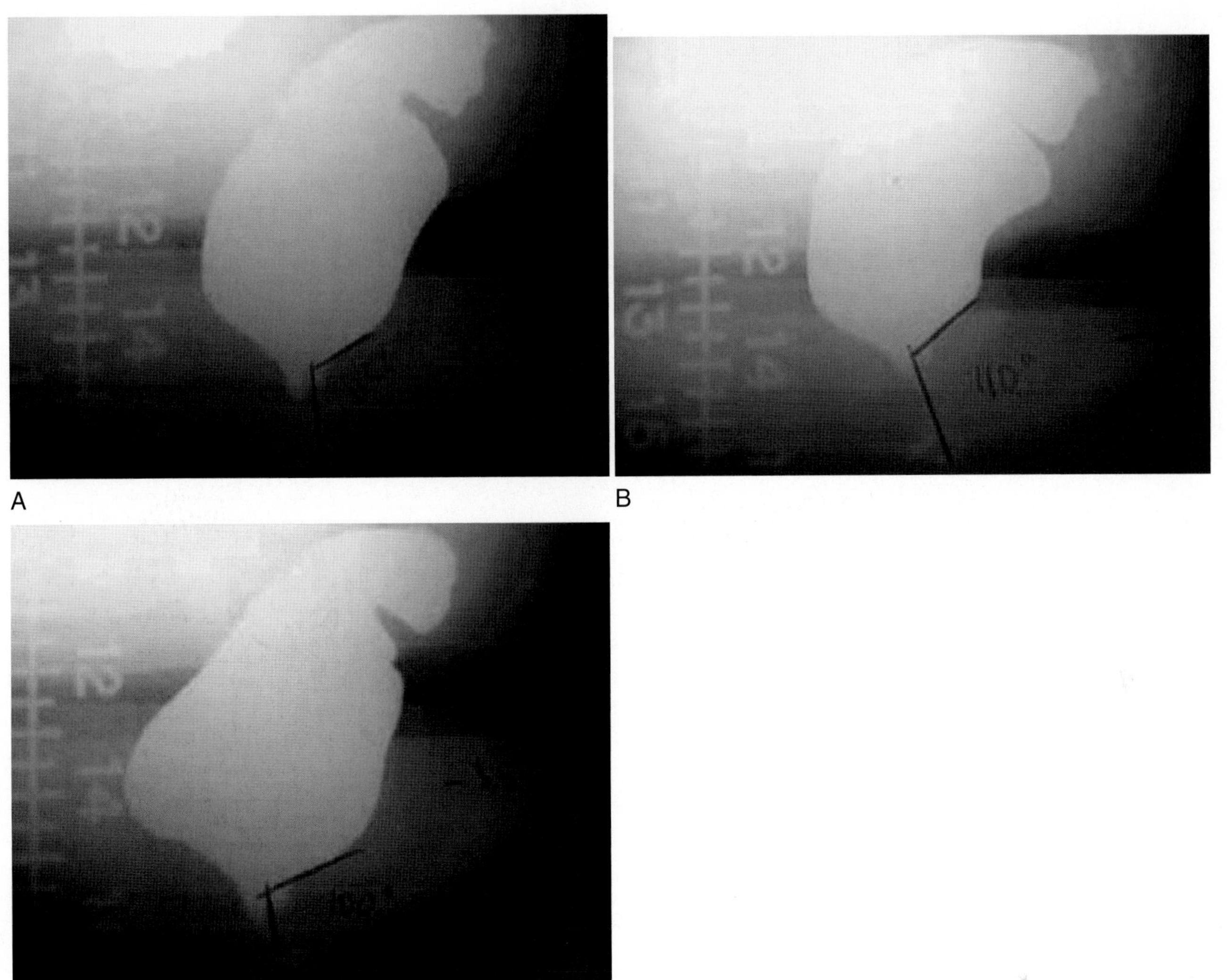

Figure 55-13 Resting (A), squeezing (B), and straining (C) phases of a defecography study.

been traditionally the study of choice for rectoceles (Fig. 55-13). A rectocele usually appears as an anterior bulge in the extrapolated line of the normal rectal wall that appears with evacuation or strain and is measured as the maximum extent of that bulge (Fig. 55-14).[10] It should be noted that, because rectoceles quite often appear as transient findings during defecography, many prefer to obtain and review the videotape of the evacuation process.[5] To evaluate for other concurrent forms of pelvic prolapse, dynamic contrast roentography or fluoroscopic cystocolpoproctography has been used by various investigators.[1,3,31,32,39] However, all of these techniques have the disadvantage of significant radiation exposure and poor visualization of soft tissues in the evaluation of the pelvic floor. MRI eliminates all of these flaws and allows superb visualization of soft tissue structures and concurrent pelvic floor pathology (Fig. 55-15). Studies seem to indicate that rectal opacification should be used to increase the detection rates of rectoceles with MRI. This usually entails the introduction of sonographic transmission gel into the rectum, which yields a high signal on T2-weighted MRI sequences. Some radiologists prefer to mix it with diluted gadolinium contrast medium for easier visualization. The only caveat to this method is the fact that it can introduce air bubbles and thus image artifacts.[4,25,32] It has been theorized that MRI fails to detect small rectoceles due to collapse of the walls of the empty rectum during the imaging study.[3,4]

Uterine Prolapse

From a surgical perspective, while evaluating high grade uterine prolapse, it is critical to rule out any kind of uterine or ovarian malignancy, in order to decide on the kind of hysterectomy to be performed. MRI is an ideal imaging modality, because it allows evaluation for all forms of pelvic pathology preoperatively (Fig. 55-16).[3]

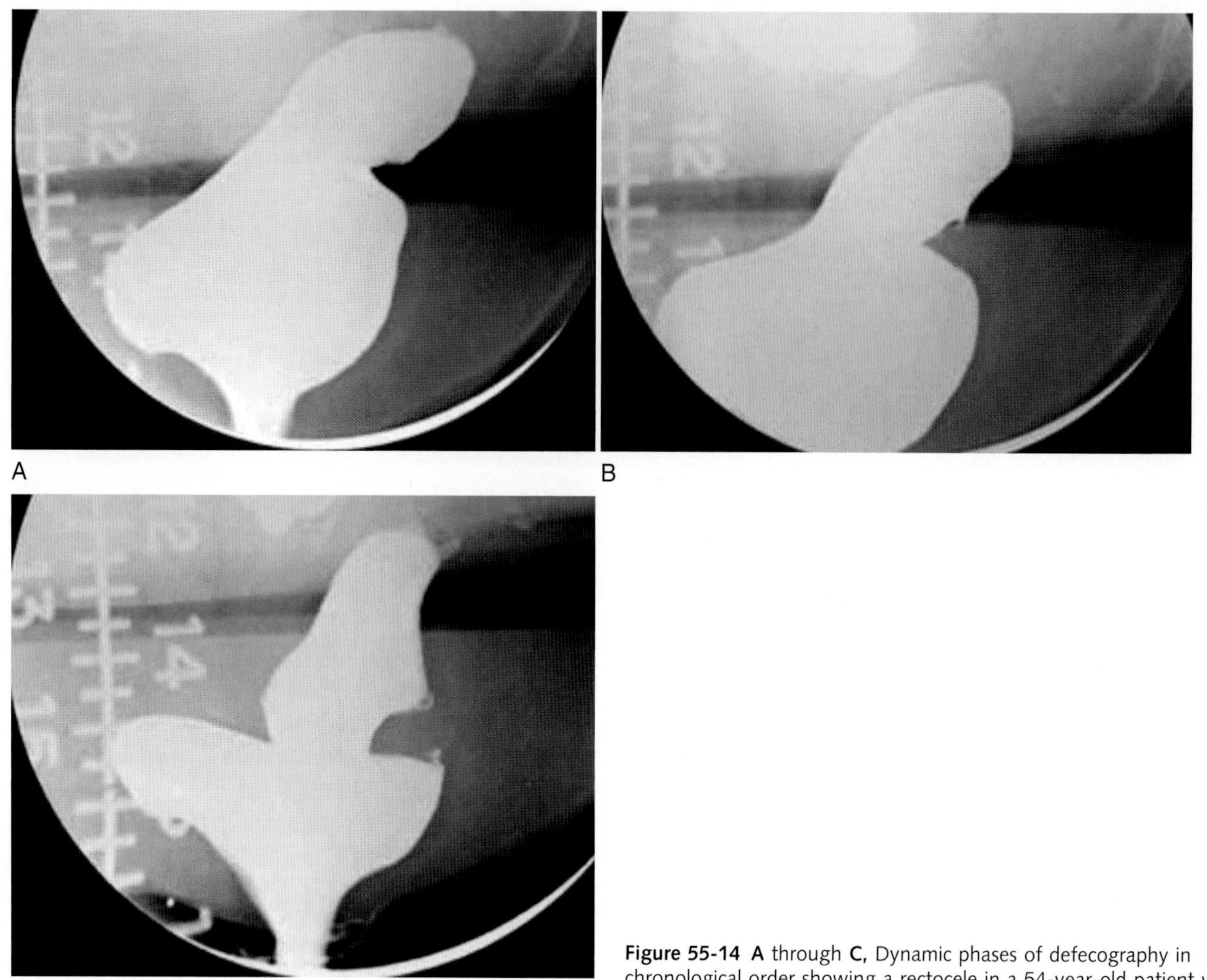

Figure 55-14 **A** through **C,** Dynamic phases of defecography in chronological order showing a rectocele in a 54-year-old patient with chronic constipation.

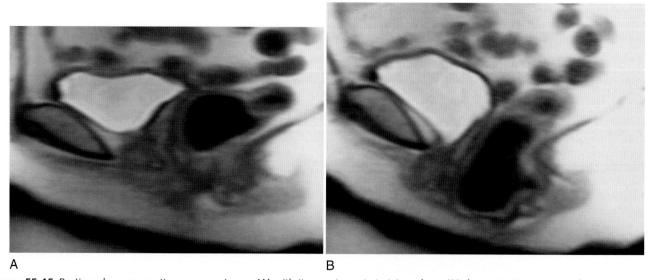

Figure 55-15 Resting phase magnetic resonance image **(A)** with its counterpart straining phase **(B)** demonstrating a rectocele.

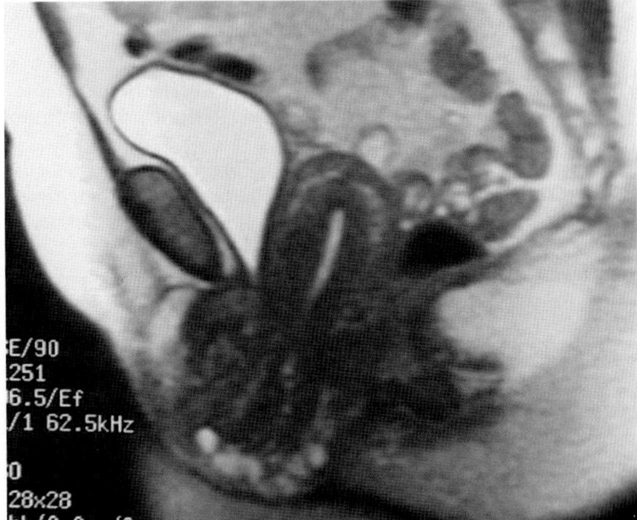

Figure 55-16 Uterine prolapse appreciated on dynamic magnetic resonance sagittal image.

References

1. Altringer WE, Saclarides TJ, Dominguez JM, et al: Four-contrast defecography: Pelvic "floor-oscopy." Dis Colon Rectum 38:695-699, 1995.
2. Maglinte DD, Kelvin FM, Fitzgerald K, et al: Association of compartment defects in pelvic floor dysfunction. AJR Am J Roentgenol 172:439-444, 1999.
3. Rodriguez LV, Raz S: Diagnostic imaging of pelvic floor dysfunction. Curr Opin Urol 11:423-428, 2001.
4. Gousse AE, Barbaric ZL, Safir MH, et al: Dynamic half Fourier acquisition single shot turbo spin-echo magnetic resonance imaging for evaluating the female pelvis. J Urol 164:1606-1613, 2000.
5. Weidner AC, Low VHS: Imaging studies of the pelvic floor. Obstet Gynecol Clin North Am 25:825-848, 1998.
6. Halligan S: Evacuation proctography. In Bartram CI, DeLancey JOL (eds): Imaging Pelvic Floor Disorders. Berlin: Springer-Verlag, 2003, pp 45-50.
7. Halligan S, Bartram CI, Park HY, Kamm MA: The proctographic features of anismus. Radiology 197:679-682, 1995.
8. Freimanis MG, Wald A, Caruana B, Bauman DH: Evacuation proctography in normal volunteers. Invest Radiol 26:581-585, 1991.
9. Ott DJ, Donati DL, Kerr RM, Chen MY: Defecography: Results in 55 patients and impact on clinical management. Abdom Imaging 19:349-354, 1994.
10. Shorvon PJ, McHugh S, Diamant NE, et al: Defecography in normal volunteers: Results and implications. Gut 30:1737-1749, 1989.
11. Hock D, Lombard R, Jehaes C, et al: Colpocystodefecography. Dis Colon Rectum 36:1015-1021, 1993.
12. Kelvin FM, Pannu HK: Dynamic cystoproctography: Fluoroscopic and MRI techniques for evaluating pelvic organ prolapse. In Bartram CI, DeLancey JOL (eds): Imaging Pelvic Floor Disorders. Berlin: Springer-Verlag, 2003, pp 51-68.
13. Frudinger A, Bartram CI, Kamm MA: Transvaginal versus anal endosonography for detecting damage to the anal sphincter. AJR Am J Roentgenol 168:1435-1438, 1997.
14. Frudinger A, Bartram CI, Halligan S, Kamm M: Examination techniques for endosonography of the anal canal. Abdom Imaging 23:301-303, 1998.
15. Bartram CI: Ultrasound. In Bartram CI, DeLancey JOL (eds): Imaging Pelvic Floor Disorders. Berlin: Springer-Verlag, 2003, pp 69-79.
16. Quinn MJ, Beynon J, Mortensen NJ, Smith PJ: Transvaginal endosonography: A new method to study the anatomy of the lower urinary tract in urinary stress incontinence. Br J Urol 62:414-418, 1988.
17. Halligan S, Northover J, Bartram CI: Vaginal sonography to diagnose enterocele. Br J Radiol 69:996-999, 1996.
18. Beer-Gabel M, Teshler M, Barzilai N, et al: Dynamic transperineal ultrasound in the diagnosis of pelvic floor disorders: Pilot study. Dis Colon Rectum 45:239-245, 2002.
19. Lienemann A, Anthuber C, Baron A, et al: Dynamic MR colpocystorectography assessing pelvic floor descent. Eur Radiol 7:1309-1317, 1997.
20. Bump RC, Norton PA: Urogynecology and pelvic floor dysfunction: Epidemiology and natural history of pelvic floor dysfunction. Obstet Gynecol Clin North Am 25:723-746, 1998.
21. Maubon A, Martel-Boncoeur MP, Juhan V, et al: Static and dynamic magnetic resonance imaging of the pelvic floor. J Radiol 81(12 Suppl):1875-1886, 2000.
22. Stoker J, Halligan S, Bartram CI: Pelvic floor imaging. Radiology 218:621-641, 2001.
23. Pannu HK, Kaufman HS, Cundiff GW, et al: Dynamic MR imaging of pelvic organ prolapse: Spectrum of abnormalities. Radiographics 20:1567-1582, 2000.
24. Comiter CV, Vasavada SP, Barbaric ZL, et al: Grading pelvic floor prolapse and pelvic floor relaxation using dynamic magnetic resonance imaging. Urology 54:454-457, 1999.
25. Maubon A, Aubard Y, Berkane V, et al: Magnetic resonance imaging of the pelvic floor. Abdom Imaging 28:217-225, 2003.
26. Schoenenberger AW, Debatin JF, Guldenschuh I, et al: Dynamic MR defecography with a superconducting, open-configuration MR system. Radiology 206:641-646, 1998.
27. Fielding JR, Versi E, Mulkern RV, et al: MR imaging of the female pelvic floor in the supine and upright position. J Magn Reson Imaging 6:961-963, 1996.
28. Yang A, Mostwin JL, Rosenshein NB, Zerhouni EA: Pelvic floor descent in women: Dynamic evaluation with fast MR imaging and cinematic display. Radiology 179:25-33, 1991.
29. Barbaric ZL, Marumoto AK, Raz S: Magnetic resonance imaging of the perineum and pelvic floor. Topics Magn Res Imaging 12:83-92, 2001.
30. Lienemann A, Anthuber C, Baron A, Reuser M: Diagnosing enteroceles using dynamic magnetic resonance imaging. Dis Colon Rectum 43:205-212, 2000.
31. Kelvin FM, Hale DS, Maglinte DD, et al: Female pelvic organ prolapse: diagnostic contribution of dynamic cystoproctography and comparison with physical examination. AJR Am J Roentgenol 173:31-37, 1999.
32. Kelvin FM, Maglinte DDT, Hale DS, Benson JT: Female pelvic organ prolapse: A comparison of triphasic dynamic MR imaging and tri-

phasic fluoroscopic cystocolpoproctography. AJR Am J Roentgenol 174:81-84, 2000.
33. Rentsch M, Paetzel CH, Lenhart M, et al: Dynamic magnetic resonance imaging defecography: A diagnostic alternative in the assessment of pelvic floor disorders in proctology. Dis Colon Rectum 44:999-1007, 2001.
34. Singh K, Jakab M, Reid WMN, et al: Three-dimensional magnetic resonance imaging assessment of levator ani morphologic features in different grades of prolapse. Am J Obstet Gynecol 188:910-915, 2003.
35. Fielding JR, Dumanli H, Schreyer AG, et al: MR-based three-dimensional modeling of the normal pelvic floor in women: quantification of muscle mass. AJR Am J Roentgenol 174:657-660, 2000.
36. Hoyte L, Fielding JR, Versi E, et al: Variations in levator ani volume and geometry in women: The application of MR based 3D reconstruction in evaluating pelvic floor dysfunction. Arch Esp Urol 54:532-539, 2001.
37. Hoyte L, Schierlitz L, Zou K, et al: Two- and 3-dimensional MRI comparison of levator ani structure, volume, and integrity in women with stress incontinence and prolapse. Am J Obstet Gynecol 185:11-19, 2001.
38. Pannu HK, Genadry R, Kaufman HS, Fishman EK: Computed tomography evaluation of pelvic organ prolapse. J Comput Assist Tomogr 27:779-785, 2003.
39. Takano M, Hamada A: Evaluation of pelvic descent disorders by dynamic contrast reontography. Dis Colon Rectum 43:S6-S11, 2000.
40. Brubaker L, Retzky S, Smith C, Saclarides T: Pelvic floor evaluation with dynamic fluoroscopy. Obstet Gynecol 82:863-868, 1993.
41. Mouritsen L: Techniques for imaging bladder support. Acta Obstet Gynecol Scand Suppl 166:48-49, 1997.
42. Gufler H, DeGreforio G, Allman KH, et al: Comparison of cystourethrography and dynamic MRI in bladder neck descent. J Comput Assist Tomogr 24:382-388, 2000.
43. Bremmer S, Ahlback SO, Uden R, Mellgren A: Simultaneous defecography and peritoneography in defecation disorders. Dis Colon Rectum 38:969-973, 1995.
44. Sentovich SM, Rivela LJ, Thorson AG, et al: Simultaneous dynamic proctography and peritoneography for pelvic floor disorders. Dis Colon Rectum 38:912-915, 1995.
45. Ekberg O: Complications after herniography in adults. AJR Am J Roentgenol 140:491-495, 1983.
46. Goei R, Kemerink G: Radiation dose in defecography. Radiology 176:137-139, 1990.

Chapter 56

DYNAMIC MAGNETIC RESONANCE IMAGING IN THE DIAGNOSIS OF PELVIC ORGAN PROLAPSE

Craig V. Comiter and Joel T. Funk

Weakness and subsequent dysfunction of the pelvic floor is common in parous women of middle or advanced age. Pelvic organ prolapse (POP) and pelvic floor relaxation are caused by anatomic abnormalities, including weakness of the muscles of the pelvic floor and the fascial attachments of the pelvic viscera. The prevalence of POP has been reported to be as high as 16% of women aged 40 to 56 years.[1] Approximately 500,000 surgeries for POP are performed in the United States each year.[2]

Women with POP present not only to the gynecologist but also to the urologist, as up to one third of patients with prolapse also suffer from urinary incontinence. POP is also associated with fecal incontinence, incomplete voiding, and constipation. A detailed knowledge of pelvic anatomy is paramount for the proper evaluation and management of such conditions. Pelvic support defects result from both neurophysiologic and anatomic changes[3] and often occur as a constellation of abnormal findings. Symptomatic individuals often have multifocal pelvic floor defects, not always evident on physical examination.[4]

Even experienced clinicians may be misled by the physical findings, having difficulty differentiating among cystocele, enterocele, and high rectocele by physical examination alone. Depending on the position of the patient, the strength of the Valsalva maneuver, and modesty of the patient, the examiner may be limited in his or her ability to accurately diagnose the various components of pelvic prolapse. Furthermore, with uterine prolapse, the cervix and uterus may fill the entire introitus, making the diagnosis of concomitant anterior or posterior compartmental prolapse even more difficult. Regardless of the etiology of the support defect, the surgeon must identify all aspects of vaginal prolapse and pelvic floor relaxation for proper surgical planning. Incorrect diagnosis of these defects may lead to inadequate surgical treatment.[5] Accurate preoperative staging should reduce the risk of recurrent prolapse, which can occur in up to 34% of patients after surgery.[6]

RADIOGRAPHIC EVALUATION

Radiographic evaluation plays an important role in the identification of these defects and should be used as an extension of the physical examination. Various methods have been used to visualize the pelvic structures and lower urinary tract, including fluoroscopy, sonography, computed tomography (CT), and, most recently, magnetic resonance imaging (MRI).

Levator Myography

Levator myography is an outdated method of visualizing the pubococcygeus and iliococcygeus via direct injection of contrast solution into the levator muscles. Originally described in 1953, this technique allows visualization of the position and supportive role of these muscle groups.[7] Widening of the levator hiatus, which often occurs after traumatic childbirth and predisposes to pelvic floor relaxation and to visceral prolapse, can be demonstrated with levator myography. Today, this information may be obtained noninvasively with CT[8] and MRI.[9,10]

Voiding Cystourethrography

Voiding cystourethrography (VCUG) is mainly used for demonstrating a cystocele, evaluating bladder neck hypermobility, and demonstrating an open bladder neck at rest (sphincteric incompetence). Dynamic lateral cystography at rest and during straining is an important adjunct to the urodynamic evaluation; it is useful for demonstrating the presence of and degree of urethravesical hypermobility and cystocele formation (Fig. 56-1).[11] In additional, dynamic fluoroscopy has been shown to be more accurate than physical examination in demonstrating an enterocele.[12,13] Other pathologic conditions detected by VCUG include

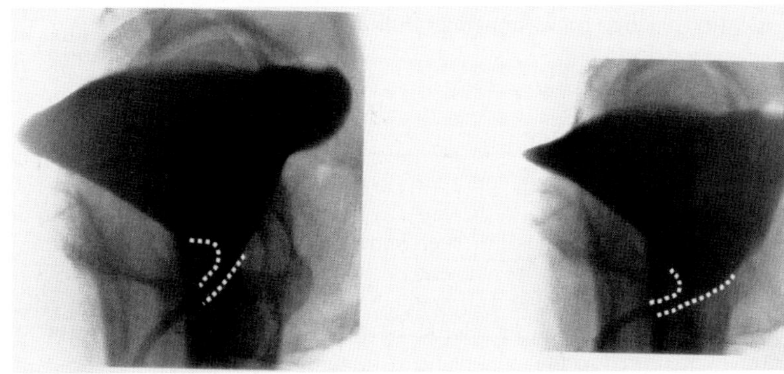

Figure 56-1 Lateral cystogram, with patient relaxed *(left)* and straining *(right)*.

vesicoureteral reflux, vesicovaginal fistula, and urethral diverticular disease.

Dynamic Proctography

Dynamic proctography, in the cooperative patient, allows precise identification and quantification of a rectocele, measured as the maximum extent of an anterior rectal bulge beyond the expected line of the rectum.[14,15] Limitations of this examination include the cumbersome and potentially painful instillation of rectal barium paste and lack of correlation between the viscosity of the paste and the individual patient's stool. Modesty makes this a difficult technique for many patients, because they are unable to defecate on command.

Colpocystourethrography

The colpocystourethrogram was first described in France in 1965 and combines opacification of the bladder, urethra, and vagina.[16] Modified and made popular in the mid 1970s, the colpocystourethrogram is a dynamic study of pelvic support and function.[17] The anatomic relationships among the bladder, urethra, and vagina may be demonstrated, and, when the study is combined with proctography, it may be even more useful in outlining the anatomy of the normal pelvis and of complex POP.

An enterocele, defined as a herniation of the peritoneum and its contents at the level of the vaginal apex, may be appreciated via straining or defecation during colpocystoproctography. This is demonstrated by a widening of the rectovaginal space.[18] The accuracy of dynamic colpocystoproctography is even further enhanced by opacification of the small bowel. The patient drinks oral barium 2 hours before the examination. With the vagina, bladder, small intestine, and rectum opacified, the vaginal axis may be measured at rest and with straining, and prolapse of the anterior, middle, and/or posterior vaginal compartment should become evident.

Sonography

Sonography offers a convenient, painless, and radiation-free technique. As with fluoroscopy, a dynamic component may be added to sonography. In particular, dynamic ultrasound allows identification of an enterocele during straining maneuver, evidenced by widening of the rectovaginal septum, diminution of the peritoneal-anal distance, and herniation of bowel contents into the cul-de-sac.[19] Ultrasongraphy using an abdominal, rectal, vaginal, or perineal transducer is also useful for demonstrating vesicourethral anatomy,[20-23] So-called contrast sonography uses echogenic material instilled into the bladder or vagina and is able to identify bladder neck funneling with straining[24] as well as paravaginal defects.[25]

Computed Tomography

CT pelvimetry is an accurate and reproducible method for measuring pelvic dimensions and the capacity of the maternal birth canal.[26,27] However, CT has not been shown to be particularly useful in the evaluation of pelvic visceral prolapse. The components of the levator plate and urogenital diaphragm are better seen in the coronal plane or sagittal view, but CT images are routinely presented in the axial plane. Although CT images can be reconstructed into a coronal view with the use of cumbersome and expensive computer software, poor image quality and distorted spatial resolution has limited the utility of this presentation technique.[8]

Magnetic Resonance Imaging

Most recently, MRI has emerged as an important diagnostic tool, both for evaluating the functional relationships among the pelvic floor viscera and supporting structures and for assessing pelvic pathology. MRI offers the advantages of being noninvasiveness, lack of exposure of the patient and examiner to ionizing radiation, and superior soft tissue contrast and multiplanar imaging without superimposition of structures. Axial images provide information about the urogenital hiatus and its contents, whereas sagittal images more easily demonstrate visceral prolapse. Because static images alone do not demonstrate relevant pelvic floor changes with activity, dynamic MRI has been used to reveal the structural functional changes that occur during stress maneuvers. Those established criteria for abnormality derived from fluoroscopy (colpocystoproctography) are directly applicable to MRI.[28]

The development of fast-scanning MRI techniques has greatly improved the ability to describe and quantify anatomic changes that have a causative role in pelvic floor relaxation. Fast-scan Valsalva imaging formatted in a pseudokinematic cine-loop provides a dynamic method to study the anatomic changes that occur with straining. Additionally, MRI offers a noninvasive method to evaluate the female pelvis without exposure to the ionizing radiation that is integral to prior modalities such as CT, colpocystoproctography, and fluoroscopy.

MRI also allows evaluation of all three pelvic compartments simultaneously for organ descent. Kelvin's group used "triphasic" dynamic MRI, consisting of a cystographic, a proctographic, and a post-toilet phase to facilitate the recognition of prolapsed organs that may be obscured by other organs that remain unemptied.[29] Fielding showed that MRI is useful for measuring levator muscle thickness,[30] demonstrating focal levator ani eventrations (outpouching) not visible with levator myography,[31] and measuring urethral length and the thickness and integrity of periurethral muscle ring.[9] Hoyte and colleagues[48] demonstrated that the anterior portion of the levator (puborectalis) is typically thinner in women with POP and/or stress incontinence compared with asymptomatic controls—possibly due to muscle atrophy caused by denervation from childbirth injuries or muscle wasting secondary to loss of insertion points for the puborectalis.

Yang and associates were the first to popularize dynamic fast MRI for the evaluation of POP,[9] using T1-weighted gradient recalled acquisition in a steady-state pulse (GRASS) sequence, with acquisition times between 6 and 12 seconds. Since then, other investigators have shown that MRI is more sensitive than physical examination for defining pelvic prolapse.[5,10,32] Whereas some advocate the use of contrast opacification of the bladder, vagina, and rectum,[29,33] others have shown that the vagina, rectum, bladder, urethra, and peritoneum are adequately visualized without any contrast administration.[5] By avoiding instrumentation of the vagina or urethra, iatrogenic alteration of the anatomy is minimized.[10]

Several years ago, Comiter and coworkers published their experience with dynamic half-Fourier acquisition, single-shot turbo spin-echo (HASTE sequence) T2-weighted MRI using a 1.5-Tesla magnet with phased array coils (Siemens) or single-

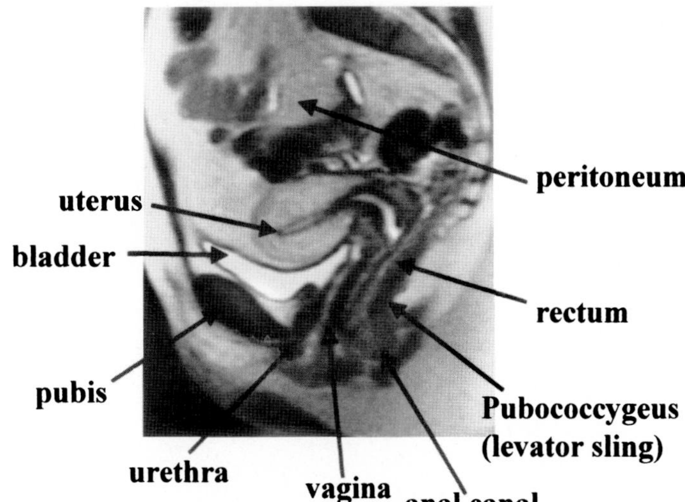

Figure 56-2 Lateral magnetic resonance image denoting normal pelvic structures.

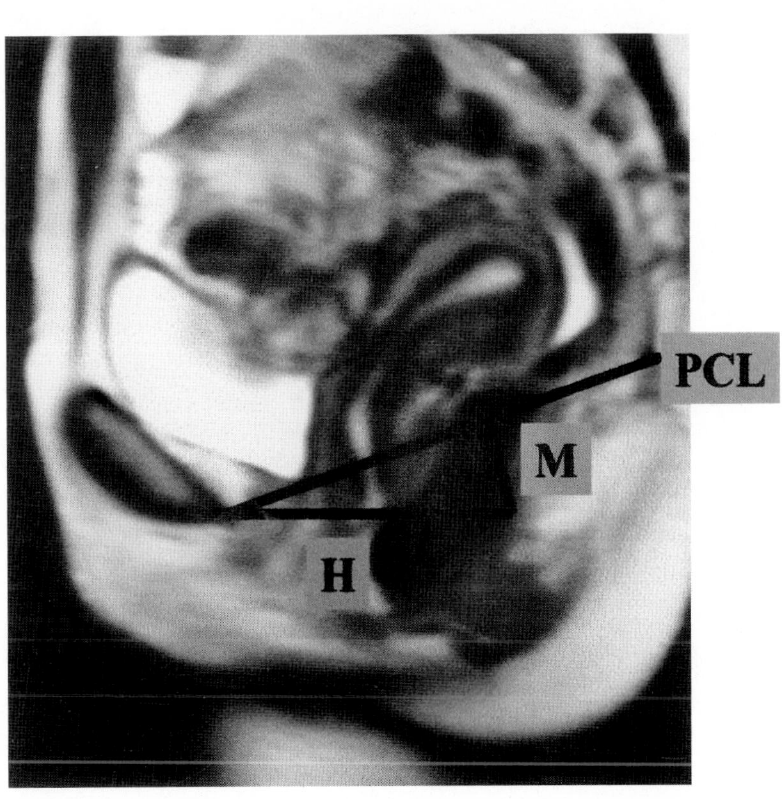

Figure 56-3 The H-line (levator hiatus width) measures the distance from the pubis to the posterior anal canal. The M-line (muscular pelvic floor relaxation) measures the descent of the levator plate from the fixed pubococcygeal line (PCL).

shot fast spin-echo (SSFSE, General Electric) for evaluating the female pelvis.[5] Midsagittal and parasagittal resting and straining supine views were obtained for the purpose of identifying the midline and for evaluating the anterior pelvic compartment (anterior vaginal wall, bladder, urethra), posterior compartment (rectum), and middle compartment (uterus, vaginal cuff), as well as the pelvic floor muscles, adnexal organs, and intraperitoneal organs (Fig. 56-2). Images were looped for viewing on a digital station as a cine stack and for measuring the relationship of pelvic organs to fixed anatomic landmarks. The first set of images comprised volumetric sagittal cuts from left to right, used to locate the midsagittal plane and to survey the pelvic anatomy. The second set of images was obtained with four cycles of repeated relaxation and Valsalva maneuver.[5,8] Total image acquisition time was 2.5 minutes, and total room time was 10 minutes per study.

This dynamic MRI technique, known as the HMO classification system, has been shown to be useful for grading pelvic visceral prolapse and pelvic floor relaxation in a simple and objective manner.[5] The size of the levator hiatus and the degree of muscular pelvic floor relaxation and organ prolapse were measured. The "H-line" (levator hiatus width) measures the distance from the pubis to the posterior anal canal. The "M-line" (muscular pelvic floor relaxation) measures the descent of the levator plate from the fixed pubococcygeal line (PCL). The PCL spans the distance from the pubis to the sacrococcygeal joint (Fig. 56-3). The "O"

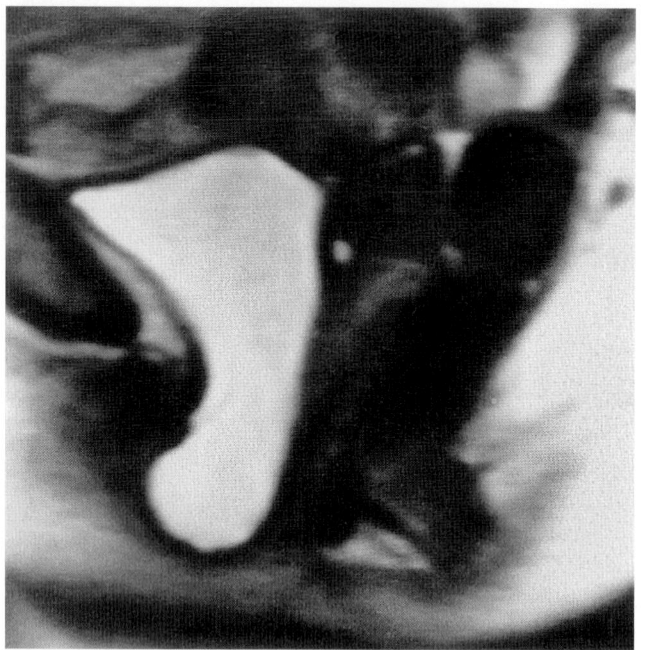

A

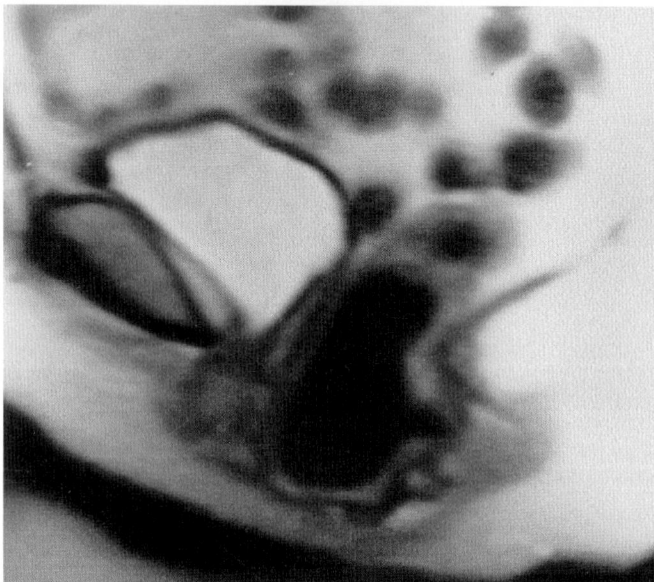

B

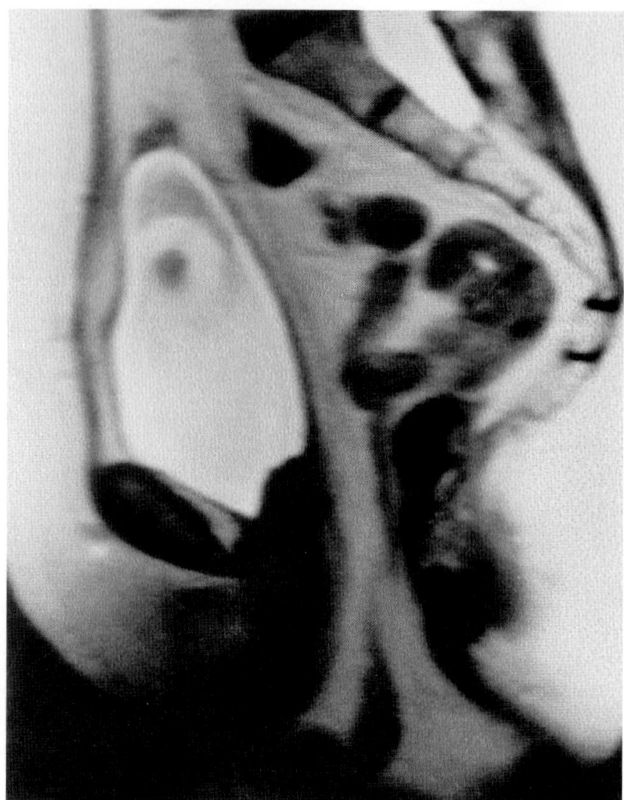

C

Figure 56-4 Organ prolapse. **A,** Cystocele. **B,** Rectocele. **C,** Enterocele.

classification (organ prolapse) describes the degree of visceral prolapse beyond the H-line. The degrees of cystocele, rectocele, enterocele, and uterine descent are graded as 0, 1, 2, or 3, corresponding to none, mild, moderate, or severe (Fig. 56-4).

In a group of women with symptomatic prolapse, the levator hiatus width (H-line) was significantly wider than in a control group (7.5 ± 1.5 cm versus 5.2 ± 1.1 cm; $P < .001$). Similarly, the levator muscular descent (M-line) was greater in the prolapse group than in the control group (4.1 ± 1.5 cm versus 1.9 ± 1.2 cm; $P < .001$).[5] These objective findings fit well with our knowledge of the pathophysiology of pelvic prolapse. Trauma to the pubococcygeus and iliococcygeus, usually from childbirth, results in widening of the levator hiatus and laxity of the musculofascial support structures.[34] This results in a sloping levator plate, with the more vertically oriented vagina and rectum tending to slide down through the widened hiatus. Therefore, the H and M lines both increase with pelvic floor relaxation. This in turn leads to organ prolapse (O classification). Because of the excellent visualization of fluid-filled viscera and soft tissues, MRI can differentiate among cystocele, enterocele, and high rectocele, which may be difficult by physical examination alone.

MRI findings were compared to physical examination and intraoperative findings. HASTE-sequence MRI was more accurate than physical examination in identifying cystocele, enterocele, vault prolapse, and pelvic organ pathology such as uterine fibroids, urethral diverticula, ovarian cysts, and Nabothian and

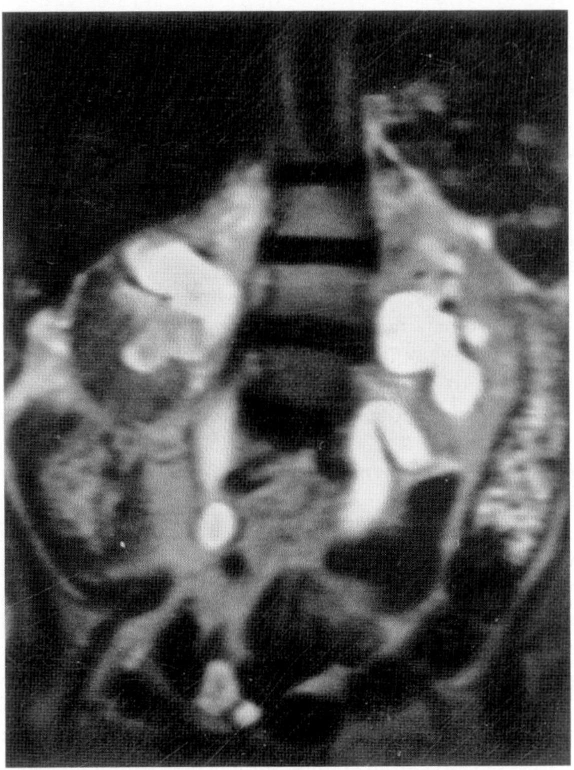

Figure 56-5 Magnetic resonance urography demonstrates hydroureteronephrosis secondary to pelvic organ prolapse obstructing the ureters.

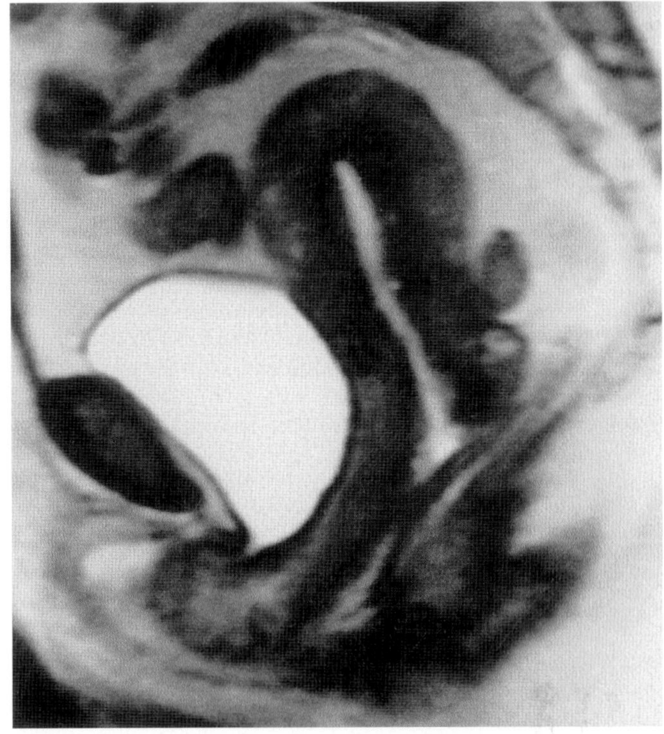

Figure 56-6 Lateral magnetic resonance image demonstrating stress urinary incontinence secondary to urethral hypermobility.

Bartholin gland cysts.[32] Comiter and colleagues found that, with dynamic MRI, surgical planning was altered in more than 30% of cases, most often because of occult enterocele not appreciated on physical examination.[35]

In patients with severe prolapse, especially if renal insufficiency is present, the surgeon must rule out obstructive hydroureteronephrosis. This may be accomplished by magnetic resonance urography, which adds only 30 seconds of examination time and no additional morbidity (Fig. 56-5). MRI may also be useful for the radiographic evaluation of stress incontinence. Hypermobility of the proximal urethra and bladder neck descent are important pathophysiologic features in the diagnosis of genuine stress urinary incontinence.[36,37] Measurement data on dynamic MRI for the bladder neck position and the extension of cystocele at maximal pelvic strain are comparable with data obtained by lateral cystourethrography (Fig. 56-6).[38]

Recent urogynecologic and radiologic publications have validated MRI as a reliable alternative to colpocystoproctography.[29,38,39] The information obtained via MRI is often superior to that obtained via colpocystoproctography, because the former allows for direct visualization of the pelvic organs and their fluid content, whereas the latter presents a silhouetted view of contrast-filled organs (complete opacification is not usually achieved). Gufler and associates demonstrated that dynamic MRI is helpful in the evaluation of persistent patient complaints after surgery for POP and is, in fact, more sensitive than physical examination.[40] Dynamic MRI is particularly sensitive for diagnosing enteroceles and is superior to colpocystoproctography or physical examination.[41] A minority of studies have shown that MRI may not be as accurate for the identification of vaginal vault prolapse or for rectocele as is colpocystoproctography.[42] Gousse's group from the University of Miami postulated that the anterior rectal wall is not well differentiated from the posterior wall on rapid-sequence MRI when the rectum is empty, because the rectal walls are collapsed.[32,43] At our institution intravaginal, intravesical, or intrarectal contrast is not instilled, but others have shown that such "triphasic dynamic" studies may even further improve the diagnostic accuracy of MRI.[29,34]

The disadvantage of MRI is that the study often must be performed with the patient in the supine position, because upright MRI scanners are not yet universally available. Colpocystoproctography is clearly more amenable to performance in a sitting position than is MRI. However, dynamic MRI with relaxing and straining views has been shown to adequately demonstrate POP during straining in the supine position.[44] Additionally, in those institutions that have access to an upright MRI scanner, sitting MRI was not shown to be superior to supine MRI for demonstrating POP. Although patients undergoing sitting MR imaging demonstrated a greater degree of visceral descent, supine studies were not inferior for demonstrating *clinically relevant* prolapse.[45]

Competition among prolapsing organs filling a finite introital space may also limit MRI, just as it may limit physical examination and dynamic fluoroscopy. This is especially true for identification of a rectocele. Additionally, claustrophobic patients and those with cardiac pacemakers or sacral nerve stimulators cannot enter the enclosed magnet. Despite these limitations, dynamic MRI has become the study of choice at our institution for evaluating POP and pelvic floor relaxation.

Alternative MRI sequences have recently been demonstrated to be as good or better than the HASTE sequence. Lienemann and colleagues recommended a true fast imaging with steady-state precession (True FISP) sequence, because it may be associated with superior image quality compared to the HASTE sequence.[41,45] Gousse's group from Miami demonstrated the utility of extended-phase conjugate-symmetry rapid spin-echo sequence (EXPRESS) as a novel and very rapid scanning technique; individual images are obtained in 0.8 seconds with the use of half-Fourier reconstruction and fast gradients with sophisticated recently available software.[43] Both the True FISP and EXPRESS dynamic MRI examinations were superior to physical examination in accuracy and completeness for the preoperative evaluation of POP.

Over the last decade, there has been an increasing interest in use of elective cesarean delivery to reduce maternal birth trauma and decrease long-term morbidity,[46,47] but reliable prepartum criteria have not been established to identify those women most likely to develop pelvic floor injuries during childbirth. Fielding's group at Harvard recently published their experience with MRI pelvimetry as a potentially important research tool.[48] Their protocol is easily performed with the patient in the supine position using a pelvic coil, fast spin-echo T2-weighted sequences, 2-mm cuts, and a 1.5-T system. Pelvimetry measurements are obtained from coronal, axial, and midsagittal images. Significant differences in mean pelvimetry measurements were demonstrated between women with and without pelvic visceral prolapse and pelvic floor relaxation. With multivariate analysis, POP patients had a wider transverse inlet diameter, and a trend toward a wider interspinous diameter. Recent CT studies have demonstrated that women with wider transverse inlet diameters have a higher prevalence of prolapse after childbirth,[26] and perhaps MRI pelvimetry may contribute to the identification of such risk factors.

SUMMARY

Most cases of incontinence and minimal pelvic floor weakness can be treated based on physical examination with or without urodynamic evaluation. On the other hand, in women with complex or recurrent POP and pelvic floor relaxation, radiographic evaluation is recommended as an extension of the physical examination. A detailed working knowledge of normal and abnormal female pelvic anatomy is necessary for the proper evaluation of pelvic visceral prolapse. However, even the most experienced gynecologist or urologist may have difficulty distinguishing among prolapsing organs competing for introital space. Accurate identification of all aspects of vaginal prolapse and pelvic floor relaxation are vital, not only to permit adequate surgical planning but also to reduce the risk of recurrent prolapse. Urography, voiding cystography, dynamic colpocystodefecography, sonography, and MRI are each useful for the evaluation of pelvic prolapse and pelvic floor relaxation.

MRI can demonstrate the levator muscles in three-dimensional fashion, providing details about herniation during straining, muscle thickness, and asymmetry. MRI allows complete analysis of the anterior, middle, and posterior pelvic compartments in a single procedure without the use of ionizing radiation. Differentiation among soft tissues is excellent, anatomic information is accurate, and no contrast agent is needed. The advent of rapid sequencing with cine stacking has enabled MRI to replace dynamic colpocystoproctography at many institutions, providing not only superb differentiation among fluid-filled, air-filled, and solid pelvic viscera but also a functional demonstration of all three pelvic compartments during relaxation and straining. As dynamic MRI becomes more widespread, standardization of the technique will become more important.

References

1. Hagstad A, Janson PO, Lindstedt G: Gynaecological history, complaints, and examinations in a middle-aged population. Maturitas 7:115-128, 1985.
2. Morren GL, Balasingam AG, Wells JE, et al: Triphasic MRI of pelvic organ descent: Sources of measurement error. Eur J Radiol 54:276-283, 2005.
3. Brubaker L, Heit MH: Radiology of the pelvic floor. Clin Obstet Gynecol 36:952-959, 1993.
4. Spence-Jones C, Kamm MA, Henry MM, Hudson CN: Bowel dysfunction: A pathogenic factor in uterovaginal prolapse and urinary stress incontinence. Br J Obstet Gynecol 101:147-152, 1994.
5. Comiter CV, Vasavada SP, Barbaric AL, et al: Grading pelvic prolapse and pelvic floor relaxation using dynamic magnetic resonance imaging. Urology 54:454-458, 1999.
6. Shull BL, Benn SJ, Kuehl TJ: Surgical management of prolapse of the anterior vaginal segment: An analysis of support defects, operative morbidity, and anatomic outcome. Am J Obstetr Gynecol 171:1429-1439, 1994.
7. Berglas B, Rubin IC: Study of the supportive structures of the uterus by levator myography. Surg Gynecol Obstet 97:677-692, 1953.
8. Weidner AC, Low VHS: Imaging studies of the pelvic floor. Obstet Gynecol Clin North Am 25:825-848, 1998.
9. Yang A, Mostwin, JL, Rosenshein NB: Pelvic floor descent in women: Dynamic evaluation with fast MR imaging and cinematic display. Radiology 179:25-33, 1991.
10. Goodrich MA, Webb M.J, King BF: Magnetic resonance imaging of pelvic floor relaxation: Dynamic analysis and evaluation of patients before and after surgical repair. Obstet Gynecol 82:883-891, 1993.
11. Kelvin FM, Maglinte DD, Hale D, Benson JR: Voiding cystourethrography in female stress incontinence. AJR Am J Roentgenol 167:1065-1066, 1996.
12. Kelvin FM, Maglinte DDT, Hornback JA, Benson JT: Pelvic prolapse: Assessment with evacuation proctography (defecography). Radiology 184:547-551, 1992.
13. Altringer WE, Saclarides TJ, Dominguez JM: Four-contrast defecography: Pelvic "flooroscopy." Dis Colon Rectum 38:695-699, 1995.
14. Kelvin FM, Maglinte DD: Dynamic evaluation of female pelvic organ prolapse by extended proctography. Radiol Clin North Am 41:395-407, 2003.
15. Shorvon PJ, McHugh S, Diamant NE: Defecography in normal volunteers: Results and implications. Gut 30:1737-1740, 1989.
16. Bethoux A, Bory S, Huguier M, Sheao SL: Le colpocystogramme. J Chir (Paris) 8:809-828, 1965.
17. Lazarevski M, Lazarov A, Novak J, Dimcevski D: Colpocystography in cases of genital prolapse and urinary stress incontinence in women. Am J Obstet Gynecol 122:704-716, 1975.
18. Shorvon PJ, Stevenson GW. Defaecography: Setting up a service. Br J Hosp Med 41:460-467, 1989.
19. Karaus M, Neuhaus P, Weidenmann B: Diagnosis of enteroceles by dynamic anorectal endosonography. Dis Colon Rectum 43:1683-1688, 2000.

20. Gordon D, Pearce M, Norton P, Stanton SL: Comparison of ultrasound and lateral chain cystourethrography in the determination of bladder neck descent. Am J Obstet Gynecol 160:12-18, 1989.
21. Bergmann A, Ballard CA, Platt LD: Ultrasonic evaluation of urethrovesical junction in women with stress urinary incontinence. J Clin Ultrasound 16:295-300, 1998.
22. Mouritsen L, Rasmussen A: Bladder neck mobility evaluated by vaginal ultrasonography. Br J Urol 71:166-171, 1993.
23. Kohorn E, Scioscia AL, Jeaty P, Hobbins JC: Ultrasound by perineal scanning for the assessment of female stress urinary incontinence. Obstet Gynecol 68:269-272, 1986.
24. Schaer GN, Koechli OR, Schuessler B: Improvement of perineal sonographic bladder neck imaging with ultrasound contrast medium. Obstet Gynecol 86:950-954, 1995.
25. Ostrzenski A, Osborne NG, Ostrzenska K: Method for diagnosing paravaginal defects using contrast ultrasonographic technique. J Ultrasound Med 16:673-677, 1997.
26. Sze EH, Kohli N, Miklos JR, et al: Computed tomography comparison of bony pelvis dimensions between women with and without genital prolapse. Obstet Gynecol 93:229-232, 1999.
27. Federle MP, Cohen HA, Rosenwein MR, et al: Pelvimetry by digital radiography: A low dose examination. Radiology 143:733-735, 1982.
28. Goh V, Halligan S, Kaplan G, et al: Dynamic MR imaging of the pelvic floor in asymptomatic subjects. AJR Am J Roentgenol 174:661-666, 2000.
29. Kelvin FM, Maglinte DDT, Hale DS, et al: Female pelvic organ prolapse: A comparison of triphasic dynamic MR imaging and triphasic fluoroscopic cystocolpoproctography. AJR Am J Roentgenol 174:81-88, 2000.
30. Fielding JR, Dumanli H, Schreyer AG, et al: MR-based three dimensional modeling of the normal pelvic floor in women: Quantification of muscle mass. AJR Am J Roentgenol 174:657-660, 2000.
31. Pannu KH, Genardry R, Gearhart S, et al: Focal levator ani eventrations: Detection and characterization by magnetic resonance in patients with pelvic floor dysfunction. Int Urogynecol J Pelvic Floor Dysfunct 14:89-93, 2003.
32. Gousse AE, Barbaric ZL, Safir MH, et al: Dynamic half Fourier acquisition, single shot turbo spin-echo magnetic resonance imaging for evaluating the female pelvis. J Urol 164:1606-1613, 2000.
33. Lienemann A, Fischer T: Functional imaging of the pelvic floor. Eur J Radiol 27:117-122, 2003.
34. Babiarz JW, Raz S: Pelvic floor relaxation. In Raz S (ed): Female Urology. Philadelphia: WB Saunders, 1996, pp 445-456.
35. Comiter CV, Vasavada S, Raz S: Pre-operative Evaluation of Pelvic Prolapse Using Dynamic Magnetic Resonance Imaging. Presented at the 29th Annual International Continence Society, Denver, CO, August, 1999.
36. Jeffcoate TN, Roberts H: Observation on stress incontinence of urine. Am J Obstet Gynecol 64:721-738, 1952.
37. Enhorning G: Simultaneous recording of intravesical and intraurethral pressure. Acta Chir Scand 276(Suppl):1-68, 1956.
38. Gufler H, DeGregorio G, Allman K-H, et al: Comparison of cystourethrography and dynamic MRI in bladder neck descent. J Comput Assist Tomogr 24:382-388, 2000.
39. Deval B, Vulierme MP, Poilpot S, et al: [Imaging pelvic floor prolapse] [French]. Gynecol Obstet Biol Reprod (Paris) 32:22-29, 2003.
40. Gufler H, CeGregorio G, Dohnicht S, et al: Dynamic MRI after surgical repair for pelvic organ prolapse. J Comput Assist Tomogr 26:724-729, 2002.
41. Lienemann A, Anthuber C, Baron A, Reiser M: Diagnosing enteroceles using magnetic resonance imaging. Dis Colon Rectum 43:205-212, 2000.
42. Cortes E, Reid WM, Singh K, Berger L: Clinical examination and dynamic magnetic resonance imaging vaginal vault prolapse. Obstet Gynecol 103:41-46, 2004.
43. Kester RR, Leboeuf L, Amendola MA, et al: Value of EXPRESS T2-weighted pelvic MRI in the evaluation of severe pelvic floor prolapse: A prospective study. Urology 61:1135-1139, 2000.
44. Lienemann A, Anthuber CJ, Baron A: Dynamic MR colpocystorectogrpahy assessing pelvic floor descent. Eur Radiol 7:1309-1317, 1997.
45. Bertshinger KM, Hetzer FH, Roos JE, et al: Dynamic MR imaging of the pelvic floor performed with patient sitting in an open-magnet unit versus with patient supine in a closed-magnet unit. Radiology 223:501-508, 2002.
46. Faridi A, Willis S, Schelzig P, et al: Anal sphincter injury during vaginal delivery: An argument for cesarean section on request? J Perinat Med 30:279-287, 2002.
47. Heit M, Mudd K, Culligan P: Prevention of childbirth injuries to the pelvic floor. Curr Womens Health Rep 1:72-80, 2001.
48. Hoyte L, Schierlitz L, Zou K, et al: Two and 3-dimensional MRI comparison of levator ani structure, volume, and integrity in women with stress incontinence and prolapse. Am J Obstet Gynecol 185:11-19, 2001.

Chapter 57

URODYNAMIC EVALUATION OF THE PATIENT WITH PROLAPSE

Sender Herschorn

Symptoms caused by pelvic organ prolapse may or may not be specific to the prolapsing compartment or compartments, and the correlation of many pelvic symptoms with the extent of prolapse is weak.[1,2] Many women with pelvic organ prolapse have no symptoms, especially if the prolapse remains inside the vagina.[3] Others present with symptoms in addition to the vaginal bulge, as a result of the associated organ dysfunction. It is recommended that symptoms be elucidated in four primary areas: lower urinary tract, bowel, sexual symptoms, and other local symptoms.[4] Documentation of symptoms not only serves as a guide to treatment but also permits an accurate assessment of post-treatment results.

There is general agreement that the aim of urodynamic testing is to reproduce symptoms of the patient under controlled and measurable conditions. Ideally, this allows diagnosis, helps with informed treatment choice, and improves treatment outcome. Specifically, the testing identifies or excludes contributing factors to incontinence or voiding dysfunction and assesses their relative importance.[5] However, the role of urodynamics in the evaluation of symptoms related to prolapse is not yet fully established. A recent Cochrane review attempted to test the hypotheses that urodynamic testing improves the clinical outcome of incontinence management, that it alters clinical decision-making, and that one type of test is better than another in these areas.[6] Only two trials were found, but the numbers of patients were too small to determine whether clinical outcomes were affected by the urodynamics. This chapter reviews the various tests that are available and may be helpful in patient evaluation.[6]

LOWER URINARY TRACT SYMPTOMS

Urinary incontinence is one of the most common symptoms associated with prolapse. Blaivas and Groutz[7] described the clinical evaluation in detail. However, the specific symptoms and their impact on the patient's quality of life should be elucidated in each case.

Urinary symptoms may include stress incontinence; symptoms of bladder overactivity, such as frequency, nocturia, urgency, and urgency incontinence; and voiding symptoms such as difficulty with bladder emptying. The mechanisms for stress incontinence include hypermobility and intrinsic sphincter deficiency. It is not unusual for patients to present with a combination of urge and stress incontinence.[8,9] If both symptoms are present, the patient has *mixed incontinence.*[10] Mixed incontinence is especially common in older women. Often, however, one symptom (urge or stress) is more bothersome to the patient than the other. Identifying the most bothersome symptom is important in targeting diagnostic and therapeutic interventions.

Many women with severe prolapse recall that, as the prolapse worsened, their stress incontinence symptoms improved. Reducing the vaginal prolapse with a pessary or a speculum during the examination by the clinician can produce stress incontinence in up to 80% of clinically continent patients with severe prolapse.[11-14] This phenomenon has been termed *latent, masked, occult, or potential* stress incontinence, and it should be elicited when considering therapy. Although the clinical experience reported refers primarily to cystocele, occult incontinence may also be unmasked in a similar manner in patients with severe middle or posterior compartment prolapse. The postulated mechanism for continence may be urethral kinking by the cystocele or external compression of the urethra.[15]

Other storage symptoms, such as frequency, nocturia, and urgency, have been listed as symptoms of prolapse,[16] although the mechanism is unknown and there are frequently other associated factors. Urge incontinence may also be present. However, urge incontinence is a common complaint in patients without organ prolapse, may or may not be the result of detrusor overactivity,[17] and becomes more prevalent with aging. Patients with advanced organ prolapse and urge incontinence have also been shown to have detrusor overactivity[15] that may resolve after surgical correction of the prolapse.[13,18] The mechanism is unclear; however, many of those patients may have outflow obstruction caused by the prolapse that is alleviated after repair. Nguyen and Bhatia reported resolution of urgency incontinence after pelvic prolapse repair in patients who had no obstruction preoperatively.[18]

A number of tools are now available to aid the clinician in elucidating the symptoms and their impact on quality of life, to gain as accurate a picture as possible. These tools include questionnaires, voiding diaries, and pad tests, which are also used to evaluate treatment outcomes.[19]

Difficult voiding symptoms are common with severe prolapse and should be elicited. Patients with prolapse may have urethral kinking or external pressure on the urethra that not only prevents incontinence but also may cause difficult voiding.[15] They occasionally have to digitally reduce the prolapse to void (splinting) or need to assume unusual positions to initiate or complete micturition.[4] Urinary splinting has been reported to be 97% specific for severe anterior prolapse.[20]

Urodynamic abnormalities with decreased uroflow, increased postvoid residual urine,[21] and bladder outlet obstruction have been reported.[15,22,23] The degree of obstruction may be related to the severity of the prolapse.[15] Acute urinary retention secondary to the prolapse is rarely seen.[24]

INITIAL EVALUATION OF URINARY SYMPTOMS

The initial evaluation includes a history, physical examination, urinalysis, and measurement of postvoid residual urine.[25] The basic evaluation may be satisfactory for proceeding with treatment, including surgery, for patients with straightforward stress incontinence associated with hypermobility and normal postvoid residual volume.[10] However, the International Scientific Committee of the Third International Consultation on Urinary Incontinence advised that urodynamic testing is highly recommended for women who desire interventional treatment,[25] although the specific chapter indicates the lack of evidenced-based medicine for this recommendation.[5] Furthermore, Diokno and coworkers[26] showed that a systematic history, vaginal speculum examination and postvoid residual measurement were 100% accurate in identifying patients who had pure type II stress incontinence on urodynamic studies. Other groups have shown a positive correlation of symptoms and urodynamic findings,[27,28] potentially bypassing the need for urodynamic studies in many patients.[29,30] Investigators have also shown that symptoms are not always related to the actual dysfunction causing the incontinence demonstrated on urodynamics.[31-35] As mentioned previously, the actual role of urodynamics in case selection and in predicting the continence outcome of surgery is still unknown.[36]

There are many instances in which a basic clinical evaluation is insufficient. The Agency for Health Care Research and Quality (formerly the Agency for Health Care Policy and Research) published guidelines in 1996 that are still relevant.[10] Criteria for further evaluation of incontinence include

- uncertain diagnosis and inability to develop a reasonable treatment plan based on the basic diagnostic evaluation
- uncertainty in diagnosis when there is lack of correlation between symptoms and clinical findings
- failure to respond or patient dissatisfaction with an adequate therapeutic trial and patient desire to pursuefurther therapy
- consideration of surgical intervention, particularly if previous surgery failed or the patient is a high surgical risk
- hematuria without infection
- the presence of other comorbid conditions, such as incontinence associated with recurrent symptomatic urinary tract infection
- persistent symptoms of difficult bladder emptying
- history of previous anti-incontinence surgery or radical pelvic surgery
- symptomatic pelvic prolapse beyond the hymen
- abnormal postvoid residual urine volume
- a neurologic condition, such as multiple sclerosis or spinal cord lesions or injury.

Additional testing includes urodynamics but may also include cystoscopy and imaging.

Urodynamics in the Patient with Prolapse

For good urodynamic practices, the reader is referred to the International Continence Society (ICS) publication that reviews current standards for carrying out uroflowmetry, filling cystometry, and pressure-flow studies.[37]

Urinary Flow Rate

A urinary flow rate is a simple urodynamic test that can provide objective and quantitative measures on both storage and voiding symptoms.[37] The curve is either continuous or intermittent. The continuous flow curve is smooth and arc-shaped or a fluctuating (if there are multiple peaks during a period of continuous urine flow). The precise shape of the curve is determined by detrusor contractility, the presence of abdominal straining, and the bladder outlet.[38]

The parameters of uroflowmetry include the following[38]:

- *Flow rate* is defined as the volume of fluid expelled via the urethra per unit time (mL/sec).
- *Voided volume* is the total volume expelled via the urethra.
- *Maximum flow rate* (Q_{max}) is the maximum measured value of the flow rate after correction for artefacts.
- *Voiding time* is the total duration of micturition (i.e., including interruptions). If voiding is completed without interruption, voiding time is equal to flow time.
- *Flow time* is the time over which measurable flow actually occurs.
- *Average flow rate* (Q_{ave}) is voided volume divided by the flow time. The average flow should be interpreted with caution if flow is interrupted or if there is a terminal dribble.
- *Time to maximum flow* is the elapsed time from onset of flow to maximum flow.

The Liverpool Nomogram (Fig. 57-1) was created in 1989 by Haylen and colleagues, who plotted voided volume against peak flow (Q_{max}) in 249 normal women.[39] Normal peak flowranges between 12 and 30 mL/sec, depending on the voided volume (Fig. 57-2). Average flow rates vary from 6 to 25 mL/sec, with a substantial overlap between normal and abnormal individuals.[40] Voiding time varies, from 10 to 20 seconds for a volume of 100 mL to 25 to 35 seconds for a volume of 400 mL. The first half of the urinary volume is rapidly evacuated in the first one third of the total voiding time, and the rest in the remaining two thirds of the voiding period.[41] Arbitrary criteria have been set by a number of authors to diagnose voiding difficulty, including peak flow less than 15 mL/sec and residual urine greater than 50 mL with a minimum total bladder volume of 150 mL before the void (volume voided + residual).[15,42] The 10th percentile curve of the Liverpool Nomogram has also been identified as a useful discriminant in the diagnosis of voiding difficulties.[43]

Bottacini and colleagues[44] reported that women with stress incontinence void with a lower flow rate than healthy women; however, other investigators have demonstrated the opposite: women with stress incontinence void with a higher flow rate because of the reduced outlet resistance.[44]

Uroflowmetry findings (peak flow rate, average flow rate, and voided volume) in prolapse have been described to be significantly lower than in normal controls.[29] Cystocoele is significantly more frequent in patients with voiding difficulties and abnormal uroflowmetry.[35] Valentini and colleagues[26] demonstrated a constrictive effect on outflow in women with varying degrees of cystocele. A poor flow rate and elevated residual urine may be associated with large cystoceles.[41]

In general, an abnormal pattern is generated in the presence of a weak detrusor, abdominal straining, or bladder outlet obstruction. Although urodynamic catheters have less effect on voiding patterns in females than in males, it is still useful to obtain a urinary flow rate on arrival of the patient, to compare

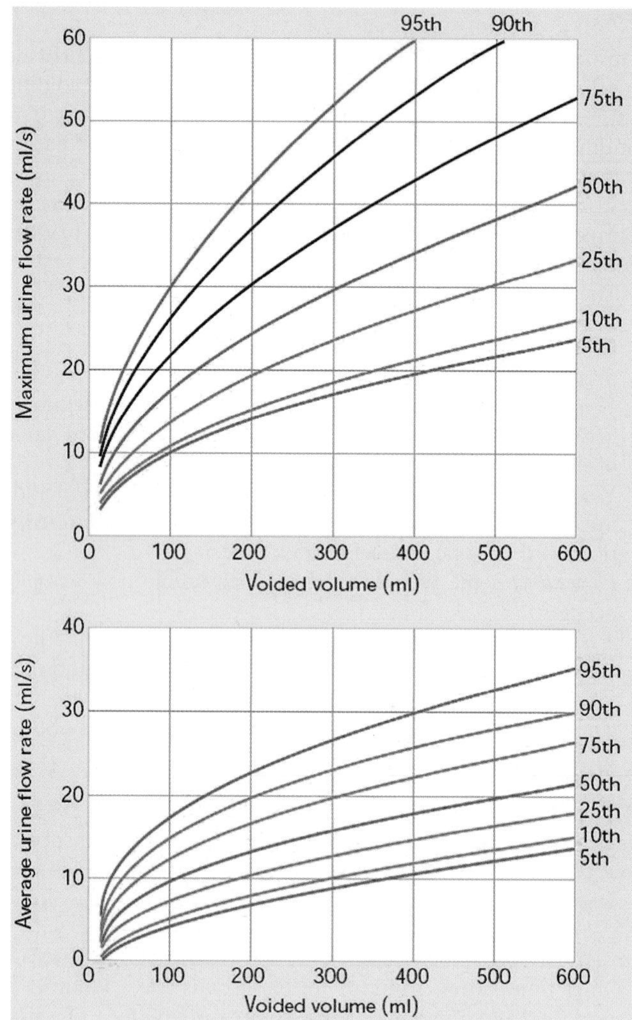

Figure 57-1 The Liverpool Nomogram showing maximum *(Top)* and average *(Bottom)* flow for women.[39]

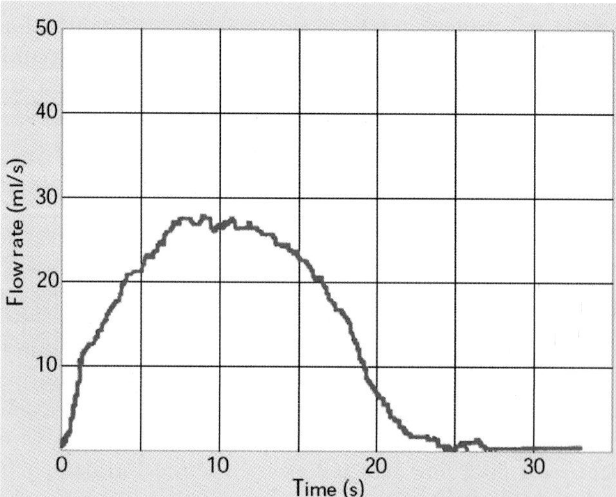

Figure 57-2 Normal flow curve for a voided volume of 350 mL with maximum flow (Q_{max}) of 27 mL/sec. (Modified from Lose G: Urethral pressure measurements. In Cardozo L, Staskin D [eds]: Textbook of Female Urology and Urogynaecology. London: Isis Medical Media, 2001, pp 215-226.)

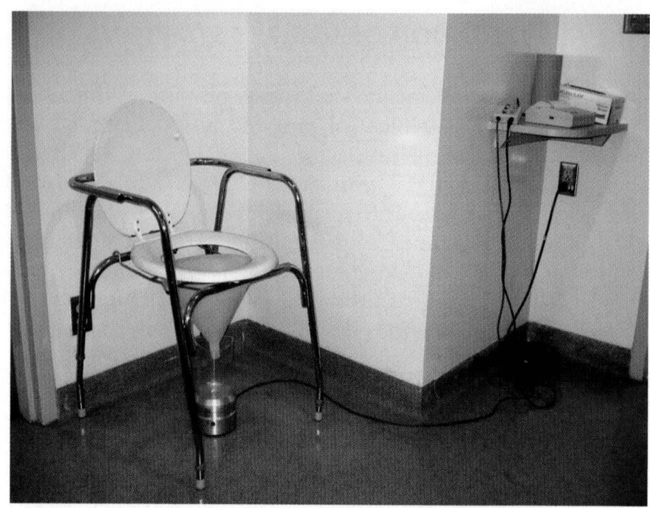

Figure 57-3 Commode chair for uroflow measurement.

with flow data generated during the subsequent urodynamic study. After the initial flow is completed, a postvoid residual can also be determined on introduction of the urodynamic catheters.

Urine Flow Meters

Flow meters are commonly of one of three types: weight, electronic dipstick, or rotating disc.[45] The first measures the weight of the collected urine; the second measures the changes in electrical capacitance of a dipstick mounted in the collecting chamber; and the third measures the power required to keep a disc rotating at a constant speed while the urine, which tends to slow it down, is directed toward it. All three can provide high sensitivity and reproducibility of data. A commode chair with uroflow measuring apparatus is shown in Figure 57-3.

Cystometry

The first part of the filling study is cystometry, the method by which the pressure-volume relationship of the bladder is measured.[38] It is used to assess detrusor sensation, capacity, and activity. The detrusor pressure (P_{det}) is calculated by subtraction of the abdominal pressure (P_{abd}), as measured by a balloon in the rectum, vagina, or bowel stoma, from the total intravesical pressure (P_{ves}), as measured by the intravesical catheter. The resulting detrusor pressure reflects the activity and pressure generated by the detrusor muscle alone. Artifacts in the P_{det} may be produced by intrinsic rectal contractions.[46]

Filling rates in the past were described as slow, medium, or fast. Currently, the filling rate is classified as physiologic or nonphysiologic, and the actual rate should be specified.[38] Most studies in non-neurologic patients are done with medium fill rates of 50 to 100 mL/min.

Bladder storage function should be noted with bladder sensation (normal; first sensation of filling; first and strong desire to void; increased, reduced, or absent bladder sensation; bladder pain; and urgency), detrusor overactivity, bladder compliance, and capacity.[38] The terminology to describe detrusor activity has been standardized by the ICS.[38] *Detrusor overactivity* is characterized by spontaneous or provoked involuntary detrusor contractions during filling. Although an involuntary contraction was originally defined as a minimum pressure rise of 15 cm H_2O,[47] there is presently no lower limit for the amplitude of an involuntary contraction (Fig. 57-4).[38] If leakage is detected in association with an involuntary detrusor contraction, it is termed *detrusor overactivity incontinence.* Detrusor overactivity can be further characterized into idiopathic and neurogenic detrusor overactivity. *Idiopathic detrusor overactivity* describes involuntary detrusor contractions of unknown etiology and has replaced the term "detrusor instability." An involunatary detrusor contraction secondary to an underlying neurologic condition is *neurogenic detrusor overactivity,* which has replaced "detrusor hyperreflexia."[38]

Another type of overactive bladder dysfunction is reduced compliance. *Bladder compliance* is defined as the change in pressure for a given change in volume. It is calculated by dividing the volume change by the change in detrusor pressure during that change in bladder volume, and it is expressed as milliliters per centimeters of water pressure (see Fig. 57-4B).[38] Normal bladder compliance is high, and in the laboratory the normal pressure rise is less than 6 to 10 cm H_2O.[48] Low bladder compliance implies a poorly distensible bladder. The actual numeric values to indicate normal, high, or low compliance have yet to be defined.[38]

The finding of detrusor overactivity on cystometry is important if it correlates with the clinical condition of the patient. Idiopathic detrusor overactivity has been reported in 30% to 35% of patients with stress incontinence undergoing surgery. It resolves in most such patients after repair and may not have a significant impact on outcome.[49,50] Alternatively, if the patient's symptoms are primarily from bladder overactivity, or other factors predisposing to abnormal bladder behavior are present, the cystometric findings will influence treatment. These predisposing factors include a history of radiation, chronic bladder inflammation, indwelling catheter, chronic infection, chemotherapy, voiding dysfunction after pelvic surgery, and other neurologic conditions.

Urethral Function Tests

The normal urethral closure mechanism maintains a positive urethral closing pressure during bladder filling, even in the presence of increased abdominal pressure. An incompetent mechanism allows leakage in the absence of a detrusor contraction.[38] Two urodynamic tests have been used to depict urethral competence: the Valsalva or abdominal leak point pressure (VLPP or ALPP) and the urethral pressure profile (UPP).

Leak Point Pressures

The VLPP is the intravesical pressure that exceeds the continence mechanism resulting in a leakage of urine in the absence of a detrusor contraction.[38] The test is performed by a progressive Valsalva maneuver or cough.[51] VLPP tests the strength of the urethra. The study is performed with the patient in the sitting or standing position with at least 150 to 200 mL of fluid in the bladder. Historically, a VLPP of less than 60 cm H_2O was evidence of significant intrinsic sphincter deficiency (ISD), between 60 and 90 cm H_2O suggested a component of ISD, and greater than 90 cm H_2O suggested minimal ISD with leakage mainly due to hypermobility.[48] Currently, no prospective studies have shown that VLPP less than 60 cm H_2O can accurately diagnose ISD. Although the VLPP may be reproducible,[52] it has not yet been standardized.[5]

There are limitations to a VLPP. If the patient's Valsalva effort is inadequate, urinary leakage may not be seen, and a VLPP measurement cannot be determined. The presence of a catheter in the urethra may prevent incontinence.[53] Furthermore, a cystocele or other prolapsing segment may produce inferior pressure on an incompetent urethra that prevents incontinence or falsely elevates the VLPP. If a cystocele is present, the VLPP should be repeated with the prolapse reduced by insertion of a vaginal pack or pessary.

The detrusor or bladder leak point pressure (DLPP) is the lowest detrusor pressure (P_{det}) on cystometry at which urinary leakage occurs during bladder filling in the absence of a detrusor contraction or increased abdominal pressure.[38] This parameter is used to investigate and monitor patients with neurogenic and low-compliance bladders. In general, patients with a DLPP greater than approximately 25 to 30 cm H_2O are at risk for upper tract deterioration from reflux or obstruction.[54,55] In these patients, it is necessary to assess compliance as well. A high DLPP indicates poor compliance with urethral obstruction, whereas a low DLPP is seen in patients with incompetent urethras. In order to demonstrate poor compliance in these patients. filling may be done with a Foley catheter to obstruct the outlet.[56]

Urethral Pressure Profile

Urethral pressure is defined as the fluid pressure needed to just open a closed urethra. The urethral pressure measurements recorded are[38]

- *urethral pressure profile* (UPP), a graph indicating the intraluminal pressure along the length of the urethra
- *maximum urethral closure pressure* (MUCP), the maximum difference between the urethral pressure and the intravesical pressure
- *functionalprofile length,* the length of the urethra along which the urethral pressure exceeds intravesical pressure in women
- *pressure transmission ratio,* the increment in urethral pressure on stress as a percentage of the simultaneously recorded increase in intravesical pressure

Intraluminal urethral pressure may be measured with the subject at rest, with the bladder at any given volume; during coughing or straining; and during voiding.[57] Measurements can be made at one point in the urethra over a period of time (continuous urethral pressure recording) or as a UPP. A mechanical retracting puller that is synchronized with the chart or digital recorder allows measurement of anatomic distances in the profile.

Two types of UPP may be measured: Resting UPP (Fig. 57-5A), with the bladder and subject at rest, and stress UPP (see Fig. 57-5B), with a defined applied stress (e.g., cough, strain, Valsalva maneuver).

The simultaneous recording of both intra-urethral (P_{ura}) and intravesical (P_{ves}) pressure enables calculation of urethral closure pressure (i.e., $P_{ura} - P_{ves}$). The three main methods for UPP measurement are perfused catheters with side holes, catheter-tip transducer catheters, and balloon catheters. Recordings of profile parameters must be repeated several times to verify reproducibility.[58]

An MUCP of less than 20 cm H_2O ("low-pressure urethra") has been reported to be predictive of poor outcome of conventional bladder neck suspension procedures[59] and has been called a predictor of ISD.[58] However, the MUCP alone does not provide any information about the integrity of the bladder neck or proximal urethra, and it can be highly variable as a result of involuntary contractions of the smooth and striated muscles of the

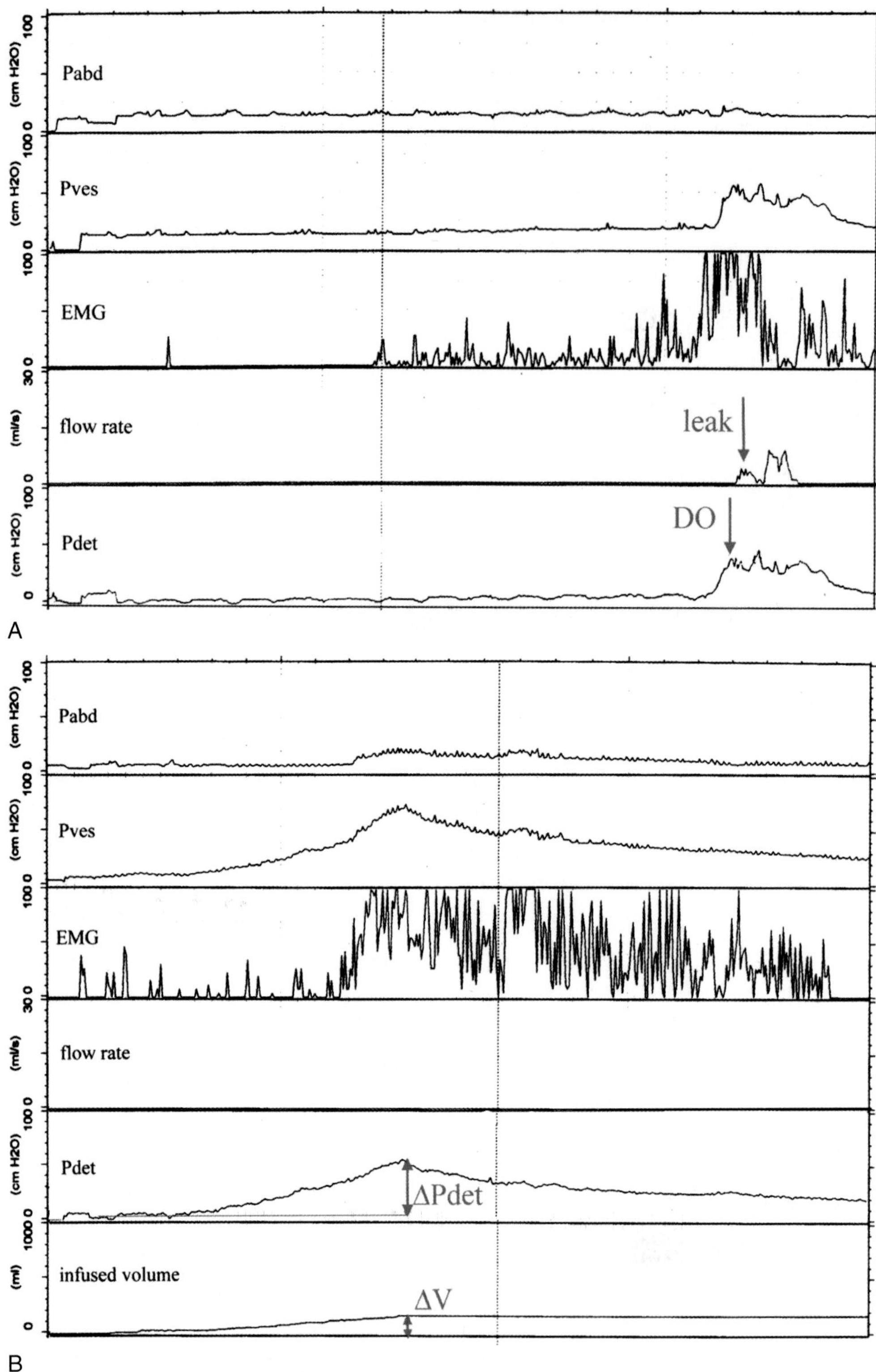

Figure 57-4 A, Detrusor overactivity. The uninhibited contraction at the end of the filling phase leads to leakage (detrusor overactivity incontinence). EMG, electromyograhic tracing; P_{abd}, abdominal pressure; P_{det}, detrusor pressure; P_{ves}, intravesical pressure. **B,** Reduced bladder compliance. As the bladder is filled, the detrusor pressure rises by 50 cm H_2O (ΔP_{det}) while the increase in bladder volume (ΔV) is 150 mL. The compliance ($\Delta V/\Delta P_{det}$) is 3 mL/cm H_2O, which is much lower than the normal range of at least 30 mL/cm H_2O. Griffiths D, Kondo A, Bauer S, et al: Dynamic testing. In Abrams P, Khoury S, Wein A (eds): Incontinence: Third International Consultation. Paris, France: Health Publications, 2005, pp 585-673.

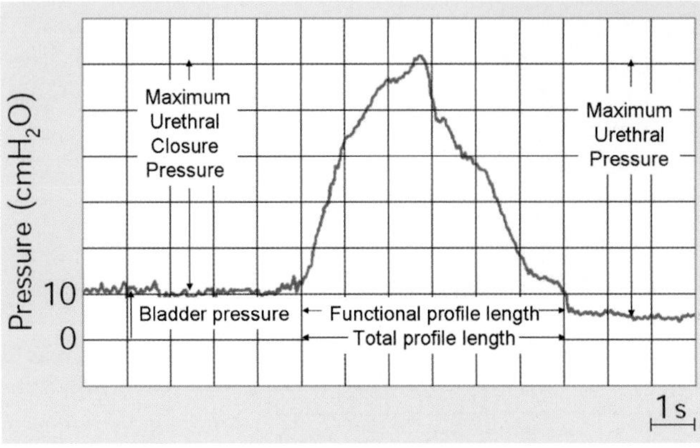

A

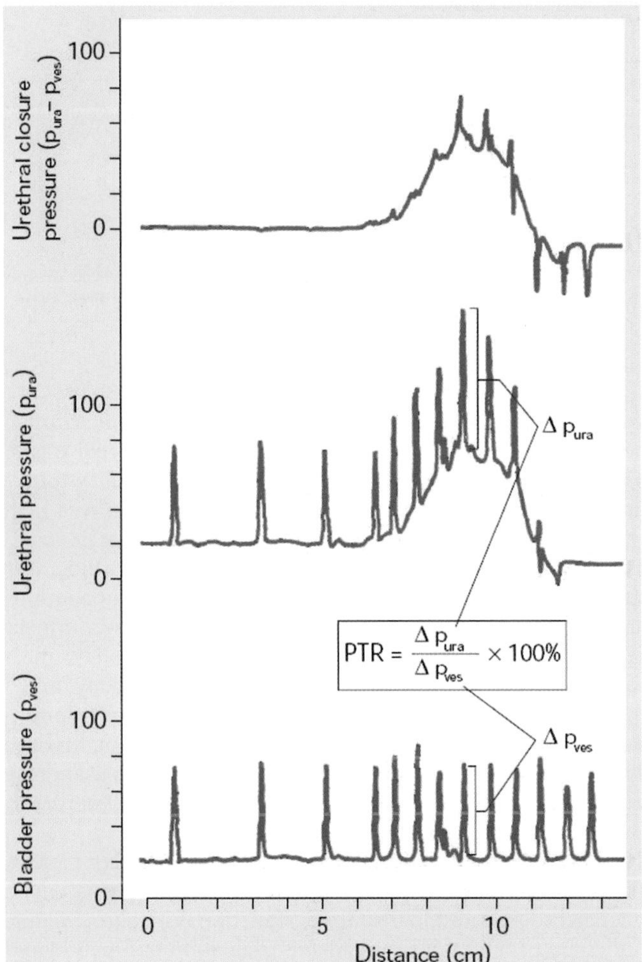

B

Figure 57-5 A, Resting urethral pressure profile. (Modified from Lose G: Urethral pressure measurements. In Cardozo L, Staskin D [eds]: Textbook of Female Urology and Urogynaecology. London: Isis Medical Media, 2001, pp 215-226.) **B,** Urethral pressure profile during coughs in a continent woman. The bottom trace shows the bladder response to a series of coughs (P_{ves}). The middle trace shows the corresponding urethral responses (P_{ura}) while the measuring catheter is slowly withdrawn out of the bladder and through the urethra. The top trace shows the difference between the middle and the bottom traces. The pressure transmission ratio (PTR) is the increment in urethral pressure on stress as a percentage of the simultaneously recorded increase in intravesical pressure: ($\Delta P_{ura}/\Delta P_{ves} \times 100\%$). (Modified from Lose G: Urethral pressure measurements. In Cardozo L, Staskin D [eds]: Textbook of Female Urology and Urogynaecology. London: Isis Medical Media, 2001, pp 215-226.)

urethral sphincter, possibly provoked by the catheter itself. Furthermore, the size, stiffness and type of catheter, rate of perfusion, patient position, and bladder volume affect the pressure readings.[5]

A variety of values of MUCP have been obtained by different authors in normal and abnormal female populations.[5] They have several notable features. The first is the intercenter variability in the values reported, with mean MUCP varying from 36 to 101 cm H_2O in subjects without stress incontinence. The second is the large intersubject standard deviation in most studies (from 10 to 52 cm H_2O). However, despite this variability, the mean MUCP was less in stress-incontinent patients than in non–stress-incontinent women, sometimes significantly so and sometimes not. Some of the variations are the result of different patient populations, and others are the result of technical errors. A weighted averaging of the mean values suggests that a normal (±SD) MUCP is about 54 ± 25 cm H_2O. In stress-incontinent women, the corresponding figure is 39 ± 24 cm H_2O. Clearly, there is so much overlap that it has been impossible to define a cutoff level that allows differentation between women with and without stress incontinence.[5]

Stress profiles show greater variability than static variables do. The within-subject standard deviation for the pressure transmission ratio varies between 13% and 18.5% (95% confidence limits up to ± 37%) in published reports. The coefficient if variation has been estimated to be 20% (95% confidence limits, ± 39%).

Maximum urethral pressure (MUP), like MUCP, also declines with aging.[60]

There clearly are limitations to the test that prevent it from providing reliable pathophysiologic information.[5]

In summary, although the VLPP under ideal circumstances may indicate the severity of stress urinary incontinence, it is not clear whether it is more useful than clincal grading,[5] and, although UPP measurements may be interesting as a research tool, their practical applicability is still to be determined.

Pressure-Flow Studies

Pressure-flow studies are designed to provide dynamic information on the emptying phase of lower urinary tract function. Obstruction is not common in women[61] but may be found after surgical correction of stress urinary incontinence or, less commonly, with detrusor sphincter dyssynergia, non-neurogenic voiding dysfunction, and, rarely, stricture disease. Interference with voiding may also be associated with pelvic organ prolapse. There are no established nomograms to depict pressure-flow relationships in women as there are in men (although one has been proposed[62]), but the pattern of high detrusor pressure and low urinary flow indicates obstruction (Fig. 57-6). Simultaneous cystography can demonstrate the level of obstruction.

Detrusor pressure during voiding is characteristically low in women. A preoperative study that demonstrates a low detrusor pressure with a low flow rate may aid in counseling the patient about postoperative urinary retention after stress incontinence surgery. The urodynamic definition of obstruction in women is

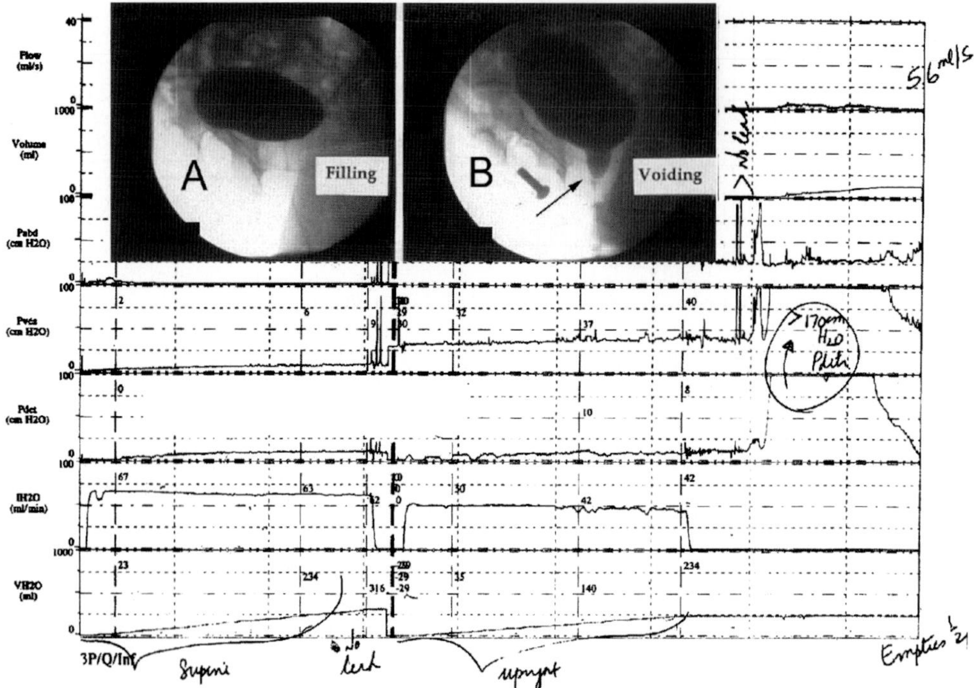

Figure 57-6 A and B, Videourodynamic study of a 62-year-old woman with urgency, frequency, and slow stream after multiple urethral dilatations. The study shows a normal bladder on filling, with no overactivity. Her voiding pressure exceeds 170 cm H_2O, and her flow rate is low. There is a urethral stricture visible (*arrow* in **B**) with proximal urethral dilatation.

different than in men. A cutoff value of 12 mL/sec or less maximum flow rate and a detrusor pressure at maximum flow of 25 cm H_2O or more, in conjunction with high clinical suspicion, provides good predictive value.[63]

Electromyography

Sphincter electromyography (EMG) during videourodynamics is used to examine striated sphincter activity during filling and voiding. These are termed *kinesiologic* studies, and they can be performed with surface electrodes, vaginal or anal probes, or needles. Normal sphincter EMG activity has characteristic audio quality that may be monitored simultaneously. Its most important role is the identification of abnormal sphincter activity in patients with neurogenic bladder dysfunction and in those with behavioral voiding dysfunction.[64] The fluoroscopy component, however, can demonstrate detrusor external sphincter dyssynergia in patients with suprasacral lesions and can show urethral obstruction in patients with dysfunctional voiding. EMG recordings are not usually necessary in routine videourodynamics for incontinence in women who have no neurologic abnormalities. Artifacts can occur secondary to room appliances, fluorescent lights, defective insulation, and patient movement.[48]

Videourodynamics

Videourodynamics is a diagnostic tool that incorporates urodynamics with simultaneous imaging of the lower urinary tract. The incorporation of radiologic visualization of the lower urinary tract during bladder filling and voiding is useful for determining the site of bladder outlet obstruction, the integrity of the sphincter mechanism, and the presence of vesicoureteral reflux, bladder diverticula, fistulas, and trabeculation.[40] Urodynamics was first synchronized with cineradiography in the early 1950s through the pioneering efforts of E. R. Miller.[65,66] The initial goal was to minimize the radiation exposure to the patient during cystourethrography. Originally, patient exposure to radiation was high when movies were taken, but with the advent of image intensifiers, video transduction, and, later, videotape recording, the patient exposure was reduced. This permitted bursts of continuous activity to be recorded during critical phases of lower urinary tract activity without overexposing the patient. Today, most studies can be done with less than 1 minute of fluoroscopy time.[48] These developments have contributed to the wealth of information about lower urinary tract function and dysfunction. Modern videourodynamic techniques incorporate fluoroscopy, and the urodynamic machine has evolved from a strip chart recorder to a microcomputer.

Videourodynamic studies are not necessary in every patient, and simpler studies frequently provide enough information to adequately delineate and treat the dysfunction. Videourodynamic studies are beneficial if simultaneous evaluation of function and anatomy is needed to provide detailed information about the whole or parts of the storage and emptying phases. Common indications well suited for videourodynamic evaluation include complex incontinence, in which the history does not fit with the findings on preliminary investigations; incontinence in women with previous anti-incontinence surgery; and incontinence in the face of a neurologic abnormality.

Aside from the minimal radiation exposure to the patient, the only disadvantage of videourodynamics is its cost. This is a result of the time and effort of the personnel required and the expense of the equipment, which may limit its utility to larger centers with larger patient populations. The cost can, however, be justified by the utility of videourodynamics in solving complicated problems.

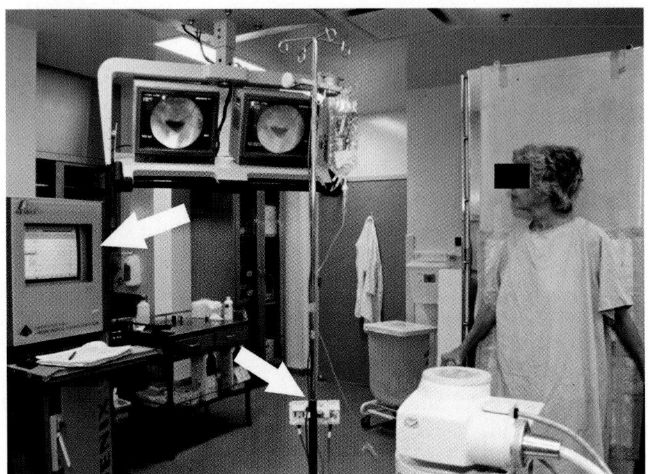

Figure 57-7 Diagram of a videourodynamic suite. The patient is in the upright position after the filling catheter has been removed. She will be asked to cough and strain to demonstrate stress incontinence and then to void. *The left arrow* indicates the multichannel recorder, and the *right arrow* indicates the transducers.

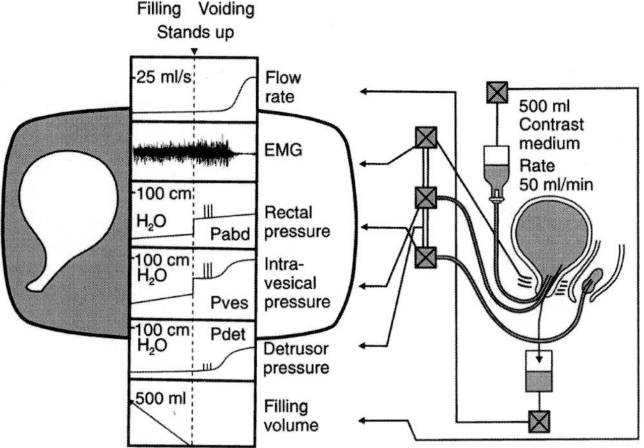

Figure 57-8 Schematic diagram of videourodynamic setup.

Components of Videourodynamics

A typical arrangement for videourodynamic studies includes a multichannel recorder, a flouroscopy unit with a table that can be positioned in the supine and upright positions, and a flow meter (Figs. 57-7 and 57-8). A commode seat attachment facilitates fluoroscopic screening of voiding in the seated position, which is ideal for women. Most modern systems are computer based, which allows for complex analysis to be performed.

Multichannel Recorder

Because the procedure involves measuring simultaneous pressures during both phases of lower urinary tract function and flow during the voiding phase, a multichannel recorder is necessary. Many systems are available,[67] most of which have dispensed with a strip chart output in favor of television monitor display of the procedure.

The choice of components of the study is up to the individual clinician. Figure 57-8 illustrates possible inclusions. The channels demonstrating volume of fluid instilled and volume voided are helpful but not essential, as these values can be measured manually. The sphincter EMG channel is not necessary for routine clinical practice but can be helpful in patients with neurologic disease; its inclusion introduces another level of complexity and sophistication.

For a review of the currently recommended urodynamic technique of pressure measurements the reader is referred to the article of Schaeffer and colleagues describing "Good Urodynamic Practices."[37]

Fluoroscopy

A good-quality fluoroscopy unit with a high-resolution image intensifier and a table that can function in both the supine and the erect position is required. Fluoroscopic images are obtained selectively during the filling and voiding study and are either superimposed on the pressure-flow tracing or displayed on a separate screen. The fluoroscopic images can be stored and reproduced individually or as continuous clips during key parts of the study. A recording of the procedure can be made for subsequent review.

Because the contrast medium instilled into bladder is unlikely to be absorbed, we use the less expensive high-osmolality contrast media. A dilute solution of 1 L of Hypaque is prepared by the pharmacy and supplied in sterile intravenous bags.

Videourodynamic Technique

The patient reports for the study with a full bladder, and a flow rate is obtained. The equipment is zeroed, and the transducer is placed at a height adjacent to the upper edge of the patient's symphisis pubis. Either a double-lumen catheter or two 8-Fr feeding tubes (one for filling, which is removed before the voiding study, and one for pressure measurements) are inserted into the bladder. Residual urine is measured. The rectal catheter is a 42-cm 14-Fr tube with a balloon over the tip. If desired, EMG recording devices may be applied to the patient.

The study is conducted by a urodynamics specialist who is present in the room, communicates with the patient throughout the procedure, and records the findings manually and electronically. A supine or semioblique filling study is carried out, various measurements are taken during the study, and responses to actions such as Credé, cough, and Valsalva maneuvers are recorded. The filling rate is no longer divided into slow, medium, or fast but rather is described as physiologic or nonphysiologic.[38] In practice, most clinicians use a medium fill rate of 50 to 75 mL/min.[46] A commonly used method is to fill the bladder supine and then stand the patient up for provocative manoeuvres.

During the study, recordings are made of bladder images in the filling phase in the supine and/or upright position (see Fig. 57-8). Anteroposterior (AP) and oblique views are obtained. The AP position permits documentation of reflux and its extent, and in the oblique position the course of the urethra can be seen separate from a cystocele. Notation is made of the bladder outline, the appearance of the bladder neck at rest, and its position relative to the inferior margin of the symphysis at rest and with straining and coughing. Leakage of urine with overactivity, decreased compliance, or leakage with various stress maneuvers is recorded. In the upright position, the presence of a cystocele and its relationship to the urethra are also noted. If the patient is able to void in front of the camera, the voiding phase (or parts of it) are recorded, along with the pressures and flow tracings. If the patient is unable to void with the catheters in place, they are removed, and a flow rate and voided volume are measured. Total fluoroscopy time is usually less than 1 minute.

Table 57-1 Radiologic Type of Stress Incontinence

Type	Description
0	Vesical neck and proximal urethra closed at rest and situated at or above the lower end of the symphysis pubis. They descend during stress, but incontinence is not seen.
I	Vesical neck closed at rest and well above the inferior margin of the symphysis. During stress, the vesical neck and proximal urethra are open and descend less than 2 cm. Incontinence is seen.
IIa	Vesical neck closed at rest and above the inferior margin of the symphysis. During stress, the vesical neck and proximal urethra open and descend more than 2 cm. Incontinence is seen.
IIb	Vesical neck closed at rest and at or below the inferior margin of the symphysis. During stress, there may or may not be further descent but as the proximal urethra opens incontinence is seen.
III	Vesical neck and proximal urethra are open at rest. The proximal urethra no longer functions as a sphincter. There is obvious urinary leakage with minimal increases in intravesical pressure.

From Blaivas JG, Olsson CA: Stress incontinence: Classification and surgical approach. J Urol 139:727-731, 1988.

The recorded study provides an opportunity for the case to be reviewed and discussed. All of the events of the study are recorded and displayed on the monitor during the study. The urodynamics machine is usually equipped with the capability of compressing the study so that it can be viewed on an ordinary letter-size sheet of paper.

Urinary Incontinence

The main advantage of fluoroscopic imaging during the urodynamic study is to obtain an anatomic view of the function or dysfunction. The technique is ideally suited to the evaluation of incontinence. A useful anatomic/radiologic classification of female incontinence, devised by Blaivas,[68] is described in Table 57-1 and illustrated in Figure 57-9. We use this classification to determine the radiologic abnormality and add to it the information from the VLPP and the position of the urethra in relation to the cystocele to describe the functional problem. Each of the urodynamic tracings in the figures described in the next few paragraphs is shown in full with annotations made during the study. The video recordings depicting parts of the studies were obtained from a video printer connected to the fluoroscopy equipment.

Type I abnormalities are illustrated in Figure 57-10; the patient had a VLPP of 62 cm H_2O and minimal hypermobility. The patient in Figure 57-11 had a VLPP of more than 120 cm H_2O on straining during upright filling. At the end of filling, a cough caused a large leak without much hypermobility and appeared to be accompanied by a small bladder contraction. This indicated that the patient had stress incontinence as well as cough-induced overactivity.

Figures 57-12 thru 57-14 demonstrate type IIa abnormalities. The patient in Figure 57-12 has a high VLPP without any appreciable cystocele. In Figure 57-13, the patient has an involuntary detrusor contraction with incontinence in the upright position and a high VLPP. The patient shown in Figure 57-14 has a grade II cystocele that appears with straining; she probably has mainly a lateral defect.

Type IIb abnormalities are shown in Figures 57-15 thru 57-17. The bladder neck in Figure 57-15 is seen well below the lower margin of the symphysis and is associated with a grade II cystocele. Because the bladder neck is above the base of the cystocele but below the lower margin of the symphysis, the patient most likely has a combined central and lateral defect. In Figure 57-16, the large cystocele is not associated with demonstrable stress incontinence, despite coughing and straining pressures greater than 100 cm H_2O. It appears to be primarily a central defect. Clinical examination must include reducing the cystocele and checking for stress incontinence. The patient in Figure 57-17 has a combined central and lateral defect. She has marked detrusor overactivity with leakage, but stress incontinence is not demonstrated, most likely because of the compressive effect of the cystocele.

Type III incontinence or pure ISD is demonstrated by the patient in Figure 57-18. Her bladder neck is open at rest, no appreciable descent is seen with coughing or straining, and her VLPP is low at 59 cm H_2O.

Videourodynamic and fluoroscopic studies, in addition to demonstrating incontinence and degree of hypermobility, may also allow characterization of the type of cystocele (see Fig. 57-15).

Obstruction

Although outflow obstruction is uncommon in females, it is occasionally seen. The patient in Figure 57-6 had an iatrogenic and functionally significant urethral obstruction that was treated with a visual internal urethrotomy and subsequent long-term self-dilation.

Pitfalls of Videourodynamics

Patient cooperation, comfort, and compliance are necessary to obtain a meaningful and relevant study. Occasionally, an apprehensive patient has a vasovagal reflex and faint when the table is moved from the supine to the upright position, and the study cannot be completed. Moreover, stress incontinence may not be demonstrated in an anxious patient.

Of 2259 studies that we reviewed in our laboratory for neurologically normal women whose chief complaint was stress incontinence, we were unable to demonstrate stress incontinence on fluoroscopy in 630 (28%). It is also difficult for many patients to void in front of the camera with catheters in the bladder and rectum and observers watching them. In our series, only 1348 patients (59.7%) were able to void, and some of these did so with abdominal straining. The others were unable to void during the procedure, and the voiding data was obtained from the uroflow measurements.

To optimize visibility of the lower urinary tract on fluoroscopy, patient positioning must be correct. However, visibility may be poor or absent with very obese patients. The clinician must also maintain a dialogue with the patient to image crucial events, because the patient must relay changes in sensation during filling and may be the first to sense incontinence.

The radiation equipment must be well maintained and undergo regular maintenance and safety inspections. The failure to maintain equipment may lead to inaccurate results. Because fluoroscopy time is short, radiation exposure to the patient is inconsequential; however, the clinician should use radiation protection, including aprons and thyroid shields.

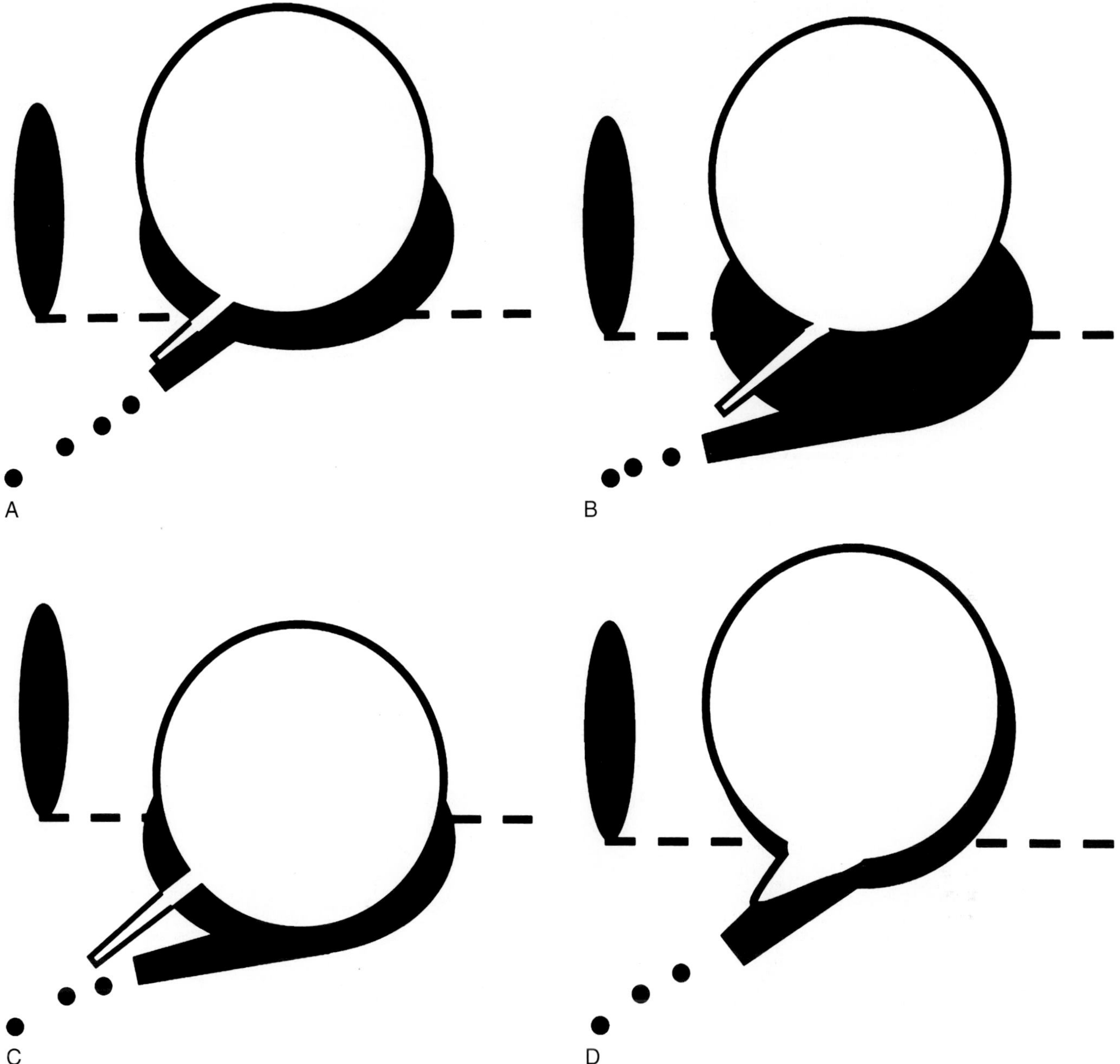

Figure 57-9 Schematic diagrams of the radiologic images obtained from women with the various types of female stress urinary incontinence. **A,** Type I. The bladder neck is closed at rest and is well above the inferior margin of the symphysis. During stress, the bladder neck and proximal urethra open and descend less than 2 cm, and incontinence is seen. **B,** Type IIa. The bladder neck is closed at rest and is above the inferior margin of the symphysis. During stress, the bladder neck and proximal urethra open and descend more than 2 cm. Incontinence is seen. **C,** Type IIb. The bladder neck is closed at rest and is at or below the inferior margin of the symphysis. During stress, there may or may not be further descent, but as the proximal urethra opens, incontinence is seen. **D,** Type III. The bladder neck and proximal urethra are open at rest. The proximal urethra no longer functions as a sphincter. There is obvious urinary leakage with minimal increases in intravesical pressure. (From Blaivas JG, Groutz A: Urinary incontinence: Pathophysiology, evaluation, and management overview. In Walsh PC, RetikAB, Vaughan ED Jr, Wein AJ [eds]: Campbell's Urology, 8th ed. Philadelphia: Saunders, 2000, pp 1027-1052.)

Other pitfalls relate to the urodynamic aspects and are similar to those previously outlined by O'Donnell.[69] Standardized terminology to communicate results and concepts should always be used.[38] The testing procedures and equipment should be compatible with commonly accepted methodologies. The value and limitations of each measurement must be realized; for example, the VLPP may not be useful in the presence of a large prolapsing cystocele. To confirm reliability within a particular laboratory, it is necessary to have a high test-retest correlation of studies. The validity of a test refers to its ability to measure what it is supposed to measure. The clinician must always be aware of the how the test in question compares to a "gold standard" test, which in urodynamics may be difficult to establish. The urodynamic studies should correlate with other clinical data. The voiding history, physical examination, endoscopic examination, and videourodynamic evaluation should serve to validate one another and strengthen the clinical assessment.

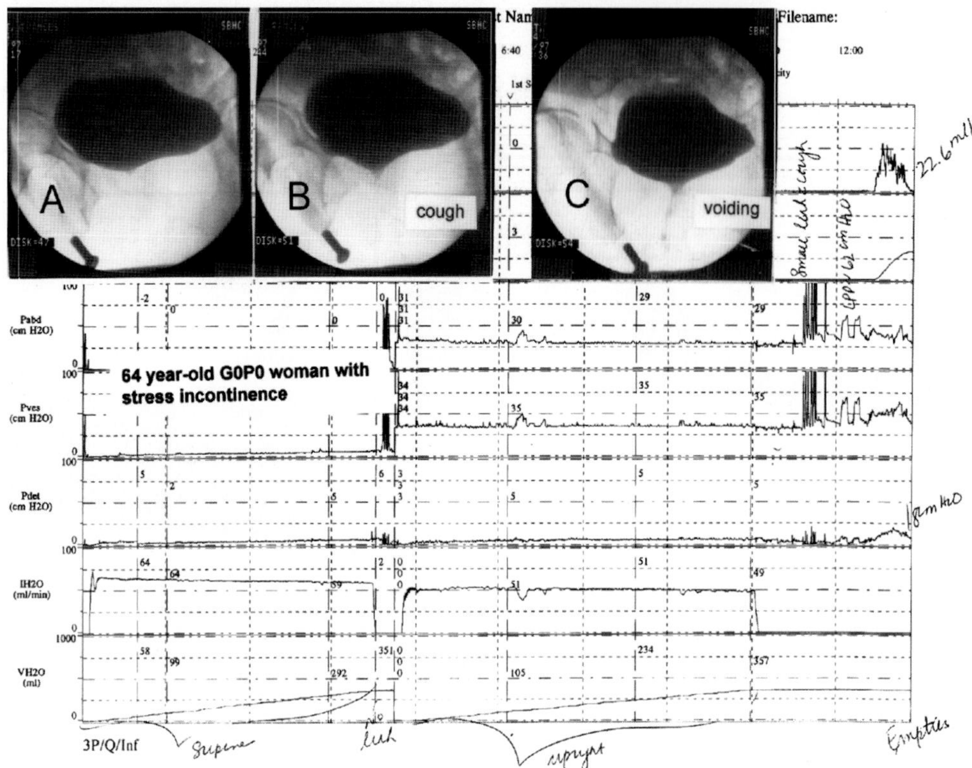

Figure 57-10 **A** through **C**, Videourodynamic study of a 64-year-old gravida 0, para 0 woman with type I stress incontinence. She had a bladder capacity of more than 300 mL. The bladder neck was slightly open at rest **(A).** With coughing, there was a small amount of descent and Valsalva leak point pressure was 62 cm H_2O. She had no apparent cystocele, and her voiding phase was normal.

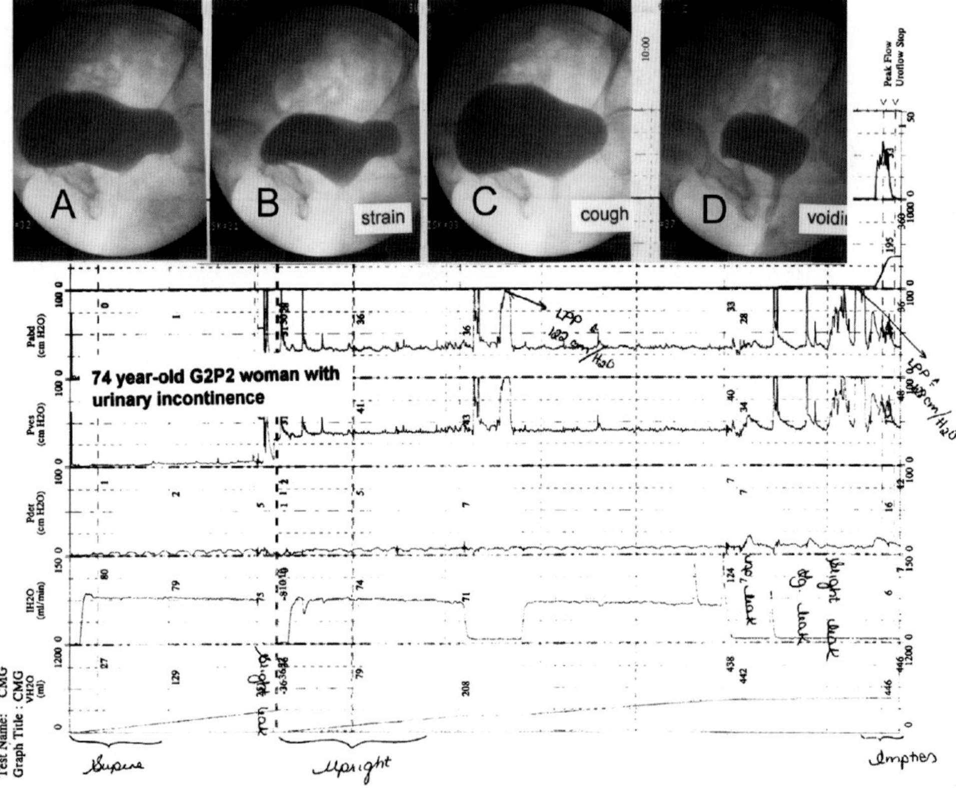

Figure 57-11 **A** through **D**, Videourodynamic study of a 74-year-old gravida 2, para 2 woman with type I stress incontinence. The bladder neck is slightly open at rest **(A).** In the upright position **(B),** leaks occur with straining and a Valsalva leak point pressure of 122 cm H_2O is recorded. On coughing **(C),** leaking is followed by a detrusor contraction (*arrow*). Voiding is normal **(D).**

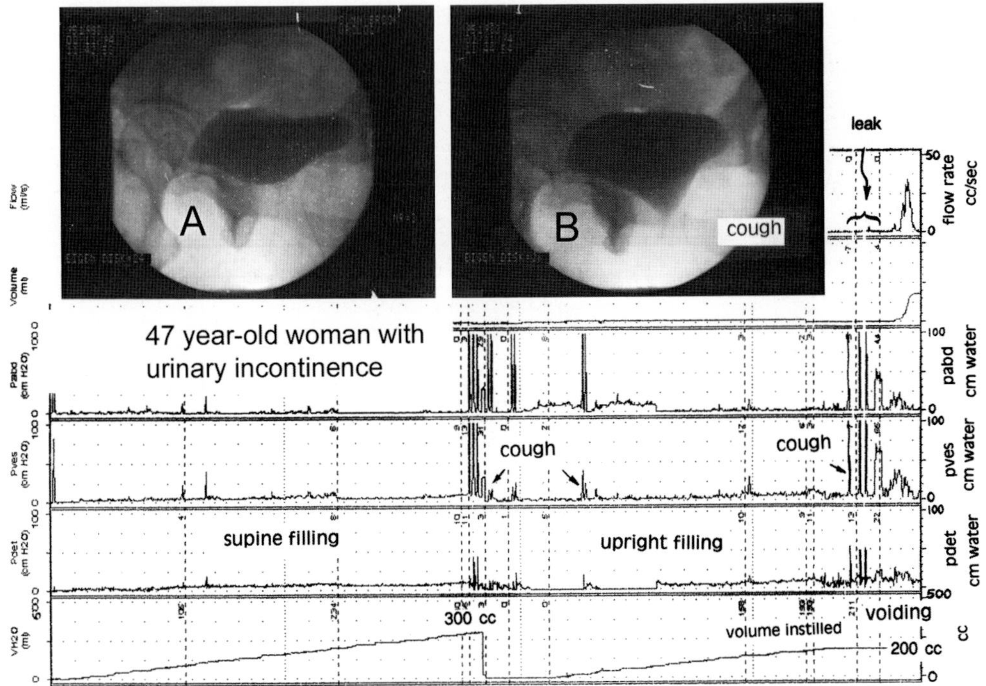

Figure 57-12 A and **B**, Videourodynamic study of a 47-year-old gravida 1, para 1 woman with type IIa stress incontinence. Her bladder neck is open at rest **(A)**. Leakage and hypermobility are seen with coughing **(B)**.

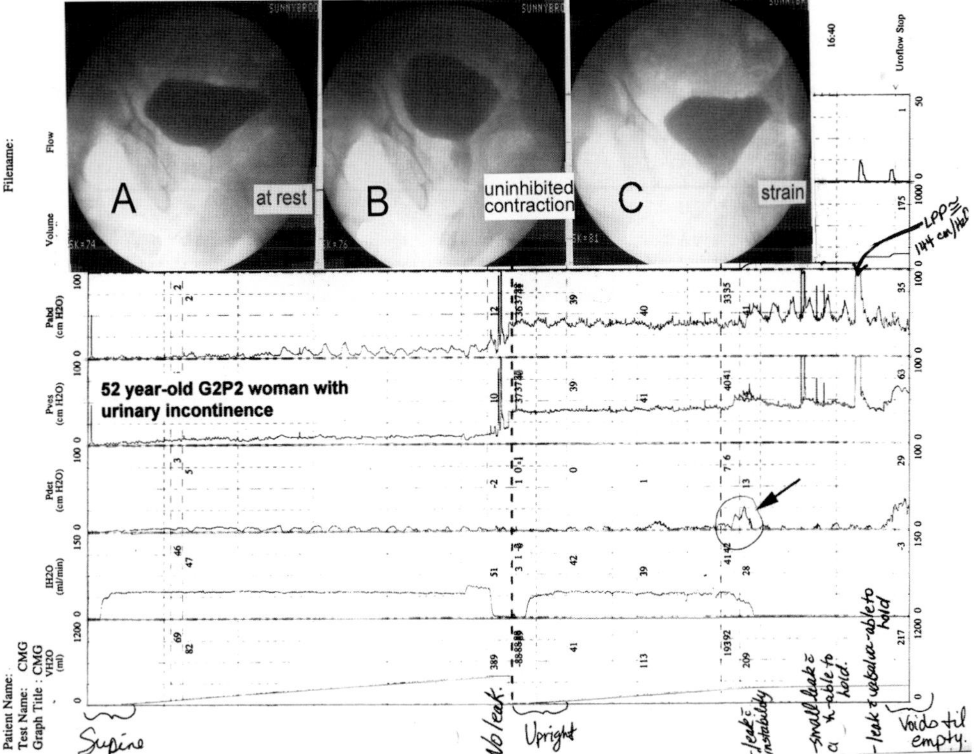

Figure 57-13 A through **C**, Videourodynamic study of a 52-year-old gravida 2, para 2 woman with a type IIa abnormality who complained of both stress and urgency incontinence. The bladder neck is slightly open at rest **(A)**. She has an involuntary detrusor contraction (*arrow*) on upright filling that results in incontinence **(B)**. With straining, leaking occurred, with a Valsalva leak point pressure of more than 140 cm H_2O **(C)**.

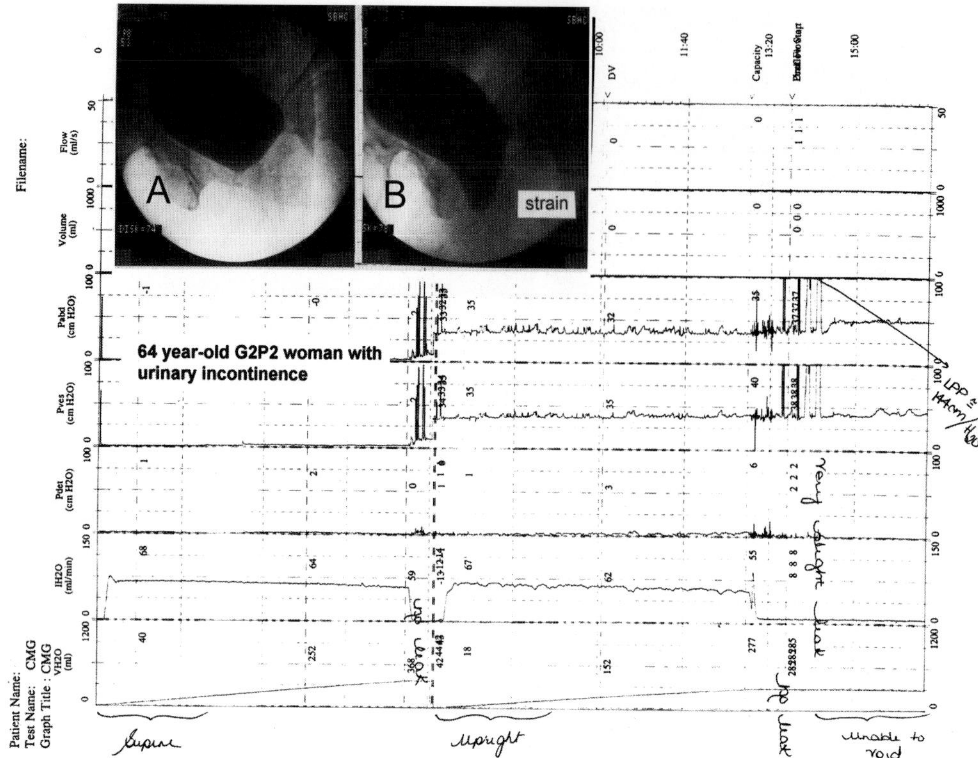

Figure 57-14 A and B, Videourodynamic study of a 64-year-old gravida 2, para 2 woman with type IIa stress incontinence. Her bladder neck is well supported on upright filling **(A).** With straining, leaking occurs with a Valsalva leak point pressure of 144 cm H_2O, and a cystocele is demonstrated **(B).** She most likely has mainly a lateral defect.

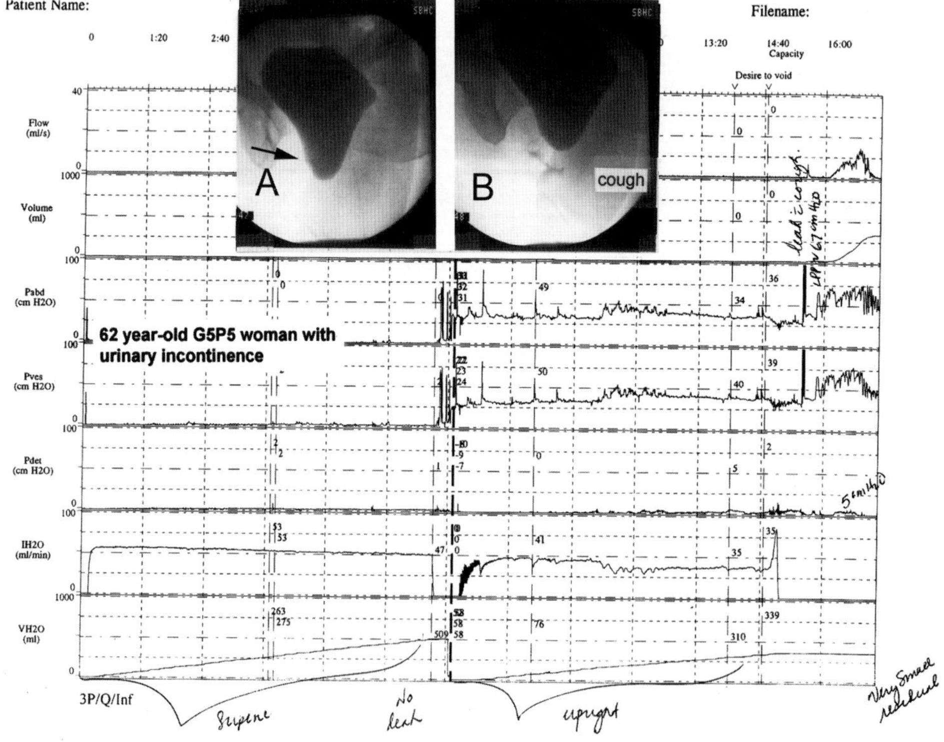

Figure 57-15 A and B, Videourodynamic study of a 62-year-old gravida 5, para 5 woman with type IIb stress incontinence. Her bladder neck (*arrow*) on filling **(A)** is below the lower margin of the inferior symphysis, and a cystocele is seen. She most likely has a combined central and lateral defect. She has leakage with coughing **(B)** and a Valsalva leak point pressure of 62 cm H_2O on straining.

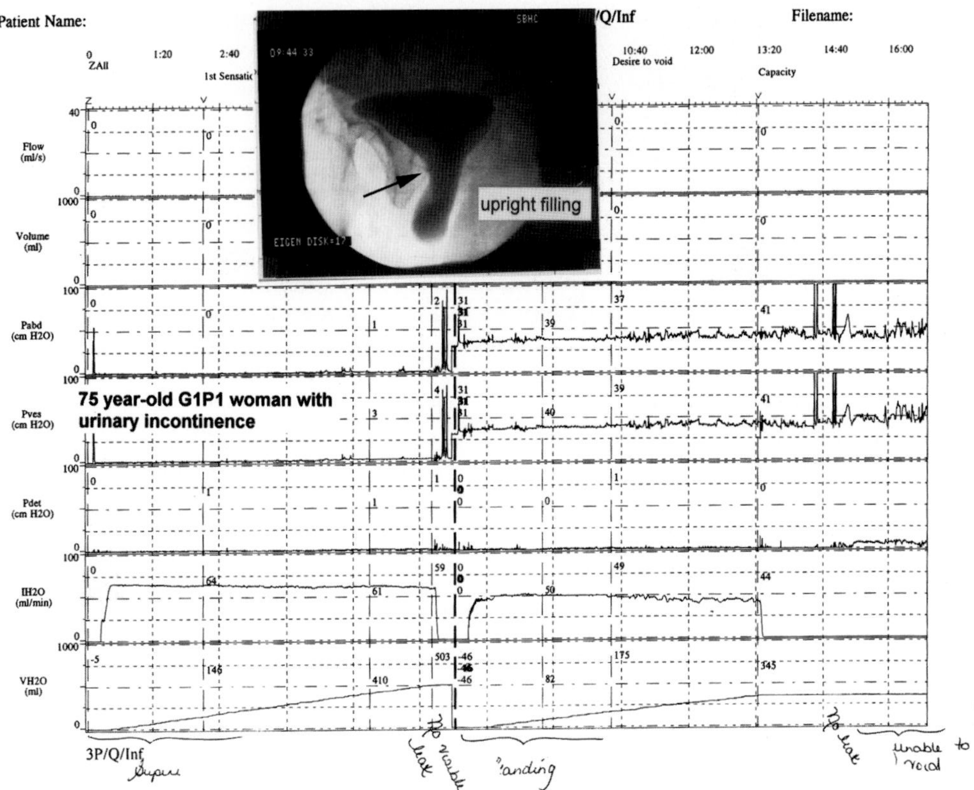

Figure 57-16 Videourodynamic study of a 75-year-old gravida 1, para 1 woman with a large cystocele. Although she complained of stress incontinence, it is not visible on this study. The bladder neck (*arrow*) is at the lower margin of the symphysis. The cystocele appears primarily to be a central defect. Clinical evaluation must include reducing the cystocele and testing for stress incontinence.

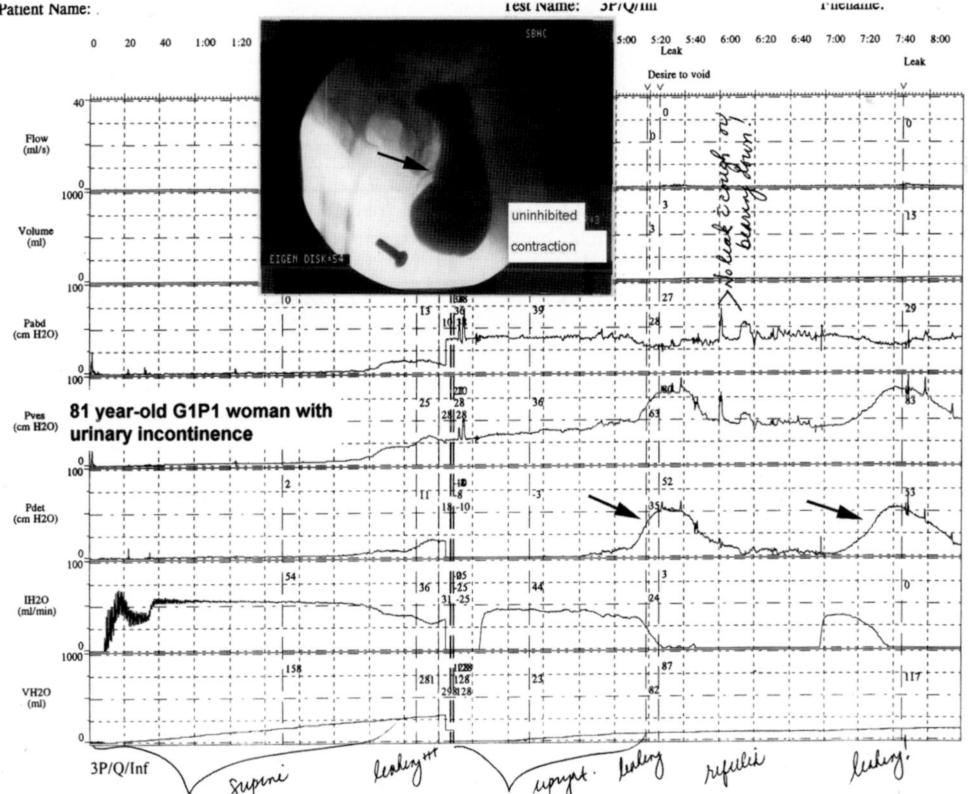

Figure 57-17 Videourodynamic study of an 81-year-old gravida 1, para 1 woman with a central and lateral defect. The bladder neck is below the symphysis (*arrow* on image). She has marked detrusor overactivity on supine and upright filling (*arrows* on graph). Although she complained of stress incontinence in addition to urge incontinence, it is not demonstrated on this study.

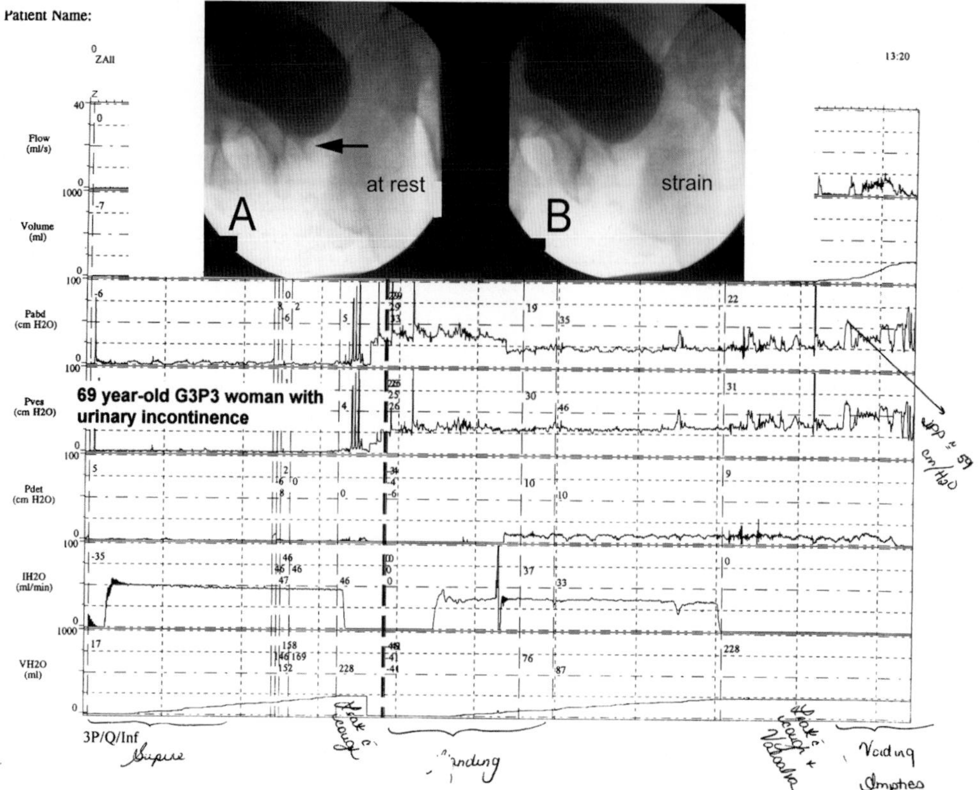

Figure 57-18 **A** and **B**, Videourodynamic study of a 69-year-old gravida 3, para 3 woman with type III abnormality after two previous stress incontinence repairs. Her bladder neck is open at rest (*arrow* in **A**). There is almost no urethral movement on straining **(B)**, and her Valsalva leak point pressure is 59 cm H_2O.

ROLE OF URODYNAMICS IN PREDICTING OCCULT STRESS INCONTINENCE IN WOMEN DUE TO BE TREATED FOR PROLAPSE

The problem of occult stress incontinence in women due to be treated for prolapse was reviewed in the recent Third International Consultation on Urinary Incontinence.[5] It has been reported that 11% to 22% of continent women undergoing vaginal repair for large cystocele develop stress incontinence after surgical repair.[70,71] Therefore, it would be helpful to have a test that predicts for the occurrence of occult stress incontinence, if stress incontinence has not been present preoperatively, either symptomatically or by reducing the prolapse. According to the literature, advanced age, incontinence before development of pelvic organ prolapse, and extensive dissection at the time of the repair seem to increase the risk of postoperative incontinence.

There are a number of studies that report the finding of unmasked stress incontinence on videourodynamic testing in 25% to 83% of patients.[72,73] Low-pressure urethras are also seen after prolapse reduction in 20% to 56% of individuals[13,73]; however, stress profiles are not particularly reliable measures. Urethral hypermobility is correlated with the degree of prolapse,[15] as is detrusor overactivity revealed by prolapse reduction.

The literature emphasizes the importance of urodynamic assessment with prolapse reduction to assess occult stress incontinence and possibly detrusor overactivity.[72,74-76] However, there are no studies assessing reproducibility or testing whether incontinence revealed by prolapse reduction occurs after surgery if no procedures are done to prevent it. The prophylactic use of the Pereyra or Kelly procedure does not reduce the risk of postoperative incontinence.[77-79] In a recently reported randomized, prospective study,[80] concomitant Burch colposuspension was shown to significantly reduce the incidence of postoperative stress incontinence after abdominal sacropcolpopexy. Before surgery, about 36% of both groups had occult stress incontinence on urodynamics. Postoperatively, the control group had an incidence of 24.5%, compared with 6.1 in the colposuspension group ($P < .0001$). In those patients with no leakage detected on urodynamics preoperatively, the Burch procedure reduced the postoperative incidence from 38.2% to 20.8% ($P = .0007$).

Questions remain about the reproducibility and predictability of urodynamics in prolapse. In the randomized controlled trial just described, Burch colposuspension significantly reduced postoperative stress incontinence regardless of the preoperative urodynamic findings.[80] Another study concluded that urodynamic testing before prolapse surgery was not cost-effective.[76] Therefore, we do not have a consistently reliable test that identifies and determines appropriate management of occult stress urinary incontinence.[5]

CONCLUSION

Detailed clinical assessment of the patient with prolapse is essential in deciding therapy. Urodynamic studies provide additional information about the various symptoms of which the patient may or may not be complaining. Uroflowmetry and postvoid residual urine measurement are good screening tests for voiding dysfunction. More invasive testing may be helpful in many cases, including those involving complex or recurrent symptoms. Although there are benefits of urodynamic studies, in that the lower urinary tract problem may be more clearly elucidated, overall there still exists a lack of evidence of reproducibility and predictive value in assigning treatments and determining outcomes.

References

1. Mouritsen L, Larsen JP: Symptoms, bother and POPQ in women referred with pelvic organ prolapse. Int Urogynecol J Pelvic Floor Dysfunct 14:122-127, 2003.
2. Burrows LJ, Meyn LA, Walters MD, Weber AM: Pelvic symptoms in women with pelvic organ prolapse. Obstet Gynecol 104(5 Pt 1): 982-988, 2004.
3. Swift SE, Tate SB, Nicholas J: Correlation of symptoms with degree of pelvic organ support in a general population of women: What is pelvic organ prolapse? Am J Obstet Gynecol 189:372-377; discussion 377-379, 2003.
4. Bump RC, Mattiasson A, Bo K, et al: The standardization of terminology of female pelvic organ prolapse and pelvic floor dysfunction. Am J Obstet Gynecol 175:10-17, 1996.
5. Griffiths D, Kondo A, Bauer S, et al: Dynamic testing. In Abrams P, Khoury S, Wein A (eds): Incontinence: Third International Consultation. Paris, France: Health Publications, 2005, pp 585-673.
6. Glazener CM, Lapitan MC: Urodynamic investigations for management of urinary incontinence in adults. Cochrane Database Syst Rev 3:CD003195, 2002.
7. Blaivas JG, Groutz A: Urinary incontinence: Pathophysiology, evaluation, and management overview. In Walsh PC, Retik AB, Vaughan ED Jr, Wein AJ (eds): Campbell's Urology, 8th ed. Philadelphia: Saunders, 2000, pp 1027-1052.
8. McGuire EJ: Bladder instability and stress incontinence. Neurourol Urodyn 7:563-567, 1988.
9. Fantl JA, Wyman JF, McClish DK, Bump RC: Urinary incontinence in community-dwelling women: Clinical, urodynamic, and severity characteristics. Am J Obstet Gynecol 162:946-951; discussion 951-942, 1990.
10. Fantl JA, Newman DK, Colling J, et al: Urinary Incontinence in Adults: Acute and Chronic Management. Clinical Practice Guideline No. 2 Update. AHCPR Publication No. 96-0682. Rockville, MD: U.S. Department of Health and Human Services, Public Health Service, Agency for Health Care Policy and Research, March 1996.
11. Fianu S, Kjaeldgaard A, Larson B: Preoperative screening for latent stress incontinence in women with cystocele. Neurourol Urodyn 4:3, 1985.
12. Bump RC, Fantl JA, Hurt WG: The mechanism of urinary continence in women with severe uterovaginal prolapse: Results of barrier studies. Obstet Gynecol 72(3 Pt 1):291-295, 1988.
13. Rosenzweig B, Pushkin S, Blumenfeld D, Bhatia N: Prevalence of abnormal urodynamic test results in continent women with severe genitourinary prolapse. Obstet Gynecol 79:539-542, 1992.
14. Romanzi LJ: Management of the urethral outlet in patients with severe prolapse. Curr Opin Urol 12:339-344, 2002.
15. Romanzi LJ, Chaikin DC, Blaivas JG: The effect of genital prolapse on voiding. J Urol 161:581-586, 1999.
16. American College of Obstetricians and Gynecologists: Pelvic organ prolapse. ACOG Technical Bulletin No. 214. Washington, DC: ACOG; 1995.
17. Fantl JA, Wyman JF, McClish DK, et al: Efficacy of bladder training in older women with urinary incontinence. JAMA 265:609-613, 1991.
18. Nguyen JK, Bhatia NN: Resolution of motor urge incontinence after surgical repair of pelvic organ prolapse. J Urol 166:2263-2266, 2001.
19. Donovan J, Bosch R, Gotoh M, et al: Symptom and quality of life assessment. In Abrams P, Cardozo L, Khoury S (eds): Incontinence 3rd International Consultation. Paris: Health Publications, 2005, pp 519-584.
20. Tan JS, Lukacz ES, Menefee SA, et al: Predictive value of prolapse symptoms: A large database study. Int Urogynecol J Pelvic Floor Dysfunct 16:203-209; discussion 209, 2005.
21. Coates KW, Harris RL, Cundiff GW, Bump RC: Uroflowmetry in women with urinary incontinence and pelvic organ prolapse. Br J Urol 80:217-221, 1997.
22. Nitti VW, Tu LM, Gitlin J: Diagnosing bladder outlet obstruction in women. J Urol 161:1535-1540, 1999.
23. Chassagne S, Bernier PA, Haab F, et al: Proposed cutoff values to define bladder outlet obstruction in women. Urology 51:408-411, 1998.
24. Klarskov P, Andersen JT, Asmussen CF, et al: Acute urinary retention in women: A prospective study of 18 consecutive cases. Scand J Urol Nephrol 21:29-31, 1987.
25. Abrams P, Andersson KE, Brubaker L, et al: Recommendations of the International Scientific Committee: Evaluation and treatment of urinary incontinence, pelvic organ prolapse and faecal incontinence. In Abrams P, Cardozo L, Khoury S, Wein A (eds). Third International Consultation on Urinary Incontinence. Paris: Health Publications, 2005, pp 1589-1630.
26. Diokno AC, Dimaculangan RR, Lim EU, Steinert BW: Office based criteria for predicting type II stress incontinence without further evaluation studies. J Urol 161:1263-1267, 1999.
27. Nitti VW, Combs AJ: Correlation of Valsalva leak point pressure with subjective degree of stress urinary incontinence in women. J Urol 155:281-285, 1996.
28. Lemack GE, Zimmern PE: Predictability of urodynamic findings based on the Urogenital Distress Inventory-6 questionnaire. Urology 54:461-466, 1999.
29. Lemack GE, Zimmern PE: Identifying patients who require urodynamic testing before surgery for stress incontinence based on questionnaire information and surgical history. Urology 55:506-511, 2000.
30. Weber AM, Taylor RJ, Wei JT, et al: The cost-effectiveness of preoperative testing (basic office assessment vs. urodynamics) for stress urinary incontinence in women. BJU Int 89:356-363, 2002.
31. Bergman A, Bader K: Reliability of the patient's history in the diagnosis of urinary incontinence. Int J Gynaecol Obstet 32:255-259, 1990.
32. Versi E, Cardozo L, Anand D, Cooper D: Symptoms analysis for the diagnosis of genuine stress incontinence. Br J Obstet Gynaecol 98:815-819, 1991.
33. Haeusler G, Hanzal E, Joura E, et al: Differential diagnosis of detrusor instability and stress-incontinence by patient history: The Gaudenz-Incontinence-Questionnaire revisited. Acta Obstet Gynecol Scand 74:635-637, 1995.
34. Amundsen C, Lau M, English SF, McGuire EJ: Do urinary symptoms correlate with urodynamic findings? J Urol 161:1871-1874, 1999.
35. Weidner AC, Myers ER, Visco AG, et al: Which women with stress incontinence require urodynamic evaluation? Am J Obstet Gynecol 184:20-27, 2001.
36. Lemack GE: Urodynamic assessment of patients with stress incontinence: How effective are urethral pressure profilometry and abdominal leak point pressures at case selection and predicting outcome? Curr Opin Urol 14:307-311, 2004.
37. Schafer W, Abrams P, Liao L, et al: Good urodynamic practices: Uroflowmetry, filling cystometry, and pressure-flow studies. Neurourol Urodyn 21:261-274, 2002.
38. Abrams P, Cardozo L, Fall M, et al. The standardisation of terminology of lower urinary tract function: Report from the Standardisation

Sub-committee of the International Continence Society. Neurourol Urodyn 21:167-178, 2002.
39. Haylen BT, Ashby D, Sutherst JR, et al: Maximum and average urine flow rates in normal male and female populations: The Liverpool nomograms. Br J Urol 64:30-38, 1989.
40. Blaivas JG: Techniques of evaluation. In Yalla SV, McGuire EJ, Elbadawi A, Blaivas JG (eds): Neurourology and Urodynamics: Principles and Practice. New York: MacMillan, 1988.
41. Kondo A, Mitsuya H, Torii H: Computer analysis of micturition parameters and accuracy of uroflowmeter. Urol Int 33:337-344, 1978.
42. Costantini E, Mearini E, Pajoncini C, et al: Uroflowmetry in female voiding disturbances. Neurourol Urodyn 22:569-573, 2003.
43. Haylen BT, Law MG, Frazer M, Schulz S: Urine flow rates and residual urine volumes in urogynecology patients. Int Urogynecol J Pelvic Floor Dysfunct 10:378-383, 1999.
44. Lemack GE, Baseman AG, Zimmern PE: Voiding dynamics in women: A comparison of pressure-flow studies between asymptomatic and incontinent women. Urology 59:42-46, 2002.
45. Massey A, Abrams P: Urodynamics of the female lower urinary tract. Urol Clin North Am 12:231-246, 1985.
46. Abrams P, Blaivas JG, Stanton SL, Andersen JT: Standardisation of of lower urinary tract function. Neurourol Urodyn 7:403-427, 1988.
47. Bates P, Bradley WE, Glen E, et al: The standardization of terminology of lower urinary tract function. Eur Urol 2:274-276, 1976.
48. Webster GD, Guralnick MS: The neurourologic evaluation. In Walsh PC, Retik AB, Vaughan ED Jr, Wein AJ (eds). Campbell's Urology, 8th ed. Philadelphia: WB Saunders, 2002, pp 900-930.
49. Awad SA, Flood HD, Acker KL: The significance of prior anti-incontinence surgery in women who present with urinary incontinence. J Urol 140:514-517, 1988.
50. McGuire EJ, Lytton B, Kohorn EI, Pepe V: The value of urodynamic testing in stress urinary incontinence. J Urol 124:256-258, 1980.
51. McGuire EJ, Fitzpatrick CC, Wan J, et al: Clinical assessment of urethral sphincter function. J Urol 150(5 Pt 1):1452-1454, 1993.
52. McGuire EJ, Leng WW: Leak-point pressures. In Cardozo L, Staskin D (eds): Textbook of Female Urology and Urogynaecology. London: Isis Medical Media, 2001, pp 225-237.
53. Maniam P, Goldman HB: Removal of transurethral catheter during urodynamics may unmask stress urinary incontinence. J Urol 167:2080-2082, 2002.
54. McGuire EJ, Woodside JR, Borden TA, Weiss RM: Prognostic value of urodynamic testing in myelodysplastic patients. J Urol 126:205-209, 1981.
55. Blaivas JG: Cystometry. In Blaivas JG (ed): Atlas of Urodynamics. Baltimore: Williams and Wilkins, 1996, pp 31-47.
56. Woodside JR, McGuire EJ: Technique for detection of detrusor hypertonia in the presence of urethral sphincteric incompetence. J Urol 127:740-743, 1982.
57. Lose G, Griffiths D, Hosker G, et al: Standardisation of urethral pressure measurement: Report from the Standardisation Sub-Committee of the International Continence Society. Neurourol Urodyn 21:258-260, 2002.
58. Lose G: Urethral pressure measurements. In Cardozo L, Staskin D (eds): Textbook of Female Urology and Urogynaecology. London: Isis Medical Media, 2001, pp 215-226.
59. Sand PK, Bowen LW, Panganiban R, Ostergard DR: The low pressure urethra as a factor in failed retropubic urethropexy. Obstet Gynecol 69(3 Pt 1):399-402, 1987.
60. Schick E, Tessier J, Bertrand PE, et al: Observations on the function of the female urethra: I. Relation between maximum urethral closure pressure at rest and urethral hypermobility. Neurourol Urodyn 22:643-647, 2003.
61. Farrar D, Warwick RT: Outflow obstruction in the female. Urol Clin North Am 6:217-225, 1979.
62. Groutz A, Blaivas JG, Chaikin DC: Bladder outlet obstruction in women: Definition and characteristics. Neurourol Urodyn 19:213-220, 2000.
63. Defreitas GA, Zimmern PE, Lemack GE, Shariat SF: Refining diagnosis of anatomic female bladder outlet obstruction: Comparison of pressure-flow study parameters in clinically obstructed women with those of normal controls. Urology 64:675-679; discussion 679-681, 2004.
64. Fowler C: Electromyography. In Blaivas JG (ed): Atlas of Urodynamics. Baltimore: Williams and Wilkins, 1996, pp 60-76.
65. Enhoerning G, Miller ER, Hinman F Jr: Urethral closure studied with cineroentgenography and simultaneous bladder-urethra pressure recording. Surg Gynecol Obstet 118:507-516, 1964.
66. Miller E: The beginnings. Urol Clin North Am 6:7-9, 1979.
67. Blaivas JG: Deciding on the right urodynamic equipment. In Blaivas JG (ed): Atlas of Urodynamics. Baltimore: Williams and Wilkins, 1996, pp 19-28.
68. Blaivas JG, Olsson CA: Stress incontinence: Classification and surgical approach. J Urol 139:727-731, 1988.
69. O'Donnell PD: Pitfalls of urodynamic testing. Urol Clin North Am 18:257-268, 1991.
70. Beck RP, McCormick S, Nordstrom L: A 25-year experience with 519 anterior colporrhaphy procedures. Obstet Gynecol 78:1011-1018, 1991.
71. Borstad E, Rud T: The risk of developing urinary stress-incontinence after vaginal repair in continent women: A clinical and urodynamic follow-up study. Acta Obstet Gynecol Scand 68:545-549, 1989.
72. Versi E, Lyell DJ, Griffiths DJ: Videourodynamic diagnosis of occult genuine stress incontinence in patients with anterior vaginal wall relaxation. J Soc Gynecol Investig 5:327-330, 1998.
73. Veronikis DK, Nichols DH, Wakamatsu MM: The incidence of low-pressure urethra as a function of prolapse-reducing technique in patients with massive pelvic organ prolapse (maximum descent at all vaginal sites). Am J Obstet Gynecol 177:1305-1313; discussion 1313-1304, 1997.
74. Ghoniem GM, Walters F, Lewis V: The value of the vaginal pack test in large cystoceles. J Urol 152:931-934, 1994.
75. Marinkovic SP, Stanton SL: Incontinence and voiding difficulties associated with prolapse. J Urol 171:1021-1028, 2004.
76. Weber AM, Walters MD: Cost-effectiveness of urodynamic testing before surgery for women with pelvic organ prolapse and stress urinary incontinence. Am J Obstet Gynecol 183:1338-1346; discussion 1346-1337, 2000.
77. Gordon D, Groutz A, Wolman I, et al: Development of postoperative urinary stress incontinence in clinically continent patients undergoing prophylactic Kelly plication during genitourinary prolapse repair. Neurourol Urodyn 18:193-197; discussion 197-198, 1999.
78. Colombo M, Maggioni A, Scalambrino S, et al: Surgery for genitourinary prolapse and stress incontinence: A randomized trial of posterior pubourethral ligament plication and Pereyra suspension. Am J Obstet Gynecol 176:337-343, 1997.
79. Bump RC, Hurt WG, Theofrastous JP, et al: Randomized prospective comparison of needle colposuspension versus endopelvic fascia plication for potential stress incontinence prophylaxis in women undergoing vaginal reconstruction for stage III or IV pelvic organ prolapse. The Continence Program for Women Research Group. Am J Obstet Gynecol 175:326-333; discussion 333-325, 1996.
80. Brubaker L, Cundiff GW, Fine P, et al: Abdominal sacrocolpopexy with Burch colposuspension to reduce urinary stress incontinence. N Engl J Med 354:1557-1566, 2006.

Chapter 58

NONSURGICAL TREATMENT OF VAGINAL PROLAPSE: DEVICES FOR PROLAPSE AND INCONTINENCE

Peggy A. Norton

NONSURGICAL TREATMENT OF VAGINAL PROLAPSE

Surgery for pelvic floor disorders such as stress urinary incontinence and pelvic organ prolapse (POP) is aimed at restoring or improving the function of the pelvic organs. By its nature, such functional surgery cannot be guaranteed to restore continence and support to its original state. Up to one third of surgeries for pelvic floor disorders fail.[1] Given these facts, many women are interested in nonsurgical options for vaginal prolapse that offer less risk and expense. Once fitted, patients are immediately aware of whether the device is comfortable and whether it is effective in treating the condition. Although use of these devices should not be viewed as a permanent solution for prolapse, many women successfully use them for many years without much bother. Such devices are widely available but require some professional intervention to determine correct use and fit, similar to fitting a contraceptive diaphragm. Little has been published on the use of vaginal devices for prolapse, possibly because there is no industry support for (or profit from) conducting properly controlled clinical trials.

Indications for Pessary Use

Indications for a pessary in the management of POP include patient desire for nonsurgical management of the condition. Traditionally, this group of patients has included those few women who are unable to undergo surgical management because of medical problems. But there are many women who might be interested in a pessary, because it manages the prolapse without the need to undergo surgery. In our practice, pessaries are used successfully in women who cannot take time off for surgery, such as mothers with small children at home and women with busy careers outside the home.

Willingness to use a vaginal device may be cultural, especially in areas where contraceptive diaphragms are used. Prashar and colleagues[2] found that only a fifth of 104 women who presented to a community continence clinic in Australia felt very comfortable about inserting a device into the vagina (and half felt uncomfortable). In our practice at the University of Utah, most women who are believed to be good candidates for a pessary trial are readily fitted and can demonstrate removal and replacement of the device. Clemons and colleagues[3] successfully fitted three-quarters of patients with POP with a pessary. It has even been suggested that use of a pessary longer than 1 year may have some therapeutic effect, in that a minority of users have an improvement in prolapse stage.[4]

Patient Selection

In addition to a patient's interest in nonsurgical management, there are physical factors that favor use of a pessary. The best clinical situation is an anterior and/or apical defect (cystocele, uterine prolapse, vaginal vault prolapse) in a woman with adequate vaginal capacity, a narrow pubic arch, and good pelvic floor strength. This is because the ventral edge of a pessary is held behind the pubic rami, and a wide arch would allow extrusion of the device. Likewise, the dorsal edge of the pessary is braced by the pelvic floor muscles. In the absence of these factors, one must consider the use of pessaries that utilize suction or inflation (see later discussion). An isolated posterior wall defect (rectocele) is more difficult to manage with a pessary, because the force vectors act to extrude the pessary. If the vaginal capacity is reduced after surgery, a narrower pessary may be needed (e.g., oval, Hodge, cube). Other reported risk factors for pessary failure include a shortened vagina and a wide levator hiatus.[3]

Selection of a Pessary

Vaginal pessaries have been used for many centuries, but improvements in materials and design have increased the usefulness of these devices for prolapse. Most are made of silicone (latex-free), are flexible to allow easier placement and removal, and should last for several years with proper care. Sources for vaginal pessaries are listed in Table 58-1.

Supportive Pessaries

Supportive pessaries (which depend on some levator muscle support to stay in place) include the Gehrung, Hodge, and Schatz designs, as well as rings and ovals with support. Although individual practices may vary, flexible ring pessaries and Gelhorn pessaries are used most commonly. Members of the American Urogynecologic Society (AUGS) were surveyed by Cundiff and colleagues,[5] and more than three quarters of respondents reported that they tailored the pessary to the defect. A ring pessary was more common for anterior and apical defects, a Gelhorn was more common for large Stage III and IV prolapse, and a donut pessary was used for posterior defects. Twenty-two percent of respondents used the same pessary, usually a ring pessary, for all support defects. One questionnaire study of gynecologists reported that ring and donut pessaries were the types most commonly used.[6] In a tertiary referral practice in Texas, Sulak and colleagues[7] used a Gelhorn pessary in 96 of 107 women with symptomatic POP. Because many of the women desiring pessary use have stage II prolapse, the pessary we use most at the

Table 58-1 Sources for Vaginal Pessaries

Web Site Address	Description
http://www.milexproducts.com/products/pessaries Milex Products Online Catalog??	Source for many continence devices, including continence dish, rings, other pessaries with knobs, and so on.
http://www.urology.coloplast.com/pelvic-organ-prolapse/evacare EvaCare formerly prod. by Mentor, not Coloplast; Mentor bought DesChutes incontinence line in 2000, maybe sold it now?; site has only breast info & press releases re these items. www.urology.coloplast.com/bladder-control/incontinence-women/index.htm??	Patient information source for EvaCare continence devices including continence dish. Source for intravaginal continence devices.
http://www.augs.org	Web site for the American Urogynecologic Society, with sites for members and patients. For bladder diaries and bladder retraining, click on information for women, diagnostic and treatment information on overactive bladder/urge incontinence. Information on pelvic floor muscle training (Kegel exercises) is also available.

University of Utah is the ring with support in sizes 3 and 4 (size refers to diameter in centimeters.)

Supportive pessaries are the easiest pessaries to use because they fold to a smaller dimension for insertion. Many of them, because they are similar to a contraceptive diaphragm, permit coitus while wearing the device. Perhaps because they are easier to manage, supportive pessaries may not be sufficient to support large prolapses. Pessaries are easiest to insert lying down, easiest to remove standing up, and may require digital bracing *per vaginum* during bowel movements. Some women have difficulty removing the pessary, and in the past some pessaries came with removal strings that became malodorous over time. Instead, we recommend tying a strand of dental floss around the ring, so that the pessary can be pulled out by the floss, and renewing the floss each time.

Space-Occupying Pessaries

Space-occupying pessaries include the cube, donut, Gelhorn, and inflatoball. These pessaries are more difficult to insert and remove, but they work in situations in which other devices would be extruded: with larger prolapse, poor pelvic floor strength, or wider pubic arch. Of these, we use the donut and the Gelhorn with the most frequency. The donut is simply pushed into the vagina quickly, and it is easiest to use in women without significant atrophy or scarring. The Gelhorn is held by the knob, aligned along an almost vertical axis (but sparing the urethra) and rapidly inserted, then adjusted so that the knob faces the introitus or posterior distal vagina. We have not found that pinching the flexible disk of the Gelhorn makes much difference to the relative discomfort with which this pessary is placed. To remove the Gelhorn, an index finger should be inserted to break the slight suction seal of the disk in the vagina, and the thumb and index finger of the other hand may grasp and pull the knob. Occasionally, we use a ring forceps to grasp the knob and bring it to the introitus. Although insertion and removal of the Gelhorn sounds daunting, it is a highly successful pessary for large prolapses, and with practice this pessary is inserted and removed on a regular basis in many patients. The cube has a relative suction effect and may be effective in cases of lax vaginal walls, but it generates significant discharge and in our experience is more prone to excoriation and ulceration than other pessaries. The inflatoball is pumped up with a small bulb and is similarly prone to excoriation unless care is taken.

Care and Long-Term Use of a Vaginal Pessary

Postmenopausal women may benefit from vaginal estrogen. This has little systemic absorption, may increase vaginal skin thickness and tolerance of the device, and is best given as a vaginal pill (Vagifem 25 μg, Novo Nordisk, Princeton, NJ) once nightly for 10 nights, then twice weekly thereafter. After an initial follow-up examination to demonstrate efficacy and self-management, women who manage their own pessary without difficulty may be seen annually. Women may need to brace the device digitally during straining for bowel movements to prevent extrusion. A device that is easily dislodged or uncomfortable is not satisfactory and should be removed and replaced.

Care of a vaginal pessary depends on the type used. Because it is easy to remove and reinsert, we recommend that women remove the ring pessary at least weekly, wash it with soap and water, leave it out overnight, and then reinsert in the morning. In our experience, women rarely encounter excessive or malodorous vaginal discharge using this approach and therefore have little use for creams other than estrogen. Space-occupying pessaries are sometimes difficult for a woman to remove on her own. In such cases, we try to individualize the intervals between insertions. We may ask a patient with a donut or Gelhorn device to return for reexamination within a few weeks. If discharge is minimal and no erosions are present, we examine next at 4 weeks and then at increased intervals. The appropriate pessary interval is either a maximum of 3 months or the interval at which foul-smelling discharge or early erosions appear.

For women who can remove and replace their own pessaries, we schedule a follow-up evaluation within 1 month of placement and then monitor the patient annually, depending on her comfort level. For women who retain the pessary for several months at a time, we believe that a visual inspection of the vagina should occur at least twice yearly. It is important to examine the anterior and posterior vaginal walls during the examination (by turning the speculum 90 degrees), as well as the obvious lateral walls that are visible when the speculum is placed in the usual fashion. This vaginal inspection is not only important in preventing erosions from the pessary, but it can offset the poor compensation for pessary placement in individual practices. If an area of redness or erosion is seen, the patient is asked to remove the device more often, use vaginal estrogen, and even consider leaving the device out for a week or two.

Clinical Outcomes

Several series have demonstrated that POP can be managed with pessary use. In one study by Wu and colleagues,[8] of the 62 women that used a pessary for more than 1 month, 66% were still using it after 12 months. In Sulak's series,[7] half of women continued to use the pessary at the time of manuscript preparation (average duration of use, 16 months).

Clemons and coworkers[9] (2004) prospectively evaluated women with symptomatic POP, and 73 of 100 women were satisfied with their pessary at 1 week. At 2 months, only 3% of women endorsed feeling a bulge, compared to 90% at baseline. Other symptoms that improved included pressure, discharge, and splinting. One third of women had urge incontinence at baseline; this improved in 54%. Twenty-three percent had voiding difficulty at baseline, which improved in half. At 2 months, 92% were either very or somewhat satisfied with their pessary. Ring pessaries were used more with stage II and III prolapse (100% and 71%, respectively), whereas Gelhorn pessaries were used more with stage IV prolapse (64%, $P < .001$). Factors associated with long-term pessary use included older age (76 versus 61 years; $P < .001$) and poor surgical risk (26% versus 0%; $P = .03$). Characteristics that were associated with women going on to surgery were sexual activity, the presence of stress incontinence (a coexisting problem that may not be helped by a vaginal pessary for prolapse), and desire for surgery at the first visit. Age 65 years was the best cutoff value for continued pessary use, with a sensitivity of 95% (95% confidence interval [CI], 84% to 99%) and a positive predictive value of 87% (95% CI, 74% to 94%). Logistic regression demonstrated that age greater than or equal to 65 years ($P < .001$), stage III-IV posterior vaginal wall prolapse ($P = .007$), and desire for surgery ($P = .04$) were independent predictors

In contrast, other researchers have found that pessary use is acceptable to women who are sexually active. Brincat and colleagues[10] reviewed 136 women who initiated pessary treatment for POP or urinary incontinence over a 2-year period. Of the 60% of women who became long-term pessary users, those who were more likely to continue pessary use were those who were using the pessary for treatment of prolapse and those who were sexually active.

Recommendations for Initiating Pessary Use

Wu and colleagues[8] recommended a simple management strategy in which a flexible ring pessary with support was the first pessary tried, and 70% of patients were successfully fitted with a size 3, 4, or 5 ring. In Utah, many urologists and gynecologists keep a few simple pessaries in their practice for fitting. A number 3 or 4 ring pessary with support can be inserted, and, if appropriate, a prescription can be written and the pessary ordered through a pharmacy. The fitting pessary can then be sterilized for refitting. Alternatively, a few high-volume urogynecologic practices keep large numbers of pessary types and sizes. Once fitted, patients return to their clinician for long-term management. This practice is more feasible for pessaries such as the Gelhorn. If the patient is postmenopausal, a 2- to 3-week course of vaginal estrogen is recommended, and a pessary may be ordered in the interval for placement in the office.

NONSURGICAL TREATMENT OF URINARY INCONTINENCE

In women, treatment of urge urinary incontinence (overactive bladder) is primarily pharmacologic and behavioral. Although stress urinary incontinence can be treated surgically, many women choose nonsurgical options such as intravaginal devices and new pharmacologic treatments. Both types of urinary incontinence may benefit from lifestyle interventions, physical therapy, biofeedback, bladder retraining, and behavioral modifications. Mixed urge and stress incontinence is sometimes treated as two separate entities, although there is increasing evidence that both components of mixed incontinence may respond to treatments aimed at a single type of incontinence, such as anticholinergics/antimuscarinics and combination selective serotonin/norepinephrine reuptake inhibitors (SSRI/NERIs). A consensus conference on urinary incontinence was sponsored by the World Health Organization in 2001, and levels of evidence for many of nonsurgical treatments were summarized by Wilson and associates[11] (Table 57-2). We consider here the use of devices for stress urinary incontinence.

Intravaginal devices work by creating a "backstop" at the level of the bladder neck. Devices that have been studied include a short super tampon inserted just inside the vagina, a Hodge pessary placed backward and upside down, and a variety of

Table 58-2 Device and Pharmacologic Treatments for Urinary Incontinence

Device or Treatment	Efficacy	Effort	Evidence
Continence devices			
Intravaginal (pessary-like) devices	Moderate to high	Low to moderate	Scant 1-2
Occlusive urethral devices (not currently marketed)	Moderate	Low to moderate	Level 3-4
Intraurethral devices (not currently marketed)	High	Moderate	Level 2-3
Pharmacologic treatments			
Of overactive bladder	Moderate	Low but expensive	Level 1
Of stress urinary incontinence	Moderate	Low, no cost estimates	Level 1
Of mixed urinary incontinence	Moderate	Low	Level 1

Adapted from Wilson D, et al., 2002.

Table 58-3 Studies of Devices for Stress Urinary Incontinence

Device and Ref. No.	*N*	Indication	Follow-up	Outcome
Smith-Hodge pessary[12]	30	Stress incontinence	None	Cough pressure profile; 24/30 patients continent
RCT of super tampon and Hodge pessary[13]	18	Exercise-induced stress incontinence	None	36% of pessary users continent; 58% of tampon users continent
Bladder neck support prosthesis[15] (no current distributor)	77	Stress and mixed Incontinence	12 wk	On subjective pad test, 29% continent, 51% decreased severity by more than half; 81% had combined subjective/objective some or maximum benefit
Bladder neck support prosthesis[16] (no current distributor)	70	Stress or mixed incontinence	4 wk	53/70 completed trial; significant improvement on pad tests, diaries; high subjective improvement and quality of life
Continence ring pessary[17]	38	Stress incontinence	1 yr	6/38 continued device use long term; improved scores on pad test, voiding diary
Variable continence pessaries[18]	100	Stress and mixed incontinence, prolapse	11 mo	59% continued use long term, with significant reduction in incontinence
Continance dish[14]	119	Stress Incontinence	6 mo	89% successful device fitting; >50% continued use for 6 mo

RCT, randomized controlled trial.
Summarized and updated from Wilson et al., 2001.

continence devices manufactured by several companies who also manufacture pessaries for prolapse (Table 57-3). Additionally, there are several disposable intravaginal devices that are not yet available for use in the United States. These devices are easy to use and seem to have moderately good efficacy, especially for the woman with predictable stress incontinence, who may use such devices when exercising or for that week of coughing from a bad cold. Use among urogynecologic and urology practices is variable: some specialists offer these devices to all women with stress incontinence, whereas others do not include intravaginal devices in their practice. The devices have not been well studied. These are low-cost devices sold in modest volumes whose manufacturers do not have research funds, and there are no sham devices for randomized controlled trials.

Types of Devices

Nonpessary Devices

Many women report use of their contraceptive diaphragm as being effective. Its mechanism is probably similar to that of other continence devices: creation of a "backstop" against which the urethra is briefly compressed during increased abdominal pressure. A short menstrual tampon may be inserted just comfortably inside the introitus; patients need to be instructed to use the tampon under dry conditions, which improves the adherence of the tampon. We instruct patients to use this "tampon trick" with a super tampon, and only on an occasional basis. The Conveen Continence Guard is a polyurethane foam cushion that is folded on its long axis and placed in the vagina. When moistened and partially unfolded, it acts as a backstop under the bladder neck. The device is available in three sizes and is worn for up to 18 hours and then discarded. It is not yet available in the United States. Several studies have documented good tolerance and significant reductions in urine loss with use.[19,20]

Supportive (Modified Pessary) Devices

The majority of continence devices have been modified from vaginal pessaries used for POP, and all recreate the supportive "backstop" effect for the urethra. These include rings with knobs placed at the bladder neck, the Hodge pessary inserted backward and upside down, the incontinence dish with support, the PelvX ring, and the Suarez ring.

Nonsupportive Devices

Nonsupportive devices include a urethral insert (Rochester Medical, Inc., Rochester, MN) and urethral suction caps (Uromed; not currently available.) Such urethral plugs and caps have been studied with some success but do not seem to be popular in clinical practice. Some women may wear these devices for activities only, whereas others need to wear them on a daily basis. Care of these pessaries is similar to that for supportive pessaries.

Clinical Use

Although use of a short super tampon may be suggested on a temporary basis, we use the incontinence dish as our main incontinence pessary. Patients can immediately see the advantages (effective, no surgery) and disadvantages (small amount of bother with insertion, need for continued use) associated with these devices. Although most women wear these devices on an as-needed basis, some patients who have daily stress incontinence prefer to wear the device on a continual basis.

Once an appropriate candidate for a supportive device has been identified, we prefer to fit the device in a separate session, often after several weeks of vaginal estrogen in postmenopausal women. It is helpful to demonstrate leakage with a standing cough stress test, then to demonstrate continence after a device is fitted. A comfortable bladder volume does not seem to impair fitting of the device. In supine lithotomy, the capacity of the vagina laterally is assessed; this may be limited in women who have had vaginal surgery. We begin with a continence dish of a similar diameter, squeezing the device to narrow its entry into the vagina. All of these devices are placed with the knob just inside the introitus, creating the support for the urethra. The best fit is that which leaves a fingerbreadth or two between the device and the pubic symphysis, is comfortable, and does not readily extrude with straining. Women with a narrow pubic arch and good pelvic floor strength are the best candidates for a supportive device, because the pessary is more easily retained. For a narrow vagina with limited capacity, a Hodge pessary (placed so that the arch is directed at the bladder neck) or a knobbed device may be preferable.

We recommend that women remove the intravaginal supportive device at least weekly, leave it out overnight, and then reinsert it in the morning. The device can be washed with simple soap and water, rinsed, and air-dried. In our experience, women rarely encounter vaginal excoriations or excessive or malodorous vaginal discharge using this approach. Postmenopausal women may benefit from vaginal estrogen. This has little systemic absorption, may increase vaginal skin thickness and tolerance of the device, and is best given as a vaginal pill (Vagifem 25 μg, Novo Nordisk) once nightly for 10 nights, then twice weekly thereafter. After an initial follow-up examination to demonstrate efficacy and self-management, women who manage their own pessary without difficulty can be seen annually. Women may need to brace the device digitally during straining for bowel movements to prevent extrusion. A device that is easily dislodged or uncomfortable is not satisfactory and should be removed and replaced.

Most studies evaluating the effectiveness of devices for stress incontinence are small in numbers and short in duration. In a prospective, randomized study by Nygaard,[13] 6 of 14 women were cured and an additional 2 improved during exercise while wearing a super-sized tampon in the vagina. Nine of 12 women had resolution of stress incontinence while wearing a contraceptive diaphragm during urodynamic testing, and 4 of 10 women wearing a contraceptive diaphragm for 1 week had improved continence.

Of 190 women presenting to a tertiary care center with symptoms of stress or mixed urinary incontinence who were offered pessary management, 63% chose to undergo fitting and 89% achieved a successful fit in the office. Of the 106 women who took a pessary home, follow-up was available on 100. Fifty-five women used the pessary for at least 6 months as their primary method of managing urinary incontinence (median duration, 13 months). Of the remaining 45 women who discontinued use before 6 months, most did so by 1 month.[14]

Intraurethral devices work through occlusion of the urethra. They are removed for voiding, and most cannot be reinserted. Several trials of several products have been conducted with favorable efficacy and low risk of side effects, but the intraurethral devices are less comfortable than the intravaginal ones. Studies of intraurethral inserts showed that most women who used them (66% to 95%) were dry or improved while the device was in place. It is not surprising that urinary tract infections may occur with these devices; however, the incidence of infection decreases after the first several months of use. These intraurethral devices have failed to gain popularity with patients and physicians. Although few women choose an intraurethral device as a first option, an occasional patient is highly satisfied with long-term use of an intraurethral device.

Use of occlusive (extra)urethral devices or patches have been reported with similar results: the devices seem to work in many patients, but acceptance by physicians and patients has been poor, and the devices are not currently marketed in the United States.

CONCLUSION

Pessaries and other devices are an important part of the treatment scheme for stress urinary incontinence. Although some patient effort is required for removal and maintenance of the devices, the risk and costs are minimal with moderate efficacy. Further research is needed to determine which women are most likely to respond to the various types of devices, and to evaluate both effectiveness and adverse events associated with these devices compared to surgery. Nevertheless, the risk-benefit ratio seems quite favorable with these devices for stress urinary incontinence.

References

1. Olsen A, Smith V, Bergstrom J, et al: Epidemiology of surgically managed pelvic organ prolapse and urinary incontinence. Obstet Gynecol 89(4):501–506, 1997.
2. Prashar S, Simons A, Bryant C, et al: Attitudes to vaginal/urethral touching and device placement in women with urinary incontinence. Int Ungynecol J Pelvic Floor Dysfunct. 11(1):4–8, 2000.
3. Clemons J, Aguilar V, Tillinghast T, et al: Risk factors associated with an unsuccessful pessary fitting trial in women with pelvic organ prolapse. Am J Obstet Gynecol 190:345-350, 2004.
4. Handa VL, Jones M: Do pessaries prevent the progression of pelvic organ prolapse? Int Urogynecol J Pelvic Floor Dysfunct 13:349-351, 2002.
5. Cundiff GW, Weidner AC, Visco AG, et al: A survey of pessary use by members of the American Urogynecologic Society. Obstet Gynecol 95:931-935, 2000.
6. Pott-Grinstein E, Newcomer JR: Gynecologists' patterns of prescribing pessaries. J Reprod Med 46:205-208, 2001.
7. Sulak PJ, Kuehl TJ, Shull BL: Vaginal pessaries and their use in pelvic relaxation. J Reprod Med 38:919-923, 1993.
8. Wu V, Farrell SA, Baskett TF, Flowerdew G: A simplified protocol for pessary management. Obstet Gynecol 90:990, 1997.
9. Clemons JL, Aguilar VC, Tillinghast TA, et al: Patient satisfaction and changes in prolapse and urinary symptoms in women who were fitted successfully with a pessary for pelvic organ prolapse. Am J Obstet Gynecol 190:1025-1029, 2004.
10. Brincat C, Kenton K, FitzGerald M, Brubaker L: Sexual activity predicts continued pessary use. Am J Obstet Gynecol 191:198-200, 2004.
11. Wilson D, Bø K, Hay-Smith E: Conservative treatment in women. In *Incontinence.* Ed P Abrams, L Cardozo, S Khoury. Health Publications, Ltd. Plymouth. pp 571-624, 2002.
12. Bhatia N, Bargman A: Pessary test in women with urinary incontinence. Obstet Gynecol 65(2):220-226, 1985.

13. Nygaard I: Prevention of exercise incontinence with mechanical devices. J Reprod Med 40:89-94, 1995.
14. Donnelly M, Powell S, Olsen A, et al: Vaginal pessaries for the management of stress and mixed urinary incontinence. Int Urogynecol J Pelvic Floor Dysfunct 15(5):302-307, 2004.
15. Kondo K, Yokoyama E, Koshiba K, et al: Bladder neck support prosthesis: a nonoperative treatment for stress or mixed urinary incontinence. J Urol 157(3):824-827, 1997.
16. Davila G, Neal D, Horbach N, et al: A bladder-neck support prosthesis for women with stress and mixed incontinence. Obstet Gynecol 93(6):938-942, 1999.
17. Robert M, Mainprize T: Long-term assessment of the incontinence ring pessary for the treatment of stress incontinence. Int Urogynecol J Pelvic Floor Dysfunct 13(5):326-329, 2002.
18. Jarrell S, Singh B, Aldakhil L: Continence pessaries in the management of urinary incontinence in women. J Obstet Gynecol Can 26(2):113-117, 2004.
19. Hahn I, Milsom I: Treatment of female stress urinary incontinence with a new anatomically shaped vaginal device (Conveen Continence Guard). Br J Urol 77:711-715, 1996.
20. Mouritsen L: Effect of vaginal devices on bladder neck mobility in stress incontinent women. Acta Obstet Gynecol Scand 80:428-431, 2001.

Chapter 59

USE OF SYNTHETICS AND BIOMATERIALS IN VAGINAL RECONSTRUCTIVE SURGERY

Fred E. Govier, Kathleen C. Kobashi, and Ken Hsiao

The surgical field encompassing vaginal reconstructive surgery and urinary incontinence is extensive and extremely complex. As opposed to many surgical disciplines that focus on a single isolated organ, we are dealing with multiple organs that interact with multiple complex supporting structures that must function as a single unit to be maximally effective. The trauma of childbirth, the ever-present effect of gravity, and the inevitable deterioration of these organs and their supporting structures with age and hormone deficiency continuously stress this intricate system. Deficiency in one or more of these components can lead to urinary incontinence, dyspareunia, pelvic pressure, or any of a multitude of other symptoms associated with pelvic floor descent and/or prolapse.

Over the last century, a variety of autologous tissues, absorbable and nonabsorbable synthetic materials, and, more recently, allografts and xenografts have been used in attempts to reconstruct the pelvic floor and its supporting structures. This chapter focuses on the relative strengths and weaknesses of each of these materials, realizing that in 2005 we still lack the perfect material for vaginal reconstructive surgery. We address urethral support, support of the anterior compartment, and support of the vaginal apex as somewhat separate topics, as well as autologous materials, allografts, xenografts, and synthetic mesh products as separate groups. Although this chapter's focus is on the materials themselves, it must be realized that failure is not limited only to the materials. Surgical technique, points of attachment, and methods of attachment can all play a crucial role in the ultimate success or failure of the operative intervention. Because the use of these materials is relatively new in reconstruction of the anterior compartment and apex, we will use our experience with urethral slings to further highlight the relative strengths and weaknesses of these materials. Even then, teasing out the exact cause of a surgical failure or a complication in this setting is challenging and at the present time there are still many unanswered questions.

PREVALENCE OF URINARY INCONTINENCE AND PELVIC FLOOR RELAXATION

Interest in women's health care issues and public awareness of stress urinary incontinence (SUI) and pelvic floor relaxation have increased substantially over the past several years. In 2000, an estimated 17 million community-dwelling individuals had daily urinary incontinence in the United States, and an additional 34 million had symptoms of overactive bladder. The costs of urinary incontinence in the United States were recently estimated at $19.5 billion, with an additional $12.6 billion for overactive bladder.[1]

A postal survey regarding urinary incontinence involving 29,500 community-dwelling women aged 18 years or older in France, Germany, Spain, and the United Kingdom was recently reported.[2] Of the women responding, 35% reported involuntary loss of urine in the proceeding 30 days, with SUI being the most prevalent type. Only 25% of the women had consulted a physician, and fewer than 5% had undergone surgery for their condition.

It is estimated that a woman's lifetime risk of needing a single prolapse surgery by 80 years of age is 11.1%, and the risk of needing reoperation for recurrent prolapse is 29.2%.[3] Undoubtedly, as the population ages, life expectancy increases, and the stigma of incontinence and pelvic prolapse is replaced by education, these numbers and their associated costs will rise.

HISTORY OF THE URINARY SLING WITH AUTOLOGOUS FASCIA

In 1907, Van Girodano introduced the concept of the urinary sling for the treatment of urinary incontinence, when he wrapped a gracilis graft around the urethra.[4] Credit for the first pubovaginal sling (PVS) goes to Goebell, who, in 1910, rotated the pyramidalis muscles beneath the urethra and joined them in the midline.[5] In 1942, Aldridge described the first fascial sling. He used rectus fascia, without muscle, passed through the retropubic space to support the proximal urethra and bladder neck.[6] Variations on this procedure over the following decades involved attempts to minimize morbidity and obtain suitable fascia from patients with multiple previous abdominal procedures and/or pelvic radiation. Ridley[7] described the use of fascia lata in 1955, followed by reports from Williams and Telinde,[8] Moir,[9] Morgan,[10] and Stanton and associates[11] involving the use of synthetic materials with variations on the approach or on anchoring sutures. Using autologous fascia and synthetic materials, these original investigators showed encouraging results, but the outcomes were plagued with urethral obstruction, erosion, fistula formation, and infections.

McGuire and Lytton revived the PVS in 1978 with their series showing an 80% success rate for intrinsic sphincter deficiency (ISD) using rectus fascia tensioned loosely around the urethra.[12] Blaivas and Jacobs modified the procedure by penetrating the endopelvic fascia, as described by Peyrera,[13] and completely detaching the rectus fascia from the abdominal wall.[14] They also stressed the importance of minimizing tension on the sling and stated that, "in the majority of patients the sling should be placed under no tension at all." Subsequent studies showed no difference in histologic or performance characteristics between free and pedicle fascia flaps for sling surgery.[15]

As the PVS was gaining acceptance, the first reports of poor long-term results from needle suspension procedures were being published. In a landmark study published in 1995, Trockman and Leach's group monitored 125 patients for a mean of 10 years after a modified Peyrera needle suspension. By questionnaire data, 51% reported that they had SUI, and only 20% reported no incontinence of any kind.[16] The American Urological Association guidelines panel for the surgical management of SUI was published in 1997 and concluded, based on cure/dry rates, that retropubic suspensions and slings were the most efficacious procedures for long-term success.[17]

Since these early reports, many authors have published long-term data that attest to the durability of the autologous fascial sling. Morgan and colleagues observed 247 patients with type II and III SUI for a mean of 51 months after autologous rectus sling placement. They reported an overall continence rate of 88% to 91% for type II and 84% for type III SUI. Among those patients with at least 5 years of follow-up, the continence rate was very durable at 85%.[18] Chaiken and coworkers reported on 251 patients with all types of anatomic incontinence treated with an autologous rectus PVS.[19] At a median follow-up of 3.1 years, 73% of patients were cured and 19% were improved. Among the 20 patients with a minimum of 10 years' follow-up, the cure rate was 95%. Brown and Govier, using autologous fascia lata, monitored 46 patients for a mean of 44 months; 90% reported overall cure of their anatomic component, and 73% described no or minimal leakage requiring no pads.[20]

The two greatest advantages of the autologous PVS were that all types of anatomic incontinence could be addressed and, if a good result were achieved at 1 year, the result would be durable. Because of these attributes, by the late 1990s most authorities agreed that the PVS using autologous fascia was the gold standard for the surgical management of anatomic incontinence. Unfortunately, harvesting this fascia from the abdominal wall or thigh adds operative time and incurs a risk of hematoma formation, wound infection, and/or hernia formation. Only relatively narrow strips of fascia can be harvested, and even then the patient requires several weeks of recovery time to achieve a normal activity level. In an effort to minimize patient morbidity and yet further improve surgical results, a variety of biomaterials (allografts, xenografts) and synthetic products (absorbable and permanent) have been introduced and are currently being used for the construction of urinary slings and vaginal reconstructions.

HISTORY AND CHARACTERISTICS OF BIOMATERIALS IN PELVIC RECONSTRUCTION

Allografts

Allografts are harvested from a human donor, usually a cadaver, and transplanted into a human recipient. The most common tissues used for pelvic floor reconstruction are fascia lata, dermis, and dura matter. Table 59-1 lists some of the companies supplying these components and their trade names. There are many advantages to the use of allografts or xenografts for pelvic floor reconstruction. Several studies have documented decreased recovery time, length of hospitalization, and postoperative pain using these materials.[21-23] Compared with permanent synthetic materials, allografts carry a lower risk of vaginal extrusion, and, if extrusion does occur, in general the graft does not require removal. Finally, larger-sized grafts for pelvic reconstructive procedures can be obtained easily without incurring additional patient morbidity.

All cadaveric donor materials in the United States are processed by licensed tissue banks regulated by the Food and Drug Administration.[24] Cadaveric donors are carefully screened by review of their medical and social history with the family, partners, and friends. Donors are excluded if the cause of death is unknown or the medical history suggests any of the following: hepatitis, bacterial sepsis, syphilis, intravenous drug abuse, cancer, collagen vascular disease, rabies, Creutzfeld-Jakob's disease (CJD), or significant risk factors for human immunodeficiency virus (HIV) infection.[25] Serologic testing is performed for HIV-1 and HIV-2 antibodies, hepatitis B surface antigen, and hepatitis C antibodies. One of the most significant problems with serologic testing is that false-negative results can occur, because it takes time after the initial infection before the immunologic response is sufficient for serologic detection. The delay can be up to 6 weeks in the case of hepatitis B, and up to 6 months for HIV.[26,27]

Tissue processing allows for the removal of most of the cellular content, along with the associated antigens, making donor and recipient tissue matching unnecessary. Additionally, tissue sterilization, while preserving the inherent collagen matrix, is required to eliminate infectious complications and ensure satisfactory graft assimilation. Although the American Association of Tissue Banks has made recommendations, no federally mandated

Table 59-1 Allografts and Xenografts

Type	Component	Trade Name (Manufacturer)
Autologous	Rectus fascia	
	Fascia lata	
	Vaginal wall	
Allograft	Fascia lata	Tutoplast (Mentor, Santa Barbara, CA)
		Faslata (Bard, Covington, GA)
	Dermis	Repliform (LifeCell Corporation, The Woodlands, TX)
		Duraderm (CR Bard, Inc., Murray Hill, NJ)
	Dura mater (no longer used)	
Xenograft	Porcine small intestine submucosa	Stratasis (Cook, West Lafayette, IN)
	Porcine dermis	Pelvicol (Bard, Covington, GA)
		IneXen (American Medical Systems, Minnetonka, MN)
	Bovine pericardium	(Braile Biomedical Industria, Brazil)

processing techniques for all tissue banks exist. Currently, allografts are prepared using a variety of proprietary processing techniques that vary depending on the vendor.

Various mechanisms are used for cellular destruction and include hypertonic solutions that osmotically rupture cells and destroy bacteria and viruses; oxidative destruction with hydrogen peroxide, which oxidatively destroys most proteins; and isopropyl alcohol to destroy cells, bacteria, and viruses by dissolving the lipids in their cell walls.[28,29] An additional method used for tissue sterilization is gamma irradiation, which kills bacteria by disrupting nucleic acids but does not guarantee sterilization of viruses or prions, even at the American Association of Tissue Banks recommended level of 1500 Gy (1.5 megarads).[27,30]

Options for long-term preservation include cryopreservation, freeze-drying (lyophilization), and solvent dehydration. Controversy exists with regards to tissue processing and how it affects tissue strength. Most of the concern regarding processing and storage revolves around two issues. The first is irradiation and how it affects the tensile strength of collagen, and the second is the ice crystal formation that occurs with cryopreservation and the freeze-drying processes and whether they adversely affect the collagen microstructure.[28,31,32]

Thomas and Gresham found no significant difference in tensile strength among fresh, frozen and freeze-dried fascia lata specimens.[33] Sutaria and Staskin found no significant difference in the tensile strength of fascias that were freeze-dried and gamma-irradiated, freeze-dried alone, or solvent-dehydrated and gamma-irradiated.[34] In contrast, Hinton and colleagues found solvent-dehydrated, irradiated fascia lata to be significantly stiffer, with a higher tensile strength than freeze-dried fascia.[32] Two studies reported that tissue irradiated after dehydration resulted in significant loss of tensile strength, and the investigators recommended that irradiation be performed before dehydration.[28,35] In an excellent review, Gallentine and Cespedes concluded that “a number of processing techniques are available that may have different adverse affects on the mechanical properties of allografts, but currently no definitive evidence is available that one technique is superior to another.”[25]

With current federal regulations in place to obtain, process, and store cadaveric materials, the risk of infectious disease transmission is extremely small. As of 1995, approximately 220,000 soft tissue transplants were being performed annually in the United States, and no cases of a transmitted infectious disease had been reported for processed cadaveric fascia lata (CFL) or dermal grafts.[24]

The risk of acquiring HIV-infected tissue from a properly screened donor is reported to be between 1 in 1,667,600 and 1 in 8 million from banked cadaveric fascia.[36-38] Seroconversion was reported in recipients of solid organs (4 of 4) and unprocessed fresh-frozen bone (3 of 3); however, 0 of 34 patients receiving other tissues, including 3 who received lyophilized tissue, became infected with HIV.[26] Still, it is alarming that intact genetic material (DNA segments) was isolated from four commercial sources of processed human cadaveric allografts.[39]

Prion transmission has gained increasing attention because of the neurodegenerative symptoms that occur in the recipient but not in the host. Prions are proteinaceous pathogens that use a novel mechanism of amino acid transposition to change the protein configuration to a that of a neurotoxic prion protein peptide, leading to cases of neurodegenerative Creutz feld–Jakob Disease. Iatrogenic cases have been reported after many types of procedures, including corneal transplants and dura mater grafting.[40] It has been described in 43 patients receiving cadaveric dural grafts after neurosurgical or orthopedic procedures, and, for this reason, dura mater is no longer being used as a biomaterial.[41] However, prion transmission has not been described with the use of cadaveric fascia or dermis for anti-incontinence or prolapse procedures. Even though no transmission has been documented in our field, the potential for infectious transmission with these allografts does exist, and all patients need to be informed of the risk before their use.

Xenografts

The most popular xenograft materials used for sling surgery are derived from porcine and bovine sources (see Table 59-1). Being from an animal source, xenografts are readily available and are devoid of the potential ethical issues associated with use of human tissue. The types most frequently used for pelvic reconstruction are porcine dermis and small intestinal submucosa (SIS) or bovine pericardium. The Food and Drug Administration has strict guidelines controlling all phases of their production.[42]

Fate of Autologous Tissue and Biomaterials

The most significant controversy involving biomaterials is the ultimate fate of the graft material itself, within the host. When autologous rectus fascia or fascia lata is used to construct a urinary sling, the results of these procedures in terms of durability are uniformly excellent.[17-20] Three studies in the literature examined the fate of autologous fascia in the host. In 1969, Crawford evaluated autologous and frozen fascia lata in rabbits by attaching strips of each from the flank to the posterior abdominal wall.[43] After killing the animals and examining the tissue, he concluded that “fresh fascia is living sutures and cadaveric tissue merely provides a bridge for host fibroblasts.” A more recent paper, in 1997, looked at free versus pedicled fascial flaps again in rabbits.[44] Strips of 7 and 15 mm of each were obtained from the abdominal wall and used to create a urethral sling. The rabbits were killed at 3 months, and all slings were found to be viable with the original histology preserved. The authors surmised that the fascia survives in the early postoperative period by diffusion. Later, neovascularization from the loose connective tissue around the flaps provides long-term vascularity. FitzGerald and colleagues evaluated the histologic appearance of autologous rectus fascial slings that were examined at revision at 3, 5, and 8 weeks for urinary retention and at 17 and 208 weeks for persistent SUI.[45] They concluded that autologous fascial slings remain viable after implantation. They did note fibroblast proliferation, neovascularization, and some remodeling of the graft, but no evidence of graft degeneration was detected. A linear orientation of the connective tissue and fibroblasts was seen in some areas, whereas other areas had remodeled to form tissue similar to noninflammatory scar.

In contrast, cadaveric fascial allografts have been extensively studied in multiple human models in the orthopedic literature as well as animal models.[43,46,47] With the use of serial biopsies, it was found that there is an initial donor fibrocyte death, which is followed by neovascularization of the graft. Fibroblast migration into the implant is then followed by remodeling and eventually by maturation of the graft.[48,49]

The maturation of xenografts is similar to that described for allografts. The processed material serves as an acellular mesh or scaffolding, which requires remodeling by the host to end up as a viable graft.

It is this need to "remodel" the graft that appears to be the Achilles heel for many or all of the allograft and xenograft products on the market today. As one examines the surgical results with these materials, it is evident that some patients quickly remodel this material to a strong durable structure. In others, it appears that the scaffolding entirely disappears. Authors have theorized that increasing age, poor vascularity, excessive scarring, diabetes, or the use of steroids can adversely affect the remodeling process; however, studies are lacking, and at this time the discrepancies in outcome are largely unexplained.

SURGICAL RESULTS OF BIOMATERIALS FOR URINARY SLINGS

Allografts

Hanada and associates,[50] in 1996, and Labasky and Soper,[51] in 1997, were the first to report on the use of cadaveric products for urinary slings. In 1998, Wright and colleagues published the first paper comparing cadaveric allograft fascia lata to autologous rectus fascia.[52] This series reported on a group of 92 patients undergoing sling procedures over a 28-month period. Fifty-nine patients received a 13 × 2 cm portion of freeze-dried allograft fascia lata, and 33 patients received autologous rectus fascia. With a mean follow-up of 9.6 months for the allograft and 16 months for the autologous fascia, no differences in surgical outcome were found. Chaikin and Blaivas described an early failure of a freeze-dried cadaveric fascia sling in which the holding sutures pulled through.[53] In 1999, FitzGerald and associates reported 35 patients who underwent PVS placement using freeze-dried irradiated CFL.[54] At the time of re-exploration in seven of the failures, "histopathologic analysis revealed areas of disorganized remodeling and graft degeneration, as well as complete absence of the graft in some patients."

In 2000, Brown and Govier compared 121 consecutive patients undergoing slings constructed with fresh-frozen CFL with 46 earlier patients undergoing the same surgical procedure with autologous fascia lata.[20] Although the mean follow-up was longer in the autologous group (44 versus 12 months), questionnaire data demonstrated no significant difference in surgical outcomes. Elliott and Boone, in 2001, reported 12-month follow-up using solvent-dehydrated CFL in 26 patients. Ninety-six percent of patients reported improvement.[55]

In 2001, Carbone and Raz's group reported on a series of irradiated freeze-dried cadaveric fascial sling procedures with a 40% failure rate and a reoperation rate of 16.9%. At the time of reoperation in 26 patients, they found the allografts to be "fragmented, attenuated or simply absent."[56] On the basis of these findings, they abandoned the use of allografts for sling construction. In 2002, O'Reilly and Govier re-examined a group of 121 patients who had slings constructed with fresh-frozen CFL; these patients had been reported earlier to have similar results to those treated with autologous slings.[57] They identified 8 patients who experienced intermediate-term failure at 4 to 13 months after they had initially been dry. This development was not noted in the autologous sling group, and, on the basis of these findings, they too abandoned the use of fresh-frozen CFL for slings.

In 2005, the debate over biografts continues, but the pendulum clearly appears to be heading away from the use of biografts for construction of urinary slings. Crivellaro and colleagues published a prospective series of 253 patients with 18-month follow-up using human dermal allografts for slings.[58] They found that 78% of the patients were improved or cured of their incontinence and were happy with their experience. Owens and Winters also looked at human dermal allografts in slings in 25 patients.[59] At a mean follow-up of 6 months, 68% of the patients were dry, but this rate fell to 32% at a mean follow-up of 14.8 months. They concluded that graft degeneration was the most likely cause of the failures. FitzGerald and coworkers looked at a longer-term follow-up in patients from a previously reported group who had undergone abdominal sacrocolpopexies (67) and/or urinary slings (35) with freeze-dried, irradiated fascia lata. They found that 83% of the sacrocolpopexy patients experienced failure at a mean follow-up of 12 months, and, at the time of reoperation in 16 patients, the graft was still present in only 3 patients.[60] In 2005, Frederick and Leach reported on 251 patients who had undergone a combined anterior repair/sling procedure for SUI using solvent-dehydrated fascia lata. They found a cure/dry rate of 56% with a cure/improved rate of 76% at a mean follow-up of 24 months. They did note that, of the failures, 56% occurred after 12 months. They concluded the late failures were of concern and are continuing to monitor this group.[61]

Xenografts

The two most commonly used xenografts in reconstructive urology are porcine dermis and porcine small intestinal submucosa (SIS). As with allografts, the results for urinary slings are controversial, and there are even fewer published reports, or fewer publications with shorter follow-up.

Porcine SIS gained increased attention after being successfully implanted in a canine model for bladder augmentation without evidence of rejection or shrinkage.[62] Histologically, the SIS-regenerated bladders demonstrated three separate layers, indicating that a regenerative healing process was occurring rather than a simple replacement with fibroblasts. During the manufacturing process, the serosa, tunica muscularis, and mucosa are removed mechanically from porcine jejunum. Intestinal submucosa is transferred into an acellular collagen matrix which, once implanted, induces local host tissue cell infiltration and is subsequently remodeled within 90 to 120 days. The biomatrix in SIS lacks cellular elements; however, collagen and other growth factors with activities similar to those of transforming growth factor-β and fibroblast growth factor 2 are present. These growth factors may act as signals for local epithelial cells to proliferate, thereby colonizing the graft and leading to tissue healing without scarring.[63]

Several groups have employed porcine SIS with good short-term results. Palma and colleagues reported that 92% of 50 patients were cured of SUI at a mean follow-up of 13 months without any serious postoperative complications.[64] Rutner and associates reported on a series of 152 patients undergoing placement of an SIS sling fixed to the pubic bone without bone anchors. Of those patients, 142 (93.4%) remained dry at a median follow-up of 2.3 years.[65] Intermediate-term failures at 9 and 11 months occurred in 2 patients.

Histopathologic studies in which porcine SIS grafts were biopsied and removed have suggested variable levels of biocompatibility. Implant site biopsies under the vaginal mucosa were taken in three cases of recurrent SUI after PVS using SIS. In all three cases, exceptional biocompatibility was demonstrated, with minimal foreign body or inflammatory reaction.[66] Ho and colleagues were less enthusiastic about the biocompatibility of porcine SIS.[67] They noted postoperative inflammatory reactions consisting of erythema and pain in 6 of 10 patients undergoing eight-ply SIS tension-free sling placement. SIS is an attractive material because of its theoretical ability to stimulate local tissue in-growth. Whether this will translate into long-term efficacy and durability remains to be seen.

As for porcine dermis, Arunkalaivanan and Barrington reported a prospective randomized trial of tension-free vaginal tape (n = 74) versus porcine dermis (n = 68).[68] With a mean follow-up of 12 months (range, 6 to 24 months), they found no difference in success for correcting SUI. In another prospective randomized trial of porcine dermis (n = 34) versus autologous rectus fascia (n = 31), Giri and colleagues demonstrated similar rates of cure and improvement between the two groups but noted significantly less morbidity for the xenograft group.[69]

In contrast, Gandhi and colleagues performed histopathologic analysis of porcine dermis sling specimens in eight patients with urinary retention and two failures.[70] Variable tissue reactions were seen, suggestive of a vigorous foreign body reaction. In cases of retention, the original graft was mostly intact, with minimal remodeling and tissue in-growth. However, surgical failures revealed minimal graft remnants left within the resected suburethral tissue.

Encapsulation of porcine dermis slings with poor tissue in-growth was also observed by Cole and coworkers.[71] They found no tissue remodeling or incorporation of porcine dermis into the host tissue at 4 months in a patient operated on for retention. This tendency of porcine dermis to encapsulate might retard host tissue infiltration and, ultimately, graft integration.

In a recent attempt to look at time-dependent variations in biomechanical properties of several types of grafts implanted into rabbits, Dora and colleagues found that cadaveric fascia, porcine dermis, and porcine SIS had a reduction in tensile strength of 60% to 89% at 2 to 6 weeks.[72] Polypropylene mesh and autologous fascia did not differ in strength from baseline over the same period.

Although the use of xenografts is appealing, the variable biocompatibility and tissue responses, combined with unpredictable clinical outcomes observed, clearly require further investigation.

HISTORY AND CHARACTERISTICS OF SYNTHETIC MATERIALS

Synthetic materials include both absorbable and nonabsorbable (permanent) materials. Other than for historical interest, all of the synthetics discussed here are mesh products, most of which are permanent. Synthetic materials have long been an attractive option for pelvic reconstruction and have many desirable attributes. The permanent mesh products are stronger than native tissue, are available in any size, and are free of any potentially infectious agents. No harvesting is necessary, limiting patient morbidity and enabling outpatient surgery under minimal anesthesia. Drawbacks include difficulty with tissue integration, infection, erosion (vaginal or other structures), and the potential for foreign body reactions.

The first use of synthetic material for construction of a female urethral sling was reported by Williams and Te Linde in 1962; they used Mersilene in 12 patients.[73] Ridley,[74] in 1966, and Morgan,[75] in 1970, reported their results using Mersilene ribbon and Marlex to construct slings. In 1985, Morgan and colleagues reported on 208 consecutive patients who had undergone Marlex sling placement with a minimum 5-year follow-up.[76] Although these early investigators showed encouraging results for control of incontinence using synthetic materials, these materials and surgical techniques were plagued with problems of erosion, infection, and fistula formation.

Silicone was introduced in 1985 and was thought to be superior to Marlex or Mersilene due to its smooth surface and its ability to promote formation of a fibrous sheath.[77] Again, initial success was good, but a high rate of sinus formation and rejection due to foreign body reaction limited its use.[78]

Ulmsten and associates were first to report the use of a polypropylene mesh around the mid-urethra, in 1996.[79] They used a loosely woven mesh placed with vaginal trocars under no tension around the midportion of the urethra. Although this procedure was controversial when first introduced, Ulmsten and many others have confirmed the incidence of infection, erosion, and extrusion of the material itself to be extremely low when used for the construction of a sling.[80-86]

Cumberland[87] and Scales[88] delineated a series of ideal properties for a synthetic biocompatible material. This material should be clinically and physically inert, noncarcinogenic, and mechanically strong and should cause no allergic or inflammatory reaction. It should be easily sterilized, must not be physically modified by body tissues, and should be available in a convenient and affordable format for clinical use. None of the synthetic meshes currently in use meet all of these criteria.

It appears that three of the most important components for a mesh product used in reconstructive urology are pore size, fiber type, and stiffness.[89] Pore size and fiber type have been used to classify the most common synthetic meshes into four types (Table 59-2; Figs. 59-1 through 59-4). Type I meshes, such as soft Prolene (Ethicon, Endosurgery Inc., Summerville, NJ) and Marlex, contain large pores (>75 µg) and are usually constructed from polypropylene. This large pore size allows the admission of macrophages and in-growth of fibroblasts (fibroplasia), blood vessels (angiogenesis), and collagen, which helps prevent infection and forms fibrous connections to the surrounding tissue.[90] Type II mesh, such as Gore-Tex (WL Gore & Associates, Inc., Flagstaff, AZ), has a pore size of less than 10 µg in at least one of three dimensions (microporous). Type III meshes, such as Mersilene, are macroporous in nature but have microporous components that often include braided and/or multifilamentous materials. Type IV materials have submicronic pore size and are not used for sling surgery.

A second important property is the composition of the fibers. Polypropylene meshes are monofilament materials, whereas many other commonly used meshes are multifilament materials. The monofilament materials have a distinct advantage in terms of pore size. Most of the multifilamentous meshes have interstices less than 10 µg wide, which allows small bacteria to infiltrate and proliferate. Theoretically, these small interstices do not allow the entry of macrophages (16 to 20 µg) or leukocytes (9 to 15 µg) to eliminate the bacteria, resulting in the potential for a higher infection rate.

Flexibility, or stiffness, is another important property that appears to be related to pore size. Marlex has a higher flexural rigidity (stiffness) than Mersilene or Teflon. Prolene is composed of knitted filaments of polypropylene, as is Marlex. However, Prolene has a pore size twice as large as Marlex (1500 versus

Table 59-2 Synthetic Fiber Types and Pore Size

Type	Component	Fiber Type	Pore Size
I	Polypropylene	Monofilament	Macro
	Gynemesh PS (Ethicon, Summerville, NJ)	Mono/multifilament	Macro
	Prolene Soft (Ethicon, Johnson & Johnson, Summerville, NJ)	Multifilament	Macro
	Marlex (Bard, Covington, GA)		
	ProLite (Atrium, Hudson, NH)		
	Polypropylene/Polyglactin 910		
	Vypro (Ethicon)		
	Polyglactin 910		
	Vicryl (Ethicon)		
II	Expanded PTFE	Multifilament	Micro
	Gore-Tex (Gore, Flagstaff, AZ)		
III	Polyethylene	Multifilament	Micro/macro
	Mersilene (Ethicon)		
IV	Polypropylene sheet	Monofilament	Submicro
	Cellgard (not used for slings)		

Macro, >75 μm; Micro, <75 μm; PTFE, polytetrafluoroethylene.

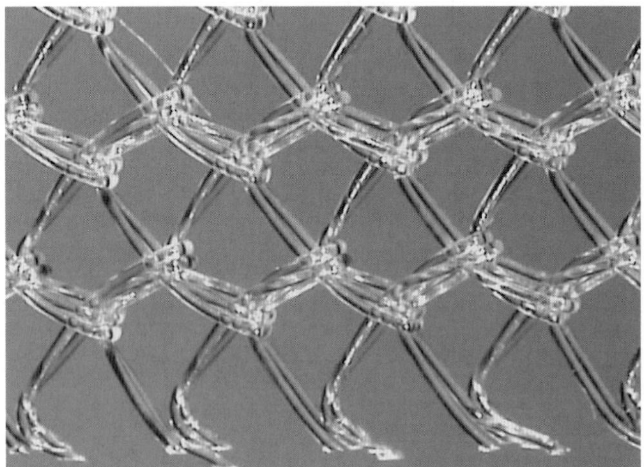

Figure 59-1 Tension-free vaginal tape (TVT). (Courtesy of Gynecare Worldwide, A Division of Ethicon, Inc., Summerville, NJ.)

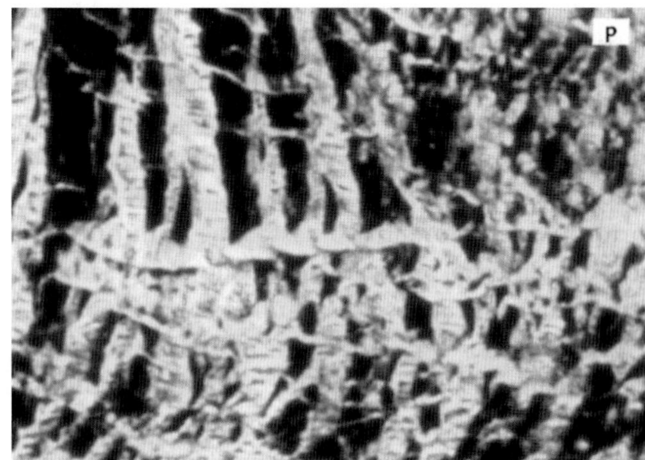

Figure 59-3 Gore-Tex mesh. (Courtesy of W.L. Gore & Associates, Inc., Flagstaff, AZ.)

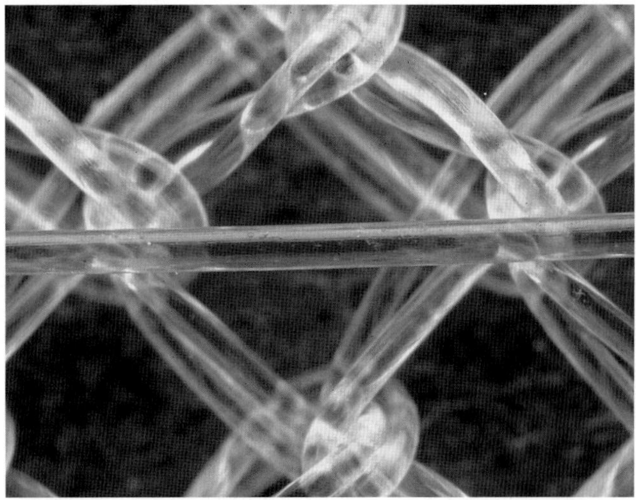

Figure 59-2 SPARC polypropylene tape. (Courtesy of American Medical Systems, Minnetonka, MN.)

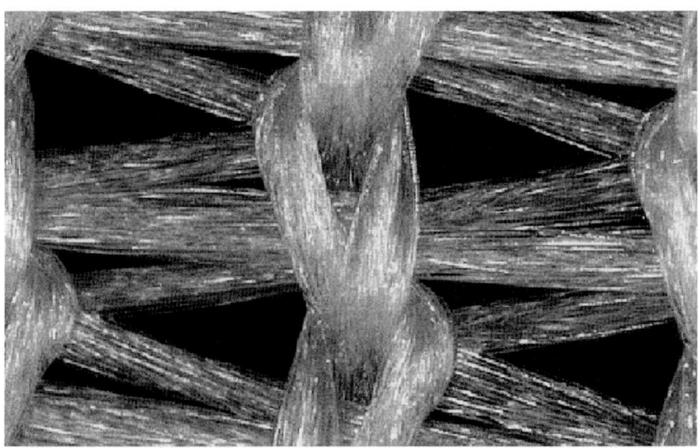

Figure 59-4 IVS Tunneller mesh. (Courtesy of U.S. Surgical, Tyco Healthcare Group Mansfield, MA.)

Table 59-3 Surgical Results for Selected Synthetics

Study (Ref. No.)	Sling Material	*N*	Follow-up (Mo)	Results
Duckett & Constantine, 2000 (93)	Solid silicone, reinforced with polyethelyne	7	3-16	100% success SUI; 71% erosion rate
Govier et al, 2005 (94)	Silicone-coated polyester (mesh)	31 prospective 20 retrospective	6-22	Prospective: 95% success SUI; 29% vaginal erosion Retrospective: 94% success SUI; 40% vaginal erosion
Barbalias et al, 1997 (95)	Gore-Tex	16	30	87.5% success SUI; 12.5% erosion
Kobashi et al, 1999 (96)	Polyester (ProtoGen)	35 (five centers)	N/A	35 erosions
Nilsson et al, 2005 (98)	Polypropylene (TVT)	90	51	81.3% objective and subjective cure of SUI; 0% erosion
Abouassaly et al, 2004 (99)	Polypropylene (TVT)	241 (six centers)	5 (range, 2-16)	5.8% bladder perforations; 4.1% reoperation for retension; 2.5% blood loss >500 mL; 1.9% pelvic hematoma; 1.0% vaginal erosion
Kobashi & Govier, 2003 (82)	Polypropylene (SPARC)	140	Not stated	1 bowel injury; 4 transfusions; 0% erosion
Delorme et al, 2004 (100)	Polypropylene, UroTape (TOT)	32	17	91% cured; 3.1% urinary retention; 0% erosion

SUI, stress urinary incontinence; TOT, transobturator tape; TVT, tension-free vaginal tape.

600 μg) and is therefore more flexible.[91] Because of this property, Prolene theoretically may have a lower erosion rate through the vagina and adjacent viscera.

SURGICAL RESULTS OF SYNTHETIC MATERIALS FOR SLINGS

In contrast to biomaterials, whose success appears to rest on the ability of the host to repopulate and remodel an acellular scaffolding, nonabsorbable synthetic mesh products are strong and permanent at the time they are placed. Assuming they are placed in the proper position, under minimal or no tension, and the fixation points are secure, the issues we should focus on are the complications of infection, erosion, and/or extrusion. As discussed earlier, it appears that the specific characteristics of the materials themselves may have a significant impact on the complication rate. Table 59-3 lists surgical success and complication rates for several synthetic materials used to construct slings. The highest rates of erosion/extrusion have been associated with polymeric silicone (Silastic),[92,93] silicone mesh,[94] polytetrafluoroethylene (Gore-Tex)[95] and polyester (ProteGen)[96] and range from 12.5% to 71%. Although this has not always been accomplished in the past, authors should either specify the structure through which the material has eroded (vagina, urethra, bladder) or use the terms "erosion" and "extrusion," with extrusion signifying vaginal exposure.

A multifactorial etiology appears to be involved in the development of erosions and extrusions. They may occur because of subclinical or delayed infection that eventually leads to separation of the vaginal incision. Excess sling tension or unrecognized urethral injury at the time of surgery may predispose to urethral erosion. As mentioned earlier, the degree of tissue in-growth and host reaction may vary according to pore size and fiber type. Mesh flexibility may also play a role, with stiffer, smaller pore materials more prone to erode or extrude. The smooth surface of silicone slings may prevent tissue in-growth, leading to poor integration into the surrounding tissues.[94]

Ulmsten and colleagues introduced tension-free vaginal tape (TVT)[79] in 1996, and it was estimated to have been used in more than 600,000 cases worldwide over the first 8 years.[97] TVT uses a large-pore, type I, monofilament, polypropylene sling placed at the mid-urethra in a tension-free manner to reconstitute the continence mechanism. SPARC (American Medical Systems, Minnetonka, MN) represents a modification of the original delivery system by directing the needles antegrade from two suprapubic incisions to the vaginal incision. Transobturator tape (TOT) delivery, the newest method of placement, leaves the mesh in a more transverse, broad-based position under the urethra from one obturator foramen to the other, completely avoiding the retropubic space.

Nilsson and associates presented 7-year follow-up data on 90 women undergoing primary TVT placement for SUI (see Table 59-3).[98] Of the patients available for evaluation, 81.3% met criteria for objective and subjective cure. No change in continence status was reported between 5- and 7-year follow-up visits in 87.5% of the patients. There was no evidence of tape erosion or tissue reaction indicative of material rejection in any of the patients. Abouassaly and coworkers performed a retrospective review of 241 patients undergoing TVT sling procedures and identified 48 (5.8%) intraoperative bladder perforations, with only 2 patients (1%) having vaginal mesh erosions.[99] Early data on the SPARC polypropylene procedure revealed one bowel injury but no mesh erosions in the first 140 patients.[82] The earliest data for polypropylene TOT demonstrated little difference in subjective and objective end points compared with TVT.[100,101] At 1-year follow-up, no sling-related complications were observed.

As shown in Table 59-3, the erosion rates of the newer polypropylene type I mesh slings have fallen dramatically, to between 0% and 1% in these four series. This was also illustrated in a recent review by Bhargava and Chapple, who looked at six centers that published data from 2002 to 2004 and found a vaginal erosion rate of only 0.6% in 2709 patients undergoing polypropylene mesh sling placement.[102]

Management of erosion or extrusion depends on the type of material, the location, and whether the patient has an erosion or an extrusion. Management varies from observation and antibiotics, to partial excision and closure, to complete removal of all synthetic materials.[95,96,103-105]

The decreased erosion rate seen with modern synthetics is most likely due to a combination of the improved biocompatibility of large-pore, monofilament mesh products; a greater emphasis on surgical technique (specifically tension-free placement); and maintenance of strict aseptic conditions. In 2005, many authorities contend that the type I, monofilament, polypropylene midurethral sling, under minimal to no tension, is the new "gold standard" for the treatment of anatomic urinary incontinence.

HISTORY OF BIOMATERIALS AND SYNTHETICS FOR THE ANTERIOR COMPARTMENT

Compromise of the structural integrity of the pelvic floor allows herniation or descent of the normally well-contained abdominal-pelvic organs. Recognition that the native tissue may no longer assume the position, strength, or functionality to repair the prolapse by simple reapproximation has prompted investigators to evaluate various techniques and materials to overcome the problem. Furthermore, recognition of the complex interplay of components of the pelvic floor has prompted investigators to view any one intervention for pelvic prolapse as a potential risk factor for further pelvic support problems. Consequently, clinicians now view the manifestations of pelvic prolapse, such as a cystocele or apical prolapse, not as an isolated defect but in a more global context and with a better understanding of what surgery a patient may require.

Although early techniques to repair anterior vaginal prolapse were theoretically sound, it quickly became clear that the use of a patient's inherently weak tissue did not provide the durability necessary to prevent recurrence. Recurrence rates after standard anterior colporrhaphy have been reported to range from 20% to 40%.[106-108] This high recurrence rate has given rise to consideration of graft reinforcement for prolapse repair.

The use of Tantalum mesh in the anterior compartment was reported in 1955 and abandoned after 4 of 10 patients had vaginal extrusion of the mesh.[109] In 1996, Julian reported vaginal extrusions in 3 of 12 patients with Marlex mesh and did not recommend its use.[110] Nicita, in 1998, reported using polypropylene mesh anchored to the arcus tendineus to correct urinary incontinence and anterior prolapse in 44 patients.[111] With a mean follow-up of 14 months, there were no recurrences and only one vaginal extrusion managed by partial excision. Also in 1998, Flood and colleagues reported on 142 patients who had anterior colporrhaphies reinforced with Marlex mesh.[112] With a mean follow-up of 3.2 years, no recurrent cystoceles were noted, and only three patients had vaginal extrusions, requiring partial excision of the mesh at 3 months, 4 years, and 7 years. The authors were enthusiastic about the use of Marlex in the anterior compartment.

In 2000, Kobashi and associates described the cadaveric prolapse repair with sling (CaPS) technique, a combined cystocele/sling procedure using a single piece of solvent-dehydrated CFL.[113] A 6 × 8 cm fascial graft was cut into a "T" configuration and attached to the vaginal apex superiorly and the levators laterally with the wings of the T, constituting the sling, secured to the pubic bone anteriorly with transvaginal bone anchors. Although this was a technique paper, follow-up at an interval of 1 to 6 months revealed no failures or allograft complications of any kind.

Since these early reports, there has been an ever-increasing number of reports of the use of allografts, xenografts, and a variety of permanent and absorbable synthetic mesh products to reinforce the anterior compartment. In addition to a myriad of materials, some authors have advocated this repair for grade 4 relaxation, and others advocate repairs for any grade 2 through 4 relaxation. Some advocate for lateral attachment directly to the arcus tendineus, the obturator fascia, or the levators, whereas others do not attach the graft to any structures at all. There are fixation techniques using absorbable sutures, permanent sutures, and bone anchors. There are centers advocating a concomitant sling in all patients and centers that continue to try to determine preoperatively who requires additional urethral support. There are those performing the combined repair through a single incision and those who advocate two separate incisions. Some authors advocate the sling and anterior repair with two separate portions of material, using separate attachment points, and some use a single piece of material to construct both, with combined attachment points. In most series, the numbers are small and the follow-up is short.

As opposed to failure of an incontinence procedure, which often prompts a return visit or can be picked up with questionnaires, mild or moderate recurrent pelvic relaxation is often largely asymptomatic and is often discovered only by repeated physical examination.

When all of these variables are combined, it is virtually impossible at this point to determine which material, if any, should be used to resupport the anterior compartment. At best, one can take what has been learned from the sling experience and make some broad generalizations.

Tables 59-4 and 59-5 summarize much of the experience to date with biomaterials and synthetics used to reconstruct the anterior compartment. For biomaterials, we would highlight the series by Kobashi and colleagues in 2000[113] and 2002[114] and by Frederick and Leach in 2005.[61] These three series used a combined cystocele/sling repair with a 6 × 8 cm portion of solvent-dehydrated CFL. The attachment points were described earlier. This is by far the largest group of allograft repairs of the anterior compartment to date and involves two separate institutions with follow-up out to 5 years in the most recent series. In the latest series, it is concerning that, in terms of continence, 56% (33 patients) of failures were initially dry and failed after 1 year. Although there are multiple possible causes, one has to consider that these patients failed to adequately remodel the allograft. On the positive side, the recurrence rate of the anterior compartment was very low, especially for symptomatic relaxation (7% at a mean follow-up of 20 months), and were no complications from the graft material itself. Perhaps even a partial remodeling of the graft supporting the anterior compartment can provide enough additional support in the most of these patients.

Among the synthetic series in Table 59-5, we would highlight the series by Sand[115] and Weber[116] and their colleagues with absorbable Vicryl mesh. If successful, the Vicryl mesh would be much less expensive than biomaterials, would put the recipient at no risk from a transmittable disease, and would have virtually

Table 59-4 Anterior Prolapse Repair Using Allograft or Xenograft Techniques

Study (Ref. No.)	N	Graft Material and Technique	Follow-up (Mo)	Outcome
*Kobashi et al, 2000 (113)	50	Combined cystocele/sling using 6 × 8 cm solvent-dehydrated CFL attached anteriorly to the pubis, laterally to the levators, and posteriorly to the vaginal apex	1-6	0% recurrence; 0% extrusion; 72% completely dry; 6% stress urinary incontinence
*Groutz et al, 2001 (120)	21	Tutoplast CFL reinforcement with 19 concomitant pubovaginal slings	20.1 (range, 12-30)	No recurrent cystoceles; 2 patients developed postoperative rectocele/enterocele; 85% patients with overt SUI cured; 100% of occult SUI cured
*Chung et al, 2002 (121)	19	Combined cadaveric dermal allograft sling and prolapse repair. Sling attached "tension free" to rectus fascia with prolene	28	1 acute graft infection requiring reoperation and rectus sling; 1 grade 1 cystocele; 1 grade 2 cystocele; 1 patient with persistent SUI; 1 patient with de novo urgency
*Kobashi et al, 2002 (114)	172	Combined cystocele/sling using 6 × 8 cm solvent-dehydrated CFL attached anteriorly to the pubis, laterally to the levators, and posteriorly to the vaginal apex	12.4 (range, 6-28)	11% grade 1 cystocele; 1.5% grade 2 cystocele; 9.8% vaginal prolapse; 10.6% SUI
Clemons et al, 2003 (127)	33	AlloDerm 3 × 7 cm portion attached anteriorly to periurethral tissues, laterally to the arcus tendineus, and posteriorly to the vaginal apex	18	36% asymptomatic grade 2 cystocele; 3% symptomatic grade 2 cystocele
*Powell et al, 2004 (123)	58	19 autologous fascia lata with 12 suburethral slings, 39 donor fascia lata with 29 slings; fascia attached at arcus tendineus.	24.7 (range, 12-57)	23% grade 2 cystocele; 16% grade 2 cystocele (autologous fascia); 27% persistent SUI
*Gomelsky et al, 2004 (124)	70	Porcine dermis graft with 65 concomitant fascia (autologous or donor) pubovaginal slings	24	4 patients with recurrent but improved SUI; 2 patients with SUI similar to preoperative; 6 grade 2 cystocele; 3 grade 3 cystocele; 6 de novo grade 2 rectoceles
Leboeuf et al, 2004 (125)	19	Porcine xenografts (Pelvicol) attached anteriorly to periurethral fascia, laterally to the arcus tendineus, posteriorly to the vaginal apex	15	6.9% recurrence
*Frederick and Leach, 2005 (61)	251	Combined cystocele/sling using 6 × 8 cm solvent-dehydrated CFL attached anteriorly to the pubis, laterally to the levators, and posteriorly to the vaginal apex	24 (range, 6-60)	7% grade 2-4 symptomatic cystocele; 45% completely dry; 76% dry/improved; 56% of sling failures occurred after 1 yr

CFL, cadaveric fascia lata; SUI, stress urinary incontinence.
*Indicates combined prolapse and incontinence procedures.

no risk of erosion. Unfortunately, one group found a substantial improvement with the mesh and one group found no difference at all.

On review of the abstracts of studies using permanent mesh products, it is clear that most authors have learned from our sling experience and have used a type I, monofilament, polypropylene mesh. Although the use of permanent mesh products clearly seems to provide a durable repair, the most significant concerns are the risk of vaginal extrusion and dyspareunia. Even with relatively short-term follow-up, the vaginal extrusion rate in these abstracts ranged from 2% to 25%, with several using polypropylene in the midrange at 8%, 8.3%, and 13%.[104,117,118] The abstract published by Milani and colleagues in 2005 showed that, in addition to a high erosion rate, 20% of the anterior repairs and 60% of the posterior repairs exhibited an increased incidence of dyspareunia.[117]

In our institution, 46 patients have undergone mesh reinforcement of the anterior compartment with polypropylene (Prolene Soft) for grade 3 and 4 defects. We are monitoring one patient who has experienced a vaginal extrusion, and we have

Table 59-5 Anterior Prolapse Repair with Synthetic Mesh Reinforcement

Study (Ref. No.)	*N*	Graft Material and Technique	Follow-up (Mo)	Outcome
Julian, 1996 (110)	12/12	Randomized study using Marlex (polypropylene) mesh reinforcement for the anterior compartment with other site-specific repairs	24	All patients had 2 or more previous failed anterior repairs. No cystocele recurrences in mesh group; 4 recurrences in control group; 25% vaginal mesh erosions
*Nicita, 1998 (111)	44	Polypropylene mesh attached taut to arcus tendineus	13.9 (range, 9-23)	1 grade 3 rectocele; 2% vaginal mesh erosion; 16% de novo urge incontinence
*Flood et al, 1998 (112)	142	Marlex (polypropylene) mesh reinforcement extended laterally into retropubic space	38	No recurrent cystocele; 2% vaginal mesh erosion; 74% success for SUI treatment
Mage, 1999 (126)	46	Polyester mesh attached at vaginal angles	26	No recurrence of cystocele; 2% vaginal mesh erosion
Migliari et al, 2000 (127)	12	Polypropylene mesh attached "tension-free" with absorbable sutures	20.5 (range, 15-32)	3 patients with asymptomatic grade 1 cystocele
Sand et al, 2001 (115)	73/70	Absorbable polyglactin 910 (Vicryl) mesh placed over plication line versus standard colporrhaphy	12	30/70 (43%) without mesh and 18/73 (25%) with mesh had grade 2-3 recurrent cystocele—40% reduced risk; 8/70 (11%) without and 2/73 (3%) with mesh had grade 3 recurrent cystocele; 13 had recurrent rectoceles
Weber et al, 2001 (116)	33/24/26	Three-armed trial of standard versus "ultralateral" versus standard plus absorbable polyglactin 910 mesh anchored to lateral limits with absorbable suture	23 (range, 5-44)	No significant difference in postoperative prolapse/urinary/sexual function symptoms between groups; all groups reported significant improvement of symptoms compared to preoperatively
De Tayrac et al, 2002 (118)	48	Polypropylene mesh placed into retropubic space "tension-free"	18 (range, 8-32)	97.9% success rate reported; 8.3% vaginal mesh erosions
*De Tayrac et al, 2004 (101)	48/26	48 polypropylene mesh with wings placed into retropubic space "tension-free" and 26 TVT	20	6.7% SUI in TVT group, 36% in no-TVT group; 6% recurrent cystocele; 8% vaginal erosion
Milani et al, 2005 (117)	32/31	32 anterior repairs polypropylene mesh attached with Maxon sutures and 31 posterior repairs polypropylene mesh	17 (range, 3-48)	32 anterior repairs—dyspareunia increased 20%, 13% vaginal mesh erosion; 31 posterior repairs—dyspareunia increased 63%, 6.5% vaginal erosions, 1 pelvic abscess. Recommended abandoning synthetic mesh for the anterior and posterior compartment.

SUI, stress urinary incontinence; TVT, tension-free vaginal tape.
*Indicates combined prolapse and incontinence procedures.

reoperated on two additional patients who failed to re-epithelialize with vaginal estrogens. All three of these patients appeared to be well healed at their 6-week examination, and extrusion occurred at a later date. Based on this early experience, we have stopped using synthetic mesh for the anterior compartment and are continuing to monitor this group.

The question we must ask ourselves as pelvic surgeons, is how much risk are we willing to accept now and for many years down the line as the patients we treat age and experience worsening atrophic vaginitis? All permanent synthetic mesh products are going to carry some risk of extrusion. Staskin and Plzak theorized that use of mesh with a higher cross-sectional area would carry

Table 59-6 Synthetic and Biomaterials for Apical Support

Study (Ref. No.)	*N*	Graft Material and Technique	Follow-up (Mo)	Outcome
Snyder et al, 1991 (137)	147	OASC: 65 Dacron, 78 polytetrafluoroethylene	43 (range, 1-204)	93% success; 2.7% graft erosion
Kohli, 1998 (133)	57	OASC: double-thickness synthetic mesh (?), nonabsorbable braided sutures	14 (range, 14-24)	12% vaginal erosion (5 mesh, 2 suture); switched to cadaveric fascia lata
Costantini et al, 1998 (138)	21	OASC: Gore-Tex	31.6 (range, 12-68)	90% (19/21) success; 2 pulmonary emboli; 0 erosions
Culligan et al, 2002 (140)	245	OASC: synthetic mesh (unspecified)	13.3 yr	Follow-up by questionnaire or physical examination; no apical failure; 15.1% failure (most anterior compartment); 2.4% vaginal mesh erosion
Brizzolara et al, 2003 (139)	124	OASC: 99 prolene mesh, 25 allograft fascia; 60 concomitant hysterectomy, 64 prior hysterectomy	55.5 (range, 0-74)	1% mesh erosion in patient with previous hysterectomy; felt primary ASC at the time of hysterectomy was no added risk
Hilger et al, 2003 (136)	38	OASC: Marlex mesh	164 (range, 120-204)	Questionnaire data plus physical examination; 10% reoperation rate "prolapse"; 16% "prolapsing tissue"; 2.6% vaginal mesh erosion
FitzGerald et al, 2004 (60)	54	OASC: freeze-dried donor irradiated fascia lata	17 (range, 3-54)	83% failure; 16 patients reoperated on with only 19% having viable graft present at 12 mo
Latini et al, 2004 (129)	10	OASC: autologous fascia lata	30.8 (range, 19-42)	30% SUI postoperative by questionnaire; 0% failure; 0% erosion
Begley et al, 2005 (134)	92	OASC and LASC:		
		• 33 Gore-Tex	29.3	9% erosion rate
		• 21 Silicone-coated polyester mesh (AMS Triangle)	15.5	19% erosion rate
		• 38 Prolene (J&J soft hernia)	9.8	0% erosion
		• 14 Fascia	18.6	0% erosion; 1% apical failure rate
Elneil et al, 2005 (141)	128	OASC and LASC: polypropylene (J&J mesh)	19 (range, 1.5-62)	Mesh not retroperitonealized; 0% bowel complication; 10% apical failure; 2.3% vaginal erosion

ASC, abdominal sacrocolpopexy; LASC, laparoscopic abdominal sacrocolpopexy; OASC, open abdominal sacrocolpopexy; SUI, stress urinary incontinence.

a higher risk of vaginal extrusion, and examination of these series appears to support that supposition.[119] Most pelvic surgeons seem to believe that the risk of vaginal extrusion with a narrow piece of a type I monofilament mesh placed around the midurethra under minimal to no tension is acceptable in most patients to prevent urinary incontinence. Whether to use a larger portion of the same mesh, which appears to carry a significantly higher risk of vaginal extrusion, for repair of the anterior compartment in an effort to prevent a recurrence (especially with a grade 2 or 3 defect), which is often minimally symptomatic, is something that pelvic surgeons need to consider very carefully.

MATERIALS USED FOR APICAL SUPPORT

A variety of surgical repairs have been described to resupport the vaginal apex. With one exception, these reports are primarily transvaginal procedures using the patient's own tissues for support and abdominal sacrocolpopexies (open or laparoscopic) that attach the apex of the vagina to the hollow of the sacrum with some type of graft. The exception is the transvaginal approach of Drs. Raz and Rodriguez, in which the arms of a type I polypropylene mesh are attached to the origin of the sacrouterine ligaments. The body of the mesh is carried down to the perineum via the posterior vaginal wall.[128] With that notable exception, we will concentrate on the open abdominal sacrocolpopexies (OASC) and laparoscopic abdominal sacrocolpopexies (LASC) for the remainder of this section.

As we have seen in the anterior compartment, there are a large number of variations in how one may perform an abdominal sacrocolpopexy (ASC). These variations, along with the reporting methodologies, make it very difficult to compare series and isolate any differences made by the materials themselves. Table 59-6 summarizes several publications looking at a variety of materials used for support. As with slings and in the anterior compartment, most of the more recent series are now using a large pore, type I polypropylene mesh. At least for the more recent series, we have to assume that a meticulous vaginal and abdominal preparation and intraoperative antibiotics were used. Most of the synthetic series used a "Y" configuration with the anterior and posterior leaflets attached to the respective portions of the vaginal wall and the main body of the graft attached to the longitudinal ligament of the sacrum or directly to the sacral bone with bone anchors. Where possible, we have tried to report the type of graft material used, whether the sutures used to attach the graft to the vaginal wall were permanent or absorbable, and whether failures occurred at the apex or involved other compartments.

The only recent report using autologous products was that of Latini and colleagues, who performed OASC on 10 patients with a mean follow-up of 30.8 months using autologous fascia lata.[129] They described harvesting adequate-size grafts through a 3-cm thigh incision and reported no vaginal erosions, apical failures, or graft complications as determined by chart review and questionnaires.

There are no published reports for biomaterials using xenografts and only a small number using allografts. The largest series to date is that of FitzGerald and associates, who recently updated their series of OASC using freeze-dried, irradiated CFL.[60] Of 54 patients undergoing OASC, 83% had experienced failure at a mean follow-up of 12 months. At the time of exploration in 16 patients, viable graft could be found in only 3 patients.

The use of synthetic materials for ASC was first reported in 1970 when Soichet reported the use of Silastic grafts in two patients.[130] Feldman and Birnbaum[131] reported on the use of Teflon in 1979, and Dewhurst and coworkers[132] used Marlex mesh in 1980. Since these early reports, a variety of synthetic products have been used. In addition to the materials themselves, there are several other controversial areas regarding the use of synthetics for ASC. The first is the type of sutures used to attach the graft to the vagina. In the past, many authors have used a permanent braided suture to minimize the risk of failure and to provide a suture that the patient and her partner would not feel. In 1998, Kohli and colleagues reported a 12% vaginal erosion rate using an unspecified type of double-thickness mesh and braided sutures.[133] Begley's group, in 2005, reported a 19% erosion rate in 21 patients using a silicone polyester mesh attached to the vagina with braided permanent suture.[134] However, most of the abstracts do not specify the type of suture used. A braided suture that is placed or erodes into the vagina is a theoretical source of infection for the graft. If that graft material has any characteristics that do not allow it to resist infection, this could be a cause of graft failure.

A second controversy is the effect of a simultaneous hysterectomy at the time of ASC. This could potentially increase the risk of infection from vaginal microbes, and, with a fresh suture line in the vagina against the graft, it could also theoretically increase the risk of vaginal extrusion. In an excellent review of ASCs published in 2004, Nygaard and coauthors found the data inconclusive but recommended that the mesh should be attached as far from the suture lines in the vaginal apex as possible.[135]

Addressing the apical failure rate in Table 59-6, one can see that, with the exception of the allograft report by FitzGerald's group, it is less than or equal to 10%; the anterior compartment appears to be an increasing concern, especially as duration of follow-up increases.

As for as longevity, a more recent abstract of a study by Hilger and colleagues using Marlex is significant.[136] Thirty-eight patients underwent OASC and had a mean follow-up of 13.7 years. By questionnaire data and chart review, there was a 26% overall failure rate, including 10% undergoing reoperation for prolapse and 16% who responded that they had "prolapsing" tissue from the vagina. It is not noted how many of these failures were apical and how many involving other compartments. The vaginal erosion rate in this series was 2.6%.

Regarding the vaginal extrusion rate, Begley and coworkers examined the use of silicone-coated mesh.[134] After noticing several vaginal erosions, with a new commercially available silicone-covered polyester mesh (AMS Triangle), they reviewed a series of 93 patients undergoing OASC or LASC with various materials. Details are shown in Table 59-6, but their vaginal erosion rates with the silicone product, Gore-Tex, polypropylene, and autologous fascia were 19%, 9%, 0%, and 0%, respectively. Among those with the silicone mesh erosions, transvaginal attempts at repair were unsuccessful in all patients, who eventually required open explorations with removal of all mesh. In contrast the Gore-Tex erosions were successfully managed by partial excision of the mesh via a transvaginal approach in most patients.

As to the vaginal extrusion rates in Table 59-6, the rates for the specific materials ranged from 0% for autologous grafts and biografts,[60,129,134,139] to 19% with the silicone coated polyester,[134] to 2.3% and 2.6% with the polypropylene (Prolene and Marlex, respectively).[136,141] In the previously mentioned review by Nygaard and associates,[135] the following vaginal erosion rates for specific materials were found: cadaveric fascia or dura mater, 0% (0/88); polypropylene (Prolene), , 0.5% (1/211); polyethylene (Mersilene, Johnson & Johnson), 3.1% (25/811); Gore-Tex, 3.4% (12/350); and Teflon (EI Dupont, deMours, and Co.), 5.5% (6/119).

In conclusion, it would appear that the risk of vaginal extrusion, from an ASC using a type I polypropylene mesh lies somewhere between that of the sling and that of anterior repair. Because it is a formidable procedure for the patient to undergo, even laparoscopically, we do not believe that most practitioners will accept the high failure rate of biomaterials. Additionally, regardless of the approach, the morbidity from harvesting autologous tissue of these dimensions is concerning. At this time, most surgeons performing this operation appear to believe that the current vaginal extrusion rates with the newer mesh products are acceptable in view of the high success rates in terms of apical support. Theoretically, there is a small risk to using a braided permanent suture to attach this graft material to the vaginal wall, and, in a case of a concomitant hysterectomy, it is prudent to keep the graft as far from the suture line in the vaginal apex as possible.

CONCLUSIONS CONCERNING THE USE OF SYNTHETICS AND BIOMATERIALS IN VAGINAL RECONSTRUCTIVE SURGERY

Tissue engineering and/or stem cell research may one day render the controversies discussed in this chapter obsolete. When that day arrives, we will have an unlimited supply of biocompatible, healthy, living fascia to use in pelvic reconstruction. Until then, it remains incumbent on pelvic surgeons to closely follow the literature, to provide informed consent, and to carefully weigh the risks and benefits of the use of these materials in our patients.

References

1. Hu TW, Wagner TH, Bentkover JD, et al: Costs of urinary incontinence and overactive bladder in the United States: A comparative study. Urology, 63:461, 2004.
2. Hunskaar S, Lose G, Sykes D, Voss S: The prevalence of urinary incontinence in women in four European countries. BJU Int 93:324-330, 2004.
3. Olson AL, Smith VJ, Berstrom JO, et al: Epidemiology of surgically managed pelvic organ prolapse and urinary incontinence. Obstet Gynecol 89:501-506, 1997.
4. Ridley JH: The Goebel-Stoeckel sling operation. In MattinglyRF, Thompson JD (eds): TeLinde's Operative Gynecology. Philadelphia: Lippincott, 1985.
5. Goebell R:. Zur operativen beseitigung der angebronen incontientia vesicase. Ztschr Gynak 2:187, 1910.
6. Aldridge AH: Transplantation of fascia for relief of urinary stress incontinence. Am J Obstet Gynecol 44:398-411, 1942.
7. Ridley JH: Surgical treatment of stress incontinence in women. JMA Georgia 94:135, 1955.
8. Williams TJ, Telinde RW: The sling operation for urinary incontinence using Mersilene ribbon. Obstet Gynecol 19:241-245, 1962.
9. Moir JC: The gauze hammock operation. J Obstet Gynecol Br Commonwealth 75:1-9, 1968.
10. Morgan JE: A sling operation using Marlex polypropylene mesh for treatment of recurrent stress incontinence. Am J Obstet Gynecol 106:369-377, 1970.
11. Stanton SI, Bringley GS, Holmes DM: Silastic sling for urethral sphincter incompetence in women. Br J Obstet Gynaecol 92:747-759, 1985.
12. McGuire EJ, Lytton B: Pubovaginal sling procedure for stress incontinence. J Urol 119:82-84, 1978.
13. Peyrera AJ: A surgical procedure for the correction of stress incontinence in women. West J Surg Obstet Gynecol 67:223, 1959.
14. Blaivas JG, Jacobs BZ: Pubovaginal sling in the treatment of complicated stress incontinence. J Urol 145:1214-1218, 1991.
15. Fokaefes ED, Lampel P, Hohenfellner M, et al: Experimental evaluation of the free versus pedicled fascial flaps for sling surgery of stress urinary incontinence. J Urol 157:1039-1043, 1997.
16. Trockman BA, Leach GE, Hamilton J, et al: Modified Pereyra bladder neck suspension: 10 Year mean follow-up in 125 patients. J Urol 154:1841-1847, 1995.
17. Leach GE, Dmochowski RR, Appell RA, et al: Female Stress Urinary Incontinence Clinical Guidelines Panel summary report on surgical management of female stress urinary incontinence. The American Urological Association. J Urol 158:875, 1997.
18. Morgan TO Jr, Westney L, McGuire EJ: Pubovaginal sling: 4-Year outcome analysis and quality of life assessment. J Urol 163:1845, 2000.
19. Chaikin DC, Rosenthal J, Blaivas JG: Pubovaginal fascial sling for all types of stress urinary incontinence: Long-term analysis. J Urol 160:1312-1216, 1998.
20. Brown SL, Govier FE: Cadaveric versus autologous fascia lata for the pubovaginal sling: Surgical outcome and patient satisfaction. J Urol 164:1633, 2000.
21. Wright EJ, Iselin CD, Carr LK: Pubovaginal sling using cadaveric allograft fascia for the treatment of intrinsic sphincter deficiency. J Urol 160:759, 1998.
22. Flynn BJ, Marinkivic SP, Yap WT: Risks and benefits of using allograft fascia lata for pubovaginal slings [abstract]. J Urol 161:310, 1999.
23. Labasky RF, Soper T: Reduction of patient morbidity and cost using frozen cadaveric fascia lata for the pubovaginal sling [abstract]. J Urol 157:459, 1997.
24. Buck BE, Malinin TL: Human bone and tissue allografts: Preparation and safety. Clin Orthop 303:8, 1994.
25. Gallentine ML, Cespedes RD: Review of cadaveric allografts in urology. Urology 59:318-324, 2002.
26. Simonds RJ, Holmberg SD, Hurwitz RL, et al: Transmission of human immunodeficiency virus type 1 from a seronegative organ and tissue donor. N Engl J Med 326:726-732, 1992.
27. Tomford WW: Current concepts review: Transmission of disease through transplantation of musculoskeletal allografts. J Bone Joint Surg Am 77A:1742-1754, 1995.
28. Maeda A, Inoue M, Shino K, et al: Effects of solvent preservation with or without gamma irradiation on the material properties of canine tendon allografts. J Orthop Res 11:181-189, 1993.
29. Singla AK: The use of cadaveric fascia lata in the treatment of stress urinary incontinence in women. BJU Int 85:264-269, 2000.
30. Food and Drug Administration: The FDA intraagency guidelines for human tissue intended for transplantation. Fed Reg 58:65514-65521, 1993.
31. DeDeyne P, Haut RC: Some effect of gamma irradiation on patellar tendon allografts. Connect Tissue Res 27:51-62, 1991.
32. Hinton R, Jinnah RH, Johnson C, et al: A Biochemical analysis of solvent-dehydrated and freeze-dried human fascia lata allografts. Am J Sports Med 20:607-612, 1992.
33. Thomas E, Gresham R: Comparative tensile strength of connective tissues. Surg Forum 14:442-443, 1963.
34. Sutaria PM, Staskin DR: Tensile strength of cadaveric fascia lata allograft is not affected by current methods of tissue preparation [abstract]. J Urol 161:1194, 1999.
35. Haut RC, Powlison AC: Order of irradiation and lyophilization on the strength of patellar tendon allografts. Proceedings of the 35th Meeting of the Orthopedic Research Society. J Bone Joint Surg 13:514, 1989.
36. Simonds RJ, Homberg SD, Hurwitz RL: Transmission of human immunodeficient virus type 1 from seronegative tissue donor. N Engl J Med, 326:726, 1992.
37. Beck RP, McCormick S, Nordstrom L: The fascia lata sling procedure for treating recurrent genuine stress incontinence of urine. Obstet Gynecol 72:699, 1988.
38. Buck BE, Resnick L, Shah SM, Malinin TI: Human immunodeficiency virus cultured from bone: Implications for transplantation. Clin Orthop 251:249, 1990.
39. Hathaway JK, Choe JM: Intact genetic material is present in commercially processed cadaveric allografts used for pubovaginal slings. J Urol 168:1040, 2002.
40. Brown P: Transmission of spongioform encephalopathy through biological products. Dev Biol Stand 93:73-78, 1998.
41. Sato T, Hoshi K, Yoshino H, et al: Creutzfeldt-Jakob disease associated with cadaveric dura mater grafts, Japan, January 1979–May 1996. MMWR Morb Mortal Wkly Rep 46:1066, 1997.
42. Birch C, Maynes MM: The role of synthetic and biological prostheses in reconstructive pelvic floor surgery. Cur Opin Obstet Gynecol 14:527, 2002.
43. Crawford JS: Nature of fascia lata and its fate after implantation. Am J Ophthalmol 67:900-907, 1969.
44. Eleftherios FD, Alexander L, Hohenfellner M, et al: Experimental evaluation of free versus pedicled fascial flaps for sling surgery of urinary stress incontinence. J Urol 157:1039-1043, 1997.
45. FitzGerald MP, Mollenhauer J, Brubaker L: The fate of rectus fascia suburethral slings. Am J Obstet Gynecol 183:964-966, 2000.
46. Arnoczky SP, Warren RF, Ashlock MA: Replacement of the anterior cruciate ligament using a patellar tendon allograft: An experimental study. J Bone Joint Surg Am 68:376-385, 1986.
47. McGregir HC, Kubdio GB: The behavior of cialit-stored and freeze-dried human fascia lata in rates. Br J Plast Surg 27:155-164, 1974.
48. Horstman JK, Ahmadu-Suka F, Norrdin RW: Anteria cruciate ligament fascia lata allograft reconstruction: Progressive histologic changes toward maturity. Arthroscopy 9:509, 1993.
49. Shino K, Inoue M, Horib S, et al: Maturation of allograft tendons transplanted into the knee: An arthroscopic and histological study. J Bone Joint Surg Br 70:556, 1988.

50. Handa VL, Jensen JK, Germain MM, Ostefard DR: Banked human fascia lata for the suburethral sling procedure: A preliminary report. Obstet Gynecol 88:1045, 1996.
51. Labasky RF, Soper T: Reduction of patient morbidity and cost using frayed cadaveric fascia lata for the pubovaginal sling [abstract 1794]. J Urol 157(Part 2):459, 1997.
52. Wright EJ, Iselin CE, Carr LK, Webster GD: Pubovaginal sling using cadaveric allograft fascia for the treatment of intrinsic sphincter deficiency. J Urol 160:759-762, 1998.
53. Chaikin DC, Blaivas JG: Weakened cadaveric fascial sling: an unexpected cause of failure. J Urol 160:2151, 1998.
54. Fitzgerald MP, Mollenhauer J, Brubaker L: Failure of allograft suburethral slings. BJU Int 84:785, 1999.
55. Elliott DS, Boone TB: Is fascia lata allograft material trustworthy for pubovaginal sling repair? Urology 56:772, 2000.
56. Carbone JM, Kavaler E, Hu JC, et al: Pubovaginal sling using cadaveric fascia and bone anchors: Disappointing early results. J Urol 165:1605, 2001.
57. O'Reilly KJ, Govier FE: Intermediate term failure of pubovaginal slings using cadaveric fascia lata: A case series. J Urol 167,1356-1358, 2002.
58. Crivellaro S, Smith JJ, Kocjancic E, Bresette JF: Transvaginal sling using acellular human dermal allograft: Safety and efficacy in 253 patients. J Urol 172:1374-1378, 2004.
59. Owens DC, Winters JC: Pubovaginal sling using Duraderm™ graft: Intermediate follow-up and patient satisfaction. Neurourol Urodyn 23:115-118, 2004.
60. FitzGerald MP, Edwards SR, Fenner D: Medium-term follow-up on use of freeze-dried, irradiated donor fascia for sacrocolpopexy and sling procedures. Int Urogynecol J 15:238-242, 2004.
61. Frederick RW, Leach GE: Cadaveric prolapse repair with sling: Intermediate outcomes with 6 months to 5 years of followup. J Urol 173:1229-1233, 2005.
62. Kropp BP, Rippy MK, Badylak SF, et al: Regenerative urinary bladder augmentation using small intestinal submucosa: Urodynamic and histopathologic assessment in long-term canine bladder augmentations. J Urol 155:2098, 1996.
63. Vyotik-Harbin SL, Brightman AO, Kraine M, et al: Identification of extractable growth factors from small intestinal submucosa. J Cell Biol 67:478, 1997.
64. Palma P, Riccoetto C, Dambros M, et al: Favorable results from the porcine small intestinal submucosa in the treatment of stress urinary incontinence. BJU Int 90:251, 2002.
65. Rutner AB, Levine SR, Schmaelzle JF: Processed porcine small intestine submucosa as a graft material for pubovaginal slings: Durability and results. Urology 62:805, 2003.
66. Wiedemann A, Otto M: Small intestinal submucosa for pubourethral sling suspension for the treatment of stress incontinence: First histopathological results in humans. J Urol 172:215, 2004.
67. Ho KV, Witte MN, Bird ET: 8-Ply small intestinal submucosa tension-free sling: Spectrum of postoperative inflammation. J Urol 171:268, 2004.
68. Arunkalaivanan AS, Barrington JW: Randomized trial of porcine dermal sling (Pelvicol™ implant) vs. tension-ree vaginal tape (TVT) in the surgical treatment of stress incontinence: A questionnaire-based study. Int Urogynecol J 14:17-23; discussion 21-22, 2003.
69. Giri SK, Clyne O, Hickey JP, et al: Prospective randomized trail of xenograft versus rectus fascia pubovaginal sling in the treatment of stress incontinence. BJU Int 93(Suppl 4):56, 2004.
70. Gandhi S, Kubba LA, Abramov Y, et al: Histopathologic changes of porcine dermal implants used for transvaginal suburethral slings. J Pelvic Med Surg 10(Suppl 1):S12, 2004.
71. Cole E, Gomelsky A, Dmochowski RR: Encapsulation of a porcine dermis pubovaginal sling. J Urol 170:1950, 2003.
72. Dora CD, Kimarco DS, Zobitz ME, Elliott DS: Time dependent variations in biomechanical properties of cadaveric fascia, porcine dermis, procine small intestine submucosa, polypropylene mesh and autologous fascia in the rabbit model: implications for sling surgery. J Urol 171:1970-1973, 2004.
73. Williams TJ, Te Linde RW: The sling operation for urinary incontinence using Mersilene ribbon. Obstet Gynecol 19:241-245, 1962.
74. Ridley JH: Appraisal of the Goebell-Frangenheim-Stoeckel sling procedure. Am J Obstet Gynecol 95:714-721, 1966.
75. Morgan JE: A sling operation using Marlex polypropylene mesh for treatment of recurrent stress incontinence. Am J Obstet Gynecol 106:369-377, 1970.
76. Morgan JE, Farrow GA, Stewart FE: The Marlex sling operation for the treatment of recurrent stress urinary incontinence: A 16-year review. Am J Obstet Gynecol 151:224, 1984.
77. Stanton SL, Brindley GS, Holmes DM: Silastic sling for urethral sphincter incompetence in women. Br J Obstet Gynaecol 92:747, 1985.
78. Duckett JRA, Constantine G: Complication of silicone sling insertion for stress urinary incontinence. J Urol 163:1835, 2000.
79. Ulmsten U, Heriksson L, Jonson P, Varhos G: An ambulatory surgical procedure under local anesthesia for treatment of female urinary incontinence. Int Urogynecol J Pelvic Floor Dysfunct 7:81, 1996.
80. Shah DK, Paul EM, Amukele S, et al: Broad based tension-free synthetic sling for stress urinary incontinence: 5-Year outcome. J Urol 170:849-851, 2003.
81. Rodriguez LV, Raz S: Prospective analysis of patient treated with a distal urethral polypropylene sling for symptoms of stress urinary incontinence: Surgical outcome and satisfaction determined by patient driven questionnaires. J Urol 170:857-863, 2003.
82. Kobashi KC, Govier FE: Perioperative complications: The first 140 polypropylene pubovaginal slings. J Urol 170:1918-1921, 2003.
83. Wilson TS, Lemack GE, Zimmerman PE: Management of intrinsic sphincteric deficiency in women. J Urol 169:1662-1669, 2003.
84. Karram MM, Segal JL, Vassallo BJ, Kleeman SD: Complications and untoward effects of the tension-free vaginal tape procedure. Obstet Gynecol 101(5 Pt 1):929-932, 2003.
85. Levin I, Groutz A, Gold R, et al: Surgical complications and medium-term outcome results of tension free vaginal tape: A prospective study of 313 consecutive patients. Neurourol Urodyn 23:7-9, 2004.
86. Tsivian A, Kessler O, Mogutin B, et al: Tape related complications of the tension-free vaginal tape procedure. J Urol 171:762-764, 2004.
87. Cumberland VH: A preliminary report on the use of prefabricated nylon weave in the repair of ventral hernia. Med J Aust 1:143-144, 1952.
88. Scales JT: Materials for hernia repair. Proc R Soc Med 46:647-652, 1953.
89. Vervigni M, Natale F: The use of synthetics in the treatment of pelvic organ prolapse. Curr Opin Urol 11:429-435, 2001.
90. White TA: The effect of porosity and biomaterial on the healing and long-term mechanical properties of vascular prostheses. ASAIO J 11:95-100, 1988.
91. Voyles CR, Richardson JD, Bland SM, et al: Emergency abdominal wall reconstruction with polypropylene mesh: Short-term benefits versus long-term complications. Ann Surg 194:219-223, 1981.
92. Chin YK, Stanton SL: A follow up of silastic sling for genuine stress incontinence. Br J Obstet Gynaecol 102:143, 1995.
93. Duckett JR, Constantine G: Complications of silicone sling insertion for stress urinary incontinence. J Urol 163:1835, 2000.
94. Govier FE, Kobashi KC, Committer C, et al: Multi-center prospective study of a transvaginal silicone coated synthetic mesh sling. Urology 66:741-745, 2005.
95. Barbalias G, Liatsikos E, Barbalias D: Use of slings made of indigenous and allogenic material (Gore-Tex) in type III urinary incontinence and comparison between them. Eur Urol 31:394, 1997.

96. Kobashi KC, Dmochowski RR, Mee SL, et al: Erosion of woven polyester pubovaginal sling. J Urol 162:2070, 1999.
97. Bhargava S, Chapple CR: Rising awareness of the complications of synthetic slings. Curr Opin Urol 14:317, 2004.
98. Nilsson CG, Falconer C, Rezapour M: Seven-year follow-up of the tension-free vaginal tape procedure for treatment of urinary incontinence. Obstet Gynecol 104:1259, 2004.
99. Abouassaly R, Steinberg JR, Lemieux M, et al: Complications of tension-free vaginal tape surgery: A multi-institutional review. BJU Int 94:110, 2004.
100. Delorme E, Droupy S, deTayrac R, Delmas V: Transobturator tape (Uratape): A new minimally-invasive procedure to treat female urinary incontinence. Eur Urol 45:203, 2004.
101. De Tayrac R, Deffieux X, Droupy S, et al: A prospective randomized trial comparing tension-free vaginal tape and transobturator suburethral tape for surgical treatment of stress urinary incontinence. Am J Obstet Gynecol 190:602, 2004.
102. Bhargava S, Chapple CR: Rising awareness of the complications of synthetic slings. J Urol 14:317-321, 2004.
103. Volkmer BG, Nesslauer T, Rinnab L, et al: Surgical intervention for complications of tension-free vaginal tape procedure. J Urol 169:570, 2003.
104. Clemens JQ, DeLancey JO, Faerber GJ, et al: Urinary tract erosions after synthetic pubovaginal slings: Diagnosis and management strategy. Urology 56:589, 2000.
105. Kobashi KC, Govier FE: Management of vaginal erosion of polypropylene mesh slings. J Urol 169:2242-2243, 2003.
106. Paraiso MFR, Ballard LA, Walter MD, et al: Pelvic support defects and visceral and sexual function in women treated with sacrospinous ligament suspension and pelvic reconstruction. Am J Obstet Gynecol 175:1423-1431, 1996.
107. Shull BL, Capen CV, Riggs MW, Kuehl TJ: Preoperative and postoperative analysis of site-specific pelvic support defects in 81 women treated with sacrospinous ligament suspension and pelvic reconstruction. Am J Obstet Gynecol 166:1764-1771, 1992.
108. Shull BL, Ben SJ, Kuehl TJ: Surgical management of prolapse of the anterior vaginal segment: An analysis of support defects, operative morbidity, and anatomic outcome. Am J Obstet Gynecol 171:1429-1439, 1994.
109. Moore J, Armstrong JR, Willis SW: The use of tantalum mesh in cystocele with critical report of ten cases. Am J Obstet Gynecol 69:1127-1135, 1955.
110. Julian TM: The efficacy of Marlex mesh in the repair of severe recurrent vaginal prolapse of the anterior mid vaginal wall. Am J Obstet Gynecol 175:1472-1475, 1996.
111. Nicita G: A new operation for genitourinary prolapse. J Urol 160:741-745, 1998.
112. Flood CG, Drutz HP, Waja L: Anterior colporrhaphy reinforced with Marlex mesh for the treatment of cystoceles. Int Urogynecol J 9:200-204, 1998.
113. Kobashi KC, Mee SL, Leach GE: A new technique for cystocele repair and transvaginal sling: The cadaveric prolapse repair and sling (CaPS). Urology 56(S6A):9-14, 2000.
114. Kobashi KC, Leach GE, Chon J, Govier FE: Continued multicenter followup of the cadaveric prolapse repair with sling. J Urol 168:2063-2068, 2002.
115. Sand PK, Koduri S, Lobel RW, et al: Prospective randomized trial of polyglactin 910 mesh to prevent recurrence of cystoceles and rectoceles. Am J Obstet Gynecol 184:1357-1362, 2001.
116. Weber AM, Walters MD, Piedmonte MR, et al: Anterior colporrhaphy: A randomized trial of three surgical techniques. Am J Obstet Gynecol 185:1299-1304; discussion 1304-1306, 2001.
117. Milani R, Salvatore S, Soligo M, et al: Functional and anatomical outcome of anterior and posterior vaginal prolapse repair with Prolene mesh. BJOG 112:107-111, 2005.
118. De Taryac R, Gervaise A, Fernandez H: [Cystocele repair by the vaginal route with a tension-free sub-bladder prosthesis] [French]. J Gynecol Obstet Biol Reprod 31:597-599, 2002.
119. Staskin DR, Plzak L: Synthetic slings: Pros and cons. Curr Urol Reports, 3:414-417, 2002.
120. Groutz A, Chaikin DC, Theusen E, Blaiva JG: Use of cadaveric solvent-dehydrated fascia lata for cystocele repair: Preliminary results. Urology 58:179-183, 2001.
121. Chung SY, Frank M, Smith CP, et al: Technique of combined pubovaginal sling and cystocele repair using a single piece of cadaveric dermal graft. Urology 59:538-541, 2002.
122. Clemmons JL, Myers DL, Aguilar VC, Arya LA: Vaginal paravaginal repair with an AlloDerm graft. Am J Obstet Gynecol 189:1612-1619, 2003.
123. Powell CR, Simsiman AJ, Menefee SA: Anterior vaginal wall hammock with fascia lata for the correction of stage 2 or grater anterior vaginal compartment relaxation. J Urol 171:264-267, 2004.
124. Gomelsky A, Rudy DC, Dmochowski RR: Porcine dermis interposition graft for repair of high grade anterior compartment defects with or without concomitant pelvic organ prolapse procedures. J Urol 171:1581-1584, 2004.
125. Leboeuf L, Mile RA, Kim SS, Gousse AE: Grade 4 cystocele repair using four-defect repair and porcine xenograft acellular matrix (Pelicol): Outcome measure using SEAPI. Urology 64:282-286, 2004.
126. Mage P: [Interposition of a synthetic mesh by vaginal approach in the cure of genital prolapse.] [French] J Gynecol Obstet Biol Reprod 28:825-829, 1999.
127. Migliari R, De Angelis M, Madeddu G, Verdacchi T: Tension-fee vaginal mesh repair for anterior vaginal wall prolapse. Eur Urol 38:151-155, 2000.
128. Rutman MP, Deng DY, Rodriquez LV, Raz S: Restoring the strength of the weakened sacrouterine ligaments (SUL) in vaginal vault prolapse and repair of pelvic floor relaxation with the use of polypropolene mesh [abstract 867]. J Urol 173(4):236, 2005.
129. Latini JM, Brown JA, Kreder KJ: Abdominal sacral colpopexy sing autologous fascia lata. J Urol 171:1176, 2004.
130. Soichet S: Surgical correction of total genital prolapse with retention of sexual function. Obstet Gynecol 36:69-75, 1970.
131. Feldman GB, Birnbaum SJ: Sacral colpopexy for vaginal vault prolapse. Obstet Gynecol 53:399-401, 1979.
132. Dewhurst J, Toplis PJ, Shepherd JH: Ivalon sponge hysterosacropexy for genital prolapse in patients with bladder extrophy. Br J Obstet Gynaecol 87:67-69, 1980.
133. Kohli N, Walsh RM, Roat TW, Karram MM: Mesh erosion after abdominal sacrocolpopexy. Obstet Gynecol 92:999-1004, 1998.
134. Begley JS, Kupferman SP, Kuznetsov DD, et al: Incidence and management of abdominal sacrocolpopexy mesh erosions. Am J Obstet Gynecol 192:1956-1962, 2005.
135. Nygaard IE, McCreery R, Brubaker L, et al: Abdominal sacrocolpopexy: A comprehensive review. Am Coll Obstet Gynecol 104:805, 2004.
136. Hilger WS, Poulson M, Norton PA: Long-term results of abdominal sacrocolpopexy. 29th Annual Meeting of the Society of Gynecologic Surgeons, Anaheim, CA, March 5-7, 2003.
137. Snyder TE, Krantz KE: Abdominal-retroperitoneal sacral colpopexy for the correction of vaginal prolapse. Obst Gynecol 77:944-949, 1991.
138. Costantini E, Lombi R, Micheli C, et al: Colposacropexy with Gore-Tex mesh in marked vaginal and uterovaginal prolapse. Eur Urol 34:111-117, 1998.
139. Brizzolara S, Pillai-Allen A: risk of mesh erosion with sacral colpopexy and concurrent hysterectomy. Obstet Gynecol 102:306, 2003.
140. Culligan PJ, Murphy M, Blackwell L, et al: Long-term success of abdominal sacral colpopexy using synthetic mesh. 28th Annual Meeting of the Society of Gynecologic Surgeons, Dallas, TX, March 4-6, 2002.
141. Elneil S, Cutner AS, Remy M, et al: Abdominal sacrocolpopexy for vault prolapse without burial of mesh: A case series. BJOG 112:486-489, 2005.

Part A
ANTERIOR VAGINAL WALL PROLAPSE

Chapter 60

MANAGEMENT OF THE URETHRA IN VAGINAL PROLAPSE

Connie S. DiMarco and Nancy B. Itano

One of the greatest challenges to the reconstructive pelvic floor surgeon is the approach to pelvic organ prolapse (POP) in the clinically continent woman. It is controversial whether the urethra should be surgically addressed at the time of vaginal prolapse repair. It has been proposed that a prophylactic anti-incontinence procedure be performed concomitantly due to the risk of developing stress urinary incontinence (SUI) once the vaginal axis has been restored. The counterargument suggests that, because only a small percentage of continent women with POP develop SUI postoperatively, many patients would undergo an unnecessary procedure with this approach. Even the most minimally invasive anti-incontinence procedures carry a potential risk of morbidity to the patient.

EFFECT OF PELVIC ORGAN PROLAPSE ON URINARY SYMPTOMS

Moderate and severe pelvic floor relaxation can present with a variety of lower urinary tract symptoms. Many urinary symptoms can be attributed to obstructive voiding. These symptoms may include frequency, urgency, nocturia, hesitancy, double-voiding, sense of inadequate emptying, stranguria, flow intermittency, and suprapubic discomfort. Elevated postvoid residual volumes can also lead to recurrent or persistent urinary tract infections. Hypothetical causes include urethral kinking, urethral compression, bladder neck elongation, and detrusor hypocontractility/dysfunction. When severe prolapse involves the bladder, patients can also present with ureteral obstruction and hydronephrosis.[1,2]

Patients with POP may be continent or incontinent. Mechanisms for continence in prolapse include urethral obstruction, anatomic urethral kinking with descent of the bladder base, and abdominal pressure dissipation.[3] These mechanisms may also contribute to obstructive voiding symptoms. Bergman and colleagues[4] proposed that, in prolapse, a large cystocele provides a "cushion effect" that absorbs some of the intraabdominal pressure, effectively lowering the abdominal pressure placed on the continence mechanism (urethral complex). Ghoniem and associates[3] proposed that the only fixed portion of the lower urinary tract in large cystoceles is the distal urethra, supported by the pubourethral ligament. They hypothesized that the pubourethral ligament may be the only supporting structure that maintains its strength in the setting of severe prolapse, allowing for urinary continence.

There are many theories on the cause of stress urinary incontinence (SUI), which are beyond the scope of this chapter. However, POP is a common coexisting condition, and prolapse reduction (surgical or manual) may reveal an underlying incompetent urethral continence mechanism.

Pelvic Organ Prolapse

Dietz and coworkers[5] reported on 223 vaginal prolapse patients with symptoms of lower urinary tract symptoms presenting in two urogynecology clinics. Urinary symptoms included SUI in 64% (142 patients), urge incontinence in 61% (134), frequency in 38% (84), nocturia in 38% (84), and obstructive symptoms (including stranguria, sense of incomplete emptying, intermittency, and hesitancy) in 56% (124).

Cystocele

Romanzi and colleagues[6] prospectively evaluated 60 women with various degrees of cystocele and found the following urinary complaints (patients could have more than one symptom): frequency/urgency, 35%; urge incontinence, 15%; stress incontinence, 60%; and difficult voiding 23%. Women with higher stages of anterior prolapse had a statistically greater likelihood of obstructive voiding than did those with lower stages of prolapse (70% in grades 3/4 versus 3% in grades 1/2). Obstruction was defined as a maximum detrusor pressure at maximum flow ($P_{det}Q_{max}$) of greater than 25 cm H_2O and a maximum flow of less than 15 mL/sec.

Uterovaginal Prolapse

Patients with uterovaginal prolapse may also present with lower urinary tract symptoms. The group at Kaohsiung Medical University[7] studied 38 clinically continent and 20 incontinent women with stage III/IV complete uterovaginal prolapse. Incontinent women were more likely to report urinary frequency, urgency, and nocturia. However, the continent women had a higher incidence of voiding hesitancy. Urodynamic parameters between the two groups were compared. The women without stress incontinence had significantly higher ($P_{det}Q_{max}$), maximum urethral closure pressures (MUCP), and urethral-abdominal pressure

Table 60-1 Urodynamic Comparison of Continent and Incontinent Women with Stage III/IV Uterovaginal Prolapse

Parameter	Continent Patients (n = 20)	Incontinent Patients (n = 38)	P Value
$P_{det}Q_{max}$ (mean, cm H_2O)	38	24	.01
MUCP (mean, cm H_2O)	84	63	.03
Urethral-abdominal pressure transmission ratio	1.02	0.66	.02

MUCP, maximum urethral closing pressure; $P_{det}Q_{max}$, detrusor pressure at maximum flow.
From Long CY, Hsu SC, Wu TP, et al: Urodynamic comparison of continent and incontinent women with severe uterovaginal prolapse. J Reprod Med 49:33-37, 2004.

transmission ratios (Table 60-1). The pressure transmission ratio should be 1.0 (ideal) when increases in abdominal pressure are transmitted equally to the abdominal transducer (usually rectal or vaginal) and the urethral transducer. With rotation of the urethra, compressive forces from the abdominal cavity are incompletely transmitted to the urethral complex, creating a ratio of less than 1.0.

Posthysterectomy Vault Prolapse and Enterocele

Wall and Hewitt[8] described urinary characteristics in 19 women with complete posthysterectomy vaginal vault prolapse. Symptoms of urgency was present in 79% (15 patients) and urge incontinence in 63% (12 patients). Occult SUI was demonstrated by prolapse reduction with a single-bladed speculum in 47% (9 patients). Urodynamic parameters included peak flow rate (Q_{max}) and $P_{det}Q_{max}$. The mean Q_{max} was 11 mL/sec, and $P_{det}Q_{max}$ was 50 cm H_2O, meeting the pressure-flow parameters for female outlet obstruction outlined by Massey and Abrams.[9]

Rectocele

Even patients with isolated posterior wall support defects can have masked SUI. Myers and colleagues[10] evaluated 90 patients with isolated posterior compartment prolapse, including 28 with grade III+ rectoceles. Fourteen percent (n = 4/28) demonstrated SUI when their prolapse was reduced with a split Pederson speculum that was not present without prolapse reduction. The mean decrease in MUCP with rectocele reduction was 7.0 cm H_2O. The authors theorized that severe posterior wall defects act to compress and support the anterior wall, artificially raising the MUCP, increasing functional length, and masking SUI.

Women with POP can present with a myriad of urinary symptoms. A thorough history must include extensive details of voiding habits, including a previous history of incontinence that improved with worsening prolapse. As with staging of prolapse severity, physical examination findings can vary with bladder volume, rectal contents, and position. The Pelvic Floor Disorders Network recently published their findings on technique modifications that can result in intraobserver variability.[11] Prolapse was graded as more severe in the standing position compared with the lithotomy supine position. The type of speculum was not standardized. Prolapse severity was consistent using either a split speculum or a manual (two-digit) reduction method. Urinalysis should be performed to rule out urinary tract infection, and a culture with sensitivities can be sent if necessary. A screening postvoid residual volume measurement, either by catheterization or by bladder ultrasound, is a simple means to identify patients with urinary retention.

OCCULT STRESS INCONTINENCE IN PROLAPSE

Many patients with significant POP are continent and demonstrate SUI only when their prolapse is reduced. There is no "gold standard" method for determining whether a patient has occult SUI. The incidence of "masked" incontinence varies with the method of prolapse reduction, with rates of 25% to 80% reported in the literature.[12-15]

The goal of prolapse reduction is to simulate surgical repair and determine whether the patient will be at risk for development of postoperative de novo SUI. Potential pitfalls include obstructing the urethra, which would lower the SUI detection rate, and mechanically widening the levator hiatus, which would falsely elevate the SUI detection rate (Table 60-2).

Several methods of prolapse reduction to detect occult SUI have been described. A positive cough stress test (CST) is determined by objective urethral leakage with increased intra-abdominal pressure. Bladder volumes vary but are commonly reported between 150 and 250 mL. Urodynamics can be employed to ensure that urinary leakage is not the result of bladder compliance abnormalities or detrusor instability. Fluoroscopy may also contribute additional anatomic information.

Pessary

The primary objective of a pessary is to reduce symptomatic vaginal prolapse. A pessary can be used temporarily to assess for underlying SUI, as described later. Patient satisfaction is also high when these devices are used for nonoperative management of prolapse. Clemons and associates[16] recently studied patient satisfaction and changes in urinary symptoms among women using either a ring or a Gellhorn pessary after 2 months. Of the initial 100 patients, 73% were successfully fitted with a pessary. SUI improved in 45% of the patients who had incontinence symptoms at baseline. Among women without incontinence at baseline, de novo SUI developed in 21%. Pessaries may be employed both in the office setting and in long-term home use to unmask SUI.

Placement of a pessary to reduce prolapse requires appropriate sizing. There should be one fingerbreadth of room around the pessary circumferentially, to prevent compression. Similarly, if the pessary is too small, the patient may extrude it when attempting to cough or perform a Valsalva maneuver. Some pessaries are designed to prevent stress incontinence (e.g., a shelf pessary) and should be avoided in this scenario. This requires a health care provider who is facile in pessary fitting and an inventory of pessaries of various shapes and sizes on hand.

In one of the earliest studies, Richardson and colleagues[13] found that 8 (80%) of 10 continent patients with uterine prolapse were incontinent after reduction with an *inflatable pessary*.

Table 60-2 Detection Rate of Occult SUI after Anti-incontinence Surgery According to Preoperative Status

Study & Ref. No.	Year	Surgery Type	*N*	Detection of Occult SUI (% [No.])	SUI after Surgery (% [No.]) Incontinent Preoperatively	Occult SUI Preoperatively	Continent Preoperatively (No Occult SUI)*
Stanton et al[21]	1982	Anterior plication	73		69 (20/29)	11 (5/44)	
Kayano et al[22]	2002	Kelly-Kennedy	33	69 (23/33)		61 (14/23)	
Chaikin et al[23]	2000	PVS	24	58 (14/24)		14 (2/14)	0 (0/10)
Gordon et al[27]	2001	TVT	30			10 (3/30)	
Barnes et al[24]	2002	PVS	38			5 (2/38)	
Meschia et al[26]	2004	TVT	25			4 (1/25)	
		Anterior plication	25			36 (9/25)	
de Tayrac et al[25]	2004	TVT		40 (19/48)	7 (1/15)	0 (0/11)	
		No sling			36 (5/14)	13 (1/8)	

PVS, bladder neck pubovaginal sling; SUI, stress urinary incontinence; TVT, tension-free vaginal tape.
*Negative cough stress test for occult SUI.

Bergman and coauthors[4] described the use of a *Smith-Hodge pessary* (size 2 or 3) to reduce prolapse in 67 women without symptoms of SUI. Twenty-four patients had a drop in abdominal pressure transmission to the urethra (<1.0) with pessary insertion. These patients were identified as having a "high likelihood" of developing SUI due to "sphincter weakness." Seventy-one percent (17/24 patients) had objective loss of urine with pessary placement. Straining Q-tip urethral angles were similar for pessary-supported patients with and without declines in pressure transmission. Urethral hypermobility did not seemingly contribute to pressure transmission.

Versi and associates,[12] using a Gehrung pessary, reported on 49 patients with stage II/III anterior wall relaxation. The radiopaque edge of the Gehrung pessary allowed visualization of pessary position during videourodynamics, ensuring that the bladder neck and urethra were not compressed. One of the 49 patients (2%) could not retain the pessary and was excluded from the study. Occult "genuine" SUI was diagnosed if there was fluoroscopic leakage of contrast into the urethra in the absence of detrusor activity. Of the 22 patients without symptoms of stress incontinence, 26% (7 patients) demonstrated genuine SUI.

A *ring pessary* may be also be used. Hextall and associates[14] demonstrated that 27% (19/70) of their subjects had objective loss of urine only when the ring pessary was placed. Patients underwent urodynamics to ensure that detrusor instability was not the cause of the incontinence.

Klutke and Ramos published their series on patients who had their prolapse reduced with a *Gellhorn pessary.*[17] A positive CST was defined as urethral leakage in the absence of detrusor instability on cystometry. All patients with a positive CST underwent a concomitant Burch colposuspension or combined needle suspension/culposuspension at the time of anterior-posterior repair. Four percent (1/23) of patients in the colposuspension group developed de novo SUI, and 30% (7/23) developed de novo detrusor instability. In the group with reconstruction only, no patients developed de novo SUI, and only 5% (1/20) developed de novo detrusor instability.

These studies show that pessaries are an effective means to reduce vaginal prolapse in the evaluation of occult SUI. A negative pessary test can predict which patients may be incontinent after prolapse repair.

Vaginal Packing

Vaginal packing does not require special equipment. Adequate packing should reduce prolapse without forcing the levator hiatus open and without obstructing the urethra. Ghoniem and associates[3] described a method using two rolls of 4 × 4 inch gauze. Fluoroscopy confirmed that the urethra was not compressed. Urodynamics confirmed that leakage was not caused by an uninhibited detrusor contraction. Vaginal packing was placed in two groups: patients with significant cystoceles ($n = 16$) and a control group of patients without prolapse ($n = 10$). In the control group, vaginal packing did not change MUCP or the proximal urethral closing pressure. Packing revealed objective urine loss in 69% (11/16) of the patients with prolapse. There was no difference in MUCP between those with occult SUI and those without SUI. The only difference was a lower proximal urethral closing pressure in those with occult SUI compared to those without SUI. The authors concluded that their technique of vaginal packing did not alter urethral pressure dynamics.

Split Speculum

The split speculum (posterior speculum blade) is also used as part of the physical examination to measure the degree of prolapse, as recommended by the International Continence Society.[18] This is easily performed when the patient is in the supine position. A split speculum can be used to reduce prolapse while asking the patient to cough or bear down. Urethral leakage can be readily visualized. Using a speculum with the patient seated or standing is technically more difficult. The handle of the split speculum may be secured on the perineum (for apical or posterior prolapse) or near the mons pubis (for anterior prolapse). Patients are often sitting or standing during urodynamic studies to recreate the conditions (i.e., positioning) during which urinary symptoms occur. If a Graves speculum (no handle) is used, it may need to be held in place manually.

Gallentine and Cespedes[19] used gauze packing in conjunction with a split speculum to detect occult SUI in patients with posthysterectomy vault prolapse. The frequency of occult SUI was 50% (6/12 patients). The mean decrease in abdominal leak point pressure was 59 cm H_2O.

Cotton Swabs

A swab (such as a Scopette or Procto-swab) may be placed at the cuff or in the posterior fornix to reduce prolapse. The non-swab end may be taped to the patient's thigh.

Veronikis, Nichols and Wakamatsu[15] prospectively evaluated the three techniques of prolapse reduction in 30 patients with massive POP. They used an intravaginal swab, a Gellhorn pessary, and the posterior blade of a Graves speculum in each patient. The pessary was dislodged in five patients and expelled completely in three patients during cystometry. The Scopette technique detected the highest rate of occult SUI (83%, 25/30). The mean MUCP was lower with the Scopette technique compared with use of a speculum or pessary and with unreduced prolapse. The swab technique diagnosed patients with a low-pressure urethra that would have been missed by the other techniques.

OUTCOME STUDIES

All of the techniques described previously attempt to predict which patients (among those without stress incontinence symptoms) might benefit from a preemptive anti-incontinence procedure. It is distressing to both the patient and the physician when a successful vaginal prolapse surgery is complicated by the development of de novo SUI. But this must be tempered by the potential urinary complications that can result from unnecessary procedures, such as de novo urge incontinence, urinary retention, and mesh erosion.

In addition to the presence of occult SUI, consideration should be given to baseline detrusor function. Many patients void by means of pelvic floor relaxation and/or Valsalva maneuvers, instead of a true detrusor contraction. Miller and colleagues[20] showed that lack of a detrusor contraction was a significant risk factor for development of urinary retention after cadaveric fascia lata bladder neck pubovaginal sling surgery. Patients with prolapse can have complicated voiding patterns. It is possible to void without detrusor activity, have incomplete emptying due to urethral kinking, and have occult intrinsic deficiency simultaneously.

Anterior Repairs

In 1982, Stanton and coworkers[21] published their prospective series of 73 patients who underwent anterior colporrhaphy and vaginal hysterectomy for a variety of reasons (prolapse, menstrual problems, elective sterilization). Eleven percent of patients (5/44) who were continent preoperatively developed objective evidence of SUI postoperatively, despite undergoing an anterior colporrhaphy; 69% (20/29) with SUI symptoms preoperatively continued to have SUI symptoms.

Another study, published in 2002,[22] sought to evaluate patients before and after vaginal hysterectomy combined with a Kelly-Kennedy anterior plication. Twenty-three of the 33 postmenopausal patients had objective loss of urine preoperatively (69%). Three months postoperatively, 14 (61%) continued to show objective SUI. The authors concluded that a Kelly-Kennedy repair was not indicated in the treatment of SUI.

Traditional Pubovaginal Sling at the Bladder Neck

Chaikin and colleagues[23] prospectively evaluated continent women undergoing surgical repair of severe urogenital prolapse. Pessary testing was performed to unmask sphincteric incontinence. Occult incontinence was discovered in 58% (14/24) of the patients. All of these patients underwent a pubovaginal sling procedure at the bladder neck in addition to anterior colporrhaphy. With a mean follow-up of 44 months, 14% (2/14) remained incontinent. The authors believed that the pubovaginal sling did not increase the risk of de novo urge incontinence. Only one woman developed urge incontinence postoperatively. None of the patients who remained continent with pessary reduction developed SUI. The authors concluded that the pessary test was a useful way to unmask clinically relevant SUI.

Barnes and associates[24] also reported on the placement of a traditional pubovaginal sling tied over the rectus fascia using autologous rectus fascia, cadaveric fascia lata, or free vaginal wall graft in 38 patients. All patients had occult SUI unmasked by vaginal packing or pessary reduction. Concomitant transvaginal site-specific repairs were performed: cystocele in 100% (38 patients), rectocele in 50% (19), enterocele in 45% (17), vault fixation in 39% (15), and vaginal hysterectomy in 21% (8). With 15 months' mean follow-up, 5% (2/38) of the patients had developed SUI. De novo urge incontinence occurred in only 9.5% (2/38). No patients developed permanent urinary retention, and mean the postoperative postvoid residual volume was 25 mL. There was only one perioperative complication, which was a wound infection. The authors concluded that the performance of a simultaneous pubovaginal sling did not cause excessive voiding dysfunction or prolonged urinary retention and should be considered as a prophylactic anti-incontinence procedure in women with occult SUI and severe urogenital prolapse.

Suburethral Synthetic Sling

In a contemporary study from de Tayrac and colleagues,[25] tension-free vaginal tape (TVT) placement was performed at the time of transvaginal prolapse repair. Prolapse was reduced (although the method of reduction was not stated), and a CST was done with a full bladder (300 to 500 mL). Forty percent of patients (19/48) had occult SUI once prolapse was reduced; 60% (29/48) had complaints of SUI at baseline. Among the patients with a positive CST (n = 19), 11 patients underwent TVT plus prolapse repair, and 8 had the prolapse repair only. No patient (0/11) with occult incontinence developed SUI after TVT. Almost one third (27%, n = 3) developed voiding dysfunction. Among the 8 patients with a positive CST who did not receive a TVT, only 1 developed stress incontinence, and none developed voiding dysfunction. Among those patients with baseline symptomatic SUI (n = 29), 15 received TVT and 14 did not. Postoperative SUI occurred in 1/15 of the TVT group (7%) versus 5/14 (36%) of the non-TVT group. Voiding dysfunction occurred in 2 (13%) of 15 patients in the TVT group 0 of 14 in the control group.

Researchers from the University of Milan[26] randomized patients with occult SUI to receive either bladder neck fascia plication or TVT in addition to prolapse repair. Occult incontinence was detected by a split Sims speculum and a CST. Clinical SUI developed in 1 patient with TVT (4%) and in 9 of 25 women with fascial plication (36%). The addition of TVT resulted in two surgical complications: a recognized bladder perforation and a retropubic hematoma. The series was not sufficiently powered to detect a significant difference in de novo urge incontinence, although the rate was higher in the TVT group than in the control group (12% versus 4%, P = .66). The authors recommended prolapse reduction by split speculum technique to detect patients at risk for development of SUI postoperatively, because 36% of their patients developed clinically significant SUI.

Gordon and colleagues[27] performed a prophylactic TVT in a series of 30 consecutive women diagnosed with occult SUI and severe prolapse. No patients developed symptomatic SUI, but 10% (3/30) had positive objective findings of SUI on CST. There was a 13% rate of de novo urge incontinence, which is within the range reported after TVT in the literature. These patients also underwent significant prolapse surgery.

The experience with suburethral slings performed via a transobturator approach is still limited. Published outcomes after transobturator sling placement are currently limited to the treatment of clinically significant SUI and do not include occult SUI in severe urogenital prolapse.

DISCUSSION

Patients with vaginal prolapse can present with a myriad of urinary symptoms. A thorough history, physical examination, and method for identifying occult SUI and detrusor function are suggested before surgical treatment of vaginal prolapse. Patients should still be counseled on the potential risks and benefits of choosing a concomitant anti-incontinence surgery. Compared with traditional procedures (e.g., Burch colposuspension, bladder neck pubovaginal slings), newer, minimally invasive midurethral slings may have the advantage of less voiding dysfunction with no added recovery time when performed along with vaginal prolapse repair.

References

1. Gemer O, Bergman M, Segal S: Prevalence of hydronephrosis in patients with genital prolapse. Eur J Obstet Gynecol Reprod Biol 86:11, 1999.
2. Beverly CM, Walter MD, Weber AM, et al: Presence of hydronephrosis in patients undergoing surgery for pelvic organ prolapse. Obstet Gynecol 90:37, 1997.
3. Ghoniem GM, Walters F, Lewis V: The value of the vaginal pack test in large cystoceles. J Urol 152:931, 1994.
4. Bergman A, Koonings PP, Ballard CA: Predicting postoperative urinary incontinence development in women undergoing operation for genitourinary prolapse. Am J Obstet Gynecol 158:1171, 1988.
5. Dietz HP, Haylen BT, Vancaillie TG: Female pelvic organ prolapse and voiding function. Int Urogynecol J 13:284, 2002.
6. Romanzi LJ, Chaikin DC, Blaivas JG: The effect of genital prolapse on voiding. J Urol 161:581, 1999.
7. Long CY, Hsu SC, Wu TP, et al: Urodynamic comparison of continent and incontinent women with severe uterovaginal prolapse. J Reprod Med 49:33-37, 2004.
8. Wall LL, Hewitt JK: Urodynamic characteristics of women with complete posthysterectomy vaginal vault prolapse. Urology 44:336, 1994.
9. Massey JA, Abrams PA: Obstructed voiding in the female. Br J Urol 61:36, 1988.
10. Myers DL, Lasala CA, Hogan JW, et al: The effect of posterior wall support defects on urodynamic indices in stress urinary incontinence. Obstet Gynecol 91:710, 1998.
11. Visco AG, Wei JT, McClure LA, et al: Effects of examination technique modifications on pelvic organ prolapse quantification (POP-Q) results. Int Urogynecol J 14:136, 2003.
12. Versi E, Lyell DJ, Griffiths DJ: Videourodynamic diagnosis of occult genuine stress incontinence in patients with anterior vaginal wall relaxation. J Soc Gynecol Invest 5:327, 1998.
13. Richardson DA, Bent AE, Ostergard DR: The effect of uterovaginal prolapse on urethrovesical pressure dynamics. Am J Obstet Gynecol 146:901, 1983.
14. Hextall A, Boos K, Cardozo L, et al: Videocystourethrography with a ring pessary in situ: A clinically useful preoperative investigation for continent women with urogenital prolapse? Int Urogynecol J 9:205, 1998.
15. Veronikis DK, Nichols DH, Wakamatsu MM: The incidence of low-pressure urethra as a function of prolapse-reducing technique in patients with massive pelvic organ prolapse (maximum descent at all vaginal sites). Am J Obstet Gynecol 177:1305, 1997.
16. Clemons JL, Aguilar VC, Tillinghast TA, et al: Patient satisfaction and changes in prolapse and urinary symptoms in women who were fitted successfully with a pessary for pelvic organ prolapse. Am J Obstet Gynecol 190:1025, 2004.
17. Klutke JJ, Ramos S: Urodynamic outcome after surgery for severe prolapse and potential stress incontinence. Am J Obstet Gynecol 182:1378, 2000.
18. Bump RC, Mattiasson A, Bo K, et al: The standardization of terminology of female pelvic organ prolapse and pelvic floor dysfunction. Am J Obstet Gynecol 175:10, 1996.
19. Gallentine ML, Cespedes RD: Occult stress urinary incontinence and the effect of vaginal vault prolapse on abdominal leak point pressures. Adult Urol 57:40, 2001.
20. Miller EA, Amundsen CL, Toh KL, et al: Preoperative urodynamic evaluation may predict voiding dysfunction in women undergoing pubovaginal sling. J Urol 169:2234, 2003.
21. Stanton SL, Hilton P, Norton C, et al: Clinical and urodynamic effects of anterior colporrhaphy and vaginal hysterectomy for prolapse with and without incontinence. Br J Obstet Gynecol 89:459, 1982.
22. Kayano C, Sartori M, Baracat E, et al: Vaginal hysterectomy allied with Kelly-Kennedy surgery and perineal repair for the treatment of patients with a prolapsed uterus and urinary stress incontinence. Clin Exp Obstet Gynecol 29:27, 2002.
23. Chaikin DC, Groutz A, Blaivas JG: Predicting the need for anti-incontinence surgery in continent women undergoing repair of severe urogenital prolapse. J Urol 163:531, 2000.
24. Barnes NM, Dmochowski RR, Park R, et al: Pubovaginal sling and pelvic prolapse repair in women with occult stress urinary incontinence: Effect on postoperative emptying and voiding symptoms. Urology 59:856, 2002.
25. de Tayrac R, Gervaise A, Chauveaud-Lambling A, et al: Combined genital prolapse repair reinforced with a polypropylene mesh and tension-free vaginal tape in women with genital prolapse and stress urinary incontinence: A retrospective case-control sutdy with short-term follow-up. Acta Obstet Gynecol Scand 83:950, 2004.
26. Meschia M, Pifarotti P, Spennacchio M, et al: A randomized comparison of tension-free vaginal tape and endopelvic fascia plication in women with genital prolapse and occult stress urinary incontinence. Am J Obstet Gynecol 190:609, 2004.
27. Gordon D, Gold RS, Pauzner D, et al: Combined genitourinary prolapse repair and prophylactic tension-free vaginal tape in women with severe prolapse and occult stress urinary incontinence: Preliminary results. Adult Urol 58:547, 2001.

Chapter 61

CADAVERIC FASCIAL REPAIR OF CYSTOCELE

Gary E. Leach and Sarah A. Rueff

Traditional anterior colporrhaphy and paravaginal repair of cystoceles are associated with recurrence rates as high as 33% and 71%, respectively.[1,2] The fascial defects responsible for anterior wall prolapse have been previously described.[3] Lateral defects, which involve detachment of the endopelvic fascia from the arcus tendineous fascia, are more common. Central defects result from a break in the pubocervical fascia, the supportive layer between the bladder and the vaginal wall. These defects are not mutually exclusive; both may be present simultaneously.

Multiple inherent problems exist with anterior colporrhaphy and paravaginal repair for anterior vaginal wall prolapse. First, as each is described, only one of the potential areas of defect, central or lateral, is addressed. Second, each involves reapproximation or plication of the patient's own tissue, which has already shown a propensity for weakness. Inevitably, reapproximation of tissue occurs under tension and can result in varying degrees of vaginal narrowing and unacceptable recurrence rates.

Cystocele repair with nonfrozen cadaveric fascia lata offers several advantages. In the technique described here, both central and lateral defects are addressed and repaired simultaneously. The repair is performed transvaginally and secured without the tension that is often necessary in traditional repairs. Avoidance of tissue plication results in minimal vaginal narrowing, which is especially important for patients who are sexually active. We use solvent-dehydrated, nonfrozen cadaveric fascia (Tutoplast, Mentor Corp., Santa Barbara, CA) and avoid the use of the patient's inherently weak tissue. Studies have shown that the tensile strength and tissue stiffness maintained by the five-step preparation process are comparable to those of native autologous rectus fascia.[4] On the other hand, freeze-dried cadaveric fascia has been shown to have less tensile strength and more tissue inconsistencies.[5]

The technique described, cadaveric prolapse repair with sling (CaPS), involves prolapse repair and simultaneous placement of a transvaginal sling to support the proximal urethra and bladder neck. The procedure is performed both in patients who complain of preoperative SUI and in those with occult SUI demonstrated with prolapse reduction. Controversy has existed in the literature regarding the need for prophylactic placement of slings at the time of prolapse repair in women who do not complain of SUI. However, studies have shown that repairing a cystocele without simultaneously supporting the urethra/bladder neck results in unacceptable rates of postoperative SUI.[6] In addition, clinically continent women with genitourinary prolapse and occult SUI are considered to be at high risk of developing symptomatic SUI once the prolapse is repaired.[7,8] Although one may worry that the prophylactic placement of a pubovaginal sling at the time of prolapse repair in women who do not complain of SUI could result in higher rates of postoperative retention, our previous published results on the CaPS have not shown this to be the case.[9-11]

PREOPERATIVE EVALUATION

Before repair of prolapse, a thorough history is obtained, which should include a gynecologic history, number of vaginal deliveries, and prior anti-incontinence procedures. The severity of a patient's symptoms is ascertained through subjective SEAPI scores (Table 61-1),[12] and the effect of the incontinence and prolapse symptoms on the patient's quality of life is measured by a validated questionnaire.[13]

A careful physical examination is performed to determine the degree of prolapse.

The patient is examined in both the dorsal lithotomy and the standing position with a full bladder. The vaginal mucosa is inspected for signs of atrophy. The posterior blade of a Graves speculum is used to retract the posterior vaginal wall, and the patient is asked to cough and to perform Valsalva maneuvers. The urethra is examined for hypermobility and stress incontinence, and descensus of the anterior vaginal wall is graded using the Baden-Walker classification (Table 61-2).[14] Incidental

Table 61-1 SEAPI Incontinence Score

Stress-related leakage ("S")	0 = No urine loss
	1 = Loss with strenuous activity
	2 = Loss with moderate activity
	3 = Loss with minimal activity
Emptying ability ("E")	0 = No obstructive symptoms
	1 = Minimal symptoms
	2 = Significant symptoms
	3 = Only dribbles or retention
Anatomy ("A")	0 = No descent with strain
	1 = Descent, not to introitus
	2 = Through introitus with strain
	3 = Through introitus at rest
Protection ("P")	0 = Never used
	1 = Certain occasions
	2 = Daily, occasional accidents
	3 = Continually, frequent accidents or constant leakage
Inhibition ("I")	0 = No urge symptoms
	1 = Rare urge urinary incontinence (UUI)
	2 = UUI once/week
	3 = UUI at least once/day

From Raz S, Erickson DR: SEAPI QNM Incontinence classification system. Neurourol Urodyn 11:187-199, 1992.

Table 61-2 Baden-Walker Prolapse Classification

Anatomic Grade	Description
1	Bladder descent toward introitus with strain
2	Bladder to the introitus with strain
3	Bladder outside of the introitus with strain
4	Bladder outside of the introitus at rest

grade 1 cystoceles found in patients who present with other complaints are not routinely repaired. The posterior and apical compartments are examined systematically for associated prolapse. Apical prolapse may not be evident with the patient in the lithotomy position, so it is important to also examine the patient standing with two fingers in the vagina to evaluate for uterine/vaginal cuff descensus. A focused neurologic examination is performed to assess for the presence of neurologic deficits.

Urodynamic evaluation is performed in all patients before surgical repair. Evaluation of SUI is performed both with and without prolapse reduction. Assessment of underlying bladder dysfunction, such as detrusor overactivity, sensory instability, poor compliance, or incomplete emptying, is important for documentation purposes. Patients with elevated postvoid residuals are counseled regarding the possible need for intermittent catheterization postoperatively.

An upper urinary tract evaluation with renal ultrasound is performed before prolapse repair. This provides a baseline study should the patient develop postoperative flank pain, and it also evaluates for preexisting hydronephrosis secondary to kinking of the distal ureters from prolapse.

PREOPERATIVE PREPARATION

Before prolapse repair is performed, the urine is confirmed to be sterile. Patients are taught self-catheterization preoperatively. In the event that a patient is unable to learn self-catheterization or has documented incomplete emptying preoperatively, consideration of placing a suprapubic tube intraoperatively should be made. Preferably, patients with vaginal wall atrophy should use estrogen vaginal cream for 4 to 6 weeks before surgery. Patients are instructed to use one third of an applicator of estrogen three times a week to improve the quality of vaginal tissue and postoperative healing properties. A povidone-iodine vaginal douche is performed the night before and on the morning of surgery. Perioperative antibiotics are given. We prefer to use a first-generation cephalosporin, ampicillin, or vancomycin (if the patient is allergic to penicillin) combined with an aminoglycoside.

Transvaginal repair of associated apical or posterior prolapse is performed with the CaPS procedure. A thorough discussion of the risks and complications of prolapse surgery is undertaken before the operation. Patients are counseled regarding the possibility of prolonged or permanent urinary retention, occult or recurrent SUI, recurrent anterior prolapse, and recurrent or de novo prolapse apically or posteriorly. All patients are counseled about the risk of persistent or de novo urgency symptoms and that either of these may require treatment in the future.

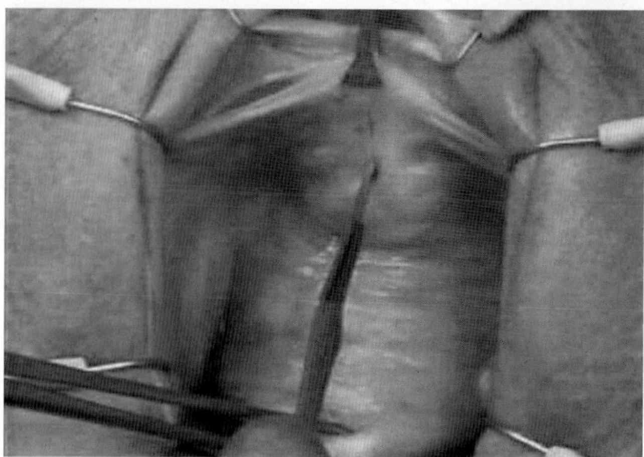

Figure 61-1 A midline incision is made from the mid-urethra to the cervix or vaginal cuff.

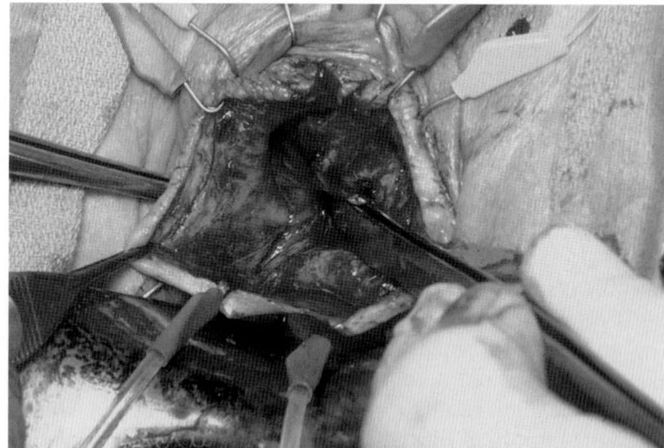

Figure 61-2 The cystocele is dissected off of the anterior vaginal wall laterally to expose the levator complex bilaterally.

OPERATIVE PROCEDURE

The procedure is performed with the patient in the dorsal lithotomy position. A Foley catheter is placed, and a Scott retractor (Lonestar, Houston, TX) is secured to the medial buttocks with towel clamps. If there is question of an enterocele within the anterior prolapse, an iodine-soaked packing is placed within the rectum before preparation and draping for the procedure. The anterior vaginal wall is infiltrated with saline, and the Foley balloon is palpated at the bladder neck. A midline incision is made from the mid-urethra to the cervix or vaginal cuff (Fig. 61-1). With the use of Metzenbaum scissors, the cystocele is dissected off of the anterior vaginal wall via dissection on the white, shiny layer of the inside of the vaginal wall. In the proper plane, there should be little or no need for use of bovie cauterization. Dissection is continued until the levator complex, consisting of the levator ani musculature and pubocervical fascia, is exposed bilaterally (Fig. 61-2).

Dissection at the level of the bladder neck is performed for sling placement. For the CaPS procedure, the pubic bone is cleared bilaterally to allow placement of transvaginal bone anchors. In patients with urethral fixation or scarring from prior

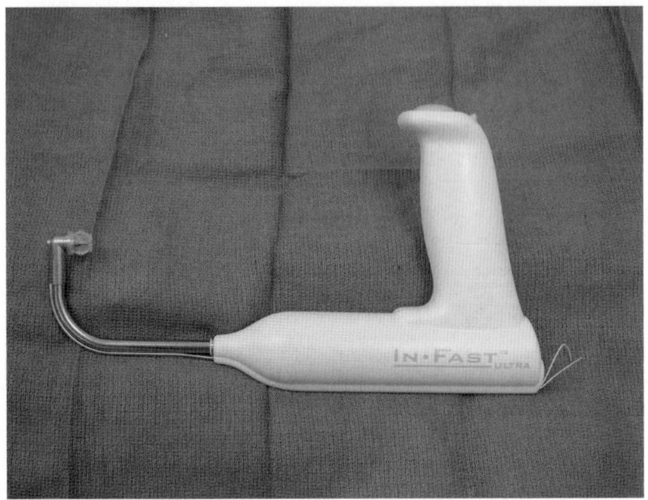

Figure 61-3 A transvaginal drill is used to place bone anchors into the pubic bone.

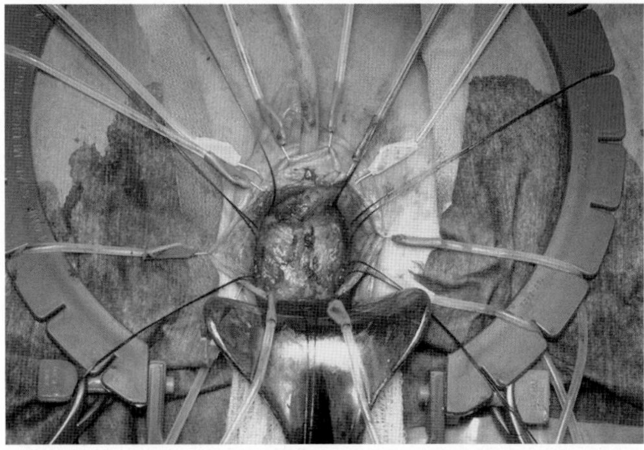

Figure 61-5 Size 1-0 polydioxanone sutures are placed into the levator complex bilaterally and the cervix or vaginal cuff proximally to provide support for the fascial patch.

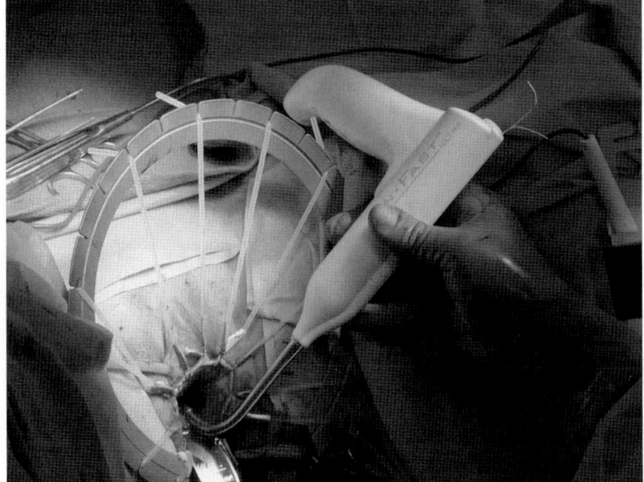

Figure 61-4 The transvaginal drill is placed on the undersurface of bone and activated until a change in tone signifies firm placement of the bone anchor.

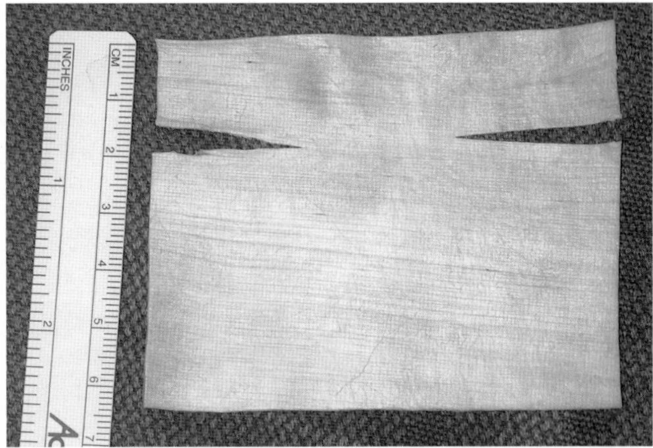

Figure 61-6 A 6 × 8 cm piece of cadaveric fascia is cut into a "T" configuration along the line of its fibers. The top portion serves as a 2-cm wide sling.

procedures, urethrolysis is performed to free the urethra and allow the sling to apply adequate urethral compression.[15] Bone anchors with polypropylene sutures attached are then placed with the use of a transvaginal drill (InFast, American Medical Systems, Minneapolis, MN) (Fig. 61-3). The bladder is placed on drainage, and the drill is positioned flush on the undersurface of the pubic bone. The drill is activated, and a change in tone signifies firm placement of the anchor into the bone (Fig. 61-4). The drill is removed, and a firm pull on the suture should confirm secure anchor placement. Bone anchor placement is repeated on the opposite side. Then, 4-0 polydiaxanone sutures (two on each side) are placed into the levator complex and tagged for the cystocele repair. A fifth suture is placed into the vaginal cuff or cervix for proximal support (Fig. 61-5).

A 6 × 8 cm piece of nonfrozen cadaveric fascia lata (Tutoplast), presoaked in antibiotic solution, is cut along the line of its fibers in a "T" configuration. The top portion serves as a 2-cm wide sling (Fig. 61-6). The edges of the sling portion are folded over, because cross-hatching of the fibers minimizes chances of pull through.[16] An 18-gauge needle is used to pass the bone anchor sutures on one side through the folded edge. The bladder neck suture is placed more medially than the distal suture to keep the fascia tight against the bladder neck (Fig. 61-7). The sutures are tied and secured in place up to the bone. The distal edge of the sling is attached to the periurethral fascia with a 2-0 absorbable suture to prevent rolling of the edge of the sling toward the bladder neck. The free edge of the fascia is folded over, and the appropriate position of the contralateral sutures is determined. The fascia should lie snug against the urethra without excessive tension. In the our experience, the use of a right angle clamp placed between the urethra and the sling while deciding proper tension can result in the sling's being tied too loosely. Once the proper position is determined, the sutures are passed through the folded fascial edge with an 18-gauge needle. The bladder neck suture is placed more medial, and the sutures are subsequently tied. The fascia is then positioned for cystocele repair. The edge of the fascial patch is folded over and held in place with Allis clamps on the top and bottom. The previously placed levator sutures are passed through the edge of the fascia bilaterally and

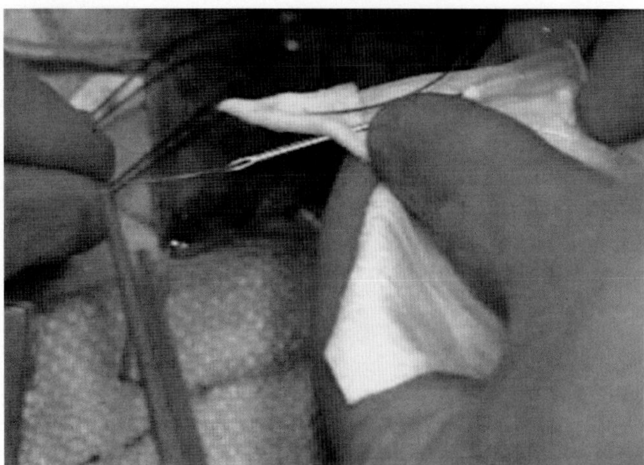

Figure 61-7 The bone anchor sutures are passed through the folded edge of the sling portion of the fascia. The bladder neck suture is placed more medial to allow the sling to lie tight against the bladder neck.

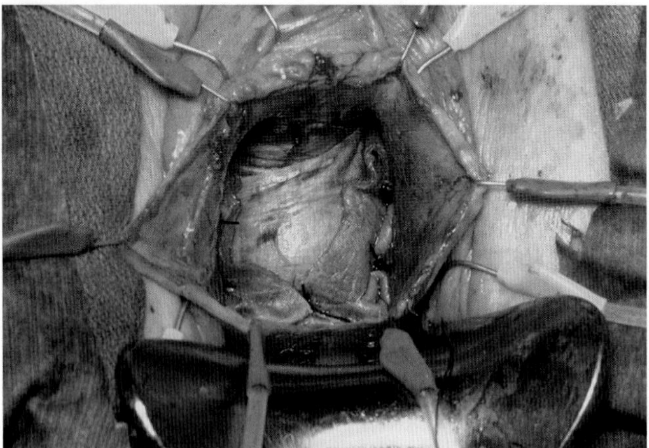

Figure 61-8 The fascial patch is secured to the previously placed sutures to repair the cystocele.

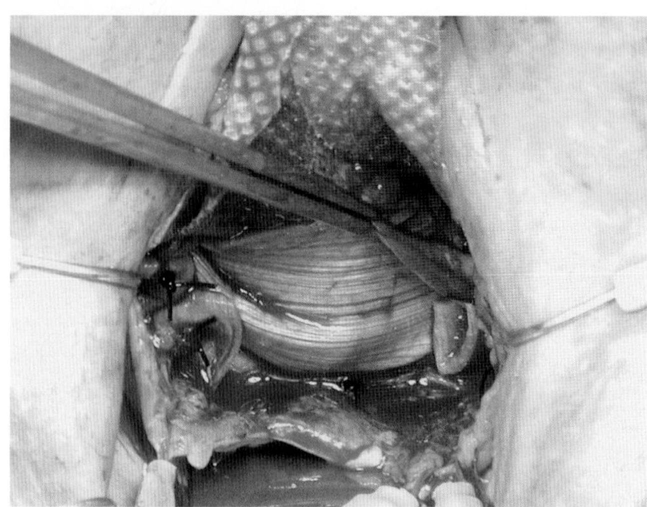

Figure 61-9 Modification of the cadaveric prolapse repair with sling (CaPS) technique. Cystocele sutures are placed within the levator complex, followed by sling passage using the transobturator technique. The synthetic sling is retracted superiorly while the fascia is attached to the levator sutures to repair the cystocele.

tied to reduce the cystocele (Fig. 61-8). Care should be taken to avoid excess tension on the levator complex that can occur with excess folding of the fascial edge. Lastly, the apical suture within the cervix or vaginal cuff is passed through to secure the proximal aspect of the fascia in place.

Cystoscopy is performed after the administration of intravenous indigo carmine. Examination with a 70-degree lens is done to ensure patency of the ureters and exclude bladder injury. Examination with a 0-degree lens is performed to exclude urethral injury. Irrigation with antibiotic-impregnated solution should be performed throughout the procedure. Once hemostasis is obtained, redundant vaginal epithelium is trimmed, and the incision is closed with a running 2-0 absorbable suture. Care should be taken to avoid excess trimming of redundant epithelium as well as excess tension on the vaginal closure, which can result in either wound separation or vaginal narrowing postoperatively. A Foley catheter and a Betadine-soaked vaginal pack are left in place.

The CaPS technique can be modified to accommodate other techniques of sling placement and alternative sling materials. We are currently investigating the utility of using a synthetic transobturator sling while continuing to use cadaveric fascia for the prolapse repair.[17] For this modification, the cystocele is dissected off of the vaginal wall to the levator complex bilaterally, as described earlier. Lateral dissection for the transobturator sling is performed before cystocele suture placement. The sling is placed using the transobturator technique, and then a 4×7 cm piece of cadaveric fascia lata (Tutoplast) is folded and attached to the levator complex, as described previously (Fig. 61-9). Proper sling tension is decided by positioning Metzenbaum scissors between the urethra and the sling and adjusting accordingly (Fig. 61-10). The vaginal epithelium is then closed with 2-0 absorbable suture, and a vaginal pack and Foley catheter are left in place.

POSTOPERATIVE CARE

The vaginal packing and Foley catheter are removed on the morning of the first postoperative day. Patients are restricted to 1500 mL of fluid per day. A voiding trial is given, and residual urine measurement is obtained via intermittent catheterization. Eighty percent of patients void to completion immediately after surgery. If residual urine measurements are greater than 100 mL, patients are reinstructed on self-catheterization. If a suprapubic tube is placed intraoperatively, residuals are checked in this manner. Patients are continued on intravenous antibiotics for 24 hours postoperatively and then begun on oral antibiotics (cephalexin or fluoroquinolone) for 1 week to minimize the risk of osteitis pubis or wound infection. Patients are routinely discharged on postoperative day 1 with oral analgesics and stool softeners in addition to antibiotics. Patients with elevated postvoid residuals are instructed to continue to monitor at home via self-catheterization or suprapubic tube until residuals are consistently less than 100 mL. If a patient is unable to learn or is uncomfortable performing self-catheterization, she can be discharged home with a Foley catheter and return for a trial of void in the office. At the time of discharge, patients are instructed to avoid heavy lifting or straining and to observe pelvic rest (i.e., no intercourse, no tampons) for 6 weeks postoperatively.

Patients are seen for follow-up at 1 week, 6 weeks, 6 months, 12 months, and yearly thereafter. Evaluation consists of urinalysis, postvoid residual urine measurement, and physical examination, as well as determination of subjective SEAPI scores. Patients are also administered a confidential, validated continence and satisfaction questionnaire every 6 to 12 months postoperatively, the results of which are entered into a prospective patient database.

RESULTS

Incontinence Outcomes

The CaPS procedure has been performed on a total of 340 patients. Eighty-four percent (287/340) now have at least 6 months of questionnaire follow-up (range, 6 to 74 months; mean, 27.4 months). Based on the patient questionnaire response, "cure" of incontinence is defined as no incontinent episodes postoperatively. "Improved" incontinence is defined as greater than 50% improvement in incontinent episodes, and "failure" is arbitrarily defined as less than 50% improvement in incontinent episodes. The overall subjective "cured/dry" rate was 29% (82/287 patients), the "cured/improved" rate was 71% (203 patients), and the "failed" rate was 29% (84 patients). In considering the type of incontinence present in "failures," 33 of the 287 patients (11%) complained of recurrent SUI, 12 (4%) complained of urge urinary incontinence (UUI), and 24 (8%) complained of mixed urinary incontinence. The remaining 5% of "failures" (15 patients) responded that they were "uncertain" as to their type of incontinence. The time-to-failure is shown in Figure 61-11: 62 (71%) of 87 incontinence "failures" occurred after 12 months of follow-up.

Of the 160 patients who complained of preoperative UUI, 51 (32%) experienced persistent UUI postoperatively. Of the 127 patients with no preoperative UUI, 12 (9.4%) developed de novo UUI.

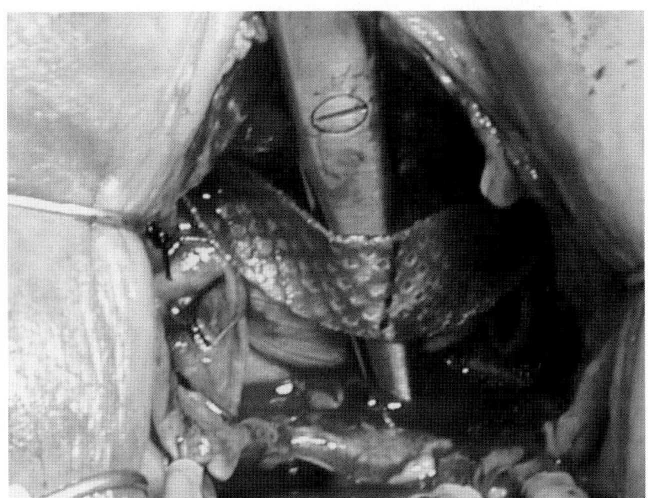

Figure 61-10 Transobturator sling tension is adjusted with Metzenbaum scissors between the sling and the urethra.

Prolapse Outcomes

With regard to cystocele recurrence, physical examination data were available for 325 (96%) of 340 patients with a mean follow-up of 18.8 months and maximum follow-up of 79 months. The symptomatic cystocele cure rate was 94% (306/325 patients). Although 42 patients (13%) had some degree of recurrent anterior vaginal wall descent, 23 (55%) had asymptomatic grade 1 cystocele, for which intervention is not recommended. The de novo grade 2-4 rectocele and apical (vaginal vault and enterocele) prolapse rates were 9% (19/207) and 7% (19/257), respectively.

There were significant changes between preoperative and postoperative SEAPI scores, as shown in Table 61-1. Significant changes were seen within each domain as well as in the overall score. A significant change was also seen in the mean prolapse quality-of-life score; with a possible score ranging between 4 and 20, the mean score decreased from 9.6 preoperatively to 5.5 postoperatively ($P < .01$).

As a measure of overall patient satisfaction with prolapse repair and continence results, patients were asked to rate their satisfaction on a visual analogue scale, with 0 being "not at all satisfied" and 10 being "completely satisfied." The distribution

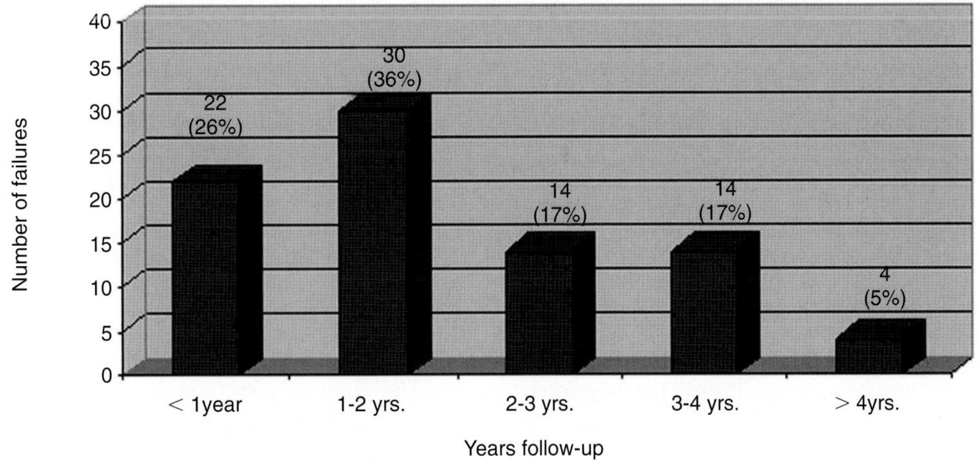

Figure 61-11 Time interval until "failure" after the cadaveric prolapse repair with sling (CaPS) procedure.

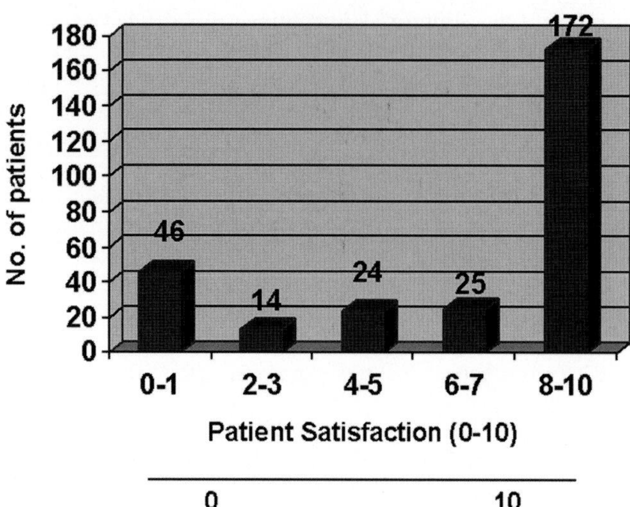

Figure 61-12 Distribution of overall postoperative patient satisfaction.

of scores is seen in Figure 61-12. The mean and median satisfaction scores were 7 and 9, respectively. Seventy-six percent (219/287 patients) had a satisfaction rate of at least 5. When patients were asked whether they would have the surgery again, 208/287 (72%) responded "yes" and 61/287 (28%) responded "no."

No mortalities have occurred with the CaPS procedure. There have been seven cases of prolonged urinary retention (>30 days), only one of which required urethrolysis. The most common complication encountered was intravaginal granulation tissue caused by extrusion of Panacryl sutures that were used for cystocele repair early in the patient series. Suture removal and fulguration of granulation tissue was performed in the office without sequelae. Once use of this suture was discontinued, no further granulation tissue developed. With regard to bone anchor fixation, there has been one case of osteitis pubis that was managed conservatively and no instances of infection requiring bone anchor removal.

CONCLUSION

The CaPS procedure, which uses nonfrozen cadaveric fascia lata for cystocele repair, has several advantages over traditional anterior repair. Both central and lateral defects can be repaired simultaneously, avoiding the use of the patient's inherently weak tissues. The procedure is performed entirely transvaginally, resulting in minimal morbidity, and avoids the use of synthetic materials in the vagina. Most patients are discharged on postoperative day 1. Sling placement at the time of cystocele repair allows simultaneous treatment of symptomatic SUI, as well as occult SUI demonstrated preoperatively with cystocele reduction, with minimal risk of urinary retention. Results of prolapse repair have been excellent and durable, with a symptomatic cure rate of 94% at long-term follow-up. Continence rates with the cadaveric fascial sling have been less durable, with failure rates approaching 30% at long-term follow-up. In order to improve continence results, we are currently exploring other materials and approaches to sling placement, as mentioned earlier, and continue to use cadaveric fascia lata for cystocele repair given its excellent long-term results.

References

1. Kohli N, Sze EHM, Roat TW: Incidence of recurrent cystocele after anterior colporraphy with and without concomitant bladder neck suspension. Am J Obstet Gynecol 175:1476-1482, 1996.
2. Benson JT, Lucente V, McClellan E: Vaginal versus abdominal reconstructive surgery for the treatment of pelvic support defects: A prospective randomized study with long-term evaluation outcome. Am J Obstet Gynecol 175:1418-1422, 1996.
3. Chopra A, Raz S, Stothers L: Pathogenesis of cystoceles: Anterior colporrhapy. In Raz S (ed): Female Urology. Philadelphia, WB Saunders, 1996.
4. Lemer ML, Chaikin DC, Blaivas JG: Tissue strength analysis of autologous and cadaveric allografts for the pubovaginal sling. Neurourol Urodyn 18:497-503, 1999.
5. Jinnah RH, Johnson C, Warden K, Clarke HJ: A biomechanical analysis of solvent-dehydrated and freeze-dried human fascia lata allografts: A preliminary report. Am J Sports Med 20:607-612, 1992.
6. Gordon D, Groutz A, Wolman I, et al: Development of postoperative stress urinary incontinence in clinically continent patients undergoing prophylactic Kelly plication during genitourinary prolapse repair. Neurourol Urodyn 18:193-198, 1999.
7. Chaikin DC, Groutz A, Blaivas JG: Predicting the need for anti-incontinence surgery in continent women undergoing repair of severe urogenital prolapse. J Urol 163:531-534, 2000.
8. Groutz A, Gold R, Pauzner D, et al: Tension-free vaginal tape (TVT) for the treatment of occult stress urinary incontinence in women undergoing prolapse repair: A prospective study of 100 consecutive cases. Neurourol Urodyn 23:632-635, 2004.
9. Kobashi KC, Mee SL, Leach GE: A new technique for cystocele repair and transvaginal sling: The cadaveric prolapse repair and sling (CaPS). Urology 56:9-14, 2000.
10. Kobashi KC, Leach GE, Chon J, Govier FE: Continued multicenter followup of the cadaveric prolapse repair with sling. J Urol 168:2063-2068, 2002.
11. Frederick RW, Leach GE: Cadaveric prolapse repair with sling: Intermediate outcomes with 6 months to 5 years of followup. J Urol 173:1229-1233, 2005.
12. Raz S, Erickson DR: SEAPI QNM Incontinence classification system. Neurourol Urodyn 11:187-199, 1992.
13. Kobashi KC, Gormley EA, Govier F, et al: Development of a validated quality of life assessment instrument for patients with pelvic prolapse [abstract]. J Urol 163:76, 2000.
14. Baden WF, Walker TA: Surgical Repair of Vaginal Defects. Philadelphia, JB Lippincott, 1992.
15. Leach GE: Urethrolysis. Urol Clin North Am 2:23-27, 1994.
16. Sutaria PM, Staskin DR: A comparison of fascial "pull-through" strength using four different suture fixation techniques [abstract]. J Urol 161:79, 1999.
17. Wein AJ: Transobturator Tape (Uratape): A new minimimally-invasive procedure to treat female urinary incontinence [abstract]. J Urol 172:1214, 2004.

Chapter 62

TRANSABDOMINAL PARAVAGINAL CYSTOCELE REPAIR

Danita Harrison Akingba, Michelle M. Germain, and Alfred E. Bent

HISTORY

In 1909, Dr. George White described a novel idea for the etiology of cystoceles based on his work with cadaver dissection.[1] He first described the supportive attachments of the vagina. He next illustrated how lateral detachment of the pubocervical fascia from the arcus tendineous fascia pelvis, or white line, results in cystocele. He also outlined the critical steps for the transvaginal paravaginal repair of these types of cystoceles. It is clear after reading the peer review section following his article that his idea was unique at the time and that a fundamental understanding of the three-dimensional relationship of female pelvic anatomy was lacking.

Three years later, White submitted a treatise in which he reviewed the three theories of that period regarding the etiology of cystocele[2]:

1. Cystocele is due to thinning out of the anterior vaginal wall and thus a hernia.
2. Ligaments suspend the bladder, like the stomach.
3. The bladder descends because its ligamentous attachments to the uterus and obliterated hypogastric arteries have been stretched or broken during labor.

In his paper, White rejected each of these theories based on clinical examination findings, lack of histologic and anatomic evidence to support the theories, and, finally, the fact that not all women having hysterectomy developed cystoceles.

White again described his technique for vaginal paravaginal repair for the management of cystocele. He acknowledged that the vaginal approach was more difficult because of limited visibility, but he believed that the surgical approach for treatment of cystocele should remain vaginal because of the then-widespread practice of concurrent perineorrhaphy. He conceded that, "to incise the peritoneum at the side of the bladder, push the bladder aside until the white line comes into view, then by the aid of an assistant's finger in the vagina, suture the anterior lateral side of the vagina to the white line, and close the peritoneum" may be "the easiest and simplest way to accomplish this."[2] However, he believed that the abdominal approach was seldom indicated, unless the patient suffered from procidentia. In that case, the patient would be best served by concurrent restoration of the broad and uterosacral ligaments.

White's papers were largely forgotten for the next 70 years. Historically, it is not clear why his ideas were not readily accepted. Perhaps it was because the approach was difficult to perform, or because his peers lacked a proficient understanding of the lateral fascial defects and their role in anterior vaginal wall prolapse. Even more significant was the almost simultaneous publication of Howard Kelly's treatise on cystocele, its repair, and the treatment of stress incontinence.[3] The Kelly plication is straightforward in its conceptualization and technically easier to perform. Failures of the Kelly plication in a large number of cystocele repairs led to a series of "new" techniques for the repair of lateral anterior wall defects, including work by John C. Burch and Cullen Richardson.[4,5]

In 1961, Burch reported his experience with colposuspension in the treatment of stress incontinence. He attached the paravaginal fascia to the white line of the pelvis in the first seven of his patients. He wrote that the maneuver "produced a most satisfactory restoration of the normal anatomy of the bladder neck . . . and a surprising correction of most of the cystocele . . . overcoming the anterior cystocele involving the neck of the bladder, but also the posterior cystocele involving the base of the bladder."[4] Despite such positive results with correction of both urethral hypermobility and bladder prolapse, Burch believed that the white line held sutures poorly and therefore sought another fixation point. Subsequently, he chose Cooper's ligament as the point of fixation.

In 1976, Richardson, Lyon, and Williams published a "new" look at pelvic relaxation. They outlined the technique for transabdominal paravaginal repair—echoing the descriptions of White and Burch. They also identified the four areas of defects or breaks in the pubocervical fascia, in their order of occurrence[5]:

1. Lateral (paravaginal), where the pubocervical fascia attaches to the arcus tendineous fascia pelvis or white line
2. Transverse, in front of the cervix, where the pubocervical fascia blends into the pericervical ring of fibromuscular tissue (or at the cuff in a woman who has had a hysterectomy)
3. Central, on anterior vaginal wall between the lateral margins of the vagina
4. Distal, where the urethra perforates the urogenital diaphragm (Fig. 62-1)

Sixty-seven percent of their patients had paravaginal defects. Typically, today, no clinical distinction is made between central and distal tears. In addition, no effort is usually made intraoperatively to distinguish among these types of defects, because Kelly-type plication procedures have been performed for both for years with good results. However, transverse defects require reapproximating the tears in the fascia.

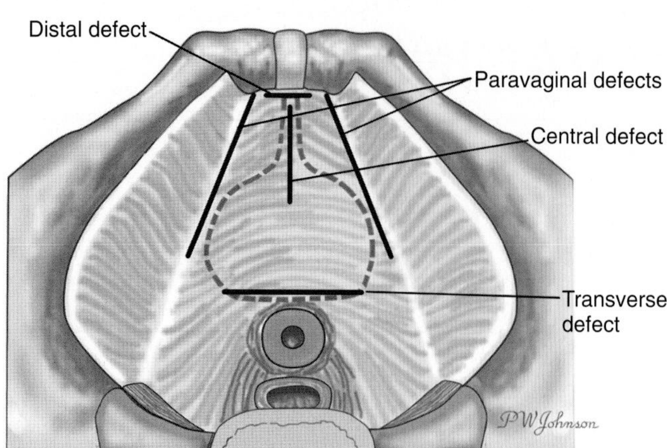

Figure 62-1 The four locations of breaks in pubocervical fascia: lateral (perivaginal), where the pubocervical fascia attaches to the arcus tendineous fascia pelvis or white line; transverse, in front of the cervix, where the pubocervical fascia blends into the pericervical ring of fibromuscular tissue (or at the cuff in a woman who has had a hysterectomy); central, on the anterior vaginal wall between the lateral margins of the vagina; and distal, where the urethra perforates the urogenital diaphragm. (From Richardson AC: Operative Techniques in Gynecologic Surgery. Philadelphia, WB Saunders, 1996.)

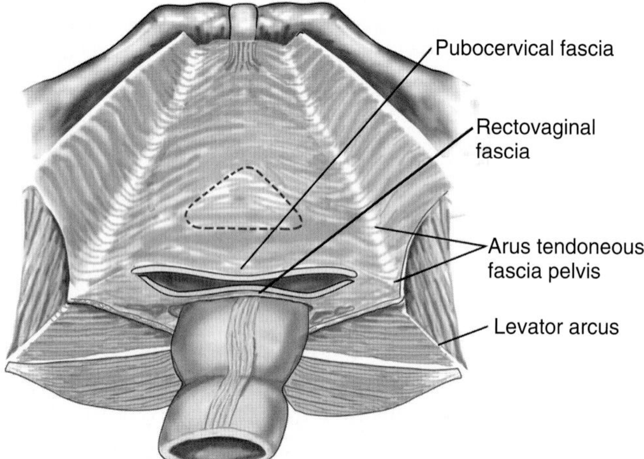

Figure 62-2 The arcus tendineous fascia pelvis extends from the inferior margin of the pubic symphysis to the ischial spine parallel to the levator arcus. Anteriorly, the bladder has been cut away. A cross-section through the vagina reveals the apposition of the rectovaginal fascia to the rectum and perirectal space. (From Richardson AC: Operative Techniques in Gynecologic Surgery. Philadelphia, WB Saunders, 1996.)

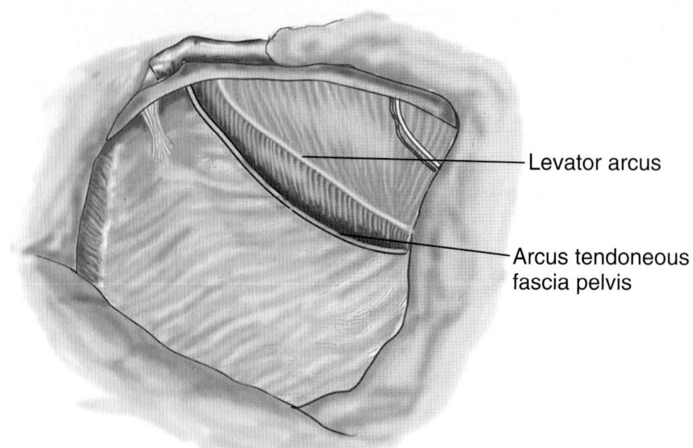

Figure 62-3 The arcus tendineous fascia pelvis has separated entirely off the pelvic sidewall. (From Richardson AC: Operative Techniques in Gynecologic Surgery. Philadelphia, WB Saunders, 1996.)

ANATOMY

The pubocervical fascia (or endopelvic fascia), a trapezoid-shaped, fibromuscular band of tissue, supports the urethra, bladder, and uterus anteriorly (Fig. 62-2). Its lateral border extends from a point just anterior to the ischial spines, along the arcus tendineous fascia pelvis or white line, to the pubic ramus anteriorly. Posteriorly, it reaches the cervix or vaginal cuff at the level of the base of the broad ligament and cardinal-uterosacral ligaments and reaches across toward the ischial spines.

Anterior vaginal wall prolapse results from herniation of the pelvic organs normally supported by the pubocervical fascia into the vaginal lumen. Many gynecologists believe that identification and repair of defects in this fascia are essential to achieve successful anterior colporrhaphy. However, the existence of fascial tissue between the vagina and bladder or vagina and rectum has never been proven histologically.[6-9] To examine the histology of surgical fascia used during anterior colporrhaphy, to compare it to rectovaginal fascia, and to determine the consistency with which this tissue is diagnosed surgically, Farrell and his colleagues examined the fascia of women who were scheduled to undergo a primary surgical correction of pelvic organ prolapse.[9] Biopsies taken of surgically identified pubocervical fascia and rectovaginal fascia during colporrhaphy failed to identify a distinct fascial layer. Instead, histologic examinations of tissue identified as fascia intraoperatively showed it to be indistinguishable from deep vaginal wall connective tissue.

It is possible to have both central and lateral defects concurrently. Lateral detachment of the pubocervical fascia may occur if the entire arcus pulls away from the pelvic sidewall (Fig. 62-3). Alternatively, the entire arcus may remain attached to the sidewall while the pubocervical fascia pulls away.[27] Finally, the arcus could split, with a portion remaining attached to the pubocervical fascia medially and another portion remaining attached to the pelvic sidewall laterally (Fig. 62-4).

Most anterior compartment prolapse results from lateral detachment of the pubocervical fascia.[5] Although Richardson and colleagues were not the first to publish on the anatomic concept of paravaginal defects, they popularized the concept of discrete isolated fascial defects in the mid-1970s. Based on this work, the overall incidence of paravaginal defects was 67%, with the great majority being right-sided defects. Some years later, Barber and Cundiff conducted a retrospective chart review of 70 patients with a preoperative diagnosis of paravaginal defect.[10] Sixty-three percent (44/70) were believed to have unilateral or bilateral paravaginal defects preoperatively, based on clinical examination. The intraoperative findings confirmed the prevalence of paravaginal defects as just 42%.

Diagnosis

A thorough physical examination in the office is the principal method of diagnosis of paravaginal defects. The patient is examined in the dorsal lithotomy position. With gentle downward traction of the posterior blade of the speculum, the anterior compartment is examined at rest and with maximum Valsalva maneuver. It is important to restore normal anatomy, so a ring forceps, Baden-Walker defect analyzer, or a wooden tongue blade should be used to gently elevate the lateral vaginal sulci, angling parallel to the white line (Fig. 62-5). Each side is checked separately, and then both together by elevating both sulci while the patient bears down. Bilateral paravaginal defects are corrected with this maneuver; central defects will prolapse around the elevating device. Suspected central defects should be supported with these instruments during Valsalva maneuver. If anterior prolapse is only partially reduced by either maneuver, then the patient is thought to have both paravaginal and central defects.

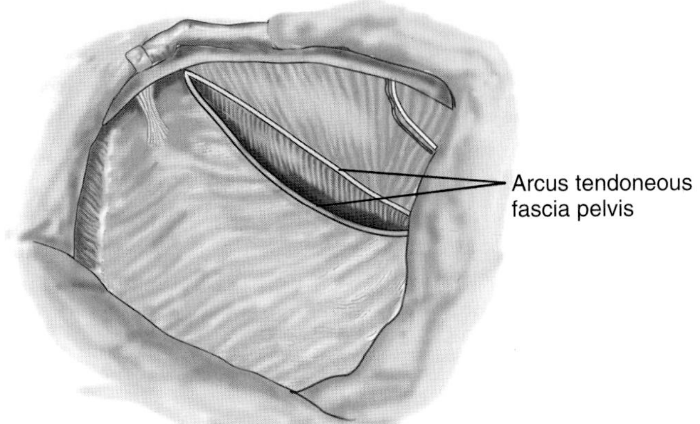

Figure 62-4 The arcus tendineous fascia pelvis has split down the middle, leaving some of its remnants attached to the pubocervical fascia and some still attached to the pelvic sidewall. (From Richardson AC: Operative Techniques in Gynecologic Surgery. Philadelphia, WB Saunders, 1996.)

Paravaginal defects can be misdiagnosed. Barber and Cundiff found that the sensitivity of physical examination for the detection of right-sided paravaginal defects was 94% and the specificity was 54%. The positive predictive value of clinical examination was 65%, and negative predictive value was 91%. For left-sided defects, the sensitivity, specificity, positive predictive value, and negative predictive value were 90%, 50%, 57%, and 88%, respectively.[10]

Ultrasound and magnetic resonance imaging have both been used for the diagnosis of paravaginal defects.[11-13] However, given the time and expense of these tests, they are not recommended for routine diagnosis of paravaginal defects in the urogynecologist's office. The clinical examination remains the standard for diagnosis.

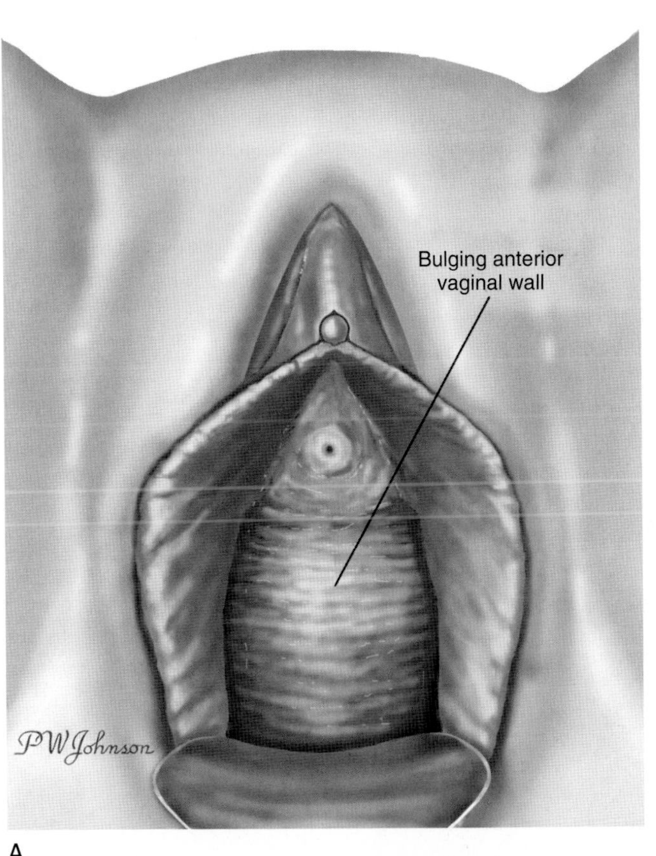

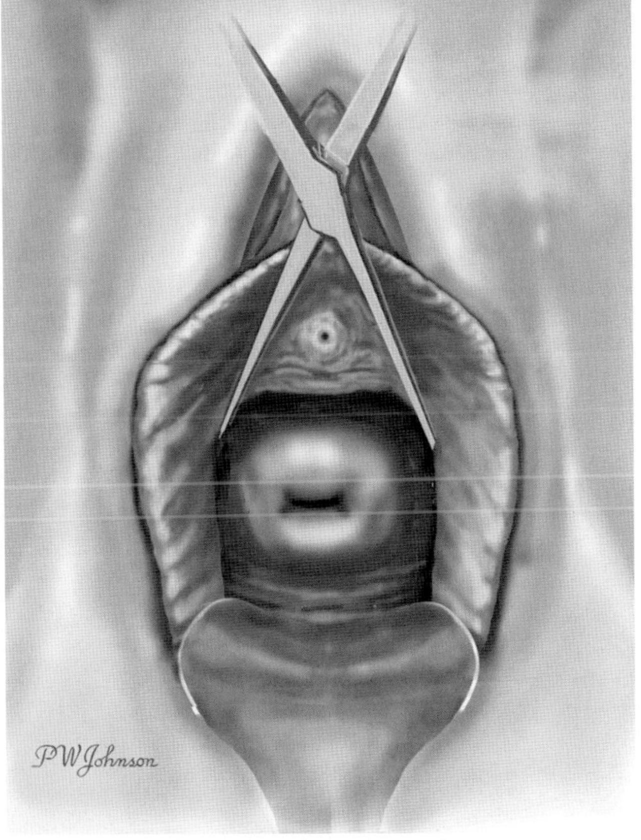

Figure 62-5 **A,** Cystocele defect seen protruding through the introitus. **B,** Lateral cystocele defect reduced with ring forceps placed laterally to elevate the pubocervical fascia toward the ischial spines. (From Retzky SS, *et al*. Urinary incontinence in women. Summit, NJ: Clinical Symposia Ciba-Geigy Corp, 47(3):22, 1995; adapted from Plate 11. Copyright 1995 ICON Learning Systems, LLC, a subsidiary of MediMedia USA Inc.)

TRANSABDOMINAL REPAIR

In 1976, Richardson described the transabdominal paravaginal repair. Although modifications have been described, the standard accepted technique has not been altered significantly from his original description. The patient is placed in low lithotomy position, and a Foley catheter is passed transurethrally. The bladder should be drained for adequate exposure and visualization into the retropubic space. If the patient has a uterus, the hysterectomy is performed first and the peritoneum is closed before proceeding with the paravaginal repair. A Pfannenstiel fascial incision is used most often. The rectus muscles are divided in the midline and held laterally by a self-retaining retractor. As with the Burch procedure, care must be taken to avoid injury to the inferior epigastric vessels. The space of Retzius is entered bluntly and developed cautiously under direct visualization to avoid injuring the large veins in this space. If the patient has had a prior Burch procedure, this space may be difficult to develop atraumatically (Fig. 62-6). Hemoclips are often required to maintain hemostasis.

Once the space is fully developed, the retropubic anatomy may be visualized, including the pubic symphysis, the bladder neck in the midline, and the obturator neurovascular bundles and Cooper's ligament laterally. The obturator fossa can usually be identified first by palpation, because it feels like a vertically positioned buttonhole. Care should be taken while dissecting around this fossa to avoid damaging the obturator nerve, artery, and vein. Finally, the white line is identified along the pelvic sidewall as it travels from the inferior border of the pubic symphysis to the ischial spine. Further, blunt dissection using a sponge on a stick or Kittner may be required to remove adipose tissue adherent to the pubocervical fascia.

The surgeon's fingers are placed inside the vagina to elevate the lateral sulcus and aid in demonstrating the white pubocervical fascia and the superior extent of the vagina (Figs. 62-7 and 62-8). It is important to plan suture locations before actual placement, to avoid undue lateral tension on the vaginal wall when the sutures are tied. Synthetic, nonabsorbable sutures are used. The first suture is placed laterally, near the apex of the vagina, through the paravesical portion of the pubocervical fascia or the detached white line if it is visible. The needle is then passed through the ipsilateral obturator internus fascia around the arcus tendineus fascia pelvis (white line) at its origin, 1 cm anterior to the ischial spine. Three to five sutures are placed sequentially through the pubocervical fascia, distal to the prior fixation point, and attached to the white line or obturator fascia at a corresponding level from the ischial spine to the lateral pubic symphysis. If the patient has bilateral paravaginal defects, the same technique is used on the opposite side. Sutures are usually tagged and held until cystoscopy is performed with the sutures both relaxed and under tension, to ensure the integrity of the bladder and the normal function of both ureters. Gelfoam may be placed into the space of Retzius for hemostasis and to aid scarification of this space. Finally, the sutures are tied so that the lateral vaginal walls are in direct contact with the obturator fascia and arcus tendineus fascia pelvis.

LAPAROSCOPIC REPAIR

Laparoscopic pelvic floor repair was described in 1995.[14] The laparoscopic paravaginal repair is similar to the laparoscopic Burch procedure. The patient is positioned in low lithotomy position, and a Foley urethral catheter is placed into the bladder. The Foley catheter should be clamped in order to partially distend the bladder and demarcate its boundaries. Some surgeons pass 30 mL of diluted methylene blue or indigo carmine transurethrally and clamp the urethral catheter so that any iatrogenic

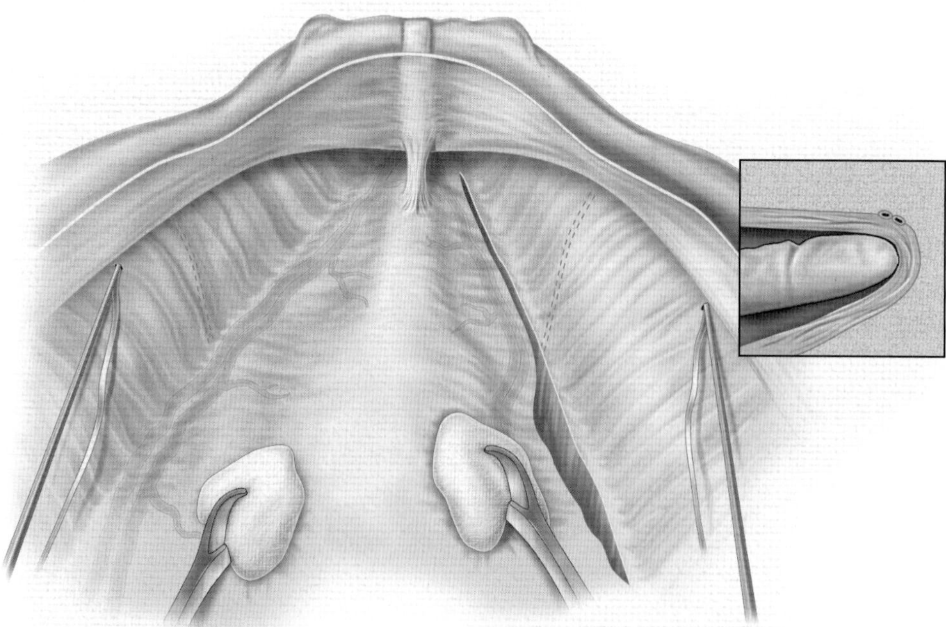

Figure 62-6 Visualization of the entire space of Retzius. (From Richardson AC: In Gershenson DM, Aronson MP (eds): Operative Techniques in Gynecologic Surgery. Philadelphia, WB Saunders, 1996, p 71.)

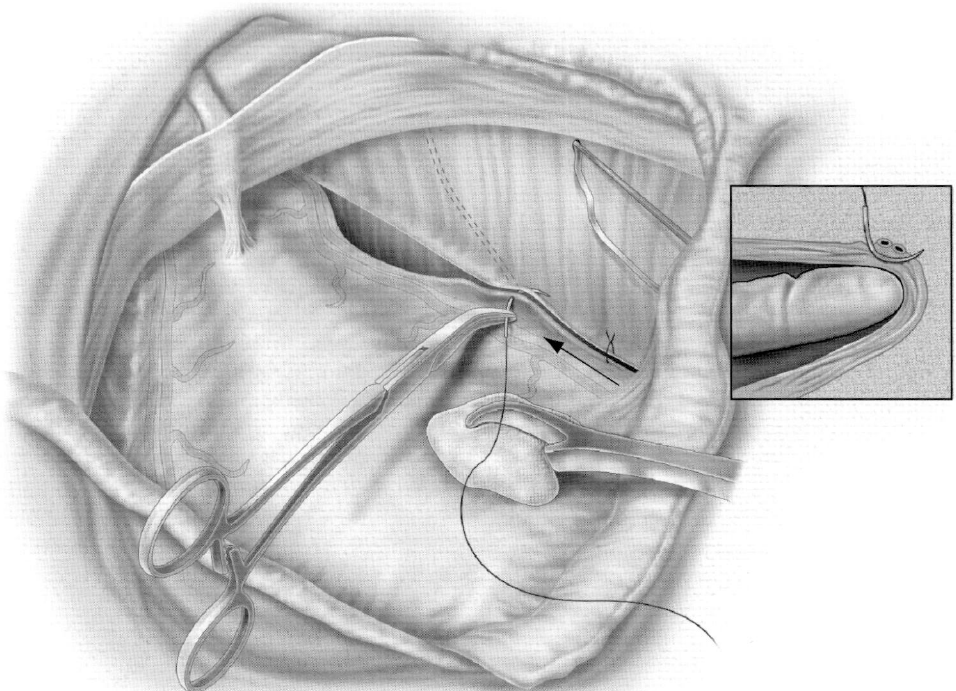

Figure 62-7 With one finger inside the vagina elevating the lateral sulcus (*insert*), a full-thickness bite of the pubocervical fascia is taken. The needle is then passed through the ipsilateral obturator internus fascia around the arcus tendineous fascia pelvis. Sutures are placed from cephalad to caudad.

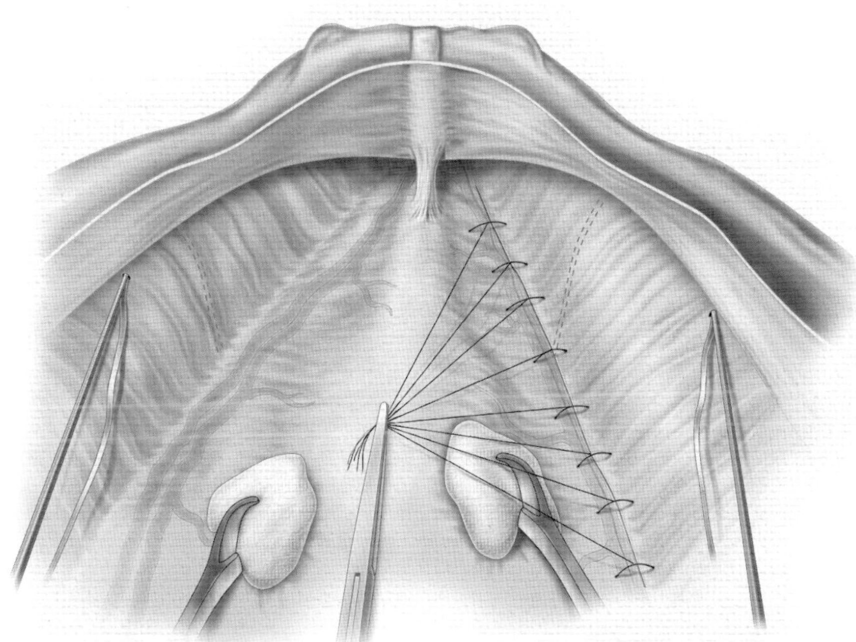

Figure 62-8 All sutures are held and tied down after cystoscopy confirms the integrity of the bladder. (From Richardson AC: In Gershenson DM, Aronson MP (eds). Operative Techniques in Gynecologic Surgery. Philadelphia, WB Saunders, 1996, p 72.)

cystotomies are recognized immediately by expression of blue into the operative field.

Placement of trocar ports is left to the discretion of the surgeon. The space of Retzius is entered by making a transverse incision 2 inches above the pubic symphysis, spanning all three obliterated umbilical ligaments, cephalad to the dome of the bladder. The bladder is then drained. The space of Retzius is dissected bluntly until the retropubic anatomy is clearly visualized. Some advocate removal of retropubic adipose tissue to aid in scarification.[15] The pubic symphysis and bladder neck are noted in the midline, and the obturator neurovascular bundle, Cooper's ligament, and the white line are noted along the pelvic sidewall. The obturator fossa is identified.

With the operator's fingers elevating the superior lateral sulcus of the vagina, the first suture is placed near the apex of the vagina, through the paravesical portion of the pubocervical fascia or the detached white line if it is visible. The needle is then passed through the ipsilateral obturator internus muscle and fascia and the white line at its origin, 1 cm anterior to the ischial spine. The lateral wall suture technique is facilitated by moving the fingers in the vagina medially to open up the sidewall compartment; this readily exposes the ischial spine and white line. The same technique is used in the open procedure. Three to five sutures are placed sequentially through the pubocervical fascia distal to the prior fixation point on each side, but in this case the sutures are tied as they are placed, using an extracorporeal knot-tying technique without a suture bridge. Often, the third and fourth sutures are placed through Cooper's ligament to support the bladder neck (Burch), and there is usually no room for a fifth suture. Cystoscopy verifies integrity of the bladder and the normal function of both ureters.

Laparoscopic paravaginal repair requires great skill, dexterity, and ingenuity. The learning curve for laparoscopic Burch or paravaginal repair is 20 to 30 procedures. There are many modifications to laparoscopic repair, but ideally the laparoscopic method should be exactly the same as the open method to achieve the same result. The laparoscope is a vehicle for performing a repair and should not be a reason to modify a technique. Seman and his colleagues described two modifications to the laparoscopic paravaginal repair[16]: simultaneous Burch colposuspension and paravaginal repair and the modified paravaginal repair, in which the sutures are placed caudad to cephalad and each one includes a third bite of the ipsilateral iliopectineal (Cooper's) ligament. The use of mesh as a bridge between Cooper's ligament and the endopelvic fascia has also been described in the literature.[17] However, there is a paucity of good data regarding long-term success and feasibility of this approach.

COMPLICATIONS

Good surgical technique should be used in gaining exposure to the retropubic space. Damage to the large veins coursing along the detrusor muscle can cause massive hemorrhage. Anatomically, there are few structures along the pelvic sidewall that contribute to complications. The obturator neurovascular bundle lies anterior to the white line, and dissection should be limited to the medial aspect of the neurovascular bundle. Cadaver dissection of the tissues underlying and adjacent to the white line reveals that there are no neurovascular structures along the white line, obturator fascia, or levators that preclude taking a full bite of tissue.[18]

Unlike procedures that create a compensatory distortion of normal anatomy, the paravaginal repair typically does not lead to postoperative problems of de novo detrusor instability or long-term urinary retention. Shull and Baden reported the rate de novo detrusor instability in their patients to be 6% in 1989. Published data reporting objective outcomes and complications of the paravaginal repair are scarce. A review of the literature revealed several articles that comment on complications. Postoperative infections, such as cystitis and wound infection, ranged from 0% to 11%; and pneumonia was reported in 4% of patients.[5,19-21] Miklos and Kohli reviewed the outcomes for 171 consecutive patients who underwent laparoscopic Burch procedure, paravaginal repair, or both concurrently. Cystotomies were noted in 2.3% of patients.[22] C. Y. Liu reported no lower urinary tract injuries, retropubic hematomas, or abscess formation with laparoscopic repair of paravaginal defects.[15]

OUTCOMES

Few studies have examined the long-term anatomic success of abdominal paravaginal repair. Much of the data focuses on correction of stress urinary incontinence rather than resolution of anterior vaginal wall prolapse. Shull and Baden reported that 97% of patients treated with paravaginal repair for lateral anterior defects and stress urinary incontinence had no postoperative complaints of stress incontinence.[19] Colombo and his group had more sobering results.[23] In 1996, they published the only prospective, randomized, controlled trial comparing Burch colposuspension to paravaginal repair for the treatment of stress urinary incontinence. The objective cure rate was 100% for Burch and 61% for paravaginal repair. Bruce and associates had similar results, with a 72% cure rate for paravaginal repair.[24] Paravaginal repair alone should not be offered for the treatment of stress incontinence. The standard of care for the treatment of stress incontinence remains a Burch or a sling procedure.

There are no good studies directly comparing abdominal paravaginal repair with laparoscopic or vaginal paravaginal repair for the treatment of anterior vaginal wall prolapse. The recurrence rate for cystocele has been reported to be 5% to 50%. Failure rates for paravaginal repair reported in several retrospective studies range from 5% to 13%.[15,20,21,25] De novo enterocele and cuff prolapse developed in 6% of patients who had abdominal paravaginal repair.[19] As far as we know, no studies have reviewed long-term major or minor complication rates of laparoscopic paravaginal repair alone.

References

1. White GR: Cystocele: A radical cure by suturing lateral sulky of vaginal to white line of pelvic fascia. JAMA 21:1707-1710, 1909.
2. White GR: An anatomic operation for the cure of cystocele. Am J Obstet Dis Women Child 65:286, 1912.
3. Kelly HA, Dumm WM: Urinary incontinence in women without manifest injury to the bladder. Surg Gynecol Obstet 18:444-450, 1914.
4. Burch JC: Urethrovaginal fixation to Cooper's ligament for correction of stress incontinence, cystocele, and prolapse. Am J Obstet Gynecol 81:281-290, 1961.
5. Richardson AC, Lyon J, Williams N: A new look at pelvic relaxation. Am J Obstet Gynecol 126:568-573, 1976.
6. Weber A, Walters MD: Anterior vaginal prolapse: Review of anatomy and techniques of surgical repair. Obstet Gynecol 89:311-318, 1997.
7. Ricci JV, Lisa JR, Thom CH, Kron WL: The relationship of the vagina to adjacent organs in reconstructive surgery: A histologic study. Am J Obstet Gynecol 74:387-410, 1947.
8. Goff BH: A histologic study of the perivaginal fascia in a nullipara. Surg Gynecol Obstet 52:32-42, 1931.

9. Farrell S, Dempsey T, Geldenhuys L: Histologic examination of "fascia" used in colporrhaphy. Obstet Gynecol 98:794-798, 2001.
10. Barber MD, Cundiff GW: Accuracy of clinical assessment of PV defects in women with anterior vaginal wall prolapse. Am J Obstet Gynecol 181:87-90, 1999.
11. Huddleston HT, Dunnihoo DR, Huddleston PM, Meyers PC: Magnetic resonance imaging of defects in DeLancey's vaginal support levels I, II, and III. Am J Obstet Gynecol 172:1778-1782, 1995.
12. Martan A, Masata J, Halaska M, et al: Ultrasound imaging of paravaginal defects in women with stress incontinence before and after paravaginal defect repair. Ultrasound Obstet Gynecol 19:496-500, 2002.
13. Nguyen JK, Hall CD, Taber E, Bhatia NN: Sonographic diagnosis of paravaginal defects: A standardization of technique. Int Urogynecol J Pelvic Floor Dysfunct 11:341-345, 2000.
14. Ross JW: Post-hysterectomy Total Vaginal Vault Prolapse Repaired Laparoscopically. Presented at the second world symposium on laparoscopic hysterectomy, American Association of Gynecologic Laparoscopists, New Orleans, April 7-9, 1995.
15. Liu CY: Laparoscopic cystocele repair: Paravaginal suspension. In Liu CY (ed): Laparoscopic Hysterectomy and Pelvic Floor Reconstruction. Oxford, UK, Blackwell Scientific, 1996, pp 330-340.
16. Seman E, Cook J, O'Shea R: Two-year experience with laparoscopic pelvic floor repair. J Am Assoc Gynecologic Laparosc 10:38-45, 2003.
17. Washington J, Somers K: Laparoscopic paravaginal repair: A new technique using staples. J Soc Laparoendoscopic Surgeons 7:301-303, 2003.
18. Scotti RJ, Garely AD, Greston WM, Olson TR: Paravaginal repair of lateral vaginal wall defects by fixation to the ischial periosteum and obturator membrane. Am J Obstet Gynecol 179:1436-1445, 1998.
19. Shull B, Baden W: A six-year experience with paravaginal defect repair for stress urinary incontinence. Am J Obstet Gynecol 160:1432-1440, 1989.
20. Shull B, Benn S, Kuehl T: Surgical management of prolapse of the anterior vaginal segment: An analysis of support defects, operative morbidity, and anatomic outcome. Am J Obstet Gynecol 171:1429-1439, 1994.
21. Ostrzenski A: Genuine stress urinary incontinence in women: New laparoscopic paravaginal reconstruction. J Reprod Med 43:477-482, 1998.
22. Miklos JR, Kohli N: Laparoscopic paravaginal repair plus Burch colposuspension: Review and descriptive technique. Urology 56:64-69, 2000.
23. Colombo M, Milani R, Vitobello D, Maggioni A: A randomized comparison of Burch colposuspension and abdominal paravaginal defect repair for female stress urinary incontinence. Am J Obstet Gynecol 175:78-84, 1996.
24. Bruce RG, El-Galley RE, Galloway NT: Paravaginal defect repair in the treatment of female stress urinary incontinence and cystocele. Adult Urol 54:647-651, 1999.
25. Larrieux JR, Noel JW, Vragovic O, Scotti RJ: Persistent site-specific defects after reconstructive pelvic surgery. Int Urogynecol J 12:151-155, 2001.
26. Burch JC: Cooper's ligament urethrovesical suspension for stress incontinence: Nine years' experience—Results, complications, technique. Am J Obstet Gynecol 100:764-774, 1968.
27. Shull B: How I do abdominal paravaginal repair. J Pelvic Surg 1:43, 1995.
28. Benson JT, Lucente V, McClellan E: Vaginal versus abdominal reconstructive surgery for the treatment of pelvic support defects: A prospective randomized study with long-term outcome evaluation. Am J Obstet Gynecol 175:1418-1422, 1996.

Chapter 63

ANTERIOR COLPORRHAPHY FOR CYSTOCELE REPAIR

Tristi W. Muir

Pelvic organ prolapse is common in women. The anterior wall of the vagina primarily provides support for the bladder and urethra. If the support for the bladder sags, a cystocele results. The lifetime risk of undergoing an operation for prolapse or urinary incontinence has been estimated to be 11.1%.[1] Of the women undergoing surgery for prolapse with and without urinary incontinence, 48% had an anterior colporrhaphy included in their surgical management. This chapter discusses the anatomy and possible causes of anterior wall prolapse. A discussion of an anterior colporrhaphy for surgical repair of a cystocele is presented.

ANATOMY AND PATHOLOGY

The anterior vaginal wall is the trapezoid of fibromuscularis and provides support to the bladder and urethra. At the apex, the broad portion of the trapezoid, the anterior vaginal wall has suspensory support provided by the cardinal-uterosacral ligaments. The lateral support is provided by a condensation of connective tissue over the levator ani muscles, the arcus tendineus fascia pelvis. The arcus tendineus fascia pelvis extends from the posterior, inferior aspect of the pubic bone to the ischial spine (Fig. 63-1). Nichols and Randall proposed that a cystocele is an end result of either distention (overstretching of the fibromuscularis of the anterior vaginal wall) or displacement (breaks in the connective tissue).[2] In 1976, A. Cullen Richardson popularized the "site-specific" approach to identifying specific breaks in the connective tissue and repairing those defects.[3]

Apical loss of support of the anterior vaginal wall may occur with an apical, transverse separation of the anterior vaginal fibromuscularis with the cardinal-uterosacral ligaments. As abdominal pressure is placed on the lateral connective tissue attachments, these attachments may fail, allowing the anterior vaginal wall to swing toward the hymen (Fig. 63-2). John DeLancey made surgical observations in 71 women undergoing a retropubic procedure for anterior wall prolapse and stress urinary incontinence.[4] He found that 88.7% of these women had a paravaginal defect and that the area of detachment was at the apex near the ischial spine. Detachment from the back of the pubic bone was rare. Although the majority of women with anterior wall prolapse and stress urinary incontinence may have a paravaginal loss of connective tissue support, the support for the anterior wall of the vagina is much more complex than a list of fascial attachments.

The support for the pelvic organs is maintained by the interaction of connective tissue attachments and innervated, intact pelvic floor musculature. The levator ani muscles provide the primary support for the pelvic floor. The pelvic organs are supported within the abdominal cavity, and the levator hiatus, through which the urethra, vagina, and rectum pass, is closed. The etiology of pelvic organ prolapse is thought to be multifactorial, including abnormalities of connective tissue, pelvic floor muscles, and/or the innervation to the pelvic floor. Norton[5] used the analogy of a boat in a dry dock to describe the interplay of the functioning pelvic floor and connective tissue supports (Fig. 63-3). The pelvic floor muscles (primarily the levator ani muscles) play the supporting role of the water. When the water level is adequate, little stress is placed on the ropes (connective tissue supports) keeping the boat in place. However, if the water level is dropped, the ropes will not be able to hold the boat for long. If the levator ani muscles no longer are able to maintain a closed levator hiatus, the stress of maintaining the pelvic organs is placed on the connective tissue supports. Direct damage to the levator ani muscle or to its innervation may open the hiatus and place the burden of support on the connective tissue of the pelvic organs. Prior damage to the connective tissue support of the anterior vaginal wall may be evident only in light of the loss of levator ani function.

DeLancey and Hurd clinically determined that the levator hiatus is larger in women with prolapse than in those without prolapse.[6] Magnetic resonance imaging (MRI) confirmed that the size of the levator hiatus and levator symphysis gap increases with increasing stage of prolapse.[7] Lennox Hoyte and colleagues evaluated the change in morphology of the levator ani muscles with two- and three-dimensional MRI images.[8] They demonstrated

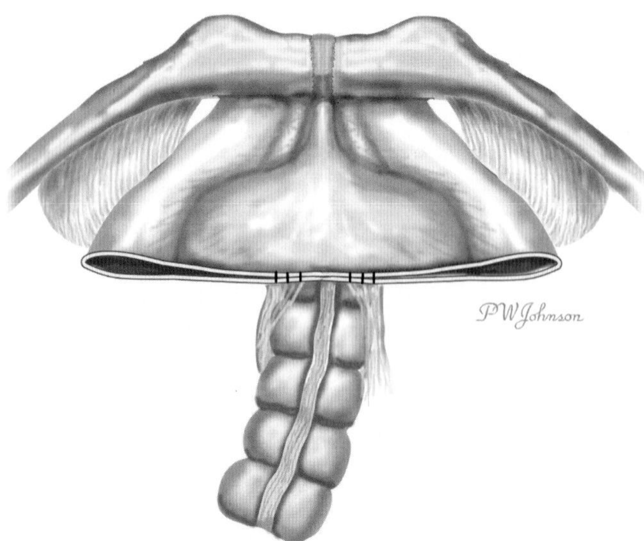

Figure 63-1 Apical and sidewall connective tissue support of the anterior vaginal wall as viewed in the retropubic space. ATFP, arcus tendineus fascia pelvis; IS, ischial spine; USL, uterosacral ligaments.

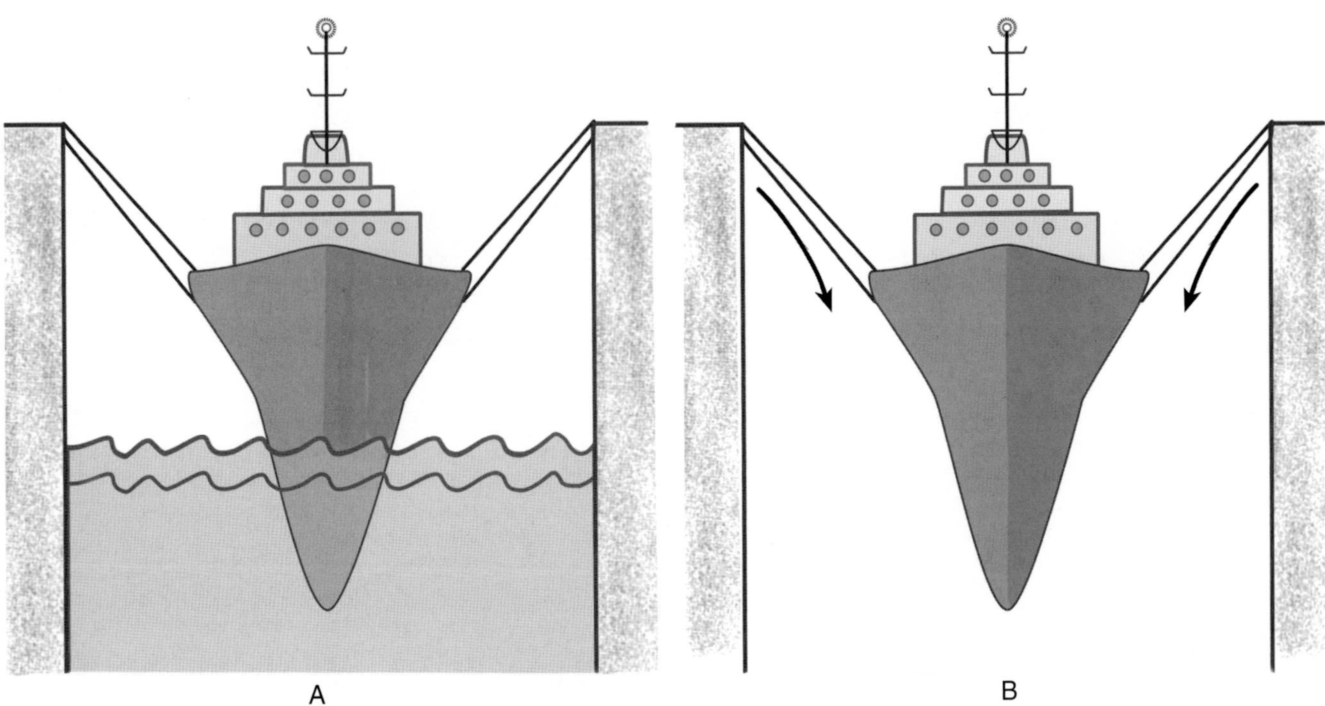

Figure 63-2 Pelvic floor disorders: the role of fascia and ligaments. The water represents functioning pelvic floor muscles, and the ropes are the connective tissue supports. **A,** With water in the dock (functioning pelvic floor muscles), the ropes can maintain the position of the boat (connective tissue supports the position of the pelvic organs). **B,** With loss of the water (loss of function of the pelvic floor muscles), the support of the boat (pelvic organs) is maintained only by the ropes (connective tissue). (From Norton PA: Pelvic floor disorders: The role of fascia and ligaments. Clin Obstet Gynecol 36:926-938, 1993.)

that women with prolapse have significantly more levator ani degradation, laxity, and loss of the integrity of the sling portion of the levator ani compared with asymptomatic controls. This change may be occur as a result of direct muscle damage associated with childbirth or chronic straining or damage to the innervation of the pelvic floor.

Abnormalities in the histology of connective tissue have also been described in women with prolapse. Abnormalities of collagen synthesis may derive from an intrinsic abnormality of collagen synthesis (due to abnormal collagen, an imbalance between synthesis and degradation, or an imbalance between collagen types). The environment (e.g., excessive straining) may also contribute to the condition of the connective tissue. Error in the repair of damaged ligaments and fascia or lack of remodeling in mature collagen may occur. Dietz and colleagues examined bladder neck descent in nulliparous twins.[9] A significant genetic contribution was proposed to contribute to the phenotype of the bladder neck mobility.

SIGNS AND SYMPTOMS

A woman with anterior wall prolapse may be asymptomatic, or she may present with symptoms related to a vaginal mass with or without changes in sexual and urinary function. Pelvic pressure, heaviness, or a bulge may occur. Women often feel that their symptoms are more significant as the day progresses and gravity allows the prolapse to fully descend. The bladder follows the anterior vaginal wall as it descends through the genital hiatus in women with an anterior wall bulge. Because the distal urethra remains fixed under the pubic symphysis, voiding difficulties due to obstruction may arise. Women who have to manually reduce their prolapse to empty their bladder are likely to have more significant prolapse than those who do not.[10] This obstructive effect on the urethra may protect a woman from leaking urine with abdominal stress (occult incontinence). Women with anterior wall prolapse extending more than 1 cm beyond the hymen are less likely to describe stress urinary incontinence than those will lesser prolapse.[10] Sexual function has also been examined in women with prolapse and appears to be similar to that in women without prolapse.[10,11]

The goal of the physical examination is to recreate the woman's symptoms. A validated measure of pelvic organ prolapse is the pelvic organ prolapse quantification (POPQ) method.[12] Measurement of the descent of the anterior vaginal wall is made at maximal strain. If a woman describes prolapse more significant than that observed in the supine or sitting positions, a standing examination may be employed. The woman's position and the degree of bladder distention (empty or full) should be documented. A full bladder may help to recreate the patient's most prominent symptoms of vaginal bulging.

Bob Shull described a method to evaluate the anterior vagina for site-specific defects.[13] Curved ring forceps are placed in the vagina, supporting the lateral anterior vaginal wall to the ischial spine. The patient is asked to bear down in a Valsalva maneuver. If the anterior vaginal wall prolapse is reduced, a paravaginal defect is diagnosed. A bilateral and a unilateral paravaginal defect may be differentiated with alternating unilateral paravaginal

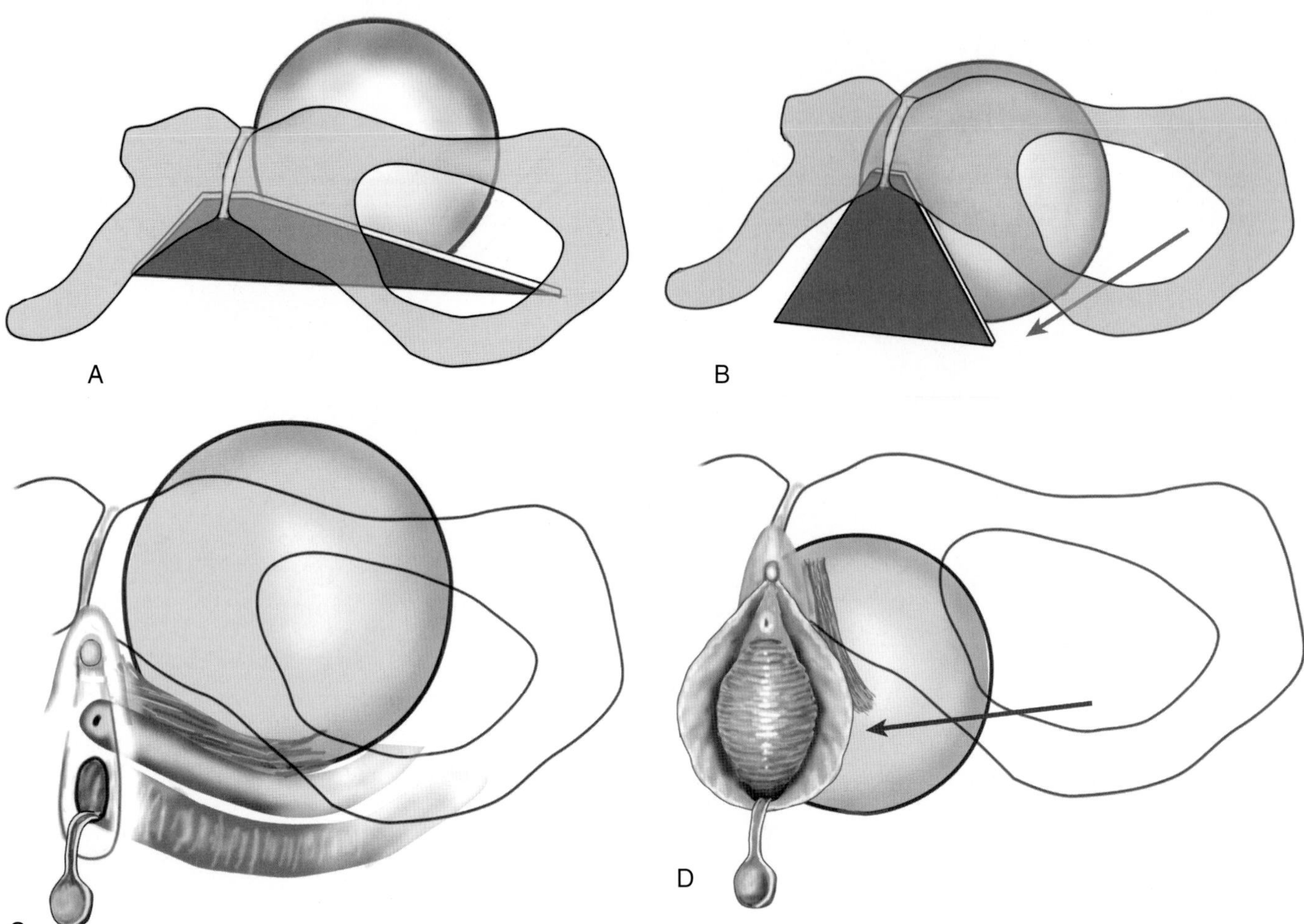

Figure 63-3 Connective tissue support of the anterior vaginal wall. **A,** Intact connective tissue support. **B,** Loss of apical and paravaginal support (beginning at the ischial spines) allows the anterior vaginal wall to swing toward the introitus. (From DeLancey JOL: Fascial and muscular abnormalities in women with urethral hypermobility and anterior vaginal wall prolapse. Am J Obstet Gynecol 187:93-98, 2002).

support. If the anterior vaginal wall continues to balloon forward despite paravaginal support, a midline defect is diagnosed. A superior or high transverse defect may be suspected if the prolapse is reduced with apical support. Loss of rugation at one of these sites is also thought to be associated with localization of the defect. Whiteside and colleagues evaluated the inter-examiner and intra-examiner reliability of site-specific defect examination.[14] They found that there was poor examiner concordance for the presence of superior, paravaginal, or central defects. Not surprising is that the reliability of the examination increased with stage of prolapse.

Evaluation of urinary function is important in women with anterior wall prolapse. A postvoid residual volume may be measured by an in-and-out catheterization, or an ultrasonic determination may be made with a bladder scan.[15] A test for hypermobility of the urethra may be performed with a sterile, lubricated cotton swab (Q-tip test). The cotton swab is inserted into the urethra to the level of the bladder neck. Measurement of the resting and straining angles from the horizontal axis may be obtained with a goniometer. Hypermobility of the bladder neck is determined if the difference between the resting and straining angles is more than 30 degrees. For patients with stage 3 or 4 anterior wall prolapse, urodynamic assessment with prolapse reduction has been suggested to identify those women with occult urinary incontinence. The method of prolapse reduction (pessary, rolled gauze, tampons, ring forceps) has not been standardized, and the reliability of this test has not been established.

TECHNIQUE

The anterior colporrhaphy involves a plication of the fibromuscularis of the anterior vaginal wall. This procedure serves to "tighten up" the overdistended support of the anterior vaginal wall or repair a midline defect. The patient is in the dorsal lithotomy position with the legs elevated. A single dose of perioperative antibiotics is administered. A weighted speculum is placed in the vagina, and a 16-Fr Foley catheter is inserted into the bladder. The epithelium of the anterior vaginal wall is incised in the midline and dissected away from the underlying fibromuscularis or "pubocervical fascia." Hydrodissection of the vaginal epithelium away from the underlying fibromuscularis with saline or an anesthetic/vasoconstrictive agent may facilitate the dissection. With traction and countertraction, the dissection is carried laterally to the levator ani muscular sidewall. It is important to continue the dissection to the apex of the anterior vaginal wall. If an

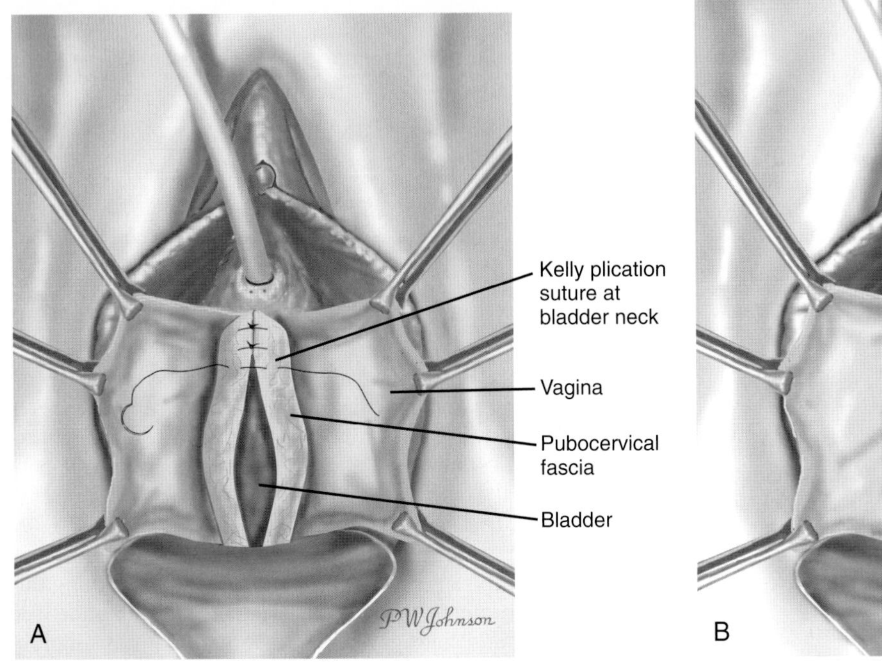

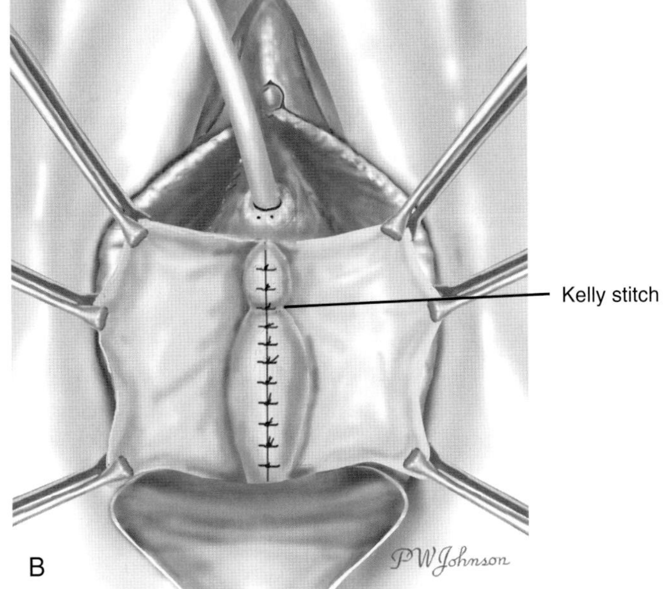

Figure 63-4 Anterior colporrhaphy with Kelly plication.

anti-incontinence procedure is included in the woman's surgery, the anterior wall dissection typically spares the mid-urethra and distal urethra. This area may be palpated with a Foley catheter in place. If the surgeon wishes to provide improved support underneath the urethra and bladder for treatment of a distal anterior wall prolapse (urethrocele), the dissection is continued distally toward the inferior aspect of the public bone.

A plication underneath the urethra and bladder neck (a Kelly plication) may be performed to provide a shelf of support underneath the urethra. The fibromuscularis associated with the inferior portion of the pubic bone, just lateral to the urethra, is grasped bilaterally. Interrupted sutures are placed to reapproximate this tissue underneath the urethra, creating a posterior urethral shelf of support. A separate suture is placed plicating the fibromuscularis underneath the bladder neck. Continuation of the midline plication is performed, reducing the width of the fibromuscular wall of the anterior vagina with interrupted sutures (Fig. 63-4).

Attention should be directed to the length of the anterior vaginal wall. In some women with prolapse, an elongated (stretched out) vaginal wall is present. Vertically oriented plication sutures tend to shorten the length of the fibromuscularis.[16] However, some women, particularly those with recurrent prolapse, may have a shortened anterior segment. Horizontally oriented plication sutures will preserve the vaginal length of the anterior segment. More than one row of plicating sutures may be required to reduce anterior wall prolapse in women with stage 3 or 4 prolapse. The aggressiveness of the plication and the longevity of the sutures are dependent on the surgeon's preference. Anne Weber and colleagues described a standard plication and an "ultralateral" plication as two different procedures in a prospective, randomized trial.[17] Placement of the plication sutures should be tailored to the prolapse anatomy of the patient.

The apex of the plicated fibromuscularis of the anterior vaginal wall must be suspended to the apical support of the vagina. If the woman has a well-supported apex, reattachment of the apical portion of the repair should be performed. If the woman is undergoing a concomitant apical suspension procedure, the apical portion of the anterior colporrhaphy should be attached to the suspension sutures. Without apical suspension of the fibromuscularis, the anterior vaginal wall will continue to sag down toward the introitus.

After plication and suspension of the anterior fibromuscularis, the vaginal epithelium may be trimmed and closed with absorbable suture. The surgeon should be cautious not to overtrim the vaginal epithelium (particularly in the postmenopausal woman with vaginal atrophy). A vaginal pack and Foley catheter are placed for 2 to 24 hours postoperatively. Voiding trials should be performed postoperatively to ensure that the patient is able to void to completion. Hakvoort and colleagues found that removal of the Foley catheter on the morning after surgery, rather than on postoperative day 4, was associated with fewer days requiring catheter drainage and a lower incidence of urinary tract infections.[18]

SURGICAL OUTCOMES

The anterior colporrhaphy has been performed for more than a century, but few studies have reported the efficacy of the procedure for the treatment of anterior wall prolapse. Most studies have addressed the efficacy (or lack thereof) of the anterior colporrhaphy in the management of stress urinary incontinence. The anatomic cure rate of the procedure for treatment of anterior vaginal wall prolapse varies between 30% and 97% (Table 63-1).[17,19-22]

Clark and colleagues monitored a cohort of women who had undergone anterior colporrhaphy and found that 7% underwent a reoperation by 71 months.[23] Risk factors for recurrent anterior wall prolapse include age less than 60 years and preoperative stage 3 or 4 prolapse.[24]

Table 63-1 Efficacy of Anterior Colporrhaphy

Study (Ref. No.)	Year	No. Patients	Mean Follow-up	Anatomic Cure (%)
Goff (19)	1933	86*	1-8 yr	93
Stanton et al (20)	1982	73	3 to 24 mo	89
Porges & Smilen (21)	1994	486 (388 with follow-up)	31 mo	97
Colombo et al (22)	2000	33	8-17 yr	97
Weber et al (17)	2001	57†	23 mo (median)	37

*Study included 31 patients who underwent excision of the vaginal wall and 55 patients with overlapping fibromuscularis.
†Study included both patients who underwent "standard" plication and patients who underwent an "ultralateral" plication.

COMPLICATIONS

Complications of anterior colporrhaphy include injury to the surrounding organs, deterioration of bladder or sexual function, and recurrence of prolapse. The routine risks of surgery inclusive of blood transfusion are uncommon with this procedure (blood transfusion occurred in 3 of 519 women undergoing prolapse surgery that included an anterior colporrhaphy, most often linked to other prolapse procedures).[25]

Injury to Ureters, Bladder, and Urethra

Injury to the lower urinary tract may occur during an anterior colporrhaphy. Kwon and colleagues reported a 2% incidence of ureteral obstruction during 346 anterior colporrhaphies, making this procedure the most common cause of unsuspected intraoperative injury to the lower urinary tract in their pelvic reconstructive procedures.[26] The cause was thought to be an aggressive lateral plication of the fibromuscularis, which kinked the ureter at the ureterovesical junction. A case report of bilateral ureteric obstruction after an anterior colporrhaphy has been described.[27] Additionally, recurrent postoperative urinary tract infections may occur because of an unrecognized intravesical suture.[28] R. Peter Beck reported 2 cases of urethrovaginal fistula among 519 women undergoing anterior colporrhaphy for prolapse with or without urinary incontinence.[25] Of note, in an attempt to improve the surgical cure of stress incontinence, Beck's group modified the bladder neck plication by attempting to be more aggressive in differential support of the urethra (to a higher retropubic position) compared with the bladder base. This more aggressive plication technique may result in ischemia or occult injury to the urethra. These cases suggest a role for universal cystoscopy in patients undergoing anterior colporrhaphy to identify and correct injury to the ureters, bladder, or urethra.

De Novo Urinary Symptoms

De novo urinary incontinence or voiding dysfunction is a known complication of prolapse and incontinence procedures. The risk of postoperative de novo urinary incontinence for women undergoing an anterior colporrhaphy for anterior wall prolapse is 10% (5% for stress urinary incontinence, 4% for overactive bladder with incontinence, and 1% for mixed urinary incontinence).[25] De novo detrusor overactivity may be the result of a number of possible postoperative changes, including outlet obstruction, and changes in detrusor innervation.

Most women who undergo an anterior colporrhaphy are able to obtain postvoid residuals of less than 100 mL by 1 week.[25] However, urethral obstruction leading to irritative voiding symptoms after an anterior colporrhaphy with Kelly plication has been described.[29] Aggressive plication under the urethra is thought to be the culprit. In some cases, a band of constriction may be palpated by vaginal examination. A vaginal approach to release of the area of constriction may be curative.

Evaluation of the effect of anterior wall dissection on innervation of the urethral sphincters was performed by measuring the terminal motor latency of the perineal branch of the pudendal nerve. Zivkovic and colleagues found that there was not a significant difference between preoperative and postoperative perineal nerve terminal motor latencies in women undergoing an anterior colporrhaphy without a needle urethropexy.[30]

Sexual Function

Sexual function in women is a complicated issue, one that may be further complicated by the presence of prolapse or incontinence. Many sexually active women with prolapse or incontinence describe preoperative dissatisfaction with their sex lives due to a variety of reasons, inclusive of decreased libido, vaginal prolapse, and fear of urinary incontinence with intercourse. Rogers and colleagues evaluated the sexual and continence functions in women preoperatively and postoperatively.[31] They found that sexual function scores declined from their preoperative values at 3 and 6 months after surgery, despite an improvement in incontinence impact scores. Gungor and colleagues also described a deterioration in sexual function, primarily related to dyspareunia, in 8 (18%) of 44 sexually active women who underwent an anterior colporrhaphy coupled with a posterior colpoperineorrhaphy.[32] However, they found an improvement in 20 (67%) of 30 sexually active women who preoperatively had dissatisfaction in their sexual life.

Sexual function remains a complicated issue in the postoperative period. Patients should be counseled that their sexual function has the potential to improve, remain unchanged, or deteriorate after prolapse surgery. In the operating room, the surgeon should make every effort to maintain vaginal caliber, to reduce the likelihood of postoperative dyspareunia.

ANTERIOR COLPORRHAPHY WITH KELLY PLICATION AS AN INCONTINENCE PROCEDURE

Most of the studies evaluating the postoperative results of anterior colporrhaphy with Kelly plication have used cure of stress urinary incontinence as the measure of success. Anterior colporrhaphy with Kelly plication has not been found to be as effective as retropubic urethropexy for the treatment of urinary incontinence, and it has largely been abandoned as a method of operative management of urinary incontinence.[33-35]

CONCLUSIONS

Anterior wall prolapse most likely develops after loss of levator ani function (through direct muscle damage or nerve damage) and breaks or attenuation of connective tissue supports. Our surgical approach to repair of prolapse focuses on connective tissue support until a time in the future when muscle and nerve regeneration are feasible. The anterior colporrhaphy has been a part of the surgeon's armamentarium for more than a century. The key to support of the anterior vaginal wall is apical support. Because the anterior vaginal wall rarely loses distal support at the posterior aspect of the pubic bone, does it matter, if the other end of the fibromuscularis hammock of support is reestablished at the apex, how the "sag" is taken out (anterior colporrhaphy versus paravaginal repair)? Even those who advocate paravaginal repair often perform a concomitant anterior colporrhaphy.[36,37] There are no studies comparing the site-specific approach to repair of the anterior vaginal wall, using a paravaginal defect repair with or without a midline defect repair (colporrhaphy), to an anterior colporrhaphy alone. The addition of graft materials in an attempt to decrease the likelihood of recurrent prolapse has been described. Comparative studies are needed to determine the risks and benefits of this practice.

Anterior wall prolapse is often associated with bladder dysfunction. Preoperative evaluation of bladder function may be necessary, especially in patients with stage 3 or 4 anterior wall prolapse. Sexual function is a complex issue. Maintenance of vaginal caliber is important in sexually active women undergoing surgical management.

References

1. Olsen AL, Smith VJ, Bergstrom JO, et al: Epidemiology of surgically managed pelvic organ prolapse and urinary incontinence. Obstet Gynecol 89:501-506, 1997.
2. Nichols DH, Randall CL (eds): Vaginal Surgery, 3rd ed. Baltimore, Williams & Wilkins, 1989, pp 241-244.
3. Richardson AC, Lyon JB, Williams NL: A new look at pelvic relaxation. Am J Obstet Gynecol 126:568-573, 1976.
4. DeLancey JOL: Fascial and muscular abnormalities in women with urethral hypermobility and anterior vaginal wall prolapse. Am J Obstet Gynecol 187:93-98, 2002.
5. Norton PA: Pelvic floor disorders: The role of fascia and ligaments. Clin Obstet Gynecol 36:926-938, 1993.
6. DeLancey JO, Hurd WW: Size of the urogenital hiatus in the levator ani muscles in normal women and women with pelvic organ prolapse. Obstet Gynecol 91:364-368, 1998.
7. Singh K, Jakab M, Reid WM, et al: Three-dimensional magnetic resonance imaging assessment of levator ani morphologic features in different grades of prolapse. Am J Obstet Gynecol 188:910-915, 2003.
8. Hoyte L, Schierlitz L, Zou K, et al: Two- and 3-dimensional MRI comparison of levator ani structure, volume, and integrity in women with stress incontinence and prolapse. Am J Obstet Gynecol 185:11-19, 2001.
9. Dietz HP, Hasell NK, Grace ME, et al: Bladder neck mobility is a heritable trait. BJOG 112:334-339, 2005.
10. Burrows LJ, Meyn LA, Walters MD, Weber AM: Pelvic symptoms in women with pelvic organ prolapse. Obstet Gynecol 104:982-988, 2004.
11. Weber AM, Walters MD, Schover LR, Mitchinson A: Sexual function in women with uterovaginal prolapse and urinary incontinence. Obstet Gynecol 85:483-487, 1995.
12. Bump RC, Mattiasson A, Bo K, et al: The standardization of terminology of female pelvic organ prolapse and pelvic floor dysfunction. Am J Obstet Gynecol 175:10-17, 1996.
13. Shull BL: Clinical evaluation of women with pelvic support defects. Clin Obstet Gynecol 36:939-951, 1993.
14. Whiteside JL, Barber MD, Paraiso MF, et al: Clinical evaluation of anterior vaginal wall support defects: Interexaminer and intraexaminer reliability. Am J Obstet Gynecol 191:100-104, 2004.
15. Paltieli Y, Degani S, Aharoni A, et al: Ultrasound assessment of the bladder volume after anterior colporrhaphy. Gynecol Obstet Invest 28:209-211, 1989.
16. Nichols DH: Anterior colporrhaphy technique to shorten a pathologically long anterior vaginal wall. Int Surg 64:69-71, 1979.
17. Weber AM, Walters MD, Peidmonte MR, Ballard LA: Anterior colporrhaphy: A randomized trial of three surgical techniques. Am J Obstet Gynecol 185:1299-1306, 2001.
18. Hakvoort RA, Elberink R, Vollebregt A, et al: How long should urinary bladder catheterization be continued after vaginal prolapse surgery? A randomized controlled trial comparing short term versus long term catheterization after vaginal prolapse surgery. BJOG 111:828-830, 2004.
19. Goff BH: An evaluation of the Bissell operation for uterine prolapse: A follow-up study. Surg Gynecol Obstet 57:763-767, 1933.
20. Stanton SL, Hilton P, Norton C, Cardozo L: Clinical and urodynamic effects of anterior colporrhaphy and vaginal hysterectomy for prolapse with and without incontinence. Br J Obstet Gynecol 89:459-463, 1982.
21. Porges RF, Smilen S: Long-term analysis of the surgical management of pelvic support defects. Am J Obstet Gynecol 171:1518-1528, 1994.
22. Colombo M, Vitobello D, Proietti, F, Milani R: Randomised comparison of Burch colposuspension versus anterior colporrhaphy in women with stress urinary incontinence and anterior vaginal wall prolapse. BJOG 107:544-551, 2000.
23. Clark AL, Gregory T, Smith VJ, Edwards R: Epidemiologic evaluation of reoperation for surgically treated pelvic organ prolapse. Am J Obstet Gynecol 189:1261-1267, 2003.
24. Whiteside JL, Weber AM, Meyn LA, Walters MD: Risk factors for prolapse recurrence after vaginal repair. Am J Obstet Gynecol 191:1533-1538, 2004.
25. Beck RP, McCormick S, Nordstrom L: A 25-year experience with 519 anterior colporrhaphy procedures. Obstet Gynecol 78:1011-1018, 1991.
26. Kwon CH, Goldberg RP, Koduri S, Sand PK: The use of intraoperative cystoscopy in major vaginal and urogynecologic surgeries. Am J Obstet Gynecol 187:1466-1472, 2002.
27. Pang MW, Wong WS, Yip SK, Law LW: An unusual case of bilateral ureteric obstruction after anterior colporrhaphy and vaginal hysterectomy for pelvic organ prolapse. Gynecol Obstet Invest 55:125-126, 2003.
28. Neuman M, Alon H, Langer R, et al: Recurrent urinary tract infections in the presence of intravesical suture material after vaginal hysterectomy and anterior colporrhaphy. Aust N Z J Obstet Gynaecol 30:184-185, 1990.
29. Erickson DR, Olt GJ: Urethral obstruction after anterior colporrhaphy: Correction by simple vaginoplasty. Urology 48:805-808, 1996.
30. Zivkovic F, Tamussino K, Ralph G, et al: Long-term effects of vaginal dissection on the innervation of the striated urethral sphincter. Obstet Gynecol 87:257-260, 1996.

31. Rogers RG, Kammerer-Doak D, Darrow A, et al: Sexual function after surgery for stress urinary incontinence and/or pelvic organ prolapse: A multicenter prospective study. Am J Obstet Gynecol 191:206-210, 2004.
32. Gungor T, Ekin M, Dogan M, et al: Influence of anterior colporrhaphy with colpoperineoplasty operations for stress incontinence and/or genital descent on sexual life. J Pak Med Assoc 47:248-250, 1997.
33. Van Geelen JM, Theeuwes AG, Eskes TK, Martin CB Jr: The clinical and urodynamic effects of anterior vaginal repair and Burch colposuspension. Am J Obstet Gynecol 159:137-144, 1988.
34. Tamussino KF, Zivkovic F, Pieber D, et al: Five-year results after anti-incontinence operations. Am J Obstet Gynecol 181:1347-1352, 1999.
35. Hutchings A, Black NA: Surgery for stress incontinence: A non-randomised trial of colposuspension, needle suspension, and anterior colporrhaphy. Eur Urol 39:375-382, 2001.
36. Shull BL, Benn S, Kuehl TJ: Surgical management of prolapse of the anterior vaginal segement: An analysis of support defects, operative morbidity, and anatomic outcome. Am J Obstet Gynecol 171:1429-1439, 1994.
37. Young SB, Daman JJ, Bony LG: Vaginal paravaginal repair: One-year outcomes. Am J Obstet Gynecol 185:1360-1367, 2001.

Chapter 64

TRANSVAGINAL PARAVAGINAL REPAIR OF HIGH-GRADE CYSTOCELE

Donna Y. Deng, Matthew P. Rutman, Larissa V. Rodriguez, and Shlomo Raz

Anterior compartment defect or cystocele is defined as anterior vaginal wall relaxation or prolapse with or without urethral hypermobility. It represents one of the most common types of genital organ prolapse. Cystoceles have been described by several different classification systems and were previously categorized based on the relative degree of bladder descent and anatomic defect. More recently, the International Continence Society (ICS) has accepted standardization of the terminology for prolapse of the lower urinary tract.[1] To ensure consistency, examiners must note the conditions of the examination findings, such as rest, strain, or supine positioning. This chapter concentrates on repair of the high-grade cystocele that has prolapsed past the vaginal introitus—grade 3/4 in the Baden-Walker classification or stage 3/4 in the pelvic organ prolapse quantification (POPQ) terminology.

The natural history of a cystocele is a continuous progression from mild to severe prolapse, but the actual risk of progression is unknown. In some patients, the progression is rapid; in others, it can be insidious, taking many years. Most lesser degrees of prolapse (stages 1 and 2) are asymptomatic except when accompanied by urinary incontinence. Pelvic prolapse does not spontaneously regress, nor does it become symptomatic until the descent reaches the introitus.[2] Cystoceles with an isolated central defect represent only 5% to 15% of all cystoceles, whereas a lateral paravaginal defect is present in 70% to 80% of patients. Stage 4 cystoceles usually manifest with both defects. Proposed risk factors for the development of a cystocele have included difficult or prolonged vaginal deliveries, elevated body mass index (BMI), parity, menopause, and previous vaginal surgery.

Cystocele may occur as an isolated defect. However, it is most commonly associated with prolapse of other genital organs, such as rectocele, enterocele, and uterine descensus. Michael and colleagues[3] observed a simultaneous enterocele in 35%, rectocele in 63%, and uterine prolapse in 38% of patients with grade 4 cystoceles. Therefore, in cases of severe anterior compartment prolapse, all of the compartments must be corrected. Treatment must involve a thoughtful and thorough evaluation plus a strong knowledge of pelvic floor anatomy The goals of surgery must be to restore vaginal depth, vaginal axis, the levator hiatus, and bladder and bowel function, while also preserving sexual function.

ANATOMY

In a well-supported woman in the standing position, the vagina forms an inverted "C" shape with two distinct vaginal angles. This can be demonstrated on a midsagittal pelvic magnetic resonance image in a patient with normal anatomy. The distal vaginal canal forms a 45-degree angle from the vertical plane, whereas the proximal vagina lies more horizontally over the posterior levator plate, forming an angle of 110 degrees. The upper vagina is held over the levator plate by the cardinal and uterosacral ligaments, and the angle is maintained by a strong levator plate and the anterior traction of the levator sling and prerectal fascia.

The bony pelvis is a scaffold from which the pelvic structures draw their support. The pelvis can be divided into posterior and anterior regions by a line traversing the ischial spines. The sacrospinous ligaments are true ligaments in that they span between bony structures, arising from the posterior aspect of the ischial spines and connecting with the anterolateral sacrum and coccyx, providing a broad support for the posterior pelvis. A linear fascial condensation arising from the obturator internus muscle, the arcus tendineus, extends from the ischial spine to the lower portion of the pubic symphysis. The arcus tendineus is also the insertion point for the semilunar-shaped levator muscles, and it provides the musculofascial support for a large portion of the anterior pelvis.

The pelvic diaphragm is the superior layer of striated muscle and fascia that provides the inferior support for the pelvic viscera. The levator ani muscle group, composed of the pubococcygeus and iliococcygeus, is a broad muscular structure that originates on each side from the arcus tendineus of the obturator fascia and the inner surface of the pubis anteriorly and sweeps medially to join its contralateral partner in the midline. The levator ani thereby forms a broad hammock upon which the bladder, proximal vagina, and intrapelvic rectum lie. The vagina, rectum, and urethra traverse the pubococcygeus through a funneled hiatus. Pubococcygeal muscle fibers entering this "U"-shaped levator hiatus form the external sphincter of the urethra. Medial fibers of the pubococcygeal portion of the levator, sometimes referred to as the puborectalis, travel posteriorly along the urethra, vagina, and rectum and fuse anterior to the rectum, forming part of the perineal support deep to the perineal body. Reflex and active contraction of the pubococcygeus elevates the urethra, vagina, and rectum, thereby helping to compress the lumens of these structures.

Like the pubococcygeus, the iliococcygeus arises from the tendinous arc, but it sweeps more posteriorly and unites with the contralateral iliococcygeus in the median raphe posterior to the rectum. The coccygeus extends from the ischial spine to the lateral aspect of the sacrum and coccyx, overlying the sacrospinous ligament. The coccygeus is a thin muscle that overlies the strong and fibrous sacrospinous ligament. These two structures are identically shaped, and when they are encountered during surgical procedures, they are approached as a single complex useful for fixation of the vaginal vault. It is important to realize that the pudendal neurovascular bundle runs in the lateral insertion of the sacrospinous ligament, near the ischial spine.

The pelvic diaphragm has investing connective tissue that is often referred to as "fascia"; it is, however, less organized and less distinct than traditional fascia (e.g., rectus abdominis fascia). This visceropelvic fascia consists of collagen, smooth muscle, and elastin. Microscopic studies suggest that it may be histologically indistinct from the deep vaginal wall and not a separate "fascia."[4] In our discussion of the musculofascial support, we will continue to refer to this tissue as "fascia" for the sake of accepted nomenclature. The pelvic fasciae have been given a confusing array of appellations by anatomists and surgeons interested in female pelvic organ prolapse. To add to the confusion, the strength of pelvic fasciae can differ significantly among individuals and races, and these differences may predispose some individuals to pelvic prolapse.[5]

The pelvic fascia consists of two leaves—the endopelvic fascia (abdominal side) and the perivesical fascia (vaginal side). The urethra, bladder, vagina, and uterus are all contained within these two layers of fascia. The two leaves fuse laterally to insert along the arcus tendineus. The pelvic fascia can be divided, distally to proximally, into four specialized areas; these areas play important roles in pelvic support and during surgical reconstruction of the female pelvis. They are not true ligaments; rather, they are condensations or a meshwork of connective tissue and smooth muscle that invests the visceral neurovascular pedicles.[1,6] The so-called pubourethral ligaments attach to the lower portion of the pubis and insert on the proximal third of the urethra; they are analogous to the puboprostatic ligaments in the male.[2] The urethropelvic ligaments provide support of the proximal urethra to the lateral pelvic sidewall.[3] The vesicopelvic fascia is the region of the pelvic fascia that attaches and supports the bladder base to the arcus tendineus. Finally, the vesicopelvic ligaments are all of the structures that support the bladder to the lateral pelvic wall. Weakness in the vesicopelvic fascia results in cystocele formation.

Cystoceles are generally classified as being caused by a central defect or a lateral defect. A central defect manifests as a midline weakness. There is good lateral support, but central herniation of the bladder base into the vagina occurs through a separation or attenuation of the vesicopelvic fascia (with separation of the cardinal ligaments). A lateral defect occurs when there is weakness or disruption of the lateral (paravaginal) attachments of the vesicopelvic ligaments to the arcus tendineus fascia pelvis. High-grade cystoceles tend to involve a combination of lateral and central defects with urethral hypermobility.[4] The cardinal-sacrouterine ligament complex attaches to the bladder base and cervix (or vaginal vault, if reapproximated during the hysterectomy).

PATHOPHYSIOLOGY

Pelvic organ prolapse is prevented by several mechanisms. The most important support is from the continuous contraction of the levator ani pelvic muscles. The activity of skeletal muscle is a combination of basic tone, reflex contraction or relaxation, and voluntary contraction or relaxation. The basic tone of the skeletal musculature is similar to that in other areas of the body. Muscles of the pelvic diaphragm contain type I (slow-twitch) fibers, which provide tonic support to pelvic structures, and type II (fast-twitch) fibers, for sudden increases in intra-abdominal pressure.[7] The continuous contraction closes the urogenital hiatus and forms a shelf for the pelvic organs to rest upon. Patients with multiple deliveries exhibit widening and descent of the levator plate. The musculature becomes less important and the "fascial" structures become the more important elements of support as the organs cross the pelvic floor.

Innervation of the muscles is primarily derived from the ventral rami of the second, third, and fourth sacral nerve roots. These pelvic somatic efferent nerves travel on the pelvic surface of the levator ani in close association with the rectum and are separated from the pelvic autonomic plexus by the endopelvic fascia. They supply the levator ani and extend anteriorly to the striated urethral sphincter.[8,9] Static support is provided by the investing connective tissue layers. Under normal conditions, the levator ani contract, and the ligaments and fasciae are under minimal stress. The fasciae stabilize the pelvic organs.

Because of the complexity of pelvic organ support, the cause of vaginal prolapse is likely to be multifactorial, including myopathic or neuropathic disorders, aging, atrophy, chronic increase in abdominal pressures, multiple deliveries, hysterectomy, and hormonal changes. Poor function of the levator ani muscles may result from direct myopathic injury or from an abnormality of innervation. Loss of tonic contraction causes the urogenital hiatus to widen, increasing the risk of organ prolapse. Pelvic relaxation decreases the angulation of the mid-vagina, so the upper vagina does not lie flat against the pelvic floor plate. Instead of an inverted "C" configuration, the vagina becomes vertically oriented and can more easily intussuscept on itself. The reason for neuropathy in a healthy woman is not clear. Childbirth has been suggested as the cause of pelvic denervation, but studies in this area have shown that uncomplicated childbirth creates only transient neurologic damage to the pelvic floor that is restored after two postpartum months.[10] The pelvic floor neuropraxia related to vaginal delivery is associated with multiple births, prolonged labor, high birth weight, and traumatic deliveries. Other risk factors for neurologic damage are congenital abnormalities, aging, chronic constipation (abdominal straining), and perineal laxity.[11,12] In a study of 50 women with prolapse, Sharf and associates performed electromyography of the levator ani and found evidence of denervation in half of the patients.[10] Other studies have also confirmed evidence of neurologic damage to the urogenital muscles in pelvic prolapse.[13,14]

The connective tissue of the pelvic floor, the endopelvic fascia, can be described as a group of collagen fibers interlaced with elastin, smooth muscle cells, fibroblasts, and vascular structures. These structures may be weakened by pregnancy, parturition, lack of estrogen, aging, diet, chronic straining, and certain connective tissue disorders (e.g., Ehlers-Danlos syndrome, Marfan's syndrome).[15] However, intrinsic collagen abnormalities and other individual predisposing factors, such as genetics, differences in pelvic architecture, inherent quality of the pelvic musculature, and tissue response to injury, might explain why many patients with known risk factors do not develop prolapse and many patients without risk factors do.

Correction of a cystocele alone, without addressing the entire pelvic floor laxity and alignment, may further alter the vaginal axis as the bladder and vesicopelvic fascia are brought anteriorly. This may increase the likelihood of uterine prolapse, enterocele, and rectocele formation.

EVALUATION

Symptoms

Cystoceles are often asymptomatic until pelvic organ prolapse is severe. The most common complaint related to anterior compartment prolapse is vaginal bulging, with or without suprapubic pressure and pain. Other symptoms include urgency, frequency, urge incontinence, recurrent urinary tract infections, back pain, renal failure, staghorn calculi, and urinary retention. Obstructive voiding symptoms are caused by urethral kinking that occurs when the bladder descends beyond the pubic ramus but the urethra remains fixed. This is commonly seen in the setting of previous surgery (bladder neck suspension, urethropexy, sling).[3] Patients may describe using unusual positions to void, such as pelvic tilting, squatting, or standing. In contrast, patients with concomitant urethral dysfunction may present with stress urinary incontinence, especially when the cystocele is manually reduced.

Clinical Evaluation

There are critical points in the evaluation of a cystocele that must be answered before treatment. The degree of cystocele and other concurrent bladder symptoms (e.g., stress incontinence, detrusor overactivity) and ability to empty the bladder to completion should be known. Surgical planning is also affected by the need to preserve sexual function and vaginal depth. The overall health of the patient must be considered, as well as the quality of vaginal tissue, presence of associated prolapse, bowel and bladder function, hormonal status, and presence of urinary tract infection. It is also important to assess the impact of the symptoms on the patient's quality of life.

Physical Examination

A thorough physical examination should be done while the patient has a full bladder, at rest and with straining, in both the standing and supine positions. The goal of examination is to determine the degree of prolapse, the specific anatomic defects, and the presence of concomitant organ prolapse. Straining and standing should accentuate the degree of descent. In the supine position, the origin of prolapse should be determined. With a half-speculum blade, the posterior vaginal wall is retracted; the patient is asked to strain while the anterior defect is evaluated. An isolated central defect is identified as bulging in the central region of the vagina (midline) with loss of vaginal rugae. However, in older patients, loss of vaginal rugae alone can be caused by smooth muscle atrophy of the vaginal wall. A lateral defect is identified by loss of the lateral vaginal sulci as the vesicopelvic fascia attenuates from the arcus tendineus fascia pelvis. There will be loss of the "M" vaginal profile (coronal view) and sliding herniation of the bladder into the vagina. After the anatomic defects have been characterized, it is important to reduce the cystocele in order to elicit occult stress urinary incontinence and hypermobility. Similarly, we retract the anterior vaginal wall to determine the presence of any posterior defect. A digital rectal examination assesses rectal tone, presence of impacted stool, attenuation of the prerectal fascia, and perineal laxity. With the use of both blades of speculum, the vaginal vault or cervix can be examined for uterine descent, vault prolapse, and enterocele.

The ICS approved the POPQ validated system for describing pelvic organ support.[1] Six points (two on the anterior vaginal wall, two in the superior vagina, and two on the posterior vaginal wall) are located with reference to the plane of the hymen. The system assigns negative numbers (in centimeters) to structures that have not prolapsed beyond the hymen and positive numbers to structures that protrude. With specific reference to the anterior compartment, point Aa is located in the midline of the anterior vaginal wall, 3cm proximal to the external urethral meatus. Point Ba represents the most dependent position of any part of the upper anterior vaginal wall, from the vaginal cuff or fornix to point Aa. Point C represents either the most distal edge of the cervix or the leading edge of the vaginal cuff after total hysterectomy. This system allows objective and reproducible documentation of the degree of prolapse.

Imaging Studies

In the setting of a large introital bulge, it may be difficult to differentiate between a severe cystocele, an enterocele, and a high rectocele by physical examination only.[16] Imaging studies should be done to specifically identify which organs are prolapsing. An ideal imaging study should provide precise information about which structures are prolapsed, the presence of urinary retention and obstruction, urethral hypermobility, and urinary incontinence.

Cystourethrography

For a cystourethrogram, the patient should be upright with a full bladder. Films should be taken during both rest and strain. This examination provides information about bladder position, bladder neck funneling, urethral mobility, stress incontinence, and postvoid residual volumes. The presence of a rectocele can also be inferred if bowel gas is identified below the pubic symphysis. This examination is static and does not provide information about other pelvic organs or soft tissues of the pelvic floor.

Dynamic Fluoroscopy

Dynamic fluoroscopy (colpocystodefecography, vaginography) relies on making the organs of interest (bladder, vagina, rectum) radiopaque and studying their positional changes with straining under fluoroscopy. This is a dynamic examination done with the patient upright. Standing recreates the setting in which the patient experiences maximal vaginal bulging. For this procedure, contrast paste must be placed into the vagina and rectum, which can be uncomfortable. Vaginography and defecography are little used now, given the increasing experience and precision of magnetic resonance imaging (MRI).

Ultrasonography

Ultrasound is an attractive imaging modality because it is easy to perform, is minimally invasive, and avoids radiation exposure. Tubo-ovarian and renal disease can also be assessed during the same examination. There is evidence that ultrasound is useful in evaluating bladder neck hypermobility; however, transvaginal imaging for pelvic prolapse does not provide adequate visualization of the soft tissues.[17] Translabial ultrasound can be used to quantify prolapse, although it appears to be better for the anterior compartment and uterine descent than for the posterior compartment.[18] This is not an imaging modality often used for prolapse.

Dynamic Magnetic Resonance Imaging

MRI is becoming a standard in the evaluation of pelvic prolapse. It is performed quickly, without contrast or ionizing radiation, and permits visualization of the soft tissues as well as the upper urinary tract. Gousse and colleagues[30] showed that, in comparison with findings at surgery, MRI had 100% sensitivity, 83% specificity, and a positive predictive value of 97% in assessing cystoceles. Compared with colpocystodefecography, MRI does not require intravesical catheterization, does not require contrast, is fast, and is noninvasive. The drawback is that MRI may underestimate the extent of cystocele and enterocele, because the examination must be performed with the patient in the supine position, which diminishes the downward forces that can be generated with abdominal straining.[19,20] Standing MRI is the ultimate modality in obtaining an even more precise study for prolapse.

Videourodynamics

A urodynamic study can be done with or without video assistance. Both methods provide information about bladder compliance, capacity, sensation of filling, detrusor instability, and contractility. An advantage in performing videourodynamics is the additional information gained in terms of anatomy by monitoring the position and funneling of the bladder neck during filling and straining. The choice to use fluoroscopy should be based on cost, availability, and familiarity with this method.

The importance of documenting the presence of urinary incontinence in patients with large cystoceles is controversial. The incidence of occult stress urinary incontinence is believed to be as high as 22% to 80% among patients with high-stage vaginal vault prolapse.[21] Because of the frequent masked urinary incontinence and the high incidence of postoperative de novo stress incontinence, many surgeons routinely perform a concomitant anti-incontinence procedure along with anterior vaginal reconstruction, independent of the continence status. A study by Barnes and colleagues[22] retrospectively reviewed the charts of 38 women who had grade 3/4 prolapse without significant symptoms of stress incontinence. None of the patients demonstrated stress incontinence during physical examination or videourodynamics studies until the prolapse was mechanically reduced. All patients subsequently had documented stress incontinence, with a mean abdominal leak point pressure of 86 cm H_2O. All patients then underwent surgical repair of the prolapse with placement of a pubovaginal sling. None of the patients developed permanent retention. Recurrent stress incontinence occurred in 5% of the patients. On the other hand, Chaikin and colleagues[23] evaluated 24 "continent" women with severe cystocele. They used a pessary to reduce the cystocele during urodynamic studies and documented incontinence in only 58% of patients. The patients with overt incontinence received an anti-incontinence procedure, and the others did not. With a mean follow-up of 47 months, none of the patients treated only by colporrhaphy developed incontinence. The authors recommended concomitant anti-incontinence procedures only for patients with overt leakage (after the cystocele is reduced). To improve the sensitivity of the urodynamic test to reveal urinary incontinence, a pessary or vaginal pack can be used to reduce the cystocele.[24,25] However, if there is significant pelvic floor relaxation, a pessary may not be able to prevent the prolapse, and it can cause artificial urethral kinking. Additionally, there is no proven correlation between pessary reduction and the reduction obtained with surgery. Therefore, the results of urodynamic testing with a pessary in place cannot be equated with the urinary symptoms after the surgical repair.

Determining the presence of bladder instability is important in preoperative counseling, because it can affect the postoperative result. In most cases (60% to 80%), urgency resolves after surgery.[26] However, some patients have no change in urgency or a worsening of their urgency with sling placement and/or bladder neck elevation. Urodynamic studies may also suggest urinary obstruction with elevated voiding pressure, low urinary flow, or radiographic evidence of urethral kinking.

Cystourethroscopy

Cystourethroscopy is performed to rule out concurrent intraurethral or intravesical pathology such as bladder carcinoma, urethral diverticulum, stones, or foreign bodies (i.e., suture material) from previous surgery. Cystoscopic illumination can also be used to differentiate an enterocele from a cystocele.[27] A pelvic examination is performed with the cystoscope in the bladder. The bladder transilluminates through the anterior vaginal wall so that the extent of the bladder prolapse is demarcated. We assess bladder neck competence both at rest and during straining. Cystourethroscopy can also be used as a bedside urodynamic examination, assessing filling sensation, postvoid residual volume, and visual cystometrics for bladder contractions. With a full bladder, a supine Valsalva stress test can be performed, looking for urethral leakage.

Upper Urinary Tract Evaluation

Patients with a stage 4 cystocele should have upper tract imaging, because there is a 4% to 7% incidence of moderate hydroureteronephrosis among patients with severe vaginal prolapse.[28,29] This risk is greater in patients with procidentia than in those with vault prolapse. Ultrasonography, excretory urography, computed tomography, or MRI may be used. An advantage of MRI is the ability to evaluate the upper urinary tract, tubo-ovarian disease, and pelvic organ prolapse simultaneously.

Laboratory Evaluations

Patients must have sterile urine before proceeding with an operative procedure. In preparation for surgery, we routinely obtain a complete blood count, basic metabolic panel, and coagulation profile in addition to the urine culture.

SURGICAL REPAIR

The goal of repair is to restore pelvic anatomic support of the anterior vaginal wall. This is rarely an independent surgery. Often, surgery entails addressing incontinence as well as prolapse of the uterus and posterior compartment. The end result must restore anatomy and function by restoring the normal vaginal axis and depth and preserving urinary, bowel, and sexual function. It must be kept in mind that anatomy does not always correlate with function.

Treatment of high-grade or symptomatic cystocele must address all defects of the pelvic floor. In the anterior compartment, we must correct urethral hypermobility as well as weakness of lateral bladder support (paravaginal), perivesical fascia (central), and the cardinal-sacrouterine ligament complex.

Transvaginal Paravaginal Repair

This technique simultaneously repairs the four defects present in patients with significant cystocele: support of the hypermobile urethra by a sling procedure, approximation of the cardinal ligaments back to the midline to form the most proximal support of the bladder, repair of the central defect by approximation of the perivesical fascia to the midline, and correction of the lateral defect by support of the bladder neck and bladder base to the obturator fascia using polypropylene mesh. The infralevator obturator "fascia" as it condenses on the pubic bone is the basis of our vaginal paravaginal defect repair; it acts as an immobile structure to secure the mesh. If only the central defect repair is performed, the cystocele may recur (due to the lack of lateral support), and de novo incontinence may ensue because of a poorly supported and hypermobile urethra. On the other hand, if only a bladder neck suspension or plication procedure is performed without correction of the cystocele, the patient may develop aggravation of the prolapse, obstructive symptoms, and urinary retention.

As mentioned, a distal urethral sling is always performed concomitantly with a stage 4 cystocele repair. The sling is placed before the cystocele repair, and the details are described in a separate chapter. Here, we concentrate on the steps of the cystocele repair. If total vaginal prolapse was present, the order of repair would be as follows: transvaginal hysterectomy, vault suspension sutures placed, enterocele repair with pursestring sutures, sling, cystocele repair, vault sutures tied, and rectocele repair.

1. Preparation includes creation of a 1 × 10 cm Prolene mesh sling and a 5 × 5 cm round Prolene mesh disc. Labial sutures are placed, and the weighted speculum is inserted. A suprapubic cystostomy tube and urethral catheter are placed. The bladder is emptied. A ring retractor with multiple hooks is used for additional exposure.
2. A vertical incision is made from the bladder neck to the vaginal cuff. The incision should be superficial enough to avoid bladder perforation but deep enough to expose the perivesical fascia.
3. The vaginal wall is dissected to expose the bladder and proximal urethra. The dissection is carried out in the avascular plane between the vaginal wall and the bladder, *laterally* toward the lateral pelvic wall and obturator fascia and *posteriorly* to expose the cardinal ligaments. The lateral dissection need only extend so far as make it easy to palpate the inferior ramus.
4. A figure-of-eight 2-0 Vicryl suture is applied to the cardinal ligaments to approximate them to the midline. The sutures are not tied at this time. The needle is left attached to the suture and will be used to anchor the mesh later. Intravenous injection of indigo carmine (5 mL) is given at this time, followed by a bolus of 500 mL saline.
5. Interrupted horizontal mattress sutures of 3-0 Vicryl are applied to plicate the attenuated perivesical and periurethral fascia to the midline (anterior colporrhaphy). The sutures are placed superficially but incorporate a wide segment of the perivesical fascia. Deep placement of the sutures should be avoided, to prevent bladder injury or ureteric obstruction. This is not the strength of the central repair but rather facilitates reduction of the defect.
6. Cystoscopy is performed to confirm that the suprapubic tube is in place, the bladder is free of injury, and the ureters excrete indigo-stained urine.
7. The bladder is retracted laterally, using the back of forceps, to facilitate placement of a 2-0 Vicryl suture (CT 1 needle) in the obturator fascia on each side. The key is to palpate the inferior ramus, then place the suture just over the periosteum, taking a strong bite of the infralevator obturator fascia. A strong tug on the suture ensures secure placement. We have found this to be a reliable, strong, nonmobile anchor. Check to make sure the suture was not placed through the vaginal flap.
8. The circular 5 × 5 cm mesh is now used to cover the perivesical fascia and secure the repair. The already placed obturator fascial sutures are used to fix the mesh laterally. Posteriorly, the mesh is fixed to the cardinal ligaments using the previously placed midline suture. Distally, two simple interrupted sutures of 3-0 Vicryl are used to secure the mesh on each side of the bladder neck, taking strong bites of the perivesical fascia. The mesh is trimmed as needed to ensure taut positioning.
9. The excess vaginal wall is trimmed and closed without tension using multiple runs of 3-0 Vicryl. A vaginal packing soaked in antibiotic cream is inserted. No urethral catheter is placed.

Postoperative Care

The antibiotic-soaked vaginal pack is kept in place until discharge. Most patients go home after 24 hours of observation. The suprapubic tube is capped and attempts at voiding are instituted before discharge. Patients are instructed in the use of the suprapubic catheter to check postvoid residuals at home. Most patients void within 24 hours, so the placement of a suprapubic tube or urethral catheter (and possible preoperative teaching of intermittent catheterization) is the surgeon's preference. We do keep the suprapubic catheter in place for at least 1 week to minimize possible urinary extravasation with its removal.

RESULTS

Our early series of 94 consecutive patients with stage 4 cystocele repair showed cure or improvement of the anatomic prolapse in 82% of patients. The range of follow-up was 8 to 22 months. The complication rate was 8%. There was transient retention in two patients and de novo urinary incontinence in 4% of the patients. Although no patient developed recurrent high-grade cystocele, two patients developed mild grade 2 cystoceles. No complications related directly to the mesh were seen; specifically, there were no erosions or graft infections. There have been no cases of permanent urinary retention to date.

CONCLUSION

Armed with a fundamental grasp of the anatomy and pathophysiology of pelvic support, once can more effectively address patients with deficiencies in pelvic support and appropriately apply the current methods of evaluation and treatment discussed in other chapters of this book.

References

1. Bump RC, Mattiasson A, Bo K, et al: The standardization of terminology of female pelvic organ prolapse and pelvic floor dysfunction. Am J Obstet Gynecol 175:10-17, 1996.
2. Zimmern PE, Leach GE, et al: The urological aspects of vaginal wall prolapse. Part I: Diagnosis and surgical indications. AUA Update Series 1993, 12 (Lesson 25).
3. Michael HS, Gousse AE, Rovner ES, et al: Four-defect repair of grade 4 cystocele. J Urol 161:587-594, 1999.
4. Farrell SA, Dempsey T, Geldenhuys L: Histologic examination of "fascia" used in colporrhaphy. Obstet Gynecol 98:794-798, 2001.
5. Zacharin RF: Pelvic Floor Anatomy and the Surgery of Pulsion Enterocele. New York, Springer-Verlag, 1985.
6. DeCaro R, Aragona F, Herms A, et al: Morphometric analysis of the fibroadipose tissue of the female pelvis. J Urol 160:707-713, 1998.
7. Gosling JA, Dixon JS, Critchley HOD, et al: A comparative study of human external sphincter and periurethral levator ani muscles. Br J Urol 53:35-41, 1981.
8. Lawson JO: Pelvic anatomy. I: Pelvic floor muscles. Ann R Coll Surg Engl 54:244-252, 1974.
9. Zvara P, Carrier S, Kour N-W, et al: The detailed neuroanatomy of the human striated urethral sphincter. Br J Urol 74:182-187, 1994.
10. Sharf B, Zilberman A, Sharf M, Mitrani A: Electromyogram of pelvic floor muscles in genital prolapse. Int J Gynecol Obstet 14:2-4, 1976.
11. Wall LL: The muscles of the pelvic floor. Clin Obstet Gynecol 36:910-925, 1993.
12. Babiarz JW, Raz S: Pelvic floor relaxation. In: Raz S (ed): Female Urology, 2nd ed. Philadelphia, WB Saunders, 1996, pp 445-456.
13. Gilpin SA, Gosling JA, Smith ARB, Warrell DW: The pathogenesis of genitourinary prolapse and stress incontinence of urine: A histological and histochemical study. Br J of Obstet Gynecol 96:15-23, 1999.
14. Smith ARB, Hosker GL, Warrell DW: The role of partial denervation of the pelvic floor in teh etiology of genitourinary prolapse and stress incontinence of urine: A neurophysiological study. Br J Obstet Gynecol 96:24-28, 1989.
15. Norton PA: The role of fascia and ligaments. Clin Obstet Gynecol 36:926-938, 1993.
16. Rodriguez LV, Raz S: Diagnostic imaging of pelvic floor dysfunction. Curr Opin Urol 11:423-428, 2001.
17. Gordon D, Pearce M, Norton PA, Stanton SL: Comparison of ultrasound and lateral chain urethrocystography in the determination of bladder neck descent. Am J Obstet Gynecol 160:182-184, 1989.
18. Dietz HP, Haylen BT, Broome J: Ultrasound in the quantification of female pelvic organ prolapse. Ultrasound Obstet Gynecol 18:511-514, 2001.
19. Kelvin FM, Maglinte DD, Hale DS, Benson JT: Female pelvic organ prolapse: A comparison of triphasic dynamic MR imaging and triphasic fluoroscopic cystocolpoproctography. AJR Am J Roentgenol 174:81-88, 2000.
20. Vandbeckevoort D, Van Hoe L, Oyen R, et al: Comparative study of copocystodefography and dynamic fast MR imaging. J Magnetic Resonance 9:373-377, 1999.
21. Gallentine ML, Cespedes RD: Occult stress urinary incontinence and the effect of vaginal vault prolapse on abdominal leak point pressures. Urology 57:40-44, 2001.
22. Barnes NM, Dmochowski RR, Park R, Nitti VW: Pubovaginal sling and pelvic prolapse repair in women with occult stress urinary incontinence: Effect on postoperative emptying and voiding symptoms. Urology 59:856-860, 2002.
23. Chaikin DC, Groutz A, Blaivas JG: Predicting the need for anti-incontinence surgery in continent women undergoing repair of severe urogenital prolapse. J Urol 163:531-534, 2000.
24. Ghoneim GM, Walters F, Lewis V: The value of the vagina pack test in large cystoceles. J Urol 152:931, 1994.
25. Bhatia NN, Bergman A: Pessary test in women with urinary incontinence. Obstet Gynecol 65:220, 1985.
26. Blaivas JG, Jacobs BZ: Pubovaginal fascial sling for the treatment of complicated stress urinary incontinence. J Urol 145:1214, 1991.
27. Vasavada SP, Comiter CV, Raz S: Cystoscopic light test to aid in the differentiation of high-grade pelvic organ prolapse. Urology 54:1085-1087, 1999.
28. Beverly CM, Walters MD, Weber AM, et al: Prevalence of hydronephrosis in patients undergoing surgery for pelvic organ prolapse. Obstet Gynecol 90:37-41, 1997.
29. Gemer O, Bergman M, Segal S: Prevalence of hydronephrosis in patients with genital prolapse. Eur J Obstet Gynecol Reprod Biol 86:11-13, 1999.
30. Gousse AE, Barberic ZL, Safir MH, et al: Dynamic half Fourier acquisition, single turbo spin-echo magnetic resonance imaging for evaluating the female pelvis. J Urol 164(8):1606-13, 2000.

Chapter 65

CYSTOCELE REPAIR USING BIOLOGIC MATERIAL

George D. Webster and Neil D. Sherman

A variety of surgical options are available to the reconstructive surgeon for treatment of anterior vaginal wall prolapse. The traditional surgical approach for cystocele repair is anterior colporrhaphy with plication of the pubocervical fascia. Despite an increased knowledge of pelvic anatomy and advances in surgical techniques, success is variable, and recurrence rates vary from 20% to 40%.[1] Recent literature has suggested that the interposition of graft material over the fascial defect to repair both central and lateral defects of the anterior vaginal wall may increase the success rate of surgery. The purpose of the graft is to allow for replacement or regeneration of fascia by providing a matrix into which in-growth of support tissue will occur.[2] A variety of graft materials are available for such pelvic floor reconstruction.

The properties of an ideal implant (graft material) were described by Cumberland[3] and Scales[4] more than 50 years ago, and the principles remain true today. These characteristics include the proposal that the implant should be elastic or supple, should be easily tailored, and it should have good tensile strength. Additionally, the implant should cause minimal foreign body reaction and allow for good tissue incorporation and collagen in-growth while promoting permanent tissue repair. Finally, the graft must be tolerated in an infected environment and cause minimal wound complications.

To date, the graft that meets all of the above criteria remains elusive. Currently available grafts are most easily classified as biologic or synthetic. Biologic grafts can be further described as autologous, allograft (cadaveric fascia and dermis), or xenograft (e.g., porcine dermis, porcine small intestine submucosa). Synthetic grafts and some biologic biomaterials are discussed elsewhere in the text; this chapter discusses the use of dermal allografts and xenografts for the treatment of anterior vaginal wall prolapse.

BIOMATERIALS

The United States National Institutes of Health (NIH) defines a biomaterial as "any substance (other than a drug) or a combination of substances, synthetic or natural in origin, which can be used for any period of time, as a whole or a part of a system which treats, augments, or replaces any tissue, organ, or function of the body."[5] Currently, there are five types of biomaterials being used in the medical environment: polymers (i.e., in catheters), composites, metals and alloys, ceramics, and biologic materials.[6] Each material offers unique capabilities and advantages based on its composition, its architecture, and whether it is biodegradable.

The concern over possible costly litigation resulted in a worldwide shortage of biomaterials in the mid-1990s. In response, the Biomaterials Access Assurance Act was passed by the U.S. Congress in July 1998 to provide some protection to manufacturers as well as encourage development of new materials.[6] In the United States, the Food and Drug Administration (FDA) regulates medical devices, but not biomaterials, unless they are a component of a medical device. In Europe, any device or apparatus intended for human use is required to have a CE mark, indicating that safety and performance criteria have been met for a particular indication.[7]

Although most would agree that the ideal biomaterial should be reproducible, biocompatible, biodegradeable, and nontoxic, less is understood about the properties required to facilitate the colonization and integration of cells into a functional tissue.[8] A principal factor in the success of a new material is its ability to perform with an appropriate host response in a specific application (i.e., its tissue biocompatibility). Tissue reactions to implanted materials vary widely, and the response determines to a great extent whether the material will be biocompatible.[9]

In the urologic and urogynecologic community, there are a broad range of uses for biomaterials. Biomaterials are used in artificial urinary sphincters, in testicular and penile prostheses, and as injectables for stress incontinence. Additionally, they can be used for the restoration of function or structure (i.e., grafts for Peyronie's disease, bladder augmentation) and for reinforcement of the vaginal wall in prolapse/reconstructive procedures.[7]

The most commonly used natural materials available for prolapse repair include autograft (rectus fascia), allograft (cadaveric fascia,) and xenografts. Xenografts may be either nonabsorbable (i.e., Pelvicol) or absorbable collagen (small intestine submucosa [SIS]).

NONABSORBABLE PORCINE COLLAGEN

Pelvicol (C.R. Bard, Covington, GA) is the most frequently researched and implanted xenograft collagen. It was developed at the University of Dundee in the United Kingdom and was designed for permanent implantation in humans for use in pubovaginal slings, vaginal wall repair, cystoplasty, and phalloplasty.[7] Pelvicol was licensed for use in Europe in 1998 and received approval from the U.S. FDA in 2000. When the tissue is used for applications outside urology and urogynecology, it is distributed under the name Permacol. Porcine collagen is 95% homologous to human collagen, and it appears to provide a strong, nonallergenic scaffold for human tissue growth.[10]

Pelvicol is derived from porcine dermis. A patented process removes all fats and cellular materials, including cells, cell components, and nucleic acids, through a series of organic and enzymatic extractions that leave the material without any DNA.[11,12] The final stage of the processing involves stabilizing the matrix with an approved cross-linking agent to maintain strength and provide permanence. Gamma sterilization of the tissue ensures sterility.

Originally, the grafts were cross-linked with glutaraldehyde. However, this agent was associated with significant calcifications,[13] so now diisocyanate, which has less graft mineralization, is used as the cross-linking agent.[10,14] Ultimately, this final product is a piece of fibrous, acellular, cross-linked porcine dermal collagen that is nonallergenic, is nontoxic, and does not elicit a foreign body response.[15] Also, the resulting material conserves the original three-dimensional architecture of the collagen matrix with a small amount of elastin.[12]

The treated tissue is free of DNA remnants as well as foot and mouth disease,[16] and the manufacturing process has been demonstrated to remove the viral and bacteriologic load from Pelvicol implants. Reoviruses are reduced by more than 12 logs and porcine parvoviruses by 6.7 logs, levels that are acceptable to both the FDA and the European United (EU) regulatory authorities.[17] Once implanted in to human tissue, the implant has been shown to be a biocompatible, sterile, and strong biologic matrix that is permanently incorporated into the host tissue.[15] The graft is available in several sizes depending on its clinical use.

There are other nonabsorbable xenograft collagens produced by other companies, but, as of this publication, human use of these grafts has not been reported. One such graft, Cytrix Soft Tissue Repair Matrix (TEI Biosciences, Boston, MA) is a bovine dermis that does not undergo cross-linking.[18] Whether this difference in processing alters graft strength remains to be seen. In a rat model, Rosenblatt showed that this graft was populated by host fibroblasts and a supporting vasculature. Over 15 months, the implant collagen was remodeled and replaced by the host into collagen that repaired the iatrogenic muscle defect.[18]

Fate of the Graft: Porcine Collagen

Although rejection of porcine dermis has not been reported, case studies suggest an unpredictable tissue response once the graft is implanted. Cole identified a completely encapsulated porcine dermis sling during urethrolysis at 6 months after surgery. Grossly, the sling was intact, and histologically, it was acellular and did not show evidence of human tissue proliferation.[19] Salomon and assocuates reported on 1 patient who underwent exploratory surgery 1 year after implantation of a transobturator Pelvicol graft for cystocele repair. At the time of surgery, there was no inflammation around the graft which was easily freed from surrounding tissues. Histologic evaluation showed colonization by fibroblasts and blood vessels with minimal inflammatory response.[17]

Gandhi and colleagues reviewed the tissue specimens of seven patients with a prior porcine dermal sling and found limited collagen remodeling and evidence of a foreign body–type reaction in patients with postoperative retention. In cases of recurrent stress incontinence, implants appeared to be completely replaced by dense fibroconnective tissue and moderate neovascularization without evidence of inflammation or graft remnants. The authors concluded that this variable tissue reaction raises questions of tolerability and efficacy and may contribute to unpredicitable clinical outcomes.[20]

After implantation, there is a migration of cells, in-growth of tissue, neovascularization, and collagen formation in and around the graft. Although it is unclear what the ultimate biomechanical properties will be like once the graft is implanted, some researchers believe that this connective tissue surrounding the implant adds to its strength.[21]

On the other hand, Dora and coworkers demonstrated in a rat model that porcine dermis and porcine SIS show a marked decreased in tensile strength and stiffness after being implanted for 12 weeks on the abdominal rectus fascia.[22] Whether this mechanical change is of clinical significance remains unknown. In still another animal study, Macleod and colleagues evaluated Permacol 20 weeks after implantation in the Sprague-Dawley rat. Although the graft maintained its thickness over the 20 weeks, there was a decrease in mean collagen density. These findings suggest an overall loss of collagen over the 20 weeks.[9]

Although it appears that there is not one specific factor that is paramount for porcine dermis graft success, attempts have been made to evaluate the integral pieces necessary for success. One belief is that the graft relies, to some degree, on its capacity to be colonized by host cells, and when recurrence occurs, it may be because of compromised native tissue and vascularity contributing to poor graft behavior.[23] In another evaluation of the tissue, Boon and coworkers implanted the graft subcutaneously in a rat model and found minimal fibroblast in-growth into cross-linked collagen. They suggested that cross-linked collagen may be considered for use in situations where neither incorporation nor dissolution of the biomaterial is desired.[24] Others have also seen a low inflammatory response to the Pelvicol.[21] This "tolerance" may contribute to a more ordered deposition of collagen,[21] perhaps allowing the graft to behave similar to autologous tissue.

With respect to vaginal examination after porcine dermis implantation, we are in agreement with the assessment by others that the Pelvicol implant is difficult to palpate postoperatively, whereas that is not always true with some mesh materials.[2] Additionally, there is minimal to no shrinkage of the material, a key factor in sexually active women and in those with preoperative vaginal stenosis.

Some authors have shown that perforating the porcine dermis improves the graft take and decreases wound infections by allowing for increased tissue in-growth and revascularization of the vaginal epithelilum overlying the graft. Tensile strength and suture pull-out strength were maintained in the perforated graft.[25]

RESULTS: PORCINE COLLAGEN

Long-term data for porcine dermis in cystocele repair are generally lacking, but early results are promising (Table 65-1). De Ridder compared the Raz classic cystocele repair using polyglactin mesh with a modified Raz technique using a Pelvicol implant as an overlay graft material. Follow-up was only 9.3 months, but there were no recurrences or erosions in the Pelvicol group.[2] Fischer used Pelvicol implant for cystocele repair in 14 patients, for rectocele repair in 80 patients, and for combined repair in 10 patients.[26] With follow-up of at least 6 months, there were no cases of extrusion, recurrence, shrinkage, induration, dyspareunia, or urgency-frequency syndrome. Gomelsky used porcine dermis for cystocele repairs with and without anti-incontinence surgery or vault suspension in 70 patients. With follow-up of at

Table 65-1 Results of Porcine Dermis Implants for the Correction of Anterior Vaginal Wall Prolapse

Study (Ref. No.)	*N*	Follow-up (Mo)	Objective Cure	Recurrence	Adverse Events	Implant Trade Name
De Ridder (2)	28	9.3		None	No erosions	Pelvicol
Fischer (26)	104	>6		Not provided	No extrusion	
Gomelsky et al (10)	70	24		8.6% grade 2, 4.3% grade 3	Superficial wound separation treated conservatively (1 case)	Intexen
Leboeuf et al (23)		15	93%	6.9% (2 pts grade 2, 1 pt grade 3)	4.7% postoperative retention; 11.7% de novo urge incontinence	Pelvicol
Steinberg et al (27)	81	8.5	69%	26% first degree (Baden-Walker); 4.9% second degree	Each preoperative stage of prolapse showed significant improvement postoperatively	Porcine dermis (company not stated)
Salomon et al (17)	27	14	81%	1 pt stage 1, 4 pts stage 2; all pts had stage 3 or 4 preoperatively	Placed via transobturator approach, combined with bilateral sacrospinous fixation; 1 graft removed because of pain at transfixing vaginal stitch	Pelvicol
Ruparelia et al (29)	48	20	85% pt satisfaction rate, 78% symptomatic improvement	2% reoperation rate	2 wound breakdowns	Pelvicol
Kocjancic et al (30)	79	6.5	73% optimal anatomic outcomes		2 poor wound healing managed as outpatient; no graft infection/rejection	Pelvicol
Verleyen et al (31)		8		1 pt stage 1	No infection, erosion, or rejection	Pelvicol
Graul et al (32)	37	6			1 expulsion; 1 small graft erosion	Pelvicol
Flam (33)	59			None	24% anaerobic infection	Pelvicol
Paparella et al (34)	45			1 pt stage 2	No infection, erosion, or rejection	Pelvicol
Cervigni et al (35)		8.8	68% anatomic cure		1 erosion	

pt, patient; pts, patients.

least 12 months, 9 patients (12.9%) had asymptomatic recurrent cystoceles that were managed conservatively.[10] Steinberg used a 6 × 12 cm trapezoid piece of porcine dermis to perform vaginal paravaginal repair. When patients were analyzed stage for stage, there was a statistically significant improvement from preoperative to postoperative stage of prolapse.[27]

Besides anatomic improvement with the use of a graft, Sundar showed that the use of porcine collagen provides a significant overall improvement in quality of life.[28]

SMALL INTESTINE SUBMUCOSA

SIS is harvested from porcine jejunum and is composed of the stratum compactum of the tunica mucosa, the tunica muscularis mucosa, and the tunica submucosa.[9] Processing leaves the extracellular collagen matrix intact, thus allowing the presence of collagen, growth factors, glycosaminoglycans, proteoglycans, and glycoproteins to promote host cell proliferation through SIS layers.[36] Theoretically, the SIS scaffold should be entirely remodeled and replaced by the host's connective tissue in 90 days.[37] SIS for pelvic reconstruction is currently available in 1-ply and 4-ply sheets for prolapse repairs (SurgiSIS and SurgiSIS ES, Cook Inc., Bloomington, IN).

To date, there are few published data available on the use of porcine SIS for the treatment of pelvic organ prolapse. In one small human study, eight patients underwent SurgiSIS-augmented vaginal prolapse surgery. At follow-up, there was adequate support of the vaginal wall, and symptom scores showed improvement.[38] Although the database for pelvic reconstruction is small, SIS has been used as a pubovaginal sling[39,40] and for the treatment of abdominal wall hernias, where it was effective in both clean and clean-contaminated repairs.[41]

As with other biologic materials, in vivo human studies for prolapse repair are lacking. Therefore, response of the implant in this application must be extrapolated from its use in pubovaginal sling surgery. In three humans requiring exploration after SIS pubovaginal sling placement, Weidemann and Otto found minimal SIS implant and no inflammatory or foreign body reaction.[42] These results were in stark contrast to the significant inflammatory reaction found after an 8-ply SIS graft was placed as a sling.[43,44] In an attempt to limit the inflammatory response, modifications to the graft and instructions for its use have been made.

A number of animal studies evaluating SIS have been performed. Other authors have used a rat model to show that SIS initially shows a moderate degree of chronic inflammation that falls to minimal levels in a 20-week period of implantation.[9]

In a rabbit model, porcine SIS was shown to decrease in surface area by 41%.[22] The clinical implications for this finding with respect to anterior vaginal wall repair were not expanded on and in reality are unknown.

In a canine model, a piece of SIS was used to replace a portion of bladder wall. Immunohistochemical examination of the regenerated bladder at 15 months showed normal histology (epithelium, muscle, and serosa) and presence of nerves and other constituents (calcitonin gene-related peptide and substance P immunoreactive nerve fibers). Of note, in vitro testing of the new bladder wall for compliance and contractility showed it to be similar in function to the original bladder wall. To date, there have been no clinical trials.[45] It remains to be seen how this knowledge can be incorporated into the use of SIS for the generation of a graft for prolapse repair.

Using a rabbit model, Claerhout and colleagues evaluated various materials including SIS and Pelvicol in abdominal wall defects. By 3 months, the SIS appeared as a thin, almost transparent membrane. For SIS, the point of weakness was determined to be the material itself, whereas for Pelvicol the maximum point of weakness was the interface between graft and native tissue.[46]

HUMAN DERMIS

The most common cadaveric dermis used in pelvic reconstructive surgery is AlloDerm (LifeCell Corp, Branchburg, NJ); Duraderm (C.R. Bard Inc, Murray Hill, NJ) has less information for prolapse repair available.[47] Cadaveric dermis is an acellular and immunologically inert biologic biomaterial that works by acting as a biologic scaffold for tissue remodeling.[48] Graft preparation involves decellularization to remove the epidermis and dermis while preserving the basement membrane complex.[49] The graft then undergoes freeze-drying such that the collagen, elastin, and proteoglycans are maintained.[48] The biomechanical properties of dermal grafts have been shown to be similar to those of autologous rectus fascia and solvent-dehydrated cadaveric fascia.[50]

Although intact DNA has been found in acellular cadaveric dermis,[51] it has not been associated with disease transmission in recipients. The American Association of Tissue Banks is the organization responsible for maintaining screening and procurement standards.

Dermal allograft has been used for many different surgical procedures,[52,53] including pelvic floor reconstruction.[54-57] One potential benefit of the tissue is its ability to maintain elasticity. However, it remains unclear whether this characteristic prevents recurrence by allowing the vaginal wall to stretch with Valsalva maneuvers and then return to its original position, or whether the elasticity contributes to failure because it may be stretched too far.[57] Histologically, it appears that dermal allograft completely incorporates into the host fibromuscular layer, with no significant inflammation and no identifiable graft 2 years after implantation.[58] Variations in processing may affect success rates with cadaveric fascia, but studies with cadaveric dermis are lacking.[59] If complications such as graft extrusion occur, they can be managed conservatively with topical estrogen cream.[60]

Human studies for anterior wall reconstruction are limited; results are shown in Table 65-2.

BOVINE PERICARDIUM

Experience with bovine pericardium for cystocele repair is extremely limited, and indeed, in our opinion, very suspect. McLennan used this graft in 61 patients undergoing vaginal paravaginal repair. With a mean follow-up of 7.25 months, 6.5% of

Table 65-2 Results of Cadaveric Dermal Graft for the Treatment of Anterior Vaginal Wall Prolapse

Study (Ref. No.)	*N*	Follow-up (Mo)	Outcome	Complications
Jelovsek et al (54)	9	18.4	44% stage 0-1	20% site granulation tissue (includes posterior repairs)
Chung et al (55)	19	28	16% objective failure	
Clemonset al (57)	33	18	41% objective failures (stage >2); 3% subjective failures	No erosion/rejection
Graul & Hurst (61)	67	10.2	2 failures defined as stage 2 or greater	1 erosion treated conservatively; 1 graft expulsion

patients had a stage 2 or greater anterior wall prolapse. There were no cases of graft erosion, and the authors noted that by 6 weeks vaginal tissue was supple and normal.[62] However, when bovine pericardium was used for pubovaginal sling procedures, the rate of erosion was much more significant.[63,64]

SURGICAL TECHINIQUE

Surgery is performed with the patient under either general or spinal anesthesia. Sequential compression devices are placed preoperatively, and prophylactic antibiotic coverage is given on call to the operating room. The patient is placed in dorsal lithotomy position with Allen stirrups.

Concominant procedures such as a hysterectomy or pubovaginal sling can be performed at the same sitting. Usually, prolapse repair is completed before anti-incontinence surgery or rectocele repair and after hysterectomy. If the patient has had a prior hysterectomy, the uterosacral ligaments are sutured and tagged for easier identification. The vaginal epithelium is injected with 0.25% Marcaine. Incision of the vaginal epithelium is usually in the midline. Lateral vaginal flaps are elevated superficial to the pubocervical fascia, all the way to the obturator fascia laterally and the uterosacral/cardinal ligaments proximally. The endopelvic fascia is perforated, and dissection is carried into the space of Retzius bilaterally. The arcus tendineus fascia pelvis is identified laterally where it attaches to the obturator internus fascia.

The native fascia may be brought together in the midline with absorbable or nonabsorbable suture depending on surgeon preference. The graft is prepared on the back table according to the manufacturer's recommendations and then brought into the vagina and trimmed to an appropriate size. Initial tapering should err on the large side so as not to foreshorten the graft. The graft is secured to the vaginal cuff and uterosacral ligaments proximally at the vaginal apex and then laterally to the obturator fascia, using interrupted 2-0 polyglycolic acid suture. Distally, the graft should be affixed to the arcus or the fascia overlying the inferior ramus of the pubis at the level of the bladder neck. Tailoring of the graft shape is accomplished as the graft fixation progresses distally. Copious antibiotic irrigation may be used throughout the procedure. Cystoscopy is performed to confirm integrity of the bladder and ureters.

After the graft has been secured in place, redundant vaginal epithelium is trimmed, and the vaginal wall is closed with interrupted absorbable suture. If an anti-incontinence procedure is necessary, it may be performed at this time via a separate incision.

CONCLUSION

Biologic biomaterials may have a valuable role in reconstructive procedures for anterior vaginal wall prolapse. When graft material is required, the surgeon must identify the positive properties of each option and determine the most appropriate material for the individual patient. Future technologic advancements may one day provide the ideal graft material that meets all the necessary criteria for long-term durability and success.

Disclaimer

The authors have been asked to review the use of particular biologic materials in the repair of anterior vaginal wall defects and to provide comment. This does not represent endorsement of use of such materials, and it should be stated that "the jury is still out" regarding the optimal approach and materials one should use to enhance the success of repairs of the anterior vaginal compartment.

References

1. Macer GA:Transabdominal repair of cystocele, a 20 year experience, compared with the traditional vaginal approach. Am J Obstet Gynecol 131:203-207, 1978.
2. De Ridder D:The use of biomaterials in reconstructive urology. Eur Urol 1(Suppl):7-11, 2002.
3. Cumberland VH: A preliminary report on the use of prefabricated nylon weave in the repair of ventral hernia. Med J Aust 1:143-144, 1952.
4. Scales JT: Materials for hernia repair. Proc R Soc Med 46:647-652, 1953.
5. National Institutes of Health: Clinical applications of biomaterials. NIH Consensus Statement 4(5):1-19, 1982.
6. Science and Technology Policy Institute: Biomaterials availability: Potential effects on medical innovation and health care. [Issue paper.] Rand IP-194:1-60, 2000.
7. Lloyd SN, Cross W: The current use of biomaterials in urology. Eur Urol 1(Suppl):2-6, 2002.
8. Kimuli M, Eardley I, Southgate J: In vitro assessment of decellularized porcine dermis as a matrix for urinary tract reconstruction. BJU Int 94:859-866, 2004.
9. Macleod TM, Williams G, Sanders R, Green CJ: Histological evaluation of Permacol™ as a subcutaneous implant over a 20week period in the rat model. Br J Plast Surg 58:518-532, 2005.
10. Gomelsky A, Rudy DC, Dmochowski RR: Porcine dermis interposition graft for repair of high grade anterior compartment defects with or without concomitant pelvic organ prolapse procedures. J Urol 171:1581-1584, 2004.
11. Oliver RF, Barker H, Cooke A, et al: Dermal collagen implants. Biomaterials 3:38-40, 1982.
12. Grosh SK, Hanke CW, DeVore DP, Gibbons DG: Variables affecting the results of xenogenic collagen implantation in an animal model. J Am Acad Dermatol 13:792-798, 1985.
13. McPherson JM, Sawamura S, Armstrong R: An examination of the biologic response to injectable glutaraldehyde cross-linked collagen implants. J Biomed Res 20:93, 1986.
14. Oliver RF: Scar and collagen implantation. Burns 13:S49-S55, 1987.
15. Harper C: Permacol™: clinical experience with a new biomaterial. Hosp Med 62:90-95, 2001.
16. Data on File: Pelvicol™ acellular collagen matrix foot and mouth disease. Tissue Science Laboratories, PLC, Manufacturers Statement, March 2001.
17. Salomon LJ, Detchev R, Barranger E, et al: Treatment of anterior vaginal wall prolapse with porcine skin collagen implant by the transobturator route: Preliminary results. Eur Urol 45:219-225, 2004.
18. Rosenblatt P: Repair of abdominal muscle defects with implants composed of xenogenic fetal collagen: Long term (15 month) in vivo evaluation of implant reconstitution and remodeling. Presented at the International Continence Society Annual Meeting, Paris, France, August, 2004.
19. Cole E, Gomelsky A, Dmochowski RR: Encapuslation of a porcine demris pubovaginal sling. J Urol 170:1950, 2003.
20. Gandhi S, Kubba LM, Abramov Y, et al: Histopathologic changes of porcine dermis xenografts for transvaginal suburethral slings. Am J Obstet Gynecol 192:1643-1648, 2005.

21. Zheng F, Lin Y, Verbeken E, et al: Host respons after reconstruction of abdominal wall defects with porcine dermal collagen in a rat model. Am J Obstet Gynecol 191:1961-1970, 2004.
22. Dora CD, Dimarco DS, Zobitz ME, Elliott DS: Time dependent variations in biomechanical properties of cadaveric fascia, porcine dermis, porcine small intestine submucosa, polypropylene mesh and utologous fascia in the rabbit model: implications for sling surgery. J Urol 171:1970-1973, 2004.
23. Leboeuf L, Miles RA, Kim SS, Gousse AE: Grade 4 cystocele repair using four-defect repair and porcine xenograft acellular matrix (Pelvicol): Outcome measures using SEAPI. Urology 64:282-286, 2004.
24. Boon ME, Ruijgrok JM, Vardaxis MJ: Collagen implants remain supple not allowing fibroblast ingrowth. Biomaterials 16:1089-1093, 1995.
25. Taylor G, Moore R, Miklos J, Mattox T: Posterior repair with perforated porcine dermal graft. Presented at International Continence Society Annual Meeting, Paris, France, 2004.
26. Fischer A: Prolapse surgery using biomaterials. Eur Urol Suppl 1:29-32, 2002.
27. Steinberg AC, Oyama IA, Feloney M, et al: Vaginal paravaginal repair with the use of porcine dermis. J Pelvic Med Surg 11:88, 2005.
28. Sundar K, Pain S, Ruparelia B: Quality of life (QOL) after pelvic floor repair with porcine collagen. Int Urogynecol J Pelvic Floor Dysfunct 12(Suppl 1):10-11, 2002.
29. Ruparelia BA, Gunasheela S, Sundar K: Anterior and posterior vaginal prolapse repairs with porcine skin collagen (Pelvicol™) implant. Int Urogynaecol J 11(Suppl 1):FDP33 S45, 2000.
30. Kocjancic E, Meshia M, Pifarotti P, et al: Multicentre randomized trial of Pelvicol™ implant in the treatment of cystocele. J Urol 173:233, 2005.
31. Verleyen P, Filip C, Bart K, et al: A prospective randomized trial comparing Pelvicol™ and Vicryl™ cystocele repair in the Razcolposuspension. Presented at Annual International Continence Society Meeting, Paris, France, August 2004.
32. Graul EA, Hurst B, Abbott T: Porcine allograft in the repair of anterior and posterior vaginal wall defects. Int Urogynecol J Pelvic Floor Dysfunct 13(Suppl 1):7, 2002.
33. Flam F: Pelvicol™ implant for the operative treatment of prolapse. Int Urogynecol J Pelvic Floor Dysfunct 13(Suppl 1):5, 2002.
34. Paparella P, Ercoli A, Marturano M, et al: The use of porcine dermal implant in the vaginal surgical repair of stage II-IV anterior vaginal wall prolapse: Feasibility, short term complications and results. Presented at the International Continence Society 33rd Annual Congress, October 2003, Florence, Italy.
35. Cervigni M, Natale F, Weir J, et al: Prospective randomized trial of two new materials for the correction of anterior compartment prolapse: Pelvicol and Prolene Soft. Presented at the 35th Annual Meeting of the International Continence Society Meeting, Montreal, Canada, September 2005.
36. Voytik-Harbin SL, Brightman AO, Kraine MR, et al: Identification of extractable growth factors from small intestinal submucosa. J Cell Biol 67:478-491, 1997.
37. Sandusky GE, Lantz GC, Badylak SF: Healing comparison of small intestine mucosa and ePTFE grafts in the canine carotid artery. J Surg Res 58:415-420, 1995.
38. Ellerkmann RM, Dunn JS, Blomquist JL, et al: Evaluation of graft biomaterial in reconstructive pelvic surgery: A pilot study. Proceedings of the 23rd annual meeting of the American Urogynecologic Society, San Francisco, CA, Oct 17-19, 2002.
39. Rutner AB, Levine SR, Schmaelzle JF: Processed porcine small intestine submucosa as a graft material for pubovaginal slings: Durability and results. Urology 62:805-809, 2003.
40. Jones JS, Cherullo EE, Abdelmalak JB, et al: Small intestine submucosa (SIS): Minimally invasive non-synthetic sling. Presented at the American Urological Association Annual Meeting, Orlando, FL, May 25-30, 2002.
41. Helton WS, Fisichella PM, Berger R, et al: Short-term outcomes with small intestinal submucosa for ventral abdominal hernia. Arch Surg 140:549-560, 2005.
42. Wiedemann A, Otto M: Small intestinal submucosa for pubourethral sling suspension for the treatment of stress incontinence: First histopathological resuls in humans. J Urol 172:215-218, 2004.
43. Ho KLV, Witte MN, Bird ET: Eight-ply small intestinal submucosa tenstion-free sling: Spectrum of postoperative inflammation. J Urol 171:268-271, 2004.
44. Kalota S: Small intestinal submucosa tenstion-free sling: Postoperative inflammatory reactions and additional data. J Urol 172:1349-1350, 2004.
45. Kropp BP, Sawyer BD, Shannon HE, et al: Characterization of small intestinal submucosa regenerated canine detrusor: assessment of reinnervation, in vitro compliance and contractility. J Urol 156(2S):599-607, 1996.
46. Claerhout F, Deprest J, Zheng F, et al: Long term evaluation of the tissue response and mechanical properties of two collagen based and polypropylene implants and a rabbit model for abdominal wall repair. Presented at the 33rd Annual Congress of the International Incontinence Society, Florence, Italy, October 2003.
47. Owens DC, Winters JC: Pubovaginal sling using Duraderm graft: Intermediate follow-up and patient satisfaction. Neurourol Urodyn 23:115-118, 2004.
48. AlloDerm regenerative tissue matrix. LifeCell Corporation. Available at: http://www.lifecell.com (accessed August 15, 2007).
49. Livesey S, Atkinson Y, Call T, et al: An acellular dermal transplant processed from human cadaver skin retains normal extracellular matrix components and ultrastructural characteristics. The American Association of Tissue Banks (AATB) Conference, Boston, Massachusetts, August 1994.
50. Lemer ML, Chaiken DC, Blaivas JG: Tissue strength analysis of autologous and cadaveric allografts for the pubovaginal sling. Neurourol Urodyn 18:497-503, 1999.
51. Choe JM, Bell T: Genetic material is present in cadaveric dermis and cadaveric fascia lata. J Urol 166:122-124, 2001.
52. Wainwright DJ: Use of an acullular allograft dermal matrix (Alloderm) in the management of full-thickness burns. Burns 21:243-248, 1995.
53. Chaplin JM, Costantino PD, Wolpoe ME, et al: Use of an acellular dermal allograft for dural replacement: An experimental study. Neurosurgery 45:320-327, 1999.
54. Jelovsek JE, Amundsen C, Addison WA, Weidner AC: Outcomes of pelvic organ prolapse surgery with Alloderm™ graft. Proceedings of the 23rd annual meeting of the American Urogynecologic Society, San Francisco, California, October 17-19, 2002.
55. Chung SY, Franks M, Smith CP, et al: Technique of combined pubovaginal sling and cystocele repair urisn a single piece of cadaveric dermal graft. Urology 59:538-541, 2002.
56. Miklos JR, Kohli N: Rectovaginal fistula repair utilizing a cadaveric dermal allograft. Int Urogynecol J Pelvic Floor Dysfunct 10:405-406, 1999.
57. Clemons JL, Myers DL, Aguilar VC, Arya LA: Vaginal paravaginal repair with an AlloDerm graft. Am J Obstet Gynecol 189:1612-1619, 2003.
58. Graul EA, Hurst B, Abbott T: Disposition of dermal allograft tissue two years after implantation. Proceedings of the 23rd annual meeting of the American Urogynecologic Society, San Francisco, California, October 17-19, 2002.
59. Crivellaro S, Smith JJ, Kocjancic E, Bresette JF: Transvaginal sling using acellular human dermal allograft: Safety and efficacy in 253 patients. J Urol 172:1374-1378, 2004.
60. Drake NL, Weidner AC, Webster GD, Amundsen CL: Patient characteristics and management of dermal allograft extrusions. Int Urogynecol J Pelvic Floor Dysfunct 16:375-377, 2005.

61. Graul EA, Hurst B: An alternative technique for the repair of pelvic prolapse. Int Urogynecol J Pelvic Floor Dysfunct 12(Suppl 1):3, 2002.
62. McLennan M, Leong FC, Melick C: Bovine pericardium augmentation graft for vaginal paravaginal defect repair of the anterior segment. Presented at the Annual Meeting of the International Continence Society, Paris, France, August 2004.
63. Martucci RC, Ambrogini A, Calado AA, et al: Pubovaginal sling with bovine pericardium for treatment of stress urinary incontinence. Braz J Urol 26:208-214, 2000.
64. Candido EB, Triginelli SA, Silva Filho AL, et al: The use of bovine pericardium in the pubovaginal sling for the treatment of stress urinary incontinence. Rev Bras Ginecol Ostet 25:525-528, 2003.

Chapter 66

TENSION-FREE CYSTOCELE REPAIR USING PROLENE MESH

Mauro Cervigni and Franca Natale

Pelvic organ prolapse (POP) is one of the emerging problems in women, considering the aging population in Western countries together with already known risk factors such as race, genetic predisposition, pregnancy, parity, obstetric trauma, menopause, and previous gynecologic surgery. Among these factors, certainly white Caucasian women have a higher odds ratio (1.0) with respect to African American and Hispanic women (0.6 and 1.2, respectively).[1]

Considering the different segments involved in the development of POP, the anterior vaginal wall, and in particular the bladder, represented the site most frequently affected in a study of 27,000 American women; the posterior segment (rectocele) was present in 19%, and uterine prolapse in 14%.[1]

Mant and colleagues, in 1997, studied a group of 17,000 women and observed that the incidence of anterior colporrhaphy was 37%, compared with a 24% rate of vaginal hysterectomy.[2]

Numerous surgical procedures have been proposed in the last century to correct all types of anterior vaginal wall defects (central, paravaginal, combined), using either an abdominal or vaginal approach. Despite improved understanding of pelvic anatomy and organ function and the advancement of surgical techniques, the long-term success rate is still variable. Recurrence rates for the various surgical procedures used to treat anterior vaginal prolapse range from 3%[3] to 20%[4] after single anterior colporrhaphy, from 22%[5] to 92%[6] if the anterior colporrhaphy is combined with other procedures (sacrospinous ligament suspension), from 2%[7] to 59%[8] after four-corner suspension, and from 5%[9] to 50%[10] after vaginal paravaginal repair. The reasons for such discrepancies are several and include poor patient selection, suboptimal surgical technique, inappropriate choice of suture material, and persistence of predisposing risk factors for prolapse (constipation, chronic respiratory disease).[11] Moreover, Farrell and colleagues emphasized that the very existence of the pubocervical fascia used during anterior colporrhaphy is doubtful. They observed in samples obtained during surgical procedures for the correction of anterior defect that the so-called fascia is adequately identified only 58% of the time and concluded that this finding calls into question techniques that rely on isolated fascia for the repair of anterior and posterior defects.[12]

In addition, recent information on the biochemical and ultrastructural composition of the connective tissue of the pelvic floor has provided new insight into its role in stabilization of the pelvic organs and in the healing processes after surgery.

EVOLUTION OF SURGICAL PROCEDURES

In the last 20 years, the repair of anterior vaginal wall prolapse has shifted from a classic anterior repair to a more detailed surgical procedure (site-specific repair) with an attempt to identify the precise localization of the tissue defect. For example, Richardson and associates proposed the vaginal paravaginal repair using native tissues to restore the anatomy.[13] These concepts were further explored in surgery of the posterior compartment. However, despite encouraging results, the anterior segment (i.e., the connective tissue supporting the bladder) remained the site of least durability.[14,15]

Moreover, the rate of complications was not insignificant (11% ureteral occlusion), and the conclusions of Barber and Bump were that a correct vaginal reconstruction is best accomplished in women with severe stress conditions (severe constipation, chronic pulmonary disease, occupation and recreational straining, severe compromise of pelvic floor neuromuscular function) with techniques that do not rely solely on the patient's native tissue for support and that this is often achieved with the use of synthetic mesh or tissue graft substitution.

CONNECTIVE TISSUE AND ITS ROLE IN THE PELVIC FLOOR

Connective tissue is analogous to a fiber-reinforced composite, containing fibrous elements (collagen and elastin) and a viscoelastic matrix including proteoglycans (large polysaccharides attached to proteins). The cells in the connective tissues, which form about 20% of the tissue volume, are embedded in the extracellular matrix. The biomechanical properties of a soft tissue are determined by the various extracellular matrix components. Collagen, which accounts for a large proportion of tissue strength, is a protein produced by fibroblasts with a specific pattern that is remarkable for its consistency. The amino acid glycine allows collagen to form a tight helix, one of its important attributes. Two other amino acids are present in its structure, namely proline and hydroxyproline. These amino acids form cross-links that stabilize the collagen chains. The collagen fibers responsible for the tensile strength of the tissue are a family of 16 different types distributed in different parts of the body. Of these, type I (the most common and strongest) and type III (smaller and randomly organized with type I), are found in tissue that requires strength and flexibility.

Elastin and laminin are two other glycoproteins that may play a role in elasticity of the ground substance. Elastin provides the ability of a tissue to be stretched and is found not only in the bladder as a component of compliance but also in the urethra. Elastin is degraded by elastase, which is part of a protease-antiprotease control mechanism found in the plasma. It has recently been demonstrated that there is an increase in the percentage activity of elastase in women with stress urinary incontinence (SUI) compared with aged-matched controls.[16] Several factors, such as age, stress, hormones, and growth factors, are involved in the regulation of connective tissue metabolism.[17]

Collagen turnover slows down with increasing age, and the concentration increases after menopause.[18-21] The changes during menopause seem to generate a connective tissue with a higher collagen concentration but with alterations in cross-linking,[22] and there is also an increase in fibril diameter in the cardinal and uterosacral ligament in patients with POP and SUI. This produces a tissue with an increased load-bearing ability but decreased elasticity.[23] Based on biochemical assays, Sayer and colleagues[24] reported modification of cross-linking in women with bladder neck prolapse and SUI. A reduction of collagen in the pubocervical fascia[25] and in nonsupportive pelvic tissue has also been observed.[26] Recent studies indicate that women of fertile age with SUI demonstrate changes in the extracellular matrix of the paraurethral connective tissue resulting in a stiffer and less supportive connective tissue and a defect in the connective tissue glue.[27-30] In women with genital prolapse after menopause, there seems to be a difference in collagen metabolism suggesting a change in the degradation of collagen related to matrix metalloproteinases and with a significant reduction in the ratio of type I to type III collagen.[31] Therefore, it is not the amount of collagen but the amount of fresh elastic collagen that is important for the mechanical strength of supporting fascia layers.

HEALING PROCESS AFTER SURGICAL REPAIR

When a wound is created, such as an anterior vaginal wall and pubocervical fascia incision, fibrous protein synthesis and remodeling reestablish tissue strength. Collagen is a central factor in wound healing. The first day after injury, immature fibroblasts synthesize and secrete collagen and proteoglycans. A weaker and more elastic flexible type III collagen is the principal type found in early wounds. After 2 weeks, the majority of regenerated tissue is composed of type III collagen, which accounts for only 7% of its final tensile strength. With maturation of the scar, a stronger type I gradually replaces the type III collagen. In this way, an organized cross-linked pattern regains some tensile strength, but the new tissue is never as strong as the original tissue.[32] The factors that influence healing and scar maturation are still incompletely understood, even though we know that the gene for type III collagen seems to be activated more than the gene for type I collagen.[33]

Elastin is a protein that the body does not seem to be able to synthesize and remodel, as it does collagen. Lack of elastin and high amounts of the less strong type III collagen may explain why new scars lack strength and elasticity.

WHAT HAPPENS WHEN A MESH IS IMPLANTED IN THE BODY

When a graft is introduced into a biologic tissue, there is a strong immediate (antibody-mediated) foreign body reaction, followed by blood flow increase, temperature rise, macrophage migration, and attempted phagocytosis of the foreign body. The graft incorporation process includes a cascade of events: first, there is a rapid activation of polymorphonuclear cells and macrophages; 60 hours later, there is fibroblast proliferation with a subsequent slow phenomenon of fibroplasia and blood vessel proliferation

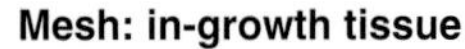

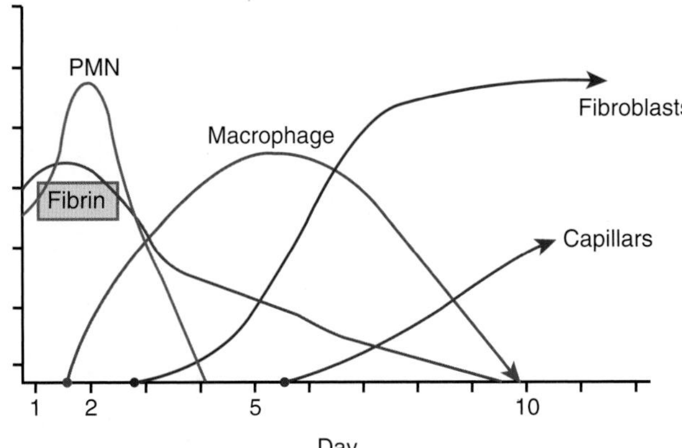

Figure 66-1 In-growth of tissue in mesh implants. PMN, polymorphonuclear cells.

(angiogenesis) with in-growth of capillaries. These modifications lead to synthesis of collagen and then to maturation of these new fibers (cross-linking).

These events happen as a result of the interaction between the graft materials (biologic or synthetic) and the tissue interface, which is of prime importance; for this reason, we need to reduce the intensity and time of the inflammatory period, in particular with regard to reducing potential complications (erosion and extrusion) (Fig. 66-1).

Once the prosthetic material has been implanted, there are four types of tissue reactions: minimal response with a thin layer of fibrosis around the implant; chemical response with a severe and chronic inflammatory reaction around the implant; physical response with an inflammatory reaction to certain materials and the presence of giant cells; and necrotic tissue, a layer of necrotic debris produced as a result of in situ exothermic polymerization.[34]

WHAT MATERIALS ARE CURRENTLY AVAILABLE FOR THE SURGICAL REINFORCEMENT OF PELVIC TISSUE?

The following materials are currently available for the surgical reinforcement of pelvic tissue: synthetic material, which acts as a substitute for natural tissue; autograft, which is tissue obtained from another area of the patient's body; allograft, which is tissue obtained from a human donor; and acellular collagen matrix, such as dermal (skin) tissue from pigs.

PROPERTIES OF SYNTHETIC BIOMATERIALS

Biocompatibility is the capability of a material to provoke a favorable reaction when introduced into a living system. Consequently, a biomaterial is any material, natural or man-made, or any biomedical device that performs, augments, or replaces a natural function. One definition of biocompatibility is "the utopian state where a biomaterial presents an interface with a physiologic environment without the material adversely affecting that environment or the environment adversely affecting the material." The biomaterials employed can come close to this utopian state, but we must accept compromises between the

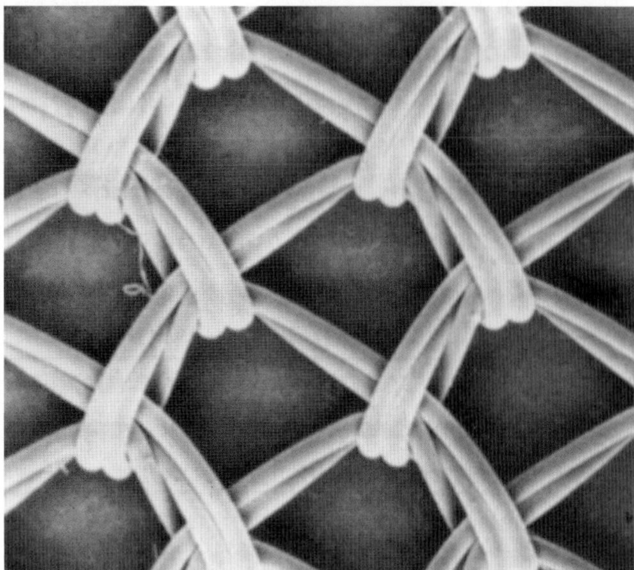

Figure 66-2 Type I synthetic mesh: monofilament polypropylene.

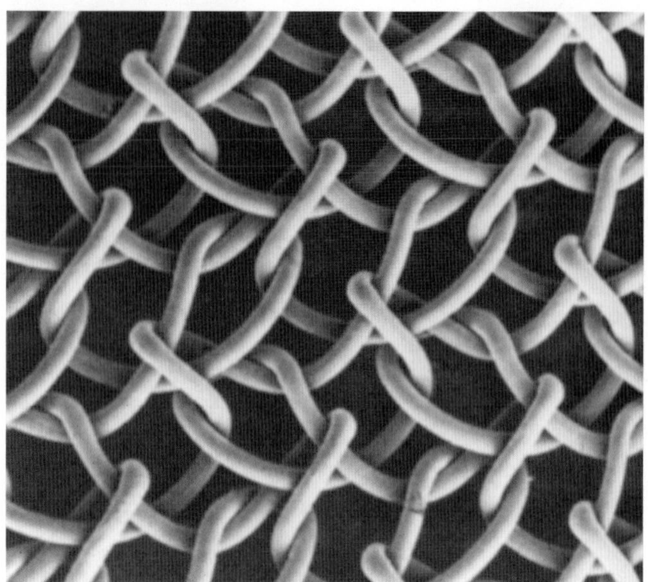

Figure 66-3 Type I synthetic mesh: Marlex.

benefits and the undesired reactions caused to the living system by the material.

Cumberland[35] and Scales[36] delineated a series of properties of an "ideal" synthetic biocompatible materials:

- Chemically and physically inert
- Noncarcinogenic
- Mechanically strong
- Does not cause allergic or inflammatory reactions
- Can be sterilized
- No physical modification by body tissue
- Convenient and affordable format for clinical use

At the present time none of the synthetic meshes meet all of these criteria.

Although from the chemical point of view all of the synthetic meshes are completely biocompatible, some physical and structural properties of the prosthesis are associated with certain complications. Prevention of biomaterial-related complications requires a profound knowledge of the physical properties of prostheses, of which the *porosity* (*pore size*) of the materials are of paramount importance.

Based on their pore size, the most common synthetic meshes can be classified into four types:

Type I: totally macroporous materials such as Atrium, Marlex, Prolene, and Trelex. These meshes contain pores larger than 75 μm (microns), which is the required size for admission of macrophages, fibroblasts (fibroplasia), blood vessels (angiogenesis), and collagen fibers into the pores (Figs. 66-2 and 66-3).[37,38]

Type II: totally microporous materials such as expanded polytetrafluoroethylene (PTFE; Gore-Tex), Surgical Membrane, and Dual-mesh. These meshes contain pores smaller than 10 μm in at least one of their three dimensions (Fig. 66-4).

Type III: macroporous materials with multifilamentous or microporous components, such as PTFE mesh (Teflon), braided Dacron mesh (Mersilene), braided polypropylene mesh (Surgipro), and perforated PTFE patch (MycroMesh) (Figs. 66-5 and 66-6).

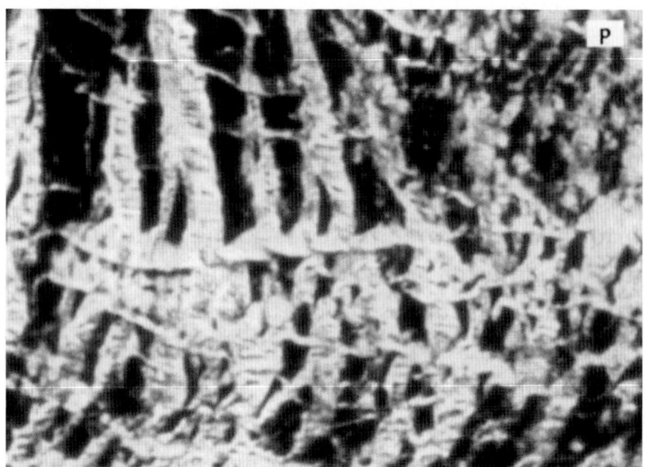

Figure 66-4 Type II synthetic mesh: Gore-Tex (expanded PTFE).

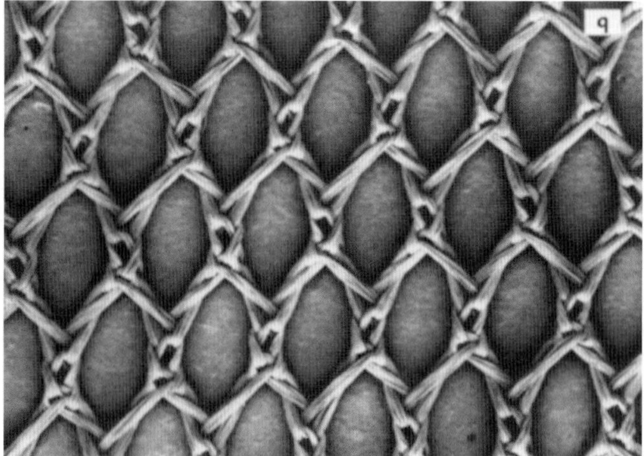

Figure 66-5 Type III synthetic mesh: polytetrafluroethylene (PTFE).

Type IV: biomaterials with submicronic pore size, such as Silastic, Cellgard (polypropylene sheeting), Preclude Pericardial membrane, and Preclude Dura-substitute.

Another important property is the *composition of fibers* (Table 66-1). Polypropylene meshes are monofilaments, whereas the other commonly used meshes are multifilaments. One theoretical disadvantage of multifilament meshes is that the interstices are smaller than 10 μm; this allows small bacteria to infiltrate and proliferate, but macrophages and neutrophilic granulocytes that could eliminate the bacteria are too large to enter a 10-μm tridimensional pore.[39-41] In addition, because of their wide pores, type I materials (but not types II and III) allow rapid in-growth of vascularized fibrous tissue, as was demonstrated by Chvapil and colleagues[42]; this leads to fibroplasia and angiogenesis, which not only prevent infection but also form fibrous connections to the surrounding tissue. Therefore, pore size is a key factor in determining inflammatory response and the growth of fibrocollagenous tissue.

Flexibility or *stiffness* is another important property that appears to be related to pore size. Marlex has higher flexural rigidity (stiffness) than Mersilene or Teflon. Marlex is also shown to wrinkle more than Mersilene. Prolene is composed of knitted filaments of polypropylene, as is Marlex; however, it has a pore size twice as large as that of Marlex (1500 versus 600 μm) and therefore is more flexible.[43] Because of this property, Prolene seems to have a lower erosion rate through the vagina and adjacent viscera, but up to now there are insufficient data to prove it. Atrium mesh, because of its intermediate pore size (800 μm), is more pliable and thinner than Marlex or Prolene. Table 66-2 reports data about mean stiffness and mean peak load of the main synthetic materials.

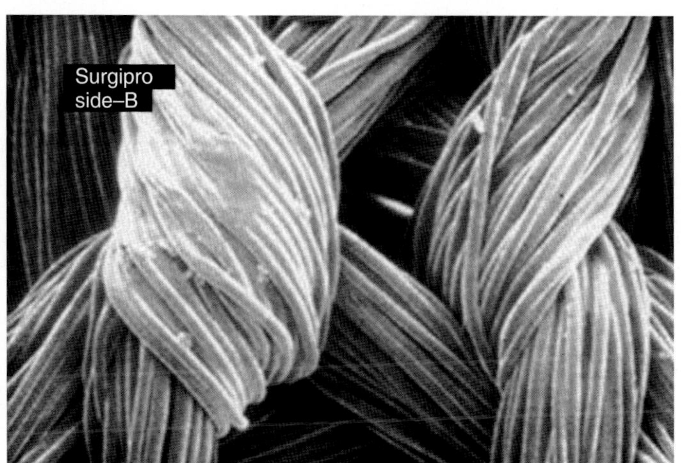

Figure 66-6 Type III synthetic mesh: multifilament mesh.

COMPLICATIONS OF SYNTHETIC MATERIALS

Biomaterial-related complications frequently encountered are infection and sinus tract formation, seroma, intestinal adhesion, erosion and fistula formation, and shrinkage.

Infection and sinus tract formation is caused by infiltration and proliferation of bacteria; it is frequently due to the use of multifilamentous suture materials for fixation of the mesh, although it may be mistaken as being caused by the mesh itself.[44-46] The reported infection rate ranges from 9.6% to 50% in type II/III prostheses,[47,48] whereas in type I it has never been reported. More important, with type I mesh, infection may be managed simply by drainage of the infected area, followed by local wound care.[49-51] On the contrary, total removal of type II and at least partial removal of type III is required to manage infection.

Prosthetic-related seroma formation is caused by the host inflammatory reaction to the prosthesis and by the dead space created between the artificial mesh and host tissue. Types I and III allow a rapid penetration of host proteinaceous materials into their pores,[52] with rapid fibrinous fixation. Therefore, the chance of seroma formation is minimized.[53] Type II, because of its inadequate pore size, has a higher rate of seroma formation ranging, from 9.6% to 14.6%.

At the present time, all available artificial meshes, absorbable or nonabsorbable, adhere to the intestine.[54-56] Covering the mesh on its intestinal side with a layer of absorbable material such as Vycril or expanded-PTFE patch partially solves this problem. Composites that combine type I and type IV mesh can prevent these complications.

A dangerous side-effect is erosion or migration of the artificial mesh when it is in direct contact with organs that do not have a serosal covering, such as rectum, bladder, and the intestinal tract.

Contraction of the mesh fibers during the scarring process leads to shrinkage of the mesh by approximately 20% compared to the original shape.

Table 66-3 shows the main complications related to each type of mesh.

Table 66-1 Composition and Types of Fibers

Chemical Component	Trade Name (Manufacturer)	Type
Polypropylene	Marlex (CR Bard, Branston, RI)	Monofilament
	Prolene (Ethicon, Sommerville, NJ)	Monofilament
	Atrium (Atrium Medical, Hudson, NH)	Monofilament
Polytetrafluoroethylene (PTFE)	Teflon (CR Bard, Haverhill, MA)	Multifilament
Expanded PTFE	Gore-Tex (WL Gore, Flagstaff, AZ)	Multifilament
Polyethylene tetraphthalate	Mersilene (Ethicon, Somerville, NJ)	Multifilament
Polyglycolic acid	Dexon (absorbable) (Davis and Geck, American Cyanamid, Danbury, CT)	Multifilament
Polyglactin 910	Vicryl (absorbable) (Ethicon, Somerville, NJ)	Multifilament

Adapted in part from Chu and Welch, John Wiley & Sons, p 907. Reprinted by permission of John Wiley & Sons, Inc.

Table 66-2 Peak Load and Stiffness of Common Synthetic Materials

Material	Mean Stiffness (N/mm)	Mean Peak Load (N)
TVT	0.23	68.1
SPARC	0.53	52.1
Prolene	0.53	56.4
Mersilene	1.17	50.3
IVS tape	1.58	46.2
Gore-Tex MycroMesh	2.61	71.3
Nylon	6.83	422.0

Adapted from Dietz HP, Vancaillie P, Svehla M, et al: Mechanical properties of urogynecologic implant materials. Int Urogynecol J 14:241, 2003.

Table 66-3 Main Complications by Type of Mesh

Complication	Type I	Type II	Type III
Infection	+	+++	++
Seroma	+	++	+
Adhesion	+++	+	++
Erosion	+++	+	++

Adapted from Debodinance P, Delporte P, Engrand JB, Boulogne M: [Development of better tolerated prosthetic materials: Applications in gynecological surgery.] [In French.] J Gynecol Obstet Biol Reprod 31:527-540, 2002.

TECHNIQUES

The Pioneers

A recent metanalysis of the European Union Hernia Trialists Collaboration compared mesh versus nonmesh methods of open groin hernia repair in 4005 patients. They concluded that mesh repair was associated with fewer recurrences (1.4% versus 4.4%; $P < .001$). This concept, using synthetic mesh applied "tension-free," and the long-term successful outcome incited researchers to transfer an analogous rationale to pelvic surgery.

Therefore, surgeons, in the early fifties, introduced synthetic materials to correct the anatomic position of the visceral organs in the pelvic cavity. In 1955, tantalum mesh was used to reinforce tissues in patients with POP.[57] In 1970, collagen mesh was proposed for the treatment of pelvic descensus.[58] The "fashion" for using polypropylene to repair prolapse started in 1992, with the first published data on Marlex appearing in 1996.[59]

Evolving Concepts

The goal of prosthetic surgery, compared with site-specific autologous tissue repair, is to replace the damaged visceral fascia, restoring cohesion between visceral and parietal fascia and rebuilding the hammock connected to the arcus tendineous fascia pelvis (ATFP), thus respecting the bladder neck and stabilizing the bladder hammock. Initial experience used an overlaid synthetic mesh reinforcing a traditional anterior colporrhaphy.[60] Meanwhile, the new concept of transvaginal suspension of pelvic floor repair was introduced by the four-corner suspension.[7] The evolution of this technique included a prosthetic reinforcement of the central segment, using a mesh applied with a double-needle suspension.[61]

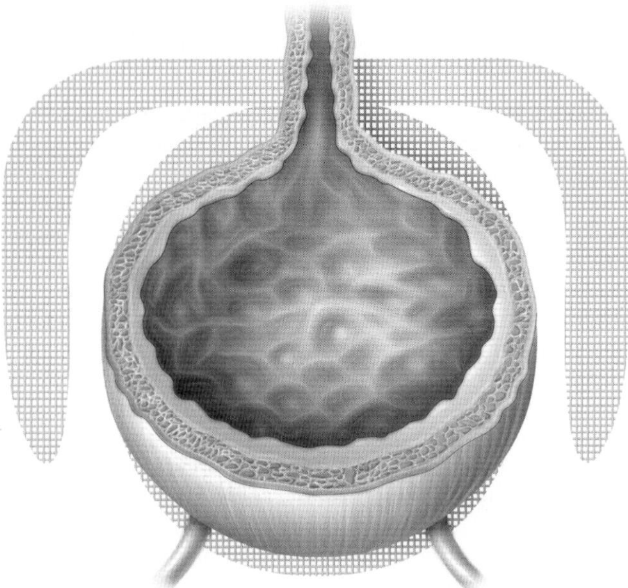

Figure 66-7 Tension-free cystocele repair.

The new "tension-free" concept acquired by general surgeons in treating abdominal hernia and the *revolution* in the treatment of female SUI brought about by the tension-free vaginal tape (TVT) were translated into POP repair. A new proposal was developed that used a Prolene mesh applied below the bladder inserted "tension-free" without any fixation.[62] Since then, other authors have proposed various transvaginal "tension-free" mesh repairs.[63-65]

In 2001, a new approach, using the transobturator route, was proposed to treat SUI patients in the same tension-free manner as TVT.[66] The excellent preliminary results incited the development of a wider concept of transperineal pelvic floor repair.[67-69] Therefore, studies employing larger meshes covering all the pelvic defects, using Prolene material (soft or traditional) applied "tension-free," extended to stronger pelvic structures: transobturator foramina and sacrospinous ligaments.

The Italian Experience

In 1998, Cervigni and coworkers developed a tension-free cystocele repair (TCR) technique applying a traditional Prolene mesh below the bladder with two wings inserted paraurethrally without any fixation.[62] The rationale of this technique was to use a wider mesh to cover all the bladder, avoiding any specific site defect evaluation, to reinforce pubocervical and endopelvic fascia. Because the mesh is applied tension-free, there is a reduction of anatomic distortion, which reduces future sequelae in the other vaginal segments (Fig. 66-7).

Nicita published a Prolene technique mesh repair that was anchored with stitches to the arcus tendineous levator ani and sacrospinous ligaments with a central hole to allow a pelvic reconstruction with the uterus in situ.[70] Migliari and Usai, using the Raz concepts, developed a four-corner suspension using a Prolene mesh to reinforce a central defect.[61]

The Australian Experience

In 1990, Petros and Ulmsten published the *Integral Theory* to explain the mechanism of incontinence and other pelvic dysfunction.[71] They postulated that all pelvic floor defects start from fascial, ligamentous, and muscular deficiency. There are forward forces (pubococcygeus and puborectalis muscles) and backward/downward forces (levator plate and ileococcygeus muscles) that could be impaired. A new surgical proposal based on this concept, developed by Farnsworth, uses a Prolene mesh with the aim to restore the normal anatomy by a complete prosthetic fascial substitution.[72] The mesh is sutured tension-free in the normal anatomic insertion of the native fasciae, restoring the three levels of vaginal support described by DeLancey.[73]

The French Experience

In 2000, a group of nine surgeons developed a transvaginal POP repair using Prolene soft, a wide mesh with four arms introduced into the transobturator canal for the anterior compartment and two arms transfixing the sacrospinous ligaments for the posterior compartment, which they inserted tension-free with the straps transferred using a long curved needle without any fixation. To reduce the risk of shrinkage, they put the four arms at the more distal part of the ATFP, and to avoid the risk of erosion, they used midline colpectomy instead of a "T" incision and the vaginal wall is not trimmed.[74] A different approach, called the "triple perineal operation," used posterior IVS for the suspension of the vaginal vault; an interposition of mesh in the vesicovaginal space for the correction of cystocele, fixed posteriorly to the cervix; and a third mesh in the rectovaginal space to treat rectocele, fixed to the posterior IVS and distally to the fibrous central nucleus of the perineum.[75]

THE NEW TRANSOBTURATOR CYSTOCELE REPAIR

Transobturator cystocele repair can be accomplished in several ways. With the transvaginal mesh repair (TVM), Prolene soft (Gynemesh) is delivered with the use of a single, reusable, long curved needle and anchored with low tension (friction) in a Velcro effect. The mesh is placed tension-free in the vesicovaginal space, the space of Retzius, and the paravesical space. The two superficial and two deeper arms are positioned apically and distally at the ATFP (Fig. 66-8).

With the Perigee transobturator repair system, polypropylene is delivered with the use of four Deschamps nonreusable needles connected with a special connector. A low-tension (friction) anchoring system is used (Velcro effect). The mesh is applied tension-free in the vesicovaginal space, the space of Retzius, and the paravesical space. The two superficial and two deeper arms are positioned apically and distally at the ATFP (Fig. 66-9).

The Avaulta system uses polypropylene covered by collagen in the central part. This is positioned like the Perigee and TVM systems, with he use of a single, reusable curved needle (Fig. 66-10).

TRANSVAGINAL MESH CYSTOCELE REPAIR

In 1996, Julian first published a study assessing the efficacy and complications of Marlex mesh in repairing severe recurrent anterior vaginal wall prolapse.[59] Twenty-four patients entered the study and were divided into control and treatment groups. Transvaginal repair was similar between groups except for reinforcement of the anterior vaginal wall with synthetic mesh. After 2 years, four patients in the control group and none in the treatment group had recurrent anterior vaginal wall prolapse ($P < .05$). A similar technique was carried out by Flood and colleague in a more consistent group of patients.[60] They obtained the same cure rate of prolapse with a longer follow-up; there was also a concomitant treatment of SUI in 74% of their patients. Mage[76] had the same results using a polyester mesh sutured to the vaginal angles. Migliari and Usai applied the same principle, using mixed fiber mesh to correct grade 4 cystocele; the mesh was positioned during a modified four-corner procedure.[61] With this technique, there was no recurrence of cystocele except in 1 patient, and 13 of 15 patients were continent.

Nicita proposed a new method to support female prolapsed pelvic organs, using a hammock-shaped Prolene mesh anchored transversally between the two arcus tendineous portions of the endopelvic fascia and between the bladder and uterine neck.[70] He treated 44 patients presenting with various degrees of incontinence and combinations of cystocele and pelvic prolapse. All patients affected by incontinence or vaginal prolapse were satisfied; uterine prolapse partially recurred in three patients.

Another original technique, the TCR, was proposed by Cervigni and associates in 1998. This approach uses a Prolene mesh in a double wing shape applied without sutures between the pubocervical fascia and vagina. The procedure was carried out in 138 women; after a mean follow-up of 18 months, there was a complete anatomic recovery in 135 patients (97.8%).[77] In a further experience with a longer follow-up, the success rate (cystocele grade <2, Baden-Walker classification) was 15.9%, and only six cases of recurrent cystocele (2.1%) were symptomatic. Erosion appeared in 7.3%. Quality of life was improved.[78] The results are reported in Table 66-4.

Table 66-5 shows the preliminary results of the use of transobturator mesh in the treatment of anterior vaginal vault prolapse.

EVIDENCE-BASED MEDICINE

In the Third International Consultation on Incontinence, held in June 2004, the 17th Committee on Prolapse Repair summarized the evidence regarding the use of mesh in prolapse repair as follows:

Level II: Transvaginal placement of permanent mesh may reduce anterior wall recurrence but has an unacceptably high rate of complications that include erosion, infection, sepsis, dyspareunia, and other functional symptoms.

Level III: Transvaginal placement of biologic graft may reduce anterior prolapse recurrence rates, although the evidence is conflicting.

Research recommendations were as follows:

Grade B: Transvaginal permanent grafts for prolapse repair have a poor risk-benefit ratio; therefore, use of these materials should occur only in approved clinical trials.

Grade D: There is no evidence to support the routine use of biologic or permanent synthetic grafts for transvaginal POP repair.

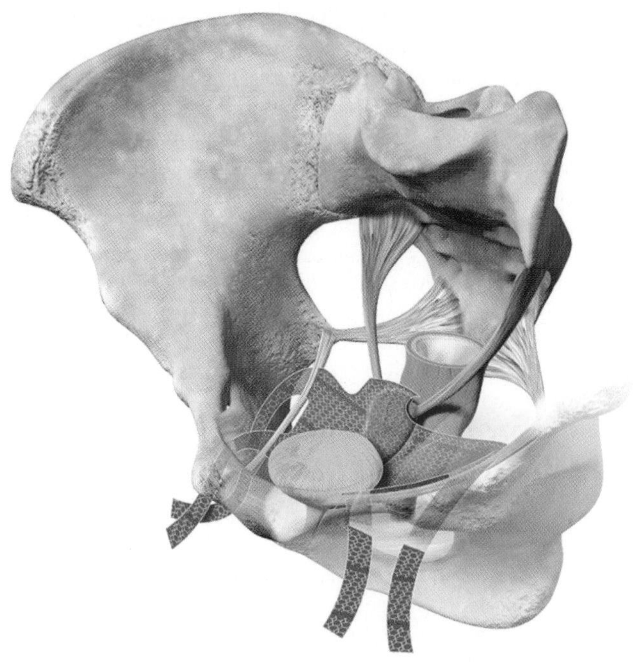

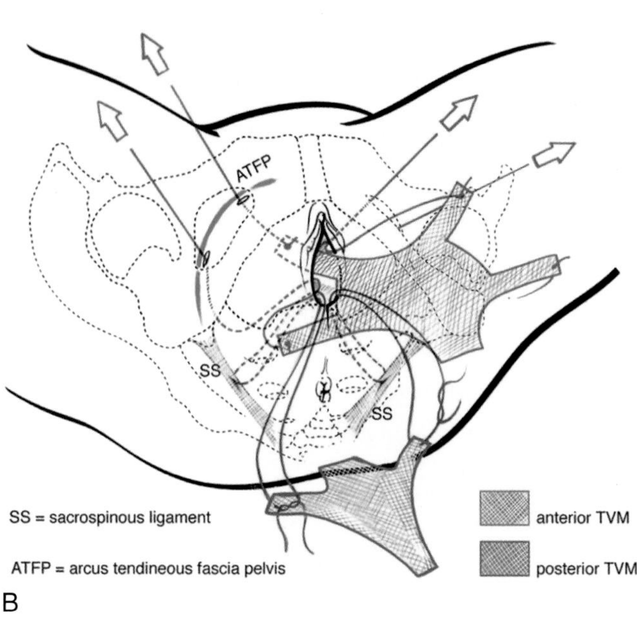

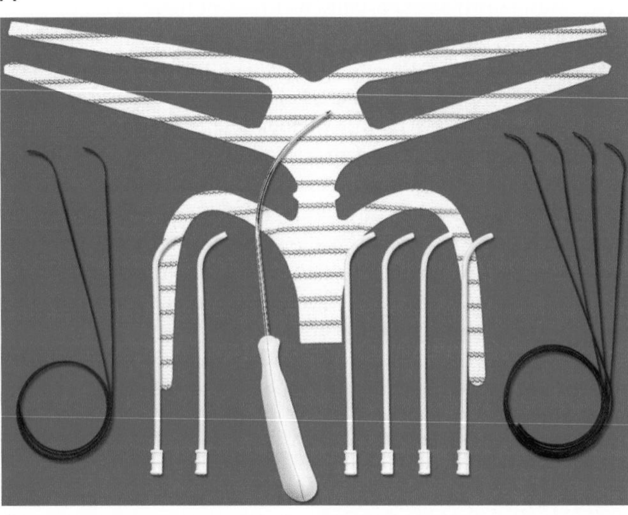

Figure 66-8 **A** through **C**, Tension-free vaginal mesh repair (TVM).

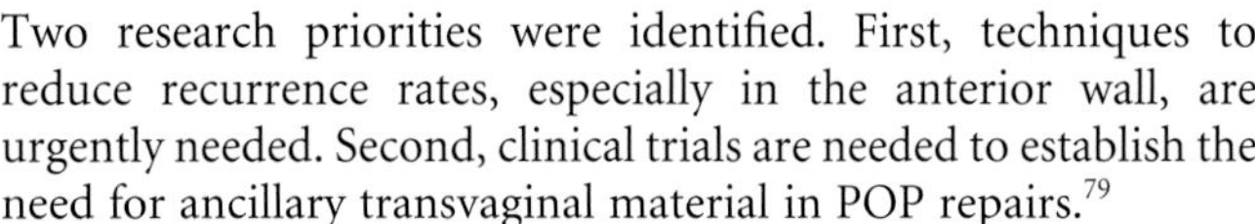

Two research priorities were identified. First, techniques to reduce recurrence rates, especially in the anterior wall, are urgently needed. Second, clinical trials are needed to establish the need for ancillary transvaginal material in POP repairs.[79]

CONCLUSIONS

The pelvic surgeon, in the past and in some instances up till now, has preferred choosing a weakened and damaged autologous tissue to treat pelvic floor defects, fearing the related complications of the use of synthetics, including foreign body reaction, infection, rejection, and erosion. In the last few years there has been an explosion in the use of prosthetic materials in the surgical approach to POP repair, stimulated either by apparent simplicity and feasibility of the new kits or by surgeon demand in order to approach complex POP cases in a more straightforward manner.

The first series of transvaginal mesh cystocele repair was promising, with low rates of recurrence and mesh erosion, even though complications occurred later. Although, up to now, no case of bladder erosion has been reported after transvaginal cystocele repair with mesh, the complications and related dysfunctional problems are not completely solved. The request of symptomatic POP patients is mainly to obtain a solution of their symptoms, because they have a strong impact on the patient's quality of life. In this sense, the more cautious recommendations proposed by Third International Consultation on Incontinence aim to reduce as much as possible any avoidable complications while maintaining reliable and long-term results.

The ideal synthetic materials for pelvic surgery have yet to be identified, but new knowledge of molecular biology will contribute to the definition of new materials, improving the management of POP and related dysfunction. Tissue engineering, at the moment one of the more promising of new medical fields, should in the near future respond to patient demands to resolve the problem without any bothersome complications.

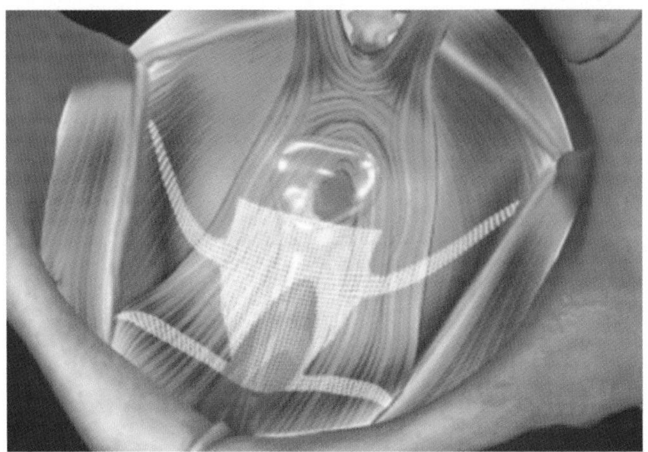
A

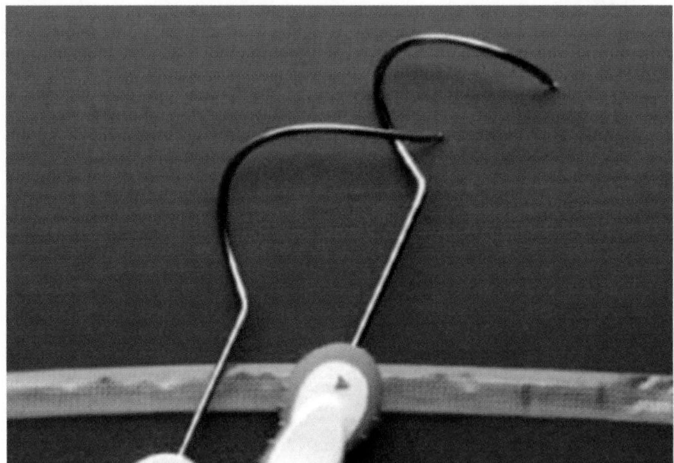
B

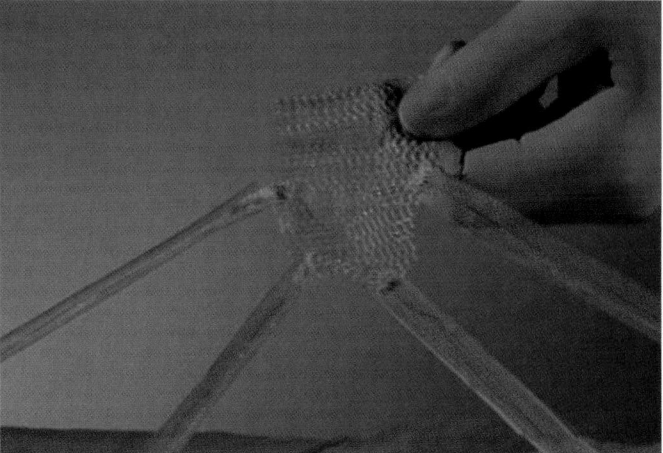
C

Figure 66-9 **A** through **C**, The Perigee transobturator repair system.

Table 66-4 Tension-free Cystocele Repair Results

Study (Ref. No.)	Year	Mesh	*N*	Follow-up	Cure (%)	Sequelae
Julian (59)	1996	Marlex	24	2 yr	100	3 mesh-related complications
Nicita (70)	1998	Prolene	44	13.9 mo	100	3 recurrent uterine prolapse
Flood et al (60)	1998	Marlex	142	3.2 yr	100	3 mesh erosions
Mage (76)	1999	Polyester	46	26 mo	100	1 mesh erosion
Migliari & Usai (61)	1999	Mixed fiber	15	23 mo	93	None
Cervigni et al (78)	2000	Polypropylene	138	18.7 mo	97	13 mesh erosion 9 dyspareunia 1 hematoma
Kobashi et al (80)	2000	Cadaveric	42	1-6 mo	100	None
Weber et al (81)	2001	Polyglactin 910	35	4.5-44 mo	42	None
		No mesh	74		36	
Sand et al (82)	2001	Polyglactin 910	81	12	75	None
		No mesh	80		57	
Clemons et al (83)	2003	Alloderm	33	18 mo	56	None
Dwyer & O'Reilly (84)	2004	Atrium	64	6-52	94	3 mesh erosions
Gomelski et al (85)	2004	Alloderm	70	24	87	None
Milani et al (86)	2005	Prolene	63	17	94	4 erosions
Gandhi et al (87)	2005	Cadaveric	76		79	None
		Anterior colporrhaphy	78		71	
De Tayrac et al (88)	2005	Polypropylene	63	24-60 mo	89.1	Shrinkage (5.5%) Erosions (9.1%) Dyspareunia (16.7%)

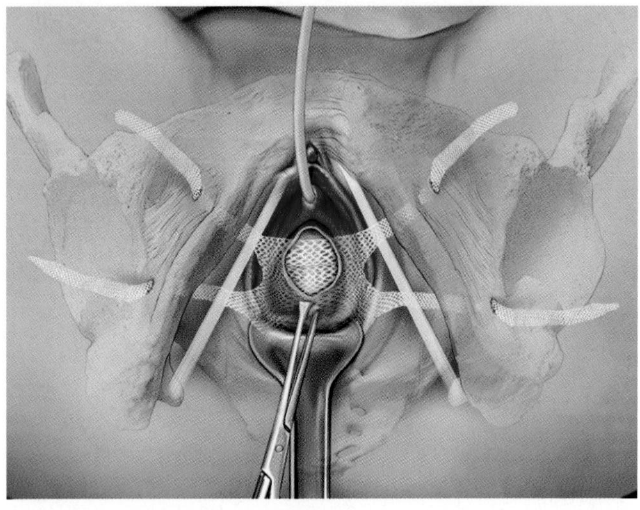

Figure 66-10 The Avaulta system for transobturator repair of cystocele.

Table 66-5 Preliminary Results of the Use of Transobturator Mesh in the Treatment of Anterior Vaginal Vault Prolapse

Study (Ref. No.)	Year	Mesh	*N*	Follow-up	Cure (%)	Sequelae
De Tayrac et al (89)	2002	Gynemesh	48	18 mo	97.9	8.3% erosion
Von Thebald & Labbè (90)	2003	Prolene mesh Posterior IVS	92			3 erosion 1 hematoma
Yan et al (91)	2004	Synthetic	30	6.7 mo	97	7% erosion 14% dyspareunia
Bader et al (64)	2004	Gynemesh	40	16.4 mo	95	2 erosions

References

1. Hendrix SL: Urinary incontinence and menopause: An evidence-based treatment approach. Dis Mon 48:622, 2002.
2. Mant J, Painter R, Vessey M: Epidemiology of genital prolapse: Observations from Oxford family Planning Association Study. Br J Obstet Gynaecol 104:579, 2007.
3. Porges RF, Smilen SW: Long-term analysis of the surgical management of pelvic support defect. Am J Obstet Gynecol 171:1518-1528, 1994.
4. Macer GA: Transabdominal repair of cystocele, a 20 years experience, compared with the traditional vaginal approach. Am J Obstet Gynecol 131:203-207, 1998.
5. Morley GW, DeLancey JOL: Sacrospinous ligament fixation for eversion of the vagina. Am J Obstet Gynecol 158:872-881, 1988.
6. Holley RL, Varner RE, Gleason BP, et al: Recurrent pelvic support defects after sacrospinous ligament fixation for vaginal vault prolapse. J Am Coll Surg 180:444-448, 1995.
7. Raz S, Klutke CG, Golomb J: Four-corner bladder and urethral suspension for moderate cystocele. J Urol 142:712-715, 1989.
8. Miyazaki FS, Miyazaki DW: Raz four-corner suspension for severe cystocele: Poor results. Int Urol J 5:94-97, 1994.
9. Richardson AC, Edmonds PB, Williams NL: Treatment of stress urinary incontinence due to paravaginal defect. Obstet Gynecol 57:357-362, 1981.
10. Benson JT (ed): Female Pelvic Floor Disorders. New York, WW Norton & Company, 1992, pp 280-294.
11. Birch C: The use of prosthetics in pelvic reconstructive surgery. Best Pract Res Clin Obstet Gynaecol 19:979-991, 2005.
12. Farrell SA, Dempsey T, Geldenhuys L: Histologic examination of "fascia" used in colporraphy. Obstet Gynecol 98(5Pt1):794-798, 2001.
13. Richardson AC, Lyon JB, Williams NL: A new look at pelvic relaxation. Am J Obstet Gynecol 126:568-573, 1976.
14. Shull BL, Bachofen C, Coates KW, Kuehl TJ: A transvaginal approach to repair of apical and other associated sites of pelvic organ prolapse with uterosacral ligaments. Am J Obstet Gynecol 183:1365-1373, 2000.
15. Barber MD, Visco AG, Weidner AC, et al: Bilateral uterosacral ligament vaginal vault suspension with site-specific endopelvic fascia defect repair for the treatment of pelvic organ prolapse. Am J Obstet Gynecol 183:1402-1410, 2000.
16. Aybek Z, Mathrubutham M, Rao S: Capacity of plasma to inhibit elastase activity is reduced in patients with stress urinary incontinence. [Abstract 57.] J Urol 159:15, 1998.
17. Kovacs EJ, Di Pietro A: Fibrogenic cytokines and connective tissue production. FASEB J 8:854-861, 1994.
18. Mays PK, McAnulty RJ, Campa JS, Laurent GJ: Age-related changes in collagen synthesis and degradation in rat tissue: Importance of degradation of newly synthesized collagen in regulation of collagen production. Biochem J 276:307-313, 1991.
19. Schultka R, Kirsche H, Peil J: Age-dependent changes of the collagen content of the human oviduct. Acta Histochem 80:41-51, 1986.
20. Hayflick L: Theories of biological aging. Exp Geront 20:145-159, 1985.
21. Peacock EE: Structure, synthesis and interaction of fibrous protein and matrix. In Peacock EE (ed): Wound Repair, 3rd ed. Philadelphia, WB Saunders, 1984, pp 56-101.
22. Falconer C, Ekman-Ordeberg G, Ulmsten U, et al: Changes in paraurethral connective tissue at menopause are counteracted by estrogen. Maturitas 24:197-204, 1996.

23. Vogel KG, Paulsson M, Heinegard D: Specific inhibition of type I and type II collagen fibrillogenesis by the small proteoglycan of tendon. Biochem J 223:587-597, 1984.
24. Sayer TR, Dixon JS, Hosker GL, Warrell DW: A study of paraurethral connective tissue in women with stress incontinence of urine. Neurourol Urodyn 9:319-320, 1990.
25. Rechberger T, Postawsi K, Jakowicki JA: Role of fascial collagen in stress urinary incontinence. Am J Obstet Gynecol 179(6Pt1):1511-1514, 1998.
26. Wong MY, Harmanli OH, Agar M: Collagen content of non-supportive tissue in pelvic organ prolapse and stress urinary incontinence. Am J Obstet Gynecol 189:1597-1599, 2003.
27. Petros P, Ulmsten U: An integral theory and its method for the diagnosis and management of female urinary incontinence. Scand J Urol Nephrol 153(Suppl):1-93, 1993.
28. Petros P, Ulmsten U: Urethral pressure increase on effort originates from within the urethra, and continence from musculovaginal closure. Neurourol Urodyn 14:337-350, 1995.
29. DeLancey JOL: Structural support of the urethra as it relates to stress urinary incontinence: The hammock hypothesis. Am J Obstet Gynecol 170:1713-1723, 1994.
30. Hukins WL, Aspden RM: Composition and properties of connective tissue. Trends Biochem Sci 7:260-264, 1985.
31. Norton P, Boyd C, Deak S: Collagen synthesis in women with genital prolapse or stress urinary incontinence. Neurourol Urodyn 11:300-301, 1992.
32. Uitto J, Perejda A (eds): Connective tissue disease: Molecular pathology of the extracellular matrix. New York, Marcel Dekker, 1986.
33. Friedman D, Boyd CD, Mackenzie JW, et al: Regulation of collagen gene expression in keloids and hypertrophic scars. J Surg Res 55:214-222, 1993.
34. Williams DF: The response of the body environment to the implant. In Williams DF, Roaf R (eds): Implants in Surgery. London: WB Saunders, 1973, 203-297.
35. Cumberland VH: A preliminary report on the use of prefabricated nylon weave in the repair of ventral hernia. Med J Aust 1:143-144, 1952.
36. Scales JT: Materials for hernia repair. Proc R Soc Med 46:647-652, 1953.
37. Bobyn JD, Wilson GJ, MacGregor DC, et al: Effect of pore size on the peel strength of attachment of fibrous tissue to porous-surfaced implants. J Biomed Mater Res 16:571-584, 1982.
38. White TA: The effect of porosity and biomaterial on the healing and long-term mechanical properties of vascular prostheses. ASAIO 11:95-100, 1988.
39. Alexander JW, Kaplan JZ, Altmaier WA: Role of suture materials in the development of wound infection. Ann Surg 165:192, 1967.
40. Elek SD, Conen PE: The virulence of *Staphylococcus pyogenes* for man: Study of the problems of wound infection. Br J Exp Pathol 38:573, 1957.
41. Neal HB III: Implants of Gore-Tex. Arch Otoryngol 109:427-433, 1983.
42. Chvapil M, Holusa R, Kliment K, Stoll M: Some chemical and biologic characteristics of a new collagen-polymer compound material. J Biomed Mater Res 3:315-322, 1969.
43. Voyles CR, Richardson JD, Bland SM, et al: Emergency abdominal wall reconstruction with polypropylene mesh: Short-term benefits versus long-term complications. Ann Surg 194:219-223, 1981.
44. Berliner SD: Biomaterials in hernia surgery. In Arregui ME, Nagan RF (eds): Inguinal Hernia: Advances or Controversies? Oxford, NY: Radcliffe Medical Press, 1994, pp 103-106.
45. Larson GM, Harrower HW: Plastic mesh repair of incisional hernias. Am J Surg 135:559-563, 1978.
46. Notaras MJ: Experience with Mersilene mesh in abdominal wall repair. Proc R Soc Med 67:45-48, 1974.
47. DeBord JR, Wyffels PL, Marshall JS, et al: Repair of large ventral incisional hernias with expanded polytetrafluoroethylene prosthetic patch. Postgrad Gen Surg 4:156-160, 1992.
48. Smith RS: The use of prosthetic materials in the repair of hernias. Surg Clin North Am 51:1387-1399, 1971.
49. Capozzi JA, Berkenfield JA, Cheaty JK: Repair of inguinal hernia in the adult with Prolene mesh. Surg Gynecol Obstet 167:124-128, 1988.
50. Matapurkar BG, Gupta AK, Agarwal AK: A new technique of "Marlex-Peritoneal Sandwich" in the repair of large incisional hernias. World J Surg 15:768, 1991.
51. Molloy RG, Moan KT, Waldron RP, et al: Massive incisional hernias: Abdominal wall replacement with Marlex mesh. Br J Surg 78:242, 1991.
52. Arnaud JP, Eloy R, Adloff M, Grenier JF: Critical evaluation of prosthetic materials in repair of abdominal wall hernias: New criteria of tolerance and resistance. Am J Surg 133:338-345, 1977.
53. Amid PK, Shulman AG, Lichtenstein IL: Selected synthetic mesh for the repair of groin hernia. Postgrad Gen Surg 4:1505, 1992.
54. Amid PK, Shulman AG, Lichtenstein IL, et al: An experimental evaluation of a new composite mesh with the selective property of incorporation to the abdominal wall without adhering to the intestines. J Biomed Materials Res 28:373-375, 1994.
55. Crist D, Gadasz T: Complications of laparoscopic surgery. Surg Clin North Am 73:265-289, 1993.
56. Soler M, Verhaeghe P, Essomba A, et al: Treatment of postoperative incisional hernias by a composite prosthesis (polyester-polyglactin 910): Clinical and experimental study. Ann Chir 47:598-608, 1993.
57. Moore J, Armstrong JT, Willis SH: The use of tantalum mesh in cystocele with critical report of ten cases. Am J Obstet Gynecol 69:1127-1135, 1995.
58. Friedman EA, Meltzer RM: Collagen mesh prosthesis for repair of endopelvic fascial defects. Am J Obstet Gynecol 106:430-433, 1970.
59. Julian TM: The efficacy of Marlex mesh in the repair of severe, recurrent vaginal prolapse of the anterior midvaginal wall. Am J Obstet Gynecol 175:1472-1475, 1996.
60. Flood CG, Drutz HP, Waja L: Anterior colporrhaphy reinforced with Marlex mesh for the treatment of systoles. Int Urogynecol J Pelvic Floor Dysfunct 9:200-204, 1988.
61. Migliari R, Usai E: Treatment results using a mixed fiber mesh in patients with grade IV cystocele. J Urol 161:1255-1258, 1999.
62. Cervigni M, Natale F, Conti Puorger C, et al: Cistopessi con protesi "tesnion-free": Esperienze preliminari. Acta Urol Ital 12(Suppl):120-121, 1998.
63. De Tayrac R, Fernandez H: Surgical repair of cystocele with mesh by the vaginal route. Am J Obstet Gynecol 186:852-853, 2002.
64. Bader G, Fauconnier A, Roger N, et al: Cystocele repair by vaginal approach with a tension-free trasversal polypropylene mesh: Technique and results. Gynecol Obstet Fertil 32:280-284, 2004.
65. Husaunndee M, Rousseau E, Deleflie M, et al: Surgical treatment of genital prolapse with a new lateral prosthetic hysteropexia technique combining vaginal and laparoscopic methods. J Gynecol Obstet Biol Reprod (Paris) 32:314-320, 2003.
66. Delorme E: Transobturator urethral suspension: Mini-invasive procedure in the treatment of stress urinary incontinence in women. Prog Urol 11:1306-1313, 2001.
67. Deval B, Ferchaux J, Berry R, et al: Objective and subjective cure rates after trans-obturator tape (Obtape) treatment of female urinary incontinence. Eur Urol 49:373-377, 2006.
68. Wang AC, Lin YH, Tseng LH, et al: Propsective randomized comparison of transobturator suburethral sling (Monarc) vs suprapubic arc (Sparc) sling procedures for female urodynamic stress incontinence. Int Urogynecol J Pelvic Floor Dynsfunct 3;1-5, 2005.
69. Davila GW, Johnson JD, Serels S: Multicenter experience with the Monarc transobturator sling system to treat stress urinary incontinence. Int Urogynecol J Pelvic Floor Dysfunct 29:1-6, 2005.
70. Nicita G: A new operation for genitourinary prolapse. J Urol 160(3 Pt 1):741-745, 1998.
71. Petros PE, Ulmsten UI: An integral theory of female urinary incontinence: Experimental and clinical considerations. Acta Obstet Gynecol Scand Suppl 153:7-31, 1990.

72. Farnsworth B: The integral theory of female urinary incontinence. Aust N Z J Obstet Gynaecol 42:99, 2002.
73. DeLancey JO: Anatomic aspects of vaginal eversion after hysterectomy. Am J Obstet Gynecol 166:1717-1724, 1992.
74. Debodinance P, Berrocal J, Clavè H, et al: Evolution des idèes sur le traitement chirugical des prolapsus gènitaux. J Gynecol Obstet Biol Reprod 33:577-588, 2004.
75. Von Theobald P, Labbè E: La triple opèration pèrinèale avec prothèses. J Gynecol Obstet Biol Reprod 32:562-570, 2003.
76. Mage P: Interposition of a synthetic mesh by vaginal approach in the cure of genital prolapse. J Gynecol Obstet Biol Reprod (Paris) 28:825-829, 1999.
77. Natale F, Marziali S, Cervigni M: Tension-free cystocele repair (TCR): Long-term follow-up. Proceedings of 25th Annual Meeting of the International Urogynecological Association, Rome, October 22-25, 2000.
78. Cervini M, Weir JM, Natale F: Tension free cystocele repair: Reliability and efficacy of a prosthetic procedure in a long-term follow-up. J Urol 171:305, 2004.
79. Abrams P, Cardozo L, Khoury S, Wein A (eds): Incontinence: Third International Consultation on Incontinence. Plymouth, England: Health Publication Ltd., 2005, pp 1397-1398 (Chapter 21).
80. Kobashi KC, Mee SL, Leach GE: A new technique for cystocele repair and transvaginal sling: The cadaveric prolapse repair and sling (CAPS). Urology 56(6 Suppl):9-14, 2000.
81. Weber AM, Walters MD, Piedmonte MR, Ballard LA: Anterior colporrhaphy: A randomized trial of three surgical techniques. Am J Obstet Gynecol 185:1299-1304; discussion 1304-1306, 2001.
82. Sand PK, Koduri S, Lobel RW, et al: Prospective randomized trial of polyglactin 910 mesh to prevent recurrence of cystoceles and rectoceles. Am J Obstet Gynecol 184:1357-1362; discussion 1362-1364, 2001.
83. Clemons JL, Myers DL, Aguilar VC, Arya LA: Vaginal paravaginal repair with an AlloDerm graft. Am J Obstet Gynecol 189:1612-1618; discussion 1618-1619, 2003.
84. Dwyer PL, O'Reilly BA: Transvaginal repair of anterior and posterior compartment prolapse with Atrium polypropylene mesh. BJOG 111:831-836, 2004.
85. Gomelsky A, Rudy DC, Dmochowski RR: Porcine dermis interposition graft for repair of high grade anterior compartment defects with or without concomitant pelvic organ prolapse procedures. J Urol 171:1581-1584, 2004.
86. Milani R, Salvatore S, Soligo M, et al: Functional and anatomical outcome of anterior and posterior vaginal prolapse repair with prolene mesh. BJOG 112:107-111, 2005.
87. Gandhi S, Goldberg RP, Kwon C, et al: A prospective randomized trial using solvent dehydrated fascia lata for the prevention of recurrent anterior vaginal wall prolapse. Am J Obstet Gynecol 192:1649-1654, 2005.
88. De Tayrac R, Deffieux X, Gervaise A, et al: Long-term anatomical and functional assessment of trans-vaginal cystocele repair using a tension-free polypropylene mesh. Int Urogynecol J Pelvic Floor Dysfunct 17:1-6, 2005.
89. De Tayrac R, Gervaise A, Fernandez H: Cure de cystocèle voie basse par protese sous-vesicale libre. J Gynecol Obstet Biol Reprod 31:597-599, 2002.
90. Von Theobald P, Labbè E: La triple opèration pèrinèale avec prothèse. J Gynecol Obstet Biol Reprod 32:562-570, 2003.
91. Yan A, Anne M, Karine A, et al: Cystocele repair by a syntheticvaginal mesh secured anteriorly through the obturator foramen. Eur J Obstet Gynecol Reprod Biol 115:90-94, 2004.

Part B

ENTEROCELE AND UTERINE PROLAPSE

Chapter 67

SACROSPINOUS LIGAMENT SUSPENSION FOR VAGINAL VAULT PROLAPSE

Sylvia M. Botros, Roger P. Goldberg, and Peter K. Sand

Several techniques are used for suspension of the vaginal vault, including the sacrospinous vaginal vault suspension, abdominal sacrocolpopexy, bilateral uterosacral vaginal vault suspension, McCall culdoplasty, iliococcygeus vault suspension, levator myorrhaphy, and many tension-free mesh techniques. The optimal surgical approach for advanced prolapse of the vaginal apex remains a subject of debate and is not well studied. Some surgeons prefer the abdominal route for younger women with advanced prolapse; however, these women are at increased risk for morbidity from the surgery, subsequent volvulus from abdominal adhesions, and foreign body reactions due to graft materials. Other surgeons prefer the vaginal route to decrease postoperative pain and morbidity and for women who are at increased operative risk.

What constitutes success or failure is not delineated in the literature, partly because indications for prolapse surgery are not uniform and the degree and site of prolapse are not always clearly defined. The Pelvic Organ Support Study (POSST) was a multicenter, observational study of 1004 women between the ages of 18 and 83 years that evaluated the prevalence of pelvic organ prolapse in a general gynecologic office setting. The investigators found that 24% of the women had stage 0 prolapse, 38% had stage I, 35% had stage II, and 2% had stage III.[1] The prevalent findings of stage II prolapse suggest that a stage II recurrence may not necessarily represent an anatomic failure after reconstructive pelvic surgery. These data support the need for the evaluation of anatomic and functional outcomes. According to some surgeons, the correction of all anatomic defects and restoration of normal anatomy should be the overarching goal. Others regard a compensatory postoperative anatomy as acceptable and perhaps even preferable in certain cases to achieve long-term functional outcomes with minimal risk of recurrent or de novo prolapse.

Sacrospinous vaginal vault suspension has the advantage of a transvaginal approach performed within the retroperitoneal space, with relatively limited dissection beyond that needed for transvaginal enterocele, rectocele, and cystocele repair. Advocates of the vaginal route argue that sacrospinous vaginal vault suspensions are fast, safe, less costly, require a shorter recovery period, lack an abdominal incision, and avoid the use of a graft. Ideally, to achieve optimal outcomes for each patient, the reconstructive surgeon should maintain a high level of skill with several techniques and tailor surgery to the individual patient.

HISTORY

The vaginal vault suspension was first described in 1892 by Zweifel,[2] who tried to suspend the vaginal vault to the sacrotuberous ligament. Richter and Albrich[3] later described successful application of this procedure. Nichols introduced the operation to the United States in 1971.[4]

Several modifications of the sacrospinous vaginal vault suspension have been described. The original technique described by Nichols involves suspension of the vaginal vault to the sacrospinous ligament through the posterior compartment. A modification of this technique was introduced by Winkler and colleagues[5] in 2000, suspending the vault to the sacrospinous ligament through the anterior compartment. This technique was developed to address the limitations of the posterior sacrospinous vault suspension by reducing postoperative proximal vaginal narrowing and lateral deviation of the upper vagina.[6] In 2003, Kearney and DeLancey[7] described the Michigan four-wall sacrospinous suspension, which suspends four points of the open vaginal apex to the sacrospinous ligament. The excess vagina is removed to avoid laxity in the anterior and posterior wall.[7] In 1993, Kovac and Cruikshank[8] described successful outcomes, even after childbirth, with sacrospinous hysteropexy, in which the uterus was suspended bilaterally to the sacrospinous ligaments.

UNILATERAL AND BILATERAL SACROSPINOUS LIGAMENT SUSPENSIONS

The anterior and posterior sacrospinous suspensions can be performed unilaterally or bilaterally; the right-sided unilateral suspension is most commonly performed. Performing the procedure on the patient's right side provides an anatomic advantage resulting from the absence of the sigmoid colon on the right. A mechanical advantage exists for right-hand–dominant surgeons as well.

Bilateral suspension has been emphasized in earlier reports.[3,9] Pohl and Frattarelli[10] reported no recurrent apical prolapse among 40 women treated with bilateral sacrospinous ligament suspension after 6 to 40 months of follow-up. Cespedes[11] reported good success after bilateral sacrospinous fixation by the anterior vaginal approach; at 17 months, no recurrent vault prolapse was seen in 27 of 28 women with grade 3 or 4 prolapse. However, there is little evidence to suggest that bilateral suspension improves outcomes compared with the unilateral approach.[12] Moreover, compared with the unilateral sacrospinous ligament suspension, the bilateral procedure entails more extensive dissection and requires generous width at the vaginal apex to avoid causing tension between fixation points. Because of these additional challenges and its lack of clear advantage, the bilateral technique is used far less often than unilateral fixation in post-hysterectomy vault prolapse.

INDICATIONS

The most common indication for sacrospinous ligament vaginal vault suspension is resuspending a symptomatic prolapsed post-hysterectomy vaginal apex. The incidence of post-hysterectomy vault prolapse requiring surgery has been estimated at 3.6 per 1000 years.[13] The risk increases from 1% to 5% 15 years after hysterectomy. The risk also increases for women who had prolapse as the primary indication for their initial surgery.[14,15] For women with pelvic ligaments and connective tissue supports that are severely attenuated or absent, the sacrospinous ligament provides a consistent and strong site for apical fixation. Sacrospinous ligament fixation may be performed at the time of hysterectomy in cases of severe apical prolapse if the uterosacral ligaments are attenuated. The use of the sacrospinous ligament fixation prophylactically at the time of hysterectomy, however, is not widely accepted. Surgeons argue that there is an increase in time and morbidity associated with the procedure, which may not be warranted by the outcomes compared with resuspension using the uterosacral ligaments. Cruikshank and Cox[16] performed sacrospinous suspensions at the time of hysterectomy on 48 of 135 women without apparent excess in morbidity. In contrast, Colombo and Milani[17] retrospectively compared 62 women who underwent sacrospinous vaginal vault suspensions with 62 women who underwent McCall culdoplasty during vaginal hysterectomy and pelvic reconstruction operations and found significant increases in operative time and blood loss in the sacrospinous group. The rate of recurrent vault prolapse was similar for the two groups.[17]

Another indication for sacrospinous suspension occurs when women desire to preserve fertility or preserve the uterus. It may also be used to decrease operative time and morbidity in elderly patients who have no evidence of endometrial hyperplasia or cancer. There is an increasing body of evidence that uterine hysteropexy may be just as effective as vaginal hysterectomy for recurrent prolapse. Sacrospinous ligament uterine suspension has been successfully used for women with symptomatic uterovaginal prolapse.[8,18,19]

Kovac and Cruikshank[8] evaluated 19 women (average age, 27 years) who underwent uterine-sparing sacrospinous ligament suspension and reported that 4 of 5 women subsequently had successful pregnancies and vaginal deliveries without recurrent apical prolapse. Hefni and colleagues[18] evaluated 109 women (61 with uterine suspension and 48 with vaginal hysterectomy and concomitant sacrospinous suspension). The mean age of these cohorts was 60 years, and after a mean follow-up period of 34 months, success rates were comparable with regard to vault prolapse and cystocele recurrences. They found significantly less blood loss, shorter operative time, and fewer complications with uterine preservation.[18] Maher and coworkers[19] retrospectively compared 34 women with sacrospinous ligament hysteropexy with 36 women with hysterectomy and sacrospinous vaginal vault suspension for symptomatic uterine prolapse. The mean follow-up was 36 months for the hysterectomy group and 26 months for the hysteropexy group. Subjective and objective success rates were similar, and they found a significant reduction in operative time and blood loss with uterine preservation.[19]

The sacrospinous hysteropexy entails fixation of the distal uterosacral ligaments and paracervical tissue to the sacrospinous ligament. Bilateral rather than unilateral suspension was performed in 15 of the 19 subjects in Cruikshank's series to avoid lateral deviation of the uterus and any adverse effect it might have on reproductive capacity.[8] Alternatively, Hefni and associates[18] performed all of their hysteropexies unilaterally.

ANATOMY

The sacrospinous ligament is an excellent support structure for the apex of the vagina. In 1992, DeLancey[20] described the anatomic aspects of vaginal eversion after hysterectomy and found that the structures supporting the vagina could be divided into three levels, primarily vertical in orientation. The first level of support, which is suspensory in nature, occurs in the upper vagina adjacent to the cervix and is suspended above by long connective tissue fibers.[20] These suspension points should lift the apex of the vagina to the level of or above the ischial spine. These apical or level I vaginal supports are increasingly recognized as a critical component in overall pelvic floor support.[21] Loss of level I support can occur after abdominal or vaginal hysterectomy in as many as 2% to 45% of patients due to failure to resuspend the vaginal cuff to the uterosacral ligaments. Resulting vaginal vault prolapse can occur with or without an enterocele.[21,22] The sacrospinous ligament provides a good option for level I support.

A good understanding of the anatomy of the sacrospinous ligament helps to minimize complications at the time of surgery. Few structures are at risk for injury in a correctly performed procedure. The sacrospinous ligament attaches laterally to the ischial spine and medially to the lateral margins of the sacrum and coccyx.[23] The pudendal nerve leaves the pelvis through the greater sciatic foramen, medial to the sciatic nerve and internal pudendal vessel, between the piriformis and coccygeus muscles and passes under the sacrospinous ligament close to its attachment to the ischial spine.[24] Verdeja found that the pudendal neurovascular bundle ranges from 0.90 to 1.30 cm medial to the ischial spine; the sciatic nerve is located 3.10 to 3.30 cm medial to the spine.[25] Based on these anatomic relationships, neurovascular injury seems most likely along the lateral third of the sacrospinous ligament when suturing. Another series of cadaver dissections, performed by Barksdale and colleagues,[26] showed the pudendal neurovascular bundle to be relatively shielded from injury by the ischial spine and sacrospinous ligament. The inferior gluteal artery—with a more perpendicular course relative to the ligament—was the vascular structure whose location appeared most vulnerable to injury. These researchers referred to three elements of the operation that may carry particular risk: suture placement along the posterior ligament, retractor placement beyond the ligament, and overly aggressive denuding of the ligament surface.[26]

PREOPERATIVE AND PERIOPERATIVE CONSIDERATIONS

The decision about which suspension procedure to perform must be individualized for every patient. The patient's age, medical history, sexual activity, specific anatomic features, prior and concomitant pelvic surgical procedures, and personal wishes for future fertility or preservation of the uterus should be taken into consideration when planning the procedure. For a patient with significant medical comorbidities, a vaginal surgical approach may benefit the patient over a procedure that would require an abdominal incision or a prolonged laparoscopic operation. For women with prior intra-abdominal surgery, pelvic adhesions, or other contraindications to abdominal surgery, the fully retroperitoneal nature of a sacrospinous vaginal vault suspension may confer advantages with respect to surgical risk, operative time, and speed of recovery. After a vaginal approach is decided on, the type of vaginal suspension should be chosen from the available options. The sacrospinous vaginal vault suspension has been studied extensively and is a reliable and safe procedure for the repair of post-hysterectomy vault prolapse.

If the patient is not sexually active, is elderly, has already failed a pelvic reconstructive procedure, or has multiple medical comorbidities and is a poor surgical candidate, an obliterative procedure such as the LeFort colpocleisis may be suitable. Alternatively, a sacrospinous vaginal vault suspension may be done under local anesthesia.

Richardson[27] has described site-specific defects in the endopelvic fascia in the anterior, posterior, and apical vaginal wall as the anatomic basis for cystocele, rectocele, and enterocele, respectively. He believed that the surgeon should be able to recognize and repair all existing pelvic floor support defects at the time of surgery. He described the post-hysterectomy enterocele as a defect in the endopelvic fascia at the vaginal apex due to failure to reconstitute pubocervical and rectovaginal fascia in this region. This allows small bowel and peritoneum to herniate into the rectovaginal septum and come in direct contact with vaginal epithelium without intervening muscle or fascia.[21,27] An unrecognized enterocele is often to blame for the rare case of recurrent apical prolapse after sacrospinous vaginal vault suspension. Cruikshank and Muniz[28] suggested the importance of the site-specific repair in a longitudinal study of 695 patients who underwent sacrospinous vaginal vault suspensions over a 16-year period. Their cohort was divided into three groups. The first group, treated between 1985 and 1990, had only sacrospinous suspensions with or without a hysterectomy ($n = 173$); the second group, treated between 1991 and 1994, had anterior and posterior colporrhaphies and high cul-de-sac closures performed concomitantly with the sacrospinous suspensions ($n = 221$); and the third group, treated between 1995 and 2000, had a more inclusive, site-specific approach with the suspensions ($n = 301$). Recurrence rates dropped significantly between the first and third groups, with the third group having the highest success rates.[28] Appropriate patient selection and flexibility in the operating room can maximize the odds of success.

Preoperative evaluation should include assessment of bony and soft tissue pelvic anatomy. Markedly foreshortened bony pelvic dimensions, such as a true platypoid pelvis, may limit the surgeon's ability to preserve adequate vaginal length and weigh against the choice of sacrospinous suspension for sexually active patients. When considering soft tissue, the length of the vaginal vault should be sufficient to avoid tension after sacrospinous fixation, which may predispose to suture pullout, anatomic distortion, and possibly unmasking potential urinary incontinence due to posterior displacement of the urethra from the pubic bone.[29] In the absence of adequate length, operative revision of the cuff or suspension to a more anterior or distal structure, such as iliococcygeus fascia, may be performed.[30] Consideration of concomitant sacrospinous vaginal suspension on the right, with an iliococcygeal suspension on the left at a slightly more distal point, may lead to improved apical support and diameter.

Preoperative planning should include assessment of estrogen status for postmenopausal women and consideration of local estrogen therapy before surgery if the vaginal cuff epithelium appears thin or poorly vascularized. Estrogen improves vaginal vascularization, epithelial thickness, and collagen in the connective tissue.[31] A well-estrogenized vaginal epithelium can facilitate healing at the site of suture fixation and reduce the likelihood of subsequent surgical failure resulting from suture pullout from the vaginal side.

Prophylactic antibiotics should be given 30 minutes before the first incision. In the operating room, the patient should be placed in the dorsal lithotomy position. Appropriate positioning is essential to avoid neurologic injury that can result from improper positioning. An examination under anesthesia should be performed to assess the pelvis, the true extent of vault prolapse, the length of the vagina, and the site of apical suture placement.

TECHNIQUE

Exposing the Ligament

Access to the sacrospinous ligament and coccygeus muscle can be achieved by several means. The most common approach, as described by Nichols,[4] involves a posterior vaginal incision and posterior colporrhaphy dissection, facilitating perforation of the rectal pillar near the ischial spine. With blunt dissection of the pararectal space medial to the ligament, the coccygeus muscle and sacrospinous ligament are exposed. The anterior sacrospinous suspension technique (Fig. 67-1)[5,6] involves perforation into the retropubic space through an anterior vaginal wall incision, as would be performed for an anterior colporrhaphy, and dissection of the ipsilateral paravesical and paravaginal area from the level of the bladder neck to the ischial spine along the arcus tendineus fasciae pelvis (Fig. 67-2). The dissection is performed in a manner similar to that for a vaginal paravaginal repair. This dissection opens a large space for the vaginal apex and avoids the narrowing often found in posterior approaches with perforation through the rectal pillars. For cases involving mainly anterior compartment defects with no rectocele, the anterior approach facilitates suspension of the vaginal apex without a posterior vaginal incision.

The Michigan four-wall technique approaches the sacrospinous ligament by resecting a diamond-shaped patch of excess epithelium at the most advanced portion of the prolapsed vaginal cuff—a region of the vaginal skin that overlies an enterocele in most cases. After the repair of the enterocele, the ligament is exposed with posterolateral dissection within the retroperitoneal plane.[7] Because this apical approach exposes the anterior vaginal epithelium with underlying pubocervical fascia and the posterior vaginal epithelium with rectovaginal fascia, sutures can be anchored through both of these cuff edges. Breisky-Navratil

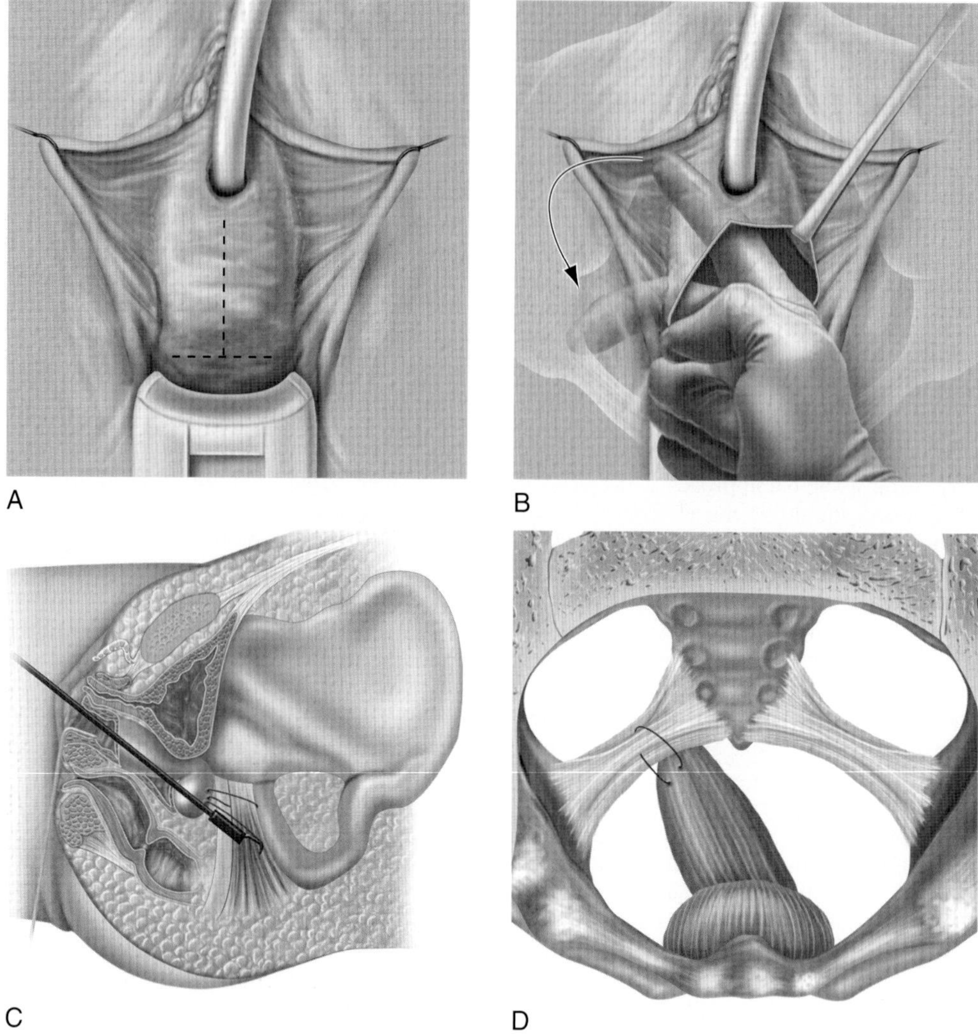

Figure 67-1 Dissection for anterior sacrospinous vaginal vault suspension. **A,** Incision; **B,** Perforation into retropubic space through anterior vaginal wall incision and dissection; **C,** Placement of suture in sacrospinous ligament with straight capiodevice; **D,** Suspension of vaginal vault to sacrospinous ligament.

retractors are well suited for exposing the coccygeus muscle and sacrospinous ligament without obstructing the surgical field. A 17 × 2.5 cm Breisky-Navratil retractor is placed medially to sweep the rectum medially off the ligament. A 12 × 3 cm Breisky-Navratil retractor is placed laterally. A Heaney retractor can then be placed posteriorly, just in front of the coccygeus muscle at the 7-o'clock position, perpendicular and on the distal edge of the coccygeus muscle for adequate retraction. Care should be taken so the tips of the retractors do not extend beyond the ischial spine. Some surgeons find retractors or suction devices mounted with a fiberoptic light source to be particularly useful for identifying the retroperitoneal anatomy.

Suture Placement

Various devices have been used to place sutures into the sacrospinous ligament, including the Deschamps ligature carrier, Miya Hook,[32] Schulte device, and Capio in-line "push and catch" suturing devices.[33] With proper assistance, some surgeons find a standard long, curved needle holder to be sufficient.

Suturing into the sacrospinous ligament should be performed with key anatomic landmarks in mind. The lateral suspension suture is placed through the ligament 1 to 2 cm medial to the ischial spine to safeguard against injury to the pudendal vessels, although the risk of injury to the pudendal complex with the newer suturing devices may be overestimated.[26] Most of these devices deliver sutures into the sacrospinous ligament and underlying coccygeus muscle over a defined arc from anterior to posterior positions and cannot reach the pudendal complex posterior to the muscles. Medial rather than lateral placement of sutures in the ligament allows for a more cephalad suspension of the vaginal vault. Medially, the rectum represents the anatomic boundary for suture placement. During placement of the sacrospinous sutures, the surgeon must ensure that all retractors maintain their proper position. Traumatic insertion of retractors beyond the ligament or excessive medial traction against the rectum and presacral area is a potential source of bleeding and neuropathy.

Fixation of the vaginal apex is most commonly performed with permanent monofilament sutures, but some surgeons prefer synthetic absorbable material to reduce the risk of suture erosion and granulation tissue formation.[34] Preparation of the vaginal apex for fixation can involve full cuff closure or a circumferential whip stitch for securing hemostasis, followed by apposition of the

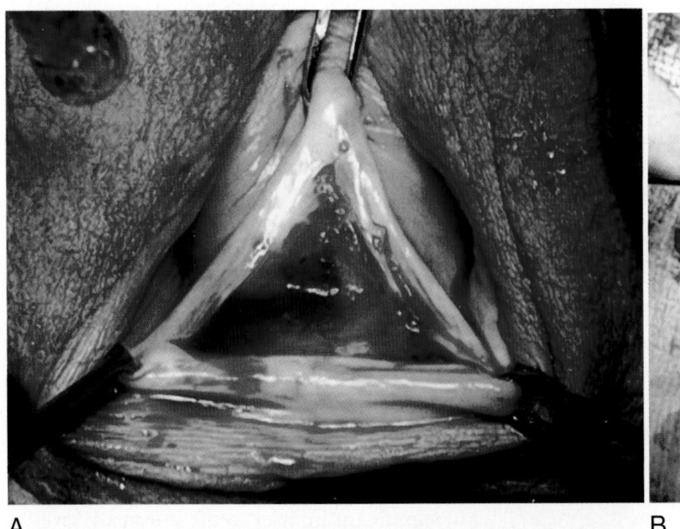
A

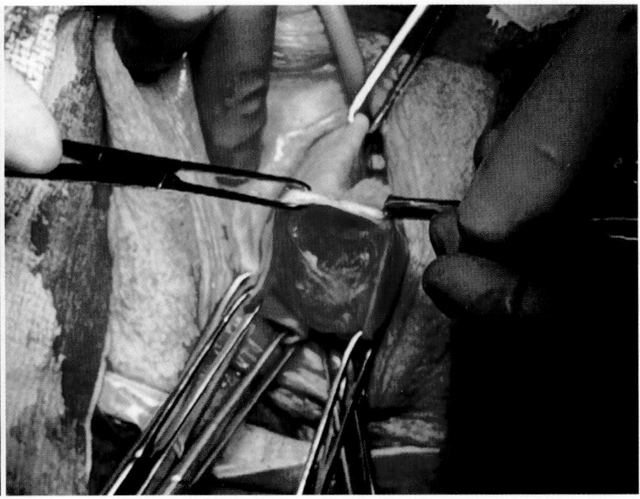
B

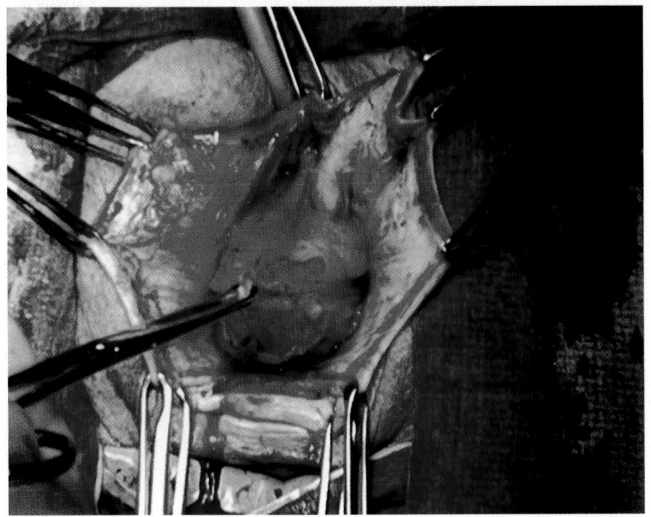
C

Figure 67-2 Schematic for an anterior vaginal vault suspension. **A,** Incision at the apex; **B,** Dissection of anterior endopelvic connective tissue from vaginal epithelium; **C,** Paravaginal dissection from level of bladder neck to ischial spine along arcus tendinous fascia pelvis.

open cuff against the ligament. Right and left anchoring sutures are secured to the undersurface of the posterior vaginal cuff epithelium for the posterior approach, to the anterior vaginal cuff epithelium for the anterior approach, or to both for the apical approach. Although scarring and fibrosis at the interface of the ligament and vaginal apex may theoretically eliminate the need for sutures after the initial healing phase, the relative advantages of permanent versus absorbable sutures have not been scientifically evaluated.

Regardless of the type of suture used or anatomic approach to the ligament, a few principles for suture placement are universal. The surgeon should avoid the creation of a suture bridge between the vagina and ligament. The use of pulley stitches (i.e., one arm of the suture placed through the vaginal cuff is tied to itself with a surgeon's knot), which attach one end of each suture to the vaginal cuff epithelium and smooth muscle, may help in applying the vagina directly against the ligament. Maintaining a width of at least 2 cm between the medial and lateral sutures at their sacrospinous origins and vaginal apex insertions can minimize the risk of constriction at the vaginal apex.

Dissection and suture placement for the uterine hysteropexy is similar to that of the anterior or posterior vault suspension and can be performed through either compartment. The difference is that after suture placement in the sacrospinous ligament, each suture is brought through the uterosacral ligaments as they insert into the cervix and then through the vaginal epithelium. If performing the technique unilaterally with a posterior approach, the sutures are placed one on either side of the cervix, with the medial suture placed on the contralateral uterosacral ligament at its insertion into the cervix. After the upper half of the vaginal wall is closed, sutures are tied down with the pulley stitch. Kovac and Cruikshank[8] and Hefni and colleagues[18] describe their techniques in detail in the original articles.

COMPLICATIONS

Numerous complications have been associated with sacrospinous vaginal vault suspensions, but most are mild and self-limited. Local neurologic complications may include pudendal, sciatic, and sacral neuropathy.[35] Cruikshank and Cox[16] found that 20 (14.8%) of 135 women experienced buttock pain after sacrospinous ligament suspension, with all cases resolving spontaneously by 6 weeks. Sciatic nerve irritation after sacrospinous suspension has been described.[12] Nerve injury is commonly cited as a complication; however, direct injury to major nerves is rare. Nichols[36] described injury to the sciatic nerve in two patients; one required reoperation, and the problem resolved spontaneously in the other.[36] Pudendal nerve entrapment may result in pain localizing in the buttocks or perineum, and it may improve after replacement of lateral fixation sutures more medially. One case of pudendal nerve entrapment was described by Alevizon and Finan.[37] The pain resoled spontaneously after release of the sacrospinous sutures. Buttock pain may occur because of the wide distribution of nerve fibers throughout the ligament, which are most concentrated in its medial portion.[38] Any evidence of direct injury to the sciatic or pudendal nerves requires reoperation in a timely fashion to remove the suture. Gluteal pain or paresthesias may occur after sacrospinous suspension, possibly due to peripheral nerve trauma.[11,39,40] Although these symptoms usually are transient and self-limited, they may persist for weeks to months postoperatively.

Serious vascular injury is a rare complication of sacrospinous ligament suspension, but it can be life threatening. Morley and DeLancey[12] reported a transfusion rate of only 4% and one infected hematoma resulting in sepsis in their review of 71 women. Various other series have reported transfusion rates ranging from 2% to 28%.[41,42] To effectively manage pelvic hemorrhage, familiarity with the surrounding anatomic landmarks is essential.

For most cases involving significant bleeding, ligation with sutures or surgical clips can be achieved under direct exposure with simple retraction. A rectal examining finger can be particularly useful for tamponade and exposure of medial vessels. Systematic inspection of the superior, inferior, and lateral surfaces of the dissected space facilitated by the slow removal of each Breisky-Navratil retractor should be performed, with particular focus on the ligament and adjacent coccygeus muscle, right medial rectal surface, and endopelvic connective tissue adjacent to the perforation of the rectal pillar. Throughout the 16-year experience of performing more than 400 sacrospinous ligament suspension procedures at our center, hemorrhage requiring vascular embolization or repeat surgery has occurred only once. In his review of the literature, Slack[43] found only 64 transfusions among 1901 reported cases.

Significant bleeding during sacrospinous vaginal vault suspension usually results from injury of small vessels along the medial aspect of the rectum[39,44] by overzealous medial dissection and retraction. Less commonly, the medial retractor can disrupt deeper vessels in the presacral area. If an individual vessel cannot be visualized with adequate retraction and lighting, the use of prolonged pressure packing may become necessary. Selective arterial embolization may be considered in hemodynamically stable patients if a defect or injured vessel cannot be localized.[26]

Infectious complications may occur. Hardiman and Drutz[45] reported a 10% incidence of febrile morbidity after vaginal reconstructive surgery that included sacrospinous ligament suspension; however, the risk of clinically significant infection resulting from the apical suspension itself appears to be low. The lack of a tissue graft eliminates the risk of foreign body infection, but suture abscesses can develop occasionally.[3,29] Proctotomy has been reported,[4,41] but significant injuries to the bowel are rare. In contrast to uterosacral vault suspension techniques, ureteral injuries are also rare, although bladder laceration has been reported.[3]

ANATOMIC OUTCOMES

Support of the Vaginal Apex

The long-term efficacy of sacrospinous ligament suspension for resuspending a prolapsed vaginal cuff has been supported in several clinical series. The success rates of the larger reports and their mean follow-up intervals are listed in Table 67-1. Although most outcomes reported for the sacrospinous ligament suspension have referred to the posterior or apical approach, later reports evaluating the anterior sacrospinous ligament suspension have found similar rates of success. Goldberg and coworkers[6] retrospectively evaluated 168 women after anterior (n = 76) or posterior (n = 92) sacrospinous vault suspension and found no measurable differences with respect to apical support, vaginal caliber according to maximum dilator size, or angle of the vaginal vault between the two groups.

Table 67-1 Sacrospinous Vaginal Vault Outcomes

Study	No. of Patients	Mean Follow-up (mo)	Success of Apical Support (%)
Richter and Albrich,[3] 1981	81		98
Nichols,[4] 1982	163	≥24	97
Morley & DeLancey,[12] 1988	71	≥12	96
Cruikshank and Cox,[16] 1990	48	8-38	83
Shull et al,[30] 1992	81	≥48	98
Pasley,[41] 1995	156	35	94.4
Hardiman and Drutz,[45] 1996	125	6-60	97.6
Paraiso et al,[51] 1996	243	73.6	93
Hoffman et al,[65] 1996	39	≥12	90
Chapin,[66] 1997	112	≥12	96
Meschia et al,[67] 1999	91	≥12	85
Winkler et al,[5] 2000	75	8.5	93
Cespedes,[11] 2000	28	17	96.4
Lantzsch et al,[68] 2001	123	57	96.7

After sacrospinous ligament suspension, the apex of the vagina is retroverted and laterally positioned—anatomic changes that appear to have no functional consequences. Morley and DeLancey[12] thought this asymmetry might confer a functional benefit postoperatively by positioning the vaginal vault away from the urogenital hiatus and over the levator muscles, lessening the intra-abdominal pressures applied to the vaginal apex. Narrowing of the vaginal apex into a conical shape, due to the excision of excess anterior or posterior vaginal epithelium, is thought by some to be a desired anatomic consequence of unilateral sacrospinous suspension.[46] After bilateral suspension, a T-shaped or Y-shaped (with concomitant enterocele repair) vaginal apex may be created, but it appears to confer no functional disadvantage.

Comparison with Abdominal Procedures

Benson and associates[47] performed the first prospective, randomized trial comparing abdominal and vaginal apical suspensions. They randomized 48 women to vaginal sacrospinous ligament suspension with paravaginal repair, and 40 women were randomized to have abdominal sacrocolpopexy, paravaginal repair, and possible retropubic urethropexy. They found after 2.5 years that the vaginal route was unsatisfactory in 33% of patients, compared with 16% of patients in the abdominal group, and they terminated the study early. Their conclusion was that the abdominal approach was more effective in treating uterovaginal prolapse than the vaginal approach.[47]

In contrast, Maher and colleagues[48] evaluated 95 women with vault prolapse in a randomized, controlled trial. Forty-seven women were allocated to abdominal sacral colpopexy and 48 women to vaginal sacrospinous colpopexy. Both groups underwent Burch urethropexies if stress urinary incontinence was present. After 2 years of follow-up, they found that subjective and objective (76% abdominal versus 69% vaginal; $P = .48$) cure rates were similar for the two groups. Abdominal surgery was associated with longer operating times, slower return to activities, and greater cost in both studies.[48]

Anterior Vaginal Wall Support

If apical support is the sole parameter by which success is measured, the success rates range from 80% to 90%. When evaluating the entire pelvic floor, however, the anterior vaginal compartment appears to represent a particularly vulnerable site. Perhaps this is a consequence of vaginal retroversion predisposing to a compensatory abnormality. Several clinical series, but not all,[49] have demonstrated an elevated risk of cystocele formation after sacrospinous ligament suspension. Recurrent cystoceles have been reported in 7.6% to 92% of women after sacrospinous ligament vaginal vault suspension, depending on the other concurrent procedures performed.[3,12,41,50]

Although early series found recurrent cystoceles in 6% of women who had satisfactory support at the apex,[12] Paraiso and colleagues[51] reported significant anterior wall defects in 26.7% of women after sacrospinous ligament suspension. Smilen and coworkers[49] evaluated 322 women and divided them into two major groups. The first group had anterior wall defects and underwent anterior repairs with or without sacrospinous vaginal vault suspensions. The second group did not have anterior wall defects, and no anterior repairs were performed, but other reconstructive procedures were performed with or without sacrospinous vaginal vault suspensions. the investigators found that the addition of sacrospinous vaginal vault suspensions did not increase the occurrence of postoperative cystoceles in either group.

Sze and associates[39] described 96 women who had pelvic organ prolapse to the hymen or beyond, and they compared women who underwent sacrospinous vaginal vault suspension with or without concomitant transvaginal needle suspension. Recurrent prolapse was observed in 33% of women when the two procedures were performed concurrently, compared with 19% of women who underwent sacrospinous suspension only. The difference did not reach statistical significance.[39] Barber and colleagues[52] reported a 21% incidence of stage III cystoceles after sacrospinous vaginal vault suspension at a mean follow-up interval of 19 months. The incidence rose to 36% when sacrospinous suspensions were performed concomitantly with endoscopic needle suspensions.[52] The increased incidence of cystoceles in these two studies might have been associated with the needle suspension alone or the specific combination of procedures. Alternatively, Goldberg and associates[53] found that bladder neck slings decreased recurrence rates of cystoceles from 42% to 19%, even when performed concomitantly with sacrospinous vaginal vault suspensions. Anterior sacrospinous vault suspensions were not independently predictive of recurrent cystoceles, and posterior sacrospinous vault suspensions were predictive of recurrent cystoceles only when combined with anti-incontinence procedures, not including slings.[53]

The precise mechanisms leading to recurrent anterior vaginal wall prolapse have yet to be outlined. It has been proposed that posterior deflection of the vaginal vault after sacrospinous vaginal vault suspension leads to increased exposure of the anterior compartment to intraperitoneal forces.[54,55] Shull and colleagues[30] suggested that underestimation of the severity of anterior prolapse on preoperative examination or overreliance on the apical suspension for compensation of anterior support defects may play a role. In their series, 16% of patients with anterior vaginal wall prolapse before surgery had no repair of the anterior vaginal wall performed during the initial surgery. Accurately identifying all areas of prolapse preoperatively and modifying the pelvic reconstruction according to intraoperative findings are key to obtaining a successful outcome.

Vaginal Anatomy and Sexual Function

Most studies of sacrospinous vaginal vault suspension have focused on anatomic outcomes, particularly on the rates of recurrent apical, posterior, and anterior vaginal prolapse. Few studies have addressed functional outcomes, such as vaginal length, caliber, axis, and sexual satisfaction. Morley and DeLancey[12] reported vaginal stenosis in 4 of 71 women evaluated at least 1 year after sacrospinous vaginal vault suspension and 1 patient with vaginal foreshortening requiring subsequent vaginoplasty. Elkins and coworkers[54] and Given and associates[56] quantified postoperative vaginal anatomy in more detail, reporting an average vaginal length after sacrospinous ligament suspension of 8.3 and 8.2 cm, respectively. Paraiso and colleagues[51] evaluated an even wider variety of outcomes after sacrospinous suspension at a mean interval of 98.8 months. Vaginal length averaged 8.0 cm, and the vaginal caliber was less than 2 fingerbreadths in 17%; new onset of vaginal constriction was reported in 7.4%.[51]

Sexual dysfunction after pelvic reconstruction with sacrospinous suspension was reported in 14% of patients by Paraiso and co-workers[51]; however, less than one half represented de novo cases. Surprisingly, vaginal length, caliber, and the presence of specific support defects did not correlate with reported sexual activity in this series. Holley and associates[50] concluded that postoperative vaginal narrowing was a significant predictor of decreased sexual activity after sacrospinous suspension and vaginal reconstruction, with 25% reporting postoperative sexual dysfunction. When vaginal narrowing did not occur, sexually active patients reported unchanged or improved sexual function.[50] These reports, in agreement with others,[17,50] concluded that vaginal narrowing and sexual dysfunction after sacrospinous ligament suspension was most often the result of anterior colporrhaphy and the repair of other concomitant defects rather than the sacrospinous suspension itself. Retroversion of the vaginal apex and deviation after unilateral sacrospinous suspension appear to have no adverse effects on coital function postoperatively.

We addressed sexual outcomes in a retrospective analysis of 133 women after sacrospinous vaginal vault suspension (76 after posterior sacrospinous suspension and 57 after anterior suspension) at a median interval of 41 months. Before surgery, 19 (33%) were sexually active in the anterior vault suspension group, with 9 (13%) reporting dyspareunia. At long-term follow-up, two patients in the anterior vault suspension group and two in the posterior vault suspension group reported new-onset dyspareunia. Three of these four cases of de novo dyspareunia were referable to severe atrophy or recurrent grade 3 prolapse; none was attributed to vaginal narrowing or shortening.[6] Sacrospinous ligament vaginal vault suspension appears to have minimal or no impact on sexual function postoperatively, and the choice of anterior or posterior technique has no discernable impact on sexual outcomes. Perhaps most encouraging was that five women in this series reported dyspareunia preoperatively that resolved after vaginal reconstruction with sacrospinous vaginal vault suspension.

PREDICTORS OF SUCCESS

The long-term success of sacrospinous vaginal vault suspension depends on a multitude of factors, including the quality of endopelvic connective tissues, postoperative convalescence, lifestyle factors, and the repair of all coexisting pelvic floor support defects at the time of surgery. Two studies have evaluated predictors of success for reconstructive surgery. Whitesides and colleagues[58] found that age older than 60 years and preoperative stage III or IV prolapse were independent predictors of recurrent prolapse. They also found that bladder neck plication and posterior colporrhaphy were associated with recurrent anterior prolapse. In contrast, Burch or bladder neck sling procedures had a lower risk of recurrent anterior vaginal wall prolapse but a greater risk of posterior vaginal prolapse. Goldberg and coworkers[53] and Cross and associates[57] found decreased risks of anterior vaginal wall prolapse with bladder neck sling procedures. Patients who had three or more concomitant procedures were more likely to have recurrent prolapse, although this factor did not reach statistical significance.[58] Nieminen and coworkers[59] identified vaginal cuff infection (OR = 6.13) and urinary tract infection (OR = 3.65) as predictors of vaginal vault recurrence.

It appears that a successful initial healing process may herald long-term success. Shull and colleagues[30] reported that among 81 women treated with sacrospinous ligament suspension and pelvic reconstruction, the absence of any pelvic support defect at the 6-week postoperative visit was associated with only a 3% likelihood that the patient would require subsequent reconstructive surgery within 2 to 5 years.[30]

ALTERNATIVE TRANSVAGINAL VAULT SUSPENSION PROCEDURES

Iliococcygeus Suspension

In 1963, Inmon[60] described iliococcygeus fixation. The iliococcygeus fascia was selected as an alternative fixation point because it required less dissection than a sacrospinous suspension, with the proposed advantage of decreasing the incidence of neurovascular injury or future cystocele.[21] One drawback of the iliococcygeus suspension, however, is the lack of level I apical support.

Shull and colleagues[61] described 42 patients in whom he performed iliococcygeus suspension, with follow-up periods of 6 weeks to 5 years, and they found only a 5% rate of recurrence. Alternatively, Maher and associates[62] compared sacrospinous suspension to iliococcygeus fixation for prolapse of the vaginal apex in matched cohorts and reported higher "patient satisfaction" scores among the sacrospinous group at a mean follow-up of 20 months. Nonsignificant trends indicated better support after the sacrospinous approach according to subjective and objective outcomes.[62]

Bilateral Uterosacral Suspension

Uterosacral suspension is another alternative to sacrospinous suspension. Karram and coworkers[22] described this procedure in women who underwent primary uterosacral suspension (at the time of hysterectomy) compared with women being treated for recurrent prolapse. Among 168 women with follow-up data, there was a 5% reoperation rate for any defect in the vagina. Only two women had recurrent, symptomatic enterocele or vault prolapse of grade 2 or greater. The investigators were unable to perform the operation in 6 of 200 cases due to exposure or because an enterocele was not found.

Barber and associates[52] described the outcomes of bilateral uterosacral suspension and found that 3 of 46 women needed reoperation. Symptomatic prolapse recurred in four women (10%), two (5%) with apical prolapse. They reported a very high (11%) ureteral occlusion rate.[52] Shull and colleagues[63] found an objective cure rate of 87% (251 of 289 patients) in his series, and Jenkins[64] reported no failures among 50 women.

Suspension of the vaginal apex to the proximal uterosacral ligaments can achieve an excellent anatomic and functional outcome. However, the uterosacral tissues occasionally lack sufficient tensile strength for an effective vault suspension, and the risk of ureteral injury may be as high as 11% when multiple fixation sutures are placed into the uterosacral ligament.

CONCLUSIONS

Based on the existing literature, it appears that each of these operations, in experienced hands, can provide excellent long-term outcomes. Prospective comparisons between sacrospinous ligament vaginal vault suspension and its alternatives will hopefully be the subject of future research.

For the surgical management of advanced prolapse of the vaginal apex, sacrospinous ligament vaginal vault suspension represents a highly reliable transvaginal alternative. Familiarity with the various methods for approaching the ligament and anchoring the vaginal apex allows the surgeon to easily combine this operation with a variety of other vaginal reconstructive procedures. Adherence to fundamental anatomic and surgical principles ensures that a functional vaginal anatomy is maintained and that complications are minimized.

References

1. Swift S, Woodman P, O'Boyle A, et al: Pelvic Organ Support Study (POSST): The distribution, clinical definition, and epidemiologic condition of pelvic organ support defects. Am J Obstet Gynecol 192:795-806, 2005.
2. Zweifel P: Vorle sungen Uber Klinische. Gynaecologie 407-415, 1892.
3. Richter K, Albrich W: Long-term results following fixation of the vagina on the sacrospinal ligament by the vaginal route (vaginaefixatio sacrospinalis vaginalis). Am J Obstet Gynecol 141:811-816, 1981.
4. Nichols DH. Sacrospinous fixation for massive eversion of the vagina. Am J Obstet Gynecol 142:901-904, 1982.
5. Winkler HA, Tomeszko JE, Sand PK: Anterior sacrospinous vaginal vault suspension for prolapse. Obstet Gynecol 95:612-615, 2000.
6. Goldberg RP, Tomezsko JE, Winkler HA, et al: Anterior or posterior sacrospinous vaginal vault suspension: Long-term anatomic and functional evaluation. Obstet Gynecol 98:199-204, 2001.
7. Kearney R, DeLancey JO: Selecting suspension points and excising the vagina during Michigan four-wall sacrospinous suspension. Obstet Gynecol 101:325-330, 2003.
8. Kovac SR, Cruikshank SH: Successful pregnancies and vaginal deliveries after sacrospinous uterosacral fixation in five of nineteen patients. Am J Obstet Gynecol 168:1778-1783; discussion 1783-1786, 1993.
9. Nichols DH: Transvaginal sacrospinous colpopexy. J Pelvic Surg 2:87-91, 1996.
10. Pohl JF, Frattarelli JL: Bilateral transvaginal sacrospinous colpopexy: Preliminary experience. Am J Obstet Gynecol 177:1356-1361; discussion 1361-1362, 1997.
11. Cespedes RD: Anterior approach bilateral sacrospinous ligament fixation for vaginal vault prolapse. Urology 56:70-75, 1997.
12. Morley GW, DeLancey JO: Sacrospinous ligament fixation for eversion of the vagina. Am J Obstet Gynecol 158:872-881, 1988.
13. Mant J, Painter R, Vessey M: Epidemiology of genital prolapse: Observations from the Oxford Family Planning Association study. Br J Obstet Gynaecol 104:579-585, 1997.
14. Swift S: The distribution of pelvic organ support in a population of female subjects seen for routine gynecologic health care. Am J Obstet Gynecol 186:712-716, 2000.
15. Brown JS, Waetjen LE, Subak LL, et al: Pelvic organ prolapse surgery in the United States, 1997. Am J Obstet Gynecol 186:712-716, 2002.
16. Cruikshank SH, Cox DW: Sacrospinous ligament fixation at the time of transvaginal hysterectomy. Am J Obstet Gynecol 162:1611-1615; discussion 1615-1619, 1990.
17. Colombo M, Milani R: Sacrospinous ligament fixation and modified McCall culdoplasty during vaginal hysterectomy for advanced uterovaginal prolapse. Am J Obstet Gynecol 179:13-20, 1998.
18. Hefni M, El-Toukhy T, Bhaumik J, Katsimanis E: Sacrospinous cervicocolpopexy with uterine conservation for uterovaginal prolapse in elderly women: An evolving concept. Am J Obstet Gynecol 188:645-650, 2003.
19. Maher CF, Cary MP, Slack MC, et al: Uterine preservation or hysterectomy at sacrospinous colpopexy for uterovaginal prolapse? Int Urogynecol J Pelvic Floor Dysfunct 12:381-384; discussion 384-385, 2001.
20. DeLancey JO: Anatomic aspects of vaginal eversion after hysterectomy. Am J Obstet Gynecol 166:1717-1724; discussion 1724-1728, 1992.
21. Flynn BJ, Webster GD: Surgical management of the apical vaginal defect. Curr Opin Urol 12:353-358, 2002.
22. Karram M, Goldwasser S, Kleeman S, et al: High uterosacral vaginal vault suspension with fascial reconstruction for vaginal repair of enterocele and vaginal vault prolapse. Am J Obstet Gynecol 185:1339-1342; discussion 1342-1343, 2001.
23. Warwick R, Williams PL: Gray's Anatomy. Philadelphia, WB Saunders Company, 1973.
24. Netter FH: Normal anatomy of the female genital tract and its functional relationships. In Oppenheimer E (ed): Reproductive System, vol 2. West Caldwell, Ciba-Geigy, 1965.
25. Verdeja AM, Elkins TE, Odoi A, et al: Transvaginal sacrospinous colpopexy: Anatomic landmarks to be aware of to minimize complications. Am J Obstet Gynecol 173:1468-1469, 1995.
26. Barksdale PA, Elkins TE, Sanders CK, et al: An anatomic approach to pelvic hemorrhage during sacrospinous ligament fixation of the vaginal vault. Obstet Gynecol 91:715-718, 1998.
27. Richardson AC: The anatomic defects in rectocele and enterocele. J Pelvic Surg 1:214-221, 1995.
28. Cruikshank SH, Muniz M: Outcomes study: A comparison of cure rates in 695 patients undergoing sacrospinous ligament fixation alone and with other site-specific procedures—A 16-year study. Am J Obstet Gynecol 188:1509-1512; discussion 1512-1515, 2003.
29. Porges RF, Smilen SW: Long-term analysis of the surgical management of pelvic support defects. Am J Obstet Gynecol 171:1518-1526; discussion 1526-1528, 1994.
30. Shull BL, Capen CV, Riggs MW, Kuehl TJ: Preoperative and postoperative analysis of site-specific pelvic support defects in 81 women treated with sacrospinous ligament suspension and pelvic reconstruction. Am J Obstet Gynecol 166:1764-1768; discussion 1768-1771, 1992.
31. Sultana CJ, Walters MD: Estrogen and urinary incontinence in women. Maturitas 20:129-138, 1994.
32. Miyazaki FS: Miya hook ligature carrier for sacrospinous ligament suspension. Obstet Gynecol 70:286-288, 1987.
33. Lind LR, Choe J, Bhatia NN: An in-line suturing device to simplify sacrospinous vaginal vault suspension. Obstet Gynecol 89:129-132, 1997.
34. Luck AM, Galvin SL, Theofrastous JP: Suture erosion and wound dehiscence with permanent versus absorbable suture in posterior vaginal surgery. In Bent AE (ed): Joint Scientific Meeting: The American Urogynecologic Society and The Society of Gynecologic Surgeons. San Diego, CA, J Pelvic Med Surg 514, 2004.
35. Carey MP, Slack MC: Transvaginal sacrospinous colpopexy for vault and marked uterovaginal prolapse. Br J Obstet Gynaecol 101:536-540, 1994.
36. Nichols DH: Fertility retention in the patient with genital prolapse. Am J Obstet Gynecol 164:1155-1158, 1991.
37. Alevizon SJ, Finan MA: Sacrospinous colpopexy: Management of postoperative pudendal nerve entrapment. Obstet Gynecol 88:713-715, 1996.
38. Barksdale PA, Gasser RF, Gauthier CM, et al: Intraligamentous nerves as a potential source of pain after sacrospinous ligament

fixation of the vaginal apex. Int Urogynecol J Pelvic Floor Dysfunct 8:121-125, 1997.
39. Sze EH, Karram MM: Transvaginal repair of vault prolapse: A review. Obstet Gynecol 89:466-475, 1997.
40. Guner H, Noyan V, Tiras MB, et al: Transvaginal sacrospinous colpopexy for marked uterovaginal and vault prolapse. Int J Gynaecol Obstet 74:165-170, 2001.
41. Pasley WW: Sacrospinous suspension: A local practitioner's experience. Am J Obstet Gynecol 173:440-445; discussion 445-448, 1995.
42. Heinonen PK: Transvaginal sacrospinous colpopexy for vaginal vault and complete genital prolapse in aged women. Acta Obstet Gynecol Scand 71:377-381, 1992.
43. Slack MC: Sacrospinous colpopexy for support of the vaginal apex. In Cardoza L, Staskin D (eds): Textbook of Female Urology and Urogynaecology. London, Martin Dunitz, 2001.
44. Morley GW: Discussion of Cruikshank SH, Cox DW. Sacrospinous ligament fixation at the time of transvaginal hysterectomy. Am J Obstet Gynecol 162:1611-1619, 1990.
45. Hardiman PJ, Drutz HP: Sacrospinous vault suspension and abdominal colposacropexy: Success rates and complications. Am J Obstet Gynecol 175:612-616, 1996.
46. Nichols DH, Randall CL: Massive eversion of the vagina. In Vaginal Surgery. Baltimore, Williams & Wilkins, 1989.
47. Benson JT, Lucente V, McClellan E: Vaginal versus abdominal reconstructive surgery for the treatment of pelvic support defects: A prospective randomized study with long-term outcome evaluation. Am J Obstet Gynecol 175:1418-1421; discussion 1421-1422, 1996.
48. Maher CF, Qatawneh AM, Dwyer PL, et al: Abdominal sacral colpopexy or vaginal sacrospinous colpopexy for vaginal vault prolapse: A prospective randomized study. Am J Obstet Gynecol 190:20-26, 2004.
49. Smilen SW, Saini J, Wallach SJ, Porges RF: The risk of cystocele after sacrospinous ligament fixation. Am J Obstet Gynecol 179:1465-1471; discussion 1471-1472, 1998.
50. Holley RL, Varner RE, Gleason BP, et al: Sexual function after sacrospinous ligament fixation for vaginal vault prolapse. J Reprod Med 41:355-358, 1996.
51. Paraiso MF, Ballard LA, Walters MD, et al: Pelvic support defects and visceral and sexual function in women treated with sacrospinous ligament suspension and pelvic reconstruction. Am J Obstet Gynecol 175:1423-1430; discussion 1430-1431, 1996.
52. Barber MD, Visco AG, Weidner AC, et al: Bilateral uterosacral ligament vaginal vault suspension with site-specific endopelvic fascia defect repair for treatment of pelvic organ prolapse. Am J Obstet Gynecol 183:1402-1410; discussion 1410-1411, 2000.
53. Goldberg RP, Koduri S, Lobel RW, et al: Protective effect of suburethral slings on postoperative cystocele recurrence after reconstructive pelvic operation. Am J Obstet Gynecol 185:1307-1312; discussion 1312-1313, 2001.
54. Elkins TE, Hopper JB, Goodfellow K, et al: Initial report of anatomic and clinical comparison of the sacrospinous ligament fixation to the high McCall culdoplasty for vaginal cuff fixation at hysterectomy for uterine prolapse. J Pelvic Surg 1:12-17, 1995.
55. Shull BL: Pelvic organ prolapse: Anterior, superior, and posterior vaginal segment defects. Am J Obstet Gynecol 181:6-11, 1999.
56. Given FT Jr, Muhlendorf IK, Browning GM: Vaginal length and sexual function after colpopexy for complete uterovaginal eversion. Am J Obstet Gynecol 169:284-287; discussion 287-288, 1993.
57. Cross CA, Cespedes RD, McGuire EJ: Treatment results using pubovaginal slings in patients with large cystoceles and stress incontinence. J Urol 158:431-434, 1997.
58. Whitesides JL, Weber AM, Meyn LA, Walters MD: Risk factors for prolapse recurrence after vaginal repair. Obstet Gynecol Surv 60:164-165, 2005.
59. Nieminen K, Huhtala H, Heinonen PK: Anatomic and functional assessment and risk factors of recurrent prolapse after vaginal sacrospinous fixation. Acta Obstet Gynecol Scand 82:471-478, 2003.
60. Inmon WB: Pelvic relaxation and repair including prolapse of vagina following hysterectomy. Am J Obstet Gynecol 56:577-582, 1963.
61. Shull BL, Capen CV, Riggs MW, Kuehl TJ: Bilateral attachment of the vaginal cuff to iliococcygeus fascia: An effective method of cuff suspension. Am J Obstet Gynecol 168:1669-1674; discussion 1674-1677, 1993.
62. Maher CF, Murray CJ, Carey MP, et al: Iliococcygeus or sacrospinous fixation for vaginal vault prolapse. Obstet Gynecol 98:40-44, 2001.
63. Shull BL, Bachofen C, Coates KW, Kuehl TJ: A transvaginal approach to repair of apical and other associated sites of pelvic organ prolapse with uterosacral ligaments. Am J Obstet Gynecol 183:1365-1373; discussion 1373-1374, 2000.
64. Jenkins VR 2nd: Uterosacral ligament fixation for vaginal vault suspension in uterine and vaginal vault prolapse. Am J Obstet Gynecol 177:1337-1343; discussion 1343-1344, 1997.
65. Hoffman MS, Harris MS, Bouis PJ: Sacrospinous colpopexy in the management of uterovaginal prolapse. J Reprod Med 41:299-303, 1996.
66. Chapin DS: Teaching sacrospinous colpopexy. Am J Obstet Gynecol 177:1330-1336, 1997.
67. Meschia M, Bruschi F, Amicarelli F, et al: The sacrospinous vaginal vault suspension: Critical analysis of outcomes. Int Urogynecol J Pelvic Floor Dysfunct 10:155-159, 1999.
68. Lantzsch T, Goepel C, Wolters M, et al: Sacrospinous ligament fixation for vaginal vault prolapse. Arch Gynecol Obstet 265:21-25, 2001.

Chapter 68

REPAIR OF VAGINAL VAULT PROLAPSE USING SOFT PROLENE MESH

Matthew P. Rutman, Donna Y. Deng, Larissa V. Rodríguez, and Shlomo Raz

Vaginal vault prolapse results from elongation or detachment of the sacrouterine-cardinal ligament complex. It commonly manifests with other vaginal defects, such as cystocele, enterocele, and rectocele. Patients typically present with symptoms similar to uterine prolapse: a mass protruding vaginally, dyspareunia, low back pain, or perineal pressure. Sometimes, patients present with symptoms of voiding dysfunction, such as incomplete emptying, retention, recurrent infections, or incontinence.

An enterocele is a hernia of the peritoneum, with its contents extending between the vagina and rectum at the level of the vaginal vault. The use of dynamic magnetic resonance imaging (MRI) has allowed routine identification of the contents: small bowel, sigmoid, fluid, or omentum. Most enteroceles are acquired as a result of prior surgery on the anterior vaginal wall altering the vaginal axis or poor closure of the cul-de-sac at the time of hysterectomy. The incidence of enterocele in patients who underwent gynecologic surgery is as high as 16%.[1] For the purposes of this chapter, we divide enteroceles into simple and complex types. A simple enterocele exists when there is no concomitant vault prolapse. The only defect is between the perivesical and prerectal fascia, which allows the peritoneum to herniate through, creating an enterocele. In a complex enterocele, there is concomitant vault prolapse. Many techniques have been described for supporting the vaginal vault after enterocele repair and hysterectomy.

APICAL VAGINAL WALL PROLAPSE: ANATOMY AND PATHOPHYSIOLOGY

The most proximal portion of the vagina, called the vaginal cuff or vault, is supported by the cardinal ligaments and uterosacral ligament complex. The cardinal ligaments are thick, anteriorly based fascial condensations originating from the greater sciatic foramen and inserting into the lateral fascia of the cervix and adjacent vaginal wall. They provide critical uterine and apical vaginal support. The uterosacral ligaments originate from the sacral vertebrae and insert into the lateral vaginal fornices, fusing with the cardinal ligaments posteriorly and stabilizing the uterus, cervix, and apical vagina in a posterior direction toward the sacrum. The broad ligaments, located more superiorly, attach the lateral walls of the uterine body to the pelvic side wall, providing additional uterine support. They contain the fallopian tubes, the round and ovarian ligaments, and the uterine and ovarian blood supply.

Lateral walls of the rectum are supported to the lateral pelvic wall and sacrum by condensations of connective tissue to the levator muscle extending to the sacrum (i.e., pillars of the rectum). The rectovaginal septum is a fascial extension of the peritoneal cul-de-sac between the vaginal apex and the anterior rectal wall. The septum consists of two distinct fascial layers: posterior vaginal fascia and prerectal fascia. The layers fuse with the cardinal-uterosacral ligament complex proximally, stabilizing the posterior vaginal apex. The two layers fuse distally and insert into the perineal body. The perineal body is a tendinous structure located in the midline of the perineum between the vagina and anus, and it provides additional pelvic support to the posterior vaginal wall and rectum. It serves as a central insertion point for the superficial and deep transverse perineal, bulbospongiosus, and external sphincter muscles. The perineal membrane consists of the distal 3 to 4 cm of the vagina and serves as an attachment point for the levator musculature. This is a critical anatomic landmark in posterior repair.

The musculature of the pelvic floor provides the main support for the pelvic viscera. It is composed of the coccygeus and levator ani muscles. The horizontal levator plate allows maintenance of the normal vaginal axis. The levator hiatus refers to the midline openings of the levator ani that allow passage of the urethra, vagina, and rectum. The proximal vagina and rectum rest on the levator floor and remain well supported with increases in intra-abdominal pressure in patients with normal pelvic support.

Pelvic floor relaxation results in vaginal wall prolapse. Multiparity, obesity, hormonal changes, increasing age, and tissue and nerve damage can play important roles in vaginal prolapse. The resulting area of prolapse depends on the location of muscular and ligamentous damage.

EVALUATION

Patients found to have small vault prolapse or enteroceles on physical examination are typically asymptomatic. As the vault prolapse increases, patients may report symptoms of vaginal and perineal fullness or lower back pain that improves with supine positioning. Other complaints include dyspareunia and symptoms of voiding dysfunction, such as incomplete emptying, retention, recurrent infections, or incontinence. Patient with voiding symptoms should be evaluated with video urodynamic studies. The physical examination is essential for diagnosis, and it usually reveals a bulging mass at the vaginal apex. An enterocele can be difficult to distinguish from a high rectocele or cystocele. Separate examination of the vaginal walls with a half-blade of a Graves speculum is routine with Pelvic Organ Prolapse Quantification measurements.

Simultaneous rectal and vaginal examination may aid in differentiating an enterocele from a high rectocele. Examination in the standing position and cystoscopic light in the bladder also may assist in making the proper diagnosis.[2] Any concomitant defects should be documented.

Many radiologic modalities have been used in the diagnosis of enterocele, including defecography, fluoroscopy, dynamic cystocolpoproctography, and MRI. Dynamic MRI provides superior imaging of all three vaginal compartments and may help differentiate introital masses.[3] In patients with severe prolapse of the anterior and apical vaginal wall, the upper urinary tract must be evaluated (e.g., renal ultrasound, pyelogram, computed tomography urography) because severe prolapse can cause severe angulation of the ureters resulting in ureteral obstruction.

CONSERVATIVE TREATMENT

Conservative treatment, which is best for early prolapse and poor surgical candidates, includes pelvic muscle rehabilitation, hormone replacement therapy, and pessary use. Patients should be instructed to avoid constipation and activities such as heavy lifting and straining. Pessary fitting can be quite challenging, and improper placement and poor hygiene can lead to erosions into the vaginal mucosa and adjacent structures. As the severity of prolapse increases, it becomes increasingly difficult to retain a pessary, which mandates formal surgical repair. Concomitant prolapse should be addressed at the same time. Colpocleisis can be performed with minimal anesthesia as an alternative to definitive repair. This is a less morbid option in the sexually inactive elderly patient with multiple comorbidities.

SURGERY

Surgical Indications

Treatment is driven by patients' symptoms. Low grades of prolapse are often asymptomatic and can be managed nonoperatively. Patients who are symptomatic and have concomitant prolapse, ulcerations, and obstructive voiding require surgical intervention. Patients with severe prolapse causing obstruction of the upper tracts and hydronephrosis also require intervention. Simultaneous repair of other vaginal prolapse should be performed.

Surgical Techniques

Numerous techniques have been described for vault prolapse and enterocele repair, including abdominal, vaginal, and laparoscopic repair. Because several of these procedures are discussed in detail in other chapters, they are mentioned briefly here as a reference only. Abdominal repair, with sacrocolpopexy or hysterectomy, closes the cul-de-sac using one of two popular techniques. The Moschcowitz repair obliterates the cul-de-sac using purse-string sutures from the bottom of the sac to the most cephalad aspect. The Halban repair obliterates the cul-de-sac by placing sutures in the sagittal plane between the anterior rectal wall and the posterior vaginal wall. Vaginal repair avoids the morbidity of a laparotomy and has the advantages of decreased hospital costs and quicker recovery time. In the following sections, we describe two techniques used for transvaginal sacrouterine fixation.

Transvaginal Sacrouterine Fixation for Vault Prolapse with Enterocele Repair

The patient is placed in the high lithotomy position after anesthesia is provided. The lower abdomen and vagina are prepared and draped in a sterile fashion. The labia minora are retracted, and a Foley catheter is placed. A ring retractor with hooks is positioned, and the enterocele is grasped with two Allis clamps. In patients undergoing concomitant hysterectomy, the peritoneal cavity is exposed. The vaginal apex is located by identifying the scar at the lateral apex. It is marked bilaterally with electrocautery. A vertical incision is made anteriorly from the base of the bladder extending posteriorly to the prerectal area. Sharp dissection is used to free the peritoneal sac from the vaginal wall. Special attention is necessary to avoid inadvertent bladder or rectal injury during the dissection. Cystoscopic illumination of the bladder can help define the bladder base.

The peritoneal sac is opened, exposing the bowel contents. After freeing any adhesions, two Betadine-soaked laparotomy pads are placed to pack the abdominal contents, and deep right-angle retractors (Haney) are used to retract for optimal exposure. This maneuver protects the bowel and bladder during the procedure. Vault suspension sutures are placed at this time to support the cuff to the sacrouterine ligaments. In patients with vault prolapse and enterocele, the procedure obliterates the cul-de-sac and suspends the vaginal cuff high on the levator plate. A 1-0 Vicryl suture is passed through the vaginal wall (apex) inside the peritoneal cavity incorporating prerectal fascia and the ipsilateral origin of the sacrouterine ligament complex (i.e., iliococcygeus muscle). The sacrum, coccyx, and the coccygeus muscle and its underlying sacrospinous ligament (i.e., strong, firm, rectangular structure) are palpated. The rectum is retracted medially, and a strong purchase is taken posterolaterally in the groove between the iliococcygeus muscle and rectal wall. We also incorporate the prerectal fascia, resulting in reduction of the rectocele. It is essential to take a strong bite of tissue in the pararectal area. The suture is brought out the vaginal wall 1 cm from the original entry point. The same maneuver is performed on the contralateral side. The culdosuspension sutures are left untied.

The enterocele (peritoneal cavity) is closed with two 1-0 Vicryl sutures in a purse-string fashion. These sutures incorporate the sacrouterine-cardinal ligament complex laterally, prerectal fascia posteriorly, and perivesical fascia anteriorly (i.e., base of the pubocervical fascia). This obliterates the potential space between the prerectal fascia and the perivesical fascia. Distal suture placement preserves adequate vaginal depth. It is important to take strong bites of the perivesical fascia, including the posterior peritoneal surface of the bladder, with careful attention to staying in the middle (i.e., ureters run laterally). This ensures closure of the enterocele and reapproximates the prerectal and perivesical fascia. The excess peritoneal sac is excised after tying the sutures. Indigo carmine is administered intravenously and cystoscopy is performed to rule out iatrogenic ureteral obstruction from suture placement.

At this point, we perform a sling or cystocele repair if required. The vault suspension sutures are tied after we reduce the vault using a weighted speculum and Allis clamp to reduce the cuff to the most posterior and deep position. This provides depth and support of the cuff and restores the normal banana-shaped vaginal axis (in the lithotomy position). Excess vaginal wall is trimmed, and the vaginal wall is closed with a running, locking 2-0 Vicryl suture.

The rectocele is repaired next. The posterior fourchette is excised, and a triangular flap of posterior vaginal wall is excised 4 cm from the hymen, exposing the perineal membrane and the levator plate. A 1-cm strip of posterior vaginal wall is excised to expose the pillar of the rectum and the prerectal fascia. The proximal vagina is repaired with 2-0 delayed absorption sutures that include the edge of the vaginal wall and the pillar of the rectum. In the distal vagina, figure-of-eight sutures are used to repair the levator hiatus by incorporating the edge of the vaginal wall and the perineal membrane (indirectly approximating the levator musculature). The perineal body repair is completed. The vagina is packed with an antibiotic-impregnated gauze.

Most vault suspension and enterocele repairs are performed as outpatient surgery. The vaginal pack is removed after 2 hours, and patients are discharged home and remain on several days of oral antibiotics.

We previously reported data for 104 patients who underwent transvaginal culdosuspension with enterocele repair or hysterectomy, or both.[4] This cohort had the procedure performed without mesh reconstruction. Concomitant prolapse was repaired in 82 patients. Perioperative complications included two patients with cuff infections, two patients with ileus and one patient with ureteral obstruction. Both patients with ileus responded to conservative management. The vaginal cuff infections did not require operative intervention and responded to antibiotics and local wound care. The patient with ureteral obstruction required ureteroneocystostomy. The patients were followed for a mean period of 17.3 months. Recurrence occurred in four patients (3.8%). All four had repeat transvaginal colposuspension, and each was free of prolapse at the last follow-up. No patients had vaginal foreshortening, urinary retention, or rectovaginal fistula. One patient had prolonged dyspareunia that resolved after 6 months.

Mesh Repair for Concomitant Vault Prolapse, Enterocele, and Rectocele

In patients with apical and posterior compartment prolapse, we restore the sacrouterine ligament complex and repair the pelvic floor with the use of a polypropylene mesh. This method also is used in patients undergoing vaginal hysterectomy. Most patients with vault prolapse have widening of the levator hiatus and descent of the levator musculature. The technique addresses reconstruction of the pelvic floor and prevents levator descent. Prior experience with anterior wall failures without the use of surrogate materials has ignited our interest in total mesh reconstruction for durable recreation of vaginal anatomy. Addressing perineal body descent is important to prevent recurrent prolapse and anorectal disorders.

A T-shaped soft Prolene mesh is cut from a sheet of 6 × 6 inch soft polypropylene mesh. The two transverse arms are measured to 4 × 1 cm, and the vertical segment is 3 × 6 cm (Fig. 68-1). The two transverse arms mimic the sacrouterine ligaments in support of the cuff. The vertical segment recreates the prerectal fascia inserting at the perineal membrane (Fig. 68-2). Vault suspension sutures are placed as described earlier, incorporating the origin of the sacrouterine ligament. The sutures are brought through the transverse arm of the mesh, and a second purchase of the sacrouterine ligament is taken (Fig. 68-3). We also incorporate the prerectal fascia, resulting in full support of the cuff by the two arms of the mesh because it mimics the normal sacrouterine ligament support. This also aids in reducing the rectocele. The enterocele closure is performed in purse-string fashion as done earlier with the posterior bites (of the prerectal fascia), including

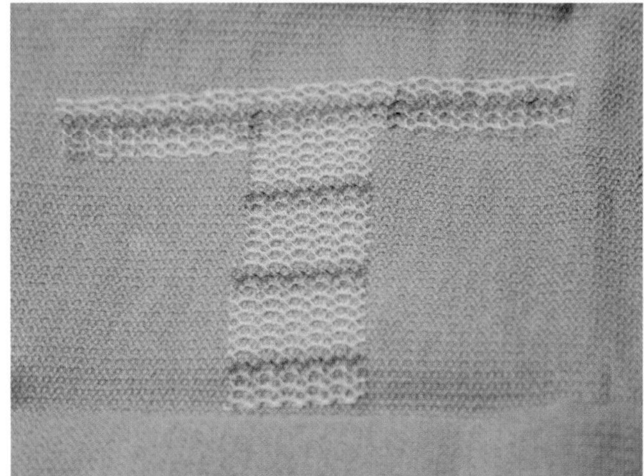

Figure 68-1 T-shaped mesh.

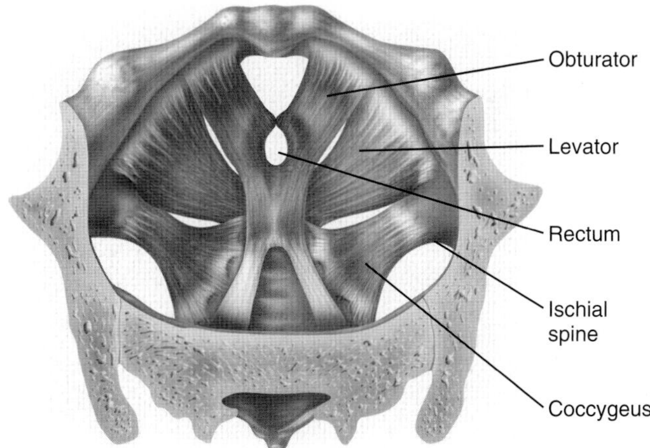

Figure 68-2 Mesh recreation of the sacrouterine ligament–prerectal fascia complex.

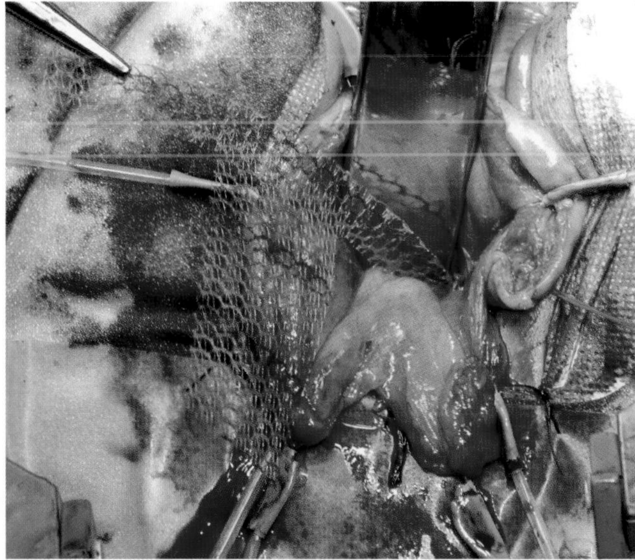

Figure 68-3 Transverse arm of mesh recreating the sacrouterine ligament origin.

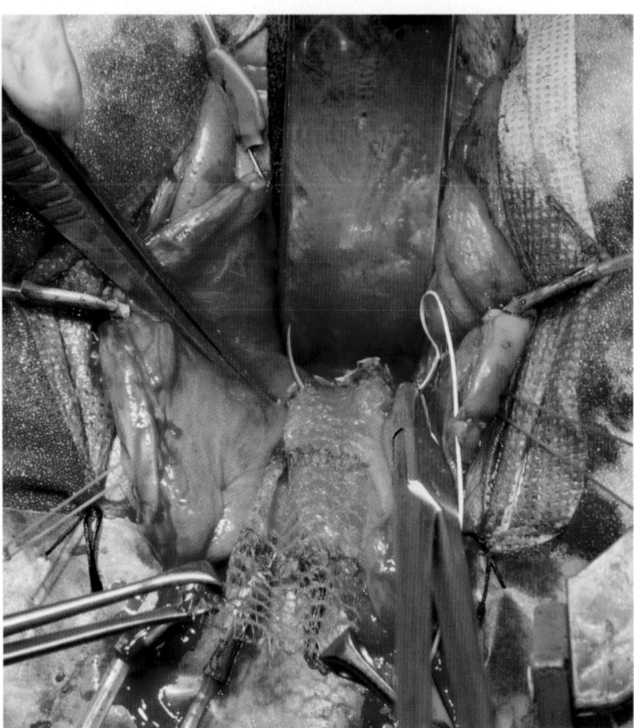

Figure 68-4 Closure of an enterocele, including mesh with prerectal fascia.

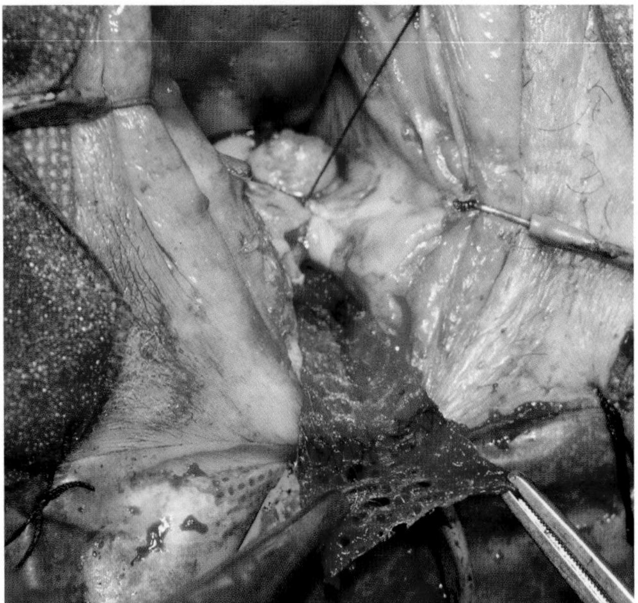

Figure 68-5 Mesh exiting at the distal vagina.

small purchases of the proximal vertical mesh segment (Fig. 68-4).The vertical segment of the mesh is then tunneled to the posterior vaginal wall for a distance of 2 to 3 cm to avoid incorporation of the mesh during the vaginal cuff closure. The mesh is eventually brought out to the distal vagina over the prerectal fascia (Fig. 68-5). The vertical segment of the mesh acts as surrogate tissue to improve the rectocele repair and prevent levator descent. The proximal vagina is repaired with 2-0 delayed absorption sutures, including the edge of the vaginal wall and the pillar of the rectum. In the distal vagina, figure-of-eight sutures are used to repair the levator hiatus by incorporating the edge of the vaginal wall, the edge of the vertical mesh segment, and the perineal membrane and levator musculature. The excess mesh is excised, and the perineal body repair is completed.

We have performed the previous procedure on more than 100 patients since February 2004. Forty percent underwent concomitant vaginal hysterectomy. We have had no intraoperative complications. Pelvic Organ Prolapse Quantification staging has revealed restoration of normal vaginal anatomy. Two patients (2.5%) have had recurrent enteroceles without vault prolapse; one required a second procedure. One patient had a small mesh erosion at the posterior vaginal wall that was cured with office excision. An additional patient had unilateral ureteral obstruction requiring ureteroneocystostomy. Longer follow-up will be reported as our data matures.

Other Techniques for Treating Vault Prolapse and Enterocele

Pelvic reconstructive surgeons have described other techniques of transvaginal uterosacral fixation for apical prolapse. Shull and colleagues[5] reported a total of 302 consecutive patients who underwent transvaginal reconstructive surgery for apical prolapse by a single surgeon. In patients with prior hysterectomy and vault prolapse, a vertical midline incision was made in the vaginal epithelium. The epithelium was dissected off the underlying enterocele sac. The pubocervical and rectovaginal fascia were identified, and the enterocele sac was found between the two planes. The enterocele sac was opened and the bowel packed. The remaining uterosacral ligaments were identified medial and posterior to the ischial spine at 4- and 8-o'clock, respectively. A double-armed nonabsorbable suture was then placed from lateral to medial aspects through the ligament on the sacral side of the ischial spine. Two additional sutures were then placed distal and medial to the initial suture. The same maneuver was then performed on the contralateral side.

At this point, six sutures were tagged and labeled. Central defects in the pubocervical and rectovaginal fascia were then repaired by plication technique. The double-armed sutures were brought through the superior aspect of the rectovaginal and pubocervical fascia, respectively. Before securing the sutures, indigo carmine was administered intravenously. The sutures were secured, resulting in the pubocervical fascia and rectovaginal fascia being anchored together at the vaginal apex. The suspensory sutures were all secured, and cystoscopy ensured ureteral patency. The vaginal epithelium was trimmed and closed with a running polyglycolic suture. Concomitant retropubic urethropexy and perineal body repair were performed if necessary. There was no closure of the peritoneal cavity in this technique.

This transvaginal technique was used in 302 patients between 1994 and 1998.[5] The means follow-up period was 1.18 years. In this cohort, 289 had at least one postoperative examination, and 87% had no subsequent support defect, with the remaining 13% having some degree of pelvic support loss. Only 5% of the patients had development of grade 2 or greater support defects. One patient required a unilateral ureteroneocystostomy for a ureteral injury discovered at the time of surgery consisting of a hysterectomy, cystocele repair, rectocele repair, enterocele repair, and vaginal cuff suspension. Three patients required homologous blood transfusion. One elderly patient with dementia died at home 4 days after release from the hospital.

High uterosacral vaginal vault suspension with fascial reconstruction for enterocele and vault prolapse was performed by Karram and coworkers[6] for a large cohort at the University of Cincinnati. Exposure was similar to the previously described technique. After the peritoneal cavity was exposed and the bowel packed, a wide retractor was used for optimal exposure. The ischial spines were palpated, and the remnants of the uterosacral ligaments were identified. An Allis clamp was placed at the 5- and 7-o'clock positions. Permanent sutures were then passed through the ligaments from side to side, incorporating the peritoneum between the two sides. A total of two to four sutures were placed. Anterior wall surgery was then performed if required. The anterior and posterior vaginal walls were suspended by their underlying fascia high to the uterosacral ligaments on each side, using four to six sutures. All other indicated repairs were performed.

Follow-up was available for 168 of the 202 women who underwent high uterosacral vaginal vault suspension.[6] Only two women (1%) had recurrent symptomatic enterocele or vault prolapse of grade 2 or greater. A total of 4.5% underwent reoperation for symptomatic anterior or posterior vaginal wall prolapse. An additional 5% had recurrent prolapse of grade 2 or greater that was asymptomatic or for which no further therapy was desired by the patient. At a mean of 21.6 months after surgery, 89% of the 168 women were "happy" or "satisfied" with their procedure. There were five cases of ureteral injury, four of which were diagnosed at the time of surgery and reversed by cutting of the suspension sutures. One case required a ureteral reimplantation due to a ureterotomy. One patient had a small bowel injury and required a laparotomy. Another patient developed a pelvic abscess requiring exploration and a diverting colostomy.

The McCall procedure and several later modifications close the cul-de-sac using an abdominal or vaginal approach. This technique plicates the uterosacral ligaments in the midline and suspends the posterior vaginal fornix to these ligaments.

The sacrospinous ligament fixation is a commonly performed procedure, particularly by urogynecologists. It is described in chapter 67 in full detail. It was initially described by Nichols[7,8] and Randall,[8] who had slight variations in their techniques. Both attach the vaginal vault to the sacrospinous ligament medial to the ischial spine, but Randall does it under visual control and Nichols under digital control. The procedure can be done unilaterally or bilaterally, and it typically uses a posterior extraperitoneal approach.[8] Several surgeons have criticized the approach for altering the vaginal axis and predisposing the patient to anterior compartment recurrences. An article with a 2.5-year follow-up reported a 29% rate of recurrent cystocele.[9] Additional complications described in the literature include hemorrhage (2%), gluteal pain (3%), pudendal nerve injury, and rarely, cystotomy or proctotomy.

Iliococcygeus fascia colpopexy involves suturing the vaginal cuff to the iliococcygeus fascia near the ischial spine bilaterally.[10,11] A similar procedure, called levator myorrhaphy, uses the levator ani fascia as the supporting structure for the vault suspension. Extraperitoneal and intraperitoneal approaches have been described, and both have had excellent reported results.[12]

Abdominal sacrocolpopexy (open or laparoscopic) is another approach advocated by some for vaginal vault prolapse. Through an intraperitoneal abdominal incision, the sacral promontory and vaginal apex are exposed. The cul-de-sac is closed. A piece of sterile mesh or fascia is then attached to the apex of the vagina and eventually fixed to the sacrum using permanent sutures. The overlying peritoneum is closed, providing coverage of the mesh. This procedure adds the morbidity of a laparotomy and does not address severe anterior and posterior wall prolapse. Nevertheless, it has consistent long-term cure rates of more than 90%.[13,14] Because the procedure does not require excision of the vaginal wall, it helps to preserve vaginal length, leading some surgeons to advocate the procedure as first-line treatment in younger patients with vault prolapse who are sexually active.[15,16]

The major complications associated with abdominal sacrocolpopexy are hemorrhage from the presacral veins and mesh erosion. Several series have reported hemorrhage rates ranging from 1.2% to 2.6 %.[16,17] Mesh erosion is reported to occur in up to 5% of cases.[17] A comprehensive review reported an overall rate of mesh erosion of 3.4%. The same review reported a 1.1% rate of small bowel obstruction requiring reoperation.[18]

Laparoscopic sacral colposuspension for apical defects has been described in numerous reports. It is done in a manner similar to the open approach, with four or five ports in the lower abdominal wall and a sponge stick in the vagina. Long-term outcomes have yet to be reported, but short-term results are in the same neighborhood as the open approach.

Although enterocele repair has been performed for approximately a century, few long-term outcomes have been reported. Previous studies report 86% to 96% cure rates at 15 and 17 months of follow-up, respectively.[4,19]

COMPLICATIONS

Intraoperative complications include bleeding, ureteric and bladder injury, and rectal injury. Ureteral injury most commonly occurs from placement of the purse-string or culdosuspension sutures. Cystoscopy after intravenous indigo carmine can establish ureteral patency. When there is lack of efflux, passage of ureteral catheters can help exclude obstruction. Delayed complications include recurrent prolapse, vaginal shortening, dyspareunia, ileus, and bowel obstruction.

CONCLUSIONS

The best approach to vaginal vault prolapse remains unknown. The surgeon's comfort and preference and proper patient selection are essential. A prospective study of 95 patients randomized to abdominal or vaginal repair showed no statistical difference in subjective or objective success. Longer operating times and longer convalescence were statistically significant in the abdominal cohort.[9] The transvaginal sacrouterine fixation for vault prolapse recreates the sacrouterine-ligament complex in support of the vaginal vault. The use of polypropylene mesh prevents levator descent, along with restoring the sacrouterine ligament complex and repairing the levator hiatus. It is a safe and effective procedure for preventing and treating enterocele and vaginal vault prolapse.

References

1. Symmonds RE, Williams TJ, Lee RA, et al: Posthysterectomy enterocele and vaginal vault prolapse. Am J Obstet Gynecol 140:852, 1981.
2. Vasavada SP, Comiter CV, Raz S: Cystoscopic light test to aid in the differentiation of high-grade pelvic organ prolapse. Urology 54:1085, 1999.
3. Barbaric ZL, Marumoto AK, Raz S: Magnetic resonance imaging of the perineum and pelvic floor. Top Magn Reson Imaging 12:83, 2001.
4. Comiter CV, Vasavada SP, Raz S: Transvaginal culdosuspension: Technique and results. Urology 54:819, 1999.
5. Shull BL, Bachofen C, Coates KW, et al: A transvaginal approach to repair of apical and other associated sites of pelvic organ prolapse with uterosacral ligaments. Am J Obstet Gynecol 183:1365, 2000.
6. Karram M, Goldwasser S, Kleeman S, et al: High uterosacral vaginal vault suspension with fascial reconstruction for vaginal repair of enterocele and vaginal vault prolapse. Am J Obstet Gynecol 185:1339, 2001.
7. Nichols DH: Types of enterocele and principles underlying choice of operation for repair. Obstet Gynecol 40:257, 1972.
8. Randall CL, Nichols DH: Surgical treatment of vaginal inversion. Obstet Gynecol 38:327, 1971.
9. Benson JT, Lucente V, McClellan E: Vaginal versus abdominal reconstructive surgery for the treatment of pelvic support defects: A prospective randomized study with long-term outcome evaluation. Am J Obstet Gynecol 175:1418, 1996.
10. Meeks GR, Washburne JF, McGehee RP, et al: Repair of vaginal vault prolapse by suspension of the vagina to iliococcygeus (prespinous) fascia. Am J Obstet Gynecol 171:1444, 1994.
11. Shull BL, Capen CV, Riggs MW, et al: Bilateral attachment of the vaginal cuff to iliococcygeus fascia: An effective method of cuff suspension. Am J Obstet Gynecol 168:1669, 1993.
12. Lemack GE, Zimmern PE, Blander DS: The levator myorrhaphy repair for vaginal vault prolapse. Urology 56:50, 2000.
13. Culligan PJ, Murphy M, Blackwell L, et al: Long-term success of abdominal sacral colpopexy using synthetic mesh. Am J Obstet Gynecol 187:1473, 2002.
14. Timmons MC, Addison WA, Addison SB, et al: Abdominal sacral colpopexy in 163 women with posthysterectomy vaginal vault prolapse and enterocele. Evolution of operative techniques. J Reprod Med 37:323, 1992.
15. Scarpero HM, Cespedes RD, Winters JC: Transabdominal approach to repair of vaginal vault prolapse. Tech Urol 7:139, 2001.
16. Winters JC, Cespedes RD, Vanlangendonck R: Abdominal sacral colpopexy and abdominal enterocele repair in the management of vaginal vault prolapse. Urology 56:55, 2000.
17. Hardiman PJ, Drutz HP: Sacrospinous vault suspension and abdominal colposacropexy: Success rates and complications. Am J Obstet Gynecol 175:612, 1996.
18. Nygaard IE, McCreery R, Brubaker L, et al: Abdominal sacrocolpopexy: A comprehensive review. Obstet Gynecol 104:805, 2004.
19. Raz S, Nitti VW, Bregg KJ: Transvaginal repair of enterocele. J Urol 149:724, 1993.

Chapter 69

USE OF A POSTERIOR SLING FOR VAGINAL VAULT PROLAPSE

Peter E. Petros

HISTORY

The first posterior sling operation was performed in 1992. Initially, the operation was used only for repair of significant vaginal vault and uterine prolapse (i.e., restoration of structure). Over the past 12 years, it was found that coexisting symptoms of abnormal emptying, nocturia, pelvic pain, urge, and frequency—a group of symptoms now described as the posterior fornix syndrome[1]—also were being improved in approximately 80% of patients (i.e., restoration of function). Although the generic name for this procedure is infracoccygeal sacropexy,[2] the operation is universally known as the posterior IVS or posterior sling operation.

RESTORATION OF STRUCTURE

Dynamic Structural Mechanism of the Uterus and Vaginal Vault

The uterus and vaginal vault are anchored passively by the suspensory ligaments, the uterosacral ligaments (USLs) and arcus tendineus fasciae pelvis (Fig. 69-1), and they are anchored actively by the three directional muscle forces that stretch the vagina against these ligaments.[3,4] The USLs, the apical segment of the vagina, rectovaginal fascia, and perineal body (see Fig. 69-1) work synergistically as a subsystem,[3] and repair of all three is often required.

Fibromuscular Supports of the Uterus and Vagina

The inherent strength of the rectovaginal fascia and its backward stretching by the levator plate are major factors in preventing prolapse, which is really a form of intussusception (Fig. 69-2). The cervix is a key anchoring point for the pubocervical fascia anteriorly and the rectovaginal fascia posteriorly, and the anterior and posterior fascial supports may need repairing in a patient with uterine or vault prolapse.

Hysterectomy may weaken the fascial side wall support and weaken the USLs, perhaps by removing a major part of the blood supply. Conservation of the uterus may be important in preventing vaginal prolapse and incontinence.[5]

Vaginal Fascia as a Tensor of the Vagina

This concept, that vaginal fascia functions as a tensor of the vagina, was originally proposed by Sturmdorf in 1916,[6] and it was confirmed by an observational radiologic study.[7] During effort, the rectovaginal fascia was stretched backward against the perineal body and downward against the USLs to compress level 2 (Fig. 69-3). In contrast, there is no compression of level 2 in the multipara with damaged tissues (Fig. 69-4), even though the muscles appear to be contracting normally, as evidenced by downward angulation of the anterior part of levator plate and forward movement of the distal urethra.

Compression of the vaginal canal appeared to be related to the angle "a" formed between the upper vagina and the horizontal at rest.[7] When the angle was more than 45 degrees to the horizontal (Fig. 69-5), only 2 of 23 patients demonstrated angulation and compression of the vagina on straining, compared with 100% when the angle was less than 45 degrees to the horizontal (n = 27). If the vaginal fascia is lax, the stretching forces (see Fig. 69-5) may not be able to grip, and there is no angulation or compression (see Fig. 69-4B). The damaged vaginal tissues become vulnerable to the forces generated by the abdomen and pelvis (see Fig. 69-5) to create cystocele, rectocele, and enterocele.

A short vagina may prevent angulation and compression (see Fig. 69-5). The vagina is a cylinder. Excising vaginal tissue during

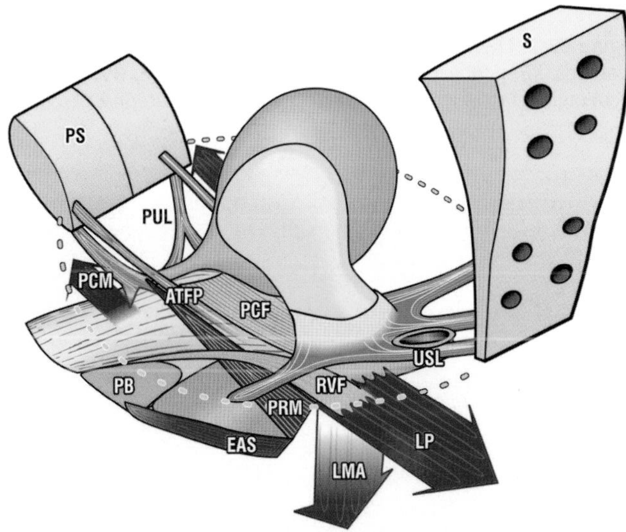

Figure 69-1 Active anchoring of the vagina, shown in a three-dimensional sagittal view from above and behind. During effort, the levator plate (LP) stretches the rectovaginal fascia (RVF) backward against the perineal body (PB). Downward contraction of the longitudinal muscle of the anus (LMA) against the uterosacral ligaments (USL) compresses the vagina. The uterus and vaginal vault are anchored passively by the suspensory ligaments (USL) and arcus tendineus fasciae pelvis and anchored actively by the three directional muscle forces *(labeled arrows)*. EAS, external anal sphincter; PCM, m. pubococcygeus; PRM, m. puborectalis; PS, pubic symphysis; PUL, pubourethral ligament; S, spine.

surgery may shorten or narrow the vagina. It is possible to conclude the following from these findings:

1. Vaginal tissue should be conserved wherever possible.
2. The vaginal fascia should be restored to its preoperative tension by approximation of the separated edges.
3. The whole system may need repair, including the USLs, rectovaginal fascia, and perineal body.

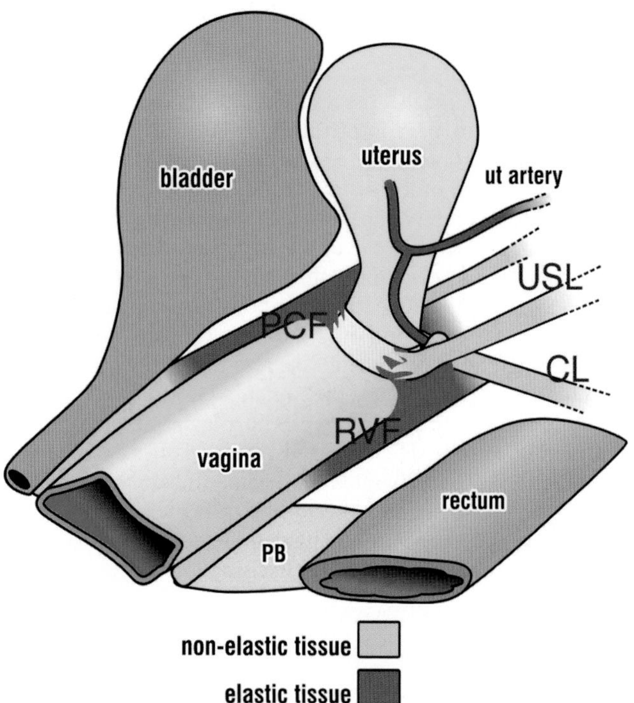

Figure 69-2 The fibromuscular supports of the vagina. CL, cardinal ligament; PB, perineal body; PCF, pubocervical fascia; RVF, rectovaginal fascia; USL, uterosacral ligament; ut, uterine.

CORRECTIVE SURGERY

The late David Nichols stated that vaginal vault prolapse is a significant longer-term complication in patients undergoing hysterectomy.[8] Nichols emphasized the need for axial repair, conservation of vaginal form and function, and the requirement to repair coexisting cystoceles, rectoceles, and enteroceles. The biomechanical rationale for this is presented in Figure 69-5.

Posterior Sling Operation

With the posterior sling operation, the aim was to create an axial procedure for cure of uterine and vaginal vault prolapse using plastic tapes to create artificial collagenous neoligaments. It was reasoned that this approach would avoid the morbidity and complications associated with alternative techniques: nerve injury and dyspareunia with sacrospinous colpopexy, bleeding from sacral veins and peritoneal adhesions with abdominal sacropexy, and ureteric injury with the McCall culdoplasty.[9]

Posterior IVS Operation for Vaginal Vault Prolapse

A more evolved technique than that originally described[2] for the posterior IVS operation is presented. Posterior IVS (i.e., infracoccygeal sacropexy) reinforces the distal part of USLs and anchors the vaginal apex to the posterior muscles of the pelvic floor with a polypropylene tape. A full-thickness incision approximately 2.5 to 3 cm long is made in the posterior vaginal wall just below the hysterectomy scar line (Fig. 69-6). Using dissecting scissors with the tip pressed against the vaginal skin, a channel is made in the direction of the ischial spine sufficient to insert the index finger. The ischial spine is located, and the point of entry through the pelvic muscles for the IVS tunneler (Tyco) is determined. If an enterocoele is opened, it is ligated with a high purse-string suture.

Bilateral skin incisions 0.5 cm long are made in the perianal skin at the 4- and 8-o'clock positions halfway between the coccyx and external anal sphincter in a line 2 cm lateral to the external

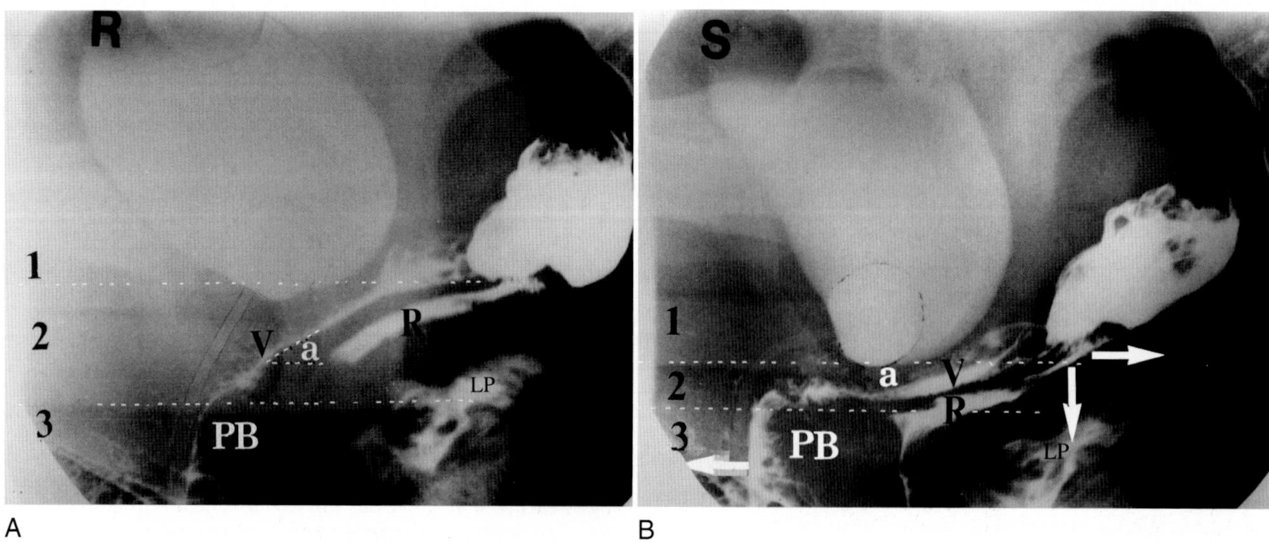

Figure 69-3 A, Nullipara at rest. The numbers 1, 2, and 3 represent the three levels of connective tissue support for the vagina. **B,** Nullipara during straining. The vagina and rectum are stretched downward and backward by directional muscle forces *(arrows)*. Note forward movement of the distal urethra. Level 2 is compressed. a, angle of the vagina compared with the horizontal; LP, levator plate; PB, perineal body; R, rectum; V, vagina.

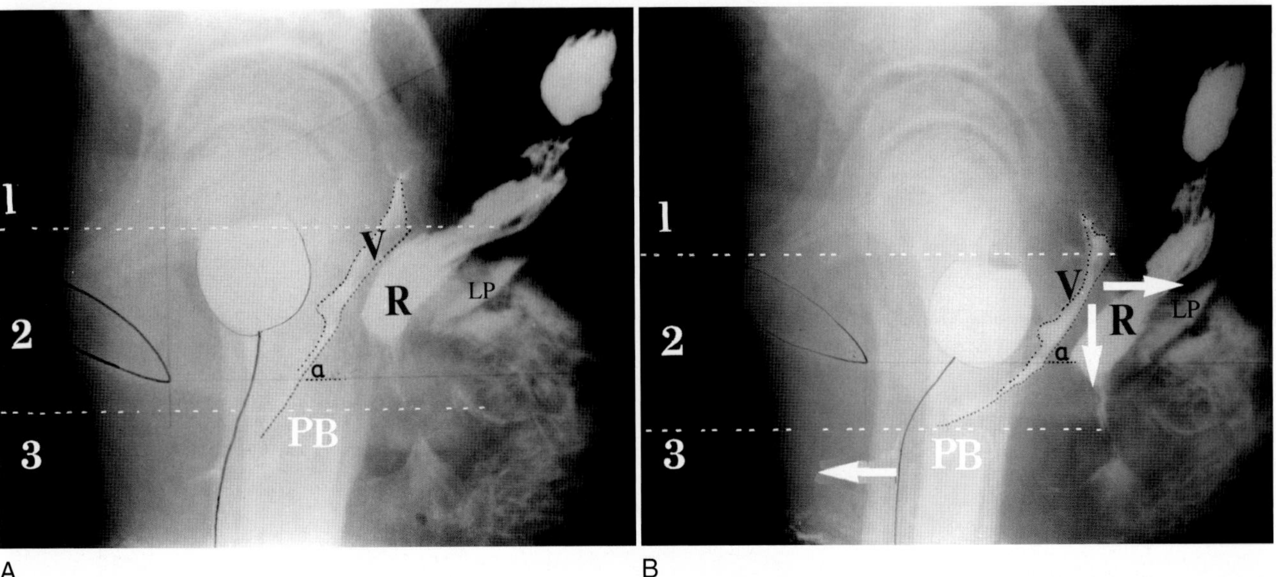

Figure 69-4 **A,** Multipara with damaged tissues. There is no angulation of the vagina around angle a. **B,** Multipara straining. The organs are directionally stretched by three forces *(arrows)*, but level 2 is not compressed, and angle a is unchanged Notice the downward bulging of the vagina. a, angle of the vagina compared with the horizontal; LP, levator plate; PB, perineal body; R, rectum; V, vagina; 1, 2, and 3, levels of connective tissue support for the vagina.

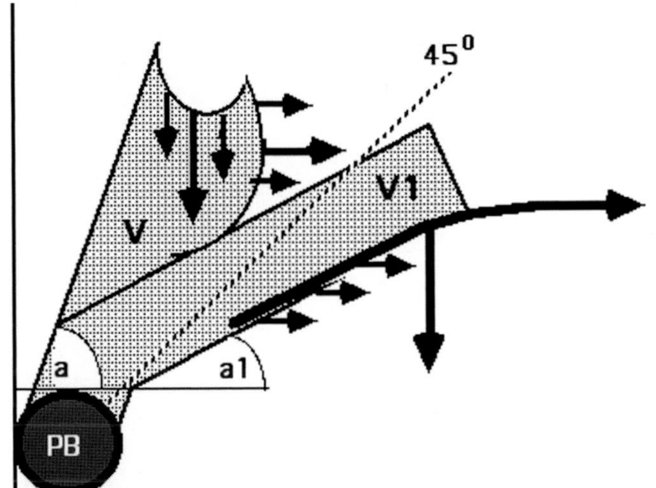

Figure 69-5 The role of the muscle forces in angulation and compression of the vagina is shown in a schematic, three-dimensional, sagittal view. The abdominal and pelvic forces *(long arrows)* act on the vagina (V) to stretch it to the V1 position, where it is compressed by the intra-abdominal forces.

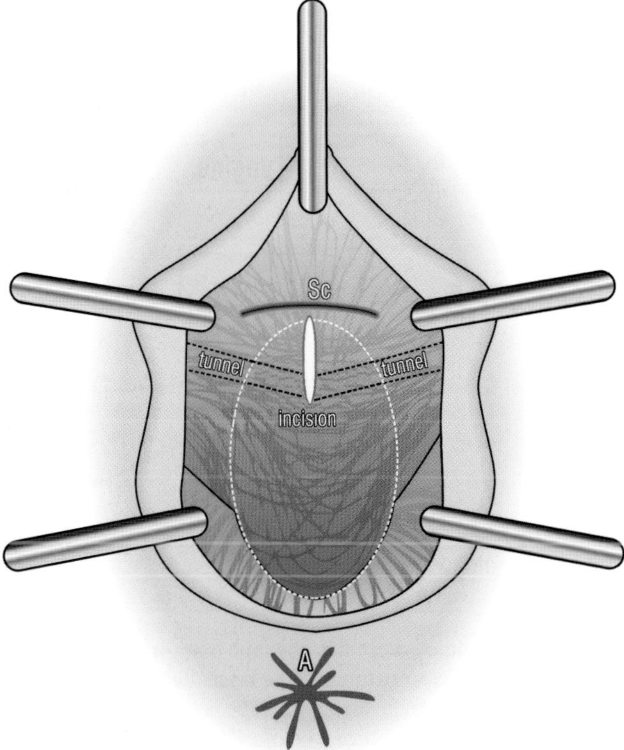

Figure 69-6 Vaginal incision, as viewed looking into the posterior vaginal wall. Sc, hysterectomy scar.

border of the external anal sphincter (Fig. 69-7). The tunneler is pushed 3 to 4 cm into the ischiorectal fossa, keeping the plastic tip parallel to the floor (Fig. 69-8). The index finger is placed into the tunnel created in the vagina to locate the tip of the tunneler, which penetrates the levator muscles 1 cm medial and dorsal to the ischial spine (Fig. 69-9). At this point, the tunneler is safely sited well away from rectum and peritoneum.

With the index finger continually applied to the plastic tip (see Fig. 69-9), the tunneler is gently inclined medially, toward the vaginal vault, and pushed through the incision. A rectal examination is made to ensure there has been no perforation. The insert is reversed. An 8-mm polypropylene tape is threaded into the eye of the plastic insert, bringing the tape into the perineal area. The procedure is repeated on the contralateral side, leaving the tape as a U-shaped configuration entirely unfixed at the perineal end.

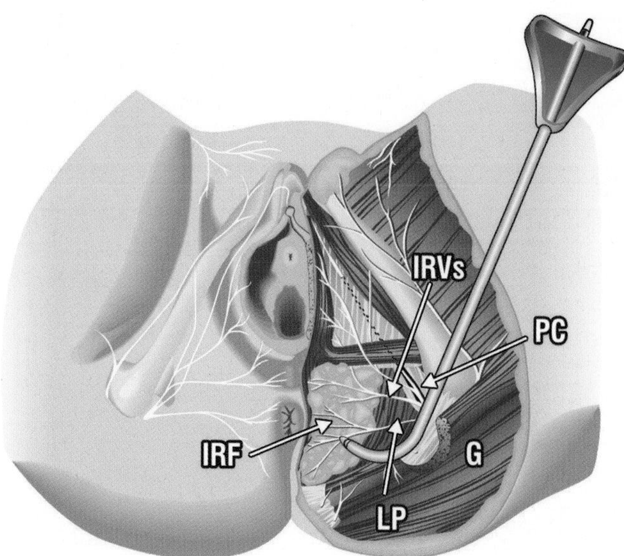

Figure 69-7 Insertion of the tunneler. G, gluteus muscle; IRF, ischiorectal fossa; IRV, inferior rectal veins; LP, levator plate; PC, pudendal canal.

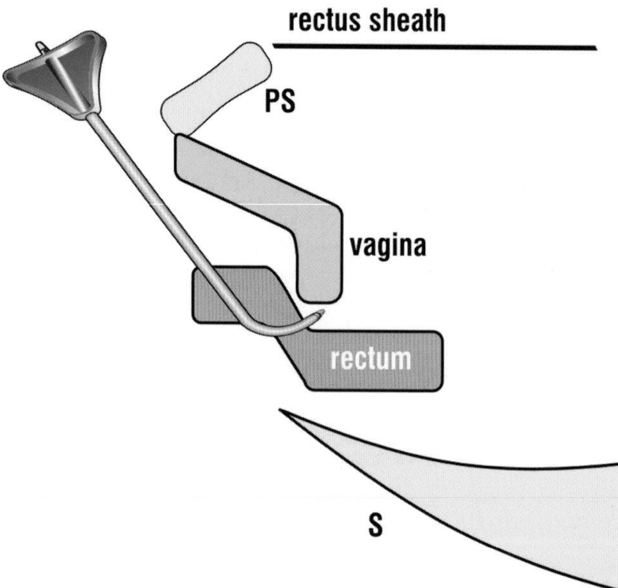

Figure 69-8 As the tunneler is inserted in a supine patient, it passes across the anterior wall of the rectum.

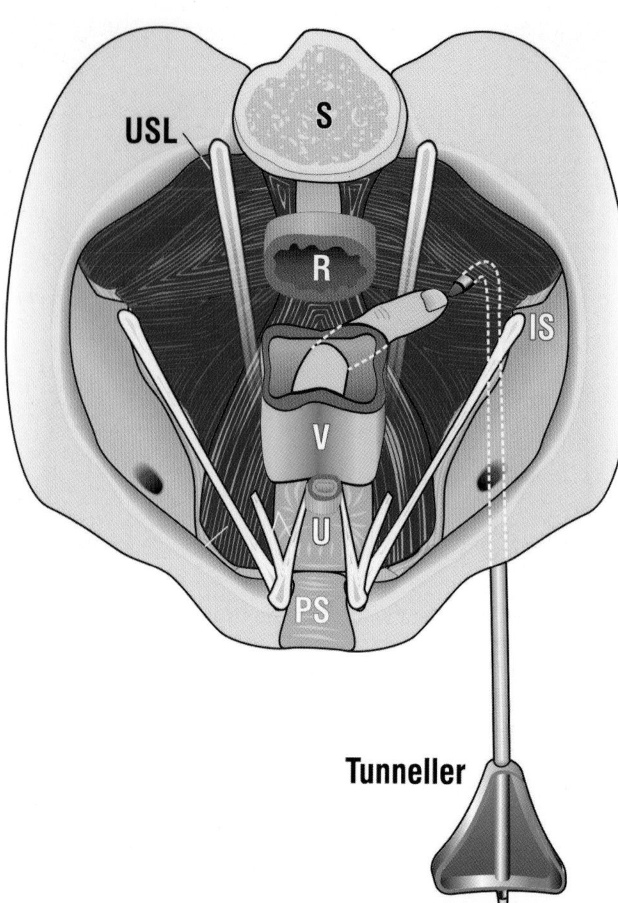

Figure 69-9 Perforating the pelvic muscles. The finger tip guides the tip through the tunnel to the vaginal incision. IS, ischial spine; PS, pubic symphysis; R, rectum; S, spine; U, urethra; USL, uterosacral ligament; V, vagina.

Ensuring the tape is kept flat, the tape is sutured securely with interrupted 2-0 Dexon sutures to the fascia behind the hysterectomy scar (Fig. 69-10), ensuring the tape is positioned well away from the incision to minimize erosion. The remnants of the USLs and attached fascia are brought across to cover the tape.

The perineal ends of the tape are pulled to full extension, cut, and left free without suturing. The skin incision may be sutured without tension or apposed with Steri-Strips. If sutures are used, it is advisable to remove them in 24 hours because this is usually the most painful part of the operation.

Posterior IVS Repair of Uterine Prolapse

In the posterior IVS repair of uterine prolapse, the principles followed are similar to those for the Manchester repair, and the

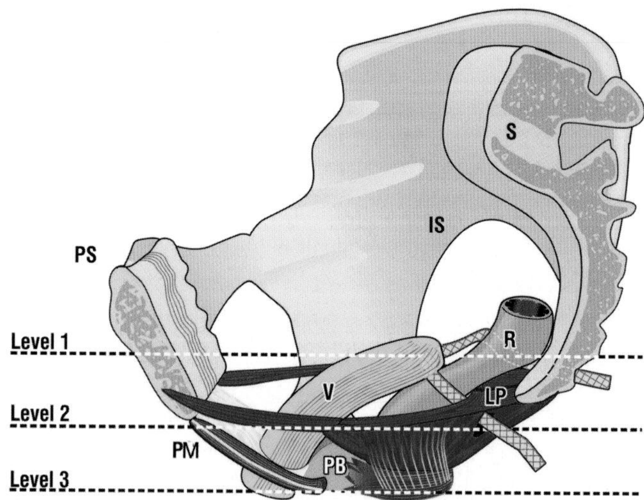

Figure 69-10 Anchoring the apex. The tape is sutured to the fascia of vagina (V). Fibrosis attaches the vagina to the posterior pelvic floor muscles, which contract to retain it in position. LP, levator plate; PB, perineal body; PM, perineal membrane; R, rectum; S, sacrum; 1, 2, and 3, levels of connective tissue support for the vagina.

approach is combined with a posterior IVS operation. An elongated cervix is amputated. An incision is made just below the junction of the vaginal skin to cervix and opened out. This brings the USLs into view. Having reconstituted the cervix, the posterior IVS tape is inserted. If possible, exit of the tunneler is directed between USLs and cervix. The tape is sutured into the USLs near their cervical insertion.

Posterior IVS with apical defect repair (enterocoele) follows the same surgical principles as vault prolapse repair. Care is taken to free the enterocoele sufficiently to locate the cardinal ligaments and USLs. The enterocoele is not routinely opened. With a large prolapse, the enterocoele is dissected clear. If entered, closure is completed with a purse-string suture. A posterior IVS operation is performed, and the tape is anchored to the USLs or behind the hysterectomy scar. The USLs and attached fascia are approximated as described previously. Excess vaginal tissue is not excised; it is instead sutured down into the approximated rectovaginal fascia.

Rectovaginal Fascia and Perineal Body Repair

The main surgical principles include conservation of vaginal tissue to prevent dyspareunia and a short vagina, and avoidance of tension during suturing. The vagina has a visceral nerve innervation, and like bowel, it is extremely susceptible to pressure. Laterally displaced fascia and perineal body are approximated. If mesh is to be used for the posterior wall, it can be set deeply below the vaginal epithelium by threading the tape through the mesh before the tape is brought through into the vagina. The mesh is then trimmed and left free, or sutured laterally and to the perineal body. Surgery on the perineal skin, which has somatic nerve innervation, should also be avoided. Confining the incisions within the vaginal epithelium makes for a far less painful operation.

Operation Characteristics of the Posterior IVS Operation

In the first reported study,[2] 75 patients were prospectively studied over 4.5 years. Preoperatively, 22 had second-degree prolapse, 45 had third-degree prolapse, and 8 had fourth-degree prolapse. Recurrence rates are detailed in Table 69-1, but no further surgery was required in two of three recurrences. The operating time for the sacropexy itself was generally less than 15 minutes. Total operating time, including posterior vaginal repair, varied between 25 and 50 minutes. Blood loss from the sacropexy itself was minimal. Mean blood loss from the posterior vaginal repair was 120 mL (range, 20 to 800 mL); the most blood lost was in a patient with undiagnosed von Willebrand's disease. No patient required transfusion. All 75 patients were discharged the day of or day after surgery without indwelling catheters. All patients returned to normal activities (including jobs) within 7 to 10 days, some within 2 to 3 days. Minor bruising was observed around the incisions in 10% of patients. No hematoma or postoperative pyrexia was reported.

Potential Complications of Posterior Sling Repair

Hematoma

Anatomically, the tunneler is inserted into the ischiorectal fossa, well away from the perirectal veins or the pudendal nerve. The blunt tip of the tunneler reduces but does not eliminate the risk of hematoma. Infection is rare. A hematoma from the vaginal repair is more likely.

Rectal Perforation by the Tunneler

Two uneventful perforations were reported in the initial series,[2] but they have not occurred since the present technique was adopted 4 years ago. Any perforation is extraperitoneal and punctate, and like a bladder perforation with the anterior sling, it is closed by smooth muscle contraction. If perforation occurs, the surgeon removes the tunneler and repeats the procedure. Any small injury is sutured with two sutures applied from the vaginal end. Fistula formation is highly unlikely and has never occurred in my personal series of more than 1500 cases.

Tape Erosion with Polypropylene Tapes

Tape erosion with polypropylene mesh tape may occur in 1% to 3 % of patients, and usually occurs centrally. The erosion is usually a simple surfacing, or it may be a foreign body reaction. The latter may extend to the perineum. Both conditions are benign. If the tape has surfaced, it is grasped, and the vaginal mucosa is pushed down around it. Under tension, the eroded segment is trimmed with scissors pushed down below the vaginal mucosa. Sometimes, the segment may need excision. Deeply burying the tape behind the hysterectomy scar at the time of surgery helps reduce the erosion rate considerably (BN Farnsworth, personal communication, 2004). A purulent discharge at the perineum usually is caused by a foreign body reaction. The patient is afebrile, with a normal white blood cell count. Bacteriologic swabs generally do not grow bacteria. Sterile pus surrounds the whole tape, and this makes removal a simple matter of finding the vaginal sinus at the apex, grasping the tape with a hemostat, and pulling it out. This is simpler and more effective than attempts to remove it through the perineum. Clinical infection is rare and is accompanied by pyrexia and an increased white blood cell count. It is advisable to perform bacteriologic swabs to identify pathogenic bacteria and to treat the patient with appropriate antibiotics before any surgical intervention.

Total Rejection of Polypropylene Tapes

Complete tissue rejection occurs rarely with polypropylene tapes. The tapes are easily removed in toto by grasping the vaginal end and pulling gently.

Risk of Rectal Perforation During Vaginal Repair

In patients with a scarred perineum, it is critical to dissect only under tension to minimize the risk of rectal perforation. Finger

Table 69-1 Cumulative Herniation Rate after Posterior IVS Operations

Condition	6 Weeks $n = 75$	1 Year $n = 71$	2 Years $n = 64$	3 Years $n = 56$	4.5 Years $n = 40$
Vault prolapse	0 (0%)	2 (2.6%)	4 (5.2%)	4 (5.2%)	4 (5.2%)
Anterior wall prolapse	0 (0%)	6 (8%)	12 (16%)	12 (16%)	12 (16%)
Partial rectocele	0 (0%)	3 (4%)	3 (4%)	3 (4%)	3 (4%)

dissection in these circumstances is especially dangerous. Hemostats placed on the edge of the vagina and on the rectal wall adhesions are stretched so that dissection is performed under tension using dissecting scissors, a prerequisite to avoid rectal perforation. An assistant creating countertension and the operator's finger in the rectum may also be helpful. If the rectum is perforated, the rectal wall must be mobilized sufficiently from the adjacent scar tissue to facilitate a tension-free repair in at least two layers.

Restoration of Posterior Zone Anatomy with a Tissue Fixation System

The tissue fixation system (TFS) posterior sling is a promising new technique, and it is similar to the McCall operation (Fig. 69-11). It uses two small anchors attached to a strip of polypropylene mesh tape as a U shape in the exact position of the USLs. It relies on adequate tissue for the anchor to grip. A full-thickness incision is made in the vaginal apex. Fine dissecting scissors create a 4-cm space between the vagina and USLs on both sides. The TFS applicator is inserted to a depth of 4 cm and set with a tug. This insertion is repeated contralaterally. The tape is tightened and trimmed 1 to 1.5 cm from the TFS. The overlying USLs and fascia are approximated and the vagina sutured. There is minimal intraoperative bleeding and postoperative pain. Mean operating time is 5 to 6 minutes.

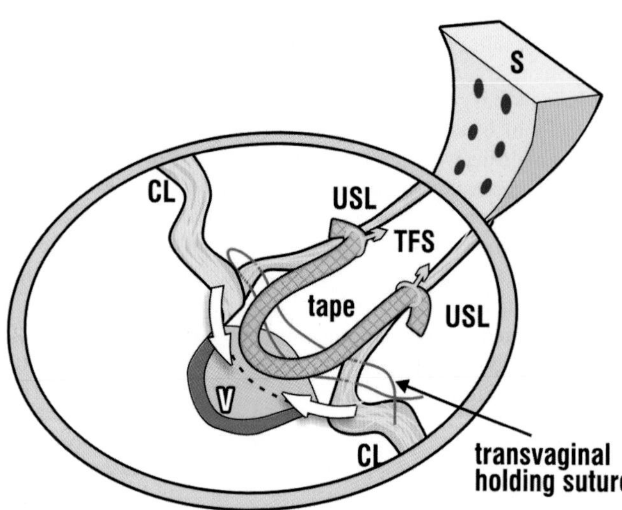

Figure 69-11 Posterior tissue fixation system, TFS viewed from above. The tape is placed along the exact position of the uterosacral ligament (USL). The *arrows* indicate that the remnants of the USL and the cardinal ligaments (CL) need to be approximated if the apex is wide to prevent enterocoele formation.

The TFS was used to treat major structural defects in 67 patients[10] (Table 69-2). The rectovaginal fascia and perineal body were repaired when required. Very few complications were seen in 67 posterior TFS operations at mean of 9 months' review.[10] In one patient, one half of the sling was found in the vagina covered by a large granuloma, with no vault prolapse and no posterior zone symptoms. This was attributed to surgeon error in not anchoring the tape sufficiently. The prolapsed part of the sling was excised and the vagina sutured. It was not possible to insert a TFS in one patient who had previously undergone pelvic clearance for extensive endometriosis. A posterior IVS operation was successfully performed. There was one vaginal infection after a standard rectocele repair. One patient reported with severe de novo urgency immediately after surgery. Transperineal ultrasound demonstrated a 2-cm–diameter hematoma at the bladder base. The symptoms settled within 6 weeks after the hematoma was absorbed.

RESTORATION OF FUNCTION

In 1993, improvement in an apparently unrelated group of symptoms grouped together as the posterior fornix syndrome[1] was observed after repair of the USLs. The symptoms were urgency, frequency, nocturia, pelvic pain, and abnormal emptying . These symptoms constitute the main body of the symptoms within the posterior zone (Fig. 69-12). Although the concept that posterior zone symptoms were potentially curable surgically was initially controversial, there has since been a growing acceptance after reports by Farnsworth[11] and others of up to 80% cure rates for urgency, nocturia, and pelvic pain after posterior IVS operations. Later data using the posterior TFS are presented in Table 69-3.

Table 69-2 Structural Outcome for Posterior Zone Prolapse Repair

Operation	No. of Patients	Recurrences
Posterior with a tissue fixation system (TFS)	67	1
Trans-TFS for rectocele	9	0
Transverse TFS plus mesh	3	0
Rectocele repair	6	0
Perineal body with a TFS	3	0
Perineal body repair	15	2

*Fourth degree (n = 2), third degree (n = 17), second degree (n = 20), and first degree (n = 28).

Table 69-3 Symptom Outcomes for 67 Patients

Frequency (>10/day)	Nocturia (>2/night)	Urge Incontinence (>2/day)	Abnormal Emptying	Pelvic Pain
n = 27 (63%)* $P < .005$	n = 47 (83%)* $P < .005$	n = 36 (78%)* $P < .005$	n = 53 (73%)* $P < .005$	n = 46 (86%)* $P < .005$

*Symptom change with surgery (percent cure in parentheses).

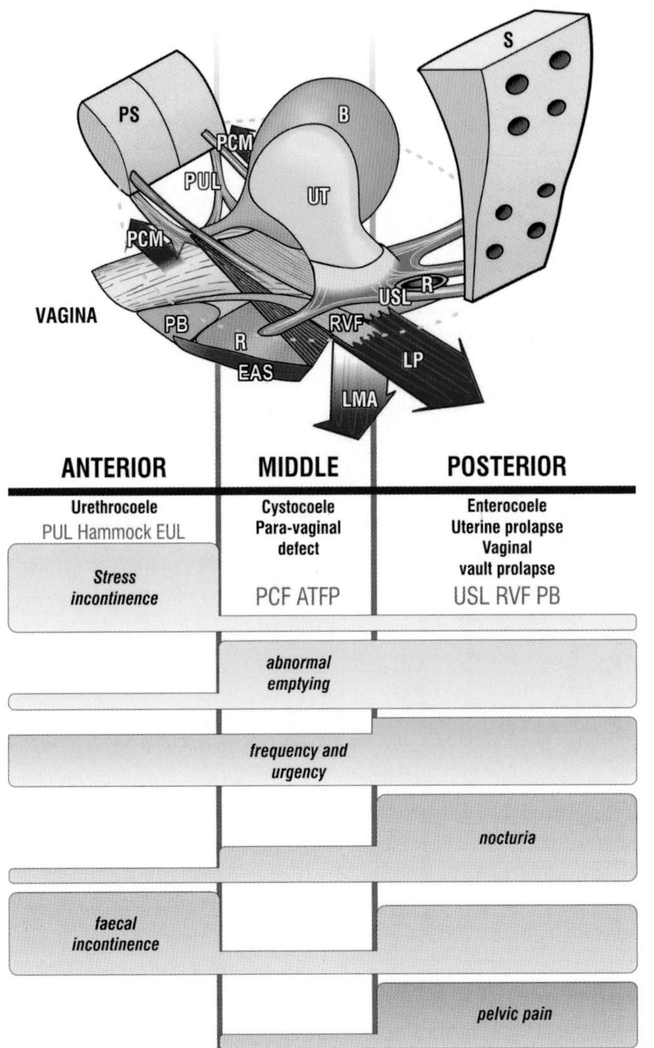

Figure 69-12 The pictorial diagnostic algorithm summarizes the relationships between structural damage in the three zones of vaginal support and symptoms. The size of the bar gives an approximate indication of the prevalence (probability) of the symptom. The same connective tissue structures in each zone may cause prolapse and abnormal symptoms. B, bladder; EAS, external anal sphincter; PB perineal body; PCM, m. pubococcygeus; PRM, m. puborectalis; PS, pubic symphysis; PUL, pubourethral ligament; R, rectum; RVF, rectovaginal fascia S, spine; USL, uterosacral ligament; UT, uterus. (From Petros P: The Female Pelvic Floor. New York, Springer-Verlag, 2004.)

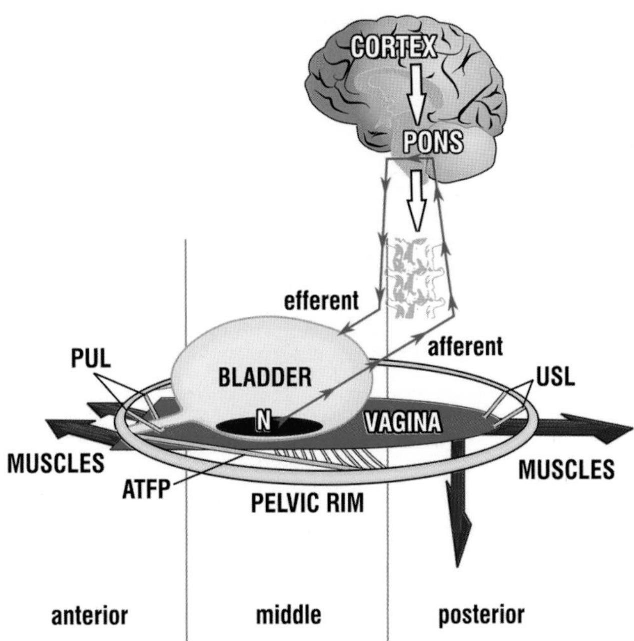

Figure 69-13 The vaginal trampoline. The vagina is suspended by the pubourethral ligaments (PUL), arcus tendineus fasciae pelvis (ATFP), and uterosacral ligaments (USL). *Red arrows* represent pelvic muscle forces. *White arrows* indicate the central inhibitory mechanism. (From Petros P: The Female Pelvic Floor. New York, Springer-Verlag, 2004.)

Twenty-eight of these patients had only minor posterior zone prolapse, Table 69-2.

Lax ligaments may cause urge, frequency, and nocturia. In the normal patient, the cortex coordinates urinary retention and micturition (Fig. 69-13).[3] As the bladder fills, the stretch receptors send afferent impulses to the cortex.[12] If it is inconvenient to micturate, the impulses are blocked by the inhibitory centers and by contraction of the three pelvic muscle forces. These stretch the vaginal membrane like a trampoline to support the hydrostatic pressure of the urine, relieving the pressure on the receptors, thereby diminishing the afferent impulses to the cortex.

Like a trampoline with loose springs, lax ligaments may not allow the muscles to tension the vaginal membrane, and the receptors (see Fig. 69-13) fire, activating the micturition reflex prematurely. The sequence of events in patients with urodynamically demonstrated detrusor instability (Fig. 69-14) was similar[13] to that in normal patients about to micturate: sensory urgency, urethral relaxation, detrusor contraction (Fig. 69-15), and urine loss.[14] This "premature micturition" may be symptomatically expressed as frequency, urgency, and nocturia. The rationale for surgical cure of these symptoms is that firm ligaments and fascia permit the vagina (see Fig. 69-13) to be stretched sufficiently to offer support. This concept can be confirmed as an office procedure using the technique of simulated operations.[15] The patient's bladder needs to be sufficiently full for her to have urge symptoms in the supine position. In its simplest form, the vagina is supported below bladder base digitally, by a ring forceps, or by gentle compression of the vaginal tissue just behind bladder neck with a Littlewood forceps.

Unmyelinated nerves run along the USLs. A lax ligament may not be able to support these nerves, and they become subjected to the force of gravity. This explains the dragging nature of the pain experienced and symptom relief on lying down.

Compared with a normal patient at rest (Fig. 69-16), it has been demonstrated radiologically and electromyographically[4] that after relaxation of the forward force, the bladder base and urethra are pulled open (i.e., funneling), apparently by pelvic contraction, during micturition (Fig. 69-17). The downward force acts against the USLs, and lax USLs diminish the opening forces. As the intraurethral resistance varies inversely with the fourth power of the radius, failure of the pelvic muscles (see Fig. 69-17) to open the urethra increases the resistance geometrically, which is perceived as obstructed micturition. For example, if the radius of the urethra in a normal patient (see Fig. 69-17) is

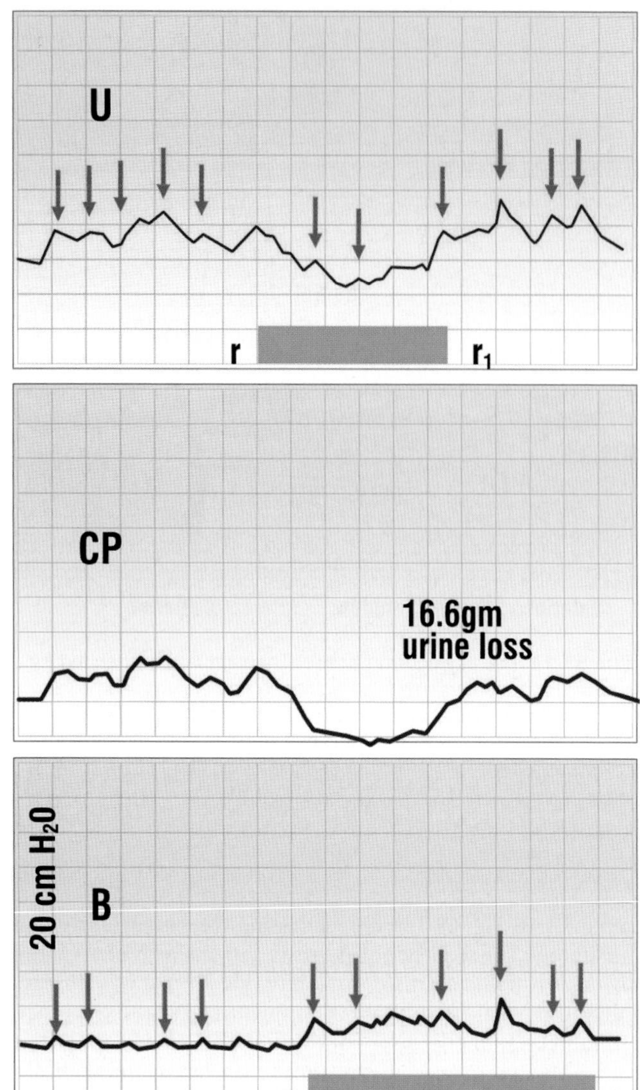

Figure 69-14 Detrusor instability: premature activation of the micturition reflex, The *arrows* indicate synchronous pressure variations in the urethra and bladder. B, bladder pressure; c to c1, rise in detrusor pressure; CP, closure pressure; r to r1, fall in urethral pressure; U, urethral pressure. (From Petros P: The Female Pelvic Floor. New York, Springer-Verlag, 2004.)

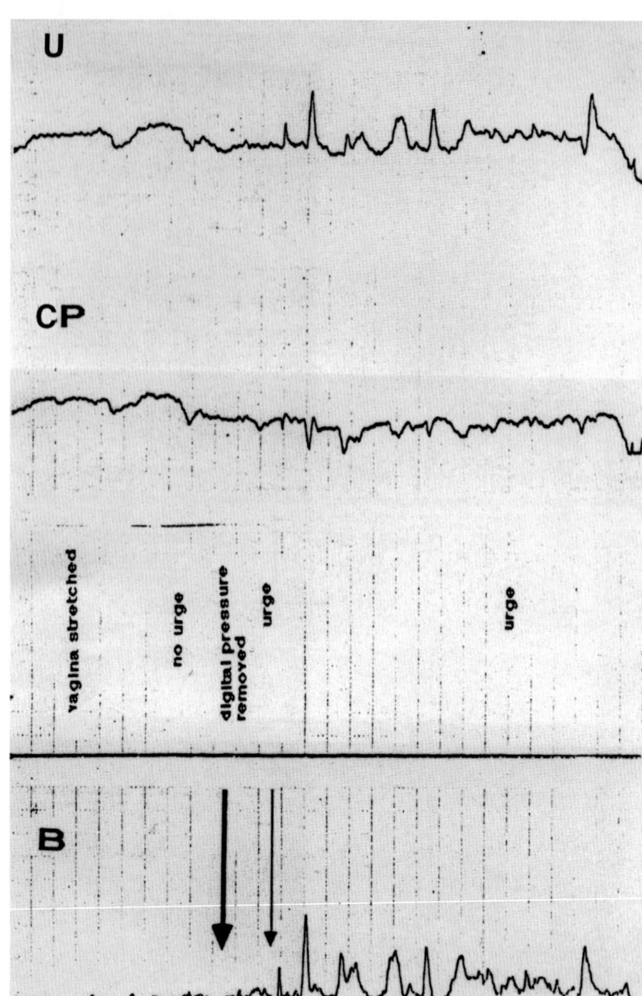

Figure 69-15 Control of detrusor instability by stretching the vagina. Some seconds after the release of vaginal tension, the detrusor begins to contract. (From Petros P: The Female Pelvic Floor. New York, Springer-Verlag, 2004.)

R, expelling urine through a urethra which can open only to a radius of R/2, will require an expulsion pressure 16 times greater than that required for R.

CONCLUSIONS AND FUTURE DIRECTIONS

The use of posterior slings for vault and uterine prolapse repair is becoming well accepted. The future challenge is to explore their use in patients with major symptoms and minimal prolapse to more accurately assess which other connective tissue structures may contributing to dysfunction and how best to repair these structures.

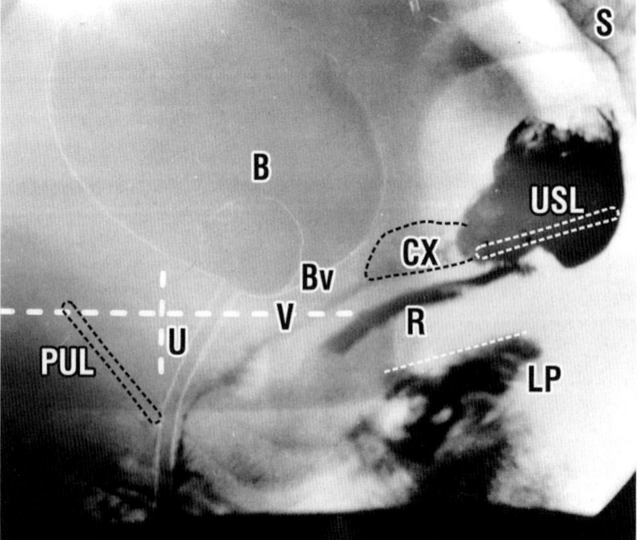

Figure 69-16 Lateral radiograph of a normal patient at rest. Bv, attachment of the bladder base to the vagina; CX, cervix; LP, levator plate; PUL, pubourethral ligament; R, rectum; U, urethra; USL, uterosacral ligament; V, vagina.

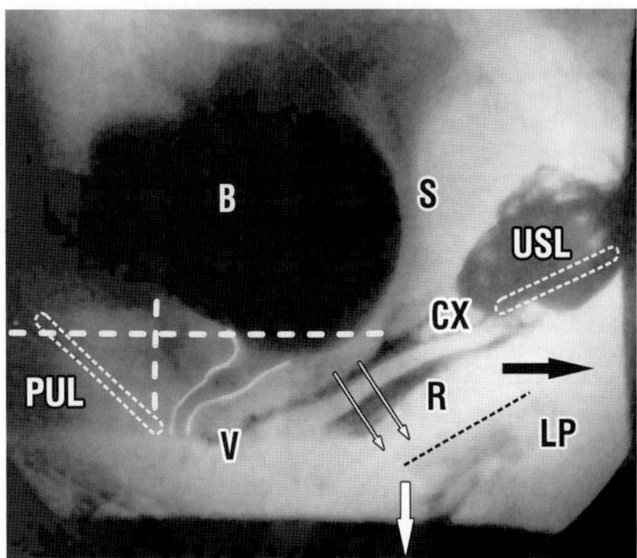

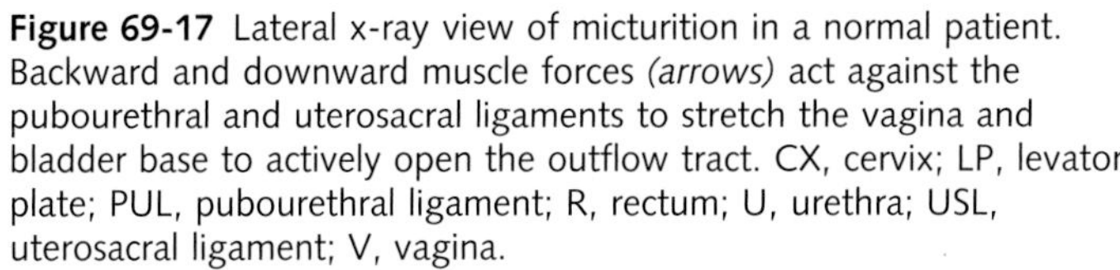

Figure 69-17 Lateral x-ray view of micturition in a normal patient. Backward and downward muscle forces *(arrows)* act against the pubourethral and uterosacral ligaments to stretch the vagina and bladder base to actively open the outflow tract. CX, cervix; LP, levator plate; PUL, pubourethral ligament; R, rectum; U, urethra; USL, uterosacral ligament; V, vagina.

References

1. Petros PE, Ulmsten U: The posterior fornix syndrome: A multiple symptom complex of pelvic pain and abnormal urinary symptoms deriving from laxity in the posterior fornix. Scand J Urol Nephrol 27(Suppl 153):89-93, 1993.
2. Petros PE: Vault prolapse. II. Restoration of dynamic vaginal supports by the infracoccygeal sacropexy, an axial day-care vaginal procedure. Int Urogynecol J Pelvic Floor Dysfunct 12:296-303, 2001.
3. Petros PEP: The Female Pelvic Floor: Function, Dysfunction and Management, According to the Integral Theory. Heidelberg, Springer, 2004, pp 14-47.
4. Petros PE, Ulmsten U: Role of the pelvic floor in bladder neck opening and closure. I. Muscle forces. II. Vagina. Int Urogynecol J Pelvic Floor Dysfunct 8:69-80, 1997.
5. Brown JS, Sawaya G, Thorn DH, Grady D: Hysterectomy and urinary incontinence: A systematic review. Lancet 356:535-539, 2000.
6. Sturmdorf A: The levator ani muscle. In Gynoplastic Technology. Philadelphia, FA Davis, 1919, pp 109-114.
7. Petros PE: Vault prolapse. I. Dynamic supports of the vagina. Int Urogynecol J Pelvic Floor Dysfunct 12:292-295, 2001.
8. Nichols DH, Randall CL: Massive eversion of the vagina. In Nichols DH & Randall CL (eds): Vaginal Surgery, 3rd ed. Baltimore, Williams & Wilkins, 1989, pp 328-357.
9. Sze EH, Karram MM: Transvaginal repair of vault prolapse: A review. Obstet Gynecol 89:466-475, 1997.
10 Petios PEP, Richardson PA: The TFS posterior sling for repair of uterine/vault prolapse—a preliminary report. ANZJOG 45:372-375, 2005.
11. Farnsworth BN: Posterior intravaginal slingplasty (infracoccygeal sacropexy) for severe posthysterectomy vaginal vault prolapse—A preliminary report. Int J Urogynecol 13:4-8, 2002.
12. Petros PE: Detrusor instability and low compliance may represent different levels of disturbance in peripheral feedback control of the micturition reflex. Neurourol Urodyn 18:81-91, 1999.
13. Petros PE, Ulmsten U: Bladder instability in women: A premature activation of the micturition reflex. Neurourol Urodyn 12:235-239, 1993.
14. Tanagho EA: The anatomy and physiology of micturition. Clin Obstet Gynaecol 5:1, 3-25, 1978.
15. Petros PEP: The Female Pelvic Floor: Function, Dysfunction and Management, According to the Integral Theory. Heidelberg, Springer, 2004, pp 48-76.

Chapter 70

TRANSVAGINAL REPAIR OF APICAL PROLAPSE: THE UTEROSACRAL VAULT SUSPENSION

Raymond T. Foster, Sr., and George D. Webster

For decades, the reconstructive treatment of uterine prolapse or post-hysterectomy vaginal cuff descent has included suspension of the vaginal apex. Reconstructive urologists and gynecologists have developed many techniques, including abdominal, laparoscopic, and vaginal routes of surgery, for the correction of apical descent.[1] Our understanding about which technique or approach is superior with regard to efficacy, safety, and durability is limited by a relative lack of level I evidence. Although many well-designed, retrospective reports (each with a large study population and long-term follow-up) exist to give us useful information about particular procedures for the correction of vault descent,[2-17] we are still unsure which procedure is best for any particular patient. The techniques used to treat pelvic organ prolapse are largely shaped by each surgeon's experience and training and not necessarily influenced by prospective, outcomes-based research.

To compound the problem of sparse well-designed and executed, randomized surgical trials, we are also handicapped by confounding, coexisting pelvic support problems. It is difficult to study apical prolapse in isolation, because most patients present for treatment with many support defects (Fig. 70-1) and associated pelvic floor dysfunction (e.g., urinary incontinence, defecatory dysfunction, pelvic pain, difficulty with sexual intercourse). We are, for example, unsure of how our choice of treatment for cystocele or urethral hypermobility may affect the outcome of our vault suspension.

Operative technique in other fields is often driven by an understanding of the cause and natural history of the surgical

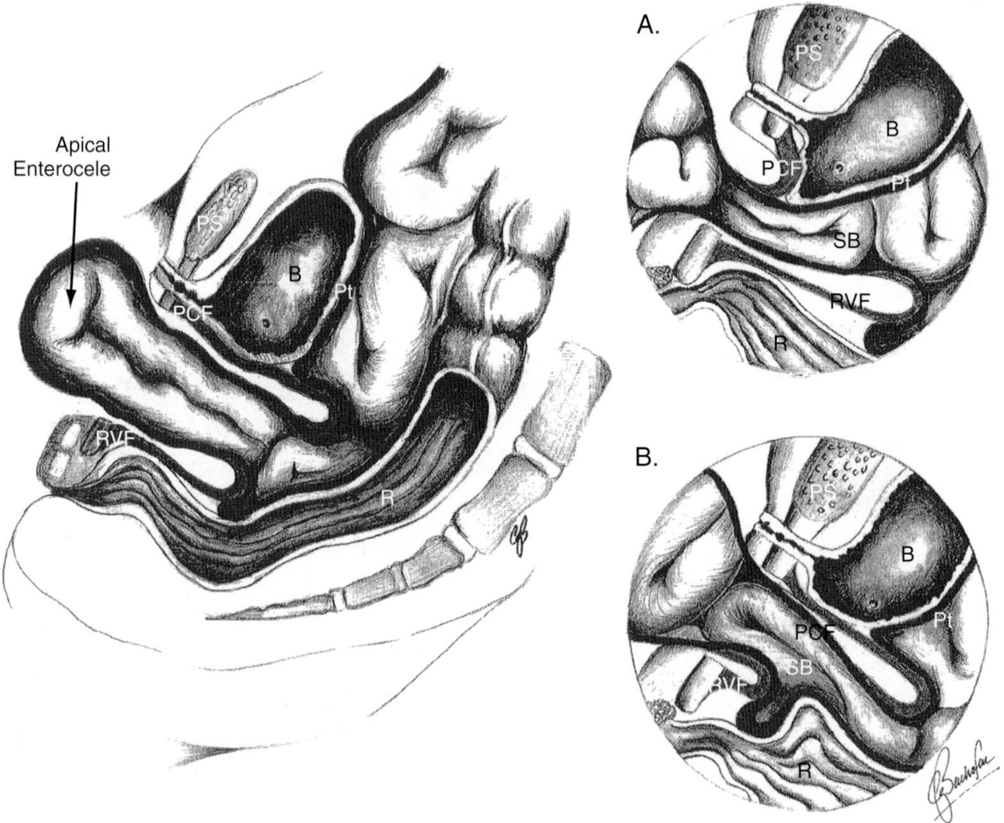

Figure 70-1 Prolapse of the vaginal vault with associated apical enterocele. **A,** Vaginal vault prolapse with cystocele. **B,** Vaginal vault prolapse with a proximal rectocele.

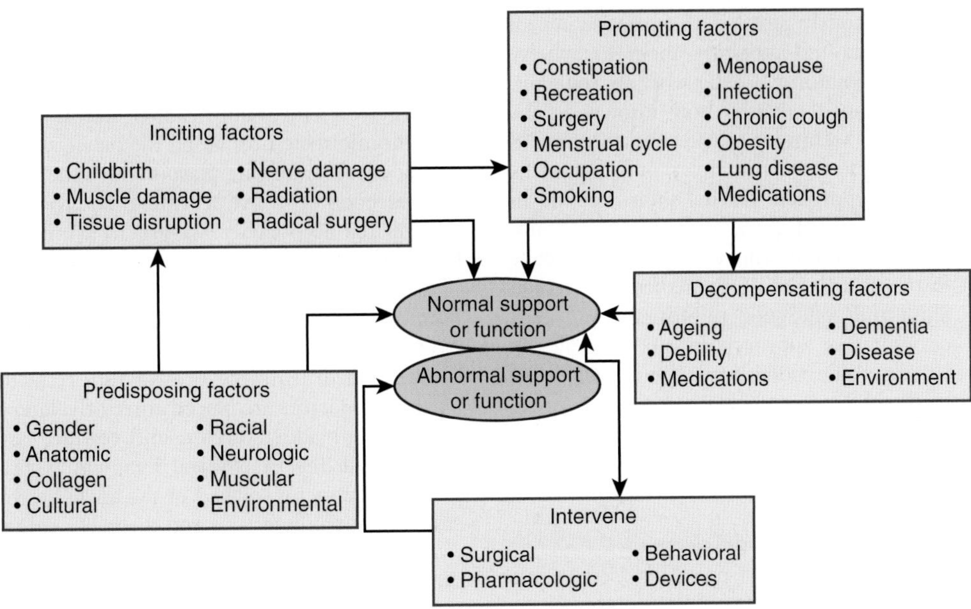

Figure 70-2 Model developed by Bump and Norton[18] to propose a mechanism for the development and progression of pelvic floor dysfunction, including pelvic organ prolapse.

problem, and this often helps guide surgical therapy. Unfortunately, we are still uncertain about these variables in pelvic organ prolapse. Bump and Norton[18] have provided a useful model with which we can consider how prolapse develops and progresses (Fig. 70-2), but in their own words, the model is "based mainly on expert opinion and supported by limited epidemiologic and clinical evidence. None of the factors has been studied in a longitudinal fashion in a representative study."

The surgical goal in treating pelvic organ prolapse is to select a technique that can maximize the chance of anatomic and functional cure and minimize the occurrence of intraoperative injury or complication, but we must recognize that surgeons have preferred techniques based on training and experience. We favor a transvaginal surgical correction of apical prolapse, and our goal is to review the history of the uterosacral ligament vault suspension, a procedure that is often considered to be the gold standard in transvaginal surgery for apical prolapse.

HISTORY

Written history of gynecologic surgery documents that uterosacral ligaments have been used in vaginal reconstructive surgery for at least the past century, but it is difficult to say who was the first person to conceive of the importance of these structures in supporting the uterus and vaginal apex. John Burns, a renowned Scottish anatomist and surgeon, was the first person to write about the importance of the uterosacral ligaments. In his 1839 book, *The Principles of Midwifery including the Diseases of Women and Children*, Burns[19] wrote:

> *By experiments made on the dead subject, we find that prolapsus is chiefly prevented by the fascia passing off from the cavity of the pelvis to the upper part of the vagina, and thence reflected to the face of the rectum. It is also prevented by the fascia of the outlet of the pelvis, and levator ani, which contribute to support the vagina. . . . The greatest aid, however, is afforded by the levator ani and the pelvic fascia, particularly that part of it which is deep in the cavity of the pelvis.*

Burns published earlier editions to this enormously popular text in 1810, 1813, 1814, 1817, 1824, 1831, 1832, and 1837. In some earlier editions (1810 and 1813), he was discouraged that apical prolapse could not be created in cadavers by disrupting the round ligaments and applying traction to the cervix through the vagina, but he and his students continued their cadaver work, and their writings became exponentially more informed.

The first mention of the use of uterosacral ligaments to suspend the vaginal apex as treatment for prolapse was by the American gynecologist Norman F. Miller, who in 1927 described the placement of a "no. 2 chromic catgut suture on a small full curved needle passed through the peritoneum and underlying fascial and muscular structures at the base of the sacro-uterine ligament, approximately 1½ inches below the promontory of the sacrum." Since this report, the use of the uterosacral ligament for apical prolapse has been described by other surgeons. McCall first described his transvaginal culdoplasty technique for treating enterocele with associated vault prolapse in 1957.[20] Lee and Symmonds[21] published what became known as the *Mayo modification* in 1972. As vaginal surgeons made developments in the treatment of apical prolapse with the uterosacral ligament (among other attachment sites, including the iliococcygeus fascia[22] and the sacrospinous ligament[23]) throughout the 20th century, parallel progress was being made in the abdominal[24, 25] and laparoscopic[26] approaches to vault prolapse. In the later half of the 20th century, less attention was attributed to a vaginal uterosacral vault suspension as other techniques and approaches became widely used with acceptable results.

Four prominent gynecologic surgeons—Cullen Richardson (1923-2001), William Saye, Tom Elkins (1950-1998), and Bob Shull—met in Atlanta in the fall of 1992 to review videos of laparoscopic support procedures and discuss surgical strategies for the treatment of pelvic organ prolapse (interview with B. Shull,

2005). Richardson had previously stressed the importance of finding specific fascial defects and repairing them to achieve optimal restoration of pelvic anatomy.[27] After working together, Richardson and Saye developed what is now known as the Richardson-Saye laparoscopic technique of enterocele repair and vault suspension, which applies the principles of site-specific repair[26] to the laparoscopic approach. During their meeting in 1992, it occurred to the assembled group that they could find specific fascial defects, repair them, and resuspend the newly reconstructed vault to the uterosacral ligaments from a vaginal approach. In 2000, Shull and colleagues[6] published their technique and experience with this approach in 302 consecutive women. With only minor modifications, this is the surgical technique that we now use for the transvaginal correction of apical prolapse, and it is this procedure that we describe in this chapter.

TECHNICAL ASPECTS OF THE UTEROSACRAL LIGAMENT VAULT SUSPENSION

We are inclined to offer transvaginal repair to most of our patients. In our hands, this route of surgery has been safe, efficacious, and durable.[3] We have developed a bias, however, in that we prefer the abdominal sacral colpopexy to treat apical prolapse in our younger and more physically active patients. We are also likely to consider abdominal sacral colpopexy in patients with complete vaginal vault inversion.

Preoperatively, we discuss with the patient the reported incidence of complications associated with such major surgery in general and with this technique in particular. The ureteral obstruction rate is between 0% and 11%.[2,4-6] Intraoperative or postoperative blood transfusion may be required in up to 1% of patients.[2,4-6] It is important that the patient have realistic expectations of what can be achieved and that recurrent prolapse of the vault or the development of other vaginal defects is not uncommon. Interference with sexual function, in particular loss of vaginal depth and caliber, is not uncommon.

Patients are placed in the dorsal lithotomy position using padded, adjustable (Allen) stirrups and wearing sequential compression hose. The rectum is packed with an open, wet Kerlix sponge to the level of the ischial spines to aid the identification of the rectum and decrease the incidence of intraoperative injury during placement of the uterosacral suspensory sutures. A self-retaining vaginal retractor (Lone Star Medical Products, Houston, TX) and a weighted speculum are used to obtain good visualization. If the patient is being treated for uterine prolapse, a vaginal hysterectomy is performed as previously described by Lee[28] with minor modifications. In patients being treated for vault descent alone, a silk marking suture is placed in the vaginal epithelium at 3-o'clock and 9-o'clock positions at the vaginal apex for later reference. At these positions, the surgeon usually can see an epithelial dimple indicating the prior attachment point of the uterosacral ligaments to the vaginal cuff.

The vaginal epithelium is incised in the midline along the extent of the prolapsed vaginal segments. The dissecting scissors are used to separate the vaginal epithelium from the underlying pubocervical and rectovaginal connective tissues as needed to expose the entire fascial defect, including the enterocele sac. With the patient in Trendelenburg position, the enterocele sac is identified and opened sharply. A wet Kerlix sponge is used to pack the bowel out of the operative field into the upper peritoneal cavity. We have learned by experience to protect the posterior peritoneum (with an instrument such as a Breisky-Navratil retractor) to avoid tearing the peritoneum during the packing process, which invariably leads to bleeding and poor visualization of anatomic structures along the pelvic side wall.

For correct and safe placement of the uterosacral suspensory sutures, good exposure is critical. To provide adequate illumination in this deep cavity, we are accustomed to using a surgical headlight or a cool lighting system adherent to our retractor that is designed to be placed within the pelvis (LightMat surgical illuminator, Lumitex, Inc., Strongsville, OH). Various techniques have been used to expose the pelvic side wall, but we have been most satisfied using Breisky-Navratil retractors. Three Breisky-Navratil retractors are placed anteriorly, laterally, and posteriorly so that the bladder, ureter, and rectum, respectively, are protected while the uterosacral ligament is easily visualized. The posterior retractor, placed in the angle between the packed and easily identifiable rectum and the pelvic side wall, can be used to sweep the rectum to the contralateral side during placement of the uterosacral suspensory suture. By placing light tension on the uterosacral ligament, by traction on the earlier placed silk suture at the dimples at the vaginal cuff, identification of this ligament becomes much easier. A no. 1 polyglactin suture is passed through the uterosacral ligament medial and cephalad to the ischial spine. We have had excellent anatomic outcomes using a single absorbable suture through each uterosacral ligament, but this procedure has been described by others with as many as three suspensory sutures through each uterosacral ligament (Fig. 70-3). Tension placed on each uterosacral suspensory suture is used to confirm placement at a sturdy location and to visualize an attachment point in the proximal uterosacral ligament.

After a suture has been placed through each uterosacral ligament, the sutures are held with a tag for later use in suspending the vaginal apex. At this point, the patient is given 5 mL of intravenous indigo carmine dye and 5 mg of intravenous furosemide. The Foley catheter is removed, and a 70-degree cystoscope is used to inspect for spill of blue urine from each ureteral orifice while the uterosacral suspensory sutures are held on tension. If ureteral obstruction is suspected, the ipsilateral suspensory suture is released to confirm ureteral efflux. If necessary, the suspensory suture is removed and replaced in a more medial position. The anterior arm of each suspensory suture is passed through the apical portion of the pubocervical connective tissue, and the posterior arm of each suture is passed through the apical portion of the rectovaginal connective tissue. A Mayo needle is used where necessary (see Fig. 70-3). Both ends of each suspensory suture are passed through the vaginal epithelium near the silk marking sutures that were placed at the outset of the procedure.

Once satisfied with placement of the uterosacral suspensory sutures, attention is directed toward site-specific repair of any remaining prolapse defects. Typically, we use an anterior colporrhaphy to correct cystocele and a posterior colporrhaphy with or without allograft material (i.e., cadaveric dermis) to correct rectocele. Anterior and posterior colporrhaphy work well to reestablish a clearly defined transverse (apical) portion of the pubocervical and rectovaginal connective tissue. Colporrhaphy also aids in the preservation of acceptable vaginal length. Besides repair of the anterior and posterior defects, we commonly perform high ligation and excision of the enterocele sac using a 2-0 polyglactin suture. If stress urinary incontinence was a preoperative complaint or if a positive stress test result or urodynamic evidence of stress urinary incontinence existed with the

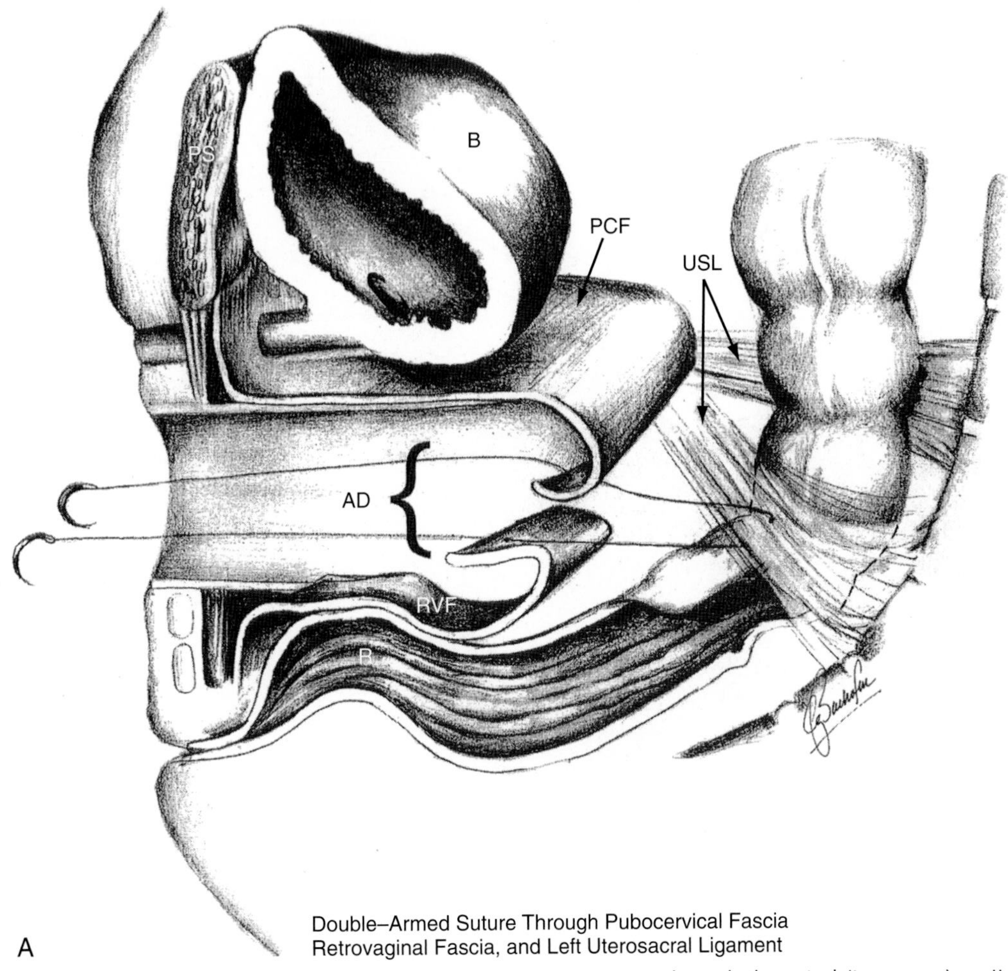

Figure 70-3 A and B, By passing one end of the each uterosacral suspensory suture through the apical (transverse) portion of the pubocervical connective tissue and the opposite end through the apical (transverse) portion of the rectovaginal connective tissue, the surgeon can elevate the vaginal cuff and reapproximate the endopelvic fascia simultaneously with two or more such sutures. AD, Apical Defect; B, Bladder; PCF, Pubocervical Fascia; USL, Uterosacral Ligament.

prolapse replaced, a pubovaginal sling also is performed. Sling tension is adjusted after the uterosacral sutures have been tied and after completion of the anterior repair.

The uterosacral suspensory sutures are then tied to close and suspend the vaginal cuff to the point of retroperitoneal uterosacral ligament fixation. The surgeon is reassured of excellent placement of these sutures if the knots seat in a posterior direction toward the sacral hollow. Redundant vaginal epithelium (after associated anterior and posterior repair by fascial plication or allograft placement) is excised and the epithelium closed. A digital vaginal examination is next performed to assess the axis and depth of the vaginal canal (Fig. 70-4). A vaginal pack is placed if deemed necessary, and a digital rectal examination is performed at completion to confirm the absence of suture material in the rectal lumen.

POSTOPERATIVE CARE AND PATIENT INSTRUCTIONS

Although patients are able to ambulate and tolerate a diet on the evening of the day of surgery, we usually leave in the Foley catheter in place until the morning of postoperative day 1. With few exceptions, we consistently use scheduled dosing of oral narcotic analgesics in lieu of intravenous narcotics (i.e., patient-controlled analgesia by intravenous morphine pump). Our typical postoperative pain control regimen includes a 12-hour dosing schedule of controlled-release oxycodone combined with a 6-hour dosing schedule of intravenous ketorolac or oral ibuprofen. Anecdotally, we observe less postoperative nausea, pruritus, and respiratory depression when we avoid using narcotics through an intravenous pump.

On the morning of postoperative day 1, the nursing staff is instructed to fill the patient's bladder with 300 mL of fluid (i.e., normal saline or sterile water) through the Foley catheter. The Foley catheter is removed, and the patient is instructed to void. The amount of urine voided is measured. If the postvoid residual urine volume exceeds the amount voided, the patient is sent home with instructions to do self-catheterization as necessary; patients are taught how to perform self-catheterization preoperatively. If the patient can spontaneously empty more than 50% of the total bladder contents, she is dismissed without an indwelling catheter or self-catheterization program.

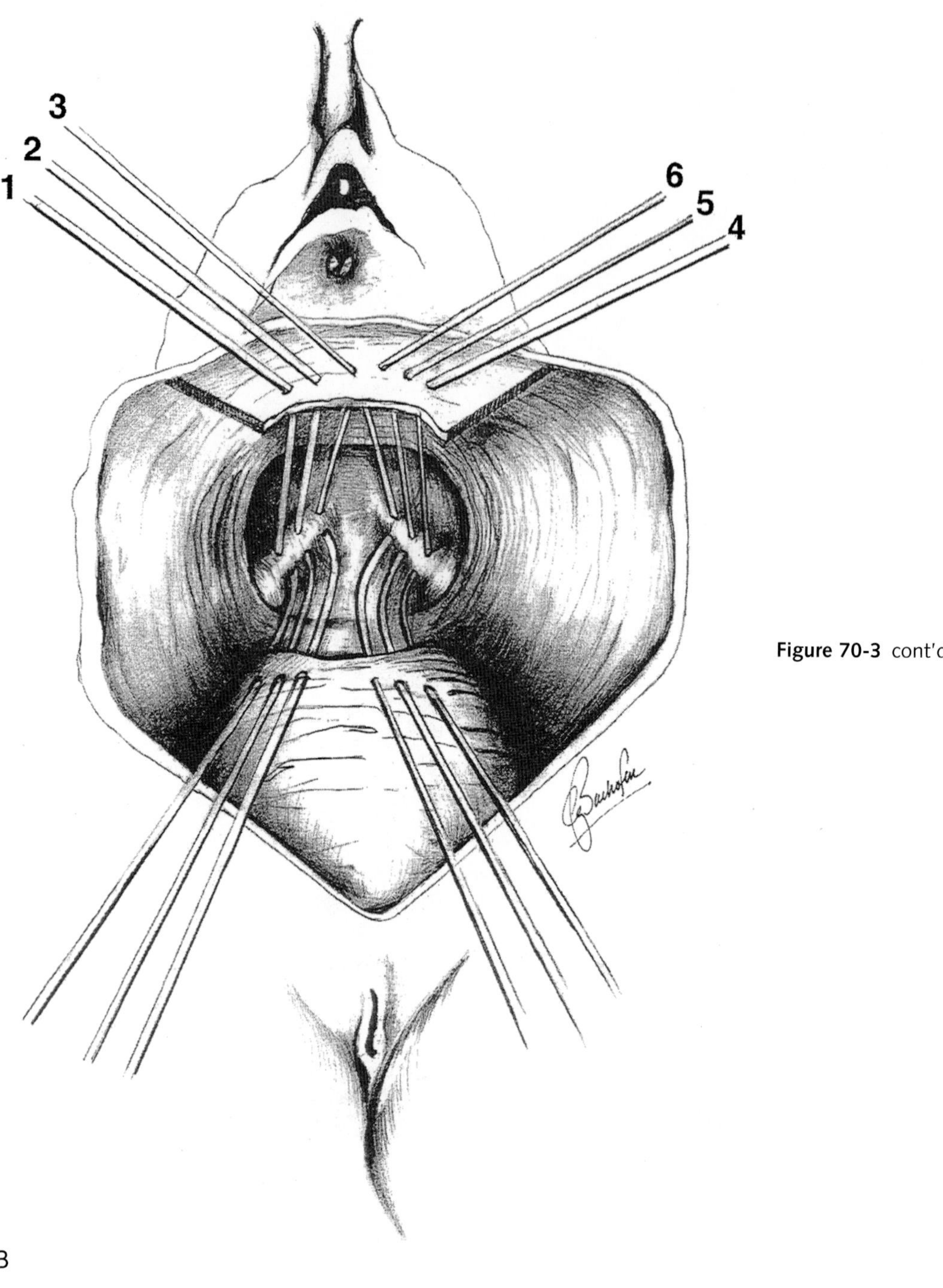

Figure 70-3 cont'd

We use printed discharge instructions that outline answers to common questions patients have in the postoperative period. The instruction sheet covers postoperative activity level (we discourage heavy lifting and straining for 90 days), constipation management, bathing, driving, vaginal bleeding, catheter program parameters, and other areas of interest and frequent concern to our patients. Patients usually are followed in the clinic after vaginal reconstructive surgery at 6 weeks, 6 months, and 1 year postoperatively. We typically allow patients to resume intravaginal intercourse and employment activities after the first postoperative visit. At the 6-month and 1-year postoperative visit, we reassess the patient's pelvic support using the Pelvic Organ Prolapse Quantification (POP-Q) scoring system.[29] The POP-Q score is compared with our preoperative evaluation so that we can assess the efficacy and durability of surgery.

CONCLUSIONS AND FUTURE DIRECTIONS

Transvaginal suspension of the vaginal vault to the uterosacral ligament for the treatment of apical prolapse is a safe, efficacious, and durable procedure.[2-6] Although reports have been published comparing the treatment of apical prolapse using the vaginal and abdominal approaches with mixed outcomes,[30,31] we believe that in our hands, transvaginal surgery affords most patients

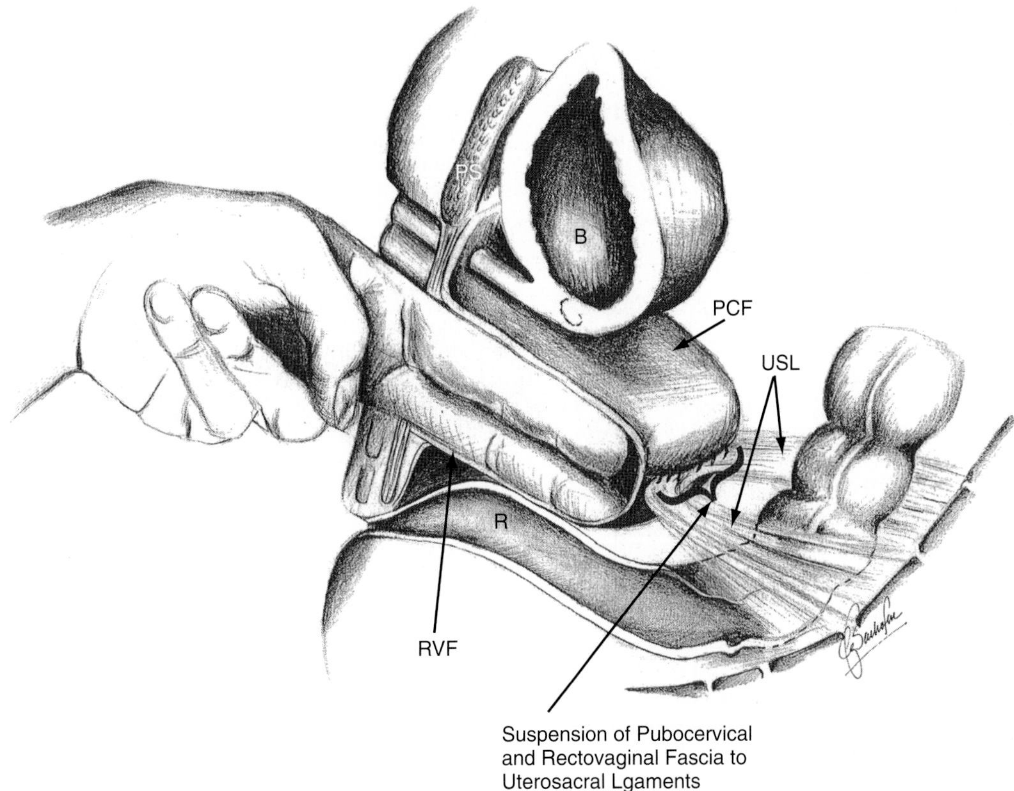

Figure 70-4 At the conclusion of the procedure, a digital vaginal examination is performed to assess the vaginal axis and depth. B, Bladder; PCF, Pubocervical Fascia; R, Rectum; RVF, Rectovaginal Fascia; USL, Uterosacral Ligament.

the best chance of cure with the least morbidity and shortest convalescence.

The care of patients with prolapse will continue to evolve as our understanding of the natural history of this disease becomes more informed. Pelvic organ prolapse, including apical prolapse, is a widespread problem among women in the United States and abroad. The lifetime risk for pelvic organ prolapse surgery in women is reported to be more than 11%.[32] Pelvic organ prolapse often coexists with urinary and fecal incontinence, sexual dysfunction, and defecatory dysfunction.

Despite myriad procedures to correct the anatomic circumstances arising with pelvic organ prolapse, there is often poor correlation between the anatomic and functional outcomes of surgery. The best operation designed to restore normal pelvic anatomic relationships can leave women with suboptimal functional outcomes. The best therapies therefore are measures taken to prevent prolapse in asymptomatic women.

The most efficient way to employ preventive measures is to identify women at risk and intervene in that group of patients. Little has been written about the epidemiology of pelvic floor dysfunction, including pelvic organ prolapse.[29] Our current understanding of the development of prolapse correlates this problem with risk factors that include vaginal parity, age, race, obesity, and chronic constipation.

Pelvic organ prolapse, urinary incontinence, and fecal incontinence have been associated with denervation injury of the pelvic floor muscles during vaginal childbirth.[33] Vaginal childbirth may be a time in the early stages of the natural history of pelvic organ prolapse when intervention could significantly prevent prolapse later in life. Some have advocated elective cesarean section as an intervention. It may be possible, however, to treat nerves damaged during vaginal childbirth so that denervation of the pelvic floor may be minimized or eliminated. We are involved in ongoing research with the squirrel monkey model of pelvic organ prolapse to define the role of parturition-induced nerve injury and to eventually propose pharmacologic intervention that would decrease the risk of permanent nerve injury after pelvic floor trauma, such as that incurred during vaginal childbirth.

Until the results of research in humans and animal models are available to help us understand the cause of prolapse, we will continue to treat prolapse with conservative, nonsurgical techniques and with invasive procedures designed to provide anatomic and functional cure. The procedure described in this chapter has a reported efficacy between 87%[6] and 100%,[5] with patients followed for up to 4 years. The morbidity and postoperative recovery associated with the transvaginal uterosacral vault suspension is acceptable and satisfying to surgeons and patients. We believe that this particular procedure will continue to be the gold standard for the treatment of apical prolapse in the hands of experienced vaginal surgeons for many years to come.

References

1. Flynn BJ, Webster GD: Surgical management of the apical vaginal defect. Curr Opin Urol 12:353-358, 2002.
2. Karram M, Goldwasser S, Kleeman S, et al: High uterosacral vaginal vault suspension with fascial reconstruction for vaginal repair of enterocele and vaginal vault prolapse. Am J Obstet Gynecol 185:1339-1342; discussion 1342-1343, 2001.
3. Amundsen CL, Flynn BJ, Webster GD: Anatomical correction of vaginal vault prolapse by uterosacral ligament fixation in women who also require a pubovaginal sling. J Urol 169:1770-1774, 2003.
4. Barber MD, Visco AG, Weidner AC, et al: Bilateral uterosacral ligament vaginal vault suspension with site-specific endopelvic fascia defect repair for treatment of pelvic organ prolapse. Am J Obstet Gynecol 183:1402-1410; discussion 1410-1411, 2000.
5. Jenkins VR 2nd: Uterosacral ligament fixation for vaginal vault suspension in uterine and vaginal vault prolapse. Am J Obstet Gynecol 177:1337-1343; discussion 1343-1344, 1997.
6. Shull BL, Bachofen C, Coates KW, Kuehl TJ: A transvaginal approach to repair of apical and other associated sites of pelvic organ prolapse with uterosacral ligaments. Am J Obstet Gynecol 183:1365-1373; discussion 1373-1374, 2000.
7. Cruikshank SH, Muniz M: Outcomes study: A comparison of cure rates in 695 patients undergoing sacrospinous ligament fixation alone and with other site-specific procedures—A 16-year study. Am J Obstet Gynecol 188:1509-1512; discussion 1512-1515, 2003.
8. Addison WA, Livengood CH 3rd, Sutton GP, Parker RT: Abdominal sacral colpopexy with Mersilene mesh in the retroperitoneal position in the management of posthysterectomy vaginal vault prolapse and enterocele. Am J Obstet Gynecol 153:140-146, 1985.
9. Cook JR, Seman EI, O'Shea RT: Laparoscopic treatment of enterocele: A 3-year evaluation. Aust N Z J Obstet Gynaecol 44:107-110, 2004.
10. Culligan PJ, Murphy M, Blackwell L, et al: Long-term success of abdominal sacral colpopexy using synthetic mesh. Am J Obstet Gynecol 187:1473-1480; discussion 1481-1482, 2002.
11. Guner H, Noyan V, Tiras MB, et al: Transvaginal sacrospinous colpopexy for marked uterovaginal and vault prolapse. Int J Gynaecol Obstet 74:165-170, 2001.
12. Lantzsch T, Goepel C, Wolters M, et al: Sacrospinous ligament fixation for vaginal vault prolapse. Arch Gynecol Obstet 265:21-25, 2001.
13. Limb J, Wood K, Weinberger M, et al: Sacral colpopexy using Mersilene mesh in the treatment of vaginal vault prolapse. World J Urol 23:55-60, 2005.
14. Nieminen K, Heinonen PK: Sacrospinous ligament fixation for massive genital prolapse in women aged over 80 years. BJOG 108:817-821, 2001.
15. Ross JW: Laparoscopic approach for severe pelvic vault prolapse. J Am Assoc Gynecol Laparosc 3:S43, 1996.
16. Timmons MC, Addison WA, Addison SB, Cavenar MG: Abdominal sacral colpopexy in 163 women with posthysterectomy vaginal vault prolapse and enterocele. Evolution of operative techniques. J Reprod Med 37:323-327, 1992.
17. Comiter CV, Vasavada SP, Raz S: Transvaginal culdosuspension: Technique and results. Urology 54:819-822, 1999.
18. Bump RC, Norton PA: Epidemiology and natural history of pelvic floor dysfunction. Obstet Gynecol Clin North Am 25:723-746, 1998.
19. Burns J: The Principles of Midwifery, including the Diseases of Women and Children. New York, CS Francis, 1839.
20. McCall M: Posterior culdeplasty; surgical correction of enterocele during vaginal hysterectomy: A preliminary report. Obstet Gynecol 10:595-602, 1957.
21. Lee RA, Symmonds RE: Surgical repair of posthysterectomy vault prolapse. Am J Obstet Gynecol 112:953-956, 1972.
22. Shull BL, Capen CV, Riggs MW, Kuehl TJ: Bilateral attachment of the vaginal cuff to iliococcygeus fascia: An effective method of cuff suspension. Am J Obstet Gynecol 168:1669-1674; discussion 1674-1677, 1993.
23. Zweifel P: Vorlesungen uber klinische Gynakologie. Berlin, Hirschwald, 1892, p 407.
24. Arthure HG, Savage D: Uterine prolapse and prolapse of the vaginal vault treated by sacral hysteropexy. J Obstet Gynaecol Br Emp 64:355-360, 1957.
25. Falk HC: Uterine prolapse and prolapse of the vaginal vault treated by sacropexy. Obstet Gynecol 18:113-115, 1961.
26. Carter JE, Winter M, Mendehlsohn S, et al: Vaginal vault suspension and enterocele repair by Richardson-Saye laparoscopic technique: Description of training technique and results. JSLS 5:29-36, 2001.
27. Richardson AC, Lyon JB, Williams NL: A new look at pelvic relaxation. Am J Obstet Gynecol 126:568-573, 1976.
28. Lee RA: Combined compartment defects: Vaginal hysterectomy with repair of enterocele, cystocele, and rectocele. In Rock JA, Thompson JD (eds): Te Linde's Operative Gynecology. Philadelphia, Lippincott-Raven, 1997.
29. Bump RC, Mattiasson A, Bo K, et al: The standardization of terminology of female pelvic organ prolapse and pelvic floor dysfunction. Am J Obstet Gynecol 175:10-17, 1996.
30. Benson JT, Lucente V, McClellan E: Vaginal versus abdominal reconstructive surgery for the treatment of pelvic support defects: A prospective randomized study with long-term outcome evaluation. Am J Obstet Gynecol 175:1418-1421; discussion 1421-1422, 1996.
31. Maher CF, Qatawneh AM, Dwyer PL, et al: Abdominal sacral colpopexy or vaginal sacrospinous colpopexy for vaginal vault prolapse: A prospective randomized study. Am J Obstet Gynecol 190:20-26, 2004.
32. Olsen AL, Smith VJ, Bergstrom JO, et al: Epidemiology of surgically managed pelvic organ prolapse and urinary incontinence. Obstet Gynecol 89:501-506, 1997.
33. Swash M, Snooks SJ, Henry MM: Unifying concept of pelvic floor disorders and incontinence. J R Soc Med 78:906-911, 1985.

Chapter 71

VAGINAL HYSTERECTOMY IN THE TREATMENT OF VAGINAL PROLAPSE

Christopher M. Rooney and Mickey M. Karram

Hysterectomy continues to be one of the most commonly performed surgical procedures in the United States, second only to cesarean section. Approximately 800,000 hysterectomies are performed annually in the United States.[1] According to the National Center for Health Statistics, 3,525,237 hysterectomies were performed in the United States between 1994 and 1999, at a rate of 5.5 per 1000 women. The most common indication for hysterectomy continues to be uterine leiomyoma, accounting for approximately 38% of all hysterectomies. Endometriosis accounts for 18% of all hysterectomies, followed by uterine prolapse (16%) and endometrial hyperplasia (4%).[1] As the population of women older than 65 years continues to rise, the practitioner can anticipate an increase in the number of women presenting with these indications.[2] Most hysterectomies are performed by the abdominal route, with the rate of vaginal hysterectomy remaining stable over the past several decades.[1] Vaginal hysterectomy in the appropriately selected patient has been reported to result in a shorter hospital stay, less operative blood loss, and less postoperative pain compared with the abdominal route of hysterectomy. Patients presenting for evaluation and surgical correction of pelvic organ prolapse are particularly appropriate candidates for vaginal hysterectomy.

ANATOMY OF PELVIC SUPPORT

Normal pelvic support is a complex interaction between the muscular and fascial structures that line the pelvic cavity, collectively known as the *pelvic floor*. The levator ani complex (i.e., coccygeus, iliococcygeus, and pubococcygeus) stretches from the coccyx to the symphysis pubis anteriorly in the erect woman. Laterally, the levator complex attaches to the arcus tendineus fasciae pelvis ("white line"). The arcus tendineus fasciae pelvis extends from the symphysis pubis to the ischial spines bilaterally. The levator ani complex is typically described in two parts: the diaphragmatic portion (i.e., coccygeus and iliococcygeus) and the pubovisceral portion (i.e., pubococcygeus). The coccygeus muscles run bilaterally from the sacrum and coccyx to the ischial spines and are associated with the sacrospinous ligaments. The iliococcygeus muscles pass laterally from the symphysis pubis to the arcus tendineus fasciae pelvis, where they attach and turn medially to join the coccygeus at the coccyx, forming the levator plate. The pubovisceral portion, or pubococcygeus, is associated with the puborectalis, arising from the posterior surface of the symphysis pubis and extending back to the ventral surface of the coccyx.[3]

Normal pelvic support is provided by the pelvic floor and by the connective tissue attachments. The pelvic organs rest on the pelvic floor and are stabilized by the connective tissues. In 1992, DeLancey described the stabilization of the vagina in levels. Level 1 support is derived from the cardinal-uterosacral complex and is responsible for holding the upper vagina and cervix in a superior position in relation to the genital hiatus. Level II support is responsible for lateral support of the midvagina to the arcus tendineus fasciae pelvis. Level III support is responsible for distal support of the lower vagina by means of connections to the perineal body and perineal membrane[4] (Fig. 71-1).

PELVIC ORGAN PROLAPSE

The cause of pelvic organ prolapse is multifactorial. Uterovaginal prolapse results from damage to the cardinal-uterosacral complex, or level I support.[5] The uterus and upper vagina normally lie over the pelvic floor and are directed to the hollow of the sacrum. Increased intra-abdominal pressure is directed toward the levator ani complex. Attenuation of the levator ani complex may result in inadequate support to the overlying pelvic organs. Such attenuation may be the result of childbirth and some connective tissue disorders. Conditions or maneuvers that result in repeated increases in intra-abdominal pressure may lead to attenuation of the pelvic floor and aggravate pelvic organ prolapse. These conditions may include occupations that require heavy lifting or medical conditions such as chronic constipation resulting in excessive straining or chronic obstructive pulmonary disease with chronic coughing.

Age also has been implicated as an etiologic factor in pelvic organ prolapse. Age is widely accepted to be associated with decreased muscle tone and decreased quality of underlying fibroblasts and collagen fibers, both of which can aggravate the underlying prolapse. Postmenopausal women who are not receiving hormone replacement therapy may also present with signs and symptoms of pelvic organ prolapse.

PELVIC ORGAN PROLAPSE

Diagnosis

Patients with uterovaginal prolapse may present with a multitude of symptoms. A carefully tailored history and physical examination are important in gaining insight into the complaint and any affect on the patient's quality of life. Patients may present with a vaginal mass, sometimes described by them as a bulge. They may complain of pelvic pain, pressure, or dyspareunia. Patients may describe urinary urgency or frequency or incontinence. In cases of severe prolapse, patients may complain of urinary retention, because of the effect of the prolapse on the anatomy of the lower urinary tract. The typical patient describes symptoms that are

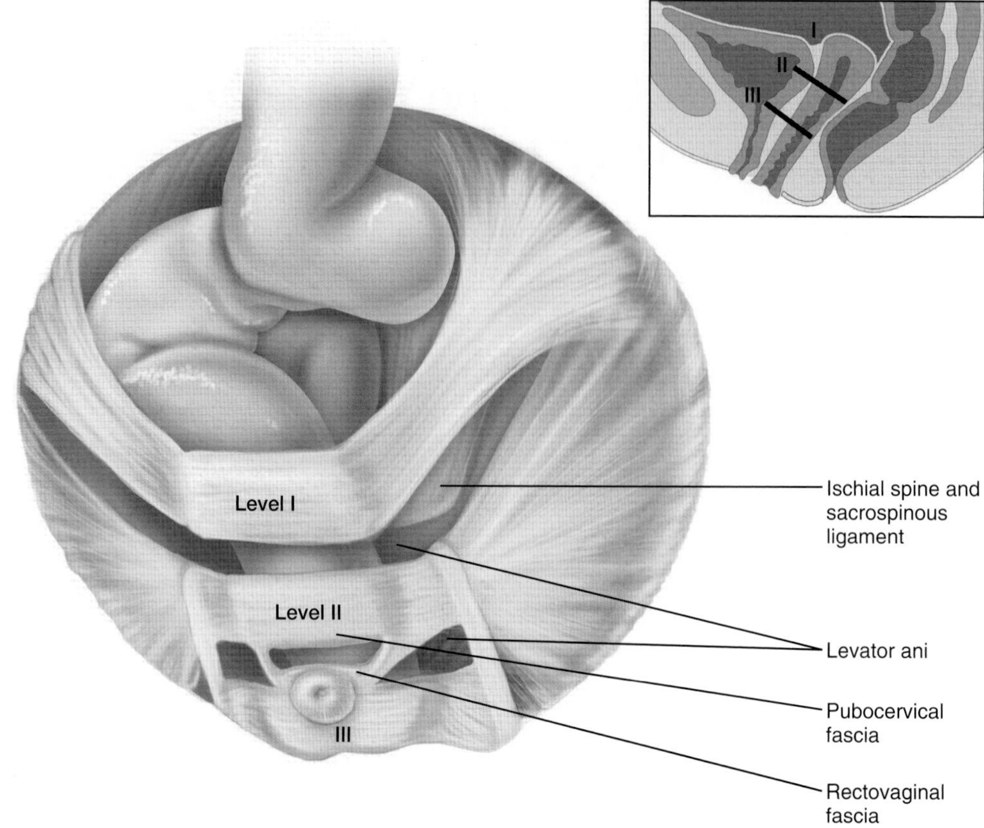

Figure 71-1 Levels of support of the upper and middle vagina. Level I support represents the apical support of the vagina by means of the uterosacral-cardinal complex. Level II support represents the lateral support of the vagina by means of attachments to the arcus tendineus fasciae pelvis. (From DeLancey JOL: Anatomic aspects of vaginal eversion after hysterectomy. Am J Obstet Gynecol 166:1717, 1992.)

worse with standing or activity and that improve on assuming a supine position. If the diagnosis of pelvic organ prolapse is obscure, it is important to consider performing the examination of the patient at the end of the day, when the prolapse is likely to be at its worst.

Physical Examination

The result of physical examination remains one of the most important pieces of information in the evaluation of pelvic organ prolapse. The diagnosis of uterovaginal prolapse is confirmed by significant descensus of the uterus on pelvic examination. A bimanual examination is important to ascertain the size and mobility of the uterus and any underlying pathology such as uterine leiomyoma or adnexal masses. The caliber of the genital hiatus is measured to predict the success of a vaginal hysterectomy. The coexistence of anterior or posterior vaginal wall prolapse should be determined. In our experience, it is advisable to evaluate the patient with uterovaginal prolapse in the supine and standing positions. The patient should be examined with an empty bladder because the prolapse may not be fully appreciated in the presence of a subjectively full bladder.[6] It is important to evaluate for the sign of stress incontinence with the bladder full and the prolapse reduced to its normal anatomic location to exclude potential or occult stress incontinence.

Classification

The severity of pelvic organ prolapse is described to standardize findings among examiners. For decades, the Baden-Walker system was used to describe the presence of pelvic organ prolapse.[7] The Baden-Walker system, still in use today, is also known as the *halfway system*. It involves description of the most dependent position of the pelvic organs during a maximum Valsalva maneuver or during standing in relation to the hymenal ring (Table 71-1).

In 1996, Bump and colleagues[8] standardized the terminology of female pelvic organ prolapse for the International Continence Society (ICS). The Pelvic Organ Prolapse Quantification (POP-Q) system involves measurement of six anatomic points (in centimeters) in relation to the hymenal ring, as well as the genital hiatus, perineal body, and total vaginal length. The hymenal ring, defined as zero, is chosen as the reference point because it is a fixed anatomic point from which interobserver variability can be standardized. Prolapse distal to the hymenal ring is described in positive centimeters from the hymenal ring. Prolapse proximal to the hymenal ring is defined in negative centimeters from the hymenal ring. The six anatomic points can be divided into two points on the anterior vaginal wall (Aa and Ba), two points on the posterior vaginal wall (Ap and Bp), and two points in the superior vagina (C and D) (Fig. 71-2).

The genital hiatus (gh) is measured from the posterior fourchette to the middle of the urethral meatus. The perineal body (pb) is measured from the posterior fourchette to the middle of the anus. Total vaginal length (tvl) is measured with point C and point D reduced to their normal anatomic positions.

Table 71-2 represents the stages of pelvic organ prolapse as defined by the POP-Q system. Because of the use of measurements revolving around fixed anatomic landmarks, the POP-Q system is a much more precise method of defining pelvic organ prolapse compared with previous systems. Interexaminer variability is markedly reduced, which is important for clinical standardization and for the purposes of research.

Table 71-1 Baden-Walker Classification of Pelvic Organ Prolapse

Cystocele	First degree: Anterior vaginal wall and bladder descend halfway to the hymen. Second degree: Anterior vaginal wall and bladder descend to the hymenal ring. Third degree: Anterior vaginal wall and bladder are outside the hymen.
Uterine or vaginal vault prolapse	First degree: Cervix or vaginal apex descends halfway to the hymen. Second degree: Cervix or vaginal apex extends to the hymen or over the perineal body. Third degree: Cervix and uterine corpus extend beyond the hymen, or the vaginal vault is everted and protrudes beyond the hymen.
Rectocele	First degree: Posterior vaginal wall descends halfway to the hymen. Second degree: Posterior vaginal wall descends to the hymen. Third degree: Posterior vaginal wall extends beyond the hymen.
Enterocele	Presence of the enterocele sac, relative to the hymen, should be described anatomically, with the patient in the supine and standing positions during a Valsalva maneuver.

VAGINAL HYSTERECTOMY AND RELATED PROCEDURES

Indications

The most frequent indication for hysterectomy is the leiomyomatous uterus. Patients with uterine fibroids may complain of pelvic pain or pressure. Other patients may complain of low back pain or urinary symptoms. Dysfunctional uterine bleeding is a common complaint of the woman with uterine fibroids. The

Table 71-2 Stages of Pelvic Organ Prolapse

Stage 0	No evidence of pelvic organ prolapse. Points Aa, Ba, Ap, and Bp are all defined at –3 cm. Points C and D are located within 2 cm of the tvl (i.e., ≤ tvl – 2 cm).
Stage 1	Most distal portion of the prolapse is > 1 cm above the level of the hymen (i.e., ≤ 1 cm).
Stage 2	Most distal portion of the prolapse within 1 cm of the hymenal ring, proximal or distal (i.e., ≥ –1cm but ≤ +1 cm)
Stage 3	Most distal portion of the prolapse is more than 1 cm distal to the hymenal ring but not more than 2 cm less than the tvl (i.e., > +1 cm but not more than tvl – 2 cm).
Stage 4	Complete eversion of the tvl

tvl, total vaginal length.

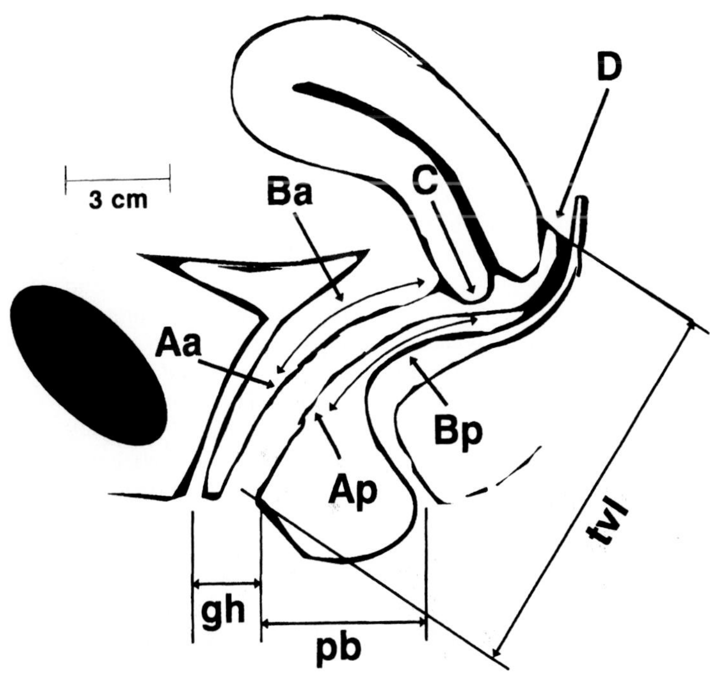

Figure 71-2 Six anatomic sites (points Aa, Ba, C, D, Bp, and Ap), the genital hiatus (gh), perineal body (bp), and total vaginal length (tvl) are used to describe the degree of pelvic organ prolapse. (From Bump RC, Mathiason A, Bo K, et al: The Standardization of Terminology of Female Pelvic Organ Prolapse and Pelvic Floor Dysfunction. Am J Obstet Gynecol 175:10, 1996.)

patient with symptomatic uterine fibroids is a safe candidate for vaginal hysterectomy assuming the uterus is mobile and the total uterine size is less than 12 weeks' gestational size.[9]

Vaginal hysterectomy is particularly appropriate for the patient with symptomatic uterine prolapse when additional pelvic reconstruction may be indicated. These patients rarely present with isolated uterine prolapse, often having coexistent prolapse of the anterior or posterior vaginal walls, requiring a tailored and thoughtful pelvic reconstruction. Other indications for vaginal hysterectomy include adenomyosis, pelvic pain, and endometrial hyperplasia.

Contraindications

With an appropriate understanding of pelvic anatomy, the experienced surgeon encounters few contraindications to the vaginal route of hysterectomy. Even the large fibroid uterus can be removed vaginally in the hands of a skilled surgeon. Uterine immobility can make a vaginal hysterectomy difficult if abdominopelvic adhesions or scarring are present. A narrow, or stenotic, vaginal introitus can complicate removal of the uterus vaginally, and consideration should be given to an abdominal approach in this case. Selected cases of endometriosis are a contraindication to the vaginal route of hysterectomy. In 1995, Kovac[10] assigned 617 women to abdominal, vaginal, or laparoscopically assisted vaginal hysterectomy based on uterine size and risk factors suggesting pelvic disease. In his series, 548 women were able to undergo successful vaginal hysterectomy. In the case of laparoscopically assisted vaginal hysterectomy, all but 2 of the 63 cases could have undergone successful vaginal hysterectomy based on laparoscopic findings. In his series, Kovac reported a 99.5% success rate for the vaginal route of hysterectomy using the techniques of morcellation, bivalving, and uterine coring (discussed later).[10] The suspicious adnexal mass and high-grade endometrial carcinoma present absolute contraindications to the urogynecologic surgeon. In some cases, low-grade endometrial carcinoma may be managed with a vaginal hysterectomy.

Technique

For a simple vaginal hysterectomy, after the patient is in the operating suite, anesthesia is administered. The patient is then appropriately placed in the dorsal lithotomy position. We prefer the use of candy cane stirrups. A careful examination of the anesthetized patient is performed to confirm the findings of the previous examination. The patient is then prepared using a povidone-iodine solution or chlorhexidine gluconate and is draped in the usual fashion. The bladder is allowed to drain after placement of a 16-Fr, 5-mL Foley catheter. After complete drainage, the catheter is clamped using a Kelly clamp.

Simms retractors are used to retract the anterior and posterior vaginal walls to fully visualize the cervix. The cervix is then grasped at the 3-o'clock and 9-o'clock positions with single-tooth tenaculums. The uterus is mobilized downward toward the introitus by traction on the tenaculums. Careful attention is paid to the location of the bladder. A solution of 1% lidocaine with epinephrine is then injected into the cervicovaginal junction in a circumferential fashion. The injection solution serves two purposes. First, it aids in hydrodissection, allowing the appropriate plane to be entered more efficiently. Second, the injection solution results in vasoconstriction, which facilitates visualization because of decreased operative blood loss.

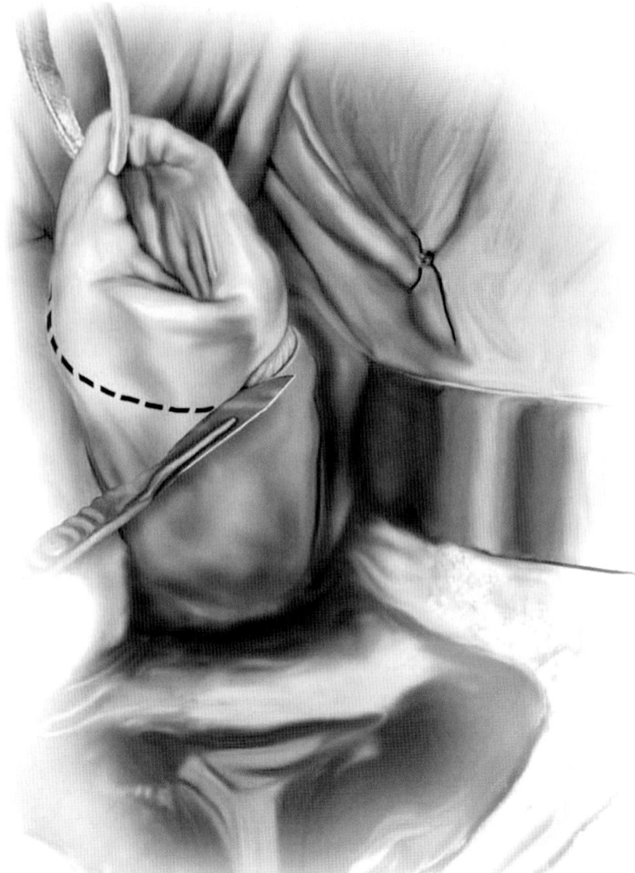

Figure 71-3 Using a scalpel, the initial incision begins circumferentially at the reflection of the vaginal mucosa and the cervix.

An incision is made from the 9-o'clock position anteriorly to the 3-o'clock position. A similar incision is made posteriorly around the cervix (Fig. 71-3). Appropriate traction is applied to the cervix in the direction opposite the incision to facilitate separation of the underlying cervical stroma from the overlying vaginal wall. Side wall retractors are used by the assistants to aid in visualization. The full-thickness vaginal mucosa is dissected off of the underlying connective tissues using curved Mayo scissors. A right angle Heaney retractor or Deaver retractor can be used to retract the anterior vagina away from the underlying cervix to correctly identify the plane of cleavage. Posteriorly, a similar dissection is undertaken, completely separating the full thickness posterior vaginal mucosa from the overlying cervix (Fig. 71-4). After the peritoneum of the posterior cul-de-sac can be palpated, a posterior colpotomy is performed, and entrance into the peritoneal cavity is confirmed using a finger (Fig. 71-5). A right-angle Heaney retractor is used to deflect the rectosigmoid colon away from the operative field.

Assuming the bladder has been sufficiently mobilized cephalad, the uterosacral ligaments can be secured to release the natural pelvic support of the cervix. We prefer the latter method because release of the uterosacral attachments facilitates anterior dissection (Fig. 71-6). Care must be taken to adequately retract the bladder away from the clamps. Heaney clamps are used to secure the uterosacral ligaments, incorporating the posterior peritoneum. The Heaney clamps are rotated laterally so that the tips of

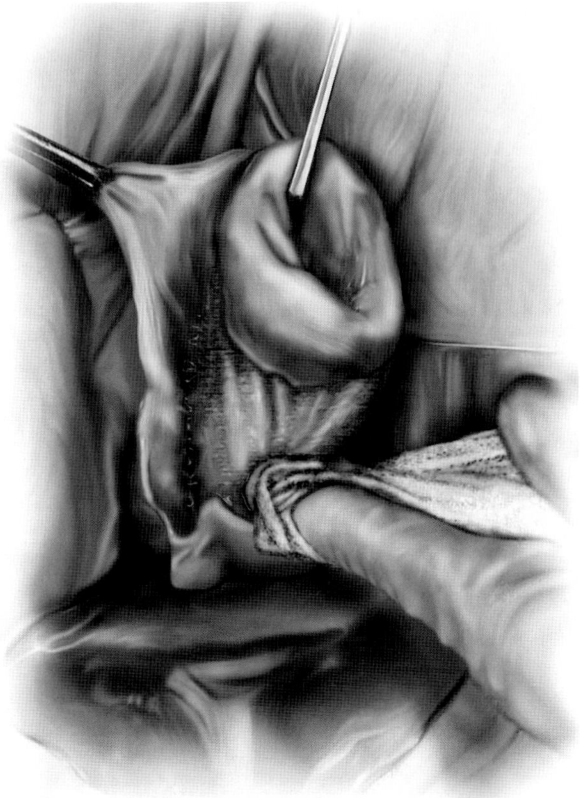

Figure 71-4 Posteriorly, the full-thickness vaginal mucosa is sharply or bluntly dissected from the cervix.

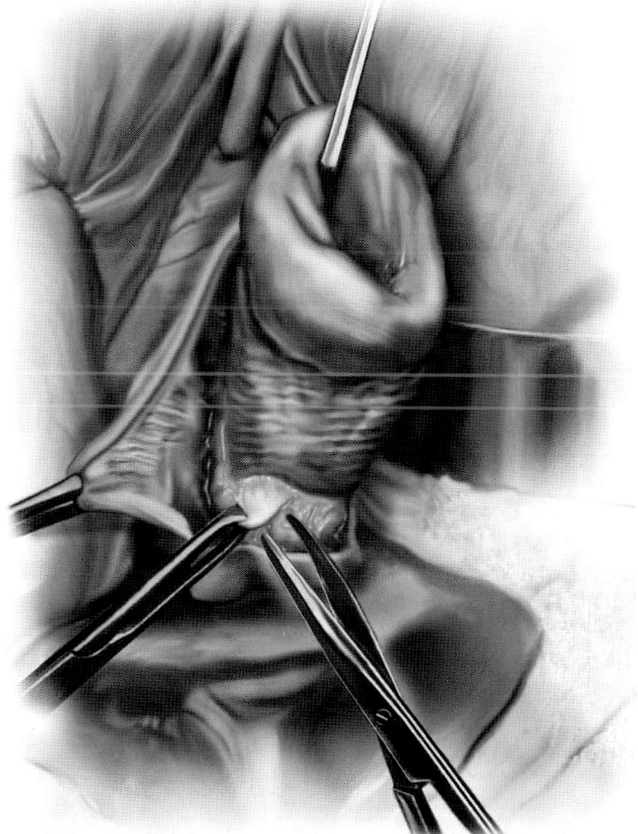

Figure 71-5 The posterior cul-de-sac is sharply entered using Mayo or Metzenbaum scissors.

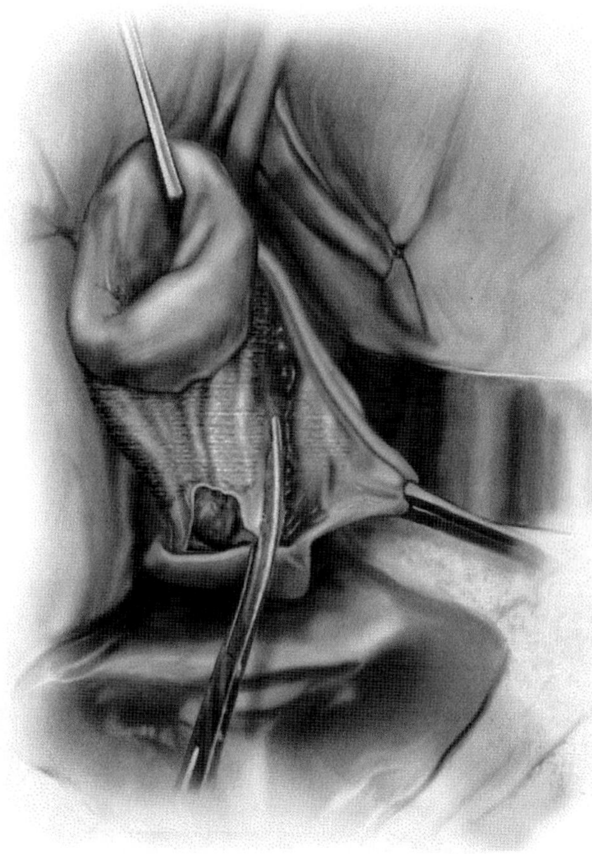

Figure 71-6 The uterosacral ligaments are clamped to gain access to the vesicouterine space.

the clamp are almost perpendicular with the plane of the cervix. The results in shortening of the uterosacral ligaments and helps avoid injury to the bladder and ureters laterally. The uterosacral ligaments are then released from the uterus using Mayo scissors. The pedicles are then secured using a suture ligature of a 1-0 absorbable suture. At this point, attention is turned anteriorly. The full-thickness vagina is separated from the underlying cervix with the Mayo scissors. The dissection ultimately leads to the vesicouterine space (Fig. 71-7). A history of cesarean section may lead to scarification. Elevating the cesarean scar with forceps allows the surgeon to separate the scar from the underlying lower uterine segment. In this fashion, the vesicouterine space is entered. A right-angle Heaney retractor or Deaver retractor is then used to deflect the bladder anteriorly to identify the vesicouterine fold. The vesicouterine fold can be visualized as a semilunar, white line. The vesicouterine fold is then elevated, and the peritoneum is incised below the level of the forceps with Mayo scissors (Fig. 71-8). Entrance into the anterior cul-de-sac is confirmed by palpation. A retractor is used to deflect the bladder away from the surgical field.

Lateral dissection using Mayo scissors aids in separation of the vaginal wall from the cervix. Heaney clamps are then used to secure the uterine vessels bilaterally as they run in the cardinal ligament. The pedicles are released from the uterus and secured using a 1-0 absorbable suture. We prefer to use a suture ligature, incorporating the previous uterosacral ligament pedicle. With this technique, the dead space between pedicles is obliterated, preventing tearing of tissue and bleeding from the small cervical

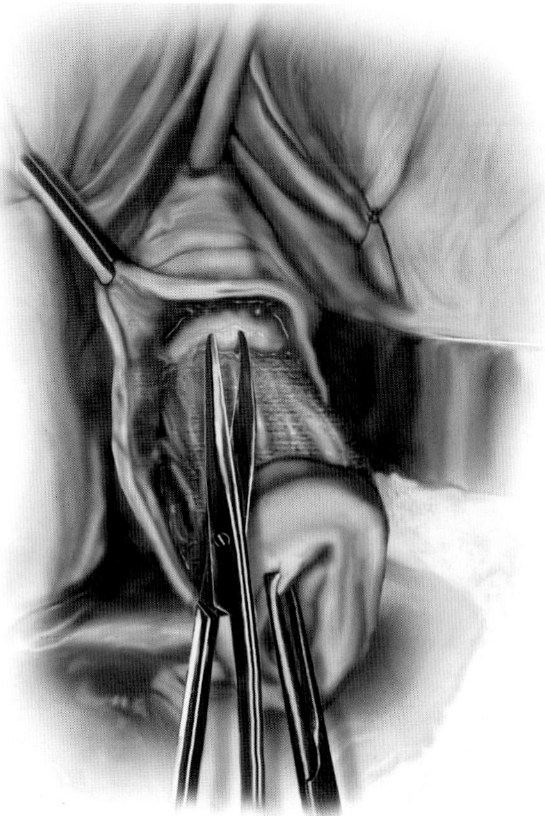

Figure 71-7 The anterior vaginal wall is dissected from the cervix using Mayo or Metzenbaum scissors. This plane will ultimately lead to the vesicouterine space.

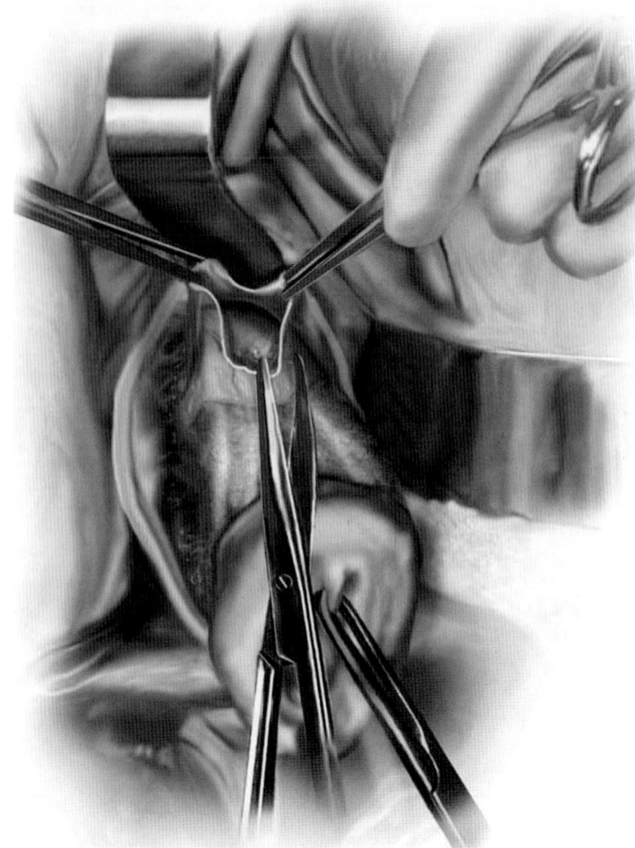

Figure 71-8 The vesicouterine fold is elevated and entered sharply using Metzenbaum scissors.

branches (Fig. 71-9). The cardinal ligament is secured in successive bites as previously described, ensuring that the anterior peritoneum and posterior peritoneum are incorporated. This technique fuses the anterior and posterior leaves of the broad ligament, preventing extensions of the peritoneal incisions into the vasculature of the broad ligament. Care must be taken to clamp medial to the previous pedicle to avoid ureteral injury. With adequate descensus, the fundus of the uterus is reached. An adequate examination should be performed to exclude pelvic adhesions or abnormal pathology. The utero-ovarian ligaments are then clamped with Heaney clamps (Fig. 71-10). The surgeon must proceed with caution to avoid bowel injury. The pedicles are released from the uterus using Mayo scissors. The uterine specimen is then submitted for pathologic analysis. The utero-ovarian pedicles are secured first using a free tie of a 1-0 absorbable suture, followed by a distal suture ligature of a 1-0 absorbable suture.

At this time, all of the pedicles are inspected for hemostasis. Packing the bowel with moist tail sponges or the use of a sponge stick can aid in visualization. The ovaries should be palpated to look for abnormal pathology.

Managing the Adnexa

The decision to proceed with vaginal oophorectomy at the time of hysterectomy is a controversial topic and should involve a thoughtful preoperative discussion with the patient. The indications for vaginal oophorectomy should be similar to the indications for oophorectomy at the time of abdominal hysterectomy. After vaginal hysterectomy, the ovaries are not as accessible, leading to a more technically difficult procedure than oophorectomy at the time of abdominal hysterectomy.[11] However, adhering to the surgical principles of mobilization and adequate visualization can lead to successful adnexectomy in more than 90% of cases, without increased morbidity.[12]

At the start of the procedure, the adnexa are identified. Using gentle traction on the round ligaments often affords the surgeon adequate visualization. Alternatively, a Babcock clamp can be used to grasp the adnexa, which are then brought into the surgical field. A finger can be used to palpate the ipsilateral ureter through the broad ligament. A curved clamp, such as a Heaney or Satinsky vascular clamp, can be used to clamp across the infundibulopelvic ligament (Fig. 71-11). Care should be taken to clamp as close to the ovary as possible to avoid ureteral injury. After adnexectomy, we prefer to secure the infundibulopelvic ligament with a free tie of 1-0 Vicryl, followed by a transfixion suture of 1-0 Vicryl placed distal to the free tie. The pedicle should be held until adequate hemostasis has been ensured to avoid retraction of an inadequately secured infundibulopelvic ligament high into the pelvis.

Vaginal Vault Suspension

After vaginal hysterectomy, the cul-de-sac should be routinely evaluated to determine if an enterocele coexists. Based on the size of the enterocele and the degree of vault prolapse, the appropriate

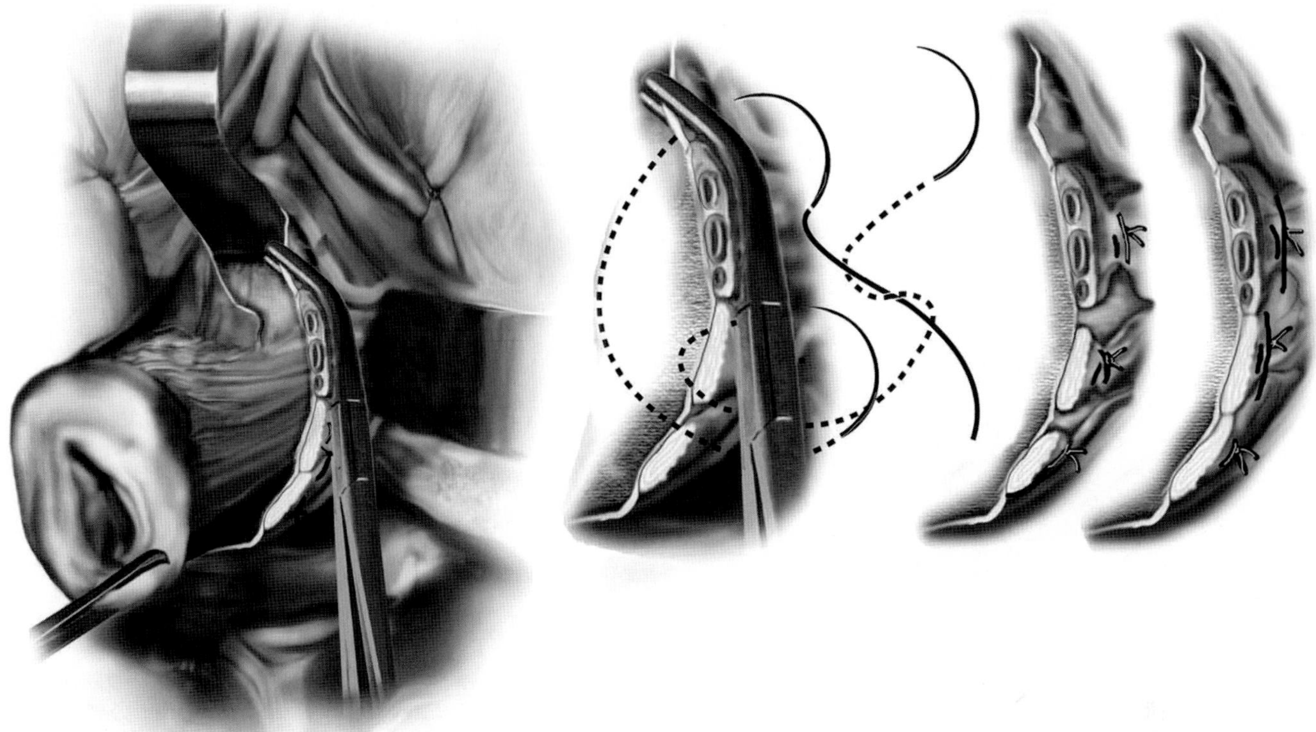

Figure 71-9 Proper technique for clamping the uterine vessels. The vascular pedicle is suture ligated to the previously ligated pedicle. This technique ensures that the dead space between pedicles is obliterated and guards against bleeding from small cervical branches.

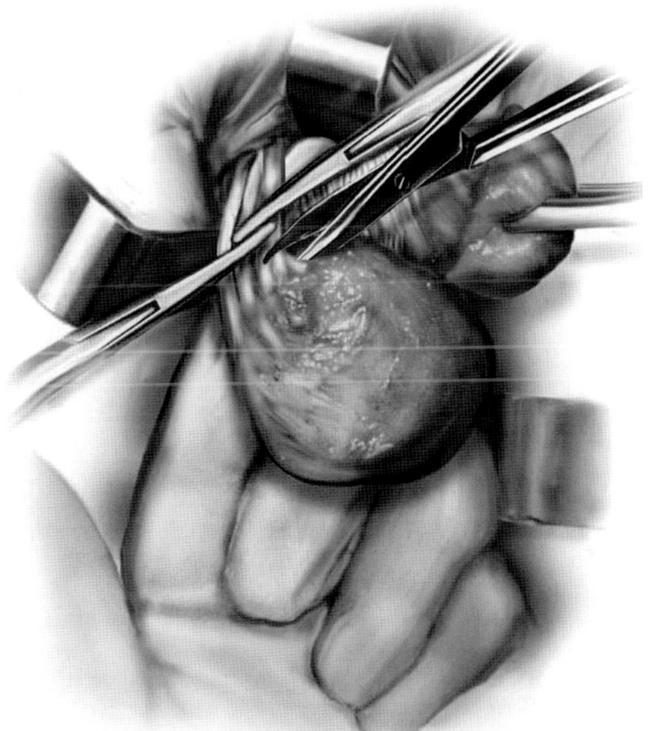

Figure 71-10 A finger is placed behind the utero-ovarian pedicle to prevent injury to the hollow viscus or other structures while the pedicle is cut with scissors.

procedure to obliterate the cul-de-sac and support or suspend the vaginal apex can be determined.

With the bowel packed away using moist tail sponges and the patient in a slight Trendelenburg position, an assessment can be made about the presence or absence of an enterocele by simple digital palpation of the posterior cul-de-sac. An identifiable pocket confirms the presence of an enterocele and determines the need for excision of redundant peritoneum and posterior vaginal wall. Subsequently, the excess vaginal mucosa and peritoneum may be removed in a wedgelike fashion using Mayo scissors or Bovie cautery (Fig. 71-12). Allis clamps are then used to grasp the peritoneum and corresponding vaginal mucosa at the 5-o'clock and 7-o'clock positions. Outward traction and elevation of the Allis clamps at a 45-degree angle in relation to the patient allow the surgeon to palpate the uterosacral ligaments coursing back toward the sacrum. With the same finger, the surgeon can palpate the position of the ipsilateral ureter in relation to the uterosacral ligament. The ureter can be found ventral and lateral to the ischial spine.

The McCall culdoplasty was first described in 1957 by Milton McCall. In the initial description, McCall used several non-absorbable sutures to plicate the uterosacral ligaments in the midline, incorporating the intervening, redundant peritoneum. This resulted in effective obliteration of the posterior cul-de-sac. External absorbable, McCall sutures were placed through the full-thickness vagina, incorporating the ipsilateral uterosacral ligament and intervening peritoneum before crossing the midline and incorporating the contralateral uterosacral ligament and passing back through the full-thickness vagina (Figs. 71-13 and

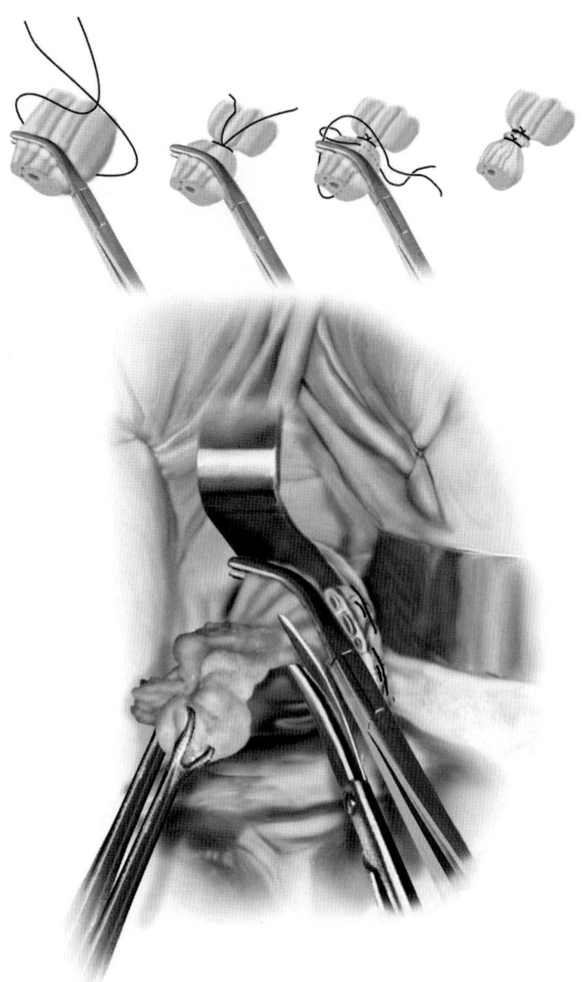

Figure 71-11 The infundibulopelvic ligament is secured using a curved Haney or Satinsky vascular clamp. The pedicle is secured first using a free tie of a =0 absorbable suture followed by a suture ligament.

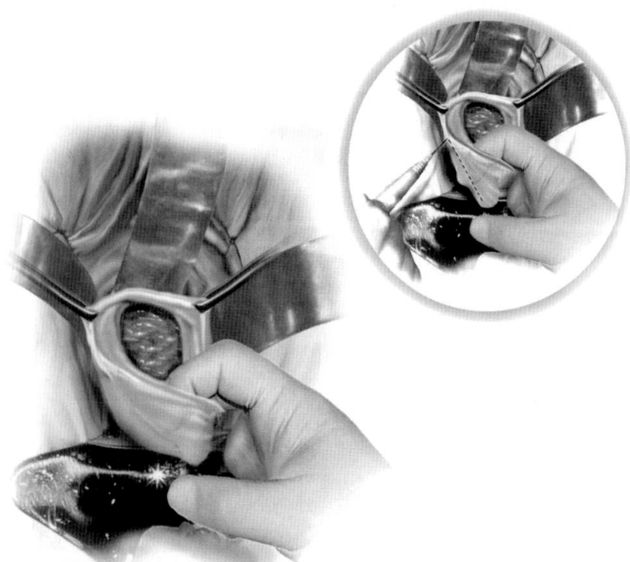

Figure 71-12 A finger in the posterior cul-de-sac can be used to confirm the presence of an enterocele. The redundant wedge of posterior vaginal wall and peritoneum can then be excised.

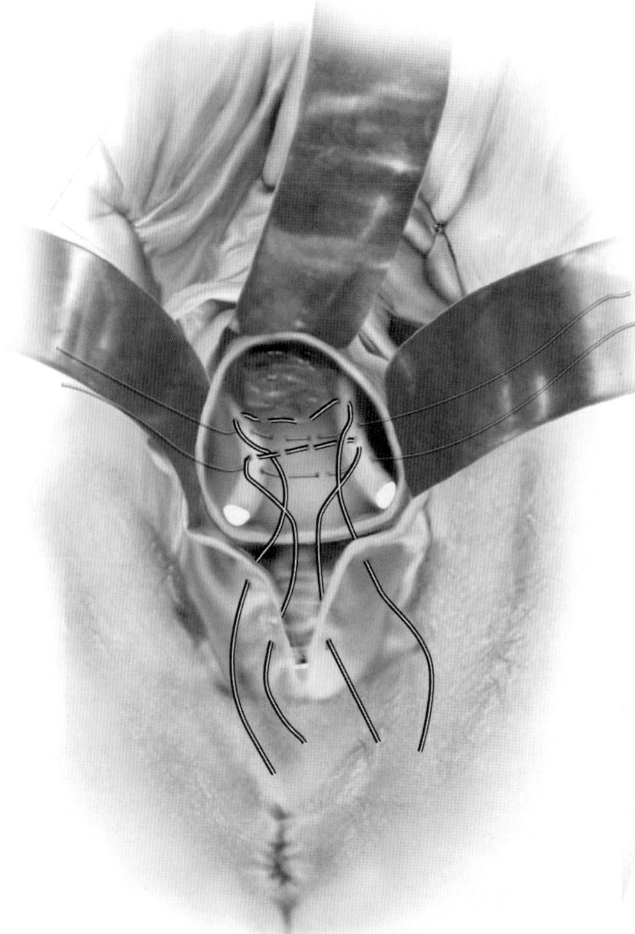

Figure 71-13 The technique of McCall culdoplasty. Two internal sutures (permanent) and two external sutures (absorbable) have been placed.

71-14). After tying the external McCall sutures, cystoscopy is performed to confirm ureteral patency.

Some patients have more advanced vaginal vault prolapse. In these cases, it may be appropriate to perform a more formal vaginal vault suspension, such as a sacrospinous fixation, high uterosacral ligament suspension, or iliococcygeus suspension.

To more adequately reestablish level I support, a high uterosacral ligament suspension can be performed. The bowel is packed away as previously described, and a Heaney retractor is used to lift the bowel out of the posterior cul-de-sac. Traction on the previously placed Allis clamps enables palpation of the remnants of the uterosacral ligaments. For the right-handed surgeon, the left index finger is used to deflect the sigmoid colon medially. As the assistant places traction on the patient's left uterosacral ligament, the surgeon places a figure-of-eight 1-0 absorbable suture through the left uterosacral ligament (lateral to medial) at the level of the ischial spine. With traction on the first suture, the surgeon then places a second figure-of-eight 1-0 absorbable suture through the left uterosacral ligament approximately 1 cm proximal to the first suture. This throw is higher and slightly more medial than the first suture because of the natural course of the uterosacral ligament. A similar procedure is performed on the opposite site, with careful attention to the location of the ureter. These four sutures are tagged and held. We prefer to use

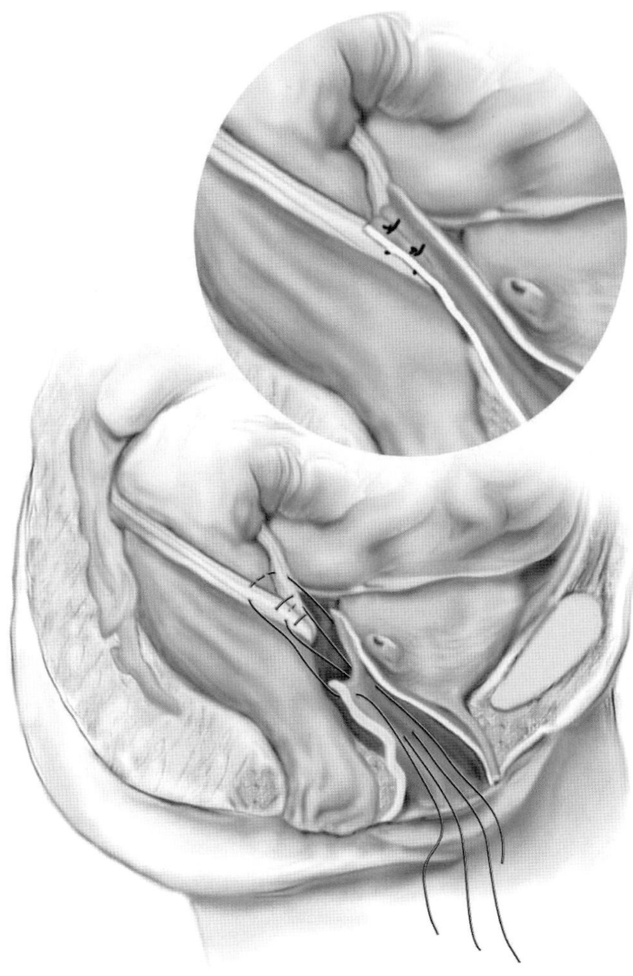

Figure 71-14 Cross section of the upper vagina before and after the McCall sutures have been tied down toward the hollow of the sacrum.

1-0 nonabsorbable sutures to obliterate the posterior cul-de-sac by plicating the distal portions of the uterosacral ligaments across the midline. The nonabsorbable sutures are then tied down, obliterating the posterior cul-de-sac. At this point, it is essential to confirm ureteral patency by cystoscopy after administration of intravenous indigo carmine.

In the absence of anterior or posterior vaginal wall prolapse, the high uterosacral ligament suspension sutures are passed out through the full-thickness vagina. The bowel packing is removed, and the vaginal cuff is closed using interrupted figure-of-eight 1-0 absorbable sutures in a transverse or longitudinal fashion. If an anterior repair is needed, the cuff is usually closed after the colporrhaphy. After hemostasis is confirmed, the vaginal mucosa is pushed toward the hollow of the sacrum, around the vault suspension sutures. The suspension sutures are then tied down. Examination should allow 2 fingerbreadths to be comfortably passed through the vaginal introitus toward the vaginal apex. The ultimate vaginal length should be a minimum of 8 cm.

THE DIFFICULT VAGINAL HYSTERECTOMY

Vaginal hysterectomy can be complicated in the face of pelvic floor relaxation or coexistent pelvic pathology.

Complete Uterine Procidentia

The technical aspects of vaginal hysterectomy in the patient with complete procidentia are the same as those for the simple vaginal hysterectomy. However, a careful preoperative evaluation must be performed to determine whether the prolapse represents a true procidentia or an elongated cervix. Severe descensus of the uterus in the case of procidentia results in anatomic distortion of the entire pelvis. The surgeon must remember that the course of the ureters is likely distorted in the wake of chronic traction associated with a large cystocele.

If it is determined preoperatively that the prolapse represents a severely elongated cervix with the uterus in a normal anatomic location, the surgeon must be careful not to amputate the cervix prematurely, because this will complicate the remainder of the procedure. Alternatively, the surgeon should take successive extraperitoneal bites until the anterior and posterior peritoneal reflections are reached (Fig. 71-15). After the anterior and posterior cul-de-sacs have been entered, the vaginal hysterectomy proceeds in a normal fashion.

Narrow Vaginal Introitus

A lack of uterine descensus or a narrow vaginal introitus, particularly in a nulliparous patient, are not contraindications to the vaginal route of hysterectomy. A thorough examination under anesthesia should be performed to determine the size and mobility of the uterus to assess the feasibility of a successful vaginal hysterectomy. A relaxing episiotomy may be necessary to afford the surgeon more room in the pelvis. If necessary, the surgeon may use a Schuchardt incision, which is made into the lateral vaginal wall and carried down to the perineal body. The Schuchardt incision resembles a sulcal tear after an operative vaginal delivery. These techniques alter the integrity of the perineal muscles and the levator muscles. The surgeon must ensure that normal anatomy has been restored after vaginal hysterectomy.

Obliterated Vesicouterine Fold

A history of multiple cesarean sections or endometriosis may complicate vaginal hysterectomy by obliterating the vesicouterine fold. As long as the bladder has been sufficiently dissected off of the cervix, anterior colpotomy is not mandatory. Alternatively, the surgeon may proceed with successive bites posteriorly until the fundus is palpated with a finger. Passing a finger around the fundus anteriorly may expose the anterior peritoneum, allowing the surgeon to safely enter the anterior cul-de-sac and effectively avoiding inadvertent cystotomy (Fig. 71-16). If the surgeon suspects an obliterated cul-de-sac based on patient history or exam under anesthesia, the dissection should proceed sharply, rather than bluntly. Blunt dissection follows the path of least resistance, tearing into the bladder.

Obliterated Cul-de-Sac of Douglas

A history of pelvic surgery, endometriosis, or pelvic inflammatory disease may result in an obliterated cul-de-sac of Douglas. This scenario predisposes to rectal injury or injury to the small bowel during attempted posterior colpotomy. If necessary, the anterior cul-de-sac should be entered first, and a finger wrapped should be around the fundus to palpate for adhesions or scarifi-

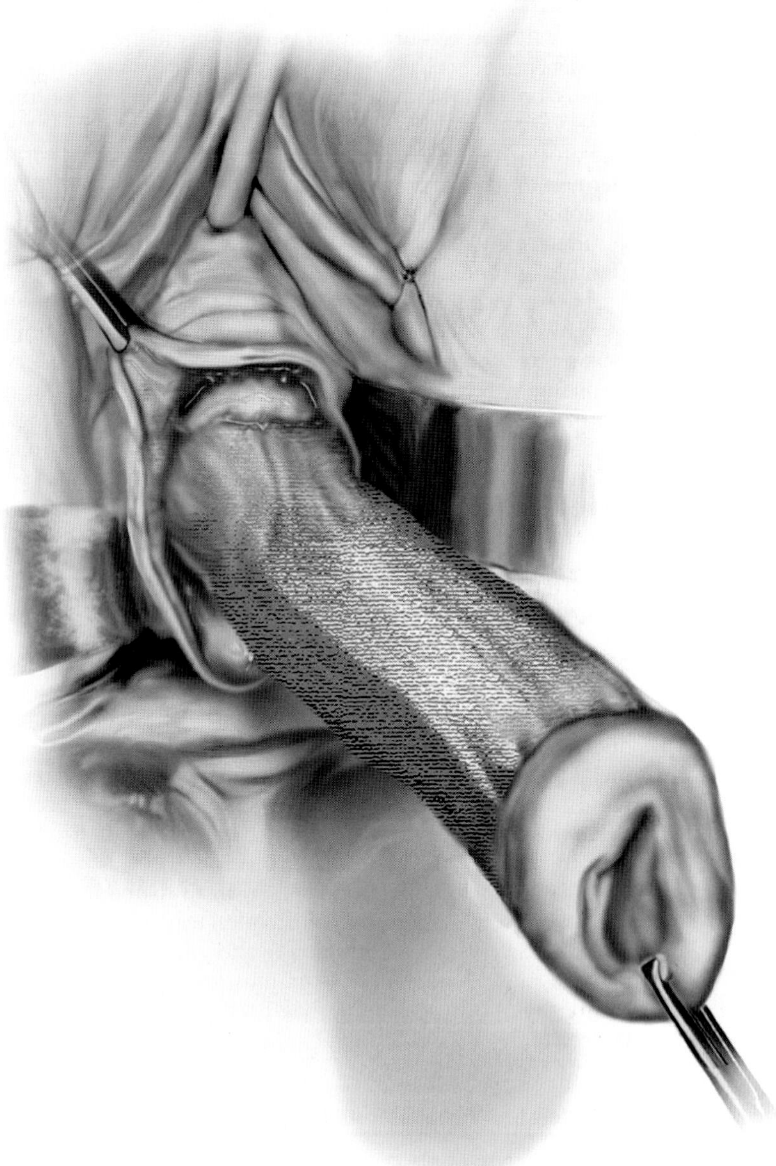

Figure 71-15 Technique of removal of an elongated cervix. Successive extraperitoneal bites are taken until the anterior and posterior peritoneal reflections are reached.

cation. In their absence, the posterior-cul-de-sac can then be entered safely without fear of rectal injury.

Massive Leiomyomatous Uterus

The uterus measuring less than 12 weeks' gestational size poses few problems for the vaginal route of hysterectomy, provided the surgical principles outlined earlier are followed. The uterus measuring more than 12 weeks' gestational size is not an absolute contraindication to the vaginal route of hysterectomy in the hands of a skilled surgeon. The large leiomyomatous uterus poses several difficulties to the surgeon.

The leiomyomatous uterus may be enlarged to the point that en bloc removal of the uterus by the vaginal route is impossible. In this situation, several techniques may be used to facilitate vaginal hysterectomy, including morcellation, bivalving of the uterus, or intramyometrial coring. Ligation of the major blood supply to the uterus, the uterine arteries, is a prerequisite for the use of these techniques. It is prudent to enter the anterior and posterior cul-de-sac to prevent injury to the bladder and rectum. After the uterine vessels have been secured, morcellation may begin. The cervix is amputated with a scalpel. Tenacula are used to grasp the posterior aspect of the uterus, which is brought down into the surgical field. A scalpel or Mayo scissors is then used to remove the tissue within the tenacula en bloc (Fig. 71-17). The entire body of the uterus is then morcellated.

After the fundus has been identified, the remainder of the uterus can be bivalved, securing the lateral pedicles as outlined earlier (Fig. 71-18). In patients with a massive uterus because of leiomyomas or adenomyosis, the fundus may not be deliverable posteriorly. In this case, intramyometrial coring is particularly appropriate (Fig. 71-19).

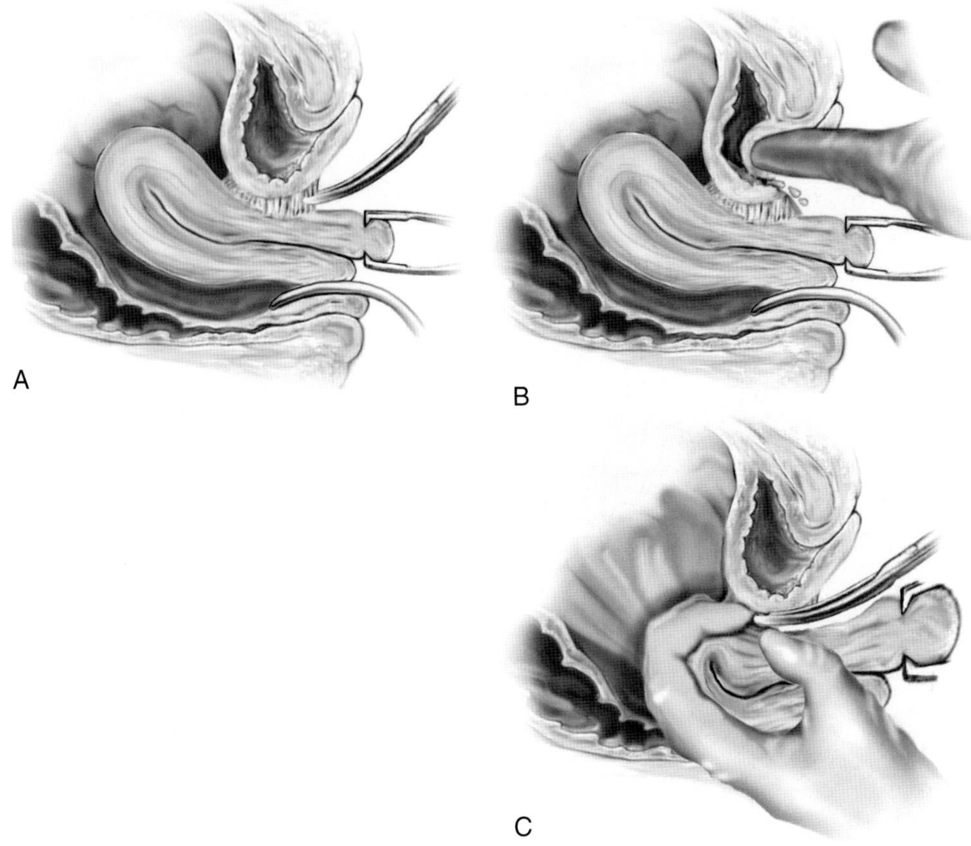

Figure 71-16 An obliterated vesicouterine fold. **A,** Adhesions are seen between the bladder and anterior cervix. **B,** Blunt dissection in this setting may lead to inadvertent cystotomy, because a finger will follow the path of the least resistance. **C,** Passing a finger around the fundus of the uterus often leads to identification of the appropriate plane of the dissection.

COMPLICATIONS OF VAGINAL HYSTERECTOMY

Complications of vaginal hysterectomy are uncommon but can include bleeding, infection, or inadvertent injury to the bladder, ureters, or bowel. Postoperative complications can include hematoma or abscess formation. Risk factors include previous abdominal surgery, a history of endometriosis or pelvic malignancy, cervical or broad ligament myomas, congenital anomalies, the presence of inflammation or pelvic adhesions, or a history of pelvic irradiation. Patient factors such as large uterine size or morbid obesity can reduce visualization. An inexperienced surgeon or inadequate retraction or lighting can add to the risks posed during the vaginal hysterectomy.

Inadvertent cystotomy remains one of the most common complications of vaginal hysterectomy. The incidence of inadvertent cystotomy during vaginal hysterectomy is reported to be between 1% and 1.8%. In 2002, Carley and colleagues[13] performed a retrospective review of 590 vaginal hysterectomies. The rate of inadvertent cystotomy was 1.9%. Cases were matched with five controls with similar procedures performed. Patients who suffered inadvertent cystotomy had a longer operative time and greater intraoperative blood loss than similarly matched controls.[13] As the rate of cesarean section continues to rise, concerns have surfaced regarding the risk of inadvertent cystotomy because of scarification in the lower uterine segment. Rooney and associates[14] performed a retrospective analysis of more than 5000 hysterectomies in 2004. They found an odds ratio of incidental cystotomy of 3.00, which approached statistical significance for women undergoing a total vaginal hysterectomy who had a history of prior cesarean section. The odds ratio for incidental cystotomy at the time of laparoscopically assisted vaginal hysterectomy in women with a history of prior cesarean section was found to be significant at a value of 7.50.[14]

One of the most serious complications of gynecologic surgery is iatrogenic injury to the ureters. The literature reports an incidence of iatrogenic ureteral injury of 0.02% to 0.8% during vaginal hysterectomy.[15] The ureters can be burned, clipped, ligated, kinked, or partially or completely transected. Intraoperative recognition is essential because of the subsequent risk of fistula formation or hydronephrosis resulting in loss of renal function. Most iatrogenic ureteral injuries occur when securing the uterine vessels. Particular care should be taken to keep the surgical clamps medial to the uterosacral ligament pedicles when performing the vaginal hysterectomy.

Iatrogenic injury to the ureter is the most common complication of the vaginal vault suspension, whether the surgeon has performed a traditional McCall culdoplasty or a high uterosacral ligament suspension. Karram and colleagues[16] reported a 2.4% risk of iatrogenic ureteral injury during 168 high uterosacral ligament suspensions. Barber and coworkers reported an 11% risk of ureteral injury during the same procedures.[16] Intraoperative cystoscopy with intravenous indigo carmine must be used to verify ureteral patency after the procedure. Webb and colleagues

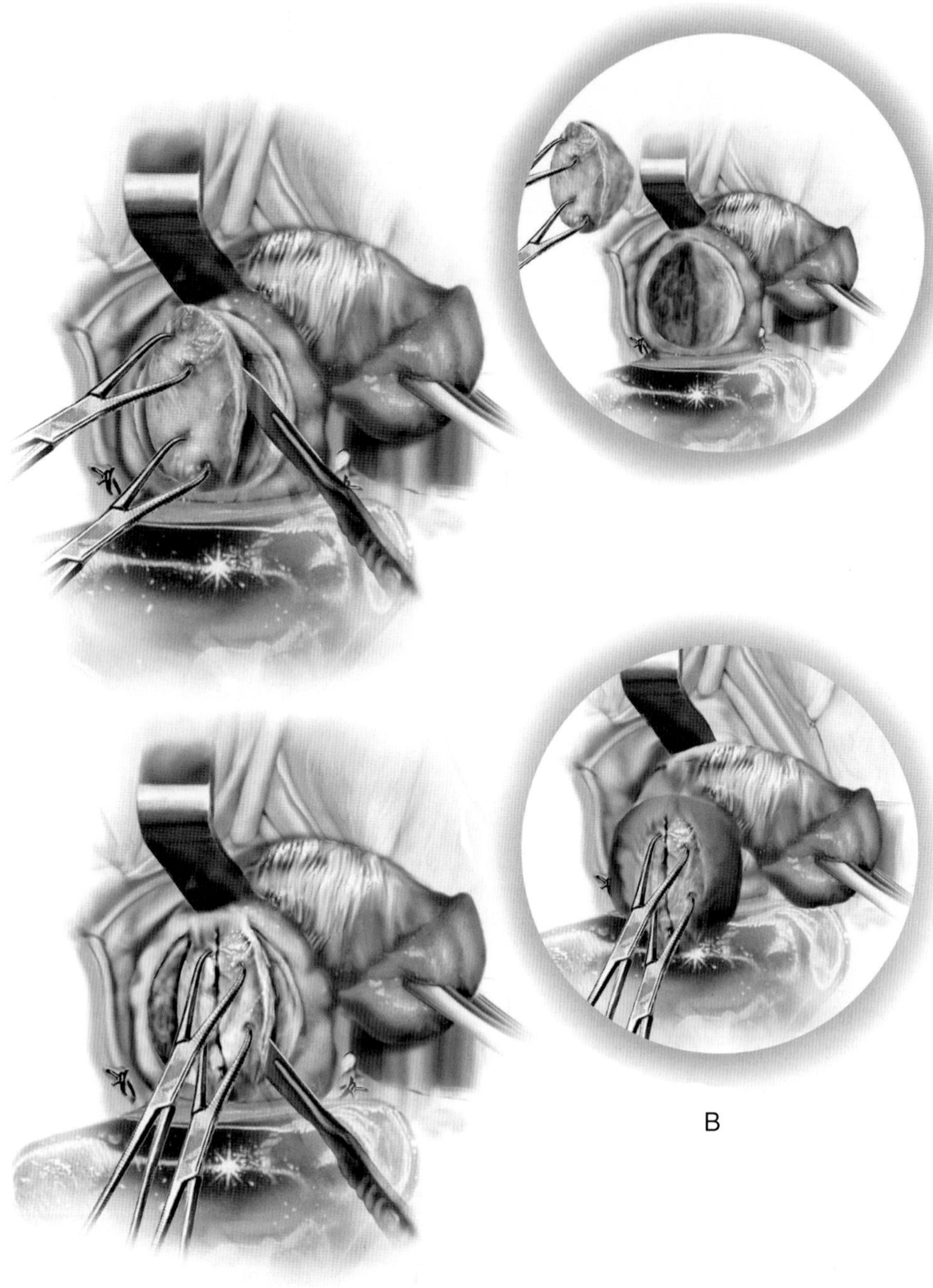

Figure 71-17 Technique of morcellation in the massively leiomyomatous uterus. **A,** An elliptical wedge of tissue is excised from the posterior uterus. **B,** The edges of the incision are brought together with the tenacula. A second wedge of tissue is removed in a similar fashion. The procedure is repeated until the fundus is reached and the uterus is delivered.

described 660 women who underwent a modified Mayo McCall culdoplasty in 1998.[16] In addition to ureteral injury, lacerations to the bowel and rectum were reported in 2.3% of cases. Other complications of the McCall culdoplasty include vault hematoma in 1.3% and cuff abscess or infection in 0.6% of patients. Webb reported a blood transfusion rate of 2.2%.[16]

Injuries to the rectum during vaginal hysterectomy are rare, with most occurring during attempted entry into the pouch of Douglas. Mathevat and colleagues[17] performed a retrospective review of more than 3000 vaginal hysterectomies with or without additional procedures. They reported five rectal injuries, all of which occurred during attempted entry to the posterior cul-de-sac.[17] Posterior colporrhaphy also poses a risk of rectal injury. In the same series, Mathevat and colleagues[17] reported 11 rectal injuries associated with posterior colporrhaphy. The overall incidence of rectal injury in their series was 0.45%.[17]

Hematoma formation is a rare complication of vaginal hysterectomy and is usually the result of inadequate hemostasis at the end of the procedure. Particular attention must be given to the pedicles in the post-hysterectomy patient to confirm hemostasis is adequate. After the vaginal hysterectomy with or without concomitant reconstructive procedures, we prefer to pack the

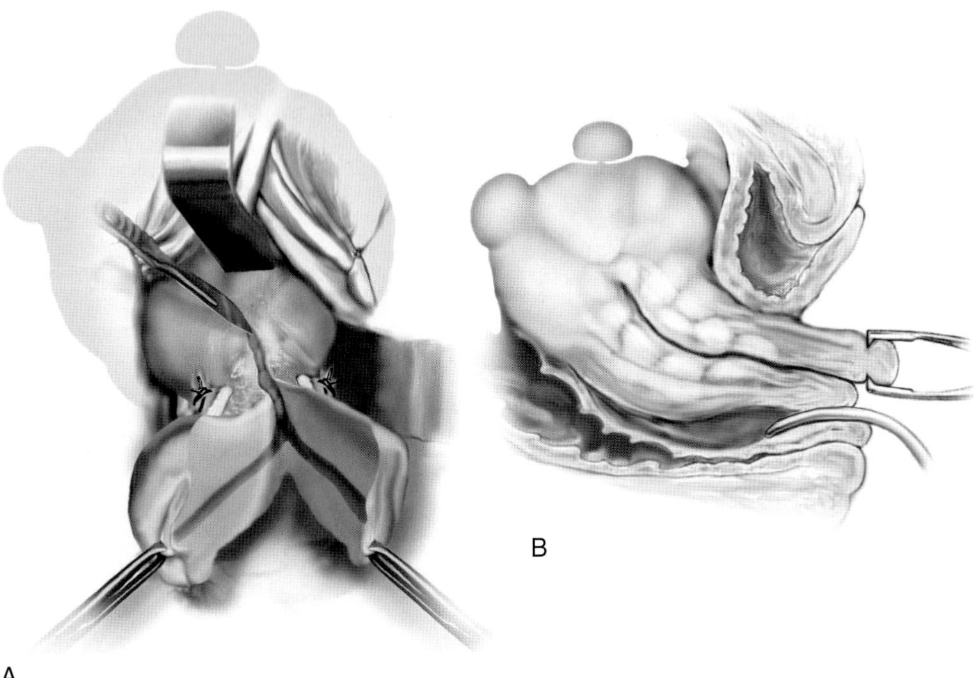

Figure 71-18 Technique of hemisection of the uterus. **A,** The midportion of the uterus. **B,** Lateral view demonstrates many uterine myomas.

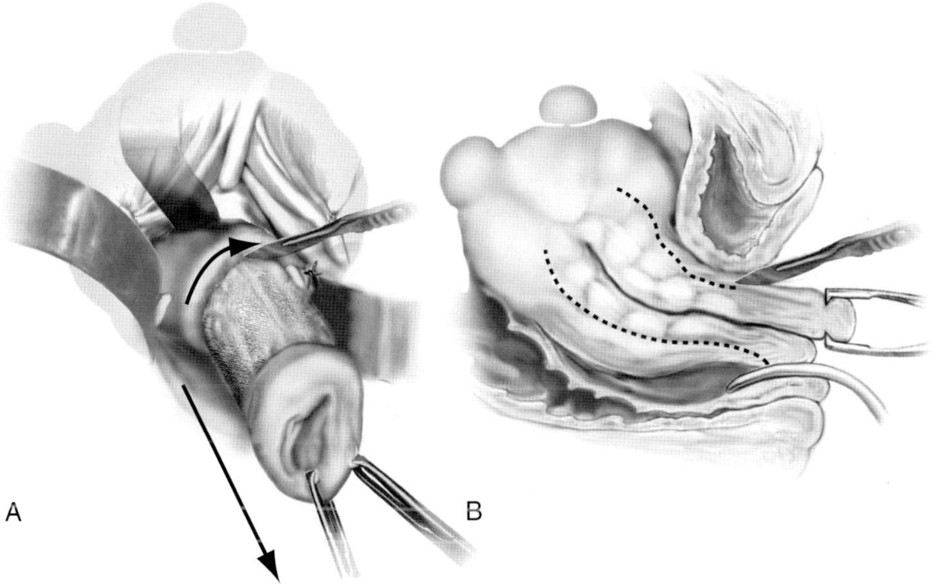

Figure 71-19 Technique of intramyometrial coring. **A,** A scalpel is used to create a cylinder of tissue. **B,** Lateral view of the technique of intramyometrial coring. Downward traction on the cervix will deliver the specimen, everting the uterine fundus.

vagina with 2-inch iodoform gauze to apply pressure to small amounts of venous oozing. The packing is removed the next morning, and hemostasis is confirmed.

CONCLUSIONS

As the population continues to increase, the gynecologist can expect a concurrent rise in the number of women presenting for hysterectomy. Currently, the rate of abdominal hysterectomy exceeds the rate of vaginal hysterectomy. Reducing the rate of abdominal hysterectomy could result in a reduction in hospital stay and postoperative recovery. With appropriate patient selection and in the hands of an experienced surgeon, vaginal hysterectomy represents a useful adjunct in the treatment of pelvic organ prolapse.

References

1. Keshavarz H, Hillis SD, Kieke BA, et al: Hysterectomy surveillance—United States 1994-1999. MMWR CDC Surveill Summ 51:1-8, 2002.
2. U.S. Census Bureau: U.S. Interim Projections by Age, Sex, Race, and Hispanic Origin. Available at http://www.census.gov/ipc/www/usinterimproj/ Accessed March 18, 2004.
3. Walters MD, Weber AM: Anatomy of the lower urinary tract, rectum and pelvic floor. In Walters MD, Karram MM (eds): Urogynecology and Reconstructive Pelvic Surgery, 2nd ed. St. Louis, Mosby, 1999, pp 3-13.
4. DeLancey JOL: Anatomic aspects of vaginal eversion after hysterectomy. Am J Obstet Gynecol 166:1717, 1992.
5. Shull BL, Bachofen CG: Enterocele and rectocele. In Walters MD, Karram MM (eds): Urogynecology and Reconstructive Pelvic Surgery, 2nd ed. St. Louis, Mosby, 1999, pp 221-234.
6. Silva WA, Kleeman SD, Segal J, et al: Effects of a full bladder and patient positioning on pelvic organ prolapse assessment. Obstet Gynecol 104:37-41, 2004.
7. Baden WF, Walker T, Lindsey JH: The vaginal profile. Tex Med 64:56, 1968.
8. Bump RC, Mattiasson A, Bo K, et al: The standardization of terminology of female pelvic organ prolapse and pelvic floor dysfunction. Am J Obstet Gynecol 175:10-17, 1996.
9. Friedman AJ, Haas ST: Reply to letter of Fruchter. Am J Obstet Gynecol 170:259, 1994.
10. Kovac SR: Guidelines to determine the route of hysterectomy. Obstet Gynecol 85:18-23, 1995.
11. Nichols DH, Randall CL: Vaginal hysterectomy. In Vaginal Surgery, 4th ed. Baltimore, Williams & Wilkins, 1996, pp 151-212.
12. Sheth SS: The place of oophorectomy at vaginal hysterectomy. Br J Obstet Gynecol 98:662-666, 1991.
13. Carley ME, McIntire D, Carley JM, et al: Incidence, risk factors and morbidity of unintended bladder or ureter injury during hysterectomy. Int Urogynecol J 13:18-21, 2002.
14. Rooney CM, Crawford AT, Kleeman SD, Karram MM: Is prior cesarean section a risk factor for incidental cystotomy at the time of hysterectomy? A case-controlled study. Am J Obstet Gynecol 193:2041-2044, 2005.
15. Visco AG, Taber KH, Weidner AC, et al: Cost-effectiveness of universal cystoscopy to identify ureteral injury at hysterectomy. Obstet Gynecol 97:685-692, 2001.
16. Karram MM, Kleeman SK: Vaginal vault prolapse. In Rock JA, Jones HW (eds): Te Linde's Operative Gynecology, 9th ed. Philadelphia, Lippincott Williams & Wilkins, 2003, pp 999-1025.
17. Mathevet P, Valencia P, Cousin C, et al: Operative injuries during vaginal hysterectomy. Eur J Obstet Gynecol Reprod Biol 97:71-75, 2001.

Chapter 72

LAPAROSCOPIC SACRAL COLPOPEXY

Marie Fidela R. Paraiso

Laparoscopic sacral colpopexy was first reported by Nezhat and colleagues in 1994.[1] Adoption of this procedure has increased in the past decade and has evolved to include robotic assistance. The possible advantages of laparoscopic surgery are improved visualization of anatomy of the peritoneal cavity because of laparoscopic magnification, insufflation effects, and improved hemostasis; shortened hospitalization resulting in potential cost reduction; decreased postoperative pain and more rapid recovery and return to work; and better cosmetic appearance of smaller incisions. Disadvantages of laparoscopic surgery include a steep learning curve in acquiring suturing skills, technical difficulty of presacral dissection, increased operating time early in the surgeon's experience, and possibly greater hospital cost because of increased operating room time and the use of disposable surgical instruments. These disadvantages, inadequate experience in advanced laparoscopy in residency and fellowship programs, surgeon preference for vaginal route surgery, and recently introduced minimally invasive apical suspension procedures have thwarted widespread adoption of laparoscopic surgery for pelvic organ prolapse.

The indications for laparoscopic vaginal apex prolapse and enterocele repair are identical to those for vaginal and abdominal routes. The choice of laparoscopic route is determined by the preferences of the surgeon and patient and by the laparoscopic skill of the surgeon. Additional factors that should be considered include history of pelvic or anti-incontinence surgery, previous failed transvaginal colpopexy, short vagina, severe abdominopelvic adhesions, the patient's age and weight, the need for concomitant pelvic surgery, and the patient's ability to undergo general anesthesia.

The technique of laparoscopic sacral colpopexy described in this chapter follows standard procedures for operative laparoscopy for access and is identical to the more proven open abdominal sacral colpopexy (see Chapter 73). Clinical outcome and complications are summarized.

ANATOMY

Thorough knowledge of the anatomy of the anterior abdominal wall is mandatory for safe and effective trocar insertion. The umbilicus is approximately at the L3-to-L4 level, and the aortic bifurcation is at the L4-to-L5 level. In obese women, the umbilicus is caudal to the bifurcation. The intraumbilical trocar should be introduced at a more acute angle toward the pelvis in thin women and closer to 90 degrees in obese women. The left common iliac vein courses over the lower lumbar vertebrae from the right side and may be inferior to the umbilicus. Common iliac arteries course 5 cm before bifurcating into the internal and external iliac arteries. The ureter crosses the common iliac artery at or above its bifurcation.

The superficial epigastric artery, a branch of the femoral artery, courses cephalad and can be transilluminated. The inferior epigastric artery branches from the external iliac artery at the medial border of the inguinal ligament and runs lateral to and below the rectus sheath at the level of the arcuate line. It is accompanied by two inferior epigastric veins.

When considering the anatomy of the repair of pelvic organ support, a surgeon must keep in mind the three levels of support of the vagina described by DeLancey in 1992.[2] The upper fourth of the vagina (level I) is suspended by the cardinal-uterosacral complex, the middle half (level II) is attached laterally to the arcus tendineus fasciae pelvis and the medial aspect of the levator ani muscles, and the lower fourth (level III) is fused to the perineal body. The endopelvic fascia laterally blends with the muscularis of the vagina. All pelvic support defects, whether anterior, apical, or posterior, represent a break in the continuity of the endopelvic fascia or vaginal muscularis and a loss of its suspension, attachment, or fusion to adjacent structures. The goals of pelvic reconstructive surgery are to correct all symptomatic defects, thereby reestablishing vaginal support at all three levels, and to maintain or restore normal visceral and sexual function.

The key anatomic landmarks of sacral colpopexy are the middle sacral artery and vein; the sacral promontory with anterior longitudinal ligament; the aortic bifurcation and the vena cava, which are at the level of L4 to L5; the right common iliac vessels and right ureter, which are at the right margin of the presacral space; and sigmoid colon, which is at the left margin. The left common iliac vein is medial to the left common iliac artery and can be damaged during dissection or retraction. The sacral foramina are only 1 to 1.5 cm from the midline, and the sympathetic chain is lateral. The ureter, which crosses over the common iliac artery bifurcation and courses along the pelvic sidewall, is approximately 1 to 1.5 cm lateral to the uterosacral ligament as it passes underneath the uterine artery.

The anatomic landmarks during laparoscopic sacral colpopexy graft attachment are the pubocervical fascia (i.e., anterior vaginal muscularis with overlying endopelvic fascia) and the rectovaginal muscularis (i.e., fibromuscular layer of the posterior vaginal wall above the rectovaginal septum). The rectovaginal septum is ideally the posterior point of attachment of the sacral colpopexy mesh, allowing continuity with the perineal body.

SURGICAL TECHNIQUE

Operative Laparoscopy for Pelvic Organ Prolapse: Setup, Instrumentation, and Trocar Placement

Ideal stirrups for combined laparovaginal cases are the Allen stirrups and Yellofins (Allen Medical Systems, Acton, MA), which have levers that can quickly convert the patient from low to high lithotomy position while preserving sterility of the field. A sterile pouch attached to each thigh is equipped with commonly used instruments such as unipolar scissors, bipolar cautery, blunt-tipped graspers, bowel graspers, and suction irrigation.

The monitor screens should be placed lateral to the legs in direct view of the surgeon standing on the opposite side of the table. The scrub nurse should be centered between the two monitor screens that are used; otherwise, the scrub nurse is located behind one surgeon and the electrosurgical unit or harmonic scalpel on the opposite side. After the three-way Foley catheter and uterine manipulator (if needed) have been placed, the vaginal tray with cystoscope can be set aside for later use.

For standard suturing technique, needle holder preference is determined by comfort of the surgeon. Conventional and 90-degree, self-righting German needle holders (Ethicon Endo-Surgery, Cincinnati, OH) have ratchet spring handles, and the Talon curved needle drivers with spring handles (Cook OB/GYN, Spencer, IN) self-right the needle at an angle of 45 or 90 degrees to the needle driver shaft, depending on the style chosen. The Storz Scarfi needle holder and notched assistant needle holder (Karl Storz Endoscopy, Culver City, CA) are most like conventional needle holders used during laparotomy. However, the handles are difficult to maintain and may pop open after extended use. The needle holder tips may become magnetized, which hampers needle grasping. Disposable suturing devices that have been introduced include the Endo-stitch (U.S. Surgical Corp., Norwalk, CT) and the Capio CL (Microvasive Boston Scientific, Natick, MA; CL refers to Cooper's ligament). Suturing devices are not recommended when performing laparoscopic sacral colpopexy because the depth of stitch placement in the vaginal muscularis is difficult to gauge tactically with these devices.

Extracorporeal knot tying is preferred because of technical facility and the ability to hold more tension on the suture, although some surgeons prefer intracorporeal suturing. When robotically assisted laparoscopic sacral colpopexy is performed, all suturing is done in an intracorporeal fashion. The choice of an open-ended or close-ended knot pusher for extracorporeal knot tying depends on surgeon preference. Our suture of choice is the single- or double-armed 1-0 Ethibond 36-inch suture on a CT-1 needle (Ethicon, Somerville, NJ). Our alternative choice for suture is 1-0 Gore-Tex (W.L. Gore and Associates, Phoenix, AZ). A 48-inch suture is preferred when suturing from ports at the level of the umbilicus. Sterile steel thimbles may be used by the surgeon or assistant when elevating the vagina while the surgeon is placing the stitches in the vaginal wall. However, vaginal manipulation when placing sutures is best achieved with endoanal anastomosis (EAA) sizers or fiberglass stents.

Intraumbilical or infraumbilical incisions depend on the anatomy of the umbilicus. Many variations of the accessory trocar sites have been described. For laparoscopic sacral colpopexy, we use three to four additional trocars: a 5- to 12-mm disposable trocar with reducer in the right and left lower quadrants lateral to the inferior epigastric vessels and a reusable 5-mm port or an additional 5- to 12-mm disposable trocar with reducer in the left upper quadrant at least 8 cm lateral to the umbilicus. Trocars are placed lateral to the rectus muscle, approximately 3 cm medial to and above the anterior superior iliac spine. Based on an anatomic study by Whiteside and coworkers[3] in 2003, we know that ilioinguinal and iliohypogastric nerve entrapment during fascial closure may be reduced if the ports are placed at least 2 cm cephalad to the anterior superior iliac spines. For more extensive reconstructive surgery, an additional 5-mm port may be placed on the principal surgeon's side so that he or she can operate with two hands. Reusable and disposable ports may be secured with circumferential screws to prevent port slippage. Versa Step Plus trocars (U.S. Surgical Corp.) allow easy introduction of needles, maintain pneumoperitoneum during extracorporeal knot tying, and prevent port slippage because of the expandable sleeve.

General Intraoperative and Postoperative Procedures

The patient is instructed to take one bottle of magnesium citrate or equivalent bowel preparation and limit her diet to clear liquids on the day before surgery. Placing an orogastric or nasogastric tube to decompress the stomach at the time of surgery is also helpful. Patients receive prophylactic intravenous antibiotic therapy 30 minutes before surgery. Pneumatic compression stockings are routinely used. The operations are performed under general anesthesia in the low lithotomy position. A 16-Fr, three-way Foley catheter with a 20- to 30-mL balloon is attached to continuous drainage, and the irrigation port is connected to sterile water or saline.

After all sutures are placed and tied, transurethral cystoscopy or suprapubic teloscopy is done to document ureteral patency and absence of sutures in the bladder. A suprapubic catheter is placed, if desired. The surgeon must again inspect the pelvis for bleeding while reducing the carbon dioxide insufflation. Routine closure of the peritoneum is performed based on the surgeon's preference. All ports are removed under direct visualization, and the peritoneum and fascia of all 5- to 12-mm incisions are reapproximated with the fascial closure instrument (Karl Storz, Tuttingen, Germany) or the Grice needle (New Ideas in Medicine, Clearwater, FL). The skin is closed in a subcuticular fashion. The fascia and subcutaneous fat can be infiltrated with a long-acting local anesthetic, such as 0.5% bupivacaine hydrochloride.

Postoperative care consists of oral pain medication (intravenous, if needed), rapid diet advancement, and ambulation. If an anti-incontinence procedure is concomitantly performed, voiding trials begin as soon as the patient is ambulatory. Intermittent self-catheterization protocols can begin immediately, especially if the patient was taught the technique preoperatively. Some patients are able to go home on the same day if adequately counseled preoperatively. Preoperative teaching includes discussion of postoperative analgesics, the need for a caretaker at home during the immediate recovery period, instruction in catheter care or intermittent self-catheterization, and explanation of goals to be reached before outpatient discharge. Patients are instructed to refrain from sexual intercourse and lifting objects heavier than 10 pounds for at least 8 weeks. They are cautioned to heed to these instructions despite rapid recovery.

Technique of Laparoscopic Sacral Colpopexy

Vaginal obturators, spongesticks, or equivalent vaginal manipulators (EEA Sizer, U.S. Surgical Corp.; CDH, Ethicon Endo-Surgery) are used for delineation of the vaginal apex and rectum. After all ancillary ports are placed, the presacral space is dissected (Fig. 72-1). If exposure of the sacral promontory and presacral space is not adequate, the patient should be tilted to her left and a reusable snake retractor (Snowden Pencer, Tucker, GA) or fan retractor (Origin Medsystems, Menlo Park, CA) placed through

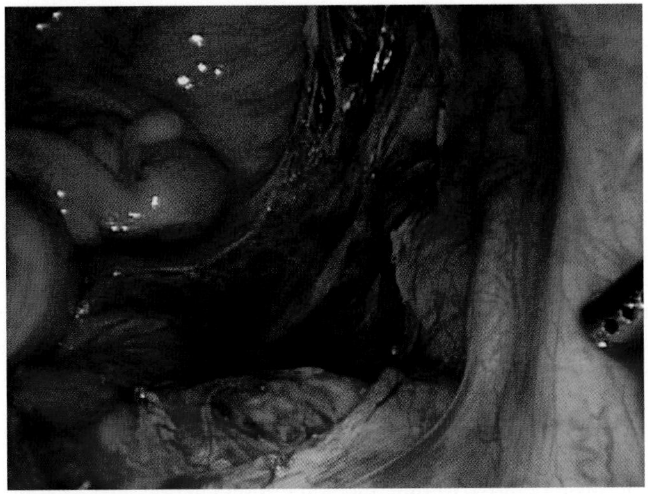

Figure 72-1 Dissection of the presacral space.

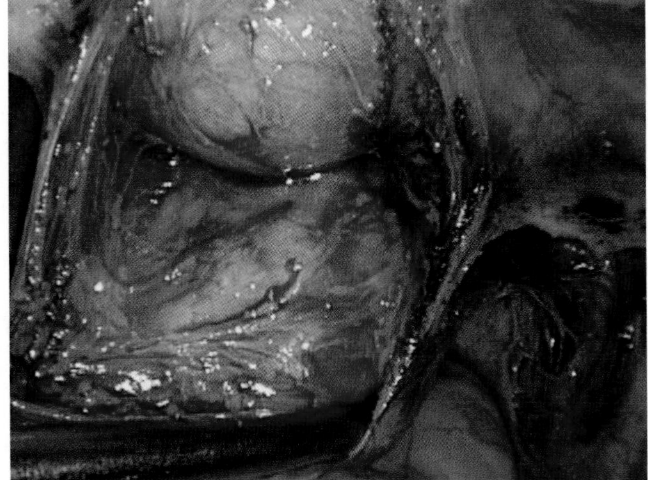

Figure 72-2 Dissection of the rectovaginal space.

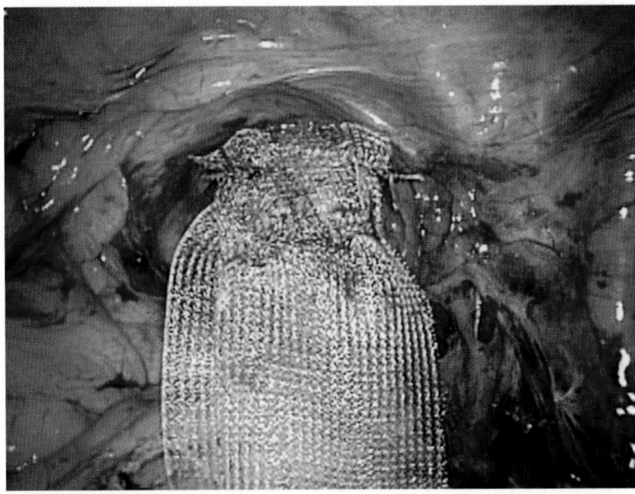

Figure 72-3 Anterior attachment of polypropylene mesh to the muscularis of the vaginal apex.

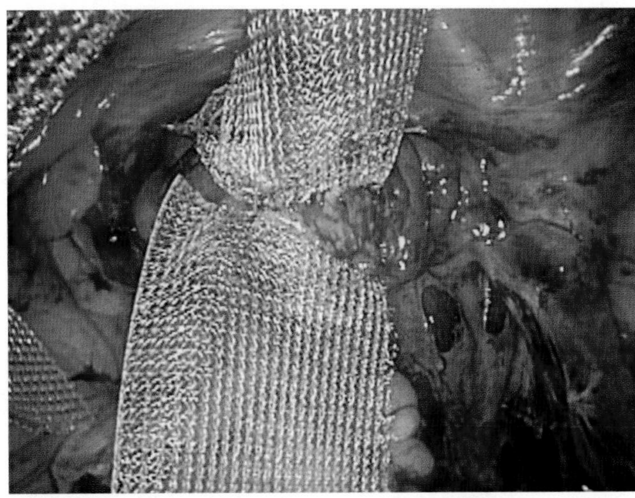

Figure 72-4 Fixation of two separate polypropylene meshes during sacral colpopexy.

an ancillary port. A suture may be placed through the sigmoid epiploicae and placed on traction outside of the abdomen lateral to the left lower quadrant port to keep the sigmoid colon retracted throughout the surgery, thereby freeing an operative port. The peritoneum overlying the sacral promontory is incised longitudinally with laparoscopic scissors or harmonic scalpel (Gynecare, Somerville, NJ) and extended to the cul-de-sac. A laparoscopic dissector or hydrodissection is used to expose the periosteum of the sacral promontory. If blood vessels are encountered during the dissection, coagulation or clip placement is used to achieve hemostasis. Some surgeons prefer to dissect the presacral space first, eliminating the most technically difficult portion of the procedure. A Halban procedure or Moschcowitz culdoplasty may be performed based on the surgeon's preference or when a deep cul-de-sac is encountered. When a concomitant culdoplasty is performed, it is completed after posterior mesh placement.

To dissect the rectovaginal septum, the peritoneum between the vaginal apex and rectum is placed on countertraction by manipulating the EAA sizers, pointing the vagina toward the pubic bone and the rectum toward the sacrum (Fig. 72-2). Anterior dissection is performed after the bladder is filled with 300 ml of sterile water. Dissection is extended to the bladder base. This dissection can be very difficult if a patient has undergone a previous anterior colporrhaphy or vaginal suspension procedure.

Our technique incorporates two pieces of 15 × 4 cm polypropylene mesh or biologic tissue. We sew the posterior mesh on first. The most caudal stitch is placed on the posterior vaginal wall and rectovaginal fascia. After placement of the first stitch, the mesh is threaded through the stitch before introducing the mesh into the peritoneal cavity. The corresponding contralateral stitch is taken and threaded through the mesh to anchor the inferior border of the mesh to the rectovaginal septum or perineum (a 15- to 18-cm mesh length may be required for laparoscopic sacral colpoperineopexy). The sutures are tied extracorporeally as they are placed. Care is taken to place the stitches through the entire thickness of the vaginal wall, excluding the epithelium. The mesh is sutured to the posterior vaginal apex and rectovaginal septum with three to four similar rows of suture and to the vaginal apex anteriorly with two to three pairs of No. 0 nonabsorbable sutures (Figs. 72-3 and 72-4). The surgeon sutures the mesh to the longitudinal ligament of the sacrum with two

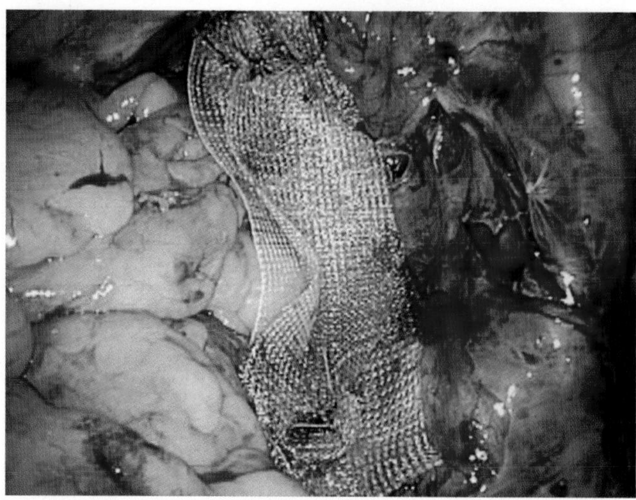

Figure 72-5 Attachment of the mesh to the anterior longitudinal ligament of the sacrum without tension.

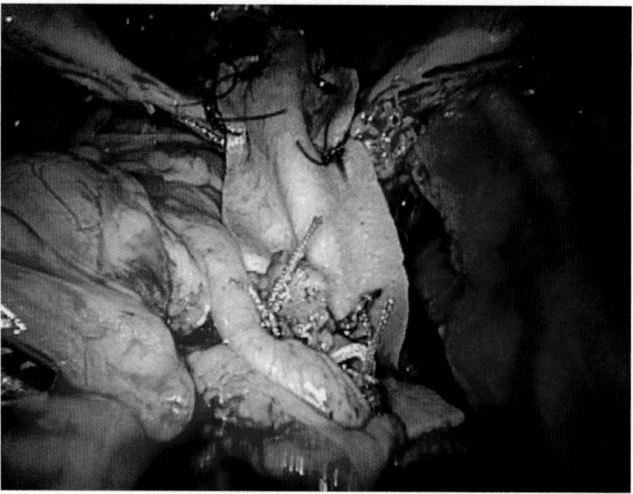

Figure 72-6 Biologic mesh implantation in sacral colpopexy.

No. 0 nonabsorbable sutures (Fig. 72-5). No undue tension is placed on the mesh. Titanium tacks or hernia staples may also be used to attach the mesh to the anterior longitudinal ligament of the sacrum. The redundant portion of the mesh is excised. Biologic tissue may also be used, especially when concomitant bowel resection is performed (Fig. 72-6). The peritoneum is reapproximated over the mesh with 2-0 polyglactin suture. If the mesh remains exposed, sigmoid epiploic fat may be sutured over it.

CLINICAL RESULTS AND COMPLICATIONS

The current gynecologic literature for laparoscopic sacral colpopexy is sparse and consists of case series from surgeons subspecializing in advanced laparoscopy and urogynecologic surgery. Comparative, adequately powered studies of laparoscopic surgery for vaginal apex prolapse do not exist.

In 1994, Nezhat and colleagues[1] reported a series of 15 patients who underwent laparoscopic sacral colpopexy for whom the mean operative time was 170 minutes (range, 105 to 320 minutes) and the mean blood loss was 226 mL (range, 50 to 800 mL). The mean hospital stay was 2.3 days, excluding a case converted to laparotomy because of presacral hemorrhage. The cure rate for apical prolapse was 100% at 3 to 40 months. In 1995, Lyons and Winer[4] reported 4 laparoscopic sacrospinous fixations and 10 laparoscopic sacral colpopexies with operative times comparable to those for vaginal and abdominal approaches. He reported less intraoperative and postoperative morbidity with the laparoscopic route; this was attributed to a superior anatomic approach and visualization of anatomic structures. Nezhat and associates[1] and Lyons and Winer[4] used mesh and suture, and they sometimes stapled the mesh into the longitudinal ligament of the anterior sacrum.

In 1997, Ross[5] evaluated 19 patients with post-hysterectomy vaginal apex prolapse prospectively with extensive preoperative and postoperative testing, including multichannel urodynamics and transperineal ultrasound. All patients underwent sacral colpopexy, Burch colposuspension, and modified culdoplasty. Paravaginal defect repair and posterior colporrhaphy were added as indicated. Ross reported seven complications: three cystotomies, two urinary tract infections, one seroma, and one inferior epigastric vessel laceration. Five patients had recurrent defects that were all less than grade 2 (two paravaginal defects and three rectoceles). Vaginal length ranged from 10.8 to 12.1 cm, and all sexually active patients reported no sexual dysfunction. All but four patients voided spontaneously, and none required more than 4 days of catheterization. All were discharged within 24 hours. The cure rate at 1 year was 100% for vaginal apex prolapse and 93% for stress incontinence, although two patients were lost to follow-up. In another study reported in 2004, Ross[6] prospectively analyzed 51 cases of laparoscopic sacral colpopexy for grade III or IV apical vaginal vault prolapse. Forty-three patients demonstrated an objective cure rate of 93% at the vaginal apex during their 5-year follow-up visit. Complications included one partial small-bowel obstruction resulting from bowel adherence to the mesh and two locally treated mesh erosions. Ross concluded that patient recovery was greatly enhanced, with most patients requiring only overnight hospitalization.

The largest series of laparoscopic sacral colpopexies is a retrospective cohort of 83 patients published by Cosson and associates[7] in the French literature. The investigators performed concomitant laparoscopic supracervical hysterectomy in 60 patients and converted six cases to laparotomy. Operative time decreased from 292 to 180 minutes with increased experience. One patient required reoperation for prolapse, and two patients underwent procedures for stress incontinence. The median length of follow-up was 343 days. In 2004, Gadonneix and coworkers[7] reported the use of two separate meshes for laparoscopic sacral colpopexy with or without Burch colposuspension in 46 consecutive patients with primary vaginal apex prolapse with or without primary stress incontinence. Mean operating time was 171 minutes, and mean hospital stay was 4 days. Median follow-up was 24 months (range, 12 to 60 months). Eleven percent of patients required conversion to laparotomy. Complications included de novo urge incontinence in 5% of patients, laparoscopically treated bladder injury in 7%, and recurrent rectoceles in 12% (occurring only in women who had undergone laparoscopic Burch colposuspension compared with no colposuspension, $P = .036$). One patient developed obstructed defecation, which the study authors attributed to excessive mesh tension.

At the Cleveland Clinic Foundation, we compared our first 56 consecutive laparoscopic sacral colpopexies with 61 consecutive open sacral colpopexies performed during the same period.[9] Mean follow-up was 14 and 16 months for the laparoscopic and open groups, respectively. Laparoscopic sacral colpopexy and concomitant procedures required a significantly longer operating room time compared with open sacral colpopexy, with mean operating room times of 269 and 218 minutes, respectively. However, mean hospital stay was significantly longer for the open group than the laparoscopic group (4 versus 1.8 days). We found similar clinical outcomes and reoperation rate. Our sample size was too small to determine differences in complications.

CONCLUSIONS

Laparoscopy is a means of achieving less invasive surgical access, and its use is expanding rapidly in all surgical specialties. The technique for laparoscopic sacral colpopexies should be as close as possible to the operative technique for open sacral colpopexy. Bladder injury is probably more common with laparoscopy, but the risk of cystotomy decreases with surgical experience. Complications associated with laparotomies, such as wound infection and hernias, are rare with the laparoscopic route.

The benefits of improved visualization of anatomic structures and the small incisions associated with the laparoscopic approach are desirable, particularly in obese patients. The advantages of less postoperative pain, shorter hospitalization, a shortened recovery period, and earlier return to work are very popular with patients, but these advantages are partially offset by increased operating time and possibly by increased cost. The operating time and cost will likely decrease as surgeons gain experience with the advanced laparoscopic techniques of suturing and knot tying. Laparoscopic approaches for pelvic organ prolapse may be somewhat underused because of the greater technical difficulty associated with surgical dissection and laparoscopic suturing. The emergence of vaginal mesh kit procedures and tunneling techniques may thwart widespread adoption of laparoscopic sacral colpopexy. However, the greatest potential for laparoscopic advances and innovations may be in operations for prolapse. We believe that laparoscopic sacral colpopexy will gain popularity because abdominal sacral colpopexy remains the most proven and effective surgery for cure of severe apical prolapse. Pelvic floor surgeons in specialized centers strive to offer their patients pelvic reconstruction by laparoscopic route, many employing robotic assistance. More comparative studies and prospective clinical trials with long-term follow-up are warranted.

References

1. Nezhat CH, Nezhat F, Nezhat C: Laparoscopic sacral colpopexy for vaginal vault prolapse. Obstet Gynecol 84:885, 1994.
2. DeLancey JO: Anatomic aspects of vaginal eversion after hysterectomy. Am J Obstet Gynecol 166:1717, 1992.
3. Whiteside JL, Barber MD, Walters MD, et al: Anatomy of ilioinguinal and iliohypogastric nerves in relation to trocar placement and low transverse incisions. Am J Obstet Gynecol 189:1574, 2003.
4. Lyons TL, Winer WK: Vaginal vault suspension. Endosc Surg 3:88, 1995.
5. Ross JW: Techniques of laparoscopic repair of total vault eversion after hysterectomy. J Am Assoc Gynecol Laparosc 4:173, 1997.
6. Ross JW: The role of laparoscopy in the treatment of severe vaginal vault prolapse: 6 to 10 year outcome [abstract]. J Am Assoc Gynecol Laparosc 11:S4, 2004.
7. Cosson M, Bogaert E, Narducci F, et al: Laparoscopic sacral colpopexy: Short-term results and complications in 83 patients. J Gynecol Obstet Biol Reprod (Paris) 29:746-750, 2000.
8. Gadonneix P, Ercoli A, Salet-Lizee D, et al: Laparoscopic sacrocolpopexy with two separate meshes along the anterior and posterior vaginal walls for multicompartment pelvic organ prolapse. J Am Assoc Gynecol Laparosc 11:29, 2004.
9. Paraiso MF, Walters MD, Rackley RR, et al: Laparoscopic and abdominal sacral colpopexies: A cohort study. Am J Obstet Gynecol 192:1752, 2005.

Chapter 73

OPEN ABDOMINAL SACRAL COLPOPEXY

Chi Chiung Grace Chen and Marie Fidela R. Paraiso

Pelvic organ prolapse is a condition that physicians are likely to encounter as women are living longer and more emphasis is placed on maintaining their physique and capacity for sexual activity. It has been estimated that more than 300,000 surgeries are being performed annually to correct pelvic organ prolapse at a cost of greater than $1 billion dollars.[1] The number of women seeking attention for these disorders is projected to increase by 45% in the future.[2]

Management of pelvic organ prolapse depends on the goals and expectations of the patient and on the patient's comorbidities. For example, women who have minimal symptoms or those with prolapse that does not extend beyond the hymen may benefit from pelvic floor exercises and behavioral modifications. Patients who have many comorbidities and are poor surgical candidates may benefit from vaginal pessaries. Women who do not desire preservation of sexual capacity may benefit from a less morbid obliterative procedure, such as colpocleisis. When contemplating the surgical correction of pelvic organ prolapse, the surgeon must also consider the existence of other support defects and any dysfunction of bladder or bowel. The surgeon must decide whether to approach these repairs abdominally, vaginally, or laparoscopically. In this chapter, we will focus on abdominal sacral colpopexy or suspension of the vagina to the sacral promontory, which is considered the gold standard procedure for correcting pelvic organ prolapse.

Abdominal sacral colpopexy should be considered if the patient has severe vaginal apical prolapse and requires concomitant pelvic or anti-incontinence surgery by the abdominal route. Other indications include previous failed transvaginal colpopexy, foreshortened vagina, weakened pelvic floor, and chronic increases in abdominal pressure as a result of medical comorbidities (e.g., chronic obstructive pulmonary disease, chronic constipation) or occupation (e.g., heavy manual labor). Some pelvic surgeons also prefer abdominal sacral colpopexy for young patients with severe apical prolapse.

"GENERAL INTRAOPERATIVE PRODURES" TO "ANATOMY AND GENERAL INTRAOPERATIVE PRODURES"

As the relevant abdominal and pelvic anatomic landmarks for open sacral colpopexy are the same as for laparoscopic sacral colpopexy, please refer to Chapter 72. Furthermore, some general intraoperative considerations are also the same and include placement of the patients in low lithotomy position under general anesthesia, prophylactic intravenous antibiotics before initiation of surgery, pneumatic compression stockings on the patients' lower extremities, and placement of a 16-Fr three-way Foley catheter to continuous drainage with the irrigation port attached to sterile water or saline to facilitate retrograde filling of the bladder to assist in dissection of the bladder off the vaginal apex during surgery.

SURGICAL TECHNIQUE

General Intraoperative Procedures

Specifically, the ideal stirrups for combined abdominovaginal cases are the Allen stirrups and Yellofins (Allen Medical Systems, Acton, MA), which have levers that can quickly convert the patient from low to high lithotomy position while preserving sterility of the field. A transverse or vertical laparotomy incision is made based on surgeon preference or concomitant procedures. For obese patients, a Maylard incision may be useful for improved exposure compared with a Pfannenstiel incision.

The patient is placed in a Trendelenburg position. The small bowel is packed upward, and the sigmoid colon is packed to the left paracolic gutter. The Bookwalter retractor or Balfour retractor is placed to hold the sides of the incision open, giving exposure to the operative field. The Bookwalter retractor is ideal for obese patients. Sterile towels are placed below the lateral points of the Balfour retractor to decrease compression of the psoas muscle, safeguarding against femoral neuropathy.

The sacral promontory is palpated, and the respective landmarks of the presacral space are delineated. The presacral peritoneum is tented and incised down to the level of the posterior cul-de-sac. The peritoneum may be retracted laterally by placing tagged 2-0 absorbable sutures, which can be tied together after the procedure is complete for closure of the peritoneum. Alternatively, a tunnel can be made in the right pararectal peritoneum from sacral promontory to the posterior cul-de-sac rather than completely incising the peritoneum. Kittners (i.e., endoscopic, blunt dissectors with radiopaque tips) are used to clear away the areolar tissue of the sacral promontory, delineating the anterior longitudinal ligament of the sacrum and the middle sacral vessels. Care must be taken to avoid trauma to the presacral vessels because these vessels retract easily, and life-threatening hemorrhage may ensue. If bleeding does occur, pressure, hemostatic clips, cautery, fibrin glue, and Gelfoam may be applied. If these measures are not successful, bone wax and sterile thumbtacks should be used. The presacral nerve should be preserved to decrease the risk of temporary postoperative urinary retention and constipation.

Manipulators are placed in the vagina and rectum for delineation. For example, fiberglass obturators or endoanal anastomosis (EAA) sizers may be placed in the vagina and rectum for traction in opposite directions to delineate the rectovaginal space. The peritoneum is incised, rectovaginal space entered, and blunt dissection performed along the length of the posterior vaginal wall. In cases of abdominal sacral colpoperineopexy, this dissection is extended to the perineum. The bladder is filled with 300 mL in a retrograde fashion with a three-way Foley catheter hooked to irrigation to delineate the superior border of the bladder. The bladder peritoneum is incised, and the bladder is sharply dissected downward to the bladder base off the vagina. Palpation of the Foley catheter bulb aids in this dissection. Care should be taken not to cauterize the bladder and vagina to a great extent. Peritoneum should be preserved at the vaginal apex if possible to decrease risk of mesh erosion.

After dissection of the bladder and preparation of the rectovaginal space, several rows of 1-0 nonabsorbable suture are stitched into the posterior vaginal muscularis. The most distally placed sutures are at the perineum during colpoperineopexy. The stitches should be placed at least halfway down the length of the posterior vagina for a sacral colpopexy. It is preferable to avoid through-and-through stitches into the vaginal epithelium. Each row of sutures should be placed 2 cm apart. The sutures are tagged, and after all sutures are placed, the ends of the suture are brought through the pores of a 4 × 15 cm polypropylene mesh. Polypropylene suture is easy to work with in this setting; when cut, it is easily passed through the pores. A longer piece of polypropylene mesh is required for the sacral colpoperineopexy. The sutures are then tied without strangulating the tissue to decrease erosion. If a Halban or Moschcowitz procedure is performed to obliterate the pouch of Douglas, these sutures can be placed before or after posterior mesh placement, but they should not be tied until the posterior mesh is placed. A 2-0 nonabsorbable suture is adequate for the culdoplasty procedures.

Approximately two or three rows of 1-0 nonabsorbable suture are placed on the anterior vaginal wall. The ends of the sutures are then brought through the pores of a second 4 × 15 cm piece of polypropylene mesh and tied. The vaginal manipulator is used to place the vagina under no tension in the right pararectal space. The securing point of the mesh to the anterior longitudinal ligament at the S1 or S2 level is then marked. Two or three polypropylene sutures are placed transversely into the anterior longitudinal ligament. The suture ends are then brought through the pores of both leafs of mesh so that each leaf can be secured without tension.

After the mesh is tied down and hemostasis ensured, the peritoneum is reapproximated over the mesh with a 3-0 absorbable suture. This is an important step to decrease risk of small-bowel obstruction below the mesh and mesh adhesion to viscera. Care must be taken not to kink the right ureter or the rectosigmoid. Sigmoid epiploica and bladder peritoneum may be used to cover the mesh. After all sutures are placed and tied, transurethral cystoscopy or suprapubic teloscopy is done to document ureteral patency and absence of sutures in the bladder. The incision is closed in the customary fashion after concomitant abdominal procedures are performed. Vaginal route procedures, if necessary, are completed after the abdominal procedures are performed (see Chapter 72 for photographs of the procedure).

Postoperative care consists of intravenous analgesia for the first 12 to 24 hours after surgery. Oral pain medication, diet advancement, and ambulation are the rule on the first postoperative day. If an anti-incontinence procedure is concomitantly performed, voiding trials begin as soon as the patient is ambulatory. Preoperative teaching includes a discussion about postoperative analgesics, the need for a caretaker at home during the immediate recovery period, instruction in catheter care or intermittent self-catheterization, and the goals to be reached before discharge. Patients are able to go home on postoperative day 2 or 3. Patients are instructed to refrain from sexual intercourse and lifting objects heavier than 10 pounds for at least 8 weeks.

Clinical Results

The effectiveness of abdominal sacral colpopexy to correct pelvic organ prolapse can be examined from two perspectives: patient satisfaction or resolution of symptoms and restoration of normal anatomy (Table 73-1). The rate of patient satisfaction or resolution of symptoms in different studies range from 85% to 100%. Unfortunately, many of these studies do not include a description of the outcome tools used to assess satisfaction. In one study, a visual analogue score using a 10-point scale was used to determine that the overall patient satisfaction rate was 85% with a follow-up interval of 3 years.[3] In another study with patient follow-up assessments ranging from 1 to 13 years (median, 4 years), 29% of patients experienced "no improvement," 39% experienced "considerable improvement," and 32% felt that they were "fully cured."[4]

To examine anatomic success, common measures of vaginal support include the Baden-Walker grading scale and the Pelvic Organ Prolapse Quantification (POP-Q) system (see Chapter 54).[5,6] In a review article by the Pelvic Floor Disorders Network, abdominal sacral colpopexy resulted in the cure of vaginal apex prolapse in 78% to 100% and the cure of prolapse in all vaginal segments in 58% to 100%, with follow-up ranging from 6 months to 3 years.[7]

The success rate of sacral colpopexy drops when it is defined as the absence of all vaginal prolapse regardless of apical, anterior, or posterior location. It is therefore important when looking at outcomes to consider recurrent or de novo anterior and posterior vaginal wall prolapse. For example, one study found that only 7% of patients after surgery experienced recurrent apical prolapse, whereas 30% developed new enterorectoceles.[8] The investigators thought that this discrepancy reflected the inconsistent use of culdoplasty and consequently recommended that this procedure be routinely performed with all sacral colpopexies. Brubaker[9] reported that 29% (19 of 65) of patients with a follow-up of 3 months had new or persistent anterior prolapse despite having undergone sacral colpopexy with a posterior graft attachment and a separate anterior compartment repair. However, only two patients were symptomatic. Sacral colpopexy is an effective method to correct apical prolapse, but its effects on other compartment defects and the optimal management of those defects remain unclear.

The need for reoperation to correct persistent, recurrent, or de novo pelvic organ prolapse may depend on factors other than surgical techniques. These factors include vaginal tissue quality, coexisting defects, and medical conditions such as chronic obstructive pulmonary disease. In one large data series, it was found that one of three patients who underwent a procedure for urinary incontinence or prolapse had to undergo reoperation within 4 years.[10] The Pelvic Floor Disorders Network reported the median reoperation rate to be 4.4%, with follow-up intervals between 6 months and 3 years.[7] The reoperations predominately were for anterior or posterior prolapse and not for apical defects.

Patients after abdominal sacral colpopexy for pelvic organ prolapse are also at risk for persistent or de novo stress urinary incontinence. The Pelvic Floor Disorders Network reported the rate of operations for stress incontinence to be 4.9% after sacral colpopexy.[7]

Table 73-1 Clinical Outcomes of Abdominal Sacral Colpopexy

Study	No. of Patients	Follow-up (mo)	Success Rate (%)	Criteria for Success
Snyder and Krantz, 1991	147	43	93	No recurrence of symptoms for at least 6 months
Sullivan et al, 2001	236	64	100	No recurrence of vaginal or rectal prolapse
Culligan et al, 2002	245	61	85	Any POPQ point < stage II
Brizzolara and Pillai-Allen, 2003	124	36	98	No recurrent vault prolapse
Timmons et al, 1992	163	33	99	Good vaginal vault support
Lecuru et al, 1994	203	33	87-100	Anatomically good results
De Vries et al, 1995	101	48	32	Fully cured (patient satisfaction based on questionnaire)
Ocelli et al, 1999	271	66	98	Cured for prolapse
Patsner, 1999	175	≥12	97	No mesh failures
Lindeque and Nel, 2002	262	≥16	99	No vaginal vault prolapse

POPQ, Pelvic Organ Prolapse Quantification system.

It is also pertinent to compare the effectiveness of open abdominal sacral colpopexy with vaginal procedures to correct pelvic organ prolapse. In a retrospective case series of 80 abdominal sacral colpopexies compared with 130 attempted vaginal sacrospinous vault suspensions (five were abandoned because of technical difficulties), the incidence of recurrent prolapse was not statistically different (1.3% and 2.4%, respectively) (Table 73-2).[11] The complication rates were similar in both groups, except that the mean estimated blood loss was higher in the abdominal sacral colpopexy group compared with the vaginal sacrospinous vault suspension group (745 versus 567 mL, $P = .04$). Moreover, in the sacral colpopexy group, one patient developed stress incontinence; this complication was not seen after sacrospinous suspension. Concomitant incontinence and other gynecologic procedures were performed with various frequencies in the different groups. The results must be interpreted in light of these inconsistencies.

Three randomized trials compared open abdominal sacral colpopexy and vaginal procedures for pelvic organ prolapse and had different results (Table 73-3). Benson and colleagues[12] and Lo and Wang found that sacral colpopexy was more effective at correcting pelvic organ prolapse than sacrospinous suspension. However, Maher and coworkers[13] found that the abdominal and vaginal approaches were equally efficacious at correcting pelvic organ prolapse. It is difficult to compare efficacy in the different studies because most of these operations were performed simultaneously with various combinations of different incontinence and gynecologic procedures. There are also no consistencies between the different studies with regard to a propensity for complications with the abdominal or vaginal approach.

COMPLICATIONS

Intraoperative complications of abdominal sacral colpopexies include those associated with any gynecologic laparotomies, such as enterotomy, proctotomy, cystotomy, and ureteral injury. The Pelvic Floor Disorders Network found that enterotomy or proctotomy occurred in 1.6%, cystotomy in 3.1%, and ureteral injury in 1.0% of operations.

Although uncommon, one of the most morbid complications associated with this procedure is hemorrhage from the presacral vessels. Hemostasis is especially difficult to achieve in this area because the vessels form a complex interlacing network above and underneath the sacral periosteum. Once lacerated, these vessels retract, making it even more impossible to isolate single vessels. The presacral vessels often form communications with adjoining pelvic vessels, especially the left common iliac vein, resulting in even more extensive hemorrhage if they are damaged. Although the incidence of presacral vascular injury in the literature has not been specifically addressed, the requirement overall rate of hemorrhage with or without transfusion is 4.4%. Management of this complication include packing the presacral space, which is often only a temporizing measure and has the added possibility of lacerating more of these delicate vessels as the pack is removed. Other measures include using electrocautery, sutures, and metallic vascular clips. These procedures are especially successful if the lacerations are small or individual vessels that can be visualized. If these strategies are not successful, other interventions include using bone wax and orthopedic bone thumbtacks.[14] To avoid this complication, some surgeons recommend minimal dissection of the presacral space by attaching the graft to the ligament,[15] and others advocate careful, extensive dissection of this space to prevent inadvertent injury to unseen vessels.

Postoperative complications include urinary tract infection, ileus and small bowel obstruction, deep venous thrombus or pulmonary embolus, extrafascial wound problems, and granulation tissue in the vagina. Urinary tract infection was the most commonly reported complication in the literature, occurring in 2.5% to 25.9% of patients. Postoperative ileus occurred in 3.6% of cases, and reoperation for small bowel obstruction occurred in 1.1% of operations. Deep venous thrombus or pulmonary embolus was reported in 3.3% of cases. Extrafascial wound complications such as hematoma, infection, or superficial separation occurred in 4.6% of operations, and 5.0% of procedures resulted in incisional hernias requiring subsequent repairs. Other uncommon complications reported in the literature include femoral, obturator and sciatic neuropathies, fascial dehiscence, vertebral osteomyelitis, and gluteal necrotizing myofascitis.

One of the most discussed but uncommon postoperative complication is mesh erosion. In one retrospective series of 155 abdominal sacral colpopexies using Mersilene mesh (Johnson & Johnson) with a median follow-up of 6.5 months (range, 1 to 87

Table 73-2 Trials of Abdominal Sacral Colpopexy and Vaginal Procedures for Pelvic Organ Prolapse

Study	Procedure	No. Patients	Follow-up (months)	Success Rate (%)	Criteria for Success
Hardiman and Drutz, 1996	Sacral colpopexy	125	47	99	No recurrence vault prolapse
	Sacrospinous vault suspension	80	26	98	
Benson et al, 1996	Sacral colpopexy and paravaginal repair	38	30	58	Asymptomatic and vaginal apex support above levator plate
	Sacrospinous vault suspension and paravaginal repair	42	30	29	
Maher et al, 2004	Sacral colpopexy	47	24	76% objective 94% subjective	Objective: no prolapse beyond the halfway point
	Sacrospinous vault suspension	48	24	69% objective 91% subjective	Subjective: no symptoms

Data from Nygaard IE, McCreery R, Brubaker L, et al: Abdominal sacrocolpopexy: A comprehensive review. Am J Obstet Gynecol 104:805-823, 2004.

Table 73-3 Erosion Rates with Different Mesh Materials

Mesh Material	Manufacture	Reported Rates of Erosion
Polypropylene	Prolene Ethicon Endo-Surgery, Inc.	0.5%
Polyethylene terephthalate	Mersilene Johnson & Johnson	3.1%
Gore-Tex	W.L. Gore & Associates, Inc.	3.4%
Teflon	E.I. DuPont de Nemours & Co.	5.5%
Polyethylene	Marlex Phillips Sumika Polypropylene Co.	5.0%

Data from Nygaard IE, McCreery R, Brubaker L, et al: Abdominal sacrocolpopexy: A comprehensive review. Am J Obstet Gynecol 104:805-823, 2004.

months), the erosion rate was 3.2%, with a median time to the appearance of erosion of 15.6 months (range, 2 to 33 months).[16] Although the true incidence of this complication is unknown because most reported studies have short follow-up intervals, the Pelvic Floor Disorders Network found that the reported rate to be 3.4% at 6 months to 3 years.[7] Moreover, the reported rate of reoperations for mesh-related complications, including erosion and infection, is 3.0%. Although mesh erosion has been reported with all available synthetic graft materials (see Table 73-3), there are no published randomized trials comparing the erosion rates of these different graft materials. Not surprisingly, case series involving nonsynthetic grafts such as autologous, cadaveric fascia or dura mater reported no cases of erosion.

References

1. Subak LL, Waetjen LE, van den Eeden S, et al: Cost of pelvic organ prolapse surgery in the United States. Obstet Gynecol 98:646-651, 2001.
2. Luber KM, Boero S, Choe JY: The demographics of pelvic floor disorders: current observations and future projections. Am J Obstet Gynecol 184:1496-1501, 2001.
3. Virtanen H, Hirvonen T, Makinen J, Kiilholma P: Outcome of thirty patients who underwent repair of posthysterectomy prolapse of the vaginal vault with abdominal sacral colpopexy. J Am Coll Surg 178:283-287, 1994.
4. de Vries MJ, van Dessel TH, Drogendijk AC, et al: Short-term results and long-term patients' appraisal of abdominal colposacropexy for treatment of genital and vaginal vault prolapse. Eur J Obstet Gynecol Reprod Biol 59:35-38, 1995.
5. Baden WF, Walker TA: Genesis of the vaginal profile: a correlated classification of vaginal relaxation. Clin Obstet Gynecol 15:1048-1054, 1972.
6. Bump RC, Mattiasson A, Bø K, et al: The standardization of terminology of female pelvic organ prolapse and pelvic floor dysfunction. Am J Obstet Gynecol 175:10-17, 1996.

7. Nygaard IE, McCreery R, Brubaker L, et al: Abdominal sacrocolpopexy: A comprehensive review. Am J Obstet Gynecol 104:805-823, 2004.
8. Geomini PM, Brolmann HA, van Binsbergen NJ, Mol BW: Vaginal vault suspension by abdominal sacral colpopexy for prolapse: A follow-up study of 40 patients. Eur J Obstet Gynecol Reprod Biol 94:234-238, 2001.
9. Brubaker L: Sacrocolpopexy and the anterior compartment: support and function. Am J Obstet Gynecol 173:1690-1696, 1995.
10. Olsen AL, Smith VJ, Bergstrom JO, et al: Epidemiology of surgically managed pelvic organ prolapse and urinary incontinence. Obstet Gynecol 89:501-506, 1997.
11. Hardiman PJ, Drutz HP: Gynecology: sacrospinous vault suspension and abdominal colposacropexy: success rates and complications. Am J Obstet Gynecol 175:612-616, 1996.
12. Benson JT, Lucente V, McClellan E: Vaginal versus abdominal reconstructive surgery for the treatment of pelvic support defects: A prospective randomized study with long-term outcome evaluation. Am J Obstet Gynecol 175:1418-1422, 1996.
13. Maher CF, Qatawneh AM, Dwyer PL, et al: Abdominal sacrocolpopexy or vaginal sacrospinous colpopexy for vaginal vault prolapse: a prospective randomized study. Am J Obstet Gynecol 190:20-26, 2004.
14. Lane FE: Modified technique of sacral colpopexy. Am J Obstet Gynecol 142:933, 1982.
15. Sanz LE, Verosko J: Modification of the abdominal sacrocolpopexy using a suture anchor system. J Reprod Med 48:496-500, 2003.
16. Visco AG, Weidner AC, Barber MD, et al: Vaginal mesh erosion after abdominal sacral colpopexy. Am J Obstet Gynecol 184:297-302,

Part C
POSTERIOR VAGINAL WALL

Chapter 74
POSTERIOR WALL PROLAPSE: SEGMENTAL DEFECT REPAIR

Tristi W. Muir

Pelvic organ prolapse is common in women. The lifetime risk for undergoing an operation for prolapse or urinary incontinence is estimated to be 11.1%.[1] The posterior wall of the vagina primarily provides support over the anterior rectum and posterior cul-de-sac. Prolapse of the posterior vaginal wall may result from the presence of an enterocele, sigmoidocele, rectocele, or a combination of these entities. This chapter focuses on the herniation of the anterior rectum into the posterior vaginal wall as the cause of the prolapse. A variety of surgical procedures are available for the management of posterior vaginal wall prolapse, including posterior colporrhaphy, site-specific defect repair, posterior fascial replacement, transanal or transperineal repair, and a sacral colpoperineopexy Posterior colporrhaphy and site-specific defect repair for surgical repair of posterior wall prolapse are discussed.

ANATOMY AND PATHOPHYSIOLOGY

The support of the vagina is provided by an interaction of the bony pelvis, pelvic floor musculature (i.e., levator ani and coccygeus muscles), and the connective tissue supports. The vagina is a fibromuscular tube, which must maintain its position but have enough mobility to accommodate urinary, sexual, and defecatory functions. This vaginal tube also must distend to allow for childbirth. The pelvic floor muscles are composed of two functional components, one horizontal and the other vertical. The coccygeus muscle and horizontal portion of the levator ani muscles provide a backstop of support of the abdominal contents. The urethra vagina and rectum exit the abdominal cavity through the levator hiatus. A muscular sling that is chronically contracted to close this hiatus but capable of relaxing open to allow for urinary, defecatory, and sexual function is provided by the puborectalis portion of the levator ani. A continually contracted levator ani muscle closes the levator hiatus and angulates the rectal and vaginal tubes toward the pubic symphysis. Anatomically, there are no native fibers of the levator ani muscles traversing the rectovaginal space.

The connective tissue supports of the posterior vaginal wall are in continuity from the apical support of the vaginal vault (originating at the sacrum) to the perineal body. The apical portion of the anterior and posterior vaginal wall is provided by the suspensory support of the cardinal-uterosacral ligaments. The cardinal-uterosacral ligaments provide a mesentery of support directed toward the sacrum (S2 to S4) and pelvic side wall. The broad posterior fan of support directs the proximal (apical) portion of the vaginal axis posteriorly, and the contracted levator ani muscles direct the midportion of the vagina and rectum anteriorly toward the pubic symphysis. This orients the proximal vagina and rectum in a horizontal plane, supported over the pelvic floor muscles rather than a vertical orientation through the levator hiatus.[2] The connective tissue attachments of the midsection of the posterior vaginal wall are directed laterally and cranially to the levator ani muscular side wall.[3] The proximal halves of the posterior and anterior vaginal wall are attached to the same condensation of endopelvic fascia on the levator ani muscles, the arcus tendineus fasciae pelvis. The distal half of the posterior vaginal wall has a separate, caudal attachment to the pelvic side wall, the arcus tendineus fasciae rectovaginalis.[4] These separate lines of attachment of the anterior and posterior vaginal wall give the distal portion of the vagina an H shape (Fig. 74-1).

The perineal body is the central connection between the two sides of the perineal membrane, which originates bilaterally on the medial portion of the ischiopubic rami. Within the perineal body lie the bulbocavernosus muscle, superficial transverse perinei muscle, and the external anal sphincter and the rectovaginal septum, or Denonvilliers' fascia. Extending from the posterior cul-de-sac to the perineal body, the rectovaginal septum is the fused, endopelvic fascial remnant of the embryonic posterior cul-de-sac.[5,6] The role of the perineal body is to resist caudally directed force provided by the rectum and provide a physical barrier between the vagina and rectum. The perineal body's mobility is limited by an intact connective tissue support within the vagina from the sacrum to the perineal body and an intact perineal membrane from ischiopubic ramus to ischiopubic ramus.[3]

An increase in intra-abdominal pressure, such as a Valsalva maneuver, flattens the horizontally oriented upper vagina against the rectum and pelvic floor musculature. In the distal vagina, a Valsalva maneuver causes an equal increase in pressure against the anterior and posterior vaginal walls. No net strain is placed on the connective tissue support of the vaginal wall (Fig. 74-2). However, if the levator hiatus is widened or not closed, two things may happen. First, the vagina may lose the horizontal orientation of its axis. As the vagina becomes more vertically oriented, intra-abdominal pressure pushes the pelvic organs through the levator hiatus and toward the genital hiatus. The

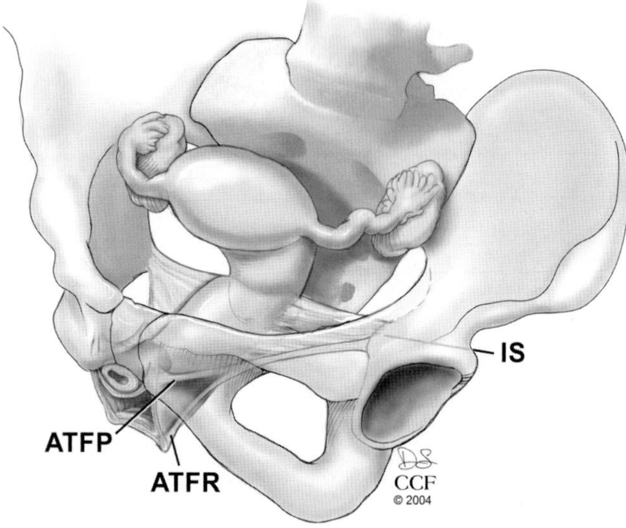

Figure 74-1 Lateral attachment of the anterior and posterior vaginal walls. The lateral support of the anterior wall fuses at the arcus tendineus fasciae pelvis (ATFP), which extends from the back of the pubic bone to the ischial spine (IS). The distal lateral connection of the posterior vaginal wall is more posterior, the arcus tendineus fasciae rectovaginalis (ATFR). The proximal connection of the posterior vaginal wall is the ATFP. (Courtesy of the Cleveland Clinic Foundation.)

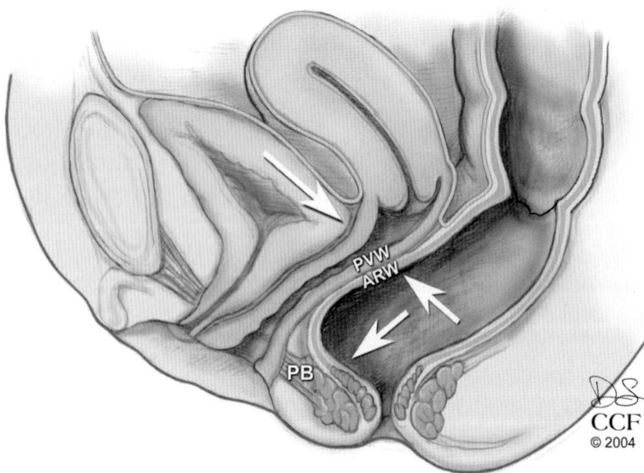

Figure 74-2 Equalization of pressure in the anterior and posterior vaginal walls *(arrows)*. The pressure on the anterior vaginal wall and the posterior vaginal wall (PVW) is equal, and no strain is placed on the connective tissue supports of the vaginal walls. The perineal body (PB) is intact and resists the downward intrarectal force. ARW, anterior rectal wall. (Courtesy of the Cleveland Clinic Foundation.)

anterior and posterior vaginal walls then do not lie in apposition. An increase in intra-abdominal or intrarectal pressure, such as that obtained with straining for a bowel movement, is not met with an equal measure of pressure of the anterior vaginal wall. Instead, the posterior vaginal wall pressure meets the atmospheric pressure present in the open vagina (Fig. 74-3). In both situations, an increase in abdominal pressure places a net force on the connective tissue supports of the posterior vaginal wall. This force on the connective tissue supports may attenuate or break

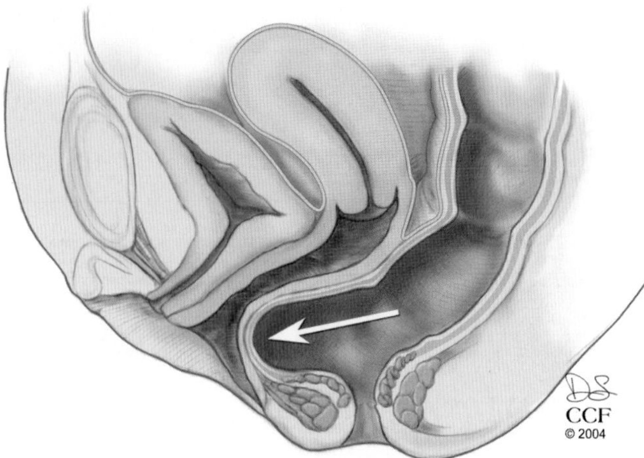

Figure 74-3 Rectocele. In a woman with an open vagina, the pressure within the rectum is met by atmospheric pressure. The anterior vaginal wall does not provide equilibrating force, and there is stress *(arrow)* placed on the posterior vaginal wall's connective tissue. This may lead to rectocele formation. (Courtesy of the Cleveland Clinic Foundation.)

the posterior vaginal wall, or it may uncover damage done by a prior event, such as childbirth.

Anything that damages the pelvic floor musculature, its innervation, or the connective tissue of the posterior vaginal wall may result in prolapse. Damage to the levator ani muscles or innervation may be traumatic (usually related to childbirth) or be a result of neuromuscular diseases or aging. Connective tissue may be damaged through trauma (i.e., childbirth or constant straining with defecatory dysfunction), congenital disease, or aging. A combination of these factors is the likely recipe for the manifestation of prolapse.

SIGNS AND SYMPTOMS

Many women with posterior wall prolapse are asymptomatic. Women who have prolapse that protrudes beyond the hymenal ring are more likely to be symptomatic.[7] This bulge may be associated with vaginal pressure or pain, which worsens as the day progresses or with abdominal straining. This bulge may affect urinary, sexual, and defecatory functions.

As the posterior vaginal wall balloons upward toward the anterior vaginal wall and outward toward the genital hiatus or beyond, urinary function may be altered. Inside the vagina, the distended posterior vaginal wall may provide additional support of the urethra and mask or decrease the severity of urinary incontinence. Urodynamic investigations, with and without reduction of the posterior wall prolapse, have demonstrated that when the posterior wall prolapse is retracted, there are significant decreases in the maximum urethral closure pressure and functional urethral length and an increase in leak volumes.[8] Beyond the genital hiatus, posterior wall prolapse may partially obstruct the external urethral meatus, altering the stream of urine.

Sexual function is a complicated issue involving both partners' psychological and physical well-being. Prolapse protruding beyond the genital hiatus may lead to an altered body image and self-esteem. This may be worsened by fear of urinary or anal incontinence. Prolapse may be significant enough to require reduction before even attempting to have vaginal intercourse. A widened genital hiatus may decrease sensation for both partners during intercourse. The woman's partner may also be concerned about causing pain or discomfort or about contributing to worsening of the prolapse.

Defecatory dysfunction and pelvic organ prolapse often coexist in women. A ballooning of the anterior rectum into the posterior vaginal wall or perineal body may alter the process of defecation. Stool may be trapped in the distended rectal pouch, leading to incomplete rectal emptying. Women may employ digitally placed pressure in the vagina, on the perineal body, or within the rectum to evacuate the stool. Some woman may perceive this as constipation (i.e., straining to have a bowel movement or an unproductive urge to defecate). However, constipation is often unrelated to a rectocele, such as that related to irritable bowel syndrome, slow-transit colon, or secondary constipation related to medications or neurologic disorders. Determining if the woman's defecatory dysfunction is related to her posterior prolapse may be difficult to discern. Weber and colleagues[9] examined bowel function and severity of posterior wall prolapse and found no correlation. If a woman's sole defecatory complaint is incomplete rectal emptying that resolves with vaginal splinting, she is likely to have functional improvement after surgical correction.

A thorough history, including direct questions about fecal incontinence, should be obtained. Fecal incontinence may also coexist with posterior vaginal wall prolapse. There is an association with a rectocele, which protrudes beyond the hymen and anal incontinence.[10] A descending perineum may provide stretch on the pudendal nerve, which innervates the external anal sphincter. This stretch injury may lead to denervation of the external anal sphincter and fecal incontinence. Prior obstetric trauma that injures the external anal sphincter may also result in fecal incontinence.

The goal of the physical examination is to recreate the woman's symptoms. A validated measure of pelvic organ prolapse is the Pelvic Organ Prolapse Quantification (POPQ) system.[11] The POPQ examination includes measures of the uterus or vaginal cuff, posterior cul-de-sac, anterior and posterior vaginal walls, perineal body, and genital hiatus at maximal strain. Total vaginal length is assessed at rest. The posterior vaginal wall may be visualized with the posterior blade of a bivalve speculum or with a Sims speculum with the woman in the dorsal lithotomy or semirecumbent position. In most women, there is excellent correlation between the dorsal lithotomy and standing positions.[12] Confirmation of the recreation of the woman's maximal protrusion can be facilitated with a hand-held mirror. If a woman describes prolapse that is more significant than that observed in the supine or sitting positions, a standing examination may be employed.

A rectovaginal examination should accompany the physical examination. The tone of the external anal sphincter at rest and with squeeze may be assessed. With digital pressure directed toward the anterior rectal wall, areas of weak support and perineal body mobility can be evaluated. The clinical examination for identifying site-specific defects through a rectovaginal examination was found to be inaccurate when compared with site-specific defects found intraoperatively.[13] However, the rectovaginal examination may help to differentiate an enterocele from a rectocele. Palpation of loops of bowel between the rectum and vagina is consistent with an enterocele. This may be more evident in the standing position or with a Valsalva maneuver. Digital pressure placed on the posterior wall of the vagina directed toward the rectum may uncover rectal prolapse.

A focused neurologic examination to evaluate S2 to S4 should accompany the physical examination. Sensation may be determined by asking the patient to discriminate between sharp and dull sensations. Pelvic floor strength may be determined with the examiner's two fingers in the vagina and asking the patient to contract the pelvic floor (i.e., perform a Kegel exercise). Strength and duration of this contraction can be determined. Tenderness or spasm of the levator ani muscles may be uncovered on clinical examination. If a woman is unable to relax the levator ani muscles, anismus may be the cause of her obstructed defecation. Anismus, or paradoxical puborectalis contraction, often responds to biofeedback or botulinum toxin.[14,15] Reflex testing of the bulbocavernosus reflex and anal wink may be performed.

Ancillary tests may be considered in the evaluation. Urodynamics with prolapse reduction may be indicated in a woman with complaints of urinary incontinence or for evaluation of potential urinary incontinence. Anorectal or colonic transit studies may help differentiate the potential causes of defecatory dysfunction. If the woman's primary complaint is related to her defecatory dysfunction rather than the bulge of the posterior vaginal wall, further defecatory testing should be performed before surgery. Incomplete emptying of the rectum may be caused by a paradoxical puborectalis contraction or slow-transit colon. Endoanal ultrasonography is useful in a woman with fecal incontinence to determine whether there is an anatomic defect in the external and internal anal sphincters. Imaging studies such as defecography and magnetic resonance imaging are used uncommonly for further elucidation of the anatomy of the prolapse.

TECHNIQUE

The vaginal epithelium is opened with a transverse incision at the posterior fourchette. The posterior vaginal epithelium is then opened in the midline to a level proximal to the bulge and dissected away from the underlying fibromuscularis. The dissection is extended laterally to the endopelvic fascial attachment of the posterior vaginal wall to the arcus tendineus fasciae pelvis and arcus tendineus fasciae rectovaginalis (Fig. 74-4).

Posterior Colporrhaphy

The underlying fibromuscularis of the posterior vaginal wall is exposed. A posterior colporrhaphy uses interrupted sutures to reduce the redundancy of the posterior fibromuscularis (Fig. 74-5). A delayed-absorbable 2-0 suture is used. A vertically oriented suture may reduce the length and width of the posterior vaginal wall. Care should be taken to maintain adequate vaginal caliber (i.e., approximately 3 fingerbreadths) and to avoid ridging of the posterior vaginal wall. If a suture constricts the vagina or creates a ridge, the suture should be removed and replaced. The vaginal epithelium is trimmed and closed with a 2-0 absorbable suture. It is important to avoid over-trimming the vaginal epithelium, particularly in a postmenopausal woman with vaginal atrophy or a woman with prior vaginal surgery and a constricted vagina. A perineorrhaphy may be performed to correct perineal body defects.

A plication of the levator muscles in the midline has been performed in conjunction with a posterior colporrhaphy in some patients. This may be indicated in a woman with a significantly widened levator hiatus. This is not the anatomic position of the

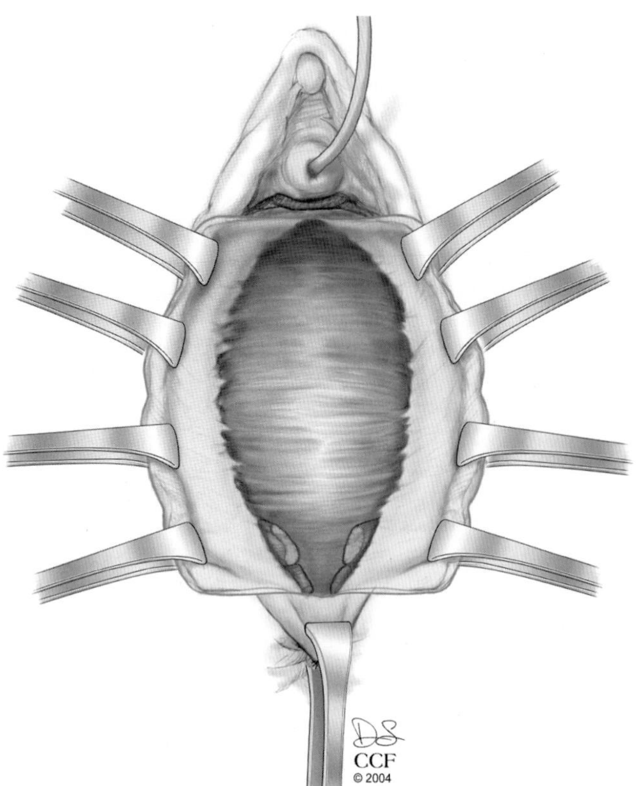

Figure 74-4 Dissection of the posterior vaginal wall epithelium. The underlying fibromuscularis of the posterior vaginal wall is exposed, and the perineal body is opened in the midline. (Courtesy of the Cleveland Clinic Foundation.)

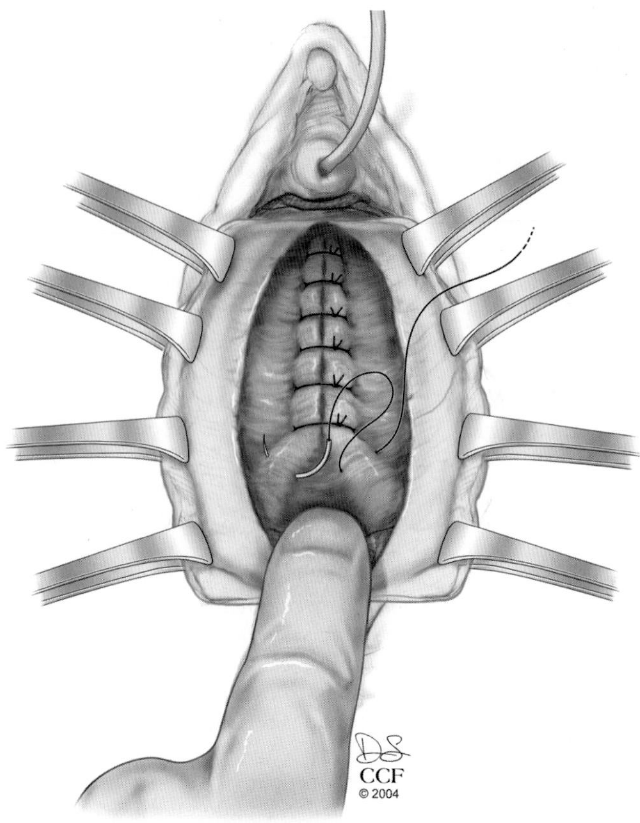

Figure 74-5 Posterior colporrhaphy. A midline plication of the fibromuscularis of the posterior vaginal wall is performed with interrupted sutures. (Courtesy of the Cleveland Clinic Foundation.)

levator ani muscles, but it may further narrow the vaginal caliber. A levator plication has been suggested to be a contributor to postoperative dyspareunia in women undergoing this procedure.[16]

A vaginal pack and Foley catheter are placed for 2 to 24 hours postoperatively. Voiding trials should be performed postoperatively to ensure that the patient is able to void adequately.

Site-Specific Defect Repair

After dissection of the posterior vaginal epithelium off the underlying fibromuscularis, the fibromuscularis (i.e., rectovaginal fascia) is carefully inspected to identify breaks. Irrigation and a digital rectal examination, placing upward pressure in the anterior rectal wall, may facilitate identification of the defects in the fibromuscularis (Fig. 74-6). Defects of the posterior vaginal wall may occur as isolated defects in the lateral, distal, midline, and superior portions of the wall or as a combination of defects (Fig. 74-7). The identified breaks are individually isolated and repaired (Fig. 74-8). Delayed-absorbable or nonabsorbable 1-0 or 2-0 suture may be used. If the fibromuscularis of the posterior wall has lost apical attachment, the fibromuscularis should be reattached to the apical support (through reattachment to a well-supported vaginal apex or attachment to the concurrent apical support procedure, such as a sacrospinous or uterosacral vaginal vault suspension). Apical lateral support may be obtained with a unilateral or bilateral iliococcygeal suspension of the fibromuscularis. The suture is placed through the iliococcygeus fascia on

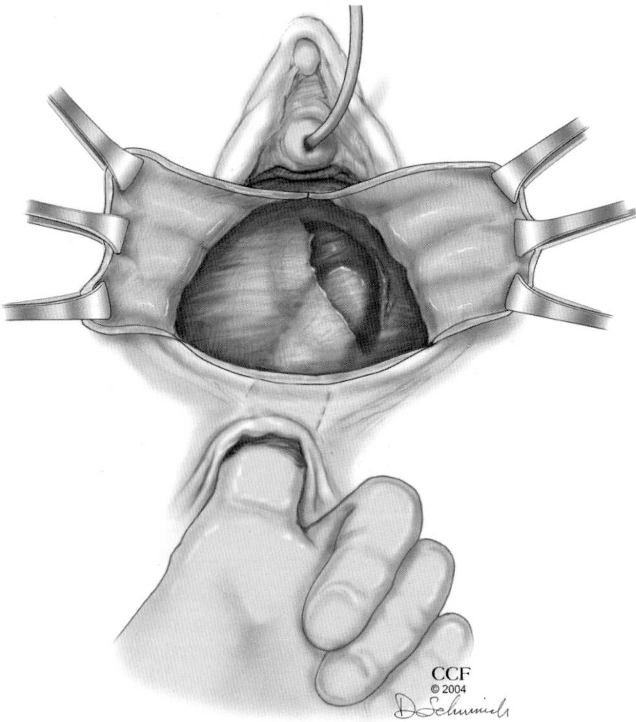

Figure 74-6 Identification of site-specific defects. After dissection of the posterior vaginal wall epithelium, a rectovaginal examination is helpful in the identification of defects in the fibromuscularis of the posterior vaginal wall. (Courtesy of the Cleveland Clinic Foundation.)

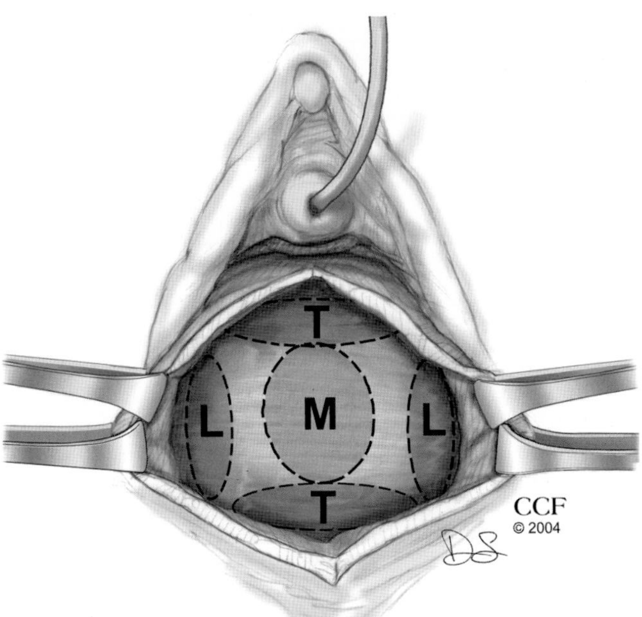

Figure 74-7 Location of site-specific defects in the fibromuscularis of the posterior vaginal wall. Transverse defects (T) may be apical or distal. Lateral defects (L) may occur as the fibromuscularis separates from its lateral attachment. Midline defects (M) may also occur. Often, a combination of these defects is found. (Courtesy of the Cleveland Clinic Foundation.)

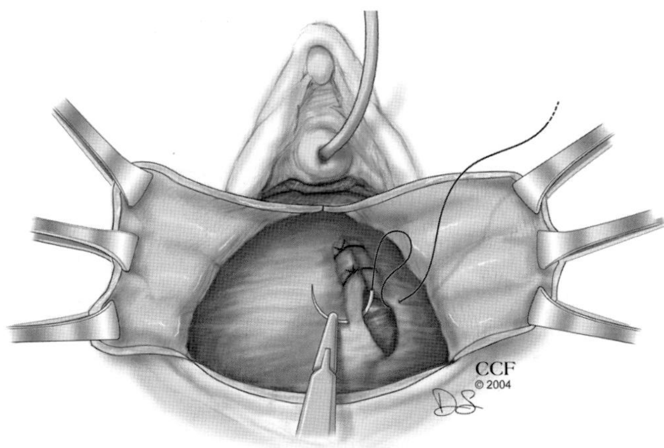

Figure 74-8 Repair of a left lateral defect with interrupted sutures. (Courtesy of the Cleveland Clinic Foundation.)

the lateral side wall (distal to the ischial spine) and then through the ipsilateral apical portion of fibromuscularis. If a distal defect is present, such as a separation of the fibromuscularis from the perineal body, the defect is repaired with absorbable suture in an attempt to reduce the incidence of postoperative dyspareunia. The vaginal epithelium is closed without significant trimming. Perineal body defects are also repaired with interrupted sutures. A levator plication is not performed.

A vaginal pack and Foley catheter are placed for 2 to 24 hours postoperatively. Voiding trials should be performed postoperatively to ensure that the patient is able to void adequately.

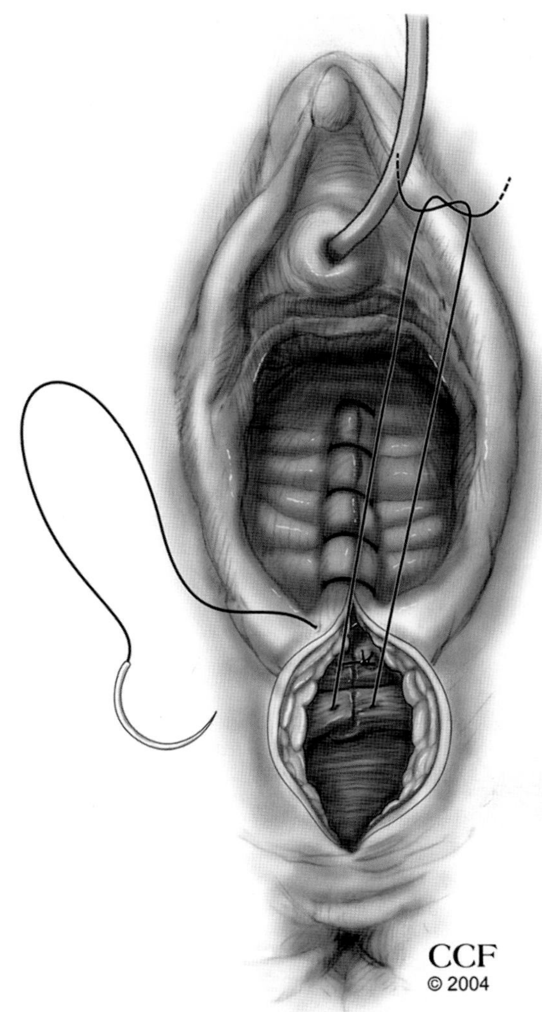

Figure 74-9 Perineorrhaphy. After the completion of the posterior repair, the perineal body is reconstructed by plicating the bulbocavernosus muscles and the transverse perinei muscles. (Courtesy of the Cleveland Clinic Foundation.)

Perineorrhaphy

The perineal body should be in continuity with the posterior vaginal wall repair. The perineal body may be opened with a midline, vertical incision. In a woman with a very short perineal body, a transverse or curvilinear incision may be made to expose the perineal body. The bulbocavernosus muscles are identified bilaterally and plicated. Similarly, the superficial transverse perinei muscles are plicated (Fig. 74-9). The plicated bulbocavernosus muscles may be reattached to the repaired rectovaginal fibromuscularis with an interrupted suture. With these sutures, the perineal membrane is reestablished, and the perineal body is in continuity with the support of the vagina.

SURGICAL OUTCOMES

The goals of pelvic reconstructive surgery are to correct the anatomic defect, improve function, and avoid complications. The difficulty in achieving these goals lies in function. The woman's defecatory dysfunction may coexist with her prolapse rather than

Table 74-1 Surgical Outcomes for Posterior Colporrhaphy

Study	No. of Patients at Follow-up	Mean Follow-up (mo)	Anatomic Cure Rate (%)	*Incomplete Evacuation*		*Sexual Dysfunction*	
				Preop (%)	Postop (%)	Preop (%)	Postop (%)
Francis and Jeffcoate, 1961	177	≥24	94			7	50
Arnold et al, (1990)*	22	≥24	77	20			23
Mellgren et al, 1995	25	12	80	48	0	6	19
Kahn and Stanton, 1997	171	42.5	76	27	38	18	27
Lopez et al, 2002†	24	9	100	68	36	18	23
Sloots et al, 2003	14	8	71	100	29	21	29§
Maher et al, 2004	38	12.5	87	100	16	37	5
Abramov et al, 2005‡	183	12	96	30¶	34¶	8	17

*Cure defined as % satisfied.
†Anatomic cure rate of 100% on clinical examination; 84% cure rate by defecography.
‡Cure defined as no prolapse beyond the hymenal ring.
§Includes one sexually inactive woman with postoperative de novo pelvic pain.
¶Defined as constipation.

Table 74-2 Surgical Outcomes for Site-Specific Defect Repair

Study	No. of Patients at Follow-up	Mean Follow-up (mo)	Anatomic Cure Rate (%)	*Incomplete Evacuation or Splinting*		*Sexual Dysfunction*	
				Preop (%)	Postop (%)	Preop (%)	Postop (%)
Cundiff et al, 1998	43	12	82	39	25	29	19
Glavind et al, 2000	65	3	100	40	5	12	6
Kenton et al, 1999	46	12	77	30	15	28	2
Porter et al, 1999	89	18	82	24	14	67	46
Singh et al, 2003*	33	18	92	57	27	31	24
Abramov et al, 2005†	124	12	89	33‡	37‡	8	16

*Cure defined as resolution of symptom of "feeling of vaginal protrusion."
†Cure defined as no prolapse beyond the hymenal ring.
‡Defined as constipation.

be a symptom of her prolapse. In this case, anatomic correction will be unlikely to improve her function. Surgical correction may interfere with defecatory and sexual functions. Historically, efficacy has been related to anatomic cure, but evaluating functional outcomes is equally important.

The posterior colporrhaphy was introduced in the 19th century. The goals of this procedure were to narrow the vaginal tube and genital hiatus and to create a shelf of support. It has remained a commonly performed surgical procedure for posterior wall prolapse. The traditional posterior colporrhaphy has an anatomic cure rate of 71% to 100% (Table 74-1).[16-23]

The site-specific defect repair approach to rectocele repair relies on theory advocated by A. Cullen Richardson, that the herniation of the rectum into the vagina is the result of identifiable defects in the fibromuscularis (rectovaginal fascia) or its attachment to the pelvic side wall.[24] The anatomic cure rate of the site-specific posterior repair is 77% to 100% (Table 74-2).[23,25-29]

The primary reason that this method of repair of posterior wall prolapse has been embraced is that it more often avoids the risk of postoperative dyspareunia. With the exception of the retrospective review by Abramov and colleagues[23] of women undergoing a site-specific posterior repair, there was no change or a decrease in dyspareunia in the series involving site-specific posterior repairs (see Table 74-2).[25-29] Abramov and colleagues[23] were the first to compare anatomic and functional outcomes in women who underwent a site-specific posterior repair (undertaken in women with specific defects identified in the fibromuscularis intraoperatively) with those who had undergone a posterior colporrhaphy without a levator plication (undertaken in women without identifiable breaks in the fibromuscularis) during the same time period.[23] Objective and subjective anatomic outcomes were better for the women undergoing a posterior colporrhaphy compared with those undergoing a site-specific repair. Functional outcomes were similar for the two groups. Improvement in defecation has also been described with this method of repair (see Table 74-2).[23,25-29]

Cundiff and coworkers[25] did not perform a perineorrhaphy in women who underwent a site-specific posterior repair. However, the perineal body was stabilized through reestablishment of the continuity of connective tissue support within the posterior vaginal wall from the sacrum to the perineal body. The stabilization of the perineal body was reflected in a significant reduction in the size of the genital hiatus despite not having performed a perineorrhaphy (4.8 cm preoperatively versus 2.5 cm postoperatively, $P < .0001$).[25]

COMPLICATIONS

Short-term complications associated with a posterior colporrhaphy or site-specific posterior repair include pain, constipation, and temporary urinary retention. Hematoma, infection, and inclusion cyst formation occasionally occur with all vaginal operations. Injury to the rectum with subsequent development of a rectovaginal or rectoperitoneal fistula is uncommon. Recurrent prolapse and de novo defecatory complaints may occur. Postoperative development of dyspareunia is widely reported after a posterior colporrhaphy (see Table 74-1).[16-23] This complication paved the road of acceptance of the site-specific posterior repair.

Postoperative sexual dysfunction related to prolapse repair, primarily dyspareunia, has been reported for decades. Francis and Jeffcoate[17] reported that 70 (50%) of 140 women who had undergone an anterior and posterior colporrhaphy with perineorrhaphy said they had apareunia or dyspareunia. Most (43 of 70)of the women with postoperative apareunia or dyspareunia were found to have a significantly narrowed postoperative vagina that would admit only one finger. Kahn and Stanton[16] found an increase in the number of women with dyspareunia from 18% (preoperative evaluation) to 27% (postoperative evaluation) after an anterior and posterior colpoperineorrhaphy. The investigators routinely plicated the levator ani muscles and proposed that pressure atrophy of the levator ani and resultant scar formation contributed to the development of postoperative dyspareunia. Haase and Skibsted[30] reported that 5 (21%) of 24 women who underwent a prolapse operation that included a posterior colpoperineorrhaphy experienced worsening or de novo dyspareunia. The appeal of the site-specific posterior repair is that ridging or excessive narrowing of the posterior vaginal wall can be avoided, which decreases the likelihood of the postoperative development of dyspareunia.

Although most studies of women undergoing a posterior colporrhaphy or site-specific defect repair have found an improvement in rectal emptying (see Tables 74-1 and 74-2), rectocele repair has been associated with postoperative fecal incontinence. Kahn and Stanton[16] reported that de novo fecal incontinence occurred in 14 (8%) of 171 women after a posterior colporrhaphy. A strong association was found between fecal incontinence and a history of more than one posterior colporrhaphy.[16]

CONCLUSIONS

The posterior vaginal wall is composed of interactions among the bony pelvis, pelvic floor muscles, and connective tissue supports. Alterations or injuries to these support units may lead to prolapse.

Posterior vaginal wall prolapse may be asymptomatic and require no treatment. Women with symptoms of vaginal protrusion, pressure or pain, defecatory dysfunction (specifically outlet obstruction leading to incomplete evacuation or need to splint to have a bowel movement), or sexual dysfunction may desire surgical management.

Surgical options commonly employed include posterior colporrhaphy (with and without a levator plication) and site-specific defect repair. Both of these posterior vaginal wall repairs may be performed with or without the addition of a perineal body repair (i.e., perineorrhaphy). Posterior colporrhaphy is effective at reducing the vaginal mass of the rectocele, but some studies have associated this anatomic improvement with an increased incidence of de novo dyspareunia and fecal incontinence. Levator plication may increase the risk of dyspareunia. It is essential to maintain adequate vaginal caliber and to avoid ridging of the vaginal tube when performing a posterior colporrhaphy. Site-specific defect repair is also effective at correcting prolapse, although Abramov and colleagues[23] suggest that it is not as anatomically successful as the posterior colporrhaphy. The vaginal caliber usually is maintained with a site-specific defect approach, and the risk of postoperative de novo dyspareunia is lower than with a posterior colporrhaphy. Augmentation of prolapse repair surgery has been performed using biologic and synthetic grafts. Prospective, randomized trials are needed to compare techniques and their outcomes, including anatomic and functional efficacy and complication rates.

References

1. Olsen AL, Smith VJ, Bergstrom JO, et al: Epidemiology of surgically managed pelvic organ prolapse and urinary incontinence. Obstet Gynecol 89:501-506, 1997.
2. Nichols DH: Posterior colporrhaphy and perineorrhaphy: Separate and distinct operations. Am J Obstet Gynecol 164:714-721, 1991.
3. DeLancey JOL: Structural anatomy of the posterior pelvic compartment as it relates to rectocele. Am J Obstet Gynecol 180:815-823, 1999.
4. Leffler KS, Thompson JR, Cundiff GW, et al: Attachment of the rectovaginal septum to the pelvic sidewall. Am J Obstet Gynecol 185:41-43, 2001.
5. Milley PS, Nichols DH: A correlative investigation of the human rectovaginal septum. Anat Rec 163:443-452, 1969.
6. Van Ophoven A, Roth S: The anatomy and embryological origins of the fascia of Denonvilliers: A medico-historical debate. J Urol 157:3-9, 1997.
7. Swift SE, Tate SB, Nicholas J: Correlation of symptoms with degree of pelvic organ support in a general population of women: what is pelvic organ prolapse? Am J Obstet Gynecol 189:372-379, 2003.
8. Myers DL, LaSala CA, Hogan JW, Rosenblatt PL: The effect of posterior wall support defects on urodynamic indices in stress urinary incontinence. Obstet Gynecol 91:710-714,1998.
9. Weber AM, Walters MD, Ballard LA, et al: Posterior vaginal prolapse and bowel function. Am J Obstet Gyencol 179:1446-1450, 1998.
10. Meschia M, Buonaguidi A, Pifarotti P, et al: Prevalence of anal incontinence in women with symptoms of urinary incontinence and genital prolapse. Obstet Gynecol 100:719-723, 2002.
11. Bump RC, Mattiasson A, Bo K, et al: The standardization of terminology of female pelvic organ prolapse and pelvic floor dysfunction. Am J Obstet Gynecol 175:10-17, 1996.
12. Swift SE, Herring M: Comparison of pelvic organ prolapse in the dorsal lithotomy compared with the standing position. Obstet Gynecol 91:961-964, 1998.
13. Burrows LJ, Sewell C, Leffler KS, Cundiff GW: The accuracy of clinical evaluation of posterior vaginal wall defects. Int Urogynecol J 14:160-163, 2003.
14. Lau CW, Heymen S, Alabaz O, et al: Prognostic Significance of rectocele, intussusception, and abnormal perineal descent in biofeedback treatment for constipated patients with paradoxical puborectalis contraction. Dis Colon Rectum 43:478-482, 2000.
15. Ron Y, Avni Y, Lukovetski A, et al: Botulinum toxin type-A in therapy of patients with anismus. Dis Colon Rectum 44:1821-1826, 2001.

16. Kahn MA, Stanton SL: Posterior colporrhaphy: Its effects on bowel and sexual function. Br J Obstet Gynaecol 104:82-86, 1997.
17. Francis WJA, Jeffcoate TNA: Dyspareunia following vaginal operations. J Obstet Gynaecol Br Commonw 68:1-10, 1961.
18. Arnold MW, Stewart WR, Aguilar PS: Rectocele repair: Four years' experience. Dis Colon Rectum 33:684-687, 1990.
19. Mellgren A, Anzén B, Nilsson BY, et al: Results of rectocele repair. Dis Colon Rectum 38:7-13, 1995.
20. López A, Anzén B, Bremmer S, et al: Cystodefecoperitoneography in patients with genital prolapse. Int Urogynecol J 13:22-29, 2002.
21. Sloots CEJ, Meulen AJ, Felt-Bersma RJF: Rectocele repair improves evacuation and prolapse complaints independent of anorectal function and colonic transit time. Int J Colorectal Dis 18:342-328, 2003.
22. Maher CF, Qatawneh AM, Baessler K, Schluter PJ: Midline rectovaginal fascial plication for repair of rectocele and obstructed defecation. Obstet Gynecol 104:685-689, 2004.
23. Abramov Y, Gandhi S, Goldberg RP, et al: Site-specific rectocele repair compared with standard posterior colporrhaphy. Obstet Gynecol 105:314-318, 2005.
24. Richardson AC, Lyon JB, Williams NL: A new look at pelvic relaxation. Am J Obstet Gynecol 126:568-573, 1976.
25. Cundiff GW, Weidner AC, Visco AG, et al: An anatomic and functional assessment of the discrete defect rectocele repair. Am J Obstet Gynecol 179:1451-1457, 1998.
26. Kenton K, Shott S, Brubaker L: Outcome after rectovaginal fascia reattachment for rectocele repair. Am J Obstet Gynecol 181:1360-1363, 1999.
27. Porter WE, Steele A, Walsh P, et al: The anatomic and functional outcomes of defect-specific rectocele repairs. Am J Obstet Gynecol 181:1353-1358, 1999.
28. Glavind K, Madsen H: A prospective study of the discrete fascial defect rectocele repair. Acta Obstet Gynecol Scand 79:145-147, 2000.
29. Singh K, Cortes E, Reid WMN: Evaluation of the fascial technique for surgical repair of isolated posterior vaginal wall prolapse. Obstet Gynecol 101:320-324, 2003.
30. Haase P, Skibsted L: Influence of operations for stress incontinence and/or genital descensus on sexual life. Acta Obstet Gynecol Scand 67:659-661, 1988.

Chapter 75

POSTERIOR REPAIR USING CADAVERIC FASCIA

Sarah A. Rueff and Gary E. Leach

Traditional posterior colporrhaphy for symptomatic rectoceles has been associated with failure rates as high as 35% and de novo dyspareunia rates ranging from 6% to 41%.[1] The technique involves midline plication of the levator muscles and rectovaginal fascia to obliterate the fascial defect and perineorrhaphy to reapproximate the central tendon and perineal body.[2] Inherent problems exist with traditional posterior repair. First, the success of the repair relies on the patient's own tissue, which has already shown a propensity for weakness. Second, by attempting to obliterate the fascial defects, the patient's anatomy is inevitably distorted, and the procedure can result in vaginal narrowing and dyspareunia. The patient may complain of constriction of the vaginal tube or may feel a ridge in the midline of the posterior wall due to suture placement.

The use of defect-specific rectocele repair is an attempt to alleviate the vaginal narrowing and dyspareunia associated with traditional repair. The technique involves identification of fascial tears and plicating nearby durable fascia over the defect. Recurrence rates of 18% to 23% with mean follow-up periods of 12 to18 months have been reported along with variable improvements in bowel habits.[3-5] As with traditional colporrhaphy, the repair relies on the patient's inherently weak tissues to repair fascial defects. By failing to address the entire posterior vaginal wall, all areas of fascial weakness may not be identified, increasing the likelihood of failure.

Rectocele repair with cadaveric fascia attempts to address the inherent problems of traditional and defect-specific rectocele repair. First, by graft interposition, all areas of weakness within the posterior compartment are addressed simultaneously. Second, the use of solvent-dehydrated, nonfrozen cadaveric fascia lata avoids the use of the patient's own weak tissues. Third, the fascia is secured to the levator complex without tension, as is often necessary with traditional repair, preventing vaginal narrowing. Fourth, avoidance of tissue plication prevents the patient from feeling a ridge in the midline and preserves the width of the introitus. For these reasons, we think rectocele repair with cadaveric fascia offers several advantages over traditional posterior vaginal reconstruction techniques.

CADAVERIC FASCIA

The choice of fascia for rectocele repair with cadaveric fascia is of utmost importance in determining surgical outcome. Fascia lata is strong, regardless of a patient's age or medical condition, and it has three to four times more tensile strength than rectus fascia.[6] Our choice of fascia is Tutoplast (Mentor Corp., Santa Barbara, CA). Tutoplast is prepared by a five-step process that involves screening of donors, cleansing, denaturization of antigens and viruses, solvent dehydration, and gamma irradiation. The tensile strength and tissue stiffness of nonfrozen cadaveric fascia lata has been investigated, and it is comparable to that of autologous fascia lata.[7] Studies have compared solvent-dehydrated and freeze-dried cadaveric fascia lata, another commercially available preparation. Solvent-dehydrated fascia lata has significantly greater stiffness, maximum load to failure, and maximum load per unit of graft compared with freeze-dried fascia lata.[8]

All commercially available cadaveric fascia lata is not the same. The method used to prepare the tissue ultimately affects its tensile strength and subsequent surgical outcomes. We prefer the use nonfrozen cadaveric fascia to commercially available synthetic mesh material, which carries inherent risks of erosion and infection. Milani and colleagues[9] described 31 women who underwent posterior repair with Prolene mesh who had an erosion rate of 6.5%. Other studies have reported similar findings, with erosion rates as high as 48%.[10]

PREOPERATIVE EVALUATION

Before undergoing rectocele repair, a thorough history is obtained focusing on the symptoms associated with posterior prolapse. Based on the results of a series of questions in the Rectocele Symptom Inventory (Table 75-1), patients are assigned a preoperative score that correlates with the degree of symptoms. Questions focus on three areas of symptoms bowel function with symptoms that include straining, stool trapping, the need to manually reduce the rectocele to facilitate defecation, or a feeling of incomplete emptying after defecation; prolapse symptoms, which include vaginal pressure or the feeling of sitting on a ball; and sexual function, which includes dyspareunia and overall sexual satisfaction. We do not routinely repair rectoceles that are asymptomatic or low grade because the theoretical risks of surgery or its side effects outweigh the benefit gained. For patients who present with constipation or bowel dysfunction that does not correlate with the severity of posterior prolapse, referral to a gastroenterologist or colorectal surgeon may be beneficial before considering surgical repair.

Physical Examination

A systematic examination of the anterior, apical, and posterior compartments is performed with the patient in the dorsal lithotomy position. The posterior blade of a Graves speculum is used to displace the anterior vaginal wall and examine the posterior wall at rest and with straining. A simultaneous rectal examination using the index finger is performed to push the posterior vaginal

Table 75-1 Rectocele Symptom Inventory

In the past month, how often have you experienced the stated symptoms?	*Scoring**				
	All of the time (4)	**Most of the time (3)**	**Some of the time (2)**	**Rarely (1)**	**Never (0)**
I have to push or strain to have a bowel movement					
I feel the stool "gets stuck" when having a bowel movement					
I assist my rectum by placing my finger in the vagina or pressing on the skin outside of the vagina to have a bowel movement					
I feel that I have not completely emptied my bowels after having a bowel movement					
I feel the sensation of pressure in my rectum or vagina or have the sensation of "sitting on a ball"					
I have pain with sexual relations					
My ability to have sexual relations is satisfactory to me	Not sexually active (0)	Most of the time (0)	Some of the time (2)	Not satisfactory (4)	

*On the Rectocele Symptoms Inventory (RSI), the total score may range between 0 and 28.

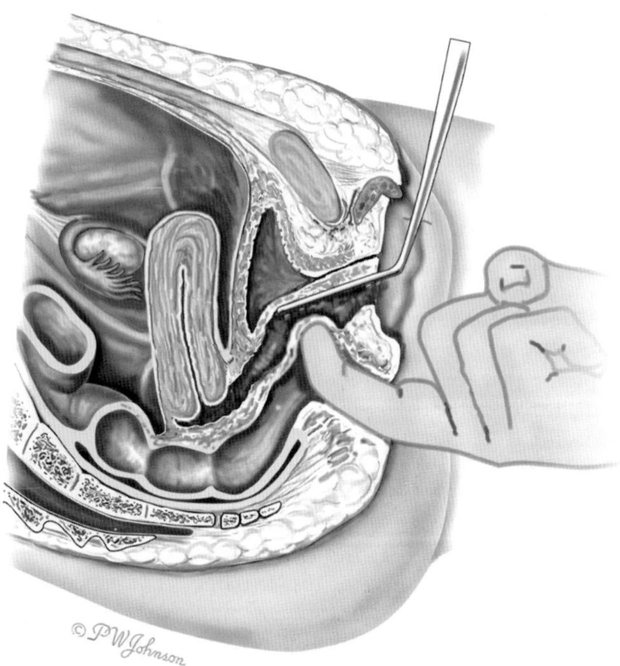

Figure 75-1 Examination of the posterior compartment with the index finger inserted into the rectum. Using the finger to push the posterior vaginal wall forward may reveal posterior wall weakness consistent with rectocele.

Table 75-2 Baden-Walker Rectocele Classification

Anatomic Grade	Description
Grade 1	Posterior wall protrusion toward introitus with strain
Grade 2	Posterior wall protrusion to the introitus with strain
Grade 3	Posterior wall protrusion outside of the introitus with strain
Grade 4	Posterior wall protrusion outside of the introitus at rest

wall forward (Fig. 75-1). Finger examination allows simultaneous assessment of the integrity of the rectovaginal fascia and the integrity of the external anal sphincter. Sphincter evaluation is especially important in patients who complain of fecal incontinence, and it can rule out other causes of defecatory dysfunction (e.g., rectal prolapse or intussusception, large hemorrhoids, skin tags). The perineal body should be evaluated for associated defects. Patients who present with a widened vaginal introitus or a shortened perineum, signified by a decreased distance between the posterior margin of the vagina and the anterior margin of the anus, may benefit from a simultaneous perineal repair.

We use the Baden-Walker system to classify rectoceles preoperatively (Table 75-2). In most cases, grade 1 rectoceles are incidental findings and asymptomatic. Only patients with grade 2 to grade 4 rectoceles and associated symptoms of stool trapping or the need to splint the vagina or perineum to facilitate defecation are considered candidates for surgical repair.

Ancillary Testing

No further evaluation is necessary in patients who present with symptomatic posterior prolapse without complicating factors. Patients with associated voiding complaints or anterior wall prolapse should undergo urodynamic evaluation before surgical intervention.

When patients have anatomic abnormalities (e.g., sigmoidocele, rectal prolapse, internal hemorrhoids) that can cause overlapping symptoms, defecating proctography may provide additional anatomic information. The study can also provide functional information regarding the efficiency of rectal emptying.[10] In other situations, given the patient's body habitus or limitations in lower extremity mobility, it may be difficult to delineate the exact compartment of prolapse. Dynamic magnetic resonance imaging (MRI)provides additional information that enables the appropriate treatment recommendation to be made. The study is performed with the patient in the standing position and consists of rapid-sequence MRI of the pelvis at rest and during Valsalva maneuvers. By simultaneous examination of all intrapelvic compartments, for example, an enterocele can be distinguished from a high rectocele and the appropriate operative procedure recommended.

PREOPERATIVE PREPARATION

Before performing prolapse repair, the urine is confirmed to be sterile. Patients are not routinely instructed on self-catheterization unless simultaneous transvaginal sling or cystocele repair is planned or the patient has incomplete emptying preoperatively. Preferably, patients should be started on stool softeners preoperatively in an attempt to regulate bowel function. Patients with vaginal wall atrophy should use estrogen vaginal cream for 4 to 6 weeks before surgery. Patients are instructed to use one third of an applicator of estrogen cream three times each week to improve the quality of tissue and postoperative healing properties. A povidone-iodine vaginal douche and a Fleet enema are performed the night before and the morning of surgery. Perioperative antibiotics are administered, preferably using a first-generation cephalosporin, ampicillin, or vancomycin (if allergic to penicillin) combined with an aminoglycoside.

When indicated, simultaneous transvaginal repair of associated anterior or apical prolapse is performed with the rectocele repair with cadaveric fascia. When multiple repairs are to be done, the rectocele repair with cadaveric fascia is performed last. A thorough discussion of the risks and complications of the procedure is undertaken with the patient before repair. Patients are counseled regarding the goals of surgery, which include restoration of anatomy, improvement of or relief from associated symptoms, and maintenance or restoration of visceral and sexual function.[11] Paraiso and coworkers[12] evaluated preoperative and postoperative symptoms that may predict outcome after a traditional posterior colporrhaphy. They found that preoperative constipation or straining to defecate predicted poor outcome after rectocele repair.[12]

OPERATIVE PROCEDURE

The procedure is performed with the patient in the dorsal lithotomy position. A Foley catheter is placed, and a Scott retractor (Lonestar, Houston, TX) is secured to the medial buttocks with towel clamps. When other procedures will be performed (e.g., transvaginal sling, cystocele repair, vaginal hysterectomy, enterocele repair, vaginal vault suspension), the procedures are completed, and the vaginal epithelium is closed before rectocele repair. To begin, a 1-0 silk suture is used to mark the apex of the rectocele, and the posterior vaginal wall is infiltrated with saline.

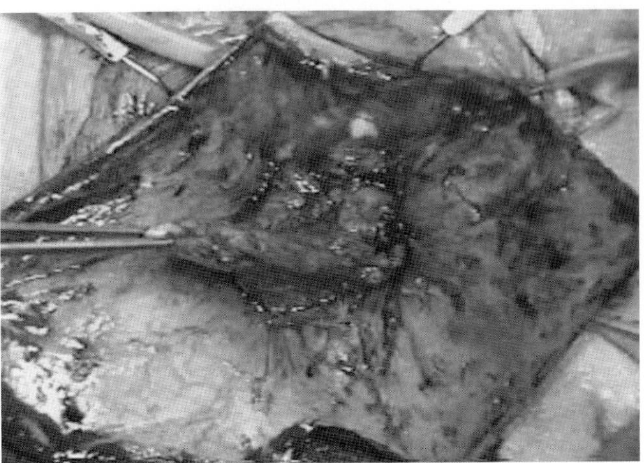

Figure 75-2 The rectum is dissected off of the posterior vaginal wall until the levator complex is exposed bilaterally.

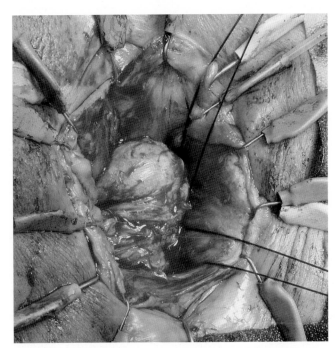

Figure 75-3 Two 1-0 polydioxanone sutures are placed within the levator complex on each side for attachment to the nonfrozen cadaveric fascia.

A midline incision is made in the posterior vaginal wall from the marking suture to the vaginal introitus. Using Metzenbaum scissors, the posterior vaginal wall is dissected off of the rectum on the white, shiny layer of the inner aspect of the vaginal wall. Dissection is continued until the levator complex, consisting of the levator ani musculature and the remaining rectovaginal fascia, is exposed bilaterally (Fig. 75-2). Four 1-0 polydioxanone attachment sutures (two per side) are placed laterally into the levator complex (Fig. 75-3), a fifth suture is placed at the apex of the rectocele near the previously placed marking suture, and a sixth suture is placed distally within the perineal body (Fig. 75-4).

A 4 × 7 cm piece of nonfrozen cadaveric fascia lata (Tutoplast), presoaked in antibiotic solution, is used to close the

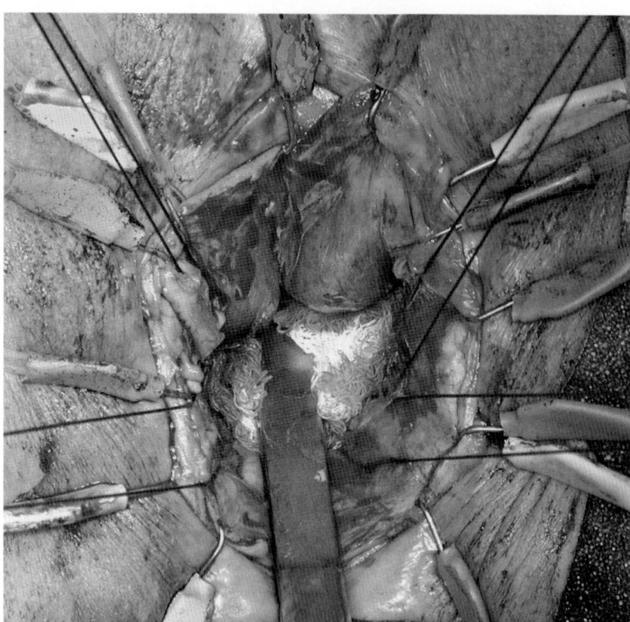

Figure 75-4 Sutures are in place within the levator complex bilaterally. Sites for apical suture and distal perineal suture are exposed.

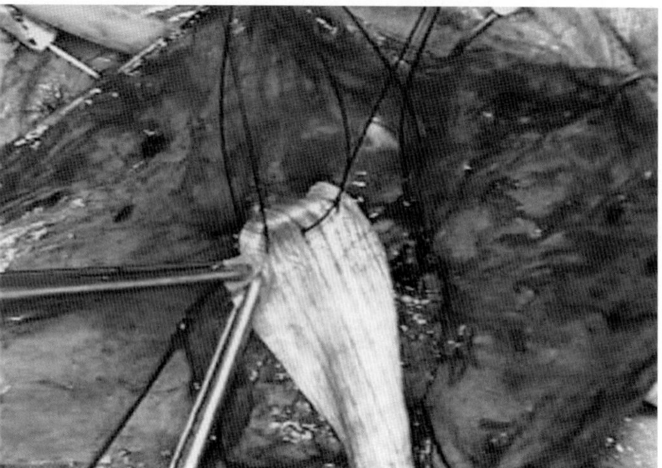

Figure 75-5 Sutures on one side are passed through the folded fascial edge and tied.

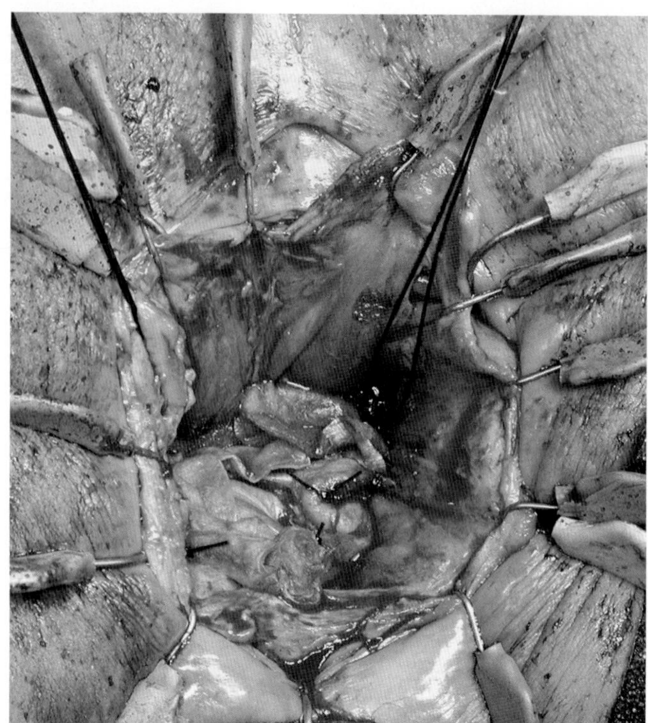

Figure 75-6 The remaining sutures are passed through the fascia and tied with the proper amount of tension.

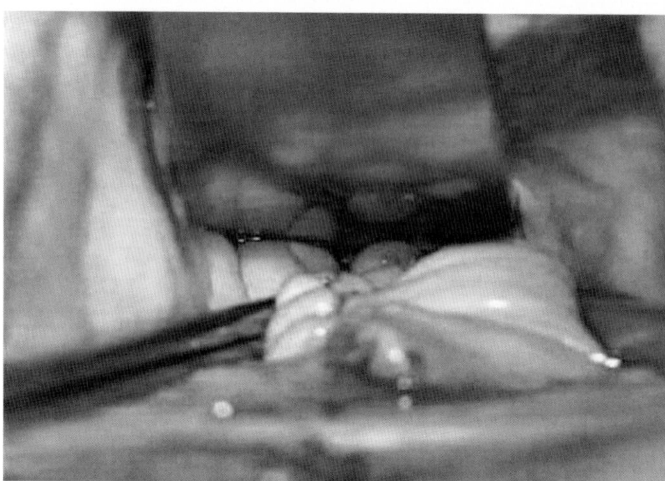

Figure 75-7 Vaginal width and depth are maintained after the rectocele repair with cadaveric fascia.

rectovaginal fascial defect. The edges of the fascia are folded over to minimize chances of suture pull-through.[13] The previously placed sutures are passed through the fascia on one side and tied (Fig. 75-5). The contralateral fascia edge is folded over, and the site for suture placement is measured to allow for proper tension. The contralateral sutures, apical suture, and distal suture are then passed through the fascia and tied (Fig. 75-6). Irrigation with antibiotic solution is performed throughout the procedure. After hemostasis is obtained, redundant vaginal epithelium is trimmed, and the incision is closed with running 2-0 absorbable suture. Care should be taken to avoid excess trimming of the vaginal epithelium and resultant tension on the vaginal closure, which can result in wound separation or vaginal narrowing postoperatively.

In patients with whom perineal reconstruction is indicated, Allis clamps are placed on the posterior fourchette at the 5-o'clock and 7-o'clock positions. The mucocutaneous junction and the underlying tissue are excised to expose the underlying perineal body. Vertical mattress sutures using 1-0 absorbable sutures are placed to reapproximate the central tendon, which is formed by the bulbocavernosus, superficial, and deep transverse perinei muscles (i.e., the urogenital diaphragm) and the external anal sphincter musculature at their junction with the levator ani musculature.[14] A subcuticular stitch is used to reapproximate the perineal skin.

At the conclusion of the repair, the vagina should comfortably admit two or three fingers (Fig. 75-7). A Foley catheter and a Betadine-soaked vaginal pack are left in place.

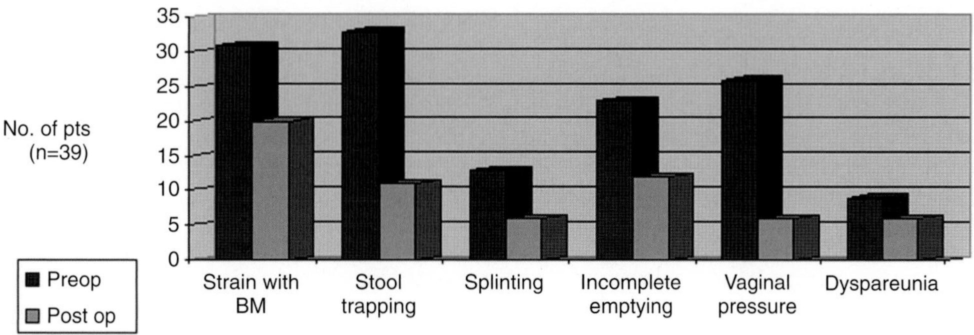

Figure 75-8 Rectocele Symptom Inventory: preoperative to postoperative changes. BM, bowel movement.

POSTOPERATIVE CARE

The vaginal packing and Foley catheter are removed on the morning of the first postoperative day. Fluid intake is restricted to 1500 mL per day. A voiding trial is administered, and residual urine measurement is obtained by means of intermittent catheterization. If residual urine measurements are more than 100 mL, patients are again instructed on self-catheterization. Urinary retention is a temporary complication reported for up to 12.5% of patients after posterior repair.[15]

Patients are continued on intravenous antibiotics for 24 hours postoperatively and then begun on an oral antibiotic (cephalexin or fluoroquinolone) for 1 week to minimize the risk of wound infection. Patients are routinely discharged on postoperative day one with oral analgesics. Stool softeners are continued for 1 month, and patients are counseled to avoid straining with defecation. Patients with elevated postvoid residual volumes are instructed to continue to monitor at home by self-catheterization until residual urine volumes are consistently less than 100 mL. If a patient is unable to learn or is uncomfortable performing self-catheterization, she can be discharged home with a Foley catheter and return for a trial of void in the office. At time of discharge, patients are instructed to avoid heavy lifting or straining and to observe pelvic rest (i.e., no intercourse, no tampons) for 6 weeks postoperatively.

Patients are seen for follow-up at 1 week, 6 weeks, 6 months, 12 months, and yearly thereafter. Evaluation consists of urinalysis, postvoid residual urine measurement, and physical examination. Patients are administered the confidential Rectocele Symptom Inventory preoperatively and at 6-month intervals postoperatively, the results of which are entered into a prospective database (see Table 75-1).

RESULTS

Prolapse Outcomes

Rectocele repair with cadaveric fascia has been performed on a total of 53 patients between the ages of 31 and 86 years (mean, 59.7 years). Forty patients (75%) had at least 6 months' follow-up (range, 6 to 54 months; mean, 19.6 months). All patients had symptomatic grade 2 to 4 rectoceles preoperatively. For 29 (72.5%) of 40 patients, rectoceles were grade 3; for 7 (17.5%) of 40 patients, rectoceles were grade 4; and for 4 (10%) of 40 patients, rectoceles were grade 2. Only 2 (50%) of 40 patients have had symptomatic rectocele recurrences (one grade 2 rectocele and one grade 3 rectocele).

Symptom Outcomes

Thirty-nine patients (74%) have at least 6 months of questionnaire follow-up (range, 6 to 50 months; mean, 25.1 months). A comparison of preoperative to postoperative symptoms based on questionnaire responses is provided in Figure 75-8. Specifically, 33 (85%) of 39 patients complained of significant symptoms of stool trapping preoperatively, and 13 (33%) of 39 complained of the need to perform vaginal or perineal splinting or postural changes to facilitate defecation preoperatively. Postoperatively, only 11 (28%) of 39 and 6 (15.4%) of 39 described stool trapping or need to splint, respectively. In regard to overall bowel function, 15 (38%) of 39 patients described their bowel function as "significantly improved," and 10 (25.6%) of 39 stated that they continued to have trouble with their bowel function.

Twenty-six patients were sexually active before the procedure. In regard to overall sexual function, 106 (38%) of 26 stated their sexual function was "significantly improved," and 12 (46%) of 26 stated their sexual function was "unchanged, not a problem," resulting in 22 (85%) of 26 of patients having stable or improved sexual function. Nine patients complained of significant dyspareunia preoperatively, which improved in 5 (55.6%) of the 9 patients. Only 2 (7.7%) of 26 developed de novo dyspareunia.

Overall, patient satisfaction with the procedure has been excellent, with 32 (82%) of 39 patients giving a satisfaction rating of 50% or more and 33 (85%) of 39 stating they would undergo the procedure again.

COMPLICATIONS

Most complications have been minor. Seven patients developed wound separation or granulation tissue, which healed with observation. Fecal urgency developed in one patient and was successfully treated with biofeedback. One patient suffered a mild cerebrovascular accident postoperatively and subsequently required transfer to a rehabilitation center. One patient had a rectotomy recognized intraoperatively that was repaired primarily. Despite intraoperative repair, the patient developed a postoperative rectovaginal fistula, which healed spontaneously with close observation and did not require operative intervention.

CONCLUSIONS

Rectocele repair with cadaveric fascia, using nonfrozen cadaveric fascia lata for posterior vaginal wall reconstruction, offers several advantages over traditional posterior colporrhaphy. Incorporation of durable graft tissue prevents a reliance on the patient's own tissue, which has an established propensity for weakness. By avoiding tissue plication and obliteration of the tissue in the midline, the degree of vaginal narrowing is minimal after rectocele repair with cadaveric fascia. In this way, complaints of postoperative dyspareunia are minimized, and patient satisfaction has been excellent. The avoidance of synthetic materials prevents subsequent graft erosion and wound infection associated with their use.

References

1. Kobashi KC, Leach GE, Frederick R, et al: Initial experience with rectocele repair using nonfrozen cadaveric fascia lata interposition. Urology 66:1203-1207; discussion 1207-1208, 2005.
2. Rosenblum N, Eilber KS, Rodriguez LV: Rectocele repair/posterior colporrhaphy. In Vasavada SP, Appell RA, Sand PK, Raz S (eds): Female Urology, Urogynecology, and Voiding Dysfunction. New York, Marcel Dekker, 2005.
3. Cundiff GW, Weidner AC, Visco AG, et al: An anatomic and functional assessment of the discrete defect rectocele repair. Am J Obstet Gyncol 179:1451-1457, 1998.
4. Porter WE, Steele A, Walsh P, et al: The anatomic and functional outcomes of the defect-specific rectocele repairs. Am J Obstet Gynecol 181:1353-1358, 1999.
5. Kenton K, Shott S, Brubaker L: Outcome after rectovaginal fascia reattachment for rectocele repair. Am J Obstet Gynecol 181:1360-1364, 1999.
6. Lemer ML, Chaikin DC, Blaivas JG: Tissue strength analysis of autologous and cadaveric allografts for the pubovaginal sling. Neurourol Urodyn 18:497-503, 1999.
7. Crawford JS: Nature of fascia lata and its fate after transplantation. Am J Opthamol 67:900, 1969.
8. Jinnah RH, Johnson C, Warden K, Clarke HJ: A biochemical analysis of solvent-dehydrated and freeze dried human fascia lata allografts. A preliminary report. Am J Sports Med 20:607-612, 1992.
9. Milani R, Salvatore S, Soligo M, et al: Functional and anatomical outcome of anterior and posterior vaginal prolapse repair with Prolene mesh. BJOG 112:107-111, 2005.
10. Birch C, Fynes M: Mesh erosion complicating vaginal surgery for the correction of posterior compartment prolapse. Poster presentation at the 34th annual meeting of the International Continence Society and the International Urogynecological Association Colloquium (ICS/IUGA), August 23-27, 2004, Paris, France.
11. Segal JL, Karram MM: Evaluation and management of rectoceles. In Vasavada SP, Appell RA, Sand PK, Raz S (eds): Female Urology, Urogynecology, and Voiding Dysfunction. New York, Marcel Dekker, 2005.
12. Paraiso MF, Weber AM, Walters MD: Anatomic and functional outcome after posterior colporrhaphy. J Pelvic Surg 129:524-529, 2001.
13. Sutaria PM, Staskin DR: A comparison of fascial "pull-through" strength using four different suture fixation techniques [abstract]. J Urol 161:79, 1999.
14. Babiarz JW, Raz S: Pelvic floor relaxation. In Raz S (ed): Female Urology. Philadelphia, WB Saunders, 1996.
15. Rovner ES, Gindsberg DA: Posterior vaginal wall prolapse: Transvaginal repair of pelvic floor relaxation, rectocele, and perineal laxity. Tech Urol 7:161-168, 2001.

Chapter 76

PERINEAL HERNIA AND PERINEOCELE

Christian Twiss and Nirit Rosenblum

Perineal hernia is an uncommon condition that was once thought to be incurable because of the difficulty in closing the hernia defect and the high recurrence rate.[1] The past century witnessed the development of a plethora of techniques to repair perineal hernias and an improved understanding of the anatomic defects, leading to their classification. Despite the knowledge gained, much remains to be discovered about perineal hernias. There are no controlled studies to guide the clinician in the choice of optimal therapy. Perineocele is an even less studied and less well-defined clinical problem. Both conditions are discussed in this chapter.

PERINEAL HERNIA

Definition and Classification

Perineal hernias occur through focal defects within the pelvic floor, and they are classified by primary cause and by anatomic region. Primary perineal hernias are focal, acquired defects within the pelvic floor that typically occur in women as a result of pelvic relaxation associated with vaginal parity or chronic conditions involving increased abdominal pressure (e.g., chronic cough, constipation, ascites). Secondary perineal hernias are true incisional hernias within the pelvic floor that result from prior pelvic (typically exenterative) surgery.

Herniation can occur through the anterior or posterior compartments of the pelvic floor. Anterior perineal hernias (i.e., pudendal hernias, pudendal enteroceles, or levator hernias) occur within the urogenital triangle anterior to the superficial transverse perineal muscles, and they occur exclusively in women; no confirmed cases in men have been reported. Anterior perineal hernias occur through the urogenital diaphragm within the triangular regions lateral to each side of the vaginal vestibule defined by the medial border of the ischiocavernosus muscle, the lateral border of the bulbocavernosus muscle, and the anterior border of the superficial transverse perineal muscle (Fig. 76-1). Posterior perineal hernias occur in within the anal triangle posterior to the superficial transverse perineal muscles and anterior to the ventral borders of the gluteus maximus muscles. They typically occur midway between the anus and the ischial tuberosity within a levator ani defect, in the space between the pubococcygeus and iliococcygeus portions of the levator ani muscle, or in the space between the levator ani and coccygeus muscles (see Fig. 76-1).

Translevator and supralevator hernias are anatomically distinct.[2] A translevator perineal hernia sac passes through the focal defect within the levator ani musculature, whereas a supralevator hernia sac remains superior to the levator ani but exists as a focal outpouching of the weakened levator ani muscle that extends beyond the plane of the levator plate. Despite the anatomic difference, the principles of hernia repair remain the same.

The hernia sac of a perineal hernia may be empty (i.e., peritoneum) or may contain one or more of the abdominopelvic viscera, including small or large bowel, bladder, omentum, ovary, and fallopian tube. Because intraperitoneal and extraperitoneal structures may herniate, a true hernia sac may not always be present.[1]

Etiology and Epidemiology

Anterior perineal hernias can be primary or secondary (i.e., after surgery or obstetric procedures). Anterior perineal hernias are rare, with fewer than 17 well-described cases in the English literature.[1,3-6] Most reported perineal hernias are posterior perineal hernias. The largest reported series of anterior perineal hernias is that of Chase in 1922, reporting 13 cases.[1] However, only 10 of these 13 cases were described in enough detail to be confirmed cases of anterior perineal hernia. All of the well-described cases of anterior perineal hernia appear to have occurred in the setting of multiple prior pelvic operations for pelvic prolapse or urinary incontinence or of difficult and prolonged labor, often requiring forceps delivery. Both causes involve direct trauma to the pelvic floor musculature, which is thought to be the primary cause of anterior perineal hernias. Most anterior perineal hernias are secondary.

Posterior perineal hernias may be primary or secondary. Primary perineal hernias are rare, and their true incidence is unknown. They typically occur between the ages of 40 and 60 years, and they occur more commonly in women, with a female preponderance of threefold to fivefold higher than for men.[7,8] This female preponderance is attributed to female pelvic floor trauma encountered during childbirth[9] and the phenomenon

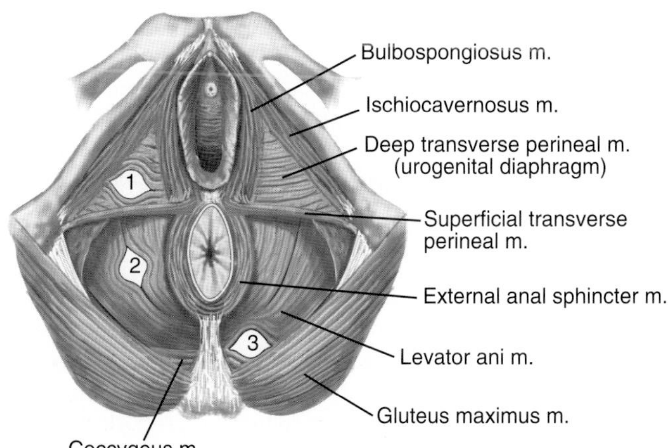

Figure 76-1 Anatomy of perineum and typical locations of perineal hernias. (Modified from Cali RL, Pitsch RM, Blatchford GJ, et al: Rare pelvic floor hernias. Dis Colon Rectum 35:604, 1992.).

Table 76-1 Risk Factors for Perineal Hernias

Primary perineal hernia
Female gender
Vaginal childbirth
Prolonged or difficult labor
Pelvic organ prolapse or pelvic floor descent
Recurrent infections of pelvic floor
Chronic cough
Chronic constipation
Obesity
Abdominal ascites
Secondary perineal hernia
Female gender
Abdominoperineal resection
Open postoperative perineal wound
Pelvic exenteration
Radical cystourethrectomy
Coccygectomy
Anti-incontinence surgery
Hysterectomy
Pelvic organ prolapse surgery
Perineal prostatectomy
Pelvic irradiation
Excessive length of small bowel mesentery

Table 76-2 Differential Diagnosis of Perineal Hernia

Diagnosis	Clinical Features
Anterior perineal masses	
Anterior perineal hernia	Labial mass reduces into pelvic floor medial to pubic ramus
Inguinal hernia	Labial mass reduces into inguinal canal across pubic ramus
Bartholin gland abscess	Labial mass irreducible, fluctuant, signs of inflammation
Lipoma or sarcoma	Labial mass, irreducible
Hematoma	Labial mass, irreducible, history or signs of perineal trauma
Cystocele, rectocele, enterocele	Introital mass, associated urinary or fecal symptoms
Posterior perineal masses	
Posterior perineal hernia	Soft, reducible, posterior to perineum
Sciatic hernia	Emerges on inferior border of gluteus maximus
Rectal prolapse	Emerges from anus, associated constipation or fecal incontinence
Perineocele	Pelvic descent, increased anovaginal distance

of pelvic relaxation.[10] A study by Gearhart and colleauges[10] demonstrated a 15% incidence of levator ani hernia in a group of 80 patients who underwent dynamic pelvic magnetic resonance imaging (MRI) for the evaluation of symptomatic pelvic organ prolapse. Forty-two percent of these patients had undergone prior pelvic surgery, and approximately 60% (or 9% of the entire group) are presumed to be primary levator ani hernias associated with symptomatic pelvic organ prolapse. Other conditions are also thought to contribute to the formation of primary perineal hernia, including recurrent pelvic floor infections and conditions involving increased abdominal pressure such as chronic cough, chronic constipation, obesity, and ascites (Table 76-1).[8,11,12]

Secondary posterior perineal hernias occur through defects in the pelvic floor resulting from surgery, and they usually manifest within 1 year after the initial surgery.[9] Most secondary perineal hernias occur after pelvic exenterative surgery, requiring corrective surgery after approximately 0.7% of abdominoperineal resections[13] and 3% of pelvic exenterations.[14] The true incidence of perineal hernia after these procedures is likely higher, and most are asymptomatic. Hullsiek[15] found a 7% incidence of perineal hernia after abdominoperineal resection by means of barium x-ray films, and most were asymptomatic.

Secondary posterior[16] and anterior[3,5,6] perineal hernias have been reported after surgery for pelvic prolapse and urinary incontinence. However, their overall incidence after prolapse and incontinence surgery is unknown. It is difficult to determine whether these hernias result from the prolapse surgery or the pathophysiologic process of pelvic prolapse itself. Presumably, it is a combination of both because a significant proportion (42%) of perineal hernias associated with symptomatic pelvic prolapse occur in the absence of a history of pelvic surgery.[10]

Table 76-1 summarizes the types of operations associated with secondary perineal hernias. Poor perineal tissue quality and factors that hinder wound healing such as diabetes and pelvic irradiation also predispose to perineal hernia. One of the most significant predisposing factors for perineal hernia after abdominoperineal resection was found to be a partial or complete open perineal wound in the postoperative period.[17]

Symptoms and Clinical Findings

Anterior perineal hernia typically manifests as a reducible labial mass, usually in the posterior aspect of the labia majora. This may be accompanied by a heavy sensation within the perineum.[4] The mass is characteristically covered with vaginal mucosa on its medial border and the labial integument on its lateral border. An anterior perineal hernia is also characteristically reducible into the pelvic floor medial and inferior to the pubic ramus, whereas an inguinal hernia within the labia reduces into the inguinal canal by crossing over the pubic ramus. The reducibility of the hernia also distinguishes it from irreducible labial masses such as Bartholin's gland abscesses or cysts, benign labial cysts, labial lipomas and sarcomas, and labial hematomas (Table 76-2). Careful vaginal and perineal examination is needed to avoid inadvertent incision into a perineal hernia that many contain bladder or bowel.

It is not uncommon for anterior perineal hernias to contain bladder because defects within the anterior pelvic floor more often contain bladder.[3] This can result in urinary sequelae, including urinary incontinence, weak urinary stream, and incomplete bladder emptying with high postvoid residual volumes.[4,6] Patients with concurrent urinary symptoms should undergo diagnostic cystoscopy and imaging of the lower urinary tract.

Posterior perineal hernias typically manifest as soft, reducible masses within the posterior perineum (posterior to the perineal body), usually occurring in the region between the anus and ischial tuberosity, but they may also emerge just ventral to the gluteus maximus, in which case they must be distinguished from a sciatic hernia, which is rare.[12] They are often asymptomatic,[10] but they may be accompanied by a heavy or dragging feeling within the perineal region and pain with sitting.

Perineal hernias usually do not incarcerate or strangulate because the pelvic floor defect is often large and the hernia remains easily reducible. However, there are reports of postoperative perineal hernia that have been accompanied by bowel obstruction and perineal skin breakdown.[18,19] Often, the bowel obstruction is intermittent and occurs because of bowel compression when the patient is sitting.

Evaluation

There is no consensus on the workup of perineal hernias beyond a careful history and vaginal, perineal, and rectal examinations. The examination should focus on diagnosing the hernia and evaluate the possibility of cystocele, rectocele, or rectal prolapse, because some perineal hernias occur in the setting of pelvic organ prolapse.

In suspected cases of anterior perineal hernia with accompanying urinary symptoms, cystourethrography and cystoscopy are recommended to confirm the presence of bladder within the hernia and to determine whether the trigone is involved in the hernia. This seems reasonable because the bladder is more commonly involved in anterior perineal hernias. If cystourethrography is performed solely to confirm presence of bladder within the perineal hernia, other modalities such as computed tomography (CT) or pelvic MRI could derive the same information.

Further imaging of the suspected hernia is warranted to confirm the diagnosis and to provide additional information for surgical planning, such as which pelvic contents are present within the hernia, where the hernia emerges from the pelvic floor, and an estimation of the size of the defect. It is arguable whether a careful physical examination can derive all this information except for the exact contents of the hernia sac. However, the most conservative approach is to obtain the most information about the hernia through careful examination and pelvic imaging before its repair.

Plain radiographs of the pelvis and barium enema are able to demonstrate bowel within the hernia sac.[20] Dynamic proctography, typically used to evaluate defecatory dysfunction, is able to demonstrate the extent and involved segment of perineal rectal herniation.[7] The presumed advantage over barium enema is applicable for cases in which the perineal herniation occurs only during straining and defecation. CT evaluation of the pelvic floor is more definitively able to identify the contents of the hernia sac and the location and extent of the associated pelvic floor defect.[11]

MRI is gaining acceptance as a preferred method of evaluation of the pelvic floor because of its excellent resolution of pelvic floor[21,22] and perianal[23] structures and the ability to visualize the prolapsing pelvic organs in real time by dynamic pelvic MRI. In addition to its utility in visualizing pelvic organ prolapse with an anatomic staging system,[24] dynamic pelvic MRI was able to detect unsuspected levator ani hernias in 15% of patients undergoing evaluation for symptomatic pelvic organ prolapse.[10] Pelvic MRI was also able to preoperatively detect a large unsuspected posterior perineal hernia associated with recurrent vaginal vault prolapse, thereby changing operative management.[2] These two studies highlight some important considerations. They confirm that perineal hernias occur in conjunction with pelvic organ prolapse and that clinicians treating these patients should maintain a degree of clinical suspicion about the diagnosis. As MRI evaluation of pelvic organ prolapse increases, the number of unsuspected perineal hernias can also be expected to increase. This ultimately presents a need and an opportunity to create patient cohorts to study and further define a protocol for the management of perineal hernia that occurs in the setting of pelvic organ prolapse.

Treatment

The treatment for perineal hernias is surgical, but there is no clearly defined protocol for their management. Because they rarely incarcerate and strangulate, the primary indication for the repair of perineal hernias is patient discomfort. The general principles remain the same as for any hernia: exposure of the sac and the musculofascial defect, opening of the sac with reduction of its contents, and high ligation of the sac followed by closure of the musculofascial defect. There remain two important caveats. First, there is not always a clearly defined sac, because not all pelvic contents (especially bladder) are completely covered by peritoneum. Second, the fascial defect encountered can be quite extensive, especially in post-exenterative perineal hernias requiring advanced reconstructive maneuvers.

There are three basic approaches to repair: perineal, abdominal, and a combined perineal and abdominal approach. Two reports described a laparoscopic mesh repair technique.[25,26] There are no controlled studies demonstrating the superiority of any one approach. However, the combined experience of several surgeons demonstrates the applicability of each approach to management.

A key concept that determines the goals and techniques of repair is whether the hernia has occurred after pelvic exenterative surgery (i.e., pelvic exenteration or abdominoperineal resection). The repair of perineal hernias in this setting typically involves the repair of a large pelvic floor defect requiring an extensive reconstruction of the pelvic floor (Table 76-3). Cancer recurrence and bowel adhesions are additional considerations that affect the operative goals at the time of repair. Perineal hernias after non-exenterative surgery are typically more localized defects in the pelvic floor that do not require advanced reconstructive techniques. Because the pelvic organs are still in place, most pelvic reconstructive techniques described for the repair of post-exenterative perineal hernias are not feasible in the absence of prior pelvic exenterative surgery. However, because pelvic relaxation and pelvic organ prolapse are predisposing factors of perineal hernias, their surgical correction needs to be considered at the time of repair.

The perineal approach (or translabial approach in the case of anterior perineal hernias) remains the least invasive one with the advantages of less morbidity and success in most cases.[17] The perineal approach also allows resection of residual perineal skin that may accompany sizable perineal hernias.[27] However, the exposure is limited, allowing less access to sac contents, adhesions, recurrent cancer, or injured viscera or vasculature.[28] Recurrences have also been reported with the perineal approach.[6,17,28] In the small series of postoperative perineal hernias reported by So and coworkers,[17] the perineal approach carried a 23% recurrence rate, compared with no recurrences after repairs using the

Table 76-3 Techniques of Perineal Hernia Repair

Year	Study	Method
1944	Cattel and Cunnigham[31]	Uterus to uterosacral ligaments
1951	Koontz[8]	Local muscle and fascia
1960	Kelly[19]	Fascia lata
1963	Cawkwell[54]	Nylon mesh
1967	Bach-Nielsen[55]	Uterus to sacrum and pelvic wall
1973	Buchsbaum and White[56]	Omental sling
1975	Alexander et al[57]	Mesenteric leaf
1980	Bell et al[58]	Gracilis myocutaneous flap
1981	Hurwitz and Walton[35]	Gluteal thigh flap
1981	Leuchter et al[59]	Bulbocavernosus myocutaneous flap
1982	Sarr et al[37]	Marlex mesh
1984	Giampapa et al[60]	Rectus abdominis muscle flap
1985	Brotschi et al[33]	Gracilis muscle sling
1987	Beck et al[28]	Marlex mesh
1987	Delmore et al[32]	Human dura
1989	Frydman and Polglase[29]	Polypropylene mesh
1995	Erdmann and Waterhouse[38]	Rectus abdominis flap
1997	So et al[17]	Gore-Tex patch
2002	Franklin et al[25]	Laparoscopic Vicryl mesh
2002	Ghellai et al[26]	Laparoscopic polypropylene mesh

Modified from Abdul Jabbar AS: Postoperative perineal hernia. Hernia 6:188, 2002.

abdominal or combined approach. Perineal repairs have been performed with[4,27,29,30] and without[5,6,17] mesh repair of the hernia defect. Because of its simplicity, the perineal approach has been recommended as the best initial approach for straightforward cases,[4,17,27] reserving the abdominal and abdominoperineal approach for recurrent cases, cases of strangulation of the hernia contents, or situations in which primary closure of the defect is complex.

The perineal technique involves a skin incision over the site of the hernia defect after sterile preparation of the perineum. In the case of anterior perineal hernias, this is directly over or alongside the involved major labium. If bladder (especially trigonal) involvement is suspected, prophylactic ureteral stents also may be placed. This is followed by careful dissection of the sac from the skin and then the margins of the hernia defect itself. In the case of post-exenterative hernias, the dissection during this step must be meticulous because it is a frequent source of bowel injuries.[18]

In cases of small hernia defects in which there is a clearly defined sac, the hernia sac is opened, the contents are reduced, and the sac is ligated and excised. Any additional nonperitonealized hernia contents, such as bladder, are also reduced. This is followed by repair of the hernia defect using a simple layered closure with or without mesh reinforcement on the pelvic side of the hernia defect.

When the pelvic viscera are in place, larger defects that cannot be closed primarily require mesh repair. Interposition of uterus has been reported.[31] In cases of large post-exenterative hernias, simple closure of the levator ani defect is usually not possible, and pelvic floor reconstruction is required using synthetic mesh, free fascial grafts, or pedicled flaps (see Table 76-3).[27-29,32-35]

The abdominal approach has been recommended as the best first approach by some surgeons,[3,8,9,12,28] primarily because of better exposure of the anatomic defect and hernia sac. This is especially true in the cases of large pelvic floor defects requiring mesh reconstruction of the pelvic floor.[9,27,28] The abdominal approach facilitates proper fixation of the mesh to the pelvic and sacral support structures, and it assists simultaneous treatment of bowel adhesions and cancer recurrence after exenterative surgery.[28] The abdominal approach also facilitates sacral resuspension of pelvic contents such as herniated rectum[36] or prolapsed vaginal vault,[2] and it permits closure of the cul-de-sac to prevent abdominal contents from accessing the area of the repaired hernia defect.[6] In cases of strangulation of the hernia contents, the abdominal approach is required to address the need for possible resection or repair of the hernia contents.

For the abdominal approach, the patient should be placed in the modified lithotomy position to allow simultaneous access to the perineum. This enables perineal traction to be applied to assist in the dissection and allows vaginal access to assist in identification of the vaginal cuff. It also permits conversion to a combined approach and possible placement of ureteral stents.[28]

Access is obtained through a lower midline incision, followed by possible exploration for recurrent cancer in post-exenterative cases. The hernia sac is identified, and the sac is dissected free from the margins of the defect. A small defect can be repaired with layered closure or mesh, whereas larger post-exenterative defects typically require more complex reconstruction of the pelvic floor as previously discussed.

The abdominoperineal or combined approach provides maximal exposure of the hernia sac and hernia defect. It is especially useful in cases in which the pelvic floor defect is difficult to access by the abdominal route[3] and in cases of large perineal hernias in which the redundant skin if the perineum must be resected.[36,37] A laparoscopic combined approach has also been described[25] in which the hernia contents are mobilized by a laparoscopic intraperitoneal approach, followed by open perineal repair of the levator defect and subsequent laparoscopic reinforcement of the repair with polypropylene mesh on the pelvic side of the repair.

The list of methods that have been used to address the hernia defect is extensive (see Table 76-3), but there are no controlled trials demonstrating the superiority of any approach. In general, small defects with healthy tissue can be addressed by closing the levator defect primarily with nonabsorbable sutures. This can also be reinforced with mesh. When this is not possible or simple closure has failed, the use of synthetic mesh has produced durable repairs regardless of the surgical approach.[6,25,28,36,37] However, when the tissue is infected, the tissue quality is poor, or the mesh has failed, the transposition of healthy, well-vascularized tissue by flap reconstruction is often required.[17] Flap repairs using gracilis,[33,34] fascia lata,[18] rectus abdominis,[38] and gluteus maximus[35] have been described.

There is no single correct approach to the repair of a perineal hernia. The choice ultimately depends on the size of the defect, the patient's surgical history, the condition of the tissues, the condition and extent of the hernia sac contents, and the comfort level of the surgeon.

PERINEOCELE

Definition

Perineocele is typically synonymous with perineal hernia.[39] However, perineal hernia is a misnomer because many perineal hernias occur as labial swellings or swellings close to the buttocks and not on the perineum. Although perineal hernias remain focal defects within the pelvic floor, there is a related but separate clinical entity involving a diffuse weakening and bulging of the entire perineum itself due to an acquired attenuation of the perineal central tendon (Figs. 76-2 and 76-3).[40,41] This has a symptom complex and treatment strategy that differs from the perineal hernias previously described. We think that *perineocele* is the term most appropriate for this condition because it is a pelvic floor herniation of the perineum itself and a clinical entity that differs from a classic perineal hernia.

The two anatomic defects associated with perineoceles are convex deformity plus descent of the perineum with abdominal straining and widening of the distance between the posterior vaginal fourchette and the anus.[40,41] Whereas the typical distance between the posterior fourchette and anus is 3 cm,[42] this distance can increase to as much as 8 to 14 cm in large perineoceles.[40,41] These defects are caused by a musculofascial disruption of the perineal body itself.

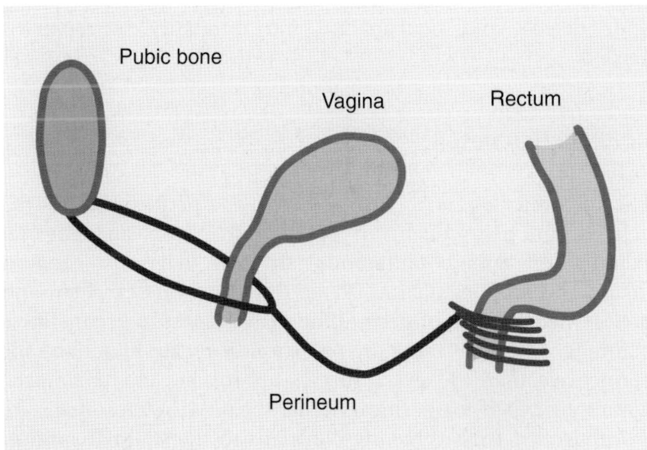

Figure 76-2 Schematic diagram of the anatomic defect of a perineocele. (Modified from Raz S: Repair of perineal hernia. In Atlas of Transvaginal Surgery, 2nd ed. Philadelphia, WB Saunders, 2002.).

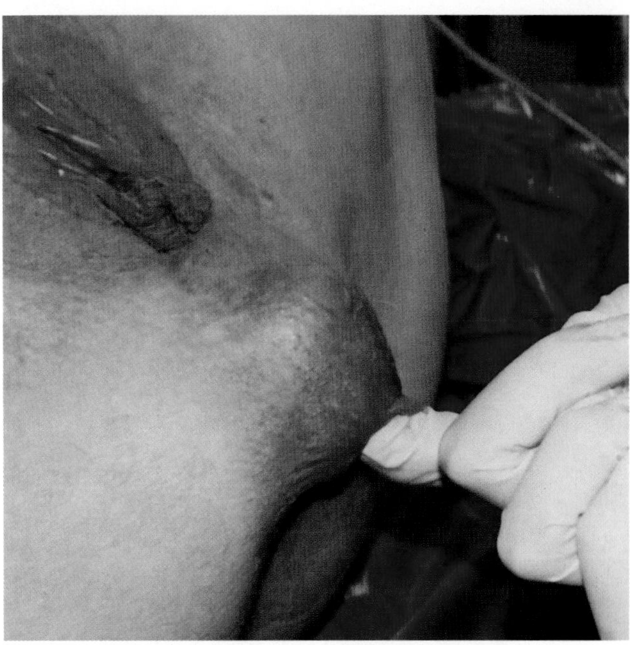

Figure 76-3 Physical examination for perineocele. (From Raz S: Repair of perineal hernia. In Atlas of Transvaginal Surgery, 2nd ed. Philadelphia, WB Saunders, 2002.).

Etiology and Epidemiology

The true incidence of perineocele has not been reported. Perineocele is thought to result from the process of pelvic floor relaxation, which is associated with the pelvic floor damage that occurs during childbirth. Lacerations to the perineum occur when the pelvic floor and perineum are stretched excessively during the second stage of labor.[43,44] Childbirth also lowers the position of the perineum,[45] which can take up to 5 years to return to its normal position.[46] It is unclear whether perineocele results from direct pelvic floor damage from childbirth or from the condition of abnormal perineal descent, or both.

Symptoms and Clinical Features

In addition to having a perineal bulge between the anus and vagina, patients with perineoceles present with additional symptoms distinct from perineal hernias. They have a feeling of perineal pressure, and they typically present with chronic constipation and a possible need to apply perineal pressure to defecate.[40,41] The descending perineum syndrome, first described by Parks and associates,[47] is characterized by downward descent of the perineum during straining efforts and is associated with chronic constipation hallmarked by excessive straining with bowel movements and perineal pain. Fecal or urinary incontinence and vaginal prolapse may also be associated. The continued downward displacement of the perineum in descending perineum syndrome causes chronic stretching of the pudendal

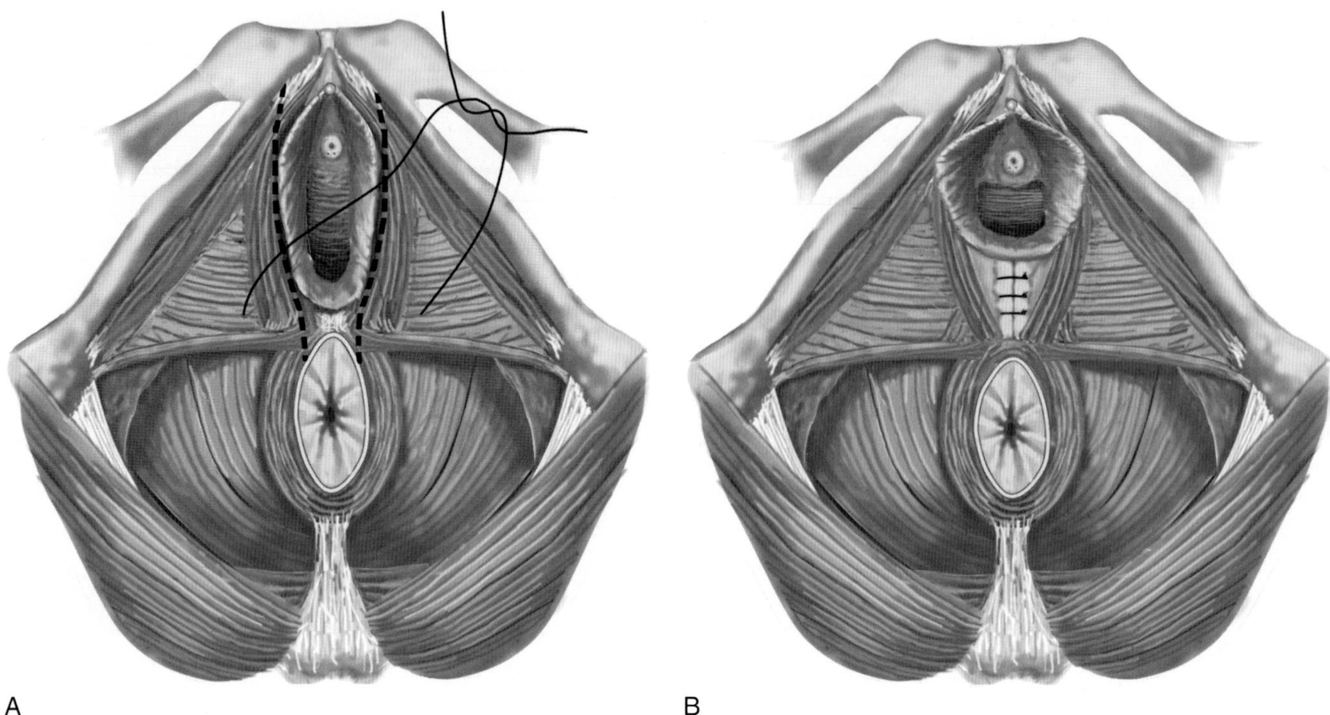

Figure 76-4 The goal of standard perineorrhaphy is to lengthen the perineum and shorten a widened genital hiatus. (Modified from Nichols DH: Posterior colporrhaphy and perineorrhaphy: Separate and distinct operations. Am J Obstet Gynecol 164:714, 1991.).

nerve, leading to worsening of the pelvic floor tone and anal tone.[48-50]

Perineocele and the descending perineum syndrome share some of the same clinical features, and it is interesting to postulate that they are in the same clinical spectrum. However, further investigation is required to determine whether perineoceles are perineal hernias with a distinct location and distinct clinical features or are dynamic defects in the pelvic floor that lead to progressive pelvic floor neuropathy and the descending perineal syndrome.

Treatment

The treatment of perineocele is surgical. Because there is no focal defect within the pelvic floor through which to reduce the sac and repair, the surgical technique differs from that of a typical perineal hernia. The goal of repair is to reconstruct the perineal body such that distance between the posterior vaginal fourchette and the anus, the perineal body length, is returned to its normal length of approximately 3 cm. This differs from the goal of standard perineorrhaphy, which is to repair the perineum in such a manner as to lengthen the attenuated perineal body while simultaneously reducing the anteroposterior length of the widened genital hiatus (Fig. 76-4).[51]

There is scant literature on the repair of perineoceles because it remains a relatively understudied clinical entity. Raz[41] has described a perineal site-specific technique for the repair of perineocele in which the levator musculature anterior to the anal sphincter is reapproximated to the transverse perineal muscles using a series of interrupted horizontal mattress sutures (Fig. 76-5). This technique is used to repair the anatomic defect and its associated symptoms, including constipation. There are no long-term data on the durability of this repair. Other investigators have made efforts to specifically address the perineum and perineal descent in the repair of pelvic floor prolapse by affixing the perineum to the sacrum with synthetic mesh while repairing vaginal vault prolapse.[52,53] However, it is not clear whether these techniques are applicable to the repair of perineocele because they correct perineal descent and its symptoms but do not address the condition of the widened perineum itself.

Perineocele, although a poorly studied condition, is a clearly defined anatomic defect of the pelvic floor that is distinct from classically described anterior and posterior perineal hernias. It is typically associated with chronic constipation, and it remains unclear whether it also carries the pelvic neuropathic sequelae of abnormal perineal descent. The study of a large group of these patients with respect to risk factors, possible associated pelvic floor defects and neuropathy, and durability of repair is needed.

CONCLUSIONS

The anatomic defects of perineal hernia and perineocele are well defined, and a careful history, clinical suspicion, and physical examination remain tantamount to their diagnosis. Modern imaging techniques such as CT and MRI provide excellent and precise visualization of perineal hernias to assist in preoperative planning. Although there are few surgical repairs described for perineocele, there are several surgical approaches and repair techniques described for perineal hernia repair. However, there are no controlled trials directing clinicians to the optimal surgical approach or repair technique. Surgical treatment remains individualized, depending on the size and nature of the hernia defect, the condition of the tissues, and the comfort level and judgment of the surgeon.

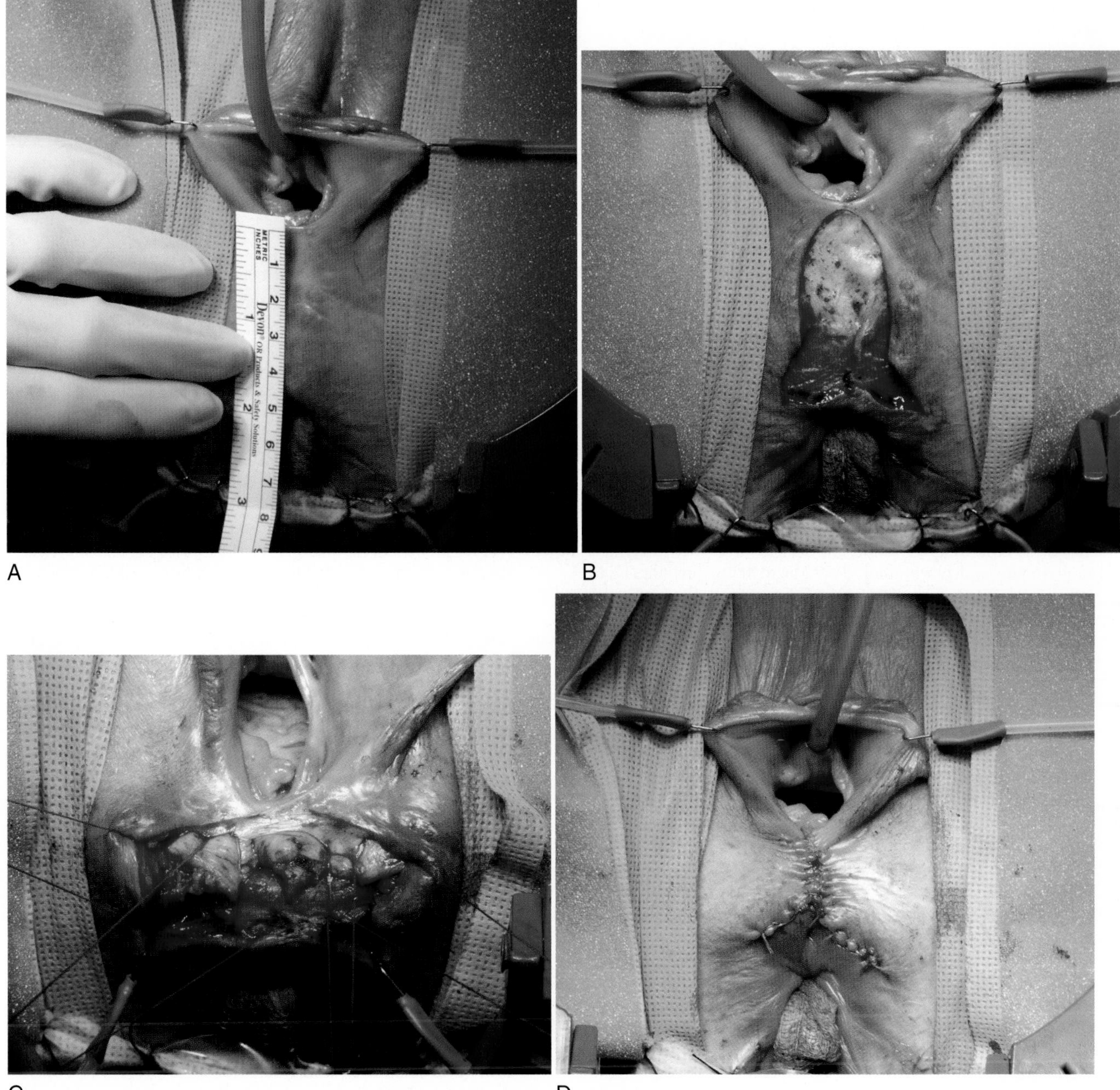

Figure 76-5 The goal of a perineocele repair is to shorten and strengthen the widened perineum by reapproximating the anal sphincter toward the superficial transverse perineal muscles. **A,** A 5-cm perineocele. **B,** Inverted Y incision to expose the defect. **C,** Suturing of the levator ani just anterior to the anus to the transverse perineal muscles. **D,** Repaired perineocele.

References

1. Chase HC: Levator hernia (pudendal hernia). Surg Gynecol Obstet 35:717, 1922.
2. Singh K, Reid WMN, Berger LA: Translevator gluteal hernia. Int Urogynecol J 12:407, 2001.
3. Hermann G: Pudendal (labial) hernia: Report of a case. N Engl J Med 265:435, 1961.
4. Anderson WR: Pudendal hernia. Unusual cause of labial mass. Obstet Gynecol 32:802, 1968.
5. Brodak PP, Juma S, Raz S: Levator hernia. J Urol 148:872, 1992.
6. Zimmern PE, Miyazaki F: Pudendal enterocele with bladder involvement. Urology 44:918, 1994.
7. Poon FW, Lauder JC, Finlay IG: Perineal herniation. Clin Radiol 47:49, 1993.
8. Koontz AR: Perineal hernia: Report of a case with many associated muscular and fascial defects. Ann Surg 133:255, 1951.
9. Pearl RK: Perineal hernia. In Nyhus LM, Condon RE (eds): Hernia, 4th ed. Philadelphia, JB Lippincott, 1995, pp 451-454.
10. Gearhart S, Pannu HK, Cundiff GW, et al: Perineal descent and levator ani hernia: A dynamic magnetic resonance imaging study. Dis Colon Rectum 47:1298, 2004.
11. Lubat E, Gordon RB, Birnbaum BA, et al: CT diagnosis of posterior perineal hernia. Am J Radiol 154:761, 1990.

12. Cali RL, Pitsch RM, Blatchford GJ, et al: Rare pelvic floor hernias. Dis Colon Rectum 35:604, 1992.
13. McMullin ND, Johnson WR, Polglase AL, et al: Post-proctectomy perineal hernia: Case report and discussion. Aust N Z J Surg 55:69, 1985.
14. Rutledge FN, Smith JP, Wharton JT, et al: Pelvic exenteration: Analysis of 296 patients. Am J Obstet Gynecol 129:881, 1973.
15. Hullsiek HE: Perineal hernia following abdominoperineal resection. Am J Surg 92:735, 1956.
16. Silva-Filho AL, Santos-Filho AS, Figueiredo-Netto O, et al: Uncommon complications of sacrospinous fixation for treatment of vaginal vault prolapse. Arch Gynecol Obstet 271:358, 2005.
17. So JB, Palmer MT, Shellito PC: Postoperative perineal hernia. Dis Colon Rectum 40:954, 1997.
18. Ego-Aguirre, E, Spratt JS, Butcher HR. et al: Repair of perineal hernias developing subsequent to pelvic exenteration. Ann Surg 159:66, 1964.
19. Kelly AR: Surgical repair of post-operative perineal hernia. Aust N Z J Surg 29:243, 1960.
20. Trackler RT, Koehler PR: The radiographic findings in posterior perineal hernia. Radiology 91:950, 1968.
21. Kelvin FM, Maglinte DDT, Hale DS, et al: Female pelvic organ prolapse: A comparison of triphasic dynamic mr imaging and triphasic fluoroscopic cystocolpoproctography. Am J Radiol 174:81, 2000.
22. Barbaric ZL, Marumoto AK, Raz S: Magnetic resonance imaging of the perineum and pelvic floor. Top Magn Reson Imaging 12:83, 2001.
23. Morren GL, Beets-Tan RG, van Engelshoven JM: Anatomy of the anal canal and perianal structures as defined by phased-array magnetic resonance imaging. Br J Surg 88:1506, 2001.
24. Comiter CV, Vasavada SP, Barbaric ZL, et al: Grading pelvic prolapse and pelvic floor relaxation using dynamic magnetic resonance imaging. Urology 54:454-457, 1999.
25. Franklin ME, Abrego D, Parra E: Laparoscopic repair of postoperative perineal hernia. Hernia 6:42, 2002.
26. Ghellai AM, Islam S, Stoker ME: Laparoscopic repair of postoperative perineal hernia. Surg Laparosc Endosc Percutan Tech 12:119, 2002.
27. Abdul Jabbar AS: Postoperative perineal hernia. Hernia 6:188, 2002.
28. Beck DE, Fazio VW, Jagelman DG, et al: Postoperative perineal hernia. Dis Colon Rectum 30:21, 1987.
29. Frydman GM, Polglase AL: Perineal approach for polypropylene mesh repair of perineal hernia. Aust N Z J Surg 59:895, 1989.
30. Venzo A, Elberg JJ, Hjortrup A: Recurrent perineal hernia repair with transperineal approach: A case report. J Pelvic Med Surg 10:205, 2005.
31. Cattell RB, Cunningham RM: Postoperative perineal hernia following resection of the rectum. Surg Clin North Am 24:679, 1944.
32. Delmore JE, Turner DA, Gershenson DM, et al: Perineal hernia repair using human dura. Obstet Gynecol 70:507, 1987.
33. Brotschi E, Noe JM, Silen W: Perineal hernias after proctectomy. Am J Surg 149:301, 1985.
34. Hansen MT, Bell JL, Chun JT: Perineal hernia repair using gracilis myocutaneous flap. South Med J 90:75, 1997.
35. Hurwitz DJ, Walton RL: Closure of chronic wounds of the perineal and sacral regions using the gluteal thigh flap. Ann Plast Surg 8:375, 1981.
36. Salum MR, Prado-Kobata MH, Saad SS, Matos D: Primary perineal posterior hernia: An abdominoperineal approach for mesh repair of the pelvic floor. Clinics 60:71, 2005.
37. Sarr MG, Stewart R, Cameron JC: Combined abdominoperineal approach to repair of postoperative perineal hernia. Dis Colon Rectum 25:597, 1982.
38. Erdmann MWH, Waterhouse N: The transpelvic rectus abdominis flap: Its use the reconstruction of extensive perineal defects. Ann R Coll Surg Engl **77**:229, 1995.
39. Spraycar M (ed): Stedman's Medical Dictionary, 26th ed. Baltimore, Williams & Wilkins, 1995.
40. Rosenblum N, Rodriguez LV, Eilber KS, et al: Central tendon defects causing abnormal perineal support: Physical exam, perineal length, and magnetic resonance image (MRI) evaluation. Paper presented at the American Urological Association meeting, Orlando, FL, 2002.
41. Raz S: Repair of perineal hernia. In Atlas of Transvaginal Surgery, 2nd ed. Philadelphia, WB Saunders, 2002.
42. Bourcier AP, Juras JC, Villet RM: Office evaluation and physical examination. In Bourcier AP, McGuire EJ, Abrams P (eds): Pelvic Floor Disorders. Philadelphia, Elsevier Saunders, 2004, pp 133-148.
43. Walfisch A, Hallak M, Harlev S, et al: Association of spontaneous perineal stretching during delivery with perineal lacerations. J Reprod Med 50:23, 2005.
44. Baessler K, Schuessler B: Pregnancy, childbirth, and pelvic floor damage. In Bourcier AP, McGuire EJ, Abrams P (eds): Pelvic Floor Disorders. Philadelphia, Elsevier Saunders, 2004 pp 33-42.
45. Small KA, Wynne JM: Evaluating the pelvic floor in obstetric patients. Aust N Z J Obstet Gynecol 30:41, 1990.
46. Snooks SJ, Swash, M, Mathers SE, et al: Effect of vaginal delivery on the pelvic floor: A 5-year follow-up. Br J Surg 77:1358, 1990.
47. Parks AG, Porter NH, Hardcastle J: The syndrome of the descending perineum. Proc R Soc Med 59:477, 1966.
48. Benson JT: Physiology of anal continence and defecation. In Benson JT (ed): Female Pelvic Floor Disorders. New York, Norton Medical Books, 1992, pp 380-389.
49. Harewood GC, Coulie, B, Camilleri M, et al: Descending perineum syndrome: Audit of clinical and laboratory features and outcome of pelvic floor retraining. Am J Gastroenterol 94:126, 1999.
50. Dominguez JM, Saclarides TJ: Preprolapse syndromes. In Brubaker LT, Saclarides TJ (eds): The Female Pelvic Floor: Disorders of Function and Support. Philadelphia, FA Davis, 1996, pp 283-288.
51. Nichols DH: Posterior colporrhaphy and perineorrhaphy: Separate and distinct operations. Am J Obstet Gynecol 164:714, 1991.
52. Link RE, Su LM, Bhayani SB, et al: Laparoscopic sacral colpoperineopexy for treatment of perineal body descent and vaginal vault prolapse. Urology 64:145, 2004.
53. Cundiff GW, Harris RL, Coates K, et al: Abdominal sacral colpoperineopexy: A new approach for correction of posterior compartment defects and perineal descent associated with vaginal vault prolapse. Am J Obstet Gynecol 177:1345, 1997.
54. Cawkwell I: Perineal hernia complicating abdominoperineal resection of the rectum. Br J Surg 50:431, 1963.
55. Bach-Nielsen P: New surgical method of repairing sacral hernia following abdominoperineal resection of the rectum. Acta Chir Scand 133:67, 1967.
56. Buchsbaum HJ, White AJ: Omental sling for management of the pelvic floor following exenteration. Am J Obstet Gynecol 117:407, 1973.
57. Alexander JC, Beazley RM, Chretien PB: Mesenteric leaf repair of pelvic defects following exenterative operations. Ann Surg 182:767, 1975.
58. Bell JG, Weiser EB, Metz P, et al: Gracilis muscle repair of perineal hernia following pelvic exenteration. Obstet Gynecol 56:377, 1980.
59. Leuchter RS, Lagasse LD, Hacker NF, et al: Management of post-exenteration perineal hernias by myocutaneous axial flaps. Gynecol Oncol 14:15, 1981.
60. Giampapa V, Keller A, Shaw WW, et al: Pelvic floor reconstruction using the rectus abdominis muscle flap. Ann Plast Surg 13:56, 1984.

Chapter 77

COMPLICATIONS OF VAGINAL SURGERY

Raymond T. Foster, Sr., Cindy L. Amundsen, and George D. Webster

Urologists and gynecologists use the vaginal approach to surgically correct many of the pelvic organ problems of women, including urinary incontinence, uterine and vaginal prolapse, vesicovaginal fistula, and urethral diverticulum. As surgeons continue to seek new ways to surgically treat women without laparotomy, it is important that vaginal surgeons remain informed about potential surgical complications, some of which are unique to this route of surgery.

In this chapter, we review the potential complications of vaginal surgery, highlight patient characteristics and specific techniques that may be associated with a higher frequency of surgical complications, and outline strategies that may reduce the likelihood of a serious intraoperative or postoperative complication. Because this textbook is dedicated to a readership interested in female urology, we focus our discussion on complications related to urologic and pelvic reconstructive procedures.

BLEEDING

Problematic bleeding is undoubtedly the most feared problem that a surgeon encounters during or immediately after a surgical procedure. During the procedure, intraoperative bleeding compromises the surgeon's ability to adequately complete the task at hand. The reported incidence of bleeding during vaginal surgery varies by specific procedure, and to some degree, reported rates of hemorrhage depend on the investigator's definition of excessive blood loss. Most surgeons consider the need for blood transfusion a reliable definition of excessive surgical bleeding, but less blood loss can still interfere with surgical outcome and prolong hospitalization. Reported rates of such intraoperative hemorrhage are between 0% and 2% for most vaginal procedures, but these rates likely underestimate the incidence of problematic bleeding.

Several investigators have reported low transfusion rates even when multiple vaginal reconstructive repairs, including hysterectomy and pubovaginal slings, are performed during the same operation. One of the largest series of patients undergoing multiple vaginal prolapse and incontinence procedures was reported by Shull and colleagues.[1] Three hundred and two patients underwent a uterosacral vault suspension in combination with other support defects involving the urethra, bladder, posterior cul-de-sac, or rectum. The mean intraoperative blood loss for all patients in this study was 243 mL, and the blood transfusion rate was 1%. Other studies have reported similarly low rates of blood transfusion and blood loss between 200 and 350 mL when performing multiple vaginal prolapse repairs with a uterosacral vault suspension.[2-5] In one report looking at a series of patients undergoing vaginal reconstructive procedures, each of which included uterosacral vault suspension, the investigator found that when he compared blood loss between those having a hysterectomy at the time of repair with patients having only reconstructive procedures, hysterectomy did not significantly increase operative blood loss or the risk of significant bleeding.[3] One of the attractive features of the uterosacral vault suspension for apical prolapse is its low incidence of troublesome bleeding. However, most published data are reported by experts in the field and may not accurately reflect the experience of the generalist surgeon.

Although the reports cited found major intraoperative blood loss to be uncommon even when an apical prolapse procedure was performed, correction of the vaginal apex with a sacrospinous ligament fixation has been often associated with the potential for increased bleeding. This procedure, originally described by Richter,[6] has been studied repeatedly in the past decade with regard to surgical complications in general and bleeding in particular. The incidence of excessive bleeding reported in most series has been between 0.5% and 3.5%.[7-9] An important aspect of these statistics, however, is that maneuvers to control bleeding in this area have been reported to promote injury to adjacent structures, including the rectum and nerves. Nieminen and Heinonen[9] reported a higher transfusion rate (28% of 25 women) when performing a sacrospinous ligament fixation in a population of patients older than 80 years.

In an attempt to define the optimal surgical strategy for controlling intraoperative hemorrhage associated with sacrospinous ligament fixation, Barksdale and coworkers.[10] conducted an anatomic study with 10 female cadavers to map the vascularity in the region of the sacrospinous ligament and propose surgical strategies for controlling hemorrhage. Their report detailed various combinations and permutations of vascular anastomoses in the area of the sacrospinous ligament (i.e., superior gluteal, inferior gluteal, internal pudendal, vertebral, middle sacral, lateral sacral, and external iliac by way of the circumflex femoral artery system). They concluded that because of the vascular anastomoses, the heroic approach of laparotomy with surgical ligation of the internal iliac artery was unlikely to be of significant benefit. They also determined the inferior gluteal artery to be the most likely artery responsible for hemorrhage related to the sacrospinous ligament fixation. Based on anatomic considerations, bleeding from the inferior gluteal artery is optimally controlled by any combination of packing and vascular clips by means of the vaginal approach or arterial embolization by invasive radiology techniques. We have become less hesitant to employ surface hemostatic factors, such as FloSeal (Baxter International, Deerfield, IL).

Very few studies have evaluated factors associated with increased blood loss during vaginal surgery, such as surgeon skill level, surgical techniques, obesity, and the impact of prior pelvic surgery. Coates and associates[11] reported surgical outcomes in 289 women undergoing a vaginal prolapse repair. In 154 of these operations, the senior staff member was the primary surgeon (mean blood loss, 248 mL), and in the remaining 135 procedures, a senior gynecology resident was the primary surgeon (mean blood loss, 234 mL). The difference in operative bleeding between the senior staff surgeon and the surgical trainee was not clinically or statistically significant. One retrospective review of surgical outcomes in obese women (i.e., body mass index [BMI] > 30 kg/m^2) compared surgical complications in 189 subjects undergoing abdominal hysterectomy and in 180 women having a vaginal hysterectomy.[12] Both groups of obese women had a mean change in hemoglobin of 1.7 g and a 13% transfusion rate, which established obesity as risk factor for hemorrhage in female pelvic surgery, regardless of the chosen surgical approach.

Besides patient characteristics and surgical experience, surgical equipment may also impact the occurrence of unacceptable bleeding. Good surgical exposure and lighting is paramount to achieving surgical goals and avoiding and controlling bleeding. The Lonestar retractor (Lone Star Medical Products, Stafford, TX) is invaluable in this regard because it retains an open introitus and allows the surgeon to maintain visualization of the vaginal apex. The use of a surgical headlight or a cool lighting system that is adherent to the retractor and placed within the pelvis (Light-Mat, Lumitex, Strongsville, OH) provides sufficient light for operating in a deep body cavity.

In addition to the traditional ways of controlling bleeding, such as suture ligation and electrocautery, other user-friendly techniques have been introduced. In the United Kingdom, Hefni and colleagues[13] randomized 116 patients to vaginal hysterectomy with traditional suture ligation (n = 59) or to vaginal hysterectomy with the LigaSure (Valleylab, Boulder, CO) vessel sealing system (n = 57).[13] Mean intraoperative blood loss was 100 mL in both groups, but perioperative bleeding complications in the suture ligation group neared statistical significance (P = .0571).

More than other approaches to surgery, the transvaginal approach may be technically challenging in the setting of previous surgery. Boukerrou and coworkers[14] reported surgical outcomes of 741 women undergoing vaginal hysterectomy. Seventy-one (9.58%) of their subjects had undergone previous cesarean section, and the remaining 670 (90.41%) had not. Mean blood loss was 181.69 mL in the group of patients with previous cesarean section and 145.96 mL in the control group (P = .05). Among women with a history of cesarean section, 11.3% had intraoperative hemorrhage (i.e., blood loss in excess of 500 mL), compared with only 2.5% of women without a history of previous cesarean section. It is intuitive to surgeons that prior procedures in the same area render subsequent operations more difficult and prone to complications such as bleeding, but few articles report this conclusion.

In addition to vaginal prolapse procedures, transvaginal incontinence procedures, such as pubovaginal slings, may also cause intraoperative bleeding. Even though the traditional bladder neck pubovaginal slings required more extensive transvaginal surgical dissection, including digital and usually blind dissection of the retropubic space, several large pubovaginal sling series have demonstrated rare intraoperative bleeding complications.[15-18] The increasingly popular minimally invasive or midurethral sling is placed by passing a trocar blindly through the retropubic or obturator space. Although there are rare reports of iliac artery injuries published on the MAUDE database, most case series report a 1% to 3% increased bleeding rate resulting in pelvic or perineal hematomas. Abouassaly and associates[19] reviewed 241 patients who had undergone placement of a tension-free vaginal tape. These patients, recruited from six medical centers, had an intraoperative hemorrhage rate of 2.5% (16 patients). Four patients (1.9%) developed a pelvic hematoma within the first 24 hours after surgery. In another series, Krauth and colleagues[20] described 604 patients undergoing placement of a minimally invasive suburethral sling by the transobturator approach. They reported a 0.8% incidence of intraoperative hemorrhage and postoperative development of two (0.33%) perineal hematomas, one of which resolved without intervention, and the other, believed to be associated with a concomitant prolapse repair (not the transobturator sling), required revision surgery.

In summary, surgeons are wise to consider each patient's individual risk factors for operative bleeding before surgery. Intuitively, obese women and women with a history of prior pelvic surgery may have an elevated risk for excessive surgical bleeding, and extra precautions should be taken in the operating room (e.g., good surgical assistants and exposure, blood products available on short notice). We evaluate bleeding time and platelet function for patients who provide us a history of prior intraoperative or postoperative hemorrhage. Any medication that can affect bleeding should be stopped 7 to 10 days before surgery when this can be safely accomplished. Surgeons who are managing patients who require some level of anticoagulation, such as a patient with a history of heart valve replacement or atrial fibrillation, are wise to obtain hematologic advice for the perioperative management of anticoagulation agents.

INJURY TO THE URINARY TRACT

Operating in the vagina places the surgeon close to the urinary tract, and great care must be taken to avoid its injury. As with any effort to avoid surgical complication, a sound surgical plan and good exposure are important, as is a thorough understanding of the anatomy within the surgical field. It is encouraging to consider that most injuries to the urinary tract during vaginal surgery are problematic only if unrecognized.

Injuries to the urethra, bladder, or ureters that are identified at the time of surgery and primarily repaired most often heal without incident or further significant consequence to the patient.[21] For this reason, we rarely perform vaginal surgery without a cystoscopic evaluation of the lower urinary tract and confirmation of bilateral ureteral spill after the administration of intravenous indigo carmine. In addition to absent ureteral spill, other abnormalities sought are suture transfixation or sling penetration of the bladder and surgical entry to the bladder, each of which would necessitate re-exploration for removal or repair. We also look for bladder wall ecchymosis, which may suggest the need for a longer period of postoperative catheterization. Several published studies have confirmed the importance of intraoperative cystoscopy when pelvic reconstructive procedures, including incontinence procedures, are performed. Harris and associates[22] reviewed the records of 224 consecutive patients undergoing urogynecologic and reconstructive pelvic surgery. Based on a 4% rate of injury to the urinary tract, which would have been unrecognized without intraoperative cystoscopy, they concluded that cystoscopy should be included in all incontinence and pelvic reconstructive procedures. Another large, prospective study, in which intraoperative cystourethroscopy was performed universally on 471 women undergoing hysterectomy, documented a 7.6% rate of injury to the urinary tract.[23] Of the patients in this report, 144 (31%) had a vaginal hysterectomy. Among those patients having vaginal hysterectomy, 11 (7.6%) experienced an injury to their urinary collecting system; 6 of the 11 had concurrent prolapse surgery. Of the 11 injuries, 2 were ligated ureters, 7 were cystotomies, 1 was a suture in the bladder, and 1 was bladder abrasion. Concurrent prolapse surgery was therefore found to be an independent risk factor for injury to the urinary system. When controlling for prolapse and incontinence surgery, there was not a significant increase in the risk of urinary tract injury based on route of hysterectomy, age, BMI, race, blood loss, uterine size, and history of previous cesarean section. However, the standard of care in community practice is to not routinely perform cystoscopy at the end of hysterectomy or pelvic organ prolapse surgery.

Transvaginal vault suspensions, specifically uterosacral vault suspensions, have been associated with urinary tract injuries, especially injuries involving one or both ureters. Because this vault suspension involves placement of sutures intraperitoneally above the level of the ischial spines, the ureter is near the suture placement. A cadaveric study by Buller and colleagues[24] demonstrated the strength of the uterosacral ligament at various locations in the pelvis and its proximity to the ureter at the site of customary suture placement. Based on their findings after necropsy of 11 female cadavers, the ureter is, on average, 2.3 ± 0.9 cm from the uterosacral ligament at the level of the ischial spine. This finding led Buller and his colleagues to claim, "The proximity of the ureter to the distal uterosacral ligament warrants concern during vaginal vault repairs that use the ligament."[24]

Several surgical series of uterosacral vault suspension have reported a 0% to 11% incidence of injury to the ureter.[1-5] In each of these series, the injuries were identified at the time of surgery after confirming an absence of ureteral spill on cystoscopic evaluation. Management usually involved removal of the uterosacral suspensory sutures with or without ureteral stent placement; however, some injuries, presumably transections, required ureteroneocystotomy. In these reports, all injuries were detected by intraoperative cystoscopy at the time of surgery, and as a result, none of the patients had permanent or long-term urinary tract sequelae. In addition to ureteral injury, cystotomy may occur during transvaginal surgical entry into the peritoneal cavity and may be repaired and the operation continued in most circumstances.[4]

Aronson and colleagues[25] reported the ureteral injury rate using a modified "deep" Mayo-McCall uterosacral ligament plication for vaginal vault suspension. The technique for placement of suture through the uterosacral ligament described by the investigators resulted in a uterosacral anchoring point much more dorsal and posterior than previously described. In this retrospective report of 411 consecutive patients, they observed three ureteral injuries, only one of which was attributable to the vault suspension procedure (0.24% [range, 0.01% to 1.35%]).

Injury to the lower urinary tract is not uncommon in vaginal procedures designed to treat stress urinary incontinence, and the data depend on the procedure used. Factors such as anesthetic technique (i.e., regional or local versus general anesthesia) and the use of hydrodissection in the retropubic space were previously thought to affect bladder injury rate, but a report from Ghezzi and coworkers[26] disputes these assumptions.

The minimally invasive techniques for placement of midurethral slings are associated with the highest rate of bladder injury, with some articles describing cystotomy rates greater than 10%.[27-29] However, in one study that surveyed members of the American Urogynecologic Society and members of the Society for Urodynamics and Female Urology, only 10% to 15% of those surveyed from both groups admitted to cystotomy rates higher than 5%. More than 90% of the members in both societies would replace the trocar at the time of surgery, and more than 80% of the members in both societies would drain the bladder transurethrally for at least 24 hours if a cystotomy was made with the trocar.[30]

Some investigators have described risk factors associated with inadvertent cystotomy. Bodelsson and associates[27], in their series of 177 patients undergoing a tension-free vaginal tape procedure, were able to show a statistically and clinically significant difference in the occurrence of cystotomy and urethrotomy among surgeons with different levels of experience. Another potential contributing factor to operative morbidity, including urinary tract injury, is obesity. However, Rafii and colleagues[29] performed a midurethral sling in 38 consecutive patients with a BMI greater than 30 and compared outcomes with 149 age- and parity-matched controls with a BMI of 30 or less.[29] They found no difference in estimated blood loss, operative times, bladder injuries, postoperative urgency, and voiding disorders. This study also found no difference between the two groups in objective and subjective cure rates. Lovatsis and coworkers[28] studied 35 patient pairs (BMI = 35 kg/m^2 versus BMI = 30 kg/m^2) undergoing placement of tension-free vaginal tape. The patients were matched according to age and history of previous incontinence surgery. In this series, obesity was protective against injury to the lower urinary tract (0% versus 14%, $P = .03$). It may be that although obesity complicates vaginal access, it protects the bladder by virtue of the fat separation of the bladder from the symphysis pubis. Rardin and associates[31] looked at surgical complications related to placement of tension-free vaginal tape as a primary procedure ($n = 157$) or as a secondary procedure for recurrent stress urinary incontinence ($n = 88$). The cystotomy rates were similar (3.2% versus 3.4%).

In summary, surgical experience appears to be related to the occurrence of injury to the urinary tract during placement of retropubic midurethral slings. However, obesity and prior incontinence surgery do not appear to increase the risk of cystotomy or urethrotomy.

We prefer to use a 70-degree cystoscope to evaluate the bladder and a 30-degree cystoscope to visualize the urethra after passing the trocars through the retropubic space but before the sling is placed. During cystoscopy, we are careful to fully expand the bladder with 400 to 500 mL of clear fluid, and we pay particular attention to the 11- and 8-o'clock and the 1- and 4-o'clock positions, which are the most likely areas to be penetrated during trocar passage. We are encouraged by failure to visualize a perforation with a fully expanded bladder and by the absence of hematuria. If a bladder perforation is identified, we remove the offending trocar and replace it, with an exaggerated emphasis on "hugging" the pubic bone during passage of the trocar. Cystoscopy is repeated to ensure adequate trocar placement is obtained on the second passage. After cystotomy, we leave a catheter for 24 to 72 hours postoperatively.

Recognizing the need for a safer suburethral sling system that may not obligate the surgeon to cystoscopy, Delorme[32] introduced a transobturator midurethral sling in 2001. Although there are few safety and efficacy data on this relatively new approach for sling placement, Cindolo and colleagues[33] experienced a single bladder neck laceration, which was repaired intraoperatively, and no occurrence of bladder perforation after placing a midurethral sling in 80 women. However, cystoscopy was not used to definitively document the absence of bladder injury. In a similar series of 71 patients, Dargent and coworkers[34] reported no instance of bladder perforation with the transobturator technique, despite cystoscopic examination at the time of surgery. Conversely, Minaglia and associates[35] reported three bladder perforations in 61 patients and concluded that "routine intraoperative cystoscopy is therefore recommended for the identification of bladder injuries during the transobturator sling procedure." Anecdotally, we have also seen a patient with an intraurethral sling after this approach.

Vesicovaginal fistula (VVF) may occur after vaginal surgery, most commonly after hysterectomy (0.5% to 2% of cases).[36,37] Examination of this occurrence shows that it more commonly follows the abdominal rather than the vaginal approach. The symptoms of continuous urinary leakage, usually developing between 1 and 6 weeks after surgery, are ominous and should lead to evaluation for fistula by vaginal examination, tampon test, and cystoscopy. Less commonly, the ureter is the source of a postoperative vaginal fistula. When suspecting a ureterovaginal fistula, usually heralded by urinary leakage emanating from the vaginal cuff, the physician should pursue further investigation with an excretory urogram.

The intraoperative events that lead to VVF remain unknown, and the fact that the cervix must be dissected from the bladder adds to the inherent risk because the bladder wall may be thinned. Inadvertent entry into the bladder during this maneuver must be carefully repaired in layers, and a Foley catheter is left for sufficient time to allow healing. This area is close to the vaginal cuff closure, and any breakdown will promote fistula formation. Suture transfixation of the bladder by the cuff closure sutures has been suggested as a factor in the genesis of fistula, although animal experiments cast doubt on this theory. The proximity of the cuff and bladder at this location make this event almost unavoidable on some occasions, particularly when the patient is obese, hemostasis is poor, or exposure, lighting, and assistance are suboptimal. Cystoscopy may help identify the bladder injury that may lead to fistula formation, but it is not performed in most cases of hysterectomy.

The timing of VVF repair has been reported to be successful at all intervals after discovery, and some advocate immediate surgical repair. However, a more judicious approach includes a period of catheterization, hoping for spontaneous healing. The size of the fistula affects the likelihood of success with this approach and how long it should be pursued. We time our intervention based on the status of the vaginal cuff tissue, and our preference is to monitor inflamed and edematous tissue at weekly intervals until the cuff reveals a healthy, mature fistulous tract. Vaginal repair usually can be performed by 6 weeks after hysterectomy.

In summary, transvaginal surgical treatment of prolapse and incontinence is a significant risk factor for injuring the urinary tract in women. We believe that careful surgical planning and intraoperative cystoscopy is an advisable element for most vaginal surgeries that seek to correct these problems. We recognize that patients experience poor long-term outcomes after urinary tract injury when the problem is undetected at the time of occurrence. However, patients are likely to recover from surgery without incident when the urinary system is repaired at the time of the primary surgery.

BOWEL INJURY

Complications involving the bowels most commonly occur during rectocele repair, although the high rectum is vulnerable during all varieties of vaginal vault suspension. For this reason, we prefer a low bowel preparation preoperatively and the placement of a rectal pack at the commencement of some procedures to aid in the identification of surgical landmarks.

Injury to the bowel is a relatively uncommon occurrence during vaginal surgery. Hoffman and coworkers,[38] at the University of South Florida, reported nine rectal injuries (0.7%) from their database of 1346 patients who underwent vaginal surgery between 1987 and 1998.[38] Of the nine, six were being treated for prolapse, one for cervical dysplasia, one for fibroid uterus, and one for gender dysphoria. In another large study from a vaginal surgery database, Mathevet and colleagues[39] reported 14 (0.45%) rectal injuries in 3076 patients undergoing vaginal surgery. Most (62.5%) of the 14 patients were undergoing surgery for the primary indication of genital prolapse. In the study of Isik-Akbay and associates[12] comparing abdominal and vaginal routes of surgery in obese women undergoing hysterectomy, the investigators found five bowel injuries in the abdominal group (2.7%) and none among women having vaginal surgery. Although the difference was not statistically significant, this report suggests fewer rectal injuries in obese patients when surgery was performed vaginally.[12]

During rectocele repair, injury is most likely to occur in women undergoing repeat surgery. When the rectum is prepared before surgery and injury occurs, it is generally appropriate to repair the defect primarily. Even though the published rate of rectal injuries is low, we routinely perform a digital rectal examination at the conclusion of vaginal prolapse procedures that involve some risk of rectal injury to ensure that there is no blood on the examining finger and that there has been no suture transfixation. As with urinary tract injury, the best time to identify injury is at the time of the primary surgery. If a rectovaginal fistula does occur postoperatively, as with vesicovaginal fistula, the timing of repair is individualized and is dictated primarily by the status of the tissues. If the fistula is large, a temporary diverting colostomy is required to afford the patient the highest probability of a successful repair. Such decisions are individualized based on severity.

INFECTION

The hallmark clinical sign of postoperative infection is fever, and in surgical training, we are taught to investigate the cause of fever with physical examination, radiographic images, and laboratory studies. Historically, surgeons have treated postoperative fever with antibiotics even in the absence of an obvious cause after a comprehensive evaluation. More contemporary evidence, however, calls into question the medical necessity of treating an unidentified postoperative infection in most patients. In 1983, Freischlag and Busuttil[40] reported their experience following 464 patients after abdominal surgery. They defined postoperative fever as a rectal temperature of 38.5°C or higher in the first 6 postoperative days. Seventy-one patients (15%) had postoperative fever. Only 19 (27%) of these 71 patients had an identifiable source of infection after a radiographic and laboratory evaluation. They concluded that routine evaluations of fever do not alter the outcome most patients and are not cost-effective.

Shackleford and associates[41] examined the predictive value of postoperative fever for infection in patients recovering from vaginal surgery. Febrile morbidity was defined in their series as an oral temperature greater than 38.0°C on two separate occasions, excluding the first 24 hours after surgery. They retrospectively examined outcomes of 431 vaginal surgery patients. Forty-three percent of these patients had vaginal hysterectomy alone, and the remaining 57% had a procedure for prolapse with (27%) or without (30%) vaginal hysterectomy. Fifty-four women (12.5%) had postoperative febrile morbidity. Thirty-five infections were definitively identified (8.1%), but only 13 of these infections occurred in the 54 patients with postoperative fever. Among the identified infections were 20 urinary tract infections (4.6%), five infections at the suprapubic catheter site (1.2%), three cases of vaginal cuff cellulites (0.7%), three "pelvic infections" (0.7%), and two cases of *Clostridium difficile* colitis. Two women had infection unrelated to their vaginal surgery; one was diagnosed with sinusitis and the other with bronchitis. Based on their findings, the investigators calculated the sensitivity of febrile morbidity for postoperative infection to be 40%, with a specificity of 98%, a positive predictive value of 26%, and a negative predictive value of 94%. Univariate analysis was performed, and they found that women with febrile morbidity were older, had longer procedures, lost more blood, were higher parity, and had lower uterine weights and longer hospital stays than women without febrile morbidity. Their data also demonstrated that women with proven infection had prolonged surgery, weighed less, had lower uterine weights, and stayed in the hospital longer than women without infections. Women who had hysterectomy done at the time of prolapse surgery were the most likely to have postoperative infection compared with women who had vaginal hysterectomy alone or prolapse surgery without hysterectomy.

Vaginal surgery is a clean-contaminated procedure. Some investigators have become interested in the vaginal flora at the time of surgery. The assumption of these clinical scientists is that an understanding of how to manipulate the vaginal flora at the time of surgery (e.g., decrease the bacterial colony count) would aid in the prevention of postoperative infection for patients undergoing vaginal procedures. Culligan and colleagues[42] published an observational study in 2003 that reported the rate of vaginal contamination (defined as an aerobic or anaerobic culture result of 5000 colony-forming units/mL) at given time intervals during vaginal reconstructive surgery. All patients in their study had preoperative antibiotic prophylaxis and a standard 5-minute surgical scrub with povidone iodine. The first set of cultures, obtained 30 minutes after the surgical scrub, revealed a 52% contamination rate in the surgical field, whereas the cultures collected at 90 minutes only had a 41% contamination rate. After this initial study that defined vaginal contamination as a surrogate end point for postoperative infection, Culligan and his group[43] published their results of a randomized trial that evaluated povidone iodine and chlorhexidine gluconate as surgical scrub solutions for vaginal surgery. Fifty patients were enrolled in the study that demonstrated a clinically and statistically significant difference between the contamination rates of surgical fields prepared with povidone iodine (63% contaminated) and chlorhexidine gluconate (22% contaminated) at 30 minutes (P = .003; relative risk = 6.12; 95% CI: 1.7 to 21.6).

Surgical infection is a problem that is often easier to prevent than to treat. In an era of prophylactic, broad-spectrum antibiotics, we are rarely confronted with wound infections at the surgical site after vaginal procedures. Postoperative febrile morbidity and postoperative infections at sites remote from the vagina remain areas of some concern, especially in elderly patients, those with above-average blood loss, and patients who undergo prolonged surgical procedures.

COMPLICATIONS RELATED TO GRAFT MATERIALS USED IN THE VAGINA

Reported rates of recurrent or de novo vaginal wall prolapse range from 15% to 30%[44] and for this reason, many clinicians implant synthetic or organic (allograft or xenograft) material to address this problem. This position is supported by the fact that surgeons have known for a long time that the efficacy and durability of hernia repair is improved by the use of a graft material. However, long-term data associated with the use of the various graft materials, including complications and success rates for prolapse repair, are limited. Vaginal surgery is performed in a clean-contaminated field, and this adds the potential risk of infection and erosion when synthetic material is used. There are also concerns about whether the inclusion of grafts or synthetics in vaginal repairs may compromise vaginal caliber or elasticity and thereby compromise sexual function. There have been few well-designed studies to provide evidence that the risks of placing the mesh are balanced by a longer durability of the vaginal repair, but this continues to be the trend.

Synthetic material may be absorbable or permanent. Two randomized studies evaluated the use of an absorbable synthetic graft to reinforce the vaginal prolapse repair, and they had opposing views on the success of the material. Neither, however, reported significant complications associated with the material. Sand and collegues[45] randomized women to polyglactin 910 mesh (with anterior colporrhaphy) or to anterior colporrhaphy alone. Thirty women (43%) without mesh and 18 women (25%) with mesh had recurrent cystocele beyond the mid-vaginal plane (P = .02). The study authors concluded that polyglactin mesh was useful in the prevention of recurrent cystoceles. In 2001, Weber and coworkers[46] compared standard colporrhaphy, standard colporrhaphy with polyglactin 910 mesh, and ultralateral anterior colporrhaphy. They analyzed 109 patients randomized to one of the three treatment arms, with a mean follow-up of 23.3 months (range, 4.5 to 44.4 months) and found no difference in the three groups with respect to the anterior vaginal wall. A single vaginal mesh erosion was the only mesh-related complication in this study. There seems not to be widespread interest in absorbable mesh to enhance prolapse repair.

The most commonly reported permanent synthetic mesh used for vaginal prolapse has been polypropylene. Randomized, controlled studies are lacking, but several published case series using polypropylene mesh report a rate of recurrent prolapse not exceeding 6%.[47-49] The same reports document mesh erosion rates between 7% and 13%, and postoperative, new-onset dyspareunia in 14% to 63% of patients. Management of vaginal exposure of the mesh should begin with conservative therapy such as intravaginal conjugated equine estrogen cream, but surgical resection of the exposed portion of mesh is commonly required.

Organic materials such as cadaveric dermal or fascia lata grafts have also been used for vaginal prolapse reinforcement. In a randomized study evaluating the success of solvent-dehydrated fascia lata versus a standard anterior colporrhaphy, 21% of the allograft-reinforced group had recurrent prolapse, compared with 29% in the control group. This finding did not reach statistical significance. No vaginal erosions were reported among the 76 patients in the allograft group.[50] We notice a surprising lack of literature to document the erosion rate of allograft material when used in transvaginal prolapse surgery, and there seems to be little evidence to guide management strategies when erosion does occur. In our own experience (69 women), we have found a 10.9% vaginal exposure rate of dermal allograft material when used in anterior or posterior repairs.[51] We also documented a 100% rate of resolution of this problem with vaginal conjugated equine estrogen cream. The median time to complete healing in our series was 13 weeks.

Xenograft material has been marketed for use in prolapse repair. Available materials include porcine dermis and porcine small intestinal submucosa. As with the materials discussed previously, there have been variable results, with recurrent prolapse reported in 8% to 39% of patients.[52,53] Vaginal exposure of the graft appears to be relatively common, similar to that seen with cadaveric dermis, with a reported incidence of 15% and a healing time of up to 3 months with conservative therapy. Porcine dermis has several suggested beneficial characteristics, including the fact that it is 95% homologous to human collagen, possibly providing a nonallergenic scaffold for human tissue ingrowth.

When considering complications such as vaginal graft erosion, infection, and postoperative dyspareunia, the physician may be wise to consider that the graft itself is not always the determining cause for these suboptimal outcomes. Surgical techniques of graft placement must always be considered, and it is inappropriate to always blame the product for a bad outcome; however, we have no way to control for the surgeon's performance.

Minimally invasive techniques used to place the material may produce complications related to blind passage of a trocar. Although the techniques are new with infrequent reports of complications, placement of augmented synthetic mesh using a trocar approach could cause rectal and bladder injury with the potential for rectovaginal fistula and vesicovaginal fistula.[54] We await development of this field, which promises to simplify the repair of vaginal organ prolapse if the techniques can achieve good functional results and prove to be safe.[55]

INJURY TO THE PERIPHERAL NERVOUS SYSTEM

Peripheral nerve injury resulting from vaginal surgery is an unexpected but reported complication after pelvic surgery. It is a potentially debilitating problem for the patient and a great concern for the surgeon. Most neuropathies that occur in reconstructive pelvic surgery are neurapraxic, and they heal with time. Physical therapy and neuroleptic medications plays a role in managing these patients, and rarely is surgery required for relief of symptoms.

The nerve injuries most commonly reported have been sciatic nerve injuries and are largely thought to be caused by positioning in free-hanging stirrups.[56-58] Injury to the sciatic nerve has been reported after sacrospinous ligament fixation in which the nerve was thought to be entrapped by the suture.[8] Symptoms are usually buttock pain radiating down the posterior thigh, and if the cause is related to sacrospinous ligament fixation, removal of the suture often resolves the pain.

We have managed patients with temporary postoperative sciatic pain after undergoing transvaginal uterosacral cuff suspension by removal of the suture or expectant management with analgesics, anti-inflammatory agents, and neuroleptic medication. Recovery time for expectant management may be several months. Use of padded Allen stirrups with an extended padded lower leg support provides a secure and stable positioning for the patient's legs, and we believe this added precaution reduces the risk of lower extremity neural injuries. Symptoms of femoral nerve injury include weakness with hip flexion, leg extension, and sensory loss over the anteromedial thigh and leg. These are uncommon but may follow prolonged lithotomy with the legs markedly abducted or a retractor blade compression injury after retropubic surgery.[59] Injury to the common peroneal nerve may occur if pressure is placed on the lateral part of the lower part of leg where the nerve wraps around the fibular head or if there is hyperflexion of the thigh. The almost routine use of sequential compression hose, which raise the lower leg from the stirrup periodically, probably reduces this complication. Common symptoms of peroneal nerve injury are footdrop and sensory loss to the anterior leg and dorsal foot.

In pelvic surgery, injury may occur to branches of the ilioinguinal and iliohypogastric nerves in the suprapubic location. These branches are susceptible to injury where the nerve runs on the undersurface of the external and internal abdominal oblique fascia above the symphysis, where they may become entrapped or involved by the fixation of pubovaginal slings. Patients present with sharp or burning pain and paresthesia in the suprapubic region that may radiate to the groin, and it can be quite problematic. Treatment may be by local injection of the trigger point, and occasionally, the site must be explored surgically to release the suture, lyse the fibrosis, or excise a neuroma.

Obturator nerve injury may occur during vaginal, paravaginal, or transobturator prolapse surgery. The patient has difficulty adducting the leg (and therefore complains about problems walking) and may have sensory loss to the medial thigh. Injury to branches of the pudendal nerve, including the dorsal genital nerve to the clitoris and the perineal branch to the urethral sphincter, perineal skin, and anal sphincter, may occur during any anterior vaginal dissection. These unfortunate injuries therefore may occur during incontinence or prolapse surgery. Common symptoms of these uncommon injuries include sharp, burning pain to the perineal area or worsening of urinary and fecal incontinence.

Important measures to reduce the incidence of neural injury include proper patient positioning, surgical technique to avoid known nerve locations, careful use of retractors and, avoidance of prolonged surgery. Even when all these preventative strategies are followed, neuropathies will occur. Postoperatively, clinical symptoms and physical examination allows the physician to make the diagnosis. If motor deficits are identified, a neurology consultation may be obtained for baseline testing and management options.

CONCLUSIONS

The possible complications associated with vaginal surgery are numerous and tend to be underestimated. Reducing complications is probably largely a product of the technical skills of the surgeon and the application of good surgical principles, but some events remain unavoidable. Variables contributing to the occurrence of adverse events in vaginal surgery that are beyond the immediate control of the surgeon include obesity, medical comorbidities, and undiagnosed bleeding dyscrasias. However, by good surgical planning and execution, the surgeon may reduce the occurrence of complications. Vaginal surgery, when performed correctly and safely, remains one of the most rewarding aspects of surgical practice for female urologists and gynecologists.

References

1. Shull BL, Bachofen C, Coates KW, Kuehl TJ: A transvaginal approach to repair of apical and other associated sites of pelvic organ prolapse with uterosacral ligaments. Am J Obstet Gynecol 183:1365-1373; discussion 1373-1374, 2000.
2. Karram M, Goldwasser S, Kleeman S, et al: High uterosacral vaginal vault suspension with fascial reconstruction for vaginal repair of enterocele and vaginal vault prolapse. Am J Obstet Gynecol 185:1339-42; discussion 1342-1343, 2001.
3. Jenkins VR 2nd: Uterosacral ligament fixation for vaginal vault suspension in uterine and vaginal vault prolapse. Am J Obstet Gynecol 177:1337-1343; discussion 1343-1344, 1997.
4. Barber MD, Visco AG, Weidner AC, et al: Bilateral uterosacral ligament vaginal vault suspension with site-specific endopelvic fascia defect repair for treatment of pelvic organ prolapse. Am J Obstet Gynecol 183:1402-1410; discussion 1410-1411, 2000.
5. Amundsen CL, Flynn BJ, Webster GD: Anatomical correction of vaginal vault prolapse by uterosacral ligament fixation in women who also require a pubovaginal sling. J Urol 169:1770-1774, 2003.
6. Richter K: The surgical anatomy of the vaginae fixatio sacrospinalis vaginalis. A contribution to the surgical treatment of vaginal blind pouch prolapse [in German]. Geburtshilfe Frauenheilkd 28:321-327, 1968.
7. David-Montefiore E, Garbin O, Hummel M, Nisand I: Sacro-spinous ligament fixation peri-operative complications in 195 cases: Visual approach versus digital approach of the sacro-spinous ligament. Eur J Obstet Gynecol Reprod Biol 116:71-78, 2004.
8. Lantzsch T, Goepel C, Wolters M, et al: Sacrospinous ligament fixation for vaginal vault prolapse. Arch Gynecol Obstet 265:21-25, 2001.
9. Nieminen K, Heinonen PK: Sacrospinous ligament fixation for massive genital prolapse in women aged over 80 years. BJOG 108:817-821, 2001.
10. Barksdale PA, Elkins TE, Sanders CK, et al: An anatomic approach to pelvic hemorrhage during sacrospinous ligament fixation of the vaginal vault. Obstet Gynecol 91:715-718, 1998.
11. Coates KW, Kuehl TJ, Bachofen CG, Shull BL: Analysis of surgical complications and patient outcomes in a residency training program. Am J Obstet Gynecol 184:1380-1383; discussion 1383-1385, 2001.
12. Isik-Akbay EF, Harmanli OH, Panganamamula UR, et al: Hysterectomy in obese women: A comparison of abdominal and vaginal routes. Obstet Gynecol 104:710-714, 2004.
13. Hefni MA, Bhaumik J, El-Toukhy T, et al: Safety and efficacy of using the LigaSure vessel sealing system for securing the pedicles in vaginal hysterectomy: Randomised controlled trial. BJOG 112:329-333, 2005.
14. Boukerrou M, Lambaudie E, Collinet P, et al: A history of cesareans is a risk factor in vaginal hysterectomies. Acta Obstet Gynecol Scand 82:1135-1139, 2003.
15. Amundsen CL, Visco AG, Ruiz H, Webster GD: Outcome in 104 pubovaginal slings using freeze-dried allograft fascia lata from a single tissue bank. Urology 56:2-8, 2000.
16. Groutz A, Blaivas JG, Hyman MJ, Chaikin DC: Pubovaginal sling surgery for simple stress urinary incontinence: Analysis by an outcome score. J Urol 165:1597-600, 2001.
17. Morgan TO Jr, Westney OL, McGuire EJ: Pubovaginal sling: 4-year outcome analysis and quality of life assessment. J Urol 163:1845-1848, 2000.
18. Carbone JM, Kavaler E, Hu JC, Raz S: Pubovaginal sling using cadaveric fascia and bone anchors: Disappointing early results. J Urol 165:1605-1611, 2001.
19. Abouassaly R, Steinberg JR, Lemieux M, et al: Complications of tension-free vaginal tape surgery: A multi-institutional review. BJU Int 94:110-113, 2004.
20. Krauth JS, Rasoamiaramanana H, Barletta H, et al: Sub-urethral tape treatment of female urinary incontinence—morbidity assessment of the trans-obturator route and a new tape (I-STOP): A multi-centre experiment involving 604 cases. Eur Urol 47:102-106; discussion 106-107, 2005.
21. Mattingly RF, Borkowf HI: Acute operative injury to the lower urinary tract. Clin Obstet Gynaecol 5:123-149, 1978.
22. Harris RL, Cundiff GW, Theofrastous JP, et al: The value of intra-operative cystoscopy in urogynecologic and reconstructive pelvic surgery. Am J Obstet Gynecol 177:1367-1369; discussion 1369-1371, 1997.
23. Vakili B, Chesson RR, Kyle BL, et al: The incidence of urinary tract injury during hysterectomy: A prospective analysis based on universal cystoscopy. Am J Obstet Gynecol 192:1599-604, 2005.
24. Buller JL, Thompson JR, Cundiff GW, et al: Uterosacral ligament: Description of anatomic relationships to optimize surgical safety. Obstet Gynecol 97:873-879, 2001.
25. Aronson MP, Aronson PK, Howard AE, et al: Low risk of ureteral obstruction with "deep" (dorsal/posterior) uterosacral ligament suture placement for transvaginal apical suspension. Am J Obstet Gynecol 192:1530-1536, 2005.
26. Ghezzi F, Cromi A, Raio L, et al: Influence of the type of anesthesia and hydrodissection on the complication rate after tension-free vaginal tape procedure. Eur J Obstet Gynecol Reprod Biol 118:96-100, 2005.
27. Bodelsson G, Henriksson L, Osser S, Stjernquist M: Short term complications of the tension free vaginal tape operation for stress urinary incontinence in women. BJOG 109:566-569, 2002.
28. Lovatsis D, Gupta C, Dean E, Lee F: Tension-free vaginal tape procedure is an ideal treatment for obese patients. Am J Obstet Gynecol 189:1601-1604; discussion 1604-1605, 2003.
29. Rafii A, Darai E, Haab F, et al: Body mass index and outcome of tension-free vaginal tape. Eur Urol 43:288-292, 2003.
30. Romero AA, Webster GD, Amundsen CL: Comparison of practice patterns when using the minimally invasive sling. J Pelvic Med Surg 11:76, 2005.
31. Rardin CR, Kohli N, Rosenblatt PL, et al: Tension-free vaginal tape: Outcomes among women with primary versus recurrent stress urinary incontinence. Obstet Gynecol 100:893-897, 2002.
32. Delorme E: Transobturator urethral suspension: Mini-invasive procedure in the treatment of stress urinary incontinence in women [in French]. Prog Urol 11:1306-1313, 2001.
33. Cindolo L, Salzano L, Rota G, et al: Tension-free transobturator approach for female stress urinary incontinence. Minerva Urol Nefrol 56:89-98, 2004.
34. Dargent D, Bretones S, George P, Mellier G: Insertion of a sub-urethral sling through the obturating membrane for treatment of female urinary incontinence [in French]. Gynecol Obstet Fertil 30:576-582, 2002.
35. Minaglia S, Ozel B, Klutke C, et al: Bladder injury during trans-obturator sling. Urology 64:376-377, 2004.
36. Hadley HR: Vesicovaginal fistula. Curr Urol Rep 3:401-407, 2002.
37. Harkki-Siren P, Sjoberg J, Tiitinen A: Urinary tract injuries after hysterectomy. Obstet Gynecol 92:113-118, 1998.
38. Hoffman MS, Lynch C, Lockhart J, Knapp R: Injury of the rectum during vaginal surgery. Am J Obstet Gynecol 181:274-277, 1999.

39. Mathevet P, Valencia P, Cousin C, et al: Operative injuries during vaginal hysterectomy. Eur J Obstet Gynecol Reprod Biol 97:71-75, 2001.
40. Freischlag J, Busuttil RW: The value of postoperative fever evaluation. Surgery 94:358-363, 1983.
41. Shackelford DP, Hoffman MK, Davies MF, Kaminski PF: Predictive value for infection of febrile morbidity after vaginal surgery. Obstet Gynecol 93:928-931, 1999.
42. Culligan P, Heit M, Blackwell L, et al: Bacterial colony counts during vaginal surgery. Infect Dis Obstet Gynecol 11:161-165, 2003.
43. Culligan PJ, Kubik K, Murphy M, et al: A randomized trial that compared povidone iodine and chlorhexidine as antiseptics for vaginal hysterectomy. Am J Obstet Gynecol 192:422-425, 2005.
44. Olsen AL, Smith VJ, Bergstrom JO, et al: Epidemiology of surgically managed pelvic organ prolapse and urinary incontinence. Obstet Gynecol 89:501-506, 1997.
45. Sand PK, Koduri S, Lobel RW, et al: Prospective randomized trial of polyglactin 910 mesh to prevent recurrence of cystoceles and rectoceles. Am J Obstet Gynecol 184:1357-1362; discussion 1362-1364, 2001.
46. Weber AM, Walters MD, Piedmonte MR, Ballard LA: Anterior colporrhaphy: A randomized trial of three surgical techniques. Am J Obstet Gynecol 185:1299-1304; discussion 1304-1306, 2001.
47. Dwyer PL, O'Reilly BA: Transvaginal repair of anterior and posterior compartment prolapse with Atrium polypropylene mesh. BJOG 111:831-836, 2004.
48. Milani R, Salvatore S, Soligo M, et al: Functional and anatomical outcome of anterior and posterior vaginal prolapse repair with Prolene mesh. BJOG 112:107-111, 2005.
49. Yan A, Anne M, Karine A, et al: Cystocele repair by a synthetic vaginal mesh secured anteriorly through the obturator foramen. Eur J Obstet Gynecol Reprod Biol 115:90-94, 2004.
50. Gandhi S, Goldberg RP, Kwon C, et al: A prospective randomized trial using solvent dehydrated fascia lata for the prevention of recurrent anterior vaginal wall prolapse. Am J Obstet Gynecol 192:1649-1654, 2005.
51. Drake NL, Weidner AC, Webster GD, Amundsen CL: Patient characteristics and management of dermal allograft extrusions. Int Urogynecol J Pelvic Floor Dysfunct 16:365-377, 2005.
52. Altman D, Lopez A, Gustafsson C, et al: Anatomical outcome and quality of life following posterior vaginal wall prolapse repair using collagen xenograft. Int Urogynecol J Pelvic Floor Dysfunct 16:298-303, 2005.
53. Gomelsky A, Rudy DC, Dmochowski RR: Porcine dermis interposition graft for repair of high grade anterior compartment defects with or without concomitant pelvic organ prolapse procedures. J Urol 171:1581-1584, 2004.
54. Jelovsek JE, Sokol AI, Walters MD, Barber MD: Anatomic relationships of infracoccygeal sacropexy (posterior intravaginal slingplasty) trocar insertion. J Pelvic Med Surg 11:60, 2005.
55. Biertho I, Dallemagne B, Dewandre JM, et al: Intravaginal slingplasty: Short term results. Acta Chir Belg 104:700-704, 2004.
56. Batres F, Barclay DL: Sciatic nerve injury during gynecologic procedures using the lithotomy position. Obstet Gynecol 62:92s-94s, 1983.
57. Burkhart FL, Daly JW: Sciatic and peroneal nerve injury: A complication of vaginal operations. Obstet Gynecol 28:99-102, 1966.
58. McQuarrie HG, Harris JW, Ellsworth HS, et al: Sciatic neuropathy complicating vaginal hysterectomy. Am J Obstet Gynecol 113:223-232, 1972.
59. Flanagan WF, Webster GD, Brown MW, Massey EW: Lumbosacral plexus stretch injury following the use of the modified lithotomy position. J Urol 134:567-568, 1985.

Section 8

DEFECATORY FUNCTION AND DYSFUNCTION

Chapter 78

PATHOPHYSIOLOGY, DIAGNOSIS, AND TREATMENT OF DEFECATORY DYSFUNCTION

Tracy Hull and Massarat Zutshi

The domain of defecatory disorders is vast, and their treatment can be frustrating for the surgeon and the patient. Except for straightforward surgically correctible disorders, most diseases in this category have many causes and need treatment that encompass medical, behavioral, and surgical modalities. These patients often go from physician to physician seeking a cure for these complex disorders.

ANATOMY

Pathogenesis of the defecatory disorders can be a function of abnormal anatomy at the outlet. The anal sphincter complex is composed of the puborectalis, the internal anal sphincter, and the external anal sphincter. The puborectalis and the external anal sphincter are striated muscles that are primarily responsible for the process of defecation by voluntary relaxation. They are innervated by the S3 and S4 nerves. The internal anal sphincter accounts for about two thirds of the resting tone and is composed of smooth muscle. It is innervated by the autonomous nervous system. The external anal sphincter accounts for one third of the resting tone. Any process that causes a change in this normal physiology can lead to defecatory disorders.

MECHANISM OF DEFECATION

Storage is a function of the transverse colon. When the sigmoid colon is filled, the process of defecation commences with the propagation of stool into the rectum. Defecation occurs in response to the sensory stimulus generated by rectal distention that is received by receptors in the pelvic floor and anal transition zone; the rectum itself is not richly innervated by sensory nerves. The sensation of filling is normally perceived at a volume of 50 mL, and the maximum tolerated volume normally is about 200 mL. Rectal pressures should be more than the anal pressures for evacuation to take place, which is usually achieved by increasing the intra-abdominal pressure. The external anal sphincter and puborectalis relax, allowing fecal contents to be evacuated. If it is socially unacceptable at that time, the external anal sphincter contracts, and the sensation of the need to evacuate disappears.

DIAGNOSIS

History and Physical Examination

A detailed history and physical examination is the first step in diagnosing any defecatory disorder. The history should be tailored to the patient's presenting symptoms. All patients should be asked about their current medications, and a history should be sought for all medical problems, especially diabetes, thyroid disorders, scleroderma, multiple sclerosis, stroke, dementia, food intolerance, and inflammatory bowel disease. The evaluation of a female patient with fecal incontinence should include a detailed obstetric history, including the number of vaginal deliveries, tears and episiotomies, unusual presentations, and prolonged labor. Other pertinent points are pad usage and number of accidents, symptoms of urinary incontinence, previous perineal surgery, back injuries, irradiation, and effect of symptoms on sexual behavior. Patients undergoing evaluation for constipation should be specifically asked about the duration of symptoms, the use of digitation to relieve symptoms, and factors that relieve or alleviate symptoms.

Physical examination of a patient with fecal incontinence should focus on the sphincters and pelvic floor. Scars are looked for, and the anal opening is assessed for any gaping. The anocutaneous reflex can be evaluated, providing a crude assessment of the nerves. The patient may then be asked to strain. Perineal descent and prolapsed hemorrhoids or prolapsed rectum should be looked for. A digital rectal examination with the patient squeezing assesses the tone, obvious defects, and muscle fatigue.

For a patient with constipation, the digital rectal examination evaluates increased tone with paradoxical contractions when straining and the presence of an internal intussusception and rectocele. In cases of rectal prolapse, inspection is important to differentiate a true rectal prolapse from prolapsing hemorrhoids, mucosal prolapse, or an anal or rectal polyp.

Enema

A tap-water enema in the office is a good and simple test to evaluate the sphincter tone in an incontinent patient. After administering the enema, the nurse documents the time the patient can hold the 100 mL of water. A patient with a suspected rectal prolapse is examined on the commode after the enema is given. The rectal prolapse may be seen while the patient strains on the commode. In a patient with irritable bowel syndrome, it may demonstrate urgency in the presence of normal tone.

Anal Physiology Testing

Anal physiology testing has two parts. The first is manometry, which records resting and squeeze pressures and evaluates rectal sensation by documenting the time of first sensation of rectal filling and maximum tolerated volume. Rectal compliance also can be calculated. Paradoxical pressures in the rectum can be

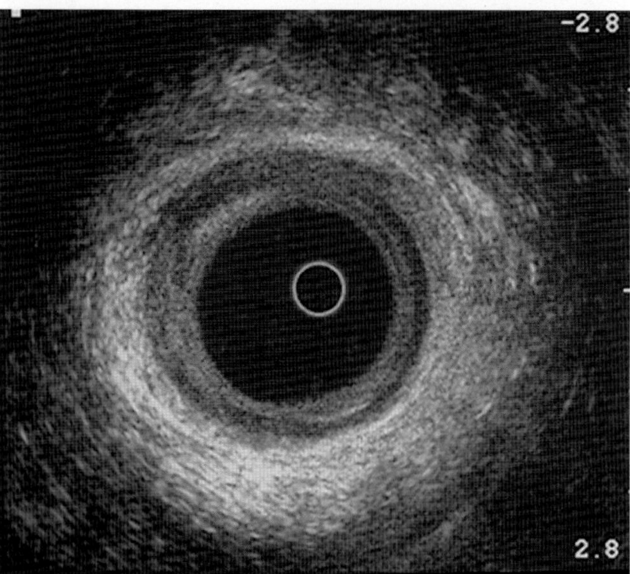

Figure 78-1 Normal anal ultrasound. EAS, external anal sphincter; IAS, internal anal sphincter.

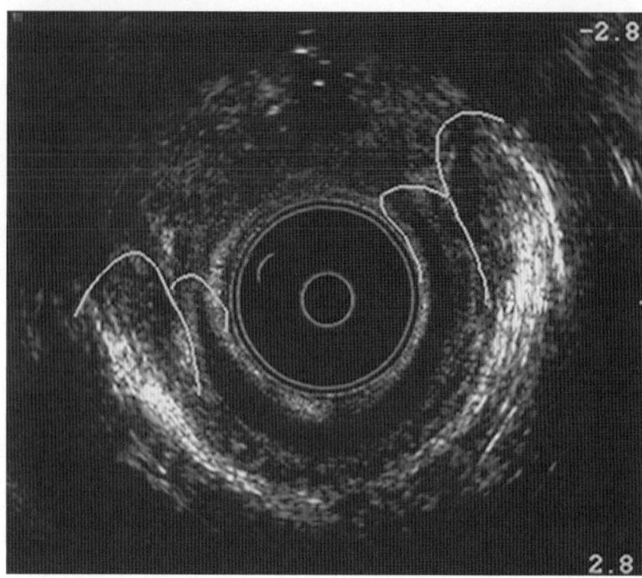

Figure 78-3 Defect in the internal and external anal sphincters.

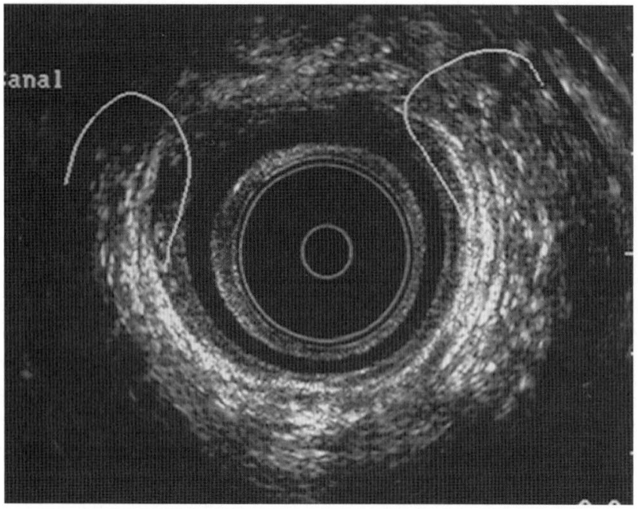

Figure 78-2 Defect in the external anal sphincter.

recorded during squeeze and strain, and they also can be demonstrated on electromyography by identifying the external anal sphincter contraction. Balloon expulsion tests can demonstrate rectal inertia or loss of coordination among the rectum, pelvic floor, and anal sphincters.

The second part of the test evaluates pudendal nerve terminal motor latency. The test uses the St. Marks electrode and records electrical impulses when the pudendal nerve is stimulated. The amplitude of the wave reflects the voltage, which is low or absent in neurologic disorders.

Anorectal Ultrasound

Endoluminal ultrasound is the single most important test to demonstrate sphincter defects. The normal sphincter is shown in Figure 78-1. Sphincter defects may be those of the internal anal sphincter or external anal sphincter (Fig. 78-2), or both (Fig. 78-3). Thinning of the internal anal sphincter is easily demonstrable. After sphincteroplasty, the repaired sphincter can be evaluated with this test.

Colon Transit Study

Transit studies specifically demonstrate slow-transit constipation. This assessment reflects motility of the colon but not the rectum. The patient swallows capsules with radiopaque markers. The markers are followed on day 1, 2, 4, and 7. Demonstration of markers in the right and left colon on day 7 indicates slow transit of the fecal matter on the right side, supporting a diagnosis of colonic inertia. If markers are aggregated on the left side, the problem may be redundancy of the left colon or outlet obstruction.

Defecating Proctogram

Patients with constipation and symptoms suggesting obstructive defecation syndrome are subjected to a test in which contrast is instilled in the rectum, small bowel, vagina, and bladder. Patients defecate in a radiolucent commode, and serial radiographs are taken to demonstrate perineal descent, cystocele, enterocele, internal intussusception, and rectal prolapse.

Dynamic Magnetic Resonance Imaging

Dynamic magnetic resonance imaging (MRI) is a test that replaces the defecating proctogram. Contrast is instilled in the vagina and rectum, and serial MR images are taken with the patient straining. Newer imaging techniques use upright MRI scans with the patient seated and evacuating in the sitting position. This test can evaluate pelvic descent, rectal diameter before and during straining, the width of the pelvic hiatus, presence of enteroceles and sigmoidoceles, and prolapse of the uterus and bladder.[1] It may become the confirmatory test for obstructive defecation. Cine radiography can give a dynamic picture of the process of evacuation, and it can demonstrate prolapse of the anterior wall of the rectum.

Colonoscopy

All colonic pathology must be excluded before undertaking formal treatment of any defecatory disorder. Colonoscopy should be part of the workup of all patients older than 50 years and patients with any suspicion of mucosal pathology.

Barium Enema

A barium enema is warranted when the anatomy of the colon needs to be defined. It may be of use in cases of rectal prolapse to demonstrate a redundant sigmoid colon, necessitating a sigmoid colectomy.

FECAL INCONTINENCE

Pathophysiology

Injury to the muscle complex or the nerves that supply them can result in a loss of continence. The most common etiologic factor is childbirth injury. Other causative factors are listed in Table 78-1.

Treatment of Fecal Incontinence

The treatment of fecal incontinence is based on the severity of symptoms, the anatomy of the sphincter mechanism, and the presence of nerve damage. An algorithm for management is provided in Figure 78-4, but treatment options depend on the availability of certain procedures and on the patient's comorbidities.

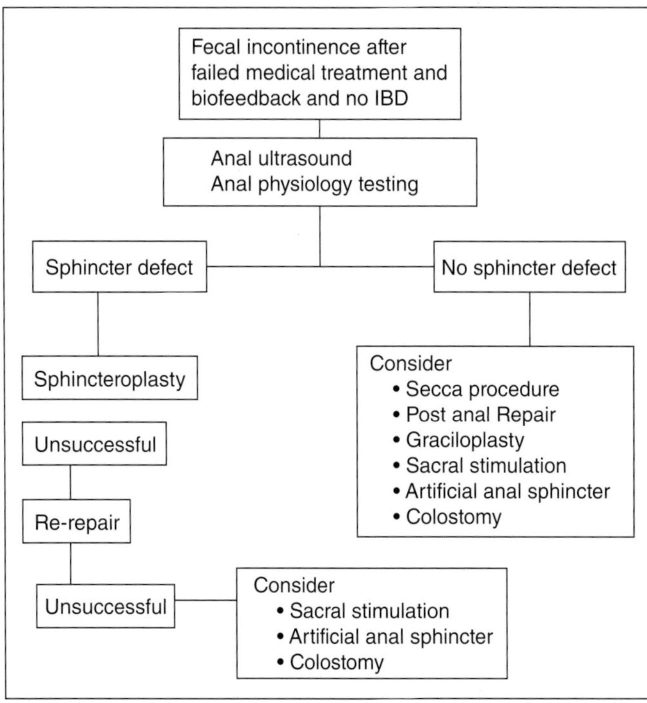

Figure 78-4 Algorithm for the management of fecal incontinence. Sacral stimulation has been used successfully in some centers. Although listed, graciloplasty no longer available in the United States. IBD, irritable bowel disease. *Sacral stimulation has been used successfully in some centers. **Not available in the US.

Table 78-1 Causes of Fecal Incontinence
Sphincter injury
Childbirth trauma
Surgical trauma
Rectal injury, traumatic
Irradiation
Congenital causes
Imperforate anus
Colonic causes
Fecal impaction
Colitis, proctitis
Rectal prolapse
Tumors
Decreased rectal compliance
Neurogenic causes
Peripheral disorders (e.g., diabetes)
Central disorders
Trauma
Stroke
Tumors
Dementia
Multiple sclerosis
Functional causes
Other causes
Diarrhea
Myopathy

Treatment of Minor Incontinence

A thorough history and physical examination are the first step in treatment to rule out inflammatory bowel disease, irritable bowel disease, and neurologic disorders. Minor incontinence can be treated with medical management[2] using bulking agents, which can change the consistency of stool and lead to evacuation as a mass movement. They are started in small doses to prevent abdominal distention and bloating, and they are gradually increased to achieve the desired effect. Other agents that are used slow the gastrointestinal motility. They tend to constipate the patients because they decrease the bulk of the stool during the increased transit time. Loperamide hydrochloride (Imodium) is the commonly used medication, and it may be started in doses of 2 mg before breakfast and advanced to a maximum of 16 mg daily as warranted. Diphenoxylate hydrochloride (Lomotil) is another drug that may be used, especially if diarrhea is the main symptom. It is started in doses of 1 tablet once or twice daily and may be advanced to 1 or 2 tablets three or four times daily.

Amitriptyline[3] has been used for idiopathic fecal incontinence. It acts through an anticholinergic mechanism, increasing intrarectal pressures. Phenylephrine cream is an α_1-adrenergic blocker that has not been approved by the U.S. Food and Drug Administration (FDA). Used in some studies in strengths of 10% to 40%, it has been shown to increase resting pressures for 1 to 2 hours.[4]

Other treatment modalities include the use of regular (even daily) enemas, which evacuate the rectum until it fills again. Bulking agents may be used in conjunction to prevent seepage between enemas.

Biofeedback and Kegel Exercises

Kegel exercises are an integral part of the treatment of fecal incontinence, but they are ineffective as the sole treatment. They may benefit to patients with very mild incontinence and those with easy fatigability of the sphincter and no sphincter defect.

Biofeedback training consists of retraining the patient's response using visual, auditory, and sensory stimuli. It consists of strength training of the external sphincter, retraining the sphincter to coordinate rectal distention with external anal sphincter contraction, and sensory training of the rectal mucosa to be able to sense earlier when the rectum receives contents. It is done in the office by a trained therapist using the electromyographic apparatus to retrain and strengthen the sphincter, and a rectal balloon is used for sensory stimulation training. Some studies have shown improvement after biofeedback therapy.[5] Biofeedback has been shown to benefit patients after sphincter repair.[6]

Treatment of Moderate Fecal Incontinence with an Intact Sphincter

Secca Procedure

The Secca procedure involves radiofrequency stimulation of the muscular layer of the anal canal and lower rectum. It has been hypothesized that the procedure causes stimulation of collagen deposition and remodeling over time, which can improve symptoms of fecal incontinence.

The procedure is done under conscious sedation. After local anesthesia is injected, radiofrequency is delivered by means of a specialized probe that contains needles that pierce the mucosa and submucosa. In about 64 separate punctures, the radiofrequency is applied beneath the mucosal surface. Contraindications to this procedure include inflammatory bowel disease, a history of depression, collagen vascular disease, acute infections, pudendal neuropathy, and a history of pelvic irradiation.[7]

Sacral Stimulation

Sacral nerve stimulation is FDA approved in the United States for stress urinary incontinence, and it is being evaluated under a research protocol for fecal incontinence. It produces constant stimulation of the sacral nerves, resulting in an increase in resting tone and squeeze pressures. In this procedure, a temporary stimulator is implanted as a first step, and if the patient improves, a permanent device is implanted. It has gained popularity in Europe, where it has been available for many years.[8]

Perianal Bulking Agents

Bulking agents instilled in the perianal area are being studied.[9] They work by increasing the internal bulk of the sphincter, preventing seepage of stool. An optimal bulking agent should be nonbiodegradable, should not migrate, and should be removable if the need arises.

Treatment of Moderate to Severe Fecal Incontinence due to a Defect in the Sphincter Mechanism

Overlapping Sphincter Repair: Sphincteroplasty

Any fixable defect of the sphincter complex should be considered for repair. Because it is difficult to determine which patient will benefit, consideration should be given to all those with a defect.

The technique involves a semicircular incision about 1 to 1.5 cm beyond the anal verge. For obstetric injuries, this arc spans about 200 degrees in a semicircular fashion, mirroring the anus. The branches of the pudendal nerves that innervate the external sphincter approach the muscle from the posterolateral position. To avoid nerve injury, the arc of the incision should not extend to the extreme posterolateral position. The rectovaginal septum is dissected, and care is taken to avoid making buttonhole defects in the anal canal or rectum. Occasionally, the only part of the perineal body that remains is the vaginal and anal mucosa, and dissection in this situation can be difficult.

The dissection is carried laterally to the ischiorectal fat. A finger placed in the vagina or rectum and dissecting from lateral to medial may facilitate the dissection. Any tears in the anal mucosa are repaired with 4-0 chromic suture. The ends of the sphincter are usually dissected with scar in the midline (or midportion of the injury). This scar is divided in the middle, leaving two ends of sphincter with scar attached. It is important to divide the scar but to not trim it from the ends of the sphincter, because this will provide tensile strength when the repair is done. If the internal and external muscles are injured, it is preferable to repair them as one unit. If the internal sphincter is intact, divide and repair only the external sphincter.

The levator ani muscles may be plicated at this point using 1-0 or 2-0 delayed absorbable sutures. This may lengthen the anal canal. The vagina should be checked after the levator plication to ensure that a ridge or narrowing did not occur with levator plication, because this may contribute to dyspareunia. If the internal anal sphincter was intact, plication can be done before the sphincteroplasty if there is redundant internal sphincter.

The sphincter ends that have been sufficiently mobilized to allow overlapping of the muscle are grasped. Some authorities[10,11] advocate merely approximating the muscles, but if possible, overlapping the muscle ends is preferred using 2-0 polyglactin sutures, placing mattress sutures for the sphincteroplasty. Approximately six sutures (three on each side) are used. The repair tightens the anal canal such that only an index finger may be admitted. During the procedure, the wound may be irrigated with antibiotic solution. The skin edges are closed in a V-Y fashion, starting laterally and leaving the center open for drainage. If there is a significant amount of dead space, a 0.5-inch Penrose drain can be inserted and then removed postoperatively.

Postoperatively, we keep patients on intravenous antibiotics for 2 to 3 days and withhold oral intake. Because sitz baths macerate the skin edges, they are avoided, but showers are permitted. We do not use constipating drugs. The Foley catheter is removed on postoperative day 2, and the patient is allowed a high-fiber diet just before discharge. At discharge, patients are placed on Metamucil, Citrucel, or Konsyl daily. Additionally, they take 1 ounce of mineral oil each morning. If they do not move their bowels by postoperative day 7, they take 1 ounce of milk of magnesia twice daily until their bowels begin to function. Because they undergo a complete bowel cleansing before surgery, patients may not move their bowels for several days after surgery.

A diverting stoma is used at the discretion of the surgeon. Preoperatively, this should be discussed with patients who have had previous failed repairs, have concomitant inflammatory bowel disease, have severe diarrhea, or need an extremely complicated repair. A stoma does not ensure success but may aid a successful outcome in such patients.[12]

Initial functional improvement can be anticipated in 80% to 90%[13-15] of patients. Pudendal nerve damage is associated with suboptimal results.[13] Age does not seem to significantly affect results,[12] although erratic bowel problems such as urgency and diarrhea may lead to continued incontinence. Wound infection occurs in up to a fourth of patients[15] but does not usually adversely affect the outcome unless the sphincter repair sutures become disrupted. Complete disruption of the skin sutures usually heals by secondary intention with adequate wound care.

Long-term follow-up suggests that about 40% of patients undergoing a repair are expected to be continent without further surgery.[16] In patients needing a repeat overlapping sphincter repair due to disruption of the initial repair, evidence suggests that satisfactory outcome can be achieved.[17]

Dynamic Graciloplasty

Graciloplasty is no longer available in the United States, because the stimulator is no longer supplied by the manufacturer. Indications for this procedure include sphincter defects from obstetric or traumatic injury, congenital defects, and idiopathic incontinence. Contraindications are diseases with a neurologic basis, such as multiple sclerosis. Dynamic graciloplasty has been an excellent choice for patients who have no alternative but to have a stoma. Success has been reported in about 40% to 65% patients undergoing this procedure.[18,19]

Treatment of Moderate to Severe Incontinence with an Intact Sphincter and No Neurologic Deficit

Postanal Repair

Postanal surgical repair is indicated in patients with an intact sphincter but no neurologic incontinence.[20] The aim of this procedure is to increase the length of the anal canal, reestablish the anorectal angle, and tighten the anal canal.

The operation is done through an inverted-V-shaped incision made 5 to 6 cm from the anal verge posteriorly. Flaps are raised, and the intersphincteric plane is identified. Dissection is carried in this plane cephalad to Waldeyer's fascia, which is divided to expose the mesorectal fat. Figure-of-eight, 2-0 polypropylene sutures are placed to draw the two sides of the iliococcygeus muscle together. The sides do not approximate because of the distance, and the sutures are tied with minimal tension to form a lattice. The pubococcygeus muscle is the next muscle encountered. Sutures are placed and tied to again to form a lattice, especially posteriorly, although anteriorly, the ends may be approximated. The last layer plicated is the puborectalis and external sphincter. The skin is closed with absorbable suture in a V-Y fashion. Postoperative care is similar to that for sphincteroplasty. Postanal repair has lost popularity because of poor overall improvement results.

Treatment of Severe Fecal Incontinence due to Failed Repairs or Neurologic Causes

Artificial Anal Sphincter

The artificial anal sphincter evolved from the artificial urinary sphincter. The device has three parts. The first is an inflatable cuff that encircles the anal orifice. The second is a pump with a valve that controls the fluid entering and exiting the cuff. It is placed in the labia or the scrotum. The third part a balloon that is placed in the space of Retzius. When the valve is activated, fluid flows from the cuff to the balloon, allowing defecation. Over the next 7 minutes, reverse flow from the storage balloon to the anal cuff produces occlusion of the anus. If evacuation is incomplete, the valve can be activated again.

Continence is restored completely in the immediate postoperative period. The main problems associated with this procedure are the rate of infections and device malfunction. These problems can affect as many as 33% of patients, even after a period of learning how to operate the device.[21,22]

Colostomy or Ileostomy

When the symptoms are severe, the quality of life is greatly affected, and all other avenues have been unsuccessfully explored, a colostomy or ileostomy is a viable option. Although this procedure may sound drastic, it improves the quality of life for these patients, who otherwise become prisoners in their homes.

CONSTIPATION

Pathophysiology

It is difficult to define constipation. It often is defined by reference to bowel frequency, because this is the most convenient way to assess and document the condition. Bowel frequency of less than three movements per week is considered to be constipation, but this is not the only criterion. Excessive straining at stools and hard stools are other symptoms that should be considered.

The pathophysiology of constipation is disordered motility of the colon and rectum rather than delayed motility. The transit time may not be vastly delayed, but the patient may be still be constipated.

The many causes of constipation are listed in Table 78-2. It is important to differentiate constipation from obstructive defeca-

Table 78-2 Causes of Constipation

Idiopathic causes
Drugs
Antidepressants
Anticholinergics
Antispasmodics
Antipsychotics
Iron supplements
Calcium
Antacids
Opiates
Antihypertensives
Anticonvulsants
Metabolic causes
Diabetes mellitus
Hypothyroid
Hypercalcemia
Pregnancy
Neurogenic causes
Hirschsprung's disease
Neurofibromatosis
Hypoganglionosis
Intestinal pseudo-obstruction
Ganglioneuromatosis
Neurologic causes
Spinal cord lesions
Parkinson's disease
Trauma to nervi erigentes
Multiple sclerosis
Collagen and vascular disorders
Dermatomyositis
Systemic sclerosis
Amyloidosis

tion syndrome because this changes the workup and treatment of these patients. A thorough history should include associated symptoms such as cramping, bloating, straining, use of digitation and pressure around the anus or in the vagina during evacuation, medications, presence of metabolic disorders, and cerebral and neurologic causes. The physical examination should include a digital rectal examination, which assesses prolapse of the anterior rectal wall, paradoxical contractions of the anal muscles, and rectal lesions.

Most patients are referred to a surgeon after exhausting all medical treatments. A full workup includes excluding all metabolic causes listed in Table 78-2. Colon transit studies using radiopaque markers (i.e., sitz markers) are ordered for all patients with long-standing constipation not responding to medical treatment. Anal manometry is ordered for patients in whom an outlet obstruction is suspected. Manometry can demonstrate paradoxical contractions of the anal muscles, which may respond to biofeedback training. For patients suspected of having rectal prolapse or obstructive defecation syndrome, a defecating proctogram or dynamic MRI may be helpful. These studies provide valuable information regarding rectal dilatation during straining, pelvic descent, and the presence of obstructing sigmoidoceles or enteroceles. In patients with suspected adult Hirschsprung's disease, a full-thickness biopsy is indicated for diagnosis if a rectal anal inhibitory reflex is not helpful (done as a part of anal manometry).

Medical Management

Recent-onset constipation may be treated with diet modification; increasing fiber with bulk laxatives (containing psyllium); saline laxatives such as magnesium citrate, magnesium sulfate, and hyperosmolar laxatives such as lactulose, sorbitol, and polyethylene glycol. Emollient laxatives such as mineral oil, docusate salts, stimulant laxatives such as castor oil, anthraquinones (e.g., senna, cascara sagrada, phenolphthalein, and bisacodyl are avoided for long-term use. Patients who have paradoxical contractions can be treated with biofeedback sessions[23] and can be taught to use the right muscles to be able to initiate the process of defecation.

Surgical Management

For patients who have exhausted medical treatment, surgical treatment requires defining the problem as colonic inertia or obstructive defecation. The algorithm for treatment is provided in Table 78-2. Long-standing constipation due to colonic inertia is treated with a total colectomy with an ileorectal anastomosis or occasionally with a cecorectal anastomosis. Because preservation of the sigmoid colon is associated with postoperative constipation,[24,25] an ileosigmoid anastomosis is not considered a good option. Laparoscopic colectomy is gaining popularity because of the decreased morbidity, shorter hospital stay, and better cosmetic result.[26,27] Patients who undergo colectomy with ileorectal anastomosis have increased number of bowel movements, although many patients complain of incontinence and persistent symptoms of abdominal pain and bloating.[28] Quality-of-life scores are usually not elevated although the symptoms of constipation are successfully treated.[29,30]

A less popular procedure is the antegrade continent enema (ACE) described by Malone in 1990. This procedure was described for children and later used in adults.[31] Through a surgically constructed retrograde appendicostomy, washout of the colon is accomplished, although it can also induce high-amplitude waves and mass movement. Although this procedure has good results, it is marred by complications such as intestinal obstruction and perforation, and it may require many surgical revisions.

A newer technique that is showing potential in treating constipation is neuromodulation. Sacral nerve stimulation, which is unavailable in the United States, has produced some promising results in studies conducted in Europe.[32] Further research and newer techniques in neuromodulation may be the future treatment of choice for colonic inertia.

Patients with obstructive defecation may respond to biofeedback,[33] relaxation therapy, and retraining. This requires a dedicated therapist and a motivated patient. Results of biofeedback therapy are encouraging in carefully selected patients.[23] Those with symptoms that do not respond to biofeedback have been improved with the stapled transanal rectal resection (STARR) procedure.[34] This is widely used in Europe and uses a circular stapler to excise a full thickness of the rectal wall at a distance of about 6 to 9 cm from the anal verge.

Surgery for constipation is appropriate for only selective patients and in patients with severe symptoms. Patients usually dictate the timing of the surgery, but they should be warned that not all preoperative symptoms are relieved. Usually, bowel frequency is a symptom that does improve.[30] Figure 78-5 is an algorithm for management of patients with chronic constipation.

IRRITABLE BOWEL SYNDROME

Pathophysiology

Irritable bowel syndrome (IBS) is a disease of symptoms with no single pathologic entity. The prevalence has been estimated at 10% to 15% in the Western population,[35,36] with only 3.3% being medically diagnosed.[37] The Rome II criteria are commonly used (Table 78-3).[38] The common symptoms are abdominal pain and altered bowel habits. Patients can develop symptoms with diarrhea (IBS-D) or constipation (IBS-C) as a predominant symptom or have a combination of diarrhea and constipation. There have been no studies that demonstrate a change in myoelectric activity in the colon and small intestine. Current studies are focusing on the role of visceral sensory abnormalities in IBS.[39]

This disease has been associated with various emotional disorders, and this has led to the speculation of being associated with a disorder of the central nervous system. However, it is uncertain whether this is a primary central nervous system disorder that affects gut motility or a primary gut disorder with inappropriate input from the central nervous system.[40] Associations between sexual and physical abuse,[41] abnormal psychiatric features,[42] and IBS have been reported. Other factors are a history of prior gastrointestinal infection, malabsorption, and food intolerance.

Treatment of Irritable Bowel Syndrome

The diagnosis of IBS is essentially one of exclusion of organic causes. A workup should include a thorough history and physical examination, a complete blood cell count, sedimentation rate, thyroid profile, and stool analysis for parasites. For patients with diarrhea-predominant symptoms, a hydrogen breath test to rule out lactose intolerance is considered. IBS has been known to remit spontaneously.

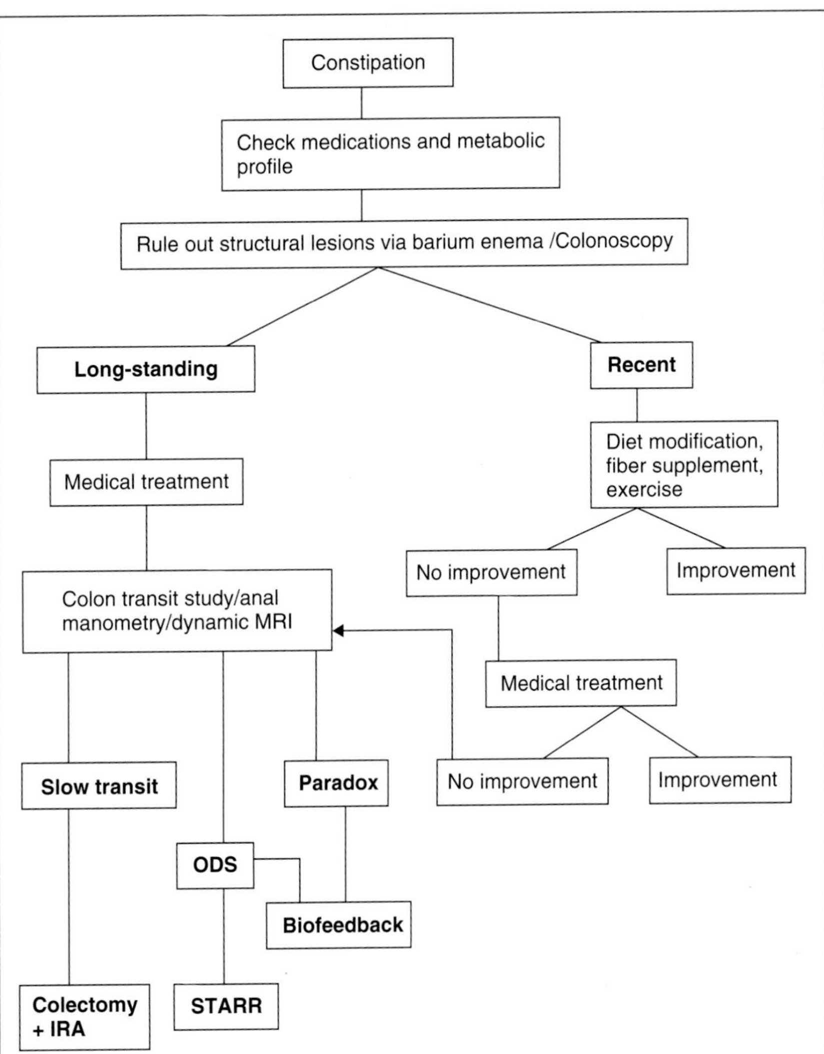

Figure 78-5 Algorithm for the management of chronic constipation. IRA, ileorectal anastomosis; MRI, magnetic resonance imaging; ODS, obstructive defecation syndrome; STARR, stapled transanal rectal resection.

Diet

The treatment of IBS is frustrating for the physician and the patient because it consists of a trial-and-error approach. The initial management is dietary guidance and counseling. It is important to have an in-depth dietary history that rules out food allergies, lactose intolerance, foods that cause increased gas production, and foods that induce an immune response, which contribute to mucosal inflammation.

Diet is modified in accordance with symptoms. Fiber may help constipation-prone patients, and limiting fiber, salads, fresh fruit, and some vegetables may help those that are diarrhea prone. However, most patients with IBS rarely adhere to a strict dietary or supplementary regimen.[43] Foods commonly found to help patients when excluded from the diet are milk, eggs, and wheat and, less commonly, coffee, nuts, and peas. Exclusion of wheat, potatoes, onions, and dairy products has been shown to decrease the amount of gas production. Lactose-free diets have not had any benefit in adult patients, except in selected groups of patients or cultures[44] (e.g., Norwegian) in which the lactose intake is high.

Drugs Causing Decreased Bowel Motility

Antidiarrheal agents have been widely used in IBS-D patients. They delay transit time, increase anal pressures, and decrease rectal sensation, causing the stool to be dehydrated. Loperamide is the most commonly used antidiarrheal and has been shown to decrease fecal urgency, borborygmi, and diarrhea.[45] Other agents commonly used are cholestyramine, which is a resin that binds bile acids, and ondansetron,[46] which is a serotonin receptor antagonist.

Antispasmodic agents have a wide application in IBS. They range from anticholinergics such as dicyclomine to calcium channel blockers and peppermint oil, which is a naturally occurring carminative.

Drugs for Irritable Bowel Syndrome with Constipation

The 5-hydroxytryptamine type 4 (5-HT_4) receptor agonist tegaserod stimulates peristaltic activity and increases small and large intestinal transit time. The dosage used has been (6 mg twice daily) has provided significant improvement of bloating, abdominal discomfort, and constipation (during first and repeated symptoms).[47,48] The common side effects are diarrhea and headaches.

Antidepressants

Amitriptyline has been used in the IBS-D patients. In addition to its mood-lifting activity, it has a physiologic effect by inhibiting the motor activity of the gut. These effects are particularly helpful in patents with pain-predominant symptoms.

Table 78-3 ROME II Criteria for the Diagnosis of Irritable Bowel Syndrome

For at least 12 weeks (which need not be consecutive) of the preceding 12 months, abdominal discomfort or pain that has two of three of the folowing features* †

1. Pain relieved with defecation
2. Onset of pain associated with a change in frequency of stool
3. Onset of pain associated with a change in form (appearance) of stool

Symptoms that cumulatively support the diagnosis of IBS

1. Abnormal stool frequency (more than three bowel movements per day; less than three bowel movements per week)
2. Abnormal stool form (lumpy or hard; loose or watery)
3. Abnormal stool passage (straining, urgency, or feeling of incomplete evacuation)
4. Bloating or feeling of abdominal distention

Symptoms are *not* typical of IBS

1. Pain that awakens or interferes with sleep
2. Diarrhea that awakens or interferes with sleep
3. Blood in the stool (visible or occult)
4. Weight loss
5. Fever

Symptoms that further aid the diagnosis of IBS

A. Fewer than three bowel movements a week
B. More than three bowel movements a day
C. Hard or lumpy stools
D. Loose or watery stools
E. Straining during a bowel movement
F. Urgency
G. Feeling of incomplete bowel movement
H. Passing mucus during a bowel movement
I. Abdominal fullness, bloating, or swelling
   Categoration of of IBS based on symptoms‡
      Diarrhea-predominant IBS: At least one of B, D, and F but none of A, C, and E, or at least two of B, D, and F plus one of A or E
      Constipation-predominant IBS: At least one of A, C, and E but none of B, D, and F, or at least two of A, C, and E plus one of B, D, and F

*Rome I criteria not included in this algorithm. The diagnosis of IBS relies on meeting Rome II inclusion criteria (updated by Rome III criteria) and excluding other illnesses based on the history, physical examination, and laboratory testing.

†In addition to meeting these positive criteria, patients have initial laboratory testing with a complete blood cell count, basic chemistry panel, and an erythrocyte sedimentation rate. The diagnostic accuracy for IBS is more than 95% when the Rome II criteria are met, the history and physical examination results do not suggest any other cause, and initial laboratory test results are negative.

‡An update to these criteria was issued at the Rome III conference and published in May 2006. The preferred terms were changed to IBS with diarrhea (from diarrhea-predominant IBS) and to IBS with constipation (from constipation-predominant IBS). In this categorical system, many people whose features place them close to a subtype boundary (e.g., IBS with alternating stool pattern) can change pattern without a major change in pathophysiology.

Other Drugs

Prokinetic drugs such as cisapride (which has been taken off the market) have been used in IBS-C patients.[49] Other drugs that have been used are anxiolytics, antigas preparations, and mast cell degranulation inhibitors such as disodium chromoglycolate. Probiotics have been studied, and the results are conflicting.[50] The probiotic commonly used is *Lactobacillus plantarum*.

Alosetron (Lotronex), a 5-HT_3 receptor antagonist, decreases small and large intestine motility and transit time. It has been used to treat severe IBS-D patients for control of diarrhea and abdominal discomfort.[51,52] The use of alosetron has been limited because of its association with ischemic colitis[53] and serious complication of constipation.[54]

Other Therapies

Other treatment modalities that have been helpful are relaxation therapy,[55] psychotherapy,[56] and hypnotherapy.[57] Patients with IBS frequently present with symptoms of constipation or fecal incontinence. These patients most often fail surgical corrections unless the symptoms of IBS are brought under control first.

RECTAL PROLAPSE

Overt rectal prolapse is the prolapse of the entire thickness of the rectal wall through the anal orifice. This is usually a problem seen in older women. A multitude of treatment modalities have been described, highlighting the fact that treatment is controversial and that no one treatment or surgery is entirely successful.

Etiopathology

The cause of rectal prolapse is unknown, but several theories have been postulated. The first of these, described by Moschowitz,[58] attributes rectal prolapse to a sliding hernia through a defect in the pelvic fascia. The second theory by Brodin and Snellman[59] postulates that rectal prolapse is an intussusception of the rectum starting about 3 inches above the anal verge. Radiologic findings that the prolapse starts well above the pelvic floor rules out the possibility of this being a sphincter disorder. Predisposing factors are intractable constipation, chronic diarrhea, neurologic diseases, anatomic defect due to pregnancies, previous surgeries, and psychiatric illness.

Rectal prolapse has been categorized as complete or full-thickness (Fig. 78-6) wall prolapse through the sphincters or intussusception that has not protruded beyond the sphincter complex. It should be differentiated from mucosal prolapse (Fig. 78-7).

Workup

The confirmatory test is a clinical demonstration of a rectal prolapse and the exclusion of prolapsing hemorrhoids. Other tests are done for associated symptoms and to rule out colonic pathology. These tests may include a barium enema to look for a redundant colon, anorectal manometry and dynamic MRI (when obstructive defecation is suspected), transit studies in patients with constipation, and a colonoscopy.

Treatment of Rectal Prolapse

The earliest operation for rectal prolapse was described by Thiersch in 1891. It involved encircling the anus with a silver

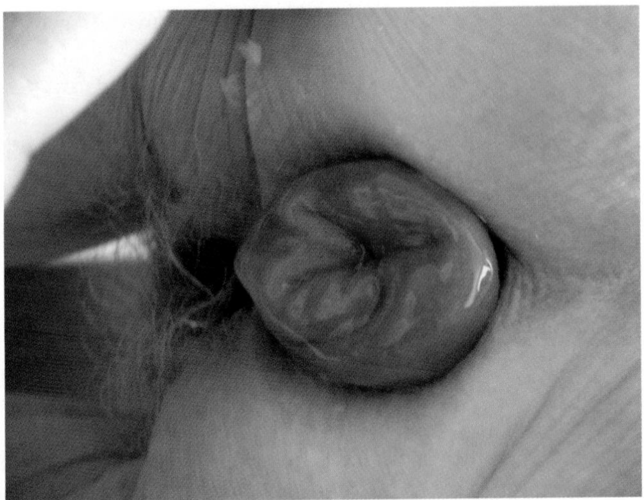

Figure 78-6 Complete rectal prolapse.

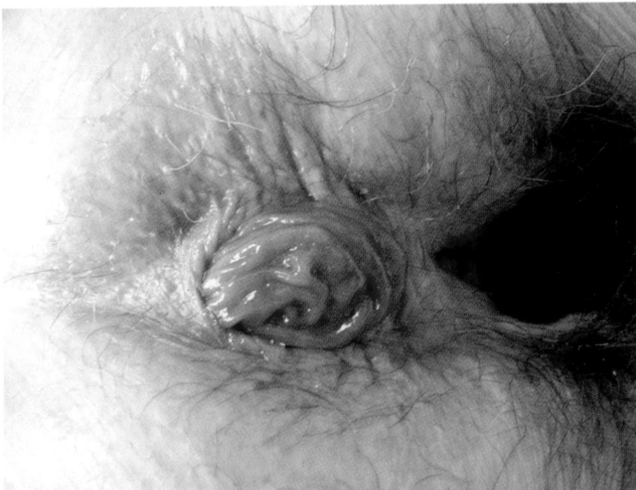

Figure 78-7 Mucosal prolapse of rectum.

wire, thereby decreasing the anal opening. This procedure has largely been abandoned.

The current operative procedures are divided into abdominal and perineal procedures. The abdominal procedures are based on fixing the rectum to the sacrum; the perineal procedures aim at excision of the prolapsed rectum.

Abdominal Procedures

The principles of abdominal procedures are based on rectal mobilization and fixation, with or without resection of the sigmoid colon based on the patient's symptoms. Rectal mobilization is described subsequently, and the various methods of rectal fixation are discussed.

Abdominal Mobilization of the Rectum

Rectal mobilization is carried out through a Pfannenstiel or midline incision. The extent varies among surgeons but usually involves posterior mobilization to the coccyx and incision anteriorly to the upper third of the vagina. Lateral mobilization is controversial, and at least one lateral stalk may be preserved to avoid new evacuation problems.

Rectal Fixation

Rectal fixation can be achieved by using mesh (i.e., Ripstein's procedure) or a foreign material (i.e., Ivalon sponge repair) or suture rectopexy.

Ripstein's procedure is more frequently done outside the United States. Ripstein and Lante[60] thought that the rectal prolapse was caused by loss of attachment of the rectum, which makes it lose its posterior curvature and become a straight tube. Massive straining causes the rectal walls to intussuscept, which begins at the rectosigmoid junction and finally protrudes through the anus. They did not believe that the pelvic defects were the primary cause and did not see the need to repair them. Rectal fixation was achieved initially by fascia lata and later changed to Marlex mesh[61] and Gore-Tex mesh.[62]

In this procedure, the rectum is mobilized to the tip of the coccyx posteriorly. The lateral stalks may be divided. The free end of a 5-cm Marlex or Gore-Tex mesh is fixed to the sacrum with nonabsorbable sutures, which are placed 1 cm from the midline, taking care to avoid any presacral bleeding. The mesh is wrapped around the rectum anteriorly, and the free end is sutured to the other side in a similar fashion. The sling should be loose enough to admit two fingers. The peritoneum is then closed over the sling.

Intraoperative complications of this procedure include presacral bleeding. Postoperative complications include hemorrhage and pelvic abscesses.[63] Late complications include persistent constipation, new onset of constipation, recurrence, erosion of the mesh, and strictures. The recurrence rate has been cited as 2% to 10%.[64,65] Some investigators[66] have recommended this procedure be performed with a sigmoid resection in patients with a longstanding history of constipation. However, others are hesitant to resect large intestine in the face of introducing mesh at the same procedure.[63]

Ivalon sponge repair was described by Wells[67] in 1959 and was popular in Europe. After rectal mobilization, a rectangular piece of Ivalon sponge is moistened and fixed to the sacrum in the midline using nonabsorbable sutures. The mobilized rectum is then pulled upward in front of the sponge, and the sponge is wrapped around the rectum and sutured to the anterior wall, leaving one third of the circumference free anteriorly. The sponge is then buried under the peritoneum.

The predominant complication is pelvic abscess, which occurs in about 16% of the patients.[68] Even though an abscess usually necessitated removal of the sponge, inflammatory scarring of the rectum on many occasions fixes the rectum to the sacrum, thereby curing the prolapse. This procedure is not performed in the United States.

Suture rectopexy was first described by Pemberton and Stalker.[69] It fixes the rectum to the sacrum posteriorly. After mobilization of the rectum posteriorly, proctopexy is achieved using two or three nonabsorbable sutures on either side to fix the rectum to the presacral fascia, taking care to avoid the presacral vessels, which can result in bleeding.

Suture rectopexy has been associated with a mortality rate of 0% to 6.7% and a recurrence rate of 0% to 20%.[70] In many, the incontinence decreases in time after rectopexy.[71]

Abdominal Rectopexy with or without Resection of the Sigmoid Colon

Sigmoid resection alone has not been popular for rectal prolapse. However, resection of the sigmoid colon has been advocated when constipation is a predominant symptom preoperatively and a redundant sigmoid colon has been demonstrated by imaging studies. In some cases, this improves after sigmoid resection.[72] Resection and the subsequent fibrosis that occurs in the area of the anastomosis may add to the fibrosis that occurs with a rectopexy.

Laparoscopic Rectopexy

The laparoscopic approach is theoretically similar to the open procedure, and results should be comparable, but the technique is still evolving. The advantage of the laparoscopic technique is a reduction in pain at the incision site and hospital stay.[73] Laparoscopically assisted rectopexy has acceptable results, with a morbidity rate of 9%, leak rate of less than 1%, and a recurrence rate of 2.5% for a full-thickness and 18% for a mucosal prolapse.[74] Studies have demonstrated that laparoscopic resection has a short-term benefit in the length of stay and is comparable to open prolapse surgery in the long term for continence and constipation and recurrence rates.[14]

Perineal Procedures

Perineal Rectosigmoidectomy

Perineal rectosigmoidectomy was initially described in 1889 and popularized by Miles[75] in 1933. Subsequently, Altemeier[76] championed its use in the United States. The indication for surgery is the high-risk individual who may not tolerate the anesthesia needed for an abdominal approach. Some institutions have advocated this approach for young men in whom the abdominal procedures may carry a higher risk of sexual dysfunction.[77]

It can be done under local, regional, or general anesthesia in the lithotomy position. The anastomosis can be hand-sewn or stapled. A circumferential incision is carried out 1 to 2 cm above the dentate line, and of the rectum is mobilized. The mesentery of the rectum is clamped and divided until the bowel cannot be pulled down anymore. The bowel is then transected and anastomosed to the distal cut end. Before the anastomosis, the levator muscles may be plicated in an effort to lengthen the anal canal to improve continence.

Complications include bleeding from the suture line, dehiscence of the suture line, anastomotic stricture, injury to the small bowel, and an increase in morbidity due to pulmonary and cardiac complications in fragile patients.[78]

Delorme Procedure

The Delorme[79] procedure is another perineal procedure. It has become more popular in recent years. A circular incision is made in the mucosa about 1 cm above the dentate line, and the mucosa is carefully lifted away, taking care to cauterize any bleeding vessels on the way. This continues until there exists no further redundancy. The redundant mucosa is amputated, and the mucosal ends are then brought together and sutured. Recurrence rates vary from 5% to 20%.[80]

Abdominal versus Perineal Procedures

The abdominal procedure is the procedure of choice for the medically fit patient in most institutions because of the lower recurrence rates. Perineal procedures are usually offered to frail patients with comorbidities. The choice of perineal procedure usually rests with the surgeon and depends on his or her level of experience. The perineal rectosigmoidectomy has a lower recurrence rate than the Delorme procedure.[81] The Delorme procedure may be a choice when there is insufficient length to do a perineal rectosigmoidectomy. Concomitant levatoroplasty after a perineal rectosigmoidectomy has been shown to improve continence.[81]

The most common abdominal procedure is rectopexy with or without resection. The abdominal procedures are associated with better continence than the perineal procedures.[82] Suture rectopexy has acceptable results, and the addition of mesh posteriorly does not seem to offer any distinct advantage. The addition of a sigmoid resection is of value in patients with a redundant colon and symptoms of constipation. The Ivalon sponge has been associated with an increase in infection and has been abandoned. The Ripstein's procedure has been associated with new-onset constipation due to the mesh configuration. Laparoscopic rectopexy is gaining popularity, and with time and development of new instruments, it will be performed more.[73]

Emphasizing the mental algorithm in approaching patients with rectal prolapse Kim and colleagues[83] reviewed 188 perineal rectosigmoidectomy and 160 abdominal rectopexy patients. They found no significant differences in morbidity but found a higher recurrence rate with perineal procedures.

Recurrent rectal prolapse is treated by a repeat repair, and both abdominal and perineal repairs have been advocated. However, care should be taken to delineate the previous anastomosis. It is important to consider all previous operations in an attempt to avoid rendering a section of bowel ischemic due to division of blood vessels at the previous repair.

CONCLUSIONS

Evaluation of the individual patient is the key to treating defecatory disorders and fecal incontinence. There is no perfect cure for these ailments, and much patience and time goes into making a diagnosis and reaching an individual treatment plan that can help these patients. Newer treatment options are emerging, and the modalities of treatment may change in the future.

References

1. Pannu HK: Magnetic resonance imaging of pelvic organ prolapse. Abdom Imaging 27:660-673, 2002.
2. Scarlett Y: Medical management of fecal incontinence. Gastroenterology 126:S55-S63, 2004.
3. Santoro GA, Eitan BZ, Pryde A, Bartolo DC: Open study of low-dose amitriptyline in the treatment of patients with idiopathic fecal incontinence. Dis Colon Rectum 43:1676-1681, 2000.
4. Cheetham MJ, Kamm MA, Phillips RKS: Topical phenylephrine increases anal canal resting pressure in patients with fecal incontinence. Gut 48:356-359, 2001.
5. Ozturk R, Niazi S, Stessman M, Rao SS: Long-term outcome and objective changes in anorectal function after biofeedback therapy for fecal incontinence. Aliment Pharmacol Ther 20:667-674, 2004.
6. Jensen LL, Lowry AC: Biofeedback improves functional outcome after sphincteroplasty. Dis Colon Rectum 40:197-200, 1997.
7. Efron JE, Corman Ml, Fleshman J, et al: Safety and effectiveness of temperature controlled radiofrequency energy delivery to the anal canal. Dis Colon Rectum 46:1606-1616, 2003.
8. Conaghan P, Farouk R: Sacral nerve stimulation can be successful in patients with ultrasound evidence of external anal sphincter disruption. Dis Colon Rectum 48:1610-1614, 2005.

9. Vaizey CJ, Kamm MA: Injectable bulking agents for treating faecal incontinence. Br J Surg 92:521-527, 2005.
10. Arnaud A, Sarles JC, Sielezneff I, et al: Sphincter repair without overlapping for fecal incontinence. Dis Colon Rectum 9:744-747, 1991.
11. Tjandra JJ, Han WR, Goh J, et al: Direct repair vs overlapping sphincter repair: A randomized controlled trial. Dis Colon Rectum 46:937-942, 2003.
12. Young C. J, Mathur MN, Eyers AA, Solomon MJ: Successful overlapping anal sphincter repair relationship to patient age, neuropathy and colostomy function. Dis Colon Rectum 41:344-349, 1998.
13. Fang DT, Nivatongs S, Vernuelen FD, et al: Overlapping sphincteroplasty for acquired anal incontinence. Dis Colon Rectum 27:720-722, 1984.
14. Solomon MJ, Young CJ, Eyers AA, Roberts RA: Randomized clinical trial of laparoscopic versus open abdominal rectopexy for rectal prolapse. Br J Surg 89:35-39, 2002.
15. Young CJ, Mathur MN, Eyers AA, Solomon MJ: Successful overlapping sphincter repair: Relationship to age, neuropathy and colostomy formation. Dis Colon Rectum 41:344-349, 1998.
16. Gutirrez AB, Madoff RD, Lowery AC, et al: Long-term results of anterior sphincteroplasty. Dis Colon Rectum 47:727-731, 2003.
17. Vaizey CJ, Norton C, Thornton MJ, et al: Long-term results of repeat anal sphincter repair. Dis Colon Rectum 47:858-863, 2004.
18. Baeten CG, Geerdes BP, Adang EMM, et al: Anal dynamic graciloplasty in the treatment of intractable fecal incontinence. N Engl J Med 332:1600-1605, 1995.
19. Wexner SD, Gonzalea-Padron A, Rius J, et al: Stimulated gracilis neosphincter operation: Initial experience pitfalls, and complications. Dis Colon Rectum 39:957-964, 1996.
20. Rainey JB, Donaldson DR, Thompson JP: Post-anal repair: Which patients derive most benefit? J R Coll Surg Edinb 35:101-105, 1990.
21. Casal E, San Ildefonso A, Carracedo R, et al: Artificial bowel sphincter in severe anal disease. Colorectal Dis 6:180-185, 2004.
22. Wong D, Jensen LL, Bartolo DC, et al: Artificial anal sphincter. Dis Colon Rectum 39:1345-1351, 1996.
23. Chiaroni G, Salandini L, Whitehead WE: Biofeedback benefits patients only patients with outlet dysfunction not patients with isolated slow transit constipation. Gastroenterology 129:86-97, 2005.
24. Pemberton JH, Rath DM, Ilstrup DM: Evaluation and surgical treatment of severe chronic constipation. Ann. Surg 214:403-411, 1991.
25. Beck DE, Fazio VW, Jagleman DG, Lavery IC: Surgical management of colonic inertia. South Med J 82:305-309, 1989.
26. Sample C, Gupta R, Bambriz F, Anvari M: Laparoscopic subtotal colectomy for colonic inertia. J Gastrointest Surg 9:803-808, 2004.
27. Wexner SD, Daniel N, Jagleman DG: Colectomy for constipation: physiological investigation is the key. Dis Colon Rectum 34:851-856, 1991.
28. Webster CMD: Results of colectomy for colonic inertia: A sixteen year experience. Am J Surg 182:639-644, 2001.
29. Fitzharris GP, Garcia-Aguilar J, Parker SC, et al: Quality of life after subtotal colectomy for slow transit constipation: Both quality and quantity count. Dis Colon Rectum 46:1720-1721, 2003.
30. Thaler K, Dinnewitzer A, Oberwalder M, et al: Quality of life after colectomy for colonic inertia. Tech Coloproctol 9:133-137, 2005.
31. Hill J, Scott S, MacLennan I, et al: Antegrade enemas for the treatment of severe idiopathic constipation. Br J Surg 81:1490-1491, 1994.
32. Malouf AJ, Wiesel PH, Nicholls T, et al: Short term effects of sacral nerve stimulation for idiopathic slow transit constipation. World J Surg 26:166-170, 2001.
33. Bassotti G, Chistolini F, Sietchiping-Nzepa F, et al: Biofeedback for pelvic floor dysfunction in constipation. Br J Surg 328:393-396, 2004.
34. Bosscanta P, Venturi M, Salamina G, et al: New trends in the surgical treatment of outlet obstruction: Clinical and functional results of two novel transanal stapled techniques from a randomised controlled trial. Int J Colorectal Dis 19:539-369, 2004.
35. Drossman DA, Cammilleri M, Mayer EA, et al: AGA technical review of irritable bowel syndrome. Gastroenterology 123:2108-2131, 2002.
36. Talley NJ: Irritable bowel syndrome: Definition, diagnosis and epidemiology. Baillieres Best Pract Res Clin Gastroenterol 13:371-384, 1999.
37. Hungin APS, Chang L, Locke GR, et al: Irritable bowel syndrome in the United States prevalence, symptoms patterns and impact. Aliment Pharmacol Ther 21:1365-1375, 2005.
38. Boyce PM, Koloski NA, Talley NJ: Irritable bowel syndrome according to varying diagnostic criteria: Are the Rome II criteria unnecessarily restrictive for research and practice? Am J Gastroenterol 95:3176-3183, 2000.
39. Poitras P, Riberdy PM, Boivin M, Verrier P: Evolution of visceral sensitivity in patients with irritable bowel syndrome. Dig Dis Sci 47:914-920, 2002.
40. Wingate DL: The irritable bowel syndrome. Gastroenterol Clin North Am 20:351-365, 1991.
41. Drossman DA, Leserman J, Nachman G, et al: Sexual and physical abuse in women with functional or organic gastrointestinal disorders. Ann Intern Med 113:828-833, 1990.
42. Walker EA, Katon WJ, Jemelka RP, et al: Comorbidity of gastrointestinal complaints, depression, and anxiety in the Epidemiologic Catchment Area (ECA) study. Am J Med 92:26S-30S, 1999.
43. Rees GA, Davies GJ, Parker M, Trevan M: Gastrointestinal symptoms and diet of members of an irritable bowel self-help group. J R Soc Health 14:222-227, 1994.
44. Bohmer CM, Tuynman HE: The clinical relevance of lactose malabsorption in irritable bowel syndrome. Eur J Gastroenterol Hepatol 8:1013-1016, 1996.
45. Cann PA, Read NW, Holdsworth CD, Barends D: Role of loperamide in the management of irritable bowel syndrome. Dig Dis Sci 1984; 29:239.
46. Steadman CJ, Talley NJ, Phillips SF, Zinsmeister AR: Selective 5-hydroxytryptamine type 3 receptor antagonism with ondansetron as treatment for diarrhea predominant irritable bowel syndrome—A pilot study. Mayo Clin Proc 67:732-738, 1992.
47. Schonfield P: Efficacy of current drug therapies in Irritable bowel Syndrome: What works and does not work. Gastroenterol Clin North Am 34:319-335, 2005.
48. Tack J, Müller-Lissner, Bytzer P, et al: A randomised controlled trial assessing the efficacy and safety of repeated tegaserod therapy in women with irritable bowel syndrome and constipation (IBS-C). Gut 54:1701-1713, 2005.
49. Van Outryve M, Milo R, Toussaint J, Van Eeghem P: Prokinetic treatment of constipation-predominant irritable bowel syndrome a placebo controlled study of cisapride. J Clin Gastroenteral 13(1): 49-57, 1991.
50. Madden JA, Hunter JO: A review of the role of gut microflora in irritable bowel syndrome and the effects of probiotics. Br J Nutr 88: S67-S72, 2002.
51. Lembo T, Wright RA, Bagby B, et al: Alosetron controls bowel urgency and provides global symptom improvement in women with diarrhea prone IBS. Am J Gastroenterol 96:2662-2670, 2001.
52. Cammilleri M, Northcutt AR, Kong S, et al: The efficacy and safety of alosetron in female patients with IBS. Am J Gastroenterol 355:1035-1040, 2000.
53. Freidel D, Thomas R, Fisher RS: Ischemic colitis during treatment with alosetron. Gastroenterology 121:231-232, 2001.
54. Cammilleri M, Chey WY, Mayer EA, et al: A randomized controlled clinical trial of the serotonin type 3 receptor antagonist alosetron in women with diarrhea-predominant irritable bowel syndrome. Arch Intern Med 61:1733-1740, 2001.
55. Heymen-Monnikes I, Arnold R, et al: The combination of medical treatment plus multicomponent behavioural therapy is superior to

medical treatment alone in the treatment of irritable bowel syndrome. Am J Gastroenterol 95:981-994, 2000.
56. Svedlund J: Psychotherapy in irritable bowel syndrome: A controlled outcome study. Acta Psychiatr Scand Suppl 306:67-86, 1983.
57. Whorwell PI, Prior A, Faragher EB: Controlled trial of hypnotherapy in the treatment of severe refractory irritable bowel syndrome. Lancet 2:1232-1234, 1984.
58. Moschowitz AV: The pathogenesis and cure of the prolapse of the rectum. Surg Gynecol Obstet 15:7-21, 1912.
59. Broden B, Snellen B: Procedentia of the rectum studied with cine radiography: A contribution to the discussion of causative mechanism. Dis Colon Rectum 11:330-347, 1968.
60. Ripstein CB, Lanter B: Etiology and surgical therapy of massive prolapse of the rectum. Ann Surg 157:259-264, 1963.
61. Keighley MR, Fielding JW, Alexander-Williams J: Results of Marlex mesh abdominal rectopexy for rectal prolapse in 100 consecutive patients. Br J Surg 70:229-232. 1983.
62. Cicconi M, Romanelli P, Cardelli M, et al: Abdominal Wells rectopexy with patch micromesh PTFE (Goretex) [in Italian]. G Chir 24:46-52, 2003.
63. Athanasidis S, Weynad G, Heilgers J, et al: The risk of infection of three synthetic materials used in rectopexy with or without colonic resection for rectal prolapse. Int J Colorectal Dis 11:42-44, 1996.
64. Gordon PH, Hoexter B: Complication of Ripstein's procedure. Dis Colon Rectum 21:277-280, 1978.
65. Biehl AJ, Pay JE, Gathright JB: Repair of rectal prolapse: Experience with the Ripstein sling. South Med J 71:923-925, 1978.
66. Tjandra JJ, Fazio VW, Church JM, et al: Ripstein's procedure is an effective procedure for treatment of rectal prolapse without constipation. Dis Colon Rectum 36:501-507, 1993.
67. Wells C: New operation for rectal prolapse. Proc R Soc Med 32:602-603, 1959.
68. Kupfer CA, Goligher JC: One hundred consecutive cases of complete rectal prolapse of the rectum treated by operation. Br J Surg 57:481-487, 1970.
69. Backer OG, Baden H: The Pemberton-Stalker rectopexy. Dis Colon Rectum 86:421-422, 1964.
70. Loygue J, Nordinger B, Cunci O, et al: Rectopexy to the promontory for the treatment of rectal prolapse. Dis Colon Rectum 27:356-359, 1984.
71. Blachford GJ, Perry RE, Thorson AG, et al: Rectopexy without resection for rectal prolapse. Am J Surg 158:574-576, 1989.
72. Mckee RF, Lauder JC, Poon FW, et al: A prospective randomized study of abdominal rectopexy with and without sigmoidectomy in rectal prolapse. Surg Gynecol Obstet 174:145-148, 1992.
73. Boccasanta P, Rosati R, Venturi M, et al: Comparison of laparoscopic rectopexy with open technique in the treatment of complete rectal prolapse: Clinical and functional results. Surg Laparosc Endosc 8:460-465, 1998.
74. Ashari LHS, Lumley JW, Stevenson ARL, Sitz RW: Laparoscopically-assisted resection rectopexy for rectal prolapse: ten year experience. Dis Colon Rectum 48:982-987, 2004.
75. Miles WE: Rectosigmoidectomy as a method of treatment for procidentia recti. Proc R Soc Med 26:1445-1452, 1933.
76. Altemeier WA, Culbertson WR, Schowengerdt C, Hunt J: Nineteen years experience with the one stage perineal repair for rectal prolapse. Ann Surg 173:993-1006, 1971.
77. Yakut M, Kayamakcioglu N, Simsek A, et al: Surgical treatment of rectal prolapse. A retrospective analysis of 94 cases. Int Surg 83:53-55, 1998.
78. Williams JG, Rothenberger DA, Madoff RD, Goldberg SM: Treatment of rectal prolapse in the elderly by perineal proctosigmoidectomy. Dis Colon Rectum 35:830-834, 1992.
79. Delorme E: On the treatment of total prolapse of the rectum by excision of the rectal mucous membranes or retrocolic. Dis Colon Rectum 28:544-553, 1985.
80. Lechaux JP, Atienza P, Goasguen N, et al: Prosthetic rectopexy to the pelvic floor and sigmoidectomy for rectal prolapse. Am J Gastroenterol 182:465-469, 2001.
81. Agachan F, Reissmann P, Pfeifer J, et al: Comparison of three perineal procedures for the treatment of rectal prolapse. South Med J 90:925-992, 1997.
82. Watts JD, Rothenberger DA, Buls JG, et al: The management of rectal procidentia: 30 years experience. Dis Colon Rectum 28:96-102, 1985.
83. Kim DS, Tsang CB, Wong WD, et al: Complete rectal prolapse: Evolution management and results. Dis Colon Rectum 42:460-466, 1999.

Section 9

FISTULAS AND DIVERTICULA

Chapter 79

URETHROVAGINAL FISTULA

Jason P. Gilleran and Philippe E. Zimmern

Urethrovaginal fistula (UVF) presents a challenging diagnostic and therapeutic dilemma for the reconstructive surgeon. Because of its uncommon occurrence, much of what is known about this entity is derived from small series and case reports. Consequently, most UVFs are seen and treated in specialized centers, whether they manifest alone or in combination with a vesicovaginal fistula. The underlying cause, number of prior repairs, and damage to the continence mechanism are key factors in approaching the patient with a UVF. This chapter reviews the common causes, diagnostic modalities, and therapeutic options for UVFs.

ETIOLOGY

Postoperative Iatrogenic Factors

Traumatic fistulas resulting from obstetric deliveries account for most UVFs in underdeveloped nations, whereas in industrialized nations,[1] UVFs occur as a complication of urethral diverticulectomy, anterior colporrhaphy, or other periurethral procedures. Some direct injuries are recognized at the time of the original surgery. In this instance, closure of the urethral lumen without verifying water-tightness, overlapping suture lines, lack of consideration for tissue interposition, insufficient bladder drainage, or a combination of these factors can contribute to the secondary formation of a UVF. Indirect mechanisms are less common but have been reported after periurethral collagen injection[2] and an anterior colporrhaphy during which tight suburethral plication resulted in tissue necrosis and secondary fistula formation.[3] An unrecognized urethral injury, which can occur during urethrolysis and particularly in the setting of dense periurethral scar tissue after a sling procedure, is another indirect mechanism. Most contemporary series on synthetic slings using tension-free vaginal tape or transobturator tape report a low incidence of urethral injuries and secondary urethral erosions, which can result in UVFs.[4-6]

Radiation Therapy

Although the incidence of vaginal fistulas occurring after irradiation for pelvic malignancies is significantly lower than in the past because of technical advances in radiation delivery, the profound long-term effects of radiation on surrounding tissues can promote fistula formation. Repair with flap interposition should be considered, but a supravesical diversion may be the only remaining option for heavily radiated tissues.

Other Causes

Vaginal lacerations after pelvic trauma, if ignored or inadequately repaired, can lead to UVF formation. Primary closure of vaginal lacerations is advocated to prevent fistula formation; regardless of the approach, these lacerations are susceptible to wound dehiscence if not properly débrided before repair.[1] Although rare, a neoplasm arising from a urethral diverticulum[7] can extend locally and manifest as a UVF. Likewise, radiation therapy for urethral cancer can lead to tumor necrosis and a secondary UVF.

DIAGNOSIS

History and Physical Examination

Presenting symptoms may provide some insight as to the location and size of a UVF. Fistulas distal to the urethral continence mechanism may be entirely asymptomatic, or they may manifest as a split urinary stream or vaginal voiding. Occasionally, recurrent urinary tract infections are the main presenting symptoms. Women with larger fistulas or with fistulas involving the proximal urethra and bladder neck region present with continuous incontinence. It is important to review the prior operative notes, evaluate tissue quality (i.e., multi-operated, densely scarred, or atrophic tissues), and look for risk factors for deficient healing (e.g., immunosuppression, malnutrition, irradiation). Physical examination should identify the size and location of the fistula and any other associated fistulas or tissue changes. However, smaller tracts may be challenging to recognize, requiring endoscopy and imaging for exact determination. In some cases, a high index of suspicion despite thorough negative investigations may lead to urethrocystoscopy under anesthesia to establish the diagnosis.

Imaging

Visualization of the fistula tract may be accomplished by voiding cystourethrography[8,9] or by double-balloon urethrography, but these techniques require high resolution to see the tract and true lateral views (Fig. 79-1). Upper tract imaging may be necessary for large or multiple fistulas to exclude ureteral obstruction or an associated ureterovaginal fistula. Urethral magnetic resonance imaging is of limited benefit to identify a fistula tract and is occasionally helpful in case of suspected residual diverticulum pocket associated with a UVF after urethral diverticulectomy.

Endoscopy

Direct visualization of the fistula opening on the floor of the urethral lumen with a short-beaked female urethroscope or a flexible scope can confirm the diagnosis.[10] It is important to document the size of the opening and its location in the urethra in relation to the continence mechanism. The status of the bladder neck, trigone, and ureteric orifices should be observed, as well as the condition of the surrounding tissues for changes

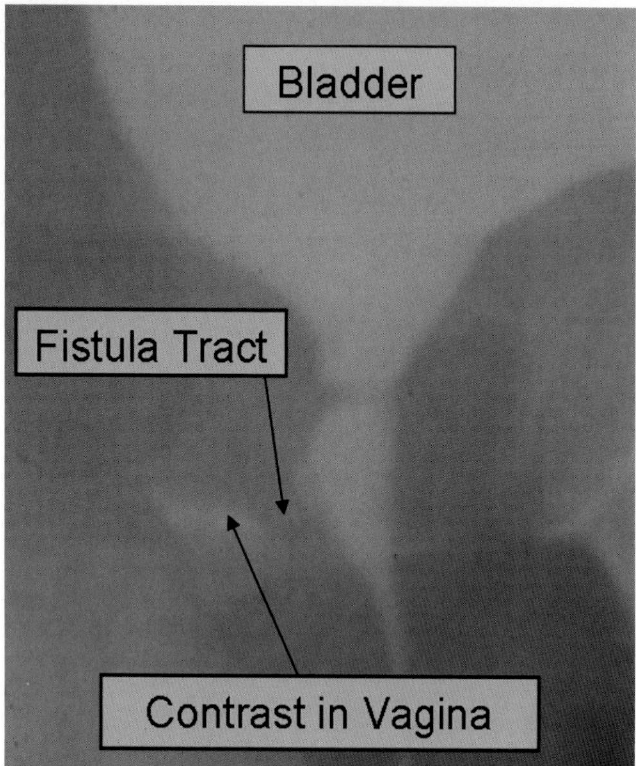

Figure 79-1 Lateral view from voiding cystourethrography (VCUG) of a woman with a urethrovaginal fistula at the mid-urethra demonstrates a fistula tract, with contrast seen in the vagina. Good resolution and true lateral voiding films are important in visualizing the tract on VCUG.

suggesting inflammation or neoplasm. A biopsy may be indicated for friable and irregular fistula edges or in case of a palpable induration around the fistula site. After vaginal laceration or urethral tear, the urethra may be completely strictured and the UVF located proximal to the site of urethral injury. Transvaginal endoscopy can help accessing the fistula tract and possibly the bladder by advancing a small flexible scope through the tract.

MANAGEMENT

The decision on how and when to best manage a UVF largely depends on the cause of the fistula, the quality of the surrounding tissues, the correction of risk factors for poor tissue healing whenever possible, and the number of prior repairs. Experience with urethral reconstruction procedures is paramount to achieving a good technical outcome. A large armamentarium of additional procedures to secure continence and prevent fistula recurrence should be available to the repairing surgeon.

Observation

Small fistulas in the distal urethra may be discovered incidentally and observed if minimally or asymptomatic. Spontaneous resolution of UVF with short-term catheter drainage has been reported.[11] Most patients, however, choose surgical repair.

Table 79-1 Perioperative Checklist

High lithotomy (or prone) position	Fine urethral instruments and sutures
Short-beaked female cystourethroscope (consider guidewire and open-ended ureteral catheter)	Access to autologous sling harvest (rectus fascia, fascia lata)
Suprapubic tube placement (Lowsley retractor or percutaneous kit)	Interposing graft (Martius labial fat pad, gracilis muscle)
Headlight	Soft urethral catheter
Vaginal retractor (Scott Lone Star, Turner-Warwick)	Magnifying loupes (optional)
Injectable saline and marking pen	Vaginal pack, antibiotics and anticholinergic medications (belladonna and opium suppository)

Surgical Repair

The goals of UVF repair are to close the tract, prevent recurrence of the fistula, and restore continence as indicated. In the case of a small distal fistula tract producing a split urinary stream with minimal or no incontinence, a simple marsupialization procedure to create a hypospadiac opening (i.e., Spence procedure) may correct the problem.[12] We review two scenarios for transvaginal repair of a UVF, one involving a simple primary closure for a small nonirradiated UVF and the other a larger UVF necessitating more advanced techniques of urethral reconstruction and flap interposition for continence and closure.

Primary Closure with a Vaginal Flap

A primary repair using layered closure was first described by Collis,[13] and it is ideal in the setting of a small to medium-sized UVF in nonirradiated tissues. Sterile urine must be obtained preoperatively, and antibiotic administration must be continued perioperatively. Several elements are necessary to facilitate a successful repair, as listed in Table 79-1. Patient positioning varies between advocates of the prone position[14] and those preferring a high lithotomy position. Maximum perioperative urinary drainage is best achieved with a urethral and a suprapubic catheter. Exposure is facilitated by a Lonestar retractor (Lone Star Medical Products, Stafford, TX) or other self-retaining retractor, a weighted vaginal speculum, a headlight, and even magnifying glasses if available. Passage of a Teflon guidewire over a 5-Fr open-ended ureteral catheter through the tract can facilitate the dissection of the tract (Fig. 79-2). Hydrodissection with normal saline can aid in separating the vagina from the urethral wall. A broad-base, inverted-U-shaped incision is made in the anterior vaginal wall. This broad-base flap permits secondary tissue interposition (e.g., autologous sling, Martius labial fat pad graft[15]) (Fig. 79-3). After raising the anterior vaginal flap, the fistula opening on the vaginal wall is closed with fine absorbable sutures. In our experience, which follows the principles recommended by Raz for a vaginal repair of a vesicovaginal fistula, the well-circumscribed UVF tract is not excised. This decision prevents enlarging the fistula site and creating further bleeding and urethral compromise. Closure of the tract is performed with two running absorbable sutures started at each corner of the fistula

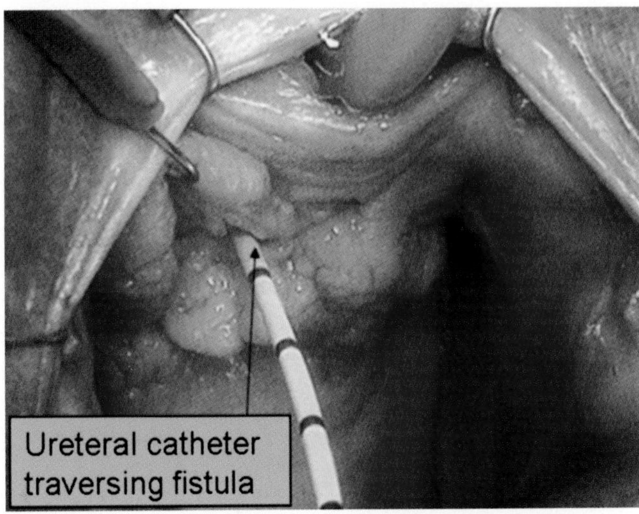

Figure 79-2 Passage of a 5-Fr ureteral catheter over a Teflon guidewire facilitates identification of the fistula tract during dissection. Additional hooks as part of the self-retaining retractor (lateral) are important to adequately visualize the surgical field.

tract and run toward the midpoint. After water-tightness of the repair is verified,[16] it is frequently necessary to interpose a layer over the urethral repair to minimize the risk of recurrence. We routinely use an autologous sling (i.e., rectus or fascia lata) interposition, which serves the dual purpose of restoring continence and minimizing recurrence. After the sling is secured in place at the undersurface of the urethra and over the UVF closed site, the initially raised anterior vaginal wall flap is advanced to complete the vaginal closure. Use of a fibrin adhesive as a protective layer between suture lines has been reported.[17] A vaginal pack with antibiotic ointment is placed for 24 hours, and anticholinergic medications are administered to avoid secondary bladder spasms.

Urethral Reconstruction

In advanced cases involving a severely damaged urethra from many previous urethral procedures, a more complex surgical repair may be necessary. At the time of consent, it is essential to explain to the patient and her family the challenges posed by repairing a large urethral defect with often scarred, thin, and poorly vascularized tissues or making a neo-urethra. A large defect always compromises the continence mechanism; closing

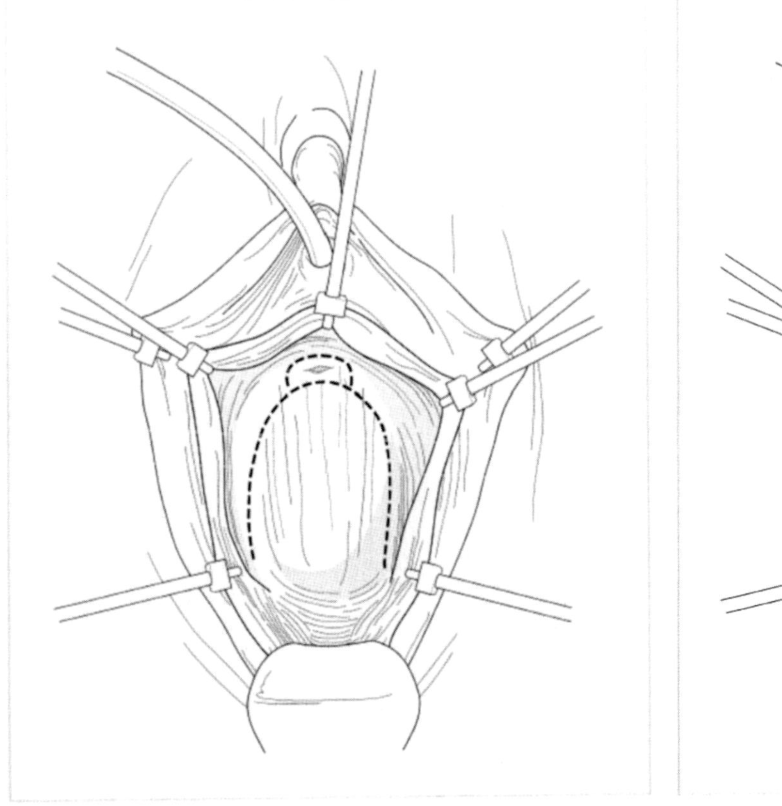

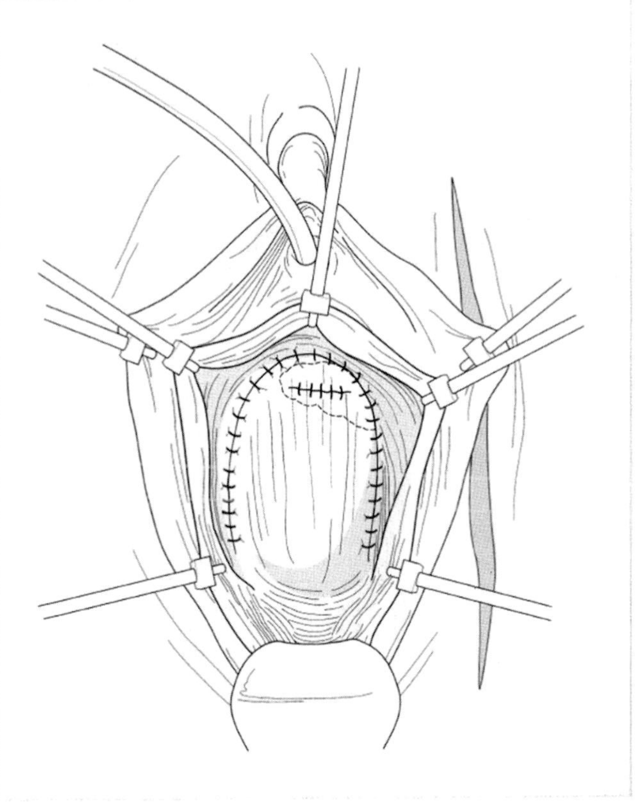

Figure 79-3 **A,** An inverted-U-shaped anterior vaginal wall flap incision is made, with the fistula *outlined*. Creating a broad vaginal flap is essential to avoid flap necrosis and allow for adequate mobilization. **B,** The flap is advanced and the fistula tract closed, with tissue interposition between the two (transparent) to prevent recurrence.

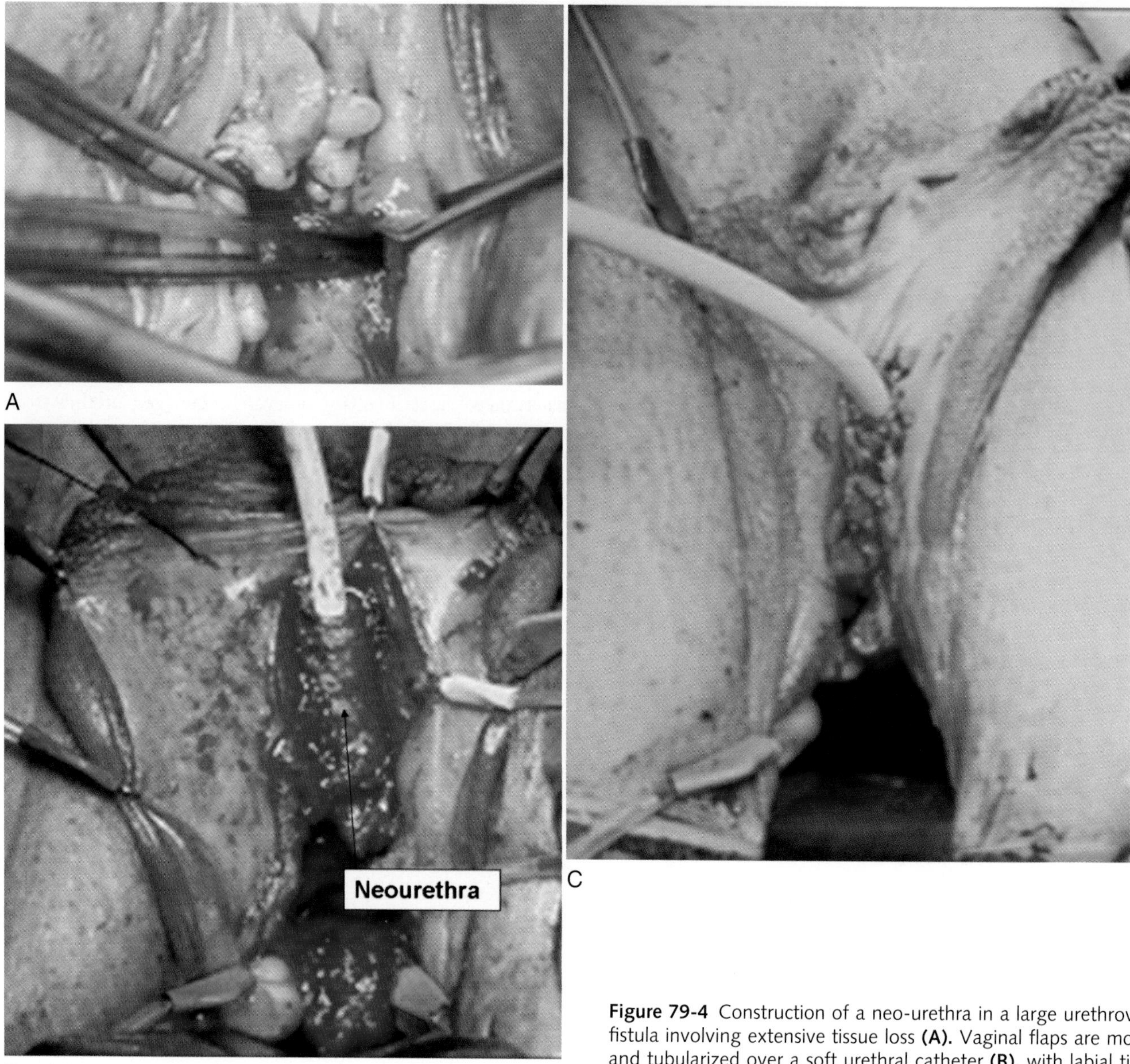

Figure 79-4 Construction of a neo-urethra in a large urethrovaginal fistula involving extensive tissue loss **(A).** Vaginal flaps are mobilized and tubularized over a soft urethral catheter **(B),** with labial tissue used for flap coverage of the neo-urethra **(C).**

the defect alone will lead to an incontinent pipe-stem urethra, and urethral support with a nonsynthetic sling can aid in restoring continence. Despite these precautions, a secondary UVF fistula can occur, and even after a technically successful repair, various degrees of stress or urge incontinence, secondary urethral narrowing, or even voiding dysfunction can remain challenging issues to manage.

Before deciding which technique to employ, a careful examination under anesthesia is needed to determine the precise location and extent of the urethral loss, the quality and length of the anterior vaginal wall, and the condition of the labia minora and the labia majora. Traditionally, the options for repair are limited to the creation of an anterior vaginal wall flap or a tube graft from the labia minora. When the defect extends into the bladder neck and trigone, placement of ureteral stents is recommended. After the tissues are adequately mobilized, our preference to create a neo-urethra or a segmental inferior urethral plate is to roll labia minora flaps medially and suture them with invagination of the mucosal layer[18] around a 14- or 16-Fr, soft, Silastic urethral catheter (Fig. 79-4). Then a second layer of tissue (i.e., Martius or sling, or both) is interposed before vaginal closure. Using the vagina to create a urethra usually is our second choice, and it can be considered when the anterior vaginal wall is long enough or the risk of foreshortening is not a concern in a patient who is not sexually active.

Beyond these two scenarios are a multitude of complex reconstructions involving poor-quality tissues, occasionally damage from radiation exposure, total or near-total urethral loss, or refractory UVFs, for which other techniques may need to be considered, including an anterior bladder wall flap, other interposition tissues (e.g., gracilis, rectus muscle,[19] omental flap), or vaginal wall closure with an island of bulbocavernous musculocutaneous flap[20] with attached skin. However, in such advanced cases, consideration should be given to transvaginal or abdominal[21] bladder neck closure or a continent or noncontinent urinary diversion.[22]

Postoperative Care

Broad-spectrum antibiotic coverage is continued, and the vaginal pack is removed after 24 to 48 hours. Uninterrupted postoperative bladder drainage with urethral and suprapubic catheters is imperative. Anticholinergic medications are administered during this period to limit bladder spasms and to prevent catheter expulsion. After approximately 3 to 4 weeks, voiding cystourethrography should be used to document urethral integrity and exclude a fistula recurrence. Return to sexual activity is delayed until complete healing of the vagina has occurred.

RESULTS

Because of the rarity of UVF, no large case-control series or randomized trials are available. Most case series consist of heterogenous UVFs managed with different techniques. One series divided 34 women into three groups based on the degree of urethral damage and type of surgical repair. In women with intact urethras who underwent a primary, transvaginal, layered closure, 23 (88%) of 26 experienced a successful anatomic and functional outcome.[12] Five women with destruction of the posterior urethra underwent extensive reconstruction, with all having successful anatomic outcomes, but only two of five were continent postoperatively. In another series of nine women with UVF, there was a 100% anatomic success rate after primary repair with a Martius labial graft interposition, with no cases of recurrent fistula or stricture.[18] However, two patients required additional surgery for stress incontinence. Similar success rates were reported in a series of 24 patients who underwent UVF repair using a Martius fat pad for reinforcement.[11]

The systematic use of a Martius labial fat pad interposition for all UVF repairs is arguable. In a report of 11 women with UVF, 7 who had undergone primary or vaginal flap closure without a Martius procedure had recurrences and subsequently underwent secondary repair with a labial fat pad.[1] The four remaining patients who underwent a Martius procedure had excellent anatomic results. In another retrospective study of 12 women with UVF, 3 of 4 patients who were repaired primarily alone had recurrences, compared with only 1 of 8 whose closures were reinforced with a Martius labial fat pad.[23] Women in this series who had multiple or recurrent UVFs and underwent Martius along with UVF repair fared better than those women repaired without a Martius flap.

Repair with a rectus abdominis muscle flap was reported for six women with refractory and complex UVFs. In this series, no patient had fistula recurrence at a mean follow-up of 23 months, and five of six women were continent and voiding to completion.[19] Similarly, a series of four "giant" vesicourethrovaginal fistulas were repaired by a suprapubic approach with fistula excision and omental interposition or a modified Tanagho bladder wall flap urethral reconstruction.[24] Two of these patients remained totally incontinent due to deficient sphincteric mechanism.

PREVENTION

"An ounce of prevention is worth a pound of cure" is applicable to urethral surgery and UVF formation. Technical considerations to help avoid this complication altogether are addressed in the following sections.

Urethral Diverticulectomy

Beyond patient positioning, adequate visualization of the tissues during urethral diverticulectomy can be facilitated by the use of a headlight and magnifying glasses. Careful dissection to limit the size of the urethral defect after complete excision of the diverticulum pocket, particularly along the inside wall of the diverticulum adjacent to the urethral lumen, can decrease the risk of fistula formation.[25] After the urethral defect is closed with fine absorbable sutures, the integrity of the closure is tested with a 5-Fr feeding tube or ureteral catheter in the lumen, occluding the distal outlet and bladder neck. Any visual leak should be further controlled with absorbable sutures. For a large defect, strong consideration should be given to tissue interposition (i.e., Martius or sling).

Pubovaginal Sling and Urethrolysis Procedures

The risk of urethral injury is of particular concern in the midurethra because the plane between urethra and vagina (Fig. 79-5A) is thinner compared with that in the proximal urethra (see Fig. 79-5B). Hydrodissection can aid in discerning this fairly avascular plane; venous bleeding from the urethral side may suggest an otherwise subtle urethral injury. Urethroscopy at the end of the vaginal dissection may be useful to identify such an injury, which should be repaired before sling placement. With a midline longitudinal incision common to many of the synthetic sling procedures, there is a risk of lateral urethral injury early in the dissection. The tips of the scissors should be pointed laterally and away from the undersurface of the urethra. In case of obstruction from a synthetic sling, it is preferable to stay lateral rather than just underneath the urethra to incise the sling.[26] Sling excision exposes the patients to urethral injury, especially when the sling is under tension and encroaches on the suburethral tissues.

Anterior Colporrhaphy

Early reports described UVF formation caused by overplication of tissues around a urethral catheter using silk sutures.[11] Although the use of permanent suture material or distal urethral plication has been abandoned for the most part, plication at the bladder neck or proximal urethra can still result in fistula formation. Palpation through the vaginal wall to identify the location of the Foley catheter balloon at the bladder neck is an important step to avoid extending the dissection underneath the urethra.

CONCLUSIONS

UVFs have different causes, locations, sizes, and associated factors. These aspects and the patient's symptoms dictate the selection of a surgical technique. Each repair is unique and challenging, and it is best performed by an experienced reconstructive surgeon. Adherence to time-honored principles of fistula repair can help ensure satisfactory anatomic results in most instances. Patients should be counseled that functional results are not always perfect in regard to continence and voiding function postoperatively.

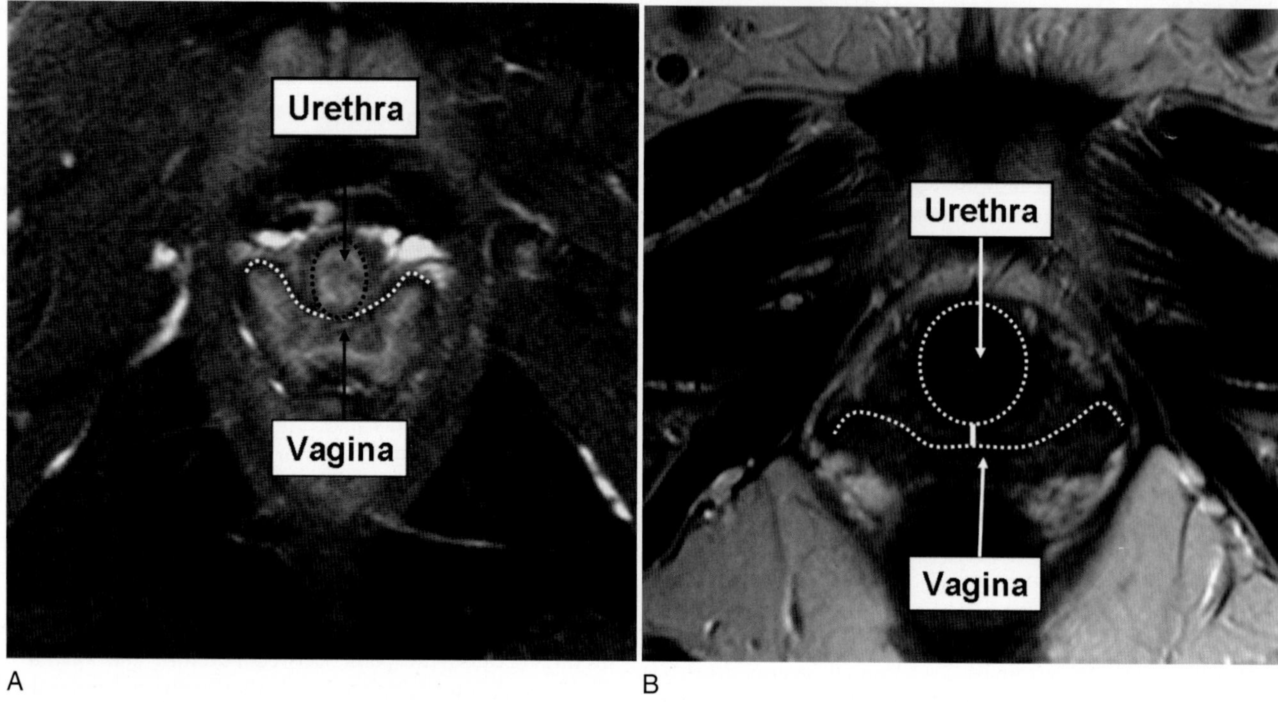

Figure 79-5 A, Transverse view on T2-weighted magnetic resonance imaging(MRI) at the mid-urethra demonstrates the proximity of the urethral and vaginal tissue *(outlined)*, with no discernible gap between the two. Dissection here is more likely to result in urethral injury and contribute to urethrovaginal fistula formation. **B,** Similar transverse MRI at the proximal urethra (one cut distal to the bladder neck) shows an identifiable gap between the urethra and vaginal tissue *(outlined)*.

References

1. Webster GD, Sihelnik SA, Stone AR: Urethrovaginal fistula: A review of the surgical management. J Urol 132:460-462, 1984.
2. Carlin BI, Klutke CG: Development of urethrovaginal fistula following periurethral collagen injection. J Urol 164:124, 2000.
3. Blaivas JG: Reconstruction of the severely damaged female urethra. In Glenn's Urologic Surgery, 5th ed. Philadelphia, Lippincott-Raven; 1998, pp 415-424.
4. Clemens JQ, DeLancey JO, Faerber GJ, et al: Urinary tract erosions after synthetic pubovaginal slings: Diagnosis and management strategy. Urology 56:589-594, 2000.
5. Madjar S, Tchetgen MB, Van Antwerp A, et al: Urethral erosion of tension-free vaginal tape. Urology 59:601, 2002.
6. Flisser AJ, Blaivas J: Outcome of urethral reconstructive surgery in a series of 74 women. J Urol 169:2246-2269, 2003.
7. Ghoniem G, Khater U, Hairston J, et al: Urinary retention caused by adenocarcinoma arising in recurrent urethral diverticulum. Int Urogynecol J Pelvic Floor Dysfunct 15:363-365, 2004.
8. Zimmern PE: The role of voiding cystourethrography in the evaluation of the female lower urinary tract. Probl Urol 5:23-41, 1991.
9. Lemack G, Zimmern PE: Voiding cystourethrography and magnetic resonance imaging of the lower urinary tract. In Corcos J, Schick E (eds): The Urinary Sphincter. New York, Marcel Dekker, 2001, pp 407-421.
10. Blander DS, Zimmern PE: Diagnosis and management of female urethral diverticula and urethrovaginal fistula. In Stanton SL, Zimmern PE (eds): Female Pelvic Reconstructive Surgery. London, Springer, 2003, pp 299-311.
11. Keettel WC, Sehring FG, DeProsse CA, et al: Surgical management of urethrovaginal and vesicovaginal fistulas. Am J Obstet Gynecol 131:425-431, 1978.
12. Tancer ML: A report of thirty-four instances of urethrovaginal and bladder neck fistulas. Surg Gynecol Obstet 177:77-80, 1993.
13. Collis MH: Further remarks upon a new successful mode of treatment for vesicovaginal fistula. Dublin Q J 31:302-316, 1861.
14. Turner-Warwick R, Chapple C: The surgical access option for urethral reconstruction. In Functional Reconstruction of the Urinary Tract and Gynaeco-Urology. Oxford, Blackwell, 2002, pp 491-498.
15. Leach GE: Urethrovaginal fistula repair with Martius labial fat pad graft. Urol Clin North Am 18:409-413, 1991.
16. Dmochowski R: Surgery for vesicovaginal fistula, urethrovaginal fistula, and urethral diverticulum. In Walsh P, Retik A (eds): Campbell's Urology. Philadelphia, Elsevier, 2002, pp 1195-1217.
17. Krogh J, Kay L, Hjortrup A: Treatment of urethrovaginal fistula. Br J Urol 63:555, 1989.
18. Patil U, Waterhouse K, Laungani G: Management of 18 difficult vesicovaginal and urethrovaginal fistulas with modified Ingelman-Sundberg and Martius operations. J Urol 123:653-656, 1980.
19. Bruce RG, El-Galley RE, Galloway NT: Use of rectus abdominis muscle flap for the treatment of complex and refractory urethrovaginal fistulas. J Urol 163:1212-1215, 2000.
20. Candiani P, Austoni E, Campiglio GL, et al: Repair of a recurrent urethrovaginal fistula with an island bulbocavernous musculocutaneous flap. Plast Reconstr Surg 92:1393-1396, 1993.
21. Litwiller SE, Zimmern PE: Closure of bladder neck in the male and female. In Graham SD, Glenn JF (eds): Glenn's Urologic Surgery, 5th ed. Philadelphia, Lippincott-Raven, 1999, pp 407-414.
22. Venn SN, Mundy TR: Diversion and bladder neck closure. In Stanton SL, Zimmern PE (eds): Female Pelvic Reconstructive Surgery. London, Springer, 2003, pp 261-273.

23. Rangnekar NP, Imdad Ali N, Kaul SA, et al: Role of the Martius procedure in the management of urinary-vaginal fistulas. J Am Coll Surg 191:259-263, 2000.
24. Bissada NK, McDonald D: Management of giant vesicovaginal and vesicourethrovaginal fistulas. J Urol 130:1073-1075, 1983.
25. Blander DS, Zimmern PE: Diagnosis and management of female urethral diverticula and urethrovaginal fistula. In Stanton SL, Zimmern PE (eds): Female Pelvic Reconstructive Surgery. London, Springer, 2003, pp 306-307.
26. Sweat SD, Itano NB, Clemens JQ, et al: Polypropylene mesh tape for stress urinary incontinence: Complications of urethral erosion and outlet obstruction. J Urol 168:144-146, 2002.

Chapter 80

RECONSTRUCTION OF THE ABSENT OR DAMAGED URETHRA

Jerry G. Blaivas and Jaspreet S. Sandhu

Damage to the female urethra requiring surgical intervention is rare. It is most commonly seen in underdeveloped countries where obstetric injuries predominate because of prolonged labor, particularly when there is maternal-fetal disproportion. It is postulated that the fetal head compresses the bladder neck and urethra against the undersurface of the pubis, causing pressure necrosis.[1] With the advent of modern obstetric techniques, the most common causes of urethral injury are shearing injuries from scarring that occurs between the urethra and cervix in response to cerclage sutures, prior cesarean section, or other sources.

In industrialized countries, surgical trauma from anti-incontinence surgery is the most common cause. Less common causes include damage from urethral diverticula, pressure necrosis from long-term indwelling catheters, pelvic fracture injury, and invasion from adjacent malignancies. Iatrogenic injuries may occur during urethral diverticulectomy, anti-incontinence surgery, anterior colporrhaphy, and vaginal hysterectomy. Erosions of synthetic slings and sutures from anti-incontinence surgery are seen with increasing frequency and may manifest years after the original surgery. This is fast becoming the most common reason for damage to the urethra, requiring various degrees of urethral reconstruction.[2-6] The most likely cause is the increased use of synthetic materials and technical issues, such as dissecting too close to the urethra or tying the sling too tightly. In our experience, urethral diverticulectomy continues to be the most common cause of extensive urethral damage.[7,8] This most likely results from failure to obtain a tension-free closure of the urethral defect that results from excision of the diverticulum. During bladder neck suspension, an inadvertent (and unrecognized) injury to the bladder or urethra may occur, or an errant suture may result in fistula formation or tissue necrosis. We have also seen several patients who sustained extensive tissue loss after a seemingly simple Kelly plication. It is postulated that the plication sutures were tied too tightly around a urethral catheter, resulting in pressure necrosis.

Long-term indwelling urethral catheters may cause pressure necrosis of the urethra, and less commonly, trauma to the pelvis may result in fracture or separation of the symphysis pubis, which lacerates the urethra or vesical neck, or both. There may be local invasion of the urethra or bladder neck from carcinoma of vagina or cervix. There can be extensive fibrosis or fistula of the urethra as a consequence of radiation treatment of adjacent cancers.

Regardless of the cause of urethral damage, the diagnostic and therapeutic challenges are considerable. The goals of surgical correction are to create a continent urethra that permits the volitional, painless, and unobstructed passage of urine. It should be of appropriate length to ensure that the patient does not void into the vagina or over the toilet bowl, which can occur if the urethra is too long. We think these goals can almost always be accomplished with a single transvaginal procedure.

DIAGNOSIS

Although urethral damage is rare, it should be suspected in certain clinical scenarios: 1) urinary incontinence after pelvic surgery, particularly urethral diverticular surgery, incontinence surgery, anterior colporrhaphy, and Kelly plication; 2) large urethral diverticula; 3) urinary incontinence or other lower urinary tract symptoms after pelvic fracture; 4) urinary incontinence that occurs around an indwelling urethral catheter; and 5) urinary incontinence or lower urinary tract symptoms in patients who have undergone pelvic irradiation. Most patients with significant damage to the urethra have urinary incontinence, but they occasionally present with overactive bladder or voiding symptoms. In patients who have undergone recent synthetic sling placement, urethral erosion should be suspected when the patient has intractable vaginal or urethral pain, recurrent urinary tract infections, vaginal discharge, or hematuria.

For patients with incontinence, the first step in diagnosis is physical examination with a comfortably full bladder; the physician should witness urethral leakage of urine with his or her own eyes before a definitive diagnosis of sphincteric incontinence is made. On more than one occasion, we have diagnosed a urethra-vagina fistula in a woman already scheduled for anti-incontinence surgery because the fistula was misdiagnosed as sphincteric incontinence. When incontinence is observed from the urethral meatus and there is reason to suspect a fistula, the examination should be repeated with a finger obstructing the meatus to observe for leakage more proximally from the fistula itself. Conversely, some women with urethrovaginal fistula have no symptoms, particularly when the fistula is in the distal half of the urethra and the vesical neck remains intact. These fistulas usually are discovered incidentally on physical examination and need no treatment. For examination, we find it best to use the posterior blade of a vaginal retractor to depress the posterior vaginal wall downward. In many instances, the anatomic deformity is obvious, or urinary leakage may be seen proximal to the urethral meatus.

The next step in diagnosis is cystourethroscopy to evaluate the extent of the fistula and to assess the remainder of the urethra, particularly the length, viability, and sphincteric function of the proximal urethra. Visualization of the urethra is best accomplished with a 0- or 30-degree lens and a cystoscope with a 90-degree beak or flexible cystoscope. Cystourethroscopy is the modality of choice for diagnosing urethral erosions after sling placement.

When a urethral injury is diagnosed, an equally high index of suspicion should be maintained for concomitant abnormalities such as vesicovaginal or ureterovaginal fistula, ureteral obstruction, vesicoureteral reflux, and sphincteric deficiency. A careful evaluation to exclude each of these conditions should be undertaken before surgery. Detrusor function may be compromised in the form of low bladder compliance, impaired detrusor contractility, or detrusor overactivity. However, it is difficult to diagnose these conditions preoperatively, and even when present, they should not be surgically treated when the damaged urethra is repaired because most subside spontaneously after successful repair of the urethra.

Urethral stricture is a rare complication of pelvic fracture or other trauma, multiple urethral dilations, prior surgery, and pelvic irradiation. This condition is usually diagnosed by cystoscopy, but it is occasionally found by urodynamic study.

MANAGEMENT

Indications for Surgery

The mere presence of extensive urethral damage is not an indication for surgery. The two main indications for reconstruction are sphincteric incontinence and urethral obstruction, but neither is an absolute indication. Urethral erosions after urethral synthetic sling surgery are a definite indication for surgery because of the presence of foreign material in contact with the urinary tract. If there is an associated condition such as a vesicovaginal fistula, it should be repaired at the same time.

Urethral reconstruction is technically demanding and requires a considerable degree of experience and skill. In inexperienced hands, the risks may be prohibitive, and when there is insufficient local tissue for reconstruction, it may be more prudent to consider urinary diversion than urethral reconstruction, particularly when complications of radiation therapy are suspected.

When sphincteric incontinence is present preoperatively, we believe that it should be surgically corrected at the time of urethral reconstruction. We prefer to construct an autologous fascial pubovaginal sling[9,10] with an interposed labial fat pad flap[7,9,11,12] between the sling and the reconstructed vesical neck. Others have recommended transvaginal bladder neck suspension,[13] but in our experience, this has a failure rate of about 50%.[9] Although it is tempting to use a synthetic sling, we do not recommend it because of the possibility of infection or erosion. It may be prudent to use allograft or xenograft tissue for the sling, but because of lack of long-term follow-up and some early failures, we have chosen these kinds of tissue grafts very selectively.[4,8]

There are three general approaches to urethral reconstruction: anterior bladder flaps,[13,14] posterior bladder flaps,[15] and vaginal wall flaps.[1,7,12,16-18] These techniques appear to be comparable with respect to creation of a neo-urethra. However, when the vesical neck and proximal urethra are involved, which is usually the case, postoperative incontinence rates of about 50% are to be expected unless a concomitant anti-incontinence procedure is performed.[13-15] We believe that vaginal reconstruction is considerably easier and faster, is much more amenable to concomitant anti-incontinence surgery, and is associated with much less morbidity than the bladder flap operations.

Timing of Surgery and Preoperative Management

In the past, much controversy surrounded the timing of surgical repair. For decades, it had been taught that surgery should be delayed for 3 to 6 months or even longer to allow adequate time for tissue inflammation and edema to subside. In our experience, surgery can be safely performed as soon as the vaginal wound is free of infection and inflammation and the tissues are reasonably pliable.

Principles of Surgical Technique

In women with damaged urethras, the vaginal tissue is often scarred, fibrotic, and ischemic. Before surgery, careful examination of the vagina is necessary to determine the actual extent of urethral tissue loss and to assess the availability of local tissue for use in the reconstruction. In most instances, there is sufficient tissue in the anterior or lateral vaginal wall that can be mobilized and used for the reconstruction.[1,7,9,12,13,16-18] Occasionally, it may be necessary to use an adjacent labial[16,19] or thigh flap.[20,21] Alternatively, an anterior bladder flap can be used.[13]

In patients undergoing urethral reconstruction for urethral erosion after synthetic sling placement, attempts should be made to remove all synthetic material, including nonabsorbable mesh and sutures.[2] When infection is absent, bone anchors can be left in place because of the difficulty in retrieving them. However, if infection exists, it is advisable and usually straightforward to identify and remove bone anchors. The urethra usually can then be reconstructed primarily.

After reconstruction of the urethra, it is often advisable to interpose a well-vascularized pedicle flap over the site of the repair. Sources include labial,[9,13,22] rectus abdominal,[17,23] gracilis,[7] and thigh tissue.[20,21] In most patients, nothing more than a labial fat pad graft is necessary (Fig. 80-1).

The most important principles of surgical repair include clear visualization and exposure of the operative site; creation of a tension-free, multilayered closure; an adequate blood supply; and adequate bladder drainage. Bladder drainage is best accomplished with a suprapubic catheter, which should be placed at the beginning of the procedure to avoid damaging the reconstructed urethra. We use a urethral catheter as a stent postoperatively. The catheter must be sewn to the anterior abdominal wall in a gentle curve to avoid putting tension of the suture line.

Surgical Technique

There are four basic techniques for urethral reconstruction: primary closure, laterally based (tube) flaps, advancement flaps, and labia minora pedicle grafts. The choice of incision depends on the local anatomy of the tissue loss and whether a pubovaginal sling or other anti-incontinence procedure is planned. If a pubovaginal sling is planned, it is best to complete the urethral reconstruction first; the sling then is completed. In our prior publications on urethral reconstruction, we made the opposite recommendation, but in subsequent operations, we encountered some instances in which the vaginal dissection for the sling interfered with subsequent incisions for the reconstruction.[7,9]

Before incising the vaginal wall for passage of the sling, it is important to select the site and shape of the initial incisions for vaginal reconstruction to be sure that no options are sacrificed. On several occasions, we inadvertently burned some bridges and hope others can learn from our mistakes. If an inverted-U-shaped

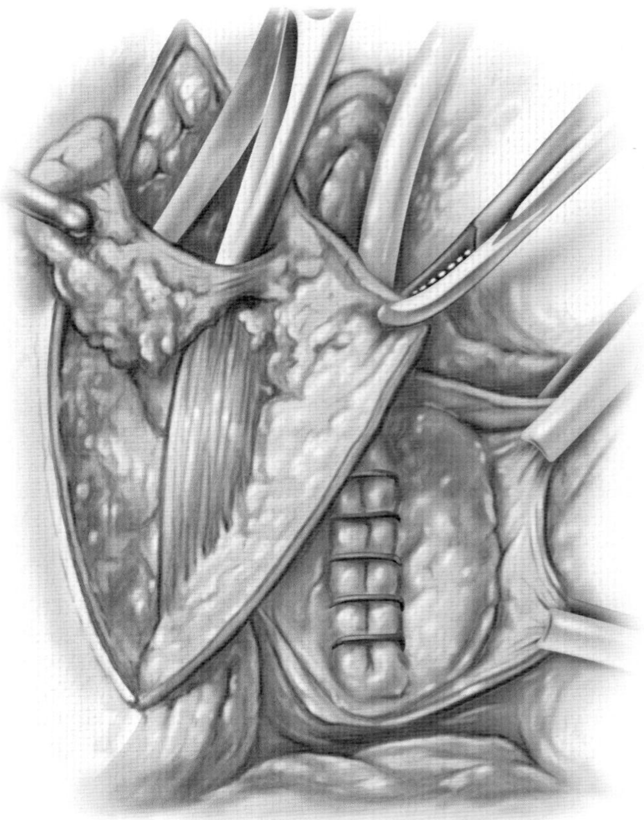

A

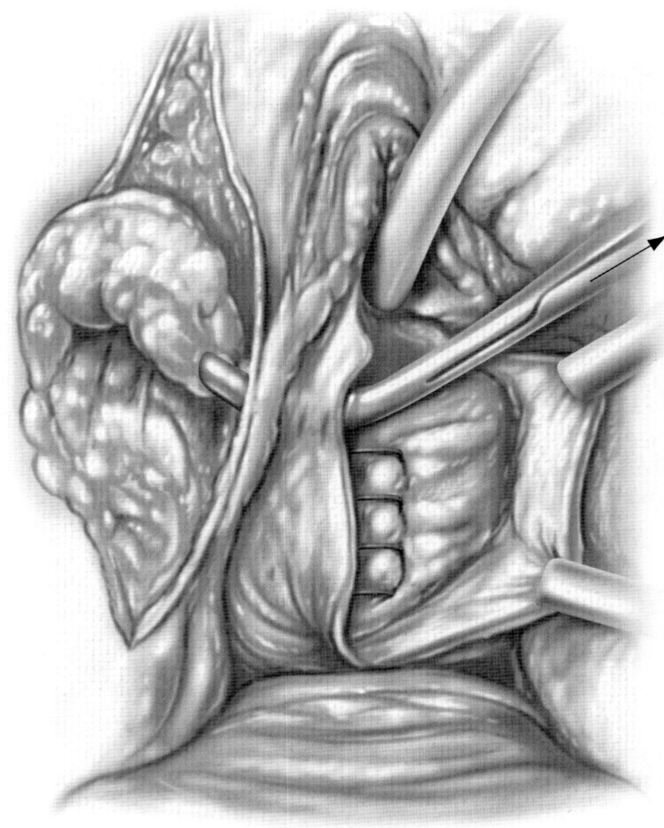

B

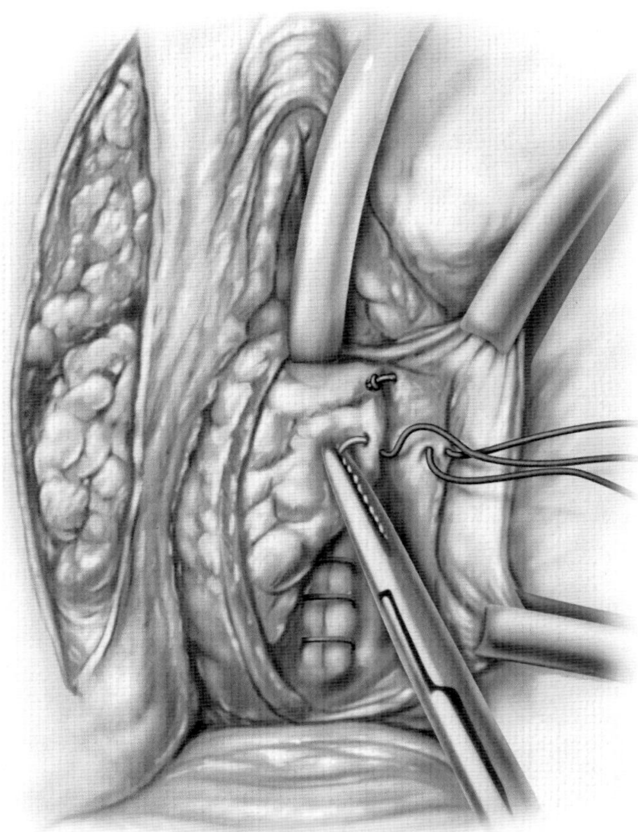

C

Figure 80-1 Labial fat pad graft—a Martius flap. **A,** A vertical incision is made over the labia majora, and the fat pad is mobilized. The initial dissection should begin beneath Scarpa's fascia. If the plane is more superficial than that, troublesome bleeding may be encountered from thin, wide, flat veins that are difficult to visualize. The fat pad is mobilized anteriorly, suture ligated and divided, and the end of the suture is left long. **B,** A tunnel is made underneath the vaginal epithelium, and the fat pad is pulled into place with the long suture *(arrow)*. **C,** It is sewn in place over the suture lines of the neo-urethra. (Modified from Mattingly RF, Thompson JD: Ch. 27. In Mattingly RF, Thompson JD [eds]: TeLinde's Operative Gynecology, 6th ed. Philadelphia, JB Lippincott, 1985, p 665.)

incision is made in the anterior vaginal wall in anticipation of advancing it to cover the reconstruction, that tissue can no longer be used as an advancement flap for urethral reconstruction if needed. Accordingly, an inverted-U-shaped incision should be made only after it is clear that an advancement flap will not be necessary. If two parallel incisions are made alongside the intended site of the urethra to roll the flaps into a tube graft, it is important to be sure that the distance between the two incisions is sufficient to allow the flaps to cover the entire circumference of the catheter and that they can be sutured together over the catheter without any tension. The tissue lateral to the incisions should not be undermined until it is clear that a laterally based flap will not be needed to cover the wound.

Primary Closure

If the defect is small and the tissue pliable enough to achieve a loose, tension-free closure over a 16-Fr catheter, primary closure should be considered (Fig. 80-2). We prefer chromic catgut to longer-acting synthetic absorbable sutures for urethral closure because the latter often make subsequent voiding or urethral instrumentation painful. Only after the repair has been completed is the decision made about how to cover the wound. In some instances, it is possible to elevate laterally based flaps and suture them in the midline over the wound, but when this is not possible, a U-shaped or inverted-U-shaped flap usually suffices. If a Martius labial fat pad graft is needed, it is prepared before closure of the wound (see Fig. 80-1); if a pubovaginal sling is also necessary, the fat pad graft is placed between the sling and urethra. The vaginal incision is closed with 2-0 or 3-0 chromic catgut (Fig. 80-3).

Advancement Flap

If there is insufficient tissue on the anterior vaginal wall at the site of the urethra to mobilize lateral flaps, it may be possible to repair the urethra and cover the repair with an advancement flap from the anterior vaginal wall cranial to the damaged urethra (see Fig. 80-3).

Tube Graft

If there is circumferential loss of the urethra and sufficient vaginal wall tissue on the anterior vaginal wall, a tube graft should be considered (Fig. 80-4). Parallel incisions are made over the site of the neo-urethra, and tissue is loosely rolled into a tube over a 16-Fr urethral catheter and closed with interrupted sutures of 3-4 chromic catgut. If there is a urethral fistula, we prefer to retain the remaining bridge of urethral tissue and close the fistula primarily to preserve local blood supply.

Labia Minora Pedicle Graft

When there is insufficient local vaginal wall tissue, a labia minora pedicle graft may be possible (Fig. 80-5). An oval incision is made in an adjacent hair-free portion of the labia minora as close to

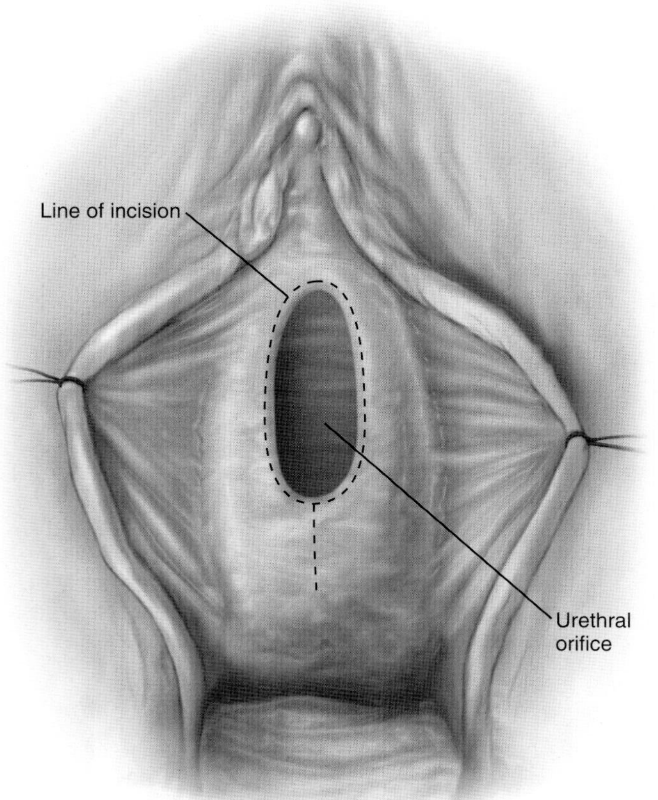

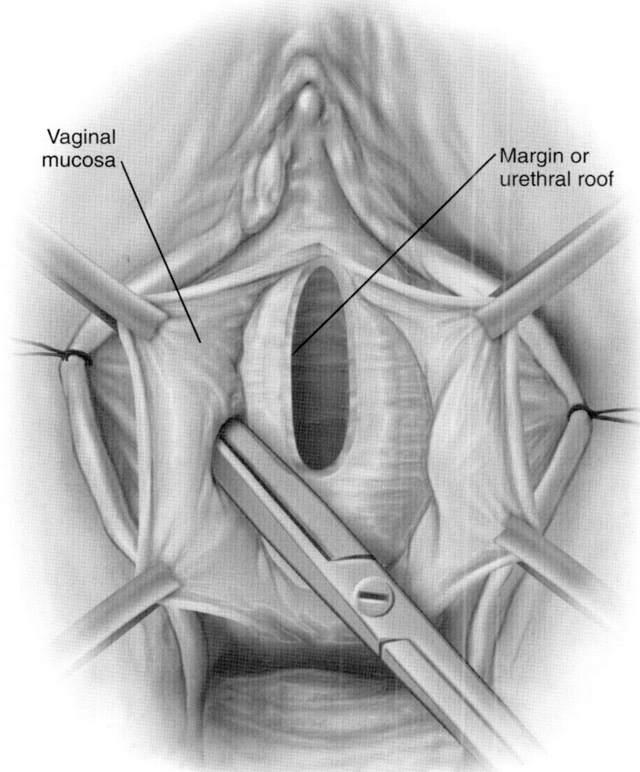

Figure 80-2 Primary closure of the urethra. **A,** The fistula is circumscribed. **B,** Lateral and cranial vaginal wall flaps are elevated, but the edges of the fistula are not excised because that would likely comprise the size of the reconstructed urethral lumen.

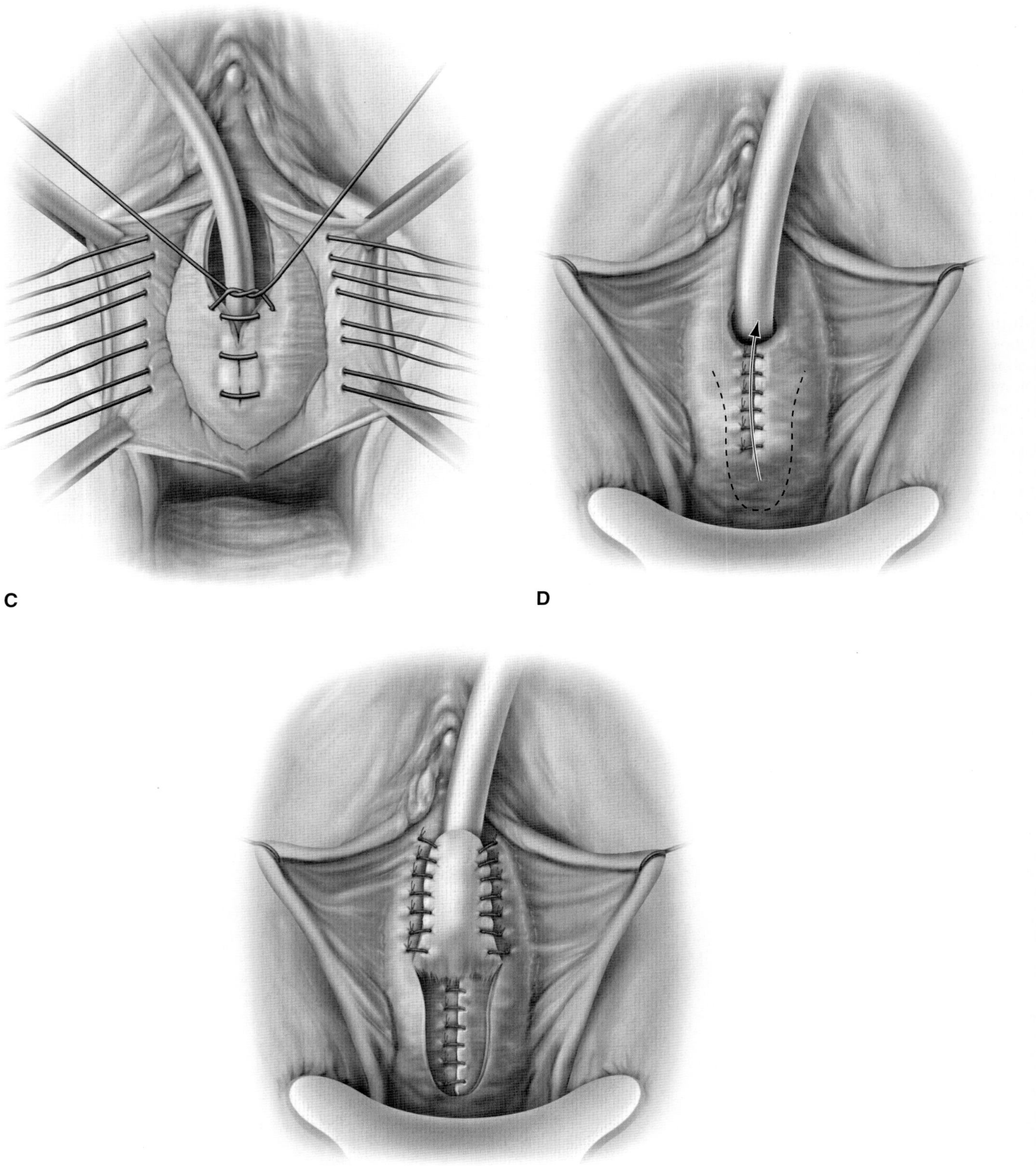

C

D

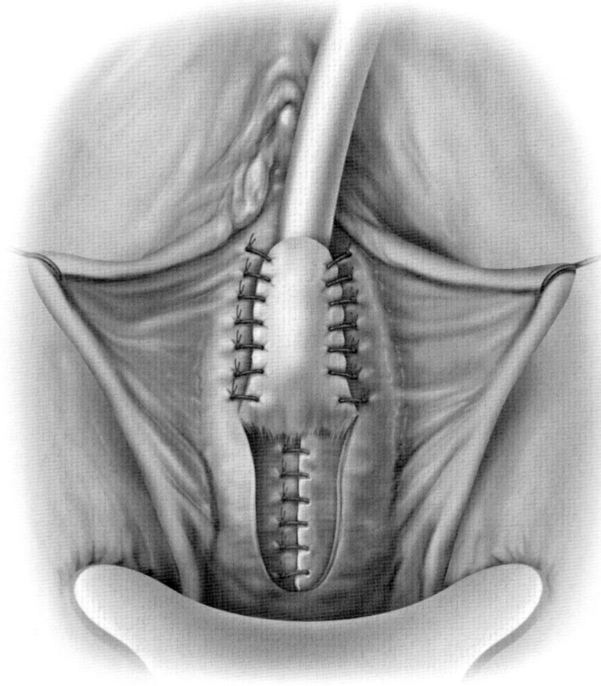

E

Figure 80-2, cont'd C, The urethra is closed primarily with interrupted sutures of 3-0 or 4-0 chromic catgut, and the vaginal wall is closed with lateral flaps. **D** and **E,** If there is insufficient mobility of the lateral tissue, an inverted-U-shaped graft of anterior vaginal wall *(arrow)* may be used. (Modified from Blaivas JG: Vaginal flap urethral reconstruction: An alternative to the bladder flap neo-urethra. J Urol 141:542-545, 1996.)

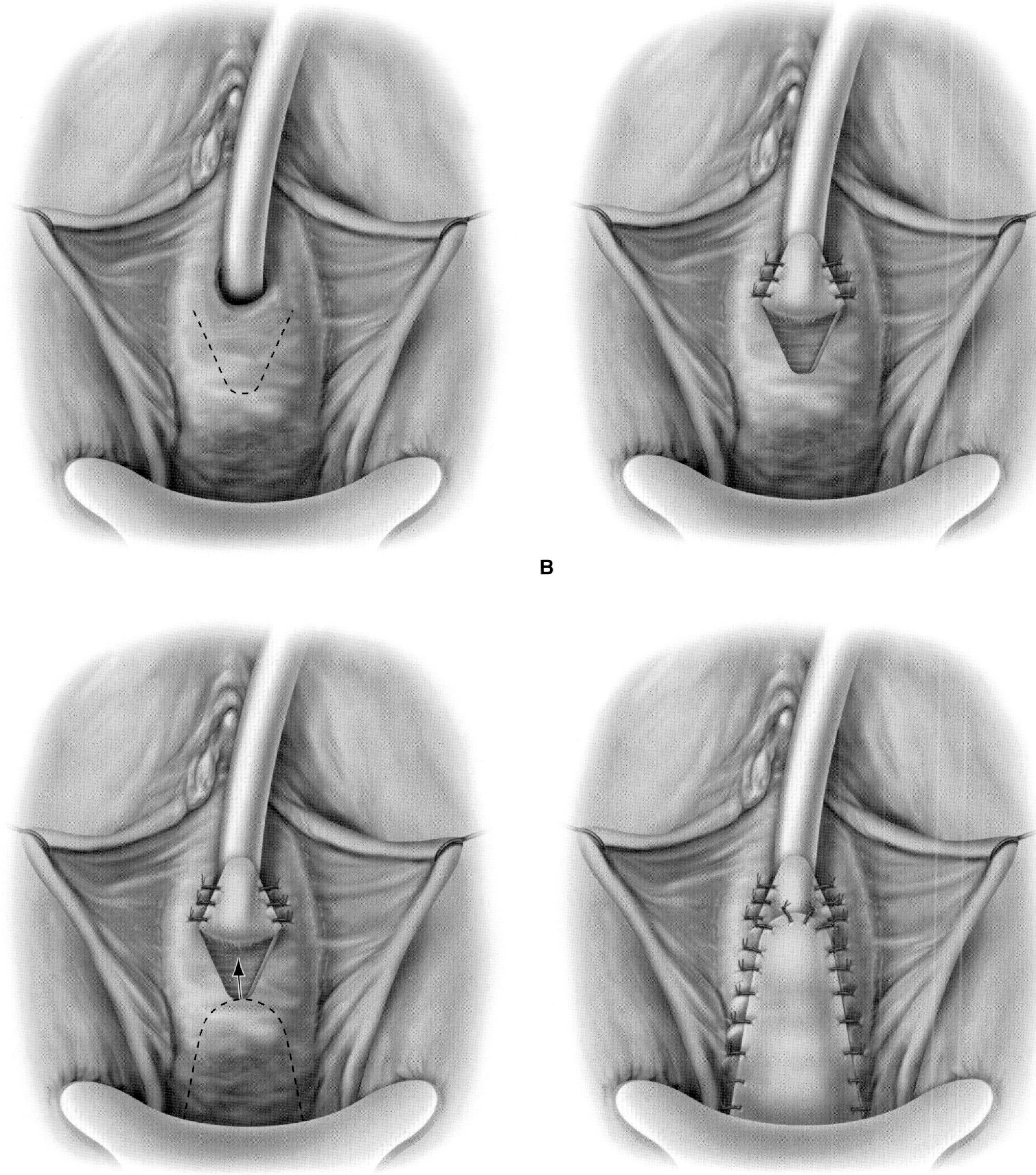

Figure 80-3 Advancement flap. **A,** The vertical distance from the planned meatus to the base of the defect should be measured, and a U-shaped incision is made so that the apex of the U reaches the site of the new meatus without any tension. **B,** The U-shaped flap is mobilized and rotated 180 degrees. Its lateral edges are sutured to the vaginal wall over the catheter for form the neo-urethral tube using interrupted sutures of 3-0 or 4-0 chromic catgut. **C,** An inverted-U-shaped graft of anterior vaginal wall is made so that its tip reaches the new meatus without tension. **D,** The flap is undermined, advanced, and sutured in place with 3-0 chromic catgut. If there is insufficient tissue for this, a full labial graft may be used (see Fig. 80-6). (Modified from O'Conor VJ, Kropp KA: Ch. 13. In Glenn JF, Boyce WH [eds]: Urologic Surgery. New York, Hoeber Medical Division, Harper & Row, 1969, p 568.)

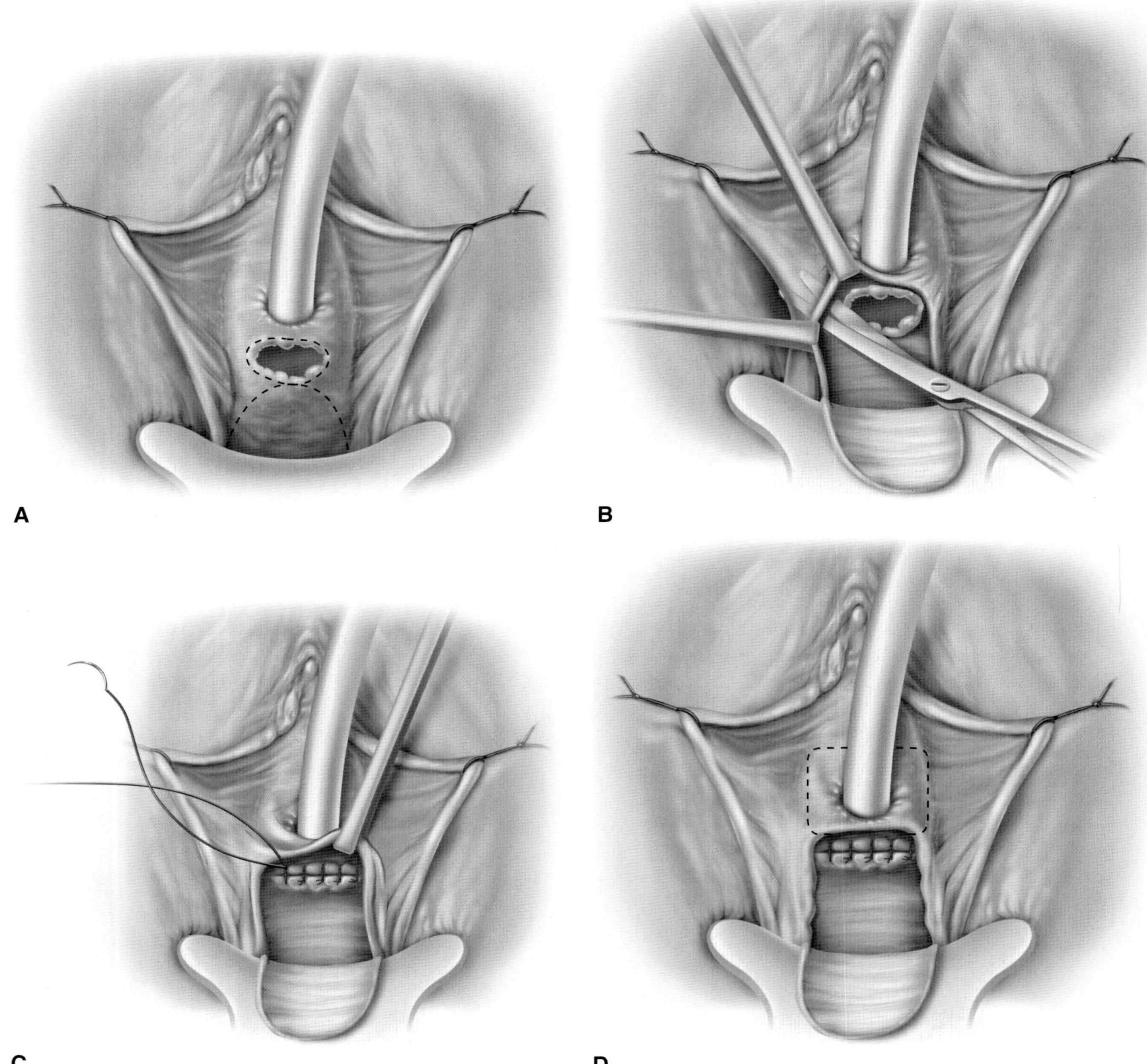

Figure 80-4 Tube graft. **A,** A bridge of tissue separates the fistula into two openings. The proximal opening is circumcised, and an inverted-U-shaped incision is made in the anterior vaginal wall with the apex of the U at the vesical neck, just proximal to first fistula. **B,** Full-thickness vaginal wall flaps are developed around the fistula. **C,** The proximal fistula is closed with interrupted sutures of 4-0 chromic catgut. **D,** A rectangular incision is made. The horizontal distance should be measured to be sure that it is wide enough to cover a 16-Fr Foley catheter. The vertical distance is defined by the site of the new urethral meatus.

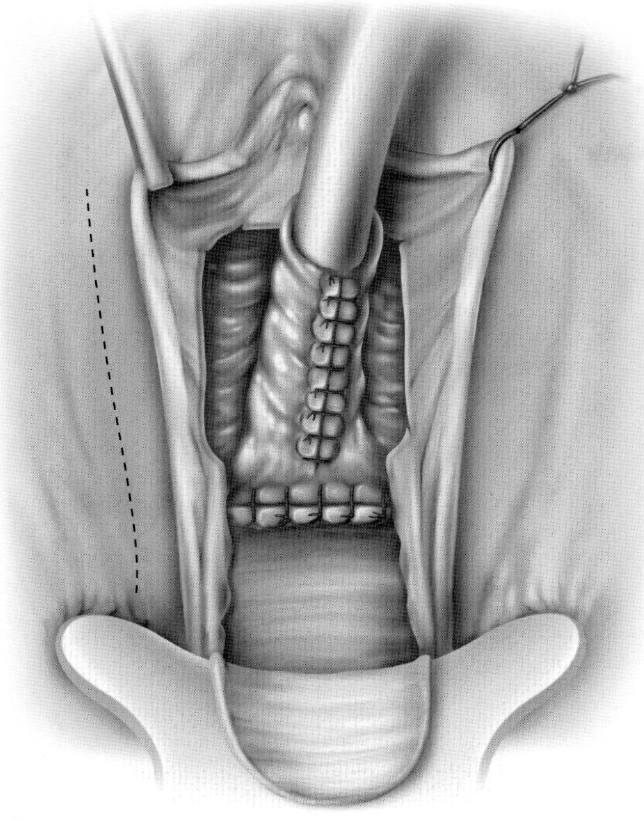

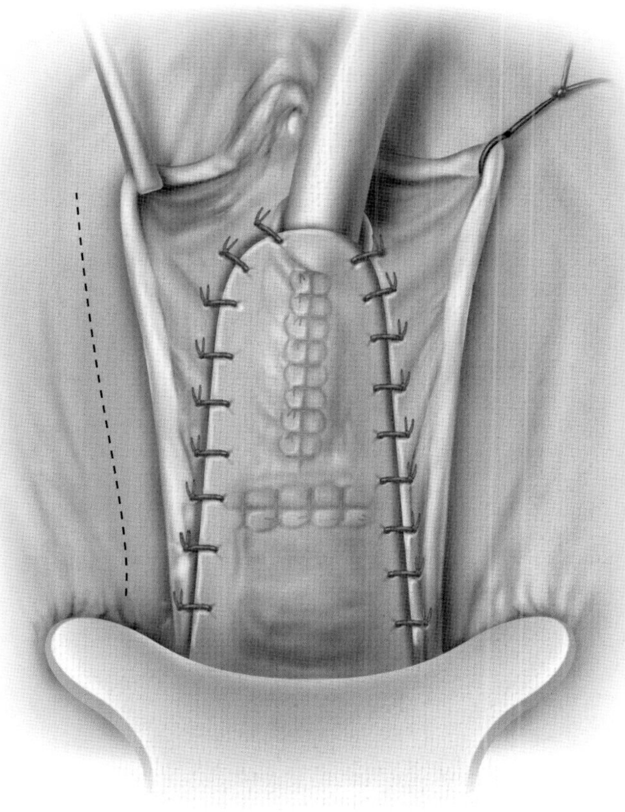

E F

Figure 80-4 E, The lateral edges of the incision are undermined medially and laterally and then rolled over and approximated in the midline over the Foley catheter, creating the neo-urethra. If necessary, A vertical incision is made over the labia majora for access to the labial fat pad graft. **F,** The vaginal wall is closed by advancing a U-shaped flap, but if this is not possible, any of the other techniques previously discussed may be used. (Modified from Blaivas JG: Vaginal flap neo-urethra: An alternative to bladder flap urethral reconstruction. J Urol 141:542 -545, 1989.)

the site of the urethra as possible (Fig. 80-6). The size of the incision should be large enough to roll into a tube around a 16-Fr catheter or to be used as a patch graft over the catheter and allow loose approximation over the catheter. The incision is deepened around labial incision, and a pedicle graft is raised on an anteriorly or posteriorly based blood supply. The graft is passed beneath the vaginal wall and rotated so that the mucosal surface forms the inner wall of the reconstructed urethra. In some patients, it is not possible to create a tunnel for passage of the graft because of extensive scarring. In this instance, an incision is made in the vaginal wall between the site of the new urethra and the graft. It is usually possible to elevate flaps to cover the graft.

Alternative Closures

If it is not possible to close the vaginal incision primarily, there are several alternatives. The most straightforward is to create an inverted-U-shaped or lateral broad-based flap (Fig. 80-2(d&e). If that is not feasible, a labia minora pedicle graft may be taken and rotated so that the skin is on the outside (Figure 80-5). Alternatively, a modification of the Martius flap using full-thickness vaginal wall can be used (see Fig. 80-6). Other techniques include gracilis myocutaneous, rectus pedicle, and Singapore flaps (19-21), but in approximately 100 cases, we have found an alternative approach to be necessary only two times.

At the conclusion of the procedure using any technique, the Foley catheter is sutured to the anterior abdominal wall with a gentle loop to ensure that undue tension is not placed on the urethra. Failure to maintain a correct position of the catheter may result in necrosis of the urethra.

Postoperative Care

If a Martius flap is used, the Penrose drain is removed as soon as there is minimal drainage, which usually is on the first or second postoperative day. The urethral wound and catheter are checked frequently to be sure that there is no tension or pressure on the suture line. The urethral catheter is removed as soon as feasible, usually within the first 2 to 5 days, but always before discharge from the hospital. Voiding cystourethrography is performed though the suprapubic catheter at about day 14. If the patient voids satisfactorily and there is no extravasation, the suprapubic tube is removed. If not, the tube is left in place, and another voiding trial is undertaken in about 2 weeks.

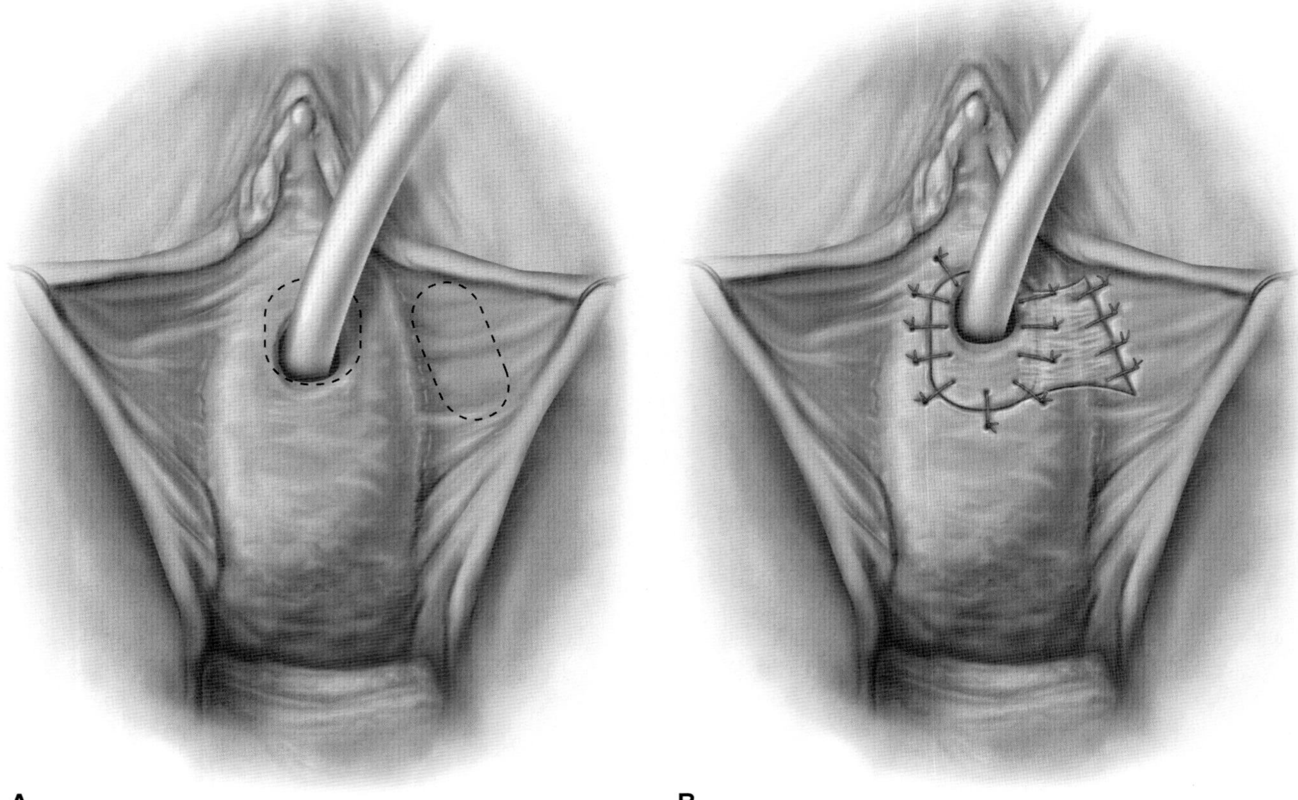

Figure 80-5 Labia minora pedicle graft for creation of a neo-urethra. **A,** An oval incision is made in the hair-free labia minora, and the incision is deepened to include a vascularized pedicle, similar to that obtained for a Marius flap, except that the labial skin is left intact. A U-shaped incision is made at the site selected for the neo-urethra. **B,** The pedicle graft is tunneled beneath the vaginal wall, and the skin surface of the pedicle flap is wrapped around the catheter and sutured to the incisions that were made in the vaginal wall to form the neo-urethra. The vaginal and labial wounds are closed primarily.

Table 80-1 Reconstruction of Damaged Urethras: Study Results

Study	No. of Patients	Continence (%)	Cure or Improved (%)	Successful Repair (%)	Obstruction (%)
Rovner and Wein,[24] 2003	9	75	88	75	13
Tanello et al,[16] 2002	2	100	100	100	—
Bruce et al,[23] 2000	6	83	100	100	0
Leng et al,[27] 1998	4	75	75	100	—
Elkins et al,[28] 1969	6	10	83	67	17
Elkins et al,[11] 1990	20	50	55	90	10
Flisser and Blaivas,[8] 2003	74	87	93	93	1
Gray,[1] 1968	10	50	50	—	—
Hamlin and Nicholson,[12] 1969	50	80	84	98	12
Morgan et al,[29] 1978	9	56	89	100	11
Patel et al,[30] 1980	9	—	78	100	0
Symmonds and Hill,[22] 1978	20	65	90	85	—

RESULTS

Because of the rarity of the condition, there have been few studies concerning reconstruction of the severely damaged urethra. Combining all the series we could find in the English language literature, there were fewer than 500 patients. Overall, successful anatomic reconstructions were reported in 67% to 100% of women (Table 80-1). Most study authors emphasized the need for well-vascularized pedicle flaps to ensure a successful outcome. Continence, however, was achieved in only 55% to 92% after a single operation, and postoperative urethral obstruction was reported in 2% to 17% of patients. In most studies, the criteria for incontinence and urethral obstruction were not specified, and in view of lack of follow-up, the results cited should be considered overly optimistic. It does seem evident that an anti-incontinence procedure should be performed at the same time

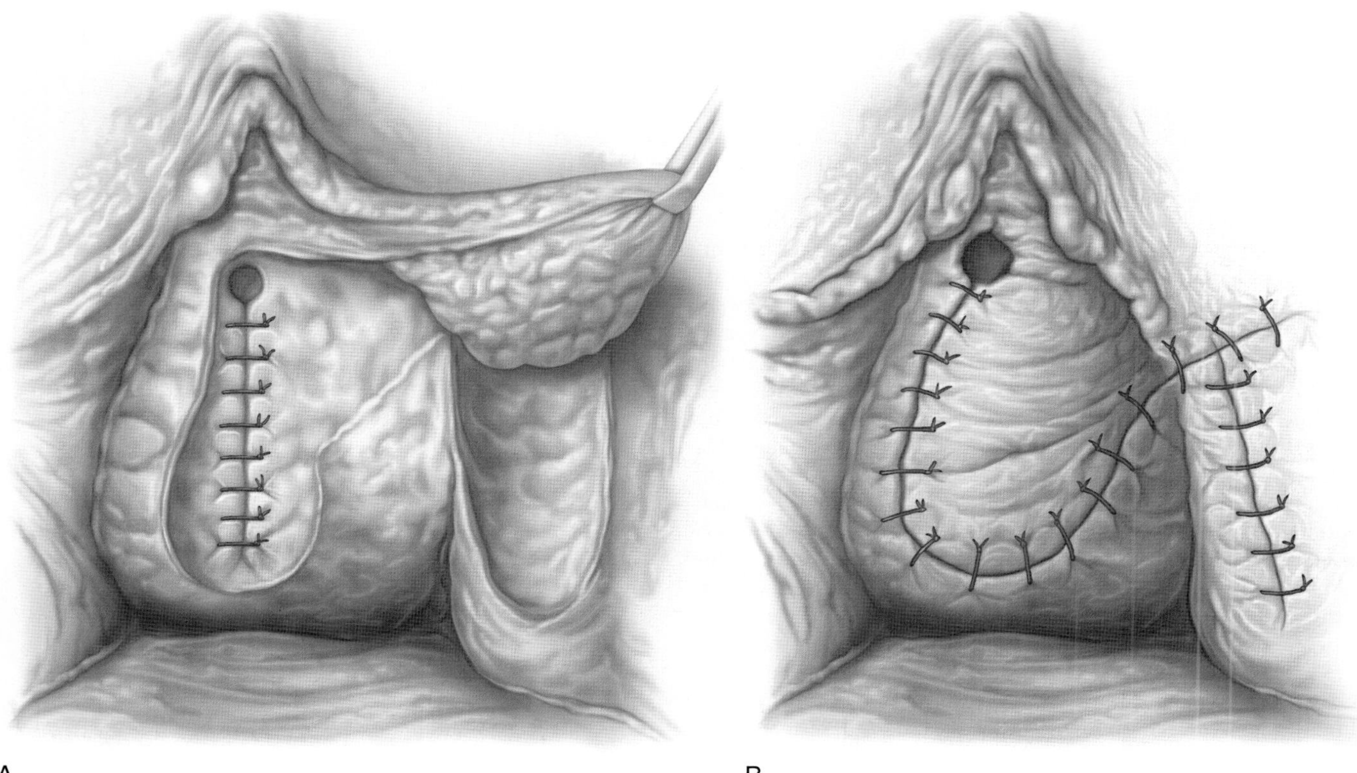

Figure 80-6 Technique of obtaining a full-thickness labial fibrofatty pedicle graft to cover the reconstructed urethra when there is insufficient local vaginal wall tissue. **A,** A U-shaped incision is made in the labia minora large enough to cover the defect. The incision is carried down through the labial fat pad (see Fig. 80-1), and the posterior end of the flap is suture ligated. **B,** The vaginal wall is closed primarily with running sutures of 3-0 or 400 chromic catgut. (Modified from Mattingly RF, Thompson JD: Ch. 27. In Mattingly RF, Thompson JD [eds]:TeLinde's Operative Gynecology, 6th ed. Philadelphia, JB Lippincott, 1985, p 665.)

as the urethral reconstruction. Failure to do so resulted in incontinence rates ranging from 50% to 84%. The results of many series indicated that secondary procedures to correct incontinence were successful in most patients.

The first report of a large series was published in 1969 by Hamlin,[12] a dedicated pioneer of fistula repair who worked in West Africa. Excellent anatomic repair was achieved in 49 of the 50 childbirth injuries, but 8 (16%) had severe incontinence, and many more had lesser degrees of incontinence. The incontinence was usually cured after a second procedure. Symmonds[22] described 50 women undergoing neo-urethra procedures using tubularized vaginal wall. Follow-up ranged from 1 to 15 years, and using an independent examiner, he reported that 37 of 50 patients were dry (i.e., no pads and said they were cured) and that 7 of 50 patients considered the operation successful, even though they had "some" stress incontinence.

We have operated on more than 100 women with extensive anatomic vesical neck and urethral defects; results for 74 have been reported.[8] The causes of the injury are given in Table 80-2. All but one patient underwent a vaginal reconstruction (one patient had a Tanagho anterior bladder flap that failed). One patient with squamous cell carcinoma of the distal third of the urethra underwent wide excision and urethral reconstruction with adjacent local flaps. In the remainder, we used a Martius flap in all except three—one had a successful repair with a gracilis flap, and two women with childbirth injuries underwent cutaneous labial pedicle grafts. One of the latter patients was successful; the other failed because of wound necrosis and underwent continent urinary diversion. A successful anatomic outcome was achieved in 93%, and continence was achieved in 87% of patients who had preoperative incontinence; no patient developed de novo incontinence. Early in our series,[7] we did not routinely perform concomitant pubovaginal slings, and 50% of the women who underwent a modified Pereyra procedure had persistent sphincteric incontinence; all were subsequently cured or improved by an autologous fascial pubovaginal sling. No patient required

Table 80-2 Causes of Urethral Pathology

Pathology	No. of Patients*
Diverticula or injury from diverticulectomy	28
Urethral injury from prior incontinence surgery	18
Anterior colporrhaphy	10
Fistula or erosion associated with synthetic material	5
Fistula from other gynecologic surgery	3
Urethral obstruction from prior surgery	3
Trauma	3
Obstetric injury	2
Ectopic ureter	1
Primary urethral stricture	1
Total	74

*Women who underwent operations because of extensive anatomic vesical neck and urethral defects.

intermittent catheterization except for the patients with anatomic failures, who underwent continent urinary diversion. One had a previously unrecognized vesicovaginal fistula.

Rovner and Wein[24] recommended that women with large, circumferential urethral diverticula undergo complete excision of the diverticulum and partial urethrectomy by transecting the urethra to gain access to its dorsal wall. Urethral continuity was restored by end-to-end urethroplasty or by tubularizing the anterior wall of the diverticulum to construct a neo-urethral segment. Autologous fascial slings were used selectively. With only short-term follow-up, they reported that six of the eight patients were dry (i.e., no pads), one was using two or three pads per day, and the remaining one reported urgency and the use of one pad each day. Complications included one distal fistula and one stricture.

Tanello and colleagues[16] described two women undergoing urethral reconstruction using a pedicle skin flap from the labia minora. They cited a 2-year follow-up and reported that both patients were dry. Bruce and coworkers[23] described six women with multiple previous urethral operations who underwent reconstruction. The surgical technique used a pedicled rectus abdominis flap interposed between the fistula closure and the vaginal suture line. The follow-up period was 23 months. Five of six patients were dry and able to void; one had urge incontinence.

Many investigators have reported the results of urethral reconstruction after urethral erosion resulting from mid-urethral sling placement. Amundesen and colleagues[2] described nine patients who presented with urethral erosion. All were repaired primarily with a multilayered closure, followed by a Martius flap in two patients. All were repaired adequately, but 66% of patients with preoperative urge urinary incontinence or stress urinary incontinence had continued incontinence. Others have reported results with similar rates of incontinence, prompting some surgeons to perform concomitant anti-incontinence procedures with interposed vascularized tissue, such as a Martius flap.[3,4]

BLADDER FLAP TECHNIQUES

We believe that bladder flap reconstructions are almost never necessary in these patients. The single patient in whom we performed this procedure failed because of refractory detrusor instability. There are two basic techniques: anterior and posterior bladder flaps. The anterior technique is depicted in Figure 80-7. More information is available in the original descriptions and the excellent work of the late Vincent O'Conor.[25]

In the latest and most extensive series, Elkins[13] and associates reported their experience with a Tanagho-like procedure in 20 West African women with extensive urethral damage after obstructed labor. These patients had large vesicovaginal fistulas, and because of extensive scarring, they were not suitable for vaginal flap techniques. The procedure was performed entirely through the vaginal approach. The anterior and lateral fistula edges are dissected sharply away from the pubic bone beneath the arch of the pubic ramus, and the retropubic space is entered from the vagina. The anterior bladder wall is then dissected free of surrounding tissues to the level of the peritoneal reflection. After the anterior bladder is mobilized, a 3 × 3 cm flap is raised and rolled into a tube over a 16-Fr catheter. The new urethra is sutured to the remaining distal urethra or at the site of the new meatus. The posterior edges of the vesicovaginal fistula are approximated and "fixation sutures are placed through the top portion of the neo-urethra to reattach the urethra to the base of

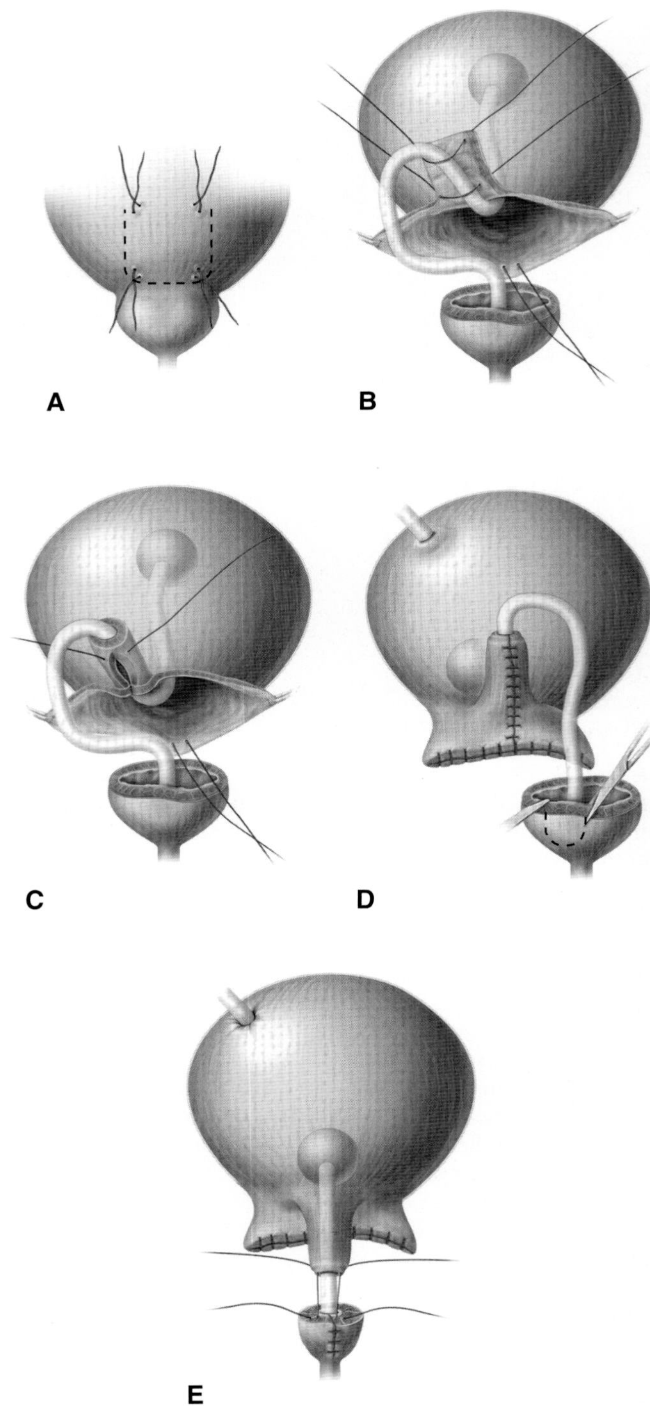

Figure 80-7 Technique of performing anterior bladder flap urethroplasty (i.e., Tanagho procedure). **A,** An anterior bladder wall flap is selected, mobilized, and held with suspension sutures. **B,** The urethra is transected at site of fistula. **C,** The bladder flap is tubularized. **D,** The posterior bladder is closed. **E,** The neo-urethra is sutured to the distal urethra. (Modified from Tanagho EA: Bladder neck reconstruction for total urinary incontinence: 10 years of experience. J Urol 125:321, 1981.)

the pubic periosteum." In the last three patients in the series, a modified Pereyra procedure was performed instead. A Martius fat pad graft was then placed beneath the suture lines. Eighteen of the 20 women so treated had a satisfactory anatomic repair of the fistula, but 4 of the 18 had persistent stress incontinence that required further surgery. Two others had refractory detrusor instability or low bladder compliance.

OTHER TECHNIQUES

Park and Hendren[26] reported a series of seven girls with severely fibrotic urethras. Urethral reconstruction was accomplished with a 2 × 4 cm full-thickness buccal mucosa graft after splitting the pubis and excising the fibrotic urethra. Causes of the urethral pathology included complications from operations for cloacal extrophy and other cloacal malformations. The investigators reported that five of seven patients were continent and that two were being treated with periurethral bulking agents. After the follow-up period of 12 to 58 months (mean, 34.7 months), all seven patients were continent, but two required bulbing agents for continence.

CONCLUSIONS

Reconstruction of the severely damaged urethra is a technically challenging undertaking that requires considerable surgical expertise and decision-making. Most women with traumatic injuries have sufficient vaginal tissue for a vaginal flap reconstruction, and we believe that the vaginal approach offers the best chance for a successful outcome. However, for those with extensive vaginal scarring that precludes a local tissue repair, bladder flap techniques or free grafts with or without gaining access by splitting the pubis may prove useful.

The most important principles to keep in mind are clear visualization and exposure of the operative site; careful selection of the initial vaginal incision to ensure that there is adequate blood supply if pedicle flaps become necessary; removal of all foreign material; creation of a tension-free, supple, multilayered closure; an adequate blood supply and soft tissue base with a Martius flap; a concomitant pubovaginal sling when anti-incontinence surgery is indicated; adequate bladder drainage; and suturing of the urethral catheter to the anterior abdominal wall and meticulous attention to catheter care to prevent pressure necrosis.

References

1. Gray LA: Urethrovaginal fistulas. Am J Obstet Gynecol 101:28, 1968.
2. Amundsen CL, Flynn BJ, Webster GD: Urethral erosion after synthetic and nonsynthetic pubovaginal slings: Differences in management and continence outcome. J Urol 170:134, 2003.
3. Clemens JQ, DeLancey JO, Farber GJ, et al: Urinary tract erosions after synthetic pubovaginal slings: Diagnosis and management strategy. Urology 56:589, 2000.
4. Kobashi KC, Dmochowski R, Mee SL, et al: Erosion of woven polyester pubovaginal sling. J Urol 162:2070, 1999.
5. Sweat SD, Itano NB, Clemens JQ, et al: Polypropylene mesh tape for stress urinary incontinence: Complications of urethral erosion and outlet obstruction. J Urol 168:144, 2002.
6. Tsivian, A, Kessler O, Mogutin B, et al: Tape related complications of the tension-free vaginal tape procedure. J Urol 171:762, 2004.
7. Blaivas JG: Vaginal flap urethral reconstruction: An alternative to the bladder flap neo-urethra. J Urol 141:542, 1996.
8. Flisser AJ, Blaivas JG: Outcome of urethral reconstruction cases in a series of 74 women. J Urol 169:2246, 2003.
9. Blaivas JG: Female urethral reconstruction. In Webster G (ed): Reconstructive Urology. Boston, Blackwell Scientific, 1993, pp 873-886.
10. Chaikin DC, Rosenthal J, Blaivas JG: Pubovaginal fascial sling for all types of stress urinary incontinence: long-term analysis. J Urol 160:1312, 1998.
11. Elkins TE, DeLancey JO, McGuire EJ: The use of modified Martius graft as an adjunctive technique in vesicovaginal and rectovaginal fistula repair. Obstet Gynecol 75:727, 1990.
12. Hamlin RHJ, Nicholson EC: Reconstruction of urethra totally destroyed in labor. Br Med J 1:147, 1969.
13. Elkins TE, Ghosh TS, Tagoe GA, et al: Transvaginal mobilization and utilization of the anterior bladder wall to repair vesicovaginal fistulas involving the urethra. Obstet Gynecol 79:455, 1992.
14. Tanagho EA: Bladder neck reconstruction for total urinary incontinence: 10 years of experience. J Urol 125:321, 1981.
15. Leadbetter GW Jr: Surgical correction of total urinary incontinence. J Urol 91:261, 1964.
16. Tanello M, Frego E, Simeone C, et al: Use of pedicle flap from the labia minora for the repair of female urethral strictures. Urol Int 69:95, 2002.
17. Ellis LR, Hodges CV: Experience with female urethral reconstruction. J Urol 102:214, 1969.
18. Symmonds RE: Loss of the urethral floor with total urinary incontinence: A technique for urethral reconstruction. Am J Obstet Gynecol 103:665, 1968.
19. Hoskins WJ, Park RC, Long R, et al: Repair of urinary tract fistulas with bulbocavernosus myocutaneous flaps. Obstet Gynecol 63:588, 1984.
20. Wee JT, Joseph VT: A new technique of vaginal reconstruction using neurovascular pudendal-thigh flaps: A preliminary report. Plast Reconstr Surg 83:701, 1989.
21. Zinman, L: Use of myocutaneous and muscle interposition flaps in management of radiation-induced vesicovaginal fistula. In MCdougal WS (ed): Difficult Problems in Urologic Surgery. Chicago, Yearbook Medical Publishers, 1989, pp 143-163.
22. Symmonds RE, Hill LM: Loss of the urethra: A report on 50 patients. Am J Obstet Gynecol 130:130, 1978.
23. Bruce RG, El-Galley RES, Galloway NTM: Use of rectus abdominis muscle flap for the treatment of complex and refractory urethrovaginal fistulas. J Urol 163:1212, 2000.
24. Rovner E, Wein AJ: Diagnosis and reconstruction of the dorsal or circumferential urethral diverticulum. J Urol 170:82, 2003.
25. O'Conor VJ Jr: Repair of vesicovaginal fistula with associated urethral loss. Surg Gynecol Obstet 146:251, 1978.
26. Park J, Hendren HJ: Construction of female urethra using buccal mucosa graft. J Urol 166:640, 2001.
27. Leng WW, Amundsen CL, Mcguire EJ, Management of Female Genitourinary Fistulas: Transvesical or Transvaginal Approach, Jurol, 160:1995, 1998.
28 Morgan JE, Farrow GA, Sims RH: The Sioughed Urethra syndrome, Am J Obstet Gynecol, 130:521, 1978.
29. Patel U, Waterhouse K, Laungani G: Management of 18 Difficult Urethrovaginal Fistula with Modified Ingelman-Sundberg and Martius Operations. J Urol, 123:653, 1980.

Chapter 81

VESICOVAGINAL FISTULA: VAGINAL APPROACH

Matthew P. Rutman, Larissa V. Rodríguez, and Shlomo Raz

Vesicovaginal fistula (VVF) is one of the most significant and distressing complications in female urology and urogynecology. A VVF is an abnormal communication between the bladder and vagina that results in continuous urine leakage from the vagina. VVFs have been recognized and described since ancient times, but successful repair was not documented until James Marion Sims' first paper in 1852.[1] He used a transvaginal technique to perform the repair, including the use of silver wire suture. Many principles he described are still applicable. Subsequent modifications and advances included the first layered repair by Mackenrodt[2] and the interposed labial fat graft of Martius[3] in the late 1920s.

In developing countries, birth trauma remains the most common cause of VVF. Prolonged and obstructed labor leads to pressure necrosis of the anterior vaginal wall and the underlying bladder neck and urethra. In industrialized nations, most fistulas result from complications of gynecologic and other pelvic surgery. Regardless of the cause, surgical repair remains the gold standard and primary treatment of VVF.

ETIOLOGY

In the United States and other developed nations, VVFs occur as a result of surgical trauma, most commonly at the time of abdominal or vaginal hysterectomy. Unrecognized suture placement into the bladder during closure of the vaginal cuff results in tissue necrosis and subsequent fistula formation. Excessive blunt dissection of the bladder can result in ischemia or an unrecognized tear in the posterior bladder wall. Approximately 75% of VVFs are reported to occur after hysterectomy for benign disease.[4] The incidence of VVF after hysterectomy is between 0.5% and 1%.[5] VVFs also occur after anterior colporrhaphy, sling procedures for stress incontinence, cystocele repair, colposuspension procedures, and urethral or bladder diverticulectomy. Approximately 90% of VVFs in North America result from gynecologic procedures. The other 10% are caused by advanced local malignancy (i.e., cervical, vaginal, and endometrial), radiation therapy, inflammatory bowel disease, foreign bodies, and infectious processes of the urinary tract.

PREVENTION

Recognizing that most VVFs are iatrogenic, it is paramount that the treating surgeon takes the necessary precautions to prevent their occurrence. Risk factors reported for fistula development include prior cesarean section, endometriosis, previous cervical conization, and radiation treatment.[6] The bladder is most often injured during the dissection of the posterior bladder wall from the anterior surface of the uterus at the level of the vaginal cuff during abdominal hysterectomy. Placement of an indwelling Foley catheter and meticulous sharp dissection can minimize inadvertent injury. Iatrogenic injuries can be unavoidable in difficult reoperations and in patients with dense adhesions that obliterate normal surgical planes. Careful attention should be paid to diagnose and repair the injury intraoperatively. Filling the Foley catheter with methylene blue dye to check for leakage is a simple and effective method of checking bladder integrity. If a bladder injury is recognized, two-layer repair is required after adequate exposure is provided. A drain should be placed. The catheter should be left in longer than the usual 1 or 2 days after hysterectomy. An interposition flap can provide an additional layer of coverage.

DIAGNOSIS

History

Patients typically present with continuous urinary drainage (day and night) from the vagina after gynecologic or pelvic surgery. Any patient with urinary incontinence immediately after pelvic surgery should be evaluated to rule out a VVF. The fistula may manifest immediately postoperatively, but it often becomes clinically apparent days to weeks later. Ureterovaginal fistulas tend to manifest later than VVFs. Ten percent of patients with a VVF have an associated ureterovaginal fistula.[7] Early in the postoperative course, patients may present with fevers, abdominal pain, hematuria, ileus, and lower urinary tract symptoms.

Patients with VVF related to prior radiation therapy may present 6 months to 20 years later.[8] Fluid draining from the vagina may be urine, lymph, peritoneal fluid, fallopian tube fluid, or vaginal secretions. Important considerations in the differential diagnosis of VVF include urethrovaginal fistula, ureterovaginal fistula, ectopic ureter, peritoneal fluid drainage, and vaginal cuff infection.

Diagnostic Tests

To confirm that the leaking fluid from the vagina is urine, the fluid can be sent for creatinine analysis. Elevated levels (relative to serum) establish the diagnosis of a communication between the vagina and urinary tract. Physical examination is paramount in the evaluation of a woman with a suspected fistula. The diameter, depth, mobility, and mucosa of the vagina must all be assessed. Concomitant prolapse, urethral hypermobility, and stress incontinence should also be evaluated. Vaginal examination with a speculum can isolate the point of leakage. The most common location for VVF (after a hysterectomy) is at the level of the vaginal cuff. Pooling of urine at the apex and the fornices is commonly seen. Surrounding vaginal mucosa may appear edematous and erythematous, making it difficult to identify the opening. Placing a Foley catheter into the bladder can assist by visualizing the balloon. If all of these measures fail to identify a fistula, dye tests can be used for confirmation. Instilling methylene blue dye through the Foley catheter, with concomitant inspection of the vagina for leakage of blue fluid, can help identify a VVF. Requesting the patient to ambulate with a vaginal pack in place may stain the packing blue. If a VVF is still not identified, the patient should be given oral phenazopyridine, which stains the urine orange. The vagina is then packed, and orange staining confirms a fistula. A positive phenazopyridine test result with a negative methylene blue test result strongly suggests a ureterovaginal fistula.

All patients with a diagnosis of a urinary fistula should undergo upper tract evaluation and cystoscopy. Upper tract evaluation can be done with intravenous pyelography (IVU) or retrograde pyelography. Ureteral involvement can be demonstrated by hydronephrosis or extravasation on IVU, although the ipsilateral kidney can appear normal with prompt drainage. Retrograde pyelography remains the most sensitive test to evaluate ureteral involvement in the presence or absence of a VVF. Cystoscopy should identify the location and size of the fistula and determine its relation to the ureteral orifices. It is important to ascertain that there is adequate bladder capacity and to rule out foreign body as the source of the fistula. Surveillance for multiple fistulas is imperative, because this finding would alter operative repair. Patients with a radiation- or malignancy-associated fistula must undergo biopsy of the site before repair. A voiding cystourethrogram (VCUG) can help identify the presence and location of a fistula. Coexisting vesicoureteral reflux, urethral diverticulum, stress incontinence, and cystocele can also be identified, which may alter the surgical plan. VCUG can help elucidate fistulas involving the rectum or uterus, and vaginoscopy can assist in identifying the vaginal communication.

TREATMENT

Conservative Management

Small VVFs may close spontaneously with continuous Foley catheter drainage (up to 10% of cases). This has usually been attempted by the time patients have sought consultation with a specialist. Three weeks of drainage is a reasonable option if the fistula is discovered early in the postoperative period. Mature fistula tracts are unlikely to resolve with this technique. Prolonged catheter drainage requires coverage with antibiotics.

Another conservative treatment option includes fulgurating the lining of the fistula tract. This should not be attempted with large fistulous tracts. Stovsky and colleagues[9] reported closure in 11 of 17 patients with fulguration of fistulas less than 3 mm long and with 2 weeks of catheter drainage. Reports have shown success with fibrin therapy in treating small VVFs.[10] Most conservative measures ultimately fail in the attempt to cure VVFs. For larger, complex, and radiation-induced fistulas, there is no role for conservative treatment, and formal repair remains the gold standard.

Operative Management

Preoperative Considerations

Before formal repair of a VVF, many factors must be considered to optimize the chances of a successful repair. Historically, most surgeons advocated waiting 3 to 6 months before surgical repair to allow the fistula to completely mature.[11,12] They theorized that this allowed maximal healing during the post-hysterectomy inflammatory stage. However, patients with VVFs experience enormous social, physical, and psychological stress during this period that greatly hinders their quality of life. Contemporary surgeons have reported excellent results with early repair, and the strategy avoided patients' distress throughout a waiting period.[13,14] Typically, early transvaginal repair is performed 2 to 3 weeks after the time of injury. This is most commonly done in women with fistulas that form after hysterectomy using an abdominal approach. Patients with vaginal cuff infections or pelvic abscesses must be treated long-term with antibiotics before any repair attempt. Patients with previously failed repairs or radiation-related fistulas are not candidates for early intervention. They should wait a minimum of several months before repair. VVFs after traumatic delivery are ischemic in origin and require a longer period of conservative management.

The most appropriate approach to formal surgical repair of a VVF is the one most familiar to the surgeon. The choice between an abdominal or vaginal approach depends on the surgeon's experience, training, and comfort level with the procedure. The highest success rates are associated with the first operation, regardless of the approach. Traditionally, the fistula's location dictated the surgical approach. Infratrigonal and bladder neck fistulas were repaired vaginally, whereas supratrigonal fistulas were repaired transabdominally. Even complex high VVFs can be repaired using a transvaginal approach with adherence to good surgical technique and tissue interposition. The advantage of an abdominal approach is the ability to perform simultaneous procedures for coexisting intra-abdominal pathology, including augmentation cystoplasty, ureteral reimplantation, and repair of bowel fistulas. The vaginal approach avoids an abdominal incision and possible bladder bivalving. It is associated with decreased morbidity, shorter hospital stay, and quicker patient convalescence. We use the transvaginal approach for most VVFs.

Many principles are integral to fistula repair, regardless of the approach chosen. Excellent exposure with watertight, tension-free closure using multiple, nonoverlapping sutures lines provide an approximately 90% chance of cure on the first attempt. Continuous catheter drainage postoperatively is mandatory. Interpositional grafts optimize the chance for cure if the integrity of the repair is in question.

Preoperative preparation includes prescribing antibiotics to clear any infection and provide a sterile environment for repair. Urine culture should document absence of infection before surgery. Broad-spectrum, intravenous antibiotics are provided preoperatively. Preoperative estrogen-containing vaginal cream is used in the postmenopausal or post-hysterectomy patient to improve the quality of the vaginal tissues.

Traditional repair of VVF included excision of the tract to provide clean and vascular edges. This was thought to increase chances for cure. Raz and associates[15,16] demonstrated excellent results without excising the fistulous tract with no adverse effects.

Excising the fistula enlarges the tract, and it may cause iatrogenic bleeding, requiring hemostatic measures that may inhibit healing. Excising fistulous tracts located near the ureteral orifices may require ureteral reimplantation.

Before surgical repair, the surgeon should be familiar with several techniques for interposition of tissue. Although these grafts are often necessary in large, complex, post-radiation, and failed primary repairs, it is difficult to accurately predict which fistulas will require the additional layer of coverage to avoid a tenuous repair.

Preoperative evaluation should attempt to identify patients who have coexisting stress urinary incontinence. Simultaneous sling procedure or bladder neck suspension can be performed, avoiding the need for a second procedure. Concomitant repair for stress incontinence does not increase the fistula recurrence rate.[17] It is also important to consider the sexual function of the patient and ensure preservation of vaginal depth in the sexually active patient. This can require rotational flaps in patients with large fistulas and vaginal stenosis. Local estrogen replacement should be used in patients with vaginal atrophy.

Vaginal Technique

We routinely repair VVFs by means of a vaginal approach and describe the technique for transvaginal repair of VVFs. The surgery is performed on an outpatient basis and avoids the morbidity of a laparotomy.

Step 1 is patient preparation. The patient is placed in the low lithotomy position and prepped in standard fashion. A headlight provides excellent visualization for the surgeon. Cystoscopy with ureteral catheterization is done when the fistula is located near the trigone and the ureteral orifices. A curved Lowsley retractor aids in placement of a 16-Fr suprapubic catheter through a small suprapubic incision. A posterolateral episiotomy (i.e., relaxing incision) may be necessary in a patient with a narrow vagina. The labia minora are sutured apart, and a ring retractor is positioned for optimal exposure. A urethral catheter is placed to ensure maximal urinary drainage. An Allis clamp is used to elevate the anterior vaginal wall, and a weighted speculum is placed posteriorly.

Step 2 is isolation of fistula. The fistulous tract is identified and catheterized with an 8- or 10-Fr Foley catheter. This aids retraction throughout the dissection. Metal sounds may be necessary to dilate the tract before catheter placement. An inverted-J incision is made with care taken to circumscribe the fistulous tract (Fig. 81-1). The long end of the J should extend to the apex of the vagina, which facilitates rotation and advancement of a posterior flap at the later stages of the procedure. Fistulas located high in the vaginal cuff may require an inverted incision, with the base of the flap facing the urethral meatus.

Step 3 is the creation of flaps. Anteriorly and posteriorly based vaginal flaps are dissected on each side of the fistulous tract, starting with healthy tissue located away from the fistula itself (Fig. 81-2). This usually provides a healthy plane of dissection and helps prevent enlargement of the fistulous tract or inadvertent bladder perforation. The ring of vaginal tissue at the opening of the fistula is left intact. The flaps should be developed at least 2 to 4 cm away from the fistulous tract, exposing the underlying perivesical fascia. The flaps are then retracted with the hooks of the ring retractor. Lateral dissection of the vaginal wall 2 to 4 cm from the fistulous tract allows complete exposure of the perivesical fascia.

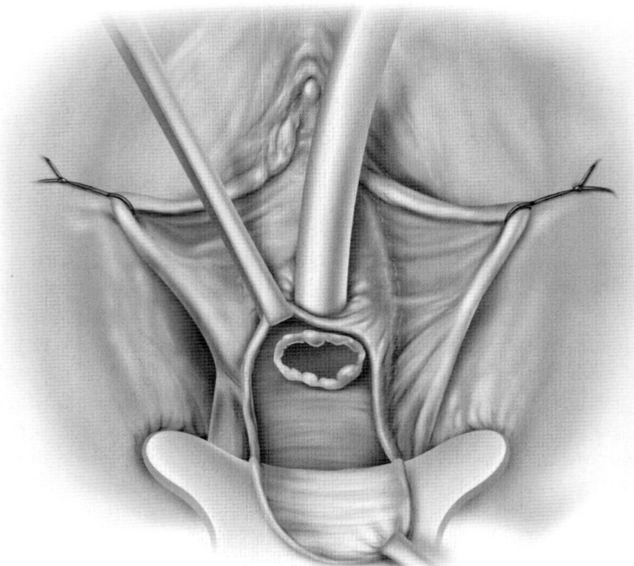

Figure 81-1 Inverted-J-shaped incision around the fistulous tract. (From Raz S, Little NA, Juma S: Female urology. In Walsh PC, Retik AB, Stamey TA, Vaughan ED Jr [eds]: Campbell's Urology, 6th ed. Philadelphia, WB Saunders, 1992, pp 2782-2828.)

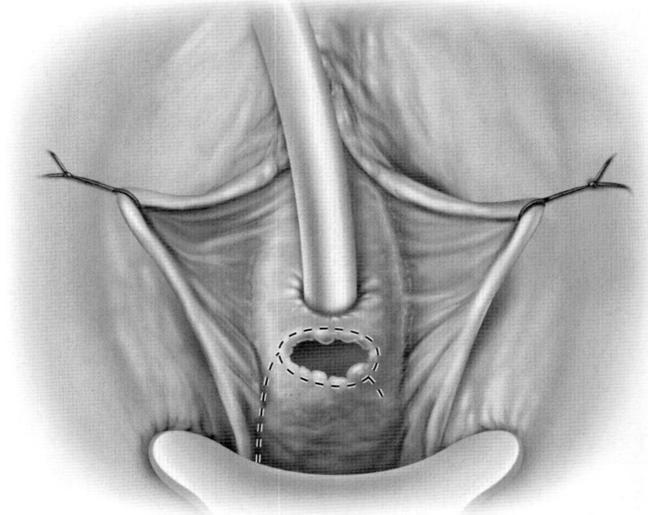

Figure 81-2 Development of vaginal flaps.

Step 4 is closure of the fistula. The standard VVF repair is done in three layers. The first layer closes the epithelialized edges of the fistula tract and a few millimeters of the surrounding tissue (including bladder wall) with interrupted, absorbable, 2-0 sutures (Vicryl or Dexon) in a transverse fashion (Fig. 81-3). The fistula catheter is removed, and the sutures are secured, closing the fistulous tract. The second layer of the repair incorporates the perivesical fascia and deep muscular bladder wall using the same suture material (Fig. 81-4). The sutures are placed at least 1 cm from the prior suture line and secured in a tension-free fashion. The sutures are placed in a line 90 degrees from the first suture

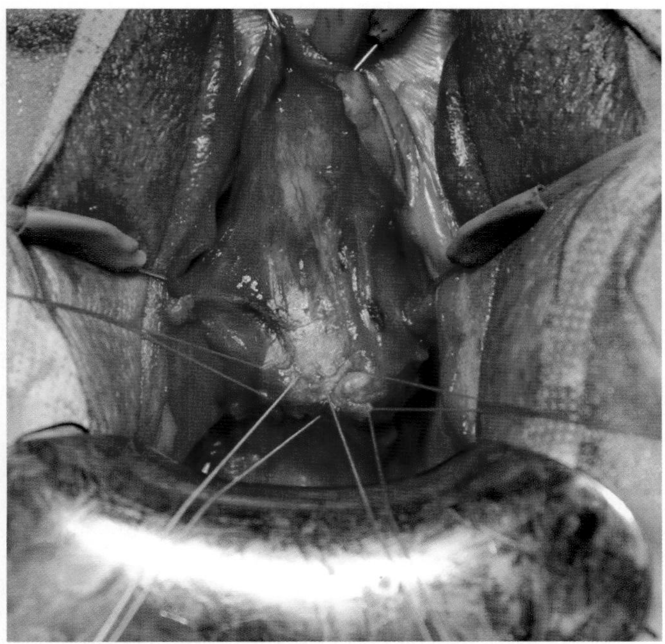

Figure 81-3 First layer of repair: transverse closure of a fistulous tract without excision.

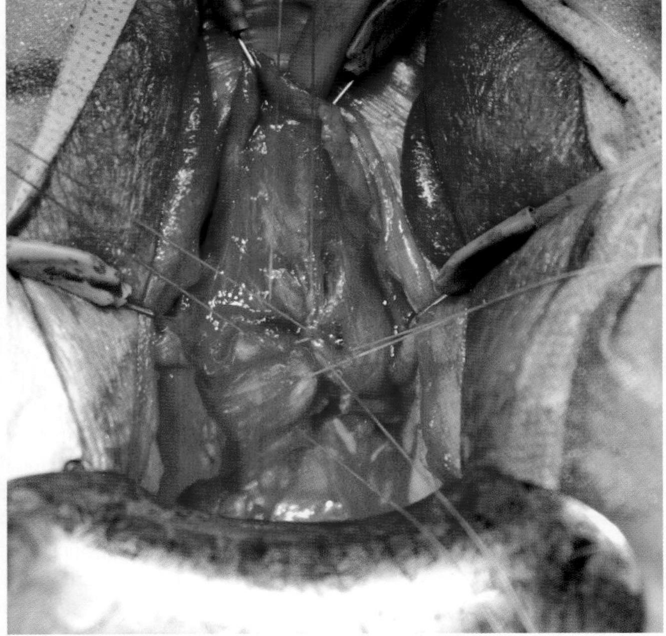

Figure 81-4 Second layer of repair: imbricated first layer with perivesical fascia.

layer to minimize overlapping suture lines. The second layer of sutures completely covers the first layer of closure. The bladder is filled with indigo carmine diluted in saline to ensure repair integrity.

Step 5 is completion of the operation. In a standard VVF repair (without interposition), the procedure is completed. The previously raised posterior flap is rotated beyond the fistula closure site by at least 3 cm. The excess vaginal flap tissue is

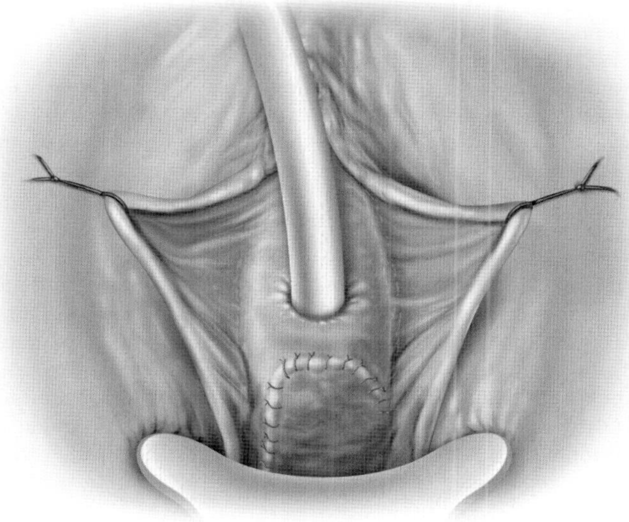

Figure 81-5 Third layer of repair: vaginal flap advancement.

excised. The vaginal wall is closed using a running, locking, absorbable, 3-0 suture (Vicryl or Dexon). This covers the tract with healthy vaginal tissue and provides a third layer of closure with no overlapping suture lines. (Fig. 81-5) An antibiotic-impregnated vaginal pack is placed, and the urethral and suprapubic catheters are left to dependent drainage.

Most cases of uncomplicated VVF require only a three-layer, tension-free repair. Complicating factors that mandate additional protection include prior irradiation, failed prior surgery, and poor tissue quality. These conditions require tissue interposition. In most cases of high VVF after hysterectomy, we perform the interposition of a peritoneal flap between the first two layers of fistula closure and the advancement of the vaginal wall flap. The tissue is readily available, requires minimal additional dissection, and creates a more secure closure of the fistulous tract.

Other Techniques

The abdominal approach is beyond the objectives of this chapter. We use the abdominal approach only in selected patients requiring concomitant abdominal procedures such as augmentation cystoplasty or ureteral reimplantation.

The Latzko operation, originally described in 1942, uses partial colpocleisis to treat the VVF.[18] The operation consists of denudement of the vaginal wall around the fistula without excising the fistulous tract. A separate layered closure is performed that includes the bladder, fistula, and vagina. A major concern with this procedure is vaginal shortening. However, success rates of 93% and 95% have been reported in two series of 43 and 20 patients, respectively, with no significant patient-reported vaginal shortening or sexual dysfunction.[19,20] Many gynecologists still use this technique because of its technical ease and minimal morbidity.

Transurethral suture cystorrhaphy without fistula tract excision has been described as a minimally invasive alternative for smaller fistulas (5 to 8 mm) located away from the ureteral orifices. The technique requires fulguration of the tract and surrounding bladder mucosa before combined transurethral and abdominal endoscopic suture placement. A minimum 2- to 3-

week period of bladder drainage is required. Eight (73%) of 11 patients treated with this technique were cured.[21]

With the recent upsurge in minimally invasive surgery, VVF repair also has been done laparoscopically.[22] The approach was first described in 1994 and has since undergone various modifications, including use of endostaplers, omental interposition, and layered closure.[23]

Management of Complex Fistulas

Complex VVFs include those associated with prior irradiation or malignancy, recurrent fistulas, fistulas of large size (>3 cm), fistulas involving the bladder neck and trigone, and those associated with poor tissue quality or difficult closure. In these cases, the standard transvaginal repair must be modified. Many techniques of tissue interposition have been described. These provide an additional layer of closure and enhance the quality of the reconstructive repair.

Radiation-Induced Fistulas

Radiation-induced VVFs require special consideration. The site of fistula formation is typically in the trigone region; it is in a relatively fixed position and radiation effects are more likely. Between 1% and 5% of patients treated for cervical or uterine carcinoma develop radiation-induced fistulas. The fistulas most commonly manifest in a delayed fashion, sometimes 15 to 20 years later.[15] Fistulas associated with prior irradiation should always be biopsied to rule out recurrence of the primary malignancy.

Radiation-induced fistulas result from obliterative endarteritis in the irradiated field.[24] The injury compromises healing. The surrounding tissues are also affected by the endarteritis, complicating an already difficult repair. Video urodynamics and cystoscopy are mandatory before surgery. They allow assessment of bladder capacity and compliance. With adequate capacity and compliance, transvaginal repair is performed with modifications, including tissue interposition and prolonged postoperative catheter drainage. If the bladder has poor compliance and small capacity, augmentation cystoplasty is required, and an abdominal approach is taken. Careful inspection of the bowel is necessary to ensure use of a nonirradiated segment for the augmentation.

Martius Graft

The Martius graft (i.e., fibrofatty labial flap) was first described in 1928.[3] This technique is commonly used in pelvic and perineal reconstructive surgery, and it has great utility in treating VVF, rectovaginal fistula, and urethrovaginal fistula and in urethral reconstruction. It has high reported success rates in complex fistula repair[25] and is a convenient source of interposition in transvaginal repair. We use a Martius flap in cases of trigonal or urethral fistula. For fistula located high in the vaginal vault (after hysterectomy), the peritoneum is our preferred source of tissue interposition in these cases.

The Martius graft is a long band of adipose tissue from the labia majora. It has excellent strength and vascularity. The blood supply is threefold. Branches of the external pudendal artery supply the graft superiorly and anteriorly. Obturator branches enter the graft at its lateral border. The inferior labial artery and vein supply the graft inferiorly. The graft may be mobilized superiorly or inferiorly, depending on the desired location of transfer.

The first two layers of the fistula are closed as described earlier. The vaginal flaps are left intact, and the labial retraction suture is removed. A vertical incision is then made over the labia majora, and the subcutaneous tissues are dissected laterally to the lateral border of the dissection, the labiocrural fold. The flap is then dissected posteriorly to the Colles fascia and medially to the labia minora and bulbocavernosus muscle. The main vascular supply is at the base, and the entire thickness of the fat pad is carefully encircled by a Penrose drain. The superior and anterior segment of the graft is clamped, transected, and suture ligated. The remaining dissection is completed, freeing the flap, except at its base (Fig. 81-6A). A tunnel is then made between the perivaginal tissues and vaginal wall. The graft is then passed from the labial area to the vaginal area (through the tunnel) with the aid of a hemostat (see Fig. 81-6B). The Martius graft is placed over the fistula site and secured with interrupted, absorbable suture in a tension-free fashion. The vaginal flap is advanced and closed as previously described, providing a fourth layer of closure. A light pressure dressing may be applied, and ice packs are routinely applied. Eilber and colleagues[26] reported a 97% cure rate with transvaginal repair using Martius graft interposition in 34 patients with complex fistulas.

We have performed an in situ technique for the creation of a Martius flap, avoiding a labial incision. After the creation of the vaginal flaps in the distal vagina, we dissect a tunnel under the vaginal wall in the direction of the fibrofatty tissue in the labia. The medial and lateral segments of the Martius flaps are isolated using a Penrose drain, the upper segment of the Martius flap is dissected free, and the flap is mobilized and transferred to cover the fistula closure.

Peritoneal Flap

We use a peritoneal flap in the repair of high fistulas located at the vaginal vault, which are seen most commonly after hysterectomy. Extending a Martius graft to this location may be difficult and inadvertently result in vaginal shortening. A peritoneal flap is an easily available, well-vascularized tissue that can be harvested without the morbidity of a second incision.

The fistula repair begins as described in the first three steps of the transvaginal technique. The fistula is circumscribed, and vaginal flaps are prepared. A catheter in the fistula can help in dissection of the flap. Sharp dissection is used to expose the peritoneum and preperitoneal fat. The fistulous tract is then closed in two layers, as previously described. The preperitoneal fat and peritoneum are advanced to cover the fistula repair and secured to the perivesical fascia with tension-free, interrupted sutures. The vaginal flap is then advanced and closed. Raz and coworkers[27] reported a 91% success rate in their initial experience using a peritoneal flap in 11 patients with VVFs. Eilber and associates[26] reported a 96% cure rate using a peritoneal flap in 83 patients who underwent complex fistula repair. This approach has high success rates, minimal morbidity, and outcomes similar to those of a Martius graft but without a second incision.

Omental Interposition

Omental interposition is primarily used in the abdominal approach for fistula repair, although it can be accessed transvaginally in women who have had previous procedures. This technique results in an omental graft that can be placed between the bladder and vagina for an additional layer of protection.

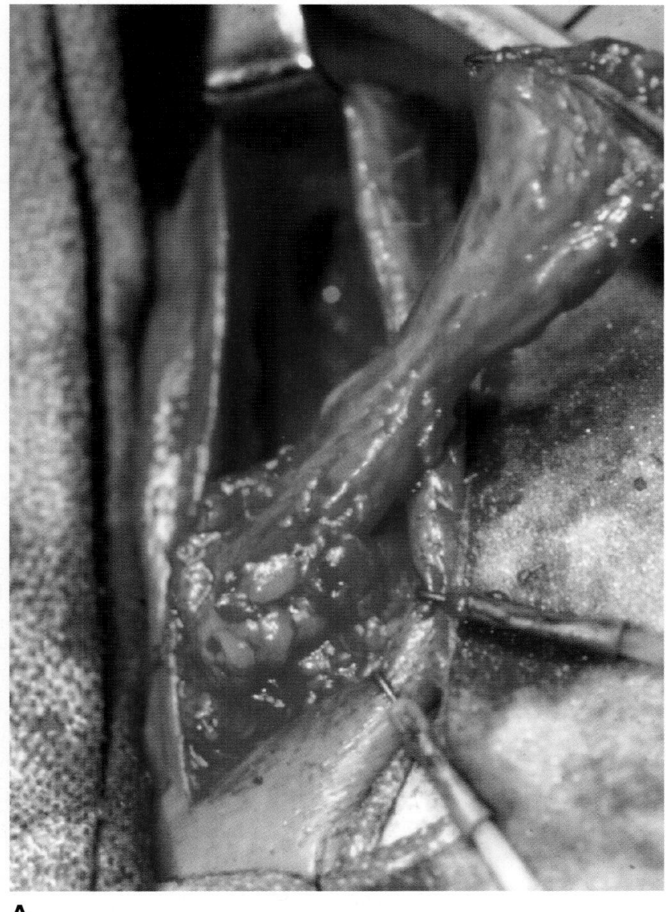

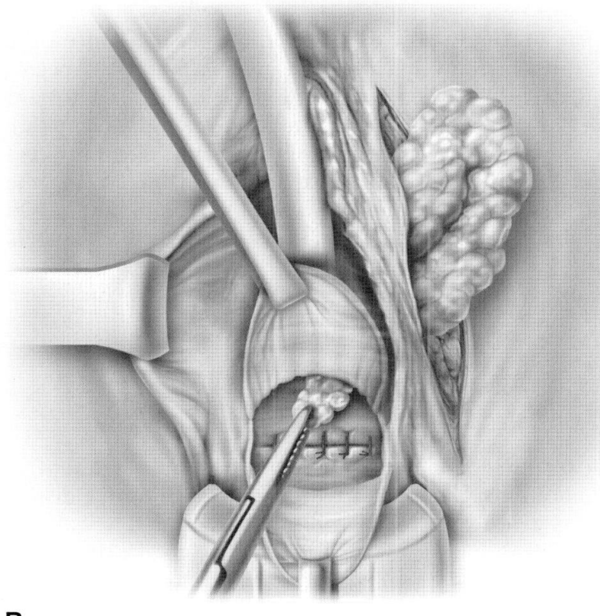

A B

Figure 81-6 A, Mobilization of a Martius flap based on an inferior pedicle. **B,** Transfer of a Martius flap to cover a fistula repair (**B,** from Raz S: Atlas of Transvaginal Surgery. Philadelphia, WB Saunders, 1992.)

Rotational Full-Thickness Labial Flap

In selected complex cases with loss of the vaginal wall, insufficient vaginal epithelium may preclude primary vaginal closure. A full-thickness labial flap can be rotated to substitute for the missing vaginal wall. The advantage of this flap is that combines the use of the fibrofatty tissue of the Martius with a well-vascularized skin flap to cover the deficient or absent vaginal wall. The fistula is closed as previously described, and the vascularized flap is rotated to provide full-thickness skin coverage.

After closure of the fistula, a U-shaped incision is made over the labia, including the lateral labial skin and underlying tissue. The apex of the flap is created at the level of the posterior fourchette and the base at the upper segment of the labia majora. The flap is dissected from the fascia overlying the pubic bone and then rotated to cover the repair. After closure of the fistula, the fatty tissue covers the fistula closure, and the skin of the labia is sutured to the edge of the vaginal flaps. Interrupted, absorbable sutures are used to secure the edges in place.[28] Small series have reported excellent results. Carr and Webster[29] reported excellent outcomes for four patients. Postoperative complications include sensory deficit at the harvest site, poor cosmetic result, wound infection, and flap sloughing.

Gluteal Skin Flap

Gluteal skin flaps are used predominantly in patients with radiation-induced fistulas or severe vaginal wall atrophy with no other viable skin source. In cases of severe radiation-induced fistula, the vaginal canal is very narrow, and access to the fistulous tract can be extremely difficult. Before the repair, a lateral episiotomy, starting at the posterior fourchette (5- or 7-o'clock) is performed and extended toward the vaginal cuff. The first two layers of the fistula are closed, and the vaginal flaps are raised as previously described. The edges of the vaginal wall incision are dissected laterally to widen the vaginal canal and make room for the flap interposition. From the end of the episiotomy incision, the incision is continued in an inverted-U-shaped fashion toward the gluteal area. The skin is then undermined, and the flap is rotated and advanced into the vaginal canal to cover the fistula. The flap contains skin and fatty tissue and is broad based. The flap is secured with interrupted, absorbable sutures, and the vaginal flaps are secured to the skin flap edges.[30] Complications include wound infection, sloughing of the flap, and injury to the anal sphincter.[31] Meticulous surgical technique is mandatory to avoid the sphincter injury.

Myocutaneous Gracilis Flap

The gracilis muscle–based myocutaneous flap is frequently described in association with repair of radiation-induced VVFs in patients with vaginal atrophy or absence. The gracilis muscle is a long, slender muscle hat extends from the inferior pubic symphysis to the medial condyle of the femur. It is an accessory muscle (used for thigh adduction and knee flexion), and it can be sacrificed with no loss in function. It sits between the adductor magnus medially and the adductor longus laterally. The blood supply is derived from the medial femoral circumflex artery, a branch of the deep femoral artery.

The flap is harvested with a tennis racquet incision on the medial aspect of the thigh over the gracilis muscle. It begins around 10 cm below the pubic tubercle and extends 20 cm toward the knee. The skin and underlying muscle are mobilized, and care is taken to preserve the vascular supply. The gracilis is transected at its distal insertion. A tunnel is then created underneath the medial aspect of the thigh and labia, and the flap is transferred to the vaginal area, providing additional coverage of the fistula tract and reconstruction of the vaginal canal. This can result in considerable cosmetic scarring, but there is no functional defect.

INTRAOPERATIVE COMPLICATIONS

Bleeding and ureteral injury represent the two major intraoperative complications. Hemostasis is critical throughout the dissection and can be controlled with fine, absorbable sutures. Electrocautery should be avoided to preserve the vascularity of the tissues and promote healing. Lack of excellent hemostasis can lead to hematoma formation and possible disruption of the fistula repair.

Ureteral catheterization is recommended for fistulas close to the trigone because of the higher risk of iatrogenic ureteral injury. Fistulas located elsewhere do not usually require this maneuver. If there is any concern about ureteral violation, cystoscopy is performed after intravenous indigo carmine is administered. Ureteral catheterization can be done if any question remains about ureteral patency.

POSTOPERATIVE MANAGEMENT

The vagina is packed with an antibiotic-impregnated gauze, which is left in place for several hours. Surgery is mostly performed on an outpatient basis. The suprapubic and Foley catheters (joined to a Y connector) are left to dependent drainage, typically for 3 weeks. Anticholinergics are given to minimize bladder spasm and increase the patient's comfort. An oral cephalosporin or quinolone is continued until the catheters are removed. Patients are instructed to resume normal activity except for strenuous exercise. Sexual intercourse is prohibited for 12 weeks. The urethral catheter is removed 3 weeks after surgery, and a suprapubic cystogram is performed. If the cystogram demonstrates no extravasation, the suprapubic catheter is removed.

OUTCOMES

Many factors must be considered when assessing patient outcomes. Morbidity, patient satisfaction, and cure rate are critical factors in determining the best approach and the likelihood of success. There have been no prospective, randomized studies comparing vaginal and abdominal approaches in VVF repair. Many series have shown success rates of 90% to 100% with both approaches.[15,32-34] The best approach remains the one with which the surgeon has the most expertise and comfort, giving the patient the best chance at cure with the first repair.

POSTOPERATIVE COMPLICATIONS

Early Complications

Vaginal bleeding, bladder spasms, and vaginal infection must be treated aggressively and immediately to prevent fistula recurrence. Secondary vaginal bleeding is treated with repacking and bed rest. Prophylactic anticholinergics should minimize bladder spasms. Belladonna and opium suppositories (e.g., B & O Supprettes) can be used if required. Perioperative antibiotics are continued in the postoperative period to prevent vaginal infections.

Delayed Complications

The most important delayed complication is fistula recurrence. Others include vaginal shortening, vaginal stenosis, and unrecognized ureteral injury. Tension-free, multilayered closure with tissue interposition (as needed) results in a greater than 95% success rate. If the fistula recurs, a second vaginal repair may be performed with a Martius graft or peritoneal flap. A minimum waiting period of 3 months after the previous repair allows for resolution of postoperative inflammation. Avoiding excessive resection of the vaginal wall minimizes the odds of significant shortening and stenosis. Secondary vaginoplasty is required in selected cases. Unrecognized ureteral injury manifests more commonly as an obstruction process than a leak. An antegrade approach with percutaneous nephrostomy is preferred to a retrograde procedure because of the possible disruption of the repair by a transurethral approach.

CONCLUSIONS

VVF remains a significant source of morbidity after gynecologic and pelvic surgery. Transvaginal VVF repair is an outpatient procedure associated with minimal morbidity, short convalescence times, and high cure rates. It is our preferred method of repair unless concomitant abdominal surgery is required.

References

1. Sims JM: On the treatment of vesico-vaginal fistula [originally published in Am J Med Sci 23:59-82, 1852]. Int Urogynecol J Pelvic Floor Dysfunct 9:236-248, 1998.
2. Mackenrodt A: Die operative Heiling grosser Blasencheindenfisteln. Zentralbl Gynakol 8:180-184, 1894.
3. Martius H: Uber die Behandlung von Blasenscheidenfisteln, insbesondere met Hilfe einer Lappenplastik. Geburtshilfe Gynakol 103:22-34, 1932.
4. Lee RA, Symmonds RE, Williams TH: Current status of genitourinary fistula. Obstet Gynecol 72:313-319, 1998.
5. Drutz HP, Mainprize TC: Unrecognized small vesicovaginal fistula as a cause of persistent urinary incontinence. Am J Obstet Gynecol 158:237-240, 1988.
6. Kursh ED, Morse RM, Resnick MI, et al: Prevention of the development of a vesicovaginal fistula. Surg Gynecol Obstet 166:409-412, 1988.
7. Symmonds RE: Incontinence: Vesical and urethral fistulas. Obstet Gynecol 27:499-514, 1984.
8. Graham JB: Vaginal fistulas following radiotherapy. Surg Gynecol Obstet 120:1019-1030, 1965.
9. Stovsky MD, Ignaroff JM, Blum MD, et al: Use of electrocoagulation in the treatment of vesicovaginal fistulas. J Urol 152:1443-1444, 1994.
10. Morita T, Tokue A: Successful endoscopic closure of radiation induced vesico-vaginal fistula with fibrin glue and bovine collagen. J Urol 162:1689, 1999.
11. O'Conor VJ: Review of experience with vesico-vaginal fistula repair. J Urol 123:367-369, 1980.
12. Wein AJ, Malloy TR, Carpiniello VL, et al: Repair of vesico-vaginal fistula by a suprapubic transvesical approach. Surg Gynecol Obstet 150:57-60, 1980.
13. Blaivis JG, Heritz DM, Romanzi LJ: Early versus late repair of vesicovaginal fistulas: Vaginal and abdominal approaches. J Urol 153:1110-1112, 1995.
14. Raz S, Little NA, Juma S: Female urology. In Walsh PC, Retik AB, Stamey TA (eds): Campbell's Urology, 6th ed. Philadelphia, WB Saunders, 1992, pp 2782-2828.
15. Zimmern PE, Hadley HR, Staskin DR, Raz S: Genitourinary fistulae: Vaginal approach for repair of vesicovaginal fistulae. Urol Clin North Am 12:361-367, 1985.
16. Leach GE, Raz S: Vaginal flap technique: A method of transvaginal vesicovaginal fistula repair. In Raz S (ed): Female Urology. Philadelphia, WB Saunders, 1992, pp 372-377.
17. Arrowsmith SD: Genitourinary reconstruction in obstetric fistulas. J Urol 152:403-406, 1994.
18. Latzko W: Postoperative vesicovaginal fistulas; genesis and therapy. Am J Surg 58:211-228, 1942.
19. Tancer ML: The post-total hysterectomy (vault) vesicovaginal fistula. J Urol 123:839-840, 1980.
20. D'Amico AM, Lloyd KL: Latzko repair of vesicovaginal fistula. J Urol 161(Suppl):202, 1999.
21. Mckay HA: Vesicovaginal fistula repair: Transurethral suture cystorrhaphy as a minimally invasive alternative. J Endourol 18:487-490, 2004.
22. Ou C, Huang U, Tsuang M, Rowbotham R: Laparoscopic repair of vesicovaginal fistula. J Laparoendosc Adv Surg Tech 14:17-20, 2004.
23. Nezhat CH, Nezhat F, Nezhat C, et al: Laparoscopic repair of vesicovaginal fistula: A case report. Obstet Gynecol 83:899-901, 1994.
24. Perez Ca, Grigsby PW, Lockett MA, et al: Radiation therapy morbidity in carcinoma of the uterine cervix: Dosimetric and clinical correlation. Int J Radiat Oncol Biol Phys 44:855-866, 1999.
25. Margolis T, Elkins TE, Seffah J, et al: Full-thickness Martius grafts to preserve vaginal depth as an adjunct in the repair of large obstetric fistulas. Obstet Gynecol 84:148-152, 1994.
26. Eilber KS, Kavaler E, Rodriguez LV, et al: Ten-Year experience with transvaginal vesicovaginal fistula repair using tissue interposition. J Urol 169:1033-1036, 2003.
27. Raz S, Bregg KJ, Nitti VW, et al: Transvaginal repair of vesicovaginal fistula using a peritoneal flap. J Urol 150:56-59, 1993.
28. Raz S: Atlas of Transvaginal Surgery. Philadelphia, WB Saunders, 2002.
29. Carr LK, Webster GD: Full-thickness cutaneous Martius flaps: A useful technique in female reconstructive urology. Urology 48:461-463, 1996.
30. Stothers L, Chopra A, Raz S: Vesicovaginal fistula. In Raz S (ed): Female Urology, 2nd ed. Philadelphia, WB Saunders, 1996, pp 490-506.
31. Wang Y, Hadley HR: The use of rotated vascularized pedicle flaps for complex transvaginal procedures. J Urol 149:590-592, 1993.
32. Langkilde NC, Pless TK, Lundbeck F, et al: Surgical repair of vesicovaginal fistulae—A ten-year retrospective study. Scand J Urol Nephrol 33:100-103, 1999.
33. Diaz CE, Calatrava GS, Caldentey GM, et al: Surgical repair of vesico-vaginal fistulae with abdominal-transvesical approach. Comments on this technique with long-term results. Arch Esp Urol 50:55-60, 1997.
34. Frohmuller H, Hofmockel G: Transvaginal closure of vesicovaginal fistulas. Urologe A 37:102, 1998.

Chapter 82

ABDOMINAL APPROACH FOR THE TREATMENT OF VESICOVAGINAL FISTULA

Mariangela Mancini and Walter Artibani

An abdominal approach can be used to repair a vesicovaginal fistula (VVF). A VVF, an abnormal communication between the bladder and the vagina, is located outside the abdomen. The peritoneum reflects over the bladder dome anteriorly and the lower third of the uterus posteriorly (Fig. 82-1). The lamina of connective tissue interposed between the bladder and the vagina, whose destruction is associated with the formation of the VVF (Fig. 82-2), is found well outside the abdominal cavity. From an anatomic perspective, it appears to be more intuitive and, indeed, to reach a VVF through the vaginal route instead of through the abdomen, specific technique for VVF repair originally was mastered by the vaginal approach. Nevertheless, the abdominal approach for treatment of the VVF has its own indications and can offer specific advantages over the vaginal route. The history of the development of this surgical technique can help us understand the part that the abdominal approach plays in VVF surgery.

HISTORY

The first surgeons who tried to correct a VVF did so through the vaginal approach. In 1663, Hendrik van Roonhuyse recommended transvaginal repair with the patient in the lithotomy position. Stiff swan quills were passed to the edges of the wound, and the bladder and surrounding tissues were widely mobilized. Van Roonhuyse's book was published in 1676.[1]

The first two successful cases treated with this technique were reported by Johann Fatio in 1675.[2] Despite these preliminary and isolated successful experiences, the presence of a VVF was commonly considered an incurable situation in the years that followed. An important innovation was introduced by Antoine Jobert the Lamballe in 1834, when he performed his first operation of transvaginal closure of a VVF by resection of the margins and coverage of the loss of substance with a cutaneous autograft obtained from the labia or the internal face of the thigh.[3] The first operation was unsuccessful because of necrosis of the graft, but the patient was successfully cured on the second attempt with the same technique. Further developing the technique, Jobert pioneered later a method of tissue mobilization that widely detached the bladder from the vagina, which he called vesicovaginal autoplasty (*autoplastie vesico-vaginale par glissement*). He used this approach to avoid traction on the margins before suturing the edges of the fistula, and thereby obtained several successes in difficult VVF cases.[4]

In 1839, George Hayward[5] reported the first cure of a VVF in the United States. He underscored the importance of accurate dissection of the vagina from the bladder before closing the fistula with stitches and pioneered the flap-splitting technique.[5] In 1852, James Marion Sims[6] published his first report of successful primary repair of a VVF, which was again performed transvaginally. This interesting paper has been recently republished in the medical literature.[6] The correct surgical technique, the use of a

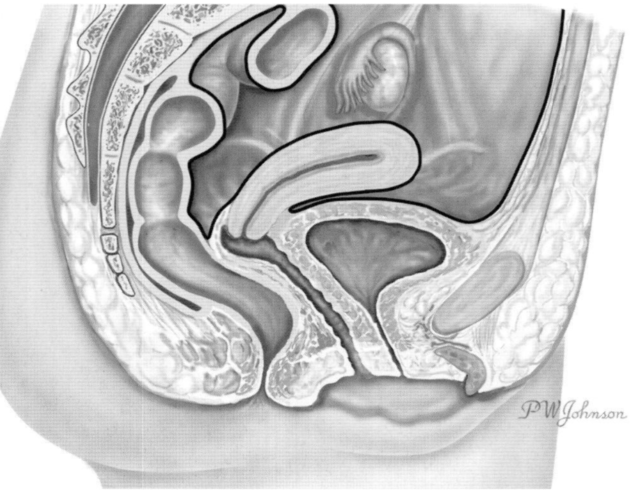

Figure 82-1 Sagittal section of the female lower abdomen and pelvis. The peritoneum *(bold line)* lines the floor of the abdominal cavity, leaving the vagina and posterior face of the bladder below it.

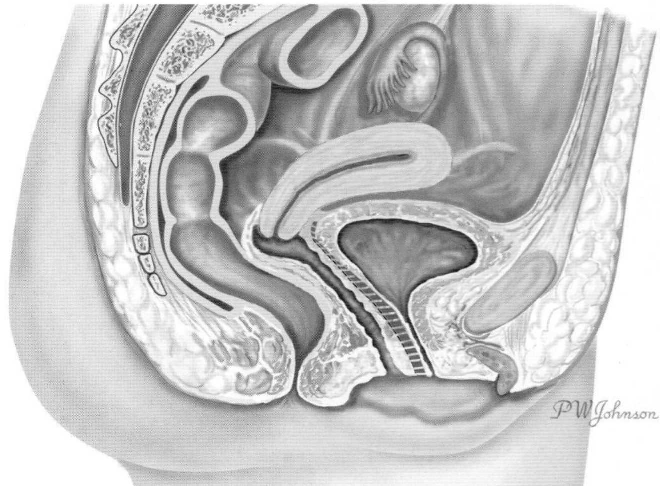

Figure 82-2 Female pelvic organs with their subperitoneal sheaths. The connective pillow layer interposed between the vagina and the bladder and urethra is indicated by *cross-hatching*. Damage to this tissue is associated with the formation of a vesicovaginal fistula.

new speculum designed by him, the search for the optimal patient position for exploration of the vagina, and an understanding of the importance of postoperative bladder drainage led to a high success rate for VVF treatment through the vaginal route and to international popularity for Sims.

This brief historical review shows that the basic principles stated by Sims and his predecessors for correct fistula treatment are still valid and that few modifications have been made by the surgeons who followed.[7] However, in 1868, Thomas Addis Emmet, who succeeded Sims as chief surgeon of the Woman's Hospital in New York, described some cases in which extensive scarring of the vagina and proximal location of the fistula compromised optimal access during transvaginal repair, indicating the need for higher access in these situations.[8,9] Some years later, the abdominal approach for the treatment of VVF was introduced. The suprapubic transperitoneal-transvesical route was first described by Friedrich Trendelenburg in 1881,[10] and in 1893, Von Dittel introduced the approach extraperitoned suprabubic for access to the VVF route.[11] In 1902, Howard Kelly recommended a transperitoneal approach in the treatment of VVFs formed after hysterectomy that were too high in the bladder to be safely reached transvaginally.[12] In 1914, Legueu[13] described in more detail the transperitoneal-transvesical approach.[13] To improve the chance of success in the most difficult cases, the omental graft technique was introduced by Hiltebrant in 1929 and further developed by Bastiaanse in the attempt to cure the challenging cases of postirradiation fistulas.[14]

In 1951, O'Conor and Sokol[15] described the complete range of possible procedures for successful treatment of VVFs, from conservative measures to vaginal or suprapubic closure to urinary diversion.[15] They emphasized the importance of careful selection of patients for each procedure. In some patients who had endured repeated previous failures, the fistulous opening was too high and too far from the bladder floor and the vagina too scarred to allow a vaginal approach. In these cases, a suprapubic procedure, preferably extraperitoneal, was described with bisection of the bladder down to the fistula opening and wide mobilization of the bladder from the vagina. A transperitoneal approach was selected when exposure was difficult because of previous operations, a history of cancer, or when the omentum needed to be used. With proper application of this technique, many successes were reported by O'Conor[16,17] in the following years. However, the suprapubic approach was not used by O'Conor[17] in 35% of his cases, for which a less invasive procedure was chosen.

This information underscores the importance of case selection. With the many possibilities available, VVF often can be treated successfully by tailing the approach to the patient's condition. It took almost 300 years of surgical research and extended practice with VVF patients, including enormous suffering and great rewards, to achieve this important goal. The history of the approaches to treatment demonstrates that flexibility is the key to successful management of this challenging pathologic condition.

ABDOMINAL APPROACH

Indications

An abdominal approach for the treatment of a VVF can be chosen for several reasons. Theoretically, the abdominal approach should be used when a less invasive approach is not feasible, but practically, this can have different meanings in different settings. At least four factors enter into the decision: the kind of fistula, the patient, the situation in which treatment takes place, and the surgeon. Fistulas are not all the same, and treatment must be individualized. Case selection is important.[18,19] The abdominal approach was developed to treat fistulas that were too high or too far from the bladder floor to be reached transvaginally. Moreover, in some cases, especially after several previous attempts, the vagina can be severely scarred and cannot be used for access to the fistula. Application of this concept depends on the surgeon's experience. Surgeons who have extensive experience with transvaginal surgery perform most repairs in this way, finding treatment of most fistulas amenable to the transvaginal approach.[20,21] Even the most complex fistulas can be repaired with the use of a peritoneal flap.[22]

There have been no abdominal repairs in the Addis Ababa Fistula Hospital in the past 4 years, during which about 4500 patients have been repaired transvaginally. However, one case of a high cervicovaginal fistula was operated on in another hospital. The patient had previously undergone a cesarean section, and in this particular case it was necessary to switch from the vaginal to the abdominal route because the fistula could not be reached safely from the vagina (A Browing, personal communication, 2005). Similarly, in patients who have been treated more than once with less invasive procedures without success, an attempt through a different route may be a reasonable choice. Some patients may express a preference for the abdominal route to increase the likelihood of cure. Some patients may need adjunctive procedures, such as ureteral reimplantation, bladder augmentation, or omental grafting, which need to be performed through the abdominal route.

The treatment setting also can influence operative decisions. In some tropical countries, for example, general anesthesia is not commonly available, which makes widespread use of the abdominal approach almost impossible.[23,24] In this situation, the technical level of hospitals encourages the use of less invasive procedures that can be performed safely under spinal anesthesia.[25,26] The surgeons' preferences are based on general surgical experience, familiarity with the procedure, and personal opinions about the case. Box 82-1 summarizes the indications for the abdominal approach that are consistently reported.

Timing

The best time to intervene and repair a fistula is unknown. Initially, treatment delay was advocated by some surgeons,[16,27,28] but later data indicate that immediate treatment is beneficial.[26] Treatment decisions are complicated by the fact that fistulas can be completely different pathologic entities, from the small, clear-cut opening produced during pelvic surgery, which is suitable for

Box 82-1 Indications for the Abdominal Approach

- Fistula too high in the bladder to be reached
- Inaccessible vagina
- Patient's preference
- Previously failed multiple attempts or failed less invasive attempt
- Necessity of other concurrent transabdominal procedures
- Hospital setting
- Surgeon's preference

immediate repair,[29] to the large, necrotic loss of substance, which results from hours of ischemic injury to the bladder during obstructed labor.[30] Timing should be tailored to the specific situation.[31,32]

It seems reasonable that a fistula should be treated as soon after diagnosis as possible, with timing modified according to the individual case. In the developed world, there often is no reason to postpone treatment.[29,31,33-35] Exceptions include the presence of infection or significant edema or a massive hematoma at the site of the fistula, which should be resolved before surgery. Taking care of coexistent problems usually requires not more than a few weeks, during which regular cystoscopic evaluation may be advisable.[36]

The possibility of spontaneous closure should be considered, especially for small, clean, postoperative fistulas, because spontaneous closure has been described in several cases after a trial of observation for 3 to 4 weeks.[26,37-39] After a conservative trial is started, we avoid using an indwelling catheter during the period, to minimize local infection and edema.

Large fistulas, fistulas recurring after previous attempts at repair, multiple fistulas, or those associated with other conditions that require surgical treatment are not prone to spontaneous closure, and there is no reason to consider a conservative approach. These cases are more often treated with the abdominal approach. Box 82-2 addresses the suggested timing of VVF management.

Preoperative Preparation

The following guidelines for the preoperative preparation of the patient are based on published data and our personal opinions and experience. Preoperative preparation should not delay surgery, unless there is infection, massive hematoma, or significant edema at the site of the fistula (see Box 82-2). The performance status and nutritional status of some patients may require time for improvement. This situation may be more common in countries with a high incidence of VVF among poor patients. In these cases, preoperative preparation to improve the general condition of the patient is indicated, as emphasized in several reports.[14,23,30,40] Box 82-3 summarizes the issues concerning preoperative preparation of VVF patients.

Box 82-2 Timing Sequence

- Diagnosis
- Cystoscopic evaluation
- Quick conservative trial (when appropriate)
- Surgery
- Postpone surgery for infection, hematoma, or significant edema

Box 82-3 Preoperative Preparation

- Improvement of patient's performance status (when necessary)
- Antibiotic prophylaxis
- Antibiotic treatment (when indicated)
- Cortisone treatment (not supported by evidence)
- Local estrogens (useful)

As soon as the patient is ready for surgery the issue of antibiotic prophylaxis must be considered. A randomized control trial, which reported the results for 79 VVF in 1998, showed that antibiotic prophylaxis (500 mg of ampicillin IV) at the start of the operation did not produce benefit in terms of success rates, but it seemed to reduce postoperative urinary infections and the need for long-term antibiotic therapy.[41] Consistent with this first experience, in a large series from Nigeria Waaldjik, reported a success rate of 98% for 1716 cases of VVF without the use of antibiotic prophylaxis.[26] Postoperative wound infection was not never seen, and antibiotic use does not seem to be mandatory according to these data. However, when economic restrains are not severe, antibiotic prophylaxis may be considered and continued postoperatively when necessary or in cases involving surgical manipulation of the intestines.

Another consideration is the use of cortisone. Collins and associates[42] reported the use of oral corticosteroids (100 mg, three times daily for 10 to 12 days preoperatively) in the treatment of fistulas to reduce edema and fibrosis. Cortisone use is not widely accepted before surgery for VVF because it may compromise healing. It is difficult on the basis of the available data to justify the use of steroids before fistula repair.

Local application of estrogen creams has been advocated as a preoperative measure.[17,43,44] Estrogens can improve the cellular proliferation rate and blood supply of the vaginal wall, which contains estrogen receptors in the epithelial layer. Estrogen receptors are also found in the connective tissue of the female pelvis between the bladder and the vagina. This tissue undergoes atrophy with hypoestrogenism. It therefore seems wise to recommend the local use of preoperative estrogen creams, particularly in postmenopausal or post-hysterectomy patients. Even in premenopausal women, the use of estrogen creams has helped in healing postcesarian VVFs soon after delivery.[45] Consistently, the use of tamoxifen, an anti-estrogen drug, has been associated with poor local healing after gynecologic surgery.[46] However, the epithelium that lines the fistulous tract itself contains estrogen and progesterone receptors in vesicouterine fistulas.[47] Estrogen stimulation in this case could antagonize spontaneous closure of the fistula by maintaining the lining epithelium. Jozwik and Jozwik[48] reported spontaneous closure of vesicouterine fistulas with hormonal suppression by induction of amenorrhea, supporting the role of estrogens in the maintenance of this kind of fistula. There are few data on the histology of VVFs. It is not known whether estrogen receptors are present in the epithelium lining VVFs. A case of persistent VVF associated with endometriosis has been reported,[49] but endometriotic tissue was not found on histologic analysis of the fistula's epithelium. In a few cases, estrogens may maintain the fistula's epithelium, but this seems more common in vesicouterine fistulas and has never been demonstrated in VVFs.

Surgical Technique

The patient is positioned supine on the operating table with the hips abducted and mildly flexed. An appropriate degree of head-down tilt is advisable. The abdomen and perineum are prepared for the operation. Even when the operative approach is through the abdomen, sterile access to the perineum should be provided for catheterization, preoperative cystoscopy (if required), access to the vagina for finger or tampon aid during separation of the vagina from the bladder, or in case a combined perineal-abdominal approach becomes necessary.

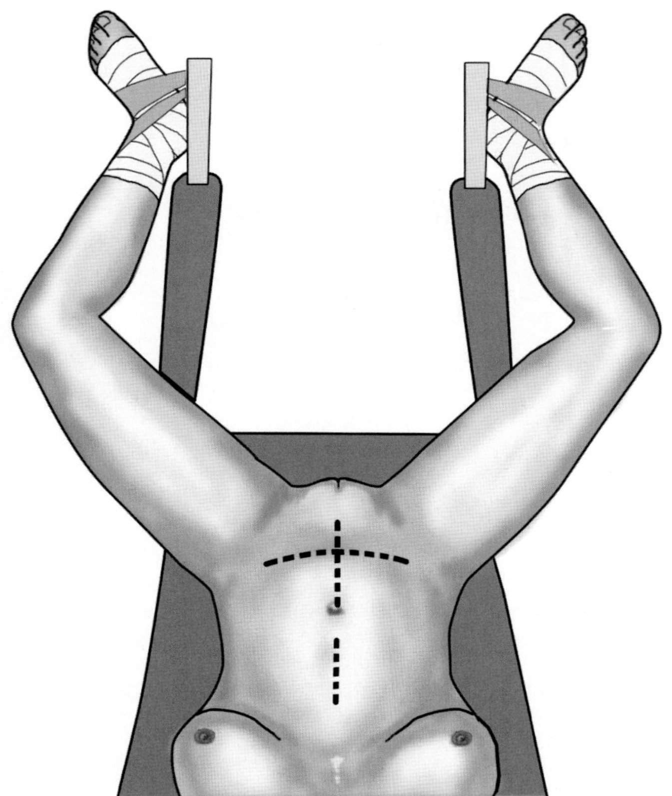

Figure 82-3 Patient position and incision lines for the abdominal approach to treating vesicovaginal fistula. Cutaneous incisions can be on the midline or horizontal (i.e., Pfannenstiel incision). The rectal fascia incision should be performed vertically on the midline in both cases. A Pfannenstiel incision can be combined with a short epigastric incision in case omental mobilization is required. The infra-umbilical median incision can be extended upward.

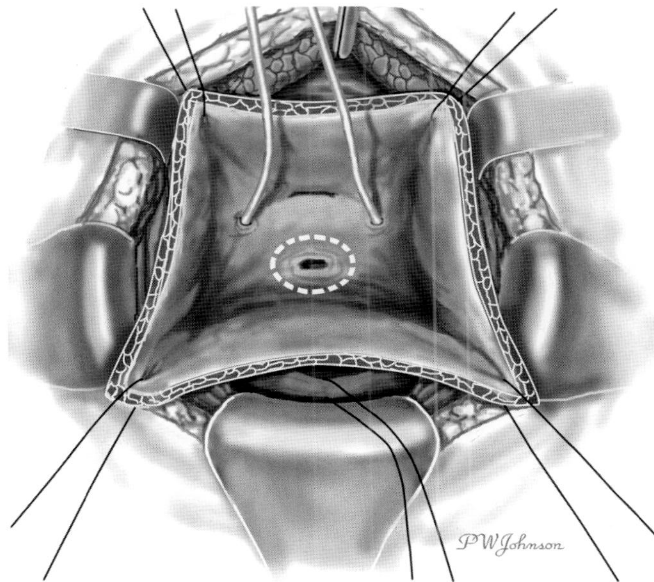

Figure 82-4 View of the internal surface of the bladder after an anterior cystotomy during the anterior transvesical approach. Suspension sutures retract the bladder walls for exposure. The ureters have been catheterized. The fistula opening is shown just behind them. The bladder wall is excised around the fistula in a racquet fashion *(dashed line)*.

A catheter is placed in the bladder. The surgical instruments are those used during classic pelvic surgery. Autostatic retractors are useful. Laparotomy can be performed by a lower midline incision or by a Pfannenstiel incision, especially when a previous operation used this route (Fig. 82-3). When needed, both incisions can be extended to the upper abdomen to obtain access for omental preparation. The median incision is extended upward, and the Pfannenstiel incision can be integrated with an extra-short epigastric median incision. Sometimes, reaccessing a previous Pfannenstiel incision may not guarantee proper exposure of the pelvis. In this case, the suprapubic cross incision or a suprapubic V-shaped incision, as described by Turner-Warvick and Chapple[50,51] and Turner-Warvick and coworkers[52] can be a suitable choice. This is particularly valid when the patient previously had surgery by the Pfannenstiel route. An additional midline incision would leave this patient with a double-cross–like scar and a long-lasting memory of the VVF. The suprapubic cross incision allows reopening of the skin though the previous incision, but after dissecting the subcutaneous tissue away from the rectal fascia, it must be transected vertically on the midline up to the umbilicus, not along the previous horizontal fascial incision. The V-shaped incision is a variant, in which after a Pfannenstiel skin incision, the rectus sheath is opened upward and laterally toward the anterior superior iliac spine; distally, the fascial incision is truncated with a 4-cm horizontal tract at the level of the pubic symphysis.

After the incision is completed, the procedure can take place through the anterior transvesical approach or the classic O'Conor technique by means of the extraperitoneal or intraperitoneal route. The former is described first.

Anterior Transvesical Approach

After the fascia is open, the Retzius space is entered. Dissection of the Retzius space allows preparation of the preperitoneal surface of the bladder, separating it from the surrounding structures. A self-retaining retractor can be placed at this point to keep the abdominal wall stabilized laterally. A vertical anterior cystotomy is performed, which allows visualization of the internal surface of the bladder with the fistula and the ureteral openings. If fistula and ureteral openings are close, ureteral catheters can be passed in the ureters at this point. A delicate retractor or suspension sutures can be used to separate the bladder walls (Fig. 82-4).

The operation proceeds with a racquet-shaped excision of the bladder wall around the fistula opening in the bladder and of the fistulous tract until clean, well-vascularized margins are obtained (Fig. 82-5). Some methods can help to gain traction on the fistula and facilitate its dissection, including use of a Foley catheter with an inflated balloon[44] and specially designed devices passed through the fistula[53,54] from the bladder opening to the vaginal opening. Dissection of the bladder from the vagina around the fistula is carried out to obtain free lateral margins, which can be then sutured without traction. Meticulous hemostasis is recommended during these maneuvers, with care taken to avoid ischemic damage to the tissue, which may compromise the repair.

At this stage, sutures are placed, starting deeply from the vaginal site. Interrupted, absorbable, 2-0 or 3-0 sutures are

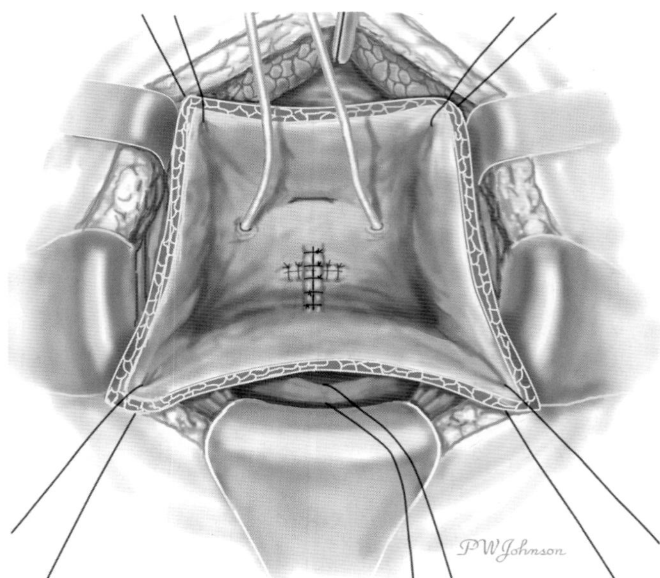

Figure 82-5 The vagina is sutured, and then the bladder is sutured. The sutures can be placed in directions perpendicular to each other, but the best strategy is to suture the vagina and the bladder according to the lines that allow the least tension on the margins.

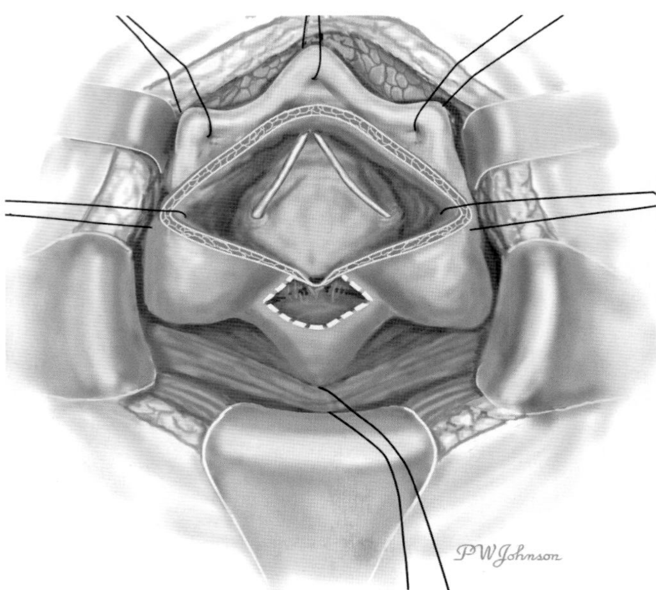

Figure 82-6 The posterior cystotomy is extended downward to include the fistula opening during the O'Conor procedure. Excision of the bladder wall is continued posteriorly widely around the fistula, which is totally excised on the vaginal side to obtain healthy free edges *(dashed line)*.

recommended. One layer is enough at the vaginal site. For fistulas located at the bladder neck, it may be feasible to close the vaginal end of the fistula from the vagina, using a combined abdomino-perineal approach.[55] The bladder end of the fistula is then closed with a double layer (muscular layer and mucosal layer) of interrupted or continuous sutures (see Fig. 82-5). Absorbable sutures should be used. The ureteral catheters are removed, and the anterior cystotomy can be closed in a similar double-layered fashion. A drain is left in the Retzius space, along with a suprapubic cystostomy or a transurethral catheter, or both. The catheter's balloon is not inflated or inflated with only 4 to 5 mL to avoid balloon compression on the suture lines.

The key points of the technique are wide excision of the fistulous tract until well-vascularized margins are achieved; generous dissection to ensure no tension on sutures; perfect hemostasis; a three-layered suture that includes the vagina, detrusor, and bladder mucosa; and a watertight suture of the bladder.

O'Conor Technique

The O'Conor technique is based on complete bisection of the bladder and wide separation of it from the vagina. In its original description, it was performed extraperitoneally, but intraperitoneal access sometimes is required.[15,16]

The bladder is exposed extraperitoneally with as much dissection as necessary to free its posterior wall. The peritoneum can be opened when the extraperitoneal posterior exposure of the bladder is insufficient, when additional procedures or omental interposition is required, or when the patient has undergone previous operations for carcinoma.[17]

After the peritoneum has been opened at the midline, the abdominal cavity can be explored. The bowel is evaluated in case an augmentation cystoplasty has been planned, and the omentum is inspected and measured to verify its ability to reach the pelvis. Adhesions can be separated, and the bladder dome and the Douglas space are reached and prepared. In the extraperitoneal and intraperitoneal approaches, the bladder is fully mobilized before incising it. A generous vertical cystotomy is performed on the posterior surface of the bladder, from the dome down to the site of the fistula, which is included in the distal part of the incision. To facilitate later closure of the cystotomy, the posterior incision of the bladder can be curved laterally so that the two edges will approximate more comfortably at the end of the operation. The bladder is practically bisected on the posterior wall with this long incision, which reaches the fistula opening. Suspension sutures can be placed along the separated bladder halves to keep them separate and guide the surgeon later during closure.

The interior surface of the bladder is inspected, and the ureters can be catheterized. The bladder wall around the fistula is sectioned circularly, and the fistula is excised to obtain free, healthy margins (Fig. 82-6). All necrotic and nonviable tissue is excised; a wide, lateral dissection of the bladder from the vagina is obtained; and the bladder is moved upward and anteriorly, with careful hemostasis to prevent postoperative ischemia (Fig. 82-7). The suturing begins at this point. Transverse vaginal closure is achieved with a single or double layer (double layer in the O'Conor's description of the procedure[15]) of absorbable continuous or interrupted sutures (Fig. 82-8). Longitudinal bladder closure is then achieved with a double layer of absorbable interrupted or continuous sutures. The bladder closure starts from the distal apex of the cystotomy and walks upward (Fig. 82-9). Interposition tissue such as peritoneum or fat can be placed over the top of the vaginal suture to reinforce it. Unlike the original description, the vaginal site of the fistula is not always closed, because some surgeons think that closure can prevent drainage of hematomas from the widely dissected intervesicovaginal space.[56] A drain is left in the retropubic space before closing the abdomen, along with a cystostomy or a transurethral catheter, or both.

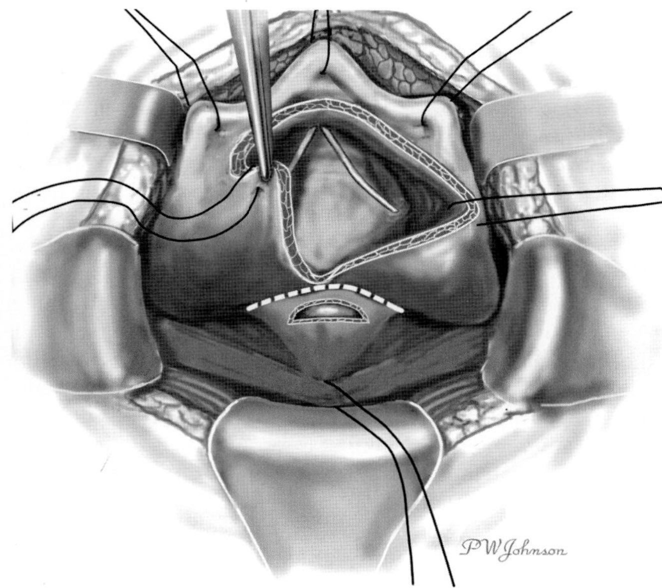

Figure 82-7 The dissection plane lies between the bladder anteriorly and the vagina posteriorly during the O'Conor procedure *(dashed line)*. This plane is carefully developed after the fistulectomy has been performed to obtain full separation of the bladder from the vagina.

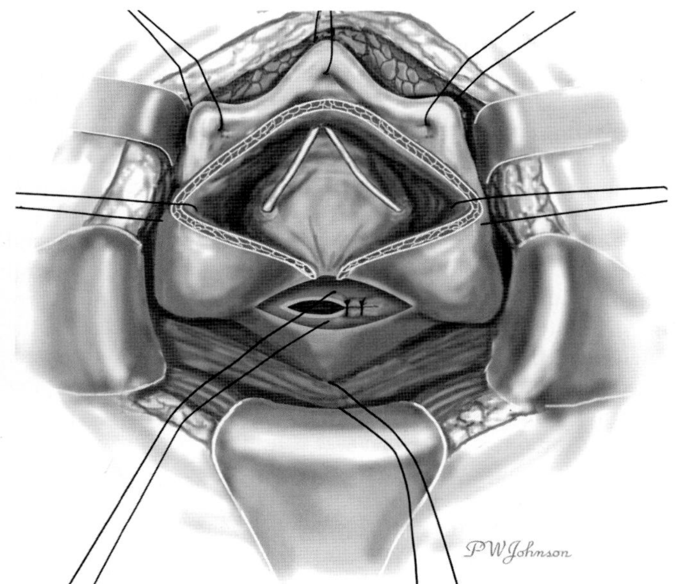

Figure 82-8 Closure of the vagina with interrupted sutures. The wide mobilization performed earlier allows closure without tension on the margins.

Interposition Grafts

Interposition grafts are used in VVF surgery because experience indicates that this tissue promotes the success of the procedure, especially in cases of multiple failures and necrotic and poorly vascularized tissues, as in postirradiation fistulas.[57,58] Another indication for interposition grafts is when the loss of substance after fistulectomy is too wide to guarantee a tension-free suture line or when proximity between the fistula and the ureteral meatus does allow primary closure of the bladder without ureteral reimplantation. Interposition grafts can be used during any abdominal surgical procedure, and they vary in terms of location, vascularization, and type of tissue used.

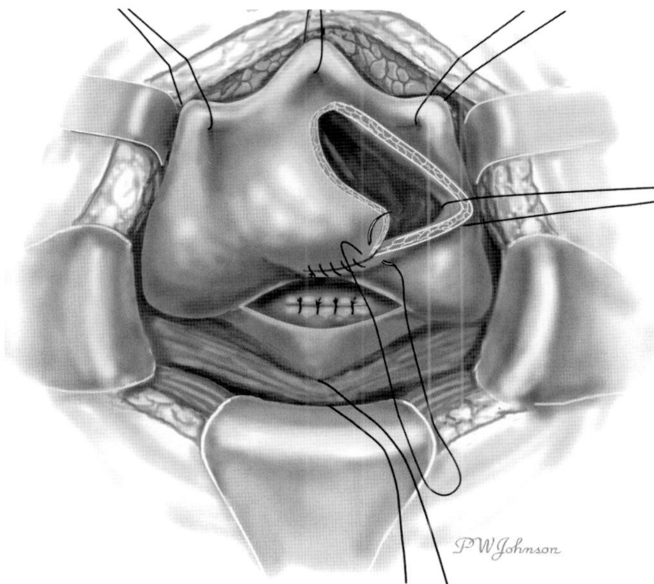

Figure 82-9 The last step of the procedure is closure of the bladder wall. This can be performed in one or two layers, starting from the distal end of the posterior cystotomy. The initial curved line of the bladder incision facilitates closure of the bladder wall without tension.

Free Bladder Mucosa

A simple procedure using free bladder mucosa can be applied easily during a limited anterior transvesical approach. A patch of bladder mucosa is harvested from the bladder dome in a size proportional to the size of the fistula, and it is then placed between the bladder and vagina, with the mucosal surface directed toward the vagina or the bladder, and it is fixed in place with a few stitches. The bladder wall is then sutured over the graft. The patch is harvested, leaving the underlying detrusor muscle intact. The donor bed fully re-epithelizes after a few weeks.[59] This method has shown good results in avoiding reimplantation of the ureters when they were close to the fistula opening in the vagina, because no attempt is made to separate the vaginal and vesicle layers of the fistula[60] or close the vaginal or bladder site of the tract.[61,62]

Sliding Bladder Wall

Gil-Vernet[63] described a technique to advance downward a portion of full-thickness bladder wall to close a large loss of substance after fistulectomy. It is a type of vesical autoplasty that has been successful in resolving complex VVFs, especially when the fistula is close to the ureteral meatus. In this procedure, a flap obtained from the posterior bladder wall is moved down to replace the mucosa excised during the fistulectomy. After closing the vaginal site, the bladder wall is bilaterally incised from the fistula opening upward, allowing a flap to be brought down to the bladder neck and sutured to the distal bladder wall in a single layer. In this way, the vaginal suture line can be completely covered. This technique is easy to perform, and it limits the need to use omentum in cases of large, complex fistulas when the bladder cannot be closed primarily. It has the advantage of replacing bladder with bladder.[64]

Dura Mater

A graft of solvent-dehydrated human dura mater can be used for interposition during the extraperitoneal approach, even in cases of limited exposure and when the fistula has not been excised. After closure of the vaginal site, the dura mater graft is placed over the suture and fixed with interrupted, absorbable suture. Subsequently, the bladder is closed in two layers.[65] The use of dura mater as a bladder or ureteral wall substitute has been successfully demonstrated.[66]

Abdominal Wall Fat

When abdominal wall fat is used for interposition, an extraperitoneal approach is undertaken in the usual fashion. The fistula is excised, and the free graft of abdominal wall fat is placed over the vaginal suture line before closing the bladder site. This simple technique can be performed easily in cases of limited exposure.[67]

Rectus Abdominis Muscle Flap

A rectus abdominis muscle flap can be raised during an extraperitoneal approach; blood for the flap is supplied by the inferior epigastric artery. This muscle has excellent vascularization, and it can be rotated easily and brought down into the pelvis in cases of complex fistulas, especially when the omentum is not available for interposition. A rectus abdominis myofascial flap has been used successfully in one patient with a large postirradiation VVF.[68] In another case of postirradiation VVF, a rectus abdominis myocutaneous flap covered a large loss of substance in the bladder after fistulectomy adjacent to the ureteral meatus, with the skin side of the graft covering the bladder inner wall.[69] Rectus abdominis myocutaneous flaps have been used successfully in a complex cases of irradiated pelvic wounds and pouch-vaginal fistulas, for which several previous transvaginal and transabdominal approaches had failed.[70] Successful use of rectus abdominis muscle flaps has been reported for four other cases of difficult, recurrent VVFs.[71,72]

Gracilis Muscle Flap

In complex cases when the omentum is not available, the gracilis muscle can be considered for tissue interposition during an abdominal repair. The access is extraperitoneal. The muscle is harvested from the thigh based on the profunda femoris artery, and the flap is transposed between the bladder and the vagina. Two cases of recurrent VVFs were successfully treated with this technique.[73]

Peritoneal Flap

When using a flap of peritoneum for interposition, access is gained through the transperitoneal route. After incision of the bladder and excision of the fistula, a flap of peritoneum with an appropriate pedicle is raised from the lateral pelvic wall. The vaginal site is closed, and the flap is placed between the bladder and the vagina and fixed with interrupted absorbable sutures. The bladder wall is closed over the flap. Care is taken at the end of the procedure to suture the peritoneal lateral edges from which the flap has been harvested, but this is not always necessary.

This simple technique can be used successfully to repair recurrent or postirradiation fistulas.[74] One possibility when using the peritoneum is to harvest a flap of the peritoneum that lines the broad ligament. A portion of the anterior surface of the broad ligament can be raised and moved medially to cover the vaginal site of a VVF in case of a large fistula.[75] An epiploic appendix can be used as interposition tissue and be brought behind the bladder when using an intraperitoneal or an extraperitoneal approach; in the latter case, access is gained by cutting a small opening in the peritoneum.[76]

Seromuscular Intestinal Graft

A patch of seromuscular intestinal graft obtained from a segment of small bowel can be used to repair VVFs. This technique requires intraperitoneal access and interruption of the bowel for harvesting the intestinal segment. The loop obtained is opened along the antimesenteric border, and the mucosal lining is mechanically removed, obtaining a seromuscular graft of small intestine. This patch is then used as interposition tissue between the bladder and the vagina, with the seromuscular face positioned toward the bladder. Complete re-epithelization of the seromuscular face of the graft with transitional epithelium occurs after a few weeks, and a 100% cure rate has been reported for treating complex postirradiation fistulas in four patients.[77]

Omentum

The omentum has excellent capacity for tissue healing, revascularization, lymphatic drainage, and anti-inflammatory activity. Unlike other tissues such as muscle, the omentum does not undergo atrophy or fibrosis after transposition. A transperitoneal approach always allows access to the omentum. However, this does not necessarily mean that the omentum can be used, because in some cases, it may be retracted or not available for interposition because of previous surgical procedures. Availability of the omentum can be established only after opening of the peritoneum. The omentum reaches directly into the pelvis in only 30% of patients.[78] In 70%, omental mobilization is required.

A complete description of the surgical technique for omental interposition was published by Turner Warwick.[50] The key point is maintenance of the vascularization of the omentum by careful preparation of its vascular pedicle. Vascularization of the omentum is based on the gastroepiploic arteries. The right artery usually is larger. The two arteries form an arch along the greater curvature of the stomach, which needs to be mobilized for elongation of the omentum when this is needed. Because mobilization should be based on the right gastroepiploic artery, the omentum should be released from the greater curvature, starting high on the left and moving down to the right. Variations of this procedure may vary from a limited tract to the entire length of the greater curvature.

The prepared omental apron is displaced in the pelvis and interposed between the bladder and the vagina, where it is secured in place with a few stitches. It is important to protect the passage of the omentum by mobilizing the ascending colon and placing the omentum behind it.[51] Suction drainage of the stomach can protect it from postoperative overdistention that could put the sutures on the small vessels along the greater curvature under tension.

Complex Repairs

Combined grafting with omentum and a gastric segment has been described in a case of postirradiation VVF with large substance loss. The gastro-omental graft was based on the right gastroepiploic pedicle. The gastric wall was used successfully to replace the posterior bladder wall, and the omentum closed the vaginal defect, which was not sutured.[79] Large postirradiation fistulas may require bladder augmentation during repair. An ileocystoplasty can be successfully performed in these cases; it can be combined with omental interposition, without closure of the vaginal site when this is not possible.[80,81]

Augmentation cystoplasty should be performed when the bladder capacity is small as a consequence of previous failed repairs, because it may prevent the necessity of urinary diversion.[82] However, urinary diversion as a final option in the treatment of VVF can be employed with good functional results. Continent diversions are more acceptable to patients, especially in countries when the local culture does not accept external diversions or the economic and clinical support for the external incontinent stoma is not available.[83] Continent urinary diversions performed with the Mitrofanoff procedure can be a valuable technique to restore continence in the most difficult patients.[84,85] When good anal continence is preserved, an ureterosigmoidostomy, such as a Mainz II pouch, can be considered.[86,87] A colon pouch can be similarly used for a continent external diversion.[88]

Laparoscopic Repair

Laparoscopic repair of a VVF fistula is a less invasive strategy than the open abdominal approach. This is especially true when the VVF resulted from a previous laparoscopic procedure. Successful laparoscopic repair of a VVF was first described by Nezhat and colleagues[89] in 1994 in a patient who had been previously treated laparoscopically for an ovarian remnant syndrome. Subsequently, more experience with this technique were published.[90-96]

Preoperative cystoscopy and ureteral catheterization are advisable before laparoscopy. During cystoscopy, a ureteral catheter or a Foley catheter can be passed through the fistula into the vagina and retrieved outside through the introitus. This helps with identification of the fistula during dissection. Leaving the cystoscope in the bladder with the light on can facilitate identification of the fistula during the operation.[96] The patient is placed in the low lithotomy position. For access, one 10-mm infraumbilical incision is made to insert the video laparoscope and the CO_2 laser, and three additional 5- to 10-mm incisions are made in the lower abdomen for the suction-irrigation probe, the grasping forceps, and the bipolar forceps.

The principles of laparoscopic surgery do not differ from those of open surgery. A classic O'Conor technique is reproducible laparoscopically.[95,96] Cystotomy on the posterior bladder wall and careful dissection of the bladder from the vagina are performed under direct vision, with the advantage of magnification provided by the laparoscopic approach. An inflated glove or a wet sponge in the vagina can help to maintain the pneumoperitoneum after the vagina has been opened. The pneumoperitoneum can also help to distend the bladder after the cystotomy has been performed After excision of the fistula and mobilization of the bladder from the vagina, the vagina and then the bladder are each sutured with one layer of interrupted or continuous absorbable sutures using extracorporeal knotting. Intracorporeal knotting has also been performed,[93] as has double-layered closure of the bladder.[94,96] A flap of parietal peritoneum can be used for interposition.[89] The omentum can be mobilized with staplers and interposed without closure of the vaginal site[91] or after the vagina has been sutured.[92-96] Patients can be discharged on the first or second postoperative day.

Additional intra-abdominal procedures, such as ureteral reimplantation or nephrectomy, can be performed during the laparoscopic approach.[93,96] Two large series of patients treated laparoscopically have been reported,[95,96] consisting of 6 (plus 2 cases of vesicouterine fistulas) and 15 cases of VVFs. Success rates of 100% and 93% were reported for these series.

Robotic Repair

A robotic system can be used as an alternative to laparoscopy in VVF repair, especially during the reconstructive period. Robotic surgical systems offer several technical advantages: high magnification, three-dimensional imaging, and a degree of freedom in movement that surpasses the possibilities of the human hand and laparoscopic instruments. Successful repair of VVFs using the Da Vinci robotic system is possible.

The first case managed with this technique was reported in 2005.[97] The patient is placed in the low lithotomy position. Preoperative cystoscopy with ureteral catheterization is performed. The patient is then moved into an extreme Trendelenburg position, and the ports are placed. Port placement does not differ from the technique used in robotic-assisted radical prostatectomy.[98]

In the first part of the operation, exposure of the bladder and cystotomy on the posterior bladder wall are performed, with identification of the fistula and excision of the fistulous tract, using a standard laparoscopic technique. The Da Vinci system is docked for the reconstructive part of the operation. The vaginal layer is closed with a single layer of sutures, and the bladder is then closed in two layers. The patient is discharged on the second postoperative day.

It is probable that robotic repair of VVFs will become more common in the future. The hope is that technologic improvements, such as the Da Vinci robot, can help surgeons successfully manage the more difficult cases with less invasive procedures and faster postoperative recovery while maintaining or improving the standards for proper surgical repair.

POSTOPERATIVE CARE

The key aspect of postoperative care in VVF surgery is continuous bladder drainage.[6] This can be accomplished by a transurethral or a suprapubic catheter, or both, placed at the end of the operation. Prevention of kinking and obstruction by blood or mucus of the catheter is crucial. The transurethral catheter balloon should not be inflated or inflated with no more than 5 mL to prevent compression on the suture lines, especially if the fistula was at the level of the bladder neck. Suprapubic and transurethral urine drainage can be beneficial in case one catheter stops functioning. Maintenance of a high urine output with adequate fluid intake is a good postoperative measure to keep the patient hydrated and prevent blockage of the catheter.[26,99] Bladder drainage should be maintained for a minimum of 10 days[100] and, more often, for 2 weeks.

The timing of catheter removal varies and must consider the patient's circumstances. More prolonged catheterization is required for extension of the bladder sutures and for poor tissue quality.[101] The transurethral catheter can be removed before or after the suprapubic catheter. The suprapubic catheter should be

Box 82-4 Postoperative Care

- Adequate bladder drainage
- High fluid intake
- Intra-abdominal fluid drainage
- Temporary gastric drainage after omentum mobilization
- Avoidance of traction on the sutures: no tampons, no sex for 2 months
- Adjuvant therapy: antibiotics, anticholinergic agents, estrogens

clamped before removal is attempted to check for effective voiding. A voiding cystogram is obtained before removing the last catheter to make sure that there is no leak from the bladder. If incomplete closure is suspected, the catheter can be left in place for 1 or 2 weeks longer. A drain in the paravesical space can be left at the end of the operation to ensure drainage of blood or fluids from the pelvis. An intraperitoneal drain can be placed during transperitoneal procedures or when the omentum has been mobilized. Drains can be removed starting 5 or 6 days after the operation. It may be advisable to leave the paravesical drains longer. Ureteral catheters can usually be removed at the end of the operation, unless the ureters have been reimplanted. After a transperitoneal procedure, especially when the omentum was mobilized, temporary gastric drainage may be advisable, to prevent gastric overdistention. Alternatively, a gastrostomy performed at the time of surgery may be a more comfortable option for the patient.[50,102] A vaginal pack is removed on the first postoperative day.

Bed rest may be advised in cases of large, necrotic fistulas and poor vascularization of surrounding tissues.[24] In other cases, ambulation on the first or second postoperative day is encouraged. Postoperative antibiotic prophylaxis is administered for 10 days or until the drains are removed, but antibiotics are not always mandatory. Oral or local estrogen treatment may be useful in postmenopausal women. Mechanical stress or tension on the suture line should be avoided. The use of vaginal tampons is discouraged for a few weeks, and sexual intercourse is not allowed for 2 months after surgery. Anticholinergic drugs may help to reduce bladder spasms that can put tension on the sutures.[99,103] These drugs should be stopped 24 hours before obtaining the voiding cystogram. Postoperative care issues are summarized in Box 82-4.

RESULTS

It is difficult and sometimes impossible to compare published series of VVF repair. In all cases, patient selection is critical, and different series may be not comparable in terms of patients, hospital setting, strategy used, and the type of fistulas involved. Cure rates are not always intended as closure at the first operation.

The relevant clinical characteristics of VVF cases are provided in Box 82-5. They should be taken into account when comparing cases and series. Tables can be found in the medical literature that compare reported series.[104,105] This approach to comparing series is common, but it sometimes is impossible to summarize in a table all the information for a reported experience. For this reason, in the next sections, we provide brief descriptions of some published experiences and our own experience with the abdominal approach to VVF repairs.

Box 82-5 Differences in Fistula Cases

- Cause
- Location of fistula
- Hospital setting
- First versus subsequent treatments
- Quality of surrounding tissue
- Associated lesions

Review of Reported Series

El-Imam and colleagues,[106] 2005: Thirty of 50 cases of VVF were selected for the abdominal approach (20 operated vaginally). The fistulas are described as large, recurrent, high fistulas occurring in older women. Causes included obstructed labor and hysterectomy. The success rate for repairs using the abdominal approach was 99%.

Vyas and coworkers,[60] 2005: Twenty-two VVFs were treated. Causes included : obstetric issues in 15 and post-hysterectomy fistula formation in 7. All were operated using the transabdominal extraperitoneal approach (some through a combined abdominoperineal approach) and free bladder mucosa autograft. Five patients had undergone previous repairs; of these, two had recurrences. The success rate was 91%.

Naru and associates,[107] 2004: Fifty-six VVFs were treated. In these cases, 72.4% had obstetric causes, and 26.4% occurred after gynecologic surgery. A transabdominal approach was chosen in 69% of the cases. In one case, a ureterosigmoid diversion was performed. The overall success rate was 83.8% (79.4% at first attempt). In this report, one ureterosigmoid diversion was done, and the patients lost at follow-up were considered as failures.

Alagol and colleagues,[65] 2004: Eleven VVFs were treated. All cases were caused by hysterectomy for benign disease. Two patients had undergone previous repair attempts. The approach was transabdominal extraperitoneal with interposition of a dura mater free graft. The success rate was 100%.

Navarro Sebastian and coworkers,[108] 2003: Eighteen VVFs and two vesicouterine fistulas were treated. Causes included postoperative formation in 83% (13 hysterectomies, 1 cesarean section) and cancer in 17% of patients. Twelve patients were operated transabdominally, nine using an intraperitoneal approach and peritoneal graft (six cases) or omental interposition (three cases), and three operations used an extraperitoneal transvesical approach. The success rate was 88.5%.

Rafique,[109] 2002: Thirty-six VVFs and two 2 vesicouterine fistulas were treated. The cause in all cases was obstetric. Twenty-nine patients were operated using a transabdominal, transvesical approach with bladder bisection. Omentum interposition was used in all cases. Two ureteral reimplantations and two hysterectomies were performed. The success rate was 89.6%.

Kam and associates,[110] 2003: Twenty VVFs were treated. Fourteen VVFs occurred after gynecologic surgery. Four patients were operated using the transvaginal approach, seven using the extraperitoneal transabdominal approach, and eight using an intraperitoneal approach with bladder bisection. In one case, a urinary diversion (i.e., ileal conduit) was performed. Interposition flaps were used in six cases. The success rate was 85%. Three failures were reoperated using the extraperitoneal approach with complete success.

Wook Bai and colleagues,[111] 2003: Twenty-six VVFs were treated. The fistulas were caused by hysterectomy or delivery. A transabdominal extraperitoneal approach was selected in 11 cases, and a combined abdominoperineal approach was used 7. The success rate for the first attempt was 90%, and for the second attempt, 80%.

Benchekroun and coworkers,[112] 2003: In this large report of 1050 cases of urogenital fistulas, 48% were VVFs. Obstetric causes accounted for 93% of the VVFs. The patients were operated preferentially transvaginally, but the abdominal route was preferred when the fistulas were high or posterior, if other procedures or omental interposition were planned, or in case of severe vaginal sclerosis. The success rate was 95%.

Sharifi and associates,[62] 2002: Fourteen VVFs were treated. Thirteen occurred after hysterectomy, and one was caused by obstructed labor. The access was transvesical extraperitoneal, and free bladder mucosa autograft was used. In 12 of 14, there was immediate success, but 2 required prolonged catheterization.

Kochakarn and colleagues,[113] 2000: The surgeons treated 230 VVFs. Known causes included hysterectomy in 195, obstructed labor in 10, and irradiation in 9. Thirty-five patients had undergone previous attempts at repair. The transvesical extraperitoneal approach was performed in 168 cases (73%), including 29 reoperations and 139 first operations. The success rates were 78% (109 of 139) for the first-operation group and 62% (18 of 29) for the reoperation group. Of the 30 failures in the first-operation group, 15 were postirradiation fistulas. The O'Conor technique with bladder bisection was performed in 30 patients (success rate of 93.3%). Twenty patients were operated transvaginally (success rate of 100%). Urinary diversion (i.e., ileal conduit, colon conduit, or bilateral ureterostomies) was performed in 10 patients.

Evans and associates,[58] 2001: Thirty-seven VVFs were treated. Twenty-five resulted from gynecologic surgery. A transperitoneal O'Connor procedure was used. In some cases, interposition flaps were used (with 100% success), and the others were operated without flaps (63% success rate).

Mondet and colleagues,[56] 2001: Thirty VVFs in 28 patients were treated. Causes included gynecologic surgery in 78%, of which 86% occurred after hysterectomy, and cesarean section in 14%. In 30% of the patients, previous procedures had been performed. A transperitoneal-transvesical approach was used. The vaginal site was not closed in 66% of the cases. In 10 cases (83% of the trigonal fistulas), ureteral reimplantation was necessary. The overall success rate was 85%; success rates were 93% for supratrigonal and 75% for trigonal fistulas. Postoperative voiding disorders were documented in 38% of the patients. The failures were treated with urinary diversion in three cases (one transileal noncontinent cutaneous ureterostomy and two ureterosigmoidostomies). In one case, a second transperitoneal operation was undertaken with ureteral reimplantation (not performed in the first procedure), and it was successful.

Flores-Carreras and coworkers,[114] 2001: The surgeons treated 153 VVFs. Fistulas resulted from hysterectomy in 90%, cesarean section in 3.9%, and Burch procedures in 1.9%. Thirty-two (20.9%) patients had been previously operated. In 113 patients (68%), a vaginal approach was chosen, with a success rate of 90% at the first attempt and 100% at the second or third attempt. Thirty-three percent pf the patients underwent a transvesical suprapubic procedure (success rate of 91% at the first attempt). Of three failures, two were reoperated, and the third patient refused reoperation (final success rate of 97%). The transperitoneal approach was used in eight patients, with two failures (75% success rate); one had a successful second operation using the transvesical approach.

Langkilde and associates,[115] 1999: Fifty-five patients VVFs were treated, 49 of whom had operations. Fistulas resulted from pelvic surgery (23 after hysterectomy) in 30 patients, cesarean section in 4, Burch procedures in 2, and radiation treatment in 19. Eight patients had undergone previous attempts. Among the 30 postoperative cases, 23 patients underwent an abdominal procedure (with transperitoneal-transvesical access), and 7 had a vaginal procedure. In four patients, reimplantation of the ureter was necessary. The success rate was 90% at the first attempt and 100% at the second (treatment of failures included two abdominal and one vaginal approach). Among those with postirradiation fistulas, 12 patients underwent urinary diversions (five ureterocutaneostomies and seven ileal conduits), 2 had an abdominal procedure, and 5 had a vaginal procedure (with a high failure rate in the postirradiation group: 6 of 7 cases).

Nesrallah and colleagues,[104] 1999: Twenty-nine VVFs were treated. All fistulas were supratrigonal in this group. Fistulas resulted from hysterectomy in 28 patients (25 operations for benign disease, 2 after irradiation plus hysterectomy, and one cesarean section). Nine (34%) of 29 had undergone previous operations. In all cases, the transperitoneal approach was used, and an O'Conor procedure was performed, often with omental interposition. Four ureteral reimplantations were added. The success rate was 100%.

Ostad and coworkers,[61] 1997: Six VVFs were treated. All fistulas resulted from hysterectomies. A transabdominal approach with free bladder mucosa graft was chosen. The success rate was 100%.

Brandt and associates,[59] 1997: Eighty VVFs were treated. Fistulas resulted from gynecologic surgery for benign disease. Three patients had undergone previous attempts at repair. The approach was extraperitoneal with free bladder mucosa autograft. The success rate was 96%, and there were no late failures.

Blaivas and colleagues,[31] 1995: Twenty-four VVFs were treated. Most fistulas resulted from previous surgery (15 from hysterectomy, 2 from anterior colporrhaphy, 2 from urethral diverticulectomy, and 1 from an anti-incontinence procedure). Procedures included 16 vaginal repairs with a Martius flap, 1 with a gracilis flap, and 7 suprapubic transvesical repairs with omentum. In two patients, the procedure was started vaginally and then switched to the abdominal route because of poor exposure. The overall success rate was 96%.

Kristensen and Lose,[116] 1994: Eighteen VVFs were treated. All fistulas were caused by hysterectomies. A total of 27 previous attempts had been performed. An O'Conor procedure with a transperitoneal approach was performed in all cases. In four, ureteral reimplantation was necessary, of which one was bilateral. Only 1 of 18 had a recurrence, with successful repair on the second attempt with interposition of omentum.

Arrowsmith,[24] 1994: Ninety-eight VVFs were treated. Fistulas resulted from obstetric causes in 93 patients, surgery in 4, and trauma in 1. Twenty-five cases were treated abdominally with the O'Conor procedure (omentum was used in nine cases), three used a combined abdominoperitoneal approach, and the rest used a vaginal approach. Nineteen percent underwent multiple procedures. The success rate was 96%. Larger fistulas did not fare worse than smaller fistulas ($P = .87$). However, treatment failure was significantly associated with bladder neck damage ($P < .015$) or severe vaginal scarring ($P < .005$).

Blandy and coworkers,[29] 1991: Twenty-five VVFs were treated. Fistulas resulted from hysterectomy in 24 patients and transvaginal uterine prolapse surgery in 1 patient. A transperitoneal transvesical approach was chosen, with interposition of omentum. The success rate was 100%.

Motiwala and associates,[117] 1991: Sixty-eight VVFs were treated. Fistulas resulted from hysterectomy in 48 patients, cesarean section in 15, and labor in 5. Fifty-one were supratrigonal fistulas. Four patients had undergone previous repairs. A transperitoneal-transvesical approach was chosen, with omentum grafts in 10 cases, and 58 used an extraperitoneal approach. Two ureteral reimplantations were necessary. The success rate was 95% for the extraperitoneal procedures and 90% for the transperitoneal cases.

Gil-Vernet and colleagues,[63] 1989: Forty-two VVFs were treated. Fistulas resulted from gynecologic operations in 28 patients, obstetric causes in 11, and irradiation in 3. All the patients had undergone previous surgical attempts at repair. An extraperitoneal approach was performed, with the sliding bladder wall technique described previously. The success rate was 100%.

Lee and coworkers,[19] 1988: The surgeons treated 182 VVFs. Fistulas resulted from hysterectomy in 156 patients, obstetric operations in 19, malignancy in 10, and trauma in 6. Ninety-one patients had undergone previous attempts at repair. The approach chosen was abdominal in 37 cases (20%) and transvaginal in 145. The success rate was 98%.

Udeh and associates,[55] 1985: Thirty-one VVFs were treated. All fistulas resulted from obstructed labor. Twenty-one patients had undergone previous attempts at repair. Two underwent elective diversion, and 29 were operated abdominally with an anterior transvesical approach. The success rate was 86%.

Personal Experience

Patients

Eighty-four patients with urinary fistulas have been operated using the abdominal approach at the Department of Urology of the University of Padova, Italy, between May 1979 and March 2003, under the chairmanship of Professor Francesco Pagano. Patients' data have been collected and analyzed retrospectively. Sixty-five of 84 patients developed a VVF after hysterectomy for benign or malignant disease; 7 of them had received adjuvant radiation treatment for cancer. Two patients had undergone radiotherapy alone. Four patients developed a VVF after vaginal delivery, one after cesarean section, one after a bladder biopsy, one after bladder diverticulectomy, one after resection of a urethral lesion, one after a vaginoplasty procedure, one after sacral colpopexy, and one after radical cystectomy and orthotopic ileal neobladder. In five cases, the patients' records were incomplete for cause. In one case, a clear reason for the fistula could not be identified. The most common onset symptoms were recorded for 82 of 84 patients: vaginal leakage with a preserved micturition pattern was present in 58 patients and complete urinary incontinence through the vagina in 24.

The patients received a preoperative evaluation, including cystoscopy, endovenous pyelography, retrograde ureterography, voiding cystography, vaginoscopy, and pressure-flow studies (for seven). Seventy-six (90%) of 84 patients presented with a VVF, 5 with a VVF and associated rectovaginal fistula, 2 with a uretero-VVF, and 1 with an orthotopic neobladder-vaginal fistula. In 56 patients, the fistula was supratrigonal; in 15, it was at the trigonal level; in 5, it was at the bladder neck; and in 3, it was on the lateral bladder wall. In five cases, fistula localization was not described. Before coming to our attention, 21 (25%) patients had received previous unsuccessful treatments in other institutions (with a median delay in this group of 25 weeks from onset of symptoms): 14 had undergone one previous attempt (2 patients had been treated endoscopically with collagen injection or diathermocoagulation of the fistulous tract), 11 had been operated using the vaginal approach, and 7 had been treated using the abdominal approach. One patient had been treated for cervical malignancy and had received an "external diversion" that was not better described. The other seven patients had undergone two previous attempts in another institution, two endoscopically with collagen or Teflon infiltration, two treated transvaginally, and three treated transabdominally.

Surgical Technique

In 64 of 84 patients, the fistula was corrected using an extraperitoneal transvesical approach, and in 14 of 84, a transperitoneal approach was used; omental interposition was performed in three of these cases. Additional intraperitoneal procedures were performed in 12 cases: augmentation ileocystoplasty in 6 cases and ureteral reimplantation in 6 cases (four bilateral and two monolateral procedures). Urinary diversion was performed as the first procedure in six patients (i.e., one continent ileal reservoir with a Mitrofanoff procedure and five external noncontinent diversions, three with colon, one with ileum, and one ureterocutaneostomy). The bladder catheter was maintained for an average period of 10 days after surgery.

Outcomes

Excluding the patients treated with urinary diversion (6 of 84), successful closure was obtained in 94% (73) of the 78 other patients in whom abdominal repair was performed. Five patients had fistula recurrences between 0 and 95 weeks; two were successfully reoperated transvaginally, with one using a Martius flap interposition. Two were treated endoscopically with collagen or silicone injection (one failed, requiring after 12 weeks a second successful abdominal repair with ureteral reimplantation and omentum interposition). One had a ureteral-sigmoid-cutaneous diversion.

Long-Term Follow-Up

Long-term follow-up was possible for 62 of 84 patients. The minimum follow-up in this group was 2 years (average, 12.5 ± 8.4 years). All patients were satisfied with their situation; 61 of 62 patients were dry, and 1 complained about mild urinary incontinence but declined further treatment.

CONCLUSIONS

The ideal treatment for a VVF is the one that provides rapidly the best result with the least invasive approach. The abdominal approach for treatment of VVF, which is an invasive approach, has several indications, and when properly selected, it can provide the definitive solution to VVFs not treatable with less invasive procedures. New techniques, such as laparoscopy or robotic surgery, can reduce the invasiveness of the open abdominal approach and make the procedure more acceptable to the patient. Some of the strategies for repair highlighted in this chapter can increase the chances of success. These strategies, which are independent of the approach used, are summarized in Box 82-6. Using these strategies, we think that major improvements can be made in the treatment of this undesirable clinical condition can be made in the near future.

Box 82-6 Strategies for Success

- Case selection
- Surgical experience, training opportunities
- Choice of less invasive procedures
- Steps taken to minimize chances of failure
- Use of interposition flaps when possible
- Prioritization of postoperative uninterrupted bladder drainage
- Correct analysis of comparable series

References

1. Von Roonhuyse H: Medico-Chirurgical Observations. London, Moses Pitt at the Angel, 1676.
2. Falk HC, Tancer ML: Vesicovaginal fistula: An historical survey. Obstet Gynecol 3:337-341, 1954.
3. Jobert A: Memoire sur les fistules vesico-vaginales et sur leur traitement par une nouvelle methode operatoire. Academie des sciences le 14 fevrier 1836. Paris, Gazette Medicale, 1836, p 193.
4. Androutsos G: Le "prince de la chirurgie," Antoine Jobert de Lamballe (1679-1867) et la premiere cure radicale des fistules vesico-vaginales par sa methode de cystoplastie par glissement. Prog Urol 13:707-710, 2003.
5. Hayward G: Case of vesico-vaginal fistula, successfully treated by an operation. Am J Med Sci 24:283-8; 1839.
6. Sims JM: On the treatment of vesico-vaginal fistula [originally published in Am J Med 23:59-82, 1852]. Int Urogynecol J 9:236-248, 1998.
7. Zacharin R: A history of obstetric vesico-vaginal fistula. Aust N Z J Surg 70:851-854, 2000.
8. Emmet TA: Vesico-vaginal fistula from parturition and other causes: With cases of recto-vaginal fistula. New York, William Wood, 1868.
9. Wall LL: Thomas Addis Emmet, the vesicovaginal fistula, and the origins of reconstructive gynecologic surgery. Int Urogynecol J 13:145-155, 2002.
10. Trendelenburg F: Uber Blasenschcidenfisteloperationen un uber Beckenhochlagerung bei Operationen in der Bauchhohle. Samml Kiln Vortr 355:3373-92, 1890.
11. Mattingly RF, Thompson JD: Vesicovaginal fistulas. In Mattingly RF, Thompson JD (eds): TeLinde's Operative Gynecology, 6th ed. Philadelphia, JP Lippincott, 1985.
12. Rutkow I: Surgery. An Illustrated History. St. Louis, Mosby–Year Book, 1993, p 417.
13. Legue F: La voie tranperitoneo-vasicale pour la cure de certaines fistules vesico-vaginales operatoires. Arch Clin Necker 1:1-3, 1914.
14. Rizvi JH: Genital fistulae. A continuing tragedy. J Obstet Gynecol Res 25:1-7, 1999.
15. O'Conor VJ, Sokol J: Vesicovaginal fistula from the standpoint of the urologist. J Urol 66:367-369, 1951.
16. O'Conor VJ Jr, Sokol JK, Bulkley GJ, Nanninga JB: Suprapubic closure of vesicovaginal fistula. J Urol 109:51-54, 1973.
17. O'Conor JV Jr: Review of experience with vesico-vaginal fistula repair. J Urol 123:367-369, 1980.
18. Hilton P: Vesico-vaginal fistula: New perspectives. Curr Opin Obstet Gynecol 13:513-520, 2001.
19. Lee RA, Symmonds RE, Williams TJ: Current status of genitourinary fistulas. Obstet Gynecol 72:313-319, 1988.
20. Raz S: Early versus late repair of vesicovaginal fistulas: Vaginal and abdominal approaches [editorial]. J Urol 153:1112, 1995.
21. Dupont M, Raz S: Vaginal approach to vesicovaginal fistula repair. Urology 48:7-9, 1996.
22. Eilber KS, Kavaler E, Rodriguez LV, et al: Ten-year experience with transvaginal vesicovaginal fistula repair using tissue interposition. J Urol 169:1033-1036, 2003.
23. Hilton P: Vesico-vaginal fistulas in developing countries. Int J Gynaecol Obstet 82:285-295, 2003.
24. Arrowsmith SD: Genitourinary reconstruction in obstetric fistulas. J Urol 152:403-406, 1994.
25. Wall LL, Karshima JA, Kirschner C, Arrowsmith SD: The obstetric vesicovaginal fistula: Characteristics of 899 patients from Jos, Nigeria. Am J Obstet Gynecol 190:1011-1019, 2004.
26. Waaldijk K: The immediate management of fresh obstetric fistulas. Am J Obstet Gynecol 191:795-799, 2004.
27. Moir CJ: Personal experiences in the treatment of vesico-vaginal fistulas. Am J Obstet Gynecol 71:476-491, 1956.
28. Mahfouz BN: Urinary fistulae in women. J Obstet Gynecol Br Emp 64:23-34, 1957.
29. Blandy JP, Badenoch DF, Fowler CG, et al: Early repair of iatrogenic injury to the ureter or bladder after gynecological surgery. J Urol 146:761-765, 1991.
30. Arrowsmith S, Hamlin EC, Wall LL: Obstructed labour injury complex: Obstetric fistula formation and the multifaceted morbidity of maternal birth trauma in the developing countries. Obstet Gynecol Surv 51:568-574, 1996.
31. Blaivas JG, Heritz DM, Romanzi LJ: Early versus late repair of vesicovaginal fistulas: Vaginal and abdominal approaches. J Urol 153:1110-1112, 1995.
32. Raz S: Early versus late repair of vesicovaginal fistulas: Vaginal and abdominal approaches [editorial]. J Urol 153: 1113, 1995.
33. Persky L, Herman G, Guerrier K: Nondelay in vesicovaginal fistula repair. Urology 13:273-275, 1979.
34. Wang Y, Hadley HR: Non-delayed transvaginal repair of high lying vesicovaginal fistula. J Urol 144:34-36, 1990.
35. Goodwin WE, Scardino PT: Vesicovaginal and uretrovaginal fistulas: A summary of 25 years of experience. J Urol 123:370-374, 1980.
36. Carr LK, Webster GD: Abdominal repair of vesico-vaginal fistula. Urology 48:10-11, 1996.
37. Waaldijk K: Immediate indwelling bladder catheterization at postpartum urine leakage. Trop Doct 27:227-228, 1997.
38. Davits RJ, Miranda S: Conservative treatment of vesico-vaginal fistulas by bladder drainage alone. Br J Urol 70:339, 1992.
39. Madjar S, Gousse A: Postirradiation vesicovaginal fistula completely resolved with conservative treatment. Int Urogynecol J Pelvic Floor Dysfuct 12:405-406, 2001.
40. Wall LL: Dead mothers and injured wives: The social context of maternal morbidity and mortality among the Hausa of Northern Nigeria. Stud Fam Plann 29:341-359, 1998.

41. Tomlinson AJ, Thornton JG: A randomized controlled trial of antibiotic prophylaxis for vesicovaginal fistula repair. Br J Obstet Gynecol 105:397-399, 1998.
42. Collins CG, Pent D, Jones FB: Results of early repair of vesicovaginal fistula with preliminary cortisone treatment. Am J Obstet Gynecol 80:1005-1012, 1960.
43. Little NA, Juma S, Raz S: Vesicovaginal fistulae. Semin Urol 7:78-85, 1989.
44. Cortesse A, Colau A: Vesicovaginal fistula. Ann Urol (Paris) 38:52-66, 2004.
45. Goh JT, Howat P, De Costa C: Oestrogen therapy in the management of vesicovaginal fistula. Aust N Z J Obstet Gynaecol 41:333-334, 2001.
46. Caputo RM, Copeland LJ: Gynecologic effects of tamoxifen: Case reports and review of the literature. Int Urogynecol J Pelvic Floor Dysfunct 7:179-184, 1996.
47. Jozwik M, Jozwik M, Sulkowska M, et al: The presence of sex hormone receptors in the vesicouterine fistula. Gynecol Endocrinol 18:37-40, 2004.
48. Jozwik M, Jozwik M: Spontaneous closure of vesicouterine fistula. Account for effective hormonal treatment. Urol Int 62:183-187, 1999.
49. Lovatsis D, Drutz HP: Persistent vesicovaginal fistula associated with endometriosis. Int Urogynecol J Pelvic Floor Dysfunct 14:358-359, 2003.
50. Turner-Warvick R, Chapple C (eds): Functional reconstruction of the urinary tract and Gyneco-Urology. Oxford, Blackwell Science, 2002.
51. Chapple C, Turner-Warwick R: Vesico-vaginal fistula. BJU Int 95:193-214, 2005.
52. Turner Warwick R, Worth P, Milroy E, Duckett J: The suprapubic V-incision. Br J Urol 46:39-45, 1974.
53. Mobilio G, Cosciani Cunico S: An instrument for the surgical repair of a vesicovaginal fistula. J Urol 117:231, 1977.
54. Landes RR: Simple transvesical repair of vesicovaginal fistula. J Urol 122:604-606, 1979.
55. Udeh F: Simple management of difficult vesicovaginal fistulas by anterior transvesical approach. J Urol 133:591-593, 1985.
56. Mondet F, Chartier-Kastler EJ, Conort P, et al: Anatomic and functional results of transperitoneal—Transvesical vesicovaginal fistula repair. Urology 58:882-886, 2001.
57. Fitzpatrick C, Elkins TE: Plastic surgical techniques in the repair of vesicovaginal fistulas: A review. Int Urogynecol J Pelvic Floor Dysfunct 4:287-295, 1993.
58. Evans DH, Madjar S, Politano VA, et al: Interposition flaps in transabdominal vesicovaginal fistula repairs: Are they really necessary? Urology 57:670-674, 2001.
59. Brandt FT, Lorenzato FR, Albuquerque CD: Treatment of vesicovaginal fistula by bladder mucosa autograft technique. J Am Coll Surg 186:645-648, 1998.
60. Vyas N, Nandi PR, Mahmood M, et al: Bladder mucosal autografts for repair of vesicovaginal fistula. BJOG 112:112-114, 2005.
61. Ostad M, Uzzo RG, Coleman J, Young GP: Use of a free bladder mucosal graft for simple repair of vesicovaginal fistulae. Urology 52:123-126, 1998.
62. Sharifi-Aghdas F, Ghaderian N, Payvand A: Free bladder mucosal autograft in the treatment of complicated vesicovaginal fistula. BJU Int 89:54-56, 2002.
63. Gil-Vernet JM, Gil-Vernet A, Campos JA: New surgical approach for treatment of complex vesicovaginal fistula. J Urol 141:513-516, 1989.
64. Couvelaire R: Les fistules vesico-vaginales complexes. J Urol 88:353, 1982.
65. Alagol B, Gozen AS, Kaya E, Inci O: The use of human dura mater as an interposition graft in the treatment of vesicovaginal fistula. Int Urol Nephrol 36:35-40, 2004.
66. Kelami A: Lyophilised human dura as a bladder wall substitute: Experimental and clinical results. J Urol 105:518-521, 1971.
67. El-Lateef Moharram AA, El-Raouf MA: Retropubic repair of genitourinary fistula using a free suporting graft. BJU Int 93:581-583, 2004.
68. Salup RR, Julian TB, Liang MD, et al: Closure of large postirradiation vesicovaginal fistula with rectum abdominis myofascial flap. Urology 44:130-131, 1994.
69. Viennas LK, Alonso AM, Salama V: Repair of radiation-induced vesicovaginal fistula with a rectus abdominis myocutaneous flap. Plast Reconstr Surg 96:1435-1437, 1995.
70. Horch RE, Gitsch G, Schultze-Seemann W: Bilateral pedicled myocutaneous vertical rectus abdominus muscle flaps to close vesicovaginal and pouch-vaginal fistulas with simultaneous vaginal and perineal reconstruction in irradiated pelvic wounds. Urology 60:502-507, 2002.
71. Perata E, Severoni S, Schietroma M, et al: Post partum vesicovaginal fistula: Abdominal muscle strip treatment. Minerva Ginecol 53:165-170, 2001.
72. Menchaca A, Akhyat M, Gleicher N, et al: The rectus abdominis muscle flap in a combined abdominovaginal repair of difficult vesicovaginal fistuale. J Reprod Med 35:565-568, 1990.
73. Fleischmann J, Picha G: Abdominal approach for gracilis muscle interposition and repair of recurrent vesicovaginal fistulas. J Urol 140:552-554, 1988.
74. Eisen M, Jurkovic K, Altwein JE, et al: Management of vesicovaginal fistulas with peritoneal flap interposition. J Urol 112:195-198, 1974.
75. Singh RB, Pavitran NM, Nanda S: Plastic reconstruction of a mega vesicovaginal fistula using broad ligament flaps—A new technique. Int Urogynecol J Pelvic Floor Dysfunct 14:62-63, 2003.
76. Lytton B: Vesicovaginal fistula: Postsurgical. In Resnick MI, Kursh E(eds): Current Therapy in Genitourinary Surgery. Philadelphia, BC Decker, 1992, pp 261-265.
77. Mraz J, Sutory M: An alternative in surgical treatment of post-irradiation vesicovaginal and rectovaginal fistulas: The seromuscular intestinal graft (patch). J Urol 151:357-359, 1994.
78. Turner-Warwick R: The use of the omental pedicle graft in urinary tract reconstruction. J Urol 116:341-347, 1976.
79. Bissada SA, Bissada NK: Repair of active radiation-induced vesicovaginal fistula using combined gastric and omental segments based on the gastroepiploic vessels. J Urol 147:1368- 1370, 1992.
80. Tabakov ID, Slavchev BN: Large post-hysterectomy and post-irradiation vesicovaginal fistulas: Repair by ileocystoplasty. J Urol 171:272-274, 2004.
81. Hsu TH, Rackley RR, Abdelmalak JB, et al: Novel technique for combined repair of postirradiation vesicovaginal fistula and augmentation ileocystoplasty. Urology 59:597-599, 2002.
82. Gan E, Li MK: Repair of complex uretrovaginal and vesicovaginal fistulas with ileal cystoplasty and ureteric reimplantation into an antireflux ileal nipple valve—A case report. Ann Acad Med Singapore 27:707-709, 1998.
83. Naude JH: Reconstructive urology in the tropical and developing world: A personal prespective. BJU Int 89:31-36, 2002.
84. Mitrofanoff P: Trans-appendicular continent cystostomy in the management of the neurogenic bladder. Chir Pediatr 21:297-305, 1980.
85. Hodges AM: Vesico-vaginal fistula associated with uterine prolapse. Br J Obstet Gynaecol 106:1127-1128, 1999.
86. Zincke H, Segura JW: Ureterosigmoidostomy: Critical review of 173 cases. J Urol 113:324-7, 1975.
87. Fisch M, Klinkowski U, Wammack R, Hohenfellner R: The sigma-rectum pouch (Mainz II). Critical analysis after 3 years of clinical experience [abstract]. J Urol 153:61A, 1995.
88. Leissner J, Black P, Fisch M, et al: Colon pouch (Meinz pouch III) for continent urinary diversion after pelvic irradiation. Urology 56:798-802, 2000.
89. Nezhat CH, Nezhat F, Nezhat C, Rottenberg H: Laparoscopic repair of a vesicovaginal fistula: A case report. Obstet Gynecol 83:899-901, 1994.

90. Phipps J: Laparoscopic repair of posthysterectomy vesico-vaginal fistula: Two case reports. Gynecol Endosc 5:123-124, 1996.
91. Von Theobald P, Hamel P, Febbraro W: Laparoscopic repair of a vesicovaginal fistula using an omental J flap. BJOG 105:1216-1218, 1998.
92. Miklos JR, Sobolewski C, Lucente V: Laparoscopic management or recurrent vesicovaginal fistula. Int Urogynecol J Pelvic Floor Dysfunct 10:116-117, 1999.
93. Nabi G, Hemal AK: Laparoscopic repair of vesicovaginal fistula and right nephrectomy for nonfunctioning kidney in a single session. J Endourol 15:801-803, 2001.
94. Ou CS, Huang UC, Tsuang M, Rowbotham R: Laparoscopic repair of vesicovaginal fistula. J Laparoendosc Adv Surg Tech 14:17-21, 2004.
95. Chibber PJ, Shah NH, Jain P: Laparoscopic O'Conor's repair for vesico-vaginal and vesico-uterine fistulae. BJU Int 96:183-186, 2005.
96. Sotelo R, Mariano MB, Garcia-Segui A, et al: Laparoscopic repair of a vesicovaginal fistula. J Urol 173:1615-1618, 2005.
97. Melamud O, Eichel L, Turbow B, Shanberg A: Laparoscopic vesicovaginal fistula repair with robotic reconstruction. Urology 65:163-166, 2005.
98. Pick DL, Lee DI, Skarecky DW: Anatomic guide for port placement of the Da Vinci robotic system radical prostatectomy. J Endourol 18:572-575, 2004.
99. Smith GL, Williams G: Vesicovaginal fistula. BJU Int 83:564-569, 1999.
100. Miller EA, Webster GD: Current management of vesicovaginal fistulae. Curr Opin Urol 11:417-421, 2001.
101. Margolis T, Mercer LJ: Vesicovaginal fistula. Obstet Gynecol Surv 49:840-847, 1994.
102. Woo HH, Rosario DJ, Chapple CR: The treatment of vesicovaginal fistulae. Eur Urol 29:1-9, 1996.
103. Carr LK, Webster GD: Abdominal repair of vesicovaginal fistulas. Urology 48:10-11, 1996.
104. Nesrallah LJ, Srougi M, Gittes RF: The O'Connor technique: The gold standard for supratrigonal vesicovaginal fistula repair. J Urol 161:566-568, 1999.
105. Angioli R, Penalver M, Muzii L, et al: Guidelines of how to manage vesicovaginal fistula. Crit Rev Oncol Hematol 48:295-304, 2003.
106. El-Imam M, El-Hassan el-HM, Adam I: Vesicovaginal fistula in Sudanese women. Saudi Med J 26:341-342, 2005.
107. Naru T, Rizvi JH, Talati J: Surgical repair of genital fistulae. J Obstet Gynaecol Res 30:293-296, 2004.
108. Navarro Sebastián FJ, García González JI, Castro Pita M, et al: Treatment approach for vesicovaginal fistula. Retrospective analysis of our data. Actas Urol Esp 27:530-537, 2003.
109. Rafique M: Genitourinary fistulas of obstetric origin. Int Urol Nephrol 34:489-493, 2002-2003.
110. Kam MH, Tan YH, Wong MY: A 12-year experience in the surgical management of vesicovaginal fistulae. Singapore Med J 44:181-184, 2003.
111. Wook Bai SW, Kim SH, Kwon HS, et al: Surgical outcome of female genital fistula in Korea. Yonsei Med J 43:315-319, 2002.
112. Benchekroun A, al Alj HA, el Sayegh H, et al: Vesico vaginal fistula: Report of 1050 cases. Ann Urol 37:194-198, 2003.
113. Kochakarn W, Ratana-Olarn K, Viseshsindh V, et al: Vesico vaginal fistula: Experience of 230 cases. J Med Assoc Thai 83:1129-1132, 2000.
114. Flores-Carreras O, Cabrera JR, Galeano PA, Torres FE: Fistulas of the urinary tract in gynecologic and obstetric surgery. Int Urogynecol J 12:203-214, 2001.
115. Langkilde NC, Pless TK, Lundbeck F, Nerstrom B: Surgical repair of vesicovaginal fistulae—A ten-year retrospective study. Scand J Urol Nephrol 33:100-103, 1999.
116. Kristensen JK, Lose G: Vesicovaginal fistulas: The transperitoneal repair revisited. Scand J Urol Nephrol Suppl 157:101-105, 1994.
117. Motiwala HG, Amlani JC, Desai KD, et al: Transvesical vesicovaginal fistula repair: A revival. Eur Urol 19:24-28, 1991.

Chapter 83

RECTOVAGINAL FISTULA

Matthew P. Rutman, Larissa V. Rodríguez, Donna Y. Deng, and Shlomo Raz

A rectovaginal fistula consists of an abnormal, epithelium-lined communication between the rectum and the vagina. It represents an extremely distressing problem for the patient and a surgical challenge for the physician. The reconstructive pelvic surgeon must have a full understanding of rectovaginal fistula to provide the patient with the most appropriate treatment option.

PATHOPHYSIOLOGY

It is important to consider the underlying cause of the rectovaginal fistula in preparing for a successful repair. The most common cause of rectovaginal fistula remains obstetric trauma,[1,2] usually caused by an unrecognized injury with traumatic vaginal delivery, wound infection, or an inadequate repair of a third- or fourth-degree perineal laceration. Up to 5% of vaginal deliveries result in these lacerations. Most heal when repaired at the time of labor. Prolonged labor and compression can result in ischemic necrosis of the vaginal septum, predisposing the delivering woman to development of a rectovaginal fistula. This is a greater concern in developing nations and likely not a large factor in industrialized countries such as the United States and Canada.

Vaginal, rectal, and pelvic operations, such as rectocele repair, low anterior resection, and hemorrhoidectomy, may lead to rectovaginal fistula as a result of intraoperative injury or postoperative infection. Rectovaginal fistula can result from nonobstetric blunt and penetrating trauma. Inflammatory processes of the bowel, such as diverticulitis, Crohn's disease, and ulcerative colitis, can produce a rectovaginal fistula.

Rectal, cervical, uterine, and vaginal malignancy and radiation therapy are known causes of rectovaginal fistulas. The incidence of rectovaginal fistula after irradiation is 0.3% to 6%.[3,4] The fistula may occur up to 2 years after irradiation because of progressive radiation damage. Any fistula associated with radiation therapy and malignancy must be biopsied to rule out recurrent malignancy before formal repair.

Inflammatory or infectious processes near the rectovaginal septum or cul-de-sac may result in formation of a rectovaginal fistula. Prolonged use of a vaginal pessary can result in a rectovaginal fistula.

The location of rectovaginal fistulas may mandate a particular surgical approach. The fistula may be in the high, middle, or low rectal region. Most fistulas associated with obstetric trauma are classified as low types. Diverticular disease and other intra-abdominal pathologic conditions are associated with higher rectovaginal fistula. The high fistula usually is associated with intra-abdominal conditions such as diverticulitis or abscess formation, and it may require a laparotomy. The low fistula of rectal origin can be repaired transvaginally, avoiding the morbidity of an abdominal approach.

EVALUATION

The diagnosis is obvious in patients with a large rectovaginal fistula because bowel content is evacuated through the vagina. Patients with a smaller fistula may be completely asymptomatic.

A thorough history and physical examination are mandatory for every patient suspected of having a fistula. The interview should include questions about prior malignancy, radiation therapy, complicated obstetric history, inflammatory bowel disease, and prior anorectal surgery. Physical examination should reveal the size, location, and number of fistulous tracts. The perineal body must be examined to determine the function and tone of the anal sphincter. Bimanual examination allows the physician to palpate the thickness of the perineal body and identify the fistula. Multiple fistulas and perianal fissures may suggest Crohn's disease. If the fistula is not easily identified, vaginal speculum examination should be performed.

If the diagnosis is still in doubt, a dye test can be performed. Methylene blue dye is instilled into the rectum, and a tampon or sponge inserted into the vagina. Staining of the pad confirms the diagnosis and can be helpful in identifying a small fistula. Proctoscopy, colonoscopy, barium examination, and computed tomography should be performed if indicated. Any area of suspicious inflammation, ulceration, or mass should be biopsied to rule out a malignant process or recurrence. Examination under anesthesia can be performed to make the diagnosis if all of the previous measures fail and the physician still suspects a fistula.

Before formal repair, it is necessary to evaluate the patient for fecal incontinence. A review of 52 patients at the University of Minnesota revealed a 48% incidence of coexistent fecal incontinence.[5] Among women who develop rectovaginal fistula after obstetric trauma, the incidence is probably much higher. It is essential to assess the function of the anal sphincter before surgical repair. Endoanal ultrasonography, anal manometry, and pudendal nerve terminal motor latency testing remain valuable tools to aid with the clinical evaluation. Ultrasound can easily identify defects in the internal anal sphincter. Defects in the external anal sphincter are more difficult to identify because of the hyperechoic pattern. Manometry can help quantify the resting and squeezing pressures of the sphincter muscle. Pudendal nerve testing helps identify underlying neuropathy.

PREOPERATIVE CONSIDERATIONS

Management of rectovaginal fistulas depends on several factors: cause, size, number, and location of the fistulas and the surgeon's preference. Anal sphincter integrity and prior operations influence the choice of treatment. Regardless of the approach chosen, several principles require consideration before repair.

Antibiotic coverage and topical hormonal replacement help optimize the health of local tissues and decrease any associated infection and inflammation. The health of the surrounding tissues influences the waiting period before surgical repair. Any inflammation or infection should be resolved. Waiting 3 to 6 months in these cases allows resolution and increases the chance of successful repair. In patients with prior failed repair, a longer waiting period may be necessary. In patients with postirradiation rectovaginal fistulas, a much longer waiting period may be required. Patients with complex fistulas (e.g., large size, radiation induced, neoplasm induced, multiple failed repairs) may require a diverting colostomy before formal repair. After diversion, a waiting period of 2 to 3 months before vaginal repair allows local tissue healing. Complete bowel preparation is given before surgery.

Excellent exposure allows good mobilization of tissue flaps. The fistulous tract should be exposed in its entirety and left intact. We tend to not excise the tract. This prevents iatrogenic enlargement of the fistula and allows us to use it in our repair. The rectal opening is closed in multiple, tension-free layers. Interposition of healthy tissue between the rectum and vagina should be used routinely. Common sources include labia fatty tissue (i.e., Martius flap), labial skin and underlying fatty tissue, gluteal skin, gracilis muscular flaps, and omentum. Case reports have described pudendal thigh fasciocutaneous island flaps and gluteal-fold flap repairs to aid in rectovaginal fistula repair.[6,7] Several common techniques of tissue interposition can be found in Chapters 81 and 82. After closure of the fistula, anal sphincter defects should be addressed to restore normal sphincter function.

SURGICAL REPAIRS

Surgical options can be divided into transvaginal repair, transanal repair, transperineal repair, and abdominal repair. Reconstructive urologists and gynecologists typically use a transvaginal approach, whereas colorectal surgeons prefer a transanal approach. An abdominal approach is often used in treating radiation-induced rectovaginal fistulas. We use a multilayered transvaginal approach, avoiding the morbidity of a laparotomy, in most rectovaginal fistula repairs.

Complete bowel preparation is done, and antibiotics are given preoperatively. The patient is given general or spinal anesthesia and placed in the high lithotomy position. A Foley catheter is placed in the bladder. Use of a surgeon's headlight and a ring retractor help to optimize exposure. A Foley catheter is inserted into the fistulous tract (Fig. 83-1). A circumferential incision is made around the Foley catheter, and the tract is dissected to the rectal wall (Fig. 83-2). A flap of distal vaginal is also prepared. The fistulous tract is then excised, leaving the rectal wall with an indwelling catheter (Fig. 83-3). The rectal wall is closed in two layers using 2-0 absorbable sutures (Fig. 83-4). The levator musculature is included in the closure.

A Martius flap is prepared. A vertical incision is made lateral to the labia, and a fibrofatty flap is developed and isolated, preserving the inferior vascular pedicle (Fig. 83-5). The flap is then tunneled through the vagina and rotated to cover the fistula. Interrupted sutures are used to fix the flap to the rectal wall. The wound is then closed in layers, advancing the vaginal wall distally and ensuring new tissue covers the area of the fistula (Fig. 83-6). Vaginal packing is left for a few hours, and the patient resumes a regular diet. Oral antibiotics are continued for 1 week. For patients who had a prior diverting colostomy, we routinely wait 3 to 6 months before takedown. Physical examination and a radiographic contrast study confirm complete healing of the fistula.

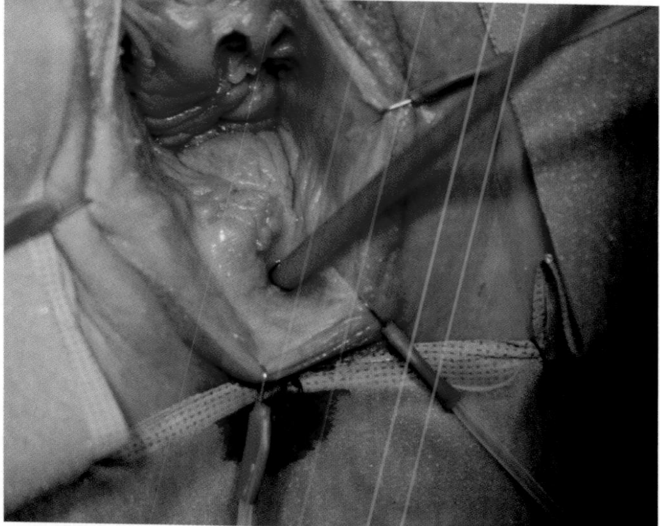

Figure 83-1 The fistulous tract is catheterized.

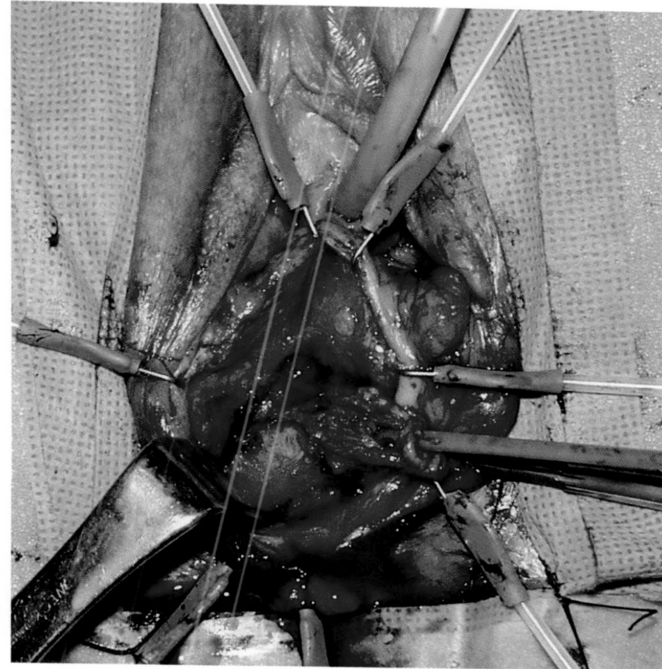

Figure 83-2 The circumferential incision is dissected to the rectal wall.

Intraoperative complications are rare. If tissue quality is poor intraoperatively (because of infection or irradiation), the surgery should be aborted and a diverting colostomy performed to allow tissue healing. Postoperative complications include recurrent

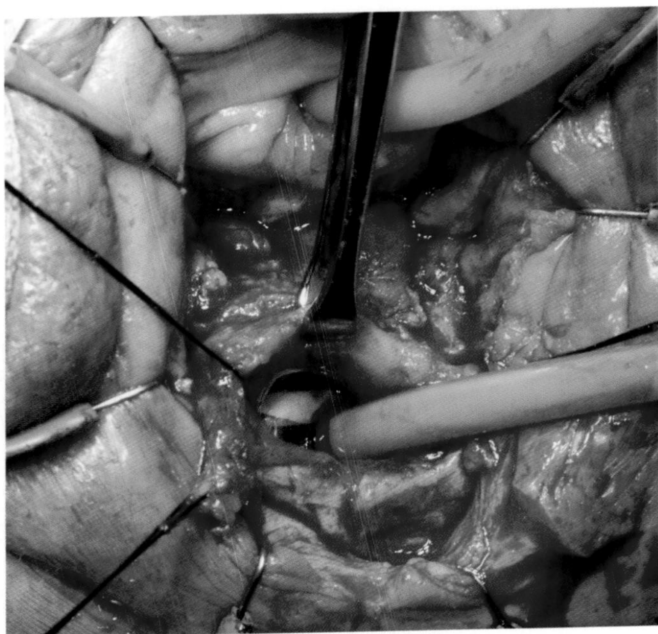
Figure 83-3 Excision of a fistulous tract.

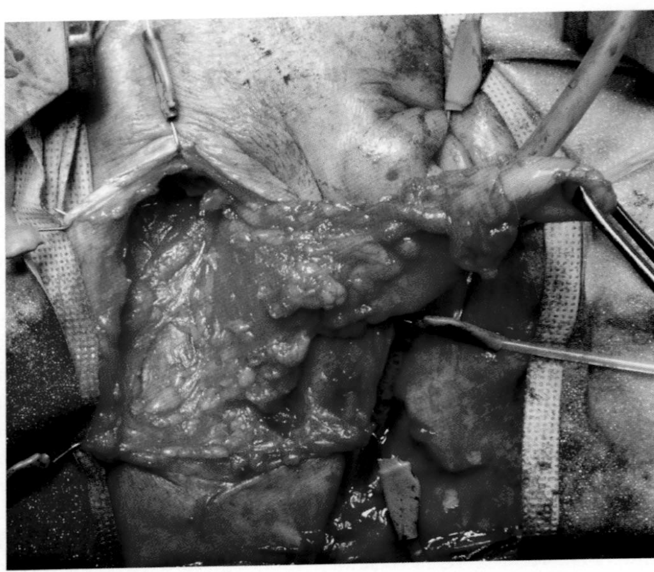
Figure 83-5 The Martius flap is based on an inferior vascular pedicle.

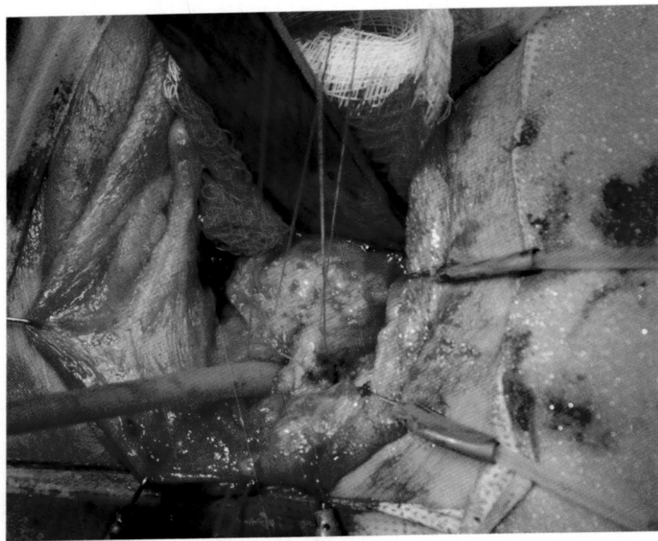
Figure 83-4 Closure of the rectal wall.

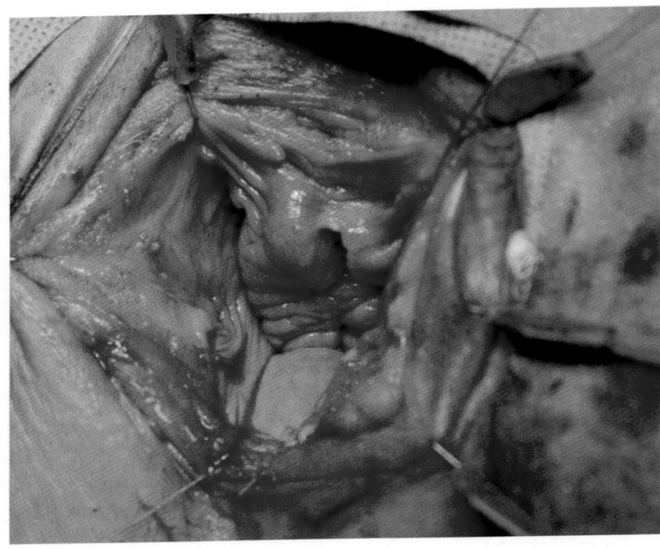
Figure 83-6 The vaginal wall flap is advanced to cover the fistula.

fistula. Recurrent fistula requires a diverting colostomy, if not previously performed, before re-exploration.

A second transvaginal approach includes inversion of the fistula. The patient is placed in the lithotomy position as described earlier. The vaginal mucosa is incised in a circumferential fashion around the fistula and mobilized in all directions. After excising the fistulous tract, a purse-string suture is placed around the opening of the rectovaginal septum, and the suture is secured, inverting the fistula into the rectum. The muscle and vaginal mucosa are then closed, resulting in three layers of repair.[8]

Case reports have reported successful use of cadaveric dermal allograft[9] interposition and porcine dermal graft interposition[10] Dexon mesh has been used to separate the suture lines between the vaginal and rectal walls.[11] These may be viable alternatives to traditional autologous flaps.

Although not commonly used by urologists and gynecologists, colorectal surgeons often advocate a transanal approach. The most common of the approaches uses an advancement flap.[12] The patient is given standard antibiotics and mechanical bowel preparation preoperatively. After general anesthesia is provided, the patient is placed in the prone jackknife position. The vagina and perineum are cleansed in standard sterile fashion. Proctoscopy identifies the fistula and allows irrigation of the lower rectum to clear any residual fecal contents. Rectal retractors help optimize exposure. Injectable Xylocaine with epinephrine is infiltrated into the dissection planes. A trapezoidal flap consisting of mucosa, submucosa, and internal sphincter (i.e., circular muscle) is raised around the fistula and mobilized 4 to 5 cm cephalad. The flap should easily advance to cover the fistula tract, and any tension should be avoided. Excess flap, including the fistula itself, is excised, and the remaining flap is advanced and sutured with 3-0 absorbable sutures. The vaginal aspect of the fistula is left open for drainage.

Layered closure can be performed transanally.[13] A transverse elliptical incision is made around the fistula through the rectovaginal septum. It is dissected circumferentially for about 3 cm. The fistula tract is excised, and a two-layer closure is performed. The rectal mucosa is then advanced distal to the deeper portion of the repair and reapproximated.

Transperineal approaches can be organized into three categories: fistulotomy, perineoproctotomy, and sphincteroplasty. Fistulotomy converts a fistula into a fourth-degree perineal laceration, resulting in fecal incontinence due to sphincter damage. This procedure is not recommended as a solo primary approach.

Perineoproctotomy with layered closure is a commonly used transperineal technique.[1] It is often used by obstetricians for repair of lower vaginal rectovaginal fistulas. The patient is prepared with standard antibiotics and bowel preparation and placed in the lithotomy position. The fistula is identified, and the bridge of skin, sphincter, and perineal body between the posterior fourchette and fistula are divided. The fistula becomes a fourth-degree perineal laceration. The fistulous tract is excised, and the defect is then closed in standard layered fashion (i.e., vaginal wall, sphincter muscle, and rectal mucosa). The perineal body is reconstructed. Postoperative complications include vaginal stenosis and dyspareunia. Fecal incontinence may result with scarring of the transected anal sphincter.

Sphincteroplasty performed through a transperineal approach allows correction of any underlying sphincter defect.[14] The patient is prepared as previously described and placed under general anesthesia. A Foley catheter is placed, and the patient is placed prone in the jackknife position. A curvilinear incision is made through the perineum. A flap of anoderm distally and mucosa and submucosa proximally is raised. The ends of the sphincter (external and internal) muscles are identified laterally and left intact. Levatoroplasty is often needed at this stage of the surgery if the injury involves the deep external sphincter muscle. The ends of the mobilized sphincter muscles are sutured in an overlapping manner using horizontal mattress sutures. This reconstructs the sphincter mechanism. Tissue is then interposed between the rectum and vagina. The endorectal flap is sutured to the reconstructed sphincter muscle, and the perineal incision is closed. The vaginal mucosa is left open to drain.

Transabdominal procedures to repair rectovaginal fistula are necessary for complex fistulas resulting from irradiation, inflammatory bowel disease, and failed previous repairs. Surrounding tissues are often poorly vascularized, and local repair is a poor option. Abdominal approaches leave the anal sphincter intact and allow easy interposition of well-vascularized tissues.

In patients with a high fistula location and normal surrounding tissues (i.e., no irradiation or inflammatory bowel disease), simple abdominal repair can be performed. A laparotomy is performed, and the rectovaginal septum is mobilized. The diseased segment is divided, and layered closure of the rectal and vaginal defects is performed. Omentum is interposed between the rectum and the vagina.

Most commonly, an abdominal approach is chosen because of poor local tissue quality. These approaches are typically performed after a primary diverting colostomy has been done or concomitantly with fecal diversion. The abdominal approach allows repair of the fistula with concomitant bowel resection. The patient undergoes complete bowel preparation, is given antibiotics, and is placed under general anesthesia. A laparotomy is performed. The splenic flexure, left colon, and sigmoid colon are fully mobilized down to the levator hiatus. The diseased bowel segment is resected. At this point, a coloanal anastomosis is performed by a pull-through[15,16] or sleeve anastamosis.[17]

A non-resectional onlay patch technique was introduced by Bricker and Johnson in 1979 for radiation-induced rectovaginal fistula.[18] The rectosigmoid colon is divided and an end-sigmoid colostomy performed. The distal end is then folded and sutured to the exposed and débrided edges of the fistulous opening in the rectum. At a later stage, after healing is confirmed, the colostomy is taken down and anastomosed to the side of the folded loop of the rectosigmoid. The major downfall of this procedure is that it leaves behind irradiated tissue, and it is rarely used today.

For patients with a fistula resulting from a neoplasm, abdominoperineal resection and vaginectomy are typically required. Patients with severe inflammatory bowel disease may ultimately require proctocolectomy. Patients with terminal malignancies or major medical comorbidities (i.e., unfit for major surgery) and symptomatic rectovaginal fistulas may be best served by a diverting colostomy.

ALTERNATIVE TREATMENTS

Alternative procedures for rectovaginal fistula have been described in the literature. Fibrin glue has been injected into the fistulous tract, with reported success rates of 74% and 80%.[19,20] In patients with Crohn's disease, several medical regimens have been studied. Sands and colleagues[21,22] reported fistula closure with infliximab infusion in 13 of 29 patients after 14 weeks of follow-up. Similar improvements have been reported with intravenous and oral cyclosporine.[23,24] Metronidazole and 6-mercaptopurine have been used to effectively treat rectovaginal fistula resulting from Crohn's disease.[25]

The Latzko technique used in vesicovaginal fistula repair can also be used to repair a high rectovaginal fistula located at the apex of the vagina. The anterior and posterior vaginal walls are denuded, and an incision is made around the fistula margins. Three layers of closure invert the fistula, close the rectal muscle and fascia, and close the vaginal mucosa.

RESULTS

The many different approaches to repair of rectovaginal fistula have various success rates and outcome measures. Success should be evaluated according to objective measures and the results of self-reported questionnaires about patient satisfaction. Successful repair of the fistula sounds great, but secondary fecal incontinence or dyspareunia may alter the outcome. The existing literature primarily reports success or failure based on healing of the rectovaginal fistula. Future reports should report on fistula healing, fecal continence, sexual function, and quality of life.

Transvaginal repairs using a layered closure have success rates of 84% to 100%.[2,26-28] Advancement flaps placed by means of a transanal approach have success rates in the range of 78% to 100%.[29-31] The rates were higher for patients undergoing initial repair.[32] Success rates of 88% to 100% have been reported for perineoproctotomy and layered closure.[1,2,8,33-35] The combination of sphincteroplasty and levatoroplasty has a success rate of 93%.[32] Transabdominal repairs also have high cure rates, in the range of 80% to 100%.[4,17,36]

CONCLUSIONS

The management of rectovaginal fistulas remains a challenge for the reconstructive pelvic surgeon. The decision-making algorithm must include the size, location, and cause of the fistula. The health of the patient and judgment of the treating physician greatly influence successful repair and a good outcome.

References

1. Mazier WP, Senagore AJ, Schiesel EC: Operative repair of anovaginal and rectovaginal fistulas. Dis Colon Rectum 38:4, 1995.
2. Hibbard LT: Surgical management of rectovaginal fistulas and complete perineal tears. Am J Obstet Gynecol 130:139, 1978.
3. Allen-Mersh, TG, Wilson, EJ, Hope-Stone, HF, et al: The management of late radiation-induced rectal injury after treatment of carcinoma of the uterus. Surg Gynecol Obstet 164:521, 1987.
4. Cooke SA, de Moor NG: The surgical treatment of the radiation-damaged rectum. Br J Surg 68:488, 1981.
5. Tsang CB, Madoff RD, Wong WD, et al: Anal sphincter integrity and function influences outcome in rectovaginal fistula repair. Dis Colon Rectum 41:1141, 1998.
6. Monstrey S, Blondeel P, Van Landuyt K, et al: The versatility of the pudendal thigh fasciocutaneous flap used as an island flap. Plast Reconstr Surg 107:719, 2001.
7. Kosugi C, Saito N, Kimata Y, et al: Rectovaginal fistulas after rectal cancer surgery: Incidence and operative repair by gluteal-fold flap repair. Surgery 137:329, 2005.
8. Given FT Jr: Rectovaginal fistula: A review of 20 years' experience in a community hospital. Am J Obstet Gynecol 108:41, 1970.
9. Miklos JR, Kohli N: Rectovaginal fistula repair utilizing a cadaveric dermal allograft. Int Urogynecol J Pelvic Floor Dysfunct 10:405, 1999.
10. Moore RD, Miklos JR, Kohli N: Rectovaginal fistula repair using a porcine dermal graft. Obstet Gynecol 104:1165, 2004.
11. Walfisch A, Zilberstein T, Walfisch S: Rectovaginal septal repair: Case presentations and introduction of a modified reconstruction technique. Tech Coloproctol 8:192, 2004.
12. Rothenberger DA, Christenson CE, Balcos EG, et al: Endorectal advancement flap for treatment of simple rectovaginal fistula. Dis Colon Rectum 25:297, 1982.
13. Greenwald JC, Hoexter B: Repair of rectovaginal fistulas. Surg Gynecol Obstet 146:443, 1978.
14. Russell TR, Gallagher DM: Low rectovaginal fistulas. Approach and treatment. Am J Surg 134:13, 1977.
15. Cutait DE, Figliolini FJ: A new method of colorectal anastomosis in abdominoperineal resection. Dis Colon Rectum 4:335, 1961.
16. Turnbull RB Jr, Cuthbertson A: Abdominorectal pull-through resection for cancer and for Hirschsprung's disease: Delayed posterior colorectal anastomosis. Cleve Clin Q 28:109, 1961.
17. Parks AG, Allen CL, Frank JD, et al: A method of treating post-irradiation rectovaginal fistulas. Br J Surg 65:417, 1978.
18. Bricker EM, Johnston WD: Repair of postirradiation rectovaginal fistula and stricture. Surg Gynecol Obstet 148:499, 1979.
19. Hjortrup A, Moesgaard F, Kjaergard J: Fibrin adhesive in the treatment of perineal fistulas. Dis Colon Rectum 34:752, 1991.
20. Abel ME, Chiu YS, Russell TR, et al: Autologous fibrin glue in the treatment of rectovaginal and complex fistulas. Dis Colon Rectum 36:447, 1993.
21. Sands BE, Blank MA, Patel K, et al: Long-term treatment of rectovaginal fistulas in Crohn's disease: Response to infliximab in the ACCENT II Study. Clin Gastroenterol Hepatol 2:912, 2004.
22. Sands BE, Anderson FH, Bernstein CN, et al: Infliximab maintenance therapy for fistulizing Crohn's disease. N Engl J Med 350:876, 2004.
23. Lichtiger S, Present DH, Kornbluth A, et al: Cyclosporine in severe ulcerative colitis refractory to steroid therapy. N Engl J Med 330:1841, 1994.
24. Present DH, Lichtiger S: Efficacy of cyclosporine in treatment of fistula of Crohn's disease. Dig Dis Sci 39:374, 1994.
25. Stein BL, Gordon PH: Perianal inflammatory conditions in inflammatory bowel disease. Curr Opin Gen Surg nv:141, 1993.
26. Lawson J: Rectovaginal fistulae following difficult labour. Proc R Soc Med 65:283, 1972.
27. Lescher TC, Pratt JH: Vaginal repair of the simple rectovaginal fistula. Surg Gynecol Obstet 124:1317, 1967.
28. Tancer ML, Lasser D, Rosenblum N: Rectovaginal fistula or perineal and anal sphincter disruption, or both, after vaginal delivery. Surg Gynecol Obstet 171:43, 1990.
29. Belt RL Jr: Repair of anorectal vaginal fistula utilizing segmental advancement of the internal sphincter muscle. Dis Colon Rectum 12:99, 1969.
30. Hoexter B, Labow SB, Moseson MD: Transanal rectovaginal fistula repair. Dis Colon Rectum 28:572, 1985.
31. Hilsabeck JR: Transanal advancement of the anterior rectal wall for vaginal fistulas involving the lower rectum. Dis Colon Rectum 23:236, 1980.
32. Lowry AC, Thorson AG, Rothenberger DA, et al: Repair of simple rectovaginal fistulas. Influence of previous repairs. Dis Colon Rectum 31:676, 1988.
33. Pepe F, Panella M, Arikian S, et al: Low rectovaginal fistulas. Aust N Z J Obstet Gynaecol 27:61, 1987.
34. Watson SJ, Phillips RK: Non-inflammatory rectovaginal fistula. Br J Surg 82:1641, 1995.
35. Thiele H, Wesch G, Nusser CJ: Surgical therapy of enterovaginal fistulae following gynecologic primary procedures [in German, author's translation]. Langenbecks Arch Chir 357:35, 1982.
36. Nowacki MP, Szawlowski AW, Borkowski A: Parks' coloanal sleeve anastomosis for treatment of postirradiation rectovaginal fistula. Dis Colon Rectum 29:817, 1986.

Chapter 84

URETEROVAGINAL FISTULA

David Ginsberg

DEFINITION AND INCIDENCE

A ureterovaginal fistula is an abnormal communication between the distal ureter and the vagina that results in urinary incontinence. Formation is often preceded by pelvic surgery, with an unrecognized ureteral injury occurring at the time of surgery. Damage to the ureter can lead to ureteral obstruction or leakage of urine at the site of injury. The urine often makes its way out through the vaginal cuff, which ultimately results in the formation of the ureterovaginal fistula.

Ureteral injury has occurred in about 0.5% to 1% of all pelvic surgeries.[1] Total abdominal hysterectomy is the most common procedure leading to injury to the ureter and subsequent ureterovaginal fistula, accounting for 75% of all cases in one study.[2] Enlarged uteri, pelvic adhesions, and significant intraoperative bleeding also appear to increase the risk of ureteral injury at the time of gynecologic surgery.[3] Other operations that may lead to ureterovaginal fistula include anterior colporrhaphy, colorectal surgery, and oophorectomy. Obstetric causes rarely lead to ureterovaginal fistula formation and are primarily attributed to cesarean section (especially after prior cesarean section),[3] although traumatic vaginal delivery has been reported as a cause of ureterovaginal fistula.[4] Other unusual causes of ureterovaginal fistula include vaginal foreign body[5] and residual stone fragments after shockwave lithotripsy.[6] Radiation therapy by itself or in conjunction with surgery can place a patient at risk for ureteral injury and subsequent formation of ureterovaginal fistula.[7] Persistent urinary leakage resulting from an injury to the ureter during any of these procedures places the patient at risk for developing an ureterovaginal fistula. Later series looking at laparoscopic pelvic surgery found a rate of ureteral injury of less than 1% to 2%, with a much lower incidence of injury associated with diagnostic laparoscopy compared with laparoscopic intervention.[8,9]

The injury to the ureter usually occurs in the distal third. Types of injury include ischemia, transaction, excision, and ligation. Ischemia is most commonly associated with radical (Wertheim's) hysterectomy, which requires the ureter to be stripped from its fascial encasement in the broad ligament. More commonly, the ureter is injured by a suture, with resultant extravasation leading to fistula formation. The left ureter is much more at risk, and most prior series reveal ureterovaginal fistula formation on the left three to five times more often than on the right side. This increased risk to the left ureter is related to its course, which places it much closer to the cervix than the right ureter. Another common site of injury is at the level of the pelvic brim, where the ureter crosses the iliac vessels. Injury at this site is thought to occur during the manipulation and division of the infundibulopelvic ligament.[3] Patients with pelvic inflammatory disease, prior pelvic surgery, and other conditions that can distort the normal pelvic anatomy may be at greater risk for ureteral injury and subsequent fistula formation.

PRESENTATION

In most series, patients with ureterovaginal fistula present 1 to 4 weeks after pelvic surgery with an acute onset of continuous incontinence. Many also void normally despite the continuous leak, because the bladder continues to fill normally through the contralateral ureter, which is usually uninvolved (bilateral ureterovaginal fistulas are rare). The presentation of ureteral injury alone in the absence of fistula formation is often missed because the symptoms are nonspecific. The most common symptoms of ureteral injury include abdominal pain, flank pain, and nausea, all of which can be easily overlooked and confused with postoperative complaints after the initial surgery or masked by postoperative narcotic use. Because symptoms of ureteral injury are nonspecific, a high degree of suspicion should be maintained for any patient with these complaints and prior pelvic surgery. Complains about urinary incontinence should result in an evaluation to look for problems such as a vesicovaginal or ureterovaginal fistula.

EVALUATION

Renal ultrasound may be helpful as a screening tool, but the result may be normal if distal obstruction is absent. The most commonly used modality to evaluate for ureteral injury is intravenous urography (IVU). It can identify n ureteral injury in most cases, and it enables evaluation of renal function and potential obstruction on the affected side (Fig. 84-1). IVU may not identify a ureterovaginal fistula in every patient. Lask and colleagues[10] evaluated iatrogenic ureteral injuries in 44 patients, 10 of whom had a ureterovaginal fistula. The fistula was identified in only 3 of 10 patients undergoing IVU.[10] These findings highlight the importance of retrograde pyelography, which may be required to identify the fistula in some patients.[11] This is especially true if the IVU result is abnormal but does not reveal ureterovaginal fistula and the patient complains of urinary incontinence after recent pelvic surgery.

Any obstruction at the level of the injury should be identified because an untreated distal blockage makes spontaneous healing of the fistula extremely unlikely. If conservative attempts at therapy are to be attempted, such as placement of a ureteral stent as discussed in the next section, the retrograde pyelogram can be done simultaneously. Computed tomography should be considered for patients who are systemically ill to evaluate for possible

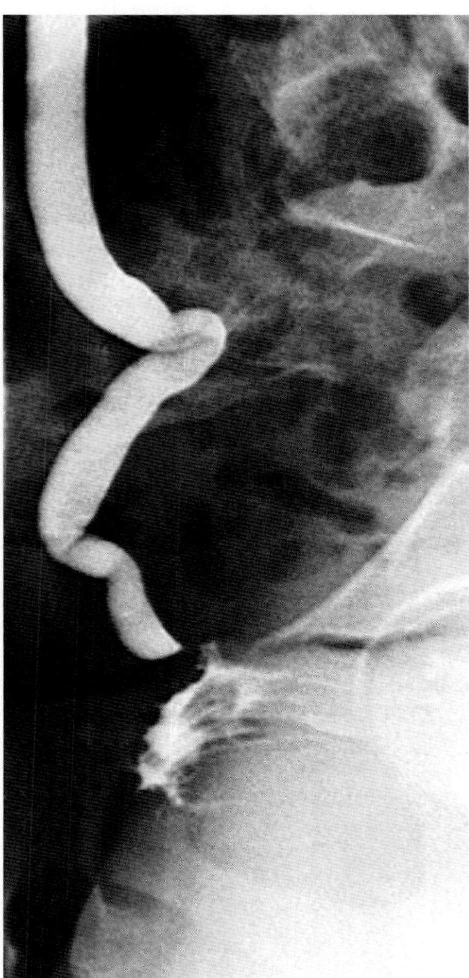

Figure 84-1 Intravenous urography (IVU), with coned down view of the pelvis. The patient underwent total abdominal hysterectomy 2 weeks earlier and now complains of flank pain and urinary incontinence. IVU demonstrates fullness of the distal ureter and an injury that has resulted in a ureteral leak and subsequent ureterovaginal fistula.

urinoma or abscess formation, which should be percutaneously drained.

In addition to radiographic evaluation, the double-dye test can be used. This was initially described using intravenous indigo carmine,[12] but it has been modified to eliminate the need for intravenous access to perform the test. With the modified test, a patient is given Pyridium orally until the urine turns orange. A tampon is placed vaginally, and the bladder is emptied with a catheter. Through that catheter, the bladder is filled with a mixture of 300 mL of normal saline and 5 mL of methylene blue dye. After 5 minutes, the bladder is emptied, and the tampon is removed and inspected. An orange stain at the top of the tampon indicates a ureterovaginal fistula, a blue stain in the middle of the tampon indicates a vesicovaginal fistula, and a blue stain at the distal tip of the vagina indicates leakage of urine through the urethra.[13]

ENDOSCOPIC THERAPY

A variety of minimally invasive therapies have been described for the management of ureterovaginal, and they have a wide range of results. The least invasive option is observation. This has been reported with periodic success in the past and was primarily used before the use of fluoroscopy and modern endoscopic equipment made ureteral stent placement commonplace.[11,14,15] Clinical and radiographic features that are likely to predict a successful outcome with nonsurgical management of a ureterovaginal fistula include minimal to moderate obstruction on the affected side, a mild degree of periureteral extravasation, upper tract improvement on subsequent follow-up studies, adequate control of urinary tract infection, and the use of absorbable suture material at the time of the initial procedure that caused the injury to the ureter.[14] The risk of expectant management is stricture formation, which may require regular dilations or, if not followed carefully, can lead to chronic obstruction, loss of kidney function, and the need for subsequent nephrectomy.[16]

Physicians had some success with a nephrostomy tube alone when a stent could not be passed by the area of ureteral occlusion. Nephrostomy tube placement protects the upper tracts if the patient is obstructed and has successfully led to ureterovaginal fistula resolution in a small number of patients.[10,11] This should be the first option if the patient is too ill to undergo anesthesia and an attempt at retrograde stent placement. This technique protects the renal unit while the patients improves and can therefore allow stent placement at a later date through an antegrade approach.[10]

The increased likelihood of fistula resolution with stent placement (and not nephrostomy drainage alone) was elucidated by Dowling and coworkers.[17] In this series, all six of the ureterovaginal fistulas that had a stent placed successfully (antegrade or retrograde) required no further therapy; all three patients managed with nephrostomy alone failed the primary mode of therapy and subsequently required surgical intervention.[17] Further evidence that nephrostomy drainage alone is insufficient was reported by Schmeller and associates[18] in a review of 11 patients with ureterovaginal fistula. With this mode of management, six patients had a persistent fistula, and two had issues of ureteral stricture.[18] It is unlikely that nephrostomy tube drainage alone will lead to spontaneous resolution of a ureterovaginal fistula if the ureter is obstructed distally.

The goal of all minimally invasive therapy should be placement of a stent across the fistula and site of injury. This protects the kidney from potential damage from distal obstruction and can lead to spontaneous healing of the fistula. Some studies have reported resolution of up to 100% of ureterovaginal fistulas if the stent was left in place for an appropriate length of time.[19,20] If the stent is successful, it is important to remember that these patients are at risk for ureteral stricture in the future, and they should be followed in the early period after stent removal with regular renal ultrasound examinations. This approach allows appropriate evaluation for the presence of de novo hydronephrosis, which can indicate stricture formation. With current endourologic techniques, it is likely that a stricture could be managed with endoscopic techniques alone, avoiding the need for open intervention.[19]

The primary difficulty with most of these patients is stent placement. The injury that led to ureterovaginal fistula formation is often obstructing and does not allow easy, retrograde passage of a ureteral stent. An antegrade approach can allow for stent passage when this cannot be done in a retrograde fashion.[21] Chang and colleagues[20] report successful resolution of ureteral fistula with an antegrade stent approach in 10 of 12 patients and recommend a stent diameter of 8 to 12 Fr to minimize the risk of subsequent ureteral stricture formation. If the stent cannot be passed by a retrograde or antegrade approach, a combined approach can be performed. Ureteroscopic assistance may be invaluable[22] and can be used in a "cut to the light" approach if the ureteral lumen is completely occluded.[23] This can be done with ureteroscopes proximal and distal to the level of the occlusion. If access to the kidney has yet to be obtained, this can be done with the patient in the prone split-leg position.[23] However, if access to the kidney has already been obtained and a percutaneous nephrostomy tube is in place, this can be done with the patient in a modified flank position to allow for simultaneous retrograde and antegrade approaches. Stents have been placed with passage of a wire from above through the strictured proximal segment and then retrieval from below with a ureteroscope; this technique requires only one ureteroscope and one surgeon, compared with cutting to the light, which is a two-surgeon procedure.[24] Fluoroscopy should be used, and after continuity is reestablished, the strictured segment should be incised proximal and distal to the lesion. All of these techniques were successful with strictures less than 2 cm long, and they should be performed by surgeons comfortable with the various endoscopic techniques that may be required.

SURGICAL THERAPY

Open surgical intervention is indicated for patients who cannot be stented or in those who have failed attempts at minimally invasive therapy. How to define a failure of conservative therapy has not been addressed in the literature. It is hard to imagine a ureterovaginal fistula spontaneously healing if leakage continues after a stent is in good position, and most fistulas that heal with drainage alone do so within 4 to 8 weeks after stent placement.[19] After it is clear that open surgery will be required, there is no reason to wait. Patients are bothered by the constant urinary leakage that occurs with this fistula, and evidence supports the success of early surgical intervention.[7,25,26] Surgical options include ureteroureterostomy, ureteroneocystostomy (often with a psoas hitch ureteral reimplant or Boari flap), ileal ureter, transureteroureterostomy, and nephrectomy.

Surgical tenets that have been recommended in the past when repairing a ureterovaginal fistula include the sacrifice of all abnormal ureter, no attempt to stay extraperitoneal, reestablishment of continuity between the ureter and bladder, and adequate postoperative drainage.[25] Excision of the affected segment of ureter and ureteroureterostomy is rarely indicated. The injury tends to be in the distal portion of the ureter, which does not lend itself to primary reanastomosis, and if done, it often results in postoperative ureteral stricture.

The most commonly performed intervention for the treatment of the ureterovaginal fistula is a ureteroneocystostomy. This allows for the injured distal area to be bypassed, obviating the need for to localize and dissect the injured portion of the ureter.

The method of ureteroneocystostomy depends on the level of ureteral injury or fistula, the level at which healthy ureter is found distally, and the degree of bladder mobility. Most patients can be managed with a psoas hitch ureteral reimplant (Fig. 84-2). This allows a tension-free anastomosis in most patients, with the psoas hitch also decreasing any risk of ureteral kinking caused by excessive bladder mobility. Goodwin and Scardino[7] had a success rate of 100% for the 16 patients in their series treated with ureteroneocystostomy. Bleland[25] found that reimplantation of the ureter with an anti-refluxing technique is preferable; however, a

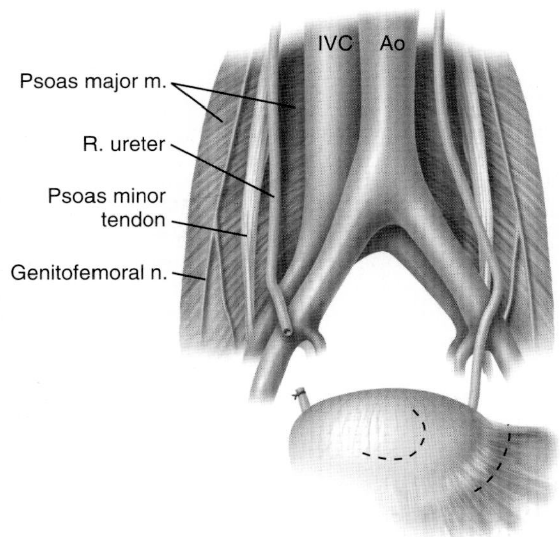

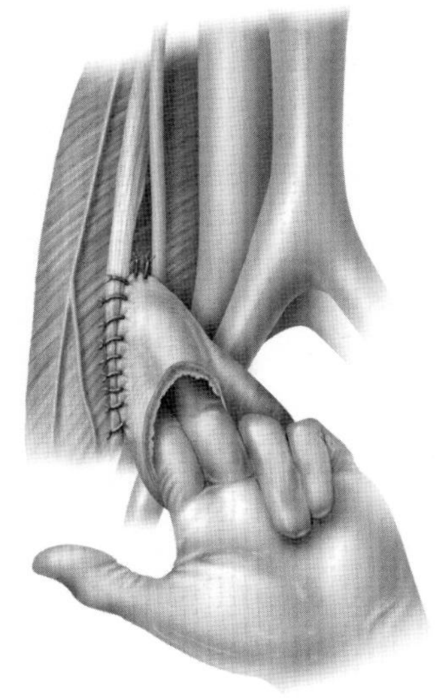

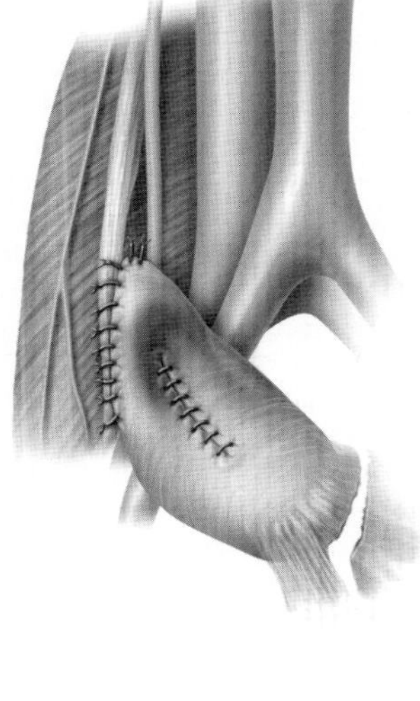

Figure 84-2 Diagram of psoas hitch ureteral reimplantation. **A,** The lateral attachments to the bladder on the side contralateral to the reimplantation side are taken down to allow for sufficient bladder mobility. A wide-based anterior bladder wall flap is made with a curvilinear incision. **B,** The bladder wall is mobilized superiorly. The posterosuperior bladder wall is secured to the psoas tendon with interrupted sutures. **C,** The ureter is reimplanted, and the bladder incision is closed. (Modified from Payne CK, Raz S: Ureterovaginal and related fistulae. In McAninch JW [ed]: Traumatic and Reconstructive Urology. Philadelphia, WB Saunders, 1996.)

ureteroneocystostomy without tunneling is unnecessary and is equally successful in regard to fistula resolution.[27,28] More important than an anti-refluxing anastomosis is a tension-free connection between the bladder and the ureter. Extra bladder mobility can be achieved with a psoas hitch by taking down the lateral attachments to the bladder on the side contralateral to the hitch.

If a psoas hitch is unable to reach the ureter without tension, another option is a Boari flap. One indication for using this primarily is the finding of a pelvic abscess at the time of reconstruction. The Boari flap allows the surgeon to perform the ureteroneocystostomy away from the infected field of the abcess.[11] More complex procedures such as transureteroureterostomy, renal autotransplantation and ileal ureter interposition are available, but they are rarely needed for this patient population.

Nephrectomy is a last resort and is rarely needed for these patients, as shown in the evolution of literature. Lee and Symonds[29] reported a nephrectomy rate of 48% in their review, with most nephrectomies performed before 1958. This rate decreased to 5% as reported by Goodwin and Scardino in 1980,[7] and in current series, the rate is essentially zero among patients able to maintain appropriate follow-up.[10,19]

CONCLUSIONS

Ureterovaginal fistula is a rare complication of pelvic surgery. It is most commonly seen after total abdominal and radical hysterectomy. Because symptoms of ureteral injury can be vague in the initial postoperative period, the physician should remain alert to the possibility, especially in patients with new-onset incontinence 1 to 2 weeks after pelvic surgery. The diagnosis can be made radiographically with IVU or retrograde pyelography or though the use of the double-dye test. Initial therapy with stent placement allows healing of the fistula in a high percentage of patients. If this is not possible, definitive therapy can be achieved with ureteroneocystostomy, usually in conjunction with a psoas hitch, with a high rate of success.

References

1. Mattingly RF, Borkowf HI: Acute operative injury to the lower urinary tract. Clin Obstet Gynaecol 5:123, 1978.
2. Symmonds RE: Ureteral injuries associated with gynecologic surgery: Prevention and management. Clin Obstet Gynecol 19:623, 1976.
3. Meirow D, Moriel EZ, Zilberman M, Farkas A: Evaluation and treatment of iatrogenic ureteral injuries during obstetric and gynecologic operations for nonmalignant conditions. J Am Coll Surg 178:144, 1994.
4. Hosseini SY, Roshan YM, Safarinejad MR: Ureterovaginal fistula after vaginal delivery. J Urol 160:829, 1998.
5. Binstock MA, Semrad N, Dubow L, Watring W: Combined vesicovaginal-ureterovaginal fistulas associated with a vaginal foreign body. Obstet Gynecol 76:918, 1990.
6. Kumar RV, Kumar A, Banerjee GK: Ureterovaginal fistula: An unusual complication of stone fragments after extracorporeal shock wave lithotripsy in situ. J Urol 152:2096, 1994.
7. Goodwin WE, Scardino PT: Vesicovaginal and ureterovaginal fistulas: A summary of 25 years of experience. J Urol 123:370, 1980.
8. Wang PH, Lee WL, Yuan CC, et al: Major complications of operative and diagnostic laparoscopy for gynecologic disease. J Am Assoc Gynecol Laparosc 8:68, 2001.
9. Harkki-Siren P, Sjoberg J, Kurki T: Major complications of laparoscopy: A follow-up Finnish study. Obstet Gynecol 94:94, 1999.
10. Lask D, Abarbanel J, Luttwak Z, et al: Changing trends in the management of iatrogenic ureteral injuries. J Urol 154:1693, 1995.
11. Mandal AK, Sharma SK, Vaidyanathan S, Goswami AK: Ureterovaginal fistula: Summary of 18 years' experience. Br J Urol 65:453, 1990.
12. Raghavaiah NV: Double-dye test to diagnose various types of vaginal fistulas. J Urol 112:811, 1974.
13. O'Brien WM, Lynch JH: Simplification of double-dye test to diagnose various types of vaginal fistulas. Urology 36:456, 1990.
14. Peterson DD, Lucey DT, Fried FA: Nonsurgical management of ureterovaginal fistula. Urology 4:677, 1974.
15. Hulse CA, Sawtelle WW, Nadig PW, Wolff HL: Conservative management of ureterovaginal fistula. J Urol 99:42, 1968.
16. Millin T: The ureter, the gynaecologist and the urologist. Proc R Soc Med 42:37, 1949.
17. Dowling RA, Corriere JN Jr, Sandler CM: Iatrogenic ureteral injury. J Urol 135:912, 1986.
18. Schmeller NT, Gottinger H, Schuller J, Marx FJ: Percutaneous nephrostomy as primary therapy of ureterovaginal fistula. Urologe A. 22:108, 1983.
19. Selzman AA, Spirnak JP, Kursh ED: The changing management of ureterovaginal fistula. J Urol 153:626, 1995.
20. Chang R, Marshall FF, Mitchell S: Percutaneous management of benign ureteral strictures and fistulas. J Urol 137:1126, 1987.
21. Lang EK: Diagnosis and management of ureteral fistulas by percutaneous nephrostomy and antegrade stent catheter. Radiology 138:311, 1981.
22. Koonings PP, Huffman JL, Schlaerth JB: Ureteroscopy: A new asset in the management of postoperative ureterovaginal fistulas. Obstet Gynecol 80:548, 1992.
23. Lingeman JE, Wong MYC, Newmark JR: Endoscopic management of total ureteral occlusion and ureterovaginal fistula. J Endourol 9:391, 1995.
24. Tsai CK, Taylor FC, Beaghler MA: Endoscopic ureteroureterostomy: long-term follow-up using a new technique. J Urol 164:332, 2000.
25. Beland G: Early treatment of ureteral injuries found after gynecological injury. J Urol 118:25, 1977.
26. Blandy JP, Badenoch DF, Fowler CG, et al: Early repair of iatrogenic injury to the ureter or bladder after gynecological surgery. J Urol 146:761, 1991.
27. Kihl B, Nilson AE, Pettersson S: Uretero-neocystostomy in the treatment of postoperative uretero-vaginal fistula. Acta Obstet Gynecol 61:341, 1982.
28. Murphy DM, Grace PA, O'Flynn JD: Ureterovaginal fistula: A report of 12 cases and review of the literature. J Urol 128:924, 1982.
29. Lee RA, Symmonds RE: Ureterovaginal fistula. Am J Obstet Gynecol 109:1032, 1971.

Chapter 85

URETHRAL DIVERTICULA

Eric S. Rovner

Diverticula of the female urethra present some of the most challenging diagnostic and reconstructive problems in female urology. These cases can be simultaneously fascinating and frustrating. Urethral diverticula have a bewildering variety of clinical manifestations, ranging from completely asymptomatic, incidentally noticed lesions identified on physical examination or radiographs to very debilitating, painful vaginal masses associated with incontinence, stones, or tumors. Anatomic variations between patients and in the location, size and complexity of these lesions ensure that each case is unique (Fig. 85-1).

Although described as early as the 19th century,[1] the modern era of diagnosing and treating female urethral diverticula began in 1956 with the advent of positive-pressure urethrography introduced by Davis and Cian.[2] Over the next several years, there was a dramatic increase in number of cases of urethral diverticula reported in the literature. Davis and Telinde's[3] series of 121 cases published in 1958 approximately doubled the number of cases reported during the previous 60 years. Development of adjuvant imaging techniques such as ultrasound and magnetic resonance imaging (MRI) during the past 3 decades has contributed greatly to understanding of urethral diverticula. With the expanding use of these imaging modalities, the diagnosis and evaluation of this condition continues to evolve. After the diagnosis is confirmed, definitive therapy often consists of operative excision and reconstruction. Successful surgical excision and reconstruction requires a detailed knowledge of the relevant operative anatomy, adherence to basic surgical tenets, and an ability to be creative and sometimes even improvisational in the operating room.

ANATOMY OF THE FEMALE URETHRA

The normal female urethra is a musculofascial tube approximately 3 to 4 cm long. It extending from the bladder neck to the external urethral meatus, and it is suspended from the pelvic side wall and pelvic fascia (i.e., tendinous arc of the obturator muscle) by a sheet of connective tissue called the urethropelvic ligament. The urethropelvic ligament is composed of two layers of fused pelvic fascia that extend toward the pelvic side wall bilaterally (Fig. 85-2). This structure can be considered to have an abdominal side (i.e., endopelvic fascia) and a vaginal side (i.e., periurethral fascia). Within and between these two leaves of fascia lies the urethra.

The urethral lumen is lined by an epithelial layer that is a transitional cell type proximally and a nonkeratinized stratified squamous cell type distally. The urethra can be considered to be a rich, vascular, spongy cylinder surrounded by an envelope of consisting of smooth and skeletal muscle and fibroelastic tissue.[4] Within the thick, vascular lamina propria-submucosal layer are the periurethral glands (Fig. 85-3). These tubuloaveolar glands exist over the entire length of the urethra posterolaterally, but they are most prominent over the distal two thirds, with most glands draining into the distal one third of the urethra. Skene's glands are the largest and most distal of these glands. These glands drain outside the urethral lumen, lateral to the urethral meatus. Most acquired female urethral diverticula originate from pathologic processes involving the periurethral glands.

The urethra has several muscular layers: an internal longitudinal smooth muscle layer, an outer circular smooth muscle layer, and a skeletal muscle layer. The skeletal muscle component spans much of the length of the urethra but is more prominent in the middle third. It has a U-shaped configuration and is deficient dorsally. Ventral to the urethra but separated from it by the periurethral fascia lies the anterior vaginal wall.

Arterial inflow to the urethra derives from two sources. The proximal urethra has a similar blood supply as the adjacent bladder, whereas the distal urethra derives its blood supply from

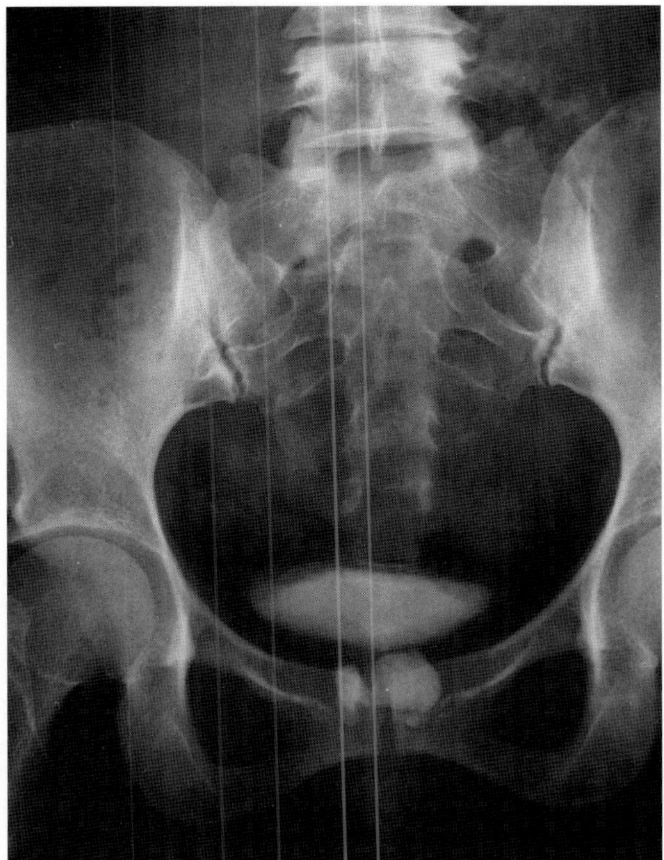

Figure 85-1 The postvoid film after voiding cystourethrography demonstrates a collection of contrast below the bladder that suggests a urethral diverticulum.

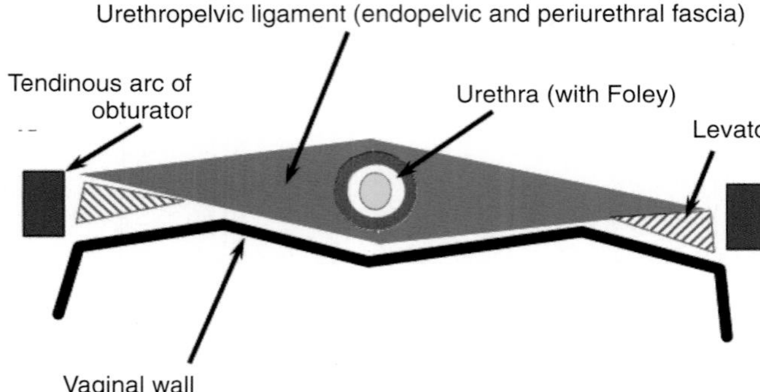

Figure 85-2 Representative anatomy of the mid-urethra in a coronal plane.

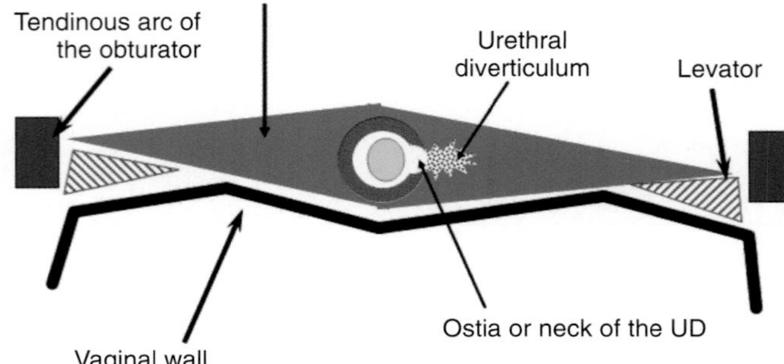

Figure 85-4 Diagram of a urethral diverticulum. The urethral diverticulum forms within and between the layers of the urethropelvic ligament.

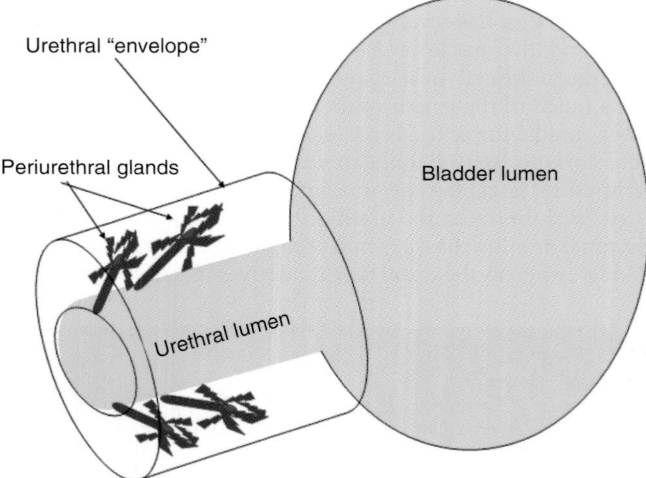

Figure 85-3 Periurethral glands are located within the submucosa of the urethra deep to the muscular envelope. They drain distally but arborize proximally.

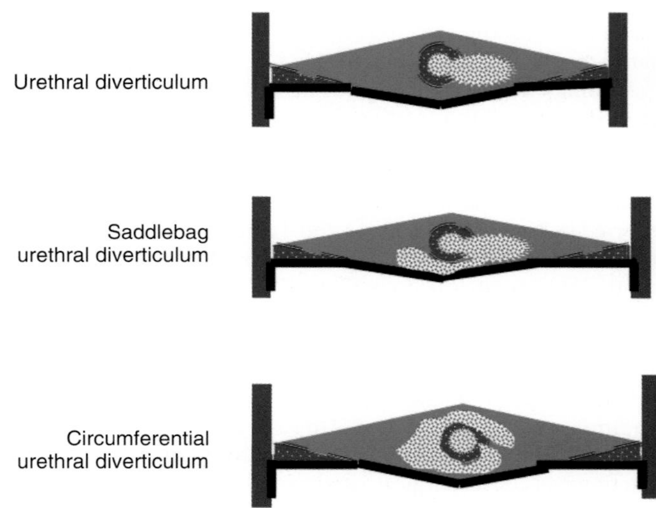

Figure 85-5 Different morphologies of urethral diverticula may exist.

the terminal branches of the inferior vesical artery through the vaginal artery, which runs along the superior lateral aspect of the vagina. Lymphatic drainage of the female urethra is to the sacral lymph nodes, internal iliac nodes, and inguinal lymph nodes. Innervation to the female urethra is from the pudendal nerve (S2 to S4), and afferents from the urethra travel by means of the pelvic splanchnic nerves.

URETHRAL DIVERTICULA

Pathophysiology and Etiology

As conceptualized by Raz and colleagues,[4] a urethral diverticulum represents an epithelialized cavity dissecting within the confines of the fascia of the urethropelvic ligament. This defect is often an isolated cystlike appendage with a single, discreet connection to the urethral lumen, called the neck or ostia (Fig. 85-4). However, complicated anatomic patterns may exist, and in certain cases, the urethral diverticula may extend partially (i.e., saddlebag urethral diverticula) around the urethra, anterior to the urethra,[5] or circumferentially about the urethra (Fig. 85-5).[6]

The exact origin of urethral diverticula is unknown. A major debate in the earlier part of the 20th century focused on whether urethral diverticula were congenital or acquired lesions.[7-9] Although this condition exists in children, it may represent a different clinical entity from adult female urethral diverticula. Scattered reports of congenital urethral diverticula in female infants have been described.[10] Marshall[11] reported five cases of urethral diverticula in young females, and three diverticula underwent spontaneous regression. Congenital anterior urethral diverticulum is a well-described entity in boys,[12-14] but this is considered to be a different clinical entity from urethral diverticula in the female. Congenital Skene's glands cysts have been reported[15,16] but are considered to be rare. Diverticula in the pediatric population have been attributed to a number of congenital anomalies, including an ectopic ureter draining into a Gartner's duct cyst and a form fruste of urethral duplication.[17-19] Most urethral diverticula are likely to be acquired and are diagnosed in female adults. In two large series of urethral diverticula, there were no patients reported who were younger than 10 years old,[20,21] arguing against a congenital origin for these lesions. Although it is possible that there exists a congenital defect in patients that results in or represents a precursor to urethral diverticula that becomes symptomatic only later in life, it remains unproven.

There are many theories regarding the formation of acquired urethral diverticula. For many years, acquired urethral diverticula were thought to be most likely caused by trauma from vaginal childbirth.[22] It was postulated that mechanical trauma during vaginal delivery resulted in herniation of the urethral mucosa through the muscular layers of the urethra, with the subsequent development of a urethral diverticula. However, 20% to 30% of patients in some urethral diverticula series are nulliparous,[23,24] which may significantly discount parity as a risk factor. Trauma with forceps delivery, however, has been reported to cause urethral diverticula,[25] as has the endoscopic injection of collagen.[26]

The periurethral glands are the probable site of origin of acquired urethral diverticula.[4] Huffman's[27] anatomic work with wax models of the female urethra were critical to the early theories regarding the pathophysiology of urethral diverticula and the involvement of the periurethral glands. By reviewing 10-μm transverse sections, he refuted earlier anatomic descriptions of the glandular anatomy of the female. He characterized the periurethral glands as located primarily dorsolateral to the urethra, arborizing proximally along the urethra and draining into ducts located in the distal one third of the urethra (see Fig. 85-3). He found that periductal and interductal inflammation was common. In support of these observations and an infectious (acquired) cause of urethral diverticula, in more than 90% of urethral diverticula cases, the ostium is located posterolaterally in the middle or distal urethra, which corresponds to the location of the periurethral glands.[28,29]

Although there are probably other factors that facilitate the initiation, formation, or propagation of urethral diverticula, infection of the periurethral glands seems to be the etiologic factor in most cases. Peters and Vaughn[30] found a strong association between concurrent or previous infection with *Neisseria gonorrhea* and urethral diverticula. However, the initial infection and especially subsequent reinfections may be caused by a variety of organisms, including *E. coli,* other coliform bacteria, and vaginal flora.

Urethral diverticula have been historically attributed to recurrent infection of the periurethral glands with obstruction, suburethral abscess formation, and subsequent rupture of these infected glands into the urethral lumen. Continual filling and pooling of urine in the resultant cavity may result in stasis, recurrent infection, and eventual epithelialization of the cavity, forming a permanent urethral diverticulum. This concept was first popularized by Routh[31] more than a century ago, and it has become the most widely accepted theory regarding the formation of female urethral diverticula. Reinfection, inflammation, and recurrent obstruction of the neck of the cavity are theorized to result in patients' symptoms and in enlargement of the diverticulum. This proposed pathophysiology appears to adequately explain the anatomic location and configuration of most urethral diverticula and is supported by the work of Huffman.[27] However, Daneshgari and colleagues[32] have reported noncommunicating urethral diverticula diagnosed by MRI. Whether this lesion represents a forme fruste of urethral diverticula or simply an obstructed urethral diverticula ostium is unclear.

Raz and colleagues[4] formulated a modern hypothesis regarding the pathogenesis of urethral diverticula through extensive clinical experience with this entity, including the diagnosis, imaging, and surgical repair of urethral diverticula. These investigators propose that acquired urethral diverticula result from infection and obstruction of the periurethral glands. These glands are normally found in the submucosal layer of the spongy tissue of the distal two thirds of the urethra. Repeated infection and abscess formation in these obstructed glands eventually result in enlargement and expansion. Initially, the expanding mass displaces the spongy tissue of the urethral wall and then enlarges to disrupt the muscular envelope of the urethra. This results in herniation into the periurethral fascia. The enlarging cavity can then expand and dissect within the leaves of the periurethral fascia and urethropelvic ligament. This expansion occurs most commonly ventrally, resulting in the classic anterior vaginal wall mass palpated on physical examination in some patients with urethral diverticula. However, the lesions may also expand laterally or even dorsally about the urethra. Eventually, the abscess cavity ruptures into the urethral lumen, resulting in the communication between the urethral diverticula and the urethral lumen. An appreciation of the anatomy and pathophysiology of urethral diverticula is important in understanding the surgical approach to the excision and reconstruction of these lesions.

Prevalence

Moore[33] stated that urethral diverticula as an entity is "found in direct proportion to the avidity with which it is sought." Although no longer considered a rare lesion, fewer than 100 cases of urethral diverticula were reported in the literature before 1950. With the development of sophisticated imaging techniques, including positive-pressure urethrography in the 1950s, the diagnosis of urethral diverticula became increasingly common.

The true prevalence of female urethral diverticula is unknown, but it is reported to occur in up to 1% to 6% of adult females in some series. Determining the true prevalence of urethral diverticula would require appropriate screening and imaging of a large number of symptomatic and asymptomatic adult female subjects in a primary care setting, which has not been done. Bruning[34] found urethral diverticula in 3 of 500 female autopsy specimens. In 1967, Andersen reported the results of positive-pressure urethrography on 300 women with cervical cancer but without lower urinary tract symptoms and found urethral diverticula in 3%.[35] Aldridge[36] reported a prevalence of urethral diverticula in 1.4% of women presenting with incontinence and related symptoms. Stewart[37] found urethral diverticula in 16 of 40 highly symptomatic females investigated with positive-pressure urethrography. Endorectal coil MRI was performed on 140 consecutive female patients with lower urinary tract symptoms, and the incidence of urethral diverticula was approximately 10%.[38] However, this represented a series of symptomatic females at a tertiary referral center, which probably did not reflect the general population.

Some series have suggested a definite racial predilection, with blacks being as much as six times as likely to develop urethral diverticula as their white counterparts.[20] The reasons for this racial distribution is not well understood. It has not been confirmed in some modern case series, and it may reflect referral bias at the urban academic centers in the original reported series.[39]

Diverticular Anatomy

Most commonly, urethral diverticula represent an epithelialized cavity with a single connection to the urethral lumen. The size of

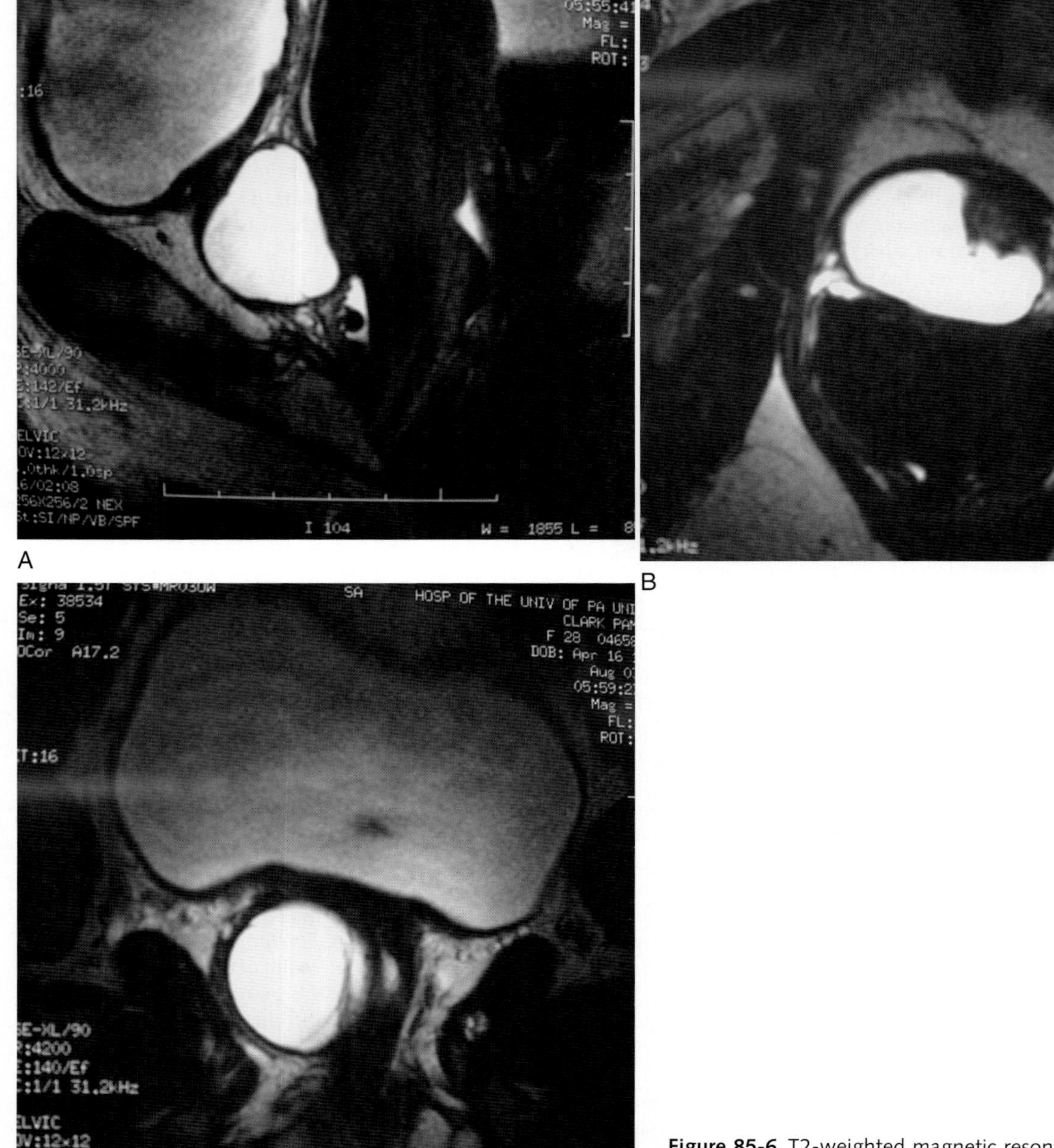

Figure 85-6 T2-weighted magnetic resonance images demonstrate a large urethral diverticulum extending to the trigone of the bladder in the sagittal **(A)**, axial **(B)**, and coronal planes **(C)**.

the lesion may vary from only a few millimeters to several centimeters. The size may vary over time because of inflammation and intermittent obstruction of the ostia with subsequent drainage into the urethral lumen.

The epithelium of urethral diverticula may be columnar, cuboidal, stratified squamous, or transitional. In some cases, the epithelium is absent, and the wall of the urethral diverticula consists of only fibrous tissue. These lesions are found within the periurethral fascia bordered by the anterior vaginal wall ventrally. Urethral diverticula are most often located in the sagittal plane, and they are centered at the level of the middle third of the urethra, with the luminal connection or ostia located posterolaterally. They may extend distally along the vaginal wall almost to the urethral meatus or proximally up to and beyond the bladder neck, underneath the trigone of the bladder (Fig. 85-6). A bewildering array of configurations can be identified on imaging and at surgical exploration (Table 85-1). In the axial plane, the urethral diverticula cavity may extend laterally along the urethral wall, and in some cases, they may extend around to the dorsal side of the urethra or wrap circumferentially around the entire urethra. Urethral diverticula may be bilobed (i.e., dumbbell shaped), extending across the midline in a so-called saddlebag configuration (see Fig. 85-5). Multiple loculations are not uncommon, and at least 10% of patients have multiple urethral diverticula at presentation. Various degrees of sphincteric compromise may exist because of the location of diverticulum relative to the

Table 85-1 Diverticular Morphology and Characteristics

Series	No. of Patients	Size Range (cm)	Axial Location (%)			Number (%)		Coronal Location	
			Anterior	Lateral	Posterior	Single	Multiple	Proximal	Mid
Lang and Davis[28]	108	N/A	N/A	N/A	N/A	N/A	N/A	11 (10)	50 (46)
Hoffman and Adams[45]	60	0.5-5.0	N/A	N/A	N/A	N/A	N/A	4 (7)	29 (48)
Pavlica et al[146]	47	0.5-6.0	3 (6)	6 (13)	38 (81)	41 (87)	6 (13)	3 (6)	39 (83)
Kim et al[147]	16	0.9-4.5	5 (31)*	N/A	11 (69)	N/A	N/A	4 (25)	10 (63)
Leach et al[99]	61	0.2-5.0	N/A	N/A	N/A	55 (90)	6 (10)	15 (25)	37 (60)

*Anterior and lateral.
N/A, not available.
Adapted from Westney OL, Leng WW, McGuire EJ: The Diagnosis and Treatment of Female Urethral Diverticulum, vol 20, lesson 37. Houston, TX, AUA Update Series, 2001, p 291.

Box 85-1 Signs and Symptoms of Urethral Diverticula

Symptoms
- Vaginal or pelvic mass
- Pelvic pain
- Urethral pain
- Dysuria
- Urinary frequency
- Postvoid dribbling
- Dyspareunia
- Urinary urgency
- Incontinence
- Urinary hesitancy
- Vaginal or urethral discharge
- Double voiding
- Sense of incomplete emptying

Signs
- Recurrent urinary tract infections
- Hematuria
- Vaginal or perineal tenderness
- Urinary retention
- Vaginal mass
- Urethral discharge with stripping of anterior vaginal wall

proximal and distal urinary sphincter mechanisms. This is a consideration for surgical repair.

Presentation

Most patients with urethral diverticula present between the third and seventh decade of life.[7,23,33,40,41] The presenting symptoms and signs of patients with urethral diverticula are protean (Box 85-1). The classic presentation of urethral diverticula has been described historically as the *three Ds*: dysuria, dyspareunia, and dribbling (postvoid). However, individually or collectively, these symptoms are neither sensitive nor specific for urethral diverticula. Although presentation is highly variable, the most common symptoms are irritative (e.g., frequency, urgency) lower urinary tract symptoms, pain, and infection.[20,21,30,42] Dyspareunia is reported by 12% to 24% of patients.[20,21] Approximately 5% to 32% of patients complain about postvoid dribbling.[20,23] Recurrent cystitis or urinary tract infection is a frequent presentation in one third of patients,[20,23] likely due to urinary stasis in the urethral diverticula. Multiple bouts of recurrent cystitis should alert the clinician to the possibility of a urethral diverticulum. Other complaints include pain, a vaginal mass, hematuria, vaginal discharge, obstructive symptoms or urinary retention, and stress or urge incontinence. Up to 20% of patients diagnosed with urethral diverticula may be completely asymptomatic. Patients may present with complaints of a tender or nontender anterior vaginal wall mass, which on gentle compression may reveal retained urine or purulent discharge through the urethral meatus. Although spontaneous rupture of these lesions is rare, urethrovaginal fistula may result under these circumstances.[43]

The size of the urethral diverticula does not correlate with symptoms. In some cases, very large urethral diverticula may result in minimal symptoms, and some urethral diverticula that are not palpable may result in considerable patient discomfort and distress. Symptoms may wax and wane and even resolve for long periods. The reasons for these exacerbations and remissions are poorly defined but may be related to periodic and repeated episodes of infection and inflammation.

Because many of the symptoms associated with urethral diverticula are nonspecific, patients may be misdiagnosed and treated for years for a number of unrelated conditions before the diagnosis of urethral diverticula is made. This may include therapies for interstitial cystitis, recurrent cystitis, vulvodynia, endometriosis, vulvovestibulitis, and other conditions. In one series of 46 consecutive women eventually diagnosed with urethral diverticula, the mean interval from onset of symptoms to diagnosis was 5.2 years.[44] In this series, women consulted with an average of nine physicians before the definitive diagnosis was made, despite the fact that 52% of women had a palpable mass on examination. This underscores the importance of a baseline level of suspicion and a thorough pelvic examination in female patients complaining of lower urinary tract symptoms or other symptoms that may be associated with urethral diverticula.

Evaluation and Diagnosis

The diagnosis and complete evaluation of urethral diverticula can be made with a combination of a thorough history; physical examination; appropriate urine studies, including urine culture and analysis; endoscopic examination of the bladder and urethra; and selected radiologic imaging. A urodynamic study may also be used in selected cases.

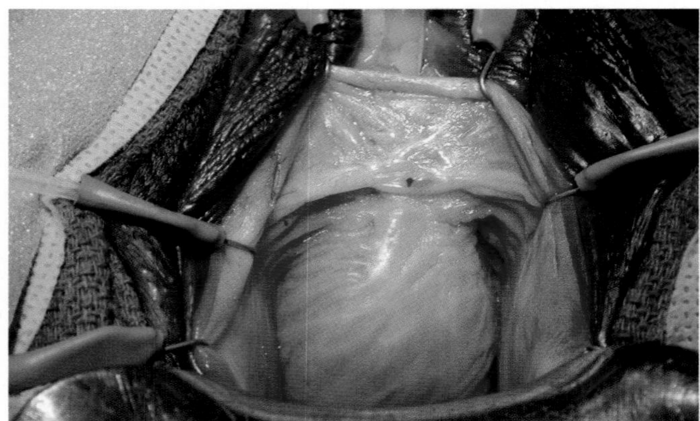

Figure 85-7 Large anterior vaginal wall mass. The urethral catheter is seen superiorly and a weighted vaginal speculum is seen inferiorly. Scott retractor hooks are seen exposing the anterior vaginal wall in this operating room photo.

Physical Examination

During physical examination the anterior vaginal wall should be carefully palpated for masses and tenderness. The location, size, and consistency of suspected urethral diverticula should be recorded. Most urethral diverticula are located ventrally over the middle and proximal portions of the urethra, corresponding to the area of the anterior vaginal wall 1 to 3 cm inside the introitus (Fig. 85-7). However, urethral diverticula also may be located anterior to the urethra or extend partially or completely around the urethral lumen. These particular configurations may have significant implications when undertaking surgical excision and reconstruction. Urethral diverticula may extend proximally toward the bladder neck. The urethral diverticula may produce distortion of the bladder outlet and trigone of the bladder on cystoscopy or on radiographic imaging, and special care should be taken during surgical excision and reconstruction because of concerns about intraoperative bladder and ureteral injury and the potential for development of postoperative voiding dysfunction and urinary incontinence. More distal vaginal masses or perimeatal masses may represent other lesions, including abnormalities of Skene's glands. The differentiation between these lesions sometimes cannot be made on the basis of a physical examination alone and may require additional radiologic imaging. A particularly hard anterior vaginal wall mass may indicate a calculus or cancer within the urethral diverticula, and it mandates further investigation. During physical examination, the urethra may be gently stripped or milked distally in an attempt to express purulent material or urine from within the urethral diverticula cavity. Although often described for the evaluation of urethral diverticula, this maneuver is not successful in producing the diagnostic discharge through the urethral meatus in most patients.[39]

The vaginal walls are assessed for atrophy, rugation, and elasticity. Poorly estrogenized, atrophic tissues are important to identify if surgical treatment is being considered. These tissues are often surgically mobilized and may be used for flaps during excision and reconstruction. The distal vagina and vaginal introitus are also assessed for capacity. These factors may influence surgical planning because a narrow introitus can make surgical exposure difficult and may mandate an episiotomy. During the physical examination, a provocative maneuver to elicit stress incontinence should be performed, and the presence or absence of vaginal prolapse should be assessed.

Urine Studies

Urinalysis and urine culture should be performed. The most common organism isolated in patients with urethral diverticula is *Escherichia coli*. However, other gram-negative enteric flora and *Neisseria gonorrhea*, *Streptococcus*, and *Staphylococcus* are often present.[3,45] A sterile urine culture does not exclude infection because these patients are often on antibiotic therapy at presentation. For patients with irritative symptoms or when a malignancy is suspected, urine cytology can be performed.

Cystourethroscopy

Cystourethroscopy is performed in an attempt to visualize the urethral diverticular ostia and to rule out other causes of the patient's lower urinary tract symptoms. A specially designed female cystoscope can be helpful in evaluating the female urethra. The short beak maintains the discharge of the irrigation solution immediately adjacent to the lens, which aids in distention of the relatively short (compared with the male) urethra, permitting improved visualization. It may also be advantageous to compress the bladder neck while simultaneously applying pressure to the diverticular sac with an assistant's finger. Luminal discharge of purulent material can often be seen with this maneuver or with simple digital compression of the urethral diverticula during urethroscopy. The urethral diverticular ostium is most often located posterolaterally at the level of the mid-urethra, but it can be very difficult to identify in some patients. The success rate in identifying a diverticular ostium on cystourethroscopy is highly variable and is reported to be between 15% and 89%.[20,23,39] Patients with urethral diverticula are often highly symptomatic, and endoscopic examination can be difficult to initiate or complete. A positive examination result may help in surgical planning, but the failure to locate an ostium on cystourethroscopy should not influence the decision to proceed with further investigations or surgical repair.

Urodynamics

For patients with urethral diverticula and urinary incontinence or significant voiding dysfunction, a urodynamic study can be helpful.[46-48] Urodynamics may document the presence or absence of stress urinary incontinence before repair. Approximately 50% of women with urethral diverticula are found to have stress urinary incontinence on urodynamic evaluation.[23,49] A video urodynamic study combines a voiding cystourethrogram and a urodynamic study, consolidating the diagnostic evaluation and decreasing the number of required urethral catheterizations during the patient's clinical workup. For patients undergoing surgery for urethral diverticula with coexistent, symptomatic stress urinary incontinence demonstrated on physical examination or by urodynamic study or for those found to have an open bladder neck on preoperative evaluation, concomitant anti-incontinence surgery can be offered. Many investigators have described successful concomitant repair of urethral diverticula and stress incontinence in the same operative setting.[23,49-51] Alternatively, on urodynamic evaluation, a small number of patients may have evidence of bladder outlet obstruction due to the obstructive or mass effects of the urethral diverticula on the urethra. Stress urinary incontinence may coexist with obstruction,[52] but both conditions can be treated successfully with a carefully planned and executed operation. Urethral pressure profilometry has also been used by some physicians to assess or diagnose patients with urethral diverticula by noticing a biphasic pattern at the level of the lesion during the study.[47,48,53]

Imaging

Critically important to the success of surgical treatment of female urethral diverticula is high-quality preoperative imaging. Along with its utility as a diagnostic entity, radiologic imaging should provide an accurate reflection of the anatomy of the urethral diverticulum, including its relationship to the proximal urethra and bladder neck.

Several imaging techniques have been applied to the study of female urethral diverticula, and no single study can be considered the gold standard for this purpose. Each technique has relative advantages and disadvantages, and the ultimate choice of diagnostic study in many centers depends on several factors, including local availability, cost, and the experience and expertise of the radiologist. Available techniques for the evaluation of urethral diverticula include double-balloon positive-pressure urethrography (PPU), voiding cystourethrography (VCUG), intravenous urography (IVU), ultrasonography, and magnetic resonance imaging (MRI) with or without an endoluminal coil (eMRI).

Positive-Pressure Urethrography, Voiding Cystourethrography, and Intravenous Urography

Classically, double-balloon PPU had been considered to be the best study for the diagnosis and assessment of female urethral diverticula.[2,21,23,54] With this technique, a highly specialized catheter with two balloons separated by several centimeters is inserted into the female urethra (Fig. 85-8). This catheter contains a channel within the catheter that exits through a side hole between the two balloons. One balloon is positioned adjacent to the external urethral meatus, and the other balloon is situated at the bladder neck. Both balloons are inflated, sealing the urethral lumen. Contrast is then infused through the channel under slight pressure, distending the urethral lumen between the two balloons and forcing contrast into the urethral diverticula, thereby opacifying the cavity. This highly specialized study provides outstanding images of the urethra and urethral diverticula, and unlike VCUG, it does not depend on the patient successfully voiding during the study. However, PPU is not widely performed clinically. It is a complicated study requiring a very specific type of modified urethral catheter and expertise in the performance and interpretation of the study by the radiologist. It is invasive, requiring catheterization of the urethra, and in the setting of acute inflammation commonly seen with female urethral diverticula, it can cause considerable patient discomfort and distress. Noncommunicating urethral diverticula[32] and loculations within existing urethral diverticula cannot be visualized with PPU because the contrast does not enter and fill these areas in the absence of a connection to the urethral lumen.

As an alternative to PPU, VCUG may provide excellent imaging of urethral diverticula (Fig. 85-9). It is widely available and is a familiar diagnostic technique to most radiologists. Sensitivity for urethral diverticula with this technique varies from 44% to 95%.[23,55] After a scout film, the bladder is filled through a urethral catheter. The catheter is removed at bladder capacity, and images of the bladder and bladder neck are obtained. Ideally, voiding images are obtained in the anteroposterior, lateral, and oblique projections. A postvoid film is obtained. Although VCUG is probably the most widely used study for the diagnosis and evaluation of patients with known or suspected urethral diverticula, it has several limitations. VCUG is invasive, requiring catheterization of the urethra for bladder filling. This can result in considerable patient discomfort and may risk translocating bacteria from an infected urethral diverticulum into the bladder during catheterization, resulting in bacterial cystitis. This is also a risk of PPU. Successful imaging of the urethral diverticulum occurs only during the voiding phase of the VCUG with subsequent filling of the urethra. Occasionally, only the postvoid film demonstrates the urethral diverticulum.[56-58] Not uncommonly, patients are somewhat inhibited or otherwise unable to void during VCUG for a variety of reasons, including pain from the initial urethral catheterization. Unfortunately, in the absence of contrast entering the urethra, opacification of the diverticulum does not occur. An inability to generate an adequate flow rate

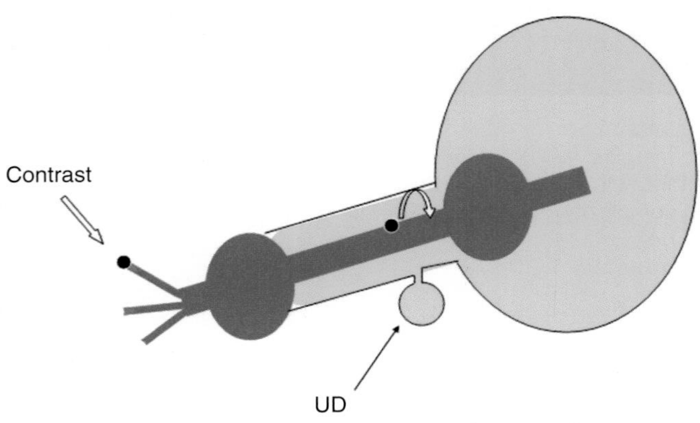

Figure 85-8 Diagram of a double-balloon catheter. Balloons are inflated at the bladder neck and external urethral meatus. Contrast is then infused through an additional port, and it exits through a side hole between the balloons, distending the urethral lumen under pressure and filling the urethral lumen and diverticulum (UD).

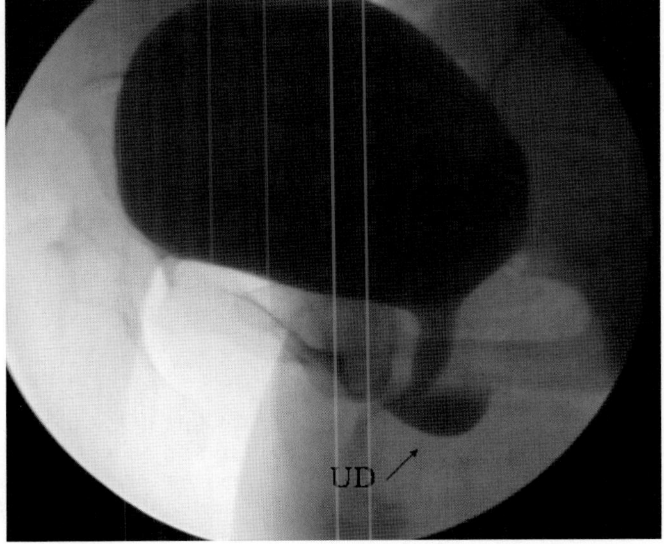

Figure 85-9 A voiding cystourethrogram demonstrates a urethral diverticulum (UD).

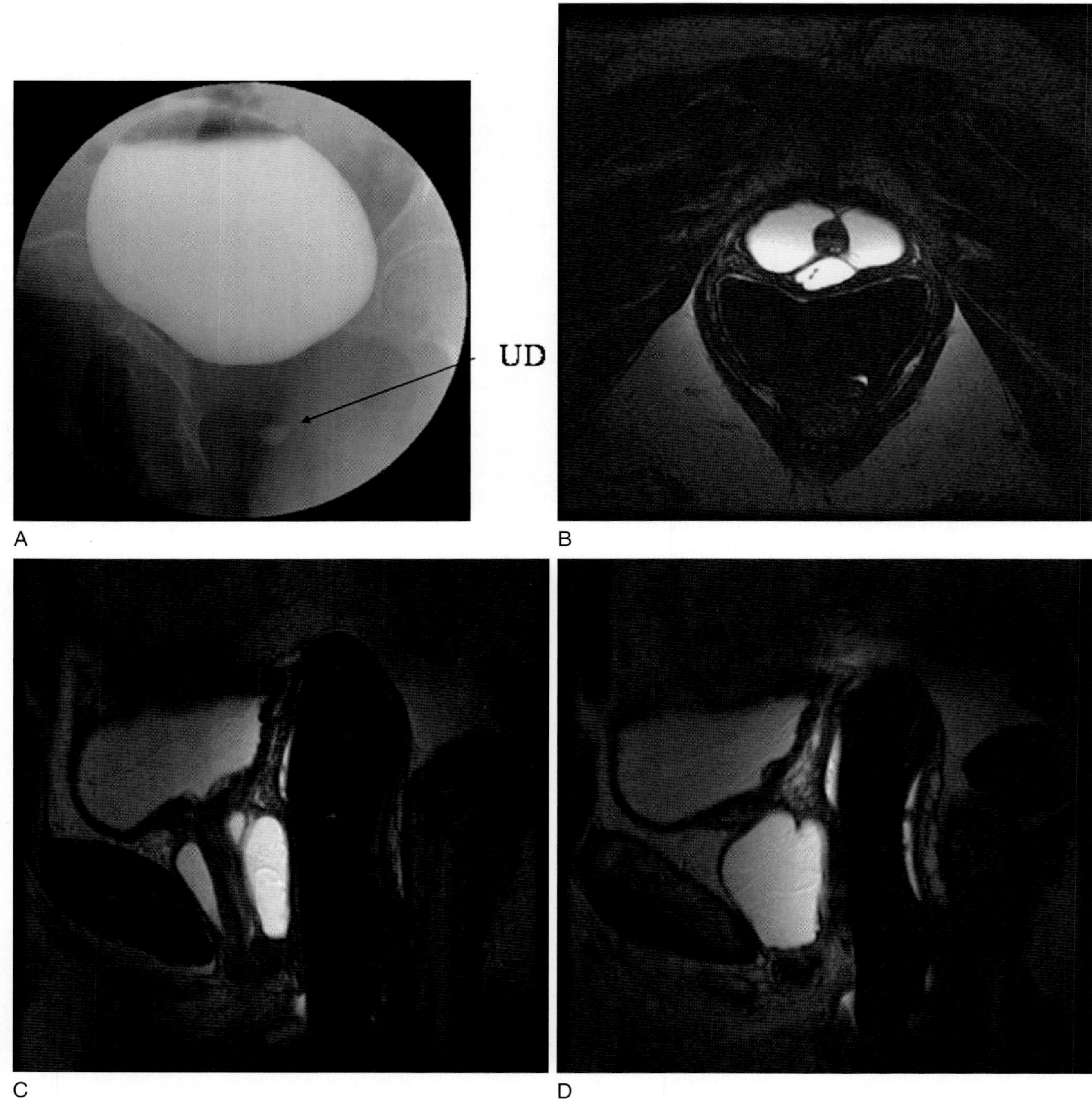

Figure 85-10 Voiding cystourethrography (VCUG) and magnetic resonance imaging (MRI) demonstrated a large, circumferential urethral diverticulum (UD). VCUG **(A)** shows poor opacification of the proximal urethra with suboptimal distention of the urethral diverticulum due to a poor voiding effort. Endoluminal MRI demonstrates the full extent and complexity of the lesion on the T2-weighted axial **(B),** midline sagittal **(C),** and parasagittal **(D)** images.

during the VCUG results in suboptimal filling of the urethral diverticulum and an underestimation of its size and complexity (Fig. 85-10). Some urethral diverticula may not opacify after a technically successful VCUG because of acute inflammation of the ostium or neck of the diverticulum or because the diverticulum does not otherwise communicate with the urethral lumen. These noncommunicating urethral diverticula exist within the urethropelvic ligament and can be successfully imaged with cross-sectioning techniques such as MRI.[32]

Three studies have compared VCUG with PPU and concluded that PPU is a more sensitive test for urethral diverticula than VCUG.[55,59,60] In one study of 32 patients, VCUG failed to demonstrate the urethral diverticula in 69% of patients, whereas PPU failed to demonstrate the lesion in only 6%.[55]

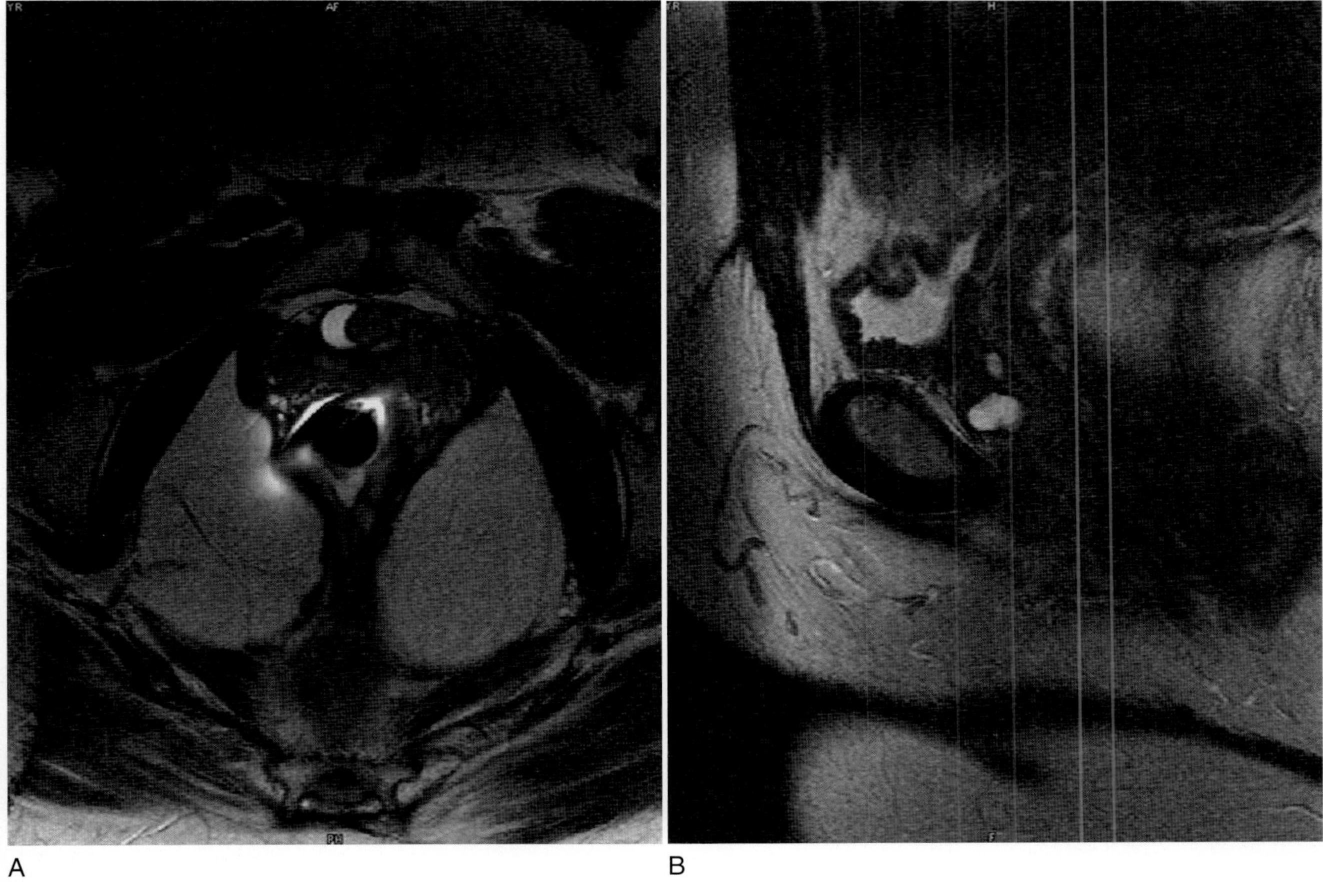

Figure 85-11 Surface coil, T2-weighted magnetic resonance imaging demonstrates a urethral diverticulum in the sagittal **(A)** and axial **(B)** planes.

IVU may be considered in patients in whom it is necessary to delineate the upper urinary tract or to rule out an ectopic ureterocele.[61] The postvoid film of the urogram can be helpful for the diagnosis of urethral diverticula in some patients.[56,57]

Ultrasound

Ultrasound has been advocated for the preoperative assessment of urethral diverticula.[62-71] Abdominal, transvaginal, translabial, and transurethral techniques have been described. Transvaginal imaging often provides information regarding the size and location of urethral diverticula. On ultrasonographic imaging, the urethral diverticulum appears as an anechoic or hypoechoic area with enhanced through transmission. Ultrasound is relatively noninvasive and does not expose the patient to radiation. Another significant advantage of ultrasound is that successful imaging of urethral diverticula does not require voiding. However, ultrasound may not produce detailed, high-resolution images that demonstrate precise surgical anatomy. This study can be somewhat operator dependent. Transurethral ultrasound techniques are evolving and may provide an incremental improvement in resolution. Similar to PPU and VCUG, the transurethral techniques are invasive because the ultrasound probe is placed per urethra and can cause patient discomfort and bacterial seeding of the lower urinary tract.

Magnetic Resonance Imaging

As an alternative to the radiologic investigations described previously, MRI permits relatively noninvasive, high-resolution, multiplanar imaging of urethral diverticula. Urethral diverticula appear as areas of decreased signal intensity on T1-weighted images compared with the surrounding soft tissues, and they have high signal intensity on T2-weighted images (see Fig. 85-10). Additional advantages of MRI compared with PPU and VCUG are that successful imaging of urethral diverticula is wholly independent of voiding and free from ionizing radiation. Surface-coil (Fig. 85-11)[72,73] and endoluminal techniques[38,60,74,75] have been described. Endoluminal imaging (eMRI) places the magnetic coil into a body cavity adjacent to the area of interest. This location produces an improved signal-to-noise ratio and high-resolution imaging of these areas.[74,75] For the evaluation of urethral diverticula, the coil is placed intravaginally or intrarectally (Fig. 85-12). Surface-coil MRI and eMRI appear to be superior to VCUG and PPU in the evaluation of urethral diverticula,[74,76,77] but the technology is expensive and not widely available. The few contraindications to MRI for urethral diverticula include metallic foreign body fragments, claustrophobia, and an inability to tolerate the endoluminal probe.

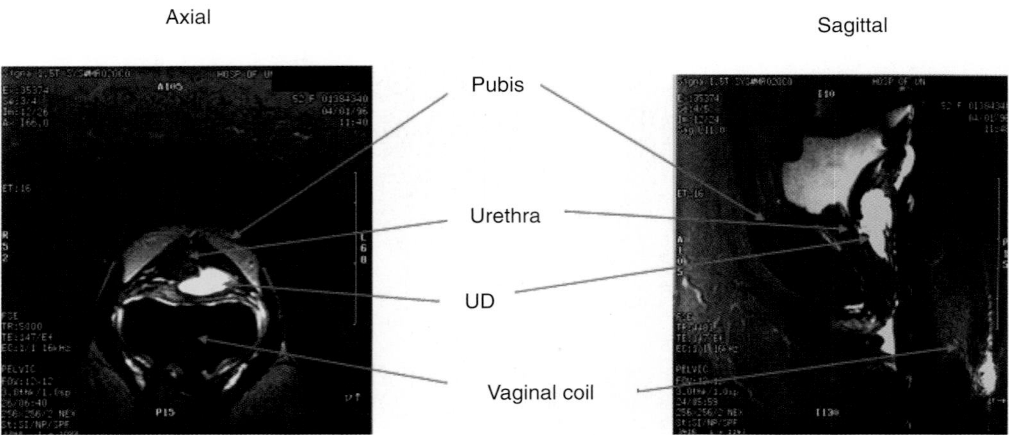

Figure 85-12 Sagittal and axial, T2-weighted endoluminal magnetic resonance images show the relevant anatomy of a patient with a urethral diverticulum (UD).

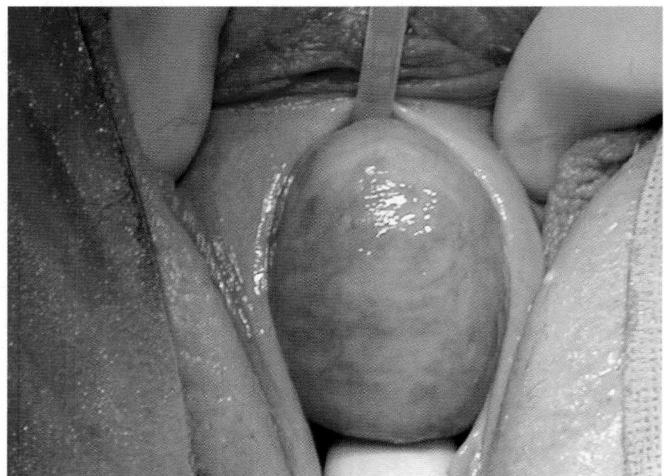

Figure 85-13 Large anterior vaginal wall leiomyoma.

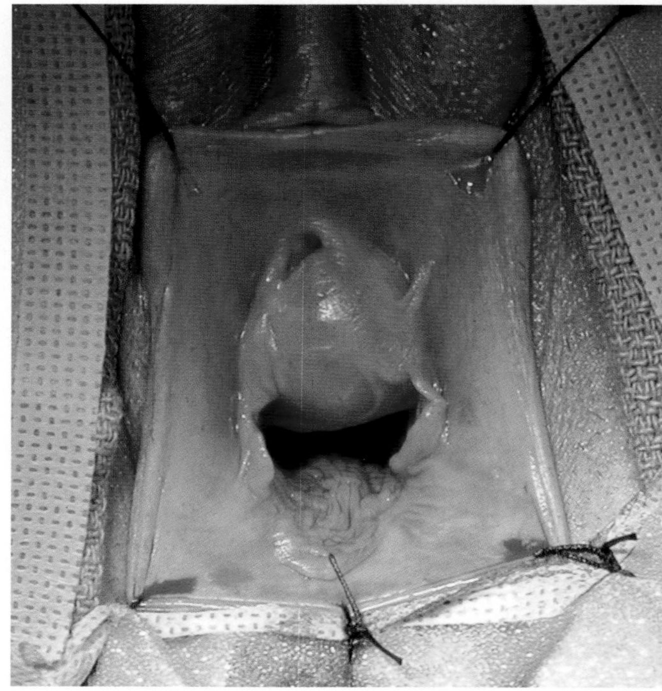

Figure 85-14 Skene's gland cyst in a 19-year-old woman. Notice the large periurethal mass with displacement of the urethral meatus.

Differential Diagnosis of Urethral Diverticula: Periurethral Masses Other Than Urethral Diverticula

Periurethral masses other than urethral diverticula comprise a wide spectrum of conditions that must be differentiated from each other and urethral diverticula. It may be possible to make a definitive diagnosis based on the history and physical examination alone; in other cases, judicious use of radiographic and cystoscopic studies is necessary to exclude urethral diverticula.

Vaginal Leiomyoma

Vaginal leiomyoma is a benign, mesenchymal tumor of the vaginal wall that arises from smooth muscle elements. It commonly manifests as a smooth, round mass on the anterior vaginal wall (Fig. 85-13). It is an uncommon lesion; approximately 300 cases have been reported in the literature.[78] In a series of 79 patients with periurethral masses, 4 (5%) were found to have leiomyoma.[79] These benign tumors were apparent on physical examination as freely mobile, nontender masses on the anterior vaginal wall. They may be misdiagnosed as urethral diverticula.[80] Symptoms, if they exist, are usually related to the size of the lesion and include a mass effect, obstruction, pain, and dyspareunia. They commonly present in the fourth to fifth decade. Like uterine leiomyomas, these lesions are usually estrogen dependent and have been demonstrated to regress during menopause.[81] Excision or enucleation[78] using a vaginal approach is often curative and is recommended to confirm the diagnosis, exclude malignant histology, and alleviate symptoms.

Skene's Gland Abnormalities

Skene's gland cysts and abscesses are similar lesions that are differentiated based on clinical findings (Fig. 85-14). Both lesions manifest as small, cystic masses just lateral or inferolateral to the urethral meatus. They may be lined with transitional or stratified squamous epithelium. Abscesses may be extremely tender and inflamed, and in some cases, purulent fluid can be expressed from the ductular orifice. Unlike urethral diverticula, these lesions do not communicate with the urethral lumen. Skene's gland cysts may be seen in neonatal girls and young to middle-aged female patients.[16] Symptoms may include dysuria, dyspareunia, obstruction, and pain. Differentiation from urethral diverticula can often be made on the basis of the physical examination, because these lesions are located relatively distally on the urethra, often distorting the urethral meatus, compared with urethral diverticula, which most commonly occur over the middle and proximal urethra. Various treatments for Skene's glands abnormalities have been described, including aspiration, marsupialization, incision and drainage and simple excision.

Adenocarcinoma arising in Skene's glands has been reported. Because of homology of these glands with the prostate, these patients may demonstrate elevated prostate-specific antigen (PSA) levels, which normalize with treatment.[82]

Gartner's Duct Cysts

Gartner's duct cysts represent mesonephric remnants and are found on the anterolateral vaginal wall from the cervix to the introitus. Because they are mesonephric remnants, they may drain ectopic ureters from poorly functioning or nonfunctioning upper-pole moieties in duplicated systems. They have been reported with single-system ectopia, although this is much less common in female patinets.[83,84] It is not clear what proportion of patients with Gartner's duct cysts have ipsilateral renal abnormalities, but upper tract evaluation is recommended. In contrast, approximately 6% of subjects with unilateral renal agenesis have a Gartner's duct cyst.[85] Up to 50% of patients with Gartner's duct cysts and renal dysplasia may also have ipsilateral müllerian duct obstruction.[86]

Treatment depends on symptoms and association with ectopic ureters. If the lesions are asymptomatic and are associated with a nonfunctioning renal moiety, they can be observed. Aspiration and sclerotherapy have been successful.[87] Simple excision or marsupialization has been recommended for symptomatic lesions. If the cyst is associated with a functioning renal moiety, treatment must be individualized.

Vaginal Wall Cysts

Vaginal wall cysts usually manifest as small, asymptomatic masses on the anterior vaginal wall.[88] They may arise from multiple cell types: mesonephric (Gartner's duct cysts), paramesonephric (müllerian), endometriotic, urothelial, or epidermoid (inclusion cyst) tissues. A specific diagnosis cannot be reliably made until the specimen is removed and examined by a pathologist. The histologic subtype is usually of little consequence, although epidermoid cysts are usually associated with previous trauma or vaginal surgery. Pradhan and Tobon[89] described the pathologic characteristics of 43 vaginal cysts removed from 41 women over a 10-year period. The derivation of the cyst was müllerian in 44%, epidermoid in 23%, and mesonephric in 11%. The others were Bartholin gland, endometriotic, and indeterminate types. As with other periurethral masses, they must be differentiated from urethral diverticula. Treatment is usually by simple excision in symptomatic patients.

Urethral Mucosal Prolapse

Urethral prolapse manifests as a circumferential herniation or eversion of the urethral mucosa at the urethral meatus. The prolapsed mucosa commonly appears as a beefy red, doughnut-shaped lesion that completely surrounds the urethral meatus. It may be asymptomatic or manifest with bleeding, spotting, pain, or urinary symptoms. It is commonly seen in two populations: postmenopausal women and prepubertal girls. Although thought to be more common in young African American girls, later series do not confirm this predilection.[90,91] In children, it is often causally related to a Valsalva maneuver or constipation. Eversion of the mucosa may occur because of a pathologically loose attachment between smooth muscle layers of the urethra.[92] The cause is much less clear for postmenopausal women, although it has been epidemiologically linked to estrogen deficiency.

Treatment may be medical or surgical. Medical treatment involves topical creams (e.g., estrogen, anti-inflammatory ointment) and sitz baths. Various surgical techniques have been described, including cauterization, ligation around a Foley catheter, and complete circumferential excision. Circumferential excision with suture reapproximation of the remaining urethral mucosa to the vaginal wall can be performed with few complications. Rudin and colleagues[91] reported outcomes for 58 girls with urethral prolapse. Medical treatment was initially successful in 20 patients, among whom there were five recurrences. The remaining 38 patients failed initial conservative management and underwent surgical excision, with four complications, including urethral stenosis in two. Jerkins and coworkers[93] found superior results in surgically treated patients compared with medical management or catheter ligation.

Urethral Caruncle

Urethral caruncle is an inflammatory lesion of the distal urethra that is most commonly diagnosed in postmenopausal women. It usually appears as a reddish, exophytic mass at the urethral meatus that is covered with mucosa. These lesions are often asymptomatic and identified incidentally on gynecological examination. When irritated, they may cause underwear spotting or become painful. Less commonly, they may cause voiding symptoms. They are etiologically related to mucosal prolapse. Chronic irritation contributes to hemorrhage, necrosis, and inflammatory growth of the tissue, which corresponds to the histology of excised lesions. If the lesion is atypical in appearance or behavior, excision may be warranted to exclude other entities. Intestinal metaplasia, tuberculosis, melanoma, and lymphoma have been reported to coexist with or mimic urethral caruncles.[94-98]

There is a paucity of literature regarding optimal treatment of urethral caruncle. Most urologists recommend initial conservative management with topical estrogen or anti-inflammatory creams and sitz baths. Large or refractory lesions may be managed with simple excision. The tip of the lesions should be grasped and traction employed to fully expose the base of the caruncle. The lesion can then easily be excised. If a large defect remains, the mucosa may be reapproximated with absorbable suture. In most instances, the urethral mucosa heals around a Foley catheter, which may be left in place for several days.

Classification of Urethral Diverticula

Although not widely adopted, a classification system for urethral diverticula has been proposed by Leach and associates.[99] This staging system for urethral diverticula, called the L/N/S/C3 classification system, is similar to that used for cancer staging and is based on several characteristics of urethral diverticula, including location, number, size, anatomic configuration, site of communication to the urethral lumen, and continence status of the patient. This system attempts to standardize description of urethral diverticula, but it has not been prospectively applied or validated by other investigators. Another proposed classification scheme uses the location of the urethral diverticula as the primary determinant of surgical approach, with distal lesions undergoing marsupialization and more proximal lesions undergoing excision and reconstruction.[40]

A classification system proposed by Leng and McGuire[100] divides urethral diverticula into two categories based on the presence or absence of a preserved periurethral fascial layer. In some patients with urethral diverticula who have undergone prior vaginal or urethral surgery, the periurethral fascial layer may be deficient, resulting in a pseudodiverticulum. These investigators suggest that the recognition of this anatomic configuration has important implications for surgical reconstruction. Patients may require additional reconstruction or interposition of a tissue flap or graft to buttress the repair and prevent recurrence or postoperative urethrovaginal fistula formation.

SURGICAL REPAIR OF FEMALE URETHRAL DIVERTICULA

Indications for Repair

Although often highly symptomatic, not all urethral diverticula mandate surgical excision. Some patients may be asymptomatic at presentation, and the lesion is incidentally diagnosed on imaging for another condition or incidentally identified on routine physical examination. Other patients may be unwilling or medically unable to undergo surgical removal. Very little is known regarding the natural history of untreated urethral diverticula. Whether these lesions will progress in size, symptoms, or complexity with time is unknown. For these reasons and because of the lack of symptoms in selected cases, some patients may not desire surgical therapy. However, there are many reports in the literature of carcinomas arising in urethral diverticula,[101-110] and it is possible that certain carcinomas arising in urethral diverticula are asymptomatic and may not be prospectively identified on radiologic imaging. Counseling and ongoing monitoring is necessary for patients who elect primary nonoperative management.

Symptomatic patients, including those with dysuria, refractory and bothersome postvoid dribbling, recurrent urinary tract infections, dyspareunia, and pelvic pain in whom the symptoms can be attributed to the urethral diverticula, may be offered surgical excision. Those with urethral diverticula and symptomatic stress urinary incontinence can be considered for a concomitant anti-incontinence procedure at the time of urethral diverticular excision (discussed later).

Techniques for Repair

Alternative Techniques

A variety of surgical interventions for urethral diverticula have been reported since 1805, when Hey[1] described transvaginal incision of the urethral diverticula and packing of the resulting cavity with lint. Approaches have included transurethral[20] and open[111,112] marsupialization, endoscopic unroofing,[113,114] fulguration,[115] incision and obliteration with oxidized cellulose[116] or polytetrafluoroethylene,[117] coagulation,[117] and excision with reconstruction. Most commonly, complete excision and reconstruction are performed as described subsequently. However, for distal lesions, a transvaginal marsupialization as described by Spence and Duckett[111,118] and Roehrborn[112] may reduce operative time, blood loss, and recurrence rate. During this procedure, care must be taken to avoid aggressively extending the incision proximally, which could result in vaginal voiding or potentially damage the proximal and distal sphincteric mechanism, resulting in stress urinary incontinence. This approach is probably applicable only to urethral diverticula in selected cases involving the distal one third of the urethra. It is not commonly performed.

Box 85-2 Principles of Transvaginal Urethral Diverticulectomy

- Mobilization of a well-vascularized anterior vaginal wall flap (or flaps)
- Preservation of the periurethral fascia
- Identification and excision of the neck of the urethral diverticulum or ostia
- Removal entire urethral diverticulum wall or sac (mucosa)
- Watertight urethral closure
- Multilayered, non-overlapping closure with absorbable suture
- Closure of dead space
- Preservation or creation of continence

Excision and Reconstruction

Excision and reconstruction is probably the most common surgical approach to urethral diverticula in the modern era. The principles of the urethral diverticulectomy operation have been well described (Box 85-2). There are a few issues about which some surgeons may disagree, including the type of vaginal incision (inverted U versus inverted T), whether it is necessary to remove the entire mucosalized portion of the lesion, and the optimal type of postoperative catheter drainage (urethra only versus urethra and suprapubic). These are, however, minor points, and they are addressed subsequently.

Complex urethral reconstructive techniques for the repair urethral diverticula have been described. Fall[119] described the use of a bipedicled vaginal wall flap for urethral reconstruction in patients with urethral diverticula and urethrovaginal fistula. Laterally based vaginal flaps have also been used as an initial approach to urethral diverticula.[120,121] Complex anatomic configurations may exist, and many novel approaches have been described for complicated, anteriorly located or circumferential lesions.[5,6,122] The technique described here is similar to that described by Leach and Raz[42] and based on earlier work by Benjamin and colleagues[123] and Busch and Carter.[124]

Preoperative Preparation

Prophylactic antibiotics can be used for a period preoperatively to ensure sterile urine at the time of surgery. Patients can also be encouraged to strip the anterior vaginal wall after voiding, thereby consistently emptying the urethral diverticulum and preventing urinary stasis and recurrent urinary tract infections. This may not be possible in those with noncommunicating urethral diverticula or in those who have significant pain related to the urethral diverticula. Application of topical estrogen creams for several weeks before surgery may be beneficial in some patients with postmenopausal atrophic vaginitis in improving the overall quality of the tissues with respect to dissection and mobilization. Preoperative parenteral antibiotics are often administered, especially for those with recurrent or persistent urinary tract infections.

Patients with symptomatic stress urinary incontinence can be offered simultaneous anti-incontinence surgery. Preoperative video urodynamics may be helpful in evaluating the anatomy of the urethral diverticula, assessing the competence of the bladder neck, and confirming the diagnosis of stress urinary incontinence. In patients with stress urinary incontinence and urethral diverticula, Ganabathi and coworkers[23] and Lockhart and associates[125] have described excellent results with concomitant needle bladder neck suspension in these complex cases. Pubovaginal fascial slings have been used in patients with urethral diverticula and stress urinary incontinence with satisfactory outcomes.[44,50,51]

Further complicating these cases may be associated symptoms such as pain, dyspareunia, voiding dysfunction, urinary tract infections, and urinary incontinence. These associated symptoms often are improved or eliminated with surgical repair. The importance of appropriate preoperative patient counseling regarding surgery and postoperative expectations of cure cannot be overemphasized.

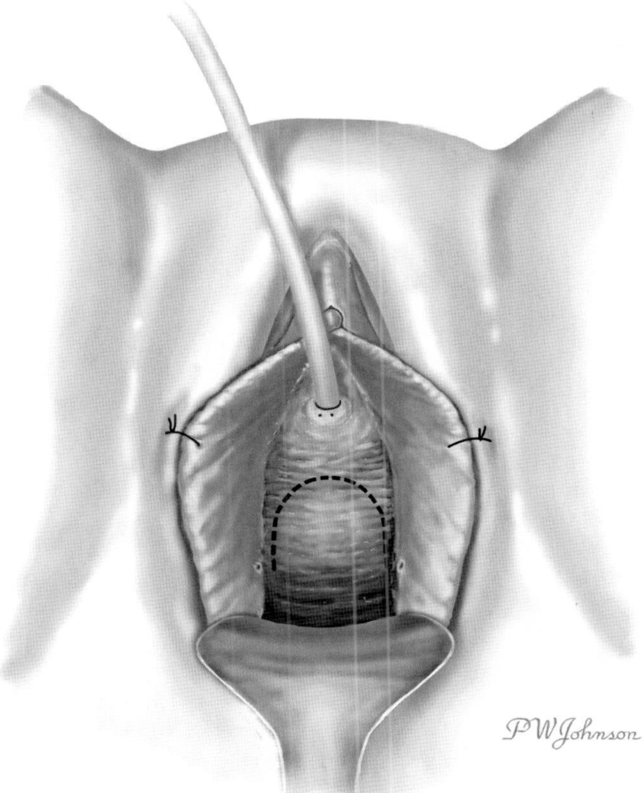

Figure 85-15 An inverted-U-shaped incision *(dashed line)* on the anterior vaginal wall. Retraction is aided by the use of Allis clamps and a ring retractor with hooks.

Procedure

The patient is placed in the lithotomy position with all pressure points well padded. The use of padded adjustable stirrups for the lower extremities greatly enhances operative access to the female perineum. A standard vaginal antiseptic preparation is applied. A weighted vaginal speculum and Scott retractor with hooks aid in exposure. A posterolateral episiotomy may be beneficial in some patients for additional exposure, although the mid-urethral (and therefore somewhat distal in the vaginal canal) location of most urethral diverticula usually precludes the need for this type of adjunctive procedure. A Foley catheter is placed through the urethra, and a suprapubic tube may be used for additional unobstructed postoperative urinary drainage. Often, a small-caliber urethral catheter is used during the case, and the placement of a suprapubic tube during the procedure ensures adequate postoperative urinary drainage. If desired, a suprapubic tube is placed at the start of the procedure using the Lowsley retractor or percutaneously under direct transurethral cystoscopic visual guidance. Placement of the suprapubic tube at the end of the case is not advisable because it requires traversing the fresh urethral suture line, which risks disruption of the repair.

An inverted U is marked out along the anterior vaginal wall, with the base of the U at the level of the distal urethra and the limbs extending to the bladder neck or beyond (Fig. 85-15). Care is taken to ensure that the limbs of the U are progressively wider proximally (toward the bladder neck) to ensure adequate vascularity at the distal lateral margins of the anterior vaginal wall flap. Unlike the inverted-T-shaped incision, the inverted-U-shaped incision provides excellent exposure laterally at the level of the midvagina, and it can be extended proximally as needed for lesions that extend beyond the bladder neck. Injectable saline can be infused along the lines of the incision to facilitate dissection. An anterior vaginal wall flap is created by careful dissection in the potential space between the vaginal wall and the periurethral fascia. The use of sufficient countertraction during this portion of the procedure is important in maintaining the proper plane of dissection. Care is taken to preserve the periurethral fascia and to avoid inadvertent entry into the urethral diverticula.

A distinct layer of periurethral fascia is usually interposed between the vaginal wall and the urethral diverticula. Preservation and later reconstruction of this layer is important to prevent recurrence, close dead space, and avoid urethrovaginal fistula formation postoperatively. Pseudo-diverticula have been described where this layer of tissue is considerably attenuated or even absent.[100] In these patients, an interpositional flap or graft such as a pubovaginal sling may be used for reconstruction.

The periurethral fascia is incised transversely (Fig. 85-16). Proximal and distal layers of periurethral fascia are carefully developed avoiding entrance into the urethral diverticula. The urethral diverticula is then grasped and dissected back to its origin on the urethra within the leaves of the periurethral fascia (Fig. 85-17). In many cases, it is necessary to open the urethral diverticulum to facilitate dissection from the surrounding tissues. The ostium or connection to the urethra is identified, and the walls of the urethral diverticulum are completely removed. Every effort should be made to remove the entire mucosalized surface of the urethral diverticulum to prevent recurrence.[23,65] This may involve removing small, adherent or inflamed portions of the urethral wall, especially in the ostial area (Fig. 85-18). All abnormal tissue in the area of the ostium should be removed if possible to ensure that no mucosal elements of the urethral diverticular wall remain, which can result in postoperative urine leakage and

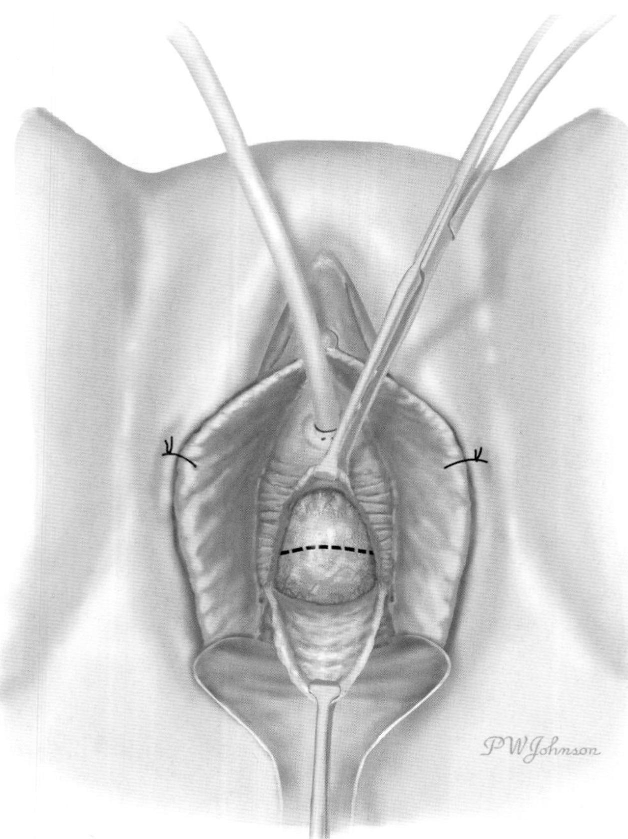

Figure 85-16 After reflection of the anterior vaginal wall, a transverse incision *(dashed line)* is made in the periurethral fascia.

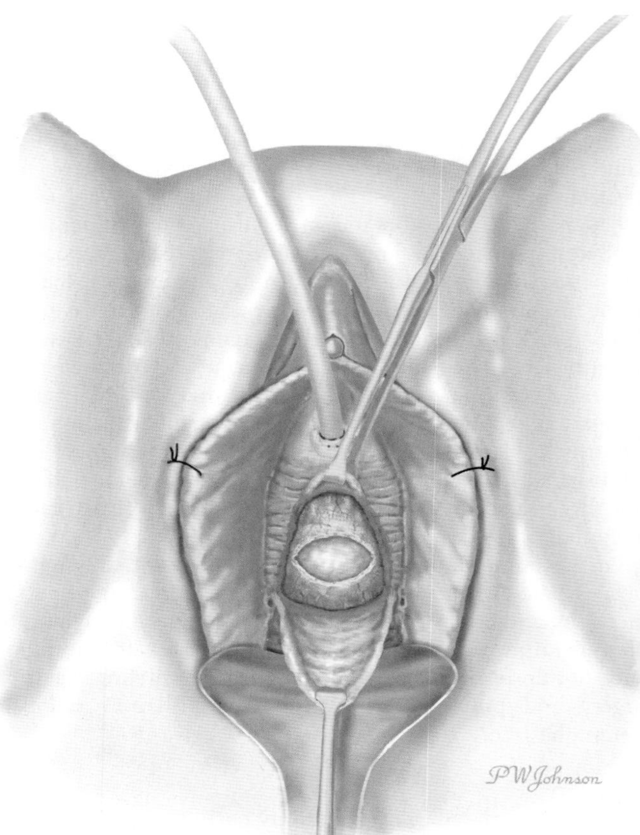

Figure 85-17 The periurethral fascia is incised and dissected from the underlying urethral diverticulum.

recurrence. Elaborate methods of identifying the full extent of the urethral diverticular cavity have been described, including catheterization of the urethral diverticulum with urinary[33,126] and Fogarty[127] catheters, packing the urethral diverticulum with gauze,[128] infusing and staining the urethral diverticulum with methylene blue,[8] and the use of silicone[129] or cryoprecipitate[130] to create a solid mass and ease dissection. However, these measures are mostly of historical interest and are usually unnecessary in modern urethral diverticular surgery.[23,39]

The Foley catheter is usually seen after complete excision of a urethral diverticulum (Fig. 85-19). The urethra can be reconstructed over as small as a 12-Fr Foley catheter without long-term risk of urethral stricture,[4] and it should be closed in a watertight fashion with absorbable suture (Fig. 85-20). The closure should be tension free. Uncommonly, a urethral diverticulum may extend circumferentially around the urethra and require segmental resection of the involved portion of the urethra and complex reconstruction.[6,131]

The periurethral fascial flaps are reapproximated with absorbable suture in a perpendicular orientation to the urethral closure line to minimize overlap and the risk of postoperative urethrovaginal fistula formation (Fig. 85-21). Care is taken to secure the periurethral fascial flaps to close all dead space.

If desired, a fibrofatty labial (Martius) flap can be harvested at this point and placed over the periurethral fascia as an additional layer of closure.[64] Indications for such a flap are not universally agreed on. However, in patients with poor-quality tissues or attenuated periurethral fascia or in whom significant inflammation is encountered intraoperatively, a well-vascularized adjuvant flap (e.g., Martius flap) may reduce the risk of wound breakdown and subsequent complications such as urethrovaginal fistula.

The anterior vaginal wall flap is then repositioned and reapproximated with absorbable suture (Fig. 85-22). This completes a three-layer closure (four layers if a Martius flap is used). An antibiotic-impregnated vaginal pack is placed.

Postoperative Care

Antibiotics are continued for 24 hours postoperatively. The vaginal packing is removed and the patient discharged home with closed urinary drainage. Antispasmodics are used liberally to reduce bladder spasms. Pericatheter VCUG is obtained at 14 to 21 days postoperatively. If there is no extravasation, the catheters are removed. If extravasation is seen, repeat pericatheter VCUG is performed weekly until resolution is documented. In most cases, extravasation resolves in several weeks with this type of conservative management.[132]

Complications

Careful adherence to the principles of transvaginal urethral diverticulectomy should minimize postoperative complications. Nevertheless, complications may arise (Box 85-3). One small series suggested that large diverticula (>4 cm) or those associated with a lateral or horseshoe configuration may be associated with

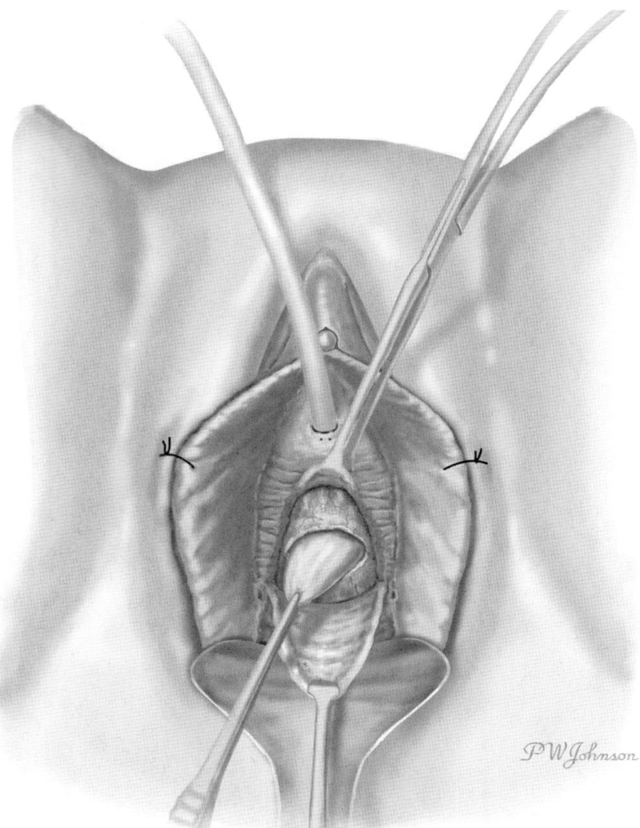

Figure 85-18 The urethral diverticulum sac is freed from the periurethral fascia.

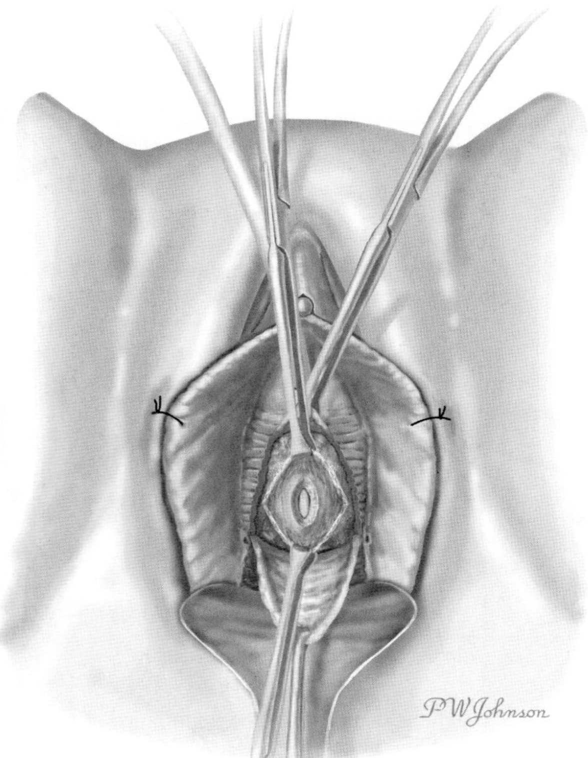

Figure 85-19 The urethral catheter is seen after complete excision of the urethral diverticulum sac.

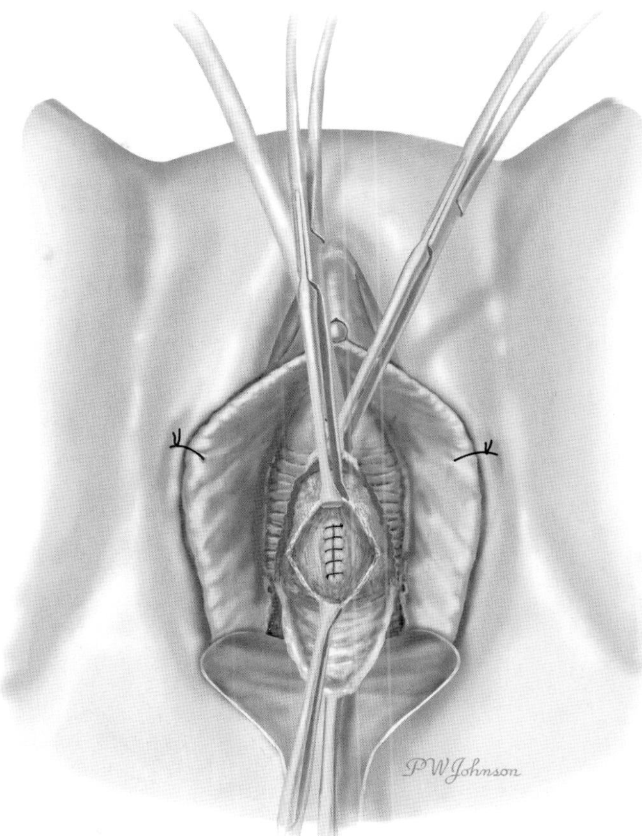

Figure 85-20 The urethra is closed with absorbable suture.

Box 85-3 Complications of Transvaginal Urethral Diverticulectomy

Urinary incontinence (1.7-16.1)*
Urethrovaginal fistula (0.9-8.3)
Urethral stricture (0-5.2)
Recurrent urethral diverticulum (1-25)
Recurrent urinary tract infection (0-31.3)
Other
  Hypospadias or distal urethral necrosis
  Bladder or ureteral injury
  Vaginal scarring or narrowing (e.g., dyspareunia)

*The range of reported incidence (%) is given within parentheses.
Adapted from Dmochowski R: Surgery for vesicovaginal fistula, urethrovaginal fistula, and urethral diverticulum. In Walsh PC, Retik AB, Vaughan ED Jr, Wein AJ (eds): Campbell's Urology, 8th ed. Philadelphia, WB Saunders, 2002, p 1214.

a greater likelihood of postoperative complications.[133] Common complications include recurrent urinary tract infections, urinary incontinence, and recurrent urethral diverticula.

Urethrovaginal fistula is a devastating complication of urethral diverticulectomy and deserves special mention. A fistula located beyond the sphincteric mechanism should not be associated with symptoms other than perhaps a split urinary stream and or vaginal voiding. As such, an asymptomatic distal urethrovaginal fistula may not require repair, although some patients may request repair. Conversely, a proximal fistula located at the

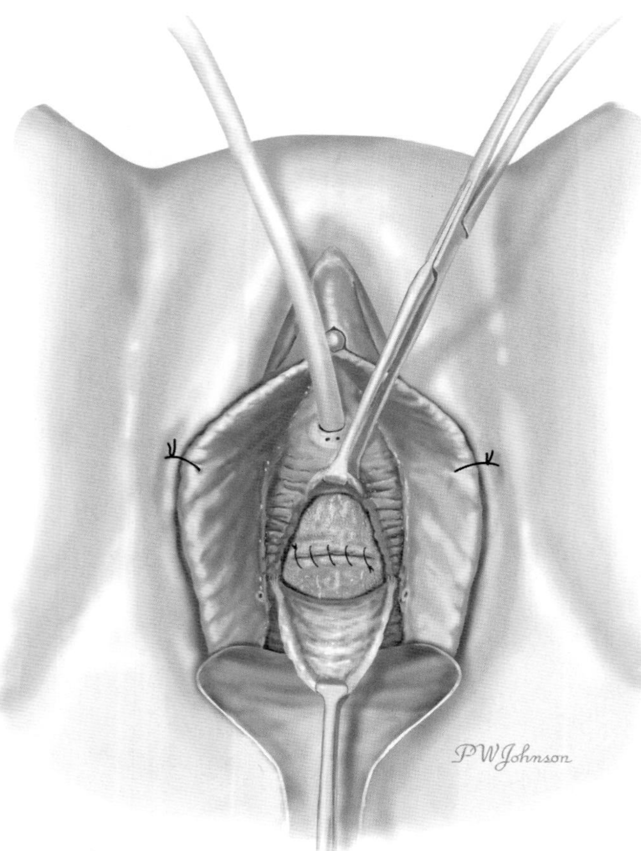

Figure 85-21 The periurethral fascia is closed with care to obliterate any dead space.

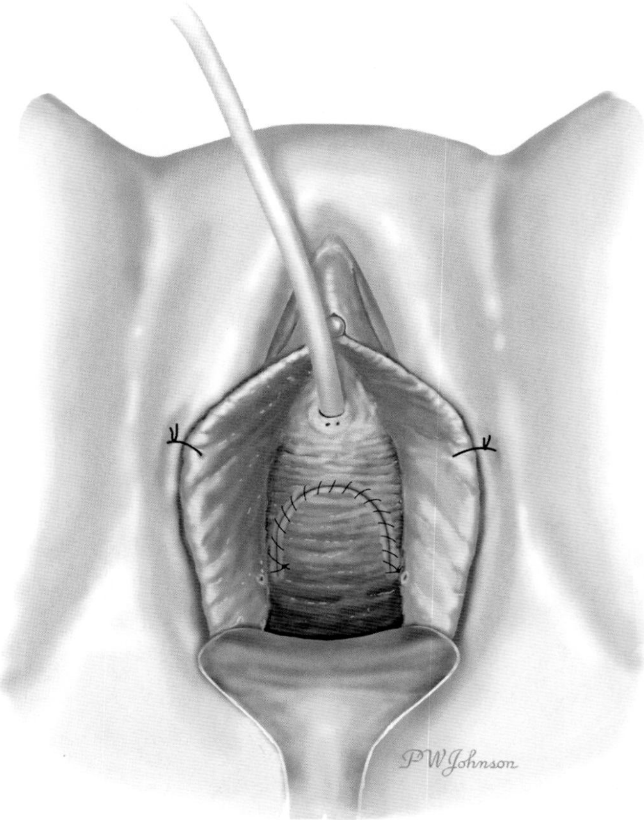

Figure 85-22 The anterior vaginal wall flap is advanced over the periurethral suture line and secured with running, interlocking absorbable suture.

bladder neck or at the mid-urethra in patients with an incompetent bladder neck will likely result in considerable symptomatic urinary leakage. These patients should undergo repair with the use of an adjuvant tissue flap such as a Martius flap to provide a well-vascularized additional tissue layer. The timing of the repair relative to the initial procedure is controversial. Meticulous attention to surgical technique, good hemostasis, avoidance of infection, preservation of the periurethral fascia (Fig. 85-23), a well-vascularized anterior vaginal wall flap, and multilayered closure with nonoverlapping suture lines should minimize the potential for postoperative urethrovaginal fistula formation.

Persistence of Symptoms after Urethral Diverticulectomy

Some patients have persistence or recurrence of their preoperative symptoms postoperatively. The finding of a urethral diverticulum after a presumably successful urethral diverticulectomy may occur as a result of a new medical problem (e.g., urinary tract infection), a new urethral diverticulum, or recurrence of the original lesion. A urethral diverticulum may recur because of incomplete removal of the urethral diverticulum, inadequate closure of the urethra or residual dead space, or other technical factors. Lee[134] identified a recurrent urethral diverticulum in 8 of 85 patients at follow-up of between 2 and 15 years from resection of the initial urethral diverticulum.[134] Repeat urethral diverticulectomy can be challenging due to altered anatomy, scarring, and the difficulty in identifying the proper anatomic planes.

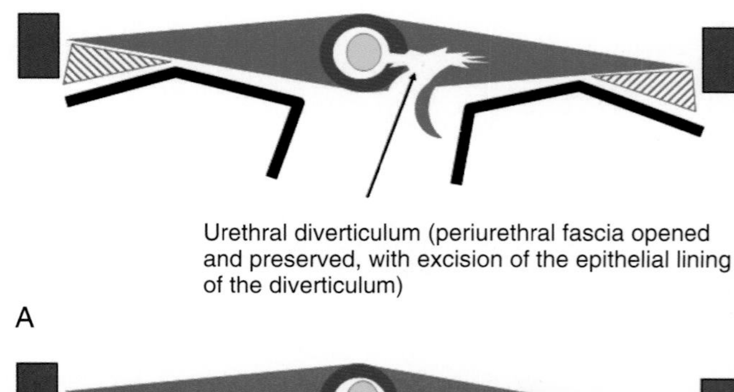

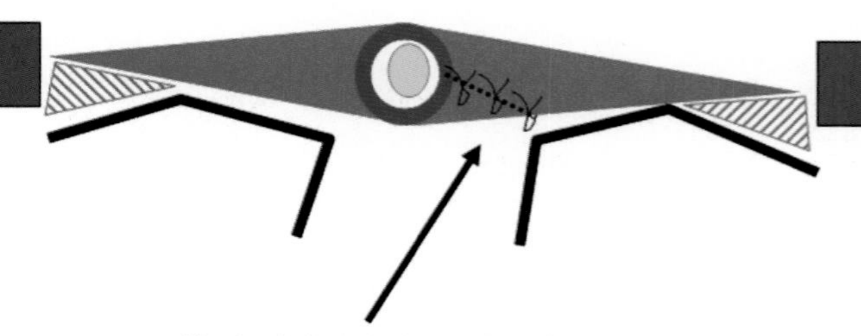

Figure 85-23 Diagrams demonstrate the importance of preserving and reconstructing the periurethral fascia. **A,** Defect in the periurethral fascia after removal of the epithelial lining of the urethral diverticulum. **B,** Closure of the urethra and periurethral fascia.

Urethral Diverticula and Associated Conditions

Malignant and benign tumors may be found in urethral diverticula. Both are rare, and fewer than 100 cases of carcinoma within urethral diverticula have been reported in the English language literature.[106] The most common malignant pathology in urethral diverticula is adenocarcinoma, followed by transitional cell and squamous cell carcinomas.[106] This contrasts with primary urethral carcinoma, in which the primary histologic type is squamous cell carcinoma. Some investigators have suggested that urethral diverticulum is associated with the development of urethral adenocarcinoma in women.[135] If this is true, nonexcisional therapy of urethral diverticula, such as marsupialization or endoscopic incision, should always be combined with a biopsy to rule out malignancy.[136] There is no consensus on proper treatment in these cases, and recurrence rates are high with local treatment alone.[106] The incidental finding of malignancy can be particularly troubling when found intraoperatively or on the postoperative pathology report. It has not been conclusively demonstrated that any particular preoperative imaging modality such as ultrasound or MRI can reliably and prospectively diagnose a small malignancy arising in a urethral diverticula. When considering curative therapy, it is unclear whether extensive surgery, including cystourethrectomy with or without adjuvant external beam radiotherapy, is superior to local excision followed by radiotherapy.[104]

Many benign lesions, including nephrogenic adenoma and endometriosis, have been described within urethral diverticula.[137-140] Pathologically, nephrogenic adenoma can be difficult to differentiate from adenocarcinoma.

Calculi within urethral diverticula may be diagnosed in 4% to 10% of cases,[44,141,142] and they are most likely caused by urinary stasis or infection. This may be suspected by physical examination findings or found incidentally on imaging evaluation. The presence of a stone does not significantly alter the evaluation or surgical approach, and it can be considered an incidental finding (Fig. 85-24).

Urethral diverticula have manifested during pregnancy. Moran[143] reported four cases of urethral diverticula diagnosed during pregnancy. Conservative treatment included antibiotics and aspiration or incision and drainage. Two women delivered vaginally, and the other two delivered by cesarean section for unrelated reasons. In one patient, drainage was performed during labor to facilitate delivery. Three of the four women had definitive repair performed after delivery. It is not known whether pregnancy is associated with formation of urethral diverticula, although patients may be more likely to become symptomatic during this period. Usually, conservative management with antibiotics may be desirable until after delivery to avoid precipitating premature labor, although successful surgical treatment during pregnancy has been reported.[144]

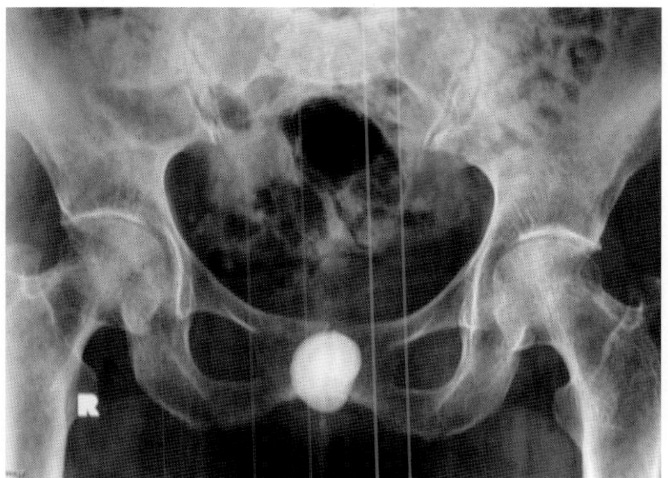

A

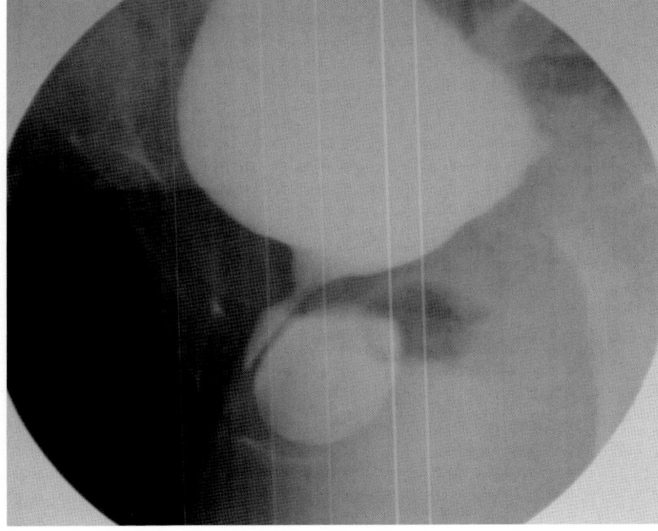

B

Figure 85-24 Large calculus within a urethral diverticulum. **A,** Voiding cystourethrographic scout film demonstrates a midline, calcified density overlying the symphysis pubis. **B,** Voiding image shows filling of the urethra and a cavity adjacent to the urethra surrounding the calcification, confirming that this represents a stone in a urethral diverticulum.

References

1. Hey W: Practical Observations in Surgery. Philadelphia, James Humphries, 1805, pp 304-305.
2. Davis HJ, Cian LG: Positive pressure urethrography: A new diagnostic method. J Urol 68:611-616, 1952.
3. Davis HJ, TeLinde RW: Urethral Diverticula: An assay of 121 cases. J Urol 80:34-39, 1958.
4. Young GPH, Wahle GR, Raz S: Female urethral diverticulum. In Raz S (ed): Female Urology. Philadelphia, WB Saunders, 1996, pp 477-489.
5. Vakili B, Wai C, Nihira M: Anterior urethral diverticulum in the female: Diagnosis and surgical approach. Obstet Gynecol 102:1179-1183, 2003.

6. Rovner ES, Wein AJ: Diagnosis and reconstruction of the dorsal or circumferential urethral diverticulum. J Urol 170:82-86, 2003.
7. Johnson CM: Diverticula and cyst of the female urethra. J Urol 39:506-516, 1938.
8. Gilbert CR, Rivera Cintron FJ: Urethral diverticula in the female: Review of the subject and introduction of a different surgical approach. Am J Obstet Gynecol 67:616-627, 1954.
9. Pinkerton JH: Urethral diverticula in women. Br Med J 5366:1204-1205, 1963.
10. Glassman TA, Weinerth JL, Glenn JF: Neonatal female urethral diverticulum. Urology 5:249-251, 1975.
11. Marshall S: Urethral diverticula in young girls. Urology 17:243-245, 1981.
12. Kaneti J, Sober I, Bar-Ziv J, et al: Congenital anterior urethral diverticulum. Eur Urol 10:48-52, 1984.
13. Kirks DR, Grossman H: Congenital saccular anterior urethral diverticulum. Radiology 140:367-372, 1981.
14. Lau JT, Ong GB: Congenital diverticulum of the anterior urethra. Aust N Z J Surg 51:305-306, 1981.
15. Kimbrough HM Jr, Vaughan ED Jr: Skene's duct cyst in a newborn: Case report and review of the literature. J Urol 117:387-388, 1977.
16. Lee NH, Kim SY: Skene's duct cysts in female newborns. J Pediatr Surg 27:15-17, 1992.
17. Boyd S, Raz S: Ectopic ureter presenting in midline urethral diverticulum. Urology 41:571-574, 1993.
18. Silk MR, Lebowitz JM: Anterior urethral diverticulum. J Urol 101:66-67, 1969.
19. Vanhoutte JJ: Ureteral ectopia into a Wolffian duct remnant presenting as a urethral diverticulum in two girls. Am J Roentgenol Radium Ther Nucl Med 110:540-545, 1970.
20. Davis BL, Robinson DG: Diverticula of the female urethra: Assay of 120 cases. J Urol 104:850-853, 1970.
21. Davis HJ, TeLinde RW: Urethral Diverticula: An assay of 121 cases. J Urol 80:34-39, 1958.
22. McNally A: Diverticula of the female urethra. Am J Surg 28:177, 1935.
23. Ganabathi K, Leach GE, Zimmern PE, et al: Experience with the management of urethral diverticulum in 63 women. J Urol 152:1445-1452, 1994.
24. Lee RA: Diverticulum of the urethra: Clinical presentation, diagnosis, and management. Clin Obstet Gynecol 27:490-498, 1984.
25. Klyszejko C, Ilnicki W, Klyszejko D, et al: Development of a urethral diverticulum after forceps delivery. Ginekol Pol 56:766-769, 1985.
26. Clemens JQ, Bushman W: Urethral diverticulum following transurethral collagen injection. J Urol 166:626, 2001.
27. Huffman JW: The detailed anatomy of the paraurethral ducts in the adult human female. Am J Obstet Gynecol 55:86, 1948.
28. Lang ED, Davis HJ: Positive pressure urethrography: A roentgenographic diagnostic method for urethral diverticula in the female. Radiology 72:410, 1959.
29. MacKinnon M, Pratt JH, Pool T: Diverticulum of the female urethra. Surg Clin North Am 39:953-962, 1959.
30. Peters W III, Vaughan ED Jr: Urethral diverticulum in the female. Etiologic factors and postoperative results. Obstet Gynecol 47:549-552, 1976.
31. Routh A: Urethral diverticula. BMJ 1:361-362, 1890.
32. Daneshgari F, Zimmern PE, Jacomides L: Magnetic resonance imaging detection of symptomatic noncommunicating intraurethral wall diverticula in women. J Urol 161:1259-1261, 1999.
33. Moore TD: Diverticulum of the female urethra. An improved technique of surgical excision. J Urol 68:611-616, 1952.
34. Bruning EJ: Die Pathologie der weiblichen Urethra und des Parurethrium. Stuttgart, Enke, 1959.
35. Andersen MJ: The incidence of diverticula in the female urethra. J Urol 98:96-98, 1967.
36. Aldridge CW Jr, Beaton JH, Nanzig RP: A review of office urethroscopy and cystometry. Am J Obstet Gynecol 131:432-437, 1978.
37. Stewart M, Bretland PM, Stidolph NE: Urethral diverticula in the adult female. Br J Urol 53:353-359, 1981.
38. Lorenzo AJ, Zimmern P, Lemack GE, et al: Endorectal coil magnetic resonance imaging for diagnosis of urethral and periurethral pathologic findings in women. Urology 61:1129-1133, 2003.
39. Leach GE, Bavendam TG: Female urethral diverticula. Urology 30:407-415, 1987.
40. Ginsburg D, Genadry R: Suburethral diverticulum: Classification and therapeutic considerations. Obstet Gynecol 61:685-688, 1983.
41. Pathak UN, House MJ: Diverticulum of the female urethra. Obstet Gynecol 36:789-794, 1970.
42. Leach GE, Schmidbauer CP, Hadley HR, et al: Surgical treatment of female urethral diverticulum. Semin Urol 4:33-42, 1986.
43. Nielsen VM, Nielsen KK, Vedel P: Spontaneous rupture of a diverticulum of the female urethra presenting with a fistula to the vagina. Acta Obstet Gynecol Scand 66:87-88, 1987.
44. Romanzi LJ, Groutz A, Blaivas JG: Urethral diverticulum in women: Diverse presentations resulting in diagnostic delay and mismanagement. J Urol 164:428-433, 2000.
45. Hoffman MJ, Adams WE: Recognition and repair of urethral diverticula: A report of 60 cases. Am J Obstet Gynecol 92:106-111, 1965.
46. Reid RE, Gill B, Laor E, et al: Role of urodynamics in management of urethral diverticulum in females. Urology 28:342-346, 1986.
47. Summitt RL Jr, Stovall TG: Urethral diverticula: Evaluation by urethral pressure profilometry, cystourethroscopy, and the voiding cystourethrogram. Obstet Gynecol 80:695-699, 1992.
48. Bhatia NN, McCarthy TA, Ostergard DR: Urethral pressure profiles of women with urethral diverticula. Obstet Gynecol 58:375-378, 1981.
49. Bass JS, Leach GE: Surgical treatment of concomitant urethral diverticulum and stress urinary incontinence. Urol Clin North Am 18:365-373, 1991.
50. Faerber GJ: Urethral diverticulectomy and pubovaginal sling for simultaneous treatment of urethral diverticulum and intrinsic sphincter deficiency. Tech Urol 4:192-197, 1998.
51. Swierzewski SJ III, McGuire EJ: Pubovaginal sling for treatment of female stress urinary incontinence complicated by urethral diverticulum. J Urol 149:1012-1014, 1993.
52. Bradley CS, Rovner ES: Urodynamically defined stress urinary incontinence and bladder outlet obstruction can coexist in women. J Urol 171:757-761, 2004.
53. Wagner U, Debus-Thiede G, Christ F: Significance of the urethral pressure profile in the diagnosis of urethral diverticulum [in German]. Geburtshilfe Frauenheilkd 46:456-458, 1986.
54. Greenberg M, Stone D, Cochran ST, et al: Female urethral diverticula: Double-balloon catheter study. AJR Am J Roentgenol 136:259-264, 1981.
55. Jacoby K, Rowbotham RK: Double balloon positive pressure urethrography is a more sensitive test than voiding cystourethrography for diagnosing urethral diverticulum in women. J Urol 162:2066-2069, 1999.
56. Stern AJ, Patel SK: Diverticulum of the female urethra. The value of the post-void bladder film during excretory urography. Radiology 121:222, 1976.
57. Goldfarb S, Mieza M, Leiter E: Postvoid film of intravenous pyelogram in diagnosis of urethral diverticulum. Urology 17:390-392, 1981.
58. Houser LM, Von Eschenbach AC: Diverticula of female urethra. Diagnostic importance of postvoiding film. Urology 3:453-455, 1974.
59. Golomb J, Leibovitch I, Mor Y, et al: Comparison of voiding cystourethrography and double-balloon urethrography in the diagnosis of complex female urethral diverticula. Eur Radiol 13:536-542, 2003.

60. Wang AC, Wang CR: Radiologic diagnosis and surgical treatment of urethral diverticulum in women. A reappraisal of voiding cystourethrography and positive pressure urethrography. J Reprod Med 45:377-382, 2000.
61. Blacklock ARE, Shaw RE, Geddes JR: Late presentation of ectopic ureter. Br J Urol 54:106-110, 1982.
62. Baert L, Willemen P, Oyen R: Endovaginal sonography: New diagnostic approach for urethral diverticula. J Urol 147:464-466, 1992.
63. Chancellor MB, Liu JB, Rivas DA, et al: Intraoperative endoluminal ultrasound evaluation of urethral diverticula. J Urol 153:72-75, 1995.
64. Dmochowski R: Urethral diverticula: Evolving diagnostics and improved surgical management. Curr Urol Rep 2:373-378, 2001.
65. Fortunato P, Schettini M, Gallucci M: Diagnosis and therapy of the female urethral diverticula. Int Urogynecol J 12:51-57, 2001.
66. Gerrard ER Jr, Lloyd LK, Kubricht WS, et al: Transvaginal ultrasound for the diagnosis of urethral diverticulum. J Urol 169:1395-1397, 2003.
67. Lee DI, Bagley DH, Liu JB: Experience with endoluminal ultrasonography in the urinary tract. J Endourol 15:67-74, 2001.
68. Martensson O, Duchek M: Translabial ultrasonography with pulsed colour-Doppler in the diagnosis of female urethral diverticula. Scand J Urol Nephrol 28:101-104, 1994.
69. Vargas-Serrano B, Cortina-Moreno B, Rodriguez-Romero R, et al: Transrectal ultrasonography in the diagnosis of urethral diverticula in women. J Clin Ultrasound 25:21-28, 1997.
70. Wexler JS, McGovern TP: Ultrasonography of female urethral diverticula. AJR Am J Roentgenol 134:737-740, 1980.
71. Lee TG, Keller FS: Urethral diverticulum: Diagnosis by ultrasound. AJR Am.J.Roentgenol 128:690-691, 1977.
72. Hricak H, Secaf E, Buckley DW, et al: Female urethra: MR imaging. Radiology 178:527-535, 1991.
73. Kim B, Hricak H, Tanagho EA: Diagnosis of urethral diverticula in women: Value of MR imaging. AJR Am J Roentgenol 161:809-815, 1993.
74. Blander DS, Rovner ES, Schnall MD, et al: Endoluminal magnetic resonance imaging in the evaluation of urethral diverticula in women. Urology 57:660-665, 2001.
75. Siegelman ES, Banner MP, Ramchandani P, et al: Multicoil MR imaging of symptomatic female urethral and periurethral disease. Radiographics 17:349-365, 1997.
76. Kim B, Hricak H, Tanagho EA: Diagnosis of urethral diverticula in women: Value of MR imaging. AJR Am J Roentgenol 161:809-815, 1993.
77. Neitlich JD, Foster HE Jr, Glickman MG, et al: Detection of urethral diverticula in women: Comparison of a high resolution fast spin echo technique with double balloon urethrography. J Urol 159:408-410, 1998.
78. Young SB, Rose PG, Reuter KL: Vaginal fibromyomata: two cases with preoperative assessment, resection, and reconstruction. Obstet Gynecol 78:972-974, 1991.
79. Blaivas JG, Flisser AJ, Bleustein CB, et al: Periurethral masses: Etiology and diagnosis in a large series of women. Obstet Gynecol 103:842-847, 2004.
80. Shirvani AR, Winters JC: Vaginal leiomyoma presenting as a urethral diverticulum. J Urol 163:1869, 2000.
81. Liu MM: Fibromyoma of the vagina. Eur J Obstet Gynecol Reprod Biol 29:321-328, 1988.
82. Dodson MK, Cliby WA, Keeney GL, et al: Skene's gland adenocarcinoma with increased serum level of prostate-specific antigen. Gynecol Oncol 55:304-307, 1994.
83. Currarino G: Single vaginal ectopic ureter and Gartner's duct cyst with ipsilateral renal hypoplasia and dysplasia (or agenesis). J Urol 128:988-993, 1982.
84. Gadbois WF, Duckett JW Jr: Gartner's duct cyst and ipsilateral renal agenesis. Urology 4:720-721, 1974.
85. Eilber KS, Raz S: Benign cystic lesions of the vagina: A literature review. J Urol 170:717-722, 2003.
86. Sheih CP, Li YW, Liao YJ, et al: Diagnosing the combination of renal dysgenesis, Gartner's duct cyst and ipsilateral mullerian duct obstruction. J Urol 159:217-221, 1998.
87. Abd-Rabbo MS, Atta MA: Aspiration and tetracycline sclerotherapy: A novel method for management of vaginal and vulval Gartner cysts. Int J Gynaecol Obst 35:235-237, 1991.
88. Deppisch LM: Cysts of the vagina: Classification and clinical correlations. Obstet Gynecol 45:632-637, 1975.
89. Pradhan S, Tobon H: Vaginal cysts: A clinicopathological study of 41 cases. Int J Gynecol Pathol 5:35-46, 1986.
90. Fernandes ET, Dekermacher S, Sabadin MA, et al: Urethral prolapse in children. Urology 41:240-242, 1993.
91. Rudin JE, Geldt VG, Alecseev EB: Prolapse of urethral mucosa in white female children: Experience with 58 cases. J Pediatr Surg 32:423-425, 1997.
92. Lowe FC, Hill GS, Jeffs RD, et al: Urethral prolapse in children: insights into etiology and management. J Urol 135:100-103, 1986.
93. Jerkins GR, Verheeck K, Noe HN: Treatment of girls with urethral prolapse. J Urol 132:732-733, 1984.
94. Atalay AC, Karaman MI, Basak T, et al: Non-Hodgkin's lymphoma of the female urethra presenting as a caruncle. Int Urol Nephrol 30:609-610, 1998.
95. Indudhara R, Vaidyanathan S, Radotra BD: Urethral tuberculosis. Urol Int 48:436-438, 1992.
96. Khatib RA, Khalil AM, Tawil AN, et al: Non-Hodgkin's lymphoma presenting as a urethral caruncle. Gynecol Oncol 50:389-393, 1993.
97. Lopez JI, Angulo JC, Ibanez T: Primary malignant melanoma mimicking urethral caruncle: Case report. Scand J Urol Nephrol 27:125-126, 1993.
98. Willett GD, Lack EE: Periurethral colonic-type polyp simulating urethral caruncle: A case report. J Reprod Med 35:1017-1018, 1990.
99. Leach GE, Sirls LT, Ganabathi K, et al: L N S C3: A proposed classification system for female urethral diverticula. Neurourol Urodyn 12:523-531, 1993.
100. Leng WW, McGuire EJ: Management of female urethral diverticula: A new classification. J Urol 160:1297-1300, 1998.
101. Gonzalez MO, Harrison ML, Boileau MA: Carcinoma in diverticulum of female urethra. Urology 26:328-332, 1985.
102. Hickey N, Murphy J, Herschorn S: Carcinoma in a urethral diverticulum: Magnetic resonance imaging and sonographic appearance. Urology 55:588-589, 2000.
103. Marshall S, Hirsch K: Carcinoma within urethral diverticula. Urology 10:161-163, 1977.
104. Patanaphan V, Prempree T, Sewchand W, et al: Adenocarcinoma arising in female urethral diverticulum. Urology 22:259-264, 1983.
105. Prudente DT, Dias Montellato NI, Arap S, et al: Carcinoma in diverticulum of female urethra. Urol Int 33:393-398, 1978.
106. Rajan N, Tucci P, Mallouh C, et al: Carcinoma in female urethral diverticulum: Case reports and review of management. J Urol 150:1911-1914, 1993.
107. Seballos RM, Rich RR: Clear cell adenocarcinoma arising from a urethral diverticulum. J Urol 153:1914-1915, 1995.
108. Tesluk H: Primary adenocarcinoma of female urethra associated with diverticula. Urology 17:197-199, 1981.
109. Thomas RB, Maguire B: Adenocarcinoma in a female urethral diverticulum. Aust N Z J Surg 61:869-871, 1991.
110. Tines SC, Bigongiari LR, Weigel JW: Carcinoma in diverticulum of the female urethra. AJR Am J Roentgenol 138:582-585, 1982.
111. Spence HM, Duckett JW Jr: Diverticulum of the female urethra: Clinical aspects and presentation of a simple operative technique for cure. J Urol 104:432-437, 1970.

112. Roehrborn CG: Long term follow-up study of the marsupialization technique for urethral diverticula in women. Surg Gynecol Obstet 167:191-196, 1988.
113. Lapides J: Transurethral treatment of urethral diverticula in women. Trans Am Assoc Genitourin Surg 70:135-137, 1978.
114. Spencer WF, Streem SB: Diverticulum of the female urethral roof managed endoscopically. J Urol 138:147-148, 1987.
115. Saito S: Usefulness of diagnosis by the urethroscopy under anesthesia and effect of transurethral electrocoagulation in symptomatic female urethral diverticula. J Endourol 14:455-457, 2000.
116. Ellick M: Diverticulum of the female urethra: A new method of ablation. J Urol 77:243-246, 1957.
117. Mizrahi S, Bitterman W: Transvaginal, periurethral injection of polytetrafluoroethylene (polytef) in the treatment of urethral diverticula. Br J Urol 62:280, 1988.
118. Spence HM, Duckett JW Jr: Motion picture: simple operation for cure of diverticula of female urethra. Trans Am Assoc Genitourin Surg 61:78-79, 1969.
119. Fall M: Vaginal wall bipedicled flap and other techniques in complicated urethral diverticlum and urethrovaginal fistula. J Am Coll Surg 180:150-156, 1995.
120. Appell RA, Suarez BC: Experience with a laterally based vaginal flap approach for urethral diverticulum. J Urol 127:677-678, 1982.
121. Woodhouse CR, Flynn JT, Molland EA, Blandy JP: Urethral diverticulum in females. Br J Urol 52:305-310, 1980.
122. Clyne OJ, Flood HD: Giant urethral diverticulum: A novel approach to repair. J Urol 167:1796, 2002.
123. Benjamin J, Elliott L, Cooper JF, et al: Urethral diverticulum in adult female. Clinical aspects, operative procedure, and pathology. Urology 3:1-7, 1974.
124. Busch FM, Carter FH: Vaginal flap incision for urethral diverticula. Paper presented at the Western Section Meeting, American Urological Association, Honolulu, June 29, 1973.
125. Lockhart JL, Ellis GF, Helal M, et al: Combined cystourethropexy for the treatment of type 3 and complicated female urinary incontinence. J Urol 143:722-725, 1990.
126. Kohorn EI, Glickman MG: Technical aids in investigation and management of urethral diverticula in the female. Urology 40:322-325, 1992.
127. Wear JB: Urethral diverticulectomy in females. Urol Times 4:2-3, 1976.
128. Hyams JA, Hyams MN: A new operative procedure for the treatment of diverticulum of the female urethra. J Urol 43:573-577, 1939.
129. Hirschhorn RC: A new surgical technique for removal of urethral diverticula in the female patient. J Urol 92:206-209, 1964.
130. Feldstein MS: Cryoprecipitate coagulum as an adjunct to surgery for diverticula of the female urethra. J Urol 126:698-699, 1981.
131. Tamada S, Iwai Y, Tanimoto Y, et al: Urethral diverticula surrounding the urethra in women: report of 2 cases [in Japanese]. Hinyokika Kiyo 46:639-642, 2000.
132. Schwab CW, Rovner ES: Utility of radiologic imaging and prolonged catheterization following complex lower urinary tract reconstruction. Paper presented at the Mid-Atlantic AUA sectional meeting, Boca Raton, FL, October 26, 2003.
133. Porpiglia F, Destefanis P, Fiori C, et al: Preoperative risk factors for surgery female urethral diverticula: Our experience. Urol Int 69:7-11, 2002.
134. Lee RA: Diverticulum of the female urethra: Postoperative complications and results. Obstet Gynecol 61:52-58, 1983.
135. Oliva E, Young RH: Clear cell adenocarcinoma of the urethra: A clinicopathologic analysis of 19 cases. Mod Pathol 9:513-520, 1996.
136. McLoughlin MG: Carcinoma in situ in urethral diverticulum: Pitfalls of marsupialization alone. Urology 6:343, 1975.
137. Paik SS, Lee JD: Nephrogenic adenoma arising in an urethral diverticulum. Br J Urol 80:150, 1997.
138. Palagiri A: Urethral Diverticulum with endometriosis. Urology 11:271-272, 1978.
139. Peterson LJ, Matsumoto LM: Nephrogenic adenoma in urethral diverticulum. Urology 11:193-195, 1978.
140. Piazza R, Aragona F, Pizzarella M, et al: Nephrogenic adenoma in urethral diverticulum: An unusual finding. Urol Int 42:69-70, 1987.
141. Ward JN, Draper JW, Tovell HM: Diagnosis and treatment of urethral diverticula in the female. Surg Gynecol Obstet 125:1293-1300, 1967.
142. Ginesin Y, Bolkier M, Nachmias J, et al: Primary giant calculus in urethral diverticulum. Urol Int 43:47-48, 1988.
143. Moran PA, Carey MP, Dwyer PL: Urethral diverticula in pregnancy. Aust N Z J Obstet Gynaecol 38:102-106, 1998.
144. Wittich AC: Excision of urethral diverticulum calculi in a pregnant patient on an outpatient basis. J Am Osteopath Assoc 97:461-462, 1997.
145. Westney OL, Leng WW, McGuire EJ: The diagnosis and treatment of female urethral diverticulum. In Ball TP Jr (ed): AUA Update Series, vol 20. Houston, TX, AUA Office of Education, 2001, pp 290-295.
146. Pavlica P, Viglietta G, Losinno F, et al: I diverticoli dell'uretra femminile: Studio radiologico ed ecografico. Radiol Med 75:521-527, 1988.
147. Kim B, Hricak H, Tanagho EA: Diagnosis of urethral diverticula in women: Value of MR imaging. AJR Am J Roentgenol 161:809-815, 1993.
148. Dmochowski R: Surgery for vesicovaginal fistula, urethrovaginal fistula, and urethral diverticulum. In Walsh PC, Retik AB, Vaughan ED Jr, et al (eds): Campbell's Urology, vol 8. Philadelphia, WB Saunders, 2002.

Section 10

PELVIC PAIN AND INFLAMMATORY CONDITIONS

Chapter 86

URINARY TRACT INFECTIONS IN WOMEN

Amanda M. Macejko and Anthony J. Schaeffer

EPIDEMIOLOGY

Urinary tract infections (UTIs) are the most common bacterial infections and account for a substantial number of office and emergency room visits as well as hospital admissions each year. Additionally, UTI is the most common cause of nosocomial infection.[1] The morbidity of UTIs varies widely, from self-limited to life-threatening conditions. The focus of this chapter is on UTI in women, who make up a significant proportion of UTI sufferers. The annual incidence among women is 12.1%. Peak incidence in women occurs between the ages of 20 to 24 years.[2] Health care costs attributed to UTIs are substantial. The estimated overall costs of UTI among ambulatory women in the United States exceeds $1 billion annually.[3]

Pathogenesis

The interaction between bacterial virulence and host defense factors can ultimately result in UTI. More virulent bacteria are necessary to infect healthy hosts with a normal urinary tract, whereas less virulent bacteria may easily infect compromised hosts.

Laboratory studies of uropathogenic strains of *Escherichia coli* (UPEC) have helped to obtain a better understanding of the pathogenesis of UTIs. The initial step is bacterial adherence to the urothelium. Type 1 pili are filamentous adhesive organelles encoded by almost all UPEC, and they are significant virulence factors associated with UTIs. FimH is an adhesin molecule at the tip of type 1 pili that specifically binds to the luminal surface of the bladder.[4] Bacterial colonization then precipitates a host inflammatory response, which includes neutrophil influx followed by apoptosis and exfoliation of the bladder's epithelial cells in an effort to rid the bladder of bacteria. Despite the host's response, however, high titers of UPEC persist in the bladder for several days.[5]

How are the bacteria able to elude the host defenses? Recent research has shown that UPEC avoids clearance by invading and replicating within the epithelial cells. They form "bacterial factories" that are refuges in which bacteria may persist and form biofilms. Bacteria within a biofilm are resistant not only to host defenses but also to typical courses of antimicrobials.[5] These bacteria may subsequently reemerge and cause recurrent acute infections.[6] Historically, the vagina and intestine have been accepted as UPEC reservoirs; however, this new paradigm demonstrates that the bladder itself may be a reservoir for UPEC.

Host Factors

Host factors include genetic, anatomic, functional, and behavioral factors that affect the host's susceptibility to uropathogens and its ability to overcome them (Table 86-1).

Vaginal Colonization

In order for a UTI to occur, the infecting organism must first obtain access to the urinary tract. In the 1960s, Stamey hypothesized that bacteria that cause UTIs originate in the rectal flora and colonize the vaginal and urethral mucosa before ascending to the bladder.[7] Vaginal colonization has proved to be a crucial step in the pathogenesis of UTI. Many factors that increase the risk of UTI do so by facilitating vaginal colonization with uropathogens.[8] Women (in comparison to men) are particularly at risk based simply on differences in anatomy. Women have a moist periurethral space, a shorter distance between the anus and urethral opening, and a shorter urethra. These factors increase exposure to uropathogens and enhance the ability of these pathogens to colonize the urinary tract.[2]

Why are some women more susceptible to vaginal colonization, and therefore recurrent UTI, than others? There is substantial evidence that vaginal colonization is determined by genetic factors. In 1977, Fowler and Stamey discovered that *E. coli*

Table 86-1 Host Factors

Genetic	Anatomic/Functional	Behavioral
Blood group antigen	Congenital abnormalities	Sexual activity
Nonsecretor status	Urinary obstruction	Diaphragm use
Density of adhesin receptors	Urinary incontinence	Spermicide use
Maternal history of UTI	Calculi	Antimicrobial use
	Residual urine	
	Catheters or foreign bodies	
	Atrophic vaginitis	

UTI, urinary tract infection.
Modified from Ronald A: The etiology of urinary tract infection: Traditional and emerging pathogens. Am J Med 113(Suppl 1A):14S-9S, 2002.

adhered more avidly to vaginal epithelial cells of women with recurrent UTI.[9] Follow-up studies by Schaeffer showed that high vaginal cell receptivity was correlated with high buccal cell receptivity, suggesting that epithelial cell receptivity is actually a genotypic trait.[10] The concept of hereditary susceptibility was further investigated by Schaeffer and associates, who demonstrated that the prevalence of the human leukocyte antigen (HLA) A3 subtype was greater in women with recurrent UTIs.[11] In addition, carbohydrate structures bound to cell membranes known as blood group antigens make up a significant component of the uroepithelial cell membrane. Certain blood group antigens have been associated with susceptibility to UTI. Sheinfeld and colleagues determined that women with Lewis blood group Le(a^-b^-) or Le(a^+b^-) (nonsecretor) had a significantly higher incidence of recurrent UTIs than women with the Le(a^-b^+) (secretor) phenotype.[12] *E. coli* bind to mannose residues, which are more available in nonsecretor mucosa.[13]

Sexual Activity

Vaginal and oral intercourse help to propagate potential pathogens into the vagina and urinary tract. Additionally, vaginal intercourse may cause trauma of the vaginal epithelium, rendering it more susceptible to bacterial adherence and vaginal colonization.[14] Several studies have linked sexual activity with vaginal colonization and UTI. Foxman and colleagues found that vaginal colonization with *E. coli* was inversely associated with the number of days since sexual activity.[15] Hooton and coworkers reported that urine cultures in the immediate postcoital period show a transient bacteriuria.[16] It has been proposed that voiding immediately after intercourse is protective, although there are no current data that support this conjecture.[1]

Spermicide and Diaphragm Use

Spermicide and diaphragm use has been found to greatly increase the risk of vaginal colonization with uropathogens and UTI, independent of sexual activity. Nonoxynol-9, the active ingredient in most spermicides, has a bactericidal effect on the normal vaginal flora and therefore enhances the growth of *E. coli.*[2,8]

Estrogen

Estrogen withdrawal in postmenopausal women alters the normal vaginal flora. In a randomized, double-blind, placebo-controlled trial of postmenopausal women with recurrent UTI, Raz and Stamm found that topically applied intravaginal estriol cream lowered the vaginal pH, restored lactobacilli in 61% of vaginal cultures, and reduced the incidence of UTI 10-fold. He concluded that intravaginal estrogen replacement restores an acidic environment that is more hospitable to premenopausal flora.[17] However, these results have not been replicated in studies evaluating oral estrogens. Cardozo and associates evaluated the effects of low-dose, oral estrogen replacement but were unable to establish a significant protective effect.[18]

Recent Antimicrobial Use

Another factor that contributes to UTI susceptibility is recent antimicrobial use. Smith and coworkers, in a prospective study, found that antimicrobial use up to 4 weeks before the onset of a UTI increased the relative risk for that UTI by 2.57 to 5.83 times. It has been proposed that recent antimicrobial use increases a woman's risk of UTI by altering the normal urogenital flora.[19] The most offending antimicrobials are β-lactams, whereas trimethoprim and nitrofurantoin seem to have much less of an effect on the normal vaginal flora.[8]

DIAGNOSTIC TOOLS

History

A thorough history is an essential component of obtaining the proper diagnosis. It is important to clarify the onset and the presence or absence of symptoms including dysuria, urinary frequency, hematuria, suprapubic tenderness, flank pain, fever, and nausea/vomiting. Has the patient had previous UTIs as a child or as an adult? If so, were her previous UTIs associated with fever?

A complete medical and surgical history is also important. Does the patient have a history of nephrolithiasis or previous urinary tract surgery? Is the patient pregnant? Does the patient diabetic? The answers to these questions will direct further workup and management.

Physical Examination

The physical examination is not considered diagnostic of UTI but can be helpful in certain cases. The findings may assist in differentiating between lower urinary tract (cystitis) and upper urinary tract (pyelonephritis) infection. Is the patient febrile? Is there costovertebral tenderness? Findings such as a urethral diverticulum may occasionally reveal a potential source of recurrent UTI. The physical examination may also help to rule out other causes of patient symptomatology. For example, the presence of vaginal discharge has a strong association with vaginal infection rather than a UTI.[20]

Urinalysis

Women should provide a midstream voided urine for analysis after spreading the labia and wiping from front to back with a clean sponge.[7] The urinalysis provides information about pyuria, bacteriuria, and hematuria. Urine dipstick analysis is a quick and inexpensive test that is often used in the clinical setting. Testing for leukocyte esterase, an enzyme produced by polymorphonuclear cells, and nitrite, a byproduct of bacterial growth, it provides an indirect measurement of both pyuria and bacteriuria.[21] If either the nitrite assay or the leukocyte esterase test is positive, the dipstick test has a sensitivity of 75% and a specificity of 82%.[22] False-negative results can occur when the infecting organism does not produce nitrites.[23] It is important to note that, although the dipstick test can be useful for screening, it is not as sensitive as microscopic examination.[7] Pyuria on microscopic examination has a high sensitivity (95%) and a relatively low specificity (71%).[24] The presence of bacteria on microscopic examination has a lower sensitivity (40% to 50%) yet a higher specificity (85% to 95%).[24]

Urine Culture

The Infectious Diseases Society of America (ISDA) defines cystitis as greater than or equal to 10^5 cfu/mL of midstream urine. However, studies by Stamm and Hooton demonstrated that greater than or equal to 10^2 cfu/mL for a catheterized urine specimen in a symptomatic patient is significant.[25] It is not necessary to obtain a urine culture in all patients. Appropriate patient selection for urine culture is addressed in a later section.

Imaging Techniques

Multiple radiographic techniques are available for imaging the urinary tract. Plain abdominal films may demonstrate radiopaque calculi. Intravenous pyelography, although not typically used in the setting of UTI, can be useful to determine the site of an obstruction.[7] Renal ultrasonography may demonstrate stone, hydronephrosis, or perirenal abscess. Advantages of ultrasound are that it does not expose the patient to radiation or contrast material; however, ultrasound results are dependent on operator experience.[7] Computed tomography (CT) and magnetic resonance imaging (MRI) demonstrate excellent anatomic detail and are more sensitive than intravenous pyelography and ultrasonography.[7] Although numerous imaging techniques are available, most UTIs do not warrant radiologic evaluation. The appropriateness of imaging in the setting of a UTI is discussed later.

TREATMENT

Antimicrobial Principles

The successful treatment of a UTI depends on two important principles. First, the treatment should result in elimination of bacteriuria. This typically occurs hours after initiation of treatment.[7] Second, the urine concentration of the antimicrobials must exceed the minimal inhibitory concentration (MIC) of the bacteria.[26] It is important to keep in mind that hospital microbiology laboratories typically report bacterial sensitivities based on serum levels that may be several-fold lower than the urine levels of a particular agent.

Antimicrobial Resistance

The most common reason for unresolved bacteriuria is bacterial resistance to the chosen antimicrobial agent. There are several ways in which bacteria may be resistant. In natural resistance, certain bacteria simply lack a drug-susceptible substrate, rendering an entire species of bacteria resistant to a particular antimicrobial. Examples include *Proteus* resistance to nitrofurantoin and *Enterococcus faecalis* resistance to cephalexin.[7] Resistance can also occur when the antimicrobial therapy actually selects for resistant mutants. This mode of resistance occurs within the urinary tract and can typically be avoided by choosing an agent with a urine concentration that exceeds the MIC by the greatest margin, adequate dosing, and stressing the importance of compliance with therapy.[7] The third mechanism of resistance is extrachromosomal plasmid-mediated resistance, also known as transferable resistance. This mode of resistance takes place within the bowel and produces multiple resistant strains. To date, transferable resistance has not been demonstrated with nitrofurantoin or fluoroquinolones, and therefore these two drugs are good options for patients exposed to other antimicrobials.[27]

Antimicrobial Selection

In selecting an antimicrobial agent, it is necessary to understand the efficacy, spectrum of activity, resistance patterns, side effects, dosing, and cost.[28] Individual antimicrobials are discussed later. Costs for a complete course of therapy of the antimicrobials based on 2001 wholesale prices are listed in Table 86-2.

Trimethoprim-sulfamethoxazole

Trimethoprim-sulfamethoxazole (TMP-SMX) blocks folic acid metabolism of bacteria, thereby preventing bacterial growth. TMP is effective as a single agent in uncomplicated UTI, has fewer side effects, and is safe for patients with sulfa allergies.[29] SMX has a synergistic bactericidal effect that improves the efficacy of the treatment of upper tract infections.[30] The combination of TMP-SMX is active against most aerobic gram-positive and gram-negative organisms. It is not active against enterococci or *Pseudomonas aeruginosa*.[23] Dosage is one double-strength tablet twice daily for 3 days for uncomplicated cystitis. Side effects may include rash, gastrointestinal upset, and photosensitivity.[31] Serious adverse events may include Stevens-Johnson syndrome.[23]

Table 86-2 Antimicrobial Cost

Antimicrobial	Dose (mg)	Cost ($)
Sulfonamides		
TMP-SMX	160/800 two times daily × 3 days	6.30-8.80
TMP	100 two times daily × 3 days	0.90-1.40
Fluoroquinolones		
Ciprofloxacin	100-250 two times daily × 3 days	17.20-25.00
Levofloxacin	250-500 daily × 3 days	21.90-25.60
Nitrofurantoin macrocrystals		
Macrodantin	100 four times daily × 7 days	47.00
Macrobid	100 two times daily × 7 days	23.00
β-lactams		
Amoxicillin	250-500 three times daily × 3 days	6.40-11.50
Cefixime	400 daily × 3 days	23.20
Cefpodoxime	100 two times daily × 3 days	18.30

SMX, sulfamethoxazole; TMP, trimethoprim.
Modified from Jancel T, Dudas V: Management of uncomplicated urinary tract infections. West J Med 176:51-55, 2002.

TMP-SMX should be avoided in pregnant patients as well as those taking warfarin.[7]

TMP-SMX has historically been the most widely used antimicrobial in the treatment of uncomplicated UTI, which may account for its high resistance rates. A recent study by Gupta and colleagues highlighted the fact that antimicrobial susceptibility patterns are dependent on geographic distribution. *E. coli* resistance to TMP-SMX ranged from 10% in the northeastern United States to 22% in the western United States.[32] Risk factors for resistance to TMP-SMX include previous use of TMP-SMX and current use of other antimicrobials, as well as diabetes and recent hospitalization.[23]

Nitrofurantoin

Nitrofurantoin inhibits several bacterial enzyme systems and is bactericidal. It is active against *E. coli* and most species of *Klebsiella, Enterobacter, Staphylococcus,* and *Enterococcus.* It is not effective against *Pseudomonas* or *Proteus* species.[33] A 7-day course of therapy is recommended for uncomplicated UTI, and it is also frequently used for UTI prophylaxis.[23] The agent does not penetrate urinary tract tissue or achieve bactericidal levels in blood and therefore is not recommended for complicated UTIs or pyelonephritis.[34] It also should not be used in patients with poor renal function, because adequate urine concentration levels will not be achieved.[7] Side effects may include gastrointestinal upset, peripheral polyneuropathy, hemolysis in patients with glucose-6-phosphate dehydrogenase deficiency, and pulmonary reactions ranging from cough to fibrosis.[7] Nitrofurantoin exhibits very low levels of resistance.[23]

β-Lactams

The β-lactam family includes penicillins, aminopenicillins, cephalosporins, and aztreonam. These antimicrobials inhibit bacterial cell wall synthesis.[23]

The aminopenicillins (ampicillin, amoxicillin ± clavulanate) are useful against *Streptococcus, Enterococcus, E. coli,* and *Proteus mirabilis.* Recommended treatment length is 7 days. The most common adverse reactions are hypersensitivity and diarrhea. Extended-spectrum penicillin derivatives including piperacillin are often active against typically ampicillin-resistant gram-negative bacilli.[7]

There are three generations of cephalosporins. Typically, the first-generation agents are active against *Streptococcus, Staphylococcus, E. coli, Proteus,* and *Klebsiella* species. Second-generation cephalosporins have similar activity to first-generation agents with additional activity against anaerobes. Third-generation cephalosporins have decreased activity against gram-positive cocci and increased activity against gram-negative bacilli. Some third-generation cephalosporins are active against *P. aeruginosa* and are often used for nosocomial infections caused by gram-negative organisms. It is important to note that none of the cephalosporins is active against enterococci. Similar to the aminopenicillins, adverse reactions include hypersensitivity and gastrointestinal upset. These agents should not be used in patients with immediate hypersensitivity to penicillins.[7]

Aztreonam is active only against gram-negative aerobes. This drug has a less than 1% incidence of cross-reactivity in penicillin-allergic patients, and its use is mainly limited to those patients with allergies to penicillin.[7]

Fluoroquinolones

Ciprofloxacin and levofloxacin are the fluoroquinolones most commonly used against UTI in the United States. They are available in both oral and intravenous forms. The mechanism of action of these drugs is to inhibit DNA gyrase. They are active against enterobacteria and *P. aeruginosa.*[7] These agents are often used as first-line therapy for UTIs in regions with high levels of bacterial resistance to ampicillin and TMP-SMX.[23] Side effects are uncommon but include gastrointestinal upset, dizziness, lightheadedness, photosensitivity, and tendon rupture. Fluoroquinolones should be avoided in pregnant women. Sucralfate should not be used concomitantly, because it decreases oral absorption.[7]

Resistance to fluoroquinolones is low in the United States,[32] but this is not the case worldwide. Spain and Portugal have high rates of resistance to ciprofloxacin, 14.7% and 5.8% respectively.[23] This is perhaps due to the wider use of fluoroquinolones in Europe. In a recent paper, Hooton and colleagues expressed concern regarding increasing fluoroquinolone resistance and recommended discouraging the routine use of fluoroquinolones for treatment of mild-to-moderate acute uncomplicated cystitis.[35]

Aminoglycosides

Aminoglycosides inhibit ribosomal protein synthesis and are active against *Staphylococcus* and most gram-negative pathogens. They are the drugs of choice in patients with urosepsis when used in combination with ampicillin.[7] Once-daily dosing at 7 mg/kg has been shown to maximize bacterial killing and to reduce nephrotoxicity, a common adverse effect.[36] These agents should be avoided in pregnant patients and in those with impaired renal function or diabetes.[7]

PRACTICAL APPROACHES TO PATIENT ASSESSMENT

Classification of Urinary Tract Infections

UTIs can be classified in several different ways. The location of the infection is one method of classification. For example, UTIs may involve the lower tract (cystitis) or the upper tract (pyelonephritis). Texts also describe UTIs as uncomplicated or complicated. Uncomplicated infections occur in healthy women who are without physiologic or anatomic urinary tract abnormalities or recent urologic surgery or instrumentation. Women with uncomplicated infections are not pregnant or immunocompromised and have not recently taken antimicrobials.[7] Complicated infections occur when there is poor response to therapy, the patient is not healthy or is otherwise compromised (e.g., pregnant), or there is a structural or functional abnormality of the urinary tract that increases the risk of therapy failure.[8] Unfortunately, the category into which a patient fits is not always readily apparent. This section attempts to help the clinician recognize patient characteristics that should guide patient categorization.

Uncomplicated Acute Cystitis

A typical patient with uncomplicated acute cystitis is a premenopausal, sexually active, nonpregnant woman. She reports recent onset of symptoms including dysuria, frequency, urgency, and possibly suprapubic discomfort and hematuria.[37] The differential diagnosis for acute cystitis includes vaginitis and sexually transmitted diseases. Some authors report that a history, physical examination, and urinalysis should be all that is needed to ascertain the appropriate diagnosis.[38] Others report that treating acute, uncomplicated cystitis in low risk women by telephone consultation to be safe and effective.[39]

Table 86-3 Pathogens Cultured in Uncomplicated Urinary Tract Infections

Escherichia coli	70-95%
Staphylococcus saprophyticus (premenopausal women)	5-20%
Klebsiella species	
Enterococcus faecalis	
Proteus mirabilis	

Modified from Hooton TM, Stamm WE: Diagnosis and treatment of uncomplicated urinary tract infection. Infect Dis Clin North Am 11:551-581, 1997.

Box 86-1 Situations in which it is Appropriate to Obtain a Urine Culture in Acute Uncomplicated Cystitis

Symptoms and/or urinalysis not consistent with cystitis
Recent antimicrobial therapy
UTI symptoms >7 days
Age >65 yr
Diabetes
Pregnancy
Recurrent UTI

UTI, urinary tract infection.
Modified from Schaeffer AJ: Infections of the urinary tract. Walsh PC, Retik AB, Vaughan ED Jr, Wein AJ (eds). Campbell's Urology. Philadelphia, WB Saunders, 2002, pp 516-602.

Box 86-2 When to use Fluoroquinolones as First-Line Therapy for Uncomplicated Acute Cystitis

Allergic to TMP-SMX
Recent antimicrobial exposure
High rate of TMP-SMX resistance in the community (>20%)
Unresolved UTI without prior fluoroquinolone therapy
Recurrent UTI

TMP-SMX, trimethoprim-sulfamethoxazole; UTI, urinary tract infection.

For the patient with uncomplicated UTI, urine cultures are usually not necessary, because most acute, community-acquired, uncomplicated infections in the United States and abroad are caused by predictable organisms (Table 86-3) and respond to empiric therapy. The routine use of urine cultures in uncomplicated cases has been shown to increase the cost of care by 39% without significant benefit to patient outcomes.[28] However, it is important to recognize situations in which it is appropriate to perform urine cultures in uncomplicated acute cystitis. These are included in Box 86-1.

Evidence-based guidelines for the treatment of acute uncomplicated cystitis were published by the Infectious Diseases Society America (IDSA) in 1999. According to these guidelines, TMP alone or TMP-SMX for 3 days is considered the current standard therapy. However, fluoroquinolones should be used as initial empiric therapy in specific situations, as outlined in Box 86-2.[7,40]

There has been renewed interest in nitrofurantoin in the treatment of uncomplicated cystitis because of its low resistance rates. However, it is not as effective as TMP-SMX or the fluoroquinolones.[41] The IDSA found that nitrofurantoin had lower cure rates (approximately 85%) than other first-line agents (90% to 95%).[40] Most women experience marked improvement in symptoms within 24 hours.[28] Response to therapy is primarily measured by clinical resolution of symptoms, and further follow-up is usually unnecessary.[7]

Unresolved Urinary Tract Infection

If the patient's symptoms do not resolve with empiric therapy, the clinician should consider these questions: Has the patient been compliant with treatment? Is the UTI caused by a resistant organism? Are symptoms due to a UTI or another diagnosis altogether? A urine culture should be obtained, and the patient should be switched to a fluoroquinolone if she is not taking one already. The patient should be monitored to ensure that her symptoms resolve and that her urine culture is negative at the end of treatment.

Recurrent Urinary Tract Infections

Recurrent UTI is noted when a premenopausal, sexually active, nonpregnant woman presents with her third episode of urgency, frequency, and dysuria in the same year. Reports show that 25% to 50% of women experience recurrent UTI, defined as three or more symptomatic UTIs in 1 year or two UTIs within 6 months.[42] Recurrent UTIs usually occur in the absence of anatomic urinary tract abnormalities and represent a new infection from bacteria outside of the urinary tract.[7] *Reinfections* typically occur at long intervals and usually are caused by different uropathogens, whereas *relapses* secondary to bacterial persistence are commonly caused by the same organism and typically occur at close intervals.[7]

A study by Scholes and colleagues aimed at determining the risk factors for recurrent UTI determined that lifetime sexual activity and sexual activity within the last year were the most important risk factors for recurrence.[42] Other risk factors included spermicide use, a new sexual partner within the past year, first UTI at 15 years of age or younger, and having a mother with a history of UTIs.[8]

As indicated in Box 86-1, when a patient has recurrent UTIs, is appropriate to obtain a urine culture, because it is vital to document that these recurrent episodes are in fact infectious. If the patient's symptoms are not caused by infection, the clinician needs to consider alternative diagnoses, including urethritis, vaginitis, interstitial cystitis, and carcinoma in situ. Further urologic workup is usually not necessary in patients with recurrent UTIs. There are three different strategies for antimicrobial prophylaxis for patients with recurrent UTIs.

Low-Dose Prophylaxis

Continuous antimicrobial prophylaxis involves daily administration of a low-dose antimicrobial such as TMP, TMP-SMX, or nitrofurantoin.[1] These agents are ideal because they have minimal adverse effects on the fecal and vaginal flora and have been shown to decrease recurrence rates by 95%.[43] Low-dose prophylaxis is well suited for patients with three or more UTIs annually and is well tolerated.[1]

Postcoital Prophylaxis

As mentioned previously, sexual intercourse is a significant risk factor for acute cystitis. Postcoital antimicrobial administration is appropriate for patients with UTI recurrence associated with intercourse. Single doses of nitrofurantoin, cephalexin, or TMP-SMX have been shown to be effective.[44]

Self-Start Therapy

A patient on self-start therapy is provided a culture kit as well an antimicrobial preparation so that she may culture her urine and begin therapy promptly after the onset of symptoms. Fluoroquinolones are typically used in self-start therapy. The patient sees her physician after therapy to assess the response. This method has been found to be safe, effective, and economical.[45]

Uncomplicated Acute Pyelonephritis

A young, sexually active woman without recent antimicrobial use or urologic instrumentation presents with symptoms of flank pain, nausea, vomiting and fever and has costovertebral angle tenderness on examination; this patient most likely has acute pyelonephritis. Treatment for acute pyelonephritis may occur in an outpatient or inpatient setting, depending on patient presentation (Table 86-4).

Table 86-4 Patient Classification in Acute Pyelonephritis

Outpatient Therapy	Inpatient Therapy
Not pregnant	Pregnant
Compliant	Noncompliant
Non–toxic-appearing	Septic
No nausea or vomiting	Unable to tolerate oral therapy

From Hooton TM, Stamm WE: Diagnosis and treatment of uncomplicated urinary tract infection. Infect Dis Clin North Am 11:551-581, 1997.

Figure 86-1 depicts the appropriate algorithm for the management of acute uncomplicated pyelonephritis, which has a similar etiologic profile to uncomplicated acute cystitis (see Table 86-3). For outpatient therapy, the ISDA recommends a 7-day course of an oral fluoroquinolone.[40] ISDA guidelines for inpatient therapy include a parenteral fluoroquinolone, an aminoglycoside with or without ampicillin, or an extended-spectrum cephalosporin with or without ampicillin. Ampicillin/sulbactam with or without an aminoglycoside is recommended if the offending species is a gram-positive organism.[40] Antimicrobials should be given for a total of 10 to 14 days. The patient may be switched to oral antimicrobials once there has been documented improvement within 72 hours.[7]

When is it Appropriate to Obtain Imaging?

If the patient does not improve clinically within 72 hours, the clinician should give serious consideration to obtaining a CT scan or ultrasound study.[46] Some patients may require intervention in addition to antimicrobials. This may include ureteral stenting or placement of a percutaneous nephrostomy to bypass an obstruction, or perhaps drainage of a perinephric abscess.

Imaging may also be helpful in determining whether there is a urologic abnormality, such as struvite stones, foreign bodies, urethral diverticula, or perivesical fistula, that is causing bacterial persistence.[7] A complete list of patient characteristics that should direct the clinician to obtain imaging is included in Box 86-3.

Complicated Urinary Tract Infection

As mentioned previously, a complicated infection is classified as either an infection that has responded poorly to therapy or one that is associated with host factors that increase the risk of therapy

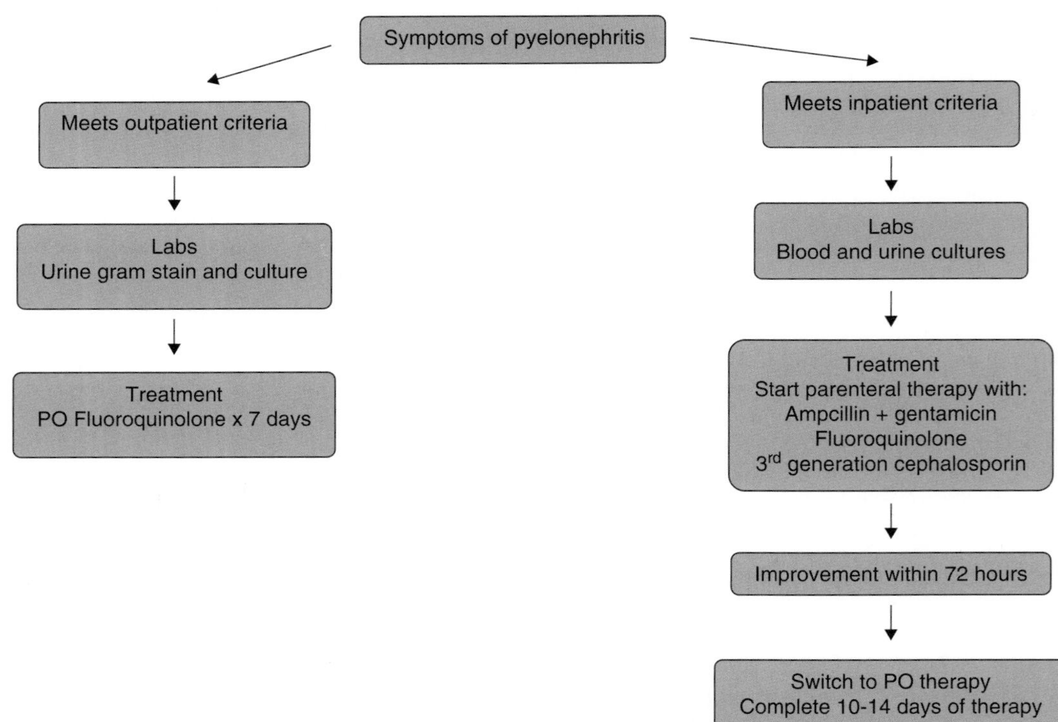

Figure 86-1 Algorithm for uncomplicated pyelonephritis. (Adapted from Schaeffer AJ: Infections of the urinary tract. In Walsh PC, Retik AB, Vaughan ED Jr, Wein AJ [eds]: Campbell's Urology. Philadelphia, WB Saunders, 2002, pp 516-602.)

Table 86-5 Host Risk Factors for Complicated Urinary Tract Infection

Structural/Functional Abnormality	Compromised Host by History	Virulent Bacteria
Obstruction	Pregnancy	Recent antimicrobial use
Congenital urinary tract abnormality	Diabetes	Hospitalized or nursing home patient
	Spinal cord injury	Recent urinary tract instrumentation

Data from Hooton TM: Pathogenesis of urinary tract infections: An update. J Antimicrob Chemother 46(Suppl 1):1-7; discussion 63-65, 2000; Bent S, Nallamothu BK, Simel DL, et al: Does this woman have an acute uncomplicated urinary tract infection? JAMA 287:2701-2710, 2002; Ronald A: The etiology of urinary tract infection: Traditional and emerging pathogens. Am J Med 113(Suppl 1A):14S-19S, 2002.

Box 86-3 When Is It Appropriate to Obtain Imaging?

On initial assessment, history or findings suggestive of:

- Ureteral obstruction (may include stone, stricture, tumor, history of genitourinary surgery, or congenital obstruction)
- Sepsis/fever
- Severe diabetes mellitus
- Neurogenic bladder
- Papillary necrosis (sickle cell, diabetes, analgesic abuse)
- Polycystic kidney disease on dialysis

After initial treatment:

- Pyelonephritis with poor response to therapy after 72 hr
- Unusual infecting organism (urea-splitting organism, tuberculosis, fungus)

Modified from Schaeffer AJ: Infections of the urinary tract. Walsh PC, Retik AB, Vaughan ED Jr, Wein AJ (eds): Campbell's Urology. Philadelphia, WB Saunders, 2002, 516-602.

Table 86-6 Pathogens Cultured in Complicated Urinary Tract Infections

Gram-negative organisms	
Escherichia coli	21-54%
Proteus mirabilis	1-10%
Klebsiella species	2-17%
Citrobacter species	5%
Enterobacter species	2-10%
Pseudomonas aeruginosa	2-19%
Other	6-20%
Gram-positive organisms	
Coagulase-negative staphylococci	1-4%
Enterococci	1-23%
Group B streptococci	1-4%
Staphylococcus aureus	1-2%
Other	2%

From Nicolle LE: Recurrent urinary tract infection in adult women: Diagnosis and treatment. Infect Dis Clin North Am 1:791-806, 1987.

failure.[8] It is important to recognize patients with complicated UTIs, because there are implications for the workup and treatment. What are the factors that lead to the classification of a complicated UTI? These factors may be classified as structural or functional abnormalities, conditions that compromise host response, and conditions that promote infection with virulent bacteria (Table 86-5).

The pathogenic organisms cultured in complicated UTIs vary from those seen in uncomplicated UTIs (Table 86-6).

If the patient is well enough to be treated as an outpatient, then a fluoroquinolone should be chosen as first-line therapy. However, if the patient has a severe infection requiring admission, then broad-spectrum antimicrobials should be initiated.[7] In general, treatment requires at least 14 to 21 days of antimicrobial therapy.[40] Individual scenarios of complicated infections are discussed in the following paragraphs.

Obstruction

Case: A 32-year-old woman with a history of nephrolithiasis presents with right-sided flank pain and fever.

Calcium oxalate stones can cause ureteral obstruction and may become secondarily colonized. Other than stones, urinary tract obstruction may also be caused by tumor, clot, or papillary necrosis.

Urea-Splitting Bacteria that Cause Struvite Stones

Case: A 25-year-old woman with recurrent UTI has recently completed a course of antimicrobials after suffering from a UTI caused by *P. mirabilis.* A post-therapy urine culture is obtained and grows the same organism. She is currently asymptomatic.

P. mirabilis causes alkalinization of the urine, leading to precipitation of calcium, magnesium, ammonium, and phosphate salts and subsequent struvite stone formation. These stones have become known as staghorn calculi because they tend to be large stones that take on the shape of the renal collecting system. Bacteria persist within these struvite stones, and bacteriuria tends to recur almost immediately on discontinuation of antimicrobial therapy. Struvite stones often contain minimal calcium and may not be evident on plain film radiographs.[7]

Congenital Urinary Tract Anomalies

Case: An 18-year-old woman with a known history of ureteropelvic junction obstruction presents with a history of recurrent UTIs.

In patients with anomalies of the urinary tract and UTI, recurrent bacteriuria with the same organism typically occurs until the anomalous structure is surgically corrected. Such anomalies include ureteral duplication with ectopic ureter, pericalyceal diverticula, urachal cysts, unilateral medullary sponge kidneys, and congenital obstructions with nonfunctioning kidneys.[7]

Pregnancy

Case: A 29-year-old pregnant woman in her third trimester presents with fever, left-sided flank pain, nausea, and vomiting.

Box 86-4 Urinary Tract Changes in Pregnancy

Collecting system
- Decreased peristalsis of the collecting system and ureters
- Mechanical obstruction of the ureters secondary to enlarging uterus

Bladder
- Displaced superiorly and anteriorly

Kidneys
- Increased glomerular filtration rate (GFR) by 30-50%

From Waltzer WC: The urinary tract in pregnancy. J Urol 125:271-276, 1981.

Although it has been shown that the incidence of bacteriuria in pregnant women is similar to that in their nonpregnant counterparts, the incidence of acute pyelonephritis is significantly increased in pregnant women compared with nonpregnant women.[47] This is perhaps due to the numerous anatomic and physiologic changes that occur in the urinary tract during pregnancy (Box 86-4). Not surprisingly, pyelonephritis is most commonly seen in the third trimester, when stasis and hydronephrosis are most evident.[7]

Before the advent of antimicrobial therapy, pregnant women with pyelonephritis had an increased rate of infant prematurity and perinatal mortality. Today, there is continued debate in the literature as to whether gestational pyelonephritis leads to prematurity and subsequent perinatal mortality. In any case, patients with pyelonephritis during pregnancy should be admitted and treated with parenteral agents.[7]Antimicrobials that are safe to use during pregnancy include penicillins, cephalosporins, and nitrofurantoin. The latter, however, should not be used in pyelonephritis, because it does not achieve adequate tissue penetration. Agents that may be harmful to the developing fetus should be avoided. Fluoroquinolones may impair cartilage development, and TMP-SMX is associated with antifolate teratogenicity in the first trimester and with neonatal hyperbilirubinemia in the third trimester.[48] After treatment, women should either be given prophylaxis or monitored closely throughout the remainder of the pregnancy, because there is an increased risk of repeated episodes of pyelonephritis.[49]

Diabetes Mellitus

Case: A 45-year-old woman with poorly controlled diabetes is admitted to the hospital with acute pyelonephritis. Despite parenteral antimicrobial therapy for 3 days, she continues to have high, spiking temperatures.

The incidence of UTI in diabetic women has been shown to be substantially higher than in nondiabetic women.[50] Treatment may be more difficult if glomerulopathy is present, because urine concentration of antimicrobials may be less than optimal.[7] Diabetes is also associated with specific entities such as intrarenal and perirenal abscess, emphysematous pyelonephritis and cystitis, xanthogranulomatous pyelonephritis, and papillary necrosis.[8] Further discussion of these entities is beyond the scope of this chapter.

Spinal Cord Injuries

Case: A 27-year-old woman with a history of a thoracic spinal cord injury presents with fevers and foul-smelling urine. She manages her bladder with clean intermittent catheterization.

The method of bladder management plays a large role in UTI in these patients. Patients with indwelling urethral or suprapubic catheters have high rates of infection.[51] Clean intermittent catheterization was introduced in 1972 and revolutionized bladder management of patients with spinal cord injury. It has been shown to reduce the risk factors for UTI by decreasing intravesical pressure and the incidence of stones.[52] Nevertheless, UTI is a common problem in spinal cord–injured patients and is often difficult to diagnose. Because of loss of sensation, patients do not present with the typical symptoms of frequency, urgency, or dysuria. Additionally, urinalysis in these patients often demonstrates bacteriuria and pyuria regardless of the presence of infection. Therefore, the diagnosis is often clinical, based on symptoms of flank, back, or abdominal discomfort; leakage between catheterizations; fever; increased spasticity; and/or cloudy, malodorous urine.[7] A urine culture must be obtained before therapy is initiated, because there is a high probability of bacterial resistance.[7] Spinal cord–injured patients with recurrent UTI should undergo urinary tract imaging, urodynamic testing, and a review of their bladder management program.[53]

SPECIAL CONSIDERATIONS

Urinary Tract Infection Prophylaxis

A nonantimicrobial treatment that prevents UTIs would be extremely useful for women who suffer from recurrent UTIs.

Cranberry

Two compounds in cranberries, fructose and proanthocyanidin, have been found to inhibit *E. coli* adhesins in vitro.[54] This finding is likely the basis for the widespread belief among laypersons that cranberries prevent UTIs. Despite a number of clinical trials, at this time there is no compelling evidence that cranberries or cranberry products prevent UTIs.[55]

Lactobacilli

Lactobacillus probiotics have been proposed as means of enhancing the natural host defenses by restoring the presence of a normal vaginal microflora.[56,57] Various properties of lactobacillus are believed to be protective against uropathogenic organisms. These include maintenance of an acidic pH, direct killing of pathogens through the production of H_2O_2, and competitive inhibition of bacterial adherence.[58]

Multiple small trials have been conducted using *Lactobacillus* species to recolonize the vaginas of women with recurrent UTI. These studies have produced mixed results, and further research in this area is needed.[57]

Vaccine

Several vaccines to provide protection against UTI caused by *E. coli* or other uropathogens are currently under development. Preliminary studies are promising for short-term protection from recurrences, but it remains to be seen whether long-term efficacy can be demonstrated.[57]

Asymptomatic Bacteriuria of Pregnancy

Asymptomatic bacteriuria occurs in 4% to 6% of both pregnant and nonpregnant women.[59]Despite these similar rates, the number of pregnant women who develop pyelonephritis is significantly higher than in nonpregnant women. It has been reported that as many as 20% to 40% of pregnant women with asymptomatic bacteriuria subsequently develop acute pyelonephritis.[60,61] Treatment of bacteriuria early in pregnancy has been shown to decrease the incidence of pyelonephritis by 90%.[62]

The American College of Obstetricians and Gynecologists currently recommends screening for asymptomatic bacteriuria in pregnancy.[60,63] Obtaining a urine culture once at the end of the first trimester is sufficient. Repeated screening of women with initial negative urine cultures is not recommended, because the risk of pyelonephritis is low.[63] If the urine culture is positive, a repeat specimen for culture should be obtained and treatment initiated. After treatment, women should have periodic urine cultures to identify recurrent bacteriuria throughout the remainder of the pregnancy.[64]

References

1. McLaughlin SP, Carson CC: Urinary tract infections in women. Med Clin North Am 88:417-429, 2004.
2. Foxman B, Brown P: Epidemiology of urinary tract infections: transmission and risk factors, incidence, and costs. Infect Dis Clin North Am 17:227-241, 2003.
3. Foxman B, Barlow R, D'Arcy H, et al: Urinary tract infection: self-reported incidence and associated costs. Ann Epidemiol 10:509-515, 2000.
4. Mulvey MA, Lopez-Boado YS, Wilson CL, et al: Induction and evasion of host defenses by type 1-piliated uropathogenic *Escherichia coli*. Science 282:1494-1497, 1998.
5. Anderson GG, Palermo JJ, Schilling JD, et al: Intracellular bacterial biofilm-like pods in urinary tract infections. Science 301:105-107, 2003.
6. Mulvey MA, Schilling JD, Hultgren SJ: Establishment of a persistent *Escherichia coli* reservoir during the acute phase of a bladder infection. Infect Immun 69:4572-4579, 2001.
7. Schaeffer AJ: Infections of the urinary tract. In Walsh PC, Retik AB, Vaughan ED Jr, Wein AJ (eds): Campbell's Urology. Philadelphia, WB Saunders, 2002, pp 516-602.
8. Hooton TM: Pathogenesis of urinary tract infections: an update. J Antimicrob Chemother 46(Suppl 1):1-7; discussion 63-65, 2000.
9. Fowler JE Jr, Stamey TA: Studies of introital colonization in women with recurrent urinary infections. VII. The role of bacterial adherence. J Urol 117:472-476, 1977.
10. Schaeffer AJ, Jones JM, Duncan JL, et al: Adhesion of uropathogenic *Escherichia coli* to epithelial cells from women with recurrent urinary tract infection. Infection 10:186-191, 1982.
11. Schaeffer AJ, Radvany RM, Chmiel JS: Human leukocyte antigens in women with recurrent urinary tract infections. J Infect Dis 148:604, 1983.
12. Sheinfeld J, Schaeffer AJ, Cordon-Cardo C, et al: Association of the Lewis blood-group phenotype with recurrent urinary tract infections in women. N Engl J Med 320:773-777, 1989.
13. Schaeffer AJ: New concepts in the pathogenesis of urinary tract infections. Urol Clin North Am 29:241-250, xii, 2002.
14. Eschenbach DA, Patton DL, Hooton TM, et al: Effects of vaginal intercourse with and without a condom on vaginal flora and vaginal epithelium. J Infect Dis 183:913-918, 2001.
15. Foxman B, Manning SD, Tallman P, et al: Uropathogenic *Escherichia coli* are more likely than commensal *E. coli* to be shared between heterosexual sex partners. Am J Epidemiol 156:1133-1140, 2002.
16. Hooton TM, Roberts PL, Stamm WE: Effects of recent sexual activity and use of a diaphragm on the vaginal microflora. Clin Infect Dis 19:274-278, 1994.
17. Raz R, Stamm WE: A controlled trial of intravaginal estriol in postmenopausal women with recurrent urinary tract infections. N Engl J Med 329:753-756, 1993.
18. Cardozo L, Benness C, Abbott D: Low dose oestrogen prophylaxis for recurrent urinary tract infections in elderly women. Br J Obstet Gynaecol 105:403-407, 1998.
19. Smith HS, Hughes JP, Hooton TM, et al: Antecedent antimicrobial use increases the risk of uncomplicated cystitis in young women. Clin Infect Dis 25:63-68, 1997.
20. Bent S, Saint S: The optimal use of diagnostic testing in women with acute uncomplicated cystitis. Dis Mon 49:83-98, 2003.
21. Semeniuk H, Church D: Evaluation of the leukocyte esterase and nitrite urine dipstick screening tests for detection of bacteriuria in women with suspected uncomplicated urinary tract infections. J Clin Microbiol 37:3051-3052, 1999.
22. Hurlbut TA 3rd, Littenberg B: The diagnostic accuracy of rapid dipstick tests to predict urinary tract infection. Am J Clin Pathol 96:582-528, 1991.
23. Nickel JC: Management of urinary tract infections: Historical perspective and current strategies. Part 2: Modern management. J Urol 173:27-32, 2005.
24. Fihn SD: Clinical practice: Acute uncomplicated urinary tract infection in women. N Engl J Med 349: 259-266, 2003.
25. Stamm WE, Hooton TM: Management of urinary tract infections in adults. N Engl J Med 329:1328-1334, 1993.
26. Klastersky J, Daneau D, Swings G, Weerts D: Antibacterial activity in serum and urine as a therapeutic guide in bacterial infections. J Infect Dis 129:187-193, 1974.
27. Schaeffer AJ: The expanding role of fluoroquinolones. Am J Med 113(Suppl 1A):45S-54S, 2002.
28. Hooton TM, Stamm WE: Diagnosis and treatment of uncomplicated urinary tract infection. Infect Dis Clin North Am 11:551-581, 1997.
29. Johnson JR, Stamm WE: Urinary tract infections in women: Diagnosis and treatment. Ann Intern Med 111:906-917, 1989.
30. Burman LG: Significance of the sulfonamide component for the clinical efficacy of trimethoprim-sulfonamide combinations. Scand J Infect Dis 18:89-99, 1986.
31. Cockerill FR, Edson RS: Trimethoprim-sulfamethoxazole. Mayo Clin Proc 66:1260-1269, 1991.
32. Gupta K, Sahm DF, Mayfield D, Stamm WE: Antimicrobial resistance among uropathogens that cause community-acquired urinary tract infections in women: A nationwide analysis. Clin Infect Dis 33:89-94, 2001.
33. Iravani A: Advances in the understanding and treatment of urinary tract infections in young women. Urology 37:503-511, 1991.
34. Wilhelm MP, Edson RS: Antimicrobial agents in urinary tract infections. Mayo Clin Proc 62:1025-1031, 1987.
35. Hooton TM, Besser R, Foxman B, et al: Acute uncomplicated cystitis in an era of increasing antibiotic resistance: A proposed approach to empirical therapy. Clin Infect Dis 39:75-80, 2004.
36. Nicolau DP, Freeman CD, Belliveau PP, et al. Experience with a once-daily aminoglycoside program administered to 2,184 adult patients. Antimicrob Agents Chemother 39:650-655, 1995.
37. Bent S, Nallamothu BK, Simel DL, et al: Does this woman have an acute uncomplicated urinary tract infection? JAMA 287:2701-2710, 2002.
38. Komaroff AL: Acute dysuria in women. N Engl J Med 310:368-375, 1984.
39. Barry HC, Hickner J, Ebell MH, Ettenhofer T: A randomized controlled trial of telephone management of suspected urinary tract infections in women. J Fam Pract 50:589-594, 2001.
40. Warren JW, Abrutyn E, Hebel JR, et al: Guidelines for antimicrobial treatment of uncomplicated acute bacterial cystitis and acute pyelo-

nephritis in women. Infectious Diseases Society of America (IDSA). Clin Infect Dis 29:745-758, 1999.

41. Hooton TM, Winter C, Tiu F, Stamm WE: Randomized comparative trial and cost analysis of 3-day antimicrobial regimens for treatment of acute cystitis in women. JAMA 273:41-45, 1995.
42. Scholes D, Hooton TM, Roberts PL, et al: Risk factors for recurrent urinary tract infection in young women. J Infect Dis 182:1177-1182, 2000.
43. Nicolle LE, Ronald AR: Recurrent urinary tract infection in adult women: Diagnosis and treatment. Infect Dis Clin North Am 1:793-806, 1987.
44. Stapleton A, Latham RH, Johnson C, Stamm WE: Postcoital antimicrobial prophylaxis for recurrent urinary tract infection: A randomized, double-blind, placebo-controlled trial. JAMA 264:703-706, 1990.
45. Schaeffer AJ, Stuppy BA: Efficacy and safety of self-start therapy in women with recurrent urinary tract infections. J Urol 161:207-111, 1999.
46. Soulen MC, Fishman EK, Goldman SM, Gatewood OM: Bacterial renal infection: Role of CT. Radiology 171:703-707, 1989.
47. Sweet RL: Bacteriuria and pyelonephritis during pregnancy. Semin Perinatol 1:25-40, 1977.
48. Weiser AC, Schaeffer AJ: The use and misuse of antimicrobial agents in urology. AUA Update Series 31:137, 2002.
49. Gilstrap LC, Leveno KJ, Cunningham FG, et al: Renal infection and pregnancy outcome. Am J Obstet Gynecol 141:709-716, 1981.
50. Ooi BS, Chen BT, Yu M: Prevalence and site of bacteriuria in diabetes mellitus. Postgrad Med J 50:497-499, 1974.
51. Tambyah PA, Maki DG: Catheter-associated urinary tract infection is rarely symptomatic: A prospective study of 1,497 catheterized patients. Arch Intern Med 160:678-682, 2000.
52. Stover SL, Lloyd LK, Waites KB, Jackson AB: Urinary tract infection in spinal cord injury. Arch Phys Med Rehabil 70:47-54, 1989.
53. Cardenas DD, Hooton TM: Urinary tract infection in persons with spinal cord injury. Arch Phys Med Rehabil 76:272-280, 1995.
54. Zafriri D, Ofek I, Adar R, et al: Inhibitory activity of cranberry juice on adherence of type 1 and type P fimbriated *Escherichia coli* to eucaryotic cells. Antimicrob Agents Chemother 33:92-98, 1989.
55. Raz R, Chazan B, Dan M: Cranberry juice and urinary tract infection. Clin Infect Dis 38:1413-1419, 2004.
56. Reid G: The scientific basis for probiotic strains of *Lactobacillus*. Appl Environ Microbiol 65:3763-3766, 1999.
57. Stapleton A: Novel approaches to prevention of urinary tract infections. Infect Dis Clin North Am 17:457-471, 2003.
58. Reid G, Bruce AW: Selection of lactobacillus strains for urogenital probiotic applications. J Infect Dis 183(Suppl 1):S77-S80, 2001.
59. Stamey TA: Pathogenesis and Treatment of Urinary Tract Infections. Baltimore, Williams & Wilkins, 1980.
60. Millar LK, Cox SM: Urinary tract infections complicating pregnancy. Infect Dis Clin North Am 11:13-26, 1997.
61. Patterson TF, Andriole VT: Detection, significance, and therapy of bacteriuria in pregnancy: Update in the managed health care era. Infect Dis Clin North Am 11:593-608, 1997.
62. Gratacos E, Torres PJ, Vila J, et al: Screening and treatment of asymptomatic bacteriuria in pregnancy prevent pyelonephritis. J Infect Dis 169:1390-1392, 1994.
63. Stenqvist K, Dahlen-Nilsson I, Lidin-Janson G, et al: Bacteriuria in pregnancy: Frequency and risk of acquisition. Am J Epidemiol 129:372-379, 1989.
64. Nicolle LE: Asymptomatic bacteriuria: When to screen and when to treat. Infect Dis Clin North Am 17:367-394, 2003.

Chapter 87

VULVAR AND VAGINAL PAIN, DYSPAREUNIA, AND ABNORMAL VAGINAL DISCHARGE

Andrea J. Rapkin and Monica Lee

DEFINITION OF VULVODYNIA AND CURRENT NOMENCLATURE

The purpose of this chapter is to outline the anatomy and physiology of vulvar and vaginal pain syndromes and to explore the differential diagnosis and management of vulvar and vaginal pain and dyspareunia (Tables 87-1 and 87-2), including the roles of medication, surgery, psychotherapy, and multidisciplinary pain management. The differential diagnosis and management of abnormal vaginal discharge is also discussed.

Vulvar pain syndromes are characterized by unexplained burning or any combination of stinging, irritation, itching, pain or rawness anywhere from the mons pubis to the anus that causes physical, sexual, and psychological distress. A multitude of terms have been used in the literature to describe vulvar pain syndromes. Vulvodynia was first described in 1889 by A. J. C. Skene[1] but received little attention until the 1970s. The International Society for the Study of Vulvovaginal Diseases (ISSVD) abandoned the term "burning vulva syndrome," first described in 1984,[2] and introduced a classification wherein the two principal divisions were vulvar vestibulitis syndrome (VVS) and dysesthetic or essential vulvodynia.[3] The most recent classification of vulvar pain, which was agreed on at the October 2003 Congress of the ISSVD, consists of two major categories[4]:

1. *Vulvar pain* related to a specific disorder
   a. Infection
   b. Inflammation
   c. Neoplasm
   d. Neurologic disease
2. *Vulvodynia:* vulvar discomfort, usually described as burning pain, occurring in the absence of a specific disorder
   a. *Generalized* (involving the entire vulva) or *localized* (involving a portion or component of the vulva, such as the vestibule, clitoris, or hemivulva)
   b. *Provoked* (i.e., by sexual and/or nonsexual contact), *unprovoked* (i.e., spontaneous), or *mixed* (provoked and unprovoked).

The term *vestibulitis* signifies the presence of inflammation, which was thought to be misleading because much evidence suggests no such presence. Therefore, the ISSVD voted to discontinue use of this term.

INCIDENCE AND EPIDEMIOLOGY OF VULVODYNIA

The typical patient with vulvodynia used to be described as a nulliparous woman in her 20s or early 30s who often may have developed symptoms suddenly.[5] The true prevalence of vulvodynia is uncertain due to its recent recognition; however, a 1991 study of 210 consecutive patients seen at a private practice for general gynecology found that 37% had some degree of positive testing for vulvar discomfort, and 15% met full criteria.[6] A survey of more than 4900 women aged 18 to 64 years reported that 16% of the 3000 respondents had experienced vulvar pain lasting at least 3 months; 7% had vulvar pain at the time of the survey, and many had seen up to five different doctors for this problem.[7] Unexplained vulvar pain was found to be of similar incidence among white and African American women. Hispanic women were 80% more likely than white women to have experienced chronic vulvar pain.

ANATOMY OF THE VULVA AND VAGINA

The vulva is the part of female anatomy located between the genitocrural folds laterally and between the mons pubis anteriorly and the anus posteriorly (Fig. 87-1).[8] It is composed of the labia majora, labia minora, mons pubis, clitoris, vestibule, urinary meatus, vaginal orifice, hymen, Bartholin's glands, Skene's ducts, and vestibulovaginal bulbs.

The labia majora form the lateral boundaries of the vulva and consist of two large folds of adipose and fibrous tissue. Anteriorly, the labia majora fuse into the mons pubis; posteriorly, they become narrower and flatter and terminate 3 to 4 cm anterior to the anus, where they are united by the posterior commissure or fourchette. The skin of the labia majora is usually darker than the adjacent skin. The skin has an outer lining of stratified squamous epithelium. Within the dermis are numerous hair follicles and sebaceous, sweat (eccrine), and apocrine glands.

The labia minora lie between the labia majora and consist of two flat folds of connective tissue containing little or no adipose tissue. They are covered by skin on their lateral aspects and partially so on their medial aspects. Hart's line separates the medial boundary of the minora from the vestibule and is the line of demarcation between the skin and mucous membrane; it runs along the base of the inner aspect of each labia minora, passes into the fossa navicularis, and separates the skin boundary of the fourchette from the mucous membrane of the hymen. The labia minora are 4 to 5 cm in length and 0.5 cm in thickness. Anteriorly, each divides into two parts, one passing over the clitoris to form the prepuce and the other joining the clitoris to form the frenulum. Posteriorly, they tend to become smaller and blend with the medial surfaces of the labia majora or unite anterior to the posterior commissure to form the fourchette. The skin and mucosa of the labia minora are extremely rich in sebaceous glands. During sexual excitement, the labia minora frequently

Table 87-1 Differential Diagnosis of Dyspareunia

Fissure	Anal fissure
	Posterior fourchette fissure
	Enteroperineal fissure (Crohn's disease)
	Lichen sclerosus
	Vaginal atrophy
	Vulvovaginitis
Pruritus	Dermatitis
	Human papillomavirus infection
	Lichen planus
	Lichen sclerosus
	Lichen simplex chronicus
	Seminal plasma allergy
	Vaginal atrophy
	Vulvovaginitis
Ulcer	Behçet's syndrome
	Chancroid
	Herpes simplex virus infection
	Lichen planus
Erythema	Bartholin's abscess
	Dermatitis
	Desquamative inflammatory vaginitis
	Hemorrhoids
	Seminal plasma allergy
	Vulvar vestibulitis
	Vulvovaginitis
Mass/tumor/swelling	Bartholin's abscess
	Bartholin's cyst
	Hemorrhoids
	Labial hypertrophy
	Radiation
	Urethral caruncle
	Urethral diverticulum
Urinary tract lesions	Urethral caruncle
	Urethral diverticulum
	Urethritis
Dryness	Inadequate sexual arousal/lubrication
	Radiation
	Vaginal atrophy
No vulvar lesions	Episiotomy scar
	Female circumcision
	Inadequate sexual arousal/lubrication
	Rigid hymeneal ring
	Vaginismus
	Vulvar neuroma
	Vulvar vestibulitis
	Vulvodynia
	Vulvovaginitis
Entry dyspareunia	Bartholin's gland cyst or abscess
	Behçet's syndrome
	Chancroid
	Dermatitis: allergy, vulvovaginitis, atopic vulvitis
	Desquamative inflammatory vaginitis
	Episiotomy scar
	Female circumcision
	Fissure: anal, posterior fourchette, enteroperineal (Crohn's)
	Hemorrhoids
	Herpes simplex or zoster
	Inadequate sexual arousal and lubrication
	Labial hypertrophy
	Lichen planus
	Lichen sclerosus
	Lichen simplex chronicus
	Mullerian abnormality
	Post-traumatic pubic symphysis pain
	Radiation damage
	Rigid hymenal ring
	Seminal plasma allergy
	Urethral caruncle
	Urethral diverticulum
	Urethritis
	Vaginal atrophy
	Vaginismus
	Vulvar vestibulitis
	Vulvodynia
	Vulvovaginitis
Deep dyspareunia	Adenomyosis
	Endometriosis
	Fixed uterine retroversion
	Inflammatory bowel disease
	Interstitial cystitis
	Irritable bowel syndrome
	Leiomyomas
	Ovarian pathology
	Pelvic adhesions
	Pelvic floor relaxation
	Pelvic inflammatory disease
	Radiation-induced vaginal scarring
	Rectocele
	Shortened vagina
	Urethral syndrome

become swollen and congested and take on the appearance of erectile tissue.

The clitoris is the female homologue of the penis. It consists of two cylindrical erectile bodies, called the corpora cavernosa, that terminate in the vestibule as the glans. The body of the clitoris is approximately 2 cm long, is formed by the fusion of the two corpora cavernosa, and extends posteriorly from the pubic arch to the glans. The glans of the clitoris is covered by a mucous membrane containing many special nerve end organs.

The vestibule is the portion of the vulva that extends from the clitoris to the fourchette and is visible on separation of the labia majora. Hart's line represents the outer perimeter of the vulvar vestibule, and the inner margin of the vestibule is the hymen. The vestibule is covered by nonpigmented, nonkeratinized squamous epithelium and is devoid of skin adnexa. It contains mucus-secreting minor vestibular glands. The ductal orifices of Bartholin's glands, the periurethral gland complexes of Skene, and the urethral meatus all empty onto the vestibular surface. The vagina opens into the vestibule. The hymen is the thin membrane of

Table 87-2 Evaluation of Patients with Vulvar or Vaginal Pain

History	Detailed pain history, obstetric/gynecologic, sexual, medical, surgical, psychosocial, medications, allergies, habits, trauma
Vulvar examination	Inspection: lesions (macules, papules, ulcers, nodules), fissures, fistulas, inflammation (edema, erythema), discharge, tumors, anatomic abnormalities (surgical, congenital, traumatic).
	Palpation: localize pain with cotton swab, identify specific neural distribution, vestibule, Bartholin's, Skene's, hymenal caliber, urethra
	Biopsy and/or culture suspicious lesions (e.g., VIN, ulcers, verrucae, white or red plaques); colposcopic magnification of lesions if indicated
Vaginal examination	Speculum examination: inspect mucosa (color, rugations, lesions)
	pH of discharge
	Wet mount saline and KOH: infection, atrophy
	Culture (fungal, bacterial): vagina, cervix
	Cystocele, rectocele, enterocele, uterine prolapse, cervical discharge, lesions
	Palpate, attempt to reproduce pain: hymen, bladder, individual pelvic floor muscles, ischial spine area for pudendal nerves, inferior hypogastric plexus (paracervical), cervical motion tenderness
	Assess ability to contract and relax muscles
Bimanual examination	Uterus: size, shape, position, mobility, tenderness, uterosacral ligament thickening/nodularity, tenderness, adnexal masses, tenderness, mobility
	Cervical motion tenderness
Rectovaginal examination	Rectal masses, stool guaiac, nodules/fibrosis in cul-de-sac
Additional diagnotic tests as needed	Pelvic floor MRI, pelvic ultrasound, pudendal nerve conduction velocity, diagnostic nerve blocks (local, pudendal, inferior hypogastric), cystourethroscopy, sigmoidoscopy, physical therapist evaluation of pelvic floor, psychological/stress/couples evaluation, HSV serology, urine analysis and culture
Create differential or specific diagnoses	Specific infectious, inflammatory, or anatomic pathology.
	Treat per diagnosis (e.g., pharmacologic, surgical)
	Neuroplastic or neuropathic/neuromuscular pain requires a multidisciplinary approach: physical therapy, psychology (cognitive/behavioral/biofeedback/sexual), series of specific nerve blocks, pharmacologic (medications to alter nerve conduction or for depression/anxiety, such as antidepressants, anticonvulsants, local anesthetics, or muscle relaxants [Botox])

HSV, herpes simplex virus; KOH, potassium hydroxide; MRI, magnetic resonance imaging; VIN, vulvar intraepithelial neoplasm.

connective tissue over the entrance of the vagina into the vestibule. Bartholin's glands lie deep beneath the fascia, one on each side of the vestibule, posterolaterally to the vaginal orifice. The cells lining the acini contain mucin, which is secreted during sexual excitement and contributes to lubrication of the vaginal orifice. The main ducts of Bartholin's glands open into the vestibule at approximately the 5 and 7 o'clock positions, outside the hymenal ring. The urethra opens into the vestibule just anterior to the vaginal introitus.

Arterial blood supply to the vulva comes from the internal pudendal artery, which derives from the internal iliac artery (hypogastric artery), and from branches of the external pudendal artery, which derives from the femoral artery. The veins of the vulva form a large plexus, which empties into the internal and external pudendal veins.

Innervation of the vulva is supplied by the cutaneous branches of the ilioinguinal nerve anterosuperiorly and by the pudendal branches of the femoral cutaneous nerve posteroinferiorly (Fig. 87-2). The three roots of the pudendal nerve derive from the second, third, and fourth sacral nerves; they unite approximately 1 cm proximal to the ischial spine, then leave the pelvic cavity by passing though the greater sciatic foramen.[9] The pudendal nerve subsequently passes posterior to the junction between the ischial spine and the sacrospinous ligament, then reenters the pelvic cavity through the lesser sciatic foramen and proceeds anteriorly through Alcock's canal. The major cutaneous nerve supply of the perineum is provided by the branches of the pudendal nerve.[9] The inferior hemorrhoidal nerve supplies the posterior portion; the superficial branch of the perineal nerve divides into medial and lateral parts known as the posterior labial nerves, and the dorsal nerve of the clitoris innervates the clitoral area.

The vagina extends from the vestibule to the uterus and is directed obliquely upward and backward at an angle approximately 45 degrees to the horizontal axis. Its long axis is parallel to the plane of the pelvic brim and at a right angle to the uterus. The upper one third of the vagina is in contact with the base of the bladder, and the entire lower two thirds is in contact with the urethra. The vagina consists of three principal layers: an outer fibrous layer that derives from pelvic fascia, a middle muscular layer, and an inner mucosal layer.

The pelvic floor muscles include the levator ani, pubococcygeus, and coccygeus muscles. All of the fasciae investing the muscles form a continuum of connective tissue that joins the fascial covering of the pelvic viscera above with the fascia of the perineum below.[9] The levator ani muscle is a broad, thin structure that is attached to the inner surface of the side of the

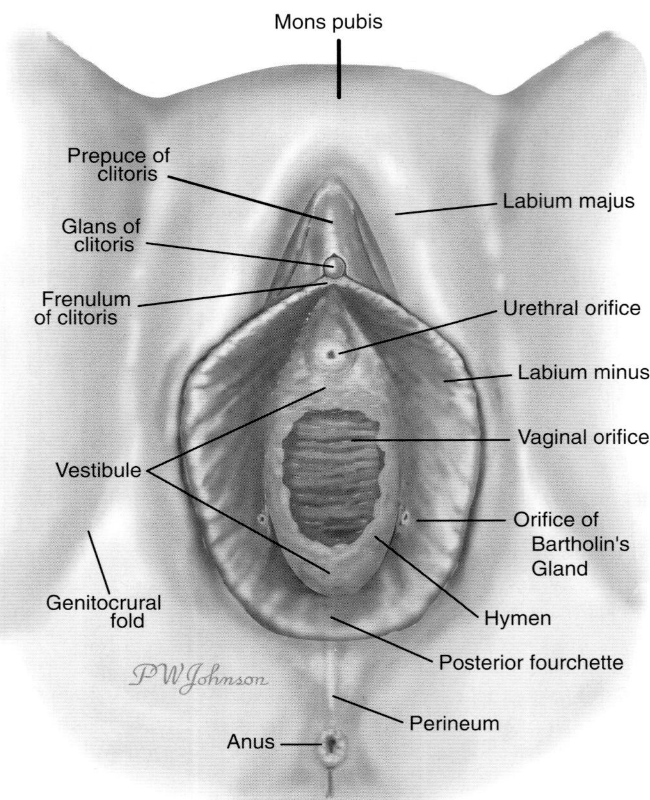

Figure 87-1 Vulvar anatomy. (Redrawn from Kaufman RH: Benign Diseases of the Vulva and Vagina, 5th ed. St. Louis, Elsevier Mosby, 2005.)

true pelvis.[9] It is attached anteriorly to the pelvic surface of the body of the pubis, lateral to the symphysis; behind, to the medial surface of the spine of the ischium; and between these two points, to the obturator fascia. Morphologically, the levator ani can be divided into the pubococcygeus and the iliococcygeus muscles.

The pubococcygeus muscle arises from the posterior surface of the pubis and from the anterior part of the obturator fascia. Its fibers are directed backward, almost horizontally, along the line of the anal canal and become attached to the front of the coccyx by a tendinous plate that is continuous with the anterior sacrococcygeal ligament. The medial coccygeal muscle arises from the ischial spine and from the posterior part of the tendinous arch of the levator ani muscle. Its fibers attach to the sides of the coccyx and to the opposite muscle in the median raphe on the undersurface of the tendinous plates of the pubococcygeus that contribute to the anococcygeal ligament. The superior or pelvic surface of the levator ani is separated by its covering fascia from the bladder, rectum, and perineum, whereas its inferior and or perineal surface forms the medial boundary of the ischiorectal fossa and is covered by the inferior fascia of the pelvic diaphragm. Its posterior border is free and is separated from the coccygeus muscle by areolar tissue, whereas the medial borders of the two muscles are separated by the visceral outlet, an interval through which the urethra, vagina, and anorectum pass from the pelvis. The nerve supply of the levator ani muscle includes a branch from the S4 nerve, a branch that arises either from the inferior rectal nerve or from the perineal branch of the pudendal nerve. The function of the levator ani muscle is constriction of the lower end of the rectum and vagina, and probably fixation of the perineal body as well. The levator ani, together with the coccygei, form a muscular diaphragm that supports the pelvic viscera and opposes itself to the downward thrust produced by any increase in intra-abdominal pressure.

The coccygeus muscle is posterosuperior in the same tissue plane as the levator ani muscle. It consists of a triangular sheath of muscular and tendinous fibers, arising by its apex from the pelvic surface of the spine of the ischium and sacrospinous ligament. It is attached at its base to the margin of the coccyx and the side of the S5 segment. The muscle receives its nerve supply through branches of the S4 and S5 spinal nerves. The coccygeus functions in pulling forward and supporting the coccyx after it has been pressed backward during defecation or parturition. The coccygeus, together with the levator ani and piriformis muscles, closes the posterior part of the pelvic outlet.

The chief sources of blood supply to the vagina are the uterine, pudendal, and middle hemorrhoidal arteries, which arise from the internal iliac arteries. They form a plexus around the vagina. The upper portion is supplied by a descending branch of the uterine artery, the cervical-vaginal artery. The lower half of the vagina is supplied by ascending branches of the middle hemorrhoidal arteries; the dorsal artery, which originates from the internal pudendal, supplies the clitoris.

EVALUATION

History

Obtaining a thorough history is critical in the evaluation and management of vulvar or vaginal pain and dyspareunia (see Table 87-2). Pain symptoms must be well characterized to assess the onset, type of pain (burning, itching, stinging, irritating), timing (constant or cyclic), associated activities (e.g., intercourse, exercise, stress), inciting agents (perfume, lotions, detergents, clothing), and relieving factors (e.g., antifungal medications). A daily pain diary may better define these characteristics. Pain should be quantified on each visit on a scale of 1 (no pain) to 10 (maximal pain imaginable). Concurrent gynecologic, genitourinary, and gastrointestinal symptoms should be identified.

In addition, past or current infections (human papillomavirus [HPV], herpes, *Candida*), medications, local and systemic dermatologic disorders, neurologic disorders (e.g., herniated disk, herpes zoster, pudendal or genitofemoral neuralgia), urologic disorders (interstitial cystitis, urethral syndrome), physical trauma (vaginal deliveries, episiotomy, vaginal surgery), and fibromyalgia should be ascertained. Sexual history evaluating arousal, lubrication, ability to achieve orgasm, whether pain is primary or secondary, and a history of sexual, physical, or emotional abuse should be addressed.[10]

Physical Examination

In many cases, the vulva appears normal. However, careful inspection should be performed to evaluate for discoloration (erythema, hypopigmentation, or hyperpigmentation), lesions (ulcers and fissures) and atrophy (white epithelium consistent with lichen sclerosis or absence of well-estrogenized tissue). On examination, tenderness (hyperesthesia) at the periurethral or

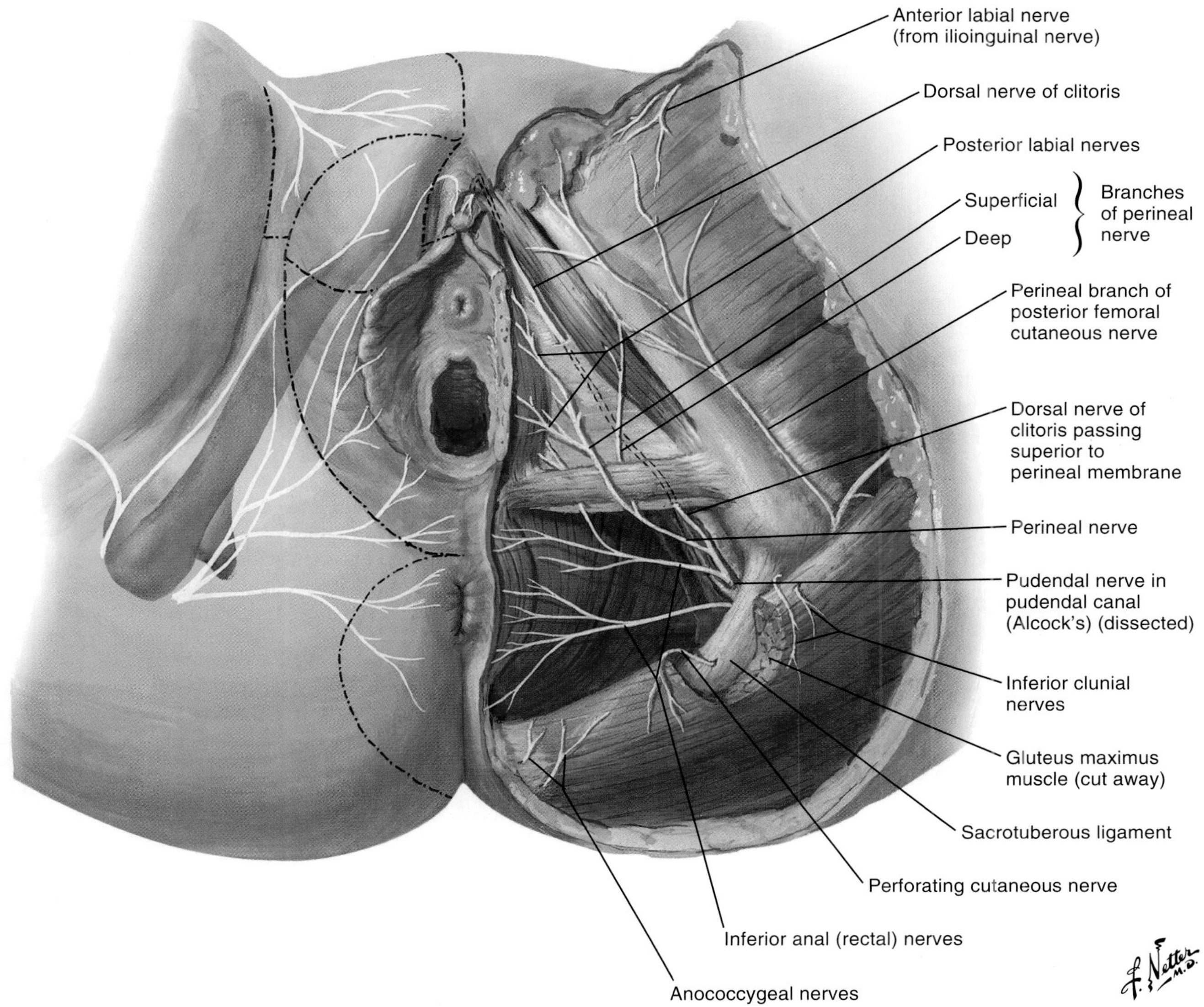

Figure 87-2 Nerves of perineum and external female genitalia. (Redrawn from © Netter images "Nerves of Perineum and External Genitalia Female." www.netter images.com).

Bartholin's glands and the vulvar vestibule should be outlined using a cotton-tipped swab, scored (on a scale from 0, no pain, to 10, severe pain), and recorded.

The hymeneal ring should be assessed for remnants or tight annular hymen which could tear with intercourse and cause dyspareunia. Tone and tenderness and trigger points of the pelvic floor muscles should be assessed. Pudendal nerves proximal to the ischial spines should be palpated for tenderness. It should be determined whether the pain is within the distribution of a particular branch of the pudendal, genitofemoral, ilioinguinal, or inferior hypogastric nerve.

Vaginal pH, whiff test, and microscopic examination of the vaginal secretions with saline and potassium hydroxide (KOH) should be performed to rule out vaginitis, vaginosis, and vaginal atrophy. Vaginal fluid may be cultured for *Candida* (because microscopic evaluation reveals candidiasis in only 50% of cases), bacterial culture and immunoglobulin E (to evaluate for local allergy). All lesions or discolorations should be further evaluated by colposcopy or biopsy to evaluate for an underlying dermatosis or an infectious or neoplastic process.[10]

DIFFERENTIAL DIAGNOSIS OF VULVAR OR VAGINAL PAIN

Vaginitis

The vaginal mucosa has only a few nerve endings needed for the sensations of pain and light touch.[11] For this reason, many vaginal infections are asymptomatic until the discharge reaches the vulva, where there is abundant somatic innervation. The problem is then perceived as vulvar itching, burning, or pain.

Vaginal Ecology

In childhood and menopause, in the absence of estrogen, the vaginal epithelium is thin and undifferentiated.[11] Estrogen causes thickening of the epithelium and a differentiation into well-recognized layers (basal, intermediate, and superficial). The percentage of superficial cells on a vaginal smear is indicative of the amount of estrogen activity. The vagina has a large amount of glycogen, second only to the liver, and it is most available in the superficial layers. Estrogen effects the formation and deposition of glycogen in the vagina.

Glycogen is important as a substrate for a series of enzymatic and fermentative processes that result in the production of lactic and acetic acid. Normal vaginal flora, consisting largely of lactobacilli and acidogenic corynebacteria, produce lactic and acetic acid from glycogen and its breakdown products. These organisms exist in a delicate balance with a small amount of *Candida.* The result of this symbiosis is a low vaginal pH, a milieu that is highly selective for bacterial growth and favors only the lactobacilli, corynebacteria, and *Candida* organisms. Changes in the vaginal flora pH or inoculum of a large amount of foreign bacteria can change this delicate equilibrium and lead to overgrowth of foreign invaders. At a low pH (3.5 to 4.1), normal vaginal flora predominate, but as the pH rises, various pathogens replace them. Interruption of the delicate balance of the vaginal flora can result from antibiotic treatments, pregnancy, oral contraceptives, intercourse, and menses. The vaginal pH is increased with vaginitis, bacterial vaginosis, and atrophy.

Vaginitis: Description, Diagnosis, Treatment

Bacterial Vaginosis

Bacterial vaginosis, the leading cause of abnormal vaginal discharge (according to the American College of Obstetricians and Gynecologists [ACOG], 1996) is a polymicrobial syndrome in which synergistic activity occurs among a characteristic set of bacterial species (*Gardnerella vaginalis* and anaerobic bacteria).[12] Risk factors for bacterial vaginosis infection include multiple or new sexual partners (male or female), early age at first coitus, douching, cigarette smoking, and use of an intrauterine contraceptive device. Approximately 50% to 75% of women who have bacterial vaginosis are asymptomatic. Symptomatic bacterial vaginosis is associated with a “fishy” odor, thin white or gray discharge, absence of pruritus, and inflammation with rare dysuria and dyspareunia.

Diagnosis of bacterial vaginosis is by clinical criteria. Three of the four Amstel criteria have been traditionally needed for diagnosis of bacterial vaginosis. However, a recent study showed that use of only two of the four criteria does not change the specificity or sensitivity of diagnosis.[13] The Amstel criteria include the following:

1. Homogeneous, grayish-white discharge
2. Vaginal pH greater than 4.5
3. Positive whiff-amine test, defined as the presence of a fishy odor when 10% KOH is added to vaginal discharge samples
4. Clue cells on saline wet mount. (Vaginal culture plays no role in diagnosis, because the organisms are detected in 50% to 60% of healthy asymptomatic women.)

Treatment of bacterial vaginosis is indicated for patients with symptomatic infection, those with asymptomatic infection before abortion or hysterectomy, and asymptomatic women with previous preterm births. It is not necessary to treat sexual partners. The condition spontaneously resolves in up to one third of women. Treatment regimens include metronidazole or clindamycin, orally or intravaginally. Metronidazole is the most successful therapy, with cure rates of greater than 90% in 1 week and 80% at 4 weeks.[14,15] The recommended dose is 500 mg twice a day for 7 days.[16] Topical vaginal therapy with 0.75% metronidazole gel, 5 g once daily for 5 days, is just as effective as the oral regimen.[16,17] A single oral dose of 2 g of metronidazole is an alternative regimen with higher relapse rate but a similar immediate rate of response.[16] Clindamycin appears to be less effective but is a reasonable alternative to metronidazole. It is available as topical vaginal therapy 2% cream, 5 g once daily for 7 days, or oral therapy at 300 mg twice daily for 7 days, or ovules 100 mg once daily for 3 days. Other, less effective therapies include triple-sulfa creams, erythromycin, tetracycline, acetic gel, povidone-iodine pouches, ampicillin, and amoxicillin.

Candida

Candida vulvovaginitis accounts for approximately one third of vaginitis cases. Studies suggest that 75% of women will suffer an attack at least once in their life.[8] The infection is less common in postmenopausal women unless they take estrogen therapy. About half of those infected experience more than one episode.

Candida albicans infection accounts for 80% to 90% of candidiasis cases; the remainder are evenly split between *Candida glabrata* and *Candida tropicalis.* The presence of estrogen, directly or indirectly, enhances candidal growth.[18] The organism thrives in many body locations, such as vaginal fluid,[19] as well as unsterile saliva.[20] In one study, one half of infected patients were found to harbor *Candida* in the mouth, and about one third had *Candida* in the anorectal tract; one fourth were found to be colonized in the vagina.[21] Besides the gut and vagina, intertriginous skin areas are especially susceptible including the vulva, groin, axillae, coronal sulcus, and the skin folds of the breast and panniculus. The organism needs warmth and moisture and does not survive long on dry skin. Tight-fitting clothing, especially if made of synthetic fabric, is more conducive to *Candida* than loose clothing is.

The mechanism by which *Candida* species cause symptomatic disease is complex, and includes the host inflammatory response to invasion and yeast virulence factors (e.g., elaboration of proteases). Factors predisposing to symptomatic infection include diabetes, immune suppression, pregnancy, oral contraceptives, antibiotics, metabolic factors (hypothyroidism, anemia, zinc deficiency), and diet. Pregnancy is the most common predisposing factor, with the incidence and severity of infection increasing with the duration of gestation. The increased glycogen content and high hormone levels constitute a favorable environment for the growth of candidal organisms. The newer oral contraceptives have lower estrogen levels and do not seem to predispose patients to *Candida* infection. Furthermore, one study found that only pill-using women with active herpetic, condylomatous, or anaerobic vaginal infections had increased prevalence of candidiasis.[22] Antimicrobials are thought to act as predisposing factors by reducing the number of protective resident bacteria. Some studies have shown that those patients who go on binges of dietary sweets suffer from recurrence of candidiasis and have high levels of urinary sugars derived from lactose and sucrose. By restricting lactose intake, 90% of these patients were able to maintain disease free intervals for longer than 1 year. If a patient has chronic refractory candidiasis, one may consider the possibility of acquired immunodeficiency syndrome (AIDS). Candidiasis has not been traditionally considered a sexually transmitted disease

(STD), especially because it does occur in celibate women. However, it may be linked to orogenital sex.[23]

Vulvar pruritus is the main symptom of candidiasis. Some women notice itching only before menses, and others complain of symptoms only after intercourse. Burning is also a common complaint, particularly on urination, and it is often experienced in those who scratch. Some patients develop reflexive urinary urgency and frequency. The combination of these symptoms can often be mistakenly diagnosed as cystitis. Dyspareunia can be present. Physical examination reveals erythema of the vulva (sometimes with erythematous papules or satellite lesions) and vaginal mucosa. The discharge is classically described as thick, adherent, and "cottage-cheese like," but it can also be thin and loose.

Diagnosis is by vaginal pH, wet-mount, KOH, and culture. Candidal vaginal pH is 4 to 4.5. A pH value of 4.7 or higher essentially limits the diagnosis to candidiasis or physiologic discharge. The diagnosis is confirmed by KOH wet mount and microscopic examination of vaginal material. The addition of 10% KOH destroys cellular elements and facilitates recognition of budding yeast and pseudohyphae. Because microscopy is negative in up to 50% of patients with confirmed vulvovaginal candidiasis, culture should be performed for patients with persistent or recurrent symptoms.

Treatment of candidiasis is indicated for relief of symptoms. Those who harbor *Candida* but are asymptomatic do not require therapy. Most patients (90%) have uncomplicated infections. The most commonly used antifungal agents are the azoles. There are both oral and vaginal preparations. The only oral preparation recommended is fluconazole: a 150-mg dose of fluconazole is as effective as multiple doses of intravaginal clotrimazole and oral butoconazole. Complicated infections occur in women with uncontrolled diabetes, immunosuppression, or a history of recurrent vulvovaginal candidiasis, and in those who are infected with *Torulopsis (Candida) glabrata,* or *C. tropicalis.* These women are less likely to respond to short courses of antimycotic drugs and may require 7 to 14 days of topical therapy or two doses of oral therapy 72 hours apart. Between 65% and 70% of those infected with *C. glabrata* respond to intravaginal boric acid (600 mg daily for 2 weeks), or a cure rate of more than 90% may be achieved with flucytosine cream (5 g nightly for 2 weeks).[24] Documented recurrent infections warrant testing for human immunodeficiency virus (HIV) infection and glucose tolerance testing and may require weekly and then monthly therapy for 4 to 6 months.

Trichomonas

The prevalence of *Trichomonas* infection depends greatly on the population studied. *Trichomonas* was found in 3% of unselected, asymptomatic college women,[25] 15% of private patients with leukhorrea,[26] 6% to 8.9% of pregnant women,[27] and 34% of pregnant inner-city adolescents.[28] Nevertheless, there seems little justification for screening low-risk, nonpregnant, asymptomatic individuals.

Trichomonas vaginalis is a unicellular protozoan flagellate, round or almond-shaped, slightly larger than a polymorphonuclear leukocyte.[8] Under high-power microscopy, four flagella can be seen to protrude from the forward end of the trichomonad. They are found in the vagina, urethra, and paraurethral glands.

This disorder is almost always sexually transmitted and can be identified in 30% to 40% of male sexual partners of infected women. The infection is associated with a high prevalence of coinfection with other STDs. There is a positive association between trichomonas infection and HIV infection.[29] Trichomonads can survive in an aqueous environment between 20 and 30 degrees and can remain infectious for up to 24 hours.[30] Women can deposit the trichomonads on toilet seats, on which the organism can survive up to 45 minutes.[31]

There are several signs and symptoms of trichomoniasis. One pathognomonic sign is abundant green, frothy, foul-smelling discharge with an alkaline pH (>6). Sometimes, generalized erythema is the only gross change in the vaginal tissue. "Strawberry vagina" is also associated with trichomoniasis, when the presence of swollen papillae project through a layer of discharge. Pruritus, or itching, is the second most common manifestation of trichomoniasis. Other symptoms include dyspareunia, urinary symptoms from urethrocystitis, discharge from the urethra and Skene's ducts, and erythema of the vulva.

The most practical and cost-effective diagnostic test available is still the saline wet mount done in a clinic setting.[8] However, motile trichomonads are found only in 50% to 70% of culture-confirmed cases. Culture on Diamond's medium is 95% sensitive and more than 95% specific but should only be used if there is a high clinical suspicion despite a negative wet mount result, or wet mount is unavailable. Diagnosis with classic Pap smears is not recommended, but diagnosis with liquid-based pap smears has been shown to be highly specific (99%) and sensitive (61%).[32]

Treatment is indicated in all nonpregnant women diagnosed with *Trichomonas* vaginitis and their sexual partners. *Trichomonas* is associated with preterm rupture of membranes and prematurity in pregnant women, but treatment has not been shown to decrease these complications.[33] Oral metronidazole is the treatment of choice; it is preferred over the vaginal route, because systemic administration achieves therapeutic drug levels in the urethra and periurethral glands, which serve as sources for endogenous recurrence. There is no need to identify the source in the male partner before treating him. It has been shown that a single 2-g dose to both sexual partners is as effective as the classic regimen, 500 mg twice a day for 7 days.[34] The advantages of the single-dose regimen include better compliance, a lower total dose, shorter period of alcohol avoidance (due to the disulfiram-like effect of metronidazole), and possibly decreased *Candida* superinfection. In the event of treatment failure, the 7-day regimen should be prescribed before resistance is suspected; many cases of "failure" result from reinfection, possibly from a different or untreated partner.[8]

Desquamative Vaginitis

Desquamative inflammatory vaginitis (DIV) is not a diagnosis in itself and may be the presentation of a range of blistering disorders, including pemphigus vulgaris, lichen planus, and mucous membrane pemphigoid.[35] The existence of an idiopathic subset of DIV remains controversial. It is a rare but disabling condition and manifests in women of any age with a history of discomfort, irritation, and dyspareunia. Women who develop DIV are different from those who typically develop STDs, being older, married, and with higher levels of education. Patients may complain of increased yellow vaginal discharge.

Examination of the vulva is normal, but erythematous regions on the vaginal walls are evident, with increased vaginal secretion. Repeated cultures are negative for pathogenic bacteria, viruses, and yeast. Microscopic examination of the vaginal discharge shows an increased number of immature epithelial cells, typical rounded parabasal cells, and an increase in polymorphonuclear leukocytes. Gram staining shows an absence of lactobacilli and occasionally increased levels of gram-positive cocci. The vaginal pH is increased from normal to 7.4. A biopsy of the erythematous portion of the vaginal wall for histology and immunofluorescence is necessary to exclude any underlying cause of DIV.

This sterile inflammatory vaginitis is difficult to treat, but successful therapy has been reported with steroids and clindamycin. Studies have found that 2% clindamycin suppositories or high-potency intravaginal steroids alone or in combination with oral clindamycin for 4-6 weeks have been effective.[36,37] Estrogen deficient women need supplementary vaginal estrogen therapy to maintain remission.

Herpes Simplex Virus

In the United States, the frequency of genital herpes simplex virus (HSV) is increasing. There are two types of HSV infection; it is reported that HSV-2 causes the most genital infections, and HSV-1 causes the most labial infections. However, HSV-1 genital infections are very common. Prevalence of HSV is high: 21.9% were positive among 13,094 individuals surveyed by the Third National Health and Nutrition Examination.[8] HSV is more commonly associated with women, African Americans, single marital status, higher number of sex partners, prior history of an STD, and urban residence.[8]

Infection is transmitted by direct sexual contact, most commonly when an active virus-secreting lesion is present. HSV has been recovered from asymptomatic male carriers and from the cervix of asymptomatic women. Subclinical shedding is common, occurring in 55% of women with HSV-2 and 29% of women with HSV-1.[38] In 70% of patients, transmission was linked to sexual contact during periods of asymptomatic viral shedding. Transmission of genital HSV was documented in 14 couples, and the risk was greater with male than female source partners (17% versus 4%).[12]

The types of genital HSV infection are primary, nonprimary first episode, and recurrent. The clinical manifestations of genital HSV are variable, depending on the type of infection.[39,40] In acute primary and recurrent infections, the initial presentation can be severe, with painful ulcers, dysuria, fever, tender inguinal lymphadenopathy, and headache. Other patients have a mild presentation or are entirely asymptomatic.[39,41] Recurrent infections are typically less severe than primary or nonprimary first-episode infections because of preexisting immunity. In turn, a nonprimary first episode is typically less severe than the primary infection, because the antibodies to one HSV type offer some protection against the other. Recurrent infections are more common with HSV-2 than HSV-1: 60% versus 14% in patients with a first symptomatic episode of genital herpes.[42] Recurrent lesions are fewer in number and are more often unilateral than bilateral.[39]

In a primary infection, the average incubation period is 4 days.[40] Patients usually have multiple, bilateral, ulcerating, pustular lesions that resolve after a mean of 9 days. Other symptoms include systemic headache, malaise, fever, and myalgia (67%); local pain and itching (98%); dysuria (63%); and tender lymphadenopathy (80%). Virus is very often isolated in the urethra and cervix of women with first-episode infection.[39] Extragenital manifestations of HSV include orolabial symptoms, aseptic meningitis, urinary bladder retention, distant skin lesions, herpetic whitlow, and proctitis. The clinical manifestations of HSV in immunocompromised patients are more extensive and include mucocutaneous involvement, variable appearance of genital lesions, and the development of chronic and recurrent ulcers. Patients may have prolonged viral shedding. In addition to genital symptoms, patients may also have more neurologic complications, such as aseptic meningitis, sacral radiculopathy, and transverse myelitis.[43]

The differential diagnoses of HSV include syphilis, chancroid, Behçet's disease, and drug eruptions. Diagnosis based on history and physical examination is often inaccurate, and laboratory testing is required. Diagnostic tests include viral culture, polymerase chain reaction (PCR), and direct fluorescence antibody (DFA). Viral cultures can be obtained with active lesions; the vesicle should be unroofed for sampling of the vesicular fluid. The overall sensitivity of viral culture is 50%,[44,45] and the highest yield is in the early vesicular stages rather than the later, crusted stages.[46] HSV PCR is a more sensitive method for samples taken from genital ulcers, mucocutaneous sites, and cerebrospinal fluid, and it is particularly useful in detecting asymptomatic viral shedding.[47-49] DFA is specific, reproducible, and less expensive than PCR. Serology is important because it is type-specific and antibodies persist indefinitely in the serum.

Because HSV is a viral disease, there is no cure; however, drug treatment can shorten the duration of symptoms, and, in patients with frequent recurrences, medicine can be used as prophylactic therapy. There are three main drugs used in the treatment of HSV: acyclovir, famciclovir, and valacyclovir. In 2002, the Centers for Disease Control published treatment guidelines for the various types of HSV infection.[16] Recommended regimens for individuals with first episode are acyclovir (400 mg PO three times daily or 200 mg PO five times a day), famciclovir (250 mg PO three times daily), or valacyclovir (1 g PO twice daily) for 7 to 10 days. Recommended regimens for individuals for suppressive therapy are acyclovir (400 mg PO twice daily), famciclovir (250 mg PO twice daily), or valacyclovir (1 g PO daily or 500 mg PO daily). Recommended regimens for individuals with recurrent episodes are acyclovir (400 mg PO three times daily or 200 mg PO five times a day or 800 mg PO twice daily), famciclovir (125 mg PO twice daily), or valacyclovir (1 g PO daily) for 5 days or valacyclovir (500 mg PO twice daily) for 3 to 5 days. Postherpetic neuralgia due to HSV has not been well documented, although the herpes virus can increase the risk of vulvodynia due to recurrent herpes prodromal symptoms or pudendal neuropathy. Prodromal symptoms may be accompanied by positive HSV immunoglobulin M antibody serology; they respond to antiviral agents, whereas the pudendal neuropathy does not.

Human Papillomavirus

HPV infection can lead to vulvar itching and pain through its anogenital manifestations. Condylomata acuminata usually manifest as single or multiple papules on the vulva, cervix, vagina, perineum, or anal region. The most common sites in women are the posterior introitus, followed by the labia majora and labia minora. External HPV lesions are frequently associated with cervical lesions. The lesions are flesh-colored, hyperkeratotic, exophytic, and either sessile or pedunculated.[50] HPV subtypes, other than the low-risk types 6 and 11, are also closely associated with squamous intraepithelial lesions of the cervix.

Diagnosis begins with a clinical examination supplemented with histologic examination of suspicious lesions. Biopsy is recommended in atypical cases or if the benign nature of the lesion is unclear.

There are several treatments for anogenital warts. For home therapy, podophyllotoxin or imiquimod may be used. For office therapy, podophyllin or 40% trichloroacetic acid may be used. Surgical options include cryotherapy, laser therapy, electrosurgery, and surgical excision.

Atrophic Vaginitis

Estrogen-deficient vaginal and vestibular epithelium can be associated with itching, burning, and dyspareunia, due not just to decreased lubrication but also to fissuring from thin epithelium and poor compliance. Perimenopause or postmenopause status, use of hormonal contraceptives, and breastfeeding are the most common circumstances leading to atrophy. The vaginal epithelium loses its glycogen-rich superficial epithelial cells; the vaginal walls loose rugation and become pale or subject to petechial hemorrhage on contact; and the vaginal pH is elevated to 5.5. A yellow discharge reveals increased intermediate and parabasal cells under saline wet mount microscopy. Treatment is with 14 days of vaginal estrogen cream or suppository, followed by therapy twice weekly or use of an estrogen-secreting vaginal ring. Improvement can be expected in 2 months, but full estrogenization may take up to 18 months. Systemic absorption is present but is minimal.

Dermatoses

Lichen Sclerosus

Lichen sclerosus is a benign, chronic, progressive dermatologic condition characterized by marked inflammation, epithelial thinning, and distinctive dermal changes.[51] This disorder usually occurs in the anogenital area (85% to 98% of cases), where it causes itching and burning.[52,53] In 20% of patients, identical lesions appear elsewhere on the body.[8] Extragenital lichen sclerosus is most commonly found on the neck and shoulders and is usually asymptomatic. Pertaining to the vulva, the disorder can involve any or all areas, including the perianal skin, the skin folds adjacent to the thighs, and the inner aspects of the buttocks approximating the anus. The disorder usually occurs in postmenopausal women. However, 10% to 15% of cases occur in children, most of which involve female genitalia.[54] Even though the disease is reported to occur mostly in white females, lichen sclerosus has also been reported in Native Africans, Asians, and dark-skinned patients.

Multiple signs and symptoms are associated with lichen sclerosus. A prodrome to the gross lesions includes nonspecific, dull, painful vulvar discomfort in some women. Other women are asymptomatic. The major symptoms of the disorder include vulvar pruritus (which can be so intense as to disrupt sleep), pruritus ani, painful defecation, anal fissures, rectal bleeding, dysuria, and difficulty voiding. Dyspareunia is associated with introital stenosis, fissures, or posterior deflection of fused labia.

On physical examination, the lesions typically begin as white papules that are irregularly outlined and may coalesce into well-defined plaques.[8] Classic lesions consist of thin, white, "cigarette paper," wrinkled skin localized to the labia minora and/or labia majora, although the whitening may extend over the perineum and around the anus in a keyhole fashion. Fissures may be found perianally, in the intralabial folds, or around the clitoris. Excoriations and lichenification may be observed, often associated with edema of the labia minora and the prepuce. Relatively minor rubbing or intercourse may lead to hemorrhage and/or petechiae with purpura and ecchymoses due to the fragility of the involved skin. Early in the course of the disease, vulvar architecture remains intact; however, phimosis of the clitoris and obliteration of the labia minora and periclitoral structures may be seen later in the course of the disease.

There is an increased risk of malignancy in patients with lichen sclerosus, of 4% to 6%. However, proof that lichen sclerosus causes cancer as a precursor lesion is lacking. The skin of patients with vulvar lichen sclerosus should be examined at least yearly. Biopsy should be performed of any thickened plaque that fails to thin with corticosteroid treatment or any persistently open or nonresolving lesion.

Diagnosis is by clinical characteristics and histologic confirmation. Before treatment is initiated, if is important that confirmation be made by histologic diagnosis. Multiple punch biopsies should be taken from the vulva, especially from sites of fissuring, ulceration, induration, and thick plaques.[8] Treatment is for relief of symptoms and discomfort, to prevent further anatomic changes, and to possibly prevent malignant transformation. Therapy comprises education, behavioral modification, support, and medication. Surgery is reserved for small subset of cases. Patients should first be educated about the chronicity of the disease and reassured that the condition is manageable. A discussion about the possibility of malignancy and the need for yearly monitoring should take place. Patients should be told about good vulvar hygiene and to stop scratching the lesion. The treatment with the best evidence of efficacy is superpotent corticosteroid ointment, clobetasol propionate 0.05% daily for 6 to 12 weeks and then one to three times a week for maintenance.[55] Long-standing treatment with clobetasol does not appear to cause untoward skin effects. With the eradication of pruritus, hyperplastic lesions may improve or disappear entirely. There is no role for estrogen, progesterone, or testosterone cream in the treatment of lichen sclerosus. Surgical intervention is indicated only for postinflammatory sequelae of the disease and when malignancy is present. Introital stenosis, posterior fissuring, and scarring of the fourchette are treated with perineoplasty. Surgical treatment for lichen sclerosus results in a recurrence rate that is extremely high, making the operation contraindicated in the absence of significant atypia.[8]

Lichen Planus

Lichen planus is a relatively common papulosquamous disorder of unknown etiology. It has its highest incidence in patients 30 to 60 years of age. It occurs most often on flexor surfaces of the extremities and the trunk. It can also affect nails, mucous membranes including the mouth, esophagus, conjunctivae, bladder, nose, larynx, stomach, and anus. It can be isolated to the vulva or be a part of a more generalized skin eruption. The prevalence of vulvar lichen planus is considered uncommon; it occurs in fewer than 10% of women who have lichen planus over a 3-year period.[56]

Patient complaints usually include irritating vaginal discharge, vulvar pruritus, burning, and dyspareunia with postcoital bleeding. Physical examination findings differ depending on the type of lesion. Papulosquamous lichen planus consists of small, intensely pruritic papules with a violaceous hue that arise on keratinized and perianal skin. Hypertrophic lichen planus is characterized by hyperkeratotic, rough lesions on the perineum and perianal region.[57] The appearance is similar to squamous cell carcinoma. Erosive lichen planus refers to glassy, brightly erythematous erosions with white striae or a white border (Wickham's striae) often visible along the margins. It can occur on the labia minora and vestibule as isolated lesions on an otherwise normal vulva or in association with marked architectural destruction, including loss of the labia minora and narrowing of the introitus. Vaginal involvement is reported in up to 70% of patients with erosive lichen planus, whereas vaginal involvement is not seen in lichen sclerosus.[57] The vaginal lining may be friable, easily bleeding. The vagina may be massively inflamed and denuded with seropurulent exudates, pseudomembrane, or serosanguineous discharge. In severe cases, adhesions and synechiae develop that can lead to narrowing or obliteration of the vagina. The vulvo-vaginal-gingival syndrome is a variant of erosive lichen planus. It involves the epithelium of the vulva, vestibule, vagina, and mouth. The lesions may not be concurrent; for example, lesions in the mouth can proceed or follow lesions in the genital area for months or years.[8]

The diagnosis of lichen planus is based on characteristic clinical manifestations. Classic histopathologic features include irregular acanthosis of the epidermis, liquefactive degeneration of the basal cell layer, and band-like dermal infiltrate of lymphocytes in the upper dermis. Hyperkeratosis is present in areas of keratinized skin. Typical histopathologic features are not found in mucosal lesions. Also, tissue biopsies are not specific except in the erosive type.

The oral and genital lesions of lichen planus, especially lichen planus, are persistent and resistant to therapy. There is no single effective therapy for erosive vulvar lichen planus, which is extremely difficult to treat. On the other hand, hypertrophic and papulosquamous lichen planus respond well to therapy. Patients should be told to maintain good vulvar hygiene and to stop scratching. The first line and mainstay of therapy is corticosteroids: topical, interlesional, and oral corticosteroids are all used. For erosive lichen planus, ultrapotent topical steroids (clobetasol or halobetasol propionate 0.05% ointment) can be applied nightly for 3 to 6 weeks, depending on the severity of disease. The ultrapotent steroid can then be reduced to twice per week, with a midpotency ointment of low potency ointment added, one to three times per week, for maintenance. It may be necessary to experiment to find the best course. Vaginal corticosteroids in the form of suppositories can be used for vaginal lesions. In one study, 16 of 17 patients improved with 25 mg hydrocortisone suppositories inserted in the vagina twice daily for 2 months.[58] In another study of 60 patients, 80% improved by taking 12.5 to 25 mg of hydrocortisone suppositories twice a day for several months, tapering to a symptom-free maintenance dose once or twice weekly.[59]

Lichen Simplex Chronicus

Lichen simplex chronicus is also called leukoplakia and hyperplastic dystrophy.[8] The condition is caused by histologic changes in the vulvar dermis after persistent rubbing or scratching, usually in women who experience chronic irritation and/or pruritus. The condition is characterized by epithelial thickening and hyperkeratosis. There is an enhancement of the normal crosshatch markings of the skin, called lichenification.[60,61] Labial skin folds appear greatly exaggerated, often edematous, and pubic hair can be broken or sparse. The lesions tend to occur on the mons pubis and labia majora.

The most important element about diagnosing lichen simplex chronicus is to perform a biopsy to distinguish it from lichen sclerosus, lichen planus, and carcinoma. Treatment is discussed in the section on allergic dermatitis.

Neoplasm

Vulvar cancer is the fourth most common gynecologic cancer (after uterine, ovarian, and cervical cancer) and comprises 5% of malignancies of the female genital tract.[62] Vulvar carcinoma is most frequently found in postmenopausal women, with the mean age at diagnosis being 55 to 65 years.

The signs and symptoms of all histologic types of vulvar malignancy are similar. Presentation usually includes a unifocal vulvar nodule, plaque, ulcer, or mass on the labia majora (40%), labia minora (20%), clitoris (10%), mons (10%), or perineum (15%). Lesions are multifocal in 5% of cases. The most common presenting symptom is pruritus. Other symptoms include vulvar bleeding or discharge, dysuria, or enlarged groin lymph node, but many patients are asymptomatic at time of diagnosis.

There are two main categories of vulvar neoplasms, that of the squamous cell type and Paget's disease.[8] In 1984 and 1987, the ISSVD further subdivided these two classifications. Squamous cell type was divided into vulvar intraepithelial neoplasm (VIN) I (mild dysplasia), VIN II (moderate dysplasia), and VIN III (severe dysplasia to carcinoma in situ). The other category included Paget's disease and melanoma in situ.

More than 90% of vulvar malignancies are squamous cell. Two subtypes exist. The first (classic or Bowenoid type, VIN) is predominantly associated with HPV-16 and -18 and is found in younger women.[63,64] Risk factors for this subtype include early coitarche, multiple sexual partners, HIV infection, and cigarette smoking. The second, more common subtype (keratinized, differentiated, or simplex type) occurs in older women and is not related to HPV infection.

The gross appearance of VIN lesions is usually quite distinct: they are well localized, delineated, slightly elevated, white, and rough. The tissues may have a red or brown hue, and both red and white patches may be noted. These changes can be seen anywhere on the vulva but are most commonly found in the region of the fourchette and perineum. Squamous cell carcinoma in situ is a superficial, noninvasive, intraepithelial carcinoma characterized by chronicity, pruritus, burning, and a variable gross appearance.

The diagnosis can be established only by histopathologic study, and biopsies should be taken from more than one site. Some sources say that the biopsy should be taken from the center of the lesion, because those taken from the leading edge do not reflect the most severe histology of the lesion. The best means of detecting an intraepithelial lesion is by careful inspection of the vulva. Surgical extirpation is the primary treatment for early-stage vulvar carcinoma.

Paget's Disease

Pruritus is the most common symptom of Paget's disease, occurring in 70% of patients. The appearance of the Paget's lesion is variable. Typically, it manifests as an erythematous, eczematoid lesion with scales and a crust scattered over the surface. It may also appear as a grayish-white lesion and frequently with moist and oozing ulcerations that bleed readily on contact. The disease is usually multifocal and occurs anywhere on the vulva, mons, perineum/perianal area, or inner thigh.

Diagnosis is by biopsy of the lesion, looking for characteristic histopathology. Vulvar biopsies should be performed for patients with suspicious lesions, including those with persistent pruritic eczematous lesions that fail to resolve with 6 weeks of therapy.

Patients should also be evaluated for invasive carcinoma: two series found a 4% to 17% rate of invasive carcinoma within or beneath the surface of the Paget's lesion.[65,66] Women with this disease should also be evaluated for synchronous neoplasms, because approximately 20% to 30% of these patients have a noncontiguous carcinoma (breast, rectum, bladder, urethra, cervix, or ovary).[67]

Treatment includes wide local excision of the disease. The local recurrence rate is high, 12% to 58%. Recurrence may occur despite negative margins, probably because of the multicentricity of the disease and microscopic extension of disease beyond clinically visible margins.[66] Recurrence after initial therapy and noncontiguous carcinoma are common.

Vulvar Infection

Folliculitis

Folliculitis is a pyoderma of the hair follicles. *Pyoderma* is defined as a localized, purulent streptococcal infection of the skin. Predisposing factors to the development of folliculitis include nasal carriage of *Staphylococcus aureus*, use of swimming pools and hot tubs, and antibiotic administration and corticosteroid therapy predisposing to *Candida*. The most common pathogens are *S. aureus, Pseudomonas aeruginosa,* and *Candida* species. Other predisposing conditions include obesity, sweating, maceration, malnutrition, diabetes, seborrhea, poor hygiene, scabies, and pediculosis.[8]

Patients usually present with pain and tenderness, depending on the depth and extent of the lesions. Folliculitis lesions are typically small, less than or equal to 5 mm. They initially appear as papules that develop into vesicles, surrounded by a ring of erythema. Folliculitis does not cause systemic toxicity, and the lesions may spontaneously drain and resolve without scarring.

Treatment includes the use of topical therapies. Warm saline compresses can accelerate pointing, at which time the lesion can be incised. Superficial folliculitis usually responds well to erythromycin-containing antibiotic lotion or cream and use of germicidal soaps. Antifungal agents are useful in the case of *Candida* infections. Mupirocin ointment should be considered for patients with frequent recurrences of folliculitis who are suspected of having nasal colonization with *S. aureus*. The ointment is applied to the anterior nares bilaterally twice a day for 5 days each month.[68]

Complications of folliculitis include recurrence and progression to furunculosis.

Bartholin's Gland Cyst or Abscess

Bartholin's duct cysts are seen in approximately 2% of new gynecologic patients.[8] They arise in the duct system, and the occlusion is usually near the opening of the main duct into the vestibule. Chronic inflammation can obstruct the orifice and lead to cystic dilation of the duct, but not the gland, proximal to the obstruction.

Bartholin's cysts average 1 to 3 cm in size and are usually asymptomatic. Larger cysts are associated with vulvar pain, dyspareunia, or difficulty sitting or ambulating. Discomfort may be associated with rapid enlargement, as might be induced by repeated or prolonged sexual stimulation.

The diagnosis is clinical and is based on the findings of a soft, painless mass in the medial labia majora or lower vestibular area. Most cysts are unilateral and are detected during a routine pelvic examination of by the woman herself.

No treatment is necessary for asymptomatic Bartholin's cysts, except in postmenopausal women, in whom a biopsy or excision should be considered to rule out carcinoma. These cysts are usually sterile and therefore do not require antibiotic therapy.[69] A cyst that is symptomatic or disfiguring requires treatment, of which there are several modes. The simplest procedure is an incision and drainage, with or without packing. However, if this procedure is done alone, there is a high likelihood of recurrence when the incised tissue edges reapproximate. Supplementation of the incision and drainage can be performed with a Word catheter. It is a balloon-tipped device that can be placed in the cavity after drainage. The bulb is inflated to keep the catheter in place for 2 to 4 weeks while the duct tract epithelializes. The end of the catheter is tucked in the vagina to minimize discomfort. An alternative procedure after failure of the Word catheter is marsupialization of the gland, whereby a new orifice is created. A fourth method involves sclerotherapy, in which silver nitrate sticks are inserted into the cyst cavity to necrotize the cyst wall after incision and drainage. Mild burning may occur. The patient returns after 48 hours for cleaning of the vulva. A randomized controlled trial found that silver nitrate insertion was as effective as excision of Bartholin's cysts or abscesses.[70] Excision of the entire Bartholin's gland is the definitive procedure for both cysts and abscesses. It is usually considered after other methods have repetitively failed, because it is not an office procedure and has higher morbidity, including excessive bleeding, hematoma formation, cellulitis, and dyspareunia.

Bartholin's gland ducts and cysts can become infected and form abscesses. They are usually the result of polymicrobial infections, with the most common organisms being *Escherichia coli, Neisseria gonorrhoeae,* and Bacteroides species.[71] Therefore, patients should have both routine cultures and those for gonorrhea and chlamydia.

Symptoms for Bartholin's abscess include pain and tenderness over the affected gland. Usually, these abscesses develop rapidly, within 2 to 3 days, and are associated with acute pain and tenderness. They tend to rupture spontaneously within 72 hours. Patients usually present with pain on intercourse or pain on walking and sitting. Examination reveals a lesion that appears as a large, tender, soft or fluctuant mass in the medial labia majora or lower vestibular area, occasionally with erythema, edema, and pointing of the abscess.

Treatment entails drainage of the abscess, which provides immediate pain relief. Incision and drainage can be performed, followed by Word catheter placement, marsupialization, or silver nitrate insertion. Antibiotic regimens include one dose of ceftriaxone (125 mg IM) or cefixime (400 mg PO) to cover *E. coli* and *N. gonorrhoeae* plus clindamycin (300 mg PO four times a day for 7 days) to cover anaerobes. If *Chlamydia trachomatis* is present, azithromycin (1 g PO in a single dose) should be administered. Treatment with broad-spectrum antibiotics may easily delay ripening of the abscess. For women older than 40 years of age, some recommend complete excision of the gland to exclude underlying carcinoma.[72]

Allergic Dermatitis

Contact dermatitis is an inflammatory reaction of the skin to a primary irritant or to an allergenic substance. Vulvar dermatitis (vulvar eczema) is the most common vulvar inflammatory skin disease in women. One third to one half of women's vulvar complaints stem from this problem.[73-75] Patients with this disorder have chronic irritation and pruritus, which leads to persistent rubbing and scratching. There are two types of vulvar dermatitis, endogenous and exogenous. Endogenous dermatitis is also called atopic dermatitis and has a familial disposition. It begins in childhood and may affect other parts of the body. Erythema found in labial folds, perianally, and in the skin between the buttocks suggests endogenous vulvar dermatitis. Exogenous dermatitis is also called contact dermatitis and results from external factors. Allergic dermatitis accounts for 20% of cases and results when an allergen induces an immune response. In irritant contact dermatitis (80% of cases), the trigger directly damages the skin.

The history is important for differentiating among atopic, allergic, and contact dermatitis. What is the intensity of the pruritus, and when is it the worst? What kind of feminine products are used? Does the patient wear occlusive clothing that predisposes to *Candida*? Does she use any type of medication or scented soaps or deodorants?

A patch test may be required to distinguish between atopic and contact dermatitis; biopsy is not helpful. Positive patch tests for relevant substances occur in 25% to 60% of women with vulvar pruritus. Biopsy, however, should be obtained to rule out other possible causes. Coexistent infections should also be diagnosed so they can be treated.

Treatment involves behavioral modification and medications. First, the patient must modify any hygiene or clothing habits that facilitate dermatitis. Then, she must eliminate known or suspected allergens and irritants. She should be warned to refrain from scratching. Wet compresses or soaking in warm water must be undertaken for a day or two in order to restore the natural physiologic environment of the vulva. After this, the patient is ready for topical application of corticosteroid cream or lotion. For mild cases, use of a low- or medium-potency steroid is usually effective (hydrocortisone or triamcinolone), twice a day for 2 to 4 weeks, then twice a week and taper to pruritic symptoms. For severe cases, high-potency steroids may be necessary (clobetasol propionate or betamethasone dipropionate) every night for 30 days and then re-evaulate. Potent steroids can be used for up to 12 weeks on the vulva without adverse effects.[76,77]

Trauma

Trauma to the vulva and vagina may lead to vulvar pain, dyspareunia, vulvar and vaginal lesions, and discharge. Accidental injuries are seldom seen in the vulva and vagina because of their anatomic location.[8] The injuries seen in prepubertal girls result most commonly from straddling objects such as bench rails, gymnasium equipment, bicycle frames, baths, and toilet seats. In adults, these injuries can be secondary to automobile and motorcycle accidents, bicycle accidents, sexual trauma, snowboarding, or physical assault. Some injuries may result from placing inanimate objects into the vagina. Most of these lesions manifest as hematomas and lacerations.

Lacerations of the vulva or vagina commonly occur from a violent fall on a slender object. Examples include falling on a stake, picket fence, handlebars of a bicycle, or the binding of a snowboard.[78] Lacerations may extend into the rectum, bladder, urethra, or the peritoneal cavity through the cul-de-sac. The area must be inspected carefully for remnants of glass, metal, or plastic. Anterior, posterior, and lateral radiographs including the vaginal area should be taken to locate metallic or other radiopaque objects. Lacerations can cause profuse hemorrhage, pain, and shock. Treatment includes restoration of normal anatomic relationships. Bleeding vessels should be ligated and tissue edges carefully reapproximated with absorbable suture. Large traumatized areas require copious irrigation and débridement. Other concomitant injuries should be ruled out.

Sexual injuries are a major source of damage to the vulva and vagina. The right and posterior fornices of the vaginal vault are frequent sites of injury for parous women, whereas lower vaginal and introital injuries are often caused by defloration.[79] Rape and insertion of foreign bodies are additional sources of vulvar and vaginal injury. Genital injuries as a result of consensual intercourse are rare.

Most introital injuries associated with consensual first coitus are minor and lead to minimal bleeding.[8] These injuries can be managed conservatively with compression. If the injury involves an extensive laceration of the hymenal ring that extends into the vagina with profuse bleeding, suturing of the laceration is indicated. It has been postulated that vigorous intercourse increases abdominal pressure, causing tensing of the cul-de-sac and decreasing the elasticity of the posterior fornix, which results in a higher likelihood of laceration. Fissuring of the posterior fourchette (vulvar granuloma fissuratum) repeatedly with intercourse may cause a nonhealing granuloma that requires primary excision and closure.[80]

Foreign objects can cause trauma of the vulva or vagina. With certain sexual techniques, patients have been known to insert molded phalluses, glass objects, tops of aerosol cans, and occasionally metal objects into the vagina, which can cause laceration. If glass objects are the cause, it is important to inspect the tissue for the presence of residual foreign bodies, with subsequent irrigation and removal. Patients also occasionally forget to remove tampons. If the tampon remains in the vagina for a long period, there is often a foul, copious, brownish discharge. A simple examination usually demonstrates the presence of the tampon. Removal of the tampon is usually sufficient unless it has been retained for more than 10 days, at which point it is appropriate to give antibiotic therapy. Vaginal pessaries are also a main culprit of vaginal trauma. They are usually used by elderly women with extensive vaginal vault prolapse and may cause erosive conditions in these patients. The patient usually complains of malodor and bloody discharge, which is indicative of abrasion and erosion of the vaginal mucosa. The use of intravaginal estrogen to prevent vaginal tissue thinning helps prevent erosion.

Prolapse

Pelvic organ prolapse refers to a hernia of one of the pelvic organs (uterus, vaginal apex, bladder, rectum) and its associated vaginal segment from its normal location. Pelvic prolapse occurs, in part, because of site-specific fascial defects that result in anterior, apical, or posterior segment weakness. Risk factors include multiparity, operative vaginal delivery, obesity, advanced age, estrogen deficiency, neurogenic dysfunction of the pelvic floor, connective tissue disorders, prior pelvic surgery, and chronically increased intra-abdominal pressure.

The displacement of the pelvic organs is graded on a scale of 0 to 4, with 0 referring to no prolapse; 1, halfway to the hymen; 2, at the hymen; 3, halfway out of the hymen; and 4, total prolapse (procidentia). There are also different prolapsed organs. Cystocele is herniation of the bladder with associated descent of the anterior vaginal segment. Cystourethrocele is cystocele combined with distal prolapse of the urethra with or without associated urethral hypermobility. Uterine prolapse is descent of the uterus and cervix into the lower vagina, to the hymenal ring, or through the vaginal introitus. Vaginal vault prolapse is descent of the vaginal apex (after hysterectomy) into the lower vagina, to the hymenal ring, or through the vaginal introitus. Rectocele is hernia of the rectum with associated descent of the posterior vaginal segment. Enterocele is herniation of the small bowel/peritoneum into the vaginal lumen, most commonly after hysterectomy in conjunction with vaginal vault prolapse.

The most common symptoms are a sensation of pressure and heaviness or protrusion of tissue from the vagina. Patients may also complain of low back pain and a feeling of heaviness that is relieved with lying down and worsens as the day progresses. Loss of anterior support can lead to urinary stress incontinence. A large anterior vaginal prolapse with vaginal vault eversion can lead to urinary retention. A rectocele can cause defecatory dysfunction. Sexual dysfunction may accompany prolapse of any of the compartments. Because there may be protrusion of the vaginal mucosa, irritation can occur and bleeding may be reported.

Diagnostic evaluation includes examination of the vaginal support from both upright and recumbent positions. The traditional speculum examination should be supplemented with a site-specific examination with a single-bladed speculum or one half of a Graves speculum. This allows for a better view of the vaginal walls when looking for specific defects of vaginal support. A rectovaginal examination should be performed with the patient in standing position for detecting an enterocele, because the small bowel, if present, can be palpated easily in the cul-de-sac between thumb and forefinger. Magnetic resonance imaging is a useful diagnostic tool.

Treatment of mild prolapse is with pelvic floor exercises, physical therapy, or behavioral modification. Women with moderate prolapse or who are not surgical candidates may benefit from a pessary. Surgical treatment is usually necessary for severe prolapse. Surgery can be associated with an up to 30% rate of recurrence/reoperation.[81]

Rigid Hymenal Ring

The hymen varies in thickness and elasticity. It may be quite elastic and easily stretched without laceration at initial sexual intercourse, or it may be tough and rigid so as to cause dyspareunia or even prevent intercourse. Attention may be drawn to this problem when the patient is unable to insert a tampon. Treatment with appropriate estrogen cream, small dilators, or hymenoplasty can correct the problem and prevent unnecessary laceration of the hymen and introitus due to trauma from intercourse.[8]

Vulvar Neuroma

Vulvar neuroma, which is usually caused by traumatic or iatrogenic transaction of peripheral nerve fibers, can cause dyspareunia and vulvar pain. It is postulated that dyspareunia related to episiotomy may be associated with disorganized proliferation of proximal nerve stumps. Patients can be in all age groups. There have been scarce case reports in the literature, but vulvar neuromas are often associated with episiotomy repairs and, in one case report, with female genital cutting.[82] The patient usually describes a deep pain of gradual onset that becomes more intense with time. The pain is usually unilateral without dyspareunia. Diagnosis is point tenderness that duplicates the pain. Frequently, a tiny nodule is palpable in the soft tissue, and most often patients can put their finger right on this area. There is no reliable efficacious treatment that ensures no recurrence. Treatment modalities include cryotherapy, chemical ablation, radiofrequency ablation, and surgical excision of the neuroma.[83]

Localized Vulvar Pain of Vestibule (Vestibulodynia or Vulvar Vestibulitis)

Vulvar vestibulitis syndrome (VVS) orvestibulodynia is characterized by discomfort and hypersensitivity in the vulvar vestibule in the absence of physical findings except for varying degrees of erythema.[84]

Some investigators have proposed that there are two forms, primary and secondary. Primary VVS refers to introital dyspareunia dating from initiation of sexual activity or intolerable pain consistently present on insertion of a tampon or vaginal speculum.[6,85] It accounts for 20% of cases.[86] Secondary VVS describes introital dyspareunia that develops after a period of comfortable sexual relations, tampon use, or speculum examinations.

The standard diagnostic criteria for VVS in the medical literature are as follows: severe pain on vestibular touch or attempted vaginal entry; tenderness to pressure localized within the vulvar vestibule; and no evidence of physical findings except for varying degrees of erythema.[87] Spontaneous pain is minimal or absent. The pain is associated with intercourse, tampon use, binding clothes, and bicycle riding. In one study, one third of women had constant burning in the vestibule, three quarters had excessive vaginal discharge, and 10% had chronic urinary tract symptoms.[88]

This phenomenon is more prominent in premenopausal women.[89] Risk factors related to some aspects of sexual reproductive history have been identified in women with VVS; they include early contraceptive use (before 17 years of age),[90] early intercourse (before 16 years), and early menarche (before 12 years). *Candida* infection and STDs, on the other hand, have not been associated with increased risk of VVS.[84] Other studies have proposed an autoimmune association between *Candida* and VVS.[91]

Excessive urinary oxalate excretion has been proposed as an etiology of vulvar pain, based upon a case report of one patient in whom complete remission of symptoms occurred with low oxalate diet.[92] A controlled study of urinary oxalate excretion, however, did not show differences in women with and without pain.[88] Another theory is that allergy causes VVS, because levels of immunoglobulin E consistent with vaginal allergy have been detected in vaginal fluid; however, treatment with antihistamines has not been effective.[88] It has been suggested that some women have a genetic deficiency that impairs their immune system's ability to stop the inflammatory response triggered by exposure to agents such as infection or chemicals.[94] VVS is also associated with interstitial cystitis, which makes sense when one considers that the vestibule, bladder mucosa, and urethra share a common embryologic derivation from the urogenital sinus.[95,96]

On examination, there is tenderness to gentle cotton swab pressure in the vestibule (allodynia). The diagnosis is made when touching the vulva with a cotton-tipped applicator produces pain only in the vestibule.[85] Some say that the Q-tip test is the sine qua non of diagnosing vestibulitis.[83] While gentle tactile stimulation is applied to specific areas of the vestibule, the patient can rate her discomfort. Starting at 12 o'clock (just below the clitoris and above the urethra) and proceeding clockwise, the most tender areas may be at 4 and 8 o'clock.

Other diagnoses must be ruled out, and estrogenization should be assessed with vaginal wet mount, looking for predominance of intermediate or parabasal cells instead of the normal, well estrogenized superficial cells. The most common conditions mimicking VVS are *Candida* infection, poor estrogenization, pudendal neuropathy, dermatitis, rigid hymen, and vaginismus/pelvic floor muscle tension myalgia.

The first step in treatment of VVS, once a diagnosis is made, is to validate the patient's pain and reassure her that it is not psychological in nature and is not caused by cancer. The next step is to ensure adequate vulvar care. Patients should avoid scents, dyes, and chemicals, including fabric softener, bubble bath, body wash, and so on. Clothing should be cotton, comfortable and loose. Activities that may be abrasive to the vulvar area, such as biking, should be eliminated. Hydration by sitz baths may help. Use of natural lubricants, such as olive oil and Astroglide, may help. For burning, ice packs may provide relief. Because anecdotal evidence has supported eliminating foods high in oxalate, the patient may want to try this avenue.

Topical anesthetics such as Xylocaine 2% jelly or 5% ointment[89] or the compounded triple therapy (prilocaine, lidocaine, tetracaine: 3.5%/2.5%/1%) in a lipoderm base can provide relief if applied three times per day and liberally 20 minutes before sexual activity. This treatment useful because it "numbs the vulva," but it probably works via its pharmacologic effect of blocking sodium channels and altering neural plasticity. Capsaicin has also been tried in a number of studies, but it has not been widely successful and is painful when first applied.[97] Another study showed great improvement with injections of methyl prednisolone acetate and lidocaine cloridrate, with complete remission in 7 of 22 women and marked improvement in 3.[98] Triple nerve block therapy using caudal, pudendal, and local anesthetic blocks over 8 weeks has also demonstrated success.[98a]

One of the first-line therapies for VVS, because it appears to be a "neuroplastic pain syndrome," are the tricyclic antidepressants, which are standard therapy for neuroplastic/neuropathic pain.[89] Amitriptyline and desipramine improve pain substantially in patients who can tolerate doses of 50-75 mg.[99] Patients should be counseled that the drug is known primarily for its antidepressant effect but is also widely used for pain, so that patients do not feel deceived. Dosing should start at 10 mg and gradually be increased to minimize side effects, until the total dose is 150 mg or the symptoms are controlled. If patients continue to experience drowsiness with amitriptyline despite decreasing doses for a week, then nortriptyline or desipramine should be substituted, using a similar dosing schedule (less sedation and fewer anticholinergic side effects). Tricyclics take at least 4 weeks to have an effect and should be tried for 3 months at 100 to 150 mg before moving on to another agent.

Gabapentin or other anticonvulsants should be considered in those who cannot tolerate tricyclics or if those medications fail.[89] Patients should be started slowly at 100 mg at bedtime of gabapentin and then increased by 100 mg every 2 days until at least 1800 mg and up to 3600 mg/day is being taken in three divided doses or nightly. Side effects include drowsiness, fatigue, dizziness, and ataxia. Up to 1200 mg can be given at night to decrease drowsiness.

Interferonα has been reported to be beneficial, primarily when injected locally.[100,101] The most common regimen is 1 million units injected three times per week for 4 weeks circumferentially at the periphery of the vestibule. Side effects include flu-like symptoms, fever, malaise, myalgias; pretreatment with acetaminophen or ibuprofen may help. These patients may also experience significant injection-site pain and may benefit from pretreatment for 20 to 30 minutes with a topical anesthetic.

Surgical excision of the vestibule (Woodruff procedure) is another treatment option for patients with VVS. The affected area is mapped and excised, then covered with undermined vaginal epithelium. Many surgeons remove all areas of the vestibule, including those areas that are not painful, because failure can recur in areas of remaining vulvar tissue. One study showed an 85% cure rate.[102] Complications include dehiscence, recurrence of symptoms, and occasionally worsening of pain. So, although vestibulectomy was once the treatment of choice for VVS, the discomfort of the procedure, the possibility of incomplete success or worsening of pain, and the success of less aggressive therapies have relegated this procedure to second- or third-line therapy.[89] One study compared group cognitive-behavioral therapy (12-week trial), surface electromyographic biofeedback (12-week trial), and vestibulectomy in the treatment of dyspareunia resulting from vulvar vestibulitis.[103] This study found that, although vestibulectomy was superior to the other treatment modalities, all three groups significantly improved on measures of psychological adjustment and sexual function. Another study by the same group demonstrated that physical therapy is a promising treatment modality for dyspareunia associated with vulvar vestibulitis.[104]

Dysesthetic Vulvodynia or Generalized Vulvodynia

It is likely that this syndrome is a variant of pudendal neuropathy or, at the least, neuropathic pain, and it is best diagnosed and treated as such.

Pudendal Neuropathy

Pudendal neuropathy, or "essential vulvodynia," was a label given to patients who complained of constant or almost constant vulvar burning and had a paucity of physical findings.[105] Pudendal canal syndrome (PCS) is induced by the compression or stretching of the pudendal nerve in Alcock's canal.[106] Causes of PCS are by sources of compression (biking, long-time sitting, horseback riding, hematoma) or stretching (descending perineum, surgery, delivery) of the pudendal nerve in the patient's history. A change in the shape or orientation of the ischial spine induced by some athletic activities may also explain some cases.[107] Pudendal neuralgia can also be found in patients with multiple sclerosis and postherpetic neuralgia.

The complete syndrome manifests with pain, hypoesthesia or hyperesthesia, and sometimes anal or urinary incontinence. However, motor symptoms are actually rare. Patients can present with an unprovoked, persistent, superficial, burning sensation that is frequently accompanied by a deep, aching component or a rare, paroxysmal lancinating pain over a large area.[105] Patients with less severe involvement may complain of an itch-burn sensation or a feeling of rawness. Some patients have burning pain with light touch and complain of dyspareunia not only on penile penetration but also during and after intercourse. Patients may also have rare, symptom-free periods that last for days or weeks. Because of the various areas supplied by the pudendal nerve, the following structures can be involved: cutaneous surfaces of the labia minora and majora, clitoris, urethral meatus, vulvar vestibule, perineum, and perianal skin.

Physical findings are sparse. There is normally no evidence of infection. Focal vestibular erythema with or without tenderness is sometimes seen. Positive findings include thickened surgical scars, presence of palpable tumor, or evidence of genital herpes. Some patients have a weak anal reflex.[108]

Pudendal neuropathy is usually a diagnosis of exclusion. However, a pudendal nerve block can be used as both a diagnostic and a therapeutic measure. The pain usually disappears for only 1 to 2 days after injection. The block is repeated every third day for a total of four blocks. Computed tomography–guided blockade may be more accurate.[109] Other tests sometimes found to be abnormal in PCS include electromyography (EMG) and pudendal nerve terminal motor latency (PNTML). There is diminished EMG activity of the external anal sphincter, external urethral sphincter, and levator ani. There is a significant increase in PNTML in women with severe PCS.

Depending on the severity of the problem, there are several modalities of treatment. Nonsteroidal anti-inflammatory agents are frequently used but are not helpful in most cases. In mild cases, tricyclic antidepressants may be helpful.[105] Anticonvulsants such as carbamazepine, phenytoin, and gabapentin have also been found to be helpful.[110] As described earlier, serial pudendal blocks with a local anesthetic can be used. However, if none of these measures are helpful, another PNMLT is abnormal, there is evidence that surgical decompression of the pudendal canal may lead to improvement.[108,111]

Pelvic Floor Muscle Disorders: Myalgia and Trigger Points

Trigger points are discrete, focal, hyperirritable spots located in a taut band of skeletal muscle.[112] The spots are painful on compression and can produce referred pain, referred tenderness, motor dysfunction, and autonomic phenomena. Acute trauma or repetitive microtrauma may lead to the development of stress on muscle fibers and the formation of trigger points. Patients may have regional, persistent pain resulting in a decreased range of motion in the affected muscles. These include muscles used to maintain body posture, such as those in the neck, shoulders, and pelvic girdle. Trigger points may also manifest as tension headache, tinnitus, temporomandibular joint pain, decreased range of motion in the legs, and low back pain. Trigger points can also be found in the pelvis, causing pelvic pain. Palpation of a hypersensitive bundle or nodule of muscle fiber of harder than normal consistency is the physical finding typically associated with a trigger point. Palpation of the trigger point elicits pain directly over the affected area and/or causes radiation of pain toward a zone of reference and a local twitch response.

Various treatment modalities, such as the spray and stretch technique, ultrasonography, manipulative therapy, and local anesthetic injection, are used to inactivate trigger points. Techniques for rehabilitation include the avoidance of perpetuating factors, rehabilitation of extrapelvic abnormalities, use of manual techniques and needling to promote resolution of connective tissue problems, closure of diastasis recti, and transvaginal/transrectal manual release of muscular trigger points and contractures.[113] Trigger-point injection has been shown to be one of the most effective treatment modalities to inactivate trigger points and provide prompt relief of symptoms.

Vaginismus

Vaginismus is an involuntary spasm of pelvic muscles that partially closes the vagina. The *Diagnostic and Statistical Manual of Mental Disorders, 4th Revision* (DSM-IV), defines vaginismus as repeated and persistent involuntary spasm of the vaginal muscles that interferes with intercourse. This condition causes penetration to be difficult and painful, or even impossible. Vaginismus is considered a sexual dysfunction although the patient may often have pain with tampon insertion and gynecologic examinations as well. It is a complex condition with several possible causes that may result from past sexual trauma or abuse, other psychological factors, or a history of discomfort with sexual intercourse. Causes can also be congenital or infectious.[114] Sometimes no cause can be determined.

Women with varying degrees of vaginismus often develop anxiety regarding coitus and penetration, and intercourse is usually painful. However, this does not mean that they cannot achieve or sustain sexual arousal. Many are very sexually responsive and can have orgasms through clitoral stimulation.

Difficulty or inability to allow vaginal penetration for intercourse is the primary symptom. Vaginal pain with attempts at intercourse or during attempted pelvic examination is common. A gynecologic examination can confirm the diagnosis of vaginismus. The health care provider will note whether there is an involuntary muscle contraction when fingers are inserted into the vagina, and this usually reproduces the pain the woman feels with intercourse. Other causes of dyspareunia should also be ruled out.

The treatment of choice with vaginismus is an extensive therapy program that combines education and counseling with behavioral exercises. Exercises include pelvic floor muscle contraction and relaxation (Kegel exercises) to improve voluntary control. Vaginal dilation exercises are recommended using plastic dilators. This should be done under the direction of a sex therapist or other health care provider, and treatment should involve the partner. This treatment should gradually include more intimate contact, ultimately resulting in intercourse.

Psychosocial Factors

Psychosocial factors are important in the management of vulvar and vaginal pain, both as a cause and as an effect of the pain. Patients with chronic vaginal or vulvar pain often experience progressively limited professional and social lives. Patients often become frustrated with the multiple physician visits, diagnostic tests, and treatment regimens including surgeries. If the medical treatment is not conclusive or successful, patients may be told it is "all in their head." This may lead to further stress, depression, and sexual dysfunction.

Most studies indicate that an average of 20% to 30% of women with pelvic pain have experienced childhood trauma or sexual abuse. If the pain is "nonsomatic" or of "unknown etiology," the frequency of abuse is found to be much higher. The impact of historical factors in causing pain is controversial but may exacerbate a patient's experience of pain.

Chronic Pelvic Pain with Resultant Dyspareunia

Chronic pelvic pain (CPP) is frequently associated with dyspareunia. CPP is a common problem, and it presents a major challenge to health care providers because of its unclear etiology, complex natural history, and poor response to therapy. A significant number of these patients have various associated problems, including bladder or bowel dysfunction, sexual dysfunction, and other systemic or constitutional symptoms. Other associated conditions, such as depression, anxiety, and drug addiction, also may coexist. Studies have shown that women with CPP are more likely to have a history of sexual and physical abuse than are other groups of women.[115] The most common causes of CPP are endometriosis, irritable bowel syndrome, interstitial cystitis, abdominal wall and pudendal neuropathy, pelvic floor muscle tension myalgia, and fibromyalgia. Residual symptomatology after accurate diagnosis and focused treatment is best managed with a multidisciplinary approach.[116] The diagnosis and management of CPP is beyond the scope of this chapter.

Abnormal Vaginal Discharge

Normal vaginal discharge is 1 to 4 mL over 24 hours, white or transparent, thick and odorless. Physiologic discharge is formed by mucoid endocervical secretions in combination with sloughing epithelial cells, normal bacteria, and vaginal transudate. Discharge may be more noticeable during pregnancy, oral contraceptive use, or at midmenstrual cycle, close to the time of ovulation. Physiologic leukorrhea has a pH of 4.0 to 4.5, has a ratio of polymorphonuclear leukocytes to vaginal epithelial cells that is less than 1, and contains many squamous cells.[117] Vaginitis and vaginosis were discussed in earlier sections of this chapter. Cervicitis can lead to abnormal vaginal discharge.

Gonorrhea Cervicitis

Gonorrhea is one of the most frequently diagnosed STDs and remains a significant cause of preventable and treatable morbidity. The peak incidence occurs in 15- to 19-year-old women.[118] *N. gonorrhoeae* is a gram-negative diplococcus, first described by Neisser in 1879.[119] The most concerning complications of gonorrhea infection relate to female reproduction. Scarring from pelvic inflammatory disease can interfere with fertilization in 20% of cases. There is also a 9% risk of ectopic pregnancy and an 18% risk of chronic abdominal pain.[120] Women can also infect newborn infants during birth, causing neonatal ophthalmia.

The incubation period for urogenital gonococcal infection is approximately 10 days in the female patient.[8] The typical symptoms are increased vaginal discharge, dysuria, intermenstrual uterine bleeding, postcoital bleeding, and menorrhagia.[50,121] Infection in women is often asymptomatic, whereas men are asymptomatic only 10% of the time.[122]

Gonorrhea in women can infect the cervix, urethra, anus, rectum, or oropharynx or can be disseminated. The most common site of infection is the cervix; approximately 50% of affected women are asymptomatic. Symptoms include vaginal pruritus and mucopurulent discharge from runny or scant to copious. Patients may also complain of new postcoital spotting or dyspareunia. On examination, the cervix may appear normal or show signs of frank discharge. The cervix may be friable, and there may be abdominal pain with upper genital tract disease. Gonococcal vulvitis and vaginitis are infrequent, because the stratified squamous epithelium of the vagina is resistant to invasion by the gonococcus.[8] The symptoms for urethritis are initially urinary frequency and burning.[8] Infection of the trigone is accompanied by increased dysuria, and the patient often has tenesmus. The urethral meatus is often edematous and erythematous with purulent discharge with the urethral epithelium everted. Patients may have severe pain from Skene's duct abscess and be unable to void. There can also be infection of Bartholin's gland, and pus may drain from that site, but if the duct is occluded, then an abscess will form. Anorectal infection can be asymptomatic or associated with clinical proctitis. In about 4% of patients with anorectal involvement, it is the sole site of infection.[123] Symptoms include anal itching, rectal discharge, rectal fullness, tenesmus, and painful defecation. Pharyngitis results from fellatio with a male partner who has gonococcal urethritis or from cunnilingus.[124] The pharynx is infected in 10% to 20% of individuals. Symptoms include fever and cervical lymphadenopathy.

There are several methods of diagnosing gonorrhea infection. The "gold standard" is culture on modified Thayer-Martin medium. This is very sensitive in symptomatic women but only 65% to 85% sensitive in asymptomatic women.[125] Cultures are 100% specific and allow testing for antibiotic resistance. Gram stains are less sensitive but allow for an earlier diagnosis and treatment. DNA probes have accuracy similar to that of culture, with high sensitivity, specificity, and positive and negative predictive values.[126] Enzyme immunoassay is not widely used, because its positive predictive value is acceptable only in populations with a high prevalence of infection. There are also commercially available nucleic acid amplification tests (NAATs). They are more rapid to perform than culture, returning results within hours, but are much more expensive. NAATs have also been shown to be more sensitive than culture, being able to detect as little as one organism per sample, whereas the threshold for conventional methods is approximately 1000 organisms.[127]

There are many accepted regimens for gonorrhea. The use of one-time, observed therapy is recommended, because compliance with multiple doses is lower. Also, because 42% of patients with gonorrhea are found to have dual infection with chlamydia,[128] concurrent treatment for both organisms is recommended. The recommended treatments of uncomplicated cervical, urethral, or anorectal infection are ceftriaxone 125 mg IM once, ciprofloxacin 500 mg PO once, ofloxacin 400 mg PO once, levofloxacin 250 mg PO once, and spectinomycin 2g IM once.[16] Pregnant women should not be treated with quinolones or tetracyclines. The partner should also be treated.

Chlamydia Cervicitis

Chlamydia is the most common agent of sexually transmitted genital infections leading to cervicitis and often abnormal vaginal discharge. Chlamydia is a true bacterium, an obligate intracellular parasite. The organism is transmitted primarily by sexual contact. The organism cannot be transmitted across intact skin or mucous membranes. Risk factors for infection are young age, black race, multiple sex partner, recent new sex partner, low rates of barrier contraception, and history of STD.[129,130]

Chlamydia has been implicated in urethritis, Bartholin's abscess, cervicitis, endometritis, salpingitis, conjunctivitis, and pneumonitis of the newborn. The ultimate sequelae in the female that may involve chlamydial infection are ectopic pregnancy, infertility, and complex salpingitis that may lead to formation of a tubo-ovarian abscess and eventually hysterectomy.[8]

Most patients with cervicitis are asymptomatic. If symptoms are present, they may include vaginal spotting with intercourse, vaginal discharge, poorly differentiated abdominal pain, or lower abdominal pain. Examination may reveal the presence of mucopus or hypertrophy of the endocervical epithelium with a copious clear discharge, or the cervix may bleed briskly when touched with cotton-tipped applicator. Approximately 30% of women with *Chlamydia* infection develop pelvic inflammatory disease if left untreated.[131]

Traditional methods of diagnosis include cervical swabs requiring a full pelvic examination, but new diagnostic techniques include cervical swabs, urine, or self-administered vaginal swabs. Antigen detection by DFA and enzyme-linked immunosorbent assay (ELISA) still requires a swab from the cervix or urethra and is 80% to 95% sensitive compared to culture. Genetic probe methods based on direct specimen swab from the cervix or urethra are also 80% to 95% sensitive compared with culture. Nucleic acid amplification, PCR, and ligase chain reaction (LCR) are being studied and have high sensitivity and specificity.[132] Clinical practice guidelines strongly recommend routine *Chlamydia* screening for sexually active women younger than 25 years of age.[16,133]

Azithromycin (1 g PO as a single dose) and doxycycline (100 mg PO twice daily for 7 days) are the two recommended regimens. Alternative regimens include 7 days of erythromycin base (500 mg PO four times daily), erythromycin ethylsuccinate (800 mg PO), ofloxacin (300 mg PO twice daily), or levofloxacin (500 mg PO once daily).[16,134] Test of cure is not recommended, except for patients with persisting symptoms and those with suspect compliance. Test of cure should be done 3 weeks after the completion of therapy.[16]

Cervical and Vaginal Lesions

Vesicovaginal Fistula

Vesicovaginal fistula is a communication between the vagina and a part of the urinary tract (ureter, bladder, or proximal urethra). Continual wetness, odor, and discomfort cause serious social problems. The main causes include obstructed labor and surgical trauma, and 10% of the cases are caused by irradiation, locally advanced pelvic tumors, and pelvic pathologies (e.g., inflammation, foreign bodies).

Classically, vesicovaginal fistulas manifest with continuous incontinence after a recent pelvic operation.[135] If the fistula is small, then watery discharge from the vagina accompanied by normal voiding may be the only symptom. Diagnostic tests can be done by passing a small ureteric catheter through the fistular tract to see if it enters the vagina. Other means of diagnosis are by retrograde and voiding cystourethrography. A high creatinine level of the discharge can confirm urinary leakage.

Colovaginal, Rectovaginal, and Coloperineal Fistulas

Colovaginal and rectovaginal fistulas are thought to be a relatively uncommon occurrence, but they can cause distressing symptoms depending on the severity, site, location, and etiology.[136] The most common cause of colovaginal fistulas is diverticular disease. They also occur as a result of irradiation, pelvic surgery, malignancy, abdominal hysterectomy, abscess formation, perforation by a foreign body, inflammatory bowel disease, and trauma. Fistulas develop in 2% of patients with diverticulitis. Most patients have colovaginal fistulas secondary to diverticular disease, Crohn's disease, or pelvic surgery, particularly hysterectomy.

The passage of feces per vagina is diagnostic of a fistula between the bowel and internal genitalia. Putting a tampon in the vagina may assist in the diagnosis. Most patients present with abnormal discharge, which may not be recognized as frank feces. Colovaginal fistula may also manifest as vaginal flatus. With small bowel–vaginal fistulas, severe excoriation may be seen secondary to the presence of digestive enzymes. Physical examination with a speculum usually reveals an opening or granular area at the apex of the vagina that appears red and is usually on the left. The next examination usually requested is a barium enema, but this is ineffective. Vaginography may be useful, however. Other diagnostic tools include colposcopy, colonovaginoscopy, and computed tomography.

References

1. Skene A: Treatise on the Disease of Women. New York, Appleton and Company; 1889.
2. Burning vulva syndrome: Report of the ISSVD task force. J Reprod Med 29:457, 1984.
3. McKay M, Frankman O, Horowitz BJ, et al: Vulvar vestibulitis and vestibular papillomatosis. Report of the ISSVD Committee on Vulvodynia. J Reprod Med 36:413-415, 1991.
4. Moyal-Baracco M, Lynch PJ: 2003 ISSVD terminology and classification of vulvodynia. International Society for the Study of Vulvovaginal Diseases (ISSVD): XVII World Congress, jointly sponsored by the American College of Obstetricians and Gynecologists, October 12-16, 2003, Salvador, Brazil. J Reprod Med 49:772, 2004.
5. Welsh BM, Berzins KN, Cook KA, Fairley CK, et al: Management of common vulval conditions. Med J Aust 178:391-395, 2003.
6. Goetsch MF: Vulvar vestibulitis: Prevalence and historic features in a general gynecological practice population. Am J Obstet Gynecol 164:1609-1615, 1991.
7. Harlow BL, Stewart EG: A population-based assessment of chronic unexplained vulvar pain: Have we underestimated the prevalence of vulvodynia? J Am Med Womens Assoc 58:82, 2003.
8. Kaufmann RH: Benign Diseases of the Vulva and Vagina, 5th ed. St. Louis, Mosby, 2005.
9. McDonald JS, Rapkin AJ: Pelvis, perineum and genitalia: General considerations. In Loeser JD (ed): Bonica's Management of Pain, 3rd ed Philadelphia, Williams & Wilkins, 2000, p 1429.
10. Rapkin AJ, Markusen TE: Chronic pelvic pain. In Rice A, Warfield C, McGrath P, et al (eds): Textbook of Clinical Pain Management: Chronic Pain. London, Arnold, 2001, pp 587-613.
11. Friedrich EG: Vulvar Disease, 2nd ed. Philadelphia, WB Saunders, 1983.
12. Joesof M, Schmid G: Bacterial Vaginosis: Clinical Evidence. London, BMJ Publishing Group, 2001.
13. Gutman RE, Peipert JF, Weitzen S, Blume J: Evaluation of clinical methods for diagnosing bacterial vaginosis. Obstet Gynecol 105:551-556, 2005.
14. Hillier S, Holmes KK: Bacterial vaginosis. In Holmes KK (ed): Sexually Transmitted Diseases, 2nd ed. New York, McGraw-Hill, 1990, p 547.
15. Joesof MR, Schmid GP: Bacterial vaginosis: Review of treatment options and potential clinical indications for therapy. Clin Infect Dis 20(Suppl 1):S72, 1995.
16. Centers for Disease Control and Prevention: Sexually transmitted diseases treatment guidelines 2002. MMWR Morb Mortal Wkly Rep 51(No. RR-6):1, 2002.
17. Hanson JM, McGregor JA, Hillier SL, et al: Metronidazole for bacterial vaginosis: A comparison of vaginal gel vs oral therapy. J Reprod Med 45:889, 2000.

18. Powell BL, Drutz DJ: Confirmation of corticosterone and progesterone-binding activity in *Candida albicans.* J Infect Dis 147:359, 1983.
19. Bisschop MP, Merkus JM, Van Cutsem J: The growth-promoting activity of vaginal fluid for *Candida albicans* (and the problem of enhanced susceptibility to vaginal candidosis). Eur J Obstet Gynecol Reprod Biol 20:107, 1985.
20. Knight L, Fletcher J: Growth of *Candida albicans* in saliva: Stimulation by glucose associated with antibiotics, corticosteroids, and diabetes mellitus. J Infect Dis 123:371, 1971.
21. Hilton AL, Warnock DW: Vaginal candidiasis and the role of the digestive tract as a source of infection. Br J Obstet Gynecol 82:922, 1975.
22. Davidson F, Oates JK: The pill does not cause "thrush." Br J Vener Dis 92:1265, 1985.
23. Rylander E, Berglund AL, Krassny C, Petrini B: Vulvovaginal candida in a young sexually active population: Prevalence and association with oro-genital sex and frequent pain at intercourse. Sex Transm Infect 80:54-57, 2004.
24. Sobel JD, Chaim W, Nagappan V, Leaman D: Treatment of vaginitis caused by *Candida glabrata*: Use of topical boric acid and flucytosine. Am J Obstet Gynecol 189:1297-1300, 2003.
25. McCormack WM, Evrard JR, Laughlin CF, et al: Sexually transmitted conditions among women college students. Am J Obstet Gynecol 139:130-133, 1981.
26. Josey WE, McKenzie WJ, Lambe DW Jr: *Corynebacterium vaginale (Haemophilus vaginalis)* in women with leukorrhea. Am J Obstet Gynecol 126:574, 1976.
27. Cassie R, Stevenson A: Screening for gonorrhea, trichomoniasis, moniliasis and syphilis in pregnancy. J Obstet Gynaecol Br Comm 80:4851, 1973.
28. Hardy PH, Hardy JB, Nell EE, et al: Prevalence of six sexually transmitted disease agents among pregnant inner-city adolescents and pregnancy outcome. Lancet 2:333-337, 1984.
29. Mason PR, Fiori PL, Cappuccinelli P, et al: Seroepidemiology of *Trichomonas vaginalis* in rural women in Zimbabwe and patterns of association with HIV infection. Epidemiol Infect 133:315-323, 2005.
30. Santler R, Thurner J: Contagiousness of *Trichomonas vaginalis.* Wien Klin Wochenschr 86:46-49, 1974.
31. Whittington MJ: Epidemiology of infections with *Trichomonas vaginalis* in the light of improved diagnostic methods. Br J Vener Dis 33:80-91, 1957.
32. Lara-Torre E, Pinkerton JS: Accuracy of detection of *Trichomonas vaginalis* organisms on a liquid-based papanicolaou smear. Am J Obstet Gynecol 188:354-356, 2003.
33. Okun N, Gronau KA, Hannah ME: Antibiotics for bacterial vaginosis or *Trichomonas vaginalis* in pregnancy: A systematic review. Obstet Gynecol 105:857-868, 2005.
34. Aubert JM, Sesta HJ: Treatment of vaginal trichomoniasis: Single two-gram dose of metronidazole as compared with a seven-day course. J Reprod Med 27:743-745, 1982.
35. Murphy R: Desquamative inflammatory vaginitis. Derm Therapy 17:47-49, 2004.
36. Jacobson M, Krumholz B, Franks A: Desquamative inflammatory vaginitis: A case report. J Reprod Med 34:647-650, 1989.
37. Murphy R, Edwards L: Desquamative inflammatory vaginitis. Br J Dermatol 145:74, 2001.
38. Wald A, Zeh J, Selks S, et al: Virologic characteristics of subclinical and symptomatic genital herpes infection. N Engl J Med 333:770-775, 1995.
39. Corey L, Adams HG, Brown ZA, Holmes KK: Genital herpes simplex virus infections: Clinical manifestations, course, and complications. Ann Intern Med 98:958, 1983.
40. Kimberlin DW, Rouse DJ: Clinical practice: Genital herpes. N Engl J Med 350:1970, 2004.
41. Whitley RJ, Kimberlin DW, Roizman B: Herpes simplex viruses. Clin Infect Dis 26:541, 1998.
42. Reeves WC, Corey L, Adamd HG, et al: Risk of recurrence after first episodes of genital herpes: Relation to HSV type and antibody response. N Engl J Med 305:315, 1981.
43. Mommeja-Marin H, Lafaurie M, Scieux C, et al: Herpes simplex virus type 2 as a cause of severe meningitis in immunocompromised adults. Clin Infect Dis 37:1527, 2003.
44. Schomogyi M, Wald A, Corey L: Herpes simplex virus-2 infection: An emerging disease? Infect Dis Clin North Am 12:47, 1998.
45. Lafferty WE, Coombs RW, Benedetti J, et al: Recurrences after oral and genital herpes simplex virus infection: Influence of site of infection and viral type. N Engl J Med 316:1444, 1987.
46. Moseley RC, Corey L, Benjamin D, et al: Comparison of viral isolation, direct immunofluorescence, and indirect immunoperoxidase techniques for detection of genital herpes simplex virus infection. J Clin Microbiol 13:913, 1981.
47. Ramaswamy M, McDonald C, Smith M, et al: Diagnosis of genital herpes by real time PCR in routine clinical practice. Sex Transm Infect 80:406, 2004.
48. Filen F, Strand A, Allard A, et al: Duplex real-time polymerase chain reaction assay for detection and quantification of herpes simplex virus type 1 and herpes simplex virus type 2 in genital and cutaneous lesions. Sex Transm Dis 31:331, 2004.
49. Kimberlin DW, Lakeman FD, Arvin AM, et al: Application of the polymerase chain reaction to the diagnosis and management of neonatal herpes simplex virus disease: National Institute of Allergy and Infectious Diseases Collaborative Antiviral Study Group. J Infect Dis 174:1162, 1996.
50. Bonnez W, Reichman R: Papillomaviruses. In Mandell GL, Bennett JE, Dolin R (eds): Principles and Practice of infectious Diseases, 5th ed. Philadelphia, Churchill Livingstone, 2000, p 1630.
51. Black MM, McKay M, Braude PR: Color Atlas and Text of Obstetric and Gynecologic Dermatology. London, Mosby Wolfe, 1995, p 119.
52. Ridley CM, Neill SM: Non-infective cutaneous conditions of the vulva. In Ridley CM, Neill SM (eds): The Vulva. Oxford, Blackwell Science, 1999, p 121.
53. Thomas RH, Ridley CM, McGibbon DH, Black MM: Anogenital lichen sclerosus in women. J R Soc Med 89:694, 1996.
54. Loening-Bucke V: Lichen sclerosus et atrophicus in children. Am J Dis Child 145:1058-1061, 1991.
55. Zellis S, Pincus SH: Treatment of vulvar dermatoses. Semin Dermatol 15:71, 1996.
56. Fischer GO: The commonest causes of symptomatic vulvar disease: A dermatologist's perspective. Australas J Dermatol 37:12, 1996.
57. Lewis FM: Vulval lichen planus. Br J Dermatol 138:569, 1998.
58. Mann MS, Kaufmann RH: Erosive lichen planus of the vulva. Clin Obstet Gynecol 34:605, 1991.
59. Anderson M, Kutzner S, Kaufmann RH: Treatment of vulvovaginal lichen planus with vaginal hydrocortisone suppositories. Obstet Gynecol 100:359, 2002.
60. Marren P, Wojnarowska F: Dermatitis of the vulva. Semin Dermatol 15:36, 1996.
61. Lynch PJ: Dermatology. Baltimore, Williams & Wilkins, 1994, p 4.
62. Jemal A, Murray T, Ward W, et al: Cancer statistics 2005. CA Cancer J Clin 55:10, 2005.
63. Hildesheim A, Han CL, Brinton LA, et al: Human papillomavirus type 16 and risk of preinvasive and invasive vulvar cancer: Results from a seroepidemiological case-study. Obstet Gynecol 90:748, 1997.
64. Iwasawa A, Nieminen P, Lehtinen M, Paavonen J: Human papillomavirus in squamous cell carcinoma of the vulva by polymerase chain reasction. Obstet Gynecol 89:81, 1997.
65. Parker LP, Parker JR, Bodurka-Bevers D, et al: Paget's disease of the vulva: Pathology, pattern of involvement, and prognosis. Gynecol Oncol 77:183, 2000.
66. Fanning J, Lambert HC, Hale TM, et al: Paget's disease of the vulva: Prevalence of associated vulvar adenocarcinoma, invasive Paget's

disease, and recurrence after surgical excision. Am J Obstet Gynecol 180:24, 1999.

67. Feuer GA, Shevchuk M, Calanog A: Vulvar Paget's disease: The need to exclude an invasive lesion. Gynecol Oncol 38:81, 1990.
68. Raz R, Miron D, Colodner R, et al: A 1-year trial of nasal mupirocin in the prevention of recurrent staphylococcal nasal colonization and skin infection. Arch Intern Med 156:1109, 1996.
69. Lee YH, Rankin JS, Alpert S, et al: Microbiological investigation of Bartholin's abscesses and cysts. Am J Obstet Gynecol 129:150-153, 1977.
70. Mungan T, Ugur M, Yalcin H, et al: Treatment of Bartholin's cyst and abscess: Excision versus silver nitrate insertion. Eur J Obstet Gynecol Reprod Biol 63:61, 1995.
71. Brook I: Aerobic and anaerobic microbiology of Bartholin's abscess. Surg Gynecol Obstet 169:32, 1989.
72. Droegemueller W: Comprehensive gynecology. Mosby, St. Louis, 1992, p 637.
73. Ball SB, Wojnarowska F: Vulvar dermatoses: Lichen sclerosus, lichen planus, and vulvar dermatitis/lichen simplex chronicus. Semin Cutan Med Surg 17:182, 1998.
74. Fischer G, Spurrett B, Fischer A: The chronically symptomatic vulva: Aetiology and management. Br J Obstet Gynaecol 102:773, 1995.
75. Fischer GO: The commonest causes of symptomatic vulvar disease: A dermatologist's perspective. Australas J Dermatol 37:12, 1996.
76. Dalziel KL, Wojnarowska F: Long-term control of vulvar lichen sclerosus after treatment with a potent topical steroid cream. J Reprod Med 38:25, 1993.
77. Dalziel KL, Millard PR, Wojnarowska F: The treatment of vulval lichen sclerosus with a very potent topical steroid (clobetasol propionate 0.05%) cream. Br J Dermatol 124:461, 1991.
78. Kanai M, Osada R, Maruyama K, et al: Warning from Nagano: Increase of vulvar hematoma and/or lacerated injury caused by snowboarding. J Trauma 50:328-331, 2001.
79. Sau AK, Dhar KK, Dhall GI: Nonobstetric lower genital tract trauma. Obstet Gynaecol 33:433-435, 1993.
80. Kennedy CM, Dewdney S, Galask RP: Vulvar granuloma fissuratum: A description of fissuring of the posterior fourchette and the repair. Obstet Gynecol 105(5 Pt 1):1018-1023, 2005.
81. Olsen AL, Smith VJ, Bergstrom JO, et al: Epidemiology of surgically managed pelvic organ prolapse and urinary incontinence. Obstet Gynecol 89:501, 1997.
82. Fernandez-Aguilar S, Noel JC: Neuroma of the clitoris after female genital cutting. Obstet Gynecol 101(5 Pt 2):1053-1054, 2003.
83. Perry PC: Vulvodynia. In Howard FM, Perry PC, Carter JE, et al (eds): Textbook of pelvic pain: Diagnosis & Management. Philadelphia, Lippincott Williams & Wilkins, 2000, pp 204-210.
84. Masheb RM, Nash JM, Brondolo E, Kerns RD: Vulvodynia: An introduction and critical review of a chronic pain condition. Pain 86:3-10, 2000.
85. Bazin S, Bouchard C, Brisson J, et al: Vulvar vestibulitis syndrome: An exploratory case-control study. Obstet Gynecol 83:47-50, 1994.
86. Witkin SS, Gerber S, Ledger WJ: Differential characterization of women with vulvar vestibulitis syndrome. Am J Obstet Gynecol 187:589, 2002.
87. Friedrich EG: Vulvar vestibulitis syndrome. J Reprod Med 32:110-114, 1987.
88. Ledger WJ, Kessler A, Leonard GH, Witkin SS: Vulvar vestibulitis: A complex clinical entity. Infect Dis Obstet Gynecol 4:269, 1996.
89. Edwards L: New concepts in vulvodynia. Am J Obstet Gynecol 189(3 Suppl):S24-S30, 2003.
90. Bouchard C, Brisson J, Fortier M, et al: Use of oral contraceptive pills and vulvar vestibulitis: A case control study. Am J Epidemiol 156:254, 2002.
91. Ashman RB, Ott AK: Autoimunity as a factor in recurrent vulvovaginal candidosis and the minor vestibular gland syndrome. J Reprod Med 34:264, 1989.
92. Solomons CC, Melmed MH, Heitler SM: Calcium citrate for vulvar vestibulitis: a case report. J Reprod Med 36:879, 1991.
93. Baggish MS, Sze EH, Johnson R: Urinary oxalate secretion and its role in vulvar pain syndrome. Am J Obstet Gynecol 177:507, 1997.
94. Jeremias MS, Ledger WJ, Witkin SS: Interleukin 1 receptor antagonist gene polymorphism is women with vulvar vestibulitis. Am J Obstet Gynecol 182:283, 2000.
95. McCormack WM: Two urogenital sinus syndromes: Interstitial cystitis and focal vulvitis. J Reprod Med 35:873, 1990.
96. Fitzpatrick CC, DeLancey JO, Elkins TE, McGuire EJ: Vulvar vestibulitis and interstitial cystitis: A disorder of urogenital sinus-derived epithelium? Obstet Gynecol 81:860, 1993.
97. Bergeron S, Binik YM, Khalife S, et al: Vulvar vestibulitis syndrome: A critical review. Clin J Pain 13:27, 1997.
98. Murina F, Tassan P, Roberti P, Bianco V: Treatment of vulvar vestibulitis with submucous infiltrations of methylprednisolone and lidocaine: An alternative approach. J Reprod Med 46:713, 2001.
98a. Rapkin AJ, McDonald JS, Morgan M: Multilevel local anesthetic nerve blockade for the treatment of vulvar vestibulitis syndrome. Am J Obstet Gynecol, 2007. In press.
99. McKay M: Dyesthetic ("essential") vulvodynia: Treatment with amitryptiline. J Reprod Med 38:9-13, 1993.
100. Horowitz BJ: Interferon therapy for condylomatous vulvitis. Obstet Gynecol 73:446-448, 1989.
101. Marinoff SC, Turner ML, Hirsch RP, Richard G: Intralesional alpha interferon: Cost-effective therapy for vulvar vestibulitis syndrome. J Reprod Med 38:19-24, 1993.
102. McCormack WM, Spence MR: Evaluation of the surgical treatment of vulvar vestibulitis. Eur J Obstet Gynecol Reprod Biol 86:135-138, 1999.
103. Bergeron S, Binik YM, Khalife S, et al: A randomized comparison of group cognitive–behavioral therapy, surface electromyographic biofeedback, and vestibulectomy in the treatment of dyspareunia resulting from vulvar vestibulitis. Pain 91:297-306, 2001.
104. Bergeron S, Brown C, Lord MJ, et al: Physical therapy for vulvar vestibulitis syndrome: A retrospective study. J Sex Marital Ther 28:183-192, 2002.
105. Turner ML, Marinoff SC: Pudendal neuralgia. Am J Obstet Gynecol 165(4 Pt 2):1233-1236, 1991.
106. Shafik A: Pudendal canal syndrome: Description of a new syndrome and its treatment—Report of 7 cases. Coloproctology 13:102-110, 1991.
107. Antolak SJJ, Hough DM, Pawlina W, Spinner RJ: Anatomical basis of chronic pelvic pain syndrome: The ischial spine and pudendal nerve entrapment. Med Hypotheses 59:349-353, 2002.
108. Shafik A: Pudendal canal syndrome as a cause of vulvodynia and its treatment by pudendal nerve decompression. Eur J Obstet Gynecol Reprod Biol 80:215-220, 1998.
109. McDonald JS, Spigos DG: Computed tomography–guided pudendal block for treatment of pelvic pain due to pudendal neuropathy. Obstet Gynecol 95:306-309, 2000.
110. Swerdlow M: Anticonvulsant drugs and chronic pain. Clin Neuropharmacol 7:51, 1984.
111. Becos J, Climov D, Bex M: Pudendal nerve decompression in perineology: A case series. BMC Surgery 4:15, 2004.
112. Alvarez DJ, Rockwell PG: Trigger points: Diagnosis and management. Am Fam Physician 65:653-660, 2002.
113. FitzGerald MP, Kotarinos R: Rehabilitation of the short pelvic floor. II: Treatment of the patient with the short pelvic floor. Int Urogynecol J Pelvic Floor Dysfunct 14:269-275; discussion 275, 2003. Epub 2003 Aug 7.
114. McDonald JS, Rapkin AJ: Pelvis, perineum and genitalia: General considerations. In Loeser JD (ed): Bonica's Management of Pain, 3rd ed. Philadelphia, Williams & Wilkins, 2000, p 1369.
115. Rapkin AJ, Kames LD, Darke LL, et al: History of physical and sexual abuse in women with chronic pelvic pain. Obstet Gynecol 76:92-96, 1990.

116. Rapkin AJ, Jolin J: Chronic pelvic pain. In Weiner RS (ed): Pain Management, 6th ed. Washington, DC: CRC Press, 2002, p 251.
117. Sobel JD. Vaginitis. N Engl J Med 337:1896-1903, 1997.
118. Gonorrhea—United States, 1998. MMWR Morb Mortal Wkly Rep 49:538, 2000.
119. Neisser ALS: Uber eine der Gonorrhea eigentumliche Micrococcusform. Abl Med Wiss 17:497, 1879.
120. Platt R, Rice P, McCormack W: Risk of acquiring gonorrhea and prevalence of abnormal adnexal findings among women recently exposed to gonorrhea. JAMA 250:3205, 1983.
121. Noble RC: Characterization of *Neisseria gonorrhoeae* from women with simultaneous infections at two sites. Br J Vener Dis 56:3, 1980.
122. Sherrard J, Barlow D: Gonorrhoea in men: Clinical and diagnostic aspects. Genitourin Med 72:422, 1996.
123. Klein EJ, Fisher LS, Chow AW, Guze LB: Anorectal gonococcal infection. Ann Intern Med 86:340, 1977.
124. Sackel SG, Alpert S, Fiumura NJ, et al: Orogenital contact and the isolation of *Neisseria gonorrhea, Mycoplasma hominis,* and *Ureaplasma urealyticum* from the pharynx. Sex Transm Dis 6:64, 1979.
125. Schink JC, Keith LG: Problems in the culture diagnosis of gonorrhea. J Reprod Med 30:244, 1985.
126. Kouman EH, Johnson RE, Knapp JS, St Louis ME: Laboratory testing for *Neisseria gonorrheae* by recently introduced nonculture tests: A performance review with clinical and public health considerations. Clin Infect Dis 27:1171, 1998.
127. Van Dyck E, Ieven M, Pattyn S, et al: Detection of *Chlamydia trachomatis* and *Neisseria gonorrheae* by enzyme immunoassay, culture, and three nucleic acid amplification tests. J Clin Microbiol 39:1751, 2001.
128. Lyss SB, Kamb ML, Peterman TA, et al: *Chlamydia trachomatis* among patients infected with and treated for *Neisseria gonorrheae* in sexually transmitted disease clinics in the United States. Ann Intern Med 139:178, 2003.
129. Gaydos CA, Howell MR, Pare B, et al: *Chlamydia trachomatis* infections in female military recruits. N Engl J Med 339:739, 1998.
130. Cook RL, St George K, Lassak M, et al: Screening for *Chlamydia trachomatis* infection in college women with polymerase chain reaction assay. Clin Infect Dis 28:1002, 1999.
131. Cates W Jr, Wasserheit JN: Genital chlamydial infections: Epidemiology and reproductive sequelae. Am J Obstet Gynecol 164:1771, 1991.
132. Marrazzo JM, Johnson RE, Green TA, et al: Impact of patient characteristics on performance of nucleic acid amplification tests and DNA probe for detection of *Chlamydia trachomatis* in women with genital infections. J Clin Microbiol 43:577-584, 2005.
133. Howell MR, Quinn TC, Gaydos CA: Screening for *Chlamydia trachomatis* in asymptomatic women attending family planning clinics. Ann Intern Med 128:277, 1998.
134. Drugs for sexually transmitted infections. Treat Guidel Med Lett 2:67, 2004.
135. Romcs I, Kelemen ZS, Fazakas ZS: The diagnosis and management of vesicovaginal fistula. BJU Int 89:764-766, 2002.
136. Bahadursingh A, Longo W: Colovaginal fistulas: Etiology and management. J Reprod Med 48:489-495, 2003.

Chapter 88

BENIGN CYSTIC LESIONS OF THE VAGINA AND VULVA

Karyn Schlunt Eilber

Benign cystic lesions of the female external genitalia are frequently encountered in gynecologic and female urologic practices. True cystic lesions of the vagina and vulva originate from vaginal and vulvar tissues, respectively, but lesions arising from the urethra and surrounding tissues can appear as cystic lesions of the vagina and vulva as well. Most cysts of the female genitalia are located within the vagina, and their prevalence has been estimated to be 1 in 200 women; however, this figure is probably an underestimation, because most cysts are asymptomatic and therefore not reported.[1] Cysts arising within the vulvar vestibulum are much less common.

Vaginal cysts typically occur in the third and fourth decades and are rarely found in prepubertal females except in countries where female circumcision in performed.[2] Pradhan and Tobon reviewed the histology of 43 vaginal cysts over a 10-year period. In their study, the incidence of cyst types in decreasing order was müllerian cysts (44%), epidermal inclusion cysts (23%), Gartner's duct cysts (11%), Bartholin's gland cysts (7%), and endometriotic type (7%).[3] The remaining types of cystic lesions include those of urethral or paraurethral origin and other rare lesions (Table 88-1).

PATIENT EVALUATION

Cysts of the vagina and vulva are usually asymptomatic, and their presence is usually noted as an incidental finding on physical examination. In patients whose cysts are discovered because of symptomatology, mild discomfort, patient detection of a mass, or urinary symptoms such as incontinence or obstructive voiding symptoms are common presenting symptoms. In most cases, the appropriate diagnosis is made by history and physical examination alone; other cases are diagnosed only after excision and histologic examination of the tissue.

Patient history should include the onset and duration of symptoms and the presence of pain, dyspareunia, voiding complaints, and prior urologic or gynecologic procedures. A history of recurrent urinary tract infections and/or intermittent incontinence may indicate the presence of a urethral diverticulum, whereas continuous incontinence may represent an ectopic ureterocele.

During physical examination, the lesion should be assessed for location, mobility, tenderness, definition (smooth versus irregular), and consistency (cystic versus solid). The presence of

Table 88-1 Vaginal Wall Cyst Location and Histology

Diagnosis	Location	Histology
Müllerian (paramesonephric) cyst	Anywhere, usually anterolateral vaginal wall	Pseudostratified columnar, mucinous
Gartner's (mesonephric) cyst	Same as müllerian cyst	Low columnar, nonciliated, nonmucinous
Skene's (paraurethral) duct cyst	Floor of distal urethra	Stratified squamous
Bartholin's gland cyst	Lateral introitus, medial to labia minora	Transitional or columnar, mucinous
Adenosis	Vaginal fornices and upper walls	Columnar, ciliated, mucinous
Cyst of canal of Nuck (hydrocele)	Superior to labia majora or inguinal canal	Flat cuboidal
Urethral caruncle	Urethral meatus	Loose connective tissue and vessels
Urethral diverticulum	Periurethral, anterior vaginal wall	Transitional or squamous epithelium
Inclusion cyst	Area of previous surgery	Stratified squamous epithelium around keratinous debris
Endometriosis	Anywhere, usually posterior fornix	Two of three: endometrial glands, stroma, hemosiderin-laden macrophages
Ectopic ureterocele	Periurethral	Transitional or squamous epithelium
Vaginitis emphysematosa	Upper two thirds of vagina	Inflammatory and giant cells
Hidradenoma	Interlabial sulcus	Papillomatous
Dermoid cyst	Paravaginal	Keratinized squamous epithelium and dermal appendages
Aggressive angiomyxoma	Vagina and vulva	Hypocellular, myxoid matrix of collagen and capillary-like vessels
Ciliated cyst	Anywhere in vagina, vulvar vestibulum	Müllerian-like columnar ciliated epithelium
Pigmented follicular cyst	Vulva	Stratified squamous epithelium with keratinization and pore

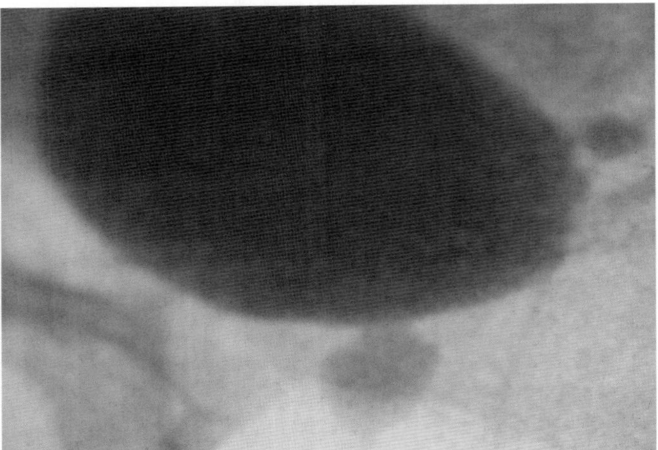

A

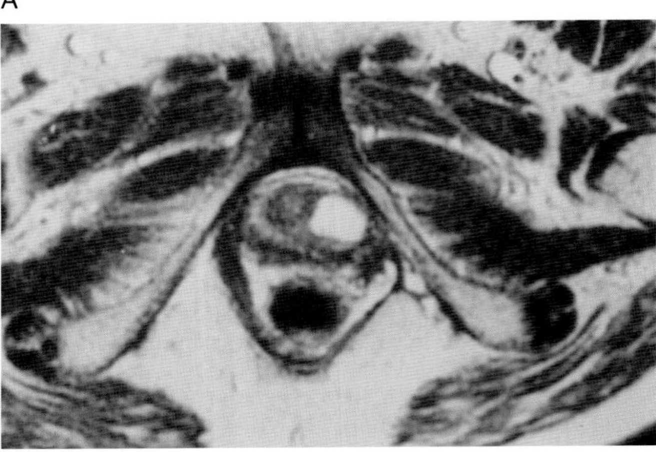

B

Figure 88-1 **A,** Voiding cystourethrogram (VCUG) demonstrates obstruction of distal urethra. **B,** Magnetic resonance imaging (MRI) confirms that the obstructing lesion is a cyst.

malignancy must always be considered. Pelvic organ prolapse, such as cystocele or enterocele, can mimic a vaginal cyst and should be ruled out.

Pelvic imaging by means of ultrasound, voiding cystourethrogram (VCUG), computed tomography (CT), or magnetic resonance imaging (MRI) may be required to characterize the lesion further (Fig. 88-1). Although each of these modalities has been useful in the diagnosis of vaginal cysts, pelvic MRI is the preferred modality for diagnosing both cystic lesions and a variety of other genitourinary abnormalities, including pelvic organ prolapse, urethral diverticula, ovarian abnormalities, and uterine pathology.

CYSTS OF EMBRYONIC ORIGIN

During the eighth week of embryologic development, the paired müllerian (paramesonephric) ducts fuse distally and develop into the uterus, cervix, and upper third of the vagina, which are lined by a pseudostratified columnar (glandular) epithelium. Wolffian (mesonephric) ducts normally regress in the female, and their remnants include Gartner's duct, epoöphoron and paroöphoron. Beginning at week 12, a squamous epithelial plate derived from the urogenital sinus begins to grow upward and replace the original pseudostratified columnar epithelium with squamous mucosa. In addition to the lower two thirds of the vagina, the urogenital sinus derivatives in the female are Skene's glands and Bartholin's glands.[4]

Müllerian Cysts

During the process of replacement of the müllerian (pseudostratified columnar) epithelium with squamous epithelium of the urogenital sinus, müllerian epithelial tissue can persist anywhere in the vaginal wall, although it typically rests within the anterolateral wall. Consequently, müllerian cysts tend to be located along the anterolateral aspect of the vagina.[5] Müllerian derivatives are the most common type of vaginal cyst; they are lined predominantly by mucinous epithelium but may be lined by any epithelium of müllerian origin: endocervical, endometrial, or fallopian.[4,6] Clinically, the distinction between müllerian and mesonephric (Gartner's duct) cysts is of little importance.

Müllerian cysts range in size from 1 to 7 cm.[4] The great majority are asymptomatic and require no treatment. Occasionally, a müllerian cyst may become large enough that symptoms warrant excision.

Gartner's Duct Cysts

Although it is clinically irrelevant to distinguish Gartner's duct cysts from müllerian cysts, true Gartner's duct cysts arise from vestigial remnants of the mesonephric (wolffian) ducts. Gartner's duct extends from the mesosalpinx via the broad ligament to the cervix, so these cysts are usually located along the anterolateral vaginal wall.[4,6] Typically, they are small, with an average diameter of 2 cm, but the cysts may enlarge to the point where they are mistaken for other structures, such as a cystocele or urethral diverticulum (Fig. 88-2A).[4] The largest Gartner's duct cyst reported was 16 × 15 × 8 cm.[7]

An association between Gartner's duct cysts and abnormalities of the metanephric urinary system exists, and cases of ectopic ureter, unilateral renal agenesis, and renal hypoplasia have all been reported in association with Gartner's duct cysts.[8-10] Currarino reported on five children with a Gartner's duct cyst and either ipsilateral renal hypoplasia or dysplasia,[9] and Sheih and colleagues found that 6% of female children with unilateral renal agenesis had a Gartner's duct cyst.[10] Although such abnormalities usually present in childhood, awareness of this association should prompt the clinician to image the urinary tract when evaluating adults who present with Gartner's duct cysts. MRI is especially useful, both for evaluation of the characteristics of the cyst and to rule out communication with the urinary tract (see Fig. 88-2B).

Gartner's duct cysts are synonymous with simple cysts and are lined by cuboidal or low columnar, nonciliated, nonmucinous cells. They can be distinguished from müllerian cysts by the presence of a basement membrane and smooth muscle layer; however, clear distinction between the two can be made only on the basis of histochemical staining: müllerian cysts are periodic acid–Schiff (PAS) and mucin positive, whereas mesonephric cysts are devoid of cytoplasmic mucicarmine or PAS-positive material.[5,6]

If a Gartner's duct cyst is large and symptomatic, excision is indicated (see Fig. 88-2C). Successful treatment with cyst aspiration and 5% tetracycline injection has been reported but without long-term follow-up.[11]

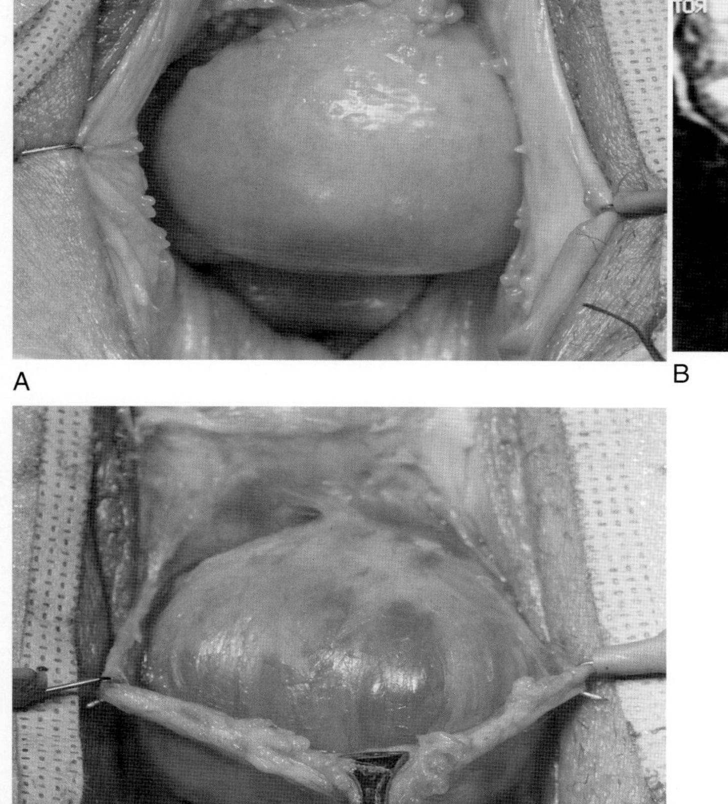

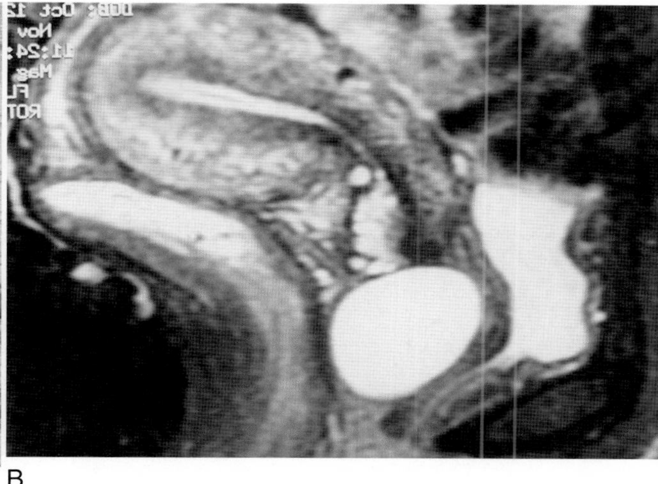

A B C

Figure 88-2 **A,** Large Gartner's duct cyst mimics a urethral diverticulum. **B,** Magnetic resonance imaging confirms cystic nature and absence of communication with the urinary tract. **C,** Excision.

Skene's Duct Cysts

Skene's (paraurethral) glands are bilateral prostatic homologues located in the floor of the distal urethra. Obstruction of the ducts is presumed to occur in response to skenitis, of which gonorrhea is the most common cause.[5,12] Because Skene's ducts are embryologically derived from the urogenital sinus, these cysts are lined by stratified squamous epithelium.[12]

Clinically significant cysts of Skene's ducts are rare, but cysts larger than 2 cm often cause patients to seek treatment for urinary symptoms such as dysuria or obstructive voiding symptoms (Fig. 88-3A).[13] In this situation, a Skene's duct cyst must be distinguished from a urethral diverticulum. Dysuria, history of urinary tract infections, and postvoid dribbling are common in the presence of a urethral diverticulum. Furthermore, on physical examination, compression of a Skene's duct cyst should not result in fluid extravasation. Both MRI and cystourethroscopy are useful to determine whether there is a communication between the lesion and the urethra (see Fig. 88-3B). It is of paramount importance to determine whether a vaginal cyst is of urethral origin. Unless a urethral diverticulum is suspected, urethral injury during cyst excision may occur, and a urethrovaginal fistula can result if the urethra is not adequately repaired and postoperative catheter drainage instituted.

Small Skene's duct cysts can be observed. Excision is recommended for larger, symptomatic cysts. Marsupialization is not necessary, and the duct itself need not be preserved.[5] Acute infection is a contraindication for excision; incision and drainage are advocated in this setting.

Bartholin's Duct Cysts

Bartholin's glands are also of urogenital sinus origin and are homologous to bulbourethral glands in males. Ductal obstruction, due to previous infection or inspissated mucus, is a prerequisite to cyst formation. Size and rapidity of growth depend on the accumulation of secretions from Bartholin's gland, which is influenced by sexual stimulation.[4] Although most patients have no symptoms or only mild dyspareunia, repeated sexual stimulation may be associated with rapidly enlarging, painful lesions. Pain may also indicate infection of the cyst.

Bartholin's gland is composed of acini lined by columnar, mucus-secreting epithelium and ducts lined by transitional epithelium. Larger ducts may contain areas of stratified squamous epithelium.[4] The origin of a Bartholin's duct cyst is indicated by its histology: cysts arising from the main duct are lined by transitional or squamous epithelium, whereas cysts originating in an acinus are lined by mucinous columnar epithelium.[5,14]

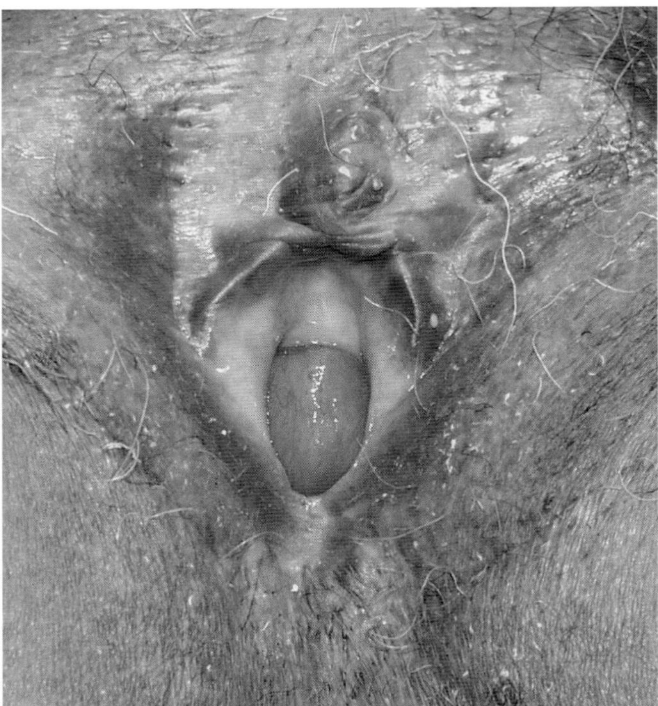

A

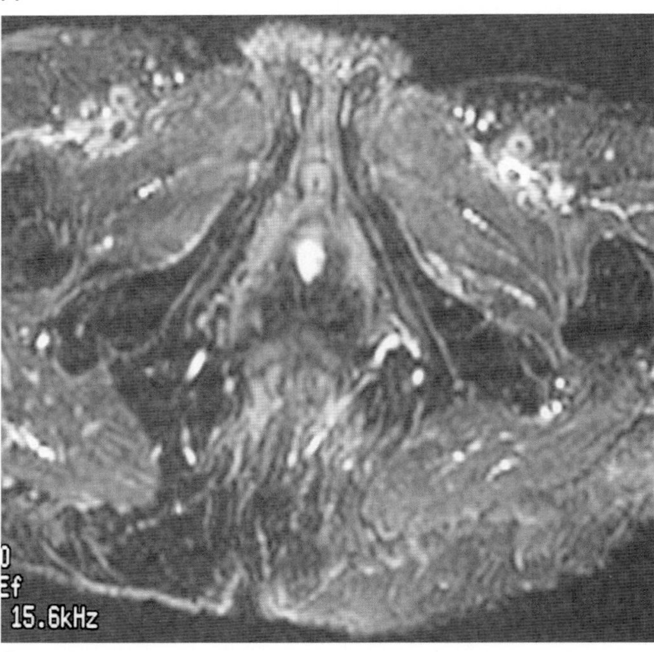

B

Figure 88-3 **A,** Vaginal mass causing distal urethral obstruction which proved to be a Skene's duct cyst. **B,** Preoperative magnetic resonance image demonstrates a cystic lesion arising in the urethra, consistent with a Skene's duct cyst.

Bartholin's duct cysts typically range from 1 to 4 cm in diameter. Most are unilateral, nontender, cystic masses located in the lateral introitus, medial to the labia minora (Fig. 88-4A). These lesions are detectable by ultrasound, CT, and MRI (see Fig. 88-4B). If small and asymptomatic, they require no treatment. Cysts associated with pain, recurrent abscess formation, or introital obstruction require surgical intervention. Excision of Bartholin's duct cysts has been described, but the preferred treatment is marsupialization to preserve function and prevent cyst or abscess reformation (see Fig. 88-4C). Incision and drainage is indicated for Bartholin's abscesses, with definitive treatment deferred until a period of quiescence.

Vaginal Adenosis

Vaginal adenosis is the presence of glandular epithelium within the vagina. It is attributed to failure of the squamous epithelium to replace the columnar epithelium in the vagina and ectocervix during embryogenesis.[15] It can be found in infants, children, and adults, and it is the most common lesion in women exposed to diethylstilbestrol (DES).[16] As with müllerian cysts, the lesions may represent any müllerian derivation and may include endocervical, endometrial, or tubal-type mucous cells (Fig. 88-5).[6,17]

Vaginal adenosis is commonly an incidental finding on examination of a DES-exposed woman and may resemble cervical ectropion. The classic appearance of adenosis is red, grape-like mucosa in the vaginal fornices and upper walls.[5] Identification of adenosis may be facilitated by its lack of staining with iodine solution.[4,5] Symptoms may include excessive mucoid vaginal discharge or mild postcoital bleeding.

No specific therapy is recommended for the treatment of adenosis, because the lesion may spontaneously regress. Routine examination of these lesions is recommended, because metaplastic conversion is well documented.

Cysts of the Canal of Nuck (Hydrocele)

The processus vaginalis, also referred to as the canal of Nuck, is a rudimentary peritoneal sac that accompanies the round ligament through the inguinal canal into the labia majora. During the first trimester, the canal of Nuck normally becomes obliterated. Persistence of the canal is associated with inguinal hernias, and occlusion at any point can lead to the formation of a cyst that is analogous to a hydrocele of the spermatic cord.

Cysts of the canal of Nuck are found in the superior aspect of the labia majora or inguinal canal. Their size may be several centimeters, and they are associated with an inguinal hernia in one third of cases.[18] Most of these cysts are diagnosed intraoperatively, but if a cyst of the canal of Nuck is suspected preoperatively, the surgical approach should be that for an inguinal herniorrhaphy.

CYSTS OF URETHRAL ORIGIN

It is important to determine whether a cystic lesion in the vagina is of urethral origin, because excision of urethral lesions requires postoperative catheter drainage to prevent fistula formation.

Urethral Caruncle

The term *caruncle* refers to a wide variety of lesions protruding from the urethral meatus. Urethral caruncles typically occur in postmenopausal women and most likely represent ectropion of the urethral wall due to postmenopausal regression of the vaginal

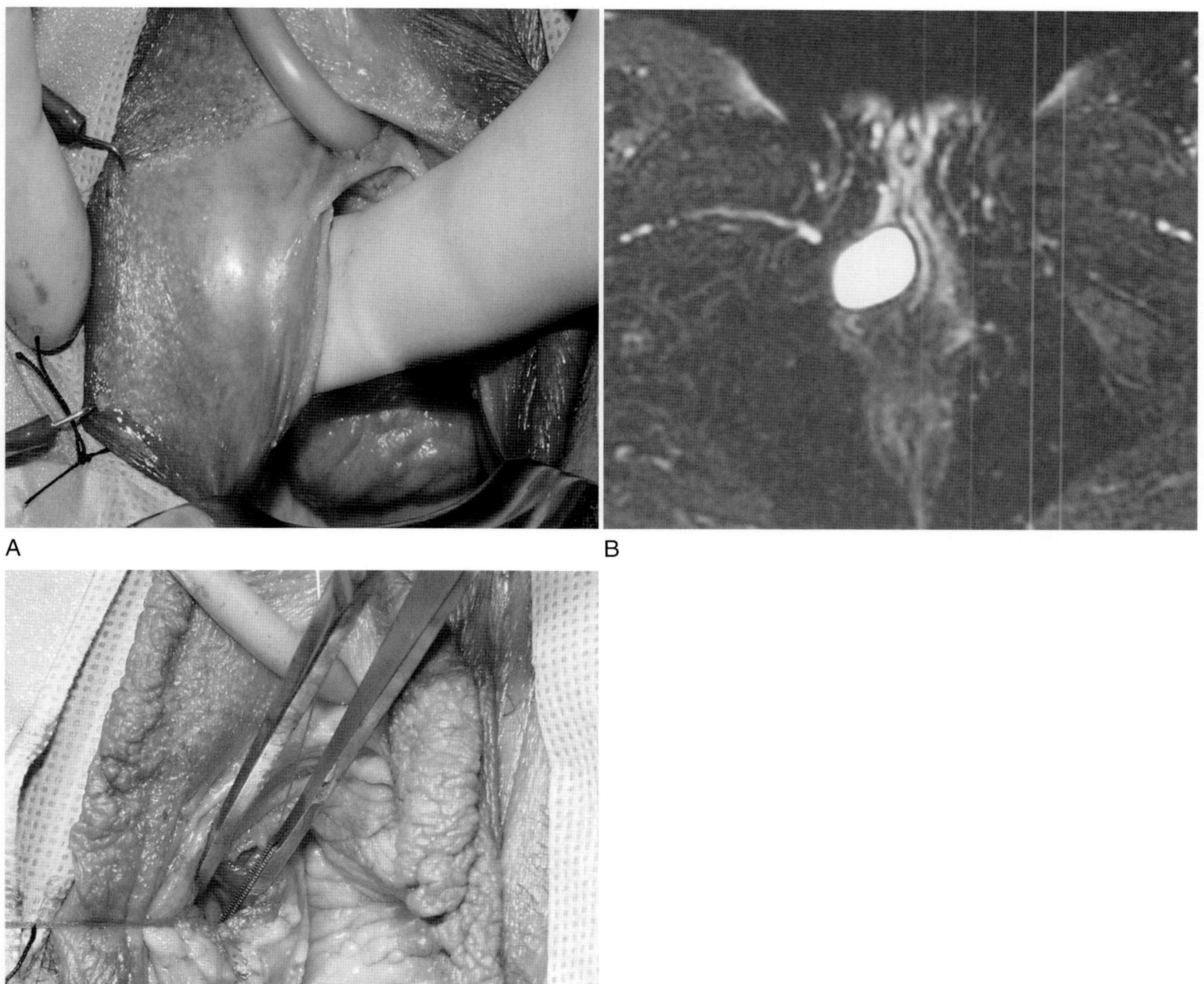

Figure 88-4 **A,** Bartholin's duct cyst on physical examination. **B,** Magnetic resonance image. **C,** Marsupialization.

mucosa. Urethral prolapse is often mistakenly diagnosed as a caruncle in a child.

On physical examination, a urethral caruncle is seen as a solitary, red, polypoid lesion protruding from one segment of the urethral meatus (Fig. 88-6). Most caruncles measure only a few millimeters in diameter. Symptoms range from mild bleeding to extreme discomfort.

Based on histology, caruncles are classified as either papillomatous, angiomatous, or granulomatous.[4] All types consist of a core of loose connective tissue and blood vessels covered by a transitional or squamous epithelium. Classification depends on the degree of associated inflammatory reaction.

Treatment is expectant for small, asymptomatic lesions. Excision is performed for lesions with significant symptoms or in cases in which carcinoma must be ruled out.

Urethral Diverticulum

A urethral diverticulum typically manifests as a cystic lesion in the anterior vaginal wall along the distal urethra (Fig. 88-7A). It most likely forms as a consequence of the rupture of infected periurethral glands into the lumen. Common symptoms include postvoid dribbling, dyspareunia, and recurrent urethritis or cystitis. Compression of the cyst may cause expulsion of urine or purulent material.

Cystourethroscopy is often the initial test when evaluating a patient with a suspected urethral diverticulum, but it may not be diagnostic if the neck of the diverticulum is small. In this case, imaging is invaluable. Neitlich and colleagues demonstrated that high-resolution, fast-spin echo technique MRI has a high sensitivity for detecting diverticula and a higher negative

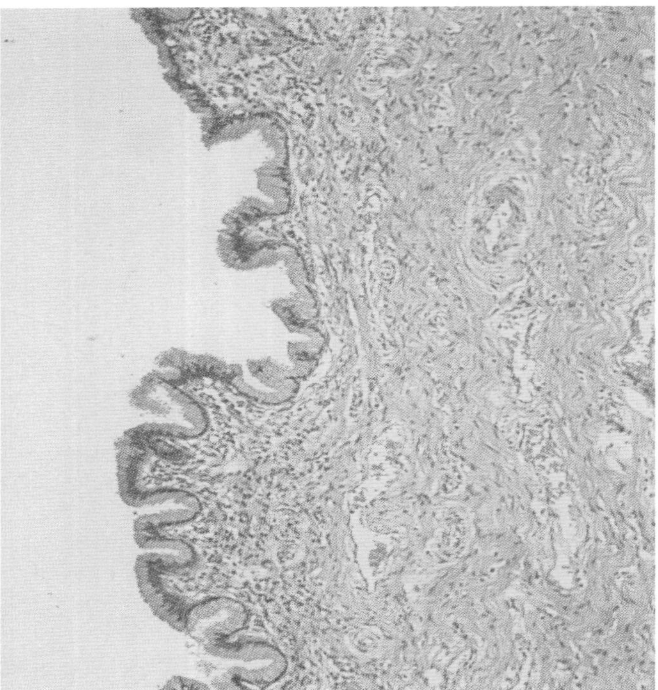

Figure 88-5 Microscopic appearance of vaginal adenosis.

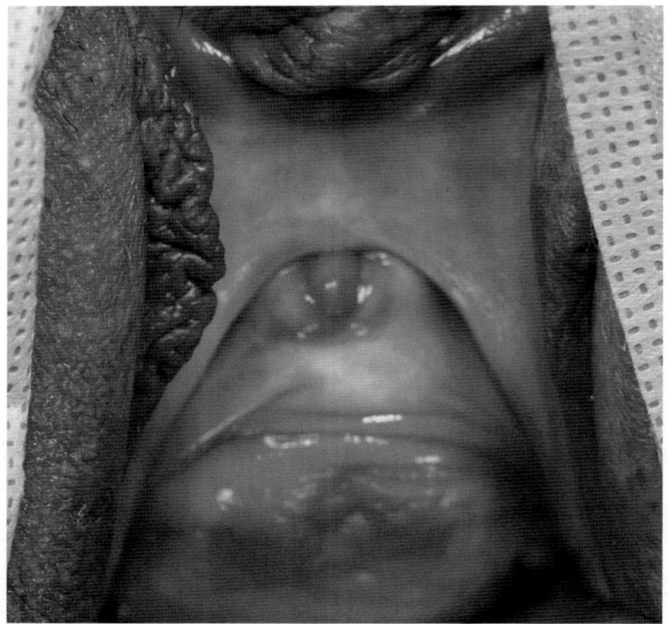

Figure 88-6 Urethral caruncle.

predictive rate than double-balloon urethrography.[19] A combination of both VCUG and MRI can be used to accurately diagnosis the condition and localize the lesion or lesions (see Fig. 88-7B,C).

Transvaginal excision with postoperative urethral catheter drainage is the preferred treatment, although endoscopic incision has been described.

EPIDERMAL CYSTS

Epidermal inclusion cysts secondary to buried epithelial fragments after episiotomy or other surgical procedures are the most common nonembryologic type of vaginal cysts.[4] In Nigeria, epidermal inclusion cysts are common in the first decade of life, and this has been attributed to the practice of prepubertal female circumcision.[2]

Inclusion cysts vary in size from a few millimeters to several centimeters in diameter. Their location correlates with an area of previous surgery, and their contents appear cheese-like and may even resemble a thick, purulent exudate. Imaging of these lesions by MRI reveals a cystic structure containing heterogeneous fluid.

On histologic examination, inclusion cysts are lined with stratified squamous epithelium and contain sebaceous-appearing material that represents desquamated epithelial cells. Cysts lined by squamous epithelium but not associated with buried skin fragments are simply termed *epidermal cysts*. Because these cysts are usually asymptomatic, they may be observed.

ENDOMETRIOSIS

Endometriosis is the ectopic implantation of endometrial glands and stroma. Primary occurrence in the vulva and vagina is rare and usually represents a secondary manifestation of pelvic disease. On gross examination, these cysts are mucoid and may appear brown or black. Nodules of endometriosis are located in the posterior fornix and appear red-blue to yellow-brown ("chocolate cyst"). The patient may complain of cyclic enlargement, dysmenorrhea, dyspareunia, pelvic pain, or dysuria.

Two of the following three characteristics must be present to make the diagnosis: endometrial glands, stroma, and hemosiderin-laden macrophages. Foreign body giant cells may be found.[4] Treatment is destruction or excision of the lesions.

ECTOPIC URETEROCELE

A ureterocele is a cystic dilatation of the distal ureter. Ureteroceles are commonly associated with the upper pole of a duplicated collecting system; if present with an ectopic ureter, they may manifest as a cystic vaginal mass. Although diagnosis is usually made at an early age, an ectopic ureterocele may manifest as incontinence in an older female child or young woman.

Clinically, most ureteroceles are diagnosed by prenatal ultrasound examination, but they may also be found as a cystic vaginal mass on physical examination. An endoscopic or open surgical approach is dictated by factors such as the presence of duplication, reflux, and parenchymal function of the upper pole associated with the ectopic ureterocele.

PELVIC ORGAN PROLAPSE

Prolapse of pelvic organs (e.g., cystocele, rectocele) can manifest as a vaginal cystic lesion. Symptoms can range from mild vaginal pressure to urinary incontinence or retention. Diagnosis is by history and physical examination. MRI is often helpful. All of the options for treatment are beyond the scope of this chapter and

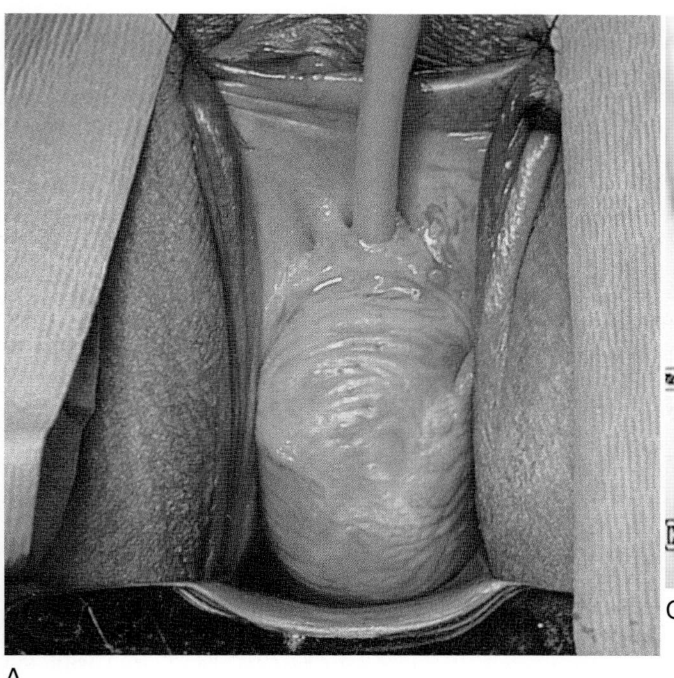

A

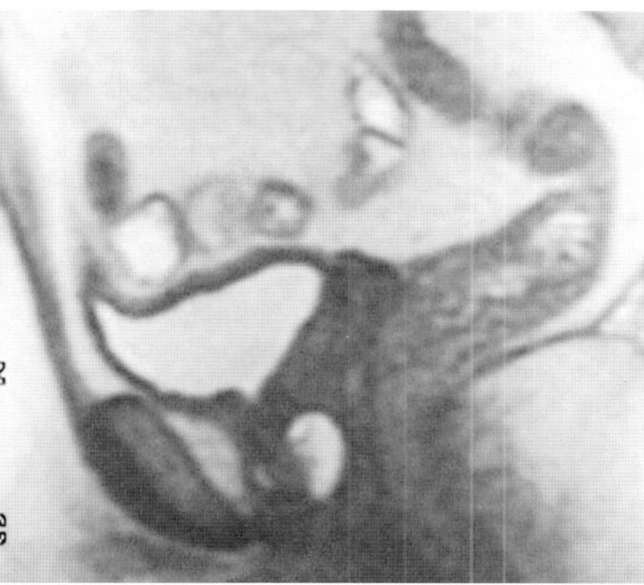

C

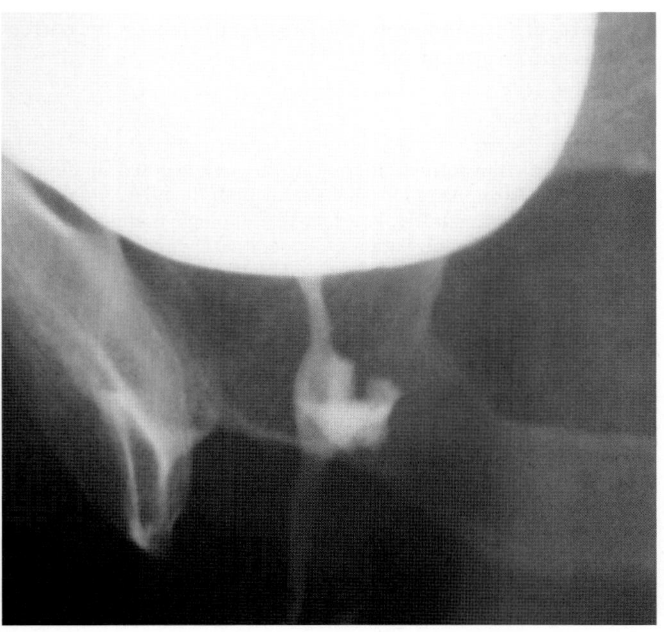

B

Figure 88-7 **A,** Large urethral diverticulum. **B,** Imaging of urethral diverticulum by voiding cystourethrogram (VCUG). **C,** Magnetic resonance image.

will not be discussed, but in general treatment depends on the patient's symptoms, health status, and degree of prolapse.

RARE CYSTIC LESIONS

Vaginitis Emphysematosa

Vaginitis emphysematosa is a rare, benign process characterized by gas-filled cysts in the vaginal wall, first described by Zweifel in 1877.[20] Fewer than 200 cases have been reported in the literature. Most patients present with symptoms of vaginitis, but an audible popping sound during intercourse has been reported by some.[21] No definitive infectious etiology has been found, but most cases are associated with *Trichomonas vaginalis.*[22]

Diagnosis can be made by physical examination. The cysts are usually found in the upper two thirds of the vagina but may extend to the lower vagina, and rarely to the vulva. On physical examination, the cysts are seen to be discrete, tense, and smooth, and they may create a popping sound when ruptured during a vaginal examination. On histologic examination, the cysts are found to contain pink hyaline-like material, and they are lined by foreign body giant cells and other inflammatory cells.[23] The condition is self-limited and does not require specific treatment.

Hidradenoma

Hidradenomas of the vagina are well-circumscribed, freely mobile nodules found mainly on the medial aspect of the labia majora in the interlabial sulcus. The majority are smaller than 1 cm. The presence of granular, papillomatous tissue is suggestive of the diagnosis. Microscopic examination is remarkable for a cystic lesion filled with papillomatous growths.[4] Treatment is by local excision.

Dermoid Cyst

Only two cases of dermoid cysts involving the vagina have been reported.[24,25] In both cases, the cyst originated in the paravaginal space and diagnosis was delayed. Histology is remarkable for a cyst lined by keratinized squamous epithelium and containing dermal appendages.

Aggressive Angiomyxoma

Aggressive angiomyxoma is a rare myofibroblastic tumor of the pelvic and genital soft tissues with just over 110 cases reported in the literature. It is typically found in women 35 to 40 years of age, although it can develop in men and children as well.[26] The term "aggressive" refers to its pattern of local infiltration and recurrent growth. Most are large (>10 cm), and surgical resection after imaging to determine the extent of disease is recommended.

Ciliated Cyst

A ciliated cyst is a cyst lined with columnar ciliated epithelium. Ciliated cysts are rare and are probably of müllerian origin. They occur in women 25 to 35 years of age and have been associated with pregnancy, exogenous progesterone, and chronic inflammation.[27] Resection is indicated for symptomatic lesions.

Pigmented Follicular Cyst

Pigmented follicular cysts are rare, occur predominantly in adult men, are composed of stratified squamous epithelium with epidermoid keratinization, and have a pore-like opening to the skin surface. Only one case of pigmented follicular cyst of the vulva has been reported, and treatment of this lesion was with CO_2 laser.[28]

CONCLUSIONS

Cystic lesions of the vagina and vulva are a relatively common occurrence and represent a spectrum of disease from embryologic derivatives to preneoplastic lesions. Familiarity with the different diagnoses is essential for any clinician involved in gynecologic or female urologic practice in order to arrive at the correct diagnosis and treatment plan.

References

1. Smith RP (ed): Netter's Obstetrics, Gynecology and Women's Health. Toronto, Canada, MediMedia, Inc., 2002.
2. Junaid TA, Thomas SM: Cysts of the vulva and vagina: A comparative study. Int J Gynaecol Obstet 19:239-223, 1981.
3. Pradhan S, Tobon H: Vaginal cysts: A clinicopathological study of 41 cases. Int J Gynecol Pathol 5:35, 1986.
4. Kaufman RH, Faro S (eds): Benign Diseases of the Vulva and Vagina. Stouis: Mosby, 1994.
5. Zaino RJ: Cysts. In Kurman RJ (ed): Blaustein's Pathology of the Female Genital Tract, 4th ed. New York, Springer-Verlag, 2001.
6. Wilkinson EJ (ed): Pathology of the Vulva and Vagina. New York, Churchill Livingstone, 1987.
7. Hagspiel KD: Giant Gartner duct cyst: Magnetic resonance imaging findings. Abdom Imaging 20:566, 1995.
8. Youssef AF (ed): Atlas of Gynecology Diagnosis. New York, Churchill Livingstone, 1984.
9. Currarino G: Single vaginal ectopic ureter and Gartner's duct cyst with ipsilateral renal hypoplasia and dysplasia (or agenesis). J Urol 128:988, 1982.
10. Sheih CP, Lu WT, Liao YJ, et al: Renal hypoplasia, Gartner's duct cyst and imperforated hemivagina: Report of a case. J Formos Med Assoc 93:531, 1994.
11. Abd-Rabbo MS, Atta MA: Aspiration and tetracycline sclerotherapy: A novel method for management of vaginal and vulvar Gartner's cysts. Int J Gynaecol Obstet 35:235, 1991.
12. Satani H, Yoshimura N, Hayashi N, et al: A case of female paraurethral cyst diagnosed as epithelial inclusion cyst. Hinyokika Kiyo 46:205, 2000.
13. Miller EV: Skene's duct cyst. J Urol 131:966, 1984.
14. Evans DM, Paine CG: Tumors of the vulva and vagina: Bartholin's cysts and paraurethral lesions. Clin Obstet Gynecol 8:997, 1965.
15. Fenoglio CM, Ferenczy A, Richart RM, Townsend D: Scanning and transmission electron microscopic studies of vaginal adenosis and the cervical transformation zone in progeny exposed in utero to diethylstilbestrol. Am J Obstet Gynecol 126:170, 1976.
16. Robboy SJ, Kaufman RH, Prat J, et al: Pathologic findings in young women enrolled in the National Cooperative Diethylstilbestrol Adenosis (DESAD) Project. Obstet Gynecol 53:309, 1974.
17. Antonioli DA, Burke L: Vaginal adenosis: Analysis of 325 biopsy specimens from 100 patients. Am J Clin Pathol 64:625, 1974.
18. Anderson CC, Broadie TA, Mackey JE, Kopecky KK: Hydrocele of the canal of Nuck: Ultrasound appearance. Am Surg 61:959, 1995.
19. Neitlich JD, Foster HE Jr, Glickman MG, Smith RC: Detection of urethral diverticula in women: Comparison of a high resolution fast spin echo technique with double balloon urethrography. J Urol 159:408, 1998.
20. Zweifel P: Die vaginitis emphysematosa ode colpo hysterplasia cystica nach winckel. Arch Gynäkol 12:39, 1877.
21. Close JM, Jesurun HM: Emphysematous vaginitis: Report of a case. Obstet Gynecol 19:513, 1962.
22. Gardner HL, Fernet P: Etiology of vaginitis emphysematosa. Am J Obstet Gynecol 88:680, 1964.
23. Kramer K, Tobon H: Vaginitis emphysematosa. Arch Pathol Lab Med 111:746, 1987.
24. Livengood CH, Addison WA, Hammond CB: Epidermoid cyst of the paravaginal space located only by computerized axial tomography: A case report. J Reprod Med 3:176, 1982.
25. Hirose R, Imai A, Kondo H, et al: A dermoid cyst of the paravaginal space. Arch Gynecol Obstet 249:39, 1991.
26. Gungor T, Zengeroglu S, Kaleli A, Kuzey GM: Aggressive angiomyxoma of the vulva and vagina. A common problem: Misdiagnosis. Eur J Obstet Gynecol Reprod Biol 112:114, 2004.
27. Hamada M, Kiryu H, Ohta T, Furue M: Ciliated cyst of the vulva. Eur J Dermatol 14:347, 2004.
28. Chuang Y, Hong H, Kuo T: Multiple pigmented follicular cysts of the vulva successfully treated with CO_2 laser: Case report and literature review. Dermatol Surg 30:1261, 2004.

Chapter 89

PATHOPHYSIOLOGY OF PELVIC PAIN

Ursula Wesselmann

Chronic pelvic pain syndromes belong to the category of visceral pain. Chronic pelvic pain is a common and debilitating problem that can significantly impair a woman's quality of life. Patients with chronic pelvic pain are usually evaluated and treated by urologists, gynecologists, gastroenterologists, and internists. The clinical presentation is often considered to be a diagnostic dilemma, because many urologic, gastrointestinal, and gynecologic disorders appear to cause or are associated with chronic pelvic pain.[1] Although these patients seek medical care because they are looking for help to alleviate their pelvic discomfort and pain, in clinical practice much emphasis has been placed on finding a specific cause and specific pathologic markers for pelvic disease. These patients typically undergo many diagnostic tests and procedures. Often, however, the examination and workup remain unrevealing and no specific cause of the pain can be identified. In these cases, it is important to recognize that pain is not only a symptom of pelvic disease, but that the patient is suffering from a chronic pelvic pain syndrome, in which "pain" is the prominent symptom of the chronic visceral pain syndrome.[2,3]

The purpose of this chapter is to review the pathophysiology of chronic nonmalignant pelvic pain, a chronic visceral pain syndrome. Because of the anatomic location of the viscera, they do not lend themselves easily to experimental manipulation, but recognition of the existence of the chronic pelvic pain syndromes has resulted in the development of novel animal models to study the pathophysiologic mechanisms of chronic pelvic pain[4] and of clinical studies to assess pain treatment options. Knowledge of the neurophysiologic characteristics of visceral pain will guide the physician in making a diagnosis of chronic pelvic pain and in sorting it out from the lump diagnosis of idiopathic pain.[3] A basic understanding of the neurobiology is paramount to gain further insights into the mechanisms of the pelvic pain disorders and contributes greatly to the development of effective clinical management strategies for patients presenting with these syndromes.

DEFINITIONS: WHAT IS CHRONIC PELVIC PAIN?

Definitions are important if a body of reliable information is to be built up in the scientific literature that will eventually lead to a better understanding of the pathophysiology of chronic pelvic pain. At present, one of the major problems of research into chronic pelvic pain is the lack of agreed definitions, which would allow comparisons among studies. On the other hand, lack of understanding of the pathophysiologic mechanisms of the pelvic pain syndromes makes it difficult to decide on criteria to define chronic pelvic pain conditions.[5]

Pain is defined by the International Association for the Study of Pain (IASP) as an unpleasant sensory and emotional experience associated with actual or potential tissue damage, or is described in terms of such damage.[6] There is no generally accepted definition of chronic pelvic pain. The IASP defines chronic pelvic pain without obvious pathology as chronic or recurrent pelvic pain that apparently has a gynecologic origin but for which no definitive lesion or cause is found.[6] This definition is problematic from a clinical perspective, because it implies absence of pathology, which might not necessarily be the case (for example, many patients with endometriosis suffer from pelvic pain). It also excludes cases in which pathology is present but not necessarily the cause of pain (for example, some patients with endometriosis do not have pelvic pain). As in many other pain conditions, the relationship of the pain complaint to the presence of pathology is often unclear in patients with chronic pelvic pain. The proportion of women with chronic pelvic pain and a specific diagnosis (or diagnoses) varies greatly in the literature. A large primary care study from Great Britain found that diagnoses related to urinary and gastrointestinal tracts are more common than gynecologic causes (30.8% urinary, 37.7% gastrointestinal, 20.2% gynecologic). Further, 25% to 50% of women with chronic pelvic pain who received medical care in primary care practices had more than one diagnosis.[7,8]

Several medical societies have recently published consensus statements revising definitions of chronic pelvic pain. The International Continence Society has defined "pelvic pain syndrome" as the occurrence of persistent or recurrent episodic pelvic pain associated with symptoms suggestive of lower urinary tract, sexual, bowel, or gynecologic dysfunction in the absence of proven infection or other obvious pathology.[9] The European Association of Urology suggested extending this definition by considering two subgroups based on the presence or absence of well-defined conditions that produce pain.[10] In the gynecologic literature, chronic pelvic pain is often referred to as pelvic pain in the same location for at least 6 months. The American College of Obstetricians and Gynecologists has proposed the following definition: chronic pelvic pain is noncyclic pelvic pain of 6 or more months' duration that localizes to the anatomic pelvis, anterior abdominal wall at or below the umbilicus, the lumbosacral back, or the buttocks and is of sufficient severity to cause functional disability or lead to medical care. A lack of physical findings does not negate the significance of a patient's pain, and normal examination results do no preclude the possibility of finding pelvic pathology.[1] Definitions of chronic pelvic pain will probably continue to be revised, as knowledge about the pathophysiology of pelvic pain is increasing based on basic science and clinical research. When reviewing literature on chronic pelvic pain, it is crucial for the reader to realize which definition of chronic pelvic was actually used for the study.

HOW COMMON IS CHRONIC PELVIC PAIN? EPIDEMIOLOGIC DATA

Chronic pelvic pain is more common than previously thought. Epidemiologic data from the United States showed that 14.7% of women in their reproductive years reported chronic pelvic pain, and the estimated number of female pelvic pain sufferers was 9.2 million in the United States alone.[11] Analysis of a large primary care database from the United Kingdom demonstrated that the annual prevalence rate of chronic pelvic pain in women was 38/1000, which is comparable to the prevalence rates of asthma and low back pain.[7] Although this study found a high prevalence of pain, many women had never had the condition diagnosed.[12]

NEUROANATOMY OF THE PELVIS

The purpose of this section is to provide an overview of the innervation of the pelvis and urogenital floor.[13,14] Although this summary attempts to derive as much information as possible from investigations involving humans, it is important to note that some generalizations are necessarily taken from animal studies, recognizing that much research in this field is still in its infancy.

All viscera, including the pelvic visceral organs, are dually innervated by both divisions of the autonomic nervous system, the sympathetic and parasympathetic divisions, as well as by the somatic and sensory nervous systems. In a broad anatomic view, dual projections from the thoracolumbar and sacral segments of the spinal cord carry out this innervation, converging primarily into discrete peripheral neuronal plexuses before distributing nerve fibers throughout the pelvis (Fig. 89-1). Interactive neuronal pathways routing from higher origins in the brain through the spinal cord add to the complexity of neuronal regulation in the pelvis. Although it is important to appreciate the influence of supraspinal centers in the coordination of pelvic organ activities, it is beyond the scope of this section to discuss these interactions in further detail; for review, see Bors and Comarr,[15] Morrison,[16] de Groat et al,[17] de Groat,[18] and Berkley and Hubscher.[19]

The nomenclature of the various plexuses, ganglia, and nerves in the pelvic cavity (see Dail[20]) is varied, and sometimes there are confusing presenting designations from both Nomina Anatomica[21] and clinical usage (see Baljet and Drukker[22]). In this review and in Figure 89-1, the anatomic nomenclature is used, with the clinical usage given in parentheses: superior hypogastric plexus (presacral nerve), hypogastric plexus (hypogastric nerve), inferior hypogastric plexus (pelvic plexus), and pelvic splanchnic nerve (pelvic nerve).

Within the pelvis, the inferior hypogastric plexus is regarded as the major neuronal integrative center. Neuroanatomic studies have confirmed its retroperitoneal location adjacent to each lateral aspect of the rectum, with interconnections between the left and right inferior hypogastric plexuses at the posterior aspect of the rectum.[23-26] It innervates multiple pelvic organs, including the urinary bladder, proximal urethra, distal ureter, rectum, and internal anal sphincter, as well as genital and reproductive tract structures.[27] The anterior part of the inferior hypogastric plexus, which is associated with the distal extent of the hypogastric plexus (hypogastric nerve), is referred to as the paracervical ganglia in females.[28] The paracervical ganglia part of the inferior hypogastric plexus in the female, situated in the parametrium lateral to the cervix and the upper part of the vagina, distributes nerve fibers to the corpora cavernosa of the clitoris, vagina, and periurethral tissues.[28]

Neuronal input to the inferior hypogastric plexuses involves dual input through the sympathetic and parasympathetic divisions of the autonomic nervous system. Sympathetic nerves originate in the thoracolumbar segments of the spinal cord (T10-L2) and condense into the superior hypogastric plexus located just inferior to the aortic bifurcation. Preganglionic efferents originate largely in the intermediolateral cell column, whereas afferents have their cell bodies located in dorsal root ganglia of these segments. Nerve fibers project from the superior hypogastric plexus as paired hypogastric plexuses (hypogastric nerves) and fuse distally before diverging bilaterally into branches destined for the inferior hypogastric plexuses. Additional sympathetic innervation to genitourinary organs may involve preganglionic nerves that synapse on postganglionic nerves originating in sympathetic chain ganglia; these postganglionic nerves join sacral nerves and course to their destinations via pelvic somatic neuronal pathways.[29] Parasympathetic preganglionic nerve efferents are thought to arise from cell bodies of the sacral parasympathetic nucleus located in the intermediolateral gray matter of the sacral spinal cord (S2-S4) and to fuse as the pelvic splanchnic nerve before entering the inferior hypogastric plexus.[30,31] Parasympathetic afferents have cell bodies located in the S2-S4 dorsal root ganglia and course also within the pelvic splanchnic nerve. In addition to its parasympathetic efferent and afferent component, the pelvic splanchnic nerve also receives postganglionic axons from the caudal sympathetic chain ganglia.[18]

A distinctive distribution of pelvic autonomic innervation is recognized at the urogenital organ level. Lower urinary tract smooth muscle, including that of the proximal urethra, urinary bladder, and lower ureter, receives direct postganglionic efferent projections from the inferior hypogastric plexus, although vesical or intramural ganglia also serve as origins for postganglionic axons.[32] The inferior hypogastric plexus additionally provides afferent input to the lower urinary tract and internal reproductive organs, with proximal afferent fibers predominantly projecting through the hypogastric plexuses (hypogastric nerves) (see Jänig and Koltzenburg[33]).

The autonomic innervation of the female genitalia has been less well studied than the male counterpart. It involves inferior hypogastric plexus projections deriving primarily from the paracervical ganglia part of the plexus. Conspicuous nerve trunks run in the adventitia of the vagina parallel to its long axis, sending off anterior branches that course to the clitoris and periurethral tissues and local branches that enter the vaginal smooth muscle walls.[22,34] A network of nerve fibers tends to follow vascular distributions and conspicuously terminates at the junction between the subepithelial connective tissue and the vaginal epithelium as well as within the epithelium.[34] Nerve density is observed to be greater in the distal vagina than in the proximal regions.[34]

Although the rectum and the anal sphincters are closely situated anatomically, their exact sources of innervation differ. Not surprisingly, a division of neural control is characterized on the basis of morphologic and functional differences. The smooth muscle of the rectum and internal anal sphincter (a thickened continuation of the circular smooth muscle fibers of the rectal wall) is influenced by the autonomic nervous system and receives innervation directly from sympathetic and parasympathetic

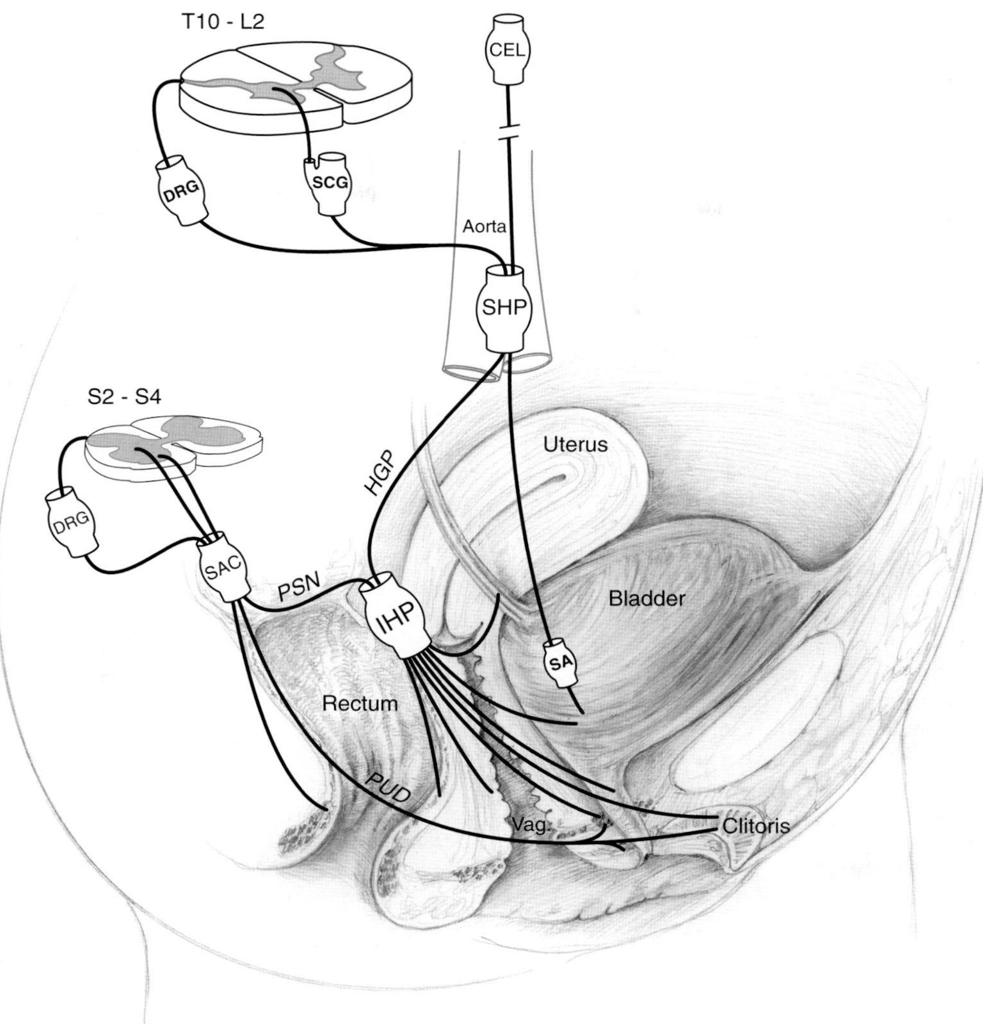

Figure 89-1 Schematic drawing showing the innervation of the pelvic area in the human female. CEL, celiac plexus; DRG, dorsal root ganglion; HGP, hypogastric plexus (hypogastric nerve); IHP, inferior hypogastric plexus (pelvic plexus); PSN, pelvic splanchnic nerve (pelvic nerve); PUD, pudendal nerve; SA, short adrenergic projections; SAC, sacral plexus; SCG, sympathetic chain ganglion; SHP, superior hypogastric plexus (presacral nerve); Vag = vagina. (From Wesselmann U, Burnett AL, Heinberg LJ: The urogenital and rectal pain syndromes. Pain 73:269-294, 1997. With permission of the International Association for the Study of Pain.)

origins coursing through or synapsing within the inferior hypogastric plexus.[35] Rectal branches from this plexus accompany the middle rectal vessels to the lateral sides of the rectum, within condensations of connective tissue referred to as the lateral ligaments of the rectum.[35] At the level of the intestinal wall, innervation continues according to the pattern observed throughout the gastrointestinal tract, which involves two ganglionic plexuses, the myenteric plexus lying between the longitudinal and circular muscle layers and the submucosal plexus.[27] In contrast, the striated muscle of both the external anal sphincter and the levator ani (including the puborectalis muscle) is generally under the control of the somatic nervous system.

Somatic efferent and afferent innervation to the pelvis is generally understood to involve the sacral nerve roots (S2-S4) and their ramifications. Somatic efferents arise within Onuf's nucleus situated in the ventral horn of the S2-S4 spinal cord, and afferents reach the dorsal horn with their cell bodies in dorsal root ganglia of these segments.[32] Central projections of somatic afferents overlap with pelvic nerve afferents within the spinal cord, which theoretically allows coordination of somatic and visceral motor activity.[29]

The sacral nerve roots emerge from the spinal cord, forming the sacral plexus,[36] from which the pudendal nerve diverges (S2-S3) along with the sciatic nerve, between an initial division of sacral nerves that branch to the levator muscle and a subsequent division of fibers that intermingle with autonomic pelvic nerves coursing to the inferior hypogastric plexus.[37-39] The pudendal nerve also receives postganglionic axons from the caudal sympathetic chain ganglia.[18] In general, the pudendal nerve runs medial to the internal pudendal vessels along the lateral wall of the ischiorectal fossa, dorsal to the sacrospinous ligament. An initial branch then splits off destined to innervate the clitoris, and the remaining pudendal nerve fibers distribute branches in various directions, which include medial branches to the anal canal (external anal sphincter and puborectalis muscle), dorsal branches to the urethral sphincter, and dorsolateral branches primarily to anterior perineal musculature (including bulbospongiosus and ischiocavernosus muscles). Nerves originating predominantly from sacral level S4 supply the posterior perineal musculature, and branches of S4-S5 nerve roots forming the coccygeal plexus distribute to perineal, perianal, and labial skin.[39]

Nociception and pain arising from within the pelvis and pelvic floor involve diverse neuronal mechanisms. In general, sensations from the pelvic viscera are conveyed within the sacral afferent parasympathetic system, with a far lesser afferent supply from thoracolumbar sympathetic origins.[33] Functionally, this dual innervation contributes to differential processing of visceral stimuli by different regions of the neuraxis. For example, in a model of colonic pain it was demonstrated that the pelvic nerve and lumbosacral spinal cord process acute or transient colorectal pain with recruitment of the splanchnic innervation during inflammation of the colon.[40,41] Pelvic nerve afferents innervate the deeper layers of hollow organs, including mucosa and submucosa as well as the muscle and serosa.[42] Receptive fields in the perineum are understood to be carried out primarily by sensory-motor discharges associated with pudendal nerve afferents.[17,33] While the interactions of sensory afferents are quite complex, likely possibilities by which these pathways exert effects on autonomic efferent function include mediatory effects on spinal cord reflexes and modulatory effects on efferent release in peripheral autonomic ganglia and in peripheral organs. These neural structures in the periphery comprise the first of numerous relays of sensory neurons that transmit painful sensations from the abdominal/pelvic cavity to the brain.

Traditionally, it was thought that ascending pathways for visceral and other types of pain were mainly the spinothalamic and spinoreticular tracts. Recently, three previously undescribed pathways that carry visceral nociceptive information have been discovered: the dorsal column pathway, the spino(trigemino)-parabrachio-amygdaloid pathway, and the spinohypothalamic pathway (see review in Cervero and Laird[43]). The dorsal column pathway plays a key role in the processing of pelvic pain, and neurosurgeons have successfully used punctate midline myelotomy to relieve pelvic pain due to cancer (see review in Willis and Westlund[44]). In addition, descending facilitatory influences may contribute to the development of maintenance of hyperalgesia, thus contributing to the development of chronic pelvic pain.[45]

VISCERAL NOCICEPTION: VISCERAL NOCICEPTORS, VISCERAL SENSITIZATION, AND REFERRED PAIN MECHANISMS

Chronic visceral pain is a much greater clinical problem than that from skin, however, until relatively recently, the focus of experimental work on pain mechanisms mainly related to cutaneous sensation. Although it was often assumed that concepts derived from cutaneous studies could be transferred to the visceral domain, there are emerging experimental data indicating that the neural mechanisms involved in pain and hyperalgesia of the skin are different from the mechanisms involved in painful sensations from the viscera.[46,47] This is supported by differences between somatic and visceral pain based on clinical observation. In contrast to somatic pain, visceral pain cannot be evoked from all viscera and is not necessarily linked to visceral tissue injury. Further, visceral pain tends to be a diffuse and poorly localized sensation, whereas somatic pain can be localized exactly. Different from somatic pain, visceral pain can be referred to other visceral structures and somatic structures of the same segmental level. For example, patients with chronic pelvic pain typically report multiple pelvic pain problems, and they present with pain radiating to the lower back and legs.[7,8]

The visceral innervation is not as dense as the somatic innervation. It is assumed that at most 5% to 8% of the total afferent input to the spinal cord is contributed by spinal visceral nerves.[48] This rather sparse afferent input to the spinal cord from the viscera is compensated for by an extensive divergence in the central nervous system. In addition, recent studies have suggested that some visceral afferents innervate more than one organ. About 20% of dorsal root ganglion cells retrogradely labeled from the colon were double-labeled from the bladder.[49] The physiologic role of the bifurcating afferents is not clear, because recordings from colon or bladder afferents failed to provide evidence of excitation of the other organ.[50,51] It is possible that these bifurcating afferents become active after inflammation. This hypothesis is supported by the observation that colonic inflammation in a rat model results in plasma extravasation in an otherwise normal bladder.[52] These neuroanatomic and neurophysiologic observations might explain why visceral pain tends to be diffuse and poorly localized, providing a diagnostic challenge to the health care provider who is trying to ascertain the origin of the pain.

There are two components of visceral pain, which were already described more than 100 years ago[53]: "true visceral pain," which is deep visceral pain arising from inside the body, and "referred visceral pain," which is pain that is referred to segmentally related somatic and also other visceral structures. Secondary hyperalgesia usually develops at the referred site.[4] Although several mechanisms have been entertained to explain the referred pain phenomenon over the last 70 years, the most convincing experimental evidence is provided by the observation of convergence. Convergence of afferent input is a typical characteristic of second-order neurons in the spinal cord that receive visceral input. These visceroceptive spinal neurons receive convergent somatic input from skin and musculature.[54] In addition, viscerovisceral convergence of input onto second-order spinal neurons is common (e.g., colon and bladder). This mechanism offers a ready explanation for the segmental nature of referred pain, but it does not address explicitly the issue of hyperalgesia in the referred zone. To interpret "referred pain with hyperalgesia," two main theories have been proposed, which are not mutually exclusive. The first is known as convergence-facilitation theory. It proposes that the abnormal visceral input produces an irritable focus in the relative spinal cord segment, thus facilitating messages from somatic structure. The second theory postulates that the visceral afferent barrage induces the activation of a reflex arc whose afferent branch is presented by visceral afferent fibers and efferent branch by somatic efferents and sympathetic efferents toward the somatic structures (muscle, subcutis, and skin). The efferent impulses toward the periphery sensitize nociceptors in the parietal tissues of the referred area, thus resulting in the phenomenon of hyperalgesia.

When examining and treating a woman with chronic pelvic pain, it is important to consider the true and referred aspects of the visceral pain syndrome, including the pain deep in the pelvic cavity and pain referred to somatic structures (lower back and legs) and other visceral organs. The mechanisms of referred viscerovisceral pain might explain the substantial overlap observed in epidemiologic studies between chronic pelvic pain and other abdominal symptoms.[12,55] Considering the concept of referred visceral pain and realizing that the visceral innervation is sparse, but compensated for by extensive divergence in the central nervous system, will allow the health care provider to look at the global picture of visceral dysfunction, rather than "chasing" one aspect of the visceral pain syndrome out of context.

The existence of visceral nociceptors has been debated for a long time, in part because of the difficulty of defining and applying physiologically relevant noxious stimuli to the viscera (for review, see Bielefeldt and Gebhart[54]). The functional properties of visceral afferent neurons have been studied by recording afferent fiber activity and responses to controlled visceral stimuli in teased fiber preparations in which one or a few axons are recorded. These experiments have shown that several kinds of sensory receptors exist in most internal organs and that different pain states are mediated by different neurophysiologic mechanisms.[56] Acute, brief visceral pain seems to be triggered initially by the activation of high-threshold visceral afferents and by the high-frequency bursts that these stimuli evoke in intensity-coding afferent fibers, which are afferents with a range of responsiveness in the innocuous and noxious ranges. However, more prolonged forms of visceral stimulation, including those leading to hypoxia and inflammation of the tissue, result in sensitization of high-threshold receptors and the bringing into play of previously unresponsive afferent fibers, termed "silent nociceptors." This is a special class of mechano-insensitive C-fiber nociceptors that has been found in almost all tissues, including in animal models of visceral pain.[57] Silent afferents are activated only in the presence of tissue damage or inflammation, which might explain why visceral pain cannot be evoked from all viscera and is not necessarily linked to every type of visceral tissue injury.

There are several potential molecular substrates that may play key roles in the peripheral sensitization of nociceptor terminals in viscera. Messengers for tetrodotoxin (TTX)-resistant sodium channels, specifically Na 1.8, are primarily found in small-diameter neurons with unmyelinated axons, which typically play an important role in nociception. Essentially all visceral sensory neurons have unmyelinated or thinly myelinated axons. Capsaicin and protons bind the vanilloid TRPV1 receptor. TRPV1 is coexpressed with calcitonin gene-related peptide (CGRP) and substance P in 60% to 80% of visceral afferents.[58] TRPV1 expression in sensory fibers was correlated positively with the degree of hypersensitivity in patients with rectal hypersensitivity.[59] In addition, urothelial cells (non-neuronal tissue) have been shown to express TRPV1 receptors as well, and these can be activated by vanilloids to produce the release of adenosine triphosphate (ATP), which then can activate P2X3 receptors in sensory afferent fibers.[60] (Birder et al. 2001). This mechanism might account for the enhanced bladder sensitivity observed in patients with interstitial cystitis. Prostaglandins are synthesized in response to tissue injury by cyclooxygenase. They sensitize sensory fibers to mechanical and thermal stimuli and contribute to spinal processing of visceral pain.[61] In studies of central contributions to visceral sensitization, the main focus has been the spinal cord. Intrathecal application of *N*-methyl-D-aspartate (NMDA) and non-NMDA receptor antagonists significantly attenuates visceral hypersensitivity in behavioral models, and spinal application of NMDA agonists increases the magnitude and duration of visceral pain responses.[62,63] NMDA receptors are expressed in primary afferents and in dorsal horn neurons.

SEX, GENDER, AND GONADAL HORMONAL STATUS

A distinguishing feature of many of the pelvic pain syndromes is the overwhelming burden reported by women in their reproductive years. For example, population prevalence estimates in patients with interstitial cystitis indicate a female-to-male ratio of 9:1.[64] Interestingly, and in support of the hypothesis that the gonadal hormonal milieu influences pain perception, several pain syndromes are more common in women than in men.[65,66] There is growing evidence from studies in animals and humans that the response to noxious stimuli may be influenced by the gonadal hormonal milieu and varies across different phases of the estrous (rodents) or menstrual (humans) cycle.[65,67-69] However, the variations observed in different studies are inconsistent[70] and cannot be linked to only one phase of the cycle.

CLINICAL IMPLICATIONS

Because epidemiologic data have confirmed the widespread existence of chronic pelvic pain in the female population in last 10 years, there is growing interest in the pharmaceutical industry to expand basic science and clinical research efforts for this underserved patient population. Controlled clinical trials are desperately needed to design improved pharmacologic treatment strategies. To date, most reports on the pharmacologic treatment of chronic pelvic pain are anecdotal. Currently used pharmacologic treatment approaches have mainly been evaluated for other chronic pain syndromes, and not specifically for chronic pelvic pain. Several different pharmacologic classes of medications have been demonstrated to be effective in alleviating pain in patients with chronic pain syndromes: nonsteroidal anti-inflammatory drugs (NSAIDs), antidepressants, anticonvulsants, local anesthetic antiarrhythmics, and opioids (for review, see Wesselmann[71]). Although clinical trials and case reports on the pharmacologic management of chronic pain syndromes provide general guidelines as to which drug to choose, currently we have no method to predict which drug is most likely to alleviate pain in a given patient. Therefore, it is a "trial and error" method of prescribing drugs.

As the pathophysiologic mechanisms of visceral pain explored in basic science research have provided explanations for some of the clinical phenomena observed in patients, additional, revived and new concepts of chronic pelvic pain have emerged. First, a spectrum of different insults might lead to chronic pelvic pain. Second, different underlying pathogenic pain mechanisms may require different pain treatment strategies for patients presenting with pelvic pain. And third, multiple different pathogenic pain mechanisms may coexist in the same patient presenting with chronic pelvic pain, requiring several different pain treatment strategies (perhaps concomitantly) to successfully treat visceral pain.[3]

Acknowledgment

Ursula Wesselmann is supported by NIH grants DK066641 (NIDDK), HD39699 (NICHD, Office of Research for Women's Health) and the National Vulvodynia Association.

References

1. American College of Obstetricians and Gynecologists: ACOG Practice Bulletin No. 51: Chronic pelvic pain. Obstet Gynecol 103:589-605, 2004.
2. Wesselmann U: A call for recognizing, legitimizing and treating chronic visceral pain syndromes. Pain Forum 8:146-150, 1999.
3. Wesselmann U: Guest Editorial: Pain—The neglected aspect of visceral pain. Eur J Pain 3:189-191, 1999.
4. Giamberardino MA, Vecchiet L: Experimental studies on pelvic pain. Pain Rev 1:102-115, 1994.
5. Wesselmann U: Obstetric and gynaecological pain. In Schmidt RF, Willis WD: Encyclopedic Reference of Pain, 1st ed. Heidelberg, Springer-Verlag, 2006.
6. Merskey H, Bogduk N: Classification of Chronic Pain. Seattle, IASP Press, 1994.
7. Zondervan KT, Yudkin PL, Vessey MP, et al: Prevalence and incidence of chronic pelvic pain in primary care: Evidence from a national general practice database. Br J Obstet Gynaecol 106:1149-1155, 1999.
8. Zondervan KT, Yudkin PL, Vessey MP, et al: Patterns of diagnosis and referral in women consulting for chronic pelvic pain in UK primary care. Br J Obstet Gynaecol 106:1156-1161, 1999.
9. Abrams P, Cardozo L, Fall M, et al: The standardization of terminology of lower urinary tract function: Report from the Standardization Sub-committee of the International Continence Society. Neurourol Urodyn 21:167-178, 2002.
10. Fall M, Baranowski AP, Fowler CJ, et al: EAU guidelines on chronic pelvic pain. Eur Urol 46:681-689, 2004.
11. Mathias SD, Kuppermann M, Liberman RF, et al: Chronic pelvic pain: Prevalence, health-related quality of life, and economic correlates. Obstet Gynecol 87:321-327, 1996.
12. Zondervan KT, Yudkin PL, Vessey MP, et al: Chronic pelvic pain in the community: Symptoms, investigations, and diagnoses. Am J Obstet Gynecol 184:1149-1155, 2001.
13. Burnett AL, Wesselmann U: History of the neurobiology of the pelvis. Urology 53:1082-1089, 1999.
14. Burnett AL, Wesselmann U: Neurobiology of the pelvis and perineum: Principles for a practical approach. J Pelvic Surg 5:224-232, 1999.
15. Bors E, Comarr AE: Neuro-anatomy and neuro-physiology. In Bors E, Comarr AE (eds): Neurological Urology. New York, Karger, 1971, pp 61-128.
16. Morrison JFB: Role of higher levels of the central nervous system. In Torrens M, Morrison JFB (ed): The Physiology of the Lower Urinary Tract. London, Springer-Verlag, 1987, pp 237-274.
17. de Groat WC, Booth AM, Yoshimura N: Neurophysiology of micturition and its modification in animal models of human disease. In Maggi CA (ed): Nervous Control of the Urogenital System. Chur, Switzerland, Harwood Academic Publishers, 1993, pp 227-290.
18. de Groat WC: Neurophysiology of the pelvic organs. In Rushton DN (ed): Handbook of Neuro-Urology. New York, Marcel Dekker, 1994, pp 55-93.
19. Berkley KJ, Hubscher CH: Visceral and somatic sensory tracks through the neuraxis and their relation to pain: Lessons from the rat female reproductive system. In Gebhart GF (ed): Visceral Pain. Vol. 5: Progress in Pain Research and Management. Seattle, WA, IASP Press, 1994, pp 195-216.
20. Dail WG: Autonomic innervation of male reproductive genitalia. In Maggi CA (ed): Nervous Control of the Urogenital System. Chur, Switzerland, Harwood Academic Publishers, 1993, pp 69-101.
21. Nomina Anatomica, 4th ed. Amsterdam, Excerpra Medica, 1977.
22. Baljet B, Drukker J: The extrinsic innervation of the pelvic organs in the female rat. Acta Anat (Basel) 107:241-267, 1980.
23. Walsh PC, Donker PJ: Impotence following radical prostatectomy: Insight into etiology and prevention. J Urol 167:1005-1010, 2002.
24. Lue TF, Zeineh SJ, Schmidt RA, et al: Neuroanatomy of penile erection: Its relevance to iatrogenic impotence. J Urol 131:273-280, 1984.
25. Lepor H, Gregerman M, Crosby R, et al: Precise localization of the autonomic nerves from the pelvic plexus to the corpora cavernosa: A detailed anatomical study of the adult male pelvis. J Urol 133:207-212, 1985.
26. Zorn BH, Watson LR, Steers WD: Nerves from pelvic plexus contribute to chronic orchidalgia. Lancet 343:1161, 1994.
27. Burnstock G: Innervation of bladder and bowel. In Bock G, Whelan J (eds): Neurobiology of Incontinence, Ciba Foundation Symposium. Chichester, UK, Wiley, 1990, pp 2-26.
28. Jänig W, McLachlan EM: Organization of lumbar spinal outflow to distal colon and pelvic organs. Physiol Rev 67:1332-1404, 1987.
29. McKenna KE, Nadelhaft I: The organization of the pudendal nerve in the male and female rat. J Comp Neurol 248:532-549, 1986.
30. Hancock MB, Peveto CA: Preganglionic neurons in the sacral spinal cord of the rat: An HRP study. Neurosci Lett 11:1-5, 1979.
31. Nadelhaft I, Booth AM: The location and morphology of preganglionic neurons and the distribution of visceral afferents from the rat pelvic nerve: A horseradish peroxidase study. J Comp Neurol 226:238-245, 1984.
32. Lincoln J, Burnstock G: Autonomic innervation of the urinary bladder and urethra. In Maggi CA (ed): Nervous Control of the Urogenital System. Chur, Switzerland, Harwood Academic Publishers, 1993, pp 33-68.
33. Jänig W, Koltzenburg M: Pain arising from the urogenital tract. In Maggi CA (ed): Nervous Control of the Urogenital System. Chur, Switzerland, Harwood Academic Publishers, 1993, pp 525-578.
34. Hilliges M, Falconer C, Ekman-Ordeberg G, et al: Innervation of the human vaginal mucosa as revealed by PGP 9.5 immunohistochemistry. Acta Anat (Basel) 153:119-126, 1995.
35. Ger R: Surgical anatomy of the pelvis. Surg Clin North Am 68:1201-1216, 1988.
36. Elbadawi A: Neuromorphologic basis of vesicourethral function: I. Histochemistry, ultrastructure and function of intrinsic nerves of the bladder and urethra. Neurourol Urodyn 1:3-50, 1982.
37. Dietemann JL, Sick H, Wolfram-Gabel R, et al: Anatomy and computed tomography of the normal lumbosacral plexus. Neuroradiology 29:58-68, 1987.
38. Juenemann KP, Lue TF, Schmidt RA, et al: Clinical significance of sacral and pudendal nerve anatomy. J Urol 139:74-80, 1988.
39. Matzel KE, Schmidt RA, Tanagho EA: Neuroanatomy of the striated muscular anal continence mechanism: Implications for the use of neurostimulation. Dis Colon Rectum 33:666-673, 1990.
40. Traub RJ: Evidence for thoracolumbar spinal cord processing of inflammatory, but not acute colonic pain. Neuroreport 11:2113-2116, 2000.
41. Traub RJ, Murphy A: Colonic inflammation induces fos expression in the thoracolumbar spinal cord increasing activity in the spinoparabrachial pathway. Pain 95:93-102, 2002.
42. Brierley SM, Jones RC 3rd, Gebhart GF, et al: Splanchnic and pelvic mechanosensory afferents signal different qualities of colonic stimuli in mice. Gastroenterology 127:166-178, 2004.
43. Cervero F, Laird JM: Visceral pain. Lancet 353:2145-2148, 1999.
44. Willis WD Jr, Westlund KN: The role of the dorsal column pathway in visceral nociception. Curr Pain Headache Rep 5:20-26, 2001.
45. Gebhart GF: Descending modulation of pain. Neurosci Biobehav Rev 27:729-737, 2004.
46. Gebhart GF: Visceral nociception: Consequences, modulation and the future. Eur J Anaesthesiol Suppl 10:24-27, 1995.
47. McMahon SB, Dmitrieva N, Koltzenburg M: Visceral pain. Br J Anaesth 75:132-144, 1995.
48. Cervero F: Sensory innervation of the viscera: Peripheral basis of visceral pain. Physiol Rev 74:95-138, 1994.

49. Bielefeldt K, Christianson JA, Davis BM: Basic and clinical aspects of visceral sensation: Transmission in the CNS. Neurogastroenterol Motil 17:488-499, 2005.
50. Sengupta JN, Gebhart GF: Characterization of mechanosensitive pelvic nerve afferent fibers innervating the colon of the rat. J Neurophysiol 71:2046-2060, 1994.
51. Sengupta JN, Gebhart GF: Mechanosensitive properties of pelvic nerve afferent fibers innervating the urinary bladder of the rat. J Neurophysiol 72:2420-2430, 1994.
52. Winnard KP, Dmitrieva N, Berkley KJ: Estrous influences about how acute inflammation of the uterus and colon affects vascular permeability of the bladder via the hypogastric nerve. Society for Neuroscience Abstract Viewer, 52.5, 2005.
53. Head H: On the disturbances of sensation with especial reference to the pain of visceral disease. Brain 16:1-133, 1893.
54. Bielefeldt K, Gebhart GF: Visceral pain: Basic mechanisms. In McMahon SB, Koltzenburg M (eds): Textbook of Pain, 5th ed. New York, Churchill Livingstone, 2006, pp 721-736.
55. Alagiri M, Chottiner S, Ratner V, et al: Interstitial cystitis: Unexplained associations with other chronic disease and pain syndromes. Urology 49:52-57, 1997.
56. Cervero F, Janig W: Visceral nociceptors: A new world order? Trends Neurosci 15:374-378, 1992.
57. Habler HJ, Janig W, Koltzenburg M: A novel type of unmyelinated chemosensitive nociceptor in the acutely inflamed urinary bladder. Agents Actions 25:219-221, 1988.
58. Hwang SJ, Oh JM, Valtschanoff JG: Expression of the vanilloid receptor TRPV1 in rat dorsal root ganglion neurons supports different roles of the receptor in visceral and cutaneous afferents. Brain Res 1047:261-266, 2005.
59. Chan CL, Facer P, Davis JB, et al: Sensory fibres expressing capsaicin receptor TRPV1 in patients with rectal hypersensitivity and faecal urgency. Lancet 361:385-391, 2003.
60. Birder LA, Kanai AJ, de Groat WC, et al: Vanilloid receptor expression suggests a sensory role for urinary bladder epithelial cells. Proc Natl Acad Sci U S A 98:13396-13401, 2001.
61. Svensson CI, Yaksh TL: The spinal phospholipase-cyclooxygenase-prostanoid cascade in nociceptive processing. Annu Rev Pharmacol Toxicol 42:553-583, 2002.
62. Rice AS, McMahon SB: Pre-emptive intrathecal administration of an NMDA receptor antagonist (AP-5) prevents hyper-reflexia in a model of persistent visceral pain. Pain 57:335-340, 1994.
63. McRoberts JA, Coutinho SV, Marvizon JC, et al: Role of peripheral N-methyl-D-aspartate (NMDA) receptors in visceral nociception in rats. Gastroenterology 120:1737-1748, 2001.
64. Jones CA, Nyberg LM: Epidemiology of interstitial cystitis. Urology 49 (Suppl 5A):2-9, 1997.
65. Berkley KJ: Sex differences in pain. Behav Brain Sci 20:371-380; discussion 435-513, 1997.
66. Unruh AM: Gender variations in clinical pain experience. Pain 65:123-167, 1996.
67. Fillingim RB, Ness TJ: Sex-related hormonal influences on pain and analgesic responses. Neurosci Biobehav Rev 24:485-501, 2000.
68. Riley JL 3rd, Robinson ME, Wise EA, et al: A meta-analytic review of pain perception across the menstrual cycle. Pain 81:225-235, 1999.
69. Wesselmann U, Garrett-Mayer E, Kaplan Gilpin AM, et al: Vulvodynia: Changes in vaginal pain perception across the menstrual cycle. Society for Neuroscience Abstract Viewer, 52.1, 2005.
70. Bradshaw HB, Temple JL, Wood E, et al: Estrous variations in behavioral responses to vaginal and uterine distention in the rat. Pain 82:187-197, 1999.
71. Wesselmann U: Chronic pelvic pain. In Turk DC, Melzack R (ed): Handbook of Pain Assessment, 2nd ed. New York, Guilford Press, 2001, pp 567-578.

Chapter 90

NEUROENDOCRINE ROLE IN INTERSTITIAL CYSTITIS AND CHRONIC PELVIC PAIN IN WOMEN

C. A. Tony Buffington

The International Association for the Study of Pain defines pain as "an unpleasant sensory and emotional experience associated with actual or potential tissue damage, or described in terms of such damage." The awareness of acute pain motivates those experiencing it toward withdrawal and guarding to permit avoidance of further injury and activation of repair processes. In some cases of chronic pain, however, the situation may be somewhat different, in that the severity of signs loses its usual tight correlation with symptoms. In chronic visceral pain states such as interstitial cystitis (IC) and chronic pelvic pain (CPP), the endocrine system also may be involved in maintaining the sensation of pain (Fig. 90-1),[1,2] although the extent to which (or in which patients) this results from an underlying genetic or developmental predisposition and to what extent it results from the etiology of the disease process cannot yet be determined.

The aims of this chapter are to describe some of the neuroendocrine abnormalities that occur in women with IC and CPP and to suggest the possibility of underlying neuroendocrine abnormalities in some of these patients.

IC is a lower urinary tract syndrome of unknown cause and no generally accepted treatment.[3] The symptoms of IC include variable combinations of pain referable to the urinary bladder, as well as increased frequency and urgency of urination. IC may affect more than 700,000 American women,[4] and a significant (potentially comparable) number of men diagnosed with sterile prostatitis or prostatodynia.[5] The quality of life of IC patients is significantly degraded; in one study, these patients scored much lower ($P < .001$) than healthy control subjects did in all eight domains of health assessed by the Medical Outcomes Study Short Form-36 Health Survey.[3]

Since 1993, my laboratory has investigated a common lower urinary tract disorder of domestic cats, feline interstitial cystitis (FIC), that represents a naturally occurring model of IC. We have found that cats with FIC meet all the criteria promulgated by the National Institutes of Health for diagnosis of IC that can be applied to animals, and we have shown that cats with FIC and humans with IC have comparable bladder, sensory afferent, central, sympathetic, and endocrine abnormalities, to the extent they have been investigated. Recent findings in these cats[3,6] are consistent with and extend the neuroendocrine abnormalities identified in humans with IC.

The National Institutes of Health classifies IC as a CPP syndrome, which has been defined as nonmenstrual pain of at least 6 months' duration that is severe enough to cause functional disability or necessitate medical or surgical treatment.[7] As many as 39% of women of reproductive age seen by primary care physicians report the presence of CPP "always," "often," or "sometimes."[8] Women with CPP use more medications, have more nongynecologic operations, and are five times more likely to have a hysterectomy than are women without CPP. These patients also are more likely to have a history of abuse and to suffer from depression, impaired sexual functioning, and reduced overall quality of life.[9]

A recent comprehensive review[7] listed some 70 disorders (15 extrauterine and 8 uterine, 11 urologic, 8 gastrointestinal, 17 musculoskeletal, and 11 "other") that may be associated with CPP in women, including IC, irritable bowel syndrome, and fibromyalgia. The comorbidity of some of these diseases was suggested by the results of a recent mail questionnaire survey in England, which found that 24% of women aged 18 to 49 years reported CPP during the previous 3 months. Of these women, 52% had CPP only, 24% had CPP and irritable bowel syndrome, 9% had CPP and urinary frequency and urgency, and 15% had all three.[10] These results suggest that patients with CPP have variable combinations of organ involvement, raising the question of the extent to which a different etiology affects each organ individually, or whether some common underlying etiology affects a variety of organs, which then respond in their own characteristic ways.

Two subtypes of IC currently are recognized based on cystoscopic evaluation of the bladder. In most patients (90%), only submucosal petechial hemorrhages (glomerulations) are observed (type I), whereas mucosal ("Hunner's") ulcers, with or without glomerulations, are identified in a minority (type II). The two types also appear to differ in patient epidemiology, histologic findings, and response to treatment, further suggesting that they

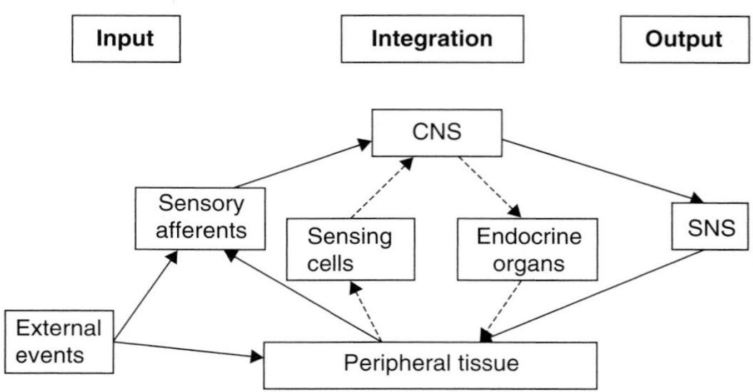

Figure 90-1 General plan of communication between the central nervous system and peripheral structures. CNS, central nervous system; SNS, sympathetic nervous system.

may be distinct entities.[11] One important difference between the two types is that many patients with type II IC report significant symptomatic relief after supratrigonal cystectomy and cystoplasty, whereas the pain in patients with type I IC is not usually diminished by this procedure.[12] This difference in patient response to removal of the bladder may provide an important clue to the underlying causes of pain associated with IC: the cause of the pain in patients with type II disease may be nociceptive, whereas the pain of patients with type I IC may be neuropathic.

Nociceptive pain results from persistent activity of sensory afferent fibers innervating the affected area and is relieved by removal of the stimulus. Examples of nociceptive pain include toothache, which is relieved by extraction, and osteoarthritis of the hip joint, which is relieved by hip replacement.[13] In contrast, neuropathic pain arises from some abnormality related to the nervous system; although generally attributed to a body structure, it can remain after desensitization of nociceptive afferents[14,15] or even removal of the structure.[16,17] Such results have been reported for endometriosis, where removal of identified abnormalities does not always lead to resolution of the CPP.[18]

THE STRESS RESPONSE SYSTEM

The presence of neuropathic pain may be related to abnormalities and imbalances of the neuroendocrine system, which is activated in response to threats to homeostasis. One commonality among some IC and CPP patients appears to be a relative predominance of activation of the sympathetic nervous system (SNS) limb of the stress response system (SRS), compared to the responses of the hypothalamic-pituitary-adrenal (HPA) and -gonadal (HPG) axes.[19] A schematic diagram of some of the features this complex system[20] is presented in Figure 90-2. Once the system is stimulated by central nervous system structures responding to sensory inputs (conscious or unconscious[21]) that are perceived as a threat to homeostasis, corticotropin-releasing factor (CRF) is released from the paraventricular nucleus of the hypothalamus. CRF acts as a neurotransmitter, to activate sympathetic premotor neurons in the pontine locus coeruleus and brainstem nuclei, and as a hormone, to stimulate the anterior pituitary. In some patients, the SNS arm of the response appears to be uncoupled from the HPA and HPG axes in that SNS outflow increases in the absence of activation of the HPA axis and in the presence of reduced HPG function.

Sympathoneural Output

Even though the neuroendocrine features of the stress response have not been thoroughly studied in humans with IC and CPP, the available data support the presence of a comparable abnormality in at least a subset of these patients. Although plasma catecholamine concentrations have yet to be reported patients with IC, the findings of abnormal vasomotor tone,[22] increased density of bladder neurons staining for tyrosine hydroxylase (the rate-limiting enzyme for catecholamine synthesis),[23,24] and increased urine norepinephrine excretion[25] that have been reported suggest increased SNS activity.

Recent studies have begun to map the pathways that transduce activation of the SRS into cellular dysfunction via the SNS. Events external to the central nervous system, from both within and without the body, are transmitted to the brain by the sensory

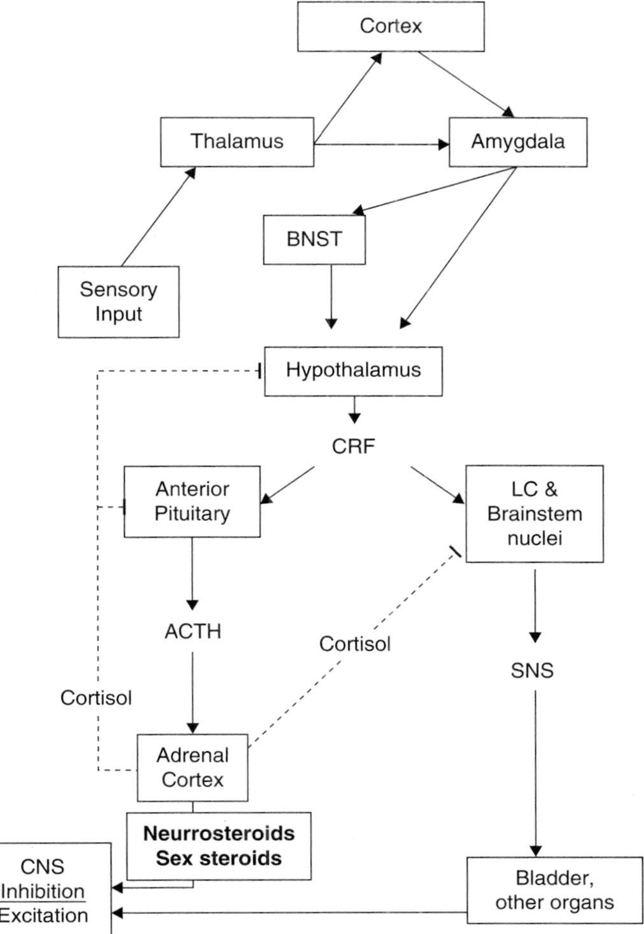

Figure 90-2 Afferent (sensory input), integrative (thalamus, cortex, amygdala, BNST, and motor (hypothalamus and beyond) components of the stress response system. ACTH, adrenocorticotropic hormone; BNST, bed nucleus of the stria terminalis; CRF, corticotropin-releasing factor; LC, locus coeruleus; SNS, sympathetic nervous system.

neurons. These signals are conveyed to the thalamus, where they are evaluated and usually forwarded to the cerebral cortex for further processing before activation of the appropriate motor program (see Fig. 90-2).[26] Potentially threatening events, however, can activate the SRS directly via the thalamic activation of the amygdala, bypassing cortical inhibitory control.[27]

Activation of the SNS results in sympathoneural release of norepinephrine. A 2003 study[28] traced this pathway from the external environment through to norepinephrine-mediated induction of the transcription factor nuclear factor kappa B (NF-κB), which is thought to play a role in mediating the urothelial inflammatory response of IC.[29] In vitro stimulation of human promonocytic (THP-1) cells with physiologic amounts of norepinephrine for 10 minutes resulted in a dose- and time-dependent induction of NF-κB and NF-κB-dependent gene expression; only norepinephrine induced this response, which was reduced by both α_1- and β-adrenergic receptor antagonists. The authors concluded that norepinephrine-mediated activation of NF-κB represented a downstream effector of the neuroendocrine response to stressful psychosocial events, linking changes in the environment to a bewildering array of cellular responses through activation of the SRS.[30]

Activation of the SRS also can increase epithelial permeability, permitting environmental agents greater access to sensory afferent neurons,[31] which could result in both increased sensory afferent firing and local inflammation. Sympathetic neural-epithelial interactions appear to play an important role in urothelial permeability. For example, Birder and colleagues showed that application of β-adrenergic receptor agonists to urinary bladder strips induced release of nitric oxide (NO) from urinary bladder epithelium, raising the possibility that norepinephrine from adrenergic nerves in the bladder (which may not be present in normal individuals)[23,24] or circulating catecholamines could influence bladder function by acting on β-adrenergic receptors in the urothelium to release NO and possibly other neurotransmitters, such as adenosine triphosphate (ATP).[32] Application of capsaicin, the pungent principle in hot peppers, also resulted in release of NO from epithelium as well as nervous tissue in the urinary bladder.[33] In light of reports that NO may increase urothelial permeability,[34,35] these results suggest that some of the sympathetically mediated alterations in permeability may be mediated by norepinephrine via this mechanism.

The increased permeability related to increased SNS activation does not require direct interaction with epithelial cells, nor is it restricted to the urinary bladder.[36] Moreover, neural release of norepinephrine[37] is but one of a variety of mechanisms whereby SRS-induced increases in efferent SNS output can activate local inflammatory cells such as mast cells, which can in turn also increase epithelial permeability.[36] Afferent sensory neurons, too, may increase epithelial permeability by releasing neurotransmitters at the peripheral process of the nerve via sympathetic-sensory coupling, dorsal root reflexes, and axon reflexes.[38] Recently, increased sensitivity to potassium chloride instillation, a test thought by some to indicate increased urothelial permeability, was reported in 244 female patients with CPP. Eighty-one percent of patients, with clinical diagnoses that included endometriosis, vulvodynia, and pelvic pain, showed a positive (painful) response to potassium instillation into the bladder.[39] However, patient's sensitivity to potassium instilled into other organs (vagina, uterus, colon, or peritoneum) was not assessed, so the specificity of the response cannot be evaluated. This may be an important control procedure, because a number of studies have reported that abnormalities in one visceral organ may affect responses in another, a process called viscerovisceral convergence.[40-42] In cats with FIC, we recently reported[43,44] sensitization and abnormal properties of dorsal root ganglion cells of axons that provide innervation not only to the bladder but throughout the lumbosacral (L4-S3) region, suggesting that generalized hypersensitivity may a mediating mechanism for viscerovisceral convergence in animals with naturally occurring as well as induced disease.

Moreover, one must recall that the presence of inflammation, or altered permeability, is not well correlated with pain, as anyone who has had a superficial bruise knows from personal experience. In the bladder, we have reported the presence of submucosal petechial hemorrhages in cats with no signs referable to the lower urinary tract,[45] and others have identified petechial hemorrhages in healthy women,[46] as well as urothelial disruption and increased presence of inducible nitric oxide synthase (iNOS), and presumably increased permeability, in elderly men with bladder outlet obstruction.[47]

Moreover, emotional and environmental factors such as stress or depression can modulate the experience of pain through descending pathways from the midbrain.[48] Therefore, even the recently reported increased firing rate of afferent nerves noted in cats with FIC[49] could result in differences in perceived sensations arising from the bladder, depending on the effects of the emotional state of the animal on descending inhibitory and facilitory balance.

Hypothalamic-Pituitary-Adrenal Axis

The HPA axis of the SRS acts at multiple levels to coordinate and modulate the body's response to perceived threats. Glucocorticoids tend to antagonize the effects of the SNS, both centrally and peripherally,[20] and they appear to play a complex role in epithelial permeability. Corticosterone has long been known to decrease capillary permeability to proteins in the brain,[50] skin,[51] and lung,[52] and cortisol has been shown to reduce in vitro permeability by enhancing tight junction integrity.[53] The effects of stress on glucocorticoid-mediated alterations in permeability are more complex and may be dose dependent. For example, stress created by a brief forced swim increased the permeability of the blood-brain barrier in adult FVB/N mice, whereas no evidence of a stress-potentiated effect was found when restraint, forced swim, or a combination of restraint and forced swim stressors were applied to Long-Evans or Wistar rats.[54] Moreover, stress-induced increases in intestinal epithelial permeability disappeared after adrenalectomy or pharmacologic blockade of glucocorticoid receptors, and dexamethasone treatment of control animals increased gastrointestinal permeability and mimicked the effects of stress.[55] Differences in tissues studied, rodent strain, type of stress, glucocorticoid studied, and the specifics of the experimental protocol all could influence interpretation of these discordant results.

The response to glucocorticoids also is likely to be hormetic (Fig. 90-3); that is, there is an inverse-U–shaped function wherein both deficiencies and excesses may produce abnormalities, which sometimes are relatively similar, further complicating interpretation of the results.[56] Glucocorticoids also tend to inhibit activation of NF-κB.[57,58] This and other adrenocortical steroid-related protective mechanisms, such as inhibition of the SRS and modulation of neuronal excitability,[59-61] may be less efficient in states of reduced function of cortisol and other steroids (see later discussion) such as IC and other stress-related bodily disorders.[62]

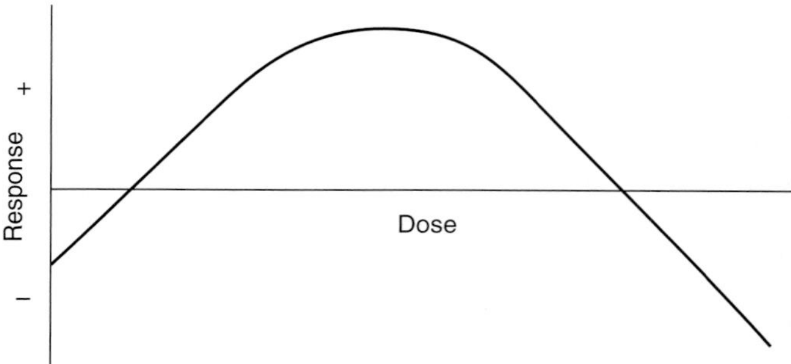

Figure 90-3 Hormetic responses are those that move from inadequate function with deficient doses of a substance, to satisfactory function at intermediate doses, to inadequate function again with excessive doses. This pattern is common to many nutrients and hormones.

In a 2002 study of IC patients and healthy controls, Lutgendorf and colleagues[63] reported that, although mean urinary or salivary cortisol did not differ between the groups, IC patients who had higher morning salivary cortisol concentrations had significantly reduced pain and urgency, and those with higher urinary free cortisol concentrations reported less overall symptomatology ($P < .05$). This relationship also was observed when comorbid conditions such as fibromyalgia, chronic fatigue syndrome (CFS), and rheumatoid arthritis were controlled for. Patients with morning salivary cortisol concentrations less than 12.5 nmol/L (0.45 μg/dL) were 12.8 times more likely to report high urinary urgency than those with values above this cutoff point. An increased ratio of adrenocorticotropic hormone (ACTH) to cortisol also was reported in women with IC by Lutgendorf and associates.[64]

Hypocortisolism has been reported in women with CPP, CFS and a variety of other disorders, often related to increased activity of the SRS.[62] The causes of the decrease in cortisol have yet to be identified in patients with IC but have been investigated in patients with CPP[62,65] and CFS.[66]

Although diagnostic laparoscopy may be normal in some patients with CPP, psychological studies have identified a high frequency of psychopathology and increased prevalence of chronic stress and traumatic life events, such as sexual and physical abuse, in women with CPP, suggesting a relationship between post-traumatic stress disorder (PTSD) and CPP. Heim and colleagues[65] explored stress history, psychopathology, and HPA axis alterations in 16 female patients with CPP and 14 pain-free, infertile controls. An increased prevalence of abuse experiences and PTSD was identified in women with CPP, as well as a higher total number of major life events, although symptoms of depression were within the normal range. Women with CPP also had normal to low diurnal salivary cortisol concentrations and normal plasma ACTH but reduced salivary cortisol response to a CRF stimulation test and enhanced suppression of salivary cortisol by dexamethasone. The authors concluded that a lack of protective properties of cortisol may be of relevance for the development of bodily disorders in chronically stressed or traumatized individuals, although other hormones were not measured. It is not necessary to show such extreme examples of abuse to find correlations between early adverse experience and disease, which also may result from environmental instability and parenting variables.[67,68]

In patients with CFS, Demitrack and associates[66] concluded, after comprehensive study of the HPA axis, that the data were most compatible with a mild central adrenal insufficiency secondary to either a deficiency of CRF (although this was not identified) or some other central stimulus to the pituitary-adrenal axis. Scott and coauthors later reported that the adrenal glands of patients with CFS were some 50% smaller than those of control subjects based on computed tomography.[69] Although they studied patients who had low cortisol responses to ACTH, these authors subsequently found comparable results in CFS patients with normal cortisol responses to ACTH.[70] A more recent study did not find any difference from normal in adrenal gland volume in another group of CFS patients,[71] leaving the question of the role of adrenal volume in the observed abnormalities still open. Additionally, Kizildere and associates[72] recently identified a β-adrenergic receptor–mediated inhibition of CRF-stimulated adrenal steroid secretion in healthy humans. They found that administration of 10 mg propranolol (a nonspecific β-adrenergic receptor antagonist) 2 hours before administration of 100 μg human CRF decreased heart rate and diastolic blood pressure by 20%. Propranolol treatment also reduced plasma ACTH concentrations by about 40% and increased serum cortisol by approximately 70%, which decreased the ACTH-to-cortisol ratio by twofold. These results suggest that increased sympathetic tone also may reduce adrenocortical responsiveness to ACTH. Moreover, ACTH release can be enhanced by α-adrenergic receptor activation, as well as by vasopressin, which also can modulate SRS activity.[73]

There is convincing evidence that the adrenal cortex is hypoactive in some circumstances in a variety of chronic disorders other than IC and CPP, including asthma, chronic fatigue syndrome, fibromyalgia, panic disorder, PTSD, and rheumatoid arthritis. Moreover, flares in disease activity in these disorders have been related to stress. Although hypocortisolism appears to be a frequent and widespread phenomenon, the nature of the underlying mechanisms and the homology of these mechanisms within and across clinical groups remain speculative. Potential mechanisms underlying the observed hypocortisolism include dysregulation of function at any level of the HPA axis, genetic vulnerability, previous stressful experiences, and individual coping and personality styles.[62]

In neuroendocrine investigations comparing healthy cats to cats with FIC in a basal state, we found higher plasma catecholamine concentrations in cats with FIC but could not identify a difference in response of ACTH and cortisol to CRF between affected and healthy cats.[74] Based on some anomalous responses to a naturalistic stressor obtained during experiments with a CRF receptor antagonist in cats with FIC,[75] we began to look more closely at adrenal function during activation of the SRS and found increased concentrations of CRF[76,77] and ACTH[75] in the absence of a comparable increase in plasma cortisol concentrations, suggesting the presence of mild primary adrenal insufficiency or decreased adrenocortical reserve. We also found that adrenal gland size was significantly smaller in cats with FIC than in healthy cats.[78] Microscopic examination of the glands did not reveal any obvious hemorrhage, inflammation, infection, fibrosis, or necrosis as causes of the reduced size. The primary abnormality identified was a reduced size of the fasciculata and reticularis zones of the adrenal cortex. These results suggest that any adrenocortical abnormality might be unmasked more readily in response to a moderate, salient stressor and may not be identifiable in patients studied under basal circumstances, a conclusion about these systems that has also been drawn by others studying human patients.[79,80]

The simplest explanation for the combination of increased CRF, ACTH, and SNS activity in the presence of reduced adrenocortical response and small adrenal fasciculata and reticularis zones without other apparent abnormalities seems to be the presence of an underlying genetic disorder or developmental anomaly (or some combination of the two). These relationships are depicted in Figure 90-4. When a woman is exposed to a sufficiently harsh stressor during pregnancy, the hormonal products of the ensuing stress response may cross the placenta and affect the course of fetal development. Prenatal and postnatal stressors can result in persistently increased central CRF activity in animals.[81] For example, in both continuous and last-trimester paradigms, prenatal dexamethasone (0.1 mg/kg) treatment increased CRF messenger RNA levels specifically in both the hypothalamus and central nucleus of the amygdala, key loci for the effects of the neuropeptide on the expression of fear and anxiety.[82]

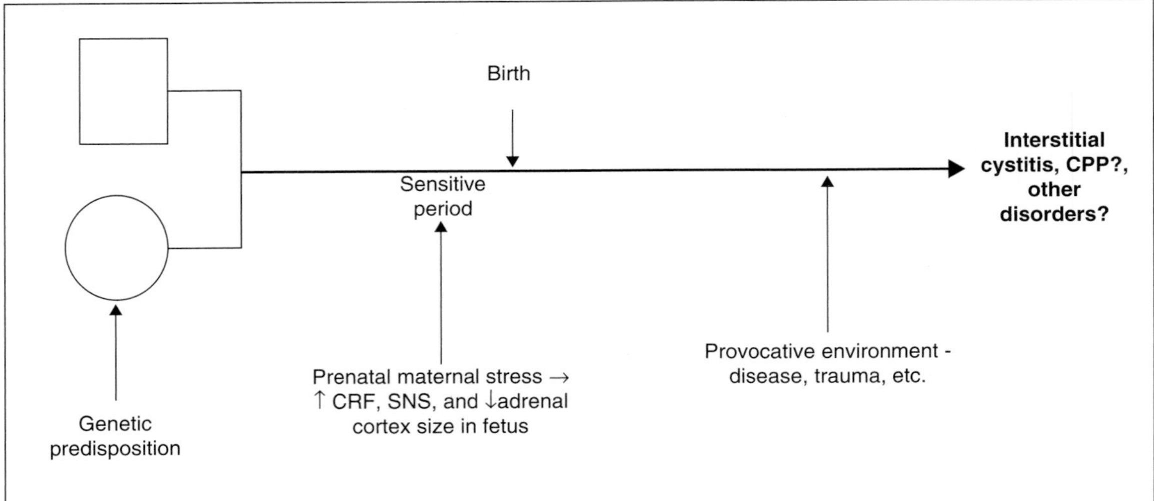

Figure 90-4 Potential trajectories to some cases of interstitial cystitis and chronic pelvic pain (CPP). Variable combinations of these factors could result in differences in disease severity among patients. CRF, corticotropin-releasing factor; SNS, sympathetic nervous system. (Adapted from Compagnone NA, Mellon SH: Neurosteroids: Biosynthesis and function of these novel neuromodulators. Front Neuroendocrinol 21:1, 2000.)

Matthews recently suggested that the biological "purpose" of transmitting this response to the fetus is to program the development of the fetal SRS and associated behaviors toward enhanced vigilance to increase the probability of survival.[83] The effects of stressors on the fetal HPA axis seem to depend on the timing and magnitude of exposure to products of the maternal stress response in relation to the developmental "programs" that determine the maturation of the various body systems during gestation and early postnatal development. If the fetus is exposed before initiation of a developmental program, there may be no effect. With exposure during the critical period while the adrenocortical maturation program is running, however, adrenal size in the developing fetus may be reduced, as shown by studies in Long-Evans rats,[84] guinea pigs,[85] blue fox,[86] rhesus monkeys,[87] and baboons.[88] If a sufficiently severe stress response occurs after the critical period of adrenocortical development, including during postnatal development, subsequent adrenocortical responses to stress and adrenal size may be increased.[83]

In either case, however, the biologic outcome might be similar. Raison and Miller[56] recently concluded from a review of the pertinent literature that inadequate biologic activity of glucocorticoids can occur either as a result of decreased hormone bioavailability or from reduced hormone sensitivity due to agonist-mediated receptor desensitization. Regardless of the cause, decreased biologic activity of adrenocortical steroids may have a variety of adverse effects on bodily function, possibly related to their role in restraining activation of the immune system and other components of the stress response, including the SNS and CRF.

The lack of long-term benefit of glucocorticoid therapy in most patients with IC[89] (but see Hosseini and colleagues[90] for results of a small, uncontrolled study of patients with type II IC given 5 mg/day oral prednisolone) suggests that the most appropriate dose has not yet been identified, that inadequate production of other steroids also might play a role in the pathophysiology of IC, and/or that SNS output needs to be attenuated. Most doses of glucocorticoid, although possibly appropriate for acute phases of the disease,[91] may be excessive for chronic therapy. As shown in Table 90-1, the daily production of cortisol in humans is in the range of 8 to 25 mg, much lower than doses of glucocorticoid sometimes suggested. In a recent open trial, 10 mg/day hydrocortisone was administered orally for 1 month to three patients with PTSD in a double-blind, placebo-controlled, crossover design. A significant treatment effect was observed in all patients, with cortisol-related reductions of at least 38% in one of the daily rated symptoms of traumatic memories, as assessed by self-administered rating scales. Although very preliminary, these results suggest that physiologic glucocorticoid replacement may have a role in some patients with CPP, if only in those with concurrent PTSD.[92]

Available evidence also suggests that part of the stress response may include maintaining production of cortisol (Δ4 pathway) at the expense of the 17,20-lyase (Δ5 pathway) products of the 17-α hydroxylase enzyme (Fig. 90-5) such as dehydroepiandrosterone sulfate (DHEAS, the longer-lived metabolite of DHEA)[72] if the stressor is severe or adrenocortical reserve is inadequate.[93,94]

DHEAS also is a neurosteroid, a term used to describe steroids that are synthesized in the central and peripheral neurons and in glial cells. The concept of neurosteroids was introduced by Baulieu in 1981[95] to describe a steroid hormone (DHEAS) he found at high levels in the brain long after gonadectomy and adrenalectomy. Androstenedione, pregnenolone, and a variety of other steroids were later also identified as neurosteroids.[96] These compounds can act as allosteric modulators of ion-gated neurotransmitter receptors, such as γ-aminobutyric acid (GABA)-A and *N*-methyl-D-aspartate (NMDA) receptors, which are the primary inhibitory and excitatory receptors, respectively, in the nervous system. Neurosteroid concentrations vary according to environmental and behavioral circumstances, such as stress, sex recognition, and aggressiveness. In the peripheral nervous system, neurosteroids also may play a role in neuronal repair after injury. Abnormal neurosteroid function may underlie some functional disturbances of the nervous system.[96-98]

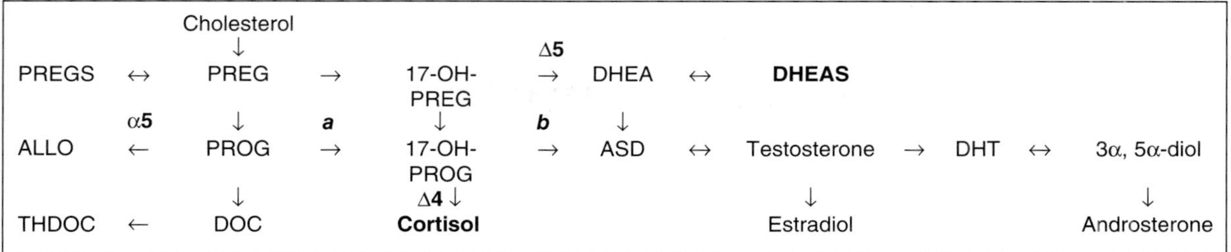

Figure 90-5 The output of the adrenal cortex includes variable combinations of glucocorticoids, sex steroids, and neurosteroids. Other sources of sex steroids and neurosteroids include the gonads and neural tissue. Some examples in women are presented in Table 90-1. The cytochrome P450 c17 enzyme (***a***) performs the 17α-hydroxylase reaction equally well using PREG or PROG as substrate, but the 17,20-lyase reaction (***b***) occurs 50 to 100 times more efficiently using 17-OH-PREG as substrate, rather than 17-OH-PROG. Therefore, conversion of 17-OH-PROG to ASD is minimal, and DHEA is the principal precursor of sex steroid synthesis. 3α,5α-diol, 3α-androstanediol; ALLO, 3α,5α-tetrahydroprogesterone; ASD, androstenedione; DOC, 11-deoxycorticosterone; DHT, dihydrotestosterone; DHEA, dehydroepiandrosterone; DHEAS, dehydroepiandrosterone sulfate; 17-OH-PREG, 17-hydroxy-pregnenolone; 17-OH-PROG, 17-hydroxy-progesterone; PREG, pregnenolone; PREGS, pregnenolone sulfate; PROG, progesterone; THDOC, 3α,5α-tetrahydrodeoxycorticosterone. (Adapted from Compagnone NA, Mellon SH: Neurosteroids: Biosynthesis and function of these novel neuromodulators. Front Neuroendocrinol 21:1, 2000.)

Table 90-1 Sources, Production Rates, and Plasma Concentrations of Selected Steroids in Women

Steroid	Source	Production (mg/day)	Plasma Concentration Range (nmol/L)
Cortisol[142]	AC zona fasciculata	8-25*	AM: 1350-5518 PM: 690-2758
DHEAS[143]	AC ZR	3.5-20* (declines with age)	3,000-12,000
DHEA[143]	AC ZR 50% Ovarian theca 20% Circulating DHEAS 30%	6-8* (declines with age)	5.6-27.8
ASD[143]	AC ZR 50% Ovarian stroma 50%	1.4-6.2	2-8
Testosterone[143]	AC ZR 25% Ovarian stroma 25% Circulating ASD 50%	0.1-0.4 (declines with age)	0.5-2.4
Allopregnanolone	AC[144] Ovary Neural tissue	—	Follicular phase: 0.8 ± 0.30 (mean ± SEM, *n* = 81)[145] Luteal phase: 3.7 ± 1.0 (mean ± SEM, *n* = 108)[145]

*No change during menses.
AC, adrenal cortex; ASD, androstenedione; DHEA, dehydroepiandrosterone; DHEAS; dehydroepiandrosterone sulfate; SEM, standard error of the mean; ZR, zona reticularis.

We recently measured serum free cortisol and DHEAS concentrations in patients with moderate to severe IC during flare and remission. During flare, the concentration of serum free cortisol was half, and that of DHEAS was 20%, of the concentration found in patients not in a flare (Fig. 90-6). During their flare, two patients were deficient in serum free cortisol, and four patients were deficient in DHEAS (adjusted for age).[99] In addition to suggesting that neuroendocrine function may be altered in IC during flare, the results of studies of cats with FIC, and of human patients with IC and other unexplained clinical conditions,[100] document that neuroendocrine abnormalities may not be identifiable by evaluation of basal neuroendocrine function and may be unmasked only by appropriate provocative testing paradigms.

Adrenocortical function also has been evaluated in patients with CFS by measuring the cortisol-to-DHEAS ratio,[101] which was twofold to threefold higher in CFS patients than in controls. Kizildere and colleagues[72] suggested that serum levels of DHEAS may be low in patients with inflammatory and noninflammatory diseases due to an activated SNS. They concluded that sympathetic hyperactivity may be a common denominator for low levels of DHEAS in both inflammatory and noninflammatory diseases. These abnormalities also suggest that some patients may have decreased availability of adrenocortical sex steroids and neurosteroids (see Fig. 90-5),[98] which could adversely affect normal neural function.[102,103]

Hypothalamic-Pituitary-Gonadal Axis

Patients with IC and CPP also may be at increased risk for inadequate biologic activity of the sex hormones, for a variety of reasons. Some patients in both groups have decreased circulating

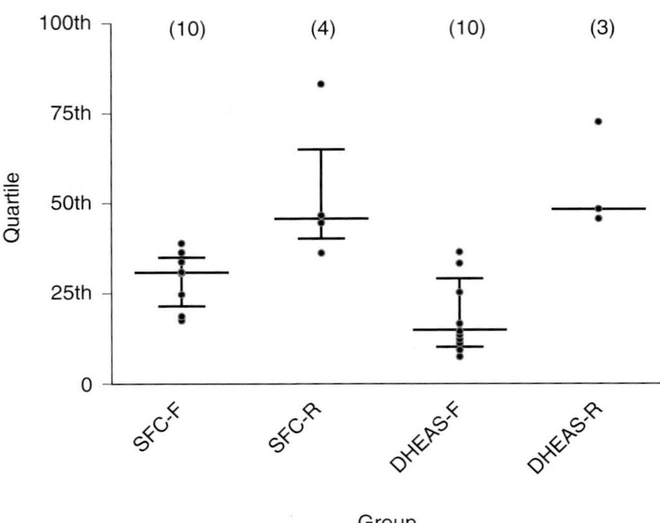

Figure 90-6 Effects of flare (F) and remission (R) of interstitial cystitis symptoms on serum free cortisol (SFC) and dehydroepiandrosterone sulfate (DHEAS). Parentheses (= no. of patients = no of dots in graph). (Adapted from Compagnone NA, Mellon SH: Neurosteroids: Biosynthesis and function of these novel neuromodulators. Front Neuroendocrinol 21:1, 2000.)

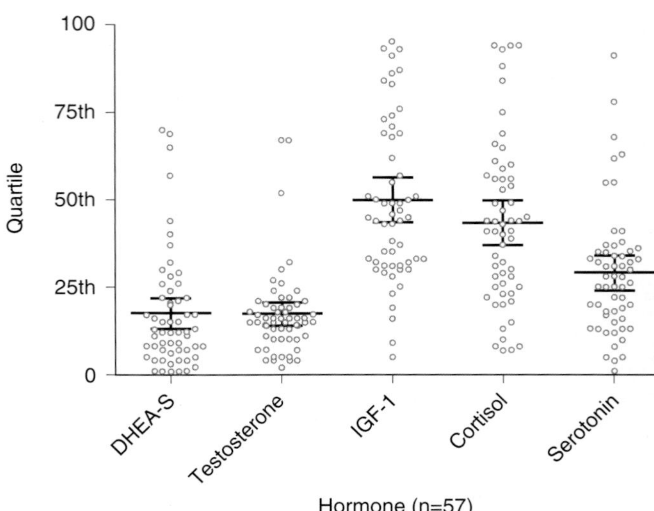

Figure 90-7 Fasting blood concentrations of selected hormones in women with fibromyalgia syndrome. DHEA-S, dehydroepiandrosterone sulfate; IGF-1, insulin-like growth factor 1. (Adapted from Dessein PH, Shipton EA, Joffe BI, et al: Hyposecretion of adrenal androgens and the relation of serum adrenal steroids, serotonin and insulin-like growth factor-1 to clinical features in women with fibromyalgia. Pain 83:313, 1999.)

glucocorticoid concentrations, suggesting decreased adrenocortical availability of sex steroid precursors[99,104]; some have undergone oophorectomy and/or hysterectomy; and some may have inadequate pituitary function. Kalantaridou and associates[105] recently reviewed the complex effects of activation of the SRS system on the female reproductive system. Increased CRF and β-endorphin release as a consequence of chronic activation of the SRS can inhibit release of gonadotropin-releasing hormone (GnRH), thus decreasing sex hormone availability. Increased glucocorticoid activity also can suppress function at all levels of the gonadal axis.[105]

Decreased estrogen activity has been recognized in some patients with CPP, as well as in patients with irritable bladder symptoms,[106] and replacement therapy may be beneficial. Androgen activity also may be inadequate in some patients.[107,108] Reported causes of androgen deficiency in women are presented in Table 90-2. Any of these causes may lead to variable combinations of the deficiency symptoms listed in Table 90-3.

Table 90-2 Causes of Androgen Insufficiency in Women

Presentation	Causes
Inadequate adrenal function	Decreased adrenal reserve, adrenal failure, surgery
Inadequate ovarian function	Oophorectomy, hysterectomy, premature menopause after radiation therapy or chemotherapy
Inadequate pituitary function	Chronic stress response, hypercortisolism
Iatrogenic	Exogenous oral estrogen, antiandrogen therapy, chronic glucocorticoid treatment
Normal aging	Low bioavailable free testosterone

Data from Cameron DR, Braunstein GD: Androgen replacement therapy in women. Fertil Steri 82: 273, 2004; and Rivera-Woll LM, Papalia M, Davis SR, et al: Androgen insufficiency in women: Diagnostic and therapeutic implications. Hum Reprod Update 10: 421, 2004.

Dessein and colleagues[109] investigated the concentrations of adrenal androgen metabolites and their relationship with health status in women with fibromyalgia, a syndrome that commonly occurs comorbidly with CPP and IC. Responses to the Fibromyalgia Impact Questionnaire and fasting blood samples were obtained from 57 women with fibromyalgia for measurement of DHEAS, free testosterone (T), cortisol, serotonin, and insulin-like growth factor-1. Normal values for DHEAS and T were obtained from 114 controls. Individual results for all patients were reported and are plotted in Figure 90-7. The individual values were divided by the uppermost value from the reference range to allow the results to be plotted as quartiles of the reference range. DHEAS concentrations were decreased significantly in both premenopausal and postmenopausal patients ($P < .0001$ and $P < .0005$, respectively). T concentrations were decreased significantly in premenopausal patients ($P < .0001$), and a trend could be identified in postmenopausal patients ($P = .06$). After adjustment for age, the only significant correlations between hormone concentrations and Fibromyalgia Impact Questionnaire scores were between DHEAS and pain ($r = -0.29$, $P < .001$), and between T and physical functioning ($r = .34$, $P = .002$). Body mass index correlated positively with pain ($r = .38$, $P < .001$) and inversely with DHEAS level ($r = -0.33$, $P = .006$).

Androgen insufficiency can occur even in regularly menstruating women. Guay recently reported measurement of total and free serum testosterone levels in 12 premenopausal women with complaints of decreased libido.[110] Eight of the women had low or immeasurable levels of both testosterones despite having regular menstrual periods. Concentrations of DHEAS and androstenedione were in the low-normal to high-normal range. Treatment

Table 90-3 Symptoms of Androgen Deficiency and Excess in Women

	Deficiency		*Excess*	
Hormone	**Signs**	**Symptoms**	**Signs**	**Symptoms**
Estrogen	Hot flashes	Depression	Breast pain	Nervousness
	Dry vagina	Minor anxiety	PMS	Irritability
	Lowered libido	Emotional instability	Irregular bleeding	Low libido
	Painful intercourse	Feelings of despair	Fluid retention	Mood swings
	Irritable bladder symptoms	Crying easily	Headache	
	Fatigue		Breast adenoma	
	Headache/migraine		Gall bladder problems	
	Night sweats		Blood sugar problems	
	Vaginal infections		Sugar cravings	
	Urinary tract infections		Fibroids	
	Incontinence		Hormonal cancers	
	Difficulty falling asleep		Heavy menstruation	
	Decreased concentration		Bloating	
	Episodes of rapid heart rate		Weight gain	
	Decreased verbal skills		Nausea	
	Irregular vaginal bleeding		Endometriosis	
			Thyroid problems	
			Sleep disturbances	
Progesterone	Breast cysts/pain	Anxiety		
	Fluid retention	Over-reacting		
	Reduced body temperature	Easily alarmed		
	Hair loss	Easily stressed		
	Heavy periods	Feelings of confusion		
	Menstrual cramps	Mood swings		
	Fibroids	Irritability		
	Hypothyroidism	Nervousness		
	Bone loss	Depression		
	Irregular cycle/Infertility	PMS		
		Headaches/migraine		
		Endometriosis		
		Sleep disturbances		
Testosterone	Decreased pubic hair	Blunted motivation	Acne/oily skin	Agitation
	Reduced lean body mass	Diminished well-being	Facial hair	Anger
	Osteopenia or osteoporosis	Flat mood	Deepened voice	Irritability
	Incontinence	Reduced libido	Ovarian cysts	
	Thinning skin		Low blood sugar	
	Genital thinning		Midcycle pain	
	Reduced muscle tone		Low HDL cholesterol	
			Thinning scalp hair	
			Increased breast cancer risk	
			Painful nipples	

HDL, high-density lipoprotein; PMS, premenstrual syndrome.

with oral DHEA, 50 to 100 mg per day, restored sexual desire in six of the eight women, gave partial improvement in one, and failed in one.

It is important to note that DHEA currently is marketed as a "dietary supplement," which means that the U.S. Food and Drug Administration does not certify the amount or quality of DHEA in the many commercially available preparations. Thompson and Carlson recently reported that determination of the DHEA content of 54 such supplements using a liquid chromatographic method revealed variation from 0% to 109.5% of the declared amount, with an overall mean value of 91%.[111] This variability suggests that circulating DHEA concentrations should be monitored in patients taking these products to ensure that intake is not inadequate or excessive. The most frequently reported side effects of excessive DHEA intake are increased facial hair and acne.[107]

Additionally, conversion of DHEA or DHEAS to androgens and estrogens may not occur normally in some patients.[112] Most of the androgens in women, especially after menopause, are synthesized in peripheral tissues from adrenal DHEA and DHEAS by 17β-hydroxysteroid dehydrogenase enzymes in a process called intracrinology.[113] Once synthesized, the sex steroids exert their action in the cells where they are synthesized without significant diffusion into the circulation, thus seriously limiting the ability to interpret serum sex steroid concentrations. They also are inactivated locally into more water-soluble compounds that diffuse into the general circulation, where they can be measured.[113,114] Dysfunctions in human 17β-hydroxysteroid dehydrogenases result in disorders of biology of reproduction and neuronal diseases, and these enzymes also are involved in the pathogenesis of various cancers. Abnormalities of this complex peripheral system may underlie some of the discordant results found in studies of DHEA and DHEAS replacement therapy.

Recently, concern has been expressed that excessive biologic activity of estrogen and testosterone, both essential hormones, can increase the risk for breast cancer in women.[115,116] On the other hand, patients with documented symptoms and laboratory evidence of hormone insufficiency have been shown to benefit from appropriate physiologic replacement therapy.[107,117] The occurrence of abnormalities with both inadequate and excessive biologic activity of hormones demonstrates the hormetic nature of the biologic response to steroid hormones (see Fig. 90-3).[118] The "dose-response" for hormones is similar to that for many essential nutrients, with deficiency signs occurring with inadequate intake, a variable plateau of satisfactory intake, and symptoms of toxicity with excessive intake.[119] The diagnosis of androgen insufficiency should be made only in adequately and satisfactorily estrogenized women, because estrogen therapy alone may be sufficient to alleviate the symptoms in some patients.[120] *Adequately* means replacement with physiologic doses that avoid potentially detrimental excesses. *Satisfactorily* means avoidance of oral preparations in this patient population, due to the effects on the liver of oral conjugated equine estrogens (or oral contraceptives). Oral forms of estrogens appear to stimulate hepatic production of both cortisol and sex hormone–binding globulin, reducing the availability of the free, biologically active forms of cortisol and testosterone. Oral conjugated equine estrogens also have been reported to increase high-density lipoproteins, triglycerides, and C-reactive protein, which may adversely affect cardiovascular health. Transdermal delivery of estradiol has not been associated with these potentially adverse changes.[121] The Princeton consensus statement[122] proposed the algorithm presented in Figure 90-8 for initiating androgen therapy in women.

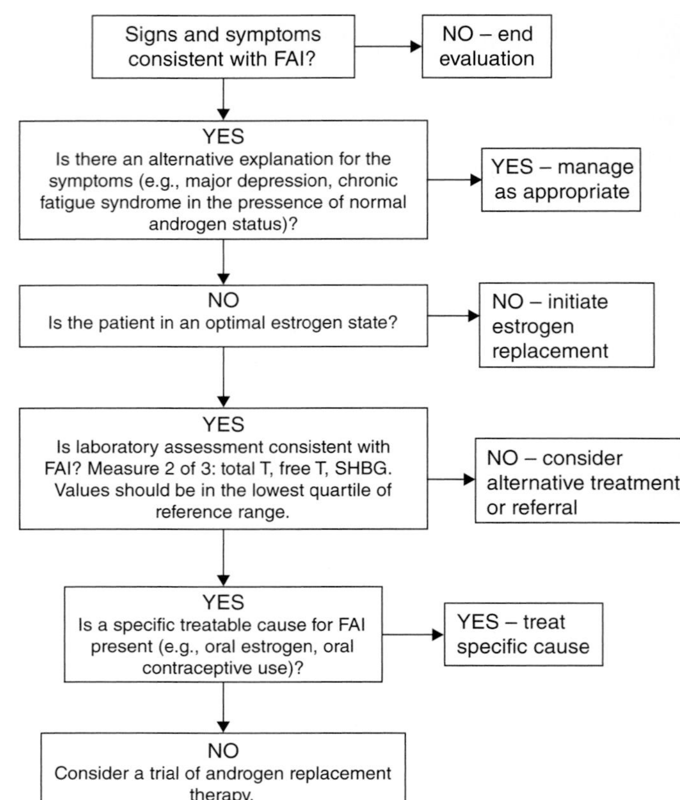

Figure 90-8 Algorithm proposed by the Princeton consensus statement for initiating androgen therapy in women. FAI, female androgen insufficiency; SHBG, sex hormone–binding globulin; T, testosterone. (Adapted from Bachmann G, Bancroft J, Braunstein G, et al: Female androgen insufficiency: The Princeton consensus statement on definition, classification, and assessment. Fertil Steril 77:660, 2002.)

The age at onset of symptoms also supports the hypothesis that hormone deficiency may play a role in IC. Prevalence was greatest in age categories 41 to 45 years and 71 to 75 years, with the highest prevalence (266 per 100,000) observed in those age 41 to 45 years.[123] Koziol also reported an average age at the time of onset of symptoms of IC of approximately 41 years, although almost 30% of patients were younger than 30 years of age at the time of onset.[124] Further support comes from the observation that some patients with IC and CPP have significant symptom improvements during pregnancy, a time when concentrations of many of the steroid hormones increase.[125]

Inadequate sex hormone biologic activity in women also may increase SNS activity. Stoney and coworkers[126] tested the effects of elective hysterectomy and/or bilateral salpingo-oophorectomy on cardiovascular risk factors, blood pressure, lipids, weight, and physiologic responses to stress in 29 middle-aged premenopausal women. After surgery, the 10 women who had undergone oophorectomy only had higher concentrations of stress-induced lipids and tended to have higher circulating concentrations of epinephrine and higher stress-induced systolic and diastolic blood pressure than did the 19 women who had undergone hysterectomy including removal of their ovaries. In rats, Ting and colleagues[127] recently reported that ovariectomy resulted in a 59% elevation in vaginal nerve density. This change was attributable to increased densities of sympathetic (70%), cholinergic parasympathetic (93%), and nociceptive sensory nerves (84%); myelinated sensory innervation did not appear to be affected. Sustained administration of 17β-estradiol reduced innervation density to an extent comparable to that of estrus, suggesting that estrogen deficiency had mediated the increments in innervation. These findings indicate that some aspects of vaginal dysfunction during menopause may be attributable to changes in innervation. Increased sympathetic innervation may augment vasoconstriction and promote vaginal dryness, and nociceptive sensory afferent proliferation may contribute to symptoms of pain, burning, and itching associated with menopause and some forms of CPP.

Documentation of widespread involvement of other organ systems[124,128-132] also suggests a role for neuroendocrine involvement in at least some patients with IC and CPP. In particular, the prominence of autonomic symptoms in some patients with type I IC provides further evidence for the presence of persistently increased SNS activity in these patients. Even the somewhat unusual bladder histopathology found in patients with IC, vasodilatation, and vascular leakage in the absence of any significant mononuclear infiltrate could be the result of high local concentrations of norepinephrine.[133,134]

IC and CPP are so complex that is seems unlikely that all, or even most, cases will be explained by a single underlying etiology. Separation of type I from type II patients in data analyses appears to be an important distinction and may suggest different underlying neuroendocrine abnormalities. Even if neuroendocrine imbalance explains only a subset of cases of IC, however, it could result in improved care for those patients. In the case of CPP, patients who have had their reproductive organs removed to treat the pain, without success, may be most likely to be affected.[104]

In susceptible individuals with IC or CPP, it may be prudent to assess adrenocortical function before elective surgical procedures or after significantly stressful experiences and to consider providing replacement therapy as indicated.[135] Although adverse addisonian-like events have not been reported in these patients to the my knowledge, studies in other patient populations have suggested that inadequate adrenocortical function in stressed patients may predispose some individuals to development of PTSD.[56,136]

The direct and circumstantial evidence that neuroendocrine abnormalities may play an important role in the etiology, pathophysiology, and therapy of IC and CPP in some patients is tantalizing and incomplete. There are so many genetic, environmental, and individual variables that finding a single "smoking gun" does not seem likely. To begin to tease apart the relative contributions of the SNS, HPA, HPG, and other systems may require measurement of a "panel" of markers of neuroendocrine function in patients, much like a serum biochemical profile. The most appropriate sample source (e.g., saliva,[137] serum[138]), timing of collection (during flare or remission periods), and assay methodology[139] for diagnosis and follow-up of neuroendocrine abnormalities remain unresolved questions, as do the amount, balance, and route of replacement therapy, when indicated. The sex and adrenal steroids arose hundreds of millions of years ago,[140] and we are left to sort out the ensuing complexity. It may be that, by broadening our perspective, at least initially, to include additional systems, we may be better able to understand syndromes that at first appear to be restricted to isolated organs but in some patients are revealed on closer inspection to be system wide.[141]

Acknowledgment

Dr. Buffington is supported by the National Institutes of Health P50 DK64539 Women's Health and Functional Visceral Disorders Center, and DK47538.

References

1. Blackburn-Munro G, Blackburn-Munro R: Pain in the brain: are hormones to blame? Trends Endocrinol Metab 14:20, 2003.
2. Bomholt SF, Harbuz MS, Blackburn-Munro G, et al: Involvement and role of the hypothalamo-pituitary-adrenal (HPA) stress axis in animal models of chronic pain and inflammation. Stress: The International Journal on the Biology of Stress, 7:1, 2004.
3. Webster DC, Dalton C, Martel RM: A nursing paradigm for interstitial vystitis. In Sant GR (ed): Interstitial Cystitis. Philadelphia, Lippincott-Raven, 1997, pp 205-213.
4. Jones CA, Harris M, Nyberg L: Prevalence of interstitial cystitis in the United States. J Urol 151:781, 1994.
5. Parsons CL, Albo M: Intravesical potassium sensitivity in patients with prostatitis. J Urol 168:1054, 2002.
6. Buffington CAT, Chew DJ, Woodworth BE: Feline interstitial cystitis. J Am Vet Med Assoc 215:682, 1999.
7. Howard FM: Chronic pelvic pain. Obstet Gynecol 101:594, 2003.
8. Jamieson DJ, Steege JF: The prevalence of dysmenorrhea, dyspareunia, pelvic pain, and irritable bowel syndrome in primary care practices. Obstet Gynecol 87:55, 1996.
9. Williams RE, Hartmann KE, Steege JF: Documenting the current definitions of chronic pelvic pain: Implications for research. Obstet Gynecol 103:686, 2004.
10. Zondervan KT, Yudkin PL, Vessey MP, et al: Chronic pelvic pain in the community: Symptoms, investigations, and diagnoses. Am J Obstet Gynecol 184:1149, 2001.
11. Peeker R, Fall M: Toward a precise definition of interstitial cystitis: Further evidence of differences in classic and nonulcer disease. J Urol 167:2470, 2002.
12. Peeker R, Aldenborg F, Fall M: The treatment of interstitial cystitis with supratrigonal, cystectomy and ileocystoplasty: Difference in outcome between classic and nonulcer disease. J Urol 159:1479, 1998.
13. McMurray A, Grant S, Griffiths S, et al: Health-related quality of life and health service use following total hip replacement surgery. J Adv Nurs 40:663, 2002.
14. Payne CK, Mosbaugh PG, Forrest JB, et al: Intravesical resiniferatoxin for the treatment of interstitial cystitis: A randomized, double-blind, placebo controlled trial. J Urol 173:1590, 2005.
15. Chen TY, Corcos J, Camel M, et al: Prospective, randomized, double-blind study of safety and tolerability of intravesical resiniferatoxin (RTX) in interstitial cystitis (IC). Int Urogynecol J Pelvic Floor Dysfunct 16:293-297, 2005. Epub 2005 Apr 8.
16. Baskin LS, Tanagho EA: Pelvic pain without pelvic organs. J Urol 147:683, 1992.
17. Dworkin RH, Backonja M, Rowbotham MC, et al: Advances in neuropathic pain: Diagnosis, mechanisms, and treatment recommendations. Arch Neurol 60:1524, 2003.
18. Abbott J, Hawe J, Hunter D, et al: Laparoscopic excision of endometriosis: A randomized, placebo-controlled trial. Fertil Steril 82:878, 2004.
19. Schommer NC, Hellhammer DH, Kirschbaum C: Dissociation between reactivity of the hypothalamus-pituitary-adrenal axis and the sympathetic-adrenal-medullary system to repeated psychosocial stress. Psychosoma Med 65:450, 2003.
20. Makino S, Hashimoto K, Gold PW: Multiple feedback mechanisms activating corticotropin-releasing hormone system in the brain during stress. Pharmacol Biochem Behav 73:147, 2002.
21. Katkin ES, Wiens S, Ohman A: Nonconscious fear conditioning, visceral perception, and the development of gut feelings. Psychol Sci 12:366, 2001.
22. Irwin PP, James S, Watts L, et al: Abnormal pedal thermoregulation in interstitial cystitis. Neurourol Urodyn 12:139, 1993.
23. Hohenfellner M, Nunes L, Schmidt RA, et al: Interstitial cystitis: Increased sympathetic innervation and related neuropeptide synthesis. J Urol 147:587, 1992.
24. Peeker R, Aldenborg F, Dahlstrom A, et al: Increased tyrosine hydroxylase immunoreactivity in bladder tissue from patients with classic and nonulcer interstitial cystitis. J Urol 163:1112, 2000.
25. Stein PC, Torri A, Parsons L: Elevated urinary norepinephrine in interstitial cystitis. Urology 53:1140, 1999.
26. Craig AD: How do you feel? Interoception: The sense of the physiological condition of the body. Nat Rev Neurosci 3:655, 2002.
27. LeDoux J: The Synaptic Self: How Our Brains Become Who We Are. New York, Penguin Books, 2002, p 406.
28. Bierhaus A, Wolf J, Andrassy M, et al: A mechanism converting psychosocial stress into mononuclear cell activation. Proc Natl Acad Sci U S A 100:1920, 2003.
29. Sadhukhan PC, Tchetgen MB, Rackley RR, et al: Sodium pentosan polysulfate reduces urothelial responses to inflammatory stimuli via an indirect mechanism. J Urol 168:289, 2002.

30. Kumar A, Takada Y, Boriek AM, et al: Nuclear factor-kappa B: Its role in health and disease. J Mol Med 82:434, 2004.
31. Veranic P, Jezernik K: The response of junctional complexes to induced desquamation in mouse bladder urothelium. Biol Cell 92:105, 2000.
32. Birder LA, Nealen ML, Kiss S, et al: Beta-adrenoceptor agonists stimulate endothelial nitric oxide synthase in rat urinary bladder urothelial cells. J Neurosci 22:8063, 2002.
33. Birder LA, Apodaca G, De Groat WC, et al: Adrenergic- and capsaicin-evoked nitric oxide release from urothelium and afferent nerves in urinary bladder. Am J Physiol Renal Physiol 44:F226, 1998.
34. Jezernik K, Romih R, Mannherz HG, et al: Immunohistochemical detection of apoptosis, proliferation and inducible nitric oxide synthase in rat urothelium damaged by cyclophosphamide treatment. Cell Biol Int 27:863, 2003.
35. Oter S, Korkmaz A, Oztas E, et al: Inducible nitric oxide synthase inhibition in cyclophosphamide induced hemorrhagic cystitis in rats. Urol Res 32:185, 2004.
36. Theoharides TC, Cochrane DE: Critical role of mast cells in inflammatory diseases and the effect of acute stress. J Neuroimmunol 146:1, 2004.
37. Elenkov IJ, Wilder RL, Chrousos GP, et al: The sympathetic nerve—An integrative interface between two supersystems: The brain and the immune system. Pharmacol Rev 52:595, 2000.
38. Wang J, Ren Y, Zou XJ, et al: Sympathetic influence on capsaicin-evoked enhancement of dorsal root reflexes in rats. J Neurophysiol 92:2017, 2004.
39. Parsons CL, Dell J, Stanford EJ, et al: The prevalence of interstitial cystitis in gynecologic patients with pelvic pain, as detected by intravesical potassium sensitivity. Am J Obstet Gynecol 187:1395, 2002.
40. Houdeau E, Larauche M, Monnerie R, et al: Uterine motor alterations and estrous cycle disturbances associated with colonic inflammation in the rat. Am J Physiol Regul Integr Comp Physiol 288: R630, 2005.
41. Giamberardino MA, Berkley KJ, Affaitati G, et al: Influence of endometriosis on pain behaviors and muscle hyperalgesia induced by a ureteral calculosis in female rats. Pain 95:247, 2002.
42. Giamberardino MA: Recent and forgotten aspects of visceral pain. Eur J Pain (London) 3:77, 1999.
43. Sculptoreanu A, deGroat WC, Buffington CAT, et al: Abnormal excitability in capsaicin-responsive DRG neurons from cats with feline interstitial cystitis. Exp Neurol 193:437, 2005.
44. Sculptoreanu A, deGroat WC, Buffington CAT, et al: Protein kinase C contributes to abnormal capsaicin responses in DRG neurons from cats with feline interstitial cystitis. Neurosci Lett 381:42, 2005.
45. Chew DJ, Buffington CA, Kendell MS, et al: Amitriptyline treatment for severe recurrent idiopathic cystitis in cats. J Am Vet Med Assoc 213:1282, 1998.
46. Waxman JA, Sulak PJ, Kuehl TJ: Cystoscopic findings consistent with interstitial cystitis in normal women undergoing tubal ligation. J Urol 160:1663, 1998.
47. Romih R, Korosec P, Jezernik K, et al: Inverse expression of uroplakins and inducible nitric oxide synthase in the urothelium of patients with bladder outlet obstruction. BJU Int 91:507, 2003.
48. Fields H: State-dependent opioid control of pain. Nat Rev Neurosci 5:565, 2004.
49. Roppolo JR, Tai C, Booth AM, et al: Bladder A-delta afferent nerve activity in normal cats and cats with feline interstitial cystitis. J Urol 173:1011, 2005.
50. Long JB, Holaday JW: Blood-brain barrier: Endogenous modulation by adrenal-cortical function. Science 227:1580, 1985.
51. Leme JG, Wilhelm DL: The effects of adrenalectomy and corticosterone on vascular permeability responses in the skin of the rat. Br J Exp Pathol 56:402, 1975.
52. Boschetto P, Musajo FG, Tognetto L, et al: Increase in vascular permeability produced in rat airways by Paf: Potentiation by adrenalectomy. Br J Pharmacol 105:388, 1992.
53. Harhaj NS, Antonetti DA: Regulation of tight junctions and loss of barrier function in pathophysiology. Int J Biochem Cell Biol 36:1206, 2004.
54. Sinton CM, Fitch TE, Petty F, et al: Stressful manipulations that elevate corticosterone reduce blood-brain barrier permeability to pyridostigmine in the rat. Toxicol Appl Pharmacol 165:99, 2000.
55. Meddings JB, Swain MG: Environmental stress-induced gastrointestinal permeability is mediated by endogenous glucocorticoids in the rat. Gastroenterology 119:1019, 2000.
56. Raison CL, Miller AH: When not enough is too much: the role of insufficient glucocorticoid signaling in the pathophysiology of stress-related disorders. Am J Psychiatry 160:1554, 2003.
57. Wen Y, Yang SH, Liu R, et al: Estrogen attenuates nuclear factor-kappa B activation induced by transient cerebral ischemia. Brain Res 1008:147, 2004.
58. Hayashi R, Wada H, Ito K, et al: Effects of glucocorticoids on gene transcription. Eur J Pharmacol 500:51, 2004.
59. Turrin NP, Rivest S: Unraveling the molecular details involved in the intimate link between the immune and neuroendocrine systems. Exp Biol Med 229:996, 2004.
60. Nadeau S, Rivest S: Glucocorticoids play a fundamental role in protecting the brain during innate immune response. J Neurosci 23:5536, 2003.
61. Koulich E, Nguyen T, Johnson K, et al: NF-kappa B is involved in the survival of cerebellar granule neurons: Association of I kappa beta phosphorylation with cell survival. J Neurochem 76:1188, 2001.
62. Heim C, Ehlert U, Hellhammer DH: The potential role of hypocortisolism in the pathophysiology of stress-related bodily disorders. Psychoneuroendocrinology 25:1, 2000.
63. Lutgendorf SK, Kreder KJ, Rothrock NE, et al: Diurnal cortisol variations and symptoms in patients with interstitial cystitis. J Urol 167:1338, 2002.
64. Lutgendorf S, Kreder K, Ratliff T, et al: Effects of stress reactivity on HPA function and symptoms in interstitial cystitis. Psychosom Med 62:1332, 2000.
65. Heim C, Ehlert U, Hanker JP, et al: Abuse-related posttraumatic stress disorder and alterations of the hypothalamic-pituitary-adrenal axis in women with chronic pelvic pain. Psychosom Med 60:309, 1998.
66. Demitrack MA, Dale JK, Straus SE, et al: Evidence for impaired activation of the hypothalamic-pituitary-adrenal axis in patients with chronic fatigue syndrome. J Clin Endocrinol Metab 73:1224, 1991.
67. Lackner JM, Gudleski GD, Blanchard EB: Beyond abuse: the association among parenting style, abdominal pain, and somatization in IBS patients. Behav Res Ther 42:41, 2004.
68. Yehuda R, Halligan SL, Bierer LM: Cortisol levels in adult offspring of Holocaust survivors: Relation to PTSD symptom severity in the parent and child. Psychoneuroendocrinology 27:171, 2002.
69. Scott LV, Teh J, Reznek R, et al: Small adrenal glands in chronic fatigue syndrome: A preliminary computer tomography study. Psychoneuroendocrinology 24:759, 1999.
70. Dinan TG: Personal communication, 2003.
71. Calis M, Gokce C, Ates F, et al: Investigation of the hypothalamo-pituitary-adrenal axis (HPA) by 1 microg ACTH test and metyrapone test in patients with primary fibromyalgia syndrome. J Endocrinol Invest 27:42, 2004.
72. Kizildere S, Gluck T, Zietz B, et al: During a corticotropin-releasing hormone test in healthy subjects, administration of a beta-adrenergic antagonist induced secretion of cortisol and dehydroepiandrosterone sulfate and inhibited secretion of ACTH. Eur J Endocrinol 148:45, 2003.
73. Aguilera G: Corticotropin releasing hormone, receptor regulation and the stress response. Trends Endocrinol Metab 9:329, 1998.

74. Buffington CA, Pacak K: Increased plasma norepinephrine concentration in cats with interstitial cystitis. J Urol 165:2051, 2001.
75. Westropp JL, Buffington CAT: Effect of a corticotropin releasing factor (crf) antagonist on hypothalamic-pituitary-adrenal activation in response to crf in cats with interstitial cystitis. Presented at the Research Insights into Interstitial Cystitis, Alexandria, VA, 2003.
76. Westropp JL, Buffington CAT: Cerebrospinal fluid corticotrophin releasing factor and catecholamine concentrations in healthy cats and cats with interstitial cystitis. Presented at the Research Insights into Interstitial Cystitis, Alexandria, VA, 2003.
77. Welk KA, Buffington CAT: Effect of interstitial cystitis on central neuropeptide and receptor immunoreactivity in cats. Presented at the Research Insights into Interstitial Cystitis, Alexandria, VA, 2003.
78. Westropp JL, Welk KA, Buffington CAT: Small adrenal glands in cats with feline interstitial cystitis. J Urol 170:2494, 2003.
79. Liberzon I, Abelson J, Flagel S, et al: Neuroendocrine and psychophysiologic responses in PTSD: A symptom provocation study. Neuropsychopharmacology 21:40, 1999.
80. Wilkinson DJC, Thompson JM, Lambert GW, et al: Sympathetic activity in patients with panic disorder at rest, under laboratory mental stress, and during panic attacks. Arch Gen Psychiatry 55:511, 1998.
81. Coplan JD, Smith EL, Altemus M, et al: Variable foraging demand rearing: sustained elevations in cisternal cerebrospinal fluid corticotropin-releasing factor concentrations in adult primates. Biol Psychiatry 50:200, 2001.
82. Welberg LAM, Seckl JR: Prenatal stress, glucocorticoids and the programming of the brain. J Neuroendocrinol 13:113, 2001.
83. Matthews SG: Early programming of the hypothalamo-pituitary-adrenal axis. Trends Endocrinol Metab 13:373, 2002.
84. Fameli M, Kitraki E, Stylianopoulou F: Effects of hyperactivity of the maternal hypothalamic-pituitary-adrenal (HPA) axis during pregnancy on the development of the HPA axis and brain monoamines of the offspring. Int J Devel Neurosci 12:651, 1994.
85. Cadet R, Pradier P, Dalle M, et al: Effects of prenatal maternal stress on the pituitary adrenocortical reactivity in guinea-pig pups. J Dev Physiol 8:467, 1986.
86. Braastad BO, Osadchuk LV, Lund G, et al: Effects of prenatal handling stress on adrenal weight and function and behaviour in novel situations in blue fox cubs (*Alopex lagopus*). Appl Ani Behav Sci 57:157, 1998.
87. Challis JRG, Davies IA, Benirschke K, et al: The effects of dexamethasone on plasma steroid levels and fetal adrenal histology in the pregnant rhesus monkey. Endocrinology 95:1300, 1974.
88. Leavitt MG, Aberdeen GW, Burch MG, et al: Inhibition of fetal adrenal adrenocorticotropin receptor messenger ribonucleic acid expression by betamethasone administration to the baboon fetus in late gestation. Endocrinology 138:2705, 1997.
89. Pontari MA, Hanno PM: Oral therapies for interstitial cystitis. In Sant GR (ed): Interstitial Cystitis. Philadelphia, Lippincott-Raven, 1997, pp 173-176.
90. Hosseini A, Ehren I, Wiklund NP: Nitric oxide as an objective marker for evaluation of treatment response in patients with classic interstitial cystitis. J Urol 172:2261, 2004.
91. Schelling G: Effects of stress hormones on traumatic memory formation and the development of posttraumatic stress disorder in critically ill patients. Neurobiol Learn Mem 78:596, 2002.
92. Aerni A, Traber R, Hock C, et al: Low-dose cortisol for symptoms of posttraumatic stress disorder. Am J Psychiatry 161:1488, 2004.
93. Scott LV, Svec F, Dinan T: A preliminary study of dehydroepiandrosterone response to low- dose ACTH in chronic fatigue syndrome and in healthy subjects. Psychiatr Res 97:21, 2000.
94. Cardoso E, Persi G, Arregger AL, et al: Assessment of corticoadrenal reserve through salivary steroids. Endocrinologist 12:38, 2002.
95. Baulieu EE: Steroid hormones in the brain: Several mechanisms? In Fuxe K, Gustafson JA, Wetterberg L (eds): Steroid Hormone Regulation of the Brain, vol 34. Elmsford, NY, Pergamon, 1981, pp 3-14.
96. Dubrovsky BO: Steroids, neuroactive steroids and neurosteroids in psychopathology. Prog Neuropsychopharmacol Biol Psychiatry 29:169, 2005.
97. Baulieu EE, Robel P: Neurosteroids: A new brain function? J Steroid Biochem Mol Biol 37:395-403, 1990.
98. Compagnone NA, Mellon SH: Neurosteroids: Biosynthesis and function of these novel neuromodulators. Front Neuroendocrinol 21:1, 2000.
99. Buffington CAT: Comorbidity of interstitial cystitis with other unexplained clinical conditions. J Urol 172:1242, 2004.
100. Adler GK, Manfredsdottir VF, Rackow RM: Hypothalamic-pituitary-adrenal axis function in fibromyalgia and chronic fatigue syndrome. Endocrinologist 12:513, 2002.
101. Kroboth PD, Salek FS, Pittenger AL, et al: DHEA and DHEA-S: A review. J Clin Pharmacol 39:327, 1999.
102. Strohle A, Romeo E, di Michele F, et al: Induced panic attacks shift gamma-aminobutyric acid type A receptor modulatory neuroactive steroid composition in patients with panic disorder preliminary results. Arch Gen Psychiatry 60:161, 2003.
103. Winter L, Nadeson R, Tucker AP, et al: Antinociceptive properties of neurosteroids: A comparison of alphadolone and alphaxalone in potentiation of opioid antinociception. Anesth Analg 97:798, 2003.
104. Heim C, Ehlert U, Hanker JP, et al: Psychological and endocrine correlates of chronic pelvic pain associated with adhesions. J Psychosom Obstet Gynecol 20:11, 1999.
105. Kalantaridou SN, Makrigiannakis A, Zoumakis E, et al: Stress and the female reproductive system. J Reprod Immunol 62:61, 2004.
106. Cardozo L, Lose G, McClish D, et al: A systematic review of the effects of estrogens for symptoms suggestive of overactive bladder. Acta Obstet Gynecol Scand 83:892, 2004.
107. Cameron DR, Braunstein GD: Androgen replacement therapy in women. Fertil Steril 82:273, 2004.
108. Rivera-Woll LM, Papalia M, Davis SR, et al: Androgen insufficiency in women: Diagnostic and therapeutic implications. Hum Reprod Update 10:421, 2004.
109. Dessein PH, Shipton EA, Joffe BI, et al: Hyposecretion of adrenal androgens and the relation of serum adrenal steroids, serotonin and insulin-like growth factor-1 to clinical features in women with fibromyalgia. Pain 83:313, 1999.
110. Guay AT: Decreased testosterone in regularly menstruating women with decreased libido: A clinical observation. J Sex Marital Ther 27: 513, 2001.
111. Thompson RD, Carlson M: Liquid chromatographic determination of dehydroepiandrosterone (DHEA) in dietary supplement products. J AOAC Int 83:847, 2000.
112. Mindnich R, Moller G, Adamski J: The role of 17 beta-hydroxysteroid dehydrogenases. Mol Cell Endocrinol 218:7, 2004.
113. Labrie F, Luu-The V, Labrie C, et al: Endocrine and intracrine sources of androgens in women: Inhibition of breast cancer and other roles of androgens and their precursor dehydroepiandrosterone. Endocr Rev 24:152, 2003.
114. Cutolo M, Giusti M, Villaggio B, et al: Testosterone metabolism and cyclosporin A treatment in rheumatoid arthritis. Br J Rheumatol 36:433, 1997.
115. Rossouw JE, Anderson GL, Prentice RL, et al: Risks and benefits of estrogen plus progestin in healthy postmenopausal women: Principal results from the Women's Health Initiative randomized controlled trial. JAMA 288:321, 2002.
116. Berrino F, Pasanisi P, Bellati C, et al: Serum testosterone levels and breast cancer recurrence. Int J Cancer 113:499, 2005.
117. Wiegratz I, Kuhl H: Progestogen therapies: Differences in clinical effects? Trends Endocrinol Metab 15:277, 2004.
118. Calabrese EJ: Estrogen and related compounds: Biphasic dose responses. Crit Rev Toxicol 31:503, 2001.
119. Mertz W: The essential trace elements. Science 213:1332, 1981.

120. Davis SR: When to suspect androgen deficiency other than at menopause. Fertil Steril 77(Suppl 4):S68, 2002.
121. Minkin MJ: Considerations in the choice of oral vs. transdermal hormone therapy: A review. J Reprod Med 49:311, 2004.
122. Bachmann G, Bancroft J, Braunstein G, et al: Female androgen insufficiency: The Princeton consensus statement on definition, classification, and assessment. Fertil Steril 77:660, 2002.
123. Clemens JQ, Meenan RT, Rosetti MC, et al: Prevalence and incidence of interstitial cystitis in a managed care population. J Urol 173:98, 2005.
124. Koziol JA: Epidemiology of interstitial cystitis. Urol Clin North Am 21:7, 1994.
125. Masi AT, Feigenbaum SL, Chatterton RT: Hormonal and pregnancy relationships to rheumatoid arthritis: Convergent effects with immunological and microvascular systems. Semin Arthritis Rheum 25:1, 1995.
126. Stoney CM, Owens JF, Guzick DS, et al: A natural experiment on the effects of ovarian hormones on cardiovascular risk factors and stress reactivity: Bilateral salpingo oophorectomy versus hysterectomy only. Health Psychol 16:349, 1997.
127. Ting AY, Blacklock AD, Smith PG: Estrogen regulates vaginal sensory and autonomic nerve density in the rat. Biol Reprod 71:1397, 2004.
128. Zondervan KT, Yudkin PL, Vessey MP, et al: The community prevalence of chronic pelvic pain in women and associated illness behaviour. Br J Gen Pract 51:541, 2001.
129. Erickson DR, Morgan KC, Ordille S, et al: Nonbladder related symptoms in patients with interstitial cystitis. J Urol 166:557, 2001.
130. Alagiri M, Chottiner S, Ratner V, et al: Interstitial cystitis: Unexplained associations with other chronic disease and pain syndromes. Urology 49:52, 1997.
131. Clauw DJ, Schmidt M, Radulovic D, et al: The relationship between fibromyalgia and interstitial cystitis. J Psychiatr Res 31:125, 1997.
132. Aaron LA, Herrell R, Ashton S, et al: Comorbid clinical conditions in chronic fatigue: A co-twin control study. J Gen Intern Med 16:24, 2001.
133. Straub RH, Cutolo M: Involvement of the hypothalamic–pituitary–adrenal/gonadal axis and the peripheral nervous system in rheumatoid arthritis: Viewpoint based on a systemic pathogenetic role. Arthritis Rheum 44:493, 2001.
134. Buffington CAT, Teng BY, Somogyi GT: Norepinephrine content and adrenoceptor function in the bladder of cats with feline interstitial cystitis. J Urol 167:1876, 2002.
135. Cooper MS, Stewart PM: Corticosteroid insufficiency in acutely ill patients. N Engl J Med 348:727, 2003.
136. Schelling G, Kilger E, Roozendaal B, et al: Stress doses of hydrocortisone, traumatic memories, and symptoms of posttraumatic stress disorder in patients after cardiac surgery: A randomized study. Biol Psychiatry 55:627, 2004.
137. Granger DA, Shirtcliff EA, Booth A, et al: The "trouble" with salivary testosterone. Psychoneuroendocrinology 29:1229, 2004.
138. Miller KK: Androgen deficiency in women. J Clin Endocrinol Metab 86:2395, 2001.
139. Holst JP, Soldin OP, Guo TD, et al: Steroid hormones: Relevance and measurement in the clinical laboratory. Clin Lab Med 24:105, 2004.
140. Baker ME: Co-evolution of steroidogenic and steroid-inactivating enzymes and adrenal and sex steroid receptors. Mol Cell Endocrinol 215:55, 2004.
141. Wessely S, White PD: There is only one functional somatic syndrome. Br J Psychiatry 185:95, 2004.
142. Greenspan FS, Gardner DG: Basic and Clinical Endocrinology, 6th ed. New York, McGraw-Hill, 2001, p 891.
143. Burger HG: Androgen production in women. Fertil Steril 77(Suppl 4):S3, 2002.
144. Corpechot C, Young J, Calvel M, et al: Neurosteroids: 3-Alpha-hydroxy-5-alpha-pregnan-20-one and its precursors in the brain, plasma, and steroidogenic glands of male and female rats. Endocrinology 133:1003, 1993.
145. Genazzani AR, Petraglia F, Bernardi F, et al: Circulating levels of allopregnanolone in humans: Gender, age, and endocrine influences. J Clin Endocrinol Metab 83:2099, 1998.

Chapter 91

FOCAL NEUROMUSCULAR THERAPIES FOR CHRONIC PELVIC PAIN SYNDROMES IN WOMEN

Rodney U. Anderson

Women have been suffering from chronic pelvic pain (CPP) syndromes presumably since the age of primate evolution. Except for endometriosis, there is little in the way of objective biologic findings to explain the pathophysiology of these complaints. In most instances, the diagnostic terms for disorders of pain in the pelvis relate to a specific organ with no identifiable mechanistic relationship. This chapter attempts to identify the common urologic/gynecologic disorders commonly considered CPP syndromes, explores the evidence for neuromuscular disorder, and reviews most of the local and focused therapeutic approaches that may be beneficial in the management of these conditions. I am specifically avoiding consideration of any pharmaceutical therapy. The objective is to suggest an integration of both physical and behavioral treatments to elicit relief from these life-altering conditions while we await more elucidation about the biologic mechanisms involved.

BIOFEEDBACK THERAPY

Biofeedback therapy for pelvic disorders has primarily been used to manage pelvic floor disorders and urinary incontinence, but it has also become quite valuable for patients with pelvic pain disorders. Biofeedback and behavioral changes can play a role in effecting clinical improvement in urologic problems including pelvic pain (vulvar vestibulitis), irritative voiding symptoms, recurrent urinary tract infections, and urinary incontinence. Biofeedback for pelvic floor dysfunction involves the use of surface internal (vaginal and rectal) electrodes that transduce muscle potentials into visual and auditory signals; by this means, patients learn to be aware and control (increase or decrease) voluntary muscle activity. Physical exercises are then used to affect the pelvic floor muscles (Fig. 91-1).

In the late 1940s, Dr. Arnold Kegel, an obstetrician/gynecologist, invented the first feedback device that was used for pelvic muscle rehabilitation to treat female urinary incontinence. The processes and procedures of biofeedback therapy have been described.[1,2] A general overview for application to pain management was summarized by Tan and colleagues.[3]

Two major subtypes of biofeedback therapy are currently in practice. The traditional form is known as peripheral or somatic feedback, which assists in teaching patients to be more physiologically aware of abnormal muscle tension and adjust accordingly. Surface electromyography (EMG), heart rate and blood

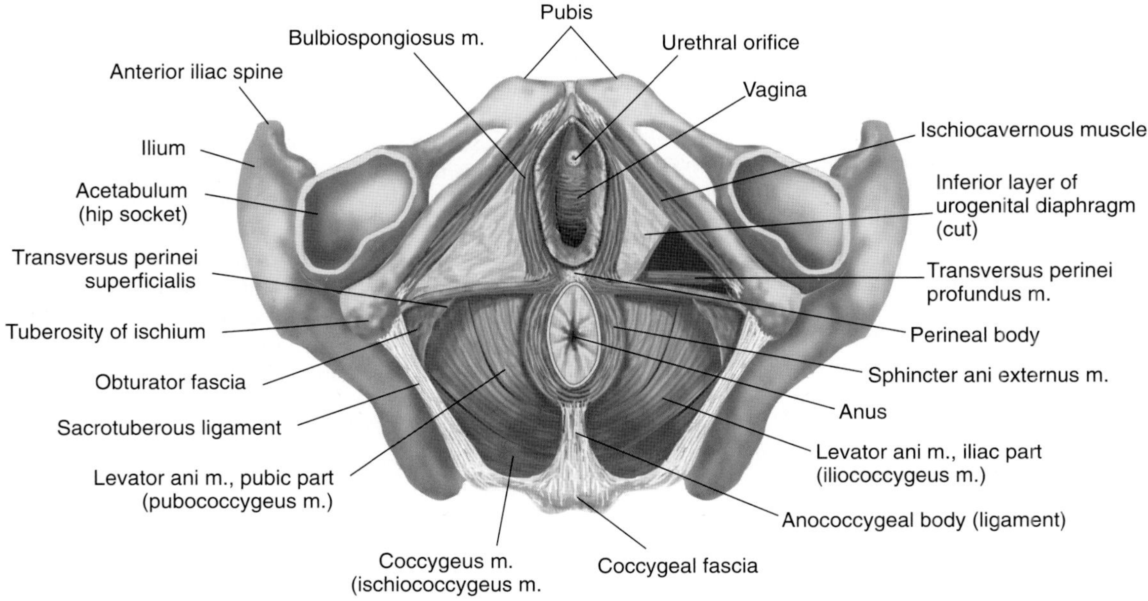

Figure 91-1 Pelvic floor muscles as seen from below in the supine female subject. (Redrawn from Travell JG, Simons DG: Myofascial Pain and Dysfunction: The Trigger Point Manual, Vol 2, 2nd ed. Philadelphia, Lippincott Williams & Wilkins, 1998.)

pressure, skin temperature, and galvanic skin responses are used. Applications of peripheral biofeedback include neuromuscular re-education (for patients after stroke), musculoskeletal therapy, urinary[4] and fecal incontinence, and pelvic pain including CPP syndromes in men,[5,6] vulvodynia,[7] and dysmenorrhea.[8,9] A second subtype of biofeedback therapy uses electroencephalography (EEG) and is classified as central biofeedback, neurofeedback, or neurotherapy. With the exception of migraine, most of the research with this therapy has been in areas other than pain, such as treatment of alcohol or additive disorders.

Glazer and coworkers reported their experience in two separate open-ended, uncontrolled studies using EMG biofeedback of the pelvic floor musculature to treat patients with vulvar vestibulitis syndrome, a subset of vulvodynia.[7,10] The rationale for study was based on the knowledge that patients with vulvar vestibulitis usually have hyperirritability of the pelvic floor muscles.[7,11] The hypothesis has been put forward that destabilization of pelvic floor muscles is a factor in perpetuating the vulvar skin disturbances and accompanying pain. Travell and Simons reported that muscle disturbances are reflected in discord of EMG recordings.[12] In the studies by Glazer and associates, patient diagnosis was confirmed by physical examination, and the initial pelvic floor EMG assessments were performed with a surface EMG single-user vaginal sensor; monthly evaluations followed during clinic visits.[7,10] A portable EMG biofeedback device and instructions for pelvic floor rehabilitation exercises were provided to each patient for twice-daily in-home practice. Patient demographics were similar in both studies; average duration of symptoms was 3.5 years (range, 2 to 6 years), and most had abstained from sexual intercourse for an average of 1 year.

In the first Glazer study of 33 women, symptoms ranged from only introital dyspareunia to chronic, intense pain provocation.[7] After 16 weeks of practice, pelvic floor contraction increased by 95%, resting tension levels decreased by 68%, and muscle instability at rest decreased by 62%. Based on subjective reporting at each evaluation, maximum pain decreased from the previous evaluation to a average of 83%. Many patients (22 [79%] of 28) resumed intercourse. Half of the women remained pain free at follow-up 6 months later. In the second study, 29 women with level 2 and 3 vulvar vestibulitis were enrolled.[10] Level 2 includes women who have pain with intercourse that requires interruption or discontinuance of coitus, and level 3 includes those who have pain with intercourse that prevents any attempt at insertion or coitus.[13] With biofeedback therapy, increased muscle stabilization was associated with decreased pain; as pain decreased, patients were more likely to resume intercourse. After therapy, 85% (24 of 29) had negligible or mild pain, and 69% resumed sexual activity.

Neuromuscular education of the pelvic floor muscles to ameliorate chronic pain has been supported by the studies in men with CPP syndromes. In a preliminary study of 19 patients using biweekly sessions of biofeedback and home exercises, significant decreases (approximately 50%) in pain and urgency scores were reported by Clemens and colleagues.[5] However, only about half of the patients completed the full course of therapy. In the study by Cornel and colleagues, biofeedback rehabilitation of 25 men with type III CPP involved verbal guidance and feedback through palpation of pelvic floor muscles and EMG measurements to teach correct muscle contraction and relaxation.[6] Significant improvements in the National Institutes of Health–Chronic Prostatitis Symptom Index (NIH-CPSI) total scores, with pain and micturition domains decreasing an average of 50%, were associated with a significant 35% decrease in pelvic muscle tonus after treatment.

MYOFASCIAL TRIGGER POINT RELEASE THERAPY

Definition and Basic Science Investigation

A long list of disorders in women has been shown to involve the musculoskeletal system; these include the levator ani syndrome, vulvodynia, vulvar vestibulitis syndrome, dyspareunia, vaginismus, coccygodynia, interstitial cystitis (IC) or painful bladder syndrome, pelvic floor tension myalgia, urge-frequency syndrome, urethral syndrome, inflammatory bowel disease, proctodynia, proctalgia fugax, and pudendal nerve entrapment,[7,14-18] and, in men, nonbacterial prostatitis and CPP syndromes.[19,20] Often overlooked and misunderstood as a musculoskeletal source of pelvic pain are myofascial trigger points (MTrPs). More than 50 years ago, Dr. Janet Travell introduced the phenomenon of referred pain and referred motor activity attributed to trigger points (TrPs) in skeletal muscles, which were later shown to be a causative factor in myofascial pain and dysfunction. Our understanding of MTrPs and their relation to myofascial pain syndromes continues to evolve, as shown in Table 91-1.

Table 91-1 Progress of Discovery and Understanding of Chronic Pain Syndromes and Myofascial Trigger Points

- 1838 Recaimer—First describes syndrome of tension myalgia of pelvic floor in "Stretching massage and rhythmic percussion in the treatment of muscular contractions"
- 1937 Thiele—Describes tonic spasms of levator ani, coccygeus, and pyriformis muscles and their relationship to pain
- 1942 Travell et al—First describes myofascial trigger points as common cause of chronic muscle pain
- 1951 Dittrich—First recognizes pelvic pain occurring as a result of referral from trigger points in subfascial fat and perifascial tissue
- 1963 Thiele—Successful uses digital massage of spastic levator muscles subsequently described as "Thiele massage"
- 1977 Sinaki et al—Consolidates various syndromes of pelvic musculature under one terminology: tension myalgia of the pelvic floor; uses combined treatment with rectal diathermy, Thiele's massage, and relaxation exercises
- 1983 Travell and Simons Publishes the first edition of *Myofascial Pain and Dysfunction: The Trigger Point Manual*; identifies external and internal muscles and areas of referred pain from myofascial trigger points
- 1984 Slocum—Treats trigger points related to the abdominal pelvic pain syndrome in women using locally injected anesthetic; indicates that emotional stress is frequently a potentiating factor, not a cause for chronic pelvic pain
- 1994 Hong—Develops rabbit animal model to identify myofascial trigger points; with colleagues, subsequently publishes 36 animal clinical and 12 basic science articles to advance understanding of myofascial trigger point
- 2004 Simons—Reviews the present understanding of myofascial trigger points as they relate to musculoskeletal dysfunction

An MTrP is defined as a highly localized and hyperirritable spot in a palpable taut band or tender nodule of skeletal muscle fibers.[16,21] MTrPs can be located in one or more muscles, and common clinical characteristics exist.[22-26] Muscles can become "knotted" and inelastic and unable to contract or relax. Stimulated by digital palpation or needling, active MTrPs characteristically elicit local pain or a referred pain similar to that of the patient's complaint of pain or aggravation of existing pain. A local twitch response is also a confirmatory sign of an MTrP. Latent MTrPs are clinically asymptomatic and do not cause pain with compression. Both active and latent MTrPs are associated with muscle weakness on active contraction and reduced range of motion, and MTrPs can be perpetuated or aggravated by mechanical stress, metabolic, endocrine, and nutritional inadequacies, as well as psychological factors.[21] Depression and chronic pain are often closely associated, and it should be appreciated that depression and anxiety are frequently consequent to unresolved symptoms.

Recent reviews present the current understanding of MTrPs and an historical summary of the development of these concepts.[27,28] An integrated hypothesis of the etiology of TrPs implicating local myofascial tissue, the central nervous system, and mechanical factors is proposed in the 1999 edition of *Travell and Simons' Myofascial Pain and Dysfunction: The Trigger Point Manual*.[29] The hypothesis postulates that a central MTrP has multiple fibers with end plates releasing excessive acetylcholine and shows histopathologic evidence of regional sarcomere shortening. The positive-feedback loop of events perpetuates these changes until the loop is interrupted. The putative steps were elegantly explained by Simons.[28] Evidence contributing to the etiology of TrPs has evolved from two early studies. Mense and Simons reported that histologic examination of biopsied muscle tissue in the vicinity of TrPs reveals large, rounded, and darkly stained muscle fibers, as well as increased muscle fiber diameters.[30] At physical examination for MTrPs, these changes are manifested as taut bands and palpable nodules. An EMG study by Hubbard and Berkoff showed greater activity in MTrPs than in adjacent nontender muscle.[31] EMG activity was significantly higher in TrPs of patients with chronic tension headaches than in normal patients and could be reduced by injection of sympathetic blockers such as phenoxybenzamine. In another study, McNutley and colleagues reported that EMG activity within an MTrP was significantly increased in subjects involved in an experimental stress test, whereas contiguous nontender muscle showed no changes.[32] This finding may have implications for the psychophysiology of stress contributing to pain and the association with MTrPs.

Physical Examination and Mapping of Trigger Points

A distinguishing feature of MTrPs is their location within a taut band of muscle or fascia as identified by palpation. They can be discovered with a careful external and internal pelvic examination. Compression of the MTrP results in a twitch response, a transient contraction from the band of fibers, and referred sensory and motor responses (e.g., tenderness, pain) occurring distant to the TrP. Two objective methods have been used to document MTrPs. Algometry provides a quantitative measurement of pressure thresholds to document the sensitivity of TrPs. Results from several studies have confirmed that MTrPs are more sensitive than contralateral muscle areas without TrPs or surrounding healthy tissue.[33,34] A difference in pressure threshold exceeding 20 newtons per square centimeter (2 kg/cm^2) between a TrP and a contralateral point is considered abnormal.[33] A second method, thermography, employs a noninvasive imaging technique to detect infrared radiation from body surfaces and heat distribution.[35] Comparative imaging of subjects with clinical TrPs and asymptomatic controls revealed discrete thermal responses in muscles with suspected TrPs. Sensory referral areas for TrPs in symptomatic subjects showed significantly reduced temperatures from precompression levels during ischemic compression; no significant temperature changes were noted in asymptomatic areas after compression. It was assumed that the colder area was caused by a reduction in blood flow due to a sympathetic autonomic change associated with the myofascial pain syndrome.

A review of the neuroanatomy of the pelvis, such as that as provided by Wesselmann and colleagues, assists in understanding the pathophysiology of urogenital and rectal pain syndromes and their management.[36] The involvement of MTrPs in CPP can thereby be taken in perspective. Travell and Simons published the first manuals on TrPs and myofascial pain and dysfunction and provided specific details of the pelvic muscles to check internally.[16,22] A subsequent edition of this manual was published in 1998.[12]

All of the muscles of the pelvis, both internal and external, must be thoroughly evaluated and subsequently treated. Muscles known to contain TrPs referring pain to an area that the patient is complaining about should be examined with extra care.

Testing for MTrPs within the pelvis depends on the palpation skills of an experienced examiner, because no diagnostic standard has been established to identify intrapelvic MTrPs. The therapist must be trained in identifying TrPs and be able to feel for superficial and deep TrPs located in the belly and the attachments of the muscles. For the purpose of locating these MTrPs, the pelvic muscles can be grouped into three categories—perineal muscles, pelvic floor muscles, and pelvic wall muscles. Examination of intrapelvic muscles for MTrPs requires a vaginal or rectal approach, as appropriate for each muscle by establishing bony and ligamentous landmarks, and relating the direction of palpation to the direction of the muscle fibers. This was explained in detail by Travell and Simons, as was the relationship between symptoms and the location of associated MTrPs.[12] Other MTrP associations have been gleaned from the experience of many physical therapists. Table 91-2 summarizes the internal pelvic muscles and external muscles referring pain to pelvis from MTrPs.

Approaches for Inactivating Myofascial Trigger Points

A variety of manual massage techniques have been reported to inactivate MTrPs.[29] Manual therapy may involve active and passive rhythmic muscle releases based on the principle that tight or poorly relaxed muscles can exhibit released tension after moderate voluntary contraction. The active and passive release maneuvers take up the slack in the muscle by stretching it to the point of beginning resistance or discomfort. This is then followed by a patient-performed isometric contraction that is held in position by the patient or therapist.

Direct transrectal massage was reported by Thiele for patients with coccygodynia with pain localized to the coccyx and the presence of spasms of the levator ani and coccygeus muscles.[14] A modified Thiele massage was used by Oyama and colleagues in 21 women to treat IC and high-tone dysfunction of the pelvic

Table 91-2 Internal and External Muscles and Referred Pain to Pelvis from Myofascial Trigger Points

Muscle	Referred Pain Site	Symptom
Pelvic floor muscles		
Levator ani	Sacrococcygeal region, perineal region	Pain in perineum, vagina, anal sphincter; pain with sitting; aggravated by lying on back and by defecation
Bulbospongiosus Ischiocavernosus Transverse perinei	Perineal region and adjacent urogenital structures	Pain in vagina, dyspareunia, perineal ache
Coccygeus	Sacrococcygeal region	Pain in coccyx, hip, or back; ischiococcygeus is likely cause of backache in late pregnancy and early labor
Sphincter ani	Poorly localized aching in anal region	Anal pain, painful bowel movement
Obturator internus	Perineal region, outward toward hip, whole pelvic floor, posterior thigh, and hamstrings	Pain in vagina, vulva, urethra, coccyx, posterior thigh; pain and feeling of fullness in rectum
Muscles referring pain into pelvis		
Piriformis	Sacroiliac joint, hip girdle, hamstrings, pelvic floor, buttock, low back	Pain in rectum during defecation, dyspareunia; pain in referred areas worsens with palpation, standing, sitting, walking
Gluteus	Hip girdle, buttock, sacrum, hamstrings	Pain in low back, hip, inguinal area
Iliopsoas	Groin, anterior thigh, low back	Pain in groin, down anterior thigh, and in low back
Quadratus lumborum	Sacroiliac joint and buttock, lower abdomen, groin	Pain in low back and with coughing, sneezing, and walking
Abdominals	Entire abdomen up into ribs	
Transverse	Groin, inguinal ligament, detrusor, and urinary sphincter	Groin pain, bladder pain, urinary frequency or retention
Rectus	Across thoracolumbar back, xiphoid process, sacroiliac joints, and low back	Somatovisceral response, nausea, vomiting, diarrhea, intestinal colic, dysmenorrhea
Pectineus Pyramidalis	Groin area, bladder, and pubis	Pain in groin, bladder, urethra, and pubic area
Thoracolumbar Paraspinals	Abdomen	Visceral pain, sacral pain, pain in middle and lower back; pain can resemble renal colic

Data from references 12, 37, 38, and 39.

floor (e.g., dyspareunia, impaired bladder and bowel evacuation, pelvic pain exacerbated by physical activity or prolonged sitting).[40] Subjects underwent 5 weeks of twice-weekly Thiele intravaginal massage, with massages of the affected hypertonic pelvic muscles, 10 to 15 times per session, from origin to insertion along the direction of muscle fibers. Additional short ischemic compression of tender points was applied as needed. IC symptom scores and pelvic floor muscle tone showed significant improvements, and pelvic tone remained improved at 4.5 months of follow-up in three of the four treated pelvic muscles, excepting the coccygeus.

Weiss reported amelioration of symptoms in 42 patients with urgency-frequency syndrome with or without urethral pain (and in some patients with IC) using manual therapy of discrete MTrPs in the pelvic floor.[18] Treatment continued one to two times weekly for 8 to 12 weeks until MTrPs and muscle tension decreased. A program of home therapy involving muscle stretches and strengthening, biofeedback, and Kegel exercises was also part of the treatment. In the 42 patients (39 women, 3 men) with urgency-frequency syndrome, 83% had moderate to marked improvements or complete resolution. Of the 10 patients with IC (6 women, 4 men), 70% had moderate to marked improvements.

Injection with local anesthetics, saline, or water has been used for inactivation of MTrPs. An important sign of precise needle placement in an MTrP is elicitation of a local twitch response. The resulting MTrP inactivation should result in immediate relief of pain and tightness.[24] Specific targeted therapy with local anesthetic injections of TrPs in the abdominal wall has been used for treatment of CPP in women.[41,42] Slocumb reported that approximately 50% of 122 women with pelvic pain had relief after treatment that consisted of TrP blocks in all patients; additional surgeries were performed in 13 women.[41] Most patients (89%) had abdominal wall TrPs; pain was relieved in 89% after anesthetic injection. Patients with only vaginal TrPs had a response rate of 85% after injections. TrP identification with needling and therapy of active MTrPs with 0.5% procaine injections was reported to provide symptomatic relief in four female patients with pelvic pain, IC, and irritative voiding symptoms.[37]

Associated Stress and Psychological Factors

CPP in women is a perplexing problem. Frequently, a physical cause of pain cannot be established, and, consequently, it is difficult to treat successfully. In the absence of a discrete physical cause, a psychopathologic causation has been considered.

Many reports have associated CPP with personality and mood disturbances, childhood events including sexual abuse, and difficulties in sexual relationships; evidence, however, is inconclusive.[43] Among the causes of CPP is tension myalgia of the pelvic floor. Recent evidence indicates that TrPs associated with myofascial problems are not the cause of CPP but a sign of somatization of neurotic or psychosomatic problems in the pelvis.[44-47] For example, Miller used stress management *alone* to effect symptom improvements in men with chronic prostatitis.[48] Eighty-six percent (110 of 218) of the patients reported that they were better, much better, or cured. Miller focused on the person and not the prostate, reinforcing the relationship between managing stress in the patients' lives and their symptoms.

One hypothesis for CPP is that acute and chronic stress induces neuroendocrine disturbances and consequent neuroinflammatory stimulus-activating receptors and cytokines via neuropeptide release that give rise to CPP symptomatology. Stress triggers a cascade of pathophysiologic events that involve activation of two pathways: the hypothalamic-pituitary-adrenal (HPA) axis and the autonomic nervous system. Chronic activation of the physiologic stress response induces putative glucocorticoid resistance and altered immunity, release of proinflammatory cytokines and prostaglandins that may contribute to pelvic tension myalgia, and, ultimately, cycling psychological distress. No systematic evaluation of the physiologic role of acute and chronic stress in pathogenesis of CPP in women has been undertaken. Over the years, clinicians have anecdotally observed that stress exacerbates symptoms, as has been shown for prostatitis,[48] and chronic stress was shown to induce inflammatory histologic changes in the prostate of a rat model.[49] Certain inherent personality traits (genetic and developmental factors) modulate reactivity to stress. Researchers at my institution have strong preliminary evidence from our male patients with CPP syndrome indicating that physiotherapeutic myofascial release and cognitive behavioral therapy, proven methods to relieve stress, can provide both curative and partial relief of pain in some patients with CPP syndrome.[50,51]

Physical and Mental Exercises Complementary to Management of Chronic Pelvic Pain

Emerging evidence suggests the influence of psychosocial factors on physiologic function and health outcomes. Mind-body therapeutic interventions, including yoga (a body-based therapy), cognitive behavioral therapy, relaxation therapy, meditation, and imagery, have shown efficacy in several common conditions. A recent systematic analysis showed that mind-body therapy can serve as an effective adjunct to conventional medical therapies for chronic low back pain, headaches, incontinence, and cardiac rehabilitation.[52] Hatha yoga has been proposed as a complimentary therapy for chronic urologic conditions involving pelvic floor dysfunction, to provide improved pain control and stress reduction. Specific yoga postures can contribute to the strengthening and relaxation of muscles that are associated with urologic symptoms resulting from hypotonicity (stress urinary incontinence) and hypertonicity (vulvodynia, IC) of pelvic floor muscles.[53]

In 1929, Edmund Jacobson published his method of "progressive relaxation," which has been used in various forms in Western medicine ever since.[54] He provided instructions to contract and relax muscles at the beginning of relaxation and, with Bell Telephone Laboratories, codeveloped the electromyograph to objectively verify the physiologic effects of tension and relaxation. He introduced the concept that relaxation of the gastrointestinal tract and arousal of the autonomic system, thought to be out of one's control, could be voluntarily reduced. A modification of progressive relaxation, the practice of "*paradoxical relaxation*" according to David Wise,[39] has been used successfully in conjunction with MTrP release therapy to produce symptomatic relief in men with CPP syndrome.[51]

Operant behavioral and cognitive-behavioral approaches to chronic pain were introduced in the 1960s and 1980s, respectively, and often serve as a component of multidisciplinary treatment dealing with anatomic and physiologic factors.[55] Aspects of these treatments include relaxation training, cognitive restructuring, interventions to change perception and emotional responses to pain, habit reversal, and maintenance and relapse prevention. These approaches are complementary for management of the psychosocial influences on a patient's response to pain. Because pain is not entirely a response to nociception, therapies such as these attempt to influence the behavior of a patient in chronic pain.

Clinical Experience with Combined Myofascial Trigger Point Release Therapy and Paradoxical Relaxation Therapy

A recent study at Stanford University has integrated physiotherapy with myofascial trigger point release therapy (MFRT) to relieve pelvic floor myalgia and paradoxical relaxation therapy to achieve autonomic and pelvic floor self regulation.[51] This study, although conducted in men with refractory CPP syndrome is nevertheless germane to both genders; it used multimodal therapy based on the potential etiology of pelvic pain as a manifestation of a neurobehavioral disorder.[7,19,20,56] A team approach to therapy included a urologist, a physical therapist experienced in pelvic pain treatment, and a psychologist.

The physiotherapist applied treatment to the patient in the lateral position. Individual muscle groups were palpated, and myofascial TrPs were identified. Positive myofascial TrPs induced pain on palpation that tends to reproduce symptoms at the site or referred to a nearby anatomic location. Pressure was held to each TrP for about 60 seconds to release.[39] Additional physiotherapy techniques also used in conjunction with MFRT sessions included voluntary contraction and release, hold and relax, contract and relax, and reciprocal inhibition as well as deep tissue mobilization including stripping, strumming, skin rolling, and effleurage. MFRT physiotherapy was given weekly for 4 weeks, then biweekly for 8 weeks.

Paradoxical relaxation therapy conducted by the psychologist coincided with physiotherapy. Patients received 1 hour of individual verbal instructions and a supervised practice session weekly for 8 weeks in progressive relaxation exercises. Training included the respiratory sinus arrhythmia breathing technique to quiet anxiety and relaxation training to have the patient focus attention on the effortless acceptance of tension in specific areas of the body. The therapy is called "paradoxical" because patients are directed to accepting their pelvic tension as a way of relaxing/releasing it.[39] Daily home practice relaxation sessions of 1 hour were recommended for a minimum of 6 months using a series of audiotaped lessons. Symptoms were assessed with a Pelvic Pain Symptom Survey and the National Institutes of Health-Chronic Prostatitis Symptom Index (NIH-CPSI). Patient-reported perceptions of overall effects of therapy were documented on a Global Response Assessment (GRA) questionnaire.

A total of 138 men with refractory chronic pain or CPP syndrome (CP/CPPS) and median disease duration of 31 months were treated; their average age 40.5 years. Symptoms were rated as markedly improved or moderately improved by 72% of patients on the GRA questionnaire at the conclusion of therapy. This was associated with commensurate clinically significant decreases in NIH-CPSI total scores of 10.5 (46%) and 6.5 (24%), respectively. The number of treatments was variable; some patients had rapid responses occurring as early as after 1 week of treatment and either further improved or remained the same. After a median of five MFRT treatments, clinical improvements (≥25% decrease in symptom scores) were first observed. A few patients had intermittent therapy, based on need, throughout recurring episodes of pelvic pain. The combined MFRT and paradoxical relaxation therapy provided an effective approach for these chronic pain patients, resulting in pain and urinary symptom relief at least comparable to or better than that achieved with traditional pharmacologic therapy.

The aspects of this treatment approach are amenable to the various expressions of pelvic pain in women. Each patient is unique in her objective and subjective clinical presentation. Thus, release of specific MTrPs that tend to recreate a patient's symptoms and behavior modification to relax the pelvic muscles and modify the habit of focusing tension in the pelvis under stress could help to ameliorate pain. The patient can also become an active participant, partnering with her therapists in the healing process.

ELECTRICAL STIMULATION FOR NEUROMODULATION

Electrical stimulation has been entertained as a modality for treating pain since the distant past, when a man stepped on an eel at the beach and experienced an electrical shock that relieved his gout pain. Multiple attempts to introduce electrical energy have arisen, from Chinese acupuncture, through surface application using transcutaneous electrical nerve stimulation (TENS), to implantation of electrodes for continuous electrical stimulation of peripheral and spinal nerve roots and electrodes applied on the surface of the spinal cord itself.

The gate control theory of controlling pain assumes that afferent nerve fibers may be influenced by continuous high-frequency electrical stimulation and thereby modulate the transmission of pain impulses. TENS has been used most successfully and was introduced for bladder urgency and urinary frequency as well as stress urinary incontinence. One disadvantage of this method may be the lack of specificity of the nerve branch or bundle of the afflicted nerve. Direct stimulation of the S3 nerve as it exits the sacrum has recently received approval from the U.S. Food and Drug Administration for management of frequency, urgency, and urge urinary incontinence refractory to medical therapy. Because pelvic pain, particularly that arising from IC, may represent a neuroinflammatory pathogenic condition, electrical modulation promises to exert favorable outcomes in pain management.

The application of intravaginal electrical stimulation to treatment of CPP in women with levator ani syndrome was evaluated in a retrospective study of 66 patients.[57] After digital vaginal palpation of the levator ani muscles for tenderness, a probe was placed in the patient's vagina and pulsed electrical stimulation was given to muscles at variable settings (up to 50 mA for up to 20 minutes per session) for one to seven sessions. Pain symptoms were reported as improved in 34 (52%) of 66 patients; benefit was sustained for more than 6 months after the last treatment. Electrical stimulation for management of vulvar vestibulitis including dyspareunia and vaginismus has been shown to be effective.[58] A group of 29 women participated in a 10-week therapy program of stimulation (20 minutes once weekly) at the vestibular area and vagina introitus. Contractile ability and resting ability of the pelvic floor muscles significantly improved; pain was significantly reduced, and half of the women with vaginismus resumed coital activity.

The therapeutic effects of high-frequency electrostimulation were also assessed in men with noninflammatory CPP syndromes using a urethroanal stimulation device.[59] This approach was based on the supposition that chronic prostate pain may represent a chronic visceral pain,[36] and the authors' speculation that electrical stimulation might block afferent nerves supplying the pelvic floor and pelvic organs, thereby providing pain relief. This premise was supported by another study showing that sacral nerve stimulation can provide a dramatic and durable improvement in pain symptoms and urgency-frequency.[60] The neuronal mechanisms associated with bladder inhibition during intravaginal electrical stimulation have been documented experimentally in the cat.[61]

Sacral neuromodulation is an approved treatment for management of refractory detrusor instability and nonobstructive voiding dysfunction; it has also been shown to be effective for amelioration of pelvic pain.[62-64] An early study with TENS indicated the possibility for treatment of the chronic painful bladder syndrome, IC.[65] Favorable responses to a percutaneous trial stimulation of the S3 sacral roots for as few as 5 days or up to 10 days have been shown for IC patients.[66,67] Significant improvements occurred in urinary dysfunction, pelvic pain, and quality of life parameters. The test neuromodulation normalized urinary levels of heparin-binding epidermal growth factor and antiproliferative factor activity—factors known to be altered in patients with IC.[66] The temporary nature of the percutaneous stimulation evaluation permits assessment of the potential efficacy and desirability of permanent sacral neurostimulation.

Neuromodulation is the physiologic process by which the activity in a neural pathway alters preexisting activity in another pathway. It is theorized that sacral neurostimulation causes afferent inhibition of sensory processing in the spinal cord. The S2-S4 nerve roots provide the primary anatomic and somatic innervations to the pelvic floor, bladder, and urethra. Comiter indicated that the mechanism associated with the effectiveness of sacral nerve stimulation for IC involves both afferent (pelvic pain and sensory urgency) and efferent (motor frequency and urgency) modulation.[68]

Comiter evaluated the efficacy of sacral nerve stimulation for treatment of refractory IC in 25 patients.[68] After a trial of nerve stimulation, 17 patients demonstrating at least 50% improvement in pain and urinary dysfunction qualified for permanent nerve stimulator implantation. Improvements were sustained in 16 of 17 patients for an average of 14 months' follow-up after permanent implantation. In a retrospective study, the efficacy of long-term sacral neuromodulation was evaluated in 21 patients with refractory IC by Peters and Konstandt.[69] Eighteen patients had used chronic narcotics for pain. After an average follow-up of 15 months after surgery for implantation of a permanent nerve stimulator, 20 patients reported marked improvements in pain, with a significant decrease (36%) in narcotic requirements; all narcotics were stopped in 4 of 18 patients.

Siegel and colleagues used sacral nerve stimulation to treat intractable pelvic pain in 10 patients (9 women, 1 man) without a primary complaint of voiding dysfunction.[70] After successful percutaneous trial nerve stimulation, a neuroprosthetic sacral nerve stimulator device was surgically implanted, with leads placed in the S3 or S4 foramen. Follow-up was after a median of 19 months. Nine of 10 patients had decreased severity and frequency of pelvic pain; 6 had significant improvements in pain symptoms. No serious device complications were reported.

Spinal cord stimulation (SCS) has been used since 1967 for the treatment of chronic lower back or lower extremity pain of diverse causes that is refractory to numerous conventional therapies. The work of Shealy and colleagues led to the development of this pain therapy, which was then used exclusively for failed back syndrome.[71] As the clinical applications of SCS expanded in the following years, the outcomes were poor due to a lack of understanding of the appropriate clinical indications, SCS equipment technical failures, and the need for a trial stimulation period to identify patients who might achieve a long-term benefit. Based on increased knowledge, SCS outcomes throughout the last 2 decades were found to provide reasonable (>45% to 60%) long-term pain relief.[72-75] There is a better understanding of the psychological factors that are predictive of SCS outcomes.[74] Avoidance of implants in patients with severe untreated depression, untreated drug abuse, or borderline personality disorder has led to improved outcomes.[76] A recent review presents the current and future trends of SCS.[77]

Technologic advances, which have widened the scope of applications for SCS, include multichannel leads, dual-lead configurations, multichannel devices, totally implantable generators, and new procedures for programming stimulators. The primary indication for treatment with SCS is neuropathic pain that has failed to be relieved by other conservative approaches. With the discovery of the dual-lead technology, the clinical applications have expanded. Acceptable relief was attained in 70% of patients with chronic axial low back and extremity pain.[78] Several patients with intractable pain of the pelvis and rectum have been treated with the dual leads.[79] SCS is a relatively simple and reversible treatment using greatly improved and clinically reliable equipment. It may serve as an option for patients with moderate to severe pain of the trunk or extremities when other pain relief methods have failed or are unacceptable. Studies of SCS for amelioration of CPP warrant further investigation.

BOTULINUM A TOXIN

Botulinum A toxin (BTX-A) is a neurotoxin derived from *Clostridium botulinum* that binds irreversibly to cholinergic, presynaptic membranes of the neuromuscular junction. When a minute amount is injected into a muscle, it prevents release of acetylcholine, thereby blocking neurotransmission and temporarily paralyzing affected muscles. It can provide symptomatic relief for up to 3 months. In the United States, BTX-A is approved for treatment of blepharospasm, strabismus, hemifascial spasm, and cervical dystonia in adults. In Europe, labeled indications are for cervical dysplasia and cerebral palsy. BTX-A has received much notoriety for its cosmetic use for facial wrinkles and in pain therapy to treat myofascial pain, low back pain, and headaches including migraine.

BTX-A has been used clinically for more than 2 decades: there is continued accumulation of evidence for its application for a variety of urologic conditions.[80] Experience with BTX-A in neurourology began in the early 1990s with treatment of neurogenic-sphincter dyssynergia after spinal cord injury, neurogenic and non-neurogenic detrusor hyperactivity, and other dysfunctional voiding disorders.[81] BTX-A injections have been used to treat voiding symptoms related to CPP syndromes in men.[82]

It has been hypothesized that interruption of the junction of somatic nerves with striated muscles may affect the central pain cycle. Zermann and coworkers used transurethral perisphinchteric injections of BTX-A in 11 patients with chronic prostatic pain.[83] Injections resulted in pelvic floor muscle weakening and relief of pelvic pain and urethral hypersensitivity.

A pilot study explored the use of BTX-A in the treatment of CPP associated with spasm of the levator ani muscles.[84] The 12 women had a minimum 2-year history of pelvic pain and pelvic floor hypertonicity. BTX-A at one of three dilutions (10, 20, or 100 IU/mL) in groups of four patients was injected bilaterally into the puborectalis and pubococcygeus muscles under conscious sedation. Visual analogue pain scale scores were significantly improved for dyspareunia and dysmenorrhea at the 12-week follow-up. Pelvic floor muscle manometry had a 37% maximal reduction at week 4 and a statistically significant 25% reduction at week 12. Marked improvement in sexual activity was associated with significant reductions in discomfort and improved habit. No differences in response were noted with different dilutions of BTX-A; no medically adverse reactions occurred.

A multicenter case series of 13 patients with recalcitrant IC was described using intravesical BTX-A.[85] This study was based on evidence from a rat somatic pain model suggesting that BTX-A may have an antinociceptive effect on both acute and chronic pain.[86] Patients were injected submucosally with 10 RA to 20 RA IU/mL of BTX-A through a cystoscope into 20 to 30 sites to target dense sensory innervations in the trigone and bladder floor. Pain, daytime frequency, and nocturia measured by visual analogue scale scores decreased significantly ($P < .01$) by 79%, 44%, and 45%, respectively. First desire to void and maximal cystometric capacity also increased by more than 50% ($P < .01$). These observations, although preliminary, suggest the potential application of BTX-A for symptomatic and functional improvements in IC.

BTX-A for treatment of urologic conditions has had a good safety profile with relatively few significant side effects. Leippold and colleagues have expressed their perspective on BTX-A as follows: "One cannot deny human ingenuity in transforming the lethal poison into a modern day therapeutic medicine."[87] Possible systemic side effects of BTX-A injection, although unusual, include nausea, vomiting, dysphagia, dry mouth, diplopia, and blurred vision, which may be due to unintentional distribution of the toxin. The incidence of systemic side effects treated in a variety of urologic conditions was reviewed by Maan and colleagues.[80] A limited number of papers have reported on localized side effects associated with toxin diffusion and possible overdosing of the targeted tissue, including temporary stress incontinence in female patients treated for chronic retention, or urinary retention, or severe generalized muscle weakness (as reviewed by Leippold and colleagues[87]). Contraindications for BTX-A injections are pregnancy, breastfeeding, myasthenia gravis, muscular dystrophy, use of aminoglycosides or any drugs that interfere with neuromuscular transmission, and hemophilia or hereditary clotting factor deficiencies.

Further research on BTX-A for treatment of CPP is warranted. Additional, larger studies are needed to explore the biologic and clinical effects of BTX-A including a placebo-control arm. Because the effects of the drug are temporary and most patients require repeat treatments, evaluation of the safety, benefits, and cost of repeated injections of the toxin are needed. In some cases, BTX-A given at high doses (>100 IU) for neurologic conditions has been shown to induce the development of antibodies (occurring in <5% of patients), making further treatment ineffective.[88] Seven serologically different types of BTX exist, each with distinct properties and actions. A new product containing botulinum B toxin has been effective in treating pain and other symptoms of cervical dystonia in patients who developed antibodies and stopped responding to BTX-A.

MANAGEMENT OF PUDENDAL NERVE ENTRAPMENT SYNDROME

Compression entrapment of pudendal nerves in the pelvis may be the cause of urogenital and anorectal pain syndromes.[89-93] Robert and colleagues conducted anatomic and clinical studies and elucidated three possible entrapment sites along the pudendal nerve: between the sacrotuberous and sacrospinous ligaments, in the pudendal canal of Alcock, and during the straddling of the falciform process of the sacrotuberous ligament by the pudendal nerve and its branches.[92] Female patients may complain of perineal, anal, and/or vaginal pain while sitting, which is diminished when standing, when in the recumbent position, or when sitting on a toilet seat. It is the positional nature of the pain and its relief when standing that are the most important diagnostic clues. Pain is not related to urination or defecation, although chronic constipation and straining with bowel movement may contribute to the condition.[93] Pudendal neuropathies secondary to pressure effects on the perineum have been reported in competitive bicyclists due to seat positions.[94] Because pudendal nerve entrapment causes symptoms similar to other pain syndromes, including coccygodynia, levator ani syndrome, urethral syndrome, and idiopathic proctalgia, misdiagnosis is possible.[95] Cases of idiopathic vulvodynia have been subsequently attributed to pudendal neuralgia.[96-98]

Physical examination of patients with symptoms of pudendal nerve entrapment typically reveals little about the cause. Reproduction of pain can be generated by digital rectal or vaginal examination along the course of the pudendal nerve deep within the pelvis. Robert and colleagues stated that the "richness of the subjective manifestation contrasts with the poverty of the clinical examination and the normality of the radiologic examination."[99] Electrophysiologic tests may be performed to measure the distal latency time of the pudendal nerve (upper limit of normal, 2.5 msec). This procedure has been described using a St. Mark's Hospital pudendal electrode that incorporates stimulating and recording electrodes on an adhesive sheet that fits on a gloved index finger for intrarectal placement.[95]

Pudendal nerve block with local anesthetics, alone or with corticosteroids, has been used for diagnosis and treatment of various perineal pain syndromes and may yield temporary pain relief. Computed tomography (CT) has been described as the best technique for good appreciation of the anatomy and precise location of anatomic points to guide blocking of pudendal nerves at potential entrapment sites.[100-103] In other instances, use of an insulated electrode to localize the pudendal nerve with electrical stimulation allows local infiltration of long-acting bupivacaine with or without corticosteroid. In some reports, the pain relief continued for 1 year after the last anesthetic block in more than 60% of patients.[92,102] McDonald and Spigos treated 26 women with severe pelvic pain with CT-guided nerve blocks once monthly for 5 months.[104] Improvement was reported by 73% (19/26), and 16 women (62%) had substantial pain reduction based on pain scale scores. The favorable results were attributed to correct placement of the local anesthetic. No response duration was reported.

Patients with pudendal neuralgia caused by involvement of the pudendal nerve may be appropriate candidates for surgical decompression after confirmation of the diagnosis by electrophysiologic tests and diagnosis and temporary pain relief with nerve block injections. Robert and coworkers reported their experience with more than 200 procedures for neurolysis and transposition over the sciatic spine of one or both pudendal nerves.[92,99,102] The success rate was 67% (45% complete pain relief and 22% significant improvement). In another series by Amarenco and colleagues, in 170 cases of perineal neuralgia treated with pudendal nerve block, 57% of patients had pain relief, but only 15% had sustained relief after 1 year.[91] Subsequent surgical decompression in 27 patients yielded a good to excellent result in 17 (62%). Shafik reported the disappearance of vulvar pain in 9 (82%) of 11 women after pudendal canal fasciotomy to release the pudendal nerve in the ischiorectal fossa.[98] An algorithm for treating pudendal neuralgia has been developed from 212 cases, approximately half of which involved surgical decompression after negative responses to nerve block; 86% of the patients were free of pain or had a significant pain reduction after 1 year of follow-up.[105]

Predictive factors related to the postoperative success of patients with pudendal nerve entrapment include duration and clinical characteristic of pain and signs of pudendal neurogenic lesions with electrophysiologic testing. From a series of patients reported by Robert and coworkers, factors associated with improved success included shorter duration of pain before surgical treatment, age younger than 50 years, and discovery of a damaged nerve.[92.102] Factors associated with decreased success were pudendal nerve distal motor latency of greater than 7.0 msec, age older than 70 years at surgery, and the finding of a normal nerve. Depression is known to be a component of pain syndromes. It has been suggested that surgery should be avoided in patients in whom a depression is manifested as chronic anal/perineal pain.[106.107] Neurolysis-transposition of the pudendal nerve failed in 5 of 6 depressed patients treated by Maullion and associates.[108]

Maullion and coworkers examined the efficacy of pudendal nerve blocks as a predictive factor for the subsequent efficacy of nerve decompression surgery.[108] Twelve patients with urogenital and rectal pain were initially treated with CT-guided injections of lidocaine/corticosteroids in the pudendal nerves. Surgical treatment was proposed if pain recurred after temporary improvements or after nerve block failure. All patients underwent surgery for decompression of the sacrotuberous and sacrospinous ligaments and either unilateral or bilateral transposition of pudendal nerves proximal to the ischial spine. After 21 months, 25% (3 of 12) patients remained asymptomatic, and one had partial improvement; eight remained in pain. The three patients cured by surgery had complete pain relief for at least 2 weeks after neurolysis repeated twice before nerve transposition. This was considered the best criterion to predict the success of surgery.

References

1. Olsen RP: Definitions of biofeedback and applied psychophysiology. In Schwartz MS, Andrasik F (eds.) Biofeedback: A Practitioner's Guide, 2nd ed. NewYork, The Guilford Press, 1995, p 29.
2. Schwartz MS: Biofeedback: A Practitioner's Guide, 2nd ed. New York, The Guilford Press, 1995.
3. Tan G, Sherman R, Shanti BF: Biofeedback pain interventions. Pract Pain Manage 3:12, 2003.
4. Sherman RA, Davis GD, Wong MF: Behavioral treatment of exercise-induced urinary continence among female soldiers. Mil Med 162:690, 1997.
5. Clemens JQ, Nadler RB, Schaeffer AJ, et al: Biofeedback, pelvic floor re-education, and bladder training for male chronic pelvic pain syndrome. Urology 56:951, 2000.
6. Cornel EB, van Haarst EP, Schaarsberg RW, Geels J: The effect of biofeedback physical therapy in men with chronic pelvic pain syndrome type III. Eur Urol 47:607-611, 2005. Epub 2005 Jan 22.
7. Glazer HI, Rodke G, Swencionis C, et al: Treatment of vulvar vestibulitis syndrome with electromyographic biofeedback of pelvic floor musculature. J Reprod Med 40:282, 1995.
8. Balick L, Elfner L, May J, et al: Biofeedback treatment of dysmenorrhea. Biofeedback Self-Regul 7:499, 1982.
9. Bennick CD, Hulst LL, Bentham JA: The effects of EMG biofeedback and relaxation training on primary dysmenorrhea. J Behav Med 5:329, 1982.
10. McKay E, Kaufman RH, Doctor U, et al: Treating vulvar vestibulitis with electromyographic biofeedback of pelvic floor musculature. J Reprod Med 46:337, 2001.
11. Glazer HI, Romanzi L, Polanecsky M: Pelvic floor muscle surface electromyography. J Reprod Med 44:779, 1999.
12. Travell J, Simons D: Myofascial Pain and Dysfunction: The Trigger Point Manual, vols 1 & 2, 2nd ed. Philadelphia, Lippincott Williams & Wilkins, 1998.
13. Marinoff SC, Turner MLC: Vulvar vestibulitis syndrome. Dermatol Clin 10:435, 1992.
14. Thiele GH: Coccygodynia: Cause and treatment. Dis Colon Rectum 6:422, 1963.
15. Sinaki M: Tension myalgia of the pelvic floor. Mayo Clin Proc 52:717, 1977.
16. Travell JG, Simons DG: Myofascial Pain and Dysfunction: The Trigger Point Manual. Vol 2. Baltimore, Williams & Wilkins, 1992.
17. Lukban J, Whitmore K, Kellogg-Spadt S, et al: The manual therapy in patients diagnosed with interstitial cystitis, high-tone pelvic floor dysfunction, and sacroiliac dysfunction. J Urol 57:121, 2001.
18. Weiss JM: Pelvic floor myofascial trigger points: Manual therapy for interstitial cystitis and the urgency-frequency syndrome. J Urol 166:2226, 2001.
19. Barbalias GA, Meares EMJ, Sant GR: Prostatodynia: Clinical and urodynamic characteristics. J Urol 130:514, 1983.
20. Hetrick DC, Ciol MA, Rothman I, et al: Musculoskeletal dysfunction in men with chronic pelvic pain syndrome type III: A case-control study. J Urol 170:828, 2003.
21. Travell JG: Myofascial trigger points: Clinical view. In Bonica JJ, Albe-Fessard D (eds): Advances in Pain Research and Therapy, vol 1. New York, Raven Press, 1976, pp 919-826.
22. Travell JG, Simons DG: Myofascial Pain and Dysfunction: The Trigger Point Manual. Baltimore, Williams & Wilkins, 1983.
23. Simons DG, Travell JG: Myofascial origins of low back pain: 1. Principles of diagnosis and treatment. Postgrad Med 73:66, 1983.
24. Hong C-Z: Consideration and recommendation of myofascial trigger point injection. J Musculoskel Pain 2:29, 1994.
25. Hong C-Z: Pathophysiology of myofascial TrP. J Formos Med Assoc 95:93, 1996.
26. Simons DG: Clinical and etiological update of myofascial pain from trigger points. J Musculoskeletal Pain 4:93, 1996.
27. Hong C-Z, Simons DG: Pathophysiologic and electrophysiologic mechanisms of myofascial trigger points. Arch Phys Med Rehabil 79:863, 1998.
28. Simons DG: Review of enigmatic MTrPs as a common cause of enigmatic musculoskeletal pain and dysfunction. J Electromyogr Kinesiol 14:95, 2004.
29. Simons DG, Travell JG, Simons LS: Travell and Simons' Myofascial Pain and Dysfunction: The Trigger Point Manual. Baltimore, Williams & Wilkins, 1999.
30. Mense S, Simons DG: Muscle Pain: Understanding its Nature, Diagnosis, and Treatment. Philadelphia, Lippincott Williams & Wilkins, 2001.
31. Hubbard DR, Berkoff GM: Myofascial trigger points show spontaneous needle EMG activity. Spine 18:1803, 1983.
32. McNutley WH, Gevirtz RN, Hubbard DR, et al: Needle electromyographic evaluation of trigger point response to a psychological stress. Psychophysiology 31:313, 1994.
33. Fischer AA, Chang CH: Temperature and pressure threshold measurements in trigger points. Thermology 1:212, 1986.
34. Reeves JL, Jaeger B, Graff-Radford SB: Reliability of pressure algometer as a measure of myofascial trigger point sensitivity. Pain 24:313, 1986.
35. Kruse RA, Christiansen JA: Thermographic imaging of myofascial trigger points: A follow-up study. Arch Phys Med Rehab 73:819, 1992.
36. Wesselmann U, Burnett AL, Heinberg LJ: The urogenital and rectal pain syndromes. Pain 73:269, 1997.
37. Doggweiler-Wiygul R, Wiygul JP: Interstitial cystitis, pelvic pain, and the relationship to myofascial pain and dysfunction: A report on four patients. World J Urol 20:310, 2003.
38. Prendergast SA, Weiss JM: Screening for musculoskeletal causes of pelvic pain. Clin Obstet Gynecol 46:1, 2003.
39. Wise D, Anderson RU: A Headache in the Pelvis: A New Understanding and Treatment for Prostatitis and Chronic Pelvic Pain Syndromes, 3rd ed. Occidental, CA, National Center for Pelvic Pain Research, 2005.
40. Oyama IA, Rejba A, Lukban JC, et al: Modified Thiele massage as therapeutic intervention for female patients with interstitial cystitis and high-tone pelvic floor dysfunction. Urology 64:862, 2004.
41. Slocumb JC: Neurologic factors in chronic pelvic pain: Trigger points and the abdominal pelvic syndrome. Am J Obstet Gynecol 149:536, 1983.
42. Ling FW, Slocumb JC: Use of trigger point injections in chronic pelvic pain. Obstet Gynecol Clin North Am 20:809, 1993.
43. Savidge CJ, Slade P: Psychological aspects of chronic pelvic pain. J Psychosom Res 42:433, 1997.
44. Rosenthal RH: Psychology of chronic pelvic pain. Obstet Gynecol Clin North Am 20:627, 1993.
45. Dellenbach P, Haeringer MT: Chronic pelvic pain: Expression of a psychological problem. [In French] Presse Med 25:615, 1996.
46. Bodden-Heidrich R, Busch M, Kuppers V, et al: Chronic pelvic pain and chronic vulvodynia as multifactorial psychosomatic disease syndromes: Results of a psychometric and clinical study taking into account musculoskeletal diseases. [In German] Zentralbl Gynakol 121:389, 1999.
47. Nijenhuis ER, Van Dyck R, Ter Kuile MM, et al: Evidence for association among somatoform disassociation, psychological dissociation and reported trauma in patients with chronic pelvic pain. J Psyhcosom Obstet Gynaecol 24:87, 2003.
48. Miller HC: Stress prostatitis. Urology 32:507, 1988.
49. Gatenbeck L, Aronsson A, Dahlgren S, et al: Stress stimuli-induced histopatho-logical changes in the prostate: An experimental study in the rat. Prostate 11:69, 1987.
50. Anderson RU: Management of chronic prostatitis-chronic pelvic pain. Urol Clin North Am 29:235, 2002.

51. Anderson RU, Wise D, Sawyer T, Chan C: Integration of myofascial trigger point release and paradoxical relaxation training for treatment of chronic pelvic pain in men. J Urol 174:155-160, 2005.
52. Astin JA, Shapiro SL, Eisenberg DM, et al: Mind-body medicine: State of science, implications for practice. J Am Board Fam Pract 16:131, 2003.
53. Ripoll E, Mahowald D: Hatha Yoga therapy management of urologic disorders. World J Urol 20:306, 2002.
54. Jacobson E: Progressive Relaxation. Chicago & London, The University of Chicago, 1929.
55. McCracken LM, Turk DC: Behavioral and cognitive-behavioral treatment for chronic pain: Outcome, predictors of outcome and treatment process. Spine 27:2564, 2002.
56. Zermann DH, Ishigooka M, Doggweiler R, et al: Neurological insights into the etiology of genitourinary pain in men. J Urol 161:903, 1999.
57. Fitzwater JB, Kuehl TJ, Schrier JJ: Electrical stimulation in the treatment of pelvic pain due to levator ani spasm. J Reprod Med 48:573, 2003.
58. Nappi RE, Ferdeghini F, Abbiati I, et al: Electrical stimulation (ES) in the management of sexual pain disorders. J Sex Marital Ther 29:103, 2003.
59. John H, Rüedi C, Kötting S, et al: A new high frequency electrostimulation device to treat chronic prostatitis. J Urol 170:1275, 2003.
60. Schmidt RA, Jonas U, Oleson KA, et al: Sacral nerve stimulation for treatment of refractory urinary urge incontinence. J Urol 162:352, 1999.
61. Lindstrom S, Fall M, Carlsson C-A, et al: The neurophysiological basis of bladder inhibition in response to intravaginal electrical stimulation. J Urol 129:405, 1983.
62. Thon WF, Raskin LS, Jonas U, et al: Neuromodulation of voiding dysfunction and pelvic pain. World J Urol 9:138, 1991.
63. Shaker HS, Hassouna M: Sacral nerve root neuromodulation: An effective treatment for refractory urge incontinence. J Urol 159:1516, 1998.
64. Weil EH, Ruiz-Cerda JL, Janknegt RA, et al: Clinical results of sacral neuromodulation for chronic voiding dysfunction using unilateral sacral foramen electrodes. World J Urol 16:313, 1998.
65. Fall M: Conservative management of chronic interstitial cystitis: Transcutaneous electrical nerve stimulation and transurethral resection. J Urol 133:774, 1985.
66. Chai TC, Zhang C-O, Warren JW, et al: Percutaneous sacral third nerve root neurostimulation improves symptoms and normalizes urinary HB-EGF levels and antiproliferative activity in patients with interstitial cystitis. Urology 55:643, 2000.
67. Maher CF, Carey MP, Dwyer PL, et al: Percutaneous sacral nerve root neuromodulation for intractable interstitial cystitis. J Urol 165:884, 2001.
68. Comiter CV: Sacral neuromodulation for the symptomatic treatment of refractory interstitial cystitis: A prospective study. J Urol 169:1369, 2003.
69. Peters KM, Konstandt D: Sacral neuromodulation decreases narcotic requirements in refractory interstitial cystitis. BJU Int 93:777, 2004.
70. Siegel S, Paskiewicz E, Kirkpatrick C, et al: Sacral nerve stimulation in patients with chronic intractable pelvic pain. J Urol 166:1742, 2001.
71. Shealy C, Mortimer J, Reswick J: Electrical inhibitors of pain by stimulation of the dorsal column: Preliminary clinical reports. Anesth Analg 46:489, 1967.
72. Spiegelmann R, Friedman WA: Spinal cord stimulation: A contemporary series. Neurosurgery 28:65, 1991.
73. North R, Kidd D, Fabarch M, et al: Spinal cord stimulation, intractable pain: Experience over two decades. Neurosurgery 32:384, 1993.
74. Burchiel KJ, Anderson VC, Wilson BJ, et al: Prognostic factors of spinal cord stimulation for chronic back and leg pain. Neurosurgery 36:1101, 1995.
75. Kumar K, Toth C, Nath RK, et al: Epidural spinal cord stimulation for treatment of chronic pain: Some predictors of success. A 15-year experience. Pain 50:110, 1998.
76. Nelson D: Psychological selection criteria for implantable spinal cord stimulators. Pain Forum 5:93, 1996.
77. Deer TR: Current and future trends in spinal cord stimulation. Curr Pain Headache Rep 5:503, 2001.
78. Burchiel KJ, Anderson VC, Brown FD, et al: Prospective, multicenter study of spinal cord stimulation for relief of chronic back and extremity pain. Spine 21:2786, 1996.
79. Alo KM, Gohel R, Corey CL: Sacral nerve root stimulation for the treatment of urge incontinence and detrusor dysfunction utilizing a cephalocaudal intraspinal method of lead insertion: A case report. Neuromodulation 4:53, 2001.
80. Maan Z, Al-Singary W, Shergill I, et al: Alternative use of botulinum toxin in urology. Expert Opin Pharmacother 5:1015, 2004.
81. Schulte-Baukloh H, Knispel HH: Botulinum toxin urology: An inventory. Urologie A 43:963, 2004.
82. Maria G, Dsito A, Lacquanit S, et al: Relief by botulinum toxin of voiding dysfunction due to prostatitis. Lancet 352:625, 1998.
83. Zermann D, Ishigooka M, Schubert J, et al: Perisphinchteric injection of botulinum toxin type A: A treatment option for patients with chronic prostatic pain? Eur Urol 38:393, 2000.
84. Jarvis SK, Abbott JA, Lenart MB, et al: Pilot study of botulinum toxin type A in the treatment of chronic pelvic pain associated with spasm of the levator ani muscles. Aust N Z J Obstet Gynaecol 44:46, 2004.
85. Smith CP, Radziszewski P, Borkowski A, et al: Botilinum toxin A has antinocioceptive effects in treating interstitial cystitis. Urology 64:871, 2004.
86. Cui M, Khanijou S, Rubino J, et al: Subcutaneous administration of botulinum toxin type A reduces formalin-induced pain. Pain 107:125, 2004.
87. Leippold, Reitz A, Schurch B: Botulinum toxin as a new therapy option for voiding disorders: Current state of art. Eur Urol 44:165, 2003.
88. Goschel H, Wohlfarth K, Frevert J, et al: Botulinum A toxin therapy: Neutralizing and nonneutralizing antibodies-therapeutic consequences. Exp Neurol 147:96, 1997.
89. Amarenco G, Savatovsky I, Budet C, et al: Perineal neuralgia and Alcock's canal syndrome. Ann Urol 23:488, 1989.
90. Robert R, Labat JJ, Lehur PA, et al: Clinical, neurophysiologic and therapeutic remarks from anatomic data on the pudendal nerve in some cases of perineal pain. Chirurgie 115:515, 1989.
91. Amarenco G, Kerdraon J, Bouju P, et al: Treatments of perineal neuralgia caused by involvement of the pudendal nerve. Rev Neurol (Paris) 153:331, 1997.
92. Robert R, Prat-Pradal D, Labat JJ, et al: Anatomic basis of chronic perineal pain: Role of the pudendal nerve. Surg Radiol Anat 20:93, 1998.
93. Shafik A: Pudendal canal syndrome: A cause of chronic pelvic pain. Urology 60:199, 2002.
94. Silbert PL, Dunne JW, Edis RH, et al: Bicycling induced pudendal nerve pressure neuropathy. Clin Exp Neurol 28:191, 1991.
95. Ramsden CE, McDaniel MC, Harmon RL, et al: Pudendal nerve entrapment as source of intractable pain. Am J Phys Med Rehabil 82:479, 2003.
96. Turner ML, Marinoff SC: Pudendal neuralgia. Am J Obstet Gynecol 165:1233, 1991.
97. McKay M: Vulvodynia: Diagnostic patterns. Dermatol Clin 10:423, 1992.
98. Shafik A: Pudendal canal syndrome as a cause of vulvodynia and its treatment by pudendal nerve decompression. Eur J Obstet Gynecol Reprod Biol 80:215, 1998.

99. Robert T, Brunet C. Faure A, et al: Surgery of the pudendal nerve in various types of perineal pain. Chirurgie 119:535, 1993.
100. Labat JJ, Robert R, Bensignor M, et al: Neuralgia of the pudendal nerve: Anatomo-clinical considerations and therapeutical approach. J Urol 96:239, 1990.
101. Thoumas D, Leroi AM, Maullion J, et al: Pudendal neuralgia: CT-guided pudendal nerve block techniques. Abdom Imaging 24:309, 1999.
102. Besignor M, Labat JJ, Robert R, et al: Perineal pain, anorectal, and urogenital. Pain 1:131, 2000.
103. Hough DM, Wittenberg KH, Pawlina W, et al: Chronic perineal pain caused by pudendal nerve entrapment: Anatomy and CT-guided perineural injection technique. AJR Am J Roentgenol 181:561, 2003.
104. McDonald JS, Spigos DG: Computed tomography-guided pudendal block for treatment of pelvic pain due to pudendal neuropathy. Obstet Gynecol 95:306, 2000.
105. Bautrant E, de Bisschop E, Vaini-Elies V, et al: Modern algorithm for treating pudendal neuralgia: 212 Cases and 104 decompressions. J Gynecol Obstet Biol Reprod (Paris) 32:705, 2003.
106. Magni G, deBertolini C, Dodi G, et al: Psychological findings in chronic anal pain. Psychopharmacology 1:170, 1986.
107. Henry C, Guenther F, Guex P, et al: Chronic anogenital and perineal pain: Clinical and psychopathological characteristics of a syndrome. Rev Med Suisse Romande 111:27, 1991.
108. Mauillon J, Thoumas D, Leroi AM, et al: Results of pudendal nerve neurolysis- transposition in twelve patients suffering from pudendal neuralgia. Dis Colon Rectum 42:186, 1999.

Chapter 92

PAINFUL BLADDER SYNDROME AND INTERSTITIAL CYSTITIS

Christopher Kennerly Payne

EVOLUTION OF TERMINOLOGY: PAINFUL BLADDER SYNDROME AND INTERSTITIAL CYSTITIS

The last 20 years has produced and explosion of interest in the diagnosis and treatment of bladder pain. Although the attention is welcomed by patients, clinicians, and researchers alike, there is a simultaneous sense of insecurity and confusion as traditional ideas are challenged. Even the name identifying the condition, interstitial cystitis (IC), has been questioned. The original description of Hunner's ulcers characterized a very small group of patients with a clearly defined disease defined by erythematous, bleeding areas on the bladder wall and physically diminished bladder capacity.[1] In 1949, Hand[2] described 223 patients, both men and women, with what would now be called IC; only 13% had severe cystoscopic findings. Nevertheless, it was left to Messing and Stamey[3] to focus attention on the disorder; they described an "early diagnosis" of IC based on cystoscopic identification of glomerulations after bladder distention. This dramatically increased the population of patients considered to have IC while simultaneously raising a question as to whether these patients really had the same underlying disease. Most patients with glomerulations have normal cystoscopic findings before distention, normal bladder capacity during distention, and relatively little inflammation on bladder biopsies. Can these patients have the same condition as those with frank ulceration? In recent years, the population has been further expanded by a move to diagnose patients based on symptoms without performing bladder distention and biopsy.

The International Continence Society (ICS) proposed useful definitions to promote clarity in discussing the problem of bladder pain.[4] First, it is recognized that bladder pain is part of a larger problem of genitourinary pain or pelvic pain syndromes. The document states, "The syndromes described are functional abnormalities for which a precise cause has not been defined. It is presumed that routine assessment (history taking, physical examination, and other appropriate investigations) has excluded obvious local pathologies such as those that are infective, neoplastic, metabolic or hormonal in nature." The term *painful bladder syndrome* (PBS) was introduced and defined as "the complaint of suprapubic pain related to bladder filling, accompanied by other symptoms such as increased daytime and night-time frequency, in the absence of proven urinary infection or other obvious pathology." It was suggested that the term *interstitial cystitis* be reserved for those with specific objective findings, stating that it is "a specific diagnosis and requires confirmation by typical cystoscopic and histological features. In the investigation of bladder pain it may be necessary to exclude conditions such as carcinoma in situ and endometriosis."

Although PBS does not have objective diagnostic criteria, it does provide a simple, unambiguous description of a disease that is useful when discussing the problem with patients. It allows for a classification of patients who chose to undergo treatment without invasive investigations. At the same time, it includes patients who undergo investigation but do not have the "typical cystoscopic and histologic features." Thus, there are actually three separate groups:

1. *Interstitial cystitis*—symptoms of PBS with typical cystoscopic and histologic features
2. *Painful bladder syndrome* (uninvestigated)—symptoms of PBS with unknown cystoscopic and histologic features
3. *Painful bladder syndrome* (investigated)—symptoms of PBS with negative cystoscopic and/or histologic features

Furthermore, patients with IC actually comprise at least three readily identifiable subgroups:

1. Bladder ulcers seen on baseline cystoscopy and confirmed by distention with biopsy
2. Normal baseline cystoscopy, glomerulations after distention, inflammation on biopsy, reduced bladder capacity
3. Normal baseline cystoscopy, glomerulations after distention, no inflammation on biopsy, normal bladder capacity

These groups may substantially overlap; at this time there is essentially no information that can be used to define distinct differences in etiology, pathophysiology, treatment, or prognosis for either subgroup of nonulcer IC patients. However, there is clearly a difference in pathophysiology between ulcer and nonulcer patients. Future studies with careful characterization of symptoms, objective findings, and longitudinal follow-up could produce important insights into the utility of these somewhat artificial distinctions.

An important limitation of the ICS terminology is that these definitions of disease do not translate readily into entry/exclusion criteria for clinical research. Ever since the National Institute of Diabetes and Digestive and Kidney Diseases (NIDDK) sponsored a conference to review the accumulated knowledge of IC in 1987, the consensus statement from this meeting[5] has been considered the "official" research definition of IC. The definition encompasses inclusion criteria (Box 92-1) that describe the syndrome and exclusion criteria (Box 92-2) that serve to create a relatively homogeneous patient population. The exclusion criteria can be subdivided into two groups: first, other diseases that, if present, could engender doubt about the source of symptoms, and second, various symptoms or patient factors used to eliminate subjects that might be problematic to evaluate in a clinical trial.

Box 92-1 NIDDK Inclusion Criteria: Two Positive Factors Are Necessary for Inclusion in the Interstitial Cystitis Study Population

Hunner's ulcer-automatic inclusion
Pain on bladder filling relieved by emptying
Pain (suprapubic, pelvic, urethral, vaginal, or perineal)
Glomerulations on endoscopy
Decreased bladder compliance on CMG

CMG, cystometrography; NIDDK, National Institute of Diabetes and Digestive and Kidney Diseases.

Box 92-2 NIDDK Exclusion Criteria for Interstitial Cystitis Study Population

Other diseases
Benign or malignant bladder tumors
Uterine, cervical, vaginal, or urethral cancer
Other cystitis: radiation, tuberculous, bacterial, or cyclophosphamide
Vaginitis
Symptomatic urethral diverticulum
Active herpes infection
Bladder or ureteral calculi
Involuntary bladder contractions (UDS)

Practical issues in research
Age <18 yr
Waking frequency <5 times in 12 hours
Nocturia <2 times per night
Symptoms relieved by antibiotics, urinary antiseptics, urinary analgesics
Duration <12 mo
Bladder capacity >400 mL, absence of sensory urgency

NIDDK, National Institute of Diabetes and Digestive and Kidney Diseases.

The NIDDK criteria were criticized in a retrospective study from the NIDDK IC Database.[6] It was observed that, when patients with a wide range of symptoms were recruited for this longitudinal study, the NIDDK criteria achieved the purpose of defining a homogeneous patient population, because 90% of the database subjects meeting NIDDK criteria were believed by the experts to have IC. On the other hand, more than 60% of the patients diagnosed clinically with IC by the same experts did not meet the strict NIDDK criteria. Because use of these criteria greatly limits the available patient population and hampers clinical research; it has been argued that research trials should draw from the full spectrum of the clinical population, so that the results will be maximally generalizable.[7]

It has been proposed that this obstacle could be overcome by using the constellation of symptoms that defines PBS as inclusion criteria. However, at this time, there have been no published clinical trials of PBS and no published criteria for selecting patients for such trials. There is also a lack of worldwide agreement on the standard diagnostic evaluation of patients with bladder pain. In the United States, patients are often diagnosed by symptoms, and even when bladder distention is performed, biopsies are often not obtained. In Europe and other parts of the world, most patients undergo distention and biopsy, and diagnosis follows ICS terminology closely.[8] Therefore, it can thus be difficult to conduct an international study. Furthermore, even when similar entry criteria are used, it may be difficult to ensure that patients from U.S. and European trials are similar, given the varying diagnostic philosophies. A recent NIDDK subcommittee charged with reviewing the literature to update the diagnostic criteria was unable find an evidence base to improve on the earlier NIDDK criteria.[9] This problem may not be solved until a reliable biomarker is developed. Until such time, the NIDDK criteria will continue to be used to provide an accepted homogeneous IC population representing a subset of the affected population; this definition is appropriate for trials of more toxic treatments for those with refractory symptoms. More inclusive criteria will be proposed to facilitate additional research, particularly for the more recently diagnosed and less severely affected patients. However, the lack of universally accepted research criteria for PBS will hamper research efforts in the short term.

EPIDEMIOLOGY, ASSOCIATIONS, AND IMPACT

The diagnosis of IC/PBS is controversial and is based primarily on symptoms; there is as yet no objective test or marker to establish the presence of the disease, so studies to define its prevalence and incidence are difficult to conduct. Such epidemiologic studies use one of three methods: patient self-reported history, physician diagnosis, or identification of symptoms that suggest IC/PBS. The estimates of prevalence obtained vary widely, depending on when the study was performed (recognition of the disease is much greater in recent years), which methodology was used (symptoms are very prevalent, physician diagnosis relatively uncommon), and where the study was performed (physician and patient attitudes differ by culture, and there may be environmental or hereditary risk factors). The major published studies examining the incidence of IC/PBS are summarized in Table 92-1. Reports employing physician diagnoses report a much lower incidence, but the methodologies of such studies still vary considerably: some consist of surveys sent to urologists,[10,11] whereas others involve review of medical records from broad, population-based samples.[12,13] Each methodology has its inherent biases and limitations. Leppilahti and colleagues[13] used a powerful technique in which patients were contacted from a representative population-based sample, diagnosed based on presence of symptoms, and then invited to participate in a physician evaluation to confirm the diagnosis. Even without including potential patients who could not be examined, the group estimated that the prevalence of IC in Finnish women was 230/100,000 for probable cases and 530/100,000 for possible/probable cases. The power of the study was limited by the facts that the population examined was very homogeneous and that only a small number of cases were actually diagnosed (three probable, four possible), but the results are informative and in marked contradistinction to the initial report of IC epidemiology by Orovisto,[14] who found only 18 cases per 100,000 women in the same type of population. Orovisto required the presence of a confirmatory biopsy.

Two studies using self-reported histories of IC/PBS employed the same definition of disease.[15,16] Participants were asked, "Have you ever had symptoms of a bladder infection (such as pain in your bladder and frequent urination) that lasted more than 3 months?" Those who answered "Yes" were then asked, "When

Table 92-1 Estimates of the Prevalence of Interstitial Cystitis

Publication	Years Surveyed	Methodology	Population	Total No. Surveyed	Prevalence (per 100,000)
Jones 1997	1988-1991	Self-report	U.S. national (overall)	20,561	501
			U.S. national (women)		865
Curhan 1999-NHS I	1994	Self-report/medical record	U.S. female nurses	91,555	52
Curhan 1999-NHS II	1995	Self-report/medical record	U.S. female nurses	93,428	67
Clemens 2005	1998-2002	Symptoms	Pacific northwest HMO		
Women				136,400	3,300-11,200
Men				120,533	1,400-6,200
Leppilahti 2005	2000	Symptoms	Finnish women	1,331	450
Oravisto 1975		Physician diagnosis	Finnish women		18
Bade 1995	NS	Physician diagnosis	Dutch women	235 urologists	8-16
Ito 2000	NS	Physician diagnosis	Japan (overall)	300 urologists	1.2
			Japan (women)		4.5
Clemens 2005	1998-2002	Physician diagnosis	Pacific northwest HMO		
Women, overall				136,400	197
Men, overall				120,533	41
Women, cystoscopy					99
Men, cystoscopy					19
Leppilahti 2005	2000	Physician evaluation	Finnish women	1,331	Word

HMO, health maintenance organization; NHS, National Health Service (U.K.).

you had this condition, were you told that you had interstitial cystitis or painful bladder syndrome?" An affirmative answer to both questions was considered to define the presence of IC/PBS. The Curhan study[15] also included review of medical records and found a much lower prevalence of disease in these records than was found by self-reported histories.

Overall, there is greater than 100-fold variation in the diagnosis of IC/PBS among studies. Whether this represents an actual difference in the presence of disease in different populations or an artifact from study design is unknown. Patient recollection is inaccurate due to confusion between IC/PBS and other forms of cystitis. At the same time, most of these studies do not capture patients who have no access to care due to economic or other social pressures and therefore may underestimate the presence of disease. Physician diagnosis similarly may underestimate the true prevalence due to selection biases.

Recent studies that assess the presence of symptoms suggestive of IC/PBS provide methods of identifying undiagnosed patients. Clemens and colleagues[17] used three different clinical definitions of IC/PBS symptoms in a study that included a questionnaire and review of medical records. Definition 1 consisted of self-reported pelvic pain along with urinary urgency or frequency lasting for at least 3 months. Definition 2 included the definition 1 criteria plus the presence of pain increasing as the bladder fills or pain relieved by urination. Definition 3 used results from a validated condition-specific questionnaire. Presence of IC/PBS for this definition was defined as a score of 12 or higher on the Interstitial Cystitis Symptom Index and Problem Index, including two or more episodes of nocturia per night and a pain score of 2 or greater. The resulting prevalence estimates were 11,200 per 100,000 women and 6,200 per 100,000 men by definition 1; 3300 and 1400, respectively, by definition 2; and 6200 and 2300, respectively, by definition 3. Interestingly, using only definition 3, a different study in Finnish women[18] demonstrated a prevalence of 450 per 100,000. Finally, investigators using a very controversial approach based on the presence of symptoms and potassium sensitivity testing in a subset of patients suggested that between 10% and 30% of women in a third-year medical school class had IC and that 25 to 30 million U.S. women could be affected.[19] Although this study was based on several questionable assumptions, there is no doubt that pelvic pain and lower urinary tract symptoms are exceedingly common and most likely are underappreciated in the general population. It is not yet clear that these patients actually have a unifying diagnosis. The need for an objective diagnostic marker for IC/PBS is obvious.

Only two investigators have estimated the incidence of IC/PBS. In a community-based study in Olmsted County, Minnesota, physician-assigned diagnoses of IC/PBS were identified using medical records from the Rochester Epidemiology Project.[20] The overall age- and sex-adjusted incidence rate was 1.1 per 100,000 per year for the interval from 1976 to 1996. The age-adjusted incidence rates were 1.6 per 100,000 women and 0.6 per 100,000 men. The median number of episodes of care-seeking for symptoms before diagnosis was 1 for women and 4.5 for men. In this study, the cumulative incidence rate (an estimate of prevalence) was 114 per 100,000 by age 80 years. A subsequent review of physician diagnoses of IC/PBS among Kaiser Permanente Northwest enrollees identified a much higher yearly incidence: 21 per 100,000 women and 4 per 100,000 men.[12] These two estimates present a rather large difference that cannot be resolved without further research. The methodologies and patient populations are quite different. It would be exciting to know that there is a substantial difference in incidence between different ethnic groups but we cannot conclude that at the present time.

Koziol and colleagues[21,22] first examined the impact of IC in a population of patients treated at a single center. The found that more than 60% of the patients were unable to enjoy usual activities or were excessively fatigued, and 54% reported depression. Travel, employment, leisure activities, and sleeping were adversely affected in more than 80% of the patients. The quality of life for these IC patients (likely a very severely affected group) was worse than that of chronic dialysis patients. Another survey of 495 IC patients in the United Kingdom demonstrated similar findings.[23] Sixty-seven percent of patients reported "considerable impact" or worse on their lifestyle, and 46% reported moderate depression or worse. Half of the patients reported at least considerable difficulties with sexual intercourse. There is no doubt that IC/PBS can greatly diminish quality of life in all domains (physical, social, emotional, relationships) and that the combination of chronic pain and lower urinary tract dysfunction places a burden that is matched by few other conditions.

An initial effort to determine the financial impact of IC/PBS on the U.S. healthcare system was produced from the Urologic Diseases in America project sponsored by the NIDDK. This endeavor compiled several national databases, including Medicare, Medicaid, and the Veteran's Administration health care system, as well as private sources. The search strategy included identifying costs associated with patients diagnosed with IC (*International Classification of Diseases, 9th Revision* [ICD-9] code 595.1) as well attempting to identify patients who may have PBS (the combination of code 788.41 for urgency-frequency with either 625.8 or 625.9, which code for female pelvic pain). Because there is no current diagnostic code for PBS, this was the first attempt to identify such patients through coding. Among the most important findings were the following:[24]

- Between 1992 and 2001, there was a twofold increase in the rate of hospital outpatient visits and a threefold increase in the rate of physician office visits related to IC. The annualized rate was 102 office visits per 100,000 population. The rate of ambulatory surgery visits for IC declined.
- A diagnosis of IC was associated with a twofold increase in direct medical costs compared with the costs for individuals without the disorder (Table 92-2).
- Between 1994 and 2000, the annual national expenditure for IC was stable at approximately $37 million, but the annual costs for PBS increased from $481 million to $750 million (Table 92-3).
- More than 80% of the outpatient care was provided by urologists.

The data are consistent with observations that fewer patients undergo procedures under anesthesia; the growing expenditures on PBS most likely represent an increased awareness of the condition combined with the trend away from performing cystoscopy, bladder distention, and biopsy. The economic impact of disease detailed in this report includes direct costs paid to the medical system and indirect costs borne by the individual and society. Direct costs include payments to physicians for inpatient and outpatient care, payments to hospitals for inpatient care, payments for outpatient procedures and tests, and the costs of prescription drugs, among others. Indirect costs include potentially measurable items such as the consequences of time away from work (borne by the individual, employers, and colleagues) and lost productivity when at work. The condition also has substantial impact through indirect costs that are more difficult to measure: work, education, and social opportunities not pursued; general decrements in quality of life; loss of family and social support; and even depression, divorce, and, for some IC/PBS patients, suicide. It is probable that these indirect costs would overwhelm the direct costs.

There are a number of intriguing associations with IC. Clauw[25] and Erickson[26] independently surveyed patients and controls for the presence of a wide variety of physical symptoms. They found

Table 92-2 Estimated Annual Expenditures of Privately Insured Employees with and without a Medical Claim for Interstitial Cystitis (Definition A) in 2002*

	Persons without IC (N = 477,339)			*Persons with IC (N = 244)*		
Subgroup	**Medical**	**Rx Drugs**	**Total**	**Medical**	**Rx Drugs**	**Total**
All	$2,993	$1,176	$4,169	$5,772	$2,648	$8,420
Age (yr)						
35-44	$2,597	$1,011	$3,608	$8,405	$1,915	$10,320
45-64	$3,352	$1,341	$4,693	$5,801	$2,987	$8,788
Gender						
Male	$2,912	$1,105	$4,017	$3,560	$2,785	$6,345
Female	$3,109	$1,278	$4,387	$5,996	$2,457	$8,453
Region						
Midwest	$2,980	$1,121	$4,101	$5,749	$2,550	$8,299
Northeast	$2,806	$1,254	$4,060	$5,414	$2,826	$8,240
South	$3,156	$1,153	$4,309	$6,088	$2,570	$8,658
West	$2,949	$1,157	$4,106	$5,688	$2,634	$8,322

*The sample consisted of primary beneficiaries, aged 18 to 64 years, who had employer-provided insurance and were continuously enrolled in 2002. Estimated annual expenditures were derived from multivariate models that controlled for age, gender, work status (active/retired), median household income (based on Zip code), urban/rural residence, medical and drug plan characteristics (managed care, deductible, coinsurance/copayments), and binary indicators for 28 chronic disease conditions. Predicted expenditures for persons aged 18 to 34 years were omitted due to small sample size.
SOURCE: Ingenix, 2002.
IC, interstitial cystitis; Rx, prescription.

Table 92-3 U.S. Expenditures for Interstitial Cystitis (Definition A) and Share of Costs, by Site of Service

	1994		*1996*		*1998*		*2000*	
Site of Service	**Expenditures**	**Share (%)**	**Expenditures**	**Share (%)**	**Expenditures**	**Share (%)**	**Expenditures**	**Share (%)**
Hospital outpatient	—	0	—	0	—	0	—	0
Physician office visit	$10,077,086	29.2	$10,974,296	28.9	$12,384,884	29.8	$17,152,667	44.4
Ambulatory surgery	$24,429,773	70.8	$26,963,811	71.1	$29,179,800	70.2	$21,439,276	55.6
Emergency room visit	—	0	—	0	—	0	—	0
Inpatient	—	0	—	0	—	0	—	0
Total	$34,506,859		$37,938,106		$41,564,684		$38,591,942	

SOURCE: National Ambulatory and Medical Care Survey; National Hospital and Ambulatory Medical Care Survey; Healthcare Cost and Utilization Project; Medical Expenditure Panel Survey, 1994, 1996, 1998, 2000.

Table 92-4 Nonbladder Symptoms Associated with Interstitial Cystitis (IC) in Two Studies*

Erickson 2001		*Clauw 1997*	
Symptom	**IC > Control**	**Symptom**	**IC > Control**
Backache	Yes	Not applicable	Not applicable
Dizziness	Yes	Dizziness	Yes
Chest pain	Yes	Chest pain	Yes
Aches in joints	Yes	Morning stiffness	Yes
		Swollen joints	Yes
Abdominal cramps	Yes	Abdominal bloating	Yes
Heart pounding	Yes	Palpitations	Yes
		Rapid heart rate	Yes
Nausea	Yes	Nausea	No
Headache	Yes	Tension headache	No
		Migraine headache	No

*Between-group significance: $P < .01$.

striking parallels, with IC patients reporting increased cardiac, gastrointestinal, and rheumatologic symptoms, but both investigators noted that these patients with chronic pain did not simply report the presence of somatic complaints in every organ system (Table 92-4). Alagiri and colleagues[27] surveyed 2405 patients with a diagnosis of IC for the presence of other diagnosed diseases plus symptoms that would suggest the presence of disease. Allergies were the most common condition, occurring at twice the rate in the general population, but more striking differences were see in dramatically increased rates of irritable bowel syndrome, fibromyalgia, Crohn's disease, and lupus. Endometriosis, incontinence, chronic fatigue, and migraines occurred in IC patients at about the same rate as in the general public. This finding is important, because the presence of anything more than mild stress incontinence is unusual in IC/PBS patients and should prompt a more comprehensive evaluation. In contrast to this large population-based study, examination of patients in a single center showed that IC and endometriosis may frequently coexist in patients with chronic pelvic pain.[28] A total of 178 female patients with chronic pelvic pain underwent both cystoscopy with bladder distention and laparoscopy. Endoscopic findings supported a diagnosis of endometriosis in 134 patients (75%), and cystoscopy confirmed a diagnosis of IC in 159 patients (89%);115 patients (65%) were diagnosed with both IC and endometriosis. The question here is whether the specific endoscopic findings are meaningful. Perhaps these patients had a generalized hypersensitivity disorder, and the glomerulations and deposits of endometriosis were not specifically related to the pathophysiology. Only more detailed research with longitudinal follow-up can answer this question.

These associated symptoms are particularly fascinating when viewed in the context of a report from Weissman and colleagues,[29] who described a genetic linkage study demonstrating associations between IC and panic disorder, thyroid disorders, mitral valve prolapse, and chronic headaches/migraines. These associations parallel the increased incidence of palpitations, heart pounding, chest pain, and rapid heart rate in the reports of Clauw[25] and Erickson.[26] These researchers, however, did not find an increase in headaches in IC patients compared with controls. Although such a genetic syndrome would likely only involve a fraction of the typical IC patients, this discovery could ultimately produce insights about the pathophysiology of disease and lead to new medical treatments. Another view on this issue was provided by Buffington[30]; in his review of published associations between IC and other disorders, he pointed out that many of the associations could be explained by a common dysregulation of the hypothalamic-pituitary-adrenal (HPA) axis. Buffington has carefully documented such abnormalities in a series of publications using the Feline Interstitial Cystitis model[31-33] and has begun studying the response to stress in these animals. Preliminary results suggest there is dissociation between the sympathetic nervous system and HPA-axis responses to stress (see Chapter 90). This is a promising area for further research, because it could lead to improved understanding of the pathophysiology and present new avenues for treatment.

A critical question in defining the future of IC/PBS and other pelvic pain syndromes is whether there are meaningful distinctions between different syndromes. Wessely and colleagues[34] performed a literature review in 1999; they found that a substantial overlap existed between the individual syndromes and that the similarities between them outweighed the differences. Similarities were apparent in case definition, reported symptoms, and nonsymptom associations such as gender, outlook, and response to treatment. They concluded that the existing definitions of these syndromes in terms of specific symptoms were of limited value and proposed that a dimensional classification would probably be more productive. They further postulated that the existence of specific somatic syndromes is largely an artifact of medical specialization; that is to say, the differentiation of specific functional syndromes reflects the tendency of specialists to focus on only those symptoms pertinent to their specialty, rather than any real differences among patients. There may be no more important question than this. For both research and treatment, it is critical to determine whether IC/PBS is really a primary disease of the bladder or part of a larger predisposition to chronic pain.

ETIOLOGY AND PATHOPHYSIOLOGY

The name "interstitial cystitis" implies a chronic bladder inflammation, and most of the theories about the pathophysiology of this disorder involve inflammation. Abnormally increased numbers of detrusor mast cells and/or abnormal mast cell function[35,36] have been suggested to be key features of the disease. The hypothesis is attractive because of the symptoms of the disease and the association with allergies and food sensitivities. However, although ulcer patients clearly have classic chronic inflammation on biopsy, the majority of subjects in the NIDDK Interstitial Cystitis Database study did not have significant histologic inflammation.[37] Moreover, treatment with mast cell inhibitors has been largely disappointing, and urinary histamine and its metabolites have not been reliable markers for the disease.[38]

Autoimmune dysregulation and chronic inflammation have also been proposed as an etiology. The demographic distribution of young female patients parallels that of other autoimmune diseases, and several autoimmune disorders are associated with IC, as discussed earlier. However, it does not seem possible that IC is an autoimmune disease in the classic sense, because many histologic studies have failed to demonstrate the expected pathologic changes. Positive clinical results from recent studies using cyclosporine have generated renewed interest in this hypothesis.

For many years, the primary theory of IC pathogenesis was a deficiency in the protective glycosaminoglycan (GAG) layer of the bladder. Parsons and others suggested that GAGs are quantitatively and qualitatively diminished. A unifying theory of urologic pelvic pain centered on epithelial cell dysfunction was proposed by Parsons.[39] The concept is that the defective urothelial barrier allows potassium and other solutes to diffuse back into the bladder, stimulating pain nerves and creating local inflammation. IC patients are clearly more sensitive to intravesical potassium (see later discussion), but actually proof of abnormal bladder permeability has been elusive. In addition, treatment aimed at restoring the GAG layer has been relatively disappointing. The clinical or basic science breakthrough that would substantiate this attractive theory has yet to arise.

The most promising scientific research in IC involves antiproliferative factor (APF). The presence of a substance in the urine of IC patients that inhibits urothelial cell growth in culture (but is not cytotoxic) was first described in 1996 by Keay and colleagues.[40] Subsequent work from the same group demonstrated that APF was found in bladder urine but not in urine taken from the renal collecting system,[41] that it was found in almost all IC patients but rarely in normal controls or in patients with other urologic disorders,[42] and that abnormally high levels of APF reverted to normal after patients were treated by bladder distention and sacral nerve stimulation.[43,44] APF activity also has been shown to correlate with other known epithelial growth factors EGF and HB-EGF.[45] The structure of APF was finally elucidated in 2004 by Keay and colleagues[46]; it belongs to the family of frizzled 8–related sialoglycopeptides and has 100% homology to the sixth transmembrane segment of the G protein–coupled Wnt ligand receptor. At this time, there is no easy test to assess APF, because the assay still depends on a cell culture. If an antibody-based assay can be developed in the future, it could have a major impact on the diagnosis of IC/PBS. This in turn would greatly facilitate both clinical and epidemiologic research. The ultimate question is whether APF is a simply a marker associated with the disease or is integrally involved in its pathophysiology.

Warren and colleagues have investigated the possibility that susceptibility to IC is inherited. One study involved a pilot mail-in study of members of the Interstitial Cystitis Association.[47] The participants were asked about the presence of IC symptoms and a diagnosis of IC in all first-degree relatives. Diagnosis was not confirmed in the probands or relatives. The survey found that women, aged 31 to 73 years, who were first-degree relatives of patients with IC, themselves had a prevalence of IC of 995/100,000. This suggests a relative risk of up to 17 times that in the general population, based on Curhan's study of IC prevalence.[15] This team also investigated IC in twins. Of the co-twins of 8 monozygotic twin respondents, 2 had probable and 3 had confirmed IC, compared with none of the co-twins of the 26 dizygotic twin respondents (including 15 female co-twins). Although this is a very small sample, the striking results suggest that there may be a genetic susceptibility to IC.[48]

CURRENT DIAGNOSTIC TESTS AND STRATEGIES

As discussed earlier, the 1988 NIDDK research criteria are the product of "expert opinion" and were intended to ensure that the populations in research studies would be comparable. The criteria were not intended for clinical practice; even in the research setting, they function suboptimally by excluding too many appropriate subjects. Because of this controversy, the NIDDK charged a subcommittee to examine the evidence supporting current diagnostic strategies and knowledge and identify the gaps to be filled. This was intended to be the first step in moving toward an evidence-based definition of IC and to include specific recommendations for future research that would create the necessary evidence. Individual participants reviewed the published data on urodynamics, biomarkers, potassium sensitivity testing, cystoscopy with distention and biopsy, and questionnaires. The conclusions of each reviewer were discussed and modified by the whole subcommittee. Each author then presented the conclusions for public comment at the 2003 NIDDK Interstitial Cystitis Research Symposium on November 1, 2003, in Alexandria, Virginia. This meeting was attended by more than 250 international experts in IC, including clinicians from many different specialties and basic science researchers. The subcommittee found that, in the 15 years since publication of the original NIDDK guidelines, no high-quality evidence had been developed to support the routine use of any diagnostic test in defining IC. The specific findings and recommendations are included in the following sections.

Urodynamics

Urodynamic studies are required to diagnose IC by the NIDDK entry criteria. Despite this fact and the many papers that purport to study IC based on the NIDDK criteria, the reviewers in 2003 identified only 10 papers that described urodynamic findings. The NIDDK criteria include the presence of noncompliant filling as a positive factor in the diagnosis and the presence of involuntary detrusor contractions (IDCs) as an exclusionary factor. However, although diminished compliance appears to occur in a subset of patients with IC/PBS, this feature of the disease has not been characterized sufficiently to be of any clinical value. At the same time, IDCs are consistently reported in a subset of IC/PBS patients and correlate with symptom severity. No data were found to suggest that these patients are different from patients who do not have IDCs. It was concluded that IDCs should not be used to exclude a diagnosis of IC/PBS. One important point presented was that most of the reports did not include any assessment of pain during bladder filling and that the standard urodynamic terms of "first desire to void" and "urgency" may not be adequate to describe urodynamics in patients with IC/PBS.[49]

My colleagues and I use urodynamic testing selectively, with the primary indications being the presence of significant incontinence, prominent voiding difficulty or high residual urine, and failure to respond to treatment. The test is adapted from the technique described by Teichman and colleagues.[50] We typically perform a baseline filling/voiding cystometrogram. This is followed by a potassium sensitivity test (PST) as described by Parsons.[51]The bladder is then anesthetized with alkalinized lidocaine, as described by Henry,[52] and cystometry is repeated. It is important that voiding be adequately evaluated before the PST and lidocaine instillation, because there is a significant incidence of voiding abnormalities, much of it related to pelvic floor dysfunction, and this may offer a separate avenue for therapy (see later discussion of pelvic floor therapy).

Cystoscopy with Bladder Distention and Biopsy

More than 50 papers including data on cystoscopy, bladder distention, and bladder biopsy were reviewed.[53] Although the presence of glomerulations after bladder distention has long been considered to be the sine qua non of IC, there is no body of evidence to support this hypothesis. The sensitivity of glomerulations as a marker for IC was questioned by Awad and colleagues.[54] This group defined patients with subjective symptoms of IC and supportive urodynamic findings. They found no difference between those who did and did not have glomerulations after bladder distention in histology or in response to treatment. The specificity of glomerulations was questioned by Waxman and associates.[55] They photographed bladder distentions performed on asymptomatic women presenting for elective tubal ligation. The photographs were reviewed by outside experts along with similar photographs taken from distentions of IC patients. The study conclusively demonstrated that the bladder mucosal lesions characteristically associated with irritative voiding symptoms and pelvic pain in patients diagnosed with IC were also observed in asymptomatic women. More recently, Erickson and colleagues[56] prospectively evaluated 36 patients undergoing bladder distention using the NIDDK cystoscopic criteria. They found no difference in symptoms or in response to the procedure between those who did and did not meet cystoscopic criteria for IC. There was no difference in histology or urine markers. They concluded that, "cystoscopic criteria do not appear to identify a distinct pathophysiologic subset of patients with IC symptoms."

It would thus appear that cystoscopy under anesthesia with bladder distention cannot be recommended as a mandatory test. At the same time, patients with chronic disease are often concerned about cancer and crave more information about their disease. Either the patient or the clinician may feel a need for further evaluation. IC does not appear to predispose patients to bladder cancer. On the other hand, several authors have published cases series of patients who were misdiagnosed with either IC or chronic pelvic pain and actually had bladder cancer or carcinoma in situ.[57-59] This is of great concern because of the trend away from examining all patients with cystoscopy. It is certainly important to maintain a high index of suspicion in these patients and to use diagnostic studies such as cystoscopy and cytology prudently. In selected patients, office cystoscopy can be well tolerated and can provide the necessary information to exclude other diseases (although the bladder can rarely be distended enough to produce glomerulations without severe pain in the absence of anesthesia). If cystoscopy is performed under anesthesia, abnormal or suspicious areas should certainly be biopsied, but there is as yet no evidence that routine biopsies of normal areas or glomerulations provide useful diagnostic or therapeutic information. At the present time, it seems rational to conclude that cystoscopy should still be used for patients with PBS and microscopic hematuria or pyuria, risk factors for bladder cancer, and for those patients for whom empiric therapy has failed. Two investigators have suggested that the likelihood of identifying any specific cause for microscopic hematuria in young women with PBS is very low.[60,61] Perhaps such low-risk patients might be initially evaluated with ultrasonography and cytology.

Biomarkers

APF was discussed in detail earlier. Currently, there is no clinically useful biomarker for IC/PBS. There is a need for large, multicenter prospective studies, including a broad spectrum of patients with lower urinary tract symptoms and pelvic pain, in which APF (and other putative biomarkers) can be tested on all patients at enrollment and correlated with eventual diagnosis and response to therapy.

Potassium Sensitivity Testing

The most controversial tool in the IC/PBS diagnostic armamentarium is the PST. First described by Parsons,[51,62] the PST has been studied more extensively than any other test. In this test, 50 mL of sterile water and 50 mL of 0.4N KCl are instilled into the patient's bladder sequentially, and the patient is asked to rate the degree of pain and urgency on a scale of 0 to 5. An increase of 2 points in either symptom is considered a positive test. It should be noted that the PST assesses sensitivity to intravesical instillation of potassium. The concentration used is pharmacologic, not physiologic. A positive test may indicate increased permeability of the urothelium to potassium, increased sensitivity of the bladder nerves, or some combination of the two.

Many investigators using very different patient populations have unanimously concluded that this test separates IC patients from normal subjects. The question is whether the test meaningfully separates patients with IC/PBS from those with other diseases. Reports document high rates of positive testing in patients with prostatitis, urethral syndrome, and a wide variety of gynecologic disorders, as well as a substantial minority of patients with detrusor overactivity (Table 92-5).[63-65] As discussed earlier, Parsons[39] has proposed that the test accurately identifies a large group of patients with undiagnosed IC/PBS who share a common uroepithelial dysfunction. Another explanation for the wide positivity of the test is the concept of neural cross-sensitization and referred pain. FitzGerald and colleagues[66,67] studied pain responses in PBS patients. They first demonstrated that subjects with PBS exhibit bladder hyperalgesia and may sense bladder discomfort at sites other than suprapubic. They were able to show that the rating of bladder discomfort and sensory mapping during cystometry usefully distinguishes between PBS subjects and controls (no pain, stress incontinent or continent). A second study examining patients with PBS, overactive bladder, or stress incontinence and normal controls found that most of the patients with PBS and some of those with overactive bladder experienced their bladder discomfort or urgency at referred sites other than suprapubic. They postulated that the etiology of widespread sensation may include an expansion of dermatomes of referral of bladder sensation, and/or the presence of associated somatic abnormalities.

Table 92-5 Results of Testing for Epithelial Dysfunction in Populations of Symptomatic Patients

Population	N	No. Positive for Epithelial Dysfunction (%)
Interstitial cystitis	1629	1285 (79)
Urethral syndrome	116	64 (55)
Chronic pelvic pain (gynecologic patients)	365	288 (79)
Category IIIA-IIIB prostatitis (chronic pelvic pain syndrome)	44	37 (84)
Lower urinary tract symptoms		
Men	526	83 (16)
Women	25	2 (24)
Acute bacterial cystitis	4	4 (100)
Detrusor instability	16	4 (25)
Radiation cystitis	9	9 (100)

Even more intriguing is the work by Pezzone and colleagues in a rat model of referred pelvic pain. In the first study, after acute bladder irritation, dramatic increases in abdominal wall electromyographic activity in response to rectal distention were observed, indicating colonic afferent sensitization. Analogously, after acute colonic irritation, bladder contraction frequency increased by 66%, suggesting sensitization of lower urinary tract afferents.[68] In the second study, colonic irritation was shown to sensitize urinary bladder afferents to noxious mechanical and chemical stimuli (including bladder distention, capsaicin, bradykinin, and substance P). Interruption of the neural input to the bladder minimized this effect, suggesting a local afferent pathway from the colon. This work suggests the stimulating hypothesis that the overlap of chronic pelvic pain disorders may be a consequence of pelvic afferent cross-sensitization.[69]

The PST was examined in two prospective double-blind trials to determine the utility of the test in predicting response to therapy aimed in improving the bladder GAG layer. A three-armed study investigating different doses of pentosanpolysulfate sodium (PPS; 300, 600, or 900 mg daily) enrolled patients based on symptoms and performed PST on all subjects at entry. In the 377 patients evaluated at baseline, the PST was positive in 302 (80.1%), negative in 51 (13.5%), and indeterminate in 24 (6.4%). The PST had no predictive value, because significant responses to treatment were seen in 92 (60%) of the 153 patients who were PST-positive at entry and in 20 (64%) of the 33 who were PST-negative.[63] In contrast, Gupta and colleagues[70] performed the PST on 36 patients who went on to receive intravesical sodium hyaluronate. They found that 20 (55%) of 36 patients reported an improvement after six doses, but 17 (74%) of those with a positive PST result improved, compared with only 5 (22%) of those with a negative test ($P = .03$). Further examination of the role of PST in identifying patients for such intravesical therapy seems appropriate.

In summary, the PST is not a physiologic test, and it assesses bladder sensitivity, not necessarily permeability; development of a practical test to conclusively measure urothelial permeability in humans would be enormously helpful in directing clinical care and research efforts. The specificity of the PST has not been established. However, the test is simple and inexpensive and clearly separates IC patients from normal controls; it is possible that further research will define a role for the test in the diagnosis of IC/PBS. In a large-scale, prospective randomized controlled trial (RCT), the PST did not predict response to PPS therapy, but in a smaller trial it did seem to predict response to intravesical sodium hyaluronate.

Questionnaires

Three questionnaires are in common use in IC/PBS: the University of Wisconsin, O'Leary-Sant, and PUF scales. Although all may be used to monitor patients longitudinally, there is no evidence that any questionnaire can be used to diagnose IC. Many epidemiologic studies are investigating the use of all or part of these instruments as screening tools to estimate prevalence in large populations.

Table 92-6 Oral Therapy Level of Evidence*

Treatment	Level of Evidence	Grade of Recommendation
Amitriptyline	2	B
Cyclosporine	4	C
Analgesics	5	C
Hydroxyzine	1	D
Cimetidine	4	D
Methotrexate	4	D
Misoprostol	4	D
Montelukast	4	D
Nifedipine	4	D
Quercetin	4	D
Behavioral modification	5	D
Dietary manipulation	5	D
IPD 1151T	4	N/A
Sodium pentosanpolysulfate	1	–C
Antibiotics	4	–C
L-Arginine	–1	–A

There are several different systems of Levels of Evidence. For example the Oxford CEBM gives:

- Level A: consistent Randomised Controlled Clinical Trial, Cohort Study, All or None, Clinical Decision Rule validated in different populations.
- Level B: consistent Retrospective Cohort, Exploratory Cohort, Ecological Study, Outcomes Research, Case-Control Study; or extrapolations from level A studies.
- Level C: Case-series Study or extrapolations from level B studies
- Level D: Expert opinion without explicit critical appraisal, or based on physiology, bench research or first principles

THERAPEUTIC OPTIONS

Overview

The inherent difficulty in managing a disease of unknown etiology characterized by chronic pain can produce a therapeutic nihilism, because there are few treatments that produce significant benefit for the majority of patients and little guidance for the physician or patient. Patient management is further compromised by the lack of quality RCTs. The evidence base supporting various treatments for IC/PBS was summarized by the International Consultation for Incontinence (ICI).[71] Oral and intravesical treatments commonly used are listed in Table 92-6, along with their associated level of evidence and grade of recommendation. The highest level of evidence comes from randomized clinical trials and the lowest level from "expert opinion." The highest grade of recommendation stems from consistent level 1 evidence (multiple RCTs or meta-analysis). These criteria follow the standards of the Oxford Centre for Evidence-Based Medicine (http://www.cebm.net).

These treatments are discussed in more detail in the following sections, along with neuromodulation techniques and surgical therapy. Although a common approach is to start with behavioral therapies, followed by oral treatment and then intravesical therapy, I prefer to give the patient significant leeway in selecting the treatment that seems most appropriate to his or her individual situation; the ICI Committee recommendations are similar. Because there are no useful comparative trials that can be used to direct therapy for an individual patient, there is considerable room to individualize treatment. Oral therapy is simple and convenient; however, the patient must accept long-term treatment and the attendant side effects. Intravesical therapy is invasive and produces considerable anxiety for many patients; this is balanced by the lack of systemic side effects as treatments are delivered directly to the bladder. The frequent trips to the doctor's office can be very inconvenient. However, many patients learn to self-administer treatments, providing a tremendous sense of control over the disease. The time required for a response to intravesical therapy is typically shorter than what may be seen with oral medications, and intravesical therapy is attractive if the diagnosis is in doubt. A clear response to intravesical therapy supports a diagnosis of IC/PBS as opposed to other causes of pelvic pain.

The hierarchy of goals in treating IC/PBS is as follows:

1. Relieve symptoms
2. Restore normal bladder function
3. Maintain response after withdrawal of treatment

Too often, only the first goal is addressed. The key to managing these cases is keeping the goal of normal bladder function in mind. The clinician should start with three pieces of information: the primary symptoms, a bladder diary with volumes, and a symptom score. These should be assessed at the outset of every new treatment and reassessed at an appropriate point during or after treatment. This, along with the presence or absence of side effects, informs the decision as to whether the treatment should be continued or abandoned and whether additional treatment is indicated. In many cases, a patient feels great relief after a particular course of therapy and has little interest in adding more treatment. The patient may not appreciate that there is room for further improvement, may be wary of potential adverse effects, or may simply not want to "rock the boat" after experiencing improvement. Regular use of the symptom scores can alert the clinician that the patient, although reporting a great response, still has significant ongoing symptoms. In other cases, the symptom score is low but the bladder diary demonstrates that the functional capacity remains small. In such cases, true bladder rehabilitation has not been achieved, and ongoing treatment is indicated, even if its focus is limited to bladder training/behavioral modification. Normalization of bladder function—achieving a normal voiding pattern, normal capacity, and normal control without pain—should be the ultimate focus. If this can be achieved and maintained, then there is a realistic chance that treatment can be withdrawn successfully and the bladder will be rehabilitated. If bladder function is not normalized, it is unlikely that treatment can be withdrawn, regardless of the symptomatic success. A rule of thumb is that medication titration can begin after 6 months with no pain and normal functional bladder capacity.

Behavioral Therapies

Behavioral therapies include bladder training and various forms of behavioral modification, including dietary restrictions, urinary alkalinization, fluid management, relaxation/stress management, and so on. Although behavioral therapies have been almost uniformly recommended as being helpful and harmless, there has been almost no useful research into the true efficacy of these treatments or the optimal way of delivering them. Bladder training was shown to be effective in at least two uncontrolled clinical studies[72,73] and should be part of the prescription for almost all patients. The initial bladder diary is used to establish baseline function and set goals. The patient should practice delaying urination for 10 to 20 minutes after experiencing a normal urge, but not holding to the point that pain is induced. Many patients have too much pain to use bladder training initially. Other treatments and general pain management can be used initially, with bladder training added after adequate pain relief has been achieved. Basic science research showing that production of APF is inhibited by bladder distention (Chai 2000)[43] suggests a mechanism by which bladder training might ultimately be instrumental in reversing the underlying pathophysiology of disease.

Dietary restriction has been recommended as a first and essential step in managing all cases of IC/PBS. However, there is no good evidence to support the efficacy of dietary management. The most common reported sensitivities are to "acidic" foods such as citrus and tomatoes, spicy foods, alcoholic beverages, and coffee/caffeine. Others have suggested that high-protein diets can induce pain through high urine urea concentrations, that food allergies stimulate the disease, and that additives such as dyes are the cause of pain. Indeed, a large proportion of these patients do report sensitivities to various foods, but there is no evidence that eating suspect foods leads to progression of disease or that restrictions improve the course of the disease. Therefore, the benefit of any dietary management must be weighed against the diminished quality of life associated with dietary restriction. The so called "IC diet" eliminates an enormous number of foods and results in a bland, unattractive regimen that does not promote good overall health. Because many patients never identify any dietary items that provoke symptoms, the diet cannot be universally recommended except as a tool to aid in the search for potential sensitivities. After 1 to 2 weeks on the restricted diet, the patient can assess any improvement and then begin adding back foods to look for reactions. If sensitivities are identified, the patient can reasonably weigh the increase in symptoms against the pleasure obtained from the particular menu item. Acid sensitivity can sometimes be managed by use of dietary supplements such as Prelief, various neutraceutical, and oral antacids. It is regrettable that many patients are forced to give up some of their favorite foods, such as tomato sauce, red wine, and spicy ethnic cuisines, due to sensitivities. It is tragic that others are forcefully instructed to give up such foods without ever experiencing any benefit.

In the same way that dietary measures are recommended in a common-sense approach without substantive data, patients are often advised to drink more water to keep the pH higher and dilute irritating components. Some patients do respond favorably, and some benefit from urinary alkalinization. However, one randomized trial[74] showed no difference in sensitivity between instillations of acidic urine and buffered urine. It would seem reasonable to examine the effect of urine alkalinization and increased free water critically for individual patients but to realize that, for many, this may only produce an increase in urinary frequency.

Stress management can be useful in most chronic pain conditions. There is an accumulating body of evidence that the hypothalamic-pituitary axis is abnormal in patients with pelvic pain and also in the spontaneously occurring feline cystitis model. Although there are no good clinical trials to support the effectiveness of these therapies, it seems reasonable to consider counseling, yoga, meditation, and other techniques that might allow the patient to reduce stress and anxiety. General pelvic muscle relaxation employing biofeedback has been used successfully (see later discussion).

Oral Therapies

The mainstay of therapy for IC/PBS has been oral medications. As pointed out earlier, the level of evidence for almost all oral medical therapies is low. The most commonly recommended agents are PPS (Elmiron), hydroxyzine (Vistaril and Atarax), and amitriptyline (Elavil). Interestingly, a survey of practice patterns from the INGENIX database indicates that anticholinergic medications are actually the most commonly prescribed drugs for IC/PBS. Although it seems logical that medications designed to treat the frequency and urgency of overactive bladder might be effective for the frequency and urgency of IC/PBS, there is no evidence that this is true. Given that patients with overactive bladder are presumed to have IDCs as the source of the symptoms and that such findings are uncommon in patients with IC/PBS patients, one might even postulate that anticholinergic medications could produce as much harm as good, by making it more difficult to empty the bladder. Antibiotics are similarly prescribed very commonly, but there is no good evidence that intensive therapy is beneficial[75] and "no evidence to suggest that antibiotics have a role in the treatment of IC in the absence of culture-documented infection."[71] There are patients who clearly have recurrent bacterial cystitis but also suffer significant bladder symptoms in the absence of infection. In such cases, a 3- to 6-month course of antibiotic prophylaxis along with supportive therapy for the lower urinary tract symptoms would seem to be appropriate.

PPS is the only oral medication that is approved by the U.S. Food and Drug Administration (FDA) for treatment of IC. It is structurally similar to components of the urothelial GAG layer and is intended to repair a postulated GAG defect that allows toxic and inflammatory components of the urine to diffuse back into the bladder. The recommended dose is 100 mg three times daily. Unlike most other medications, it has been examined in a number or RCTs of reasonable quality. The ICI committee concluded that the evidence shows that PPS is ineffective in treatment of IC/PBS with a C level recommendation. The results of the three placebo-controlled, randomized clinical trials are summarized in Table 92-7. The results are reasonably consistent, with three of the four studies demonstrating efficacy or a strong trend toward efficacy for PPS over placebo. The overall utility is not great, with only about one third of patients responding, but the low response rate is balanced by a low incidence of side effects. In the RCTs, the overall incidence of adverse events with PPS was similar to that with placebo. Hair loss is an infrequent but potentially distressing problem affecting 2% to 3% of patients. It can sometimes be managed by reducing the dose and is reversible when the drug is discontinued. Safety has been confirmed in long-term, open-label continuation studies, and the benefit obtained by responders appears to be durable.[76,77] Van Ophoven and colleagues reported that patients with a minor response to PPS might see additional benefit from the addition of subcutaneous heparin, also an analogue of the bladder GAG layer.[78]

PPS should be administered for a minimum of 3 and preferably 6 months before it is abandoned as ineffective. If a clear effect is seen, then the response can be cumulative and improvement may continue gradually over 1 year or longer. It is therefore

Table 92-7 Results of Three Placebo-Controlled, Randomized Clinical Trials of Pentosanpolysulfate Sodium (PPS) for Treatment of Interstitial Cystitis

Author	Year	Design	*N*	Dosage	Duration	Outcome Measure	Results
Holm-Bensten	1987	Double-blind, placebo, RCT	114	200 mg bid	4 mo		
Mulholland	1990	Double-blind, placebo, RCT	110	100 mg tid	3 mo	More than "slight improvement"	28% vs 13%
Parsons	1993	Double-blind, placebo, RCT	148	100 mg tid		50% Overall improvement	32% vs 16%
Sant	2003	2 × 2 with hydroxyzine and PPS	121	100 mg tid			34% vs 18%

RCT, randomized controlled trial.

critically important to establish baseline symptoms clearly and to define the treatment plan at the outset of therapy, because many patients are confused as to whether to persist on medications, and some inappropriately continue the medication for years in the absence of any benefit. In summary, PPS is a safe medication that offers a reasonable chance of improving the symptoms of IC/PBS, and it can be offered to those patients who are willing to commit to a fairly long course of therapy. It is, again, the only oral medication specifically approved by the FDA for IC/PBS and certainly should be offered to all patients at some point in their treatment. PPS was developed specifically to cure the proposed pathophysiology of IC. As such, clinical results with the drug have been quite disappointing. However, new research is providing insights into the pharmacology of the drug and may ultimately lead to improved efficacy. PPS is a heterogeneous mixture of molecules with varying sizes and charges. Only recently has a reliable laboratory assay been developed to track PPS excretion. Erickson and colleagues[79] determined that the median urine PPS level in 34 patients with IC was 1.2 μg/mL (range, 0.5 to 27.7 μg/mL) and that all PPS recovered from the urine patients with IC who were taking oral PPS comes only from the low-molecular-weight fraction.[79] In contrast, rabbit studies have shown that the high-molecular-weight fraction of PPS is recovered in small amounts from urine after intravenous administration but not at all after oral administration. The authors concluded that the low-molecular-weight fraction has greater gastrointestinal absorption and urine excretion. They speculated that IC patients with low PPS levels could have achieved better symptom relief if their PPS levels had been higher and that improved PPS bioavailability might come from using only the LMW fraction of PPS or by placing PPS into different vehicles. The same group went on to test this theory by attaching galactosyl residues to PPS to promote binding to the endogenous lectins in the bladder.[80] The hypothesis is that increased binding may improve efficacy for treating IC. They were able to show that only 2% to 4% of PPS and heparin binds to the bladder but that this can be substantially increased by using lactose-PPS and lactose-heparin. In the future, clinical trials of modified drugs may demonstrate improved effectiveness for IC than the parent compounds. Another group examined a different approach, putting PPS into a novel formulation with a lyotropic liquid and an absorption enhancer. The liquid converts to mucoadhesive gel with water. In a rat model, the absolute bioavailability increased from 1.9% at baseline to 46.4% with the new model. Again, the ultimate test is whether improved bioavailability will improve outcome, but the preliminary research is very promising.[81]

Amitriptyline and other tricyclic antidepressants have been commonly used in the treatment of IC/PBS as well as for a wide variety of other chronic pain syndromes. Although individual clinicians may have "favorite" drugs from this category, only amitriptyline has strong evidence to support its efficacy. Several uncontrolled studies suggested that amitriptyline was effective for those patients who were able to tolerate it,[82-84] although discontinuation of therapy due to adverse events was common. Van Ophoven[78] reported a single-center RCT demonstrating a greater than 30% reduction in symptom score for 42% of patients treated with amitriptyline, compared with only 13% for those treated with placebo. Surprisingly, the dropout rate was only 1 of 25 in each arm of the study. A National Institutes of Health–sponsored clinical research group is investigating the use of amitriptyline in the treatment of newly diagnosed PBS.

Amitriptyline is typically started at either 10 or 25 mg taken nightly at bedtime and titrated up to a maximum of 75 mg as tolerated. The mechanism of action is not known, but it does not appear that the effect is due to treatment of an underlying mood disturbance; the dose used for depression is usually greater than 150 mg. Most clinicians do not monitor blood levels when these lower doses are used. Amitriptyline has strong antihistaminic effects (see later discussion) and has central antinociceptive actions. The primary side effects are sedation along with other central nervous system problems, constipation, dry mouth, and weight gain. Palpitations and arrhythmias are associated with this class of medication, and the drug should be used cautiously, if at all, in patients with underlying cardiac rhythm disturbances. Careful, slow dose titration can provide an opportunity for patients to accommodate to the side effects and continue therapy. Sedation can be beneficial for patients with problematic nocturia, and constipation can generally be prevented or easily managed if it is anticipated. Some patients respond favorably to very low doses of 10 to 20 mg but, I recommend continuing titration to side effects then dropping back to the comfortable dose. The goal, as always, is to get the most out of every treatment and to aim for not only relief of symptoms but normalization of bladder function. Once the optimal dose is determined, about 6 to 8 weeks should be allowed to see a response before discontinuing treatment. It is safest to titrate down when discontinuing the drug, although this can be done more rapidly than when titrating up. Amitriptyline is a good choice for IC/PBS patients with pain as a predominant symptom, for those with bothersome nocturia, and, of course, for those with concomitant depression (although collaboration with a psychiatrist in choosing the dose is recommended).

Hydroxyzine and other antihistamines are commonly used to treat IC/PBS, based on the theory that abnormal mast cell function is a key part of the disease pathophysiology. However, the quality of research and evidence to support the effectiveness of these drugs is lacking. Hydroxyzine has been touted as the most effective mast cell–stabilizing agent. It was reported to be effective in a series of IC patients selected because of associated problems with allergies[85] but was not superior to placebo (31% versus 20%) in the one multicenter RCT that has been performed.[86] Hydroxyzine is typically dosed at 50 mg every night and 25 mg during the day. Some patients respond to lower doses, and some physicians prescribe a single 75-mg dose to be taken at bedtime. Dose titration is usually employed, starting at 25 mg nightly. The most common side effect is sedation but nighttime dosing can convert this into an advantage for those patients with nocturia and/or difficulty sleeping. Other side effects are generally mild. A 6- to 8-week course of therapy after full-dose titration is recommended. Although there are anecdotal reports of success with diphenhydramine and with the selective (nonsedating) antihistamines, there is a paucity of data, and these agents should probably be reserved for patients who are intolerant of hydroxyzine. The histamine 2 blocker, cimetidine, has been reported to be effective in some uncontrolled studies, and one RCT comparing cimetidine at 400 mg twice daily to placebo suggested that cimetidine was superior in reducing pain and frequency.[87] Although more data are needed before the drug can be recommended routinely, it is a generally safe medication and does not cause sedation, so it might be useful if other antihistamines are not tolerated. It is particularly appropriate for the large group of IC patients with seasonal allergies, hay fever, and other atopic disorders. Cimetidine can affect the metabolism of many other medications, and this needs to be considered, because many IC/PBS patients suffer from polypharmacy. When patients do have a complete response, they can often titrate the dose down, but it seems less likely that they will be able to completely stop therapy without experiencing a relapse.

As noted in the ICI report,[71] many other oral medications have been used in treating IC/PBS. Nonsteroidal anti-inflammatories, steroids, and other agents that modulate inflammation, such as quercetin, montelukast, and misoprostol, have all been associated with anecdotal success. There is special interest in immune system–modulating agents, because it has been postulated that IC may have an autoimmune etiology. Small case series have been reported using prednisone and other agents, but a controlled study comparing cyclosporine to PPS has stimulated interest in this form of treatment.[88] Sixty-four patients were recruited and were randomly assigned to receive either cyclosporine at 3 mg/kg (twice daily in divided dosing) or PPS 100 mg three times daily in an open-label study. Cyclosporine was clearly superior to PPS, with a clinical response rate (according to a patient global response assessment) of 75%, compared with 19% for PPS ($P < .001$) after 6 months of treatment. It should be noted that these were relatively severely affected patients; their mean symptom index was 16 out of 20, 15 of the 64 subjects had ulcers, and their mean age was 56.2 ± 14.7 years. The quality of the response was also impressive, with an increase in awake bladder capacity of 81 mL, a decrease in symptom score of 7.9 points from baseline 15.7, and a decrease in nocturia of 2.2 episodes from a baseline of 3.9—all clearly clinically meaningful changes. A previous uncontrolled series by the same author[89] reported that 11 of 20 responders stopped taking their cyclosporine, but symptoms recurred within months in 9 of them. The primary toxicity of cyclosporine is hypertension and diminished renal function, so careful monitoring is required. All immunosuppressive agents can potentially expose patients to opportunistic infections and even malignancies, but the risk is probably much less than in the transplant population, in whom multiple agents are used simultaneously. There is clearly a need for a great deal more work to confirm and expand these results to other agents and even combination therapy. In the meantime, cyclosporine appears to be a reasonable treatment option for patients with refractory disease if regular follow-up and careful monitoring can be assured.

Intravesical Therapies

Intravesical therapy is an attractive option for the treatment of IC because of the opportunity to deliver therapy while minimizing side effects. Treatments are limited by patient discomfort, expense, and the relatively poor absorption of most drugs through the bladder. Nevertheless, intravesical therapy is an important part of the therapeutic armamentarium and still presents a great opportunity for further research. Intravesical therapy is preferred by some patients and is an important second-line tool for those who do not respond to oral agents.

Although many agents and combinations of drugs have been given in the bladder for IC/PBS, the only agent specifically FDA-approved for intravesical therapy is dimethylsulfoxide, or DMSO (RIMSO-50). The mechanism of action of DMSO is unknown, although the drug has a number of properties that could be beneficial, including anti-inflammatory, analgesic, muscle relaxation, and collagen dissolution. There has been little quality research on DMSO because it is an older drug and it also has a strong odor that makes blinding very difficult, if not impossible. Perez-Marrero and colleagues[90] performed a placebo-controlled, crossover study involving 33 patients. They found that 53% of DMSO-treated patients were markedly improved, compared with 18% of the placebo-treated patients. Of the DMSO group, 93% had objective improvement, compared with 35% of the placebo group. Peeker and colleagues[91] compared DMSO to bacillus Calmette-Guérin (BCG) in 21 patients using a crossover trial, finding some response to DMSO but none to BCG. However, this study was criticized for not allowing adequate time for BCG to take effect. Many other uncontrolled studies have suggested that more than 60% of patients with IC/PBS will respond to intravesical DMSO, although the relapse rate is high, perhaps up to 50% in the first year. My colleagues and I typically use a cocktail of DMSO with alkalinized lidocaine and steroids, giving six weekly treatments. It seems reasonable to add steroids to the DMSO solution, because it is unlikely that they can be absorbed without DMSO. Patients are assessed with the use of symptom scores and voiding diaries. Those with objective and subjective responses then continue on monthly maintenance therapy and may be gradually titrated off therapy. It is common for patients to have a mild increase in symptoms during the first two treatments, and they should be counseled about this possibility. Most patients tolerate the treatments quite well; those who do not have usually been given "straight" DMSO instead of a "cocktail," which reduces the initial pain, or they have been instructed to hold the solution for an extended period of time. Absorption of DMSO is rapid, and retaining the solution for 15 minutes is probably more than adequate.

Many other agents have been proposed for intravesical use. Heparin, PPS, and hyaluronic acid/sodium hyaluronate are all

GAG layer analogues that have been used with anecdotal success. However, two large controlled trials of sodium hyaluronate apparently showed no efficacy,[92] and no controlled studies have been done with the other agents. We typically use 20,000 units of heparin with alkalinized lidocaine administered daily to three times per week for patients who are intolerant of DMSO or who like the ability to gain symptom control with daily self-instillations. It is essential that the clinical utility of intravesical GAG therapy be carefully analyzed, because oral bioavailability of GAGs is poor. It is critically important to determine whether GAG therapy can actually be used to treat most patients with IC/PBS. At this time, essentially nothing is known about the optimal agent or combination of agents, the optimal dose or dosing schedule, or the long-term safety and efficacy of treatment. These questions are amenable to RCTs if a collaborative group with adequate funding would take up the challenge.

Most other intravesical therapies fall into the category of initial hope followed by disappointment. Intravesical BCG showed promise in a controlled pilot study[93] and seemed to produce a durable response in a few patients.[94] However, a multicenter randomized study conducted by the NIDDK research network did not confirm the early work. A total of 265 patients were randomized to receive six weekly BCG instillations or saline instillation. The adjudicated response rates, based on the patient's global response assessment plus medication usage, were 12% for placebo and 21% for BCG ($P = .062$). The primary reason for the observed difference in response rates was that 15 of the patients taking BCG reported being "markedly improved," compared with only 5 of those taking placebo.[95] Similarly, capsaicin and its ultrapotent analogue, resiniferatoxin (RTX), appeared to offer great promise in the laboratory and in uncontrolled pilot trials,[96-98] but RTX failed in a pivotal phase II study. A randomized, double-blind, placebo-controlled study was conducted in 163 patients with IC; the participants were randomly assigned to receive a single intravesical dose of 50 mL of RTX at 0.01 µmol/L, 0.05 µmol/L, or 0.10 µmol/L or placebo. At the primary end point, RTX did not improve overall symptoms, pain, urgency, frequency, nocturia, or average void volume during 12 weeks of follow-up. RTX resulted in a dose-dependent increase in the incidence of instillation pain but was otherwise generally well tolerated.[99] Both of these studies had a significant effect on the IC research community in directing efforts away from these areas.

Currently, there has been interest in using botulinum toxin for IC/PBS, based on excellent results in patients with detrusor overactivity and the possibility of similar activity on sensory nerves. A small, uncontrolled pilot study included 13 patients in the United States and Poland who received either 100 or 200 units of botulinum A toxin (BTX-A) or Dysport. Nine (69%) showed a subjective response, and there was no urinary retention. In contrast, Kuo[100] injected 10 IC patients with either 100 units into the detrusor or 100 units in the detrusor plus an additional 100 units into the trigone. None of the patients was symptom free, and only limited improvements in bladder capacity and pain score were achieved in 2 patients. In this group, 7 of the 10 patients had subjective emptying symptoms, although there was no overt retention. In my own experience, one woman required intermittent self-catheterization for 2 months after a single injection. Although there is ample scientific rationale to be interested in botulinum toxin for treating IC/PBS, the ICI group concluded that, "Botox cannot be recommended for clinical use outside of carefully controlled studies."[71]

Physical Therapies

There is a clear clinical association between IC/PBS and muscular abnormalities of the pelvic floor.[101] It is not clear whether the pelvic floor myofascial abnormalities are primary or secondary, but the presence of such physical findings has encouraged a number of investigators to pursue pelvic floor physical therapies, including biofeedback, myofascial release, and trigger point injections. Vaginal and anorectal biofeedback therapy has sometimes shown beneficial effect,[102] but the current focus is on active internal physical therapy aimed at specific trigger points. Most preliminary studies have been very positive (Table 92-8). The NIDDK clinical trials group is currently preparing a controlled feasibility study to further investigate the possibility of using PT in men and women with PBS/IC and chronic pelvic pain.

Table 92-8 Published Effectiveness of Transvaginal Manual Physical Therapy (PT) for Painful Bladder Syndrome

Author & Year	Subjects & Intervention	Success Rate	How Determined
Weiss, 2002*	52 with IC or urgency/frequency, treated with manual PT to pelvic floor weekly for 8-12 wk	70% of IC patients and 83% of urgency/frequency patients had moderate to marked improvement	Subjective rating of percent improvement over baseline
Lukban, 2001 (abstract only, Whitmore group)	16 female IC with high-tone pelvic floor dysfunction and sacroiliac (SI) dysfunction treated with manual PT of SI joints, hip girdle, and pelvic floor for 2-15 visits	"94% improvement" in Oswestry disability score, symptom score; mean ICSI fell from 16 to 8	Modified Oswestry disability index, symptom scores, ICSI.
Oyama, 2004	21 female IC with high-tone pelvic floor dysfunction, treated with transvaginal Thiele massage† twice weekly for 5 wk	Overall rate not reported.	ICSI/ICPI decreased from 9 to 7; urgency VAS decreased from 4 to 3; pain VAS decreased from 5 to 3

*The methods reported by Weiss are typical of most pelvic floor physical therapists working in this field.
†Thiele massage does not require advanced pelvic floor PT training.
IC, interstitial cystitis; ICPI, IC problem index; ICSI, IC symptoms index; VAS, visual analogue score.
Data courtesy of MaryPat FitzGerald.

Physical therapy presents a very promising avenue for alleviation of symptoms in patients with chronic pelvic pain. A great deal of research is needed to confirm initial results, to refine patient selection, and to determine the optimal and necessary treatment regimen. At this time, there is a severe shortage of qualified physical therapists with interest and expertise in pelvic pain. Only by proving the efficacy of the treatment can more therapists be attracted to the field.

Nerve Stimulation

Neuromodulation is the most promising new avenue for treatment of refractory IC, and several different techniques are under active investigation. Sacral neuromodulation is clearly the best established treatment modality. Although it has not been formally studied for IC, the Medtronic InterStim device has been approved by the FDA for urinary urgency and frequency since 1997, and many IC patients have benefited from implants. Maher and coauthors[103] first reported on the use of the device in 15 patients with IC. The patients were older (mean, 62 years) and had a dramatic acute response, with 73% going on to receive a permanent implant. Mean bladder pain decreased from 8.9 to 2.4 on a 10-point scale, and mean voided volume increased from 90 to 143 mL. Similar improvements were seen in bladder diary and symptom scores. Results of chronic stimulation were not reported. Comiter[104] described the results in 25 IC patients (mean age, 47 years) who had a trial of percutaneous nerve stimulation or a staged technique. Seventeen (68%) were successful and went on to a permanent implant. Success was much higher with the staged technique (13 of 15 patients) than with the percutaneous evaluation (4 of 10 patients). Striking improvement was seen in symptom scores, pain, and bladder diary variables. Peters[105] also compared the standard percutaneous approach to the new staged implantation technique with similar conclusions. In a separate report, Peters[106] examined the results of sacral neuromodulation for IC after 6 months. Moderate or marked improvement in pain was reported by 20 of 21 patients, and 4 of 18 became free of narcotics. For those taking narcotics at the outset, the morphine dose equivalent decreased from 82 to 52 mg/day. There is a great need to determine the durability of sacral neuromodulation in the IC population and to identify optimal candidates. I recommend patients who have primary urge-frequency and adequate bladder capacity under anesthesia for this therapy, but better data would be welcome.

Other forms of nerve stimulation have not been as impressive. Posterior tibial stimulation was ineffective in 14 patients with refractory IC,[107] and a randomized study of transdermal pulsed laser therapy to the posterior tibial nerve showed no difference between active and sham devices in the treatment of IC.[108] An exciting technology under development is pudendal nerve stimulation. Although no device is yet approved for this use, Peters[105] conducted a randomized trial in which 30 patients underwent simultaneous placement of electrodes at S3 and the pudendal nerve. Twenty-four (80%) of the subjects responded and had a permanent implant placed. The pudendal nerve was chosen as a superior lead in 79.2%; the sacral site was superior in 20.8%. The order in which the leads were simulated had no impact on the final lead implanted, and no carryover effect was seen. Overall reduction in symptoms was 63% for the peripheral nervous system and 46% for the sympathetic nervous system ($P = .02$). This is particularly exciting work, because devices are being tested that could be placed percutaneously in an office setting.

Surgical Therapies

Surgery is often employed early in the management of IC/PBS; traditionally, bladder distention has been the first treatment most IC patients experience, with the "diagnosis" of IC made by cystoscopy, distention, and biopsy. However, as discussed earlier, the role of cystoscopy in the diagnosis of IC is undergoing a major reevaluation; this, in turn, forces bladder distention to be considered more on its own merits as an IC treatment. Overall, it appears that bladder distention is a marginally effective therapy. Although the quality of reporting is generally poor and dominated by retrospective, highly selected case series, there is general agreement that hydrodistention has a modest and transient value in the treatment of IC/PBS symptoms, with 20% to 60% of patients experiencing partial or complete resolution of symptoms, almost always for less than 6 months.[79,109-111] Because bladder distention is the most expensive and invasive of the primary IC treatments, it seems reasonable to employ it selectively rather than universally.

I recommend selecting patients for distention who either are more likely to benefit from the procedure or may benefit from the diagnostic and prognostic information obtained. There is weak evidence that patients with a large bladder capacity under anesthesia (>600 mL) are less likely to respond to distention.[109] Although functional bladder capacity by voiding diary correlates poorly with bladder capacity under anesthesia, some patients with IC symptoms have fairly normal maximum void volumes on diary (>250 mL). These patients seem to be more likely to have a large capacity under anesthesia and are therefore less likely to benefit from the procedure. In addition, it is probable that these patients might be adequately assessed by office cystoscopy when an evaluation is required for hematuria or some other reason. Patients with very small capacities on void diary (<150 mL) are less likely to tolerate office cystoscopy and somewhat more likely to benefit from a bladder distention. Bladder distention allows the clinician to stratify the findings, giving some objective sense of severity of disease. Although one cannot say that the objective findings directly correlate with prognosis in an individual patient, they do allow for identification of a subgroup of patients with severe disease that might be treated more aggressively and provide some reassurance for those with clearly normal bladder capacity under anesthesia.

Regarding the technique of distention, the critical issues are to adequately characterize the baseline cystoscopy, the findings on distention, and the bladder capacity under anesthesia. Our method is delineated as follows, but it is most important that the clinician be internally consistent in technique.

1. The distention should be performed with the patient under a deep general or regional anesthesia. Local anesthesia and sedation do not allow for a full therapeutic distention. The patient experiences the trauma of the procedure without the potential benefit.
2. The entire urothelium is carefully visualized before distention. Abnormalities present at this time usually represent ulcers that will crack and tear during distention. If abnormal areas are seen, bladder wash cytology and bladder biopsies should be obtained.
3. We distend the bladder for 7 minutes under direct vision at 80 cm H_2O pressure. In women, digital pressure at the bladder neck may be required to prevent leakage around the cystoscope, which would both produce inaccurate information about the bladder capacity and lessen the

potential therapeutic impact of the procedure. Linear cracking seen during distention after an initially normal cystoscopy is an intermediate-level finding indicating more severe disease with loss of elasticity.
4. The bladder is then drained. At least the first part of the drainage procedure should be done under direct vision through the side port of the cystoscope. Capillary bleeding (glomerulation) may be dramatic but transient and is best seen during the drainage. If possible, photographs taken sequentially during this time help to document the findings for future reference and provide validating information for the patient. The cystoscopic fluid is collected and measured. Terminal hematuria is subjectively graded.
5. If any lesions were seen on the initial cystoscopy, they are biopsied at this time. Ulcers should be completely fulgurated, because this may provide the patient a dramatic response with relief of pain. The value of biopsy when the initial cystoscopy is normal is unclear. Many clinicians prefer to look for detrusor mastocytosis and to treat such patients aggressively with antihistamines. Patients often appreciate the objective data removing the fear of cancer. On the other hand, biopsy adds trauma and risk of complication and has not been shown to affect outcome.
6. A complete report of the procedure includes the baseline findings, the findings during distention, subjective grading of glomerulations and terminal hematuria, and the bladder capacity under anesthesia.

Although the role of cystoscopy and bladder distention has been markedly diminished, it is still an important procedure with some diagnostic, prognostic, and therapeutic value. It does not need to be the initial procedure or treatment, but it should always be performed if the picture is confusing or there is no response to standard treatments.

Special attention is directed to the treatment of ulcers. As mentioned earlier, patients with ulcers often respond dramatically to a variety of local treatments; in fact, Hunner advocated partial cystectomy in such cases.[1] One danger related to the declining role of cystoscopy in the diagnosis of IC is the possibility of overlooking this group of patients, who actually have an excellent prognosis for at least intermediate- to long-term pain relief. Almost all reports agree that complete treatment of ulcers by any of a variety of techniques (partial cystectomy, endoscopic resection, cauterization) produces almost uniform pain relief. Laser treatment without distention has been advocated for ulcer patients, with 13 of 24 subjects having a mean response duration of 19 months after only a single treatment.[112] I agree that ulcer treatment can be performed without distention, but I have not seen any advantage in using the laser over standard electrocautery.

Despite the wide variety of treatment options already discussed, a substantial minority of IC patients suffer from severe frequency and debilitating pain that is refractory to all therapy. Many are disabled by their disease. These patients are candidates for radical surgery. As with other IC treatments, the options are myriad and confusing, and the data to support any particular treatment are suspect. Reasonable minimum requirements for considering radical surgery include the following:

1. An adequate trial of all standard IC treatments and appropriate secondary therapies
2. A concerted effort at pain management, ideally by a specialist in the field
3. Realistic understanding of the nature of the surgical procedure, the risks of the procedure itself, and the possibility that pain may persist even after diversion or complete cystectomy

There is a general sense that patients with objectively severe disease (reduced capacity under anesthesia) are better candidates for surgery. A capacity of less than 350 mL clearly represents a major (and possibly irreversible) change in the bladder. The bladder has lost elasticity and may become progressively fibrotic. If sequential hydrodistentions demonstrate progressive loss of capacity, the picture is even more ominous. Very low capacity can be associated with hydronephrosis, reflux, and intractable frequency and/or pain. Even as new treatments for IC are developed, it is not clear that these bladders can be salvaged. If the bladder capacity is greater than 600 mL under anesthesia, the patient clearly has the potential for complete rehabilitation, and radical surgery should be approached with trepidation. Although the published literature lacks adequate detail and power, there is a strong suggestion that a bladder capacity of less than 350 mL is a predictor for success with surgery. If a surgical approach is chosen, there are a number of options. Some of the published data on the various operations are reviewed in Table 92-9. These approaches are briefly reviewed here, with the key decision making factors for each.

1. *Supratrigonal cystectomy and augmentation:* For a period of time, this procedure was considered standard treatment for severe IC, and there is much more data about it than about other operations. Most of the early enthusiasm has waned, despite good published results. The primary advantage of this approach is simplicity, because there is no need for ureteral reimplantation. Risks include the development of urinary retention and ureteral reflux. Patients should be willing to accept self-catheterization, because the development of retention is unpredictable.
2. *Conduit diversion with or without cystectomy:* I consider conduit urinary diversion to be the standard surgical treatment for patients with refractory IC. The patients can be assured of relief of urinary frequency. Pain relief should be at least as high as with any other surgical therapy, and the risk of recurrent symptoms may be the lowest. It is probable that mere diversion of the urine will produce adequate pain relief in most cases; cystectomy is not routinely required. Some surgeons believe that the diseased organ must be removed to prevent other local complications.[113] The negative aspects of conduit diversion include problems related to the stoma (e.g., skin complications, hernia formation) and the altered body image.
3. *Total cystectomy and neobladder:* The primary alternative to conduit diversion is total cystectomy plus neobladder. The obvious advantage is the possibility of a completely normal lifestyle—normal voiding and a normal body image. On the other hand, this operation is technically more demanding; cystectomy is required and must be carefully performed to provide an appropriate field for the neobladder. The short-term complications of the procedure are therefore higher than with a conduit. The long-term complications are probably less, except for the possibility of recurrent pain. It has been theorized that contact between IC urine and intestine can lead to disease in the intestinal segment; this is not well supported by data, but if it is true, the contact time is much greater with a

Table 92-9 Radical Surgery for Interstitial Cystitis

Author	Year	Operation	*N*	Initial Response	Follow-up (Mean [Range])	Comments
Begany and Politano	1995	Neobladder	5	100% pain free	52 mo (3-78 mo)	All had <250 mL anesthetic capacity and were continent; 2 were on self-catheterization
Nurse et al.	1991	Neobladder	8	NR	NR	Offered to patients with IC in trigone by biopsy, one patient with SUI
Costello et al.	2000	Supratrigonal cystectomy and ileocystoplasty	5	100% pain free	18 mo (3-69 mo)	Anesthetic capacity 120-350 mL, all patients continent, 2 patients on self-catheterization; only 2 had follow-up >3 mo
Webster and Maggio	1989	Supratrigonal cystectomy and augmentation	19	12 no symptoms, 4 pain free but with frequency, 2 self-catheterization	39 mo (12-76 mo)	Anesthetic capacity 150-550 mL, 16/19 right colon, some not detubularized, 4 with reflux
Peeker et al.	1998	Supratrigonal cystectomy and ileocystoplasty	13	10/10 with classic disease successful, but all with nonulcer disease failed	5 yr (6 mo-8 yr)	7/10 voided, 3 self-catheterized; all nonulcer patients successfully treated with Kock pouch and resection of trigone
Nurse et al.	1991	Supratrigonal cystectomy and augmentation	24 unselected	16 successful, 8 with persistent frequency/urgency	NR	—
			12 selected by biopsy	10 successful	Less than above	Only patients without disease on trigone biopsy offered procedure
Kontturi et al.	1991	Supratrigonal cystectomy and colocystoplasty	12	9 successful	4.7 yr (1.2 to 11 yr)	2 cystectomy/conduit (persistent pain, SUI); 3 BNI for retention; 2 urge incontinence
Nielsen et al.	1990	Supratrigonal cystectomy and ileocystoplasty	8	2 successful, 6 with recurrent pain; 4/6 with retention requiring self-catheterization	10 mo (8-22 mo)	Median bladder capacity 435 mL (range, 200-675 mL); all failures >400 mL; 5/6 failures had cystectomy and diversion
Lotenfoe et al.	1995	Cystectomy and continent diversion	22	73% "surgical cure"; 7 patients with persistent pain postoperatively	NR	14/17 (82%) success if <400 mL, 1/5 if >400 mL; recommend epidural to localize pain & psychological evaluation

SUI, stress urinary incontinence.

continent form of diversion than with a conduit. As with supratrigonal cystectomy and augmentation, this form of reconstruction must be strictly limited to patients who are willing to perform self-intermittent catheterization. I have performed six neobladder operations in women with IC and contracted bladders. Five of the six are continent and pain free but have to self-catheterize three to six times per day due to incomplete voiding. The other patient developed persistent pain and stress incontinence very early in the postoperative period.

4. *Continent diversion with or without cystectomy:* Continent urinary diversion is the most complex reconstructive procedure and has the highest complication rate. The catheterizable stoma requires revision due to problems with catheterization or incontinence in approximately 20% to 30% of patients. The procedure is primarily indicated for the patient who seeks a more normal body image, without an external appliance, but is not able to perform self-catheterization (due to urethral pain). The same issue as to whether a cystectomy should be performed applies as with a conduit diversion.

In summary, radical surgical procedures offer tremendous relief to a small subset of IC patients with severe, refractory disease. These patients must be carefully screened in order to select those with the highest likelihood of benefit. There is no clear "best" reconstructive procedure, so the decision must be made based on individual patient preferences and the judgment of the surgeon.

Pain Management

Not all patients with IC complain of pain. Some describe an uncomfortable "pressure" in the bladder that generates urinary frequency while denying any "pain." Nonetheless, most IC patients suffer from some degree of pain, and for many the pain is debilitating. Given that IC is not a curable disease at the current time, pain control becomes a legitimate and important goal in and of itself. Nevertheless, pain management tends to be poorly handled in IC (as in many chronic diseases) for a variety of reasons, some legitimate and some not. The impediments to proper pain control and strategies for improving pain management in IC/PBS are discussed in this section.

Physicians are often reluctant to prescribe pain medication to IC patients. In contrast, most physicians feel comfortable prescribing pain medication to their postsurgical patients. This simple dichotomy highlights some of the important issues about pain in IC. Surgeons are trained in the management of acute pain. They understand the disease process, the expected course, and the range of responses that might be expected with various medications. Still, postoperative pain is often undertreated due to individual variation. Surgeons are much less comfortable treating chronic pain. Even when the disease process is understood, there is a reluctance to use adequate doses of chronic analgesics; this is in large part due to a lack of training and relatively limited exposure to this type of patient. The IC patient faces an even greater hurdle, the hurdle of "invisible disease." In our current state of knowledge, IC is a diagnosis of exclusion, raising the specter of the patient as a malingerer and/or drug seeker. This is relevant because urologists have long been the target of such behavior, in the guise of the recurrent stone patient. Suspicion of motive, uncertainty of diagnosis, and a feeling of inadequacy can interfere with the physician's role. Finally, although lip service is paid to the importance of adequate pain control, physicians continue to see colleagues cited for improper prescription of controlled substances. Lawsuits have been filed for inadequate pain treatment but also for contributing to addiction. Many states place significant additional burdens on providers of common therapeutic narcotics.

At the same time, we must acknowledge that treatment of acute pain in IC is quite difficult. Narcotics and nonsteroidal medications are often ineffective. It is therefore incumbent on the patient to try and address the issue of pain control proactively. In many instances, the "best" arrangement is for the patient to be referred to a pain specialist, typically an anesthesiologist or oncologist skilled in the evaluation and management of chronic pain. In this setting, the urologist continues to work with the patient with standard bladder treatments while the pain specialist uses alternative approaches. In the best of cases, this involves multimodality therapy, including narcotic and non-narcotic analgesics, physical therapy, and psychological counseling, nerve blocks, and so on.

Some of the principles used in working with chronic pain are as follows.

1. Long-acting narcotics are preferable to short-acting narcotics. The dose of the long-acting drug is titrated up to a satisfactory level, and the patient is given a small amount of short-acting medication for breakthrough pain.
2. Combination medical therapy is usually superior to narcotics alone. Nonsteroidal anti-inflammatory medications, tricyclic antidepressants, and a wide variety of novel medications (often anticonvulsants) can be used to achieve a synergistic response.
3. Analgesic medications should be tied to concrete, functional outcomes. It is unlikely that a medication will provide complete resolution of the problem. Objective improvements can be assessed in any of a variety of role functions (e.g., work, home, sexual) as well as in urinary frequency and pain control.

The most important principle is for the physician to care for the patient as a family member, using all diagnostic skill, all reasonable therapeutic modalities, and the utmost compassion.

CONCLUSIONS

IC presents a formidable challenge to the urologist. The disease continues to create diagnostic problems and to defy the development of universally effective therapy. Although it is easy for the clinician and patient to become frustrated, most patients can achieve substantial amelioration of their symptoms over time.

Teamwork is required in the management of IC, more so than in almost any other disease faced by the urologist. The clinician must respect the integrity of the patient and the burden faced by those living with "invisible disease." The patient must actively participate in seeking effective therapy. Although it is always reasonable to hope for a cure, realistic goals must be set with an aim to maximizing function.

If behavioral techniques such as dietary modification, stress reduction, and bladder training fail to control the symptoms of IC, medical treatment is indicated. First-line therapies include bladder distention, DMSO bladder instillations, PPS, amitriptyline, and hydroxyzine. Most patients respond to one of these treatments. New treatments being investigated for refractory disease include instillations of BCG and hyaluronic acid and sacral nerve stimulation. The role of therapy directed at the pelvic floor muscles (myofascial release and biofeedback) is also being defined. Pain management is an underutilized tool for a disease in which daily pain is a common symptom. A multidisciplinary approach using the skills of a urologist, a physical therapist, and a pain specialist can produce excellent results. Ultimately, a small percentage of patients will go on to radical surgical treatment. Limited evidence suggests that those with a low bladder capacity under anesthesia (<350 mL) do especially well with surgery, although the optimal method of urinary tract reconstruction has not been established.

High-quality RCTs are desperately needed in the study of IC. Only through this type of research will we be able to make progress in discovering which therapies work for which patients and to counsel patients accordingly. Clinicians are encouraged to work together to develop clinical protocols, and patients are urged to participate in research studies whenever possible.

References

1. Hunner GL: A rare type of bladder ulcer in women: Report of cases. Boston Med Surg J 172:660-664, 1915.
2. Hand JR: Interstitial cystitis: Report of 223 cases (204 women and 19 men) J Urol 61:291-310, 1949.
3. Messing EM, Stamey TA: Interstitial cystitis: Early diagnosis, pathology, and treatment. Urology 12:381-392, 1978.
4. Abrams P, Cardozo L, Fall M, et al: The standardisation of terminology of lower urinary tract function: Report from the Standardisation Sub-committee of the International Continence Society. Neurourol Urodyn 21:167-178, 2002.
5. Gillenwater JY, Wein AJ: Summary of the National Institute of Arthritis, Diabetes, Digestive, and Kidney Diseases workshop on interstitial cystitis. Bethesda, Maryland, National Institutes of Health, August 28-29, 1987. J Urol 140: 203-206, 1988.
6. Hanno PM, Landis JR, Matthews-Cook Y, et al: The diagnosis of interstitial cystitis revisited: Lessons learned from the National Institutes of Health Interstitial Cystitis Database study. J Urol 161:553-557, 1999.
7. Propert KJ, Payne C, Kusek JW, Nyberg LM: Pitfalls in the design of clinical trials for interstitial cystitis. Urology 60:742-748, 2002.
8. Payne CK, Terai A, Komatsu K: Research criteria versus clinical criteria for interstitial cystitis. Int J Urol 10:S7-S10, 2003.
9. Payne CK: Oral presentation of the report of the clinical Subcommittee on the Diagnosis of Interstitial Cystitis and Painful Bladder Syndrome, NIDDK IC Research Forum, Alexandria, Virginia, October 30-November 1, 2003.
10. Ito T, Miki M, Yamada T: Interstitial cystitis in Japan. BJU Int 86:634-637, 2000.
11. Bade JJ, Rijcken B, Mensink HJA: Interstitial cystitis in The Netherlands: Prevalence, diagnostic criteria and therapeutic preferences. J Urol 154:2035-2037; discussion 2037-2038, 1995.
12. Clemens JQ, Meenan RT, O'Keeffe Rosetti MC, et al: Prevalence and incidence of interstitial cystitis in a managed care population. J Urol 173:98-102; discussion 102, 2005.
13. Leppilahti M, Sairanen J, Tammela TL, et al: Prevalence of clinically confirmed interstitial cystitis in women: A population based study in Finland. J Urol 174:581-583, 2005.
14. Orovisto KJ: Epidemiology of Interstitial Cystitis Ann. Chir Gynecol Fenn 64(2):75-77, 1975.
15. Curhan GC, Speizer FE, Hunter DJ, et al: Epidemiology of interstitial cystitis: A population based study. J Urol 162:500, 1999.
16. Jones CA, Nyberg L: Epidemiology of interstitial cystitis. Urology 49:2-9, 1997.
17. Clemens JQ, Meenan RT, O'Keeffe Rosetti MC, et al: Prevalence of interstitial cystitis symptoms in a managed care population. J Urol 174:576-580, 2005.
18. Leppilahti M, Tammela TL, Huhtala H, Auvinen A: Prevalence of symptoms related to interstitial cystitis in women: A population based study in Finland. J Urol 168:139-143, 2002.
19. Parsons CL, Tatsis V: Prevalence of interstitial cystitis in young women. Urology 64:866-870, 2004.
20. Roberts RO, Bergstralh EJ, Bass SE, et al: Incidence of physician-diagnosed interstitial cystitis in Olmsted County: A community-based study. BJU Int 91:181-185, 2003.
21. Koziol JA, Clark DC, Gittes RF, Tan EM: The natural history of interstitial cystitis: A survey of 374 patients. J Urol 149:465-469, 1993.
22. Koziol JA: Epidemiology of interstitial cystitis. Urol Clin North Am 21:7-20, 1994.
23. Tincello DG, Walker AC: Interstitial cystitis in the UK: Results of a questionnaire survey of members of the Interstitial Cystitis Support Group. Eur J Obstet Gynecol Reprod Biol 118:91-95, 2005.
24. Clemens JQ, Joyce GF, Wise M, Payne CK: Interstitial cystitis and painful bladder syndrome. In Litwin MS, Saigal CS (eds): Urologic Diseases in America. U.S. Department of Health and Human Services, Public Health Service, National Institutes of Health, National Institute of Diabetes and Digestive and Kidney Diseases. NIH Publication No. 07-5512. Washington, DC: U.S. Government Printing Office, 2007.
25. Clauw DJ, Schmidt M, Radulovic D, et al: The relationship between fibromyalgia and interstitial cystitis. J Psychiatr Res 31:125-131, 1997.
26. Erickson DR, Morgan KC, Ordille S, et al: Nonbladder related symptoms in patients with interstitial cystitis. J Urol 166:557-561; discussion 561-562, 2001.
27. Alagiri M, Chottiner S, Ratner V, et al: Interstitial cystitis: Unexplained associations with other chronic disease and pain syndromes. Urology 49(5A Suppl):52-57, 1997.
28. Chung MK, Chung RP, Gordon D: Interstitial cystitis and endometriosis in patients with chronic pelvic pain: The "Evil Twins" syndrome. JSLS 9:25-29, 2005.
29. Weissman MM, Gross R, Fyer A, et al: Interstitial cystitis and panic disorder: A potential genetic syndrome. Arch Gen Psychiatry 61:273-279, 2004.
30. Buffington CA: Comorbidity of interstitial cystitis with other unexplained clinical conditions. J Urol 172(4 Pt 1):1242-1248, 2004.
31. Buffington CA, Pacak K: Increased plasma norepinephrine concentration in cats with interstitial cystitis. J Urol 165(6 Pt 1):2051-2054, 2001.
32. Buffington CA, Teng B, Somogyi GT: Norepinephrine content and adrenoceptor function in the bladder of cats with feline interstitial cystitis. J Urol 167:1876-1880, 2002.
33. Westropp JL, Welk KA, Buffington CA: Small adrenal glands in cats with feline interstitial cystitis. J Urol 170(6 Pt 1):2494-2497, 2003.
34. Wessely S, Nimnuan C, Sharpe M: Functional somatic syndromes: One or many? Lancet 354:936-939, 1999.
35. Peeker R, Enerback L, Fall M, Aldenborg F: Recruitment, distribution and phenotypes of mast cells in interstitial cystitis. J Urol 163:1009-1015, 2000.
36. Theoharides TC, Sant GR, el-Mansoury M, et al: Activation of bladder mast cells in interstitial cystitis: A light and electron microscopic study. J Urol 153(3 Pt 1):629-636, 1995.
37. Tomaszewski JE, Landis JR, Russack V, et al: Biopsy features are associated with primary symptoms in interstitial cystitis: Results from the interstitial cystitis database study. Urology 57:67-81, 2001.

38. Erickson DR, Xie SX, Bhavanandan VP, et al: A comparison of multiple urine markers for interstitial cystitis. J Urol 167:2461-2469, 2002.
39. Parsons CL: Prostatitis, interstitial cystitis, chronic pelvic pain, and urethral syndrome share a common pathophysiology: Lower urinary dysfunctional epithelium and potassium recycling. Urology 62:976-982, 2003.
40. Keay S, Zhang CO, Trifillis AL, et al: Decreased 3H-thymidine incorporation by human bladder epithelial cells following exposure to urine from interstitial cystitis patients. J Urol 156:2073-2078, 1996.
41. Keay S, Warren JW, Zhang CO, et al: Antiproliferative activity is present in bladder but not renal pelvic urine from interstitial cystitis patients. J Urol 162:1487-1489, 1999.
42. Keay S, Zhang CO, Marvel R, Chai T: Stretch-activated release of adenosine triphosphate by bladder uroepithelia is augmented in interstitial cystitis. Urology 57(Suppl 6):9-14, 2001.
43. Chai TC, Zhang C-O, Shoenfelt JL, et al: Bladder stretch alters urinary heparin-binding epidermal growth factor and antiproliferative factor in patients with interstitial cystitis. J Urol 163:1440-1444, 2000.
44. Chai TC, Zhang C, Warren JW, Keay S: Percutaneous sacral third nerve root neurostimulation improves symptoms and normalizes urinary HB-EGF levels and antiproliferative activity in patients with interstitial cystitis. Urology 55:643-646, 2000.
45. Keay S, Kleinberg M, Zhang CO, et al: Bladder epithelial cells from patients with interstitial cystitis produce an inhibitor of heparin-binding epidermal growth factor-like growth factor production. J Urol 164:2112-2118, 2000.
46. Keay SK, Szekely Z, Conrads TP, et al: An antiproliferative factor from interstitial cystitis patients is a frizzled 8 protein-related sialoglycopeptide. Proc Natl Acad Sci U S A. 101:11803-11808, 2004. Epub 2004 July 28.
47. Warren JW, Jackson TL, Langenberg P, et al: Prevalence of interstitial cystitis in first-degree relatives of patients with interstitial cystitis. Urology 63:17-21, 2004.
48. Warren J, Jackson T, Meyers D, Xu J: Concordance of interstitial cystitis (IC) in identical twins: Preliminary data. Urology 57(6 Suppl 1):126, 2001.
49. Bushman W: Oral presentation of the report of the clinical Subcommittee on the Diagnosis of Interstitial Cystitis and Painful Bladder Syndrome. NIDDK IC Research Forum, Alexandria, Virginia, October 30-November 1, 2003.
50. Teichman JM, Nielsen-Omeis BJ, McIver BD: Modified urodynamics for interstitial cystitis. Tech Urol 3:65-68, 1997.
51. Parsons CL, Stein PC, Bidair M, Lebow D: Abnormal sensitivity to intravesical potassium in interstitial cystitis and radiation cystitis. Neurourol Urodyn 13:515-520, 1994.
52. Henry R, Patterson L, Avery N, et al: Absorption of alkalized intravesical lidocaine in normal and inflamed bladders: A simple method for improving bladder anesthesia. J Urol 165(6 Pt 1):1900-1903, 2001.
53. Pontari MA: Oral presentation of the report of the clinical Subcommittee on the Diagnosis of Interstitial Cystitis and Painful Bladder Syndrome, NIDDK IC Research Forum, October 30-November 1, 2003, Alexandria, Virginia.
54. Awad SA, MacDiarmid S, Gajewski JB, Gupta R: Idiopathic reduced bladder storage versus interstitial cystitis. J Urol 148:1409-1412, 1992.
55. Waxman JA, Sulak PJ, Kuehl TJ: Cystoscopic findings consistent with interstitial cystitis in normal women undergoing tubal ligation. J Urol 160:1663-1667, 1998.
56. Erickson DR, Tomaszewski JE, Kunselman AR, et al: Do the National Institute of Diabetes and Digestive and Kidney Diseases cystoscopic criteria associate with other clinical and objective features of interstitial cystitis. J Urol 173:93-97, 2005.
57. Utz DC, Zincke H: The masquerade of bladder cancer in situ as interstitial cystitis. J Urol 111:160-161, 1974.
58. Tissot WD, Diokno AC, Peters KM: A referral center's experience with transitional cell carcinoma misdiagnosed as interstitial cystitis. J Urol 172:478-480, 2004.
59. Nickel JC, Ardern D, Downey J: Cytologic evaluation of urine is important in evaluation of chronic prostatitis. Urology 60:225-227, 2002.
60. Gomes CM, Sanchez-Ortiz RF, Harris C, et al: Significance of hematuria in patients with interstitial cystitis: Review of radiographic and endoscopic findings. Urology 57:262-265, 2001.
61. Stanford EJ, Mattox TF, Parsons JK, McMurphy C: Prevalence of benign microscopic hematuria among women with interstitial cystitis: Implications for evaluation of genitourinary malignancy. Urology 67:946-949, 2006.
62. Parsons CL: Potassium sensitivity test. Tech Urol 2:171-173, 1996.
63. Parsons CL, Dell J, Stanford EJ, et al: The prevalence of interstitial cystitis in gynecologic patients with pelvic pain, as detected by intravesical potassium sensitivity. Am J Obstet Gynecol 187:1395-1400, 2002.
64. Parsons CL, Rosenberg MT, Sassani P, et al: Quantifying symptoms in men with interstitial cystitis/prostatitis, and its correlation with potassium-sensitivity testing. BJU Int 95:86-90, 2005.
65. Philip J, Willmott S, Irwin P: Interstitial cystitis versus detrusor overactivity: A comparative, randomized, controlled study of cystometry using saline and 0.3 M potassium chloride. J Urol 175:566-570; discussion 570-571, 2006.
66. FitzGerald MP, Kenton KS, Brubaker L: Localization of the urge to void in patients with painful bladder syndrome. Neurourol Urodyn 24:633-637, 2005.
67. FitzGerald MP, Koch D, Senka J: Visceral and cutaneous sensory testing in patients with painful bladder syndrome. Neurourol Urodyn 24:627-632, 2005.
68. Pezzone MA, Liang R, Fraser MO: A model of neural cross-talk and irritation in the pelvis: Implications for the overlap of chronic pelvic pain disorders. Gastroenterology 128:1953-1964, 2005.
69. Ustinova EE, Fraser MO, Pezzone MA: Colonic irritation in the rat sensitizes urinary bladder afferents to mechanical and chemical stimuli: An afferent origin of pelvic organ cross-sensitization. Am J Physiol Renal Physiol 290:F1478-F1487, 2006.
70. Gupta SK, Pidcock L, Parr NJ: The potassium sensitivity test: A predictor of treatment response in interstitial cystitis. BJU Int 96:1063-1066, 2005.
71. Hanno P, Keay S, Moldwin R, Van Ophoven A: Forging an international consensus: Progress in painful bladder syndrome/interstitial cystitis. Report and abstracts. International Consultation for Incontinence, Rome, September 2004. Int Urogynecol J Pelvic Floor Dysfunct 16(Suppl 1):S2-S34, 2005.
72. Chaiken DC, Blaivas JG, Blaivas ST. Behavioral therapy for the treatment of refractory interstitial cystitis. J Urol 149:1445-1448, 1993.
73. Parsons CL, Koprowski PF: Interstitial cystitis: Successful management by increasing urinary voiding intervals. Urology 37:207-212, 1991.
74. Nguan. 2005.
75. Warren JW, Horne LM, Hebel R, et al: Pilot study of sequential oral antibiotics for the treatment of interstitial cystitis. J Urol 163:1685-1688, 2000.
76. Hanno PM: Analysis of long-term Elmiron therapy for interstitial cystitis. Urology 49(Suppl 5A):93-99, 1997.
77. Jepsen JV, Sall M, Rhodes PR, et al: Long-term experience with pentosanpolysulfate in interstitial cystitis. Urology 51:381-387, 1998.
78. van Ophoven A, Heinecke A, Hertle L: Safety and efficacy of concurrent application of oral pentosan polysulfate and subcutaneous low-dose heparin for patients with interstitial cystitis. Urology 66:707-711, 2005.

79. Erickson DR, Sheykhnazari M, Bhavanandan VP: Molecular size affects urine excretion of pentosan polysulfate. J Urol 175(3 Pt 1): 1143-1147, 2006.
80. Muthusamy A, Erickson DR, Sheykhnazari M, Bhavanandan VP: Enhanced binding of modified pentosan polysulfate and heparin to bladder: A strategy for improved treatment of interstitial cystitis. Urology 67:209-213, 2006.
81. Dong L, Yum A, Nguyen J, Wong P: Enhanced ileal absorption of a hydrophilic macromolecule, pentosan polysulfate sodium (PPS). J Biomater Sci Polym Ed 15:671-682, 2004.
82. Hanno PM, Buehler J, Wein AJ: Use of amitriptyline in the treatment of interstitial cystitis. J Urol 141:846-848, 1989.
83. Kirkemo AK, Miles BJ, Peters KM: Use of amitriptyline in treatment of interstitial cystitis. J Urol 143:279A, 1990.
84. Pranikoff K, Constantino G: The use of amitriptyline in patients with urinary frequency and pain. Urology 51(5A Suppl):179-181, 1998.
85. Theoharides TC: Hydroxyzine in the treatment of interstitial cystitis. Urol Clin North Am 21:113-118, 1994.
86. Sant GR, Propert KJ, Hanno PM, et al; Interstitial Cystitis Clinical Trials Group: A pilot clinical trial of oral pentosan polysulfate and oral hydroxyzine in patients with interstitial cystitis. J Urol 170:810-815, 2003.
87. Thilagarajah R, Witherow RO, Walker MM: Oral cimetidine gives effective symptom relief in painful bladder disease: A prospective, randomized, double-blind placebo-controlled trial. BJU Int 87:207-212, 2001.
88. Sairanen J, Tammela TL, Leppilahti M, et al: Cyclosporine A and pentosan polysulfate sodium for the treatment of interstitial cystitis: A randomized comparative study. J Urol 174:2235-2238, 2005.
89. Sairanen J, Forsell T, Ruutu M: Long-term outcome of patients with interstitial cystitis treated with low dose cyclosporine A. J Urol 171(6 Pt 1):2138-2141, 2004.
90. Perez-Marrero R, Emerson LE, Feltis JT: A controlled study of dimethyl sulfoxide in interstitial cystitis. J Urol 140:36-39, 1988.
91. Peeker R, Haghsheno MA, Holmang S, Fall M: Intravesical bacillus Calmette-Guerin and dimethyl sulfoxide for treatment of classic and nonulcer interstitial cystitis: A prospective, randomized double-blind study. J Urol 164:1912-1915; discussion 1915-1916, 2000.
92. Interstitial Cystitis Association: Physician Perspectives. Rockville, MD, Interstitial Cystitis Association, 2004.
93. Peters K, Diokno A, Steinert B, et al: The efficacy of intravesical Tice strain bacillus Calmette-Guerin in the treatment of interstitial cystitis: A double-blind, prospective, placebo controlled trial. J Urol 157:2090, 1997.
94. Peters KM, Diokno AC, Steinert BW, Gonzalez JA: The efficacy of intravesical bacillus Calmette-Guerin in the treatment of interstitial cystitis: Long-term followup. J Urol 159:1483, 1998.
95. Mayer R, Propert KJ, Peters KM, et al; Interstitial Cystitis Clinical Trials Group: A randomized controlled trial of intravesical bacillus calmette-guerin for treatment refractory interstitial cystitis. J Urol 173:1186-1191, 2005.
96. Craft RM, Carlisi VJ, Mattia A, et al: Behavioral characterization of the excitatory and desensitizing effects of intravesical capsaicin and resiniferatoxin in the rat. Pain 55:205, 1993.
97. Craft RM, Cohen SM, Porreca F: Long-lasting desensitization of bladder afferents following intravesical resiniferatoxin and capsaicin in the rat. Pain 61:317, 1995.
98. Lazzeri M, Beneforti P, Spinelli M, et al: Intravesical resiniferatoxin for the treatment of hypersensitive disorder: A randomized placebo controlled study. J Urol 164:676, 2000.
99. Payne CK, Mosbaugh PG, Forrest JB, et al; ICOS RTX Study Group (Resiniferatoxin Treatment for Interstitial Cystitis). Intravesical resiniferatoxin for the treatment of interstitial cystitis: A randomized, double-blind, placebo controlled trial. J Urol 173:1590-1594, 2005.
100. Kuo HC: Preliminary results of suburothelial injection of botulinum a toxin in the treatment of chronic interstitial cystitis. Urol Int 75:170-174, 2005.
101. FitzGerald MP, Kotarinos R: Rehabilitation of the short pelvic floor. I: Background and patient evaluation. Int Urogynecol J Pelvic Floor Dysfunct 14:261-268, 2003. Epub 2003 Aug 2.
102. Cornel EB, van Haarst EP, Schaarsberg RW, Geels J: The effect of biofeedback physical therapy in men with chronic pelvic pain syndrome type III. Eur Urol 47:607-611, 2005. Epub 2005 Jan 22.
103. Maher CF, Carey MP, Dwyer PL, Schluter PL: Percutaneous sacral nerve root neuromodulation for intractable interstitial cystitis. J Urol 165:884-886, 2001.
104. Comiter CV: Sacral neuromodulation for the symptomatic treatment of refractory interstitial cystitis: A prospective study. J Urol 169:1369-1373, 2003.
105. Peters KM, Carey JM, Konstandt DB: Sacral neuromodulation for the treatment of refractory interstitial cystitis: Outcomes based on technique. Int Urogynecol J Pelvic Floor Dysfunct 14:223-228; discussion 228, 2003.
106. Peters KM, Konstandt D: Sacral neuromodulation decreases narcotic requirements in refractory interstitial cystitis. BJU Int 93:777-779, 2004.
107. Zhao J, Nordling J: Posterior tibial nerve stimulation in patients with intractable interstitial cystitis. BJU Int 94:101-104, 2004.
108. O'Reilly BA, Dwyer PL, Hawthorne G, et al: Transdermal posterior tibial nerve laser therapy is not effective in women with interstitial cystitis. J Urol 172(5 Pt 1):1880-1883, 2004.
109. Hanno PM, Wein AJ: Conservative therapy of interstitial cystitis. Semin Urol 9:143-147, 1991.
110. Payne CK, Azevedo KA, Marotte J: A new look at the role of bladder distension in treatment of interstitial cystitis [abstract]. J Urol 167(Suppl):64, 2002.
111. Ottem DP, Teichman JM: What is the value of cystoscopy with hydrodistension for interstitial cystitis? Urology 66:494-499, 2005.
112. Rofeim O, Hom D, Freid RM, Moldwin RM: Use of the neodymium:YAG laser for interstitial cystitis: A prospective study. J Urol 166:134-136, 2001.
113. Eigner EB, Freiha FS: The fate of the remaining bladder following supravesical diversion. J Urol 144:31-33, 1990.

Section 11

GERIATRIC UROLOGY

Chapter 93

EPIDEMIOLOGY OF INCONTINENCE AND VOIDING DYSFUNCTION IN THE ELDERLY

Virgilio G. Petero, Jr., and Ananias C. Diokno

The understanding of epidemiology—the study of the distribution and determinants of disease—is critical in the search for the risk and protective factors that lead to primary or secondary disease prevention. This is especially true of urinary incontinence and voiding dysfunction, conditions that are multifactorial in origin. Although there is still a major gap in our knowledge about the issues involved in the epidemiology of these conditions, there has been a significant advance in the procurement of epidemiologic information in many parts of the world. This new-found enthusiasm led to the to the realization that urinary incontinence and voiding dysfunction are highly prevalent and that the consequences can be devastating for the afflicted women and have a tremendous impact on the nation's health care system. Largely because of these research initiatives, treatment and preventive strategies have emerged.

This chapter addresses the epidemiology of incontinence and voiding dysfunction. Although these conditions affect women of all ages, they are generally considered health concerns of the older age group. This review places special emphasis on elderly women.

URINARY INCONTINENCE

The International Continence Society defines *incontinence* as "the complaint of any involuntary leakage of urine."[1] The *prevalence* of urinary incontinence is defined as the probability of incontinence within a defined population group within a specified time period. The concept is important for establishing the distribution of the condition in the population and for projecting the need for health and medical services. The prevalence of all cases of urinary incontinence is estimated as the ratio of the number of incontinence respondents identified in a cross-sectional survey of continent and incontinent subjects. The prevalence of specific types and severity levels is estimated in an analogous manner. Any studies on the epidemiology of incontinence and voiding dysfunction or any condition or disease depend significantly on the definition of the condition and on the method used to obtain the information. The lack of a uniform definition of urinary incontinence is a fundamental problem in assessing and comparing the findings in different studies.

Prevalence of Urinary Incontinence in the Community

The pioneering studies on the prevalence of incontinence were done in Europe and mainly included subjects living in the community. From these early investigations, it was established that urinary incontinence is much more prevalent among the elderly than in any other age group living in the community. The sentinel paper published in 1968[2] was followed by a comprehensive study by Thomas and colleagues[3] in 1980. The group carried out a postal survey of two London boroughs and assessed 22,430 female subjects 5 years old or older. The survey team defined regular incontinence as two or more episodes of urinary incontinence occurring in the past month, whereas occasional incontinence was defined as less than two incontinence episodes per month. The group reported the prevalence of incontinence in all age groups (5 to more than 85 years) to be 8.5%. The prevalence rates of urinary incontinence in the different age groups are shown in Table 93-1.

When incontinence was correlated with previous pregnancy and with the number of pregnancies, nulliparous women were found to have a lower prevalence than those who had one or more babies. The number of pregnancies did not make any

Table 93-1 Prevalence of Urinary Incontinence in Women Living in London

Age Group (Years)	Regular Urinary Incontinence (%)	Occasional Urinary Incontinence (%)
5-14	5.1	11.2
15-24	4.0	11.9
25-34	5.5	20.0
35-44	10.2	20.7
45-54	11.8	21.9
55-64	11.9	18.6
65-74	8.8	14.6
75-84	16.0	13.6
≥85	16.2	16.2
Total	16.6	8.5

From Thomas TM, Plymat KR, Blannin J, et al: Prevalence of urinary incontinence. BMJ 281:1243, 1980.

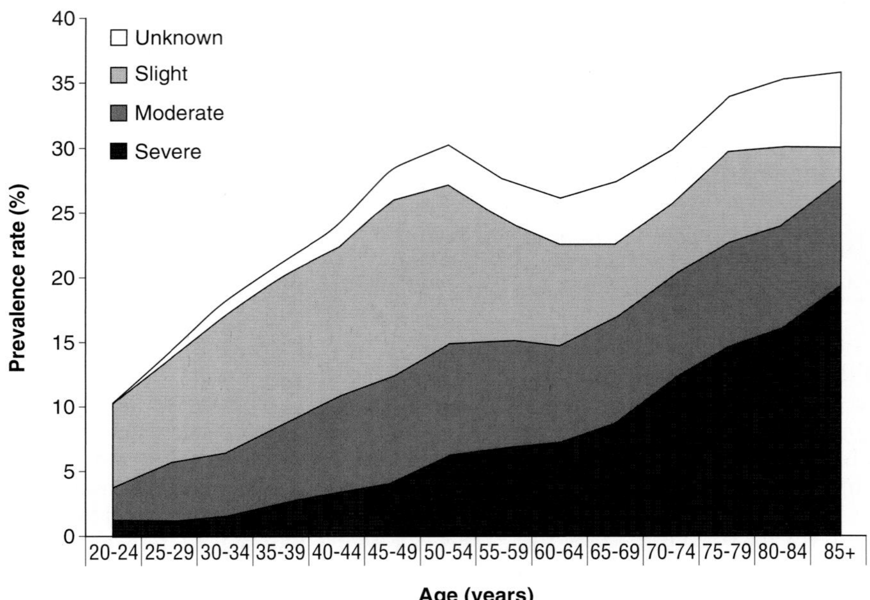

Figure 93-1 Prevalence of urinary incontinence by age group and severity in the Norwegian EPINCONT study. (From Hannestad YS, Rortveit G, Sandvik H, et al: A community-based epidemiological survey of female urinary incontinence: The Norwegian EPINCONT study. J Clin Epidemiol 53:1150-1157, 2000.)

difference among the incontinent respondents, except those in the 45- to 54-year age group, in which those who had had four or more babies were most likely to report regular incontinence. Incontinence was also reported to be moderate or severe in approximately 20% of the respondents, of whom less than one third received health or social services for the condition.

A European epidemiologic study was conducted by Hunskaar and coworkers[4] in four countries. Based on a mail survey of 29,000 households representing the general population of adult women 18 years or older (mean, 46.3 years) and on incontinence defined as any leakage or involuntary loss of urine during the preceding 30 days, the group reported the prevalence of incontinence to be 15% for women in Spain, 32% in France, 32% in the United Kingdom, and 34% in Germany. The survey also determined the type of incontinence. *Stress urinary incontinence* symptoms were defined as a leak or loss of urine caused by sneezing, coughing, exercising, lifting, or physical activity. *Urge urinary incontinence* symptoms were defined as an urge to urinate but being unable to reach the toilet before leaking or having a strong sudden urge to go to the toilet to urinate with no advance warning. *Mixed urinary incontinence* symptoms were defined as at least one stress and one urge symptom. Among the adult women in four countries, stress (37%) and mixed (33%) types were shown to be more predominant than urge incontinence (20%) and other (10%) types. In the subpopulation of women 60 years old or older, the mixed type predominates (41%), followed by stress incontinence (31%), urge incontinence (22%), and other types (6%).

The prevalence of any type of urinary incontinence by age shows an intriguing pattern. A survey of Norwegian women 20 years old or older found a gradual increase of prevalence across adulthood until age 50, when the prevalence reaches 30%, and then a stabilization or even slight decrease until age 70, when prevalence starts increasing again. The severity of incontinence also increases regardless of the type of incontinence with advancing age (Fig. 93-1).[5]

In the United States, the first comprehensive epidemiologic study on urinary incontinence in the elderly living in the community was the Medical Epidemiologic and Social Aspect of Aging (MESA) survey, which was conducted in 1983 in Washtenaw County, Michigan, by Diokno and colleagues.[6] This was a cross-sectional and longitudinal study of elderly respondents 60 years old or older sponsored by National Institute of Aging. A multistage stratified area probability sample of the Washtenaw County identified 13,912 households that were screened by household interviewers to identify households containing one or more persons 60 years old or older. The prevalence of urinary incontinence among all women 60 years old or older interviewed was 38%. The severity of urinary incontinence was analyzed according to the quantity of urine loss per day and the frequency of urine loss in 365 days (Table 93-2). The clinical type of urinary incontinence was also detailed in the MESA study. The result showed the mixed type of incontinence was the most prevalent, involving 55% of the incontinent responders, followed by stress (27%), urge (9%), and the other category (9%).

A more recent epidemiologic study in the United States was reported by Kinchen and associates[7] in 2002. The team conducted a national, cross-sectional, mailed survey of 45,000 households to determine the prevalence of urinary incontinence in adult women 18 years old or older. Among the 24,443 female respondents, 37% reported urinary incontinence in the past 30 days. The type of incontinence also depicts a higher prevalence rate for mixed (45%) and stress (41%) incontinence than for urge incontinence (12%). Age of onset differs by the type of incontinence. The median age of women was 48 years old for those reporting stress incontinence, 55 years for mixed incontinence, and 61 years for urge incontinence.[7]

In Asia, an epidemiologic study (cross-sectional, mailed survey) was done by the Asian Society for Female Urology (ASFU) to determine prevalence of overactive bladder symptoms and incontinence in 11 Asian countries.[8] The questionnaire used to establish the prevalence of incontinence, however, was different from the American and European surveys in that it was more focused on urge incontinence than on any type of incontinence. The prevalence of urinary incontinence ranged from 17% for Thailand and 13% for the Philippines to 4% for Singapore and

Table 93-2 Severity of Urinary Incontinence by Volume and Frequency of Urine Loss in Women 60 Years or Older

Volume of Urine Loss in 24 Hours	No. of Days with Urine Loss 1 to 9 (%)*	10 to 49 (%)*	50 to 299 (%)*	300 to 365 (%)*	Total (%)*
Drops to 0.5 teaspoon	16.1	11.6	5.6	3	36.3
0.5 teaspoon to 1 tablespoon	9.7	9.7	7.5	3.2	30.1
1 tablespoon to 0.25 cup	4.6	4.6	5.4	3.2	17.8
0.25 cup or more	2.4	2.4	4.3	6.7	15.8
Total	32.8	28.3	22.8	16.1	100.0

*Percent of women affected.
From Diokno AC, Brock BM, Brown MB, et al: Prevalence of urinary incontinence and other urological symptoms in the noninstitutional elderly. J Urol 136:1022, 1986.

China. The Asian survey also reported a much higher prevalence of mixed incontinence of 64%, with urge incontinence at 23% and stress incontinence at 13%.

The discrepancy between the prevalence rates of incontinence in Europe, America, and Asia may be attributed to the study methods and questions used. It is also possible that these differences reflected cultural variations, race, and ethnicity.

Prevalence of Urinary Incontinence in Institutions

The prevalence of urinary incontinence is much higher among institutionalized women. A survey sponsored by the United States Department of Health, Education, and Welfare about long-term facilities reported that 55% of patients surveyed had some problems with urinary control and that an additional 5% of patients were using a catheter or some collecting device.[9] Similarly, the National Nursing Home Survey sponsored by the National Center for Health Statistics confirmed the prevalence of incontinence of 50% among the more than 1.5 million nursing home facility residents in the United States.[10] Willington[11] estimated that 30% of unselected elderly admissions have urinary incontinence.

Some studies suggest institutional prevalence ranges between 6% and 72%.[12] Several reviews from around the world, some of which sample of institutions rather than individual institutions, suggests a prevalence of 50% or higher.[13-20] The range of prevalence in institutions is probably a consequence of the definition of urinary incontinence and criteria for admission to residential care, which vary within countries and among facilities.[21] The process that results in the relatively high prevalence of urinary incontinence in residential care facilities remains unclear. Thom and colleagues[22] reported that the relative risk of admission to a nursing home was two times greater for incontinent women after adjustments for age, cohort factors, and comorbid conditions. These findings suggest that incontinence may contribute to institutionalization. However, an alternative explanation of residential care contributing in some way to the development of incontinence cannot be excluded with confidence.

Racial and Ethnic Differences

Most epidemiologic studies of urinary incontinence have been conducted on white populations. The data available on black women indicate that they are less susceptible to urinary incontinence than white women.[23] However, in those who were incontinent, the severity was not significantly different between the two racial groups.[23,24]

It was suggested that black and white women have different factors promoting urinary incontinence.[25] The clinical data in the United States indicate that black women have higher urethral closure pressure, larger urethral volume, and greater vesical mobility compared with white women.[26] This difference in physiologic subtypes was supported by data confirming a significant difference in the predominance of stress incontinence in white women.[27] Black South African women rarely develop stress incontinence and the related disorder of pelvic floor prolapse, at a rate 80 times lower than whites.[28] Later studies later attempted to explain these observations as a function of different urethral pressures and lengths and pubococcygeal muscle strength.[29,30]

The prevalence of urinary incontinence among the Hispanic women 65 years old or older in the United States is lower than the general population. Using a methodology similar to the MESA study, Espino and coworkers[31] reported a prevalence rate of 15%. Similarly, mixed incontinence predominates at a rate of 42%, urge at 33%, and stress incontinence at 10%.

Incidence and Remission Rates

The incidence of urinary incontinence is the probability of becoming incontinent during a defined period of time. The concept is helpful in determining the onset and in understanding the risk factors for the condition. There are few epidemiologic data on the development or natural history of urinary incontinence and its transition to various levels of severity and type of incontinence. Campbell and associates[32] reported an incidence rate of incontinence among women 65 years old or older in New Zealand to be about 10% in a 3-year period. Moller and colleagues[33] and Samuelsson and coworkers[34] reported an incidence of 6% and 3% in young and middle-aged women, respectively. During the 5-year follow-up, the annual incidence was 2.9%, with severe incontinence at occurring at a rate of 0.5%. The remission rate (i.e., women who were incontinent at baseline and became incontinent at the end of study) was 5.9%.

In the MESA survey, the incidence of elderly women who were continent at the initial baseline interview and became incontinent a year later (i.e., second interview) was 22.4%. The incidence at the third interview of respondents who were still continent during the second interview was 20.2%. The remission rate during the second interview was 11.2%. Similarly, 13.3% of the incontinent respondents at the second interview became continent by the third interview. When a continent woman becomes incontinent the subsequent year, the most likely pattern is a mild form of incontinence. About one half of the cases of mild incontinence at the beginning of survey remained mild; few became severe. Women with severe incontinence usually remained severely incontinent after 1 year of follow-up. One half of the cases of moderate incontinence remained moderate, and the rest became mild or severe. In terms of the type of incontinence, women who originally had stress incontinence remained the same or developed the mixed type. Women with the mixed type usually stayed the same. Most continent women who became incontinent developed the stress type or a mixed stress-urge type of incontinence.

The current interpretation of the data indicates that the substantial incidence rates are paralleled by equally substantial remission rates. However, it is not clear whether the level of remission reflects active treatment or intervention or it is part of the natural course of incontinence.[35]

Correlates of Urinary Incontinence

Urinary incontinence is a condition of multifactorial origin. The MESA study investigated and reported the many suspected correlates of incontinence. The factors investigated extended beyond the medical correlates into social and psychological aspects. Among women, the measures of depression, negative affect balance, and life satisfaction reflect to a statistically significant degree the effect of incontinence.[36] Continent older women reported the highest levels of psychological well-being (i.e., the least depression and negative affect balance) and the most life satisfaction. Psychological well-being declines with increasing severity of urinary incontinence; the more severely incontinent women experience higher depression and negative affect balance and lower life satisfaction than the less severely incontinent women or continent women. Changes in the measures of happiness and positive affect balance are not as clear. Herzog and colleagues[37] suggested that these relationships are partly explained by the fact that incontinent respondents are less healthy than the continent respondents.

Miller[38] presented data from the New Haven Established Populations for the Epidemiologic Study of the Elderly (EPESE) study showing that respondents who reported difficulty holding their urine "all the time" or "most of the time" scored highest on a scale of depressive symptoms, followed by respondents who had difficulty "sometimes" or "hardly ever." Continent respondents scored the lowest of the three groups. This pattern persisted when functional disabilities and chronic disabilities were controlled.

Study of the medical correlates of urinary incontinence confirmed that incontinence in elderly individuals is associated with many debilitating medical conditions.[39] Surveys showed that physical mobility problems, specific neurologic symptoms, lower urinary tract problems, bowel problems, respiratory problems, and a history of genital surgery are more prevalent among those who are incontinent than those who are not. Other factors associated with female geriatric incontinence include a history of parent or sibling incontinence, incontinence during pregnancy or postpartum, hearing problems, use of female hormones, and vaginal infections. Mobility problems among the elderly were identified by the use of a wheelchair or walking aids, the presence of diagnosed arthritis or rheumatism, and whether the respondent fell during past year. The results showed that the proportion of respondents who reported mobility limitations was significantly greater among those who were incontinent than among those who were not. Among incontinent women, those with urge symptoms reported more difficulty with mobility than those with other symptoms. For example, among women with urge incontinence, 28.2% had mobility problems, in contrast to only 6.8% of those with stress incontinence.

Incontinence was associated significantly more often with neurologic factors (i.e., disease of the nerves or muscles or numbness in any part of body). Bowel problems, including lost control of stools in the past year, and problems with constipation were significantly more prevalent among the incontinent respondents than among their continent counterparts. Similarly, vaginal infections were reported more frequently by incontinent women. With regard to respiratory symptoms, incontinent women cough or sneeze more often than continent women. More incontinent than continent respondents reported urinary tract problems. The largest differences were found among those who reported urinary tract infections; the presence of blood, cloudiness, or foul smell in the urine; slow and weak stream of urine; and the presence of pain, burning, or stinging during urination.

The MESA respondents were followed for several years to identify causal relationships between urinary incontinence and its correlates. The data suggest a clear relationship among the onset of poor health, mobility problems, and urinary symptoms. These factors appear to be significant risk factors for the development of urinary incontinence in the elderly.

The widespread use of diuretics among the elderly population was also confirmed by the MESA study.[40] One in three women 60 years or older uses a diuretic. Wells and coworkers[41] reported that diuretics were used in 29% of incontinent elderly women seen in a continence clinic. Ouslander,[42] in his study of nursing home patients, observed no significant difference in the use of diuretics between continent and incontinent patients. Shimp and colleagues[43] reported the influence of diuretics on bladder symptoms in a study of 200 incontinent women recruited from a continence program clinic. Incontinent women taking diuretics had a positive correlation with nocturia and a trend toward significant urge incontinence ($P = .056$) compared with incontinent women not taking diuretics.

The MESA study showed that there was no significant difference in the prevalence of incontinence in users and nonusers of diuretics. However, it was found that diuretic users who had uninhibited bladder contractions on cystometry had a significantly higher prevalence of urinary incontinence (85%) compared with nonusers with similar bladder abnormalities (25%). Among respondents who did not have uninhibited bladder contractions on cystometry, the use or nonuse of diuretics resulted in no difference between the two groups ($P = .085$). Although these comparisons were made in men because there were not enough women with uninhibited bladder contraction to compare, there is no reason not to expect similar relationships in women.

The correlation between diuretics and the presence of uninhibited bladder contractions has significant implications. When confronted with an elderly patient who has recently experienced the onset of urinary incontinence, especially the urge type, the physician should specifically ask about the concomitant use of diuretics. If diuretic use correlates with the onset of incontinence, the physician can discontinue the diuretic and change to a nondiuretic therapy if medically feasible. If the diuretic cannot be discontinued, the use of bladder relaxants should be considered as long as the patient has adequate detrusor contractility and can empty the bladder adequately. As part of the overall management of incontinence in patients with mobility and dexterity, easier access to the toilet should be considered; otherwise, provisions for toilet supplements, such as commodes or urinals should be encouraged.

Urodynamic Parameters for the Continent and Incontinent Elderly

The MESA survey performed urodynamic studies among 167 women who volunteered to undergo the study a the household interview followed by a clinic visit for a free examination, including urinalysis. One hundred incontinent and 67 continent women were studied.

The uroflow measures of peak and average flow rates showed no difference between continent and incontinent subjects or between the different clinical types of incontinence. The mean noninstrumented peak flow rate among women voiding 300 mL or more was 23.3 mL/sec, whereas the mean noninstrumented peak flow rate for a voided volume between 200 and 299 mL was 18.2 mL/sec. The mean average flow rates were 12.0 mL/sec and 8.8 mL/sec, respectively.

The postvoid residual urine volume showed no significant difference between continent and incontinent women respondents. The prevalence of postvoid residual urine volume of 101 to 150 mL among continent women was 9.7%, and for incontinent women, it was 3.5%. The prevalence of uninhibited detrusor contraction on cystometry among the continent respondents was 4.9%, and for the incontinent respondents, it was 12.2%. The overall prevalence rate was 7.9%. The difference in prevalence rates between continent and incontinent subjects was not statistically significant. These rates are more in line with the prevalence of uninhibited detrusor contractions among hospitalized women without urologic symptoms reported by Jones and Schoenberg,[44] but they are lower than the 39% reported by Hilton and Stanton.[45] The difference appears to be related to the general health status of the individual. Healthier subjects are less likely to have uninhibited detrusor contractions.

The urethral pressure profile parameters in the MESA study revealed that assessment performed in the supine position did not reveal any significant difference between the continent and incontinent subjects. However, static and dynamic urethral pressure profilometry performed in the in the standing position showed a significant difference in the values between continent and incontinent subjects. Although a significant difference existed, there was considerable overlap in the values, and it was impossible to adopt a specific range of values that could be used to identify urethral insufficiency in elderly subjects.

On the lateral stress cystography, the posterior urethra–vesical angle was strongly associated with continence status. However, there was significant overlap in the posterior urethra–vesical angle values that made it impossible to assign a specific value for the diagnosis of incontinence. It appears that this test is of value in the assessment of the type of stress incontinence and in assessing the type of repair to be used.

Patient Strategies to Control Urine

Because urinary incontinence is not life threatening, many incontinent individuals have found ways of managing their own conditions. Part of the MESA study was to determine how incontinent elderly women manage their urine loss condition.[37] The survey revealed that 69% of incontinent women were using one or more methods to control urine loss. For most incontinent women, absorbent products such as sanitary napkins, toilet tissue, and absorbent garments were the most popular means, as reported by 55% of women respondents. The second most common means of controlling incontinence was to locate a toilet on arrival at an unfamiliar place. Forty-two percent of women reported using this strategy as part of controlling their incontinence. Voiding manipulation such as scheduled urination, urination before leaving home, and other conscious efforts to plan urination was practiced by 28% of female incontinent respondents who altered their diet and fluid intake to control incontinence and 12% who did pelvic muscle exercises. Only 6% of women reported taking medications for their incontinence.

Forty-two percent of those with severe incontinence had talked with their physicians in the past year, whereas only 25% of those with moderate incontinence and 19% of those with mild incontinence had done so. With regard to the type of incontinence, 30% of those with the mixed type of incontinence had talked with their physicians in the past year, whereas only 20% of those with urge or stress incontinence had done so.

Continent Surgery and Its Outcomes

An estimated 126,000 operations for incontinence are performed annually in the United States.[46] A review of the literature demonstrates that the median proportion of women cured or improved by surgery at 1 to 2 years was 78% for anterior repair, 86% for retropubic suspension, and 91% for sling procedures.[47] Realizing the value of patient satisfaction as an outcome of continence surgery, the National Family Opinion (NFO) world group panel evaluated the prevalence and outcome of continence surgery among community dwelling women.[48] The group reported that 4% of women living in the community and 8% of women 60 years old or older had a history of continence surgery. One third of the women had their surgery within the past 5 years. The initial satisfaction of surgery was high, but it then decreased as time progressed. Of those who had surgery within the past 3 years, 64% were currently satisfied. Of those who had surgery more than 3 years, satisfaction rates between 42% and 45% were reported. Seventy-three percent of the women who had surgery reported incontinence in the preceding month, 58% had incontinence in the preceding week, and 53% used pads regularly. Of those with recurrent urinary incontinence, 83% continued to have stress urinary incontinence, although 62% experienced stress and urge symptoms, and 14% had urge symptoms only.

Prevention of Urinary Incontinence

Urinary incontinence is a preventable condition.[49] Behavioral techniques, including pelvic muscle training and bladder training, are safe and effective for stress, urge, and mixed urinary incontinence.[50-53] Only a few randomized, controlled trials have sought to prevent incontinence. Until recently, the randomized, controlled trials assessing a behavioral modification program for prevention of urinary incontinence have been limited to pregnant and postpartum women. None of the randomized, controlled trials previously reported tested the preventive effects of bladder training and pelvic muscle training in older women.[54,55]

Diokno and colleagues[56] reported the first successful randomized, controlled trial of a group behavioral modification program to prevent incontinence in postmenopausal women living in community who were 55 years old or older, compared with the usual care. The program consisted of a 2-hour classroom presentation, followed 2 to 4 weeks later with an individualized evaluation to test knowledge, adherence, and skills in behavioral techniques and to provide a brief re-enforcement of technique as needed. Both groups (i.e., treated and control or no treatment) were followed for 12 months. Continence status, pelvic muscle strength, voiding frequency, and intervoid interval were significantly better in the treatment group.[56] The result of this trial suggest that women with stronger pelvic muscles have increased awareness of pelvic muscle function, which translates into greater voluntary contraction of the pelvic muscles at the onset of increased physical activity, maintaining or improving continence.[57]

Socioeconomic Issues

As is true for any chronic health condition, the burden of urinary incontinence reflects experiences of the incontinent individual and those around her, and it puts significant strain on society and the health care system. Between 1984 and 1995, the estimated number of persons 65 years old or older with urinary incontinence increased by 218%.[58] Urinary incontinence is a costly condition, with the annual expenditure similar to other chronic diseases in women, such as osteoporosis, Alzheimer's disease, and arthritis, that vary in their effects on morbidity, mortality, and quality of life.[59]

The estimated cost of urinary incontinence in 1995 for persons 65 years old or older in the United States, based on the calculated 6.32 million community-dwelling and 1.06 million institutionalized elderly patients,[59] was $24.3 billion, of which direct costs accounted for 97% ($23.6 billion).[58] The single biggest contributing cost was for routine care among older adults living in the community; this represented 29.4% of total costs. The cost per individual was $3565, an increase of 174% from $2052 in 1984.

The indirect costs include income from work lost. Among all workers with urinary incontinence, 23% of women missed work, whereas only 8% of men did so. The reported average annual work absence for women totaled 28.7 hours for inpatients (7.1 hours) and outpatients (21.6 hours). Although women and men have similar numbers of outpatient visits for urinary incontinence, average work loss associated with outpatient care was greater for women, probably because of the availability of outpatient procedures for women.[60]

VOIDING DYSFUNCTIONS

Few studies have examined the prevalence of urinary symptoms other than incontinence among women. The prevalence of urinary symptoms has been infrequently reported in detail among women of different ages. For example, there are few data for normal values of daytime and nighttime voiding frequencies for women of different ages. Voiding dysfunction is perceived less commonly as an important urinary symptom in women, despite evidence that detrusor function may become less efficient with age.[61]

Normal Voiding Parameters

The distribution of frequency of voiding among the elderly women in the United States was reported by the MESA survey. It appears that the normal voiding frequency was no more than eight times per day; 88% of all women respondents who were asymptomatic (i.e., no self-reported incontinence or irritative or obstructive symptoms) and 70% of incontinent women reported this daily frequency. In terms of nocturia, 93% of asymptomatic women and 83% incontinent women void no more than two times at night. The frequency of nocturia increased among women with bladder symptoms. Nocturia of three times or more was reported by 25% of women with irritative bladder symptoms and 24% of women with difficult bladder-emptying symptoms. The increased frequency reported among symptomatic respondents compared with asymptomatic respondents was statistically significant.

Fitzgerald and coworkers[62] reevaluated the definition of urinary frequency by assessing 300 healthy, asymptomatic volunteer women between the ages of 18 and 91 years (median, 40 years). They found a median of 8.3 voids in 24 hours, with 95% of subjects recording fewer than 13 voids per 24 hours. Ninety-two percent of the women voided no more than once per night, including 36% who voided once. Two or more nocturnal voidings were reported by 8% of the volunteers. Among the 133 (44%) subjects who had nighttime voiding, 39% of them did so because they were awakened by the need to void. The group concluded that 8 voids or more per 24 hours as the definition of *frequency* may be inappropriate and suggested that a value 13 voids or more may be more appropriate. However, it can be argued that because the information came from a self-selected group of volunteers who reside in a large metropolitan area, the figures obtained may not be representative of the true voiding frequency in the general community.

Lower Urinary Tract Symptoms in Women

Using the validated Bristol Female Lower Urinary Tract Symptoms (BFLUTS) questionnaire,[63] it was demonstrated that lower urinary tract symptoms were prevalent among and troublesome to a group of community-dwelling women.[64] In the MESA survey, the prevalence of lower urinary tract symptoms (i.e., hesitancy, poor stream, interrupted stream, straining to void, and use of catheter to drain the bladder) among women 60 years old or older was 10.9%. Men of a similar age group reported a 22.1% prevalence. Other surveys report prevalence rates of 18% for women 65 years old or older[65] and 8% for women 81 years old or older.[66] It is believed that the difficult bladder-emptying symptoms in women are more likely a consequence of an underactive bladder, whereas in men, the most likely cause is outlet obstruction.[6]

Voiding symptoms other than poor stream have seldom been assessed in women, although hesitancy has been described as occurring in a small population of younger women.[67] Using the BFLUTS questionnaire, Swithinbank and colleagues[68] reported the age-specific prevalence of voiding symptoms among women, including the character of the stream (i.e., intermittency, hesitancy, and slow stream), incomplete emptying, dysuria, and straining (Fig. 93-2). With the exception of weak stream, these symptoms were more commonly described by younger women.[68]

The high prevalence of lower urinary tract symptoms among women is not surprising. Many other investigators have reported similar prevalence rates for these symptoms in age-matched men and women when testing the International Prostate Symptom Score (I-PSS) as a diagnostic tool.[69-71] As in the case with men, storage symptoms appear to be much more bothersome than voiding symptoms.

Overactive Bladder Syndrome

Overactive bladder is a common disabling condition that affects health-related quality of life. The International Continence

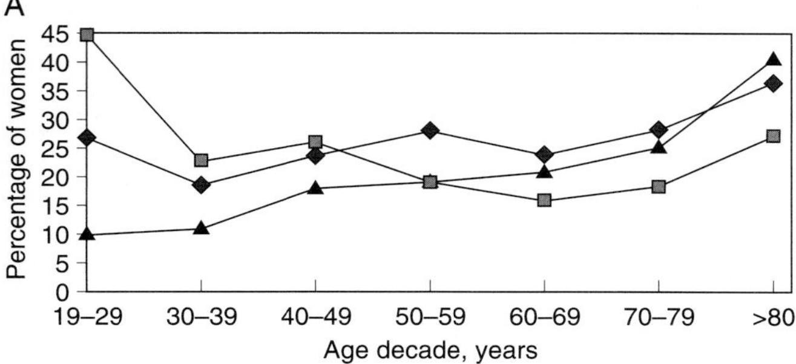

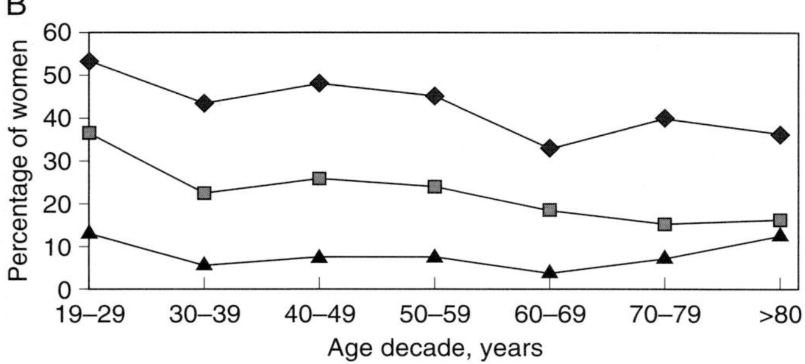

▲ (A) slow/poor stream; (B) straining

◆ (A) intermittency; (B) incomplete emptying

■ (A) hesitancy; (B) dysuria

Figure 93-2 Relationships between age and type of stream **(A)** and bladder emptying symptoms **(B)** in women. (From Swithinbank LV, Abrams P: A detailed description, by age, of lower urinary tract symptoms in a group of community-dwelling women. BJU Int 85(Suppl2):19-24, 2000.)

Society (ICS) derived a consensus symptomatic definition of *overactive bladder syndrome* as urinary urgency, with or without urge incontinence, usually with urinary frequency and nocturia, in the absence of pathologic and metabolic factors that would explain the symptoms.[1] Urodynamically, overactive bladder is characterized by the presence of involuntary bladder contractions that occur during bladder filling despite the patient's attempt to suppress them.

The National Overactive Bladder Evaluation (NOBLE) study was initiated to better understand the prevalence and impact of overactive bladder in a broad spectrum of the U.S. population.[72] Using a clinically validated, computer-assisted telephone interview questionnaire, a sample population of adults, who were 18 years old or older and representative of the main population by sex, age, and geographic region, was surveyed.

A surprising result from this study is the equal prevalence of urgency-related bladder control problems in men and women (16.0% and 16.9%, respectively), although more women (13.4%) suffer from overactive bladder with incontinence than men (2.6%). The prevalence and prevalence ratios were inversely related to increasing education, a pattern that was more apparent among women who had overactive bladder with urge incontinence. In women, but not in men, the prevalence of overactive bladder with urge incontinence increased in relation to increasing body mass index.

The age-specific prevalence of overactive bladder was similar for men and women, but age patterns differed by sex and type of overactive bladder. The age-specific prevalence of overactive bladder without incontinence appears to plateau after age 44 years for women and after age 54 years for men. In contrast, age-specific prevalence of overactive bladder with urge incontinence continues to increase with increasing age, with women having a steeper age-related increase than men. These contrasting patterns suggest that overactive bladder without incontinence may precede the onset of overactive bladder with urge incontinence. Moreover, in the older ages, the transition rate from overactive bladder without to overactive bladder with urge incontinence may exceed the rate of occurrence of new cases of overactive bladder without incontinence. This may explain the plateau in prevalence of overactive bladder without incontinence. Longitudinal studies will be required to test this hypothesis. If confirmed, the incidence of overactive bladder with urge incontinence may be mitigated through secondary prevention efforts directed toward overactive bladder without urge incontinence.

Women and men who have overactive bladder, with or without urge incontinence, have significantly poorer scores for health-related quality of life, mental health, and quality of sleep compared with sex- and age-matched controls. These differences were significant after adjusting for other covariates, including comorbid illnesses.

CONCLUSIONS

Urinary incontinence and voiding dysfunctions are prevalent conditions that can affect women of all ages. The incidence is especially high among the elderly, whether they are living in the community or in institutions. These conditions are associated with many medical correlates and have a tremendous effect on the psychological well-being of the afflicted. Urinary incontinence and voiding dysfunctions are very costly, with the expenditure similar to the more popularly recognized health concerns of the aging woman.

The explosion of epidemiologic data has led to novel treatment and prevention strategies, although patient satisfaction about the outcome of surgery may not be as high as previously believed. Epidemiologic information about different racial and ethnic populations is now being reported. Our knowledge about the different issues of voiding dysfunctions is still inadequate, and our understanding of normal voiding parameters is still far from complete.

References

1. Abrams P, Cardozo L, Fall M, et al: The standardization of terminology in lower urinary tract function: Report from the Standardization Sub-committee of the International Continence Society. Neurol Urodyn 21:167. 2002.
2. Brocklehurst JC, Dillane JB, Griffiths, et al: The prevalence and symptomatology of urinary infection in an aged population. Gerontol Clin 10:242, 1968.
3. Thomas TM, Plymat KR, Blannin J, et al: Prevalence of urinary incontinence. BMJ 281:1243, 1980.
4. Hunskaar S, Gunnar L, Lars V, et al: Prevalence of stress incontinence in women in four European countries. Neurol Urodyn 21:275, 2002.
5. Hannestad YS, Rortveit G, Sandvik H, et al: A community-based epidemiological survey of female urinary incontinence:

The Norwegian EPINCONT study. J Clin Epidemiol 53:1150, 2000.

6. Diokno AC, Brock BM, Brown MB, et al: Prevalence of urinary incontinence and other urological symptoms in the noninstitutional elderly. J Urol 136:1022, 1986.
7. Kinchen K, Gohier J, Obenchain R, Bump R: Prevalence and frequency of stress incontinence among community-dwelling women. Eur Urol 85(Suppl 1):85, 2002.
8. Lapitan MC, Chye PL: Asia-Pacific Continence Advisory Board. The epidemiology of overactive bladder among females in Asia: A questionnaire survey. Int Urogynecol J 12:226, 2001.
9. U.S. Department of Health, Education and Welfare: Long-term Care Facility Improvement Study. Washington, DC, US Government Printing Office, 1975.
10. Van Nostrand JF, Zappolo A, Hing E, et al: The National Nursing Home Survey: Summary for the United States. DHEW publication no. 79-1794. Vital and Health Statistics, series 13, no. 43. Washington, DC, National Center for Health Statistics, Health Resources Administration, 1977.
11. Willington FL: Significance of incompetence of personal sanitary habits. Nurs Times 71:340, 1975.
12. Cheater FM, Castleden CM: Epidemiology and classification of Urinary incontinence. Clin Obstet Gynaecol 14:183, 2000.
13. Aggazzotti G, Pesce F, Grassi D, et al: Prevalence of urinary incontinence among institutionalized patients: A cross-sectional epidemiologic study in midsized city in northern Italy. Urology 56:245, 2000.
14. Brandeis GH, Baumann MM, Hossain M, et al: The prevalence of potentially remediable urinary incontinence in frail older people: A study using the minimum data set. J Am Geriatr Soc 45:179, 1997.
15. Sgadari A, Topinkova E, Bjornson J, et al: Urinary incontinence in nursing home residents: A cross-sectional comparison. Age Ageing 8:47, 1996.
16. Toba K, Ouchi H, Iimura O, et al: Urinary incontinence in elderly inpatients in Japan: A comparison between general and geriatric hospital. Aging 8:47, 1996.
17. Borie M, Davidson H: Incontinence in institutions: Costs and associated factors. Can Med Assoc J 147:322, 1992.
18. Ouslander JG, Palmer MH, Rovner BW, et al: Urinary incontinence in nursing homes: Incidence, remission and associated factors. J Am Geriatr Soc 41:1083, 1993.
19. Fonda D, for the Victorian Geriatricians Peer Review Group: Improving management of urinary incontinence in geriatric centres and nursing homes. Aust Clin Rev 10:1063, 1995.
20. Peet SC, Castleden CM: The prevalence of urinary and faecal incontinence in hospitals and residential and nursing homes for older people. BMJ 311:1063, 1995.
21. Hunskaar S, Arnold EP, Brugio K, et al: Epidemiology and natural history of urinary incontinent. In Abrams P, Khoury S, Wein A (eds): Incontinence. Plymouth, UK, Scientific International, 1999, p 197.
22. Thom DH, Haan MN, Van Den Eeden S: Medically recognized urinary incontinence and risks of hospitalization nursing home admission and mortality. Age Aging 26:237, 1997.
23. Fultz NH, Herzog AR, Raghunathan TE, et al: Prevalence and severity of urinary incontinence in older African American and Caucasian women. J Gerontol A Biol Sci Med Sci 54:M299-M303, 1999.
24. Dolan LM, Casson K, McDonald P, et al: Urinary incontinence in Northern Ireland: A prevalence study. BJU Int 83:760, 1999.
25. Bump RC, Norton PA: Epidemiology and natural history of pelvic floor dysfunction. Obstet Gynecol Clin North Am 25:723, 1998.
26. Howard D, Davies PS, Delancey JO, et al: Differences in perineal lacerations in black and white primiparas. Obstet Gynecol 96:622-624, 2000.
27. Peacock LM, Wiskind AK, Wall LL: Clinical features of urinary incontinence and urogenital prolapse in a black inner city population. Am J Obstet Gynecol 171:1464, 1994.
28. Heyns OS: Bantu Gynaecology. Johhanesburg, Witwaterstrand University Press, 1956, p 98.
29. Skinner DP: Stress incontinence: A comparative racial study. Med Proc 9:189, 1963.
30. Knobel J: Stress incontinence in the black female. S Afr J Obstet Gynaecol 49:430, 1975.
31. Espino DV, Palmer RF, Miles TP, et al: Prevalence and severity of urinary incontinence in elderly Mexican-American women. J Am Geriatr Soc 51:1580, 2003.
32. Campbell AJ, Reinken J, McCosk L: Incontinence in the elderly: Prevalence and prognosis. Age Ageing 14:65, 1985.
33. Moller LA, Lose G, Jorgensen T: The prevalence and bothersomeness of lower urinary tract symptoms in women 40-60 years of age. Acta Obstet Gynecol Scand 79:298, 2000.
34. Samuelsson EC, Victor FT, Svardsudd KF: Five-year incidence and remission rates of female urinary incontinence in a Swedish population less than 65 years old. Am J Obstet Gynecol 183:568, 2000.
35. Hunskaar S, Burgio K, Diokno A, et al: Epidemiology and natural history of urinary incontinence in women. Urology 62(Suppl 4A):16, 2003.
36. Herzog AR, Fultz NH, Brock BM, et al: Urinary incontinence and psychological distress among older adults. Psychol Aging 3:115, 1988.
37. Herzog AR, Fultz NG Normolle DP, et al: Methods used in to manage urinary incontinence by older adults in the community. J Am Geriatr Soc 37:339, 1989.
38. Miller RL: Urinary incontinence in the community elderly: Functional status, cognitive function and depressive symptoms: Findings from the Yale Health and Aging study. Paper presented at the 113th annual meeting of the American Public Health Association, Washington, DC, 1985.
39. Diokno AC, Brock BM, Brown MB, et al: Medical correlates of urinary incontinence in the elderly. Urology 36:129, 1990.
40. Diokno AC, Brown MB, Herzog AR: Relationship between use of diuretics and continence status in the elderly. Urology 38:39, 1991.
41. Wells TJ, Brink CA, Diokno AC: Urinary incontinence in the elderly women: Clinical findings. J Am Geriatr Soc 35:933, 1987.
42. Ouslander JG: Diagnostic evaluation of geriatric urinary incontinence. Geriatr Med 2:715, 1986.
43. Shimp LA, Wells TJ, Brink CA, et al: Relationship between drug use and urinary incontinence in elderly women. Drug Intel Clin Pharmacol 22:786, 1988.
44. Jones KW, Schoenberg HW: Comparison of the incidence of bladder hyperreflexia in patients with benign prostatic hyperplasia and age-matched female controls. J Urol 133:425, 1985.
45. Hilton P, Stanton SL: Algorithmic method for assessing urinary incontinence in elderly women. BMJ 282:940, 1981.
46. Brown JS, Waetjen LE, Subak LL, et al: Pelvic organ prolapse surgery in the United States. Am J Obstet Gynecol 186:712, 2002.
47. Leach GE, Dmowhowski RR, Appell RA, et al: Female stress urinary incontinence clinical guidelines panel summary report on surgical management of female stress urinary incontinence. J Urol158:875, 1997
48. Diokno AC, Burgio K, Fultz NH, et al: Prevalence and outcomes of continence surgery in community dwelling women. J Urol 170:507, 2003.
49. The Simon Foundation: Vital Issues. Consensus Statement of First International Conference for Prevention of Incontinence. Available at *www.simonfoundation.org*
50. Fantl JA, Wyman JF, McCish DK, et al: Efficacy of bladder training in older women with urinary incontinence. JAMA 265:609, 1991.
51. Fantl JA: Behavioral intervention for community dwelling individuals with urinary incontinence. Urology 51(Suppl):30, 1998.
52. Doherty MC, Dwyer JW, Pendergrast JF, et al: A randomized trial of behavioral management for continence with older rural women. Res Nurs Health 25:3, 2002.

53. Diokno AC, Yuhico M Jr: Preference, compliance and initial outcome of therapeutic options chosen by female patients with urinary incontinence. J Urol 154:1727, 1995.
54. Hay-Smith J, Herbison P, Morkved S: Physical therapies for prevention of urinary and faecal incontinence in adults. Cochrane Database Syst Rev (2):CD003191, 2002.
55. Morkved S, Bo K: Effect of postpartum pelvic floor muscle training in prevention of and treatment of urinary incontinence: A one-year follow-up. BJOG 107:1022, 2000.
56. Diokno AC, Sampselle CM, Herzog AR, et al: Prevention of urinary incontinence by behavioural modification program: A randomized, controlled trial among older women in the community. J Urol 171:1165, 2004.
57. Miller JM, Ashton-Miller JA, Delancey JO: A pelvic muscle precontraction can reduce cough-related urine loss in selected women with mild SUI. J Am Geriatr Soc 46:870, 1998.
58. Wagner TH, Hu TW: Economic costs of urinary incontinence in 1995. Urology 51:355, 1998.
59. US Dept of Health and Human Services. National Hospital Discharge Survey. Data from Vital and Health, series 13, no. 12. Hyattsville, MD, National Center for Health Statistics, 1994.
60. Liwin MS, Saigal CS (eds): Urologic Diseases in America. US Department of Health and Human Services, National Health Institute, National Institute of Diabetes and Digestive and Kidney Disease. Washington, DC, US Government Printing Office, pp 94-98, 2004.
61. Elbadawi A, Yalla SV, Resnick NM: Structural basis of geriatric voiding dysfunction. II. Aging detrusor: Normal versus impaired contractility. J Urol 150:1657, 1993.
62. Fitzgerald MP, Stablein U, Brubaker L: Urinary habits among asymptomatic women. Am J Obstet Gynecol 187:1384, 2002.
63. Jackson S, Donovan J, Brookes S, et al: Bristol Female Lower Urinary Tract Symptoms questionnaire: Development and psychometric testing. Br J Urol 77:805, 1996.
64. Swithinbank LV, Donovan JL, du Heaume JC, et al: Urinary symptoms and incontinence in women: relationships between occurrence, age and perceived impact. Br J Gen Pract 49:897, 1999.
65. Teasdale TA, Tuffet GE, Luchi RJ, Adam E: Urinary Incontinence in a community-residing population. J Am Geriatr Soc 36:600, 1988.
66. Brocklehurst JC, Fry J, Griffiths L, Kalton D: Dysuria on old age. J Am Geriatr Soc 19:582, 1971.
67. Somner P, Bauer T, Nielsen KK, et al: Voiding patterns and prevalence of incontinence in women. A questionnaire survey. Br J Urol 66:12, 1990.
68. Swithinbank LV, Abrams P: A detailed description, by age, of lower urinary tract symptoms in a group of community-dwelling women. BJU Int 85:19, 2000.
69. Lepor H, Machi G: Comparison of AUA symptom index in unselected males and females between fifty-five and seventy-nine years of age. Urology 42:36, 1993.
70. Chancellor MB, Rivas DA: American Urological Association symptom index specificity for benign prostatic hyperplasia. J Urol 150:1706, 1993.
71. Chai TC, Belville WD, McGuire EJ, Nyquist L: Specificity of American Urological Association voiding symptom index: Comparison of unselected and selected samples of both sexes. J Urol 150:1710, 1993.
72. Stewart WF, Van Rooyen JB, Cundiff GW, et al: Prevalence and burden of overactive bladder in the United States. World J Urol 20:327, 2003.

Chapter 94

LOWER URINARY TRACT DISORDERS IN THE ELDERLY FEMALE

Theodore M. Johnson, II, and Joseph G. Ouslander

Aging is a continuous and inevitable process that affects everyone. It occurs at various rates in different individuals and in different organ systems within the same individual. The individual organism's responses to the aging process are diverse and depend on many complex factors. The lower urinary tract, as much as any other organ system, is greatly influenced by the interactive and additive effects of age-related changes and the accumulation of many pathologic entities with increasing age. Symptoms of lower urinary tract dysfunction are common in elderly women.

This chapter focuses on the age-related and age-associated changes that underlie lower urinary tract dysfunction in this population. We review in some detail the two most common disorders of the lower urinary tract in elderly women—urinary incontinence and urinary tract infection (UTI).

AGING AND THE FEMALE LOWER URINARY TRACT

When considering the effects of increasing age on any organ system, a crucial distinction must be made between true age-related changes that occur in everyone and age-associated changes resulting from the accumulation of pathologic conditions that do not occur in everyone. Table 94-1 lists age-related changes and age-associated factors that can influence lower urinary tract function and symptoms in elderly women. Because determining true

Table 94-1 Aging and the Female Lower Urinary Tract

Change or Effect	Potential Effects
Age-related changes	
Altered cell function	Altered interstitial tissues and mucosal surfaces Increased likelihood of pelvic prolapse and urinary infection
Decreased estrogen level	Thinner and more friable mucosa and interstitial tissues Increased likelihood of pelvic prolapse, urinary symptoms, and infection
Altered concentrations of central nervous system neurotransmitters; altered nerve conduction	Increased likelihood of bladder and urethral dysfunction
Altered immune function	Increased susceptibility to infection
Altered bladder function Decreased capacity Increased uninhibited contractions Increased residual volume	Increased likelihood of urinary symptoms, incontinence, and infection
Lower urethral pressure	Increased likelihood of incontinence
Age-associated factors	
Cognitive and sensory impairment	Decreased ability to relate symptoms
Locomotor disturbances and immobility Stroke Hip fracture Peripheral vascular disease Parkinson's disease	More difficulty getting to a toilet; increased likelihood of fecal impaction and incontinence
Poor fluid intake	Increased likelihood of fecal impaction and bacteriuria
Central nervous system diseases affecting bladder function Stroke Dementia Parkinson's disease	Increased likelihood of incontinence
Other diseases affecting bladder function Malignancy Atherosclerotic vascular disease	Increased likelihood of bladder dysfunction
Drug usage (see Table 94-2)	Increased likelihood of bladder or urethral dysfunction

age-related changes in the female lower urinary tract would involve invasive procedures (e.g., catheterization for urodynamic studies, cystoscopy) in continent elderly women without urinary symptoms, this type of information is rarely sought. Despite these difficulties in obtaining data, several types of age-related changes are known to have a prominent influence on lower urinary tract function.

One of the most important age-related changes affecting the female lower urinary tract is the postmenopausal decline in estrogen. This remains true, even though evidence has suggested that oral estrogen supplementation is linked to worse continence outcomes.[1] The bladder, urethra, and genital tract have a common embryologic origin, and the epithelium of all of these tissues responds to hormonal changes. When the influence of estrogen declines, the epithelium and supporting tissues of the pelvic area atrophy, resulting in a friable mucosa and a tendency toward prolapse. The lower glycogen content in the vaginal epithelium results in less lactic acid metabolism by Doderlein's bacilli and an increase in the pH of vaginal secretions that may increase susceptibility to infection. Changes occur in the concentration of certain neurotransmitters in various locations in the central nervous system with increasing age. Given the important influence of the central nervous system on human bladder function, these age-related changes in central neurotransmitters may play a role in disorders of micturition in the elderly. Alterations in immune function also occur with increasing age. Although these changes have been seen mainly in cellular immunity, age-related changes in immune function, especially local immune activity in the lower urinary tract, may play an important role in susceptibility to bacteriuria and symptomatic UTI in older women.

Certain functional changes appear to occur in the bladder and urethra with increasing age. In one study, abnormal cystometrographic results were found for 15 of 24 continent elderly women who were free of neurologic disease.[2] Twelve of these 15 showed uninhibited contractions; 10 had a bladder capacity of less than 250 mL. Other studies have shown prevalence rates of 5% to 11% of abnormalities in continent older women.[3,4]

Some work has attempted to elucidate in the underlying anatomic basis of these changes. In a series of investigations in symptomatic and asymptomatic adults older than 65 years using urodynamics and electron microscopy of bladder biopsy specimens, investigators found that patients with detrusor activity had specific anatomic abnormalities, including a dysjunction pattern with protrusion junctions and ultraclose abutments. These changes are believed to be the anatomic explanation for the propagation of involuntary detrusor contractions in older patients.[5-7]

Maximal urethral pressure and functional urethral length are decreased in continent elderly women.[8,9] In one study, the maximal urethral pressure in continent women fell from a mean of 87 cm H_2O in the third decade to 42 cm H_2O in the seventh decade, a value that overlapped that of younger women with stress incontinence.[8] These age-related changes in lower urinary tract function should be considered when evaluating urodynamic findings in elderly women. One postmortem study of 25 bladders from women between the ages of 74 and 102 years revealed marked trabeculation, diverticula, and cellular formation.[10] Another study demonstrated continuous loss of striated muscle cells of the rhabdosphincter due to apoptosis, which eventually may reach a critical mass, leading to reduced function of the muscle with resultant urinary incontinence.[11] Histologic section of the bladder outlet showed a high incidence of chronic inflammation, edema, and fibrosis, presumed to be related to chronically infected residual urine. The trabeculation in these bladders was thought to be the result of loss of elastic tissue and coalescence of muscle fiber and of muscle hypertrophy resulting from bladder outlet obstruction or frequent uninhibited bladder contractions against a closed sphincter, or both. Other investigators have reported that the bladder in elderly women is more often decompensated and thin walled and that hypertrophy does not occur with uninhibited contractions.[12] Further research on the anatomic changes that occur in the aging lower urinary tract will help to clarify these issues.

Several age-associated factors (Table 94-1) can have an important influence on lower urinary tract function and symptoms in elderly women. Although most elderly individuals are generally active and healthy, the incidence of several disorders does increase with age. Impairments of cognitive and sensory function are more common in the elderly than in younger populations. These impairments may make it difficult for the elderly to interpret and relate symptoms of lower urinary tract dysfunction accurately. Poor nutritional and fluid intake can predispose the elderly to fecal impaction and urinary infection. The prevalence of asymptomatic bacteriuria increases with age (discussed later), and this situation predisposes to symptomatic urinary infection. Locomotor disturbances are common in the elderly. The incidence of stroke, arthritis, osteoporosis with resultant hip fractures, peripheral vascular disease with claudication or resultant amputations, Parkinson's disease, and other gait disorders increase with age. These disorders can make it difficult for the elderly to reach a toilet, especially in the setting of urinary frequency and urgency. Impaired mobility may play a prominent role in the development of incontinence in elderly women (discussed later). The incidence of diseases of the central nervous system, such as stroke, dementia, and Parkinson's disease, increases with age. Given the important role of higher centers in the control of micturition, these diseases are frequently involved in urinary dysfunction in the elderly.

An associated problem is that as a result of the high prevalence of so many diseases among the elderly, they are also likely to be taking a wide variety of drugs (often several different agents in complex dosage schedules), many of which can affect lower urinary tract function (Table 94-2). An important component of the assessment of older women with lower urinary tract symptoms is evaluation of the potential role of medications in causing or contributing to their symptoms. It is important to understand the potential effects of acetylcholinesterase inhibitors, given for dementia to stabilize cognitive decline, because these procholinergic agents can worsen or cause incontinence. Bladder relaxant agents may worsen cognition in some older adults.[13]

URINARY TRACT INFECTION IN ELDERLY WOMEN

Asymptomatic and symptomatic UTIs are common in the elderly. The overall expenditures for the treatment of UTIs in women in the United States, excluding spending on outpatient prescriptions, were approximately $2.47 billion in 2000.[14] The estimated lifetime risk for a woman to have a UTI is greater than 50%.[14] The prevalence of bacteriuria increases with age; it is more common in elderly women than in men and in patients in nursing homes and hospitals than in elderly people residing at home. Compared with younger women, elderly women are at higher risk for hospitalization from a UTI[14] and have twice the risk for

Table 94-2 Medications That Can Negatively Affect Continence

Type of Medication	Potential Effects on Continence
Diuretics	Polyuria, frequency, urgency
Anticholinergics	Urinary retention, overflow incontinence, impaction
Acetylcholinesterase inhibitors (for dementia)	Urgency, urge urinary incontinence
Psychotropics	
Antidepressants	Anticholinergic actions, sedation, rigidity, immobility
Antipsychotics	Anticholinergic actions, sedation
Sedatives and hypnotics	Sedation, delirium, immobility, muscle relaxation
Narcotic analgesics	Urinary retention, fecal impaction, sedation, delirium
α-Adrenergic blockers	Urethral relaxation
α-Adrenergic agonists	Urinary retention
β-Adrenergic agonists	Urinary retention
Calcium channel blockers	Urinary retention
Alcohol	Polyuria, frequency, urgency, sedation, delirium, immobility

Table 94-3 Prevalence of Bacteriuria in Elderly Women

Setting of Population	Women Affected (%)
Community	11-17
Nursing home	23-27
Hospital	32-50

developing bacteruria after urodynamic procedures,[15] Table 94-3 summarizes several studies of the prevalence of bacteriuria in the elderly.[16-26] Longitudinal studies of bacteriuria among older women have documented that the organisms change over time and that bacteriuria resolves and returns spontaneously in many women.[20,24-26] Several factors have been implicated in the increased prevalence of bacteriuria in the elderly, including atrophic mucosal changes as a result of estrogen deficiency, increased residual urine volumes, immobility, the prevalence of fecal and urinary incontinence, and the relatively common use of indwelling catheters.[27] Risk factors for bacteruria and UTIs in postmenopausal women include sexual activity, diabetes, urinary incontinence, and past UTIs.[28] Symptoms common in elderly women that are usually associated with UTI, such as frequency, urgency, dysuria, and incontinence, do not reliably predict whether the urine is infected.[17-19,21] Midstream urine specimens from elderly women are highly unreliable in predicting true bladder infection. The white blood cell count on urinalysis correlates poorly with bladder infection,[10] and there is at least a 17% incidence of false-positive cultures when midstream urine specimens are repeated or compared with suprapubic aspirates.[20,29] Growth of between 10^4 and 10^9 colonies/mL and contaminated specimens are also more common with midstream specimens. Taking two consecutive midstream specimens increases the reliability substantially. These factors can make the accurate diagnosis of true bladder infection difficult in elderly women.

Asymptomatic bacteriuria is generally considered a benign condition in the elderly who are free of catheters. Studies have, however, shown a substantial incidence of potentially correctable lower urinary tract disease that can contribute to bacteriuria in asymptomatic elderly patients.[22] One study found that bacteriuric elderly nursing home residents had a 30% to 50% lower survival rate (deaths from a variety of causes) when followed for 10 years compared with nonbacteriuric residents matched for age, blood pressure, smoking habits, hematocrit, and blood cholesterol levels.[30] A second study of community-dwelling elderly also showed an association between bacteriuria and mortality,[31] but a cause-and-effect relationship has not been documented. Two studies of treated asymptomatic bacteriuria in older institutionalized[32] and ambulatory[33] women have not documented substantial effects on mortality. In summary, therapy for asymptomatic bacteruria in older individuals has not produced improvements in survival or amelioration of genitourinary symptoms, but it has correlated with increased antimicrobial resistance and adverse drug effects. For these reasons, guideline consensus statements have recommended against the routine screening for and treatment of asymptomatic bacteriuria in older persons resident in the community elderly institutionalized residents of long-term care facilities.[34]

Symptomatic UTIs in elderly women should be treated with an antimicrobial that achieves a high concentration in the urine. Consensus guidelines recommend that trimethoprim/sulfamethoxazole (TMP/SMX) DS twice daily be first line therapy for UTIs, based on cost and efficacy considerations. Floxacins (i.e., ciprofloxacin and others) should be reserved for situations in which there are high rates of resistance (10% to 20%) to TMP/SMX.[34] In younger women, a 3-day regimen is associated with a 93% eradication rate. Longer courses are associated with higher eradication rates, which must be weighed against higher rates of adverse drug events.[35] Because of the acknowledged higher rates of failure in 3-day treatment for older women, the consensus statement recommends a 7-day treatment course for uncomplicated symptomatic infections. Drug selection should be modified based on such factors as allergy, renal function, cost, and bacterial sensitivities (especially when infections are recurrent). Although age-related changes do occur in the kidney's ability to eliminate these drugs, dosage adjustments usually are unnecessary unless the serum creatinine level is above 2.0 mg/dL.

Compliance with drug regimens may be a problem for many elderly patients and should be kept in mind as a potential cause of treatment failure. Recurrent infections in elderly women usually are caused by reinfection with a different organism. Relapse with the same organism should prompt a search for a structural abnormality in the lower urinary tract. When relapse

Table 94-4 Prevalence of Urinary Incontinence Among Older Women

Setting of Population	Women Affected (%)
Community	Approximately 33%: any incontinence* 4-6%: severe incontinence†
Acute care hospital	Approximately 40%
Nursing home	50-70%

*Positive response to questioning about any uncontrolled urine loss in the past year.
†Incontinence that occurs more than once per week or requires the use of pads.

occurs in the absence of a structural abnormality, a 3- to 6-week course of drug therapy should be given. Infrequent symptomatic reinfections should be treated as separate episodes; frequent symptomatic infections can be managed by long-term prophylaxis. Nitrofurantoin (100 mg/day) and TMP/SMX (½ of a single strength (40 mg/200 mg) tablet/day) have been shown to prevent recurrent symptomatic infections[36] and appear to be cost-effective, especially in women who have three or more symptomatic infections per year.[37]

URINARY INCONTINENCE IN ELDERLY WOMEN

Scope of the Problem

Incontinence is a common, disruptive, and potentially disabling condition in the elderly. The prevalence of urinary incontinence is illustrated in Table 94-4. Incontinence is a heterogeneous condition among older women, ranging in severity from occasional episodes of dribbling small amounts of urine to continuous urinary incontinence with concomitant fecal incontinence. The prevalence of urinary incontinence among women increases with increasing age. The likelihood of having severe urinary incontinence also increases with increasing age; compared with 8% of women between 30 and 39 years old reporting severe urinary incontinence, 33% of women between 80 and 90 years old reported severe urinary incontinence.[38] Although these general trends are clear, there are more subtle trends. The overall prevalence of urinary incontinence increases with rising age, but the prevalence of stress incontinence may peak at age 50 and then decrease slightly.[39] Parity, which is a significant risk factor for stress incontinence in younger women, is a much less important risk factor for stress incontinence in older women.[40,41]

Not all incontinent elderly women are severely demented, bedridden, and in nursing homes. Many in institutions and in the community are ambulatory and have good mental function. Physical health, psychological well-being, social status, and the costs of health care can be adversely affected by incontinence. Physical consequences can include skin breakdown, UTIs, and fractures, which may result if patients fall when they are forced to get up in the middle of the night to urinate. The psychosocial effects can be even more devastating; many elderly patients may suffer intense embarrassment, loss of self-esteem, and feelings of helplessness, depression, and anxiety, resulting in a withdrawal from vital social contacts or at least a reluctance to go places or engage in activities that are not close to toilet facilities.[42] The financial impact of incontinence is also significant. It has been estimated that the cost of managing incontinence in elderly nursing home residents alone is close to $3 billion per year.[43] Estimates put the U.S. Medicare cost of inpatient and outpatient treatment of urinary incontinence in women at $234.4 million (1998). Urinary incontinence as the main reason for physician care for a Medicare visit rose from 845 per 100,000 in 1992 to 1845 per 100,000 persons in 2000.[39]

Urinary incontinence is curable in many elderly patients, especially those who have adequate mobility and mental function. There is growing literature suggesting that for some individuals, urinary incontinence can be prevented or delayed by exercises and behavioral strategies.[44] Even when urinary incontinence is not curable, incontinence can always be managed in a manner that keeps patients comfortable, makes life easier for caregivers, and minimizes the cost of caring for the condition and its complications.

Acute, Reversible Incontinence versus Persistent Incontinence

The distinction between acute, reversible forms of incontinence and persistent incontinence is clinically important in older women because incontinence is often contributed to or caused by factors outside the lower urinary tract in this population. *Acute incontinence* refers to situations in which the incontinence is of sudden onset, usually related to an acute illness or an iatrogenic problem, and subsides after the illness or medication problem has been resolved. *Persistent incontinence* refers to incontinence that is unrelated to an acute illness and persists over time. The causes of acute and reversible forms of urinary incontinence can be remembered by the acronym DRIP (Table 94-5). Many of the reversible factors listed in this table can also play a role in patients with persistent forms of incontinence. A search for these factors should be undertaken in all incontinent geriatric patients.

Persistent forms of incontinence can be classified clinically into four basic types in the geriatric population: stress, urge, overflow, and functional. These types can overlap each other, and an individual patient may have more than one type simultaneously. Although this classification does not include all of the neurophysiologic abnormalities associated with incontinence (e.g., reflex or "unconscious" incontinence), it is helpful in approaching the clinical assessment and treatment of incontinence in the elderly.[45]

Stress incontinence is the most common type among women younger than 75 years, especially in ambulatory clinic settings.[46-48] It may be infrequent and involve very small amounts of urine, and it may need no specific treatment in women who are not bothered by it. However, it may be so severe or bothersome that it requires surgical correction. It is most often associated with weakened supporting tissues and consequent hypermobility of the bladder outlet and urethra caused by lack of estrogen or by previous vaginal deliveries or surgery. Older adults with stress incontinence, compared with their continent older counterparts, are more likely to be white, have arthritis, be using oral estrogen therapy, have chronic obstructive pulmonary disease, and be obese.[49] Parity appears to be a somewhat weaker risk factor among women 60 years old or older than among women younger than 60 years.[30] Many older women also develop stress incontinence because of intrinsic urethral dysfunction after one or more lower urinary tract surgical procedures.

Table 94-5 Reversible Factors That May Contribute to Urinary Incontinence

DRIP Acronym	Definition	Description
D	Delirium	New-onset urinary incontinence (UI) may be associated with delirium because of acute underlying conditions requiring diagnosis and treatment.
R	Restricted mobility Retention	Acute conditions causing immobility may precipitate UI; environmental manipulation and scheduled toileting are appropriate until the condition resolves. Urinary retention may be precipitated by many drugs (see Table 94-2) or may occur acutely because of anatomic obstruction; immobility and large fecal impactions may also contribute.
I	Infection Inflammation Impaction	Acute cystitis may precipitate urge UI. Otherwise asymptomatic bacteriuria may contribute to urinary frequency and should be eradicated before any urodynamic evaluations are carried out. Atrophic vaginitis and urethritis can cause irritative voiding symptoms, including UI. Fecal impaction and fecal incontinence may be associated with UI.
P	Polyuria Pharmaceuticals	Poorly controlled diabetes with glucosuria can contribute to urinary frequency and UI. Edema due to congestive heart failure or venous insufficiency can cause nocturia and exacerbate nocturnal UI (see Table 94-2)

Urge incontinence is the most common symptomatic and urodynamic type of incontinence in women older than 75 years, especially those in institutions, and it is commonly a component of the overactive bladder syndrome.[50-52] Urge incontinence can be caused by a variety of lower genitourinary and neurologic disorders. Older incontinent individuals with urge incontinence are more likely than their older, continent counterparts to be white, have arthritis, be using oral estrogen therapy, have insulin-treated diabetes, have depression, be older (within a 70- to 79-year-old cohort), and have poor lower extremity physical performance.[49] It is most often associated with detrusor motor instability or detrusor hyperreflexia. Some patients have a poorly compliant bladder without involuntary contractions (due to radiation or interstitial cystitis, both of which are unusual conditions in older women). Other patients have symptoms of urge incontinence but do not exhibit detrusor motor instability on urodynamic testing. This is usually called *sensory instability* or *hypersensitive bladder*; it is likely that some of these patients have detrusor motor instability in everyday life that is not documented at the time of the urodynamic study. However, some patients with neurologic disorders have detrusor hyperreflexia on urodynamic testing but may not have urgency and are incontinent without any warning symptoms (i.e., unconscious incontinence). These patients are generally treated as if they have urge incontinence if they can empty the bladder and do not have other correctable genitourinary pathology (discussed later). A subgroup of very elderly incontinent patients with detrusor hyperreflexia has been described who also have impaired bladder contractility; they empty less than a third of the bladder volume with involuntary contractions on urodynamic testing.[51-53] The implications of this urodynamic finding for the pathophysiology and treatment of incontinence in the elderly are unclear and are being investigated.

Urinary retention with overflow incontinence is relatively unusual among older women and can result from anatomic or neurogenic outflow obstruction, a hypotonic or acontractile bladder, or both (Box 94-1). Several types of drugs can also contribute to this type of incontinence (see Table 94-2).

Stress, urge, and overflow incontinence can occur in combination. About one third of older women with stress incontinence also have symptoms of urge incontinence and detrusor instability. Similarly, about one third of women with urge incontinence also have symptoms or signs of stress incontinence.[46-48,54] These mixed types of incontinence can have important therapeutic implications, especially in decisions about surgery for stress incontinence.

Functional incontinence results when an elderly person is unable or unwilling to reach a toilet on time. Distinguishing this type of incontinence from other types of persistent incontinence is critical to appropriate management. Factors that cause functional incontinence (e.g., inaccessible toilets, psychological disorders) can exacerbate other types of persistent incontinence.

Box 94-1 Causes of Urinary Retention in Elderly Women

- Bladder outlet obstruction
  - Mechanical compression
    - Gynecologic malignancy
    - Uterine fibroids
    - Ovarian cyst
    - Fecal impaction
  - Fibrosis of bladder outlet (uncommon) secondary to chronic inflammation
- Urethral obstruction
  - Stricture
  - Prolapse and urethral distortion
- Hypotonic bladder
  - Peripheral neuropathy
    - Diabetes
    - Alcoholism
  - Mechanical interruption of motor innervation
    - Tumor
    - Herniated disk
    - Trauma
  - Overdistention injuries
- Detrusor-sphincter dyssynergy
- Drug-induced retention (see Table 94-2)

Box 94-2 Diagnostic Evaluation of Urinary Incontinence in Older Women

All Patients
Focused history
Targeted physical examination
Urinalysis
Postvoid residual determination

Selected Patients
Simple urodynamic test
Complex urodynamic tests
- Dual-channel cystometrogram
- Pressure-flow study
- Urethral pressure profilometry
- Sphincter electromyography
- Video urodynamic evaluation

Laboratory studies
- Urine culture
- Renal function tests
- Blood glucose
- Serum calcium
- Urine cytology

Radiologic studies
- Renal ultrasound
- Voiding cystourethrography

Urologic or gynecologic evaluation
- Cystourethroscopy

Patients with incontinence that appears to be predominantly related to functional factors may also have abnormalities of the lower genitourinary tract such as detrusor hyperreflexia. In some patients, it can be very difficult to determine whether the functional factors or the genitourinary factors predominate without a trial of specific types of treatment. It is therefore appropriate to consider functional incontinence as a diagnosis of exclusion among older patients. Cognitive impairment or impaired mobility should not preclude a trial of specific treatment for incontinence when indicated.

Evaluation

In patients with a sudden onset of incontinence (especially one associated with an acute medical condition and hospitalization), the possible causes (see Table 94-5) can be determined by a brief history, physical examination, and basic laboratory studies (e.g., urinalysis, culture, serum glucose or calcium level).

Box 94-2 lists the basic components of the evaluation of persistent urinary incontinence. All patients should have a focused history, targeted physical examination, urinalysis, and a determination of postvoid residual urine volumes. The history should focus on the characteristics of the incontinence, current medical problems and medications, and the impact of incontinence on the patient and caregivers. Bladder records or voiding diaries are often helpful. Physical examination should focus on abdominal, rectal, and genital examinations and on evaluation of lumbosacral innervation. During the history and physical examination, special attention should be paid to factors such as mobility, mental status, medications, and accessibility of toilets that may be causing incontinence or interacting with urologic and neurologic disorders to make the condition worse. A clean urine sample should be collected for urinalysis to exclude glucosuria, pyuria, bacteriuria, and hematuria. Persistent sterile microscopic hematuria (>5 red blood cells/high-power field) is an indication for further evaluation to exclude a tumor or other urinary tract abnormality.

A series of simple tests of lower urinary tract function can be carried out in a clinic, hospital, nursing home, or even at home. They include observation of voiding, a pad test for stress incontinence, and simple cystometry.[55] These tests are not necessary for all patients (discussed later). Like other diagnostic tests, they should be performed only if the results will change the patient's management. When they are performed, they must be carried out and interpreted carefully in light of other information from the history and physical examination. Bladder capacity and stability as determined by simple cystometry are highly correlated with results of formal multichannel cystometrograms.[56] Simple cystometry may be unnecessary to make a reasonable treatment plan in many elderly patients, such as those who have sterile urine and no atrophic vaginitis, meet none of the criteria given in Table 94-6, and who reliably give a history of stress incontinence without irritative or obstructive voiding symptoms, leak with stress maneuvers, and can empty the bladder completely (they can be treated for stress-type incontinence) or who reliably give a history of urge incontinence without symptoms of stress incontinence or voiding difficulty and can empty the bladder completely (they can be treated for urge-type incontinence). These tests are not essential for patients who are going to be treated initially with behavioral therapy alone, which can be used for stress, urge, mixed, and functional incontinence. The criteria for referral for further evaluation given in Table 94-6 have been shown to be reasonably sensitive but not very specific for identifying patients who require further evaluation for appropriate treatment.[50]

Management

Several therapeutic modalities are used in managing incontinent older women. Special attention should be paid to the management of acute forms of incontinence, which are most common in elderly patients in acute care hospitals. These forms of incontinence are often transient if managed appropriately; however, inappropriate management may lead to a permanent problem. The most common treatment for incontinent elderly patients in acute care hospitals is indwelling catheterization. In some instances, this therapy is justified by the necessity for accurate measurement of urine output during the acute phase of an illness. In many instances, however, it is unnecessary and poses a substantial and unwarranted risk of catheter-induced infection. Although it may be more difficult and time consuming for caregivers, making toilets and toilet substitutes accessible combined with some form of scheduled toileting is probably a more appropriate approach to the treatment of patients who do not require indwelling catheters. Launderable or disposable and highly absorbent bed pads and undergarments may also be helpful in managing these patients. These products may be more costly than catheters but probably result in less morbidity and therefore lower overall cost in the long run. Specially designed incontinence undergarments and pads can be very helpful for many nonhospitalized patients but must be used appropriately. They are being marketed on television and are readily available in retail stores. Although they can be effective, several caveats should be

Table 94-6 Criteria for Referral of Elderly Incontinent Women for Urologic, Gynecologic, or Urodynamic Evaluation

Criteria	Definition	Rationale
History		
Recent history of lower urinary tract or pelvic surgery or irradiation	Surgery or irradiation involving the pelvic area or lower urinary tract within the past 6 months	A structural abnormality related to the recent procedure should be sought.
Relapse or rapid recurrence of a symptomatic urinary tract infection	Onset of dysuria, new or worse irritative voiding symptoms, fever, suprapubic or flank pain associated with growth of more than 100,000 colony-forming units of a urinary pathogen; symptoms and bacteriuria that return within 4 weeks of treatment	A structural abnormality or pathologic condition in the urinary tract predisposing to infection should be excluded.
Physical examination		
Marked pelvic prolapse	Pronounced uterine descent to or through the introitus; prominent cystocele that descends the entire height of the vaginal vault with coughing during speculum examination	Anatomic abnormality may underlie the pathophysiology of the incontinence and may require surgical repair.
Severe stress incontinence*	Prominent, bothersome stress incontinence that has failed to respond to adequate trials of nonsurgical therapy	Bladder neck suspension procedures are generally well tolerated and successful in properly selected elderly women who have stress incontinence that responds poorly to more conservative measures.
Severe hesitancy, straining, or interrupted urinary stream	Straining to begin voiding and a dribbling or intermittent stream when the patient's bladder feels full	Signs suggest obstruction or poor bladder contractility.
Postvoid residual		
Difficulty in passing a 14-Fr straight catheter	Catheter passage impossible or requires considerable force or a larger or more rigid catheter	Anatomic blockage of the urethra or bladder neck may exist.
Postvoid residual volume >200 mL†	Volume of urine remaining in the bladder within 5 to 10 minutes after the patient voids spontaneously in as normal a fashion as possible	Anatomic or neurogenic obstruction or poor bladder contractility may exist.
Urinalysis		
Hematuria (sterile)	More than five red blood cells/high-power field on microscopic examination in the absence of infection	A pathologic condition in the urinary tract should be excluded.
Failure to respond to nonsurgical management	After behavioral or drug therapy, or both, incontinence persists and the patient desires further evaluation and treatment.	A formal urodynamic evaluation may help to better define and reproduce the symptoms associated with the patient's incontinence and target treatment more effectively.

*If medical conditions preclude surgery or the patient is adamantly opposed to considering surgical intervention, the patient should not be referred.
†Some patients with lesser degrees of urinary retention may require evaluation, depending on other findings.

mentioned. Garments and pads are a nonspecific treatment. They should not be used as a first response to incontinence or before some type of diagnostic evaluation is done. Many patients are curable if treated with specific therapies, and some have potentially serious factors underlying their incontinence that must be diagnosed and treated. Pants and pads can interfere with attempts at certain types of behaviorally oriented therapies (discussed later).

Supportive measures are critical in managing all forms of incontinence and should be used in conjunction with other more specific treatment modalities. A positive attitude, education, environmental manipulations, appropriate use of toilet substitutes, avoidance of iatrogenic contributions to incontinence, modifications of diuretic and fluid intake patterns, and good skin care are all important.

To a large extent the optimal treatment of persistent incontinence depends on identifying the types of incontinence that exists. Table 94-7 outlines the primary treatments used for the basic types of persistent incontinence found among older incontinent women. Each treatment modality is briefly discussed in the following sections.

Drug Treatment

The efficacy of drug treatment has not been as well studied in the elderly as in younger populations,[56,58] but for many patients, especially those with urge or stress incontinence, drug treatment

Table 94-7 Primary Treatments for Different Types of Urinary Incontinence in Elderly Women

Type of Incontinence	Primary Treatment
Stress	Pelvic muscle (Kegel) exercises
	α-Adrenergic agonists
	Estrogen
	Biofeedback, bladder training
	Surgical intervention
Urge	Bladder relaxants
	Estrogen topically (if vaginal atrophy is present)
	Behavioral intervention (e.g., bladder training, biofeedback)
	Surgical removal of pathologic lesions
Overflow*	Surgical removal of obstruction
	Intermittent catheterization (if practical)
	Indwelling catheterization
Functional	Behavioral therapies (e.g., prompted voiding, habit training)
	Environmental manipulations
	Incontinence undergarments and pads
	External collection devices
	Bladder relaxants (selected patients)†
	Indwelling catheters (selected patients)‡

**Overflow incontinence* is no longer a recommended term (since 2002) by the International Continence Society, which favors the terminology of *acute* or *chronic retention of urine.*[57]

†Many patients with functional incontinence also have detrusor hyperreflexia, and some may benefit from bladder relaxant drug therapy.

‡See Box 94-3.

may be very effective. Drug treatment can be prescribed in conjunction with one or more of the behavioral interventions discussed in the following section. Head-to-head comparisons of drug and behavioral therapy have shown that both are efficacious for treatment of urinary incontinence,[59] and in practice. they often complement each other. Treatment decisions should be made on an individual basis and depend in a large part on the characteristics and preferences of the patient and the physician.

For urge incontinence, drugs with anticholinergic and bladder smooth muscle–relaxing properties are used. All of them may cause bothersome systemic anticholinergic side effects, especially dry mouth, in the elderly, and they can precipitate urinary retention in some patients. The advantages of extended-release preparations (e.g., tolterodine LA, oxybutynin XL, oxybutynin transdermal) and newer drugs (e.g., trospium, darifenacin, solefenacin) for overactive bladder over older, cheaper, immediate-release oxybutynin are more favorable side effect profiles (but no more efficacy). In animal models, these agents demonstrate more selectivity for the bladder than for the salivary glands, but some insist that the tolerability and effectiveness of agents are related to their antimuscarinic activity. Although use of immediate-release oxybutynin in older patients who are tolerant of side effects is possible, consensus guidelines recommend against immediate-release oxybutynin.[60] One newer agent, tolterodine, has been shown to have a slight decrease in efficacy and no decline in tolerability.[61]

The potential for severe anticholinergic side effects is much more likely in older adults than in younger adults. Patients with Alzheimer's disease must be followed for the development of drug-induced delirium. Patients with cognitive impairment may be taking cholinesterase-inhibitor agents (i.e., medications for dementia that offer small gains in cognition and slower rates of cognitive decline). The potential interaction can be clinically evident at times; patients may have a worsening of their cognition with bladder relaxants (i.e., anticholinergic effect)[13] or may have a worsening in their continence with acetylcholinesterase inhibitors (i.e., procholinergic effects). Research has shown that receptor targeting or properties that prevent a drug from crossing the blood-brain barrier may be important considerations in whether a medication will have effects on cognition. One study using darifenacin demonstrated in 129 nondemented patients that active drug did not have any significantly greater effect on cognition compared with placebo.[62] Drugs specifically indicated for use in urinary incontinence or overactive bladder likely offer some advantage over other drugs with more pronounced systemic anticholinergic side effects.[63] Several studies suggest that cognitive and physical functional impairments are associated with poor responses to bladder-relaxant drug therapy.[64-66] The results of these studies should not preclude a treatment trial in this patient population. Some patients may respond, especially in conjunction with scheduled toileting or prompted voiding. The goal of treatment in these patients may not be to cure the incontinence but to reduce its severity and prevent discomfort and complications.

For stress incontinence, drug treatment involves a combination of an α-adrenergic agonist, duloxetine[67] (approved in Europe but not in the United States for treatment of stress incontinence), a selective serotonin reuptake inhibitor (SSRI) medication used in the treatment of depression, or topically applied estrogen, or both. Drug treatment is appropriate for motivated patients who have mild to moderate degrees of stress incontinence, do not have a major anatomic abnormality (e.g., large cystocele), and do not have any contraindications to these drugs. Although there are few published data on duloxetine in older patients, its inclusion here is merited because of the dearth of other medications for the treatment of stress urinary incontinence. Duloxetine generally enhances urine storage by facilitating the vesical sympathetic reflex pathway and inhibiting the parasympathetic voiding pathway. Duloxetine has been shown to increase significantly bladder capacity and sphincter tone without interfering with the normal voiding cycle. Duloxetine has also been evaluated for depression and lower urinary tract disease.[67]

α-Agonist medications that may be given for stress urinary incontinence have an effect on hypertension. The most commonly used over-the-counter medication previously used for stress urinary incontinence was phenylpropanolamine, which was removed from the market in 2000 because it was shown in women to be highly associated with intracranial hemorrhage when used as a dietary aid, which leaves pseudoephedrine as the over-the-counter agent. Pseudoephedrine may exacerbate hypertension and contribute to insomnia in some older patients. These patients may also respond to behavioral treatments (discussed later), and some data suggest that the two treatment modalities are roughly equivalent, with about three fourths of patients reporting improvement.[68] A combination of these modalities can be a reasonable approach for some patients.

Estrogen alone is not as effective as it is in combination with an α-agonist for stress incontinence. Estrogen is also used chronically or intermittently (i.e., 1- to 2-month courses) for the treatment of overactive bladder symptoms and urge incontinence in women with atrophic vaginitis and urethritis.

Given that lack of estrogen results in conditions that make urinary incontinence more likely, several studies have examined estrogen as a preventive agent or therapy for urinary incontinence. In a large study of more than 20,000 women, oral estrogens (0.625 mg of conjugated equine estrogen, with and without progesterone) were shown to increase the risk of developing urinary incontinence at 1 year. Among women who were incontinent, estrogen treatment worsened the frequency of urinary incontinence.[1] Despite the pessimism about using oral estrogens, there may still be a role for topical estrogen. Its administration has been shown to yield significant improvements in colposcopic findings, statistically significant increases in mean maximum urethral pressure and mean urethral closure pressure, and improvements in the abdominal pressure transmission ratio to the proximal urethra. The continence outcomes are less well understood.[69] It is not possible to infer that because low estrogen levels are associated with physiologic changes, hormone replacement will reverse these changes, restore function, or reduce symptoms.

Drug treatment for chronic overflow incontinence using a cholinergic agonist or an α-adrenergic antagonist is usually not effective, although anecdotal reports suggest α-blockers may be useful in some female patients. Bethanechol may be helpful when given for a brief period subcutaneously in patients with persistent bladder contractility problems after an overdistention injury, but it is generally not effective when given orally over the long term.[70]

Symptomatically and urodynamically, many elderly women have a combination of urge and stress incontinence. In theory, a combination of estrogen and imipramine may be appropriate for these patients because imipramine has both anticholinergic and α-adrenergic effects. When urge incontinence is the predominant symptom, a combination of estrogen and oxybutynin would be appropriate. Behavioral interventions are also a reasonable approach to women with mixed incontinence.

Behavioral Interventions

Many types of behavioral procedures have been described for the management of urge and stress urinary incontinence.[71,72] The nosology of these procedures has been somewhat confusing, and in much of the literature, the term *bladder training* is used to encompass a wide variety of techniques. It is important to distinguish between procedures that are patient dependent (i.e., require adequate function and motivation of the patient), in which the goal is to restore a normal pattern of voiding and continence, and procedures that are caregiver dependent and can be used for functionally disabled patients, in which the goal is to keep the patient and environment dry (Table 94-8).

Pelvic muscle (Kegel) exercises consist of repetitive contractions of the pelvic floor muscles. This procedure is taught by having the patient interrupt voiding. This technique should be

Table 94-8 Behavioral Interventions for Urinary Incontinence in Elderly Women

Procedure	Definition	Types of Incontinence	Comments
Patient dependent			
Pelvic muscle (Kegel) exercises	Repetitive contraction of pelvic floor muscles	Stress Stress and urge	Requires adequate function and motivation
Biofeedback	Use of bladder, rectal, or vaginal pressure recordings to train patients to contract pelvic floor muscles and relax bladder		Requires equipment and trained personnel
Bladder training	Use of educational components of biofeedback, bladder records, pelvic muscle, and other behavioral exercises	Stress and urge	Requires trained therapist, adequate cognitive and physical function, and patient motivation
Bladder retraining	Progressive lengthening or shortening of intervoiding interval, with adjunctive techniques* Intermittent catheterization used in patients recovering from overdistention injuries with persistent retention	Acute (e.g., postcatheterization with urge or overflow, poststroke)	Goal is to restore normal pattern of voiding and continence; requires adequate cognitive and physical function and patient motivation
Caregiver dependent			
Scheduled toileting	Fixed toileting schedule	Urge and functional	Goal is to prevent wetting episodes
Prompted voiding	Regular opportunities to toilet with behavioral reinforcement		Can be used in patients with impaired cognitive or physical functioning
Habit training	Toileting based on established individual pattern with behavioral reinforcement		Requires staff or caregiver availability and patient motivation

*Techniques to trigger voiding (e.g., running water, stroking thigh, suprapubic tapping), completely emptying the bladder (e.g., bending forward, suprapubic pressure), and alterations of fluid or diuretic intake patterns may be helpful for some patients.

used only to identify the proper muscles, and patients should be discouraged from doing this repeatedly because of the potential risk of teaching patients dysfunctional voiding habits. To get a sense of the muscles used, the patient is asked to squeeze the examiner's fingers during a vaginal examination (without doing a Valsalva maneuver, which is the opposite of the intended effect). One exercise consists of a several-second squeeze and a several-second relaxation. Once learned, the exercises should be practiced many times throughout the day (usually 75 exercises per day, broken down into three sessions of 25 exercises each), and they should be used in everyday life during situations (e.g., coughing, running water) in a variety of positions (e.g., sitting, standing, lying down) that can precipitate incontinence. Pelvic muscle exercises may be taught in conjunction with biofeedback procedures and can be especially helpful for women who bear down (i.e., increasing intra-abdominal pressure) when they attempt to contract the pelvic floor muscles. Vaginal cones (weights) may be useful adjuncts to pelvic muscle exercises in some patients.

Biofeedback procedures involve the use of bladder, rectal, or vaginal pressure or electrical activity recordings to train patients to contract the pelvic floor muscles and relax the bladder. Studies have shown that these techniques can be very effective for managing stress and urge incontinence, even in the elderly.[73] The use of biofeedback techniques may be limited by requirements for equipment and trained personnel; some of these techniques are relatively invasive and require the use of bladder or rectal catheters, or both. Some newer biofeedback techniques use surface electrodes and are less invasive. Electrical stimulation vaginally or rectally has also been used in the management of stress and urge incontinence. Research suggests that excellent results can be achieved in some older women in treating stress and urge incontinence without the use of electrical stimulation or computer-assisted biofeedback.[74,75] In contrast to medication therapy, the degree of continence achieved with pelvic muscle exercises is not as highly correlated with an increase in bladder capacity.[76]

Other forms of patient-dependent training procedures include various forms of bladder training and bladder retraining. Bladder training procedures involve the educational components taught during biofeedback but not the use of biofeedback equipment. Patients are taught how to do pelvic muscle exercises, provided strategies for managing urgency, and instructed to regularly use bladder records. These techniques are highly effective in selected community-dwelling patients, especially women.[77] Investigators have attempted to identify baseline characteristics that predict clinical success with behavioral techniques. It is probably more important to discuss factors that *do not* predict worse outcomes: greater age, greater parity, lower levels of education, and previous surgery (the latter two may actually predict greater success).[78]

The goal of caregiver-dependent behavioral interventions, such as prompted voiding and habit training, is to prevent incontinence episodes rather than restore the normal pattern of voiding and complete continence. These procedures have been shown to be effective in reducing incontinence in selected nursing home residents. In its simplest form, scheduled toileting involves toileting the patient at regular intervals, usually every 2 hours during the day and every 4 hours during the evening and night. Habit training involves a schedule of toiletings or prompted voidings that is modified according to the patient's pattern of continent voids and incontinence episodes as demonstrated by a monitoring record. Positive reinforcement is offered for continent voids and neutral reinforcement when incontinence occurs. Adjunctive techniques to prompt voiding (e.g., running tap water, stroking the inner thigh, suprapubic tapping) and to help empty the bladder completely (e.g., bending forward after completion of voiding) may be helpful for some patients. Prompted voiding has been the best studied of these procedures. It is a simple behavioral procedure that combines several of the elements mentioned earlier.[79] The success of these procedures is largely dependent on the knowledge and motivation of the caregivers implementing them, rather than on the physical functional and mental status of the incontinent patient. These techniques are not feasible in home settings without available caregivers. For these types of procedures to be feasible and cost-effective in the nursing home setting, the amount of time generally spent by the nursing staff in changing patients after incontinence episodes should not be exceeded by the time and effort needed to implement such training procedures. Targeting these procedures to selected patients, such as those with less frequent voiding and larger bladder capacities or voided volumes, may enhance their cost-effectiveness.[79] Quality assurance methods, based on principles of statistical quality control used in industry, have been shown to be helpful in maintaining the effectiveness of prompted voiding in nursing homes.[80]

Surgery

Surgical interventions are described in detail in other chapters in this textbook. Surgery should be considered for elderly women with stress incontinence that continues to be bothersome after attempts at nonsurgical treatment have been made and in women with a significant degree of pelvic prolapse or intrinsic urethral dysfunction. As with many other surgical procedures, patient selection and the experience of the surgeon are critical to success. Several case series have demonstrated that with proper patient selection, even elderly adults can successfully undergo surgery, but the number of overall incontinence procedures in older women remains low. All women being considered for surgical therapy should have a thorough evaluation, including urodynamic tests, before undergoing the procedure. Women with mixed stress incontinence and detrusor motor instability may also benefit from surgery, especially if the clinical history and urodynamic findings suggest that stress incontinence is the predominant problem. Modified techniques of bladder neck suspension can be done with minimal risk and are highly successful in achieving continence, even in the elderly. Urinary retention can occur after surgery, but it is usually transient and can be managed by intermittent catheterization. Injection of bulking agents appears to be effective in older women, and age does not appear to correlate with outcomes.[81] This procedure may be especially helpful for frail older women who have stress or mixed incontinence that has not responded to behavioral or drug therapy.

Catheters and Catheter Care

Three basic types of catheters and catheterization procedures are used for the management of urinary incontinence: external catheters, intermittent straight catheterization, and chronic indwelling catheterization. An external catheter for use in women is commercially available, but its safety and effectiveness have not been well documented in the elderly. Intermittent catheterization can help in the management of patients with urinary retention and overflow incontinence. The procedure can be carried out by the patient or a caregiver, and it involves straight catheterization two to four times daily, depending on residual urine volume. In

Box 94-3 Indications for and Principles of Chronic Indwelling Catheter Use

Indications

1. Urinary retention that
   Is causing persistent overflow incontinence, symptomatic infections, or renal dysfunction
   Cannot be corrected surgically or medically
   Cannot be managed practically with intermittent catheterization
2. Skin wounds, pressure sores, or irritations that are being contaminated by incontinent urine
3. Care of terminally ill or severely impaired patients for whom bed and clothing changes are uncomfortable or disruptive
4. Preference of patient or caregiver when patient has failed to respond to more specific treatments

Catheter Care

1. Maintain sterile, closed, gravity drainage system; change the catheter every 4 to 8 weeks.
2. Avoid breaking the closed system.
3. Use clean techniques in emptying and changing the drainage system; wash hands between patients in institutionalized settings.
4. Secure the catheter to the upper thigh or lower abdomen to avoid perineal contamination and urethral irritation due to movement of the catheter.
5. Avoid frequent and vigorous cleaning of the catheter entry site; washing with soapy water once each day is sufficient.
6. Do not irrigate routinely.
7. If bypassing occurs in the absence of obstruction, consider the possibility of a bladder spasm, which can be treated with a bladder relaxant.
8. If catheter obstruction occurs frequently, increase the patient's fluid intake and acidify the urine if possible.
9. Do not routinely use prophylactic or suppressive urinary antiseptics or antimicrobials.
10. Do not perform routine surveillance cultures to guide management of individual patients because all chronically catheterized patients have bacteriuria (which is often polymicrobial), and the organisms change frequently.
11. Do not treat infection unless the patient develops symptoms; symptoms may be nonspecific, and other possible sources of infection should be carefully excluded before attributing symptoms to the urinary tract.
12. If a patient develops frequent symptomatic urinary tract infections, a genitourinary evaluation should be considered to rule out pathology such as stones, periurethral or prostatic abscesses, or chronic pyelonephritis.

the home, the catheter should be kept clean (but not necessarily sterile). Studies conducted largely among younger paraplegics have shown that this technique is practical and reduces the risk of symptomatic infection compared with chronic catheterization.

Self-intermittent catheterization has been shown to be feasible for elderly women outpatients who are functional and are willing and able to catheterize themselves.[82] However, studies carried out in young paraplegics and elderly female outpatients cannot automatically be extrapolated to frail elderly women or the institutionalized population. The technique may be useful in certain patients in acute care hospitals or nursing homes, such as those who have undergone bladder neck suspension, or in certain situations, such as after removal of an indwelling catheter in a bladder-retraining protocol. Nursing home residents, however, may be difficult to catheterize, and the anatomic abnormalities commonly found in elderly patients' lower urinary tracts may increase the risk of infection because of repeated straight catheterizations. Use of this technique in an institutional setting (which may have an abundance of organisms that are relatively resistant to many commonly used antimicrobial agents) may yield an unacceptable risk of nosocomial infections, and the use of sterile catheter trays for these procedures would be very expensive. It therefore may be extremely difficult to implement such a program in a typical nursing home setting.

Chronic indwelling catheterization is overused in some settings, and when used for periods of up to 10 years, it has been shown to increase the incidence of a number of other complications, including chronic bacteriuria, bladder stones, periurethral abscesses, and even bladder cancer. Elderly female nursing home residents managed by this technique are at relatively high risk for developing symptomatic infections.[83] Given these risks, it seems appropriate to recommend limiting the use of chronic indwelling catheters to certain specific situations and to follow sound principles of catheter care when using indwelling catheterization to attempt to minimize complications (Box 94-3).

References

1. Hendrix SL, Cochrane BB, Nygaard IE, et al: Effects of estrogen with and without progestin on urinary incontinence [see comment]. JAMA 293:935-948, 2005.
2. Brocklehurst JC, Dillane JB: Studies of the female bladder in old age. I. Cystometrograms in non-incontinent women. Gerontol Clin 8:285-305, 1966.
3. Jones KW, Schoenberg HW: Comparison of the incidence of bladder hyperreflexia in patients with benign prostatic hypertrophy and age-matched female controls. J Urol 133:425-426, 1985.
4. Diokno AC, Brown MB, Brock BM, et al: Clinical and cystometric characteristics of continent and incontinent noninstitutionalized elderly. J Urol 140:567-571, 1988.
5. Elbadawi A, Yalla SV, Resnick NM: Structural basis of geriatric voiding dysfunction. I. Methods of a prospective ultrastructural/urodynamic study and an overview of the findings. J Urol 150(Pt 2): 1650-1656, 1993.
6. Elbadawi A, Yalla SV, Resnick NM: Structural basis of geriatric voiding dysfunction. III. Detrusor overactivity. J Urol 150(Pt 2): 1668-1680, 1993.
7. Elbadawi A, Hailemariam S, Yalla SV, Resnick NM: Structural basis of geriatric voiding dysfunction. VI. Validation and update of diagnostic criteria in 71 detrusor biopsies. J Urol 157:1802-1913, 1997.
8. Edwards L, Malvern J: The urethral pressure profile: Theoretical considerations and clinical application. British J Urol 46:325-335, 1974.

9. Hendriksson L, Andersson KE, Ulmsten U: The urethral pressure profiles in continent and stress-incontinent women. Scand J Urol Nephrol 13:5-10, 1979.
10. Brocklehurst JC: The bladder. In Brocklehurst J (ed): Textbook of Geriatric Medicine and Gerontology. New York, Churchill Livingstone, 1992, pp 629-646.
11. Strasser H, Tiefenthaler M, Steinlechner M, et al: Urinary incontinence in the elderly and age-dependent apoptosis of rhabdosphincter cells [see comment]. Lancet 354:918-919, 1999.
12. McGuire EJ: Urinary dysfunction in the aged: Neurological considerations. Bull N Y Acad Med 56:275-284, 1980.
13. Tsao JW, Heilman KM: Transient memory impairment and hallucinations associated with tolterodine use. N Engl J Med 349:2274-2275, 2003.
14. Griebling TL: Urologic diseases in America project: Trends in resource use for urinary tract infections in women [see comment]. J Urol 173:1281-1287, 2005.
15. Yip SK, Fung K, Pang MW, et al: A study of female urinary tract infection caused by urodynamic investigation. Am J Obstet Gynecol 190:1234-1240, 2004.
16. Romano JM, Kaye D: UTI in the elderly: Common yet atypical. Geriatrics 36:113-115, 1981.
17. Akhtar AJ, Andrews G, Cairo F, et al: Urinary tract infection in the elderly: A population study. Age Ageing 1:48, 1972.
18. Brocklehurst JC, Dillane JB, Griffiths L, Fry J: The prevalence and symptomatology of urinary infection in an aged population. Gerontol Clin 10:242-253, 1968.
19. Brocklehurst JC, Fry J, Griffiths LL, Kalton G: Dysuria in old age. J Am Geriatr Soc 19:582-592, 1971.
20. Brocklehurst JC, Bee P, Jones D, Palmer MK: Bacteriuria in geriatric hospital patients its correlates and management. Age Ageing 6:240-245, 1977.
21. Garibaldi RA, Brodine S, Matsumiya S: Infections among patients in nursing homes: Policies, prevalence, problems. N Engl J Med 305:731-735, 1981.
22. Gladstone JL, Friedman SA: Bacteriuria in the aged: A study of its prevalence and predisposing lesions in a chronically ill population. J Urol 106:745-749, 1971.
23. Jewett MA, Fernie GR, Holliday PJ, Pim ME: Urinary dysfunction in a geriatric long-term care population: Prevalence and patterns. J Am Geriatr Soc 29:211-214, 1981.
24. Sourander LB, Kasanen A: A 5-year follow-up of bacteriuria in the aged. Gerontol Clin 14:274-281, 1972.
25. Boscia JA, Kobasa WD, Knight RA, et al: Epidemiology of bacteriuria in an elderly ambulatory population. Am J Med 80:208-214, 1986.
26. Abrutyn E, Mossey J, Levison M, et al: Epidemiology of asymptomatic bacteriuria in elderly women. J Am Geriatr Soc 39:388-393, 1991.
27. Sobel JD, Kaye D: Host factors in the pathogenesis of urinary tract infections. Am J Med 76:122-130, 1984.
28. Hu KK, Boyko EJ, Scholes D, et al: Risk factors for urinary tract infections in postmenopausal women. Arch Intern Med 164:989-993, 2004.
29. Moore-Smith B: Bacteriuria in elderly women. Lancet 2:827, 1972.
30. Dontas AS, Kasviki-Charvati P, Papanayiotou PC, Marketos SG: Bacteriuria and survival in old age. N Engl J Med 304:939-943, 1981.
31. Nordenstam GR, Brandberg CA, Oden AS, et al: Bacteriuria and mortality in an elderly population. N Engl J Med 314:1152-1156, 1986.
32. Nicolle LE, Mayhew WJ, Bryan L: Prospective randomized comparison of therapy and no therapy for asymptomatic bacteriuria in institutionalized elderly women. Am J Med 83:27-33, 1987.
33. Boscia JA, Kobasa WD, Knight RA, et al: Therapy vs no therapy for bacteriuria in elderly ambulatory nonhospitalized women. JAMA 257:1067-1071, 1987.
34. Nicolle LE, Bradley S, Colgan R, et al: Infectious Diseases Society of America guidelines for the diagnosis and treatment of asymptomatic bacteriuria in adults. Clin Infect Dis;40:643-654, 2005.
35. Warren JW, Abrutyn E, Hebel JR, et al: Guidelines for antimicrobial treatment of uncomplicated acute bacterial cystitis and acute pyelonephritis in women. Infectious Diseases Society of America (IDSA). Clin Infect Dis 29:745-758, 1999.
36. Stamey TA, Condy M, Mihara G: Prophylactic efficacy of nitrofurantoin macrocrystals and trimethoprim-sulfamethoxazole in urinary infections. Biologic effects on the vaginal and rectal flora. N Engl J Med 296:780-783, 1977.
37. Stamm WE, McKevitt M, Counts GW, et al: Is antimicrobial prophylaxis of urinary tract infections cost effective? Ann Intern Med 94:251-255, 1981.
38. Melville JL, Katon W, Delaney K, Newton K: Urinary incontinence in US women: A population-based study. Arch Intern Med 165:537-542, 2005.
39. Thom DH, Nygaard IE, Calhoun EA: Urologic diseases in America project: Urinary incontinence in women-national trends in hospitalizations, office visits, treatment and economic impact [see comment]. J Urol 173:1295-1301, 2005.
40. Grodstein F, Fretts R, Lifford K, et al: Association of age, race, and obstetric history with urinary symptoms among women in the Nurses' Health Study. Am J Obstet Gynecol 189:428-434, 2003.
41. Rortveit G, Hannestad YS, Daltveit AK, Hunskaar S: Age- and type-dependent effects of parity on urinary incontinence: The Norwegian EPINCONT study. Obstet Gynecol 98:1004-1010, 2001.
42. Ouslander JG, Abelson S: Perceptions of urinary incontinence among elderly outpatients. Gerontologist 30:369-372, 1990.
43. Hu TW: Impact of urinary incontinence on health-care costs. J Am Geriatr Soc 38:292-295, 1990.
44. Diokno AC, Sampselle CM, Herzog AR, et al: Prevention of urinary incontinence by behavioral modification program: A randomized, controlled trial among older women in the community. J Urol 171:1165-1171, 2004.
45. Ouslander JG: Geriatric urinary incontinence. Dis Mon 38:65-149, 1992.
46. Ouslander JG, Hepps K, Raz S, Su HL: Genitourinary dysfunction in a geriatric outpatient population. J Am Geriatr Soc 34:507-514, 1986.
47. Wells TJ, Brink CA, Diokno AC: Urinary incontinence in elderly women: Clinical findings. J Am Geriatr Soc 35:933-939, 1987.
48. Diokno AC, Wells TJ, Brink CA: Urinary incontinence in elderly women: Urodynamic evaluation. J Am Geriatr Soc 35:940-946, 1987.
49. Jackson RA, Vittinghoff E, Kanaya AM, et al: Urinary incontinence in elderly women: Findings from the Health, Aging, and Body Composition Study. Obstet Gynecol 104:301-307, 2004.
50. Ouslander J, Leach G, Staskin D, et al: Prospective evaluation of an assessment strategy for geriatric urinary incontinence. J Am Geriatr Soc 37:715-724, 1989.
51. Resnick NM, Yalla SV, Laurino E: The pathophysiology of urinary incontinence among institutionalized elderly persons [see comment]. N Engl J Med 320:1-7, 1989.
52. Pannill FC 3rd, Williams TF, Davis R: Evaluation and treatment of urinary incontinence in long term care. J Am Geriatr Soc 36:902-910, 1988.
53. Resnick NM, Yalla SV: Detrusor hyperactivity with impaired contractile function. An unrecognized but common cause of incontinence in elderly patients. JAMA 257:3076-3081, 1987.
54. Fantl JA, Wyman JF, McClish DK, Bump RC: Urinary incontinence in community-dwelling women: Clinical, urodynamic, and severity characteristics. Am J Obstet Gynecol 162:946-951; discussion 951-952, 1990.
55. Ouslander JG, Leach GE, Staskin DR: Simplified tests of lower urinary tract function in the evaluation of geriatric urinary incontinence. J Am Geriatr Soc 37:706-714, 1989.

56. Ouslander JG, Sier HC: Drug therapy for geriatric urinary incontinence. Clin Geriatr Med 2:789-807, 1986.
57. Abrams P, Cardozo L, Fall M, et al: The standardisation of terminology of lower urinary tract function: report from the Standardisation Sub-committee of the International Continence Society. Neurourol Urodyn 21:167-178, 2002.
58. Agency for Health Care Policy and Research: Urinary incontinence in adults. Clin Pract Guidel Quick Ref Guide Clin (2)QR1-27, 1992.
59. Burgio KL, Locher JL, Goode PS, et al: Behavioral vs drug treatment for urge urinary incontinence in older women: A randomized controlled trial [see comment]. JAMA 280:1995-2000, 1998.
60. Fick DM, Cooper JW, Wade WE, et al: Updating the Beers criteria for potentially inappropriate medication use in older adults: results of a US consensus panel of experts [see comment] [erratum appears in Arch Intern Med 164:298, 2004]. Arch Intern Med 163:2716-2724, 2003.
61. Michel MC, Schneider T, Krege S, Goepel M: Does gender or age affect the efficacy and safety of tolterodine? J Urol 168:1027-1031, 2002.
62. Lipton RB, Kolodner K, Wesnes K: Assessment of cognitive function of the elderly population: Effects of darifenacin. J Urol 173:493-498, 2005.
63. Ouslander JG, Blaustein J, Connor A, et al: Pharmacokinetics and clinical effects of oxybutynin in geriatric patients. J Urol 140:47-50, 1988.
64. Castleden CM, Duffin HM, Asher MJ, Yeomanson CW: Factors influencing outcome in elderly patients with urinary incontinence and detrusor instability. Age Ageing 14:303-307, 1985.
65. Zorzitto ML, Jewett MAS, Fernie GR, et al: Effectiveness of propantheline bromide in the treatment of geriatric patients with detrusor instability. Neurourol Urodyn 5:133, 1986.
66. Tobin GW, Brocklehurst JC: The management of urinary incontinence in local authority residential homes for the elderly. Age Ageing 15:292-298, 1986.
67. Yoshimura N, Chancellor MB: Current and future pharmacological treatment for overactive bladder. J Urol 168:1897-1913, 2002.
68. Wells TJ, Brink CA, Diokno AC, et al: Pelvic muscle exercise for stress urinary incontinence in elderly women. J Am Geriatr Soc 39:785-791, 1991.
69. Dessole S, Rubattu G, Ambrosini G, et al: Efficacy of low-dose intravaginal estriol on urogenital aging in postmenopausal women [see comment]. Menopause 11:49-56, 2004.
70. Finkbeiner AE: Is bethanechol chloride clinically effective in promoting bladder emptying? A literature review. J Urol 134:443-449, 1985.
71. Burgio KL, Burgio LD: Behavior therapies for urinary incontinence in the elderly. Clin Geriatr Med 2:809-827, 1986.
72. Hadley EC: Bladder training and related therapies for urinary incontinence in older people. JAMA 256:372-379, 1986.
73. Burgio KL, Whitehead WE, Engel BT: Urinary incontinence in the elderly. Bladder-sphincter biofeedback and toileting skills training. Ann Intern Med 103:507-515, 1985.
74. Goode PS, Burgio KL, Locher JL, et al: Effect of behavioral training with or without pelvic floor electrical stimulation on stress incontinence in women: A randomized controlled trial [see comment]. JAMA 290:345-352, 2003.
75. Burgio KL, Goode PS, Locher JL, et al: Behavioral training with and without biofeedback in the treatment of urge incontinence in older women: A randomized controlled trial [see comment]. JAMA 288:2293-2299, 2002.
76. Goode PS, Burgio KL, Locher JL, et al: Urodynamic changes associated with behavioral and drug treatment of urge incontinence in older women. J Am Geriatr Soc 50:808-816, 2002.
77. Fantl JA, Wyman JF, McClish DK, et al: Efficacy of bladder training in older women with urinary incontinence. JAMA 265:609-613, 1991.
78. Burgio KL, Goode PS, Locher JL, et al: Predictors of outcome in the behavioral treatment of urinary incontinence in women. Obstet Gynecol 102(Pt 1):940-947, 2003.
79. Schnelle JF: Managing Urinary Incontinence in the Elderly. New York, Springer-Verlag, 1991.
80. Schnelle JF, Newman D, White M, et al: Maintaining continence in nursing home residents through the application of industrial quality control. Gerontologist 33:114-121, 1993.
81. Griebling T: Geriatric urology. In: Solomon DH, LoCicero J 3rd, Rosenthal RA, eds. New Frontiers in Geriatrics Research: An Agenda for Surgical and Related Medical Specialties. New York, American Geriatrics Society, 2004, pp 269-302.
82. Bennett CJ, Diokno AC: Clean intermittent self-catheterization in the elderly. Urology 24:43-45, 1984.
83. Warren JW, Damron D, Tenney JH, et al: Fever, bacteremia, and death as complications of bacteriuria in women with long-term urethral catheters. J Infect Dis 155:1151-1158, 1987.

Chapter 95

URODYNAMICS EVALUATION IN THE ELDERLY

Pat O'Donnell

Urodynamic studies are the most comprehensive objective clinical measures of bladder and urethra function available for the clinical evaluation of elderly women with urinary incontinence or any other voiding dysfunction. Although urodynamic studies have many limitations, the clinical information derived from these studies is invaluable for making reasonable long-term management decisions in the treatment of urinary incontinence in older women. Comprehensive urodynamic studies are accepted well by older women, and discomfort or complications related to the studies do not preclude performing studies, even in frail elderly women.

Elderly incontinent women represent a group of patients who derive the most clinical benefit from urodynamic studies because of the complexity of voiding dysfunctions in this patient population and the impact that these voiding dysfunctions have on the quality of life in older women. Although the consequences of urinary incontinence in younger women are debilitating and life changing, it is primarily the elderly women who are placed in nursing homes because of it. Urodynamic studies represent a diagnostic evaluation available that has the potential to change the outcome of long-term incontinence therapy in older women. Successful treatment of voiding dysfunctions in older women has a profound impact on the quality of life of these patients, which emphasizes the importance of the diagnostic clinical information from urodynamic studies. Urodynamic studies provide the clinician with a basic understanding of the pathophysiology of the complex condition of incontinence in older women.

The clinical value of urodynamic studies in elderly women reflects the magnitude of the problem of incontinence in this patient population. The incidence of incontinence is higher among older women than younger women. The personal impact of urinary incontinence on quality of life is so powerful that it can potentially take an older woman away from her home in a community-dwelling environment to the chronic-care environment of a nursing home. The life-changing consequences of incontinence are so great that aggressive evaluation should be considered as an initial part of management of these older patients.

Changes in the bladder and urethral function, along with the changes in physical and mental function, that are associated with aging significantly complicate the diagnosis and management of incontinence in older women. Although voiding dysfunctions in this group represent a survival risk related to complications such as urinary tract infections or hip fractures associated with nocturia and urge urinary incontinence, the most common reasons to consider initial comprehensive urodynamic studies in elderly women are the quality-of-life concerns of the patient about activities that matter most in her daily life. These are the activities she needs to do each day to care for herself and the activities that she enjoys and that make life worthwhile. The long-term choices about evaluation and management are personal decisions by the individual patient that are based on the information provided to her by the physician, the recommendations made to her by the physician, and how she chooses to use that information to live the rest of her life the best way possible. The diagnostic information provided by urodynamic studies is necessary for the physician to counsel the patient about the many decisions that she must make over time regarding the long-term management of her bladder symptoms.

The mental functional status and physical functional status of an elderly individual determine to some extent to how she can participate in the choices about evaluation and therapy. The choices may be different if an elderly woman is in a community-dwelling, assisted-living, or chronic-care environment. The availability of family support is important in decisions about urodynamic studies and long-term management of urinary incontinence. If family members and the patient understand the value of urodynamic studies in clinical management decisions, the patient can commit to maximum personal participation in the procedure. The commitment by the patient and her family to the choice that she makes about comprehensive evaluation and long-term therapy is an essential component of the quality of the urodynamic studies and the clinical value of the information provided by the studies for the physician.

Occasionally, family members of older women may have unrealistic expectations about treatment outcomes. The patient also may have treatment expectations that are not realistic. This situation is even more difficult for the physician when the family or the patient does not have a commitment to working through complications of therapy or treatment failure. In these circumstances, the urodynamic studies can be very helpful in providing objective information about the complexity of the clinical problem that can be communicated to the patient and her family. Urodynamic studies provide objective clinical information that allows realistic expectations about therapy and provide a basis for a personal commitment to therapy that needs to be made by the patient and her family.

Urodynamic studies help the physician advise an older woman about her condition, explain the treatment choices that are reasonable, and help her to understand the possible treatment outcomes so that her expectations are realistic and she can become an active participant with the physician in the long-term management process. Because of the complexity of incontinence in older women, the partnership between the physician and the patient in the long-term management of urinary incontinence is an extremely important relationship. Complex urodynamic studies that are well performed have a positive impact on the relationship between the physician and the elderly patient. As a result, the physician is better able to recommend a practical approach to therapy, and the patient can become a confident partner in a process that is usually a long-term relationship. Urinary incontinence in older women rarely has a single therapeutic modality that results in complete resolution of bladder problems. Instead, voiding dysfunctions in older women usually require long-term treatment with a therapeutic goal of decreasing the severity of symptoms over time. Therapeutic choices and periodic changes in treatment need to be based on the best urodynamic studies available. Repeating the urodynamic studies during long-term management of older women can be valuable to the physician in altering the course of therapy.

URODYNAMICS LABORATORY

A laboratory for urodynamic evaluation of incontinence in elderly women needs to have the highest diagnostic capabilities possible and to be a very comfortable and congenial experience for the patient. The ambience of a urodynamics laboratory for older women is one of the most important aspects of the evaluation. Because the performance of the measurements alters the very functions that are being measured, the environment needs to feel as much like home to the patient as possible to minimize the measurement effect on the study results. A comfortable environment can make it possible for an older woman to be an active participant in the studies, and it enables the study results to provide the best possible information about her bladder and urethral function relative to symptoms experienced during her daily life.

Another important aspect of the urodynamics laboratory is the relationship between the urodynamicist and the patient. Scheduling extra time in the laboratory before the studies is helpful in developing a personal relationship that is nurturing and congenial to minimize any feelings of fear and anxiety that the older patient may experience during the studies. Older women are often more difficult to engage in active participation in the studies than younger women. Because the complexity of bladder dysfunctions and functional impairment is greater in older women compared with younger women, the studies are considerably more difficult to perform and usually require more time to complete.

When performing urodynamic studies in older women, the urodynamicist sometimes may feel like a flight attendant who says, "In the event of a sudden loss in cabin pressure, place the oxygen mask over your nose and mouth and breathe normally." It is not likely that anyone would breathe normally under those conditions. Although it is necessary to recognize the artificial conditions of the urodynamics laboratory, the goal is to create an environment and testing experience that allows the measured behavior of the bladder in elderly women to be as normal as possible. It is one of the primary objectives during testing of older women to minimize the measurement effects of the urodynamic studies on normal bladder and urethral function.

Comprehensive urodynamic studies in older women are not like an electrocardiogram of the bladder in the way the studies are performed and interpreted. Much of the information required for interpretation of urodynamic studies is recorded by the urodynamicist as the studies are being done by describing events and sensations experienced by the older patient. The training and experience of the urodynamicist is an integral part of the diagnostic capabilities of the urodynamics laboratory.

The symptoms experienced by the older woman are less predictive of urodynamic findings than those in younger women.[1] The voiding history and physical examination do not provide enough clinical information to make decisions about treatment in older women without the additional information provided by urodynamic studies. However, the urodynamicist needs to know the clinical history and the observations made on physical examination to perform the best studies possible for the patient. Because urodynamic studies are more difficult to perform in older women and the results are so important in clinical management decisions for these patients, measurements often need to be repeated during the initial testing procedure to ensure that the clinical information provided is as complete and accurate as possible.

It is a goal of the urodynamicist to duplicate the clinical symptoms described by the patient in the urodynamics laboratory. However, the symptoms experienced during the daily life of an older woman often do not occur during the urodynamic studies. In the elderly population, another approach to evaluation may be necessary. If the clinician can identify the symptoms experienced by the patient during her daily activities as completely and thoroughly as possible, the urodynamic studies can be used to better understand why she experiences those symptoms and what can be done to treat the symptoms based on the information provided by the studies.

The diagnostic capabilities of the urodynamic testing equipment are frequently a concern of the physician. Physicians do not want to be limited in their diagnostic capabilities by the limitations of the equipment in the urodynamics laboratory. Although midlevel equipment from most manufacturers can provide the basic information needed for most patients, higher-level equipment is preferred for elderly women because of the complexity of the clinical problems. However, the most expensive equipment does not ensure high-quality studies. The ambience of the laboratory and the skill of the urodynamicist are as important as the capabilities of the equipment. Because elderly women usually have more complex voiding dysfunctions than younger women, the higher-level equipment is often required to meet the performance needs of the clinician in testing these patients.

Urodynamic studies are objective measurements that require a significant knowledge of lower urinary tract function and clinical experience for interpretation. Similar knowledge and experience are required to clinically use the urodynamic studies to make reasonable recommendations for treatment in older women. Each study or test can provide only a fraction of the clinical data, and to see the complete clinical picture and make treatment decisions, especially for older patients, the physician needs comprehensive urodynamic studies.

Urodynamic studies of older women are needed when considering pharmacologic, behavioral, or surgical therapy. It is much easier to change medications or combine pharmacologic therapy with behavioral therapy than it is to revise an operation. However, any long-term treatment needs to be based on the most complete clinical information available. Without urodynamic studies, the clinician is voluntarily relinquishing the most comprehensive objective measurements of bladder and urethral function that are available. Without urodynamic studies in this population, the opportunity of providing the most appropriate initial treatment is significantly decreased, even when nonsurgical therapy is recommended. An ineffective trial of pharmacologic therapy without urodynamic studies is rarely harmful in the long term, but the cost to the elderly woman is time and money at a moment in her life when she often feels she has little of either.

NONINVASIVE URINARY FLOW STUDIES

Noninvasive urinary flow studies are relatively easy to perform in younger women but can be difficult to perform in older women for many reasons. Older patients with urinary incontinence often have an impaired ability to inhibit involuntary detrusor contractions and an impaired ability to voluntarily initiate a bladder contraction.[2] The older woman is usually instructed to arrive at the urodynamics laboratory with her bladder as full as possible so that the noninvasive urinary flow study can be done. She might have "had to go" just before coming to the urodynamics laboratory, or she might have had an "accident" just before arrival. She may be unable to voluntarily void even though she has not voided for hours. Catheterization of the bladder in an elderly woman who is unable to void often demonstrates a relatively large amount of urine in the bladder. The volume of urine obtained in this case is not a postvoid residual urine volume because the patient was unable to void. It is common for older women with urinary incontinence to be unable to prevent or initiate a bladder contraction. In contrast, young women can usually voluntarily void at almost any time.

It is helpful to have a urinary flow unit in the office so that measurement of urinary flow rate can be done many times for older women to determine as closely as possible the urinary flow characteristics of the patient. An ultrasound postvoid residual volume measurement unit in the office allows the assessment to be done with each office visit to obtain multiple determinations. Ultrasound bladder volume measurements have been shown to have a high correlation with catheterized volume measurements in elderly patients.[3] Although the measurement of the postvoid residual urine volume is a simple method to evaluate bladder emptying in elderly patients, it is not possible to predict the type of bladder dysfunction that the patient has without additional studies.[4]

Urethral Pressure Profile

The maximum urethral pressure and urethral length decrease in continent women with increasing age.[5] Clinical evaluation of urethral function in older women is one of the most important aspects of assessment of lower urinary tract function. However, urethral function remains one of the most elusive measurements of lower urinary tract function. Urethral dysfunction of some type is usually a component of urinary incontinence in older women. The urethral pressure profile (UPP) measurements in women significantly correlate with incontinence episodes and absorbent pad use.[6] Although the UPP measurements have a significant correlation with incontinence severity, the UPP is a measurement of resting urethral pressure and not a direct measurement of continence. This distinction is important when using the UPP measurement in clinical decisions.

Assessment of urethral sphincter dysfunction may require a composite of historic, urodynamic, anatomic, and clinical severity criteria.[7] The composite of intrinsic sphincter deficiency has been suggested to include a maximum urethral closure pressure less than or equal to 20 cm/H_2O, a Valsalva leak point pressure of less than or equal to 50 cm/H_2O, and a stress urethral axis less than or equal to 20.[7]

The concept that intrinsic functional properties of the urethra exist that contribute to the integrity of the urethral continence mechanism resulted from many years of clinical work by McGuire and others.[8,9] During the 1970s, McGuire and Lytton[8] observed that women who had failed previous incontinence procedures had poor urethral function indicated by low urethral pressure. McGuire and colleagues[9] subsequently categorized women who have poor urethral function as having type III incontinence. Type III incontinence refers to a poorly closed proximal sphincter identified by video urodynamics and leak point pressure measurement. Intrinsic sphincter deficiency refers to a low-pressure urethra identified using UPP measurements recorded in the mid-urethral high-pressure zone. The UPP and abdominal leak point pressure (ALPP) assessments are performed differently and identify different characteristics of urethral function. Although the low-pressure urethra and the type III urethra identify different aspects of urethral function, the clinical objective of both studies is to recognize women who have severely compromised urethral function. Because clinical evaluation of urethral function in older women is important in the management of incontinence, the UPP and ALPP measurements can be used to better characterize urethral dysfunction. Although the UPP has many limitations, the measurements can contribute to the information obtained from ALPP assessment if the UPP is used appropriately. Elderly women who have intrinsic sphincter deficiency based on the UPP should be clinically identified and counseled about treatment because of the higher risk for failure of any therapeutic approach in this group.[10,11]

The maximum urethral closure pressure and the Valsalva leak point pressure are significantly decreased with increasing severity of the incontinence grade.[13] Some studies have suggested a statistically significant relationship between the UPP and ALPP.[12-15] From a clinical management perspective, the UPP and ALPP are different measurements of urethral function that can be useful in combination, but they are not comparable measurements.

UPP measurements are usually performed using micro tip transducers. Although many techniques have been used, the microtip transducer remains the clinical standard for UPP measurements. A dual-channel microtip catheter is preferred. It has a microtip transducer located at the tip of the catheter for bladder pressure measurement and a microtip transducer located approximately 5 cm proximally for measurement of urethral pressure. The subtraction of intravesical pressure from urethral pressure produces the urethral closure pressure profile.[16] The dual-channel microtip transducer allows the urodynamicist to perform stress UPP measurements. An electronic catheter puller is used to ensure a constant rate as the catheter passes through the urethra. Because of measurement variations in the UPP, many measurements are done to determine the maximum resting urethral pressure. The UPP measurement in older women is usually performed in the supine position because of measurement artifact that occurs in the standing position.

A stress UPP is a measure of the difference between the intravesical pressure and intraurethral pressure during stress maneuvers such as coughing. A stress pressure profile is performed in the same way as a resting UPP with additional instructions for the patient to cough during the urethral pressure measurement. Usually, the patient is instructed to cough approximately six or more consecutive times as the UPP catheter is pulled through the functional urethra at a rate of approximately 1 mm per second. The pressure transmission ratios of a stress pressure profile measurement have been found to be sufficiently reproducible to be useful in characterizing stress sphincteric function.[17]

During coughing, an increase in urethral pressure occurs that is usually greater in magnitude than the increase in abdominal pressure, which indicates that active and passive compensatory pressure mechanisms are involved in continence. Denervation of the urethra, hypermobility of the urethra, and intrinsic dysfunction of the urethra are some of the reasons that the normal compensatory pressure mechanisms fail. A negative pressure gradient between the urethra and bladder during coughing indicates that the pressure compensatory mechanisms of the urethra are not functioning normally. Urethral function studies in healthy women compared with women having genuine stress incontinence show that the active closure mechanisms at the bladder neck and mid-urethra are significantly weakened in women with genuine stress incontinence, and the results do not support the concept that impaired passive pressure transmission to the urethra is an important pathophysiologic factor in genuine stress incontinence.[18] A dynamic active closure mechanism has been demonstrated at the bladder neck in addition to the dynamic closure mechanism that is located in the middleurethra.[18] Increases in urethral closure pressure during coughing probably occur because the urethra is compressed against a hammock supportive layer, rather than the urethra being truly intra-abdominal.[19] These observations do not support the concept of passive abdominal pressure transmission to an intra-abdominal urethra as the mechanism of urethral continence.

Pelvic organ prolapse can produce obstructive symptoms and prevent or reduce urinary leakage.[20] The resting urethral pressure is often higher than expected in women who have a cystocele. The resting UPP measurement is usually done initially without cystocele reduction. Repeat urethral pressure measurements are done after cystocele reduction. Results of the Scopettes (Birchwood Laboratories, Eden Prairie, MN) reduction technique to reduce prolapse revealed a 56% incidence of low-pressure urethra and stress urinary incontinence in 83% of patients with grade 4 vaginal prolapse.[21] A statistically significant relationship exists between urethral incompetence and hypermobility of the urethra.[22] If a significant decrease in resting urethral pressure occurs with reduction of the cystocele, surgical reduction of the cystocele can be expected to produce an even greater decrease in resting urethral pressure.

The effect of a cystocele on the UPP can indicate relatively good urethral function even though the actual urethral function after surgical repair of the cystocele may be significantly compromised. The change in urethral pressure with cystocele reduction in the laboratory setting can be helpful for indicating changes in urethral function after surgical repair of the cystocele. However, in some older women, surgical reduction of a cystocele can result in a profound decrease in urethral function compared with preoperative manual reduction of the cystocele in the urodynamics laboratory.

Abdominal Leak Point Pressures

An ALPP is a measure of the lowest total bladder pressure at a known volume at which leakage occurs during prompted increases in abdominal pressure.[23] The total bladder pressure is equal to the sum of the detrusor pressure and the abdominal pressure measured in the bladder. If the bladder compliance is normal, the abdominal pressure is usually approximately the same as the total bladder pressure at a low intravesical volume in the absence of a detrusor contraction.

A simplified office technique for measuring ALPP in older women can be done during filling cystometry. The patient is placed in a semi-erect position, and bladder filling is stopped at 200 mL. The patient is instructed to strain progressively to the maximum abdominal pressure possible or until leaking occurs. The external urethral meatus is visually observed. When leaking is observed, the intravesical pressure is recorded. If leaking does not occur, the patient is instructed to cough progressively to a maximum coughing pressure. The point at which leaking occurs with coughing is recorded. If leaking does not occur, the maximum abdominal pressure measured is recorded, and the absence of leaking is documented. At this point, filling cystometry is continued. This technique is particularly suited to office-based urodynamic studies in older women. The ALPP measured using this technique may have measurement error causing a higher ALPP value because the patient is not in a full standing position.[12] It is more difficult to identify leaking using a visual technique compared with a fluoroscopic technique.

If fluoroscopy is available, the measurement can be done in the semi-erect position or the standing position using the smallest catheter that is practical. A 5-Fr, double-lumen catheter can be used. One lumen is used to fill the bladder, and the other lumen is used to measure intravesical pressure. A 3-Fr microtip catheter can be used to measure ALPP fluoroscopically, but it is expensive and requires filling of the bladder with a separate catheter, which may not be practical for most urodynamics laboratories. A 20% iodinated contrast medium typically is used, although a 60% contrast medium can be used when better visualization of the urethra is required as in obese patients. An anteroposterior view of the urethra is often used, although a lateral view may provides better visualization of the bladder neck and mid-urethral continence mechanisms. When a lateral view is used, positioning the patient about 10 degrees off a line perpendicular to the x-ray table places the femoral heads out of alignment and allows a better radiographic view of the urethra. In this position, the urethra is usually centered between each femur, which makes leaking much easier to visualize.

The measurement of ALPP in elderly women is an essential urethral function study. During the urodynamic studies, older women occasionally are unable physically to generate an abdominal pressure of 60 cm H_2O, which is needed to identify type III incontinence if no leaking is seen. Some frail elderly women may have low abdominal pressures during most daily activities.

Because women who have stress incontinence usually leak in the standing position, it is preferable to measure the ALPP in the standing position. Some older women may have difficulty standing and performing straining maneuvers at the same time. Although a semi-erect position is a compromise in the measurement technique, it is often a more feasible position to perform the ALPP measurement for older women.

A cystocele can cause an error in the ALPP measurement, resulting in a higher abdominal pressure required for leaking. The ALPP can be measured with cystocele reduction using Scopettes, vaginal gauze packing, or a vaginal speculum.[24] It is sometimes difficult to reduce the cystocele in older women enough in the urodynamics laboratory to be confident that the ALPP measurement accurately indicates urethral function. Women who demonstrate stress incontinence with the vaginal prolapse reduced and the urethra supported normally should be suspected of having type III incontinence.[25] Placement of a pessary to reduce vaginal vault prolapse can obstruct the urethra and result in a measurement error.

The clinical objective of ALPP measurement in older women is to determine the functional status of the urethra so that a reasonable clinical management recommendation can be made. Many older women have very complicated combinations of urethral dysfunction, bladder dysfunction, and vaginal prolapse. Vaginal vault prolapse can significantly complicate the measurement of urethral function. The ALPP is an essential piece of the clinical puzzle, and without the leak point pressure measurements, clinical evaluation of urethral function in older women is not complete.

Cystometrogram

The cystometrogram is a measure of the response of the bladder to being filled.[26] Cystometry is the method by which the pressure-volume relationship of the bladder is measured.[16] A medium filling rate typically is used when obtaining a cystometrogram in elderly women. A medium fill rate ranges from 10 to 100 mL per minute, which is a relatively wide range for older women. A lower filling rate in the medium filling range is preferred in older women to better evaluate the response of the bladder to filling. A filling rate of 30 mL per minute is usually satisfactory for older women. A slow filling rate of 10 mL per minute requires a long time to fill the bladder if the capacity is normal. Repeat filling of the bladder using a slow filling rate is a consideration for women who have severe detrusor instability or a very small bladder capacity.

A common filling technique uses a small (5 to 7 Fr), double-lumen urethral catheter attached to a perfusion pump, and water or saline is the infusion medium. A 5-Fr urethral catheter is preferred because of the small size, although the small lumen may decrease the pump flow rate during filling. A larger urethral catheter (e.g., 6 Fr) has been shown to decrease the maximum urinary flow rate during pressure flow studies in women.[27] The 5-Fr, double-lumen catheter allows filling cystometry and pressure flow studies to be done consecutively using the same catheter, which is an advantage for older women.

A rectal catheter is a common method for measurement of abdominal pressure in older women. The intravesical catheter is a much more reliable initial measure of intra-abdominal pressure than the rectal catheter measurement. For this reason, the rectal catheter recording is adjusted to equal the bladder pressure recordings during resting and straining maneuvers at baseline before filling. Using a cough and strain maneuver, the rectal catheter recording usually can be adjusted to almost exactly match the bladder pressure recording at baseline. When the rectal pressure channel and the bladder pressure channel are reading as close to the same as possible during straining maneuvers, bladder filling is begun. During filling, small fluctuations in abdominal pressure can be seen that result from respiration, which assures the urodynamicist that both channels are working properly. Occasionally, a rectal contraction may cause the differential pressure measurement to have a negative value, which usually can be disregarded. Spontaneous rectal contractions usually disappear as the study progresses.[28] Rectal contractions of some type occur in approximately 29% of patients having urodynamic studies, regardless of age.[29] Persistent rectal contractions are a relatively uncommon event while obtaining the cystometrogram in older women.

Bladder sensation during filling cystometry can be difficult to evaluate in older women because of the subjective nature of the measurement. The relationship of bladder sensation to bladder activity needs to be recorded, and identifying bladder sensation requires the patient to understand the importance of communicating awareness of bladder sensation to the urodynamicist.

Unstable detrusor contractions may occur during the filling phase of cystometry in older women. The pressure resulting from involuntary detrusor contractions, the duration of the contractions, and the number of contractions during filling varies considerably among patients. When an involuntary detrusor contraction occurs during filling, involuntary loss of urine usually occurs. A sensation of urinary urgency may precede an involuntary detrusor contraction, or the sensation of urgency may occur during the contraction. However, older women who have a history of urge urinary incontinence may not exhibit unstable detrusor contractions during filling.

Elderly women who have had a previous stroke with residual neurologic deficits may exhibit detrusor hyperreflexia during filling cystometry. Suprapontine lesions in elderly patients can result in involuntary detrusor contractions during filling cystometry with associated electromyographic activity that has the appearance of detrusor sphincter dyssynergia. Involuntary loss of urine has occurred during phases of electromyographic relaxation in older patients who were studied using telemetry (Fig. 95-1).[30]

When continuous involuntary detrusor contractions occur during filling cystometry, the problem in some patients can be obtaining any further useful information from the studies. At that point, measurement of pressure flow studies during voluntary voiding would be useful, although measurements requiring voluntary voiding may not be possible. Further filling of the bladder should be discontinued during continuous involuntary contractions. After the bladder has stabilized, a slow filling rate of 10 mL per minute can sometimes allow filling to a volume adequate for voluntary voiding. Older women who cannot inhibit bladder contractions often have an inability to voluntarily initiate a bladder contraction. Sometimes, it is impossible to obtain a pressure flow study in older women who have continuous involuntary detrusor contractions, regardless of the techniques used for filling the bladder to a higher capacity. Same-session repeat cystometry and pressure flow studies have shown an increase in volume for the first desire to void and normal desire to void, whereas the maximum cystometric capacity remained unchanged in healthy women.[31] However, for some older women who have a small capacity or detrusor instability, changing to a slow filling rate can increase the maximum cystometric capacity.

If detrusor activity during filling cystometry remains stable, the first or normal desire to void is recorded, a strong desire to void is recorded, and the maximum cystometric capacity is recorded. At the maximum cystometric capacity, the passive bladder pressure is measured to determine compliance. Compliance is a measure of the change in volume per unit of change in pressure, and it is expressed in milliliters per centimeter of water.[16] From a clinical management perspective, compliance is a measurement of the ability of the bladder to stretch without increasing pressure inside the bladder. A normal bladder can be filled to the maximum cystometric capacity with minimal change in the passive pressure within the bladder. In a study to determine the relationship of detrusor instability with changes in compliance in 270 women, 75% of the patients showed a compliance of greater than 130 mL/cm, 95% showed a compliance greater than 40 mL/cm, and women having compliance less than 40 mL/cm had a 16 times greater incidence of detrusor instability.[32]

Low bladder compliance can be a serious problem in older women who have had radiation therapy or previous pelvic surgery.[33] Older women with abnormal bladder compliance often present with severe stress urinary incontinence. Although a significant abnormality in bladder compliance is relatively uncommon in older women, it is extremely important to recognize it. A sling procedure in an elderly woman with stress incontinence and low bladder compliance can result in increased bladder outlet resistance and passive bladder pressures of more than

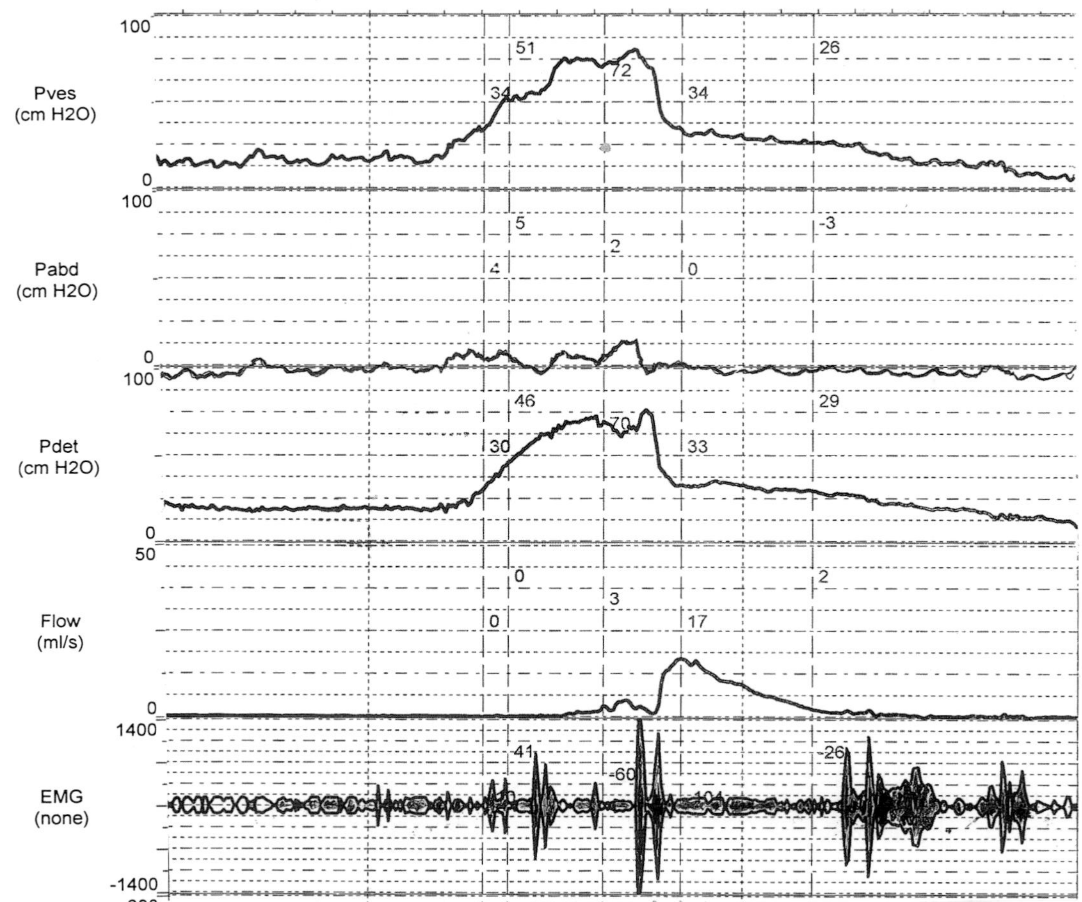

Figure 95-1 This 90-year-old woman has no known neurologic disease. She has detrusor instability with a high-pressure contraction and increased electromyographic activity. There is a delay in the onset of involuntary urine loss. The highest peak of electromyographic activity correlated with decreased the urinary flow, which was caused by outlet obstruction that resulted in an increase in detrusor pressure. The increased detrusor pressure appeared to overcome the opposing electromyographic activity, resulting in a sustained decline in electromyographic activity and an increase in urine flow that decreased bladder outlet resistance and decreased bladder pressure because of the outflow of urine. This pattern was previously observed during telemetric monitoring of incontinent elderly men.[30]

40 cm H_2O, which can cause hydronephrosis and deterioration of renal function.

Voiding Pressure Flow Studies

Voiding pressure flow studies are useful for assessing older women. However, the clinical importance of pressure flow studies is not often emphasized in the management of older women. Voiding pressure flow studies identify three fundamental voiding states[34]:

1. Low detrusor pressure and high urinary flow rate (unobstructed)
2. High detrusor pressure and low urinary flow rate (obstructed)
3. Low detrusor pressure with low urinary low rate (poor detrusor contractility)

Older women present with problems ranging from mixed incontinence with vault prolapse to recurrent urinary tract infections with incomplete bladder emptying. Although these are not precise categories, most older women with incontinence can be classified by the results of pressure flow studies. These categories often are associated with similar symptoms but represent different clinical entities, and the approach to management usually is different for the three pressure flow categories.

Older women who have had previous incontinence surgery usually present with complex combinations of lower urinary problems. For example, it is common for older women who have had a urethral suspension procedure to experience symptoms of mixed incontinence and symptoms of bladder outlet obstruction. Some degree of vaginal vault prolapse is a common physical finding in women with these symptoms. Only pressure flow studies can differentiate high detrusor pressure with a low urinary flow rate from low detrusor pressure with a low flow rate.

Minimally invasive surgical procedures for the treatment of stress incontinence in women have reduced the morbidity of incontinence surgery enough that operative procedures often are offered to elderly women. Successful surgical treatment is available to many older women who would not have been advised to consider a surgical option in the past. However, older women with urinary incontinence are a complicated group of patients, especially when surgical options are being considered, because the results of surgery in older women can be disappointing.

Older women often have very poor urethral function (ALPP less than 60 cm H_2O) with minimal urethral mobility. Although a pubovaginal sling placed without tension usually results in continence for women with good urethral function, a compressive sling is required to achieve continence in women with very poor urethral function. Pressure flow studies are important in the preoperative evaluation of bladder function in older women with urinary incontinence and poor urethral function because urinary retention can be a complication of a compressive sling procedure.

The advent of minimally invasive surgery for urinary incontinence in older women has resulted in clinical diagnoses after surgical procedures in this population that were uncommon in the past. Pressure flow studies are invaluable in elucidating the pathophysiology of these unique clinical problems that occur after minimally invasive incontinence surgery in elderly women. When persistent voiding symptoms occur in these patients, comprehensive urodynamic studies performed preoperatively are invaluable for comparison with postoperative studies. The pressure flow studies are among the most valuable studies for clinical evaluation and formulating management strategies for these complicated clinical problems. Persistent voiding symptoms after minimally invasive surgical procedures in older women should be evaluated with comprehensive urodynamics studies.

Bladder outlet obstruction in older women may occur after minimally invasive procedures for treatment of stress urinary incontinence, and pressure flow studies are the most important studies in the postoperative evaluation of these patients. The measurement parameters for bladder outlet obstruction in older women after incontinence surgery have not been well defined. Voiding dysfunctions in elderly women after incontinence surgery need prompt urodynamic evaluation to plan long-term management. If bladder outlet obstruction is identified, a significant delay in urethrolysis after a sling procedure is associated with persistent bladder symptoms after urethrolysis,[35] which suggests that changes in bladder activity after prolonged obstruction may not be reversible. De novo urge incontinence after minimally invasive sling procedures in older women needs to be evaluated with pressure flow studies to be sure that the overactive bladder symptoms are not caused by bladder outlet obstruction.

The urethra has a different role in maintaining continence from that of the bladder. However, when considering the dynamics of voiding, the bladder and urethra appear to behave as a functional unit. Abnormalities of urethral function can affect bladder function, and abnormalities of bladder function can affect urethral function. Pressure flow studies are a measure of the dynamic functional unit of the bladder and urethra. Pressure flow studies are reproducible and provide consistent urodynamic measurements in women.[36]

Aging significantly alters the function of the urethra and the bladder. Elderly women who experience symptoms of stress urinary incontinence may have urinary flow rates that are considerably lower than would be expected based on the measured bladder pressure, even when the bladder pressure is low (Fig. 95-2). In these older women, it appears that the intrinsic urethral closing properties and the intrinsic urethral opening properties are deficient. The aging urethra seems to lose some of the dynamic properties that maintain continence and those required for normal voiding.

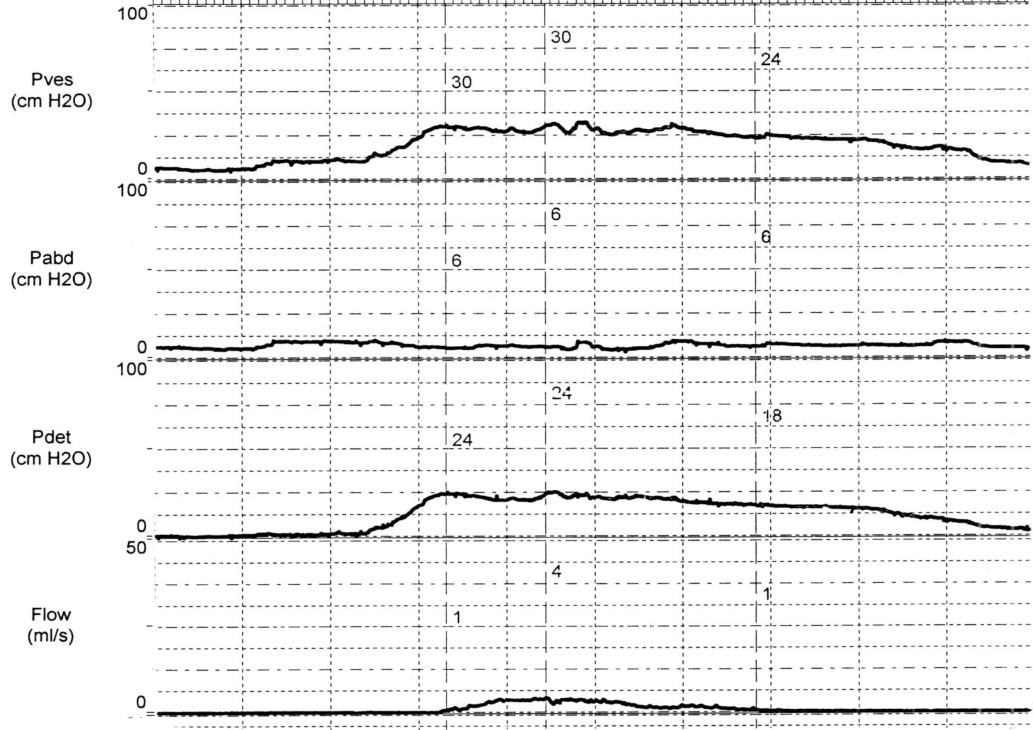

Figure 95-2 This elderly woman has severe symptoms of stress incontinence. The physical examination shows minimal hypermobility, no cystocele, and atrophic vaginitis. Her bladder is stable during filling. The urinary flow rate is low relative to the detrusor pressure. It appears as if the urethra has compromised dynamic properties related to voiding and continence.

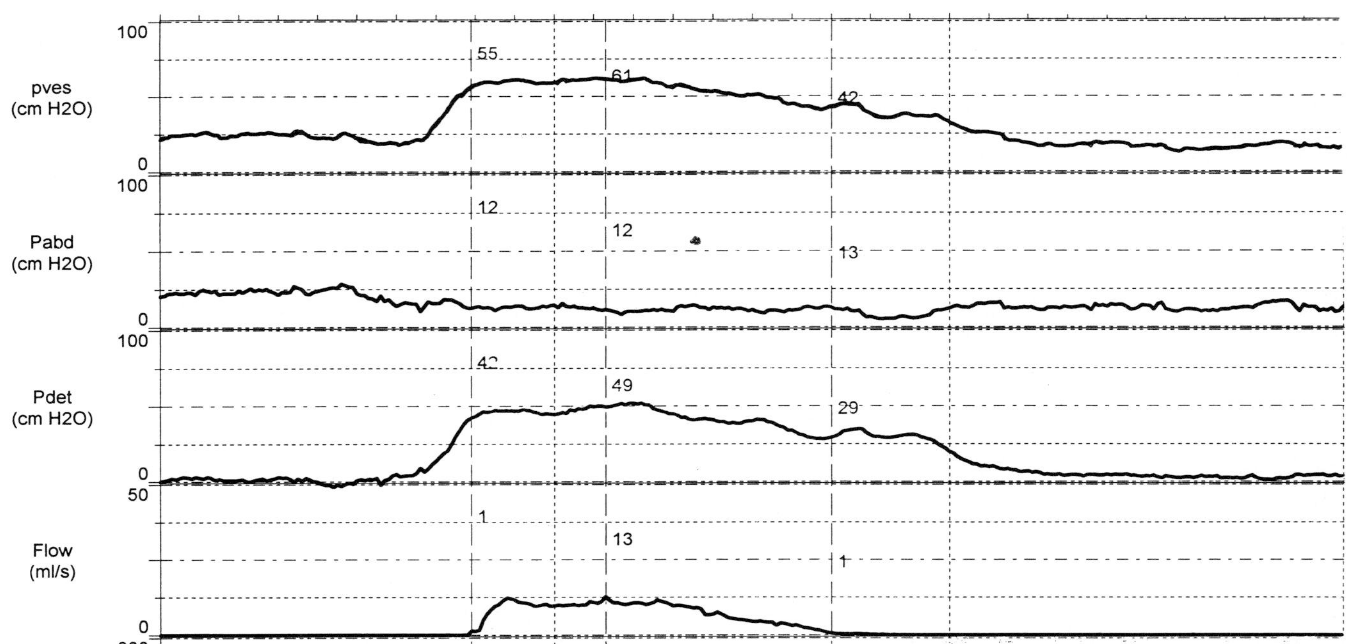

Figure 95-3 This older woman has symptoms of mixed urinary incontinence. Her bladder is stable during filling. She has bladder outlet obstruction that appears to be caused by a cystocele.

Voiding pressure flow studies allow the clinician to identify the dynamic relationships within the voiding functional unit of the bladder and urethra in elderly women. These studies are essential for any management decision, especially if a surgical procedure that could alter the functional dynamic relationship between the urethra and bladder is being considered.

Bladder outlet obstruction is the association of a low urinary flow rate with a detrusor contraction of sufficient magnitude, duration, and speed to empty the bladder.[34] This is an important definition because it requires the clinician to examine the pressure flow studies to assess the voiding dynamics of the patient. However, well-established parameters for voiding pressure flow studies in elderly women are not available. Bladder outlet obstruction can occur in women who have a cystocele (Fig. 95-3), and a low urinary flow rate may result from low detrusor pressure (Fig. 95-4).

Voiding Pressure Flow Techniques

A 5- to 7-Fr, double-lumen catheter is placed into the bladder for measurement of bladder pressure and infusion of fluid into the bladder. A balloon catheter is placed into the rectum for measurement of intra-abdominal pressure. Except in elderly women with severe physical or mental impairment, the pressure flow studies can be performed without significant discomfort or difficulty. Even though older women may have the neurologic capacity to voluntarily initiate voiding, that ability is often significantly impaired, and the patient may be unable to voluntarily initiate voiding in the urodynamics laboratory. Turning on a faucet in the room to allow the patient to hear the sound of running water can sometimes assist the patient to voluntarily initiate voiding. When an elderly woman is unable to voluntarily void for a study, it does not mean that she has an acontractile bladder.

The measurement of voiding pressure flow studies should be done during voluntary voiding. Elderly people who experience urge urinary incontinence usually void voluntarily most of the time.[2,37] It may be possible to obtain a voluntary voiding pressure flow study by using a lower filling rate and allowing the patient a longer time to initiate voiding. Every effort should be made to obtain voluntary voiding pressure flow studies because the information has immense clinical value.

The urodynamicist sometimes instructs the patient to voluntarily void as an involuntary detrusor contraction is in progress. This should not be considered a true voluntary voiding pressure flow study. Although it may be the best measurement that can be obtained under the circumstances, the information should be used carefully, and the limitations of the study should be recognized when making clinical decisions about management.

Involuntary detrusor contractions in elderly patients do not appear to be normal bladder contractions that are uninhibited.[2] Involuntary detrusor contractions in elderly people appear to be abnormal bladder contractions. In elderly patients with urinary incontinence due to detrusor hyperreflexia, cystometric measures of contractility vary considerably on repeating the study on the same occasion.[38] Voiding pressure flow studies measured during an involuntary detrusor contraction therefore provide limited clinical information about the dynamics of normal voiding in that individual. Because the goal of treatment in elderly women is improvement of quality of life, the clinical objective is to incorporate the information obtained from urodynamic studies into reasonable, practical, and feasible clinical management decisions.

Electromyography

Measurement of the sphincteric electromyography in elderly women is important clinically, but the measurement can be

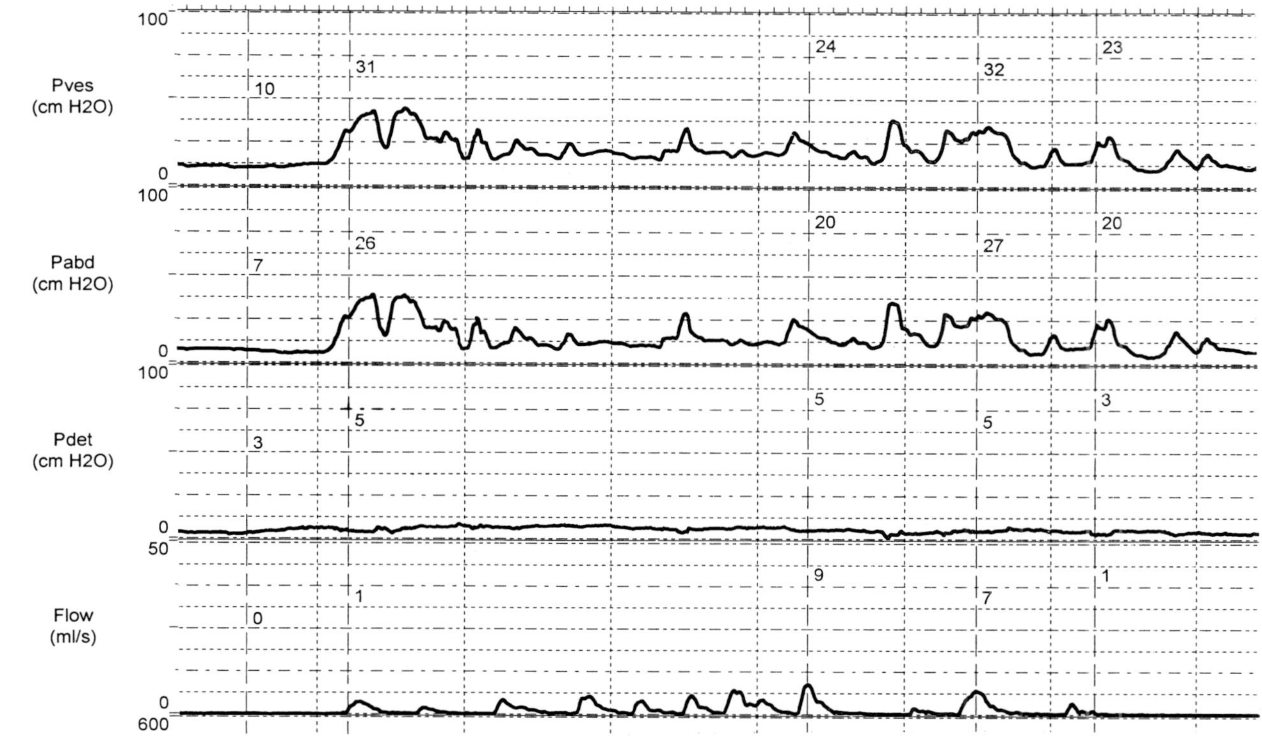

Figure 95-4 This elderly woman has symptoms of mixed incontinence. She has a low urinary flow rate because of poor bladder function.

technically difficult to perform. Although it is of immense clinical value to identify abnormal electromyographic activity, it is useful for the clinician to know that the sphincteric electromyographic activity during voiding is normal in elderly patients. For example, older patients may have central nervous diseases that result in an electromyographic appearance of detrusor sphincter dyssynergia.[30] Older women who have had long-standing urge urinary incontinence caused by involuntary detrusor contractions may have a highly developed voluntary sphincteric contraction in response to the sensation of urinary urgency that has the appearance of detrusor sphincter dyssynergia. Although it may not be possible to differentiate these entities without neurourologic testing, both can be treated with biofeedback.

Routine electromyographic measurement in elderly women is relatively uncomplicated after the technique has been developed and established for a particular urodynamics laboratory. The signal source is usually the external anal sphincter. Because the amplitude and frequency of electromyographic activity is usually lower in older women compared with younger women, the external anal sphincter is considered the best location for the signal source. Intravaginal surface electrodes and intraurethral surface electrodes are less reliable for electromyographic measurement[39] and rarely provide an adequate signal for clinical evaluation in older women. Well-placed surface electrodes are preferred in elderly patients.[40] Although needle electrodes are considered superior to surface electrodes in patients who may have neurologic disease, surface electrodes are more practical and desirable for electromyographic studies in older women. Because needle electrodes easily become dislodged during the study, many attempts to replace a needle electrode are very uncomfortable for older women.

Preparation of the skin and correct placement of surface electrodes are important to ensure an adequate signal is obtained.[41] After the surface electrodes have been placed and the electromyographic activity is being monitored by the urodynamicist, the patient is instructed to perform a mild cough. If the electromyographic electrodes are properly placed, a mild cough will result in a sharp increase in electromyographic activity and an immediate return to baseline. With the bladder empty at rest, the gain on the electromyographic amplifier can be adjusted in response to a mild cough by the patient. Increasing the gain on the electromyographic amplifier is often required because of the low baseline electromyographic activity in this patient population. If the electronic gain on the amplifier becomes too high, a mild cough will produce a full-scale response on the electromyographic display. As the gain is increased, baseline electrical activity increases, which is usually caused by background electrical activity rather than the baseline sphincteric electromyographic activity. This baseline electromyographic artifact is usually caused by 60-cycle interference from the electrical power source. Interference from external electrical power sources is a much greater problem in these studies of older women because the electromyographic activity of the muscles measured is usually lower than in younger women, and it requires a higher electromyographic amplifier gain.

References

1. Ouslander J, Staskin D, Raz S, Su HL, Hepps K: Clinical versus urodynamic diagnosis in an incontinent geriatric female population. J Urol 137:68, 1987.
2. O'Donnell PD: Pathophysiology of urinary incontinence in elderly men. In Geriatric Urology. Boston, Little, Brown, 1994.
3. Chan H: Noninvasive bladder volume measurement. J Neurosci Nurs 25:309, 1993.
4. Starer P, Libow LS: The measurement of residual urine in the evaluation of incontinent nursing home residents. Arch Gerontol Geriatr 7:75, 1988.
5. Rud T: Urethral pressure profile in continent women from childhood to old age. Acta Obstet Gynecol Scand 59:331, 1980.
6. Theofrastous JP, Bump RC, Elser DM, et al: Correlation of urodynamic measures of urethral resistance with clinical measures of incontinence severity in women with pure genuine stress incontinence. The Continence Program for Women Research Group. Am J Obstet Gynecol 173:407; discussion 412, 1995.
7. Bump RC, Coates KW, Cundiff GW, et al: Diagnosing intrinsic sphincteric deficiency: Comparing urethral closure pressure, urethral axis, and Valsalva leak point pressures. Am J Gynecol 177:303, 1997.
8. McGuire EJ, Lytton B: Pubovaginal sling procedure for stress incontinence. J Urol 199:82, 1978.
9. McGuire EJ, Lytton B, Kohorn EI, Pepe V: The value of urodynamic testing in stress urinary incontinence. J Urol 124:256, 1980.
10. Kilicarslan H, Gokce G, Ayan S, et al: Predictors of outcome after in situ anterior vaginal wall sling surgery. Int Urogynecol J Pelvic Floor Dysfunct 14:339, 2003.
11. Rezapour M, Falconer C, Ulmsten U: Tension-Free vaginal tape (TVT) in stress incontinent women with intrinsic sphincter deficiency (ISD): A long-term follow-up. Int Urogynecol J Pelvic Floor Dysfunct 12(Suppl 2):S12, 2001.
12. Nguyen JK, Gunn GC, Bhatia NN: The effect of patient position on leak point pressure measurements in women with genuine stress incontinence. Int Urogynecol J Pelvic Floor Dysfunct 13:9, 2002.
13. Nager CW, Schuz JA, Stanton SL, Monga A: Correlation of urethral closure pressure, leak-point pressure and incontinence severity measures. Int Urogynecol J Pelvic Floor Dysfunct 12:395, 2001.
14. McLennan MT, Melick CF, Bent AE: Leak-point pressure: Clinical application of values at two different volumes. Int Urogynecol J Pelvic Floor Dysfunct 11:136, 2000.
15. Almeida FG, Bruschini H, Srougi M: Correlation between urethral sphincter activity and Valsalva leak point pressure at different bladder distentions: Revisiting the urethral pressure profile. J Urol 174(Pt 1)1312, 2005.
16. Abrams P, Blaivas JG, Stanton SL, Andersen JT: The standardization of terminology of lower urinary tract function. Scand J Urol Nephrol 114(Suppl):5, 1988.
17. Cundiff GW, Harris RL, Theofrastous JP, Bump RC: Pressure transmission ratio reproducibility in stress continent and stress incontinent women. Neurourol Urodyn 16:161, 1997.
18. Lose G: Urethral pressure and power generation during coughing and voluntary contraction of the pelvic floor in females with genuine stress incontinence. B J Urol 67:580, 1991.
19. DeLancey JO: Structural support of the urethra as it relates to stress urinary incontinence: The hammock hypothesis. Am J Obstet Gynecol 173:346, 1995.
20. Long CY, Hsu SC, Wu TP, et al: Urodynamic comparison of continent and incontinent women with severe uterovaginal prolapse. J Reprod Med 49:33, 2004.
21. Veronikis DK, Nichols DH, Wakamatsu MM: The incidence of low-pressure urethra as a function of prolapse-reducing technique in patients with massive pelvic organ prolapse (maximum descent at all vaginal sites). Am J Obstet Gynecol 177:1305; discussion 1313, 1997.
22. Schick E, Jolivet-Tremblay M, Tessier J, et al: Observations on the function of the female urethra. III. An overview with special reference to the relation between urethral hypermobility and urethral incompetence. Neurourol Urodyn 23:22, 2004.
23. O'Connell HE, McGuire EJ: Leak point pressures. In O'Donnell PD (ed): Urinary Incontinence. St. Louis, Mosby, 1997.
24. Gallentine ML, Cespedes RD: Occult stress urinary incontinence and the effect of vaginal vault prolapse on abdominal leak point pressures. Urology 57:40, 2001.
25. Wall LL, Hewitt JK: Urodynamic characteristics of women with complete post hysterectomy vaginal vault prolapse. Urology 44:336; discussion 341, 1994.
26. Nitti VW: Cystometry and abdominal pressure monitoring. In Nitti VW (ed): Practical Urodynamics. Philadelphia, WB Saunders, 1998, pp 38-51.
27. Baseman AG, Baseman JG, Zimmern PE, Lemack GE: Effect of 6F urethral catheterization on urinary flow rates during repeated pressure-flow studies in healthy female volunteers. Urology 59:843, 2002.
28. Wall LL, Hewitt JK, Helms MJ: Are vaginal and rectal pressures equivalent approximation of one another for the purpose of performing subtracted cystometry? Obstet Gynecol 85:488, 1995.
29. Combs AJ, Nitti VW: Significance of rectal contractions noted on multichannel urodynamics. Neurourol Urodyn 14:73, 1995.
30. O'Donnell PD, Hannish H: Telemetric electromyographic monitoring in elderly inpatient men. J Neurourol Urodyn 11:115-121, 1992.
31. Brostrom S, Jennum P, Lose G: Short-term reproducibility of cystometry and pressure-flow micturition studies in healthy women. Neurourol Urodyn 21:457, 2002.
32. Harris RL, Cundiff GW, Theofrastous JP, Bump RC: Bladder compliance in neurologically intact women. Neurourol Urodyn 15:483, 1996.
33. Zoubek J, McGuire EJ, Noll F, DeLancey JO: The late occurrence of urinary tract damage in patients successfully treated by radiotherapy for cervical carcinoma. J Urol 141:1347, 1989.
34. Kim YH, Boone T: Voiding pressure flow studies In Nitti VW (ed): Practical Urodynamics. Philadelphia, WB Saunders, 1998, pp 52-64.
35. Leng WW, Davies BJ, Tarin T, et al: Delayed treatment of bladder outlet obstruction after sling surgery: Association irreversible bladder dysfunction. J Urol 172 (Pt 1):1379, 2004.
36. Digesu GA, Hutchings A, Salvatore S, et al: Reproducibility and reliability of pressure flow parameters in women. BJOG 110:774, 2003.
37. O'Donnell PD: The volume-interval relationship of incontinence episodes in elderly inpatient men. Urology 41:334-337, 1993.
38. Lord A, Eastwood H: Detrusor hyperreflexia? Are there two types? Age Ageing 23:32, 1994.
39. Brostrom S, Jennum P, Lose G: Motor evoked potentials from the striated urethral sphincter: A comparison of concentric needle an surface electrodes. Neurourol Urodyn 22:123, 2003.
40. O'Donnell PD, Beck C, Eubanks C: Surface electrodes in perineal electromyography. Urology 32:375, 1988.
41. O'Donnell PD: Pitfalls of urodynamic testing. Urol Clin North Am 18:257, 1991.

Section 12

RECONSTRUCTION

Chapter 96

USE OF BOWEL IN LOWER URINARY TRACT RECONSTRUCTION IN WOMEN

Christoph Wiesner and Joachim W. Thüroff

The use of small and large bowel for bladder augmentation or substitution has been reported by surgeons since the first experimental report by Tizzoni and Foggi in 1888.[1] Bladder enlargement by augmentation enterocystoplasty is predominantly offered to women with neuropathic and non-neuropathic bladder dysfunction who have not responded to pharmacologic regimens. Female patients in whom complete removal of bladder and urethra is mandatory because of urologic or gynecologic malignancies and those who have a bladder problem and irreparable loss of the functional urethra are candidates for urinary diversion. The underlying disease and the patient's preference must be considered when deciding on the type of urinary reconstruction or diversion, such as bladder augmentation or orthotopic bladder substitution to the trigone or bladder neck, orthotopic bladder substitution to the urethra, continent cutaneous urinary diversion, or continent anal urinary diversion.

Preoperative preparation in all female patients includes ultrasound of the upper urinary tract, evaluation of the renal function to judge the renal reserve to compensate for reabsorption of acids from an intestinal reservoir (i.e., renal isotope clearance >50% of the age-specific norm, serum creatinine level <2.0 mg/dL), and a colonic contrast study or coloscopy to exclude bowel pathology when large bowel segments are used. In patients with a history of previous irradiation encompassing the bowel segments required to construct the planned reservoir, previous resection of longer segments of ileum, or chronic inflammatory bowel disease (e.g., Crohn's disease, ulcerative colitis), the urinary diversion must be tailored according to the bowel pathology. Postoperative care comprises follow-up of acid-base balance, renal ultrasound, and pouchoscopy starting from the fifth postoperative year.

HISTORY OF AUGMENTATION ENTEROCYSTOPLASTY AND ORTHOTOPIC BLADDER SUBSTITUTION

Augmentation enterocystoplasty is considered the last resort of functional bladder reconstruction before urinary diversion is required. Females with benign diseases such as intractable idiopathic or neurogenic detrusor overactivity incontinence, low-compliance bladder from irradiation, or interstitial cystitis may benefit from enlarging the organ with bowel segments or removing the diseased bladder tissue and substituting it with bowel segments.[2-6]

The cup-patch technique for bladder augmentation was first reported by Goodwin and colleagues for small bowel[7] (Fig. 96-1) and for large bowel[8] in 1959. A 20- to 25-cm ileal segment serving as the cup is opened at its antimesenteric border before it is formed to a U-shaped patch, folded over, and sutured to the bladder dome. When supratrigonal cystectomy is required (i.e., in interstitial cystitis or detrusor hyperreflexia), the resection line runs just above the trigone, leaving the ureteral orifices in place for preservation of the natural anti-reflux mechanism and avoiding potential complications of ureteral reimplantation into bowel.

Bladder substitution to the bladder neck may become necessary in female patients with interstitial cystitis because of inflammation of the remnant trigone and when preexisting ureteral reflux or obstruction is apparent. Bladder augmentation or substitution can be performed with different bowel segments, such as ileum only,[9] ileum combined with cecum,[10] or sigmoid colon only.[11] An additional sling procedure or colposuspension may be required when coexisting stress incontinence is apparent.[6]

Flood and coworkers[6] reported the long-term outcomes of 106 patients, including 82 women, who underwent augmentation enterocystoplasty. Preoperatively, all patients had reduced bladder compliance or detrusor overactivity caused by different underlying benign diseases. The overall success rate was 95% for all patients. Postoperative bladder capacity increased significantly from 108 to 438 mL. Urodynamic evaluation revealed stress incontinence in 15 patients (14%). Six of these patients had occasional leakage and did not require further treatment, and five were successfully treated by a sling procedure or collagen injection.

Complete relief of clinical symptoms of bladder pain and frequency was reported for 73% to 100% of patients in several series when enterocystoplasty was performed for intractable forms of interstitial cystitis.[2-4] Between 66% and 86% of female patients were able to void spontaneously; the remainder had to empty their bladders by intermittent self-catheterization.

Linn and associates[12] reported the clinical outcomes of 23 patients, including 22 women and 1 man, who underwent subtrigonal ($n = 17$) or supratrigonal ($n = 6$) cystectomy and orthotopic bladder substitution with the ileocecal pouch (i.e., Mainz pouch I) for interstitial cystitis. Postoperative bladder capacity was significantly increased, and urinary frequency was significantly decreased in all patients. Complete relief of clinical symptoms was achieved in 82% of the patients with subtrigonal cystectomy and in 100% of the patients with supratrigonal cystectomy. All patients who underwent supratrigonal cystectomy were able to void spontaneously, whereas 41% of the patients in whom the trigone was resected had to empty their bladder by intermittent self-catheterization.

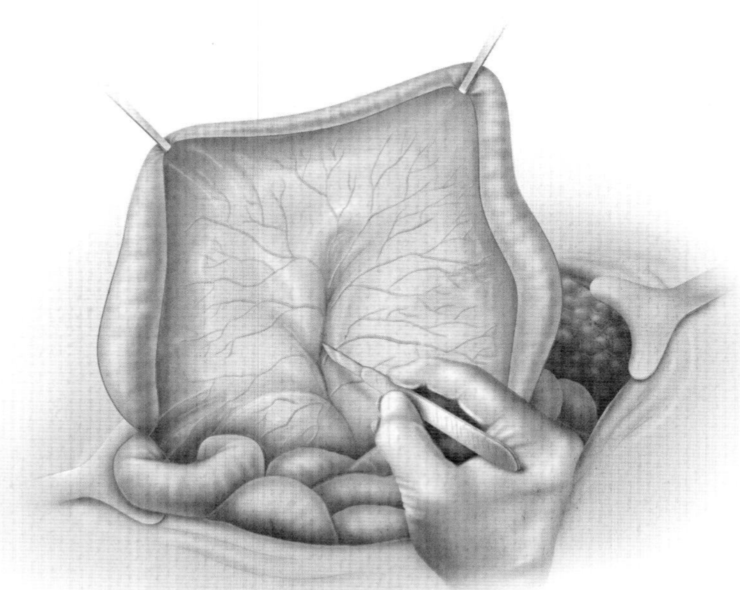

A

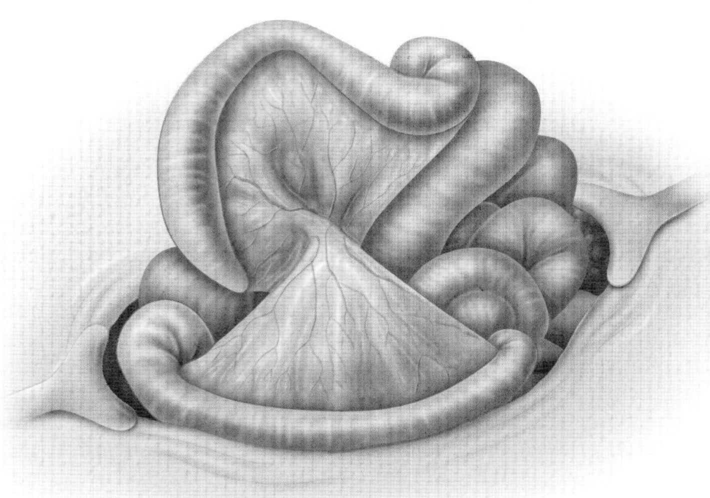

B

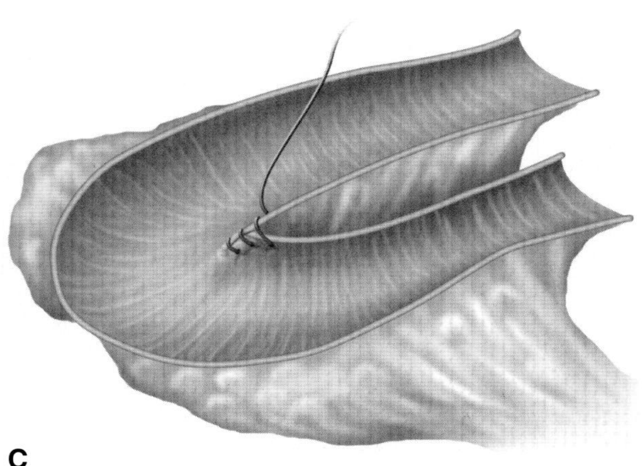

C

Figure 96-1 Augmentation enterocystoplasty by the cup patch technique. **A,** A 20- to 25-cm ileal segment is isolated, serving as the cup. **B,** Continuity of the ileum is reestablished by ileoileostomy. **C,** The isolated ileal segment is opened at its antimesenteric border and formed to a U-shaped patch.

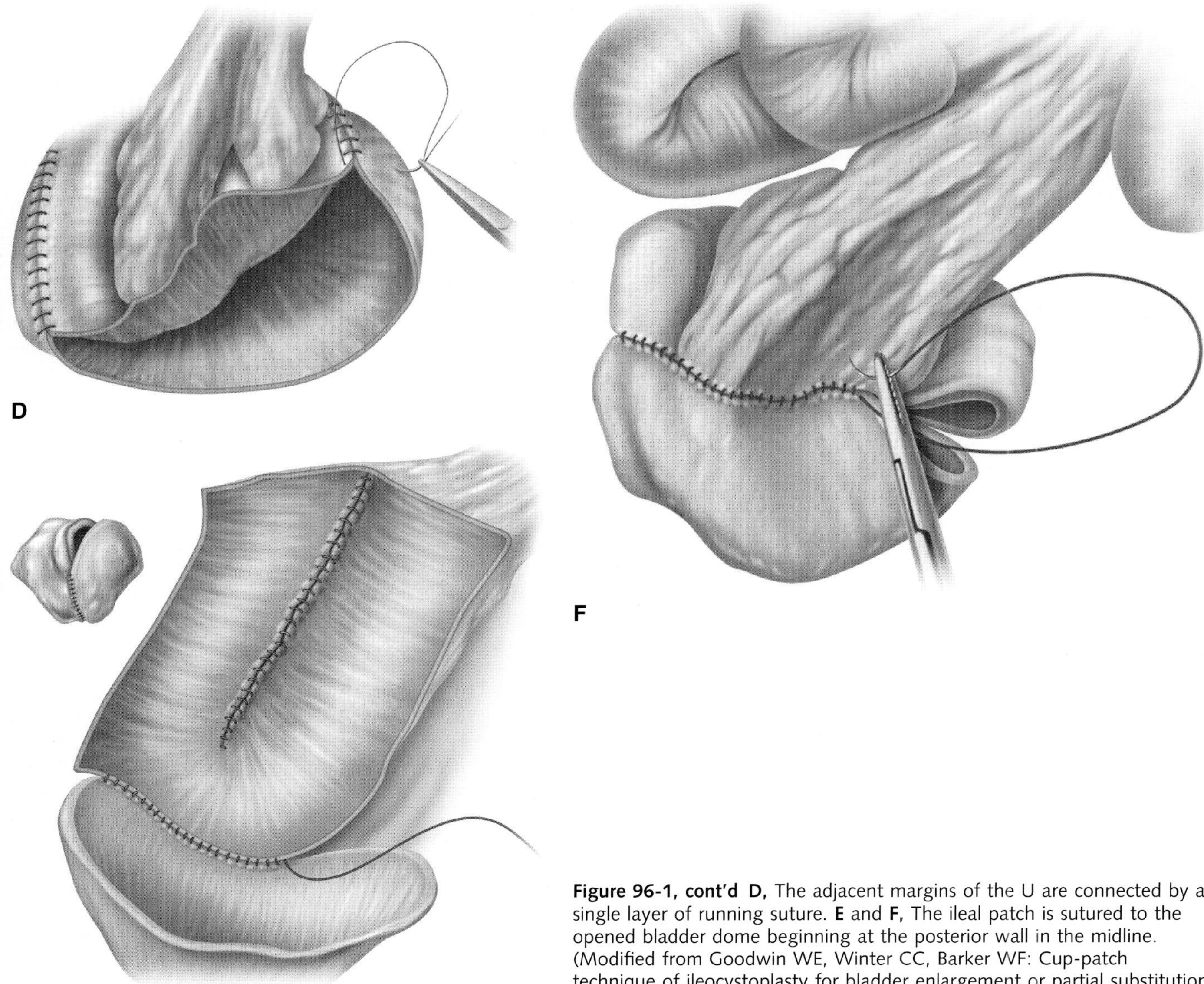

Figure 96-1, cont'd D, The adjacent margins of the U are connected by a single layer of running suture. **E** and **F,** The ileal patch is sutured to the opened bladder dome beginning at the posterior wall in the midline. (Modified from Goodwin WE, Winter CC, Barker WF: Cup-patch technique of ileocystoplasty for bladder enlargement or partial substitution. Surg Gynecol Obstet 108:240-244, 1959.)

ORTHOTOPIC BLADDER SUBSTITUTION

The first radical cystectomy in combination with an orthotopic bladder substitution for treatment of bladder cancer in a woman was reported by Tscholl in 1987,[13] but before 1990, orthotopic urinary diversion was mostly limited to male patients when radical cystoprostatectomy was performed.[14] Removal of the urethra was considered mandatory in female patients with bladder cancer to provide an adequate surgical margin. It was considered impossible to achieve urinary continence with the remaining short female urethra. Studies of cystectomy specimens that were removed for bladder cancer and a better anatomic understanding of the continence mechanism made it likely that urinary diversion to the urethra could be applied to selected female patients.[15-17]

Intraoperative frozen section analysis of the distal urethral margin is mandatory to exclude tumor involvement when orthotopic diversion is planned for bladder cancer or gynecologic malignancies. Preoperatively, competence of the external rhabdosphincter must be proved to ensure postoperative continence and to allow spontaneous voiding through the urethra. The choice of the reservoir depends on the surgeon's preference when orthotopic bladder substitution in the female patient can be performed by using any segments of the gastrointestinal tract for constructing the reservoir.

Ileal Bladder Substitutes

In 1987, Ghoneim and colleagues[18] described the urethral Kock pouch, which used 45 to 50 cm of the distal ileum.[18] The proximal third of ileum is preserved for the reflux-preventing valve. The reservoir is created by the distal two thirds of bowel, which is opened along its antimesenteric border before folding it into a U-shape and performing a side-to-side anastomosis of the adjacent margins with a single layer of running suture. A nipple valve is created by isoperistaltic ileal intussusception and fixed by three or four rows of metal staples. Its position is secured by interrupted seromuscular sutures at the base of the nipple valve. The intestinal plate is folded over and closed by a single layer of running suture. The reservoir is rotated such that the posterior aspect is brought anteriorly and positioned into the pelvis with the apex facing toward the urethral stump, where the pouch is opened and anastomosed to the urethra by interrupted sutures. Ureterointestinal reimplantation is performed by end-to-side anastomosis of the ureters to the afferent limb of the nipple valve.

The T-pouch ileal neobladder was established in 1998 as a modification of the urethral Kock pouch diversion (Fig. 96-2).[19] The afferent segment is created by an 8- to 10-cm segment of the proximal ileum. Its distal portion of 3 to 4 cm is tapered and tunneled into a serosa-lined tunnel, which is created at the midline anastomosis of the back wall of the pouch.

The ileal neobladder was established in 1987 by using a 60- to 70-cm ileal segment and leaving the distal portion of the terminal ileum and Bauhin's valve intact (Fig. 96-3).[20] The ileum is folded in a W-shaped manner and opened at its antimesenteric border except over a 5-cm segment, where the incision is made close to the anterior mesentery to create a posterior flap, which serves as the new bladder neck and to which the urethra is anastomosed. The reservoir is accomplished by side-to-side anastomosis of the posterior walls before the anterior wall is folded over and closed. Anti-refluxive ureteral reimplantation was initially favored using the LeDuc technique of creating a mucosal sulcus[21] or by using the Abol-Enein technique of serosa-lined extramural tunnels.[22] Since 1996, the technique of ureterointestinal implantation is predominantly performed by a refluxive ileoureteral end-to-side anastomosis into two 3- to 5-cm chimneys of ileum serving as afferent segments.[23]

Studer's ileal neobladder was established in 1985 by using 60 to 65 cm of terminal ileum and leaving the proximal 25 cm intact for creation of an isoperistaltic afferent limb (Fig. 96-4).[24] The distal 40 cm of ileum is folded into a U-shape and opened antimesenterically before the medial borders of the U are anastomosed to each other by a single layer of running suture. The ureterointestinal anastomoses are performed by direct end-to-side anastomosis to the proximal portion of the afferent limb. The reservoir is finalized by folding the bottom of the U over the proximal end. Before complete closure, an incision is placed into the most dependent part of the reservoir for the ileourethral anastomosis.

Ileocecal Bladder Substitute: Orthotopic Mainz Pouch

For creation of the orthotopic ileocecal reservoir (i.e., orthotopic Mainz pouch), a 10- to 15-cm segment of cecum in continuity with 20 to 30 cm of terminal ileum is isolated. The bowel is opened along its antimesenteric border. The opposing margins of the bowel are anastomosed to each other by a single row of running suture to create the posterior pouch wall. Originally, the ureters are implanted through a submucosal tunnel into the ascending colon to prevent reflux. Urethrointestinal anastomosis is performed by an incision at the base of the cecum. The reservoir is closed by side-to-side running sutures. In 2003, El-Mekresh and coworkers[25] reported a modified technique of ureterointestinal reimplantation into the terminal ileum with the ileocecal valve serving as an anti-reflux-mechanism by using an end-to-end anastomosis (Wallace) for the left ureter and end-to-side anastomosis (Nesbit) for the right ureter with the afferent ileal limb (Fig. 96-5).

Clinical studies that included long-term follow-up predominantly reported outcomes for male patients who underwent orthotopic bladder substitution. However, some reports are available on the outcomes of female patients with a specific focus on voiding patterns.

The rates of ileal neobladder–related early and late complications in a large series of 363 male patients were reported to be 15.4% and 23.4%, respectively.[26] Early pouch-related complications included urinary leakage (7.7%), pyelonephritis (7.4%), and early obstruction of the ureteroileal anastomosis (3.0%). Late complications were associated with the ileoureteral anastomosis and upper urinary tract, including stenosis (9.3%), acute pyelonephritis (6.3%), and reflux (3.3%). Ileourethral anastomotic strictures were seen in 2.2%, 96.1% of the patients were able to void spontaneously, and daytime continence was achieved in 95%.

Ghoneim and associates[27] reported the clinical outcomes of 185 male patients treated with the urethral Kock pouch diversion. Deterioration of the upper urinary tract occurred in 13.7% of the renal units, with 9% due to reflux and 4.7% due to anastomotic strictures. Calculus formation was recognized in 18%, and urethral anastomotic strictures were encountered in 5.1%. Daytime and nighttime continence rates were 92% and 73%, respectively.

Perimenis and colleagues[13] evaluated the long-term outcomes of male patients treated with Studer's ileal neobladder with an afferent tubular segment. Nine (3.5%) of 254 renal units were treated for ureterointestinal anastomotic strictures. At the latest follow-up, renal parenchyma was normal in 246 units (97%), and serum creatinine levels remained unchanged compared with preoperative values in all patients. Daytime continence rates were 94% and 91% at 5 and 10 years, respectively, whereas nighttime continence rates were 72% and 60%, respectively. Residual urine volumes greater than 100 mL were recognized in 8% and were associated with urethrointestinal anastomotic strictures or protrusion of the intestinal mucosa into the urethra.

Cancrini and coworkers[28] reported their 2-year experiences of orthotopic urinary diversion by Studer's ileal neobladder in seven female patients.[28] The rate of urinary continence was 100% during the day and 71% at night. Urodynamic studies 12 months postoperatively revealed a good neobladder capacity of 320 mL and no evidence of stress incontinence or significant levels of residual urine.

Stenzl and associates[29] performed radical cystectomy with nerve-sparing dissection of the bladder neck and proximal urethra by leaving the lateral vaginal walls and the tissue next to the bladder neck intact. The technique was based on their previous studies of anatomic and histologic studies of the urethra in female cadavers. Daytime and nighttime continence was achieved within 6 months in all patients, and the residual urine volume was between 0 and 150 mL.

Ali-El-Dein and colleagues[30] reported the clinical outcomes of 136 female patients who underwent radical non–nerve-sparing cystectomy and orthotopic bladder substitution by ileal neobladders (n = 120) or hemi-Kock pouch reservoirs (n = 16).[30] Early pouch-related complications included development of vaginal fistulas in four patients, who were treated by open surgical revision. Calculi developed in seven patients, who were treated endoscopically. One hundred patients were evaluable by urodynamic

Text continued on page 983

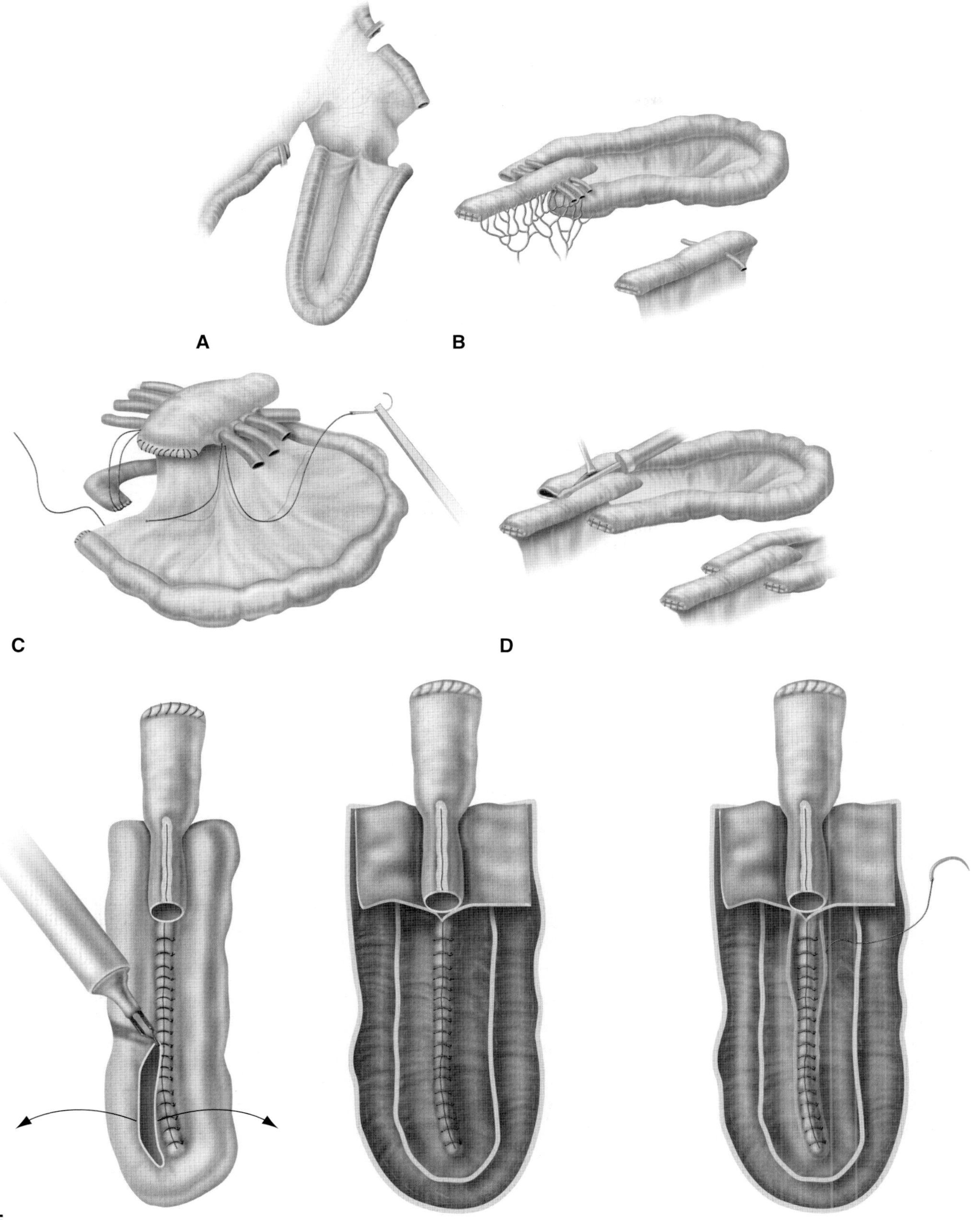

Figure 96-2 T-pouch ileal neobladder. **A,** The T-shaped pouch is constructed using a 44-cm ileal segment, which is placed as a V, and a more proximal 8- to 10-cm ileal segment for the anti-refluxive afferent limb. **B,** Windows of Deaver are created to the distal 3 to 4 cm of the afferent segment. **C,** The serosa of the adjacent 22-cm V-shaped limbs is connected by sutures passing through the window of Deaver. **D,** The anchored portion of the afferent limb is tapered at the antimesenteric border. **E,** The ileal segments are opened *(arrows)* adjacent to the mesentery until the ostium of the afferent limb is reached and continued upside toward the antimesenteric border, providing ileal flaps on both sides.

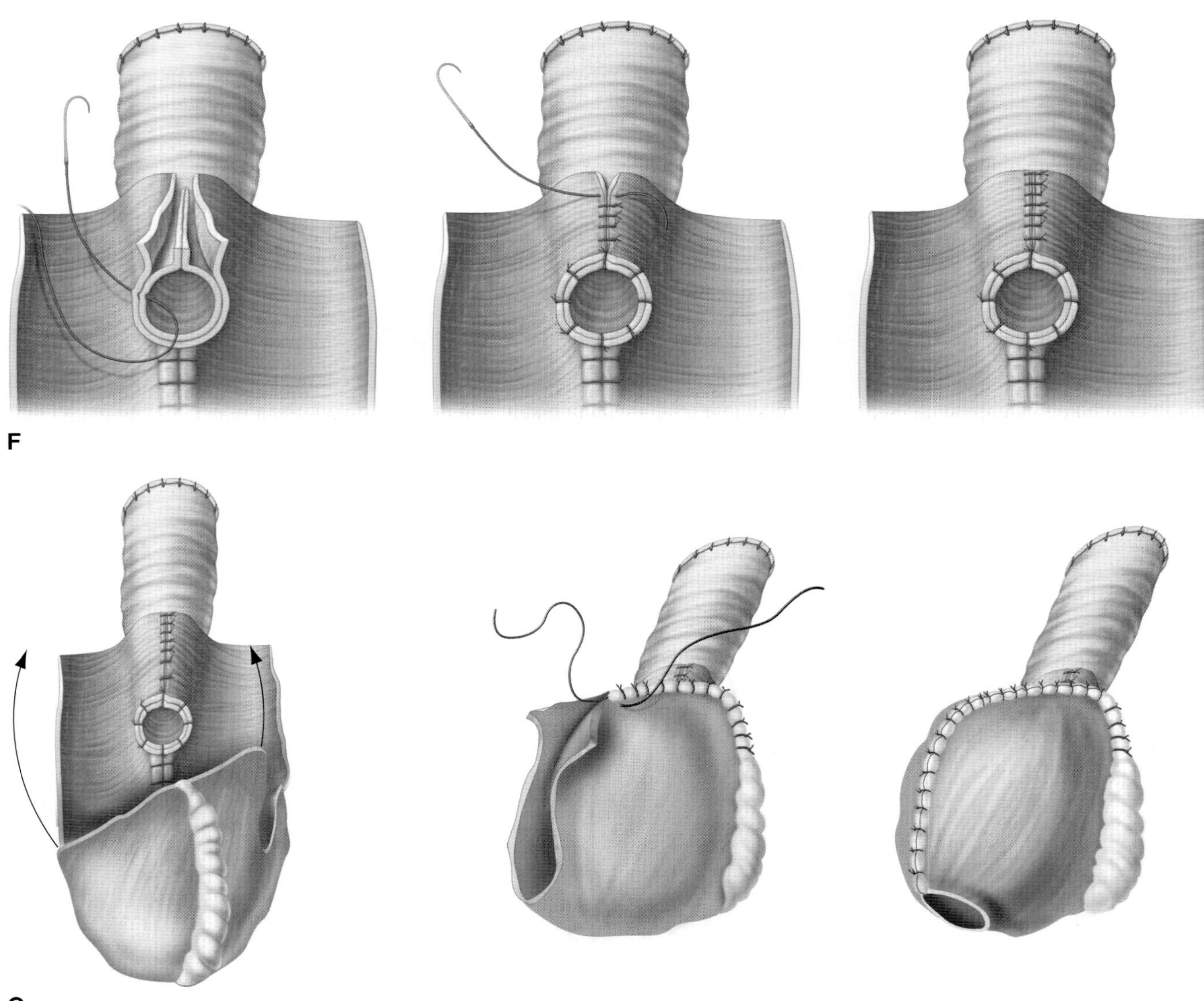

Figure 96-2, cont'd F, The tapered afferent segment is covered by the ileal flaps to provide the anti-refluxive flap-valve mechanism. **G,** The reservoir is folded *(arrows)* and closed in the opposite direction from which it was opened, except a short portion at the anterior right side for the urethral anastomosis. (Modified from Stein JP, Lieskovski G, Ginsberg DA, et al: The T-pouch: An orthotopic ileal neobladder incorporating a serosal lined ileal antireflux technique. J Urol 159:1836-1842, 1998.)

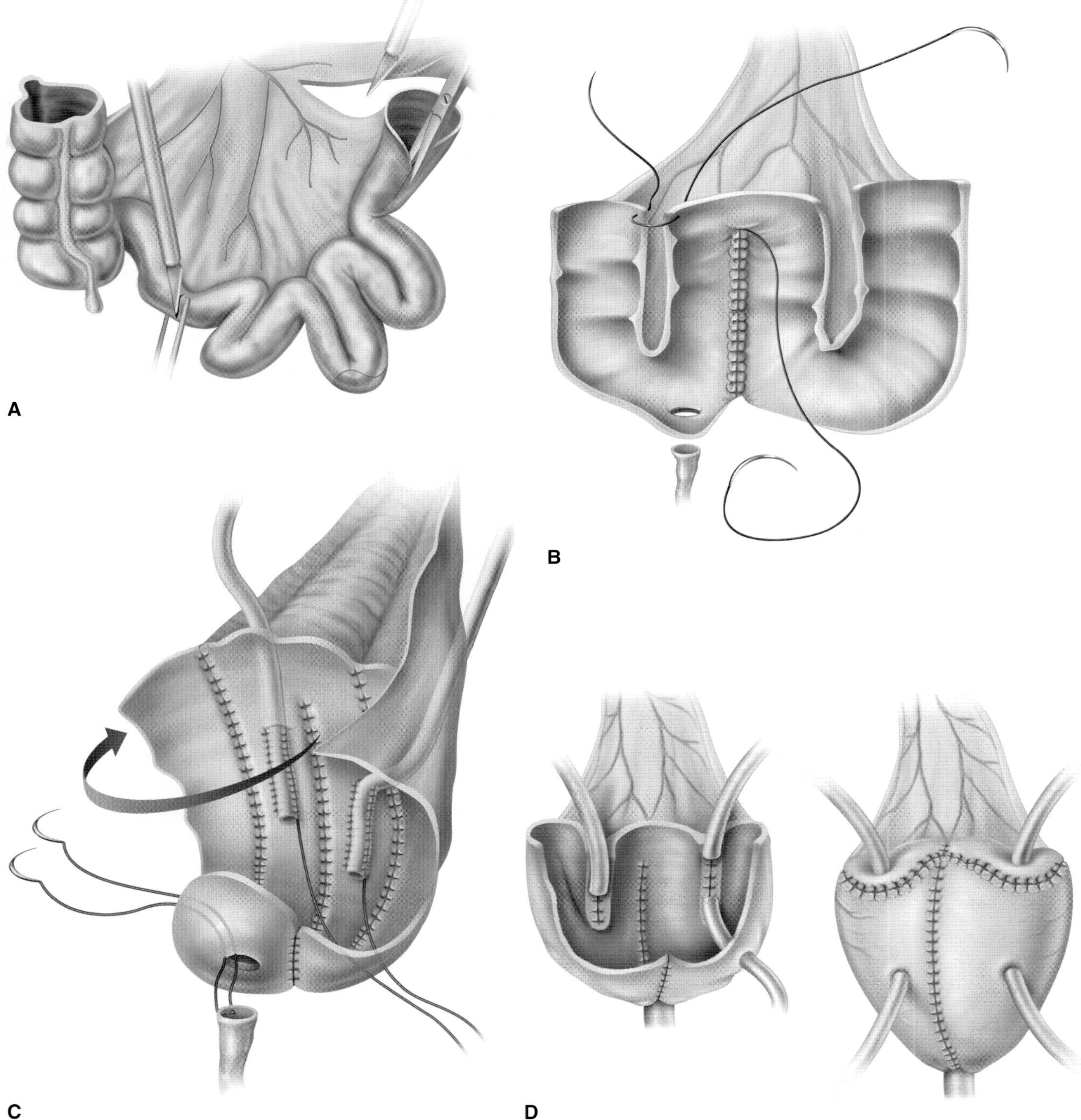

Figure 96-3 Ileal neobladder. **A,** A 60- to 70-cm ileal segment is folded in a W-shaped manner and opened at its antimesenteric border, except for a 5-cm portion that serves as the new bladder neck. **B,** The reservoir is accomplished by side-to-side anastomosis of the posterior walls before the anterior wall is folded over and closed. **C,** Ureteral reimplantation was initially performed by the LeDuc technique of creating a mucosal sulcus *(arrow)*. **D,** Alternatively, the Abol-Enein technique of serosa lined extramural tunnels was established. Since 1996, ureterointestinal reimplantation is performed by a refluxive ileoureteral end-to-side anastomosis into two 3- to 5-cm chimneys of ileum serving as afferent segments (not shown). (Modified from Campbell's Urology, 8th Edition, Saunders Philadelphia, 2002).

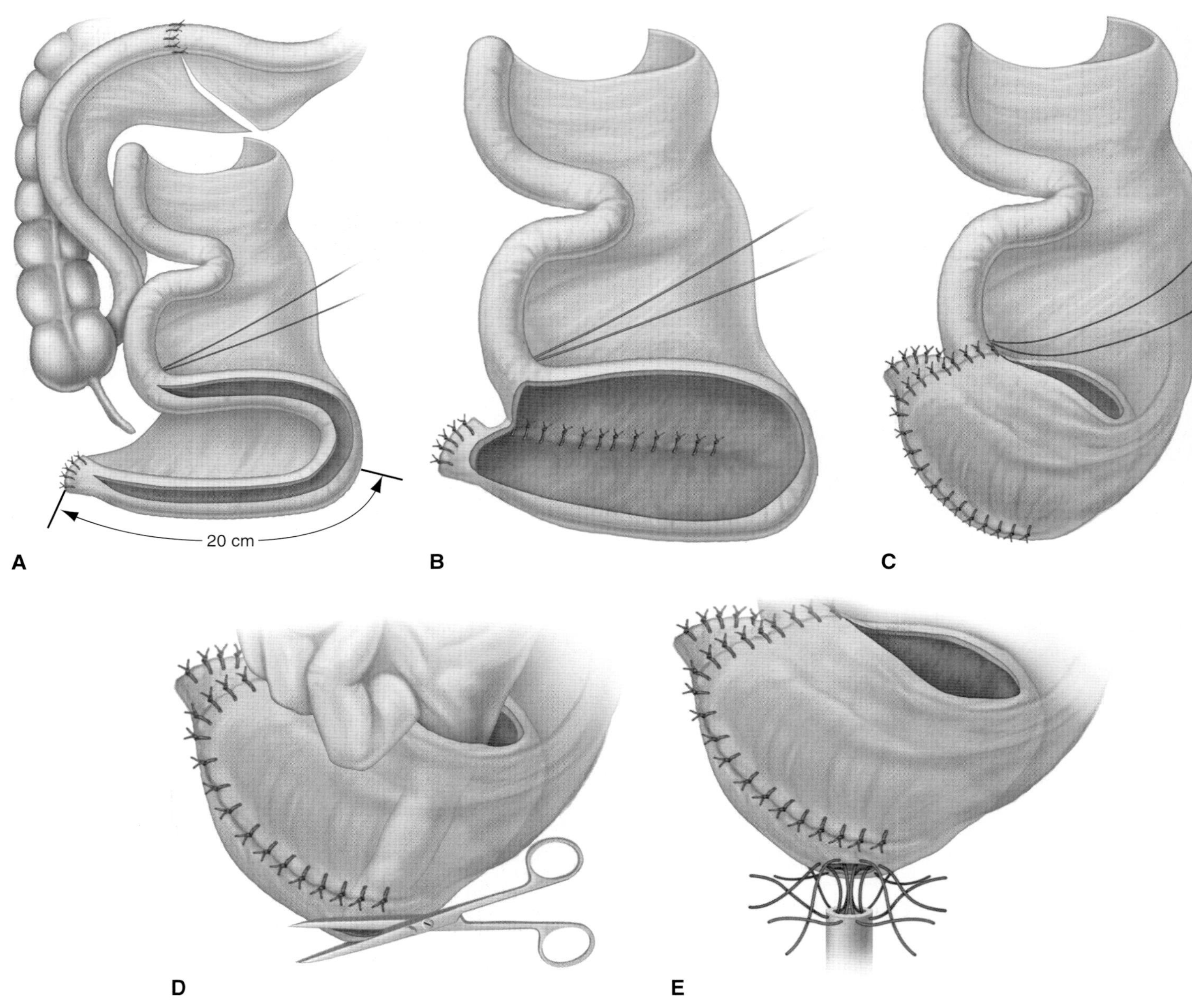

Figure 96-4 Studer's ileal neobladder with afferent tubular segment. **A,** A 60- to 65-cm segment of the terminal ileum is isolated about 25 cm proximal to the ileocecal valve and folded into a U-shape. The distal 40 cm of the ileal segment are opened along the antimesenteric border. The proximal 25 cm are left intact for the isoperistaltic afferent limb. **B,** The medial borders of the U are anastomosed to each other by a single layer of running suture. The ureterointestinal anastomosis is performed by direct end-to-side anastomosis to the proximal portion of the afferent limb. **C,** The reservoir is folded and oversewn. **D** and **E,** A buttonhole is made at the caudal portion of the reservoir and anastomosed to the urethra. (Modified from Perimenis P, Studer UE: Orthotopic continent urinary diversion an ileal low pressure neobladder with an afferent tubular segment: How I do it. Eur J Surg Oncol 30:454-459, 2004.)

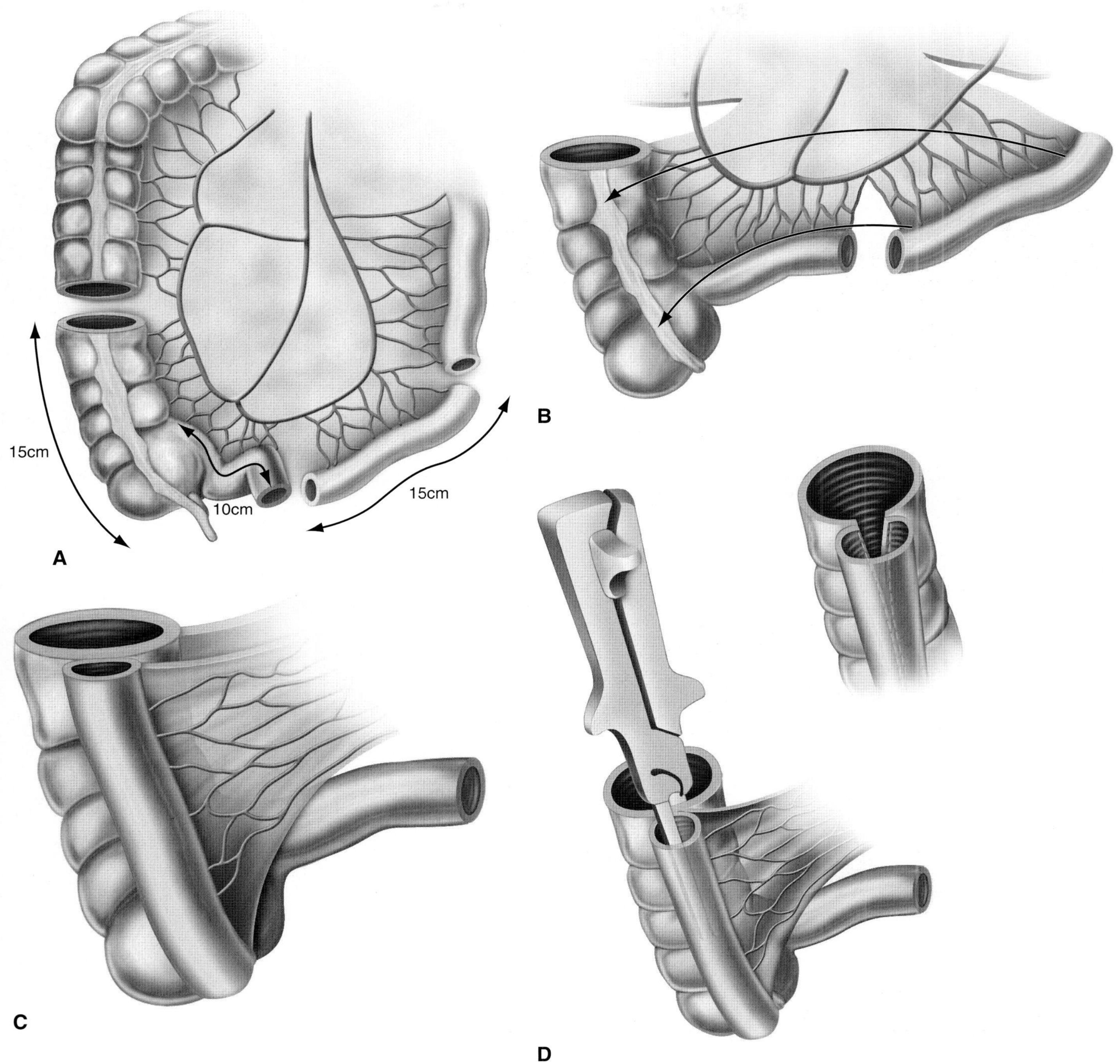

Figure 96-5 Simplified orthotopic ileocecal pouch. **A,** The orthotopic ileocecal reservoir (orthotopic Mainz pouch) is created by a 10- to 15-cm segment of cecum in continuity with 20- to 30-cm of the terminal ileum. The aboral 10 cm of the ileal segment is in continuity with the cecum, serving as the afferent loop. The ileocecal valve is left intact to prevent reflux. **B** to **E,** A stapled side-to-side anastomosis of the oral 15 cm of the isolated ileal segment with the cecum is performed to achieve a spherical reservoir.

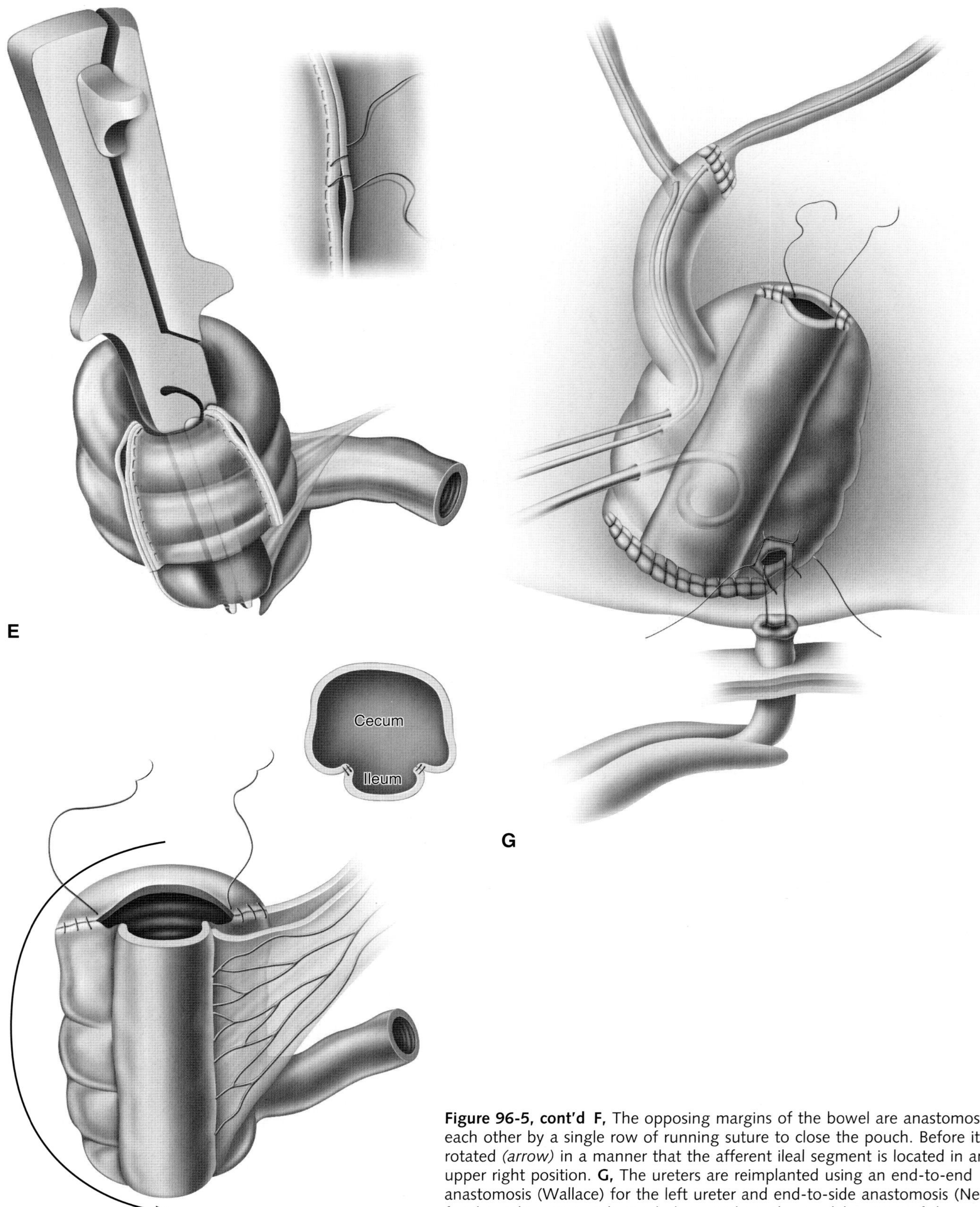

Figure 96-5, cont'd **F,** The opposing margins of the bowel are anastomosed to each other by a single row of running suture to close the pouch. Before it is rotated *(arrow)* in a manner that the afferent ileal segment is located in an upper right position. **G,** The ureters are reimplanted using an end-to-end anastomosis (Wallace) for the left ureter and end-to-side anastomosis (Nesbit) for the right ureter. A buttonhole is made at the caudal portion of the reservoir and anastomosed to the urethra.

studies. The rate of daytime continence was 95%, and that of nighttime continence was 86%. Of the female patients, 12% were incontinent during the night. Total incontinence occurred in 2%. Stress incontinence was documented by urodynamic studies in 3%, and it was related to negative urethral pressure transmission. Chronic urinary retention was seen in 16% of female patients. The lateral pouch–urethra angle, which was evaluated by voiding radiography, was between 90 and 160 degrees before and during voiding in females without voiding difficulties. Voiding radiography showed a smaller pouch–urethra angle of 61 to 103 degrees and concomitant posterior herniation of the anterior vaginal wall or pouchocele formation in female patients with significant postvoiding urinary retention. Treatment of voiding dysfunction included conversion into a continent cutaneous diversion in two women with total incontinence, pharmacotherapy with imipramine when nocturnal incontinence was diagnosed, clean intermittent self-catheterization in cases of chronic urinary retention, and pouch revision with correction of the posterior angle for significant overflow incontinence with pouchocele. The investigators conclude that chronic urinary retention in female patients with orthotopic urinary diversion is caused by a mechanical problem, not neurogenic factors. They concluded from their investigations that an autonomic nerve-sparing procedure, which compromises on the radicality of cystectomy, is not necessary for a satisfactory functional outcome.

Another study evaluated the long-term outcomes of 18 female patients with urethral substitution by the ileal neobladder.[31] Pouch-related complications occurred in two, including one with urethroileal stenosis and one with ureteroileal stenosis. Seventy percent of the patients were hypercontinent and emptied their neobladder by clean intermittent self-catheterization because of significant residual urine or complete voiding incompetence. A difference in voiding pattern was not observed when comparing resection lines located at the proximal urethra and at the bladder neck.

Volkmer and colleagues[32] investigated the impact of urinary diversion by orthotopic ileal neobladder on sexuality in 29 female patients (8 with benign and 21 with malignant diseases) by questionnaires. Influencing factors were age (<60 years), benign disease, partnership at surgery, and current partnership. Sexuality was not influenced by the necessity of pouch catheterization, urinary stress incontinence, and hormonal therapy. The study authors concluded that orthotopic urinary diversion did not influence female sexuality postoperatively.

CONTINENT CUTANEOUS DIVERSION

A catheterizable cutaneous stoma represents an alternative continent urinary diversion that provides an intact body image. It can be offered to patients who experience radical cystectomy, including urethrectomy. Benign indications include irreparable loss of the sphincteric urethra and severe cases of interstitial cystitis. Careful patient selection for motivation, compliance, and manual dexterity to perform a self-catheterization is necessary to ensure success of the continent diversion in the long term. Exclusion criteria are inadequate manual dexterity, reduced intellectual capacity, or decreased motivation to perform self-catheterization.

Continent cutaneous urinary diversion is achieved by creation of a urinary reservoir, which is to be emptied by intermittent self-catheterization; preservation of the upper urinary tract; and provision of continence by a specific outlet. Several surgical techniques use different bowel segments and different mechanisms to provide continence.

Kock Pouch

Kock developed the first continent ileal reservoir using 60 to 70 cm of ileum for pouch formation and construction of two nipple valves (Fig. 96-6).[33] At the proximal and distal ends of the ileum, which is excluded from intestinal continuity for pouch formation, 10- to 12-cm of bowel segments are left intact for creation of the afferent and efferent nipple valves. The remaining 40 cm of ileum is incised antimesenterically, sutured side to side in a U-shape, folded over, and closed to create a spherical pouch. For the final position, the reservoir is rotated such that the posterior aspect is brought anteriorly. Staple fixation of the intussusception nipple to itself and to the wall of the reservoir is crucial to secure the afferent anti-reflux-valve and the efferent continence valve and to prevent nipple gliding or eversion. The ureters are implanted end to side into the afferent ileal limb.

Overall complication rates between 32% and 53% are reported in the literature.[34-40] Early pouch-related complications at a rate of up to 25% include pouch rupture, pouch sepsis, pouch abscess, and pinhole fistula at the efferent segment.[34] Late complications are mostly associated with dysfunction of the efferent segment, including stoma incontinence (17% to 23%), nipple prolapse or nipple gliding (7% to 10%), stoma stenosis (0% to 10%), and calculus formation (8% to 15%). Complications of the afferent segment are less common and mostly related to strictures of the ureteral-intestinal anastomosis (2% to 5%), ureteral reflux (2% to 13%), and afferent nipple stones (5.2%).[40] Continence rates vary between 78% and 94%.

ILEOCECAL POUCH: MAINZ POUCH I

The Mainz pouch I procedure was established in 1983. It uses 10 to 15 cm of cecum and ascending colon and two terminal ileal segments of equal length for reservoir construction (Fig. 96-7).[10] The surgical procedure comprises antimesenteric incision of ileum, cecum, and ascending colon and side-to-side anastomosis of the ascending colon with the terminal ileal loop and of the latter with the proximal ileal loop. The anterior wall of the pouch is closed by a single row of running sutures.

Both ureters are implanted in an anti-refluxive manner into the large bowel using the submucosal tunnel technique described by Goodwin.[41] The Abol-Enein technique was introduced for preoperatively dilated ureters.[22] The technique entails fashioning two serosa-lined, extramural tunnels. The buttonhole technique implies oblique, end-to-side, refluxive ureteral implantation.[42]

Originally, the continent outlet was created using 12 to 15 cm of terminal ileum, which is left intact and is intussuscepted isoperistaltically over a length of about 5 cm through the ileocecal valve and stapled to itself, the ileocecal valve, and the wall of the pouch (Fig. 96-8A to C). Since 1990, the submucosally embedded, in situ appendix is used for construction of the continent outlet when possible (see Fig. 96-8D and E).[43] The submucosal tunnel is created by seromuscular incision of the free tenia. The seromuscularis layer is closed over the embedded appendix. Seromuscular and full-thickness bowel-flap tubes were described in

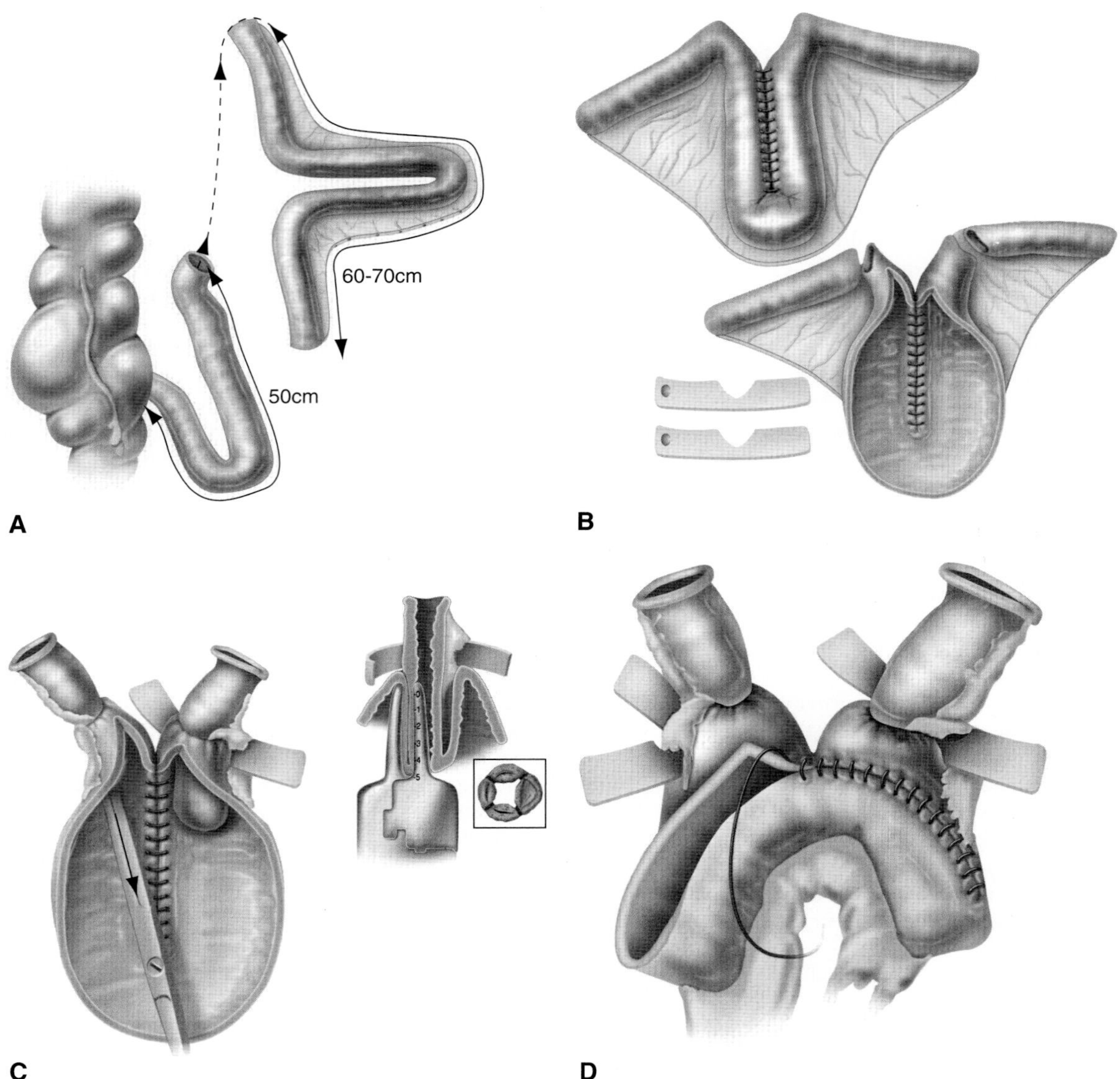

Figure 96-6 Kock pouch cutaneous diversion. **A,** A 60- to 70-cm segment of ileum is isolated approximately 50 cm above the ileocecal valve. The bowel is positioned in a U-shape. **B,** The ileum is incised along its antimesenteric border and sutured in a side-to-side manner into a U-shape. **C,** The nipple valves are fixated by ileal intussusception with three rows of staples. The afferent valve serves as anti-reflux mechanism to ureteral implantation, the efferent valve as continent outlet. **D,** Closure of the reservoir is performed by 2 inverting running sutures. (Modified from Kock NG, Nilson AE, Nilsson LO, et al: Urinary diversion via a continent ileal reservoir: Clinical results in 12 patients. J Urol 128:469-475, 1982.)

1995 as alternative procedures for patients in whom the appendix was not available (Fig. 96-9).[44]

Most reported complications are related to the continent outlet. Calculus formation is more often reported for the stapled intussuscepted ileal nipple valve (3% to 5.5%).[45,46] Major complications such as nipple necrosis, nipple prolapse, and nipple gliding are seen in 3.8% to 6.6% of patients.[45,46] Complications of the appendix stoma include necrosis of the appendix in 2.1% to 2.5% and stoma stenosis in 14.6% to 21% of patients.[45-48] Continence rates are between 98% and 100%.[45,46,48] Anti-refluxive ureteral implantation through the submucosal tunnel technique is associated with a 5.7% ureteral obstruction rate for preoperatively nondilated ureters and a 16% obstruction rate for preoperatively dilated systems at long-term follow-up.[49] When direct ureterointestinal implantation was performed in 30 patients (i.e., 10 patients with direct ureteral reimplantation and 20 patients with primary direct ureteral implantation), no deterioration of kidney function and no evidence of obstruction were seen at a median follow-up of 50.7 months.[42] Reflux occurred in one renal unit, without necessity for reintervention.

Transverse Colonic Pouch: Mainz Pouch III

The transverse colonic pouch (i.e., Mainz pouch III or the transverse ascending or transverse descending pouch) was created for continent urinary diversion in patients who had prior pelvic irradiation (Fig. 96-10).[50] About 20 cm of transverse colon and ascending or descending colon are used. The outlet is created by a full-thickness colonic tube of about 8 cm, 6 cm of which are embedded into a submucosal tunnel. The ureteral implantation

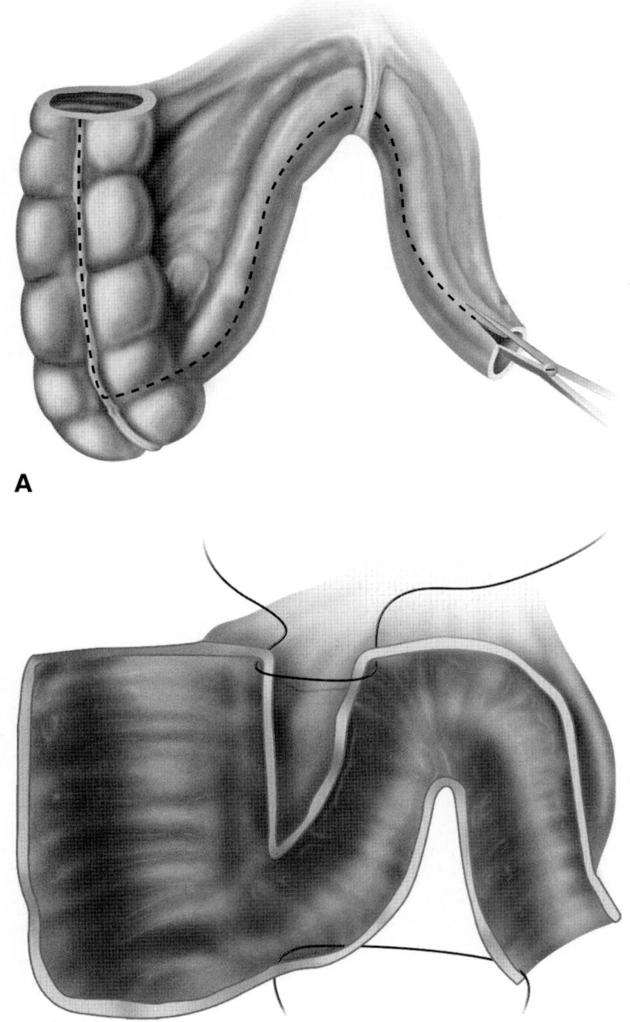

Figure 96-7 Cutaneous ileocecal pouch (MZ-pouch I). A 10- to 15-cm segment of cecum and ascending colon and two terminal ileal segments of equal length are used for reservoir construction. The ileum, cecum, and ascending colon are incised antimesenterically. The posterior wall of the pouch is done by anastomosis of the ascending colon with the terminal ileal loop, and the latter with the proximal ileal loop by a single row of running sutures. The anterior wall of the pouch is also closed by a single row of running sutures. (Modified from Hohenfellner R: Ausgewählte Urologische OP-Techniken, 2. Auflage Stuttgart, New York, Thieme Verlag, 1997).

follows the Goodwin technique or the serosa-lined extramural tunnel technique. Eighteen percent of complications of the transverse colonic pouch (i.e., Mainz III) are related to the efferent colonic outlet, with stoma incontinence occurring in 5% and stoma stenosis developing in 14%.[50]

Indiana Pouch

The Indiana pouch was developed 1984 as a modification of the Gilchrist procedure (Fig. 96-11).[51] An 8- to 10-cm segment of terminal ileum and 25- to 30-cm of cecum and ascending colon are isolated, and the large bowel is opened along the antimesenteric border. The distal end of the opened colon is folded down to the apex of the incision. The reservoir is closed with a single layer of sutures. For a reservoir constructed by mechanical stapling, a 2- to 3-cm incision at the antimesenteric border of the cecum opposite the ileocecal valve is performed. The distal end of the colonic segment is folded down to the cecal incision, fixed by holding sutures, cut open, and stapled between the holding sutures using the GIA stapler with absorbable staples until complete detubularization of the colonic segment is achieved. The edges of the opposing colonic segments are closed by absorbable TA55 staples. Originally, ureteral implantation was performed in an anti-refluxive manner through a submucosal tunnel. Currently, an end-to-side direct anastomosis is employed. The efferent segment is constructed by tapering the terminal ileum, allowing easy passage of an 18-Fr catheter. A modification encompasses embedding the tapered ileal segment into a submucosal tunnel.[52]

Complication rates range between 10.8% and 52.0%.[53-55] Pouch-related complications are pouch rupture (2.5% to 3.2%) and calculus formation (3.7% to 10.5%). Complications of the efferent segment are stoma stenosis (3.7% to 15.2%) and stoma incontinence (1.2% to 28.2%). Obstruction of the ureteral anastomosis is reported in up to 7.2%. Preoperative radiotherapy negatively influences the postoperative outcome.[56] Ureteral obstruction was seen in 15% of patients with preoperative irradiation, compared with 4% without preoperative irradiation. Stoma incontinence developed in 4% of patients, all whom had undergone preoperative radiotherapy.

Right Colonic Reservoir with a Stapled Ileal Outlet

Davidsson and colleagues[57] reported a right colonic reservoir with a stapled ileal (Lundiana) outlet in 1992. The reservoir is created by a 30-cm, right colonic segment and a 10-cm segment of the terminal ileum serving as the outlet. The colonic segment is opened along the anterior tenia down to the level of the ileocecal valve. The incision is extended transversely to the base of the valve.

The edges of the cecal wall incision are grasped together with the ileocecal valve using a Babcock clamp. The ileal segment is tapered over a 10-Fr catheter with a TA55 stapler in a position that allows the edges of the cecal wall and part of the ileocecal valve to be incorporated. The staple line closes the cecum, tapers the valve on the catheter, and tethers the narrowed ileocecal valve to the cecal wall. The ureters are implanted in an anti-refluxive manner following the LeDuc technique of creating a mucosal sulcus or the technique of making a submucosal tunnel before the reservoir is closed.

At a mean follow-up of 58 months, clinical outcome was investigated in 99 patients, who received a right colonic reservoir with the Lundiana outlet.[58] Early pouch-related complications included partial pouch necrosis (1%), pouchovaginal fistula (1%), ureteral implantation stenosis (1%), and acute pyelonephritis (2%). Late pouch-related complications were diagnosed in 25% of the patients, including calculus formation (10%), stomal stenosis (7%), ureteral implantation stenosis (5%), acute pyelonephritis (4%), and perforation of the pouch (3%).

Florida Pouch

In 1987, Lockhart[59] described an alternative colonic reservoir (i.e., Florida pouch) that included the cecum, ascending colon,

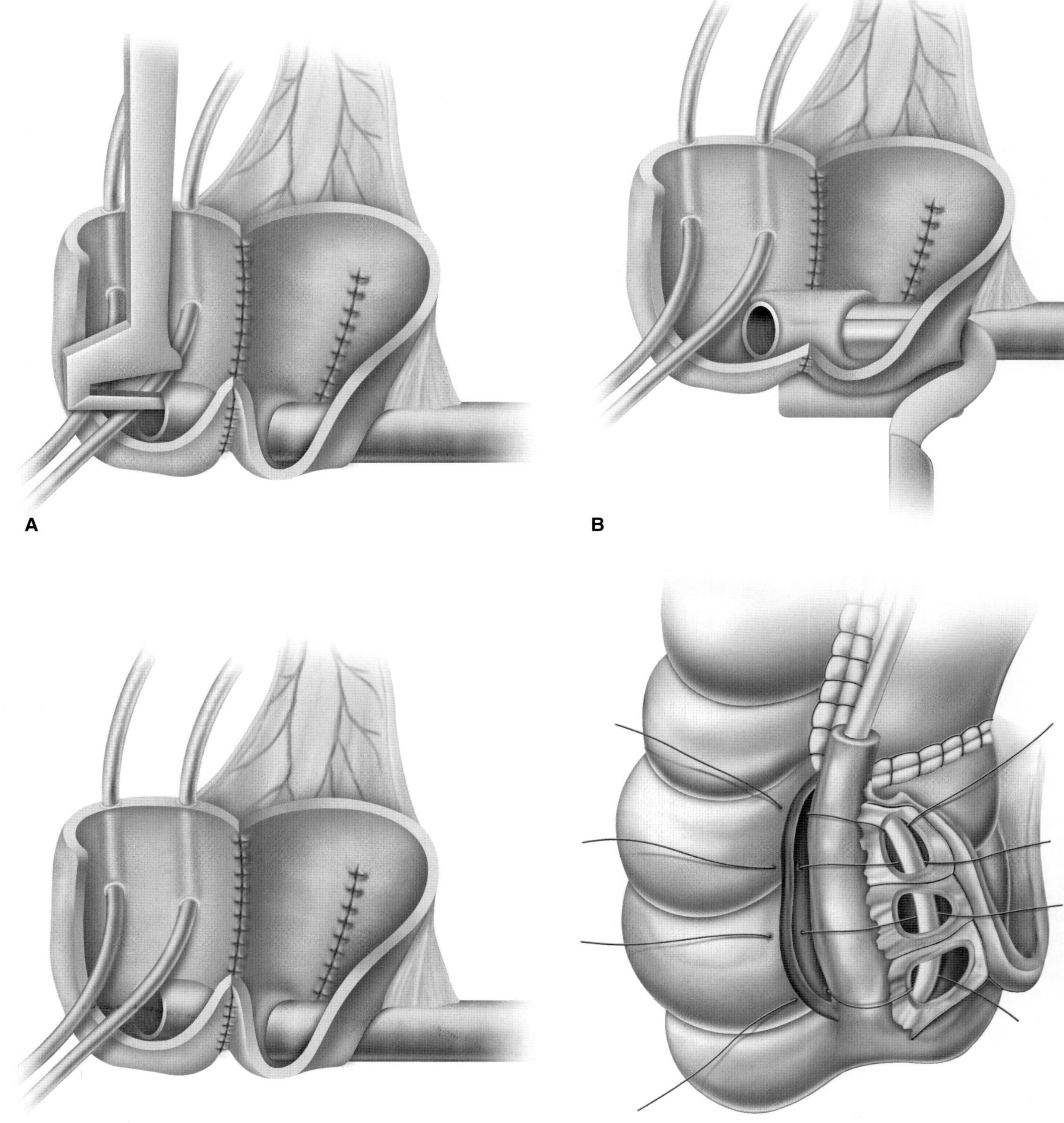

Figure 96-8 Intussuscepted ileal nipple and appendix stoma. **A** to **C,** The intussuscepted ileal nipple is created by using 12- to 15-cm of terminal ileum, which is left intact and is intussuscepted isoperistaltically over a length of about 5 cm through the ileocecal valve and stapled to itself, the ileocecal valve, and the wall of the pouch. **D,** The submucosally embedded in situ appendix is created by seromuscular incision of the free tenia.

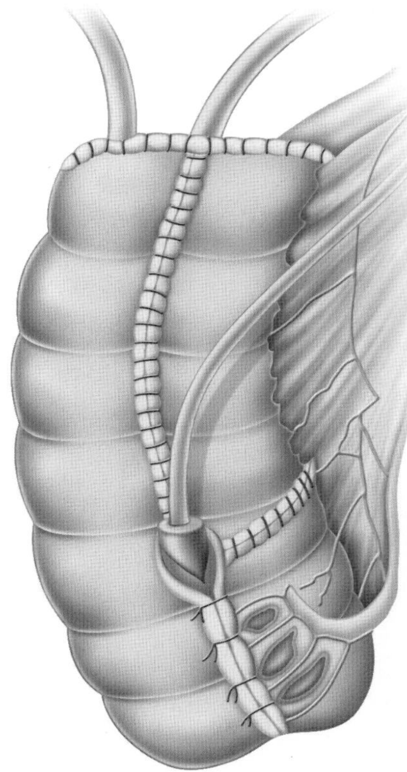

Figure 96-8, cont'd E, The seromuscularis layer is closed over the embedded appendix. (Modified from Hohenfellner R: Ausgewählte Urologische OP-Techniken, 2. Auflage Stuttgart, New York, Thieme Verlag, 1997).

one third of the right transverse colon, and 10 to 12 cm of the terminal ileum for the outlet. The colon is folded in a U-shape, fully detubularized, and closed by a locking running suture. Ureteral implantation was originally performed using the LeDuc anti-refluxive ureteroileal implantation (described earlier)[21] or by the Goodwin technique (described earlier).[41] It was later modified to a direct anastomosis of the ureters to the colon, avoiding an anti-refluxive implantation.[60] The terminal ileum is used as the efferent segment. The ileum is left attached to the reservoir and plicated with two parallel rows of sutures placed longitudinally into the ileum and ileocecal valve.

Complication rates for ureter implantation were evaluated for the ureteral implantation technique (tunneled by LeDuc or Goodwin or nontunneled end-to-side anastomosis).[60,61] Ureteral obstruction occurred in 13.3% with tunneled implantation and in 4.9% with end-to-side implantation of the ureters, but the rate of refluxing units was higher in the latter group (7.0% versus 3.3%). Complications of the efferent segment were stoma incontinence in 3.0% to 6.7% and stoma stenosis in 4.0% to 10.0%.[21] Pouch stones were seen in 3.0% to 5.4% of patients.[38,62]

Ureterosigmoidostomy and Rectosigmoid Pouch: Mainz Pouch II

Intestinal urinary diversion by ureterosigmoidostomy was introduced by Simon in 1852[63] and was followed by numerous modifications of the anti-refluxive ureterointestinal anastomosis.[64-66] The rectosigmoid pouch (i.e., Mainz pouch II) was established in 1990 (Fig. 96-12).[67] It provides a low-pressure reservoir and decreases the risk for the upper urinary tract. The rectosigmoid functions as a urinary reservoir, and the anal sphincter functions as a continence mechanism. The procedure can be offered to female patients who require radical cystectomy including the urethra and to those with benign or malignant conditions who have irreparable loss of the sphincteric urethra. It provides continence without a stoma and the need for intermittent self-catheterization.[67-69] Women with an incompetent anal sphincter and dilatation of the upper urinary tract are not candidates for this procedure. A volume of 250 mL of saline should comfortably be accommodated for 2 hours in a preoperative test. Additional evaluation of the anal sphincter competence by anal pressure profilometry is recommended.

For construction of the rectosigmoid pouch, about 20 to 25 cm bowel are opened antimesenterically down to the peritoneal reflection of the rectum and folded to an inverted U-shape. The posterior wall of the pouch is created by side-to-side anastomosis of the medial margins of the inverted U. Non-refluxing uretero-intestinal anastomosis is performed through a 4-cm submucosal tunnel. Alternatively, ureterointestinal reimplantation can be performed by a serosa-lined extramural tunnel, especially with preoperatively dilated ureters[22] or by LeDuc's implantation technique.[21] Before closure, the back wall of the pouch is fixed to the promontory to avoid displacement of the pouch and ureteral kinking. Closure is achieved by side-to-side anastomosis of the lateral margins of the inverted U.

Early complications occurring within 3 months after the surgery are reported in up to 10% of patients.[67,68,70] Complications include mechanical or paralytic ileus, suture leakage, and dislocation of ureteric stents with development of urinoma, peritonitis, or urinary fistulas. Late complications comprise pyelonephritis in up to 6% of patients, ureteric implantation stenosis in 1% to 7%, metabolic acidosis in up to 70%, and development of secondary tumors in up to 22%.[67,68,70,71] Continence rates range between 95% and 100%.[68]

Volkmer and coworkers[72] reported four pregnancies in three women after ureterosigmoidostomy. During pregnancy, monthly urologic examinations included renal ultrasound and resistance index; levels of serum electrolytes, urea, and creatinine; and blood gas analysis. Antibiotics and sodium-potassium-hydrogen citrate were administered prophylactically in all pregnant women. Delivery was achieved by cesarean section in three (one with preeclampsia at week 36) and vaginally in one.

CONCLUSIONS

A variety of surgical techniques and their modifications offer a broad spectrum of possible solutions to female patients when reconstruction of the lower urinary tract by bowel segments becomes necessary. Augmentation enterocystoplasty and orthotopic substitution to the trigone or bladder neck is reserved for women with benign diseases, such as low-capacity or low-compliance bladders caused by neurogenic and non-neurogenic diseases or chronic inflammation that is refractory to conservative treatment regimens. Women in whom radical cystectomy becomes necessary because of a malignant disease require total bladder substitution. Surgical techniques of ureterosigmoidostomy or rectosigmoid pouch diversion provide continence through the anal sphincter. These techniques can be offered to

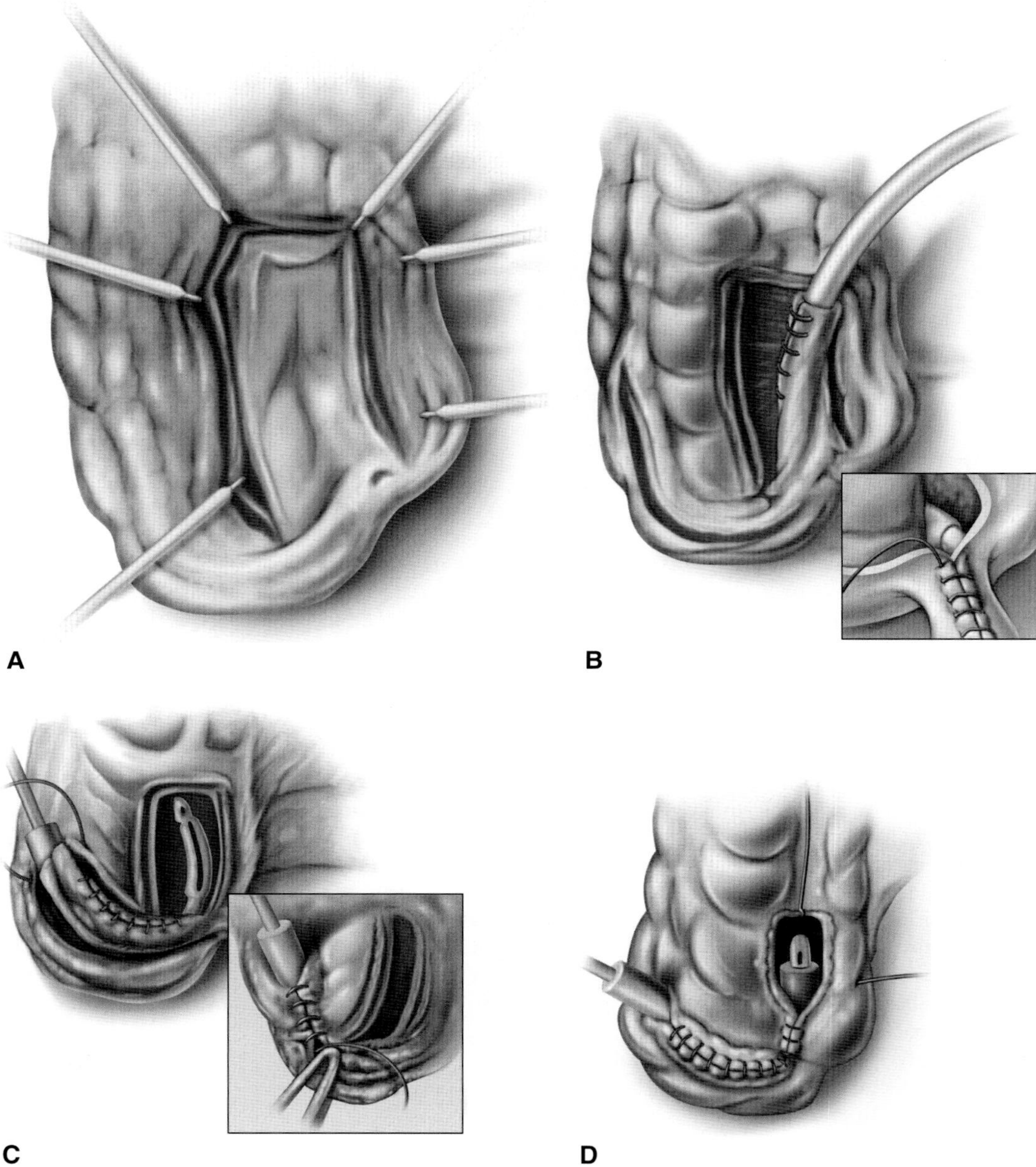

Figure 96-9 Full-thickness bowel flap. **A** and **B,** The full-thickness bowel flap tube is created by an inverted-U-shaped incision along the tenia libera of the cecum and tubularized. **C,** The tube is embedded into a submucosal tunnel at the tenia omentalis. **D,** The tunnel is finished by closing the lateral margins of the seromuscularis. (Modified from Hohenfellner R: Ausgewählte Urologische OP-Techniken, 2. Auflage Stuttgart, New York, Thieme Verlag, 1997).

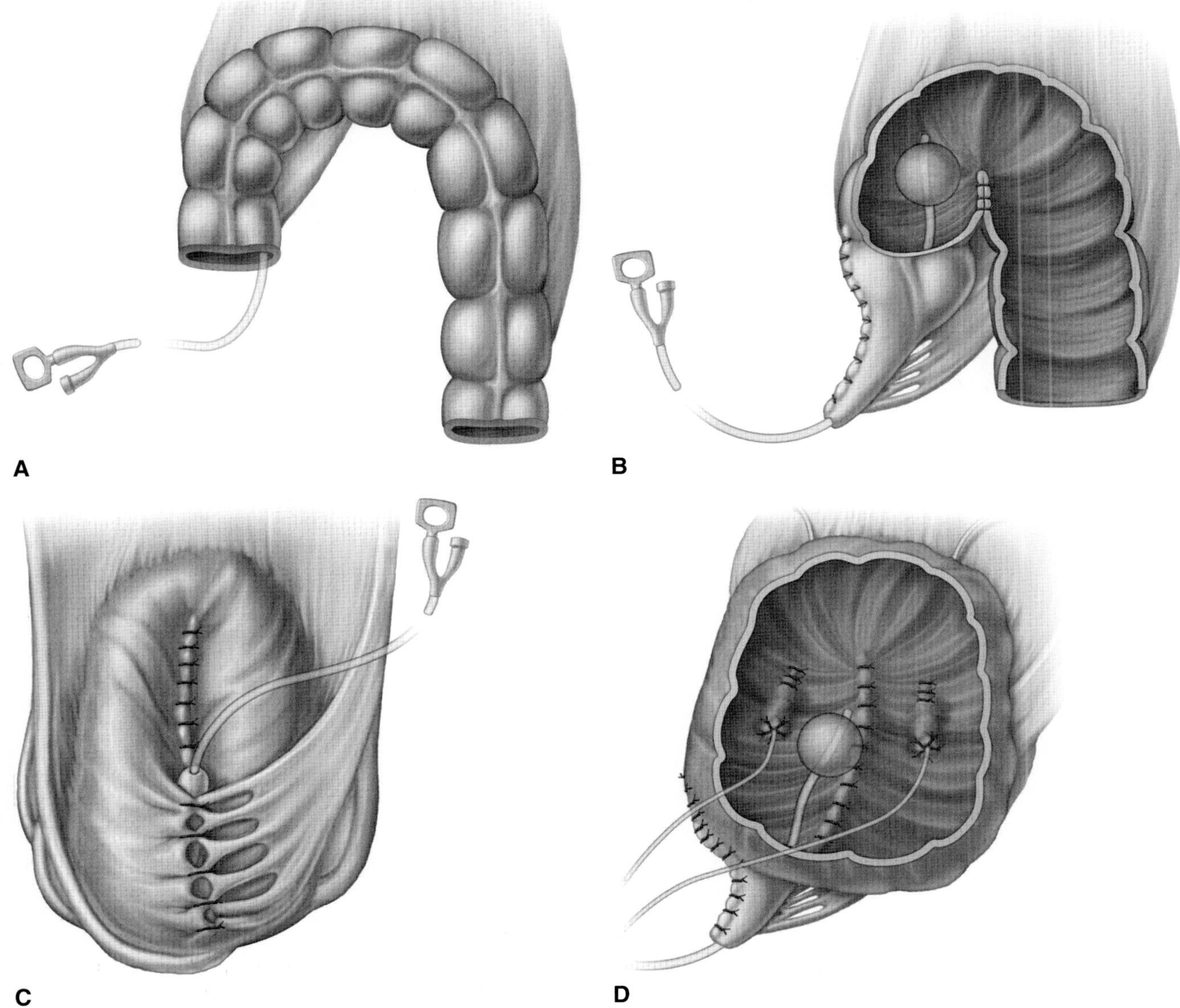

Figure 96-10 Transverse colonic pouch diversion (Mainz pouch III). **A,** A 20-cm segment of transverse colon and ascending or descending colon are isolated. **B,** The outlet is created by a full-thickness colonic tube of about 8 cm. **C,** The colonic tube is embedded into a submucosal tunnel. **D,** The ureters are implanted by the Goodwin technique (shown) or by a extramural serosal tunnel. (Modified from Leissner J, Black P, Fisch M, et al: Colon pouch (Mainz pouch III) for continent urinary diversion after pelvic irradiation. Urology 56:798-802, 2000).

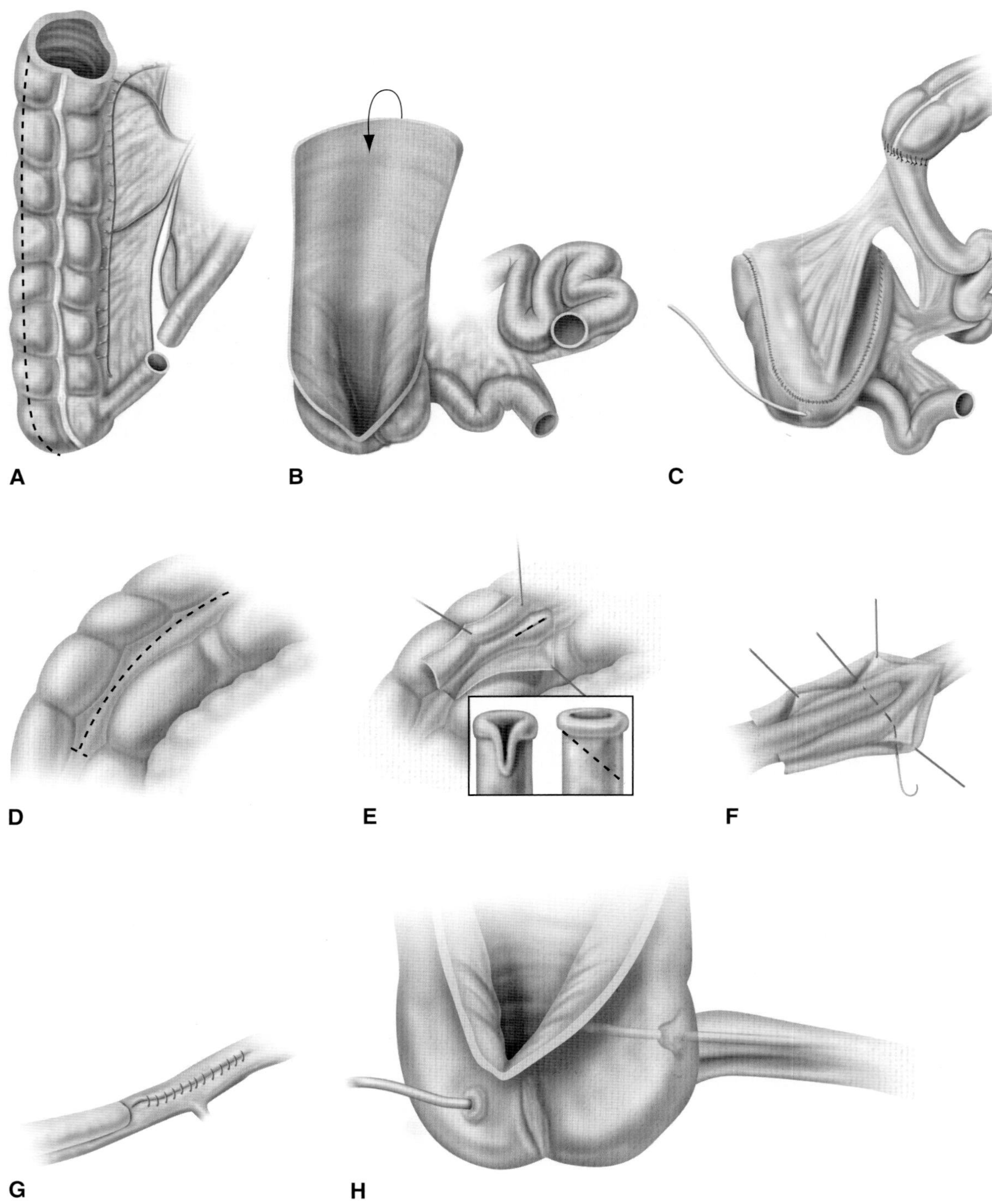

Figure 96-11 Indiana pouch. **A,** A 8- to 10-cm segment of terminal ileum and 25- to 30-cm of cecum and ascending colon are used for construction of the Indiana pouch, and they are opened along the antimesenteric border. **B** and **C,** The aboral end of the opened colon is folded down *(arrow)* to the apex of the incision and closed with a single layer of sutures. **D,** Ureteral implantation is performed through a T-shaped incision of the colonic tenia, leaving the mucosa intact. **E,** The ureteral orifice is established after mucosal incision. **F** and **G,** The spatulated ureter is anastomosed to the bowel mucosa by single sutures, and the seromuscularis is closed over it. **H,** The efferent segment is established by tapering the terminal ileum using absorbable GIA staples, leaving a caliber of ileum for passage of an 18-Fr catheter. The outlet is imbricated by sutures at the junction of ileum and cecum. (Modified from Rowland RG: Present experience with the Indiana pouch. World J Urol 14:92-98, 1996.)

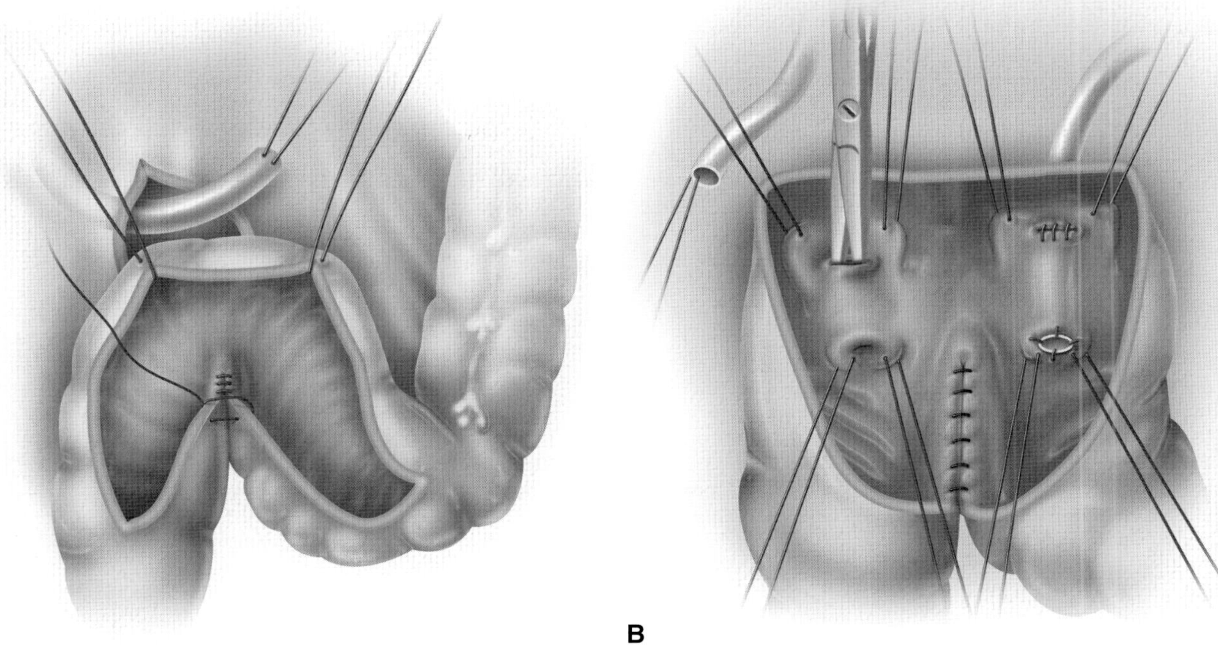

Figure 96-12 **A,** Sigma rectum pouch (Mainz pouch II). A 20- to 25-cm segment of bowel is chosen and opened antimesenterically down to the peritoneal reflection of the rectum and folded to an inverted U-shape. **B,** The posterior wall of the pouch is created by side-to-side anastomosis of the medial margins of the inverted U. Non-refluxing ureterointestinal anastomosis is performed through a 4-cm submucosal tunnel. (Modified from Fisch M, Wammack R, Hohenfellner R: The sigma-rectum pouch [Mainz pouch II]. In Hohenfellner R, Wammack R [eds]: Continent Urinary Diversion. Edinburgh, Churchill Livingstone, 1992, pp 165-166.)

patients with irreparable loss of the functional urethra or if urethrectomy is required in radical tumor surgery.

Continent cutaneous diversion with a catheterizable cutaneous stoma is a practicable and safe alternative when diversion or orthotopic urinary diversion to the urethra is not feasible or desired. To ensure success of continent cutaneous diversion, careful patient selection is required for motivation, compliance, and the manual dexterity necessary to perform selfcatheterization. Orthotopic bladder substitution to the urethra is simple to perform and can be offered to selected female patients. Intraoperatively, frozen sections of the distal urethral stump and surrounding tissues are sampled to ensure complete tumor excision. Sparing the autonomic nerves is questioned because of the possibility of compromising the radicality of tumor excision. Patients should be educated about postoperative functional problems, including incontinence and chronic urinary retention requiring clean, intermittent self-catheterization. Intermittent self-catheterization should be practiced preoperatively to ensure acceptance and compliance with the maneuver after surgery.

References

1. Tizzoni G, Foggi A: Die Wiederherstellung der Harnblase. Centralbl Chir 15:921-923, 1888.
2. van Ophoven A, Oberpfenning F, Hertle L: Long-term results of trigone-preserving orthotopic substitution enterocystoplasty for interstitial cystitis. J Urol 167:603-607, 2002.
3. Costello AJ, Crowe H, Agarwal D: Supratrigonal cystectomy and ileocystoplasty in management of interstitial cystitis. Aust N Z J Surg 70:34-38, 2000.
4. Chakravarti A, Ganta S, Somani B, Jones BS: Caecocystoplasty for intractable interstitial cystitis: Long term results. Eur Urol 46:114-117, 2004.
5. Awad SA, Al-Zahrani HM, Gajewski JB, Bourque-Kehoe AA: Long-term results and complications of augmentation ileocystoplasty for idiopathic urge incontinence in women. Br J Urol 81:569-573, 1998.
6. Flood HD, Malhotra SJ, O'Connell HE, et al: Long-term results and complications using augmentation cystoplasty in reconstructive urology. Neurourol Urodyn 14:297-309, 1995.
7. Goodwin WE, Winter CC, Barker WF: Cup-patch technique of ileocystoplasty for bladder enlargement or partial substitution. Surg Gynecol Obstet 108:240-244, 1959.
8. Goodwin WE, Winter CC: Technique of sigmoidocystoplasty. Surg Gynecol Obstet 108:370-372, 1959.
9. Hanley HG: Ileocystoplasty: A clinical review. J Urol 82:317-320, 1959.
10. Thüroff JW, Alken P, Riedmiller H, et al: The Mainz pouch (mixed augmentation ileum and cecum) for bladder augmentation and continent diversion. J Urol 136:17-26, 1986.
11. Deleveliotis A, Macris SG: Replacement of the bladder with an isolated segment of sigmoid: Achievement of physiological urination in patients with carcinoma of the bladder. J Urol 85:564-568, 1961.
12. Linn JF, Hohenfellner M, Roth S, et al: Treatment of interstitial cystitis: Comparison of subtrigonal and supratrigonal cystectomy combined with orthotopic bladder substitution. J Urol 159:774-778, 1998.

13. Perimenis P, Burkhard FC, Kessler TM, et al: Ileal orthotopic bladder substitute combined with an afferent tubular segment: Long-term upper urinary tract changes and voiding pattern. Eur Urol 46:604-609, 2004.
14. Stein JP, Ginsberg DA, Skinner DG: Indications and technique of the orthotopic neobladder in women. Urol Clin North Am 29:725-734, 2002.
15. Stein JP, Cote RJ, Freeman JA, et al: Indications for lower urinary tract reconstruction in women after cystectomy for bladder cancer: A pathological review of female cystectomy specimens. J Urol 154:1329-1333, 1995.
16. Stenzl A, Draxl H, Posch B, et al: The risk of urethral tumors in female bladder cancer: Can the urethra be used for orthotopic reconstruction of the lower urinary tract? J Urol 153:950-955, 1995.
17. Colleselli K, Stenzl A, Eder R, et al: The female urethral sphincter: A morphological and topographical study. J Urol 160:49-54, 1998.
18. Ghoneim MA, Kock NG, Lycke G, El-Din ABS: An appliance-free sphincter-controlled bladder substitute: The urethral Kock pouch. J Urol 138:1150-1154, 1987.
19. Stein JP, Lieskovski G, Ginsberg DA, et al: The T-pouch: An orthotopic ileal neobladder incorporating a serosal lined ileal antireflux technique. J Urol 159:1836-1842, 1998.
20. Hautmann RE, Egghart G, Frohneberg D, Miller K: The ileal neobladder. J Urol 139:39-42, 1988.
21. LeDuc A, Camey M, Teillac P: An original antireflux ureteroileal implantation technique: Long term follow-up. J Urol 137:1156-1158, 1987.
22. Abol-Enein H, Ghoneim MA: A novel uretero-ileal re-implantation technique: The serous lined extramural tunnel. A preliminary report. J Urol 151:1193-1198, 1994.
23. Hautmann RE: The ileal neobladder: Atlas. Urol Clin North Am 9:85, 2001.
24. Studer UE, Ackermann D, Casanova GA, Zingg EJ: Three years experience with an ileal low pressure bladder substitute. Br J Urol 63:43-52, 1989.
25. El-Mekresh M, Franzaring L, Wöhr M, et al: Simplified orthotopic ileocecal pouch (Mainz pouch) for bladder substitution. Aktuelle Urol 34:226-223, 2003.
26. Hautmann RE, De Petriconi R, Gottfried HW, et al: The ileal neobladder: Complications and functional results in 363 patients after 11 years of followup. J Urol 161:422-428, 1999.
27. Ghoneim MA, Shaaban AA, Mahran MR, Kock NG: Further experiences with the urethral Kock pouch. J Urol 147:361-365, 1992.
28. Cancrini A, De Carli P, Fattahi H, et al: Orthotopic ileal neobladder in female patients after radical cystectomy: 2-year experience. J Urol 153:956-958, 1995.
29. Stenzl A, Colleselli K, Poisel S, et al: Rationale and technique of nerve sparing radical cystectomy before an orthotopic neobladder procedure in women. J Urol 154:2044-2049, 1995.
30. Ali-El-Dein B, El-Sobky E, Hohenfellner M, Ghoneim MA: Orthotopic bladder substitution in women: Functional evaluation. J Urol 161:1875-1880, 1999.
31. Hautmann RE, Paiss T, De Petriconi R: The ileal neobladder in women: 9 years of experience with 18 patients. J Urol 155:76-81, 1996.
32. Volkmer BG, Gschwend JE, Herkommer K, et al: Cystectomy and orthotopic ileal neobladder: The impact on female sexuality. J Urol 172:2353-2357, 2004.
33. Kock NG, Nilson AR, Norlen L, et al: Urinary diversion via a continent ileum reservoir: Clinical experience. Scand J Urol Nephrol Suppl 49:23, 1978.
34. Soulie M, Seguin P, Martel P, et al: A modified intussuscepted nipple in the Kock pouch urinary diversion: Assessment of perioperative complications and functional results. Br J Urol 90:397-402, 2002.
35. Jonsson O, Olofsson G, Lindholm E, Törnquist H: Long time experience with Kock ileal reservoir for continent urinary diversion. Eur Urol 40:632-640, 2001.
36. Skinner DG, Lieskovski G, Boyd S: Continent urinary diversion. J Urol 141:1323-1327, 1989.
37. Okada Y, Shichiri Y, Terai A, et al: Management of late complications of continent urinary diversion using the Kock pouch and the Indiana pouch procedures. Int J Urol 3:334-339, 1996.
38. Carr LK, Webster GD: Kock versus right colon continent urinary diversion: Comparison of outcome and reoperation rate. Urology 48:711-714, 1996.
39. Bander NH: Initial results with slightly modified Kock pouch. Urology 37:100-105, 1991.
40. Stein JP, Freeman JA, Esrig D, et al: Complications of the afferent antireflux valve mechanism in the Kock ileal reservoir. J Urol 155:1579-1584, 1996.
41. Goodwin WE, Winter CC, Turner RD: Replacement of ureter by small intestine: Clinical application and results of the ileal ureter. J Urol 81:406-418, 1959.
42. Hohenfellner R, Black P, Leissner J, Allhoff EP: Refluxing ureterointestinal anastomosis for continent cutaneous urinary diversion. J Urol 168:1013-1017, 2002.
43. Riedmiller H, Bürger R, Müller S, et al: Continent appendix stoma: A modification of the Mainz pouch technique. J Urol 143:1115-1116, 1990.
44. Lampel A, Hohenfellner M, Schultz-Lampel D, Thüroff JW: In situ tunneled bowel flap tubes: 2 new techniques of a continent outlet for Mainz pouch cutaneous diversion. J Urol 153:308-315, 1995.
45. Gerharz EW, Köhl U, Weingärtner K, et al: Complications related to different continence mechanisms in ileocecal reservoir. J Urol 158:1709-1713, 1997.
46. Fichtner J, Fisch M, Hohenfellner R: Appendiceal continence mechanisms in continent urinary diversion. World J Urol 14:105-107, 1996.
47. Lampel A, Fisch M, Stein R, et al: Continent diversion with the Mainz pouch. World J Urol 14:85-91, 1996.
48. Gerharz EW, Köhl UN, Melekos MD, et al: Ten years experience with the submucosally embedded in situ appendix in continent urinary diversion. Eur Urol 40:625-631, 2001.
49. Stein R, Pfitzenmaier J, Behringer M, et al: The long-term results (5-16 years) of Mainz pouch I technique at a single institution. J Urol Suppl 165:88, 2001.
50. Leissner J, Black P, Fisch M, et al: Colon pouch (Mainz pouch III) for continent urinary diversion after pelvic irradiation. Urology 56:798-802, 2000.
51. Rowland RG, Mitchell ME, Bihrle R, et al: Indiana continent urinary reservoir. J Urol 137:1136-1139, 1987.
52. Chanturaia Z, Pertia A, Managadze G, et al: Right colonic reservoir with submucosally embedded tapered ileum—Tiflis pouch. Urol Int 59:113-118, 1997.
53. Rowland RG, Present experiences with the Indiana pouch. World J Urol 14:92-98, 1996.
54. Holmes DG, Trasher JB, Park GY, et al: Long term complications related to the modified Indiana pouch. Urology 60:603-606, 2002.
55. Aria Y, Kawakita M, Terachi T, et al: Long-term followup of the Kock and Indiana pouch procedures. J Urol 150:51-55, 1993.
56. Wilson TG, Moreno JG, Weinberg A, Ahlering TE: Late complications of the modified Indiana pouch. J Urol 151:331-334, 1994.
57. Davidsson T, Barker SB, Mansson W: Tapering of intussuscepted ileal nipple valve or ileocecal valve to correct secondary incontinence in patients with urinary reservoir. J Urol 147:144-146, 1992.
58. Mansson W, Davidsson T, Könyves J, et al: Continent urinary tract reconstruction—The Lund experience. BJU Int 92:271-276, 2003.
59. Lockhart JL: Remodeled right colon: An alternative urinary reservoir. J Urol 138:730-734, 1987.
60. Helal M, Pow-Sang J, Sanford E, et al: Direct (non tunneled) ureterocolonic reimplantation in association with continent reservoirs. J Urol 150:835-837, 1993.
61. Lockhart JL, Pow-Sang JM, Persky L, et al: A continent colonic urinary reservoir: The Florida pouch. J Urol 144:864-867, 1990.

62. Webster C, Bukkapatnam R, Seigne JD, et al: Continent colonic urinary reservoir (Florida pouch): Long term surgical complications (greater than 11 years). J Urol 169:174-176, 2003.
63. Simon J: Ectropia vesica (absence of the anterior walls of the bladder and pubic abdominal parities): Operations for directing the orifices of the ureters into the rectum; temporary success; subsequent death; autopsy. Lancet 2:568, 1852.
64. Goodwin WE Harris AP, Kaufmann JJ, et al: Open transcolonic uretero-intestinal anastomosis: A new approach. Surg Gynecol Obstet 97:295-298, 1953.
65. Hohenfellner R, Planz C, Wulff HD, et al: Die transsigmoidale Ureterosigmoidostomie (Sigma-Rectum-Blase): Operationstechnik und Gesamtkaliumbestimmung. Urologe 6:275-281, 1967.
66. Leadbetter WF: Consideration of problems incident to performance of ureteroenterostomy: Report of a technique. J Urol 65:818-825, 1951.
67. Fisch M, Wammack R, Müller SC, Hohenfellner R: The Mainz pouch II. Eur Urol 25:7-15, 1994.
68. D'Elia G, Pahernik S, Fisch M, et al: Mainz pouch II technique: 10 years' experience. BJU Int 93:1037-1042, 2004.
69. Bastian PJ, Albers P, Hanitzsch H, et al: Health-related quality-of-life following modified ureterosigmoidostomy (Mainz pouch II) as continent urinary diversion. Eur Urol 46:591-598, 2004.
70. Bastian PJ, Albers P, Hanitzsch H, et al: The modified ureterosigmoidostomy (Mainz pouch II) as a continent form of urinary diversion. Urologe A 43:982-988, 2004.
71. Gilja I, Kovacic M, Radej M, et al: The sigmoidorectal pouch (Mainz pouch II). Eur Urol 29:210-215, 1996.
72. Volkmer BG, Seidl EM, Gschwend JE, et al: Pregnancy in women with ureterosigmoidostomy. Urology 60:979-982, 2002.

Chapter 97

TRANSVAGINAL CLOSURE OF THE BLADDER NECK IN THE TREATMENT OF URINARY INCONTINENCE

R. Duane Cespedes

The treatment of urinary complications in the female patient with advanced neurologic disease is a challenging problem. Unlike their male counterparts, reliable urinary collection devices do not exist, limiting the available options. Most of these patients are treated with a long-term indwelling Foley catheter, which frequently causes severe complications, including a small and contracted bladder, recurrent infections, bladder stones, and a destroyed urethra. The long-term indwelling catheter and Foley balloon may produce urethral erosion and bladder neck pressure necrosis, resulting in spontaneous urethral expulsion with bladder spasms. In many cases, after the problems of detrusor compliance and bladder storage have been addressed, the patient is left with a fixed, open, and severely damaged urethra. Many options have been proposed for treatment of the destroyed urethra, including transvaginal closure, transabdominal closure, combined transvaginal and transabdominal approaches, a tight pubovaginal sling, or an artificial urinary sphincter. For milder cases with a partially intact urethra, a sling procedure can adequately close the bladder neck of most incontinent patients, but for the more severe cases, a bladder neck closure and suprapubic diversion are often necessary. Bladder neck closure methods remain the therapy of last resort, but they must occasionally be used because not all patients can be successfully managed with minimally invasive therapies.

HISTORICAL PERSPECTIVE

For urethras that are not totally destroyed, a pubovaginal sling has been used successfully to close the urethra. Chancellor and associates[1] used a combined "tight" autologous pubovaginal sling and enterocystoplasty in 10 female patients with urethras destroyed by long-term Foley use. At 24 months, the investigators reported excellent results with minimal incontinence or other complications. They remarked that at least 1 cm of normal urethra was required for proper functioning of the sling and that the sling must be pulled tighter than normal. Mesh may not be applicable in this circumstance because the sling is purposely pulled very tight, possibly leading to a catastrophic erosion. Overall, this method is appealing because it reduces the fistula risk, allows a relief valve if the suprapubic diversion becomes obstructed, and allows alternative catheter access if needed.

There are few published reports on the techniques and outcomes of transvaginal bladder neck closure in female patients. Reid and colleagues[2] described five female patients (three procedures were performed transabdominally, and two were performed transvaginally) with an overall 80% cure rate. Fenely[3] reported 24 female patients with neurologic disease who underwent transvaginal bladder neck closure and suprapubic tube placement. A vesicovaginal fistula developed in four patients, resulting in persistent incontinence. Zimmern and colleagues[4] described six female patients with closure of the bladder neck. At 21 months of follow-up, no fistulas or cases of incontinence had occurred. In 1994, Levy and associates[5] reported a 40% success rate using a transvaginal bladder neck closure. They subsequently modified their approach by using a combined transvaginal-transabdominal approach and reported a 100% success rate at a mean of 16 months' follow-up for their subsequent 10 patients. Shpall and Ginsberg[6] reported 39 patients who underwent a combined transabdominal bladder neck closure and continent cutaneous diversion. At a mean of 37 months, six patients (15%) had developed fistulas, and four patients were successfully repaired.

As illustrated by this historical perspective, the risk of complications, specifically a vesicovaginal fistula, is real, and they are difficult to repair. A bladder neck closure is much different from simple closure of the bladder wall, and the risk of a fistula should not be underestimated. Several principles should be understood before performing a bladder neck closure. The bladder neck is usually hyperactive in patients with neurologic disease because most of them have detrusor hyperreflexia, and every voiding reflex includes active opening of the bladder neck. Active opening and closing of the bladder neck therefore forcibly attempts to destroy the bladder neck closure. To reduce this risk, postoperative suppression of the voiding reflex using prolonged, continuous catheter drainage (3 weeks) and liberal use of anticholinergics is imperative.

For a fistula to form, leakage must occur. The repair must be watertight from the beginning, and this requires a precise mucosal closure using a running suture, with multiple additional layers above it to reinforce the strength of the repair. The urethral mucosa sutures lines and the vaginal epithelial suture lines should not overlap the bladder neck closure. For added protection, a drain should be placed through an abdominal incision.

INDICATIONS FOR THE PROCEDURE

A transvaginal bladder neck closure is an uncommon surgical procedure. The main indication is for patients with a neurogenic bladder who have a urethra destroyed by prolonged Foley catheter drainage. The usual clinical scenario is a progressive increase in leakage around the catheter, necessitating progressively larger catheters and more fluid in the Foley balloon. This eventually results in a wide, patulous, and severely damaged urethra.

Management of these patients often requires transvaginal closure of the bladder neck and simultaneous urinary diversion using a continent catheterizable augmentation, incontinent ileovesicostomy, or suprapubic catheter.

Other possible indications for a bladder neck closure include a urethra destroyed by disease or injury, such as a urethral diverticulum, recurrent urethrovaginal fistula after surgical procedures, and severe urethral trauma.

PREOPERATIVE EVALUATION

Pelvic examination of the urethra usually reveals an enlarged, shortened, patulous urethra with overt visualization of the bladder neck or bladder itself in severe cases. Cystoscopy is performed to confirm the absence of other pathology in the bladder, such as foreign bodies, stones, cancer, or diverticula, which may accompany long-term Foley catheter drainage. Evaluation of the upper urinary tracts is indicated to assess for stones, hydronephrosis, or ureteral obstruction.

The choices for urinary diversion must be comprehensively discussed with the patient and family. If a continent diversion will be performed in conjunction with bladder neck closure, the patient must demonstrate sufficient manual dexterity to perform self-catheterization. If the patient has a reliable caregiver, this may be sufficient, although this does introduce additional risk for complications because a high-pressure system may develop if catheterizations are delayed.

In many cases, an incontinent ileovesicostomy to the skin ("chimney") is the safest long-term option because it reliably creates a low-pressure system and largely avoids the inflammatory and infectious complications of an indwelling catheter. This method also provides an easy, inexpensive, and reliable bag-on-stoma situation for caregivers. Two different methods for performing an incontinent ileovesicostomy diversion have been described.[7,8] When performing a diversion that entails opening of the bladder, it is preferable in some situations to close the bladder neck transabdominally. Khoury and colleagues[9] have reported an effective method of transabdominal closure.

Suprapubic catheter drainage is perhaps the most commonly used diversion because it is initially the least invasive, but it is not without complications. Although a suprapubic tube minimizes the urethral complications and allows the use of larger catheters, the problems with bladder inflammation, infection, bladder fibrosis, stone formation, and upper tract deterioration can still occur. In many cases, a suprapubic tube is used temporarily until the definitive diversion can be performed. Suprapubic tube placement is facilitated by using a transurethral Lowsley retractor to tent up the anterior bladder wall to the rectus and subsequently pull the Foley down into the bladder.[10] The urine should be routinely cultured and broad-spectrum antibiotics, matched to the culture, used before surgery.

SURGICAL TECHNIQUE

The patient is placed in the dorsal lithotomy position and then prepared and draped to allow access to the lower abdomen and vagina. If a suprapubic tube will be used postoperatively, a large (20- to 24-Fr) tube is placed first using a Lowsley retractor to elevate the bladder to the anterior abdominal wall. Normal saline is injected into the vaginal wall to develop a subepithelial plane

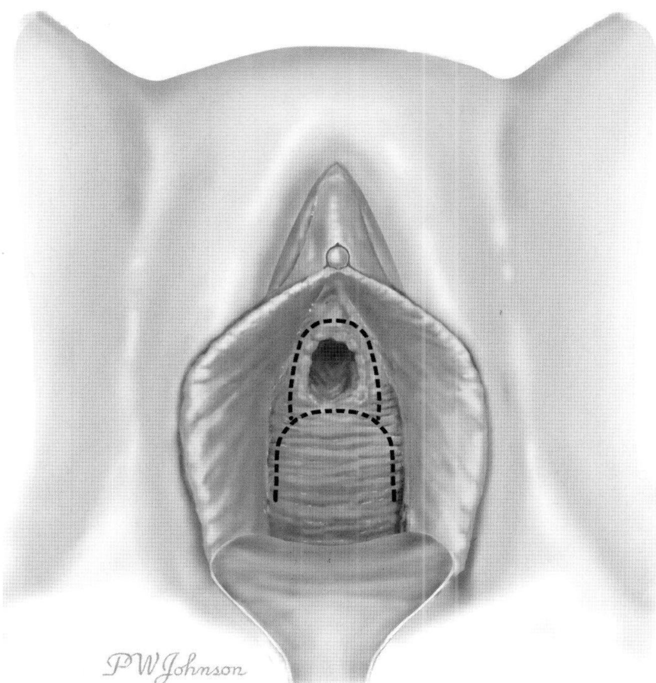

Figure 97-1 After injection of normal saline into the anterior vaginal wall, an incision is made around the urethral opening to create the vaginal wall flap.

around the urethra and to develop a mucosal flap for coverage. A circumscribing incision is made around the urethral opening, and an inverted-U-shaped incision is made in the anterior vaginal wall below the urethra (Fig. 97-1). The vaginal flap is created by sharp dissection in the anterior vaginal wall, separating the epithelium from the underlying fascia. The dissection is carried laterally and superiorly around the open bladder neck (Fig. 97-2). The dissection is continued deeper around the bladder neck, freeing the bladder from its attachments to the symphysis pubis and lateral pelvic side wall. This invariably requires entering the retropubic space by detaching the urethropelvic ligaments on either side of the bladder neck and the pubourethral ligaments superior to the urethra. If the urethra is more than about 1 cm long, the distal portion should be resected to ensure that it can be folded in without leaving any exposed mucosa. Indigo carmine is injected to ensure identification of the ureteral orifices to prevent injury during bladder neck closure.

The bladder neck is closed in three layers. The first two layers are vertically closed, and the third layer is closed horizontally. The mucosal layer is precisely closed with a running 3-0 polyglycolic acid suture to ensure a watertight closure. If any tension exists on this or a subsequent suture line, further dissection is required to ensure that it is tension free. The muscular layer is then closed over the mucosa with a running 2-0 polyglycolic acid suture, incorporating the urethral muscle and distal bladder neck region (Fig. 97-3). The bladder neck and anterior bladder wall should be closed horizontally (to prevent overlapping suture lines) over the previous layers using interrupted 1-0 polyglycolic acid sutures. At this point, the bladder neck closure should be elevated somewhat back into the retropubic space behind the pubic symphysis (Fig. 97-4). A Martius flap may be placed at this time to advance another layer over the repair, although it is rarely

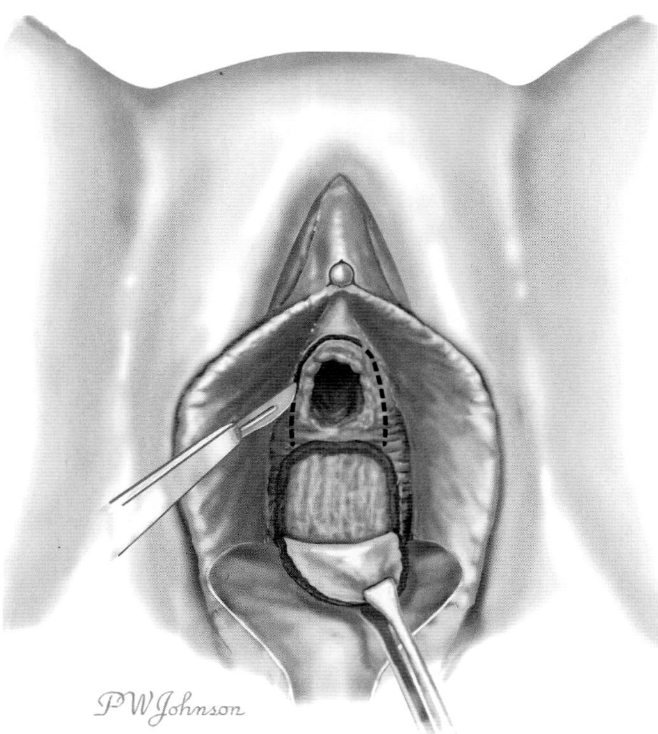

Figure 97-2 The urethral meatus is dissected free, and the vaginal wall flap is created.

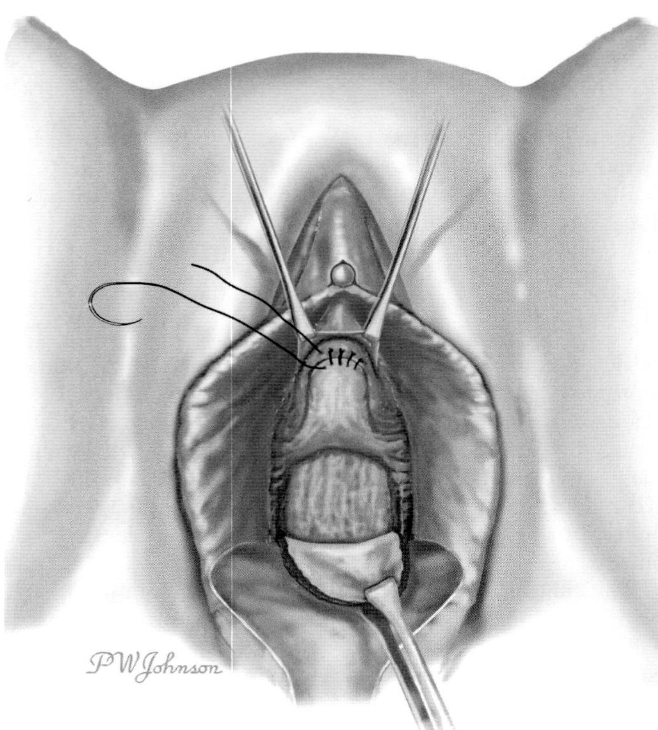

Figure 97-4 The final muscular layer is closed in a horizontal fashion and rotated superiorly behind the pubis.

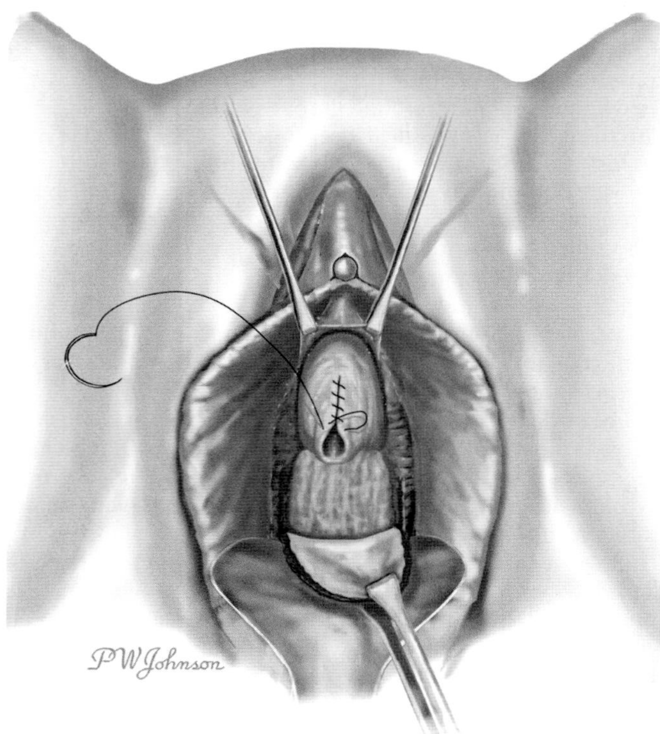

Figure 97-3 The bladder neck wall musculature is vertically closed in a running fashion after the mucosal layer has a watertight closure.

needed unless the patient has poor tissue or has been irradiated.[11] A retropubic drain is usually placed and advanced out through a suprapubic incision. The vaginal wall flap is advanced over the entire bladder neck closure, ensuring that it covers the original urethral opening (Fig. 97-5).

POSTOPERATIVE CARE AND COMPLICATIONS

A vaginal pack is placed in the vagina for tamponade purposes and to place pressure on the tissue layers to facilitate adhesion between them. I usually leave the pack in place for 24 hours. The drain is removed when drainage is less than 50 mL per day. The suprapubic tube is carefully secured and irrigated routinely until all hematuria subsides. Antibiotics are used postoperatively for 2 weeks during the healing period. After 3 weeks, a cystogram is performed to ensure the bladder neck is completely closed.

The most significant complication of transvaginal bladder neck closure is postoperative vesicovaginal fistula. This may occur early or late in the healing period. Several steps can be taken to prevent the development of fistulas: using several watertight closure layers; positioning the bladder neck high in the retropubic space; minimizing suture overlap; avoidance of postoperative bladder spasms with anticholinergics; using a drain such that inadvertent urine leakage does not fistulize to the vagina; use of a Martius flap for irradiated or poor tissue; and ensuring low-pressure drainage during the healing process. If a fistula does form despite these measures, a secondary repair may be performed after the inflammation has subsided, which is

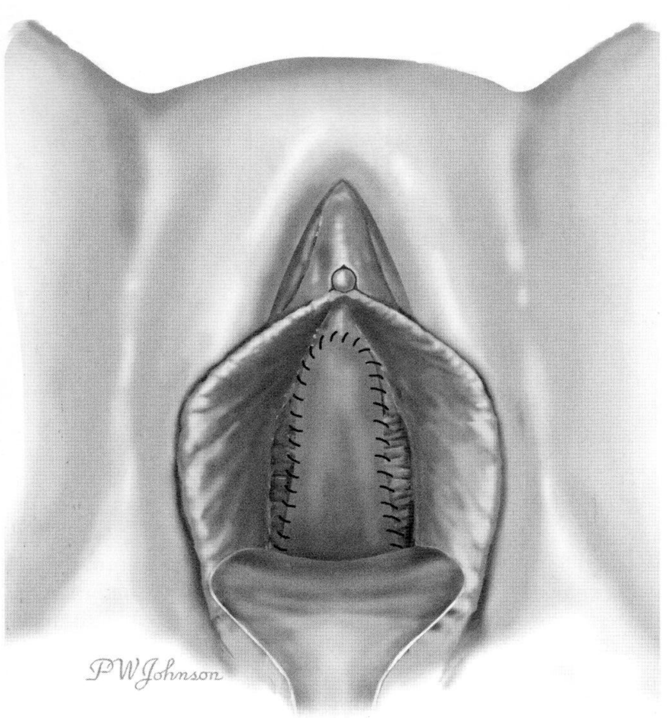

Figure 97-5 The vaginal epithelium is advanced over the entire defect and closed with a running suture.

approximately 3 months. In some cases, a pedicled graft may be required to bring good tissue into the area, or an abdominal approach can be used to allow an omental interposition flap to cover the repair.

CONCLUSIONS

Bladder neck closure is an uncommon procedure and is typically used in patients with urethras destroyed by long-term Foley usage. A successful closure can be performed by using the principles of watertight, non-overlapping suture lines and by ensuring low-pressure drainage during healing. There are many choices for urinary diversion, and these should be discussed with the patient, keeping the long-term goals in mind.

Acknowledgments

The opinions contained herein are those of the authors and are not to be construed as reflecting the views of the Air Force or the Department of Defense.

References

1. Chancellor MB, Erhard MJ, Kilholma PJ, et al: Functional urethral closure with pubovaginal sling for destroyed female urethra after long-term urethral catheterization. Urology 43:499-503, 1994.
2. Reid R, Schneider K, Fruchtman B: Closure of the bladder neck in patients undergoing continent vesicostomy for urinary incontinence. J Urol 120:40-42, 1978.
3. Feneley RCL: The management of female incontinence by suprapubic catheterization, with or without urethral closure. Br J Urol 55:203-207, 1963.
4. Zimmern PE, Hadley HR, Leach GE, Raz S: Transvaginal closure of the bladder neck and placement of a suprapubic catheter for destroyed urethra after long-term indwelling catheterization. J Urol 134:554-558, 1985.
5. Levy JB Jacobs JA, Wein AJ: Combined abdominal and vaginal approach for bladder neck closure and permanent suprapubic tube: Urinary diversion in the neurologically impaired woman. J Urol 152:2081-2082, 1994.
6. Shpall AI, Ginsberg DA: Bladder neck closure with lower urinary tract reconstruction: Technique and long-term follow-up. J Urol 172:2296-2299, 2004.
7. Mutchnik SE, Hinson JL, Nickell KG, Boone TB: Ileovesicostomy as an alternative form of bladder management in tetraplegic patients. Urology 49:353-357, 1997.
8. Schwartz SL, Kennelly MJ, McGuire EJ, Faerber GJ: Incontinent ileo-vesicostomy urinary diversion in the treatment of lower urinary tract dysfunction. J Urol 152:99-102, 1994.
9. Khoury AE, Agarwal SK, Bagli D, Mergurian P, McLorie GA: Concomitant modified bladder neck closure and Mitrofanoff urinary diversion. J Urol 162:1746-1748, 1999.
10. Zeidman EJ, Chiang H, Alarcon A, Raz S: Suprapubic cystostomy using Lowsley retractor. Urology 32:54-55, 1988.
11. Blaivas JG, Heritz DM: Vaginal flap reconstruction of the urethra and vesical neck in women: A report of 49 cases. J Urol 155:1014-1017, 1996.

Chapter 98

TISSUE ENGINEERING FOR RECONSTRUCTION OF THE URINARY TRACT AND TREATMENT OF STRESS URINARY INCONTINENCE

Daniel Eberli and Anthony Atala

Urinary incontinence is associated with impairment of quality of life, social isolation, and depressive symptoms.[1] A conservative estimate is that urinary incontinence affects approximately 20% of women. However, the prevalence may be as high as 50% among older women, with a peak at 47 years old.[2-4] In the United States the estimated annual direct cost of caring for patients with urinary incontinence is more than $16 billion.[5]

In general, treatment plans are usually directed toward the specific type of urinary incontinence, and the treatment option with the lowest risk for adverse complications is usually offered. Lifestyle intervention, pelvic floor muscle training, vaginal devices (i.e., pessaries), and pharmacologic treatments are usually considered before surgical intervention.[1]

Surgical options include endoscopic injection of bulking agents, colposuspension (e.g., Burch procedure), sling operations, traditional transvaginal needle suspension, and tension-free vaginal tape. However, many of the current surgical treatment options only offer short-term relief of urinary incontinence, and the overall success of these therapies is limited by the complications, including infection, graft erosion, bladder and bowel perforation, prolonged catheterization, and vascular injury.[2] The shortcomings of current therapies have led to the application of regenerative medicine and tissue engineering to the field of urinary incontinence.

Regenerative medicine encompasses various areas of technology, such as tissue engineering, stem cells, and cloning. Tissue engineering, one of the major components of regenerative medicine, follows the principles of cell transplantation, materials science, and engineering toward the development of biologic substitutes that can restore and maintain normal function. Tissue engineering strategies generally fall into two categories: the use of acellular matrices, which depend on the body's natural ability to regenerate for proper orientation and direction of new tissue growth, and the use of matrices with cells. Acellular tissue matrices are usually prepared by manufacturing artificial scaffolds or by removing cellular components from tissues by mechanical and chemical manipulation to produce collagen-rich matrices.[6-9] These matrices tend to slowly degrade on implantation and are generally replaced by the extracellular matrix (ECM) proteins that are secreted by the ingrowing cells. Cells can also be used for therapy by injection alone or with carriers such as hydrogels.

When cells are used for tissue engineering, a small piece of donor tissue is dissociated into individual cells. These cells are implanted directly into the host or are expanded in culture, attached to a support matrix, and then reimplanted into the host after expansion. The source of donor tissue can be heterologous, allogeneic, or autologous (Table 98-1). Ideally, structural and functional tissue replacement will occur with minimal complications. The preferred cells to use are autologous cells. For this method, a biopsy of tissue is obtained from the host, the cells are dissociated and expanded in culture, and the expanded cells are implanted into the same host.[9-12] The use of autologous cells, although it may cause an inflammatory response, avoids rejection, and the deleterious side effects of immunosuppressive medications can be avoided.

Most strategies for tissue engineering depend on a sample of autologous cells from the diseased organ of the host. However, for many patients with extensive end-stage organ failure, a tissue biopsy may not yield enough normal cells for expansion and transplantation. In other instances, primary autologous human cells cannot be expanded from a particular organ, such as the pancreas. In these situations, stem cells are envisioned as being an alternative source of cells from which the desired tissue can be derived. Stem cells can be derived from discarded human embryos (i.e., human embryonic stem cells), from fetal tissue, or from adult sources (e.g., bone marrow, fat, skin). Therapeutic cloning has also played a role in the development of the field of regenerative medicine. Therapeutic cloning, which has also been called nuclear transplantation and nuclear transfer, involves the introduction of a nucleus from a donor cell into an enucleated oocyte to generate an embryo with a genetic makeup identical to that of the donor. Stem cells can be derived from this source, which may have the potential to be used therapeutically.

Major advances have been achieved within the past decade. Regenerative medicine may extend the treatment options for urinary incontinence. However, like every new field, regenerative medicine and tissue engineering are expensive. Several of the

Table 98-1 Origin of Tissue

Source of Donor Tissue	Definition
Autologous	Same individual
Homologous (allogeneic)	Same species, different individual
Heterologous	Different species (bovine)

clinical trials involving bioengineered products have been placed on hold because of the costs involved with the specific technology. With a bioengineered product, costs are usually high because of the biologic nature of the therapies involved. As with any therapy, the costs allowed by the medical health care system for a specific technology must be limited. The costs of bioengineered products must be lowered for them to have an impact clinically. This issue is being addressed for many tissue-engineered technologies. As the technologies advance over time and the volume of the application is considered, costs will naturally decrease.

NATIVE CELLS

One of the limitations of applying cell-based regenerative medicine techniques to organ replacement has been the inherent difficulty of growing specific cell types in large quantities. By studying the privileged sites for committed precursor cells in specific organs and by exploring the conditions that promote differentiation, researchers may be able to overcome the obstacles that limit cell expansion in vitro. For example, urothelial cells have been grown in an institutional setting in the past, but only with limited expansion. Several protocols developed over the past 2 decades identified the undifferentiated cells and kept them undifferentiated during their growth phase.[13-16] Using these methods of cell culture, it is possible to expand a urothelial strain from a single specimen that initially covered a surface area of 1 cm^2 to one covering a surface area of 4202 m^2 (the equivalent of one football field) within 8 weeks.[13]

These studies indicated that it should be possible to collect autologous bladder cells from human patients, expand them in culture, and return them to the donor in sufficient quantities for reconstructive purposes.[13,15-20] Major advances have been achieved within the past decade on the possible expansion of a variety of primary human cells, with specific techniques that make the use of autologous cells possible for clinical application.

ANGIOGENIC FACTORS

The engineering of large organs requires a vascular network of arteries, veins, and capillaries to deliver nutrients to each cell. One possible method of vascularization is the use of gene delivery of angiogenic agents such as vascular endothelial growth factor (VEGF) with the implantation of vascular endothelial cells to enhance neovascularization of engineered tissues. Skeletal myoblasts from adult mice were cultured and transfected with an adenovirus encoding VEGF, and these cells were combined with human vascular endothelial cells.[21] The mixtures of cells were injected subcutaneously in nude mice, and the engineered tissues were retrieved up to 8 weeks after implantation. The transfected cells formed muscle with neovascularization, as determined by histology and immunohistochemical probing, with maintenance of their muscle volume, whereas engineered muscle of nontransfected cells had a significantly smaller mass of cells, with loss of muscle volume over time, less neovascularization, and no surviving endothelial cells. These results indicate that a combination of VEGF and endothelial cells may be useful for inducing neovascularization and volume preservation in engineered tissue. The use of angiogenic factors may support cell-based therapy in patients with postirradiation incontinence or patients with large fibrotic degeneration of the urinary sphincter.

BIOMATERIALS

For cell-based tissue engineering, the expanded cells are seeded onto a scaffold synthesized with the appropriate biomaterial. In tissue engineering, biomaterials replicate the biologic and mechanical function of the native ECM found in tissues in the body by serving as an artificial ECM. Biomaterials provide a three-dimensional space for the cells to form into new tissues with appropriate structure and function, and they allow the delivery of cells and appropriate bioactive factors (e.g., cell-adhesion peptides, growth factors) to desired sites in the body.[22] Because most mammalian cell types are anchorage dependent and will die if no cell-adhesion substrate is available, biomaterials provide a cell-adhesion substrate that can deliver cells to specific sites in the body with high loading efficiency. Biomaterials can provide mechanical support against in vivo forces such that the predefined three-dimensional structure is maintained during tissue development. Bioactive signaling agents, such as cell-adhesion peptides and growth factors, can be loaded along with cells to help regulate cellular function.

The ideal biomaterial should be biodegradable and bioresorbable to support the replacement of normal tissue without inflammation. Incompatible materials are destined for an inflammatory or foreign body response that eventually leads to rejection and necrosis. Degradation products, if produced, should be removed from the body by means of metabolic pathways at a rate that keeps the concentration of these degradation products in the tissues at a tolerable level.[23] The biomaterial should also provide an environment in which appropriate regulation of cell behavior (i.e., adhesion, proliferation, migration, and differentiation) can occur such that functional tissue can form. Cell behavior in the newly formed tissue is regulated by many interactions of the cells with their microenvironment, including interactions with cell-adhesion ligands[24] and with soluble growth factors.[25]

Biomaterials provide temporary mechanical support while the cells undergo spatial tissue reorganization. The properly chosen biomaterial should allow the engineered tissue to maintain sufficient mechanical integrity to support itself in early development, and in late development, it should have begun degradation so that it does not hinder further tissue growth.[22] Three classes of biomaterials have been used for engineering tissues (Table 98-2): naturally derived materials (e.g., collagen and alginate), acellular tissue matrices (e.g., bladder submucosa, small intestinal submucosa), and synthetic polymers such as polyglycolic acid (PGA), polylactic acid (PLA), and poly(lactic-co-glycolic acid) (PLGA). These classes of biomaterials have been tested in terms of their biocompatibility.[26,27] Naturally derived materials and acellular tissue matrices have the potential advantage of biologic recognition. However, synthetic polymers can be produced on a large scale with controlled properties of strength, degradation rate, and microstructure.

Table 98-2 Classes of Biomaterials

Class	Example
Naturally Derived Materials	Collagen and Alginate
Acellular tissue matrices	Bladder submucosa or small intestinal submucosa
Synthetic polymers	Polyglycolic acid (PGA), polylactic acid (PLA), and poly(lactic-co-glycolic acid) (PLGA)

Naturally Derived Materials

Collagen is the most abundant and ubiquitous structural protein in the body, and it can be readily purified from animal and human tissues with an enzyme treatment and salt or acid extraction.[28] Collagen implants degrade through a sequential attack by lysosomal enzymes. The in vivo resorption rate can be regulated by controlling the density of the implant and the extent of intermolecular cross-linking. The lower the density, the greater the interstitial space and the larger the pores for cell infiltration, leading to a higher rate of implant degradation. Collagen contains cell-adhesion domain sequences (e.g., RGD) that may assist to retain the phenotype and activity of many types of cells, including fibroblasts[29] and chondrocytes.[30]

Alginate, a polysaccharide isolated from seaweed, has been used as an injectable cell-delivery vehicle[31] and a cell-immobilization matrix[32] because of its gentle gelling properties in the presence of divalent ions such as calcium. Alginate is relatively biocompatible, and it is approved by the U.S. Food and Drug Administration (FDA) for human use as material to dress wounds. Alginate is a family of copolymers of D-mannuronate and L-guluronate. The physical and mechanical properties of alginate gel are strongly correlated with the proportion and length of polyguluronate block in the alginate chains.[31]

Acellular Tissue Matrices

Acellular tissue matrices are collagen-rich matrices prepared by removing cellular components from tissues. The matrices are often prepared by mechanical and chemical manipulation of a segment of tissue.[6-9] The matrices slowly degrade on implantation, and they are replaced and remodeled by ECM proteins synthesized and secreted by transplanted or ingrowing cells.

Synthetic Polymers

Polyesters of naturally occurring α-hydroxy acids, including PGA, PLA, and PLGA, are widely used in tissue engineering. These polymers have gained FDA approval for human use in a variety of applications, including sutures.[33] The ester bonds in these polymers are hydrolytically labile, and the polymers degrade by nonenzymatic hydrolysis. The degradation products of PGA, PLA, and PLGA are nontoxic natural metabolites and are eventually eliminated from the body in the form of carbon dioxide and water.[33] The degradation rate of these polymers can be tailored from several weeks to several years by altering crystalinity, initial molecular weight, and the copolymer ratio of lactic to glycolic acid. Because these polymers are thermoplastics, they can be easily formed into a three-dimensional scaffold with a desired microstructure, gross shape, and dimension by various methods, including molding, extrusion,[34] solvent casting,[35] phase-separation techniques, and gas-foaming techniques.[36] Many applications in tissue engineering require a scaffold with high porosity and ratio of surface area to volume. Other biodegradable synthetic polymers, including poly-anhydrides and poly-ortho-esters, can be used to fabricate scaffolds for tissue engineering with controlled properties.[37]

TISSUE ENGINEERING OF SPECIFIC STRUCTURES

Investigators around the world, including those at our institution, have been working toward the development of several cell types and tissues and organs for clinical application. In the following sections, we describe the engineering of tissues that may have an impact on the reconstructive strategies for urinary incontinence.

Urethra

The urethra consists of layers of longitudinal and circular smooth muscle. Weakening of the urethral muscle wall by compression damage during delivery or trauma can result in incontinence.[2] Various biomaterials without cells, such as PGA and acellular collagen-based matrices from small intestine and bladder, have been used in animal models for the regeneration of urethral tissue.[6,38-42] Some of these biomaterials, such as acellular collagen matrices derived from bladder submucosa, have also been seeded with autologous cells for urethral reconstruction. Our institution has been able to replace tubularized urethral segments with cell-seeded collagen matrices.

Acellular collagen matrices derived from bladder submucosa by our institution have been used experimentally and clinically. In animal studies, segments of the urethra were resected and replaced with acellular matrix grafts in an onlay fashion. Histologic examination showed complete epithelialization and progressive vessel and muscle infiltration, and the animals were able to void through the neo-urethras.[6] These results were confirmed in a clinical study of patients with hypospadias and urethral stricture disease.[43] Decellularized cadaveric bladder submucosa was used as an onlay matrix for urethral repair in patients with stricture disease and hypospadias. Patent, functional neo-urethras were confirmed in these patients, with up to 7 years of follow-up. The use of an off-the-shelf matrix appears to be beneficial for patients with abnormal urethral conditions, and it obviates the need for obtaining autologous grafts, decreasing operative time and eliminating donor site morbidity.

These techniques are not applicable for tubularized urethral repairs. The collagen matrices are able to replace urethral segments only when used in an onlay fashion. However, if a tubularized repair is needed, the collagen matrices should be seeded with autologous cells to avoid the risk of stricture formation and poor tissue development.[44,45] Tubularized collagen matrices seeded with autologous cells can be used successfully for urethra replacement.

Bladder

Gastrointestinal or colon segments are commonly used as tissues for bladder replacement or repair. However, both tissues are designed to absorb specific solutes, whereas bladder tissue functions as a barrier to prevent resorption of waste products. Because of the problems encountered with the use of gastrointestinal segments, numerous investigators have attempted using alternative materials and tissues for bladder replacement or repair.

The success of cell transplantation strategies for bladder reconstruction depends on the ability to use donor tissue efficiently and to provide the right conditions for long-term survival, differentiation, and growth. Urothelial and muscle cells can be expanded in vitro, seeded onto polymer scaffolds, and allowed to attach and form sheets of cells.[46] These principles were applied in the creation of tissue-engineered bladders in an animal model that required a subtotal cystectomy with subsequent replacement with a tissue-engineered organ in beagle dogs.[47] Urothelial and muscle cells were separately expanded from an autologous bladder biopsy and seeded onto a bladder-shaped biodegradable polymer scaffold. The results from this study showed that it is possible to tissue engineer bladders that are anatomically and functionally normal. Clinical trials for the application of this technology are being conducted.

Vagina

Several pathologic conditions, including congenital malformations and malignancy, can adversely affect normal vaginal development or anatomy. According to the hammock hypothesis, the vagina provides a firm backdrop for the urethra to rest against when the intra-abdominal pressure increases, preventing urinary leakage.

Vaginal reconstruction has been challenging because of the paucity of available native tissue. The feasibility of engineering vaginal tissue in vivo has been investigated.[48] Vaginal epithelial and smooth muscle cells of female rabbits were harvested, grown, and expanded in culture. These cells were seeded onto biodegradable polymer scaffolds, and the cell-seeded constructs were then implanted into nude mice for up to 6 weeks. Immunocytochemical, histologic, and Western blot analyses confirmed the presence of vaginal tissue phenotypes. Electrical field stimulation studies in the tissue-engineered constructs showed similar functional properties to those of normal vaginal tissue. When these constructs were used for autologous total vaginal replacement, patent vaginal structures were confirmed in the tissue-engineered specimens, whereas the non–cell-seeded structures were stenotic.[49]

Uterus

Congenital malformations of the uterus may have profound implications clinically. Patients with cloacal exstrophy and intersex disorders may not have sufficient uterine tissue for future reproduction. We investigated the possibility of engineering functional uterine tissue using autologous cells.[50] Autologous rabbit uterine smooth muscle and epithelial cells were harvested and then grown and expanded in culture. These cells were seeded onto preconfigured uterine-shaped biodegradable polymer scaffolds, which were used for subtotal uterine tissue replacement in the corresponding autologous animals. On retrieval 6 months after implantation, histological, immunocytochemical, and Western blot analyses confirmed the presence of normal uterine tissue components. Biomechanical analyses and organ bath studies showed that the functional characteristics of these tissues were similar to those of normal uterine tissue. Breeding studies using these engineered uteri are being performed.

Additional Treatment Options

Bulking Agents

Injectable bulking agents can be endoscopically placed in the treatment of urinary stress incontinence. The advantages in treating urinary incontinence with this minimally invasive approach include the simplicity of a quick outpatient procedure and the low morbidity associated with it. Several investigators are seeking alternative implant materials that would be safe for human use.[51]

The ideal substance for the endoscopic treatment of incontinence should be injectable, nonantigenic, nonmigratory, volume stable, and safe for human use. Toward this goal, long-term studies were conducted to determine the effect of injectable chondrocytes in vivo.[52] It was initially determined that alginate, a liquid solution of gluronic and mannuronic acid, embedded with chondrocytes could serve as a synthetic substrate for the injectable delivery and maintenance of cartilage architecture in vivo. Alginate undergoes hydrolytic biodegradation, and its degradation time can be varied depending on the concentration of each of the polysaccharides. The use of autologous cartilage for the treatment of stress urinary incontinence in humans would satisfy all the requirements for an ideal injectable substance.

Chondrocytes derived from an ear biopsy can be readily grown and expanded in culture. Neocartilage formation can be achieved in vitro and in vivo using chondrocytes cultured on synthetic biodegradable polymers. In these experiments, the cartilage matrix replaced the alginate as the polysaccharide polymer underwent biodegradation. This system was adapted for the treatment of vesicoureteral reflux in a porcine model.[53]

Patients with urinary incontinence were treated endoscopically with injected chondrocytes at three different medical centers. Phase I trials showed an approximate success rate of 80% at follow-up 3 and 12 months postoperatively.[54] These studies showed that chondrocytes can be easily harvested and combined with alginate in vitro, the suspension can be easily injected cystoscopically, and the elastic cartilage tissue formed is able to correct urinary stress incontinence.

Restoration of Functional Urinary Sphincter Muscle

The pelvic diaphragm prevents urinary incontinence by providing resting urethral tone by means of slow-twitch fibers and rapid refectory contraction by means of fast-twitch fibers if the abdominal pressure rises. The external striated urethral sphincter is mostly responsible for preventing stress urinary incontinence. The use of injectable cultured myoblasts (i.e., muscle precursor cells) for the treatment of stress urinary incontinence has been investigated, and it has the potential to become the first treatment to restore sphincter muscle function.[55,56] Labeled myoblasts were directly injected into the proximal urethra and lateral bladder walls of nude mice with a microsyringe in an open surgical procedure. Tissue harvested up to 35 days after injection contained the labeled myoblasts and had evidence of differentiation of the labeled myoblasts into regenerative myofibers. The study authors reported that a significant portion of the injected myoblast population persisted in vivo. Myoblasts were further investigated using sciatic nerve–transected rats, which showed a significant improvement of the fast-twitch muscle contraction amplitude 2 weeks after myoblast injection.[57] The study authors report a minimal inflammation response with a low number of CD4-activated lymphocytes at the injection site, confirming the immunologic acceptance of the autologous cells. A subsequent study showed a significant improvement in leak point pressure when the sciatic nerve–transected rats where treated with myoblast injections.[58]

The fact that myoblasts (Fig. 98-1) can be labeled, survive after injection, and begin the process of myogenic differentiation further supports the feasibility of using cultured cells of muscular origin as an injectable bioimplant. The use of injectable muscle precursor cells has also been investigated for use in the treatment of urinary incontinence due to irreversible urethral sphincter injury or maldevelopment. Muscle precursor cells are the quiescent satellite cells found in each myofiber that proliferate to form myoblasts and eventually form myotubes and new muscle tissue.

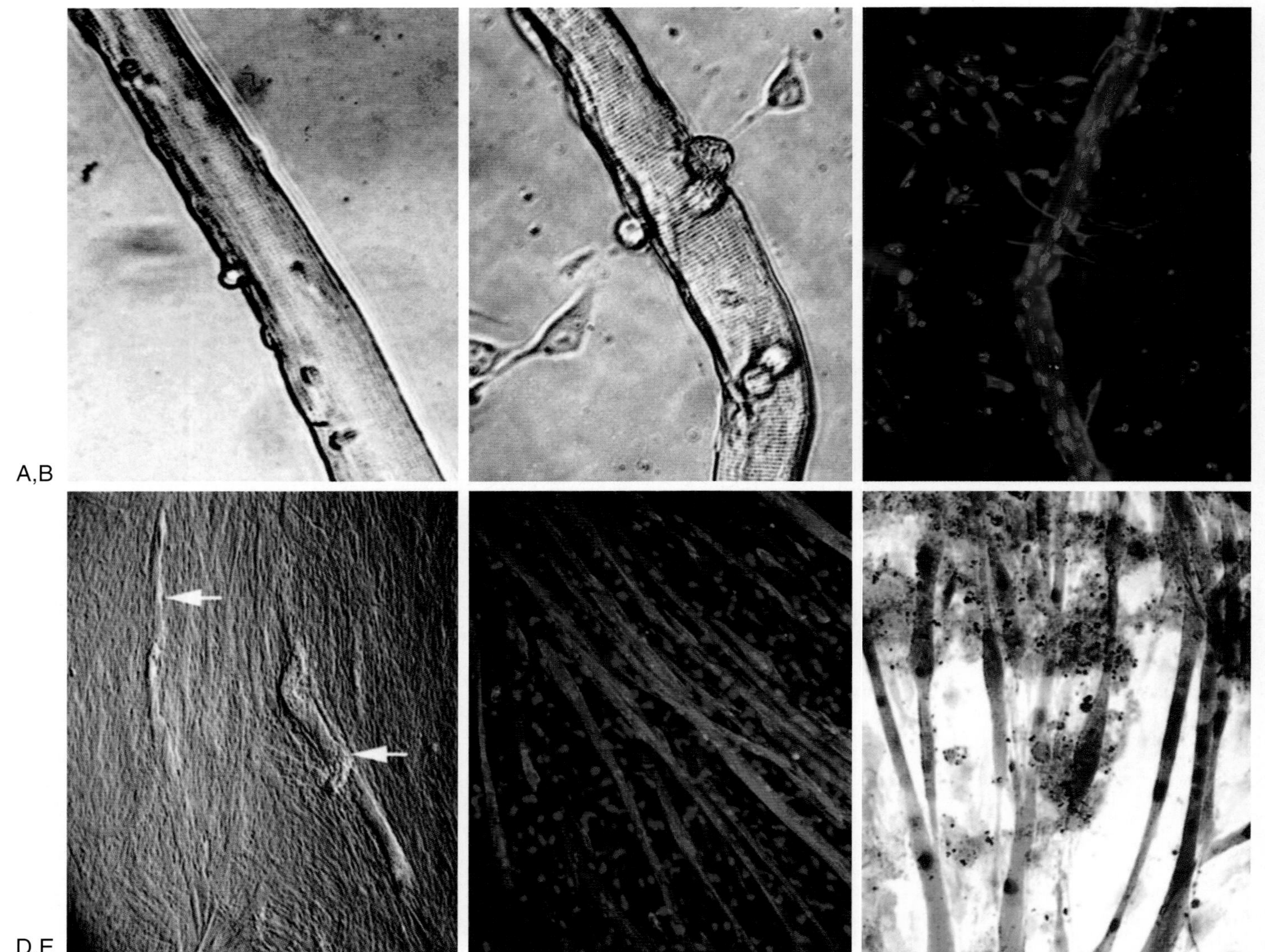

Figure 98-1 Characterization of the muscle precursor cells (i.e., satellite cells) obtained using the myofiber explant culture technique. **A,** Aspect of a single myofiber of the flexor brevis muscle immediately after isolation. **B,** After 2 days in culture, satellite cells are detached from the native myofibers. **C,** Immunofluorescence staining showed that the activated satellite cells emerging from the myofibers were desmin positive (*red*, Texas red stain). The nuclei are counterstained *(blue)* with 4′,6-diamidino-2-phenylindole (DAPI). **D,** On day 7, satellite cells had proliferated around the native myofibers *(arrows)* and started to fuse into myotubes. **E,** On day 15, mature myotubes expressing α-actinin-2 were present. **F,** The muscle precursor cells expressing β-galactosidase formed myotubes *(blue)* with the X-Gal staining on day 15 (magnification ×100). (Courtesy of Anthony Atala, MD, Wake Forest Institute for Regenerative Medicine, Winston Salem, NC.)

Intrinsic muscle precursor cells have previously been shown to play an active role in the regeneration of injured striated urethral sphincter.[59] In a subsequent study, autologous muscle precursor cells were injected into a rat model of urethral sphincter injury, and replacement of mature myotubes and restoration of functional motor units were confirmed in the regenerating sphincteric muscle tissue (Fig. 98-2).[60] The urethral sphincter contraction force was measured 5 and 30 days after injection and showed a significant improvement for the group with the muscle precursor cell injection (Fig. 98-3). This is the first demonstration of the replacement of sphincter muscle tissue and its innervation by the injection of muscle precursor cells. The innervation is crucial for muscle contraction, for activation of the satellite cells,[61] and for the maturation of the regenerated myotubes.[62]

Preclinical trials for the application of this technology are being conducted in large animals. Sphincter-derived muscle cells have been used for the treatment of urinary incontinence in a pig model.[63] The damaged sphincter was visualized by transurethral ultrasound, and the muscle precursor cells and fibroblasts were injected into the damaged zone. Our institution is performing a preclinical study in dogs. Animals that received a muscle precursor cell injection after damage to the sphincter showed a significant improvement in leak point and sphincter pressure compared with controls.

In summary, these results are promising, and the first clinical trials are within reach. Muscle precursor cells may be a minimally invasive solution for urinary incontinence in patients with irreversible urinary sphincter muscle insufficiency.

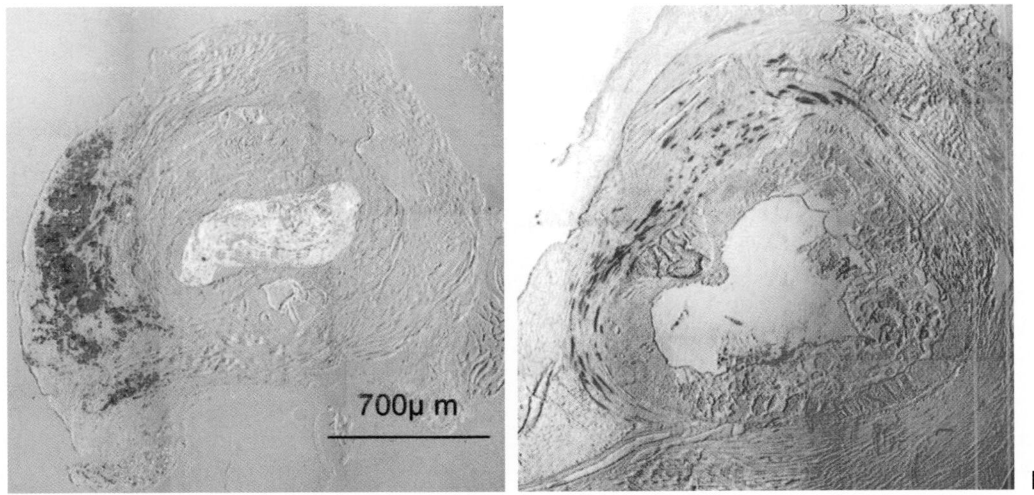

Figure 98-2 Muscle formation after injection of muscle precursor cells (MPCs). Aspect of the urethral sphincter stained with X-Gal solution on day 5 **(A)** and day 30 **(B)** after autograft of β-galactosidase–expressing MPCs. On day 5, numerous β-galactosidase–expressing cells were found in the injured side. On day 30, they had migrated toward each boundary of the injured side and had formed myotubes. (Courtesy of Anthony Atala, MD, Wake Forest Institute for Regenerative Medicine, Winston Salem, NC.)

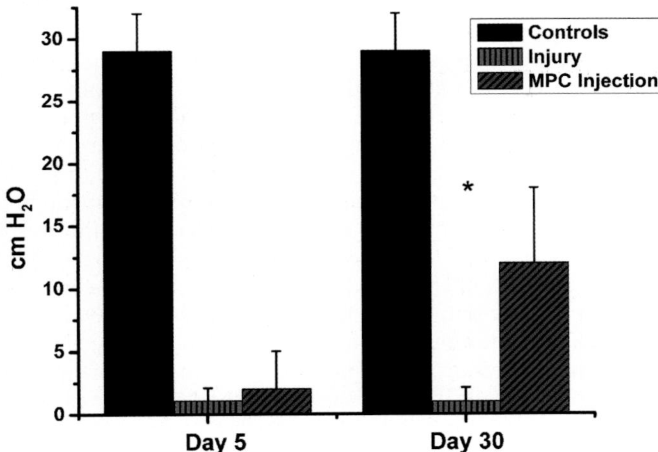

Figure 98-3 Comparison of urethral sphincter contraction force within each group at different times. The urine leak point pressure was measured with (p2) and without (p1) electrical stimulation of the striated urethral sphincter. The graph shows the difference (p2 – p1 in cm H_2O), reflecting the maximal bladder pressure that the urethral sphincter can sustain. Significant differences between normal and injured sphincters were seen at all times (P = .0001) and between injured groups with and without injection of muscle precursor cells on day 30 (P = .0028). The difference between the two injured groups was not significant on day 5 (P = .3817). (Courtesy of Anthony Atala, MD, Wake Forest Institute for Regenerative Medicine, Winston Salem, NC.)

ALTERNATE CELL SOURCES: STEM CELLS AND NUCLEAR TRANSFER

Human embryonic stem cells exhibit two remarkable properties: the ability to proliferate in an undifferentiated but pluripotent state (i.e., self-renewal) and the ability to differentiate into many specialized cell types.[64] They can be isolated by immunosurgery from the inner cell mass of the embryo during the blastocyst stage (5 days after fertilization), and they are usually grown on feeder layers consisting of mouse embryonic fibroblasts or human feeder cells.[65] Later reports showed that these cells could be grown without the use of a feeder layer,[66] thereby avoiding exposure of the human cells to mouse viruses and proteins. These cells have demonstrated longevity in culture by maintaining their undifferentiated state for at least 80 passages when grown using current protocols.[67,68]

Human embryonic stem cells have been shown to differentiate into cells from all three embryonic germ layers in vitro. Skin and neurons have been formed, indicating ectodermal differentiation.[69-72] Blood, cardiac cells, cartilage, endothelial cells, and muscle have been formed, indicating mesodermal differentiation.[73-75] Pancreatic cells have been formed, indicating endodermal differentiation.[76] As further evidence of their pluripotency, embryonic stem cells can form embryoid bodies, which are cell aggregations that contain all three embryonic germ layers while in culture, and they can form teratomas in vivo.[77]

Although there has been tremendous interest in the field of nuclear cloning since the birth of Dolly in 1997, the first successful nuclear transfer was reported more than 50 years ago by Briggs and King.[78] Cloned frogs, which were the first vertebrates derived from nuclear transfer, were subsequently reported by Gurdon in 1962,[79] but the nuclei were derived from nonadult sources. Since 2000, tremendous advances in nuclear cloning technology have been reported, indicating the relative immaturity of the field. Dolly was not the first cloned mammal to be produced from adult cells; live lambs were produced in 1996 using nuclear transfer and differentiated epithelial cells derived from embryonic discs.[80] The significance of Dolly was that she was the first mammal to be derived from an adult somatic cell using nuclear transfer.[81] Since then, animals from several species, including cattle,[82] goats,[83,84] mice,[85] and pigs,[86-89] have been grown using nuclear transfer technology.

Two types of nuclear cloning—reproductive cloning and therapeutic cloning—have been described, and a better understanding of the differences between the two types may help to alleviate some of the controversy that surrounds these technologies,[90,91] Banned in most countries for human applications, *reproductive cloning* is used to generate an embryo that has genetic material identical to that of its cell source. This embryo can be implanted into a uterus to give rise to an infant that is a clone of the donor. *Therapeutic cloning* is used to generate early-stage embryos that are explanted in culture to produce embryonic stem cell lines whose genetic material is identical to that of its source. These autologous stem cells have the potential to become almost any type of cell in the adult body and are therefore useful in tissue and organ replacement applications.[92] Therapeutic cloning, which has also been called somatic cell nuclear transfer, may provide an alternative source of transplantable cells.

According to data from the Centers for Disease Control and Prevention (CDC), an estimated 3000 Americans die every day of diseases that could have been treated with stem cell–derived tissues.[93] With current allogeneic tissue transplantation protocols, rejection is a frequent complication because of immunologic incompatibility, and immunosuppressive drugs are usually administered to treat or prevent graft-versus-host disease.[92] The use of transplantable tissue and organs derived from therapeutic cloning may enable avoidance of immune responses that typically are associated with transplantation of non-autologous tissues.[94]

Although promising, somatic cell nuclear transfer technology has certain limitations that require further improvements before therapeutic cloning can be applied widely in replacement therapy. The efficiency of the overall cloning process is low. Most embryos derived from animal cloning do not survive after implantation.[95-97] In practical terms, many nuclear transfers must be performed to produce one live offspring for animal cloning applications. The potential for cloned embryos to grow into live offspring is between 0.5% to 18% for sheep, pigs, and mice.[98] However, greater success (80%) has been reported in cattle,[99] which in part may reflect the availability of advanced bovine supporting technologies, such as in vitro embryo production and embryo transfer, which have been developed for this species for agricultural purposes. To improve cloning efficiency, further improvements are required in the many complex steps of nuclear transfer, such as enucleation and reconstruction, activation of oocytes, and cell cycle synchronization between donor cells and recipient oocytes.[100]

Common abnormalities have been found in newborn clones, including enlarged size with an enlarged placenta (i.e., large-offspring syndrome),[101] respiratory distress, and defects of the kidney, liver, heart, and brain.[102] They are also affected by obesity[103] and premature death.[104] These problems may be related to the epigenetics of the cloned cells, which involve reversible modifications of the DNA or chromatin, whereas the original DNA (genetic) sequences remain intact. Faulty epigenetic reprogramming in clones, in which the DNA methylation patterns, histone modifications, and overall chromatin structure of the somatic nuclei are not being reprogrammed to an embryonic pattern of expression, may explain these abnormalities.[97] Reactivation of key embryonic genes at the blastocyst stage is usually not present in embryos cloned from somatic cells, whereas embryos cloned from embryos consistently express early embryonic genes.[105,106] Proper epigenetic reprogramming to an embryonic state may help to improve the cloning efficiency and reduce the incidence of abnormal cloned cells.

Nuclear transfer has the potential to be used for functional reconstruction of the urinary sphincter, especially when muscle biopsies are not suitable or will not yield a sufficient amount of precursor cells. Decline of tissue regenerative potential is a hallmark of ageing, and several studies have shown the decline in muscle precursor cells with age.[107,108] Because most patients with stress urinary incontinence are elderly women, nuclear transfer may offer a tool to overcome the donor problem.

We applied the principles of tissue engineering and therapeutic cloning in an effort to produce genetically identical skeletal muscle tissue in a large animal model, the cow *(Bos taurus)*.[109] Bovine skin fibroblasts from adult Holstein steers were obtained by ear notch, and single donor cells were isolated and microinjected into the perivitelline space of donor enucleated oocytes (i.e., nuclear transfer). The resulting blastocysts were implanted into progestin-synchronized recipients to allow further in vivo growth. After 12 weeks, cloned cells were harvested, expanded in vitro, and seeded onto biodegradable scaffolds. The constructs, which consisted of the cloned muscle cells and the scaffolds, were then implanted into the subcutaneous space of the same steer from which the cells were cloned to allow tissue growth, and they were retrieved 12 weeks after implantation. The cloned skeletal explants showed spatially orientated tissue bundles with elongated multinuclear muscle fibers. The skeletal muscle was further identified by immunohistochemistry staining that was positive for sarcomeric tropomyosin and by Western blot using antibodies against desmin and myosin. Histologic analysis found extensive vascularization and little inflammation.

Because previous studies have shown that bovine clones harbor the oocyte mitochondrial DNA,[110-112] the donor egg's mitochondrial DNA (mtDNA) was thought to be a potential source of immunologic incompatibility. Differences in mtDNA-encoded proteins expressed by cloned cells may stimulate a T-cell response specific for mtDNA-encoded minor histocompatibility antigens when the cloned cells are implanted back into the original nuclear donor.[113] We used nucleotide sequencing of the mtDNA genomes of the clone and fibroblast nuclear donor to identify potential antigens in the muscle constructs. Only two amino acid substitutions distinguished the clone and the nuclear donor, and as a result, a maximum of two minor histocompatibility antigens could be defined. Given the lack of knowledge regarding peptide-binding motifs for bovine major histocompatibility complex class I molecules, there is no reliable method to predict the impact of these amino acid substitutions on bovine histocompatibility.

Oocyte-derived mtDNA was thought to be a potential source of immunologic incompatibility in the cloned renal cells. Maternally transmitted minor histocompatibility antigens in mice have been shown to stimulate skin allograft rejection in vivo and cytotoxic T-lymphocyte expansion in vitro[113] that could prevent the use of these cloned constructs in patients with chronic rejection of major histocompatibility matched human renal transplants,[114,115] We tested for a possible T-cell response to the cloned skeletal muscle using delayed-type hypersensitivity testing in vivo and Elispot analysis of interferon-γ– secreting T cells in vitro. Both analyses revealed that the cloned muscle cells showed no evidence of a T-cell response, suggesting that rejection will not necessarily occur in the presence of oocyte-derived mtDNA. This finding may represent a step forward in overcoming the histocompatibility problem of stem cell therapy.[116]

These studies demonstrated that cells derived from nuclear transfer can be successfully harvested, expanded in culture, and transplanted in vivo with the use of biodegradable scaffolds on which the single suspended cells can organize into tissue structures that are genetically identical to that of the host. These studies were the first demonstration of the use of therapeutic cloning for regeneration of tissues in vivo.

CONCLUSIONS

Regenerative medicine techniques are being employed experimentally for virtually every type of tissue and organ in the human body. Because regenerative medicine incorporates the fields of tissue engineering, cell biology, nuclear transfer, and materials science, personnel who have mastered the techniques of cell harvest, culture, expansion, transplantation, and polymer design are essential for the successful application of these technologies. Various tissues are at different stages of development, with some already being used clinically, a few in preclinical trials, and some in the discovery stage. Recent progress suggests that engineered tissues may have expanded clinical applicability in the future and may represent a viable therapeutic option for those who require tissue replacement or repair.

References

1. Holroyd-Leduc JM, Straus SE: Management of urinary incontinence in women: Scientific review. JAMA 25;291:986-995, 2004.
2. Nygaard IE, Heit M: Stress urinary incontinence [review]. Obstet Gynecol 104:607-620, 2004.
3. Brown JS, Nyberg LM, Kusek JW, et al: Proceedings of the National Institute of Diabetes and Digestive and Kidney Diseases, International Symposium on Epidemiologic Issues in Urinary Incontinence in Women. Am J Obstet Gynecol 188:77-78, 2003.
4. Burgio KL, Matthews KA, Engel BT: Prevalence, incidence and correlates of urinary incontinence in healthy, middle-aged women. J Urol 146:1255-1259, 1991.
5. Wilson L, Brown JS, Shin GP, et al: Annual direct cost of urinary incontinence. Obstet Gynecol 98:398-406, 2001.
6. Chen F, Yoo JJ, Atala A: Acellular collagen matrix as a possible "off the shelf" biomaterial for urethral repair. Urology 54:407-410, 1999.
7. Dahms SE, Piechota HJ, Dahiya R, et al: Composition and biomechanical properties of the bladder acellular matrix graft: Comparative analysis in rat, pig and human. Br J Urol 82:411-419, 1998.
8. Piechota HJ, Dahms SE, Nunes LS, et al: In vitro functional properties of the rat bladder regenerated by the bladder acellular matrix graft. J Urol 159:1717-1724, 1998.
9. Yoo JJ, Meng J, Oberpenning F, Atala A: Bladder augmentation using allogenic bladder submucosa seeded with cells. Urology 51:221-225, 1998.
10. Yoo JJ, Park HJ, Lee I, Atala A: Autologous engineered cartilage rods for penile reconstruction. J Urol 162:1119-1121, 1999.
11. Atala A, Lanza RP: Preface. In Atala A, Lanza RP (eds): Methods of Tissue Engineering. San Diego, Academic Press, 2001.
12. Atala A, Mooney D: Preface. In Atala A (ed): Tissue Engineering. Boston, Birkhauser Press, 1997.
13. Cilento BG, Freeman MR, Schneck FX, et al: Phenotypic and cytogenetic characterization of human bladder urothelia expanded in vitro. J Urol 152:665-670, 1994.
14. Scriven SD, Booth C, Thomas DF, et al: Reconstitution of human urothelium from monolayer cultures. J Urol 158:1147-1152, 1997.
15. Liebert M, Hubbel A, Chung M, et al: Expression of mal is associated with urothelial differentiation in vitro: Identification by differential display reverse-transcriptase polymerase chain reaction. Differentiation 61:177-185, 1997.
16. Puthenveettil JA, Burger MS, Reznikoff CA: Replicative senescence in human uroepithelial cells. Adv Exp Med Biol 462:83-91, 1999.
17. Nguyen HT, Park JM, Peters CA, et al: Cell-specific activation of the HB-EGF and ErbB1 genes by stretch in primary human bladder cells. In Vitro Cell Dev Biol Anim 35:371-375, 1999.
18. Tobin MS, Freeman MR, Atala A: Maturational response of normal human urothelial cells in culture is dependent on extracellular matrix and serum additives. Surg Forum 45:786-789, 1994.
19. Solomon LZ, Jennings AM, Sharpe P, et al: Effects of short-chain fatty acids on primary urothelial cells in culture: Implications for intravesical use in enterocystoplasties. J Lab Clin Med 132:279-283, 1998.
20. Lobban ED, Smith BA, Hall GD, et al: Uroplakin gene expression by normal and neoplastic human urothelium. Am J Pathol 153:1957-1967, 1998.
21. Nomi M, Atala A, Coppi PD, Soker S: Principals of neovascularization for tissue engineering. Mol Aspects Med 23:463-483, 2002.
22. Kim BS, Mooney DJ: Development of biocompatible synthetic extracellular matrices for tissue engineering. Trends Biotechnol 16:224-230, 1998.
23. Bergsma JE, Rozema FR, Bos RR, et al: In vivo degradation and biocompatibility study of in vitro pre-degraded as-polymerized polylactide particles. Biomaterials 16:267-274, 1995.
24. Hynes RO: Integrins: Versatility, modulation, and signaling in cell adhesion. Cell 69:11-25, 1992.
25. Deuel TF: Growth factors. In Lanza RP, Langer R, Chick WL (eds): Principles of Tissue Engineering. New York, Academic Press, 1997, pp 133-149.
26. Pariente JL, Kim BS, Atala A: In vitro biocompatibility assessment of naturally derived and synthetic biomaterials using normal human urothelial cells. J Biomed Mater Res 55:33-39, 2001.
27. Pariente JL, Kim BS, Atala A: In vitro biocompatibility evaluation of naturally derived and synthetic biomaterials using normal human bladder smooth muscle cells. J Urol 167:1867-1871, 2002.
28. Li ST: Biologic biomaterials: Tissue-derived biomaterials (collagen). In Bronzino JD (ed): The Biomedical Engineering Handbook. Boca Raton, FL, CRS Press, 1995, pp 627-647.
29. Silver FH, Pins G: Cell growth on collagen: A review of tissue engineering using scaffolds containing extracellular matrix. J Long Term Eff Med Implants 2:67-81, 1992.
30. Sams AE, Nixon AJ: Chondrocyte-laden collagen scaffolds for resurfacing extensive articular cartilage defects. Osteoarthritis Cartilage 3:47-59, 1995.
31. Smidsrod O, Skjak-Braek G: Alginate as immobilization matrix for cells. Trends Biotech 8:71-78, 1990.
32. Lim F, Sun AM: Microencapsulated islets as bioartificial endocrine pancreas. Science 210:908-910, 1980.
33. Gilding DK: Biodegradable polymers. In Williams DF (ed): Biocompatibility of Clinical Implant Materials. Boca Raton, FL, CRC Press, 1981, pp 209-232.
34. Freed LE, Vunjak-Novakovic G, Biron RJ, et al: Biodegradable polymer scaffolds for tissue engineering. Biotechnology (N Y) 12:689-693, 1994.
35. Mikos AG, Thorsen AJ, Czerwonka LA, et al: Preparation and characterization of poly(L-lactic acid) foams. Polymer 35:1068-1077, 1994.
36. Harris LD, Kim BS, Mooney DJ: Open pore biodegradable matrices formed with gas foaming. J Biomed Mater Res 42:396-402, 1998.
37. Peppas NA, Langer R: New challenges in biomaterials. Science 263:1715-1720, 1994.
38. Bazeed MA, Thuroff JW, Schmidt RA, Tanagho EA: New treatment for urethral strictures. Urology 21:53-67, 1983.
39. Atala A, Vacanti JP, Peters CA, et al: Formation of urothelial structures in vivo from dissociated cells attached to biodegradable polymer scaffolds in vitro. J Urol 148:658-662, 1992.

40. Olsen L, Bowald S, Busch C, et al: Urethral reconstruction with a new synthetic absorbable device: An experimental study. Scand J Urol Nephrol 26:323-326, 1992.
41. Kropp BP, Ludlow JK, Spicer D, et al: Rabbit urethral regeneration using small intestinal submucosa onlay grafts. Urology 52:138-142, 1998.
42. Sievert KD, Bakircioglu ME, Nunes L, et al: Homologous acellular matrix graft for urethral reconstruction in the rabbit: Histological and functional evaluation. J Urol 163:1958-1965, 2000.
43. El-Kassaby AW, Retik AB, Yoo JJ, Atala A: Urethral stricture repair with an off-the-shelf collagen matrix. J Urol 169:170-173, 2003.
44. De Filippo RE, Pohl HG, Yoo JJ, et al: Total penile urethral replacement with autologous cell-seeded collagen matrices [abstract]. J Urol 167:S152-S153, 2002.
45. De Filippo RE, Yoo JJ, Atala A: Urethral replacement using cell seeded tubularized collagen matrices. J Urol 168:1789-1793, 2002.
46. Atala A, Freeman MR, Vacanti JP, et al: Implantation in vivo and retrieval of artificial structures consisting of rabbit and human urothelium and human bladder muscle. J Urol 150:608-612, 1993.
47. Oberpenning F, Meng J, Yoo JJ, Atala A: De novo reconstitution of a functional mammalian urinary bladder by tissue engineering. Nat Biotechnol 17:149-155, 1999.
48. De Filippo RE, Yoo JJ, Atala A: Engineering of vaginal tissue in vivo. Tissue Eng 9:301-306, 2003.
49. De Filippo RE, Yoo JJ, Atala A: Engineering of vaginal tissue for total reconstruction. J Urol 169:A1057, 2003.
50. Wang T, Koh CJ, Yoo JJ, et al: Creation of an engineered uterus for surgical reconstruction [abstract]. Presented at the Proceedings of the American Academy of Pediatrics Section on Urology, New Orleans, LA, 2003.
51. Kershen RT, Atala A: New advances in injectable therapies for the treatment of incontinence and vesicoureteral reflux. Urol Clin North Am 26:81-94, 1999.
52. Atala A, Cima LG, Kim W, et al: Injectable alginate seeded with chondrocytes as a potential treatment for vesicoureteral reflux. J Urol 150:745-747, 1993.
53. Atala A, Kim W, Paige KT, et al: Endoscopic treatment of vesicoureteral reflux with a chondrocyte-alginate suspension. J Urol 152:641-643, 1994.
54. Bent A, Tutrone R, McLennan M, et al: Treatment of intrinsic sphincter deficiency using autologous ear chondrocytes as a bulking agent. Neurourol Urodyn 20:157-165, 2001.
55. Yokoyama T, Chancellor MB, Watanabe T, et al: Primary myoblasts injection into the urethra and bladder as a potential treatment of stress urinary incontinence and impaired detrusor contractility: Long-term survival without significant cytotoxicity. J Urol 161(Suppl):307, 1999.
56. Chancellor MB, Yokoyama T, Tirney S, et al: Preliminary results of myoblast injection into the urethra and bladder wall: A possible method for the treatment of stress urinary incontinence and impaired detrusor contractility. Neurourol Urodyn 19:279-287, 2000.
57. Cannon TW, Lee JY, Somogyi G, et al: Improved sphincter contractility after allogenic muscle-derived progenitor cell injection into the denervated rat urethra. Urology 62:958-963, 2003.
58. Lee JY, Cannon TW, Pruchnic R, et al: The effects of periurethral muscle-derived stem cell injection on leak point pressure in a rat model of stress urinary incontinence. Int Urogynecol J Pelvic Floor Dysfunct 14:31-37; discussion 37, 2003.
59. Yiou R, LaFleuchuer J, Atala A: The regeneration process of the striated urethral sphincter involves the activation of intrinsic satellite cells. Anat Embryol 206:429-435, 2003.
60. Yiou R, Yoo JJ, Atala A: Restoration of functional motor units in a rat model of sphincter injury by muscle precursor cell autografts. Transplantation 76:1053-1060, 2003.
61. Koishi K, Zhang M, McLennan IS, Harris AJ: MyoD protein accumulates in satellite cells and is neurally regulated in regenerating myotubes and skeletal muscle fibers. Dev Dyn 202:244-254, 1995.
62. Dedkov EI, Kostrominova TY, Borisov AB, Carlson BM: Reparative myogenesis in long-term denervated skeletal muscles of adult rats results in a reduction of the satellite cell population. Anat Rec 263:139-154, 2001.
63. Strasser H, Marksteiner R, Eva M, et al: Transurethral ultrasound guided injection of clonally cultured autologous myoblasts and fibroblasts: Experimental results. Paper presented at the Proceedings of the 2003 International Bladder Symposium, Arlington, VA, 2003.
64. Brivanlou AH, Gage FH, Jaenisch R, et al: Stem cells: Setting standards for human embryonic stem cells. Science 300:913-916, 2003.
65. Richards M, Fong CY, Chan WK, et al: Human feeders support prolonged undifferentiated growth of human inner cell masses and embryonic stem cells. Nat Biotechnol 20:933-936, 2002.
66. Amit M, Margulets V, Segev H, et al: Human feeder layers for human embryonic stem cells. Biol Reprod 68:2150-2156, 2003.
67. Reubinoff BE, Pera MF, Fong CY, et al: Embryonic stem cell lines from human blastocysts: Somatic differentiation in vitro [erratum in Nat Biotechnol 18:559, 2000]. Nat Biotechnol 18:399-404, 2000.
68. Thomson JA, Itskovitz-Eldor J, Shapiro SS, et al: Embryonic stem cell lines derived from human blastocysts [erratum in Science 282:1827, 1998]. Science 282:1145-1147, 1998.
69. Reubinoff BE, Itsykson P, Turetsky T, et al: Neural progenitors from human embryonic stem cells. Nat Biotechnol 19:1134-1140, 2001.
70. Schuldiner M, Eiges R, Eden A, et al: Induced neuronal differentiation of human embryonic stem cells. Brain Res 913:201-205, 2001.
71. Schuldiner M, Yanuka O, Itskovitz-Eldor J, et al: Effects of eight growth factors on the differentiation of cells derived from human embryonic stem cells. Proc Natl Acad Sci U S A 97:11307-11312, 2000.
72. Zhang SC, Wernig M, Duncan ID, et al: In vitro differentiation of transplantable neural precursors from human embryonic stem cells. Nat Biotechnol 19:1129-1133, 2001.
73. Kaufman DS, Hanson ET, Lewis RL, et al: Hematopoietic colony-forming cells derived from human embryonic stem cells. Proc Natl Acad Sci U S A 98:10716-10721, 2001.
74. Kehat I, Kenyagin-Karsenti D, Snir M, et al: Human embryonic stem cells can differentiate into myocytes with structural and functional properties of cardiomyocytes. J Clin Invest 108:407-414, 2001.
75. Levenberg S, Golub JS, Amit M, et al: Endothelial cells derived from human embryonic stem cells. Proc Natl Acad Sci U S A 99:4391-4396, 2002.
76. Assady S, Maor G, Amit M, et al: Insulin production by human embryonic stem cells. Diabetes 50:1691-1697, 2001.
77. Itskovitz-Eldor J, Schuldiner M, Karsenti D, et al: Differentiation of human embryonic stem cells into embryoid bodies compromising the three embryonic germ layers. Mol Med 6:88-95, 2002.
78. Briggs R, King TJ: Transplantation of living nuclei from blastula cells into enucleated frogs' eggs. Proc Natl Acad Sci U S A 38:455, 1952.
79. Gurdon JB: Adult frogs derived from the nuclei of single somatic cells. Dev Biol 4:256-273, 1962.
80. Campbell KH, McWhir J, Ritchie WA, Wilmut I: Sheep cloned by nuclear transfer from a cultured cell line. Nature 380:64-66, 1996.
81. Wilmut I, Schnieke AE, McWhir J, et al: Viable offspring derived from fetal and adult mammalian cells [erratum in Nature 386:200, 1997]. Nature 385:810-813, 1997.
82. Cibelli JB, Stice SL, Golueke PJ, et al: Cloned transgenic calves produced from nonquiescent fetal fibroblasts. Science 280:1256-1258, 1998.

83. Baguisi A, Behboodi E, Melican DT, et al: Production of goats by somatic cell nuclear transfer. Nat Biotechnol 17:456-461, 1999.
84. Keefer CL, Keyston R, Lazaris A, et al: Production of cloned goats after nuclear transfer using adult somatic cells. Biol Reprod 66:199-203, 2002.
85. Wakayama T, Perry AC, Zuccotti M, et al: Full-term development of mice from enucleated oocytes injected with cumulus cell nuclei. Nature 394:369-374, 1998.
86. Betthauser J, Forsberg E, Augenstein M, et al: Production of cloned pigs from in vitro systems. Nat Biotechnol 18:1055-1059, 2000.
87. Polejaeva IA, Chen SH, Vaught TD, et al: Cloned pigs produced by nuclear transfer from adult somatic cells. Nature 407:86-90, 2000.
88. Onishi A, Iwamoto M, Akita T, et al: Pig cloning by microinjection of fetal fibroblast nuclei. Science 289:1188-1190, 2000.
89. De Sousa PA, Dobrinsky JR, Zhu J, et al: Somatic cell nuclear transfer in the pig: Control of pronuclear formation and integration with improved methods for activation and maintenance of pregnancy. Biol Reprod 66:642-650, 2002.
90. Colman A, Kind A: Therapeutic cloning: Concepts and practicalities. Trends Biotechnol 18:192-196, 2000.
91. Vogelstein B, Alberts B, Shine K: Genetics: Please don't call it cloning! Science 295:1237, 2002.
92. Hochedlinger K, Jaenisch R: Nuclear transplantation, embryonic stem cells, and the potential for cell therapy. N Engl J Med 349:275-286, 2003.
93. Lanza RP, Cibelli JB, West MD, et al: The ethical reasons for stem cell research. Science 292:1299, 2001.
94. Lanza RP, Cibelli JB, West MD: Prospects for the use of nuclear transfer in human transplantation. Nat Biotechnol 17:1171-1174, 1999.
95. Solter D: Mammalian cloning: Advances and limitations. Nat Rev Genet 1:199-207, 2000.
96. Rideout WM III, Eggan K, Jaenisch R: Nuclear cloning and epigenetic reprogramming of the genome. Science 293:1093-1098, 2001.
97. Hochedlinger K, Jaenisch R: Nuclear transplantation: Lessons from frogs and mice. Curr Opin Cell Biol 14:741-748, 2002.
98. Tsunoda Y, Kato Y: Recent progress and problems in animal cloning. Differentiation 69:158-161, 2002.
99. Kato Y, Tani T, Sotomaru Y, et al: Eight calves cloned from somatic cells of a single adult. Science 282:2095-2098, 1998.
100. Dinnyes A, De Sousa P, King T, et al: Somatic cell nuclear transfer: Recent progress and challenges. Cloning Stem Cells 4:81-90, 2002.
101. Young LE, Sinclair KD, Wilmut I: Large offspring syndrome in cattle and sheep. Rev Reprod 3:155-163, 1998.
102. Cibelli JB, Campbell KH, Seidel GE, et al: The health profile of cloned animals. Nat Biotechnol 20:13-14, 2002.
103. Tamashiro KL, Wakayama T, Akutsu H, et al: Cloned mice have an obese phenotype not transmitted to their offspring. Nat Med 8:262-267, 2002.
104. Ogonuki N, Inoue K, Yamamoto Y, et al: Early death of mice cloned from somatic cells. Nat Genet 30:253-254, 2002.
105. Bortvin A, Eggan K, Skaletsky H, et al: Incomplete reactivation of Oct4-related genes in mouse embryos cloned from somatic nuclei. Development 130:1673-1680, 2003.
106. Boiani M, Eckardt S, Scholer HR, McLaughlin KJ: Oct 4 distribution and level in mouse clones: Consequences for pluripotency. Genes Dev 16:1209-1219, 2002.
107. Conboy IM, Conboy MJ, Smythe GM, Rando TA: Notch-mediated restoration of regenerative potential to aged muscle. Science 302:1575-1577, 2003.
108. Conboy IM, Rando TA: The regulation of Notch signaling controls satellite cell activation and cell fate determination in postnatal myogenesis. Dev Cell 3:397-409, 2002.
109. Lanza RP, Chung HY, Yoo JJ, et al: Generation of histocompatible tissues using nuclear transplantation. Nat Biotechnol 20:689-699, 2002.
110. Evans MJ, Gurer C, Loike JD, et al: Mitochondrial DNA genotypes in nuclear transfer-derived cloned sheep. Nat Genet 23:90-93, 1999.
111. Hiendleder S, Schmutz SM, Erhardt G, et al: Transmitochondrial differences and varying levels of heteroplasmy in nuclear transfer cloned cattle. Mol Reprod Dev 54:24-31, 1999.
112. Steinborn R, Schinogl P, Zakhartchenko V, et al: Mitochondrial DNA heteroplasmy in cloned cattle produced by fetal and adult cell cloning. Nat Genet 25:255-257, 2000.
113. Fischer Lindahl K, Hermel E, Loveland BE, Wang CR: Maternally transmitted antigen of mice: A model transplantation antigen. Annu Rev Immunol 9:351-372, 1991.
114. Hadley GA, Linders B, Mohanakumar T: Immunogenicity of MHC class I alloantigens expressed on parenchymal cells in the human kidney. Transplantation 54:537-542, 1992.
115. Yard BA, Kooymans-Couthino M, Reterink T, et al: Analysis of T cell lines from rejecting renal allografts. Kidney Int 39:S133-S138, 1993.
116. Auchincloss H, Bonventre JV: Transplanting cloned cells into therapeutic promise. Nat Biotechnol 20:665-666, 2002.

Chapter 99

VAGINOPLASTY—CONSTRUCTION OF NEOVAGINA

Malcolm A. Lesavoy

Reconstruction of the female perineum is indicated for congenital absence of the vagina, lymphedema, vaginal defects, previous ablative surgery for various perineal malignancies, relief of pain after radiation therapy, and repair of labial hypertrophy. Vaginal reconstruction has become a standard procedure performed by plastic surgeons, gynecologists, and urologists. The most common indication for vaginal reconstruction is congenital absence of the vagina.

In general, the results of vaginal reconstruction are satisfactory. However, problems may include inadequate genital wound coverage because of foreshortened graft or flap harvest, fecal contamination if preoperative bowel preparation has not been adequate, adjacent urethral injuries during dissection of the new vaginal pocket, and difficult immobilization of the patient in the postoperative period.

Counseller[1] reported that congenital absence of the vagina occurs in approximately 1 of every 4000 births and that these abnormalities usually coexist with uterus and urinary tract abnormalities. Usually, the ovaries are not affected, and the secondary sex characteristics develop normally. Embryologically, because the cervix and vagina initially form a solid unit, the lack of cavitation and cell death needed to form a vagina is the reason for vaginal agenesis.[1] However, the hormonal factors that stimulate cavitation are unknown.

Patients with labial hypertrophy undergo labioplasty for functional, aesthetic, and social reasons. Hypertrophy of the labia minor or labia majora may be congenital or acquired. Patients with this condition may experience inflammation, poor hygiene, and self-consciousness during sexual activity and when wearing tight pants. Reduction of the labia minora or labia majora is a relatively minor outpatient procedure that yields satisfactory results for many patients.

VAGINAL RECONSTRUCTION

History

In 1573, a student of Vesalius, Realdus Colombus, first reported vaginal agenesis, and it was not until 1872 that Heppner described vaginal reconstruction using the labia.[2] However, the landmark report for vaginal reconstruction is credited to Abbe in 1898.[3] In one patient, Abbe described dissecting a canal and lining it with split-thickness skin grafts.

These skin grafts were placed over a rubber stent packed with gauze. After 10 days, the stent was removed, and the skin grafts were completely vascularized. The patient was asked to wear a vaginal conformer postoperatively, and evidently, intercourse was possible. However, Abbe's report was lost for almost 40 years, until McIndoe[4] popularized the Abbe technique by lining the new vaginal canal with partial-thickness skin grafts. McIndoe reported an impressive array of 63 repairs,[5] and in 1948, Counseller reported 70.[1] Other methods of vaginal reconstruction have been attempted, but most have had undesirable effects, especially when segments of the gastrointestinal tract have been used for lining the new vaginal canal. In 1953, Conway and Stark[6] described use of the rectum; earlier, Sneguireff,[7] Popow,[8] and Schubert[9] had described the same thing. In 1904, Baldwin[10] even described using a loop of ileum. However, obvious difficulties with bowel transposition such as necrosis, infection, and abscess formation occurred. If the procedure was successful, the secretions arising from the bowel lining were mostly inappropriate and unwanted. The added morbidity of an intra-abdominal procedure, various bowel anastomoses, the possibility of vascular compromise, and undesired mucosal secretions account for the lack of popularity of these procedures.

The Frank procedure, a nonoperative technique, has been successful in some instances of incomplete vaginal atresia. In 1927, Frank and Geist[11] demonstrated the use of intermittent pressure at the perineal dimple between the anus and the urethra in the normal location of the vagina. This pressure is applied until the patient feels mild discomfort by a series of graduated obturators in the form of increasing sizes of test tubes. The pressure is relieved and then reapplied. The skin is inwardly stretched in the same way that a skin expander works with an outward force. This process continues for weeks until the largest dilator can be introduced within the neovagina and worn comfortably. This procedure requires a very compliant and persistent patient and an anatomy that is consistent with incomplete vaginal agenesis. The skin lining the new vagina is cutaneous squamous epithelium, and it must be lubricated externally to allow intercourse.

Surgical Techniques

Abbe-McIndoe Procedure

Over the years, the Abbe-McIndoe procedure evolved to become the easiest and most successful method of vaginal reconstruction, avoiding the risks and disadvantages of laparotomy (Figs. 99-1 and 99-2). The procedure must be performed under general or spinal anesthesia. A Y-shaped incision is made along the median raphe between the urethra and the anus. A catheter is placed in the urethra, and dissection is carried cephaloposteriorly. This dissection can be done relatively bluntly, and safety is ensured by keeping a gloved finger in the rectum for tactile ease of dissection. The Y incision allows three cutaneous flaps to be enfolded into the vaginal canal so that circumferential scar contraction can be avoided. The depth of dissection should be somewhat exaggerated and is in the range of 10 to 14 cm in the adult. The surgeon

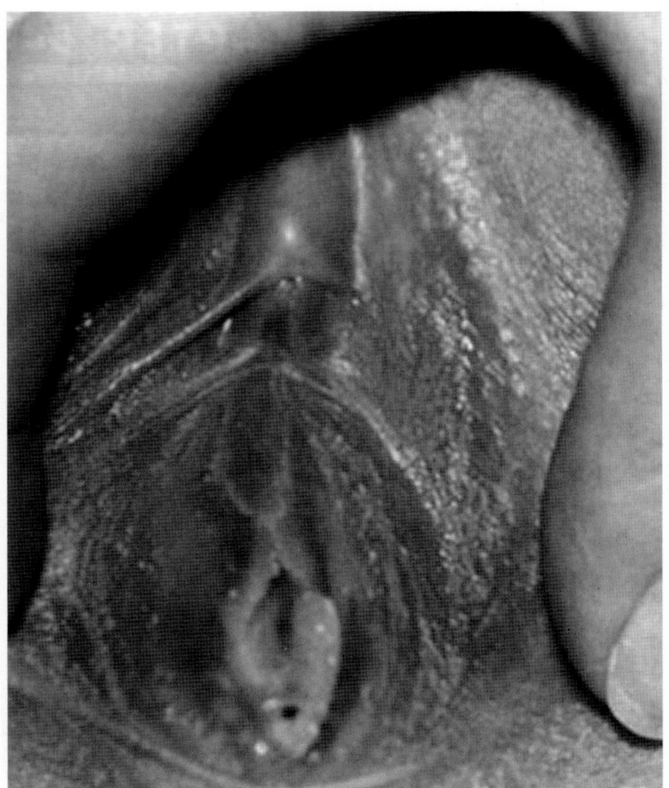

Figure 99-1 Congenital vaginal aplasia with an enlarged urethral meatus below the clitoris. (From Lesavoy MA, Carter EJ: Vaginal reconstruction. In Raz S [ed]: Female Urology, 2nd ed. Philadelphia, WB Saunders, 1996, pp 605-616.)

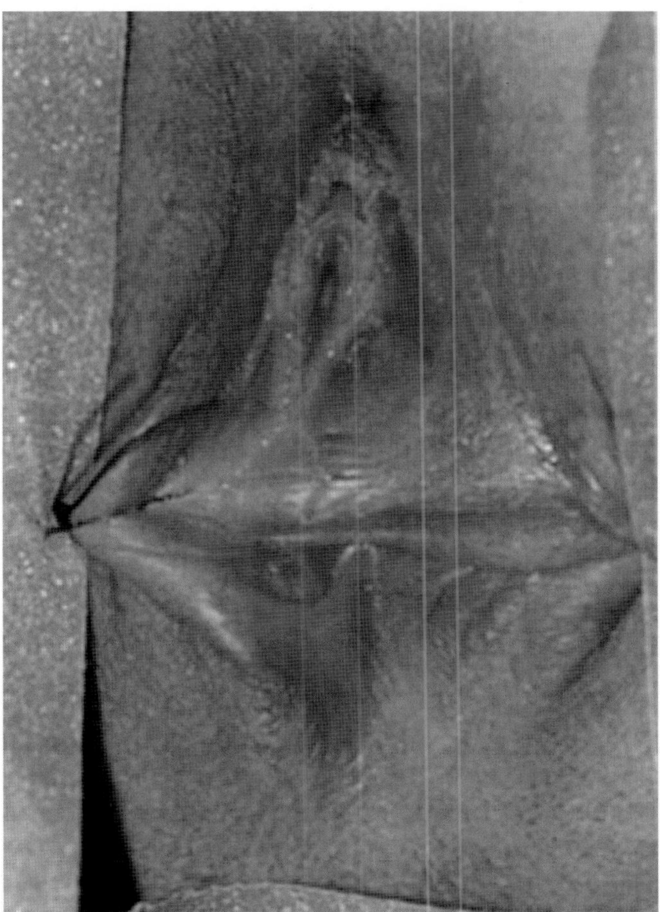

Figure 99-2 Sutures holding the labia majora. (From Lesavoy MA, Carter EJ: Vaginal reconstruction. In Raz S [ed]: Female Urology, 2nd ed. Philadelphia, WB Saunders, 1996, pp 605-616.)

must overcorrect somewhat because of the expected subsequent contraction (Fig. 99-3).

After the vaginal canal has been bluntly dissected, a partial-thickness skin graft is harvested from the buttock-hip area. The surgeon must keep in mind the subsequent scar that will ensue from this partial-thickness skin graft and therefore should avoid harvesting the graft from an area low on the thigh. The skin graft can be taken with any type of dermatome, and two or three sheets of skin may be needed to achieve a total dimension of approximately 14 × 7 cm.

Several techniques have been developed to apply the skin graft to the vaginal canal. Historically, candle wax, carved balsa wood, gauze packing, syringe casing, dental wax, and hard plastic conformers have been used. The Heyer-Schulte Company has produced a soft, pliable, and expandable vaginal conformer that works very well. This stent has a central semirigid foam core and a surrounding silicone envelope that can be expanded with air or saline (Fig. 99-4). There is a central drain site through the core of the stent. After the graft has been harvested, the vaginal stent should be inflated with air and lubricated with mineral oil.

The skin graft sheets are sutured to each other and placed over the stent with the raw dermal sides out (Fig. 99-5). The epidermal side of the skin is adjacent to the stent. Subsequently, hemostasis is checked in the neovaginal canal, and the stent and overlying skin grafts are eased into the canal (Fig. 99-6). It may be necessary to deflate the vaginal stent while slowly rotating and pushing the stent and skin graft into the vaginal canal, but after the stent is seated to the depth of the dissection, it should again be inflated to spread out the skin graft, ensure direct apposition to the raw walls, and provide an excellent bolster for the ensuing neovascularization of the skin graft.

The flaps from the Y incision are sutured to the superficial ends of the skin graft in a tacking fashion with absorbable sutures. Fluff gauze is then packed around the perineum under compression, and the labia majora are sutured to each other to ensure that the stent does not slide out of the canal.

Postoperatively, the patient remains in bed for a minimum of 5 days and is medically constipated (a lower bowel preparation is required preoperatively). On the fifth or sixth postoperative day, the patient is sedated in bed, and the labial sutures are removed. The skin graft can then be checked by aspirating the outer lumen of the Heyer-Schulte vaginal stent and deflating it, gently removing the stent, and leaving the skin graft intact within the vaginal vault. If there is any difficulty with this maneuver, mineral oil can be injected between the stent and the skin graft using a soft rubber catheter. This lubricates the interface between the stent and the skin graft so that disruption and shearing of the skin graft are avoided when the stent is removed. The perineum can be cleansed, and the stent can be washed and replaced immediately. Subsequently, a perineal binder can be applied, and the

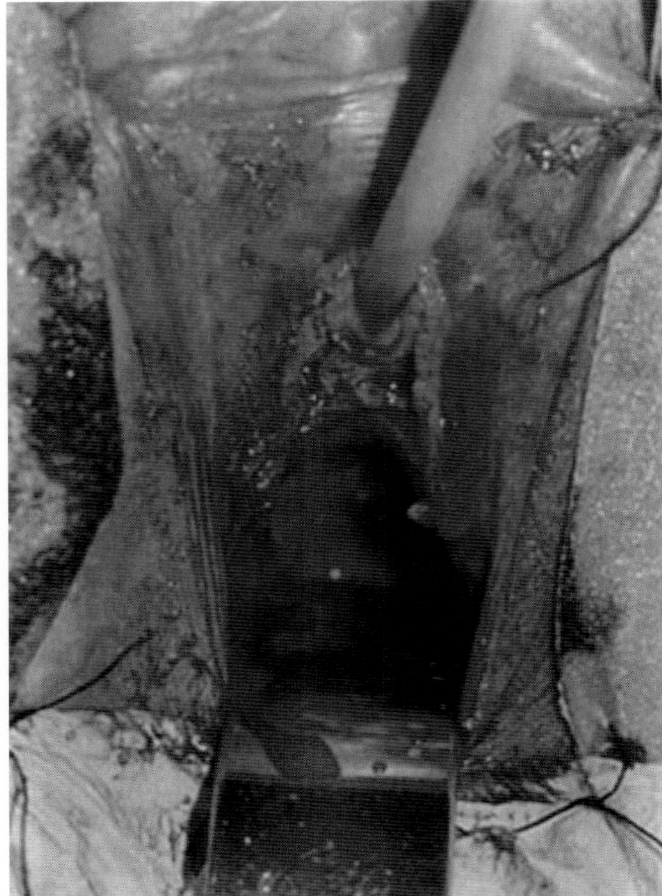

Figure 99-3 Catheter in the urethra and dissection of the neovaginal canal. (From Lesavoy MA, Carter EJ: Vaginal reconstruction. In Raz S [ed]: Female Urology, 2nd ed. Philadelphia, WB Saunders, 1996, pp 605-616.)

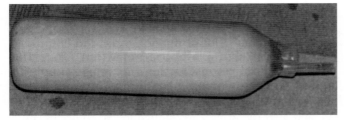

Figure 99-4 Heyer-Schulte inflatable vaginal stent. (From Lesavoy MA, Carter EJ: Vaginal reconstruction. In Raz S [ed]: Female Urology, 2nd ed. Philadelphia, WB Saunders, 1996, pp 605-616.)

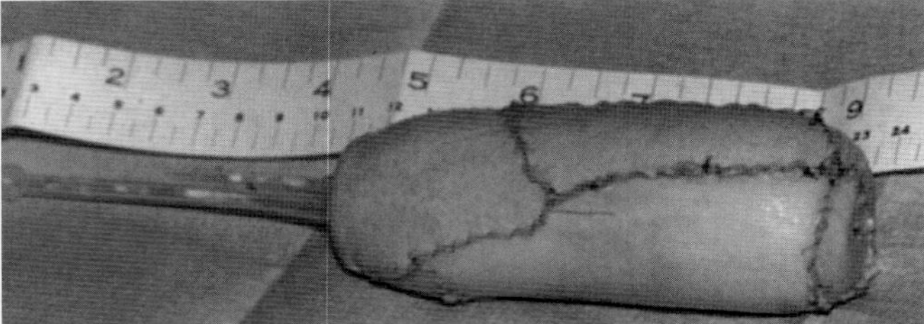

Figure 99-5 Split-thickness skin graft sutured around the vaginal stent, with the epithelial side inward next to the stent and the raw side out. (From Lesavoy MA, Carter EJ: Vaginal reconstruction. In Raz S [ed]: Female Urology, 2nd ed. Philadelphia, WB Saunders, 1996, pp 605-616.)

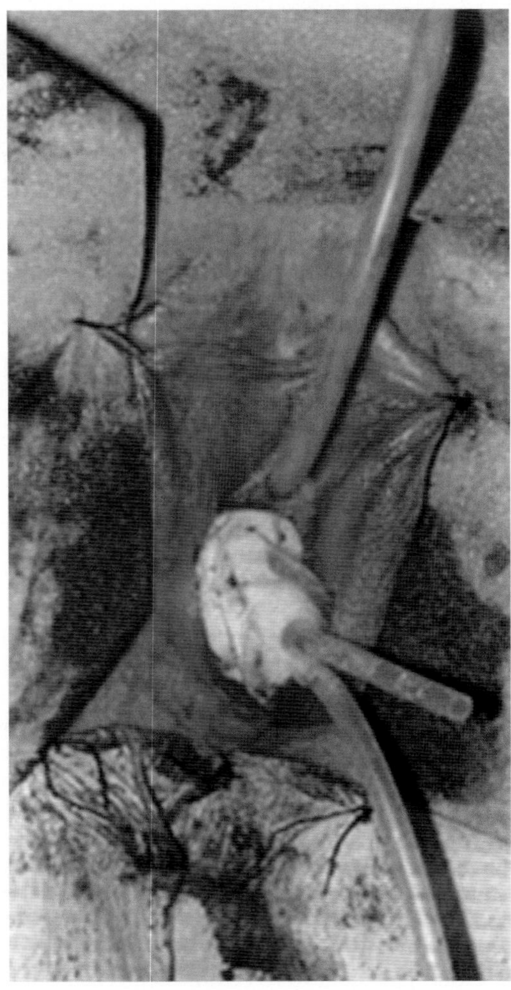

Figure 99-6 Vaginal stent with the skin graft invaginated into the neovaginal canal. (From Lesavoy MA, Carter EJ: Vaginal reconstruction. In Raz S [ed]: Female Urology, 2nd ed. Philadelphia, WB Saunders, 1996, pp 605-616.)

patient can be allowed to ambulate; the constipating medicine is then discontinued.

The vaginal stent is checked every other day, and the patient is usually discharged on the seventh or eighth postoperative day. The patient should be fully aware of the mechanics of the stent so that she can remove, wash, and reintroduce the stent daily while at home.

After vaginal reconstruction, a conformer must be worn for a minimum of 6 months postoperatively. If this is not done, contraction of the vaginal vault will ensue. After 3 or 4 months, as the skin graft matures, vaginal intercourse should be encouraged. This procedure should not be done unless intercourse is anticipated. Intercourse provides an excellent obturator and conformer. After 6 months, the conformer can be eliminated during the day but should be worn at night. If the patient is active

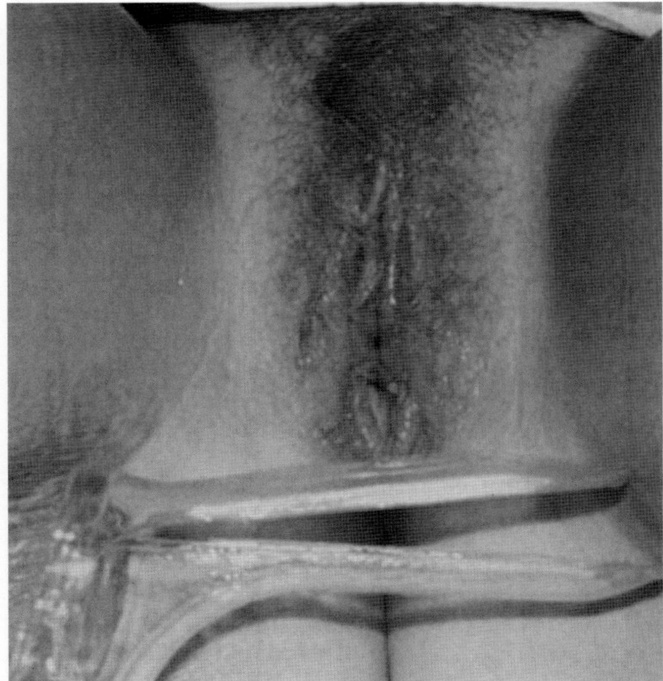

Figure 99-7 A photograph taken 3 months postoperatively shows the normal-looking vulva and the size of the speculum that can be inserted into the vagina. (From Lesavoy MA, Carter EJ: Vaginal reconstruction. In Raz S [ed]: Female Urology, 2nd ed. Philadelphia, WB Saunders, 1996, pp 605-616.)

sexually and has intercourse two to three times per week, the conformer can be eliminated. However, if there is a time when intercourse is not anticipated for weeks or months, the conformer should be worn at night (Figs. 99-7 to 99-10). Because the skin grafts do not have the same properties as normal vaginal mucosa and do not have secretory abilities, most patients require the application of lubricants before intercourse.[30,31]

Full-Thickness Skin Grafts

Full-thickness skin grafts are important for certain types of vaginal reconstruction, such as for vaginal aplasia, vaginal stenosis, intersex conditions, and iatrogenic disease. One advantage of these grafts is that they allow reconstruction at an earlier age (any time after puberty), providing psychological reassurance as the child develops that she is normal. They also reduce postoperative stenting time and minimize vaginal stenosis by decreasing postoperative vaginal contraction. They improve the cosmesis of the donor site, and a full-thickness skin graft grows with the body proportionately.[12,13] Inguinal donor sites are used for full-thickness skin grafts, and the donor site closure occurs primarily.

Flaps

Vulvobulbocavernosus Myocutaneous Flap

The vulvobulbocavernosus myocutaneous flap was described by Knapstein and colleagues[14] in 1990. This flap is based on the skin fat and underlying vulvobulbocavernosus erectile muscle tissue, and it is useful because of the low axis of the flap. It is not easily used for transfer into the upper pelvis, but it is best for reconstruction of the vagina after a pelvic exenteration that removes the perineal body and the anus (i.e., a lower pelvic defect). This

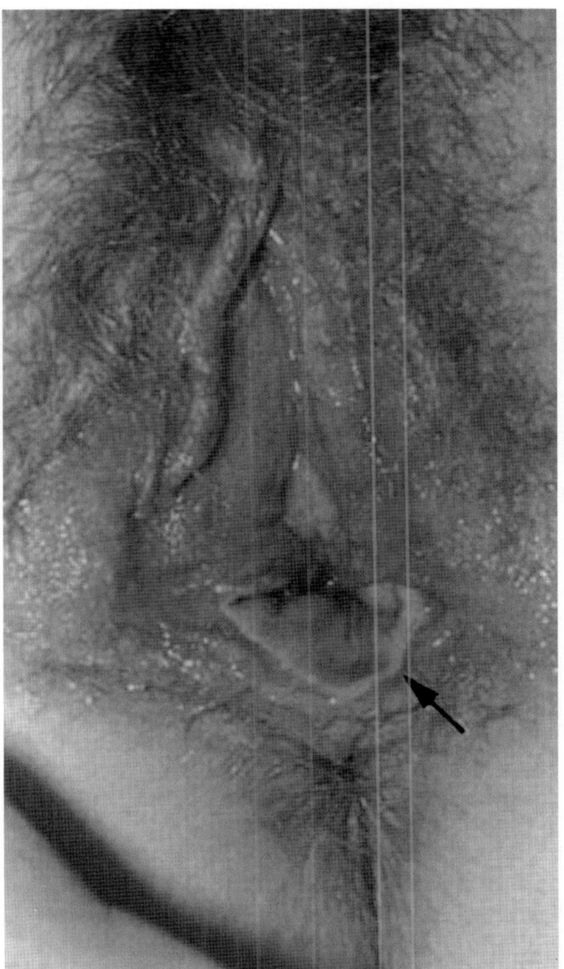

Figure 99-8 Discrepancy in the skin graft color of the neovagina. (From Lesavoy MA, Carter EJ: Vaginal reconstruction. In Raz S [ed]: Female Urology, 2nd ed. Philadelphia, WB Saunders, 1996, pp 605-616.)

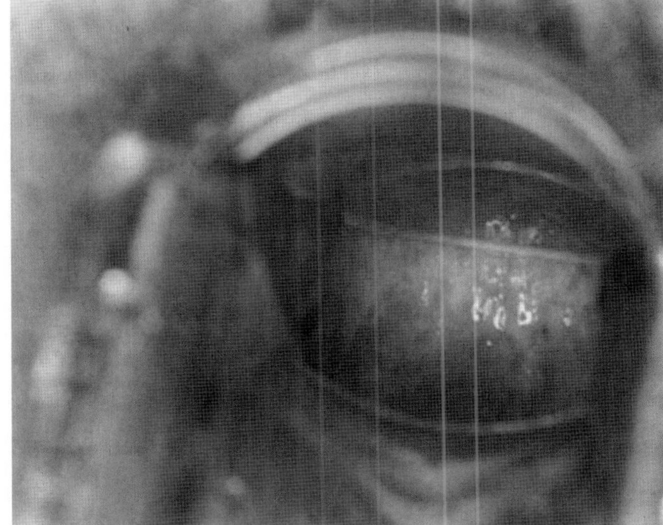

Figure 99-9 Depth of the neovagina as seen through the plastic speculum. (From Lesavoy MA, Carter EJ: Vaginal reconstruction. In Raz S [ed]: Female Urology, 2nd ed. Philadelphia, WB Saunders, 1996, pp 605-616.)

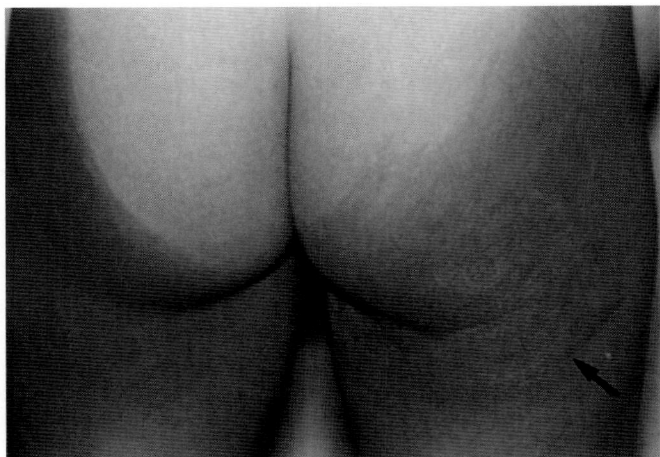

Figure 99-10 Donor site on the right buttock. (From Lesavoy MA, Carter EJ: Vaginal reconstruction. In Raz S [ed]: Female Urology, 2nd ed. Philadelphia, WB Saunders, 1996, pp 605-616.)

is a relatively new procedure and should be considered for patients with anterior or total exenteration with low rectal anastomosis.

The vulvobulbocavernosus myocutaneous flap usually is not large enough to form a complete vaginal canal. The anterior edges of the flap are sewn together to form the anterior margins of the newly formed vaginal cylinder. Its disadvantage is the retention of vulvar hair, which results in vaginal discharge and a strong odor. The blood and nerve supply comes from the pudendals.[15]

Gracilis Myocutaneous Flaps

The gracilis muscle is the most common flap used after pelvic exenteration for vaginal reconstruction.[16,17] After pelvic exenteration. an abdominoperineal resection, or vaginal irradiation (Fig. 99-11), the patient is usually left with a large vaginal defect. Use of a gracilis island myocutaneous flap can enhance vaginal reconstruction. It also provides adequate vaginal length and is an expendable muscle for the most part.

The gracilis myocutaneous flap provides sufficient bulk to fill the empty pelvic space and simultaneously brings its own blood supply, leading to a softness and pliability not achievable with skin graft techniques. The disadvantage of the gracilis may include a loss of approximately 10% to 20% of the flap due to vascular compromise of the flap resulting from potential tension of its small-caliber vascular pedicle when transposed into the pelvic defect. Residual scarring on the legs is commonly a source of minor complaints.[18-20]

The principle of employing muscle with its overlying skin, vascularized by the muscular perforators, has been well documented in the plastic and reconstructive surgical literature by Owens (1955),[21] Bakamjian (1963),[22] Hueston and McConchie (1968),[23] and McCraw and colleagues (1976).[24] McCraw and associates were the first to describe the principle of the skin island over the muscle unit, and this principle is applicable to vaginal reconstruction. McCraw's paper on vaginal reconstruction was one of the landmark works in the plastic surgery literature, and the findings revived the use of myocutaneous flaps.

The operation begins with the patient in the lithotomy position (Fig. 99-12). Unilateral or bilateral island gracilis myocutaneous flaps are harvested (Fig. 99-13) based on their superior neurovascular pedicles (Fig. 99-14). The flap can then be tunneled (Fig. 99-15) under intact perineal skin (Fig. 99-16) and invaginated into the neovaginal canal. A conformer is not needed, and the donor sites are closed in a linear fashion with primary approximation along the medial thigh area (see Fig. 99-15).

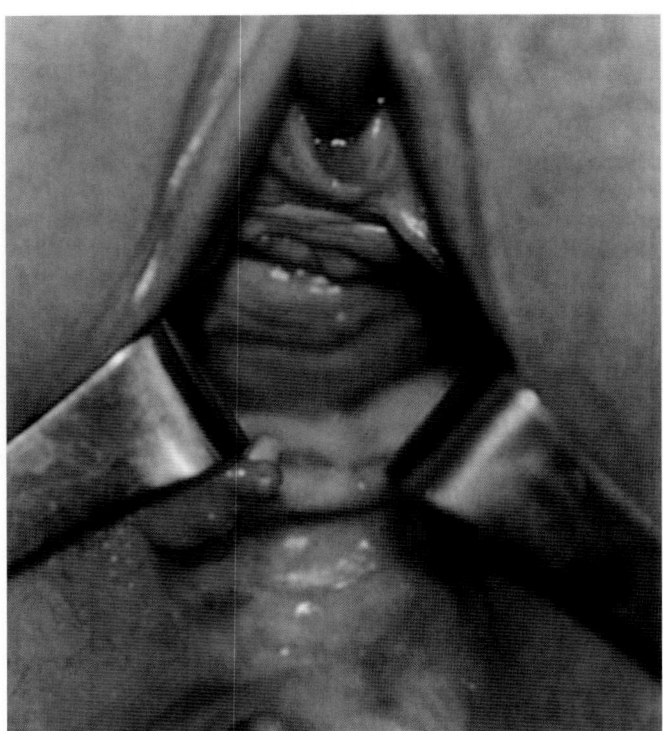

Figure 99-11 A patient with radiation vaginitis had severe pain, drainage, fibrosis, and contraction. (From Lesavoy MA, Carter EJ: Vaginal reconstruction. In Raz S [ed]: Female Urology, 2nd ed. Philadelphia, WB Saunders, 1996, pp 605-616.)

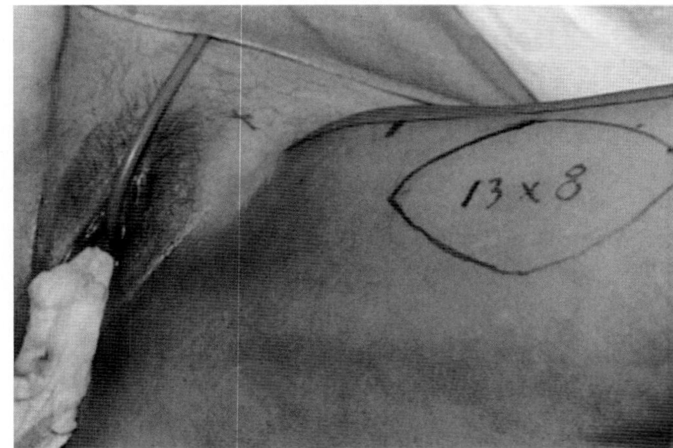

Figure 99-12 After excision of radiation-damaged tissue and a pack in the vaginal vault, a 13 × 8 cm gracilis myocutaneous island flap is outlined on the left medial thigh. (From Lesavoy MA, Carter EJ: Vaginal reconstruction. In Raz S [ed]: Female Urology, 2nd ed. Philadelphia, WB Saunders, 1996, pp 605-616.)

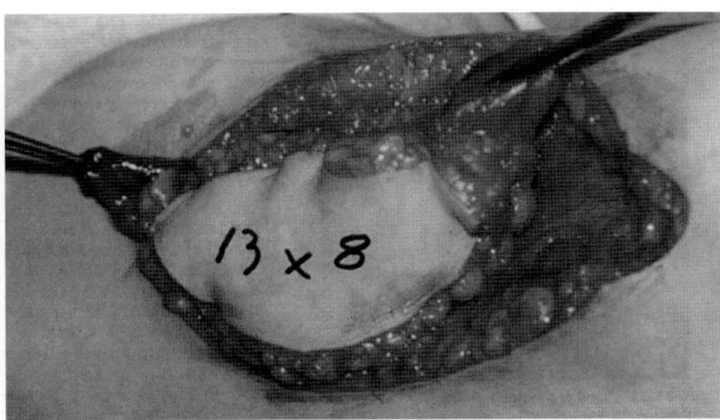

Figure 99-13 The gracilis muscle and island skin flap are isolated. (From Lesavoy MA, Carter EJ: Vaginal reconstruction. In Raz S [ed]: Female Urology, 2nd ed. Philadelphia, WB Saunders, 1996, pp 605-616.)

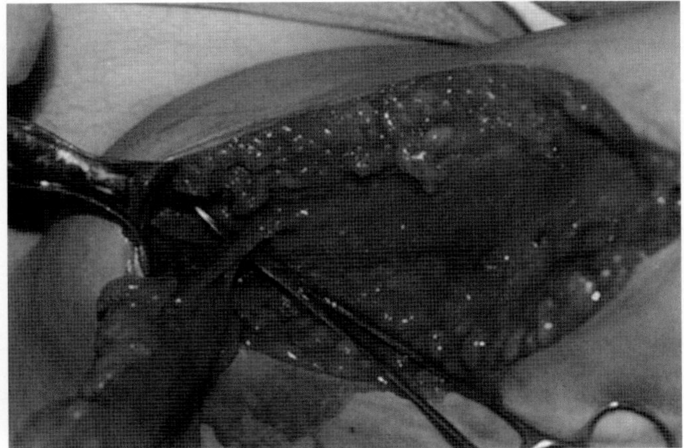

Figure 99-14 The undersurface of the gracilis myocutaneous island flap and its neurovascular bundle. (From Lesavoy MA, Carter EJ: Vaginal reconstruction. In Raz S [ed]: Female Urology, 2nd ed. Philadelphia, WB Saunders, 1996, pp 605-616.)

A unilateral gracilis myocutaneous flap may be used for radiation contracture and pain of the vaginal vault (see Figs. 99-11 to 99-17) Sensibility of the skin of the gracilis myocutaneous island is maintained through the sensory branches of the obturator nerve as described by Lesavoy and colleagues.[25] However, sensitivity of the transposed skin is not the same as that of a normal vagina. Sensitivity to pressure is excellent, but tactile sensitivity is diminished.[26] Sexual sensitivity is mostly cerebral.

Rectus Abdominis Myocutaneous Flap

Because of its success in breast reconstruction, the rectus abdominis myocutaneous flap can also be used for vaginal reconstruction. Its primary arterial blood supply is the inferior epigastric vessels. Two island flaps can be harvested: the horizontally oriented lower abdominal myocutaneous flap[27] or the vertically oriented upper abdominal myocutaneous flap.[28] The transverse and vertical rectus abdominis myocutaneous flaps, because of the extended length of their vascular pedicels, allow a high arc of rotation. The axis is determined by the vascular supply, and the flap is transferred intra-abdominally through the posterior rectus

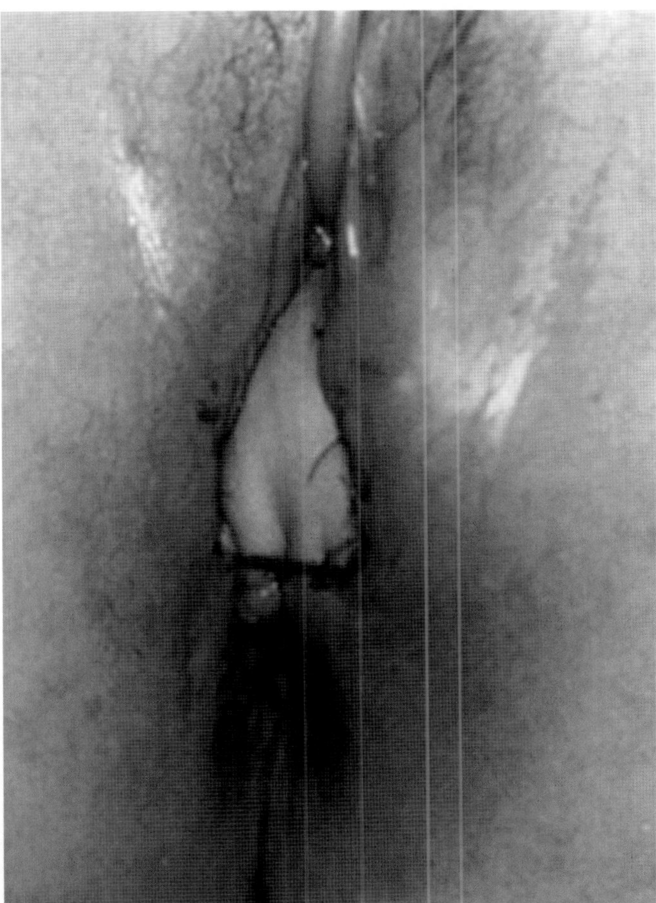

Figure 99-15 The flap is set into the vaginal defect. The donor site is closed primarily.

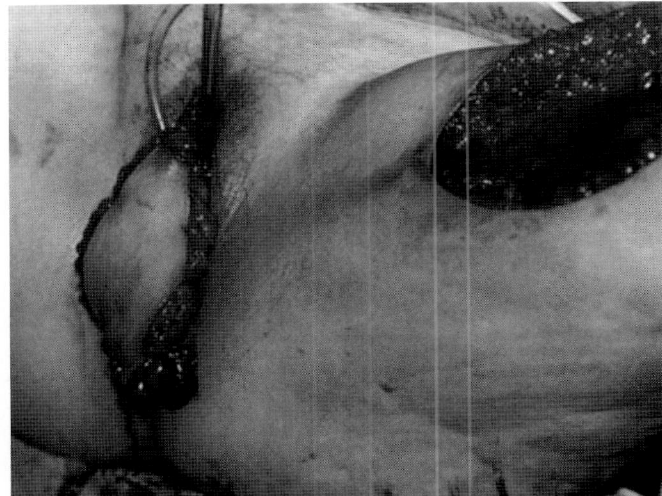

Figure 99-16 The myocutaneous island flap is transferred to subcutaneously to be inset. (From Lesavoy MA, Carter EJ: Vaginal reconstruction. In Raz S [ed]: Female Urology, 2nd ed. Philadelphia, WB Saunders, 1996, pp 605-616.)

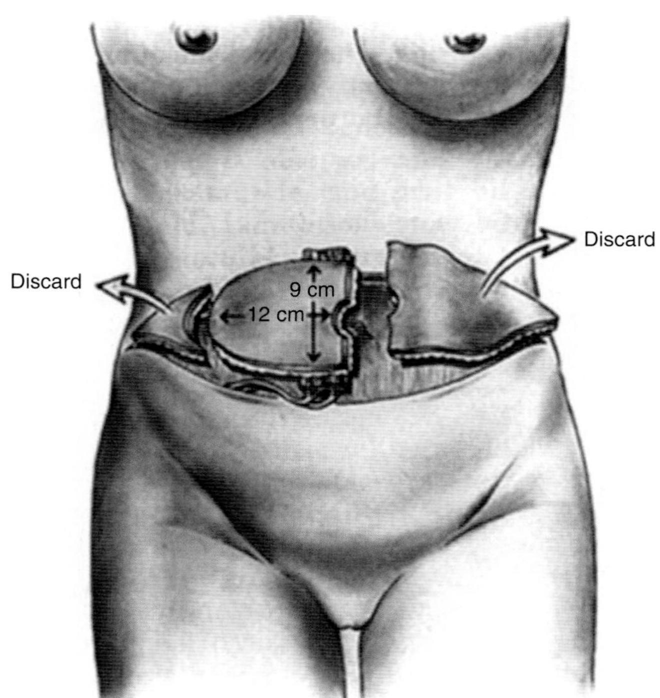

Figure 99-17 Harvesting of right rectus abdominis myocutaneous flap for vaginal reconstruction.

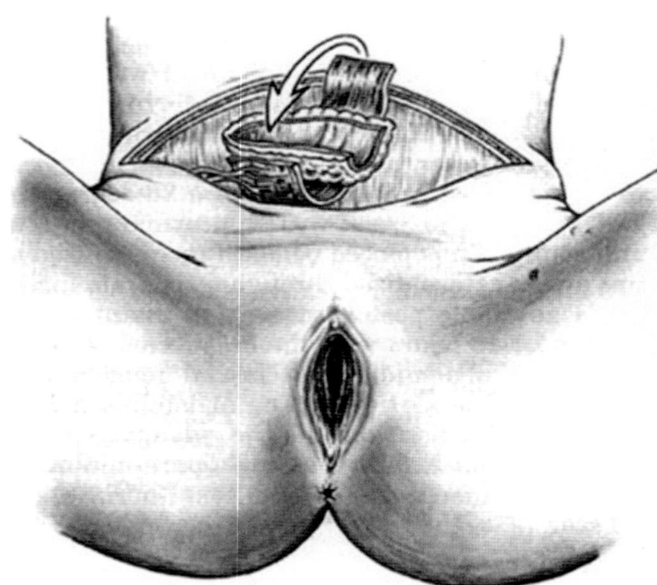

Figure 99-18 The flap is mobilized and formed into a tube. (From Lesavoy MA, Carter EJ: Vaginal reconstruction. In Raz S [ed]: Female Urology, 2nd ed. Philadelphia, WB Saunders, 1996, pp 605-616.)

sheath. This need for laparotomy is a negative aspect of this procedure. A vertically oriented flap may be preferred when it is necessary to maintain an intact lower abdominal rectus muscle for exit sites of stomas on the contralateral side.

Among the many advantages of this flap are a very reliable blood supply[19] and the ability to resurface a defect with a single flap. This flap also provides ease of mobilization without tension and is associated with a low incidence of vascular compromise.[18,29] In a series of 22 patients, there was little tissue loss and an acceptable donor site, and return to sexual activity was possible for 80% of patients.[28]

After completion of the exenteration procedure, attention is directed toward harvesting the myocutaneous flap from the abdomen. Centered just to the left or right of the umbilicus, a transverse rectus abdominal myocutaneous (TRAM) flap is harvested measuring approximately 9 cm long by 12 cm wide. The flap should include skin, subcutaneous tissue, a strip of anterior rectus sheath, and the rectus muscle itself (see Fig. 99-17). The initial incision should commence at the lateral apex of the TRAM (which corresponds to the anterior axillary line) and should extend medially to include all of the abovementioned flap components. The rectus muscle is identified and carefully dissected laterally to the region of the deep inferior epigastric perforating vessels, with identification of the inferior epigastric vascular pedicle at its origin on the external iliac vessels. This ensures adequate flap mobilization when the flap is isolated. At this point, the superior and inferior margins of the rectus muscle are divided (Fig. 99-18). A vaginal tube is formed from the flap by means of continuous and interrupted sutures to approximate the superior and inferior margins of skin and muscle with the raw side out (Fig. 99-19).

The manually formed vaginal cone is then mobilized and transferred through the posterior rectus sheath after a laparotomy incision is made through the peritoneum at the origin of the deep inferior epigastric vessels into the pelvis to reach the vaginal defect (Fig. 99-20). The lateral-most portion of the flap becomes the apex of the vagina. Care must be taken when placing the flap to ensure that no tension is placed on the vascular pedicle. The neovagina is then attached to the introitus with interrupted

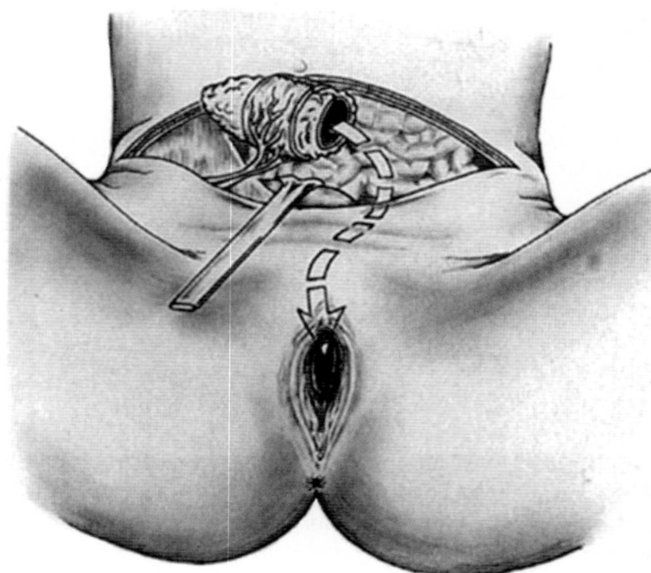

Figure 99-19 The mobilized myocutaneous flap is sutured together to form a blind tube of sufficient length and diameter to serve as a functional vagina. It is then transferred through the posterior rectus sheath to reach the vaginal defect. (From Lesavoy MA, Carter EJ: Vaginal reconstruction. In Raz S [ed]: Female Urology, 2nd ed. Philadelphia, WB Saunders, 1996, pp 605-616.)

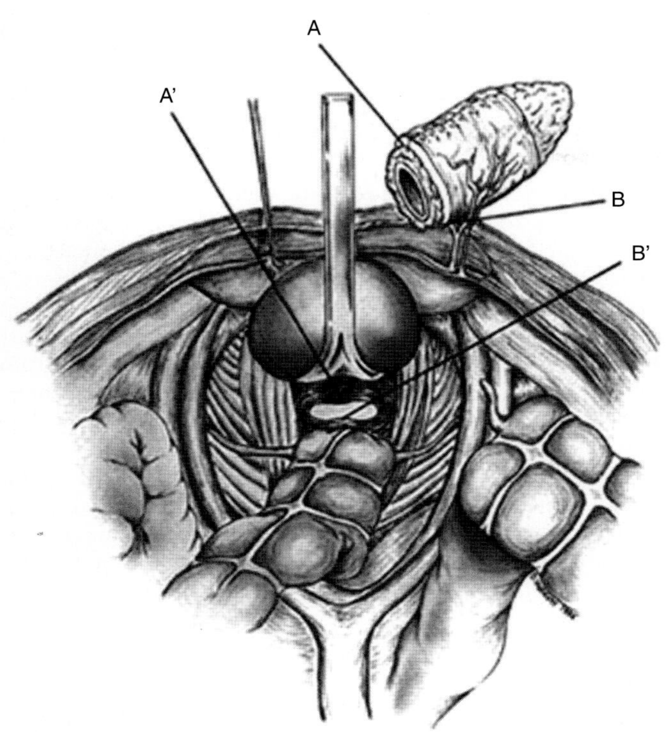

Figure 99-20 View after a laparotomy incision is made through the peritoneum at the origin of the deep inferior epigastric vessels into the pelvis to reach the vaginal defect. (From Lesavoy MA, Carter EJ: Vaginal reconstruction. In Raz S [ed]: Female Urology, 2nd ed. Philadelphia, WB Saunders, 1996, pp 605-616.)

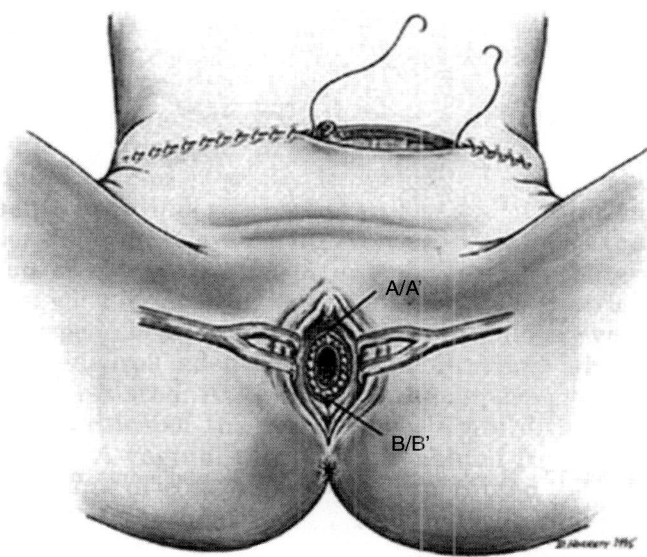

Figure 99-21 The myocutaneous flap is transposed into the pelvis and sutured to the perineal (introital) incision.

sutures (Fig. 99-21).[15,18] An estrogen cream is spread on the mold, which is placed in the vagina and sutured in place.[18] On day 5, the mold is removed, and a vaginal dilator is worn three times per week for 3 months in conjunction with the application of estrogen cream.[18]

The initial procedure is concluded with primary closure of the fascial defect with interrupted or continuous permanent sutures. The closure of subcutaneous tissue after a horizontal (TRAM) harvest is best achieved with the patient in a 30-degree, semi-Fowler position to assist with approximation. A subcutaneous drain is placed beneath the mobilized skin flaps and is externalized through a separate incision.

It is advisable postoperatively to maintain strict bed rest for 48 hours. The hips are flexed 30 degrees to decrease abdominal wall fascial tension at the repair site. The vertical rectus abdominis myocutaneous (VRAM) flap has all the advantages of the TRAM flap, but it leaves a single para-midline scar at closure rather than the additional horizontal lateral scar.

Intestinal Flaps

Other methods of vaginal reconstruction, such as flaps of small intestine, ascending colon, sigmoid colon, and sigmoid and lower rectum, are briefly described because they have been used with various degrees of success for vaginal reconstruction. The patient requires hospitalization 2 days before the operation to allow time to prepare and sterilize the bowel adequately.

With the patient in the lithotomy position, a vaginal tract is dissected from the perineum into the peritoneum, and the tract is widened laterally. When hemostasis is satisfactory, the vaginal tract is packed and the abdomen opened. The sigmoid usually is mobile enough to allow a satisfactory vascular pedicle to be developed. With proper planning, an adequate length of intestine (12 to 15 cm) can be isolated, an oblique end-to-end anastomosis is performed, and the bowel segment is drawn through the vaginal tract. The patient is returned to a lithotomy position. The end of the bowel is incised on an angle to gain additional room, and it is then attached to the introitus.

Advantages of the intestinal neovagina include the absence of a need for frequent dilatation or stent wearing. However, the disadvantages include excessive mucus formation, especially when the small intestine is used, and a mortality rate between 1% and 2%.[12]

Summary of Vaginal Reconstruction

Vaginal reconstruction can be an uncomplicated and straightforward procedure when attention to detail is maintained.[30,31] The Abbe-McIndoe procedure of lining the neovaginal canal with split-thickness skin grafts has become the standard. Use of the inflatable Heyer-Schulte vaginal stent provides comfort for the patient and ease for the surgeon in maintaining skin graft approximation.

For large vaginal and perineal defects, myocutaneous flaps such as the gracilis island flap have been extremely useful for correction of radiation-damaged tissue to the perineum and for the reconstruction of large ablative defects. Minimal morbidity and scarring ensue because the donor site can be closed primarily.

The gracilis has sufficient bulk to fill the pelvis, decreasing the incidence of herniation or obstruction. It also provides vaginal length, is an expendable muscle, and generally is out of the irradiated field. Limitations may be its 10% to 20% incidence of vascular compromise due to the vessel's small caliber, which results in tension as the flap is moved into the pelvic defect.

The TRAM flap is used to form a functional vagina. Its advantage over the gracilis is its variable vascular pedicle caliber and length. Its reliable blood supply and potentially long vascular pedicle provide flap versatility, with a resulting low incidence of vascular compromise. This flap augments the surgical options available for pelvic and vaginal reconstruction.

An absolute contraindication to rectus harvest is a history of vascular disruption of the inferior epigastric vessels. Obesity may be a relative contraindication because the thick subcutaneous tissue prohibits flap flexibility and mobilization into the pelvic space.

There is a wide range of procedures from which to choose for the correction of congenital absence of the vagina. Unfortunately, no consensus has been reached about which is best. Each patient must be evaluated on an individual basis.

For the success of all types of vaginal reconstruction, a compliant patient is a necessity. The patient must wear a vaginal obturator for a minimum of 3 to 6 months postoperatively and is encouraged to use intercourse as an obturator. Vaginal reconstruction can be a gratifying procedure that enhances the functional and emotional well-being of these patients. Reconstruction can be successful in patients with congenital or ablative vaginal absence, and it can be a functional and emotional advantage for all concerned. Attention to detail and support are necessary for all patients.

LABIAL REDUCTION: LABIOPLASTY

Congenital, traumatic, or neoplastic deformities can affect the labia minora and labia majora in some women. Congenital or traumatic hypertrophy of the labia minora has been an increasing concern to some women, and the defect can be relatively easily corrected. The labia minora that protrude beyond the confines of the labia majora can be functionally and aesthetically unsatisfactory, and some women may experience irritation from clothing during athletic exercise, cosmetic or functional interference with sexual intercourse, and embarrassment and self-consciousness with tight undergarments.[32,33]

Surgical indications for reduction of the labia minora are for patient satisfaction with functional and aesthetic characteristics. The surgical procedure for reduction of the labia minora is relatively straightforward and can be performed on an outpatient basis.[34,35]

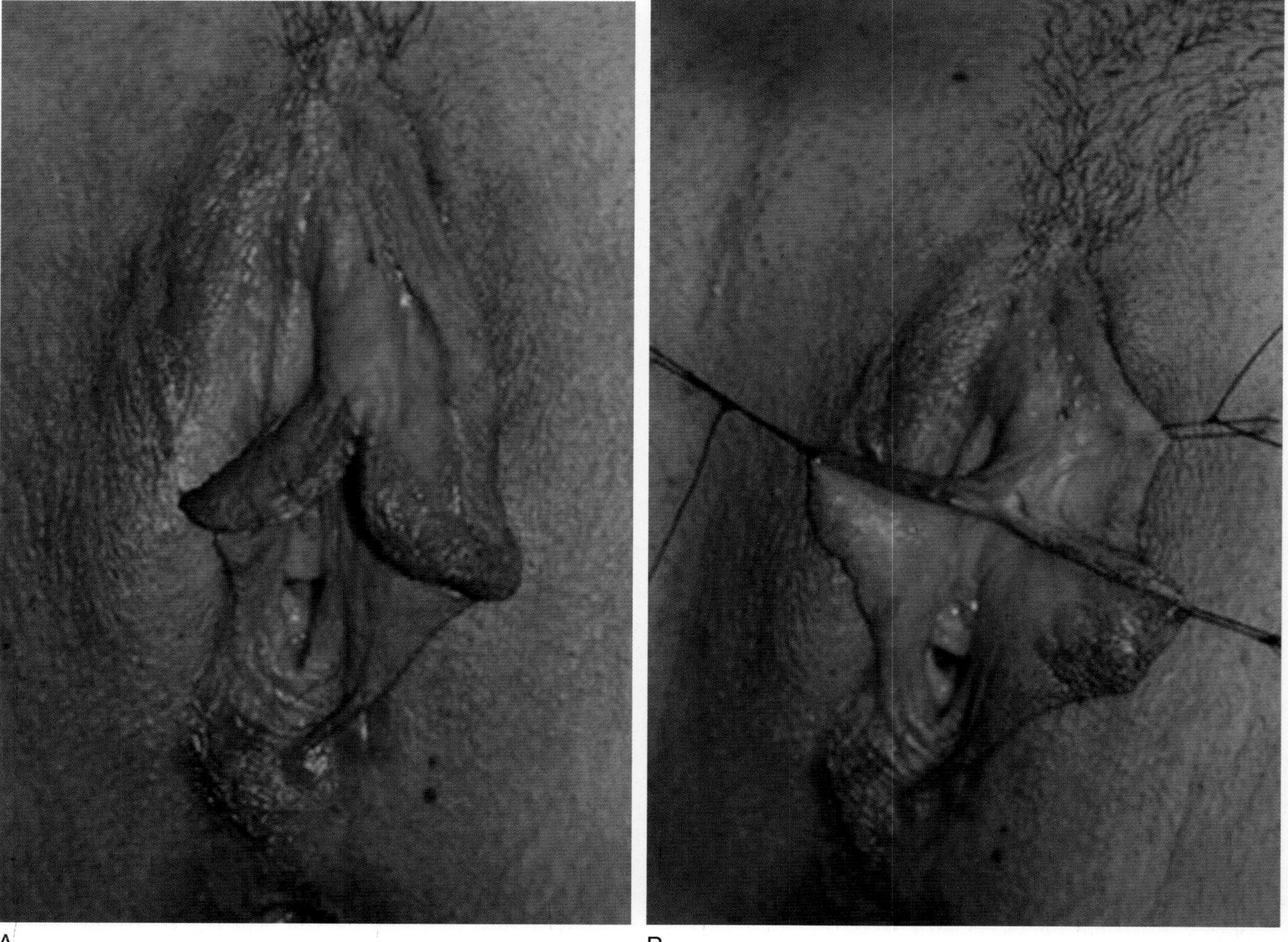

Figure 99-22 A, Preoperative view of a large and patulous labia minora exhibiting symptoms of irritation from sports, clothing, and aggressive sexual activity. **B,** Intraoperative retraction of the labia minora.

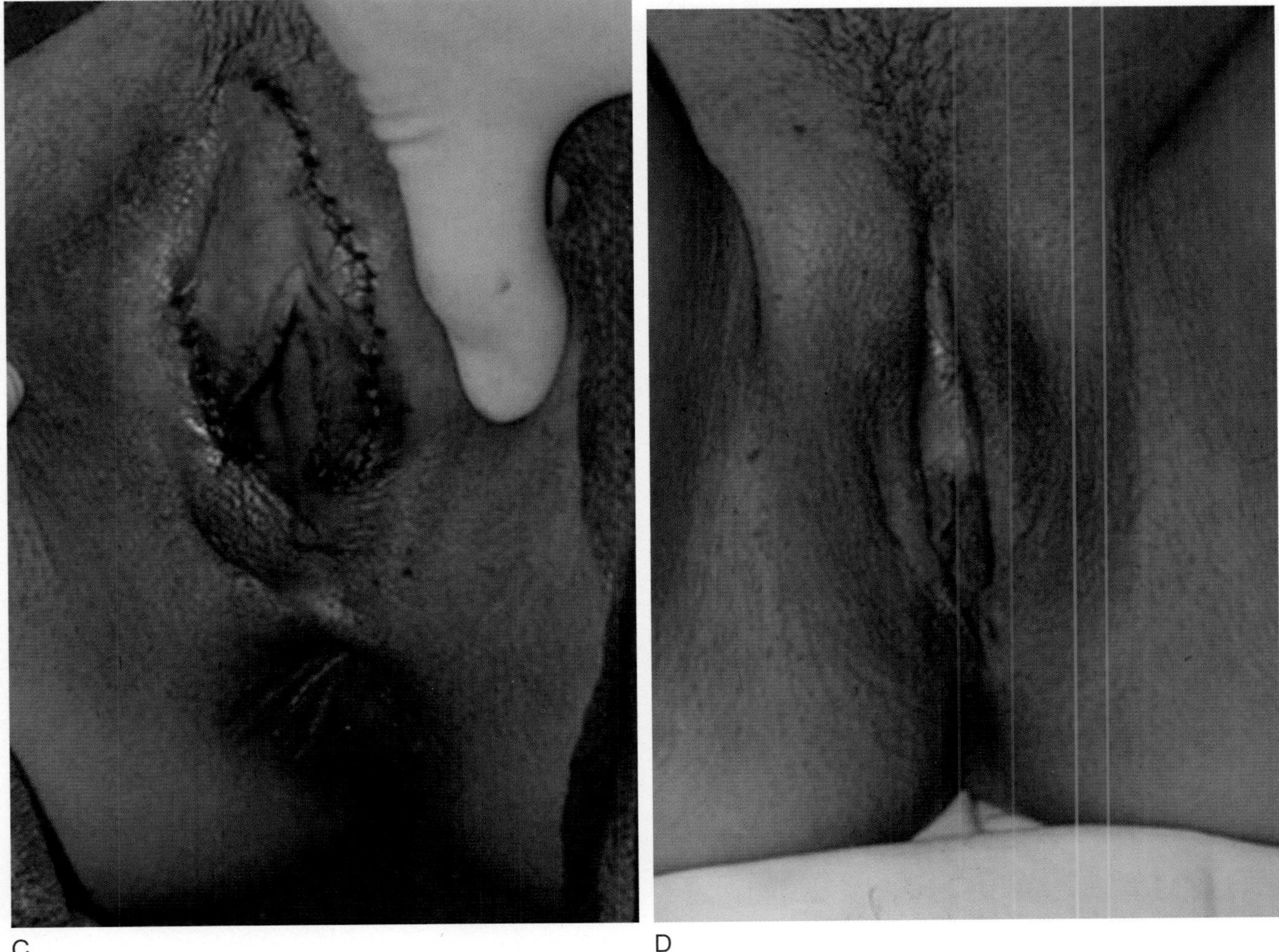

Figure 99-22, cont'd **C,** Immediate postoperative indications of asymmetric resection and closure of labia minora. **D,** Postoperative result.

The surgical contour should be explicitly discussed with the patient before surgery, and the excision should avoid eversion of mucosal surfaces so that the superficial squamous epithelium is turned inward. In this way, the scars are inconspicuous, and mucosal irritation from eversion does not occur. Infiltration with local anesthetic and epinephrine can reduce postoperative pain, intraoperative bleeding, and postoperative bruising, but it should be done in conjunction with general anesthesia. The protuberant area is excised, and the remaining edge is sutured with absorbable material (Figs. 99-22 to 99-25).

Surgical reduction of the labia minora often improves the physical comfort and psychological aspects of hypertrophy. If the hypertrophied labia interfered emotionally and physically with intercourse, the sexual satisfaction of these patients will be improved. Patients undergoing labia minora reduction usually are pleased with the aesthetic and functional results.

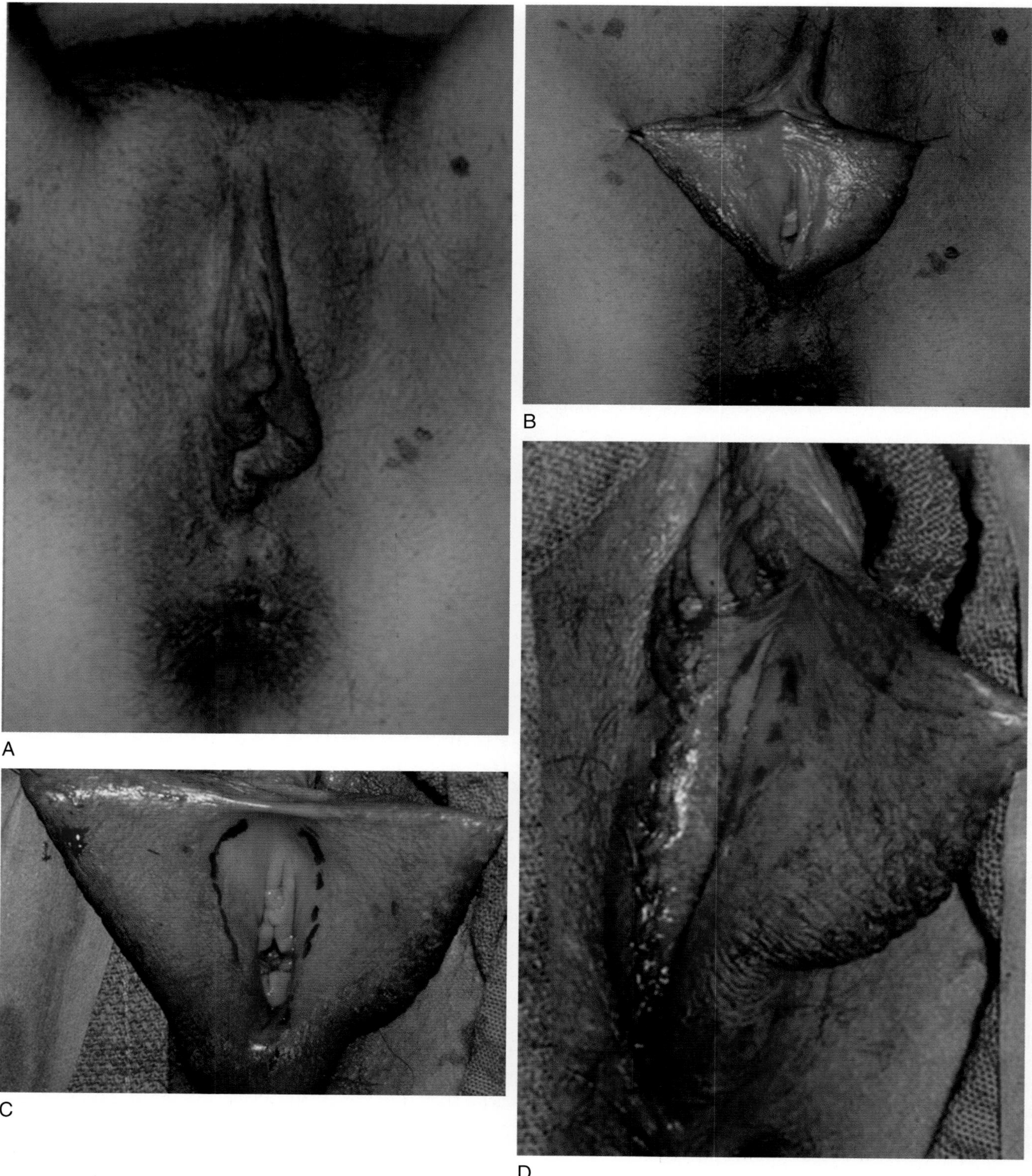

Figure 99-23 **A,** Preoperative hypertrophy of the labia minora. **B,** Intraoperative retraction of the labia minora. **C,** Intraoperative markings of resection of bilateral labia minora. **D,** The right labium minus has been resected; the left labium minus has not yet been resected.

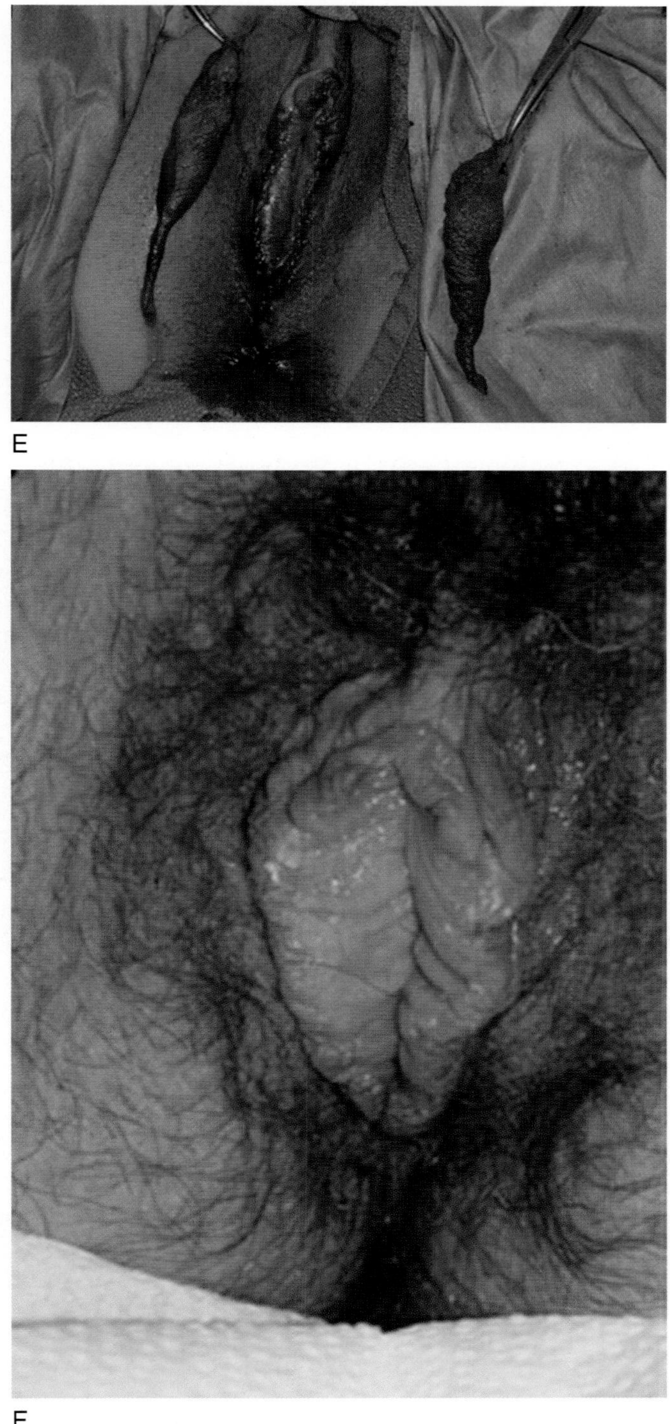

Figure 99-23, cont'd E, Resected tissue of the labia minora. **F,** Postoperative result.

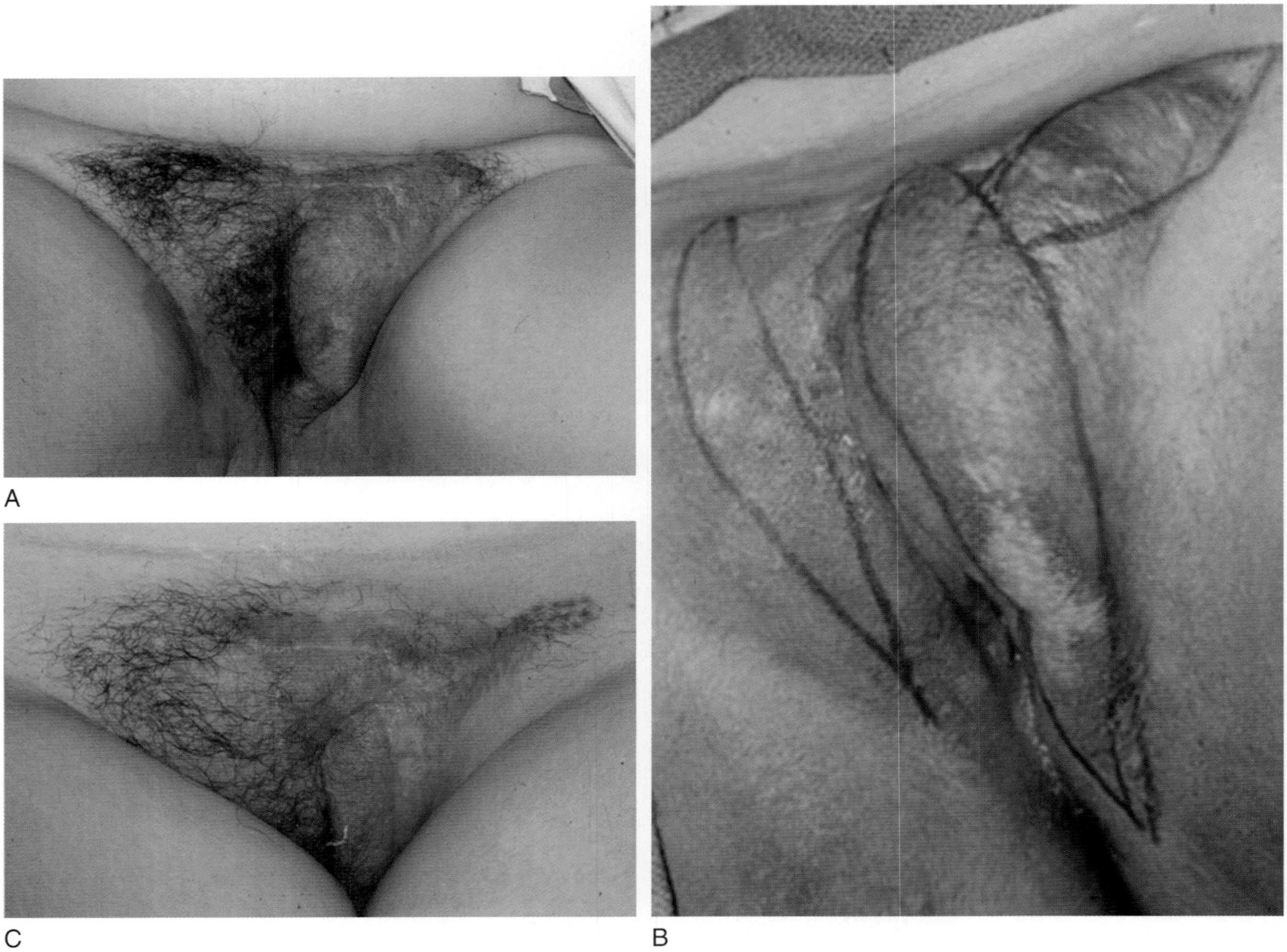

A

C

B

Figure 99-24 A, Hemangioma of the left labium majus and suprapubic area with areas of previous biopsies. **B,** Markings for excision of bilateral labia majora hemangioma. **C,** Postoperative result.

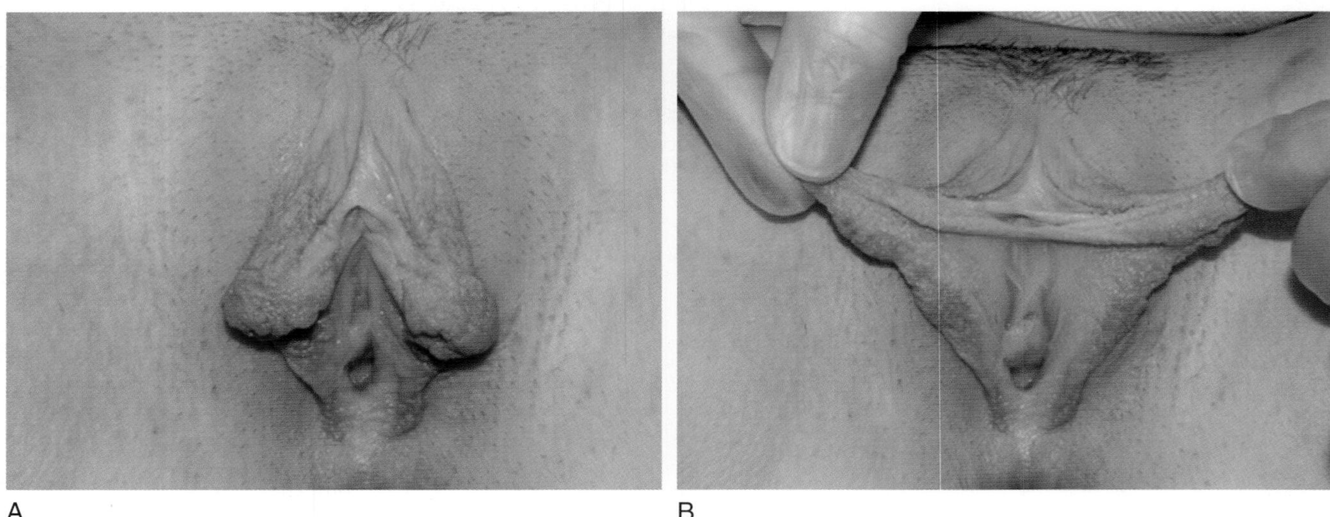

A B

Figure 99-25 A to **E,** Six days after labia minora reduction, the tissue shows minimal swelling.

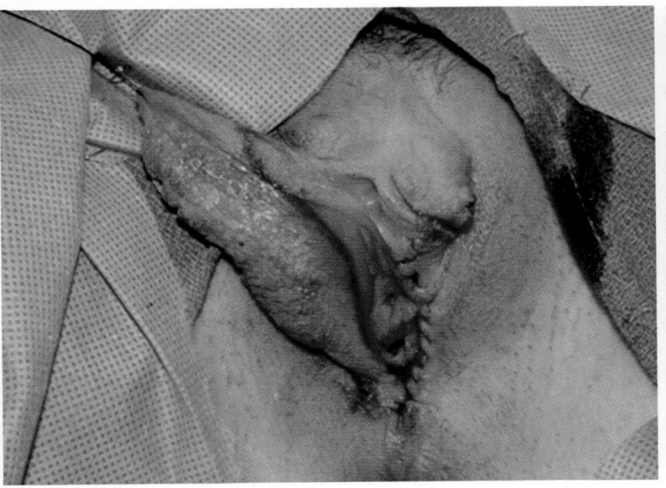

C

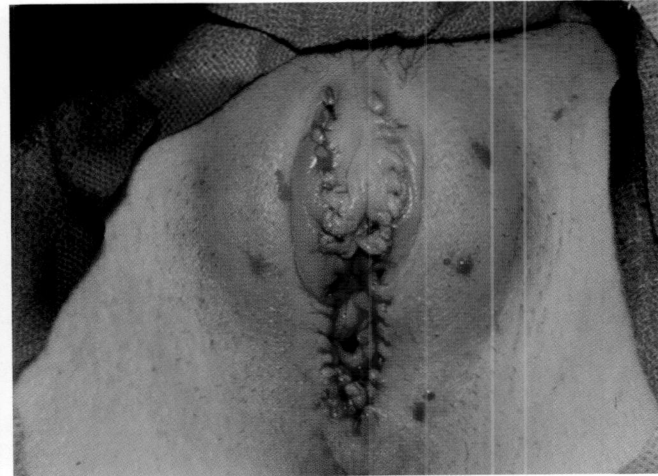

D

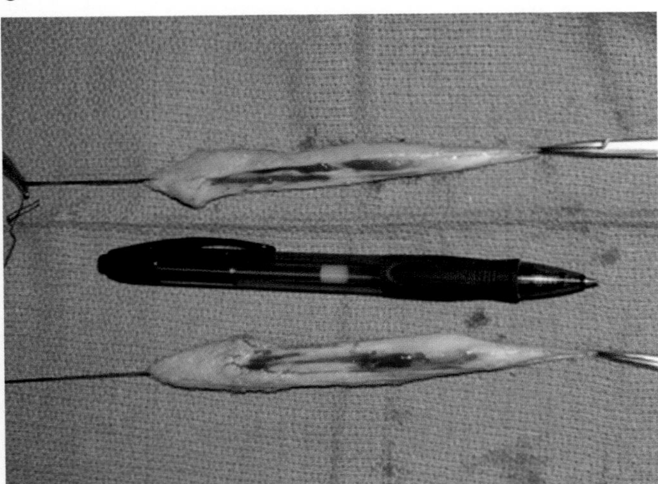

E

Figure 99-25, cont'd A to **E,** Six days after labia minora reduction, the tissue shows minimal swelling.

References

1. Counseller VS: Congenital absence of the vagina. JAMA 136:861, 1948.
2. Paunz A: Formation of an artificial vagina to remedy a congenital defect [citation of Heppner, 1872]. Zentralbl Gynakol 47:833, 1923.
3. Abbe R: New method of creating a vagina in a case of congenital absence. Med Rec.
4. McIndoe A: The application of cavity grafting. Surgery 1:535, 1937.
5. McIndoe A: The treatment of congenital absence and obliterative conditions of the vagina. Br J Plast Surg 2:254, 1950.
6. Conway H, Stark RB: Construction and reconstruction of the vagina. Surg Gynecol Obstet 97:573, 1953.
7. Sneguireff WF: Zewei neu Faile von Restitutio Vaginiae per Transplantationen Ani et Recti. Zentralbl Gynakol 28:772, 1904.
8. Meyer HW: Kolpo-plastik [citation of Popow DD, 1910]. Zentralbl Gynakol 37:639, 1918.
9. Schubert G: Concerning the formation of a new vagina in the case of congenital malformation. Surg Gynecol Obstet 193:376, 1914.
10. Balwin JF: The formation of an artificial vagina by intestinal transplantation. Ann Surg 40:398, 1904.
11. Frank RT. Geist SH: Formation of an artificial vagina by a new plastic technique. Am J Obstet Gynecol 14:712, 1927.
12. Horton CE, Sadove RC, McCraw JB: Reconstruction of female genital defects. Plast Surg 6:4203, 1990.
13. Sadove RC. Horton CE: Utilizing full thickness skin grafts for vaginal reconstruction. Clin Plast Surg 15131:443, 1988.
14. Knapstein PG, Friedberg V, Sevin BU: Reconstructive Surgery in Gynecology. New York, Georg Thieme, 1990, pp 30-32.
15. Hatch KD: Construction of a neovagina after exenteration using the vulvobulbocavernosus myocutaneous graft. Obstet Gynecol 63:110, 1984.
16. Wee JT, Joseph VT: A new technique for vaginal reconstruction using neurovascular pudendal thigh flaps: A preliminary report. Plast Reconstr Surg 83:701, 1989.
17. Soper JT, Berchuck A, Creasman WT, et al: Pelvic exenteration: Factors associated with major surgical morbidity. Gynecol Oncol 35:93, 1989.
18. Carlson JW, Soisson AP, Fowler JM, et al: Rectus abdominis myocutaneous flap for primary vaginal reconstruction. Gynecol Oncol 51:323, 1993.
19. Benson C, Soisson AP, Carlson J, et al: Neovaginal reconstruction with a rectus abdominis myocutaneous flap. Obstet Gynecol 81(Pt 2):871, 1993.

20. Lacey MD, Jeffery L, Stern MD, et al: Vaginal reconstruction after exenteration with use of gracilis myocutaneous flaps. The University of California, San Francisco experience. Am J Obstet Gynecol 158(Pt 1):1278, 1988.
21. Owens N: A compound neck pedicle designed for the repair of massive facial defects. Plast Reconstr Surg 15:369, 1955.
22. Bakamjian V: A technique for primary reconstruction of the palate after radical maxillectomy for cancer. Plast Reconstr Surg 31:103, 1963.
23. Hueston JJ, McConchie IH: A compound pectoral flap. Aust N Z J Surg 38:61, 1968.
24. McCraw J, Massey F, Shankin K, Horton C: Vaginal reconstruction using gracilis myocutaneous flaps. Plast Reconstr Surg 58:176, 1976.
25. Lesavoy MA, Dubrow TJ, Korn HN, et al: Sensible flap coverage for pressure sores in patients with meningomyelocele. Plast Reconst Surg 85:390, 1990.
26. Hatch KD: Neovaginal reconstruction. Cancer 71(Suppl):1660, 1993.
27. McCraw J, Kemp G, Givens F, Horton CE: Correction of high pelvic defects with the inferiorly based rectus abdominis myocutaneous flap. Clin Plast Surg 15:449, 1988.
28. Pursell SH, Day TG Jr, Tobin GR: Distally based rectus abdominis flap for reconstruction in radical gynecologic procedures. Gynecol Oncol 37:234, 1990.
29. Tobin GR, Day TG: Vaginal and pelvic reconstruction with distally based rectus abdominis myocutaneous flaps. Plast Reconstr Surg 81:62, 1988.
30. Lesavoy MA: Vaginal reconstruction. Clin Obstet Gynecol 12:515, 1985.
31. Lesavoy MA: Vaginal reconstruction. Urol Clin North Am 12:369, 1985.
32. Caparo VJ: Congenital anomalies. Clin Obstet Gynecol 14:988, 1971.
33. Radman HM: Hypertrophy of the labia minora. Clin Obstet Gynecol 48(Suppl 1):78S, 1976.
34. Hodgkinson DJ, Hait G: Aesthetic vaginal labioplasty. Plast Reconstr Surg 74:414, 1984.
35. Alter GJ: A new technique for aesthetic labia minora reduction. Ann Plast Surg 40:287, 1998.
36. Wierrani F, Grünberger W: Vaginoplasty using deepithelialized vulvar transposition flaps: The Grünberger method. J Am Coll Surg 196:159, 2003.

INDEX

Note: Page numbers followed by f refer to figures; page numbers followed by t refer to tables; page numbers followed by b refer to boxes.

D